TUBERCULOSIS

SECOND EDITION

TUBERCULOSIS

SECOND EDITION

Editors

WILLIAM N. ROM, M.D., M.P.H.

Sol and Judith Bergstein Professor of Medicine and Environmental Medicine
Director, Division of Pulmonary and Critical Care Medicine
Department of Medicine
New York University School of Medicine
Director, Bellevue Chest Service
New York, New York

STUART M. GARAY, M.D.

Clinical Professor of Medicine
Associate Director, Division of Pulmonary and Critical Care Medicine
Department of Medicine
New York University School of Medicine
Attending Physician
New York University Tisch Hospital
Bellevue Hospital Center
New York, New York

Foreword by

BARRY R. BLOOM, PH.D.

Dean
Harvard School of Public Health
Boston, Massachusetts

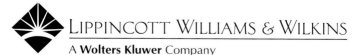

LIPPINCOTT WILLIAMS & WILKINS
A **Wolters Kluwer** Company
Philadelphia · Baltimore · New York · London
Buenos Aires · Hong Kong · Sydney · Tokyo

Acquisitions Editor: Danette Somers
Developmental Editor: Julia Seto
Production Editor: Jonathan Geffner
Manufacturing Manager: Colin W. Warnock
Cover Designer: David Levy
Compositor: Lippincott Williams & Wilkins Desktop Division
Printer: Edwards Brothers

Library of Congress Cataloging-in-Publication Data
Tuberculosis / editors, William N. Rom, Stuart M. Garay ; foreword by Barry R.
    Bloom.—2nd ed.
    p. ; cm.
  Includes bibliographical references and index.
  ISBN 0-7817-3678-1
  1. Tuberculosis. I. Rom, William N. II. Garay, Stuart M.
  [DNLM: 1. Tuberculosis, Pulmonary. 2. Antitubercular Agents—pharmacology. 3.
Mycobacterium tuberculosis—drug effects. 4. Tuberculosis, Multidrug-Resistant. WF
300 T8843 2003]
RC311.T8243 2003
616.9'95—dc21

                                                      2003047698

Care has been taken to confirm the accuracy of the information presented and to describe generally accepted practices. However, the authors, editors, and publisher are not responsible for errors or omissions or for any consequences from application of the information in this book and make no warranty, expressed or implied, with respect to the currency, completeness, or accuracy of the contents of the publication. Application of this information in a particular situation remains the professional responsibility of the practitioner.

The authors, editors, and publisher have exerted every effort to ensure that drug selection and dosage set forth in this text are in accordance with current recommendations and practice at the time of publication. However, in view of ongoing research, changes in government regulations, and the constant flow of information relating to drug therapy and drug reactions, the reader is urged to check the package insert for each drug for any change in indications and dosage and for added warnings and precautions. This is particularly important when the recommended agent is a new or infrequently employed drug.

Some drugs and medical devices presented in this publication have Food and Drug Administration (FDA) clearance for limited use in restricted research settings. It is the responsibility of the health care provider to ascertain the FDA status of each drug or device planned for use in their clinical practice.

10 9 8 7 6 5 4 3 2 1

CONTENTS

CONTRIBUTING AUTHORS

June E. S. Abadilla, M.D. Clinical Assistant Instructor, Department of Medicine, State University of New York Health Science Center; Division of Pulmonary and Critical Care Medicine, Downstate Medical Center, Brooklyn, New York

Steven B. Abramson, M.D. Professor of Medicine and Pathology, Department of Medicine, New York University School of Medicine; Chairman, Rheumatology and Medicine, New York University Hospital for Joint Diseases, New York, New York

Peter S. Andersen, D.Sc., DVM Head, Department of Infectious Disease Immunology, Statens Serum Institut, Copenhagen, Denmark

Stephen K. Baker, M.D. (Deceased) Assistant Professor of Medicine, Northwestern University Medical School, Chicago, Illinois

Sayera Banu, Ph.D., M.D. Staff Scientist, Immunology Laboratory, International Centre for Diarrhoeal Disease Research, Bangladesh, Dhaka, Bangladesh

Clifton Barry III, Ph.D. Senior Investigator, National Institute of Allergy and Infectious Diseases, National Institutes of Health, Rockville, Maryland

Joseph H. Bates, M.D., M.S. Associate Dean, University of Arkansas for Medical Science College of Public Health; Chief Medical Officer, Arkansas Department of Health, Little Rock, Arkansas

Marcel A. Behr, M.D. Assistant Professor, Department of Medicine, McGill University; Assistant Physician, Department of Medicine, Montreal General Hospital, Montreal, Quebec, Canada

William Borkowsky, M.D. Professor, Department of Pediatrics, New York University School of Medicine, New York, New York

Arthur D. Boyd, M.D. Professor, Department of Surgery, New York University School of Medicine; Attending Surgeon, Department of Surgery, New York University Medical Center, New York, New York

Rena S. Brand, M.D. Clinical Associate Professor and Associate Attending Professor, Department of Dermatology, New York University Medical Center, New York, New York

Patrick J. Brennan, Ph.D. University Distinguished Professor, Department of Microbiology, Immunology and Pathology, Colorado State University, Fort Collins, Colorado

Roland Brosch, Ph.D. Research Scientist, Department of Microbial Pathogenics, Pasteur Institute, Paris, France

Susan Burgin, M.D. Assistant Professor, Department of Dermatology, New York University School of Medicine; Clinical Assistant Attending, Department of Dermatology, Bellevue Hospital, New York, New York

William J. Burman, M.D. Associate Professor, Department of Medicine, Division of Infectious Diseases, University of Colorado Health Sciences Center; Director, Infectious Diseases Clinic, Denver Public Health, Denver, Colorado

Joseph N. Burzynski, M.D., M.P.H. Instructor in Clinical Medicine, Department of Pulmonary Medicine, Columbia University College of Physicians and Surgeons; Physician-in-Charge, Washington Heights Chest Center, New York City Department of Health and Mental Hygiene, New York, New York

Ellen Buschman, Ph.D. McGill Centre for the Study of Host Resistance, McGill University Health Center, Montreal, Quebec, Canada

Kenneth G. Castro, M.D. Director, Division of Tuberculosis Elimination, Centers for Disease Control and Prevention, Atlanta, Georgia

Edward D. Chan, M.D. Associate Professor, Department of Medicine, University of Colorado School of Medicine; Assistant Staff Physician, Department of Medicine, National Jewish Medical and Research Center, Denver, Colorado

John Chan, M.D. Associate Professor, Departments of Medicine and Microbiology and Immunology, Albert Einstein College of Medicine; Attending Physician, Department of Medicine, Division of Infectious Diseases, Montefiore Medical Center, Bronx, New York

Delphi Chatterjee, Ph.D. Associate Professor, Department of Microbiology, Immunology, and Pathology, Colorado State University, Fort Collins, Colorado

Chen-Yuan Chiang, M.D., M.P.H. Chief, Section of Chest Disease, Center for Chest Disease, Department of Health, Tainan, Taiwan

Stewart T. Cole, Ph.D. Professor, Unit of Genetic Molecular Bacteriology, Pasteur Institute, Paris, France

Rany Condos, M.D. Assistant Professor, Division of Pulmonary and Critical Care Medicine, New York University School of Medicine, New York, New York

Bernard K. Crawford, Jr., M.D. Assistant Professor, Department of Cardiothoracic Surgery, New York University School of Medicine; Attending Surgeon, Department of Thoracic Surgery, New York University Tisch Hospital, New York, New York

Dean C. Crick, Ph.D. Associate Professor, Department of Microbiology, Immunology and Pathology, Colorado State University, Fort Collins, Colorado

Charles L. Daley, M.D. Associate Professor of Clinical Medicine, Department of Medicine, University of California at San Francisco; Chief, Chest Clinic, Division of Pulmonary and Critical Care Medicine, San Francisco General Hospital, San Francisco, California

Karl Drlica, Ph.D. Public Health Research Institute at the International Center for Public Health, Newark, New Jersey

Sabine Ehrt, Ph.D. Assistant Professor, Department of Microbiology and Immunology, Joan and Sanford I. Weill Medical College of Cornell University, New York, New York

Donald A. Enarson, M.D. Adjunct Professor, Department of Medicine, University of Alberta, Edmonton, Alberta, Canada; Director, Scientific Activities, International Union Against Tuberculosis and Lung Disease, Paris, France

Steven Field, M.D. Clinical Assistant Professor, Department of Medicine, New York University School of Medicine; Assistant Attending, Department of Medicine, New York University Tisch Hospital, New York, New York

JoAnne L. Flynn, Ph.D. Associate Professor, Department of Molecular Genetics and Biochemistry, University of Pittsburgh School of Medicine, Pittsburgh, Pennsylvania

Dorothy Nahm Friedberg, M.D., Ph.D. Clinical Associate Professor, Department of Ophthalmology, New York University School of Medicine; Attending Physician, Department of Ophthalmology, New York Eye and Ear Infirmary, New York, New York

Kenneth F. Garay, M.D. Vice President, Medical Affairs, Director of Otolaryngology and Head and Neck Surgery, Department of Otolaryngology, Meadowlands Hospital Medical Center, Secaucus, New Jersey

Stuart M. Garay, M.D. Clinical Professor, Department of Medicine, Associate Director, Division of Pulmonary and Critical Care Medicine, New York University School of Medicine; Attending Physician, Department of Medicine, New York University Tisch Hospital, Bellevue Hospital Center, New York, New York

Brigitte Gicquel, Ph.D. Professor, Head of the Unit, Mycobacterial Genetics Unit, The Pasteur Institute, Paris, France

Lawrence Glassman, M.D. Department of Cardiothoracic Surgery, North Shore University Hospital, Manhasset, New York

Jeffrey Glassroth, M.D. George R. and Elaine Love Professor and Chair, Department of Medicine, University of Wisconsin School of Medicine; Chair, Department of Medicine, University of Wisconsin Hospitals and Clinics, Madison, Wisconsin

David S. Goldfarb, M.D. Associate Professor, Department of Medicine, New York University School of Medicine; Assistant Chief, Nephrology Section, New York Harbor Department of Veterans Affairs Medical Center, New York, New York

James E. Gomez, Ph.D. Postdoctoral Fellow, Laboratory of Infection Biology, The Rockefeller University, New York, New York

Bruce A. Hanna, Ph.D. Associate Professor, Departments of Pathology and Microbiology, New York University School of Medicine; Director, Clinical Microbiology, Department of Pathology, Bellevue Hospital, New York, New York

George Haralambou, M.D. Clinical Instructor, Department of Medicine, Division of Pulmonary and Critical Care Medicine, New York University Medical Center, New York, New York

Timothy J. Harkin, M.D. Assistant Professor, Department of Medicine, New York University School of Medicine; Assistant Director, Chest Service, Bellevue Hospital Center, New York, New York

Leonid B. Heifets, M.D., Ph.D. Professor, Department of Microbiology, Colorado University Health Science Center; Professor and Director, Mycobacteriology Clinical Reference Laboratory, National Jewish Medical and Reserach Center, Denver, Colorado

Michael Henry, M.D. Fellow, Department of Internal Medicine, Division of Infectious Diseases, New York University Medical Center, New York, New York

Albert E. Heurich, M.D. Associate Professor, Department of Medicine, State University of New York Health Science Center at Brooklyn; Medical Director of Respiratory Care, Department of Medicine, Kings County Hospital Center, Brooklyn, New York

Robert S. Holzman, M.D.   Professor of Medicine and Environmental Medicine, Department of Medicine, New York University School of Medicine; Chief of Infectious Diseases, Department of Medicine, Bellevue Hospital, New York, New York

C. Robert Horsburgh, Jr., M.D., M.U.S.   Professor, Departments of Epidemiology, Biostatistics, and Medicine, Boston University Schools of Public Health and Medicine; Physician, Department of Medicine, Boston Medical Center, Boston, Massachusetts

Yoshihiko Hoshino, M.D., Ph.D.   Research Scientist, Department of Medicine, New York University School of Medicine, New York, New York

Kris Huygen, Ph.D.   Head of Laboratory, Department of Mycobacterial Immunology, Pasteur Institute of Brussels, Brussels, Belgium

Michael F. Iademarco, M.D., M.P.H.   Assistant Professor, School of Medicine and Rollins School of Public Health, Emory University; Associate Director for Science, Division of Tuberculosis Elimination, National Center for HIV, STD, and TB Prevention, Centers for Disease Control and Prevention, Atlanta, Georgia

Michael D. Iseman, M.D.   Professor, Department of Medicine, University of Colorado School of Medicine; Chief, Mycobacterial Disease Service, Department of Medicine, National Jewish Medical and Research Center, Denver, Colorado

Jaishree Jagirdar, M.D.   Professor, Department of Pathology, University of Texas Health Science Center, San Antonio; Director of Anatomic Pathology, Department of Pathology, University Hospital, University of Texas, Health Science Center, San Antonio, Texas

Stephan L. Kamholz, M.D.   David J. Greene Professor of Medicine, Department of Medicine, New York University School of Medicine, New York, New York; Chairman, Department of Medicine, North Shore University Hospital, Manhasset, New York; Long Island Jewish Medical Center, New Hyde Park, New York

Stefan H. E. Kaufmann, Ph.D.   Director, Department of Immunology, Max-Planck-Institute for Infection Biology, Berlin, Germany

Joseph Keane, M.D.   Lecturer in Medicine, Dublin Molecular Medicine Center, Trinity College Dublin; Consultant Respiratory Physician, St. James's Hospital, Dublin, Ireland

Hardy Kornfeld, M.D.   Professor, Department of Medicine, University of Massachusetts Medical School, Worcester, Massachusetts

Sara B. Kramer, M.D.   Clinical Assistant Professor, Department of Medicine, New York University School of Medicine; Assistant Attending, New York University Medical Center, New York, New York

Carl N. Kraus, M.D.   Clincal Associate, Tuberculosis Research Section, National Institute of Allergy and Infectious Diseases, National Institutes of Health, Rockville, Maryland

Barry N. Kreiswirth, Ph.D.   Adjunct Assistant Professor, Department of Medicine, New York University School of Medicine, New York, New York; Director, Public Health Research Institute Tuberculosis Center, Public Health Research Institute at the International Center of Public Health, Tuberculosis Center, Newark, New Jersey

Suman Laal, Ph.D.   Assistant Professor, Department of Pathology, New York University School of Medicine; Research Microbiologist, VA Medical Center, New York, New York

Sicy H. S. Lee, M.D.   Clinical Assistant Professor, Department of Medicine, Division of Rheumatology, New York University School of Medicine, Hospital for Joint Diseases, New York, New York

Eric Leibert, M.D.   Assistant Professor, Department of Medicine, Division of Pulmonary Disease and Critical Care Medicine, New York University School of Medicine; Deputy Director, Chest Service, Bellevue Hospital, New York, New York

Thomas Lennon   Lennon Documentary Group, New York, New York

Stuart Lewis, M.D.   Adjunct Professor, Department of Environmental Medicine, New York University School of Medicine, New York, New York

Monica Lorenzo-Latkany, M.D.   Clinical Instructor, Department of Ophthalmology, New York University School of Medicine, New York, New York

Joseph Lowy, M.D.   Assistant Professor, Department of Medicine, Division of Pulmonary and Critical Care Medicine, New York University School of Medicine, New York, New York

Tao Lu, Ph.D.   Public Health Research Institute at the International Center for Public Health, Newark, New Jersey

Muhammad Malik, Ph.D.   Public Health Research Institute at the International Center for Public Health, Newark, New Jersey

Barun Mathema, M.P.H.   Research Epidemiologist, Public Health Research Institute at the International Center for Public Health, Newark, New Jersey

Georgeann McGuinness, M.D.   Associate Professor, Co-Director, Thoracic Imaging, Department of Radiology, New York University Medical Center, New York, New York

John D. McKinney, Ph.D.   Assistant Professor, Head of Laboratory, Laboratory of Infection Biology, The Rockefeller University, New York, New York

Michael R. McNeil, Ph.D. Professor, Department of Microbiology, Immunology and Pathology, Colorado State University, Fort Collins, Colorado

Robert L. Modlin, M.D. Professor of Dermatology, Microbiology, and Immunology, Department of Medicine, University of California at Los Angeles; Chief, Division of Dermatology, Department of Medicine, University of California at Los Angeles Medical Center, Los Angeles, California

Marisa Moore, M.D., M.P.H. Chief, Surveillance Section, Surveillance and Epidemiology Branch, Division of Tuberculosis Elimination, Centers for Disease Control and Prevention, Atlanta, Georgia

Thomas M. Moran, Ph.D. Associate Professor, Department of Microbiology and Immunology, Mt. Sinai School of Medicine, New York, New York

André L. Moreira, M.D., Ph.D. Assistant Professor, Department of Pathology, New York University School of Medicine; Assistant Professor, Department of Pathology, New York University Medical Center, New York, New York

John F. Murray, M.D. Professor Emeritus, Department of Medicine, University of California at San Francisco; Senior Faculty, Department of Pulmonary Critical Care Medicine, San Francisco General Hospital, San Francisco, California

Edward A. Nardell, M.D. Associate Professor, Harvard Medical School, Harvard School of Public Health; Director, Tuberculosis Research, Program in Infectious Disease and Social Change, Department of Social Medicine, Harvard Medical School; Chief, Pulmonary Medicine, The Cambridge Hospital, Cambridge, Massachusetts

Carl F. Nathan, M.D. Chairman, Department of Microbiology and Immunology, Joan and Sanford I. Weill Medical College of Cornell University, New York, New York

Richard J. O'Brien, M.D. Chief, Research and Evaluation Branch, Division of Tuberculosis Elimination, Centers for Disease Control and Prevention, Atlanta, Georgia

Philip Orbuch, M.D. Clinical Associate Professor and Associate Attending Professor, Department of Dermatology, New York University Medical Center, New York, New York

Mark Parta, M.D., M.P.H.T.M. Attending Physician, AIDS Program, Bellevue Hospital Center, New York, New York

Miriam Keltz Pomeranz, M.D. Assistant Professor, Department of Dermatology, New York University School of Medicine; Associate Attending, Department of Dermatology, Bellevue Hospital, New York, New York

Bindu Raju, M.D. Assistant Professor, Department of Medicine, Division of Pulmonary and Critical Care Medicine, New York University School of Medicine; Clinical Assistant Attending, Department of Chest Medicine, Bellevue Hospital Center, New York, New York

Joan Reibman, M.D. Associate Professor, Department of Medicine, Division of Pulmonary and Critical Care Medicine, New York University School of Medicine, New York, New York

Mona Rigaud, M.D., M.P.H. Clinical Assistant Professor, Department of Pediatrics, New York University Medical Center; Department of Pediatrics, Bellevue Hospital–Tisch Hospital, New York, New York

William N. Rom, M.D., M.P.H. Sol and Judith Bergstein Professor of Medicine and Environmental Medicine, Director, Division of Pulmonary and Critical Care Medicine, Department of Medicine, New York University School of Medicine; Director, Bellevue Chest Service, New York, New York

Stephen G. Rothstein, M.D. Clinical Associate Professor, Department of Otolaryngology, New York University Medical Center; Associate Attending, Department of Otolaryngology, Tisch Hospital, New York, New York

Ami N. Rubinowitz, M.D. Assistant Professor, Department of Radiology, New York University Medical Center, New York, New York

Lisa Saiman, M.D. M.P.H. Associate Professor of Clinical Pediatrics, Department of Pediatrics, Columbia University College of Physicians & Surgeons; Assistant Hospital Attending, Department of Pediatrics, New York Presbyterian Medical Center, New York, New York

Larry S. Schlesinger, M.D. Samuel Saslaw Professor, Department of Internal Medicine, Division of Infectious Diseases, Ohio State University; Division Director, Department of Infectious Diseases, Ohio State University Medical Center, Columbus, Ohio

Neil W. Schluger, M.D. Associate Professor of Medicine and Public Health, Department of Medicine, Columbia University College of Physicians and Surgeons; Clinical Chief, Division of Pulmonary, Allergy, and Critical Care Medicine, Department of Medicine, Columbia Presbyterian Medical Center, New York, New York

Erwin Schurr, Ph.D. Associate Professor, Departments of Medicine and Human Genetics, McGill University; Medical Scientist, Department of Medicine, McGill University Health Centre, Montreal, Quebec, Canada

Kent A. Sepkowitz, M.D. Associate Professor, Department of Medicine, Weill Medical College of Cornell University; Director, Infection Control, Memorial Sloan–Kettering Cancer Center, New York, New York

Alex Sherman, M.D. Clinical Assistant Professor, Department of Medicine, New York University School of Medicine; Attending Physician, Department of Medicine, New York University Medical Center, New York, New York

Jerome L. Shupack, M.D. Professor, Department of Dermatology, New York University School of Medicine; Attending, Tisch Hospital, New York, New York

Peter A. Sieling, Ph.D. Associate Professor, Department of Medicine, Division of Dermatology, David Geffen School of Medicine at University of California at Los Angeles, Los Angeles, California

Andrew G. Sikora, M.D., Ph.D. Teaching Assistant, Department of Otolaryngology, New York University School of Medicine; House Staff, Department of Otolaryngology, Bellevue Hospital, New York, New York

Emil Skamene, M.D., Ph.D. Professor, Departments of Medicine and Human Genetics, Director, McGill Centre for the Study of Host Resistance, McGill University; Director of Research, McGill University Health Centre, Montreal, Quebec, Canada

Mark F. Sloane, M.D. Assistant Professor of Clinical Medicine, Division of Pulmonary and Critical Care Medicine, New York University School of Medicine; Director, Medical Intensive Care Unit, Division of Pulmonary and Critical Care Medicine, New York University Medical Center; New York Pulmonary Associates, New York, New York

Issar Smith, Ph.D. Tuberculosis Center, Public Health Research Institute at the International Center for Public Health, Newark, New Jersey

Ruth Spiegel, D.M.D. (Deceased) Clinical Associate Professor of Dentistry, Department of Oral Pathology, Biology and Diagnostic Science, University of Medicine and Dentistry of New Jersey, Piscataway, New Jersey

Ralph M. Steinman, M.D. Professor, Laboratory of Cellular Physiology and Immunology, The Rockefeller University; Senior Physician, Rockefeller University Hospital, New York, New York

Hillel Tobias, M.D., Ph.D. Clinical Professor, Department of Medicine, New York University School of Medicine; Attending Physician, Medical Director, Liver Transplant Service, New York University Medical Center, New York, New York

Timo Ulrichs, M.D. Fellow, Department of Immunology, Max-Planck-Institute for Infection Biology; Fellow, Institute for Infection Medicine of the Free University of Berlin, Berlin, Germany

Andrew A. Vernon, M.D., M.H.S. Clinical Assistant Professor of Medicine, Adjunct Professor of Epidemiology, Emory University Schools of Medicine and Public Health; Associate Director of Science (OD), National Center for HIV, STD, and TB Prevention, Centers for Disease Control and Prevention, Atlanta, Georgia

Richard J. Wallace, Jr., M.D. Chairman, John Chapman Professorship in Microbiology, Professor of Medicine, Department of Microbiology, The University of Texas Health Center at Tyler, Tyler, Texas

Michael Weiden, M.D. Assistant Professor, Department of Medicine, Division of Pulmonary and Critical Care Medicine, New York University School of Medicine; Assistant Attending, Department of Pulmonary Medicine, Bellevue Hospital, New York University School of Medicine, New York, New York

David Zagzag, M.D., Ph.D. Associate Professor, Departments of Pathology and Neurosurgery, New York University School of Medicine; Associate Attending, Department of Pathology, New York University Medical Center, New York, New York

Ying Zhang, Ph.D. Associate Professor, Department of Molecular Microbiology and Immunology, Johns Hopkins Bloomberg School of Public Health, Baltimore, Maryland

Xilin Zhao, Ph.D. Research Scientist, Public Health Research Institute at the International Center for Public Health, Newark, New Jersey

FOREWORD

Tuberculosis has probably been responsible for more deaths than any other disease. After decades of complacency resulting from the belief that tuberculosis and other infectious diseases were no longer major health problems, we now are obliged to recognize that "the global unfinished agenda" of infectious disease has emerged as the greatest threat to global health—and perhaps to economic and political security in the world. Tuberculosis is responsible for the deaths of over 2 million people annually worldwide, and is the major attributable cause of death from human immunodeficiency virus/acquired immunodeficiency syndrome (HIV/AIDS). One-third of the world's population is infected with *Mycobacterium tuberculosis* and share a 10% lifetime risk of developing the disease, which becomes an almost 10% annual risk in immunocompromised infected individuals. The new edition of *Tuberculosis* could not be more timely, because it is the co-epidemics of HIV/AIDS and tuberculosis that now challenge the world to devise means of preventing the greatest loss of human life in history.

This book summarizes the current state of our knowledge and how it could be used more effectively to combat tuberculosis. It brings together information from many sources on the pathology and pathogenesis of the disease, its multiple manifestations, and principles of treatment. At the scientific level, it also reveals our remaining wealth of ignorance about the fundamental disease processes, about the strategies used by the pathogen to elude both immune responses and drug therapies, and provides ideas from many of the best experts in the world, both on how to use the tools we have and also how to develop new strategies on a global scale to reduce or eliminate tuberculosis as a major public health problem.

It is ironic that as tuberculosis is fanned by the HIV/AIDS epidemic to take an increasing toll in the developing countries and Eastern Europe, tuberculosis in the United States—after a major increase in the early 1990s—has declined to its lowest recorded level ever, from 26,673 cases in 1992 to 16,377 in 2002. This constitutes a major achievement in a 10-year period. What has made such a dramatic decline possible is the reduction in the rate of active transmission of infection in the United States, since rates of reactivation appear not to have declined significantly. The lesson is that we now have effective—if not ideal—tools to cure tuberculosis, as compared with those

we have for HIV/AIDS. This is not only important for the individual patient but is, at the same time, the best public health intervention to block transmission. However, the experiences of many countries indicate that we have much to learn about how to use the drugs and strategy of directly observed treatment, short course (DOTS) more effectively. There are major lessons regarding the consequences of not using the drugs that are available in the most effective way, with the alarming emergence of multi-drug resistance in 72 countries and all continents of the world. In this context, there is a serious concern that the tools that are effective now may not be effective in future.

A realistic assessment of our current state in controlling this disease would be that there remains a great need for new knowledge and new tools. Since the publication of the first edition of *Tuberculosis*, there indeed has been an explosion of new knowledge that offers great hope not only for greater scientific understanding of the pathogen, the immune response, and the disease, but also for the development of new drugs and vaccines that are urgently needed. Perhaps the greatest of the scientific breakthroughs is the uncoding of the genome of the pathogen, *M. tuberculosis*. Everyone in the scientific community has access to the DNA sequence, and information about every gene, protein, antigen, and potential drug target. This is a gigantic scientific advance, and knowledge of the genome is available to all. A second advance is the knowledge of the human genome. This knowledge offers not only new opportunities to understand the mechanisms by which the pathogen stimulates immune responses but also possibilities for new diagnostic tests. Together, these advances provide a new basis for understanding the two key questions in pathogenesis, latency and virulence. They offer possibilities of rational design of new drugs that are able to act on new targets to deal with emerging resistant strains and, most importantly, that may be effective against the persistent or latent form of the organism and prevent reactivation. These breakthroughs also have brought to light knowledge about the newly discovered innate immune responses, conserved from fruit flies to humans, that together with acquired cell-mediated immune responses offer insights into developing safer and more effective vaccines than bacille Calmette–Guérin.

Ultimately, controlling of tuberculosis—which for over a century has engaged some of the best minds in medical science, including Pasteur, Villemin, Calmette, Waksman, Styblo, and many others—may not be so much a scientific problem as one of commitment and political will. The common perception is that health is a matter of individual responsibility. But individual perceptions of health are highly socially conditioned—by social stigmatization as well as fear and denial, and also by positive social action and political commitment. There are extraordinary new institutions recently created to address many of the problems of tuberculosis that neither poor countries nor individuals themselves have been in a position to accomplish. There is a Global Fund for AIDS, Tuberculosis, and Malaria seeking to raise funds on a scale never before contemplated to make resources available to poor countries that have a commitment and a national plan to combat these diseases. The Global Tuberculosis Drug Facility was created under the World Health Organization with the mission of increasing access to existing tuberculosis drugs for millions of people and making them available to countries that need them.

The Global Alliance for Tuberculosis, a new public/private partnership, seeks to develop new and more effective tuberculosis drugs for which there are not sufficient market incentives for the major pharmaceutical companies to invest.

Since infectious diseases do not respect national borders, we must recognize that a global commitment to address the burden of tuberculosis is almost certainly the most effective form of enlightened self-interest. Beyond self-interest, it is possible not only that we are at a crossroads in mounting an effective scientific response to tuberculosis, but also that we are at the threshold of a new era in which civil society in a globalizing world is recognizing its responsibility to protect all people around the world against the major infectious disease killers. How we address the problems of tuberculosis and HIV/AIDS will determine how our generation is judged by history.

Barry R. Bloom, Ph.D.
Dean, Harvard School of Public Health

PREFACE

In the future the battle against this plague of mankind (tuberculosis) will not just be concerned with an uncertain something but with a tangible parasite, about whose characteristics a great deal is known and can be explored.

Robert Koch, 1882

Since 1903, the Bellevue Chest Service has served as a major provider of medical care to New York City's tuberculosis patients. Primary therapy then was fresh air provided from a boat moored in the East River or in tents atop Bellevue's roof, surrounded by a foot of snow during wintertime. From 1938 through the 1960s, the Bellevue Chest Service pioneered the training of physicians in the specialty of tuberculosis and other respiratory diseases. Superb teacher/clinicians, namely James Alexander Miller (1903–1938), J. Burns Amberson (1938–1955), John McClement (1955–1983), and H. William Harris (1983–1989), have graced the Chest Service since its first days. These men trained hundreds of physicians in the art and science of caring for patients with tuberculosis. Out of this lively atmosphere came the 1956 Nobel Prize to Drs. André Cournand and Dickinson Richards for assessment of cardiopulmonary physiology with venous catheters.

In the mid 1980s, after many years of decline, tuberculosis reemerged in epidemic form in New York City, hastened by the onset of acquired immunodeficiency syndrome (AIDS), the increase in drug abuse and homelessness, and a failing public health infrastructure. Tuberculosis cases began to increase nationally, reversing a 30-year declining trend. The magnitude of the global tuberculosis problem is even more staggering. With approximately 1.8 billion people (one third of the world's population) already infected with *Mycobacterium tuberculosis*, the World Health Organization predicted that 90 million new cases of tuberculosis will occur per decade and 30 million people will be expected to die of tuberculosis. The changing epidemiology related to promulgating Directly Observed Therapy (DOT) is described in the second edition of *Tuberculosis*.

To combat this menace, we have assembled chapters by leading authorities in every aspect of the disease. The first half of *Tuberculosis*, Second Edition, continues to present the new epidemiology and is followed by detailed sections on the biochemistry of the mycobacterium and host immune responses. New in the second edition is a chapter on the newly sequenced genome of *M. tuberculosis* and a chapter comparing bacille Calmette–Guérin to *Mycobacterium bovis*. Genetic pathways and individual genes and their function are rapidly becoming unraveled and are described in subsequent chapters. With the human genome sequenced, we are learning much more about innate immunity and the host immune response. We have endeavored to include as much of this evolving knowledge as possible. The second half of the text covers the entire clinical spectrum of tuberculosis; it was written by expert clinicians, including many New York University physicians who care for Bellevue's tuberculosis patients. Although we have attempted to reduce the number of chapters, most of the clinical topics have remained to keep the textbook a value for both basic scientists and clinicians. *Tuberculosis*, Second Edition, concludes with discussions of current and future public health issues. Our contributors' expertise has substantially eased our editorial burden.

During the course of writing the first edition of *Tuberculosis*, the tuberculosis patient population at Bellevue peaked at more than 500 new patients and has now declined to 100 patients per year by the time of publication of the second edition. The scourge of multidrug-resistant tuberculosis has declined significantly and is now residing in foreign countries (The Dominican Republic, the Baltics) or hot spots such as Russian prisons. Now the challenge with the new multidrug-resistant strain, fingerprinted and labeled W, which proved deadly to tuberculosis/human immunodeficiency virus–1 (TB/HIV-1) co-infected patients, is that it remains latent in hundreds of contacts. Understanding the biology of latency, both the genes of *M. tuberculosis* and the host's response, has become an exciting area of research. Several new chapters address this topic. Many hospitals, including ours, have installed new ventilation systems, ultraviolet lights, and high-efficiency particulate filters and mandated tight-fitting respirators. Directly observed therapy has become the standard of care in New York City and throughout the world.

We now know practically all mechanisms of action for antimycobacterial drugs. Pharmacogenomics has targeted numerous pathways for drug disruption, yet drug development and clinical trials of new therapeutics proceed at a snail's pace. Use of the polymerase chain reaction test could revolutionize rapid diagnosis; however, new technologies need to be inexpensive to radically change the course of this disease due to its concentration among developing countries. The HIV-1 epidemic has expanded in Africa, South Asia, and Russia, providing more fertile soil for tuberculosis. The combination of HIV-1 infection and latent TB infection increases the risk for active TB by 200-fold; in this context, DOT short course, which works so well in curing TB, will be overwhelmed by the number of new cases. Implementation of the antiretroviral therapy in developing countries can reduce TB incidence by up to 80%. The second edition of *Tuberculosis* attempts to capture these themes in sections on treatment and public health.

Tuberculosis investigation has become an exciting new discipline after nearly a half century of quiescence. Because of this rekindled interest and proliferation of knowledge, we hope that *Tuberculosis*, Second Edition, will continue to stimulate interest in this centuries-old, dreaded disease. We thank our many colleagues who have contributed their valuable time to this effort and ask their understanding for our editorial suggestions and revisions.

Finally, our wives, Holly and Adrienne, were once again extraordinarily tolerant of us during this work, and we dedicate this volume to them and our children, Nicole and Meredith, and Jordan, respectively.

William N. Rom, M.D., M.P.H.
Stuart M. Garay, M.D.

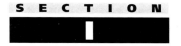

SECTION

I

HISTORY AND EPIDEMIOLOGY

THE WRITER'S VOICE: TUBERCULOSIS IN THE ARTS

JOAN REIBMAN
THOMAS LENNON

Doctors and scientists who specialize in a disease often compile the names of famous people who contracted it. Curiosity, and perhaps a certain prurience, drives us. More than that, we compile such lists because doing so argues for the importance of the disease. It makes the abstract and anonymous concept of an illness more human by putting an individual face and name and experience to it.

The list of writers struck with tuberculosis (TB) is astonishing: Samuel Johnson, John Keats, Percy Bysshe Shelley, the Brontë sisters, Robert Louis Stevenson, Maxim Gorky, Masaoko Shiki, Anton Chekhov, Franz Kafka, and George Orwell (1,2) are among the most famous of a much larger group (see Table 1.1 on page 9). These writers serve us, because it is a writer's function to make his or her experience accessible. This chapter will explore five authors and their differing responses to TB: bewilderment, secretiveness, irrational hope, and protest. Their lives span this past century. Each of the five artists had boundaries to cross, whether of race or tradition, gender or ideology, and their disease, while it often thwarted their work, also at times inspired them.

It was 1899, the turn of the century, when Paul Laurence Dunbar was first told of his "pneumonia," and fluid was drained from his lungs. Dunbar was an American poet (Fig. 1.1). What makes this description so improbable was that he was the son of slaves. No African American had ever presumed such a career for himself. Dunbar was writing poems before he was a teenager; John Keats was an early hero. Like the Romantic poet he so admired, Dunbar would have only a few years in which to find his voice.

The only black person in his class in Dayton, Ohio, he headed the literary society, wrote romances and westerns for

money, and launched with his friend, the future aviator Orville Wright, a newspaper aimed at the town's black population. Even his friend rated a poem (3):

> Orville Wright is out of sight
> In the printing business
> No other mind is half so bright
> As his'n is.

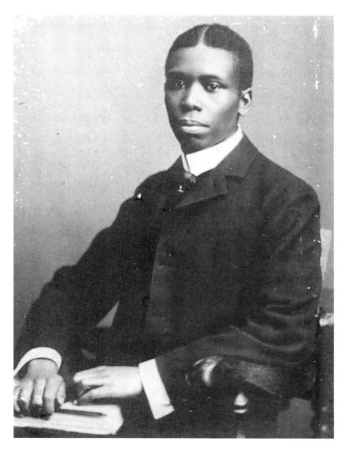

FIGURE 1.1. Portrait of Paul Laurence Dunbar. (From Ohio Historical Society, Columbus, OH, U.S.A., with permission.)

Presented at the Nobel Symposium on Tuberculosis, Stockholm, Sweden, 2000

J. Reibman: Department of Medicine, New York University, New York, New York.

T. Lennon: Lennon Documentary Group, New York, New York.

Dunbar graduated from school in 1891, convinced that he was destined for great things, to the only job he could find: bellhop, an elevator operator, in downtown Dayton (4–8). For 2 years, Dunbar composed poetry while shuttling passengers from floor to floor; on a moment's notice he would turn out verse celebrating any occasion, for any audience, in any style. If finding a voice is hard for all writers, it was especially so for a black man in this time and place. These were the years of segregation laws, lynchings, and the Ku Klux Klan. In his first book of poems, self-published and sold door-to-door, Dunbar writes in two distinct voices, as if he were two different poets, alternating between romantic Keats-like poems in classic English and plantation poems in slave dialect.

For this educated and urbane young man, the images of happy folk singing in the cotton fields were almost as foreign as the harps and angels of the English romantic style. But his plantation poems would earn him his fame, his livelihood, and his stature as a national figure. Blacks loved the handsome young man dressed in fine clothes; the ease with which he turned a phrase put the lie to black inferiority. And whites embraced him, too. They anointed him "Poet Laureate" of the Negro race (5). In these odes to an imaginary and benign Southern past, the American public found a balm for its racial conscience. And so the dialect voice that made Dunbar his fortune posed his great dilemma. That he was diagnosed with tuberculosis gave him few years in which to solve it.

By 1899, when he had turned twenty-seven, Dunbar's episodes of hemoptysis were so severe that he was sent to the mountains near Denver, Colorado. "It is yet a terrible thing to be forced away from home, from all one loves," he wrote "to an unknown, uncared-for country, there to fight, hand to hand with death, an uncertain fight" (9). Dunbar's race meant that he could not enter most sanatoriums, hospitals, or clinics. At least he was spared the treatment of many African Americans with TB, who were sent to prisons or mental asylums (10).

Short of money, Dunbar criss-crossed the country reading his poems, taking whatever treatment was on hand for his hemoptysis. From Florida he wrote, "Creosote, creosote, creosote, early retiring, no running around..." (11). His literary output remained prodigious. He wrote lyrics for the musical "In Dahomey." He wrote scathing novels about black urban life. But he hated it when, at every reading, his audiences demanded his dialect poems, their plantation favorites. He spoke for himself and his race when he wrote (3):

> I know why the caged bird sings, ah me
> When his wing is bruised and his bosom sore,
> When he beats his bars and he would be free.

To be a truly great poet, Dunbar would have had to bridge the divide between black and white cultures, with no precedents or models to guide him. He would have had to take the language of his parents and the language of the Romantic poets and fuse them into something that was his own. Tuberculosis cut those efforts short. But there were intimations of what might have been. In his poem *We Wear The Mask* (3), he gave voice to a central theme of African American life: the duality and disguise imposed by racial prejudice.

WE WEAR THE MASK

> We wear the mask that grins and lies,
> It hides our cheeks and shades our eyes
> The debt we pay to human guile;
> With torn and bleeding hearts we smile,
> And mouth with myriad subtleties.
>
> Why should the world be overwise
> In counting all our tears and sighs?
> Nay let them only see us, while
> We wear the mask.

Before he died at age 34, Dunbar returned to Ohio (3).

> Kind o'nice to set aroun'
> On the old familiar groun'
> Knowin' that when Death does come,
> That he'll find you right at home.

For Mori Ogai, one of Japan's great doctors and great modern writers, the mask was a lifelong preoccupation, imposed not by race but by disease. This brilliant man waged a lifelong campaign in medicine and literature to strip away the superstitions and stigmas of traditional Japan. Yet for reasons of social tradition and modern science, Mori Ogai never unmasked his own secret: tuberculosis.

When Mori Ogai began his studies at Tokyo University in 1872, Japanese medicine was a backwater. The new Emperor Meiji had called on his subjects to seek knowledge from all over the world to remake Imperial Japan into a great and modern nation. It was a call to arms for Japan's elite of which this young man knew himself to be a part. However, in his last year of medical school, Mori Ogai contracted pleurisy; his studies suffered and he graduated at the bottom of his class. He was only able to get himself abroad as a lieutenant in the army medical corps; his assignment, in the great modernization of Japan, would be nutrition and hygiene. In 1887, just 5 years after Koch's description of the tuberculous bacillus, Mori Ogai found himself at the Hygienic Institute of Berlin University, in the laboratory of the great man himself. Now with full comprehension of the disease as infectious, Mori Ogai would face all the public and personal dilemmas of TB.

He returned to Japan, a professor in the Army Medical School, impatient to modernize Japanese medicine. Self-confident, erudite, an angry young man, he called for internationalism in science as well as the use of rational scientific theory, and he ridiculed the country's medical establishment. "In the world today, there is only one medicine, modern medicine. Anything which does not have this foundation is on a par with the acupuncture of the priests, the old cure for ringworm and herbalists" (12) (Fig. 1.2). But his modern mission was also rooted in an ancient Confucian concept of the responsibility of a country's elite to care for those under them. The most up-to-date methods in nutrition, sanitation, and health education would enable the state to meets its traditional moral obligations. In the course of his rise to Surgeon General, Mori Ogai promoted such eclectic public health measures as the licensing of prostitutes, a looser fit for female corsets, and a traditional diet to prevent beriberi. He saw the link between housing conditions and contagion, and agitated for low-density housing for the poor, a reconstructed water supply, and a sewer system. In addition, the medical journal that he founded

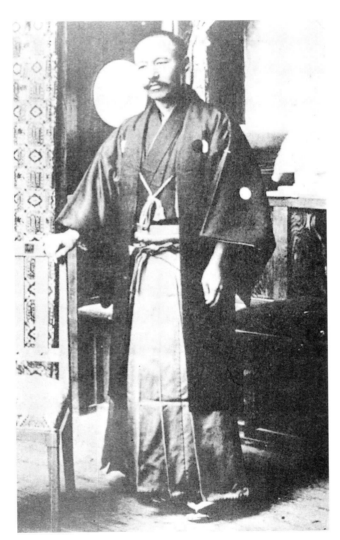

FIGURE 1.2. Mori Ogai, Surgeon General. (From Rimer JT. In: *Mori Ogai*. Boston: Twayne Publishers, a division of G.K. Hall & Co., 1975, with permission.)

played a key role in introducing tuberculin, Koch's new treatment for TB (12–14).

At the turn of the century, TB was exploding, as Japanese abandoned the countryside and crowded into slums. Tuberculosis was the cause of one in every seven Japanese deaths (14). Factory laborers, clustered in close quarters, were especially vulnerable. When the mostly female textile laborers were found to have the disease, they were driven from their jobs and homes and banished to villages where they died alone, behind closed doors (14). This illness was not just a death sentence but also a moral transgression, a source of shame. The entire family would find itself ostracized; even members of the next generation would be unable to marry. Not surprisingly, many of the infected concealed their disease. Mori Ogai, so visible on so many public health issues, was relatively quiet on the subject of TB. And he kept his own disease entirely hidden. It was only in his fiction that he dared reveal his experience.

This eminent physician was also a leading figure in modern Japanese literature. He published Japan's foremost literary journal; championed young authors; translated Strindberg, Ibsen, and Oscar Wilde; and in his own plays and novellas brought a new realism and psychology to Japanese writing (12,13,15). That realism extended to the treatment of disease. In his play *Masks*, he tells the story of a young student who approaches a physician about a cough (16). The physician gives the diagnosis of "chronic bronchitis." A Japanese audience would have understood that chronic bronchitis was one of many euphemisms for TB, such as bronchial catarrh, pneumonial catarrh, and caseous pneumonia. Such euphemisms spared the patient's stigma; what's more, they kept the physician in practice, since no one would consult a doctor known to diagnose TB (14). In *Masks*, the student inadvertently sees his medical record, which reads "diagnosis positive." And so the doctor, to console the student, confesses the presence of his own disease: "The slide is dated today . . . you can see the bacteria, the scattered filament-like ones are *Mycobacterium tuberculosis*. They appear red against the blue field. It's called Ziehl–Neelsen carbolfuchsin stain, and that's pretty much the way it's done these days. Whose tubercle bacilli do you think those are? . . .They're mine. . . . For seventeen years, until I told you, I have never told this to a soul" (16). The doctor goes on to explain a philosophy he has created to rationalize his secrecy. His posture is to "stand aloof from the common herd, to strengthen his resolve and place himself high above them in an aristocratic position of lonely eminence. Such eminent beings wear masks and those masks are to be respected. . . ." (16).

Mori Ogai wore his mask because the disease forced unacceptable choices on him. The scientist would have banished himself to a life of isolation. The human being was not prepared for such a life and so he rationalized a personal philosophy of resignation and transcendence in which the rules and routines imposed on the sick simply did not apply to him. In real life, this writer concealed his diagnosis even from his own family, covertly coughing and burning his tissues in his garden, persisting in his work and refusing all care. The cause of his death in 1922 was listed as "atrophy of the kidney." However, before dying, he had allowed a personal friend to examine him; the results were disclosed 30 years later. "[The] phlegm . . . was chock full of tuberculosis bacilli," his colleague had said, "It was just like examining a culture" (12). Mori Ogai's secret life reminds us of what it means to live with full understanding of an infectious disease for which there is no cure.

Secrecy, silence, and resignation were not in Katherine Mansfield's repertoire. One of New Zealand's great short-story writers, the free-spirited Mansfield carried out a tireless search for a cure for her TB, and her letters and journal helped convey to the public the human experience of this disease.

"I am so keen upon all women having a definite future, are not you?" Mansfield wrote when she was 18. "The idea of sitting still and waiting for a husband is absolutely revolting. . . ." (17). She fled New Zealand at the first opportunity. Living on the fringes of the London literary scene, she tried out hashish, bisexuality, and occultism. She became pregnant and was dispatched to Bavaria by her family, in the hopes that she would mend her ways. "I was soaped and

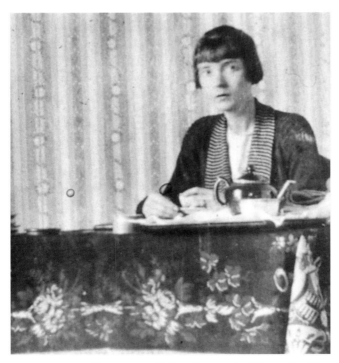

FIGURE 1.3. Katherine Mansfield at her work table, at the Villa Isola, Menton, France, 1920. (Photographer: Ida Baker. Reproduced with permission from the Alexander Turnbull Library, Wellington, New Zealand.)

smacked and sprayed and thrown in a cold water tank," she wrote (17); it became the source of her first book of stories, *In a German Pension*, published in 1911. By the time she was diagnosed with TB in 1917, she was a writer of some reputation, the voice of women with wasted lives, women disappointed, women betrayed (Fig. 1.3).

She married John Middleton Murry, an avant-garde literary journalist, and they became members of the Bloomsbury circle of writers, which included T. S. Eliot, Virginia Woolf, and the consumptive D. H. Lawrence. But her true literary model, the man she revered, was the great Russian doctor, writer, and TB patient: Anton Chekhov. Like Chekhov, Katherine Mansfield would spend years traveling from place to place in a futile search for a cure. "I don't want to find this is real consumption," she wrote, "Perhaps it's going to gallop—who knows—and I shan't have my work written. *That's what matters. . . .*" (18). She wrote to her husband, "The program seems to be to sit tight, pack, and make for the sun. . . . Although I am still snapping up fishes like a sea lion, steaks like a land lion, milk like a snake . . . and eggs, honey, cream, butter and nourishing trimmings galore, they seem to go to a sort of Dead Letter Office. . . ." (18).

Refusing to stay in a sanatorium, Mansfield traveled to the Italian Riviera, the South of France, England, and the South of France again. She was separated from her husband, communicating through letters. "I have been ill for nearly four years—and I'm changed changed—not the same. . . . I don't want dismissing as a masterpiece. . . . I haven't anything like as long to live as you have. I've *scarcely any time I feel. . . .* Praise [others] when I'm dead—Talk to ME. I'm lonely. I haven't ONE single soul. . . ." (18). She is afraid her husband is repelled by her illness. "Life is getting a new breath, nothing else counts. And Murry is silent, hangs his head, hides his face with his fingers AS THOUGH it were unendurable. . . ." (17). She wrote, "I am stuck in bed—by my old doctor. . . . I hate bed. I shall never to bed in Heaven. . . . If a cherubim and a seraphim come winging their way towards me with some toast and jelly I shall pop like a chestnut into Hell and be roasted" (17).

She published two more collections of stories, *Bliss* and her last, *The Garden Party*, in 1922. She sought help from a Dr. Manoukhine who promised a cure using x-ray therapy to her spleen, "After five doses of x-rays one is hotted up inside like a furnace and one's very bones seem to be melting. I suppose this is the moment when real martyrs break into song but I can think of nothing but fern grots, cucumbers, and fans. . . ." (18). As modern medicine failed her, she turned to the mystic Gurdjieff and moved to his retreat in France, the Institute for the Harmonious Development of Man. "This *is* the place, and here at last one is understood entirely, mentally and physically. I could never have regained my health by any other treatment and all my friends accepted me as a frail half-creature who migrated towards sofas. . . ." (18). Here, in touch with the earth and caring for the cows, she feels she is finding her true self. And here, at age 34, she dies, leaving her letters to testify to the loneliness and terror of TB.

In 1937, a 24-year-old French Algerian, on his way to the mountains, wrote, "This fever beating in my temples. I spent all my time thinking of K. Mansfield, about that long, painful, and tender story. . . . What awaits me in the Alps is, together with loneliness and the idea that I shall be there to look after myself, the *awareness* of my illness" (19). His name, of course, was Albert Camus, and 5 years later he would come to prominence with the publication of *The Stranger*.

Camus was raised by his widowed mother in Belcourt, a working-class section of Algiers. His passion was soccer; he and the classmates he played with were destined to leave school in their teens and enter the nearby factories. But Camus's teacher begged his mother to keep Albert in school. When he was 17 and beginning his advanced studies, Camus presented with hemoptysis and was diagnosed with tuberculosis. His therapy was red meat, overeating, and pneumothorax treatments every 2 weeks. Rarely written about and never given its due, tuberculosis shaped Camus's life, and the moral and political arguments for which he became renowned (Fig. 1.4).

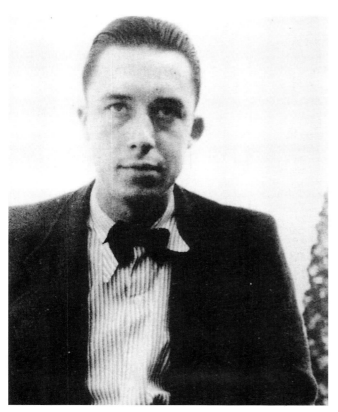

FIGURE 1.4. Albert Camus as a young man. (From Todd O. In: *Albert Camus: a life*. New York: Alfred A. Knopf, with permission. Archives A. Camus/Imec.)

Camus intended to support himself by teaching. However, his medical report read "pulmonary tuberculosis . . . infiltrated into almost the entire left lung, with infection beginning at the top of the right lung," (20) and the Algerian Surgeon General refused to license him. He became a journalist, first for *Alger Republicain* and later for *Paris-Soir*. In 1936, his health prevented him from joining the Spanish Civil War, the great crusade of the day. Three years later, when World War II broke out, he tried to enlist and was again exempted from the army (21). His illness, painful and debilitating, freed him to pursue his writing career.

The Nazi occupation of France and its territories forced hard moral choices from which Camus was not exempt. He received ongoing pneumothorax treatments from a Jewish pulmonologist in Algeria, Dr. Cohen, whom he visited covertly since the doctor's practice was banned. Meanwhile, he agreed to omit his chapter on Kafka, a Jew, in order to publish his book, *The Myth of Sisyphus*. That same year, he moved to the mountains near Le Chambon-sur-Lignon, in France. "Keep quiet lung!" he wrote. "Fill yourself with this icy pure air. . . . May I cease being forced to listen to your slow rotting away. . . ." (19). Although this region was a center of resistance, Camus remained disengaged. His diaries and letters reveal his intense literary ambition and a longing to rejoin his wife. The drama of the war, except as it impinged on his family, was secondary (21). But in this village Camus found inspiration for his book, *The Plague*. "Illness is a convent," he wrote, "which has its rule, its austerity, its silences, and its inspirations" (19). This novel, called "a major novel of World War II," is the chronicle of a deadly epidemic and the responses of those quarantined in the town (22). The narrator is a doctor, who continues to care for his patients even though he lacks any ability to cure them.

If the plague is clearly a metaphor for the Nazi occupation, the imagery is derived from Camus's own illness. And the novel contains a portrait of Camus himself, in the character of a journalist who remains selfishly focused on his own escape to join his loved one, but who finally renounces his personal desires and participates in the great struggle. And finally, in late 1943, Camus left the mountains and joined the Resistance as editor of its newspaper, *Combat*. Now a recognized author, he became a voice of the French intellectual resistance, even as he continued to receive biweekly pneumothorax treatments.

In 1947, as he toured the United States and South America, he again coughed up blood. He wrote in his notebooks, "After such a long certainty of being cured, this back-sliding ought to crush me . . . it rather makes me laugh. In the end, I am liberated. Madness too is a liberation" (19). He added, "Those moments when one yields to anguish . . . lying down, motionless, devoid of will and of future, listening only to the long twinges of pain. . . . But anguish is just that, the thing to which one is never superior" (19).

He first received chemotherapy for his tuberculosis at the end of 1949: 3 months of streptomycin and paraaminosalicylic acid. Improved, he wrote a series of books—*The Rebel, The Fall,* and *Exile and the Kingdom*—that consolidated his moral and political opinions. He engaged the most painful problems of postwar France: the treatment of collaborators, the culpability of the French Communist party of which he had once been part, and the civil strife in Algeria. Having lived his adult life as a condemned man, Camus could not sanction taking the life of another. And so, he opposed the death penalty, even for collaborators; he condemned Stalin; and he opposed the Algerian independence movement because of their use of terrorist tactics. These views brought denunciation from both the left and the right, he was savaged in the intellectual journals of Paris, and he lost almost every literary friend he had. In his speech accepting the Nobel Prize in 1957, he answered back: "Our craft will always be rooted in two commitments, difficult to maintain: the refusal to lie about what one knows and the resistance to oppression" (23).

By the time Camus lost his life in a car crash in 1960, isonazid was in full use and rifampin only a few years away. Our story should end here, the tuberculous writer now a relic of history. But, to quote the doctor in *The Plague*, "What those jubilant crowds did not know but could have learned from books [is] that the plague bacillus never dies or disappears for good; . . . and that perhaps the day would come when, for the bane and enlightening of men, it would rouse up its rats again and send them forth. . . ." (24).

In preparing this chapter, we searched for written testimony about the disease that today infects one third of the world's population. We contacted physicians, writers, artists, arts organizations, libraries, booksellers, hundreds of people. We got wonderful responses from people around the globe, and almost no testimony. Many, as in Haiti and South Africa, said TB was a disease of the poor, those who do not have the means to write. For all the science, these people live like Dunbar and Mansfield, bewildered, with no prospect of a cure. And TB retains its stigma. We spoke with a physician from Iran; he knew of artists with TB and promised he would talk to them. We never heard back. In Brazil, the response was the same. A doctor from Russia explained that admission of TB could result in one's legal and permanent removal from a job, the loss of one's livelihood. These people are afraid to speak. They still wear the mask.

Camus, in his Nobel Prize acceptance speech, said that the artist's job was "to [stir] the greatest number of people by offering them a privileged picture of common joys and sufferings" (23). Artists have done just this with TB. And now, with the most stigmatized version of the disease, TB associated with acquired immune deficiency syndrome (AIDS), artists continue to fulfill this role.

Writer, artist, filmmaker, Derek Jarman was from an early age an unrestrained advocate of what he liked to call the

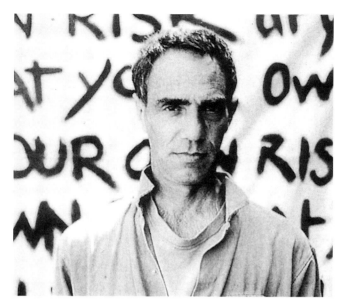

FIGURE 1.5. Derek Jarman, 1992. (Photograph by Howard Sooley.)

"queer life." Active in all aspects of the English art scene from the 1960s on, he wrote, painted, and directed films, including the flamboyant "Caravaggio." By 1981, his American friends were writing to him of their ailments. By 1982, his English friends were dying. By 1986, he had his diagnosis: "The young doctor who told me this morning I was a carrier of the AIDS virus was visibly distressed. I smiled and told her not to worry, I had never liked Christmas. . . ." (25). He planned. "On December 1986, finding I was body positive, I set myself a target: I would disclose my secret and survive Margaret Thatcher. I did. Now I have my sights on the millennium and a world where we are all equal under the law." He stated, "The one thing I could do was to carry on working so other people in the same circumstances could see it was possible" (Fig. 1.5). In the last 7 years of his life, he directed six feature films, wrote five books, painted, and created a garden at Dungeness, where, he said, he "intended to celebrate our corner of Paradise, the part of the garden the Lord forgot to mention" (25).

Tuberculosis was his first human immunodeficiency virus–associated infection and it galvanized his efforts on gay rights and AIDS. He became a member of the activist group, OutRage, and by his outrageous art and writings, he insisted on being seen and heard, fully human and without shame. For his efforts, he was canonized by his friends, the Sisters of Perpetual Indulgence, as "St. Derek of Dungeness." He painted illness, a single thermometer, crumpled bags, and a mask, asking "TB or not TB." His disease progressed: *Pneumocystis carinii*, cytomegalovirus, wasting. He completed his last script and film, "Blue," released in 1994 (26).

TABLE 1.1. ARTISTS WITH TUBERCULOSIS

Name	Dates	Field	Country
Thomas Bernhard	1931–1989	Writer	Austria
Franz Kafka	1883–1924	Writer	Czechoslovakia
Norman Bethune	1890–1939	Writer/physician	Canada
Sara Jeanette Duncan	1861–1922	Writer	Canada
Teresa Stratas	1939–	Opera singer	Canada
Norval Morrisseau	1932–	Painter	Canada (Native American)
Aubrey Beardsley	1872–1898	Painter	England
Quentin Bell	1910–1996	Writer	England
Charlotte Brontë	1816–1855	Writer	England
Anne Brontë	1820–1849	Writer	England
Emily Brontë	1818–1848	Writer	England
Elizabeth Barrett Browning	1806–1861	Poet	England
Steven Georgiou (Cat Stevens)	1947–	Musician	England
Leigh Hunt	1784–1859	Writer	England
Derek Jarman	1942–1994	Writer Painter/visual artist	England
Samuel Johnson	1709–1784	Writer	England
John Keats	1795–1821	Poet	England
John Keegan	1934–	Historian	England
D.H. Lawrence	1885–1930	Writer	England
George Orwell	1903–1950	Writer	England
Alexander Pope	1688–1744	Poet	England
Sir Walter Scott	1771–1832	Writer	England
Percy Bysshe Shelley	1792–1822	Poet	England
Elizabeth Siddal	1829–1862	Painter	England
Alan Sillitoe	1928–	Writer	England
Robert L. Stevenson	1850–1894	Writer	England
Anthony Trollope	1815–1882	Writer	England
Lili Boulanger	1893–1918	Musician	France
Frederic Chopin	1810–1849	Composer	France
Jules Laforgue	1860–1887	Poet	France
Alphonse de Lamartine	1790–1868	Poet/politician	France
Amedeo Modidgliani	1884–1920	Painter	France/Italy
Romain Rolland	1866–1944	Writer	France
Jean Jacques Rousseau	1712–1778	Writer/philosopher	France
Antoine Watteau	1684–1721	Artist	France
Simone Weil	1909–1943	Writer	France
Albert Camus	1913–1960	Writer	France (Algerian)
Johann Wolfgang Von Goethe	1749–1832	Writer	Germany
Christian Grabbe	1801–1836	Dramatist	Germany
Friedrich Schiller	1759–1805	Writer	Germany
Carl Maria von Weber	1786–1826	Composer	Germany
Castera Bazile	1923–1966	Painter	Haiti
Nicolo Paganini	1782–1840	Musician	Italy
Giovanni Battista Pergolesi	1710–1736	Musician	Italy
Luigi Boccherini	1743–1804	Musician	Italy
Ishikawa Takuboku	1886–1912	Poet	Japan
Futabatei Shimei	1864–1909	Writer	Japan
Kunikida Doppo	1871–1908	Writer	Japan
Higuchi Ichiyo	1868–1912	Writer	Japan
Shunsuke Matsumoto	1912–1948	Writer	Japan
Mori Ogai	1862–1922	Writer/physician	Japan
Yasuds Yukihiko	1884–1978	Painter	Japan
Masaoko Shiki	1867–1902	Poet	Japan
Katherine Mansfield	1888–1923	Writer	New Zealand
Edvard Grieg	1843–1907	Composer	Norway
Rikard Noraak	1842–1866	Composer	Norway
Maksim Gorky	1868–1936	Writer	Russia
Anton Chekhov	1860–1904	Writer	Russia
Fedor Dostoyevesky	1821–1881	Writer	Russia
Igor Stravinsky	1882–1971	Composer	Russia
Lesya Ukrainka	1871–1913	Poet/dramatist	Russia

TABLE 1.1. *(continued)*

Name	Dates	Field	Country
Galina Vishnevskaya	1926–	Singer	Russia
Feni Dumile	1939–1991	Artist	South Africa
Azaria Mbatha	1941–	Artist	South Africa
Tobias Smollett	1721–1771	Writer	Scotland
Antonio Machado	1875–1939	Poet	Spain
August Bebel	1840–1913	Writer	Switzerland
Oscar Ivar Levertin	1862–1906	Poet	Switzerland
Carlos Bulosan	1911–1956	Writer	US/Philippines
Judy Collins	1939–	Singer/musician	US
Stephen Crane	1871–1900	Writer	US
Paul Lawrence Dunbar	1872–1906	Writer	US (African American)
Dashiell Hammett	1894–1961	Writer	US
Hans Hofman	1880–1966	Visual artist	US/Germany
Oscar Howe	1915–1983	Visual artist	US (Native American)
Ring Lardner	1885–1933	Writer	US
Vivian Leigh	1914–1967	Actress	US
Janet Lewis	1899–1998	Writer	US
Eugene O'Neill	1888–1953	Writer	US
Timothy O'Sullivan	1840–1882	Photographer	US
Walker Percy	1916–1990	Writer	US
Bud Powell	1924–1966	Jazz pianist	US
Eleanor Roosevelt	1884–1962	Writer/columnist	US
Carlos Santana	1947–	Musician	US (Mexican)
Frederick Sommer	1905–1999	Photographer	US
Thurman, Wallace	1902–1934	Writer	US (African American)
Walt Whitman	1820–1892	Poet	US
Thomas Wolfe	1900–1938	Writer	US

The virus rages fierce. I have no friends now who are not dead or dying. Like a blue frost it caught them. At work, at the cinema, on marches and beaches. In churches on their knees, running, flying, silent or shouting protest.

As they fought for breath TB and pneumonia hammered at their lungs, and Toxo at the brain. Reflexes scrambled—sweat poured through hair matted like lianas in the tropical forest. Voices slurred—and then were lost forever. My pen chased this story across the page tossed this way and that in the storm. . . .

Our name will be forgotten
In time
No one will remember our work
Our life will pass like the traces of a cloud
And be scattered like
Mist that is chased by the
Rays of the sun
For our time is the passing of a shadow
And our lives will run like
Sparks through the stubble
I place a delphinium, Blue, upon your grave.

ACKNOWLEDGMENTS

We give special thanks to Jean Reibman, without whose diligence this project never would have been completed. We also thank those who offered support and assistance: Ernest B. Gilman, Ph.D., New York University; Aliye Bill, New York University; Patrick Moore, Estate Project; Ruth Divinagracia, M.D., Philippines; Mary Bassett, M.D., Zimbabwe; Ana Krieger, M.D., Brazil; Cheryl Dax, South Africa; Sue Williamson, South Africa; Tom Frieden, M.D., World Health Organization (WHO); Ian Smith, M.D., WHO, Stop TB Initiative; Bill Bower, M.D., U.S.A.; Peter Cegielski, M.D., Centers for Disease Control and Prevention (CDC); Louise Gubb, South Africa; Paul Farmer, M.D.; Mohammad M. Feizabadi, V.M., Ph.D., Iran; Eric Bateman, ED, South Africa; Judith Grodd, U.S.A.; Mark Veitch, M.D., Australia; Aleksander Feoktistov, M.D., Russia; Richard Morse, Haiti; Attie de Lange, Ph.D., South Africa; Hein Viljoen, Ph.D., South Africa; Cora Agatucci, Ph.D., U.S.A.; Malcolm Hacksley, National English Literary Museum, South Africa; William Johnston, Ph.D., U.S.A.; Peter Horn, South Africa; Paulette Coetze, South Africa; Bernard Fourie, M.D., South Africa; Andrey Mariandyshev, M.D., Russia; Fukuda Mahito, Ph.D., Japan; Gay Men's Health Crisis; PEN; Ohio Historical Society; Turnbull Library of New Zealand; Nagasaki University Library; Howard Sooley, England; Tom Semkow, New York University.

REFERENCES

1. Dubos R, Dubos J. *The white plague.* New Brunswick, NJ: Rutgers University Press, 1987.

2. Ryan F. *The forgotten plague*. Boston: Little, Brown and Company, 1992.
3. Dunbar PL. *The collected poetry of Paul Laurence Dunbar*. Charlottesville, VA: University Press of Virginia, 1996.
4. Brawley B. *Paul Laurence Dunbar: poet of his people*. Port Washington, NY: Kennidat Press, 1936.
5. Wiggins I. *The life and works of Paul Laurence Dunbar*. Nashville, TN: Winston-Derek Publishers, 1992.
6. Hudson GH. *A biography of Paul Laurence Dunbar*. Columbus, OH: Ohio State University Press, 1970.
7. Cunningham V. *Paul Laurence Dunbar and his song*. New York: Dodd, Mead and Company, 1947.
8. Lawson V. *Dunbar critically acclaimed*. Washington, DC: Associated Publishers, 1941.
9. Dunbar PL. *The love of Landry*. Salem, NH: Ayer, 1991.
10. Ott K. *Fevered lives: tuberculosis in American culture since 1870*. Cambridge, MA: Harvard University Press, 1996.
11. Dunbar PL. *Letters to Alice Dunbar*. Dayton, OH: Ohio Historical Society, 1898.
12. Bowring RJ. *Mori Ogai and the modernization of Japanese culture*. Cambridge, UK: Cambridge University Press, 1979.
13. Rimer JT. *Mori Ogai*. Boston: Twayne Publishers, a division of GK Hall & Co., 1975.
14. Johnston W. *The modern epidemic: a history of tuberculosis in Japan*. Cambridge, MA: Harvard University Press, 1995.
15. Ogai M. *The historical fiction of Mori Ogai*. Honolulu: University of Hawaii Press, 1991.
16. Ogai M. *Youth and other stories*. Honolulu: University of Hawaii Press, 2000:1994.
17. Boddy G. *Katherine Mansfield: the woman and the writer*. Victoria, Australia: Penguin Books, 1988.
18. 1991. *Letters between Katherine Mansfield and John Middleton Murry*. New Amsterdam: New Amsterdam Books, 1991.
19. Camus A. *Notebooks 1935–1951*. New York: Marlowe and Company, 1998.
20. Todd O. *Albert Camus: a life*. New York: Alfred A. Knopf, 1999.
21. Lottman HR. *Albert Camus: a biography*. Corte Madera, CA: Gingko Press, 1997.
22. Bonner SE. *Camus: portrait of a moralist*. Minneapolis: University of Minnesota Press, 1998.
23. Camus A. *Nobel acceptance speech*. Stockholm, Sweden: Nobel Foundation, 1957.
24. Camus A. *The plague*. New York: Vintage Books, 1991.
25. Peake T. *Derek Jarman*. London: Little, Brown and Company, 1999.
26. Jarman D. *Blue*. Woodstock, NY: Overlook Press, 1993.

GLOBAL EPIDEMIOLOGY OF TUBERCULOSIS

DONALD A. ENARSON
CHEN-YUAN CHIANG
JOHN F. MURRAY

The epidemiology of tuberculosis encompasses not only an evaluation of the distribution and determinants of the disease, but also an evaluation of the methods used for its control and their impact on the geographic distributions and trends of tuberculosis (1). Accordingly, this chapter on the global epidemiology of tuberculosis has several components. We begin by defining how the size of the tuberculosis problem is measured and by reporting the worldwide magnitude of the disease. Then we describe the determinants of tuberculous infection and disease and their geographic and social distributions. Next, we document the secular trends that have been observed during the last 30 to 40 years in high- and low-risk populations and the recent changes that have dramatically distorted these trends. Then we comment on the reasons for the recent resurgence of tuberculosis that includes many countries with a high burden of the disease. Finally, we conclude by considering how available control measures can deal with the rapidly growing number of patients with the disease. Because other authors deal with geographic and evolutionary epidemiology and the epidemiology of tuberculosis in the United States and in its inner cities, we concentrate here on the evolving situation in industrialized countries other than the United States, and in the more impoverished countries that collectively constitute the "developing nations" of the world.

SIZE OF THE PROBLEM

Documenting the size of the tuberculosis burden in a given community is not as easy as it sounds. The definition of what constitutes a case of tuberculosis varies among coun-

tries and sometimes within countries, the extent of surveillance differs enormously, and the validity of reported data is often questionable. These uncertainties pertain to each of the following measurement indices and are amplified when data from the more than 170 countries of the world are compiled.

Measuring Tuberculosis in the Community

When tuberculosis was common and specific antituberculosis treatment was not available, the *mortality rate* was a good indicator of the magnitude of the tuberculosis problem in a community. Before the introduction of chemotherapy and under stable conditions, the mortality rate was about one half of the incidence rate. Cohort studies were first made in Norway (2), then in the United States (3), followed by Great Britain (4), other European countries, Japan (5), and Taiwan (6). However, because statistics concerning mortality from tuberculosis derived from death certificates are extremely imprecise when the disease becomes less common (7) and because so few patients with tuberculosis die of the disease in countries with good control programs, the mortality rate has ceased to be a reliable indicator of either the size or the trend of the tuberculosis problem.

Also, surveys of the *prevalence of the disease tuberculosis* in representative samples of the general population, using chest radiology and sputum bacteriology, have been conducted in certain countries and in some instances have been repeated periodically (8,9). Under stable conditions and in the absence of specific treatment, this prevalence rate is a reasonable indicator of the magnitude of the tuberculosis problem in a community. In the prechemotherapy era, the ratio of prevalence to incidence of disease in a community was 2:1 (i.e., the average duration of a case was 2 years). However, the introduction of specific and effective antituberculosis treatment completely disrupted the usual ratio of prevalence to incidence. Nevertheless, these prevalence sur-

D.A. Enarson: Department of Medicine, University of Alberta, Alberta, Edmonton, Canada; International Union Against Tuberculosis and Lung Disease, Paris, France.

John F. Murray: University of Alberta, Edmonton, Alberta, Canada.

C.-Y. Chiang: Section of Chest Disease, Center for Chest Disease, Department of Health, Tainan County, Taiwan.

veys provide a good measure of the density of infectious sources of tuberculosis at a single moment in time and indicate the frequency of chronic infectious cases.

A third measure of the burden of tuberculosis in a community is the measurement of tuberculous infection using the tuberculin skin test. Initially introduced as a form of therapy, tuberculin proved more useful as a means of identifying the *prevalence of infection with Mycobacterium tuberculosis* independent of clinical disease. Serial tuberculin skin test surveys have provided valuable information and remain a widely used means of monitoring changes over time in the prevalence of tuberculous infection in countries where such surveys have been undertaken.

The epidemiologic concept of the *annual risk of tuberculous infection* was developed from the results of skin testing of new recruits to the military service of the Netherlands (10). This estimate reflects the probability of becoming infected in a given year. The mathematical calculation of the annual risk of infection (ARI) is determined by the formula: $ARI = 1 - (1 - p)^{1/a}$, where p is the prevalence of infection and a is the average age of the group tested. The average annual risk of infection estimated from a single prevalence survey is an insensitive measure of short-term changes in the trend of tuberculosis because it represents an average estimate over the whole life span of the individuals tested, centered on a point half the age of the population tested. When tuberculosis becomes very uncommon, the intrinsic problems of the tuberculin test, particularly bias caused by the prevalence of infection with mycobacteria other than *M. tuberculosis,* create serious difficulties.

In countries where notification of newly diagnosed cases of tuberculosis is extremely thorough, the *incidence of active tuberculosis* can be approximated, and such data have been used to monitor the epidemiologic situation. This measure is only reliable in the few countries where both supervision and review of all notifications are undertaken by tuberculo-

sis experts to ensure the validity and completeness of the registration of cases. Where this expertise is not part of the procedure, the information is much less useful for epidemiologic monitoring. Annual risk of infection has been used to estimate annual incidence of active cases (11). Various "benchmarks" of tuberculosis may be identified as follows (in rates per 100,000/year): Above 1,000, tuberculosis can be said to be "epidemic"; above 100, groups can be defined as at "high risk" for tuberculosis; below 10, groups can be defined as at "low risk" for tuberculosis; below 1, tuberculosis programs are entering the elimination phase; at 0.1 tuberculosis can be said to be eliminated (12).

Another way of measuring the magnitude of tuberculosis in a community is to calculate its economic impact. The World Bank used this approach in 1993 (13) in its "World Development Report," which included an estimate of the *disability-adjusted life years* (DALYs), or the years that are consumed by various diseases, including tuberculosis.

Current Global Estimates

In 1992, the World Health Organization (WHO) published estimates of the prevalence of tuberculous infection, the incidence of the disease tuberculosis, and the number of deaths from tuberculosis that presumably occurred worldwide in 1990; these data were based on results of tuberculin skin test surveys, case notifications, estimates of health services coverage, and tuberculosis mortality rates reported by member countries and were calculated using simple epidemiologic models (14). The estimates for existing cases per country were revised in 1997, taking into account all existing published and unpublished materials and incorporating a consultative process with national experts to arrive at a consensus on an estimate (15). The prevalence of tuberculous infection from the 1990 exercises (Table 2.1) was estimated by these methods to be 1.7 billion (thousand mil-

TABLE 2.1. WORLD HEALTH ORGANIZATION (WHO) ESTIMATES OF THE WORLDWIDE PREVALENCE OF TUBERCULOUS INFECTION, 1990

Region	Prevalence (%)	No. of Infected (millions)	Percentage of Total
Africa[a]	33.8	171	9.9
Americas[b]	25.9	117	6.8
Eastern Mediterranean[a]	19.4	52	3.0
Southeast Asia[a]	34.3	426	24.7
Western Pacific[c]	43.8	195	11.3
China	33.7	379	22.0
Europe[a] and others[d]	31.6	382	22.2
All regions	32.8	1,722	100

[a]Includes all the countries in the WHO region.
[b]Includes all the countries of the American region of WHO, except United States and Canada.
[c]Includes all the countries of the western Pacific region of WHO, except China, Japan, Australia, and New Zealand.
[d]United States, Canada, Japan, Australia, and New Zealand.
From Sudre P, ten Dam G, Kochi A. Tuberculosis: a global overview of the situation today. *Bull WHO* 1992;709:149–159, with permission.

TABLE 2.2. WORLD HEALTH ORGANIZATION (WHO) ESTIMATES OF THE NUMBER OF CASES AND INCIDENCE OF TUBERCULOSIS IN THE WORLD IN 1997, BY WHO ADMINISTRATIVE REGION[a]

Region	Case Number	Incidence per 100,000 Population	Percentage of All Cases
Africa	1,586,000	259	19.9
The Americas	411,000	52	5.2
Eastern Mediterranean	615,000	129	7.7
Europe	440,000	51	5.5
Southeast Asia	2,948,000	202	37.0
Western Pacific	1,962,000	120	24.6
Total	7,962,000	136	100

[a]The distribution of HIV-related tuberculosis cases by region is as follows: 515,000 cases in Africa (80.5%); 25,000 cases in the Americas (3.9%); 10,000 cases in Europe (1.6%); 16,000 cases in eastern Mediterranean (2.5%); 64,000 cases in Southeast Asia (10.0%); and 9,000 cases in the western Pacific regions (1.4%).
From Dye C, Scheele S, Dolin P, et al. Global burden of tuberculosis: estimated incidence, prevalence, and mortality by country. *JAMA* 1999;282(7):677–686, with permission.

lion) persons, or approximately one third of the world's population. The annual incidence of new cases of tuberculosis from the 1997 exercises (Table 2.2) was estimated to be slightly less than 8 million patients; an estimated 1.87 million deaths occurred that year. As shown in the two tables, there are striking geographic variations in these data. Estimates by WHO of the number of new cases of tuberculosis expected in years to come indicate a steadily growing problem (16). By 2000, WHO estimated that the number of cases had risen to 8.7 million (17).

From the 1997 estimates, 22 countries have been identified that collectively account for 80% of all existing cases worldwide (Table 2.3).

Although these figures are in general agreement with those reported in 1990 by Murray et al. (18), and even earlier values of Styblo and Rouillon (19), all estimates of the global size of the tuberculosis problem and its regional variations are based on a number of assumptions that have inherent problems. Thus, these numbers are at best imperfect projections.

TABLE 2.3. WORLD HEALTH ORGANIZATION (WHO) ESTIMATES OF BURDEN OF TUBERCULOSIS IN THE 22 COUNTRIES CONTAINING 80% OF EXISTING CASES IN 1997

Country	Case Number	Incidence per 100,000 Population	Percentage of All Cases
India	1,799,000	187	23
China	1,402,000	113	18
Indonesia	583,000	285	7
Bangladesh	300,000	246	4
Pakistan	261,000	181	3
Nigeria	253,000	214	3
Philippines	222,000	314	3
South Africa	170,000	392	2
Russian Federation	156,000	106	2
Ethiopia	156,000	260	2
Vietnam	145,000	189	2
Democratic Republic of Congo	129,000	269	2
Brazil	122,000	75	2
Tanzania	97,000	308	1
Kenya	84,000	297	1
Thailand	84,000	142	1
Myanmar	80,000	171	1
Afghanistan	74,000	333	1
Uganda	66,000	320	1
Peru	65,000	265	1
Zimbabwe	63,000	538	1
Cambodia	57,000	539	1

WHO, World Health Organization.
From Dye C, Scheele S, Dolin P, et al. Global burden of tuberculosis: estimated incidence, prevalence, and mortality by country. *JAMA* 1999;282(7):667–686, with permission.

DISTRIBUTION AND DETERMINANTS OF TUBERCULOSIS

Tuberculosis differs from many other infectious maladies in having particular social and geographic distributions. Moreover, tuberculosis is an infectious disease, like many other scourges of mankind, but it has its own unique determinants.

Distribution

Geography

The geographic distribution of tuberculosis has changed considerably over time. In comparing different locations at different times, it is necessary to transform all values into comparable measures; in this comparison we have used the average annual risk of infection, according to the relationships developed by Styblo (11). Among the highest rates of tuberculosis ever recorded in human society were those of the aboriginal peoples of North America (20), who had annual risk of infection values greater than 10%. Next in rank were the populations of North America (3) and northern Europe (21), both with annual risk of infection values about 10%. The highest recorded levels in Asia (5) and Latin America (22) were substantially lower, below 10%.

The present situation is considerably different (15): The highest annual risk of infection rates in the world, about 2% to 5%, are encountered in the Andes, Himalayas, Cambodia, Indonesia and the Philippines, Haiti, and sub-Saharan Africa. Rates in North America and northern Europe, where the highest levels were once observed, are now around 0.1%. Using all sources, it has been possible to estimate the trend in tuberculosis in the various regions in the world from 1960 to 1990. Average rates in East Asia have declined from 6.2% to 1.7%; in Africa south of the Sahara, from 4.2% to 2.5%; in the Middle East, from 3.5% to 0.4%; in India and China, from 2.0% to 1.5%; in Latin America, from 1.3% to 0.4%; and in Europe, from 1.0% to 0.3%. However, as discussed subsequently, these downward trends have changed dramatically during the last few years in some locations.

Social Factors

The social distribution of tuberculosis has always been extremely uneven. Tuberculosis is strikingly associated with poverty, particularly urban poverty (23). Even where tuberculosis is uncommon in the general population, the disease persists in groups with a low socioeconomic level. Because tuberculosis changes slowly within a population, when that population moves from one place to another, it carries the risk of tuberculosis with it for the duration of the lifetime of the persons who moved. The World Bank estimated social cost of tuberculosis using DALYs. The uneven distri-

bution of cases noted above is even further exaggerated when one considers the distribution of social cost. Thus, the social cost in DALYs is highest in Asia (other than India and China), where 5.1% of all DALYs are related to tuberculosis, followed by Africa with 4.7%, India with 3.7%, China with 2.9%, Middle East with 2.8%, Latin America with 2.5%, formerly socialist economies of Europe (FSE) with 0.6%, and industrialized countries with only 0.2%.

Determinants

There are two distinct stages in the development of tuberculosis: infection and disease. Each has its own set of risk factors that must be considered separately. Although the various factors that contribute to the development of tuberculous infection and progression to the disease tuberculosis are discussed in detail in other chapters of this book, certain important aspects are briefly reviewed here because of their probable roles in the global resurgence of tuberculosis that is underway.

Infection

Tubercle bacilli are usually transmitted from one person to another as an infectious aerosol, but it may be passed in contaminated milk, in milk products, or by direct inoculation. Sharing the same breathing space with an infectious patient is clearly the most important risk factor for acquiring infection (24). The infectiousness of a given source case depends on the type and extent of that patient's tuberculosis; whether or not that person is coughing, sneezing, or otherwise generating an infectious aerosol; and whether or not the diagnosis has been made and suitable treatment instituted. These fundamental considerations explain why some patients are much more infectious than others. Virtually all spread of *M. tuberculosis* in a community is caused by patients with pulmonary tuberculosis, as opposed to those with extrapulmonary involvement; most contagious are persons whose sputum contains acid-fast bacilli on direct microscopic examination (i.e., are "smear positive"), which means their secretions contain more than 10^4 organisms/mL; and particularly, those who are undiagnosed and hence untreated. Accordingly, these patients, who usually represent about half of all newly discovered cases of tuberculosis, are the chief targets of tuberculosis control programs. Identifying and treating patients with smear-positive tuberculosis is the quickest and most efficient way of breaking the chain of transmission of the disease.

The length of exposure, proximity of contact, and the degree of ventilation of the ambient environment also influence the probability of becoming infected with tuberculosis (25). These factors explain (a) why intimate household contacts are more likely to become infected than are casual contacts to the same source patient, and (b) why socioeconomic conditions that favor crowding and close association among persons in poorly ventilated enclosures predispose to the spread of tubercle bacilli.

Not every previously uninfected person acquires tuberculous infection after inhaling viable *M. tuberculosis* into their lungs. Resistance to infection in the previously unexposed contact must depend largely on innate defense mechanisms (i.e., those everyone is born with that do not depend on specific sensitization), but the nature of these factors is poorly understood. It is very difficult to document how often new infection actually occurs after exposure; however, because only about one fourth of close household contacts of smear-positive index patients were estimated to have been infected by their exposure (26), this value can be viewed as the average rate of infection from prolonged, heavy exposure. Recent observations by Stead (27) suggest a significant role for genetic factors in innate resistance to infection by *M. tuberculosis;* moreover, it appears that infection with the human immunodeficiency virus (HIV) favors the development of tuberculous infection (28), presumably by impairing innate resistance.

Disease

The fate of otherwise healthy contacts who become infected with tubercle bacilli has been thoroughly studied. But it is not well appreciated that the great majority (possibly as many as 90%) of infected persons do not develop clinically significant tuberculosis during their lifetime. These persons have *tuberculous infection* but they do not have the *disease tuberculosis.* They can be relatively easily identified because they have a positive response to the tuberculin skin test. In the remaining 10% the disease tuberculosis does occur, and in about half of these persons, or 5% of the total, progression to disease occurs during the first few years after exposure. In the other 5% there is a long interval, often several decades, between the occurrence of infection and the onset of disease; this sequence defines what is called *reactivation of latent,* or *remotely acquired,* tuberculous infection. Estimates for these risks are derived from studies of the fate of infected individuals, in the setting of contact with active cases, when tuberculosis rates were low and declining (29).

The most important factor—by far—that determines whether infection, new or old, will progress to disease is the adequacy of the host's immune response, especially cell-mediated immunity, to the presence of *M. tuberculosis.* Youmans (30) stated succinctly, "Progression of tuberculous disease can only take place in the presence of inadequate cellular immunity to infection." Thus, tuberculosis has been linked to putative cellular immune deficiencies associated with age, undernutrition, genetic factors, the administration of immunosuppressive drugs, and the presence of diseases such as diabetes mellitus, lymphoreticular malignancies, chronic renal insufficiency, silicosis, and, most notably, HIV infection.

The length of time that has elapsed since becoming infected is the most important determinant of the risk of developing the disease tuberculosis in an immunocompetent person; the risk appears to decrease exponentially during the first few years after infection and then reaches a low level for the rest of the person's lifetime, unless immunologic abnormalities intervene. Other modifiers of the risk of disease are age, with greater risk during infancy and adolescence, and gender, with young women more likely than young men to develop disease soon after infection (2–4,31). The explanation for the high rates in young people lies in the fact that the greatest likelihood of developing the disease is within the first several years after infection (29). In communities with high annual rates of infection, virtually everyone is infected by tubercle bacilli by the age of 20 years (32). If the major portion of the risk of disease occurs within the first 5 years after infection, the highest rates of disease would occur at ages 20 to 25, as is the case (Fig. 2.1). The reason for the higher rates in young women as compared with young men is unknown, and the gender difference appears to be reversed in patients with tuberculosis in sub-Saharan Africa, although this might, to some extent, reflect undernotification of cases in women. However, as the annual risk of infection within a population decreases, the incidence of new cases of tuberculosis also decreases and there is a shift in the age peak from young adults, especially women, to older adults, especially men (Fig. 2.2). This change reflects the absence of new infection, with its rapid progression to disease among the young, and the presence of latent infection that was acquired during childhood and adolescence, with late reactivation among the elderly. It does not represent postponement of maximal risk from young age to a later period; it is a cohort effect of the higher rate of tuberculous infection in the earlier life of the elderly (3). In lifelong residents of industrialized countries today, the prevalence of tuberculous infection is much higher among old persons than among young persons because of

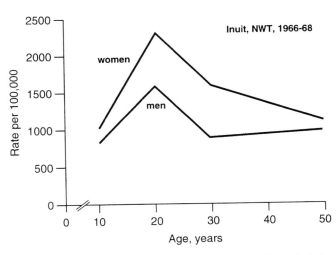

FIGURE 2.1. Annual notification rate of active tuberculosis by age and gender in Inuit of Nunavut, Canada, 1966 to 1968.

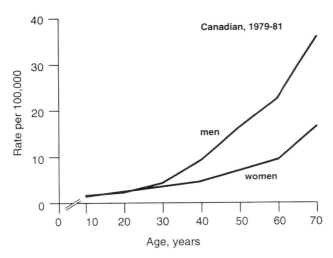

FIGURE 2.2. Annual notification rate of active tuberculosis by age and gender in persons born in Canada, excluding aboriginal Indians, 1979 to 1981.

the steady decline in the annual risk of infection during past decades.

SECULAR TRENDS

Given the uncertainties about the size of the worldwide tuberculosis burden, it follows that much doubt exists regarding the long-term epidemiologic changes that may have occurred. Sufficient data are available, however, to allow reasonable inferences about recent secular trends of the disease in selected countries.

Expected Findings

A conceptual model of the epidemiologic course of tuberculosis in a previously unexposed human population has been proposed (21). After introduction of *M. tuberculosis* to a group without prior exposure to the organism (i.e., no immunologic "experience"), the incidence of active tuberculosis in the population rises rapidly and reaches a peak that reflects the high rate of new clinical disease that occurs soon after initial infection. Thereafter, because most of the community has already become infected, fewer persons are at risk of developing primary tuberculosis and the incidence of disease must decrease from its early high peak and may stabilize or continue a steady decline, often at a rate of 3% to 5% per year. After the introduction of chemotherapy, the rate of decline of the incidence of active tuberculosis should increase to approximately 10% per year, according to data from many industrialized countries from 1970 to 1985. When incidence rates reach low levels, the rate of decline ordinarily slows owing to the contribution of new cases from high-risk groups (discussed subsequently).

The clinical and epidemiologic features of tuberculosis vary at different stages during the course of tuberculosis in the population (33). When tuberculosis case rates are extremely high, most cases result from recent infection and the disease is most common in young people. Annual incidence rates are very high (more than 100 per 100,000) and high-risk groups are absent. In contrast, when tuberculosis is uncommon in the community, most cases are the result of remote infection and the disease affects the elderly. Moreover, those cases of tuberculosis that do occur arise chiefly from among high-risk groups whose risk is determined mainly by the likelihood of having been infected in the past. The clinical picture of tuberculosis changes from the "early" forms to the "late" forms. The radiographic extent of pulmonary disease also diminishes; consequently, a higher proportion of patients have disease limited to small areas of the lungs (34); moreover, tubercle bacilli are less numerous in these patients, which results in a low proportion of infectious cases. As the appearance of disease in an infected individual and its progression in the diseased person is closely associated with the immunologic status of that individual, these changes might reflect a change in such status within the population. It is also possible that earlier case detection might occur, although the loss of vigilance for tuberculosis as the disease declines is notorious (35), suggesting that this is not the entire explanation.

High-Risk Populations

The rising limb of the proposed epidemiologic model has rarely been validated in human populations. However, one example was observed among the prairie Indians of Canada (36). Immediately following the institution of the reservation system, mortality rates from tuberculosis rose from 1% per year in 1881 to 9% per year in 1886 and only slowly declined again to 1% per year by 1900. In the early 1900s, large numbers of young, healthy Sudanese recruits to the Egyptian army (37) and Senegalese recruits to the French army (38), none of whom had been previously exposed to tubercle bacilli, rapidly developed fulminant disease and died after coming into contact with people with infectious tuberculosis. More information will undoubtedly come from studies of tuberculosis in sub-Saharan Africa where the rise in tuberculosis associated with the HIV epidemic is spectacular.

In contrast to the paucity of evidence concerning the ascending limb of the conceptual epidemiologic curve, the descending limb is well established, although the rates of decline have varied from one population to another. For example, in the Inuit population who live in the far north of Canada, the situation was precisely documented from 1962 to 1985 with detailed information regarding tuberculosis status on more than 80% of the entire population (39). In the early 1960s the annual notification rates of active tuberculosis in the entire community were between 1,000 and 2,000 per 100,000 (i.e., 1% to 2% per year). The incidence was highest among young adults, particularly women, as is usual in such situations (Fig. 2.1). This changed dramatically by the 1980s when the overall notification rates had decreased substantially and the highest incidence was seen among the elderly, especially old men.

The decline in rates of active tuberculosis in this group is the most rapid decline ever documented (at points exceeding 20% per year). In 1964, a minority of children had been immunized with bacille Calmet–Guérin (BCG) vaccine; by 1984, the vaccination coverage had increased to over 80% of all children. At the same time, the prevalence of previous tuberculosis in adults, as shown by the presence of fibrotic lesions in chest radiographs, had increased from 35% to 42%. During this period in addition to active case finding and case holding until cure, there was an aggressive program of preventive therapy that was most active between 1968 and 1972. Preventive treatment, which often consisted of 12 to 18 months of fully supervised, two-drug therapy, was given to eligible individuals (40). By 1984, 43% of those with previous tuberculosis (fibrotic lesions) and 34% of those without evidence of previous disease, but who had been infected with tuberculosis, had been treated. From 1970 to 1972, the greatest number of cases and highest incidence rate of active tuberculosis (1,330 per 100,000 per year) was in the group with previous tuberculosis. Lower rates were seen in those who were previously uninfected (200 per 100,000 per year) and in those who had been vaccinated (250 per 100,000 per year). By 1980 to 1982, incidence rates in all groups had fallen but the decline was most dramatic in the group with previous disease. Within this group, only a small number of cases were observed (70 per 100,000 per year). Moreover, those cases that did develop occurred only among patients who had not been given preventive chemotherapy.

Low-Risk Populations

The main reason for the very low rate of disease in low-prevalence countries is the restriction of transmission of tuberculous infection to increasingly smaller high-risk groups resulting from extremely thorough case finding, along with successful treatment of patients with infectious disease in the general population, leading to a declining likelihood of effective contact between uninfected persons and those few remaining with infectious disease. Tuberculosis, in such settings, is almost a "noninfectious" disease. In Canada, which changed from a high-risk to a low-risk country during the last 60 years, complete case finding and effective treatment reached the whole population by about 1957. Although the notification rate of active tuberculosis was not immediately affected, it subsequently did decline at a more rapid rate than previously, increasing to 10% per year compared to the earlier rate of around 3% per year. The reason why the rate did not decline promptly after the

introduction of effective chemotherapy for tuberculosis is that a large number of persons with tuberculous infection remained at risk of disease from late reactivation; this risk continues throughout the lifetime of the infected persons, and disease among this group will only completely disappear when all the cohort has died.

With the decline in tuberculosis rates, certain groups at high risk for the disease have emerged; these have been studied in detail in Canada (41,42) and in the United States (43). The segments of the general population that experienced rates of active tuberculosis at least ten times higher than the national average were considered "high-risk" groups in these reports; the actual rates exceeded 100 per 100,000 per year in each of the groups. The relative risks (i.e., the ratio of the rate in the particular group as compared with that in the general population) in high-risk groups in the Canadian study were as follows: 62 for contacts of patients with active disease, 38 for previous cases (fibrotic lesions), 39 for patients with silicosis, 20 for residents of urban slums, 15 for Asian-born Canadians, and 13 for aboriginal populations. Since 1982, a new high-risk group has emerged with the highest relative risk for tuberculosis ever recorded, namely, patients with HIV infection. In the 1970s and 1980s in Canada, collectively, high-risk groups accounted for 80% of all the cases diagnosed during that period: 33% occurred in Canadians born in Asia, 17% in individuals who had previously had tuberculosis, 12% in aboriginal Canadians, 8% in contacts of patients with active disease, 7% in residents of urban slums, and 3% in patients with HIV infection.

In low-prevalence countries, which comprise most of the industrialized world, high-risk groups remain the source of most of the new cases of tuberculosis that continue to develop. Thus, as will be discussed further, these groups have contributed disproportionately to the present resurgence of tuberculosis that is occurring in these countries.

Current Findings

In striking contrast to the steady downward trend in the incidence of tuberculosis that was observed during the 1960s, 1970s, and into the 1980s throughout virtually the entire world, although at greatly differing rates in different countries, a leveling off occurred in the mid-1980s in many places that was subsequently followed by an increase in notifications of the disease. This was documented in a recent update of tuberculosis notifications published by WHO (15), shown in Figure 2.3, giving a comparison with previous reports. Globally, 3.7 million cases of tuberculosis were reported in 2000: 20% in the Africa region, 6% in the Americas region, 4% in the eastern Mediterranean region, 10% in the Europe region, 38% in the Southeast Asia region, and 22% in the western Pacific region.

These figures must be interpreted with caution because they depend on the completeness and accuracy of case find-

Rate per 100,000

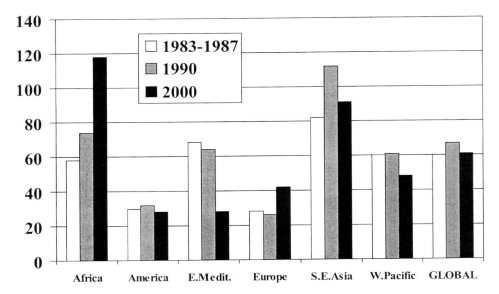

FIGURE 2.3. Comparison of the notification rates of active tuberculosis in 1990 with the average rates for 1983 to 1987, according to World Health Organization region and overall. (From the Tuberculosis Programme, World Health Organization. Tuberculosis notification update. *WHO/ TB*/92:169, with permission.)

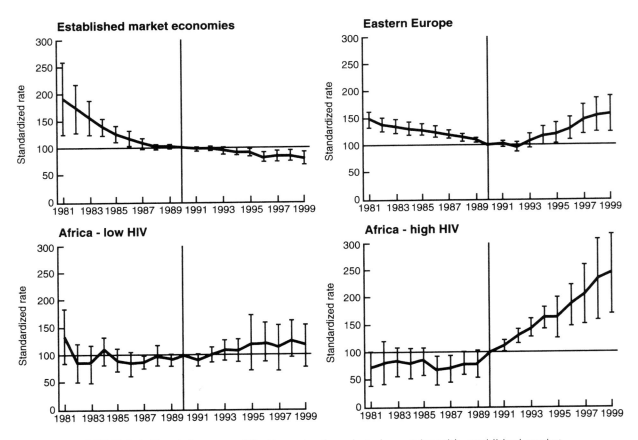

FIGURE 2.4. Trends in case notification rates for selected countries with established market economies, in eastern European and African countries with low and high prevalence rates of human immunodeficiency virus infection. The rates for all countries have been expressed relative to an arbitrary standard of 100 in 1990. *Vertical bars* show 95% confidence limits. (From WHO Report 2001. Global tuberculosis control. *WHO/CDS/TB* 2001;287:17, with permission.)

ing and reporting activities. The 3.7 million tuberculosis cases reported in 2000 represent 42% of the 8.74 million new cases estimated by WHO. Nevertheless, in some countries of eastern Europe and in a number of African nations (Fig. 2.4) with long-established and reliable programs, the recent increase in tuberculosis notifications indicates a definite increase in incidence of the disease. A number of European countries that had noted increases from the 1980s to the early 1990s (Switzerland, Norway, Netherlands, United Kingdom, Ireland, Austria, Finland, and Sweden) have subsequently displayed a declining trend once again. By contrast, in Denmark and Italy the increase has continued (17). Although the exact numbers cannot be precisely determined, there now seems no doubt about the fact that during the last 5 to 10 years there has been a resurgence of tuberculosis in a number of locations in the world. Available evidence indicates that the number of cases will continue to increase in the foreseeable future (16).

REASONS FOR THE RESURGENCE

The projected recrudescence of tuberculosis from 8.0 million new cases in 1997 to 10.2 million in 2005 will worsen existing disparities in the global distribution of the disease; some regions will be considerably more affected than others. Figure 2.4 reproduces data collected and published by WHO (44) that document the prevailing trends in case notification rates of tuberculosis in four different regions of the world, and that reveal some important epidemiologic developments. First, the rate of notification continues downward in rich industrialized countries, those with "established market economies," but at a slower pace after 1988 than before. Second, the regular downward trend in eastern Europe abruptly reversed itself in 1992. Third, two patterns are evident in African countries: in those with low prevailing seroprevalence rates of HIV infection, notifications of tuberculosis are creeping upward slowly; by contrast, in countries with high prevalence of HIV infection, notifications are soaring at a phenomenal rate. The reasons for these striking differences are discussed in this section.

Human Immunodeficiency Virus Infection and Other Conditions

Many physicians and health care professionals from prosperous countries are unaware that—worldwide—tuberculosis is the most common opportunistic infectious complication and the most common cause of death among patients with HIV infection. Coinfection with *M. tuberculosis* and HIV is truly a devastating partnership, with each component exacerbating and quickening the progression of the other (45). First recognized in a small number of cases in the United States during the early 1980s, HIV infection has now infected more than 60 million people throughout the world, of whom 24 million have died. Sub-Saharan Africa has long been and remains the most heavily burdened region, and the powerful interaction between HIV and tubercle bacilli has greatly worsened the previously prevailing alarmingly high incidence of tuberculosis. Overall, 32% of all cases of tuberculosis in Africa, the worst afflicted region in the world, are associated with HIV infection (44). But as shown in the bottom two panels of Figure 2.4, there is a huge difference between those countries in which the prevalence rates of HIV infection in adults aged 15 to 49 years are below and above 5%. The message is clear: wherever HIV abounds, tuberculosis prospers, which explains why most of the millions of new cases of tuberculosis projected during the year 2005 will be HIV related and will occur in Africa.

The presence of HIV infection appears to enhance and accelerate the development and progression of tuberculosis at virtually every stage in its natural history, from implantation of *M. tuberculosis* in the lungs to death from advanced disease. Although obviously difficult to establish unequivocally, it appears that persons with HIV infection are more likely than those without it to develop tuberculous infection after exposure to tubercle bacilli, a conclusion that was drawn from a detailed study of an outbreak of tuberculosis among residents of a housing facility for HIV-infected persons (45).

What is proven beyond doubt is that HIV infection is the mightiest risk factor ever identified that increases the likelihood of progression of tuberculous infection, whether recently or remotely acquired, to clinically active disease; the risk has been estimated at 5% to 10% *per year* among persons with HIV infection compared with 5% to 10% *per lifetime* in persons without HIV infection (45). The appearance of HIV-associated tuberculosis usually follows one of two distinct pathways: either from rapid progression of newly acquired tuberculous infection, which follows the recent inhalation and inoculation of *M. tuberculosis* in the lungs; or from reactivation of latent tuberculous infection, which arises from viable tubercle bacilli implanted in the body many years, even decades, earlier. The contribution of each sequence to the total number of cases of HIV-associated tuberculosis is unknown and must vary from one community to another, depending on the local prevalence of tuberculous infection, the number of persons with contagious disease, and the use and extent of antituberculosis chemoprophylaxis.

Recent studies using molecular fingerprinting have documented that tuberculosis may also supervene through two other less common sequences in HIV-infected persons who have previously been treated for the disease. One pathway is relapse of tuberculosis from recurrence of the same strain of tubercle bacilli that caused the original infection; the other is the development of a new unrelated episode of tuberculosis from exogenous reinfection by a different strain of *M. tuberculosis*, including multidrug-resistant bacilli, from the one that caused the initial infection (47). Exogenous reinfection has also been demonstrated in non-HIV-infected persons who had been treated for and cured of a previous bout of pulmonary tuberculosis (48).

Tuberculosis is fostered by the presence of HIV-induced depressed cell-mediated immune function, and its severity influences the clinical and radiographic manifestations of the disease. However, it is important to recognize that these differences, when they occur, are nearly always associated with the presence of advanced HIV infection, as reflected in low levels of circulating CD4$^+$ T lymphocytes, and that in the majority of cases it is impossible to tell who is HIV infected and who is not. The only reliable way to make the distinction is to perform an HIV serologic test. The increasing likelihood of developing "unusual" manifestations of tuberculosis, such as extrapulmonary disease and mycobacteremia, as HIV-induced immunosuppression worsens has been nicely documented by Jones et al. (49) and is shown in Table 2.4.

Perhaps the only aspect of tuberculosis that is not exaggerated by the presence of HIV infection is the contagiousness of the dually infected person, both because of the high proportion of patients with extrapulmonary disease, who are usually noninfectious, and because of the increased number of patients with HIV-associated pulmonary tuberculosis who have negative sputum smears for acid-fast bacilli (50,51). Quantitative studies also show lower bacillary counts in sputum from persons with pulmonary tuberculosis who are HIV coinfected compared with those who are not (52). It needs to be emphasized, though, that patients with pulmonary tuberculosis who do not have acid-fast bacilli in their sputum, regardless of HIV status, should not be regarded as *non*infectious: they are *less* infectious than smear-positive patients (53).

The adverse effect of HIV-induced cell-mediated immunodepression on tuberculosis is straightforward and widely recognized; much less well known is the stimulating effect of tuberculosis on the progression of HIV infection. The results of both epidemiologic and clinical studies have convincingly established the exacerbating role of cellular activation—induced by stimulation of the immune system—in the initiation and propagation of HIV infection. Ongoing immune activation associated with specific immune responses directed at persistent infection, with resulting increased HIV replication, was proposed to explain the faster rate of progression of HIV disease in sub-Saharan Africa and similar regions burdened by endemic parasitic and other chronic infections, including tuberculosis (54). Direct evidence of the detrimental interaction between HIV and tubercle bacilli was provided by Goletti et al. (55) who showed that the onset of tuberculosis in HIV-infected patients caused an increase in plasma viremia associated with a 5- to 160-fold increase in HIV replication, and that this, in turn, was correlated with the level of cellular activation.

Other Disorders

Workers with silicosis have a greatly increased risk of tuberculosis, which reflects the fact that respirable silica particles deposited in the lungs directly impair the function of alveolar macrophages, thereby inhibiting their ability to combat organisms such as mycobacteria (56). Before the advent of HIV infection, silicosis was the most potent risk factor known to predispose to tuberculosis; today in some parts of the world, particularly in South African gold mines, where both HIV infection and silicosis are rampant, the rates of tuberculosis and other mycobacterial diseases are colossal (57). People with immunosuppressive disorders other than HIV infection (e.g., lymphoproliferative diseases or chronic renal failure) or persons who are receiving certain drugs that depress the immune system (e.g., corticosteroids or cytotoxic agents) also have an increased likelihood of developing clinical tuberculosis (58). In addition, patients with diabetes mellitus or gastric resection or plication are at increased risk of tuberculosis, although the mechanisms underlying their susceptibility are not well understood. Collectively, all of these conditions that favor the occurrence of tuberculosis, with the important exception of HIV infection, contribute little or not at all to the current worldwide resurgence of the disease.

TABLE 2.4. CLINICAL FEATURES OF PATIENTS WITH DIFFERENT CD4$^+$ CELL COUNTS, NUMBER (%)

	CD4$^+$ T Lymphocytes/μL			
	<100	101–200	201–300	>300
Number	43	20	16	18
Mean CD4$^+$ count (SD)	43(29)	155(31)	238(31)	569(492)
Extrapulmonary disease	30(70)	10(50)	7(44)	5(28)
Mycobacteremia	18(49)	3(20)	1(7)	0(0)

Modified from Jones PL, Young SMM, Antoniskus D, et al. Relationship of the manifestations of tuberculosis to CD4 cell counts in patients with human immunodeficiency virus infection. *Am Rev Respir Dis* 1993;148:1292–1297.

Socioeconomic Conditions

During its heyday in Europe and North America, tuberculosis was so prevalent among rich and poor alike that it was impossible to discern any socioeconomic predilection. However, as the disease began to wane, the link between socioeconomic disadvantage and the disease became evident; indeed, much of the decline in mortality from tuberculosis that began long before the availability of effective antituberculosis chemotherapy has been attributed to improved living conditions, better nutrition, and less overcrowding (59). Moreover, it has been suggested that part of the recent recrudescence of tuberculosis may be related to a worsening of the socioeconomic circumstances that prevail among certain segments of the world's population (60).

Poverty

Poverty and tuberculosis have long gone hand in hand (23), a partnership that was recently reconfirmed (60) and persists today. In the United Kingdom, for example, tuberculosis is at least ten times more common in the poorest communities than in the richest (61). Although two studies from sub-Saharan Africa failed to show an association between low socioeconomic status and active tuberculosis (62,63), overall, tuberculosis is much more common in poor countries than in rich ones (15). Moreover, within many affluent countries, including the United States, the cases of tuberculosis that still occur are generally concentrated in inner-city ghettoes within urban areas. Poor people generally live in crowded areas. An increasing number are homeless, and malnutrition is common—both of which may foster the development of tuberculosis. Two other contributing factors are the role of selective settlement of immigrants from high-prevalence countries into the poorest neighborhoods of urban communities and the influence of the concomitants of poverty—ignorance, fear, alcoholism, drug abuse, mental illness, and debility from other illness—on the failure to seek medical attention when it is needed, and on the problem of poor compliance with therapy when it is available. Studies of the transmission of tuberculosis in the United States by molecular typing have shown clustering among young African American men who are substance abusers and who live in poor areas (64). This phenomenon undoubtedly reflects the greater likelihood of exposure and attendant risk of acquiring tuberculous infection in certain community settings, but it also raises the possibility of some decrease in host defenses among newly infected persons as well.

Because poverty is such a multifaceted condition, it has proved impossible to disentangle and quantify its various elements. Nevertheless, the relationship (Fig. 2.5) between the average annual incidence rate of tuberculosis and the median income in the districts in which the patients resided when their disease was diagnosed is striking (65). All the

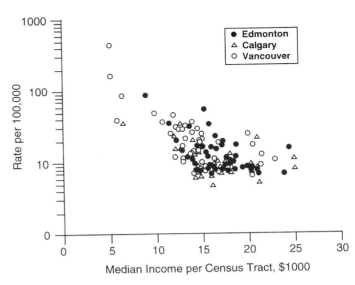

FIGURE 2.5. Notification rate of active tuberculosis in selected cities of western Canada in 1981 in the population born in Canada, excluding aboriginal Indians, by individual census tract and median income in the census tract.

pathogenic processes that are set in motion by economic destitution and that favor the development of tuberculosis, though not precisely explained, are present and amplified in the developing nations of the world where half the people must subsist on the equivalent of $2 per day or less. The extreme poverty of the people in these countries is compounded by that of the governments, which explains why health care resources, including those for tuberculosis, are often nonexistent and, when present, are nearly always inadequate.

Crowding and Homelessness

We have already emphasized that the essential circumstances for the spread of tuberculosis include the presence of one or more infected persons who are discharging viable *M. tuberculosis*, exposure of uninfected contacts, and lack of adequate tuberculosis control and treatment. Airborne transmission of bacilli from infectious patients to susceptible hosts is obviously enhanced by crowded living conditions and prolonged exposure. Although this type of spread is typically found in close family units, miniepidemics of tuberculosis have been observed among U.S. Navy personnel who were quartered on ships where there was also an infectious person in a bunkroom (66,67). Tuberculin skin tests converted from negative to positive in 20% to 80% of those exposed, with most of the variation in conversion rates being accounted for based on where the sailors slept and the patterns of shipboard ventilation. Transmission of tuberculosis has also been well documented to occur in other restricted environments, such as hospitals (68), nursing homes (69), hospices (70), and prisons (71).

At first glance, homelessness appears like the exact opposite of crowding and thus might be viewed as possibly protective against the occurrence of tuberculosis. Unfortunately, this is not the case: homeless persons represent an inordinately high-risk population (72). The substantial increase of homelessness during the last 25 years in the United States and other industrialized countries has created the need for emergency shelters in which crowding is extreme and, because of the high prevalence of tuberculosis among the homeless, exposure to *M. tuberculosis* is common. Contributing factors to the high prevalence rates of active tuberculosis among homeless persons, which have been estimated to be 150 to 300 times higher than those in the general population (73), are the presence of coexisting substance abuse and malnutrition. Mental illness is also highly prevalent and contributes to problems in the recognition and treatment of tuberculosis when it occurs. High rates of tuberculous infection has been documented among the homeless in San Francisco (74) and New York (75); in both studies the risk of infection correlated with the length of time spent in shelters, and in San Francisco with the total time homeless. Molecular fingerprinting has demonstrated higher rates of clustering among the homeless than in other persons with tuberculosis in New York (76). In a recent prospective investigation in San Francisco the high rate of tuberculosis among the homeless was largely attributable to recent transmission and/or rapid progression to disease in persons who were HIV positive and nonwhite (77). One homeless person with highly infectious tuberculosis infected as many as 41 of 97 contacts in a neighborhood bar, 14 of whom developed active disease (78).

Malnutrition

Morbidity and mortality from bacterial respiratory infections are worsened by low body weight and poor nutritional status, although in patients with severe tuberculosis, it may be unclear whether malnutrition predisposes to or results from the disease (79). The powerful biologic effect of inadequate nutrition on the development of disease was nicely demonstrated by studies showing that weight loss, even though slight (mean 1.5 kg in 6 months), among Rwandan women was a significant risk factor for HIV seroconversion (80). Underweight recruits in the U.S. Navy with positive tuberculin skin test reactions and normal-appearing chest radiographs were 3.4 times more likely to develop tuberculosis than were overweight sailors (81). Malnutrition accompanies famine and the unavailability of food, poverty and the lack of means to purchase food, substance abuse and the neglect of food, and the presence of debilitating diseases that affect caloric intake, absorption of foodstuffs, or energy expenditure. Tuberculosis is common in all of these circumstances, but exactly how malnutrition favors the development of the disease is unknown. Presumably, various components of the immune system, including T-lymphocyte function and cell-mediated immunity, are impaired. It is also not known which dietary elements (proteins, vitamins, micronutrients, or other substances) are necessary to protect against the occurrence of tuberculosis; most probably, multiple factors are involved. Experimental studies suggest an important contributory role for protein undernutrition (82).

Immigration

At first glance, notification rates of tuberculosis in countries with established market economies (upper left-hand panel, Fig. 2.4) are reassuring in that they show a fairly regular 2% to 3% annual decrease. But the method of summarizing data from several countries totally obscures a vital epidemiologic fact: within many of the included countries, a steadily increasing proportion of all new cases of tuberculosis is diagnosed in immigrants, refugees asylum seekers, and foreign workers (i.e., non-native-born persons). For example, the percentage of foreign-born persons among all cases of tuberculosis in the United States increased from 22% in 1986 to 48% in 1998 (83,84); in Canada the percentage rose from 20% in 1965 to nearly 40% in 1985 (85) and currently accounting for over 70% of cases. Rising rates have also been reported from many countries in Europe (86).

One obvious reason for the changing proportions of tuberculosis between foreign-born and native-born persons is that immigration provides an ongoing steady supply of people from low-income high-prevalence countries who, as is customary in their locale, develop tuberculous infection at an early age; once infected, they take their viable tubercle bacilli with them wherever they go. Therefore, the development of tuberculosis in immigrants is likely to be of the reactivation variety. A corollary but less obvious reason is illustrated in Figure 2.6, which shows the age-profile of foreign-born and native-born persons with newly diagnosed tuberculosis in Switzerland: the former are apt to be young persons between the ages of 20 to 45 years, whereas the latter are usually elderly adults. This means that, as the years go by, new immigrants replace earlier ones and their age profile remains much the same; by contrast, the progressively older persons who harbor *M. tuberculosis* slowly die off and are not replaced, thus reducing the pool of vulnerable native-born candidates.

Because of the steady increase in the proportion of foreign-born persons among all persons with tuberculosis, there has been great interest in determining to what extent immigrants spread their disease to others, particularly to native-born people, who otherwise might never be exposed to someone with infectious tuberculosis. Only two studies have addressed this important issue, and the results are remarkably different. The first study from the Netherlands by Borgdorff et al. (87) showed that approximately half the cases of tuberculosis among Dutch nationals resulted from

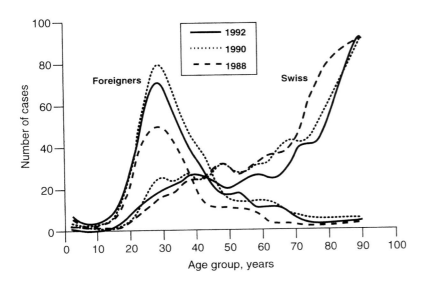

FIGURE 2.6. Number of reported cases of tuberculosis by 5-year age groups among Swiss and foreigners living in Switzerland in 1988, 1990, and 1992. (The curves are smoothed, and data from individuals 85 years and older are lumped.) (From l'Office Fédéral de la Santé Publique. La tuberculose en Suisse 1988–1922. *Bull Office Fed Sante Publique* 1993;41:739–745, with permission.)

transmission of *M. tuberculosis* from immigrants. Later, a similar analysis, also carried out by Borgdorff et al. (88), of all cases of tuberculosis arising in San Francisco revealed that U.S.-born persons with tuberculosis generated nearly three times more cases of tuberculosis than foreign-born persons (transmission index 0.59 versus 0.21, respectively). This conclusion confirmed that of a previous study using less sophisticated techniques: in San Francisco, native-born tuberculars propagate tuberculosis to a much greater extent than do foreign-born (89). Clearly, these contrasting results call for further investigations to sort out transmission dynamics of tubercle bacilli in communities in which there is epidemiologic evidence of similar rates of recent spread of infection and progression to disease ("clustering").

Many immigrants are poor and hence are obliged to settle in low-income areas, particularly in inner cities, where housing is densely crowded. Reactivation of tuberculosis in these circumstances results in heavy exposure to household members. This problem is worsened by the presence of illegal immigrants, who are moving in increasing numbers from high-prevalence to industrialized countries, taking their tuberculous infections with them. Because identification is often perceived to result in deportation, these persons are loath to seek medical attention, including care for infectious tuberculosis, for fear of being found by the authorities; this may greatly lengthen the period of transmission of tubercle bacilli to household and other contacts.

Poor Tuberculosis Control

As already pointed out, the incidence of tuberculosis in a given community is influenced by several factors acting individually or in concert. However, regardless of the nature and magnitude of these factors, they can be mitigated to a large extent by a well-organized and efficient tuberculosis control program, the essential elements of which are

reviewed in the next section and discussed in detail in the last section of the book. Suffice it to say that much of the persistence of tuberculosis in some parts of the world and its increase in others can be attributed—sadly—to inadequate (or absent) regional tuberculosis control programs. The remarkable rise in multidrug-resistant strains of *M. tuberculosis* in the East Coast of the United States during the 1980s is a striking example of the failure of community control programs to deal with the complex problems presented by growing numbers of homeless, substance abusers, legal and illegal immigrants, and fueled by HIV infection (90). Clinically significant drug resistance is always a man-made phenomenon, and its presence and magnitude have long been regarded as measures of the effectiveness of the local control system. It has now become clear, however, that the interaction between HIV infection and tuberculosis can result in increased transmission of drug-resistant tubercle bacilli even in regions where there are effective control programs (91).

Knowledge, medications, and techniques for the effective prevention and control of tuberculosis have been available for decades. Failure to apply what has been shown to work well results primarily from lack of funds, but in the final analysis, this omission derives from lack of political commitment and financial appropriations. The immense problems created by poor control are extremely well documented by the resurgence of tuberculosis in the Harlem area of New York City during the 1980s (92); the convergence of HIV infection and tuberculosis in a subpopulation with high rates of substance abuse and homelessness at a time when funding for public health programs, including those for tuberculosis, were being drastically curtailed, resulted in an increase in incidence rates of tuberculosis from 50.2 per 100,000 in 1979 to 169.2 per 100,000 in 1989. This scandalous occurrence is yet another example that the presently available, potent antituberculosis drug regimens are powerless unless a system exists that ensures first, that all patients with tuberculosis are diagnosed; then, that a satisfactory treatment regimen is prescribed; and finally, that each patient takes his or her medications for the full course of therapy. Evaluation of whether sufficient resources, commitment, and know-how are being employed and their impact on local tuberculosis control programs can be enhanced by adding molecular-based epidemiologic techniques to conventional ones (93).

CONTROL OF TUBERCULOSIS

There are important programmatic considerations that greatly affect the results of antituberculosis treatment and hence the epidemiology of disease. These are briefly reviewed here. BCG vaccination and treatment of latent tuberculous infection are dealt with elsewhere.

Treatment Outcome

The outcome of tuberculosis treatment differs according to the conditions of the program under which therapy is administered. The importance of the program is illustrated by the results of three different approaches (Fig. 2.7): no chemotherapy, good chemotherapy, and haphazard chemotherapy (94). When no chemotherapy is given, 25% of the patients die within 2 years and 49% die within 5 years; 33% are spontaneously cured; the remaining 18% remain smear positive and sources of infection within the community. When standardized chemotherapy is given, taking into

account the results of susceptibility tests to determine the continuation phase of treatment (e.g., in British Columbia, Canada in the early 1980s), 8% of the patients die while on treatment, 90% are cured, and only 2% remain smear positive at the end of treatment. When chemotherapy is not standardized and thus haphazard (with a wide array of treatment regimens prescribed, many of them inappropriate—a practice frequently occurring in the private sector) (95), the fatality rate is dramatically reduced to only 10% and the proportion of patients cured is also increased to 60%; however, 30% remain smear positive (as illustrated from results of treatment in Korea and Taiwan in the 1970s). Thus, the net effect of such programs is to *increase* the number of sources of infection within the community compared with the results of a "good" program.

Under some program conditions, what should be good chemotherapy becomes poor chemotherapy. Two factors account for this change: poor adherence to treatment and resistance to antituberculosis medications. Poor adherence is the most important reason for lack of success of many chemotherapy programs. Resistance to chemotherapeutic agents is very uncommon in such countries as Canada (96), Algeria (97), and Tanzania (98) where initial resistance to one or more drugs occurs in less than 10% and acquired resistance in less than 40%. In some other countries, however, the problem is considerably greater. In Korea, for example, in a national prevalence survey, initial resistance was present in 24% of patients and acquired resistance in 74% (99); in China, the corresponding figures were 27% and 72% (100). In Korea 53% and in China 62% of all patients discovered in the prevalence surveys had previously been treated; these patients with "residual" disease, which represented failures of the national program, had become sources of infection with drug-resistant *M. tuberculosis* in the community. A mathematical model estimated that the relative infectiousness of patients with chronic disease is greater than that of patients with new disease (101), and the importance of such cases in transmission has been recently demonstrated in molecular epidemiologic investigations (102).

In most cases, drug resistance is a problem created either by errors made by an individual physician in caring for the patient or, less frequently, by incorrect program practices [particularly failing to observe the swallowing of medications (103)] and can be avoided by strictly adhering to good public health practice.

In Tanzania, primary resistance to any antituberculosis drug occurs in approximately 6% and acquired resistance in about 40% of patients who are diagnosed with tuberculosis (98). These figures have not changed for 30 years despite the introduction and widespread use of rifampicin-containing regimens throughout the country. Careful control of the availability of rifampicin through the program alone, use of combined tablets of isoniazid and rifampicin, restriction of the use of rifampicin to the initial intensive phase of treat-

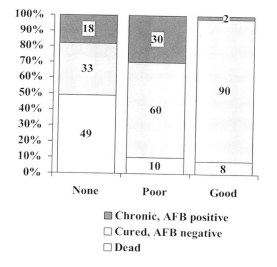

FIGURE 2.7. Outcome for patients with pulmonary tuberculosis according to the type of treatment they received. *AFB,* acid-fast bacillus. (Plotted from data obtained in Grzybowski S, Enarson DA. The fate of cases of pulmonary tuberculosis under various treatment programmes. *Bull Int Union Tuberc Lung Dis* 1978;53: 70–75.)

ment (usually 2 months), and strict observance of every dose swallowed have prevented the emergence of resistance to the drug.

Good public health practice, outlined in the WHO policy package termed "DOTS," can be expected to have a substantial impact on reducing the probability of infection, rapidly reducing the prevalence of tuberculosis cases and slowing reducing their incidence (104) where health services are maintained and HIV infection is not increasing.

SUMMARY AND CONCLUSION

Here is where we are in the global fight against tuberculosis. We know that it is possible to drastically reduce the problem in a whole population, as we have seen most dramatically in the Inuit population and to a lesser extent in many countries of northwestern Europe and North America, and now in some communities in low-income countries. We know that we can achieve the desirable rates of case detection of infectious sources of *M. tuberculosis* (70%) and cure of these patients (85%) even under the most difficult socioeconomic constraints. We know that the number of cases worldwide will dramatically increase in the next few years because of the HIV epidemic.

Where do we go from here? In very low prevalence countries, such as Canada, the Netherlands, and Norway, we know that the transmission of *M. tuberculosis* has virtually ceased but that we will continue to see cases of tuberculosis in foreign-born persons and in increasingly older native-born persons for at least several decades, owing to the cohort effect of high rates of tuberculous infection in the remote past. In such countries, the greatest emphasis must be placed on diagnosing and treating high-risk patients with sporadic disease to avoid the tragedy caused by inadequate knowledge of tuberculosis due to decreasing experience with the disease. In addition, if it were possible to accurately determine who, among all those infected with tuberculosis, is highly likely to develop subsequent disease, it would be possible to provide cost-efficient treatment of latent tuberculous infection, which is at present not possible because we are not able to adequately identify those in the population with the highest risk of future disease.

In countries where tuberculosis is still common—and especially in countries where HIV infection will dramatically increase the number of cases in the near future—all efforts must be placed on stopping both the transmission of HIV infection and the transmission of tubercle bacilli in the community (through rigorous application of the DOTS strategy). We know this can be accomplished where the community is highly mobilized and well-organized national programs are in place. Such programs are urgently required wherever they do not yet exist, and to accomplish this, significant commitments are required. Tuberculosis control is the most *cost-effective* of all health interventions in develop-

ing countries; every person in the world should have access to an effective tuberculosis control program.

REFERENCES

1. Styblo K. *Epidemiology of tuberculosis.* Jena: Gustav Fischer, 1984:77–161.
2. Andvord KF. Hvad kan vi laere ved av folge tuberkulosens gang frå generasjon til generasjon? *Norsk Magasin Laengevidenskaben* 1930;91:642–660.
3. Frost WH. The age selection of mortality from tuberculosis in successive decades. *Am J Hyg* 1939;30:91–96.
4. Springett VH. An interpretation of statistical trends in tuberculosis. *Lancet* 1952;262:521–525, 575–580.
5. Chiba Y. *Development of tuberculosis.* Tokyo: Hokendojinsha, 1959:1–664.
6. Lin HT. The tuberculosis problem and its control in East Asia and South Pacific area. *Bull Int Union Tuberc Lung Dis* 1986;61: 28–39.
7. Epifranio C. Mortalidad: certificados de defuncion. *Al Medico* 1973;76:1–9.
8. Nationwide random survey for the epidemiology of pulmonary tuberculosis conducted in 1979. *Chin J Respir Dis* 1981;5: 67–71.
9. Korean National Tuberculosis Association. *Report on the Third Tuberculosis Prevalence Survey in Korea.* Seoul: Korean National Tuberculosis Association, 1975.
10. Bleiker MA, Griep WA, Beunders BJW. The decreasing tuberculin index in Dutch recruits. *KNCV Selected Papers* 1964;8: 38–49.
11. Styblo K. The relationship between the risk of tuberculous infection and the risk of developing infectious tuberculosis. *Bull Int Union Tuberc Lung Dis* 1985;60:117–119.
12. Clancy L, Rieder HL, Enarson DA, et al. Tuberculosis elimination in the countries of Europe and other industrialized countries. *Eur Respir J* 1991;4:1288–1295.
13. World Bank. *World Development Report 1993: investing in health.* Oxford: Oxford University Press, 1993:1–329.
14. Sudre P, ten Dam G, Kochi A. Tuberculosis: a global overview of the situation today. *Bull WHO* 1992;70:149–159.
15. Dye C, Scheele S, Dolin P, et al. Global burden of tuberculosis. Estimated incidence, prevalence, and mortality by country. *JAMA* 1999;282:677–686
16. Dolin PJ, Raviglione MC, Kochi A. Global tuberculosis incidence and mortality during 1990–2000. *Bull WHO* 1994;72: 213–220.
17. WHO Report 2002. Global tuberculosis control: surveillance, planning, financing. *WHOCDSTB* 2002;295:21.
18. Murray CJL, Styblo K, Rouillon A. Tuberculosis in developing countries: burden, intervention and cost. *Bull Int Union Tuberc Lung Dis* 1990;65:2–20.
19. Styblo K, Rouillon A. Estimated global incidence of smear-positive tuberculosis. Unreliability of officially reported figures on tuberculosis. *Bull Int Union Tuberc Lung Dis* 1981;56:118–126.
20. Fellows DS. Mortality in the native races of the Territory of Alaska, with special reference to tuberculosis. *Public Health Rep* 1934;49:289–299.
21. Grigg ERN. The arcana of tuberculosis. *Am Rev Tuberc* 1958; 78:151–172.
22. PAHO Tuberculosis, Maternal and Child Health Program. Epidemiological assessment of tuberculosis: trends in some countries of the Americas. *Epidemiol Bull* 1987;8:1–5.
23. Terris M. Relation of economic status to tuberculosis mortality by age and sex. *Am J Public Health* 1948;38:1061–1070.

24. Shaw JB, Wynn-Williams N. Infectivity of pulmonary tuberculosis in relation to sputum status. *Am Rev Tuberc* 1954;69:724–732.

25. Riley RL. Transmission and environmental control of tuberculosis. In: Reichman L, Hershfield E, eds. *Tuberculosis: a comprehensive international approach.* New York: Marcel Dekker, 1993:123–136.

26. Grzybowski S, Barnett GD, Styblo K. Contacts of cases of active pulmonary tuberculosis. *Bull Int Union Tuberc Lung Dis* 1975;50:90–106.

27. Stead WW. Genetics and resistance to tuberculosis. Could resistance be enhanced by genetic engineering? *Ann Intern Med* 1992;116:937–941.

28. Nunn P, Mungai M, Nyamwaya J, et al. The effect of human immunodeficiency virus type-1 on the infectiousness of tuberculosis. *Tubercle Lung Dis* 1994;75:25–32.

29. Ferebee SH. Controlled chemoprophylaxis trials in tuberculosis. A general review. *Adv Tuberc Res* 1969;17:39–106.

30. Youmans GP. *Tuberculosis.* Philadelphia: WB Saunders, 1979:323.

31. Grzybowski S, Allen EA. The challenge of tuberculosis in decline. *Am Rev Respir Dis* 1964;90:707–720.

32. Grzybowski S. Ontario studies of tuberculin sensitivity. 1. Tuberculin testing of various population groups. *Can Med Assoc J* 1965;56:181–192.

33. Grzybowski S, Enarson DA. Tuberculosis. In: Simmons DH, ed. *Current pulmonology.* Chicago: Year Book Medical, 1986:73–96.

34. Enarson DA, et al. Tuberculosis and human immunodeficiency virus infection in Africa. In: Reichman L, Hershfield E, eds. *Tuberculosis: a comprehensive international approach.* New York: Marcel Dekker, 1993:395–412.

35. Xie HJ, Enarson DA, Chao CW, et al. Deaths in tuberculosis patients in British Columbia, 1980–1984. *Tuber Lung Dis* 1992;73:77–82.

36. Ferguson RG. *Studies in tuberculosis.* Toronto: University of Toronto Press, 1955:6–9.

37. Cummins SL. Tuberculosis in primitive tribes and its bearing on tuberculosis of civilized communities. *Int J Public Health* 1920;1:10–171.

38. Borrel A. Pneumonie et tuberculose chez les troupes noires. *Ann Inst Pasteur* 1920;34:7–148.

39. Grzybowski S, Styblo K, Dorken E. Tuberculosis in Eskimos. *Tubercle* 1976;57 (Suppl 4):1–58.

40. Dorken E, Grzybowski S, Enarson D. Ten year evaluation of a trial of chemoprophylaxis against tuberculosis in Frobisher Bay, Canada. *Tubercle* 1984;65:93–99.

41. Enarson DA, Wade JP, Embree V. Risk of tuberculosis in Canada. Implications for programs directed at specific groups. *Can J Public Health* 1987;78:305–308.

42. Enarson DA, Fanning EA, Allen EA. Case-finding in the elimination phase of tuberculosis: high risk groups in epidemiology and clinical practice. *Bull Int Union Tuberc Lung Dis* 1990;65:73–74.

43. Rieder HL, Cauthen GM, Comstock GW, et al. Epidemiology of tuberculosis in the United States. *Epidemiol Rev* 1989;11:79–98.

44. WHO Report 2001. Global tuberculosis control. *WHOCDSTB* 2001;287:17.

45. Murray JF. Tuberculosis and HIV infection: A global perspective. *Respiration* 1988;65:335–342.

46. Daley CL, Small PM, Schecter GF, et al. An outbreak of tuberculosis with accelerated progression among persons infected with the human immunodeficiency virus. An analysis using restriction-fragment length polymorphism. *N Engl J Med* 1992;326:231–235.

47. Small PM, Shafer RW, Hopewell PC, et al. Exogenous reinfection with multidrug-resistant *Mycobacterium tuberculosis* in patients with advanced HIV infection. *N Engl J Med* 1993;328:1137–1144.

48. Caminero JA, Pena MJ, Campos-Herrero MI, et al. Exogenous reinfection with tuberculosis on a European island with a moderate incidence of disease. *Am J Respir Crit Care Med* 2001;163:717–720.

49. Jones BE, Young SMM, Antoniskis D, et al. Relationship of the manifestations of tuberculosis to CD4 cell counts in patients with human immunodeficiency virus infection. *Am Rev Respir Dis* 1993;148:1292–1297.

50. Samb B, Sow PS, Kony S, et al. Risk factors for negative sputum acid-fast bacilli smears in pulmonary tuberculosis: results from Dakar, Senegal, a city with low HIV seroprevalence. *Int J Tuberc Lung Dis* 1999;3:330–336.

51. Colebunders R, Bastian I. A review of the diagnosis and treatment of smear-negative pulmonary tuberculosis. *Int J Tuberc Lung Dis* 2000;4:97–107.

52. Elliott AM, Namaambo K, Allen BW, et al. Negative sputum smear results in HIV-positive patients with pulmonary tuberculosis in Lusaka, Zambia. *Tubercle Lung Dis* 1993;74:191–194.

53. Behr MA, Warren SA, Salamon H, et al. Transmission of *Mycobacterium tuberculosis* from patients smear-negative for acid-fast bacilli. *Lancet* 1999;353:444–449.

54. Whalen C, Horsburgh CR, Hom D, et al. Accelerated course of human immunodeficiency virus infection after tuberculosis. *Am J Respir Crit Care Med* 1995;151:129–135.

55. Goletti D, Weissman D, Jackson RW, et al. Effect of *Mycobacterium tuberculosis* on HIV replication. Role of immune activation. *J Immunol* 1996;157:1271-1278.

56. Snider DE. The relationship between tuberculosis and silicosis. *Am Rev Respir Dis* 1978;118:455–460.

57. Corbett EL, Churchyard GJ, Clayton TC, et al. HIV infection and silicosis: the impact of two potent risk factors on the incidence of mycobacterial disease in South African miners. *AIDS* 2000;14:2759-2768.

58. Murray JF. Tuberculosis in the immunocompromised host. In: Revillard J-P, Wierzbicki N, eds. *Immune disorders and opportunistic infections.* Suresnes: Fondation Franco-Allemande, 1989:250–265.

59. McKeown T, Record RG. Reasons for the decline of mortality in England and Wales during the nineteenth century. *Popul Studies* 1962;16:94–122.

60. Spence DPS, Hotchkiss J, Davies PDO. Tuberculosis and poverty. *BR MED J* 1993;307:759–761.

61. Bhaatti N, Law MR, Morris JK, et al. Increasing incidence of tuberculosis in England and Wales: a study of the likely causes. *BR MED J* 1995;310:967–969.

62. Schoeman JH, Westaway MS, Neethling A. The relationship between socioeconomic factors and pulmonary tuberculosis. *Int J Epidemiol* 1991;20:435–440.

63. Glynn JR, Warndorff DK, Malema SS, et al. Tuberculosis: associations with HIV and socioeconomic status in rural Malawi. *Trans R Soc Trop Med Hyg* 2000;94:500–503.

64. McConkey SJ, Williams M, Weiss D, et al. Prospective use of molecular typing of *Mycobacterium tuberculosis* by use of restriction fragment-length polymorphism in a public tuberculosis-control program. *Clin Infect Dis* 2002;34:612–619.

65. Enarson DA, Wang J-S, Dirks JM. The incidence of active tuberculosis in a large urban area. *Am J Epidemiol* 1989;129:1268–1276.

66. Ochs CW. The epidemiology of tuberculosis. *JAMA* 1962;179:247–252.

67. Houk VN, Baker JH, Sorensen K, et al. The epidemiology of

tuberculosis infection in a closed environment. *Arch Environ Health* 1968;16:26–35.

68. Zaza S, Blumberg HM, Beck-Sague C, et al. Nosocomial transmission of *Mycobacterium tuberculosis*: role of health care workers in outbreak propagation. *J Infect Dis* 1995;172:1542–1549.

69. Stead WW, Lofgren JP, Warren E, et al. Tuberculosis as an endemic and nosocomial infection among the elderly in nursing homes. *N Engl J Med* 1985;312:1483–1487.

70. Daley CL, Small PM, Schecter GF, et al. An outbreak of tuberculosis with accelerated progression among persons infected with the human immunodeficiency virus. *N Engl J Med* 1992;326:231–235.

71. Centers for Disease Control and Prevention. Transmission of multidrug-resistant *Mycobacterium tuberculosis* among immunocompromised persons in a correctional system—New York. 1991. *MMWR Morb Mortal Wkly Rep* 1992;41:507–509.

72. Barnes PF, Yang Z, Presotn-Martin S, et al. Patterns of tuberculosis transmission in central Los Angeles. *JAMA* 1997;278:1159–1163.

73. Barry MA, Wall C, Shirley L, et al. Tuberculosis screening in Boston's homeless shelters. *Public Health Rep* 1986;101:487–494.

74. Zolopa AR, Hahn JA, Gorter R, et al. HIV and tuberculous infection in San Francisco's homeless adults. *JAMA* 1994;272:455-461.

75. Paul EA, Lebowitz SM, Moore RE, et al. Nemesis revisited: tuberculosis infection in a New York City men's shelter. *Am J Publ Health* 1993;83:1743-1745.

76. Frieden TR, Woodley CL, Crawford JT, et al. The molecular epidemiology of tuberculosis in New York City: the importance of nosocomial transmission and laboratory error. *Tuber Lung Dis* 1996;77:407–413.

77. Moss AR, Hahn JA, Tulsky JP, et al. Tuberculosis in the homeless. A prospective study. *Am J Respir Crit Care Med* 2000;162:460–464.

78. Kline SE, Hedemark LL, Davies SF. Outbreak of tuberculosis among regular patrons of a neighborhood bar. *N Engl J Med* 1995;333:222–227.

79. Berkowity FE. Infections in children with severe protein-energy malnutrition. *Pediatr Infect Dis J* 1992;11:750–759.

80. Moore PS, Allen S, Sowell AL, et al. Role of nutritional status and weight loss in HIV seroconversion among Rwandan women. *J Acquir Immune Defic Syndr* 1993;6:611–616.

81. Edwards LG, et al. Height, weight, tuberculous infection and tuberculous disease. *Arch Environ Health* 1971;22:106–112.

82. McMurray DN, Bartow RA. Immunosuppression and alteration of resistance to pulmonary tuberculosis in guinea pigs by protein undernutrition. *J Nutr* 1992;122:738–743.

83. McKenna MT, McGray E, Onorato I. The epdemiology of tuberculosis among foreign-born persons in the United States, 1986 to 1993. *N Engl J Med* 1995;332:1071–1076.

84. CDC. Tuberculosis elimination revisited: obstacles, opportunities, and a renewed commitment. Advisory Council for the Elimination of Tuberculosis (ACET). *MMWR Morb Mortal Wkly Rep* 1999;48(No. RR-9):1–13.

85. Enarson DA, Wang JS, Allen EA. Case-finding in the elimination phase of tuberculosis: tuberculosis in displaced people. *Bull Int Union Tuberc Lung Dis* 1990;65:71–72.

86. Rieder HL. Epidemiology of tuberculosis in Europe. *Eur Respir J* 1995;8(Suppl 20):620–632.

87. Borgdorff MW, Nagelkerke N, Van Soolingen D, et al. Analysis of tuberculosis transmission between nationalities in the Netherlands in the period 1993–1995 using DNA fingerprinting. *Am J Epidemiol* 1998;147:187–195.

88. Borgdorff MW, Behr MA, Nagelkerke N, et al. Transmission of tuberculosis in San Francisco and its association with immigration and ethnicity. *Int J Tuberc Lung Dis* 2000;4:287–294.

89. Chin DP, DeRiemer K, Small PM, et al. Differences in contributing factors to tuberculosis incidence in U.S.-born and foreign-born persons. *Am J Respir Crit Care Med* 1998;158:1797–1803.

90. Frieden TR, Sterling T, Pablo-Mendez A, et al. The emergence of drug-resistant tuberculosis in New York City. *N Engl J Med* 1993;328:521–526.

91. Bradford WZ, Martin JN, Reingold, et al. The changing epidemiology of acquired drug-resistant tuberculosis in San Francisco, USA. *Lancet* 1996;348:928–931.

92. Brudney K, Dobkin J. Resurgent tuberculosis in New York City. Human immunodeficiency virus, homelessness, and the decline of tuberculosis control programs. *Am Rev Respir Dis* 1991;144:745–749.

93. Jasmer RM, Hahn JA, Small PM, et al. A molecular epidemiologic analysis of tuberculosis trends in San Francisco, 1991–1997. *Ann Intern Med* 1999;130:971–978.

94. Grzybowski S, Enarson DA. The fate of cases of pulmonary tuberculosis under various treatment programmes. *Bull Int Union Tuberc Lung Dis* 1978;53:70–75.

95. Uplekar M, Juvekar S, Morankar S, et al. Tuberculosis patients and practitioners in private clinics in India. *Int J Tuberc Lung Dis* 1998;2: 324–329.

96. Wang JS, Allen EA, Chao CW, et al. Tuberculosis in British Columbia among immigrants from five Asian countries, 1982–85. *Tubercle* 1989;70:179–186.

97. Boulahbal F, Khaled S, Tazir M. The interest of follow-up of resistance of the tubercle bacillus in the evaluation of a programme. *Bull Int Union Tuberc Lung Dis* 1989;64:23–25.

98. Chonde TM. The role of bacteriological services in the National Tuberculosis and Leprosy Programme in Tanzania. *Bull Int Union Tuberc Lung Dis* 1989;64:37–39.

99. Kim SJ, Hong YP. Drug resistance of *Mycobacterium tuberculosis* in Korea. *Tubercle Lung Dis* 1992;73:219–224.

100. Nationwide random survey for the epidemiology of pulmonary tuberculosis conducted in 1979. *Chin J Respir Dis* 1981;5:67–71.

101. Schulzer M, Enarson DA, Grzybowski S, et al. An analysis of pulmonary tuberculosis data from Taiwan and Korea. *Int J Epidemiol* 1987;16:584–589.

102. Van Rie A, Warren R, Richardson M, et al. Classification of drug-resistant tuberculosis in an epidemic area. *Lancet* 2000;356:22–25.

103. Weiss SE, Slocum PC, Blais FX, et al. The effect of directly observed therpay on the rates of drug resistance and relapse in tuberculosis. *N Engl J Med* 1994;330:1179–1184.

104. Zhang L-X, Tu D-H, Enarson DA. The impact of directly-observed treatment on the epidemiology of tuberculosis in Beijing. *Int J Tuberc Lung Dis* 2000;4: 904–910.

EPIDEMIOLOGY OF TUBERCULOSIS IN THE UNITED STATES

C. ROBERT HORSBURGH, JR.
MARISA MOORE
KENNETH G. CASTRO

DESCRIPTIVE EPIDEMIOLOGY OF TUBERCULOSIS DISEASE

A national surveillance system for tuberculosis (TB) cases was established in 1953 and is maintained by the Centers for Disease Control and Prevention (CDC). This system collects information on cases of active TB diagnosed in the United States, Puerto Rico, and associated jurisdictions. Between 1953 and 1985, states reported cases of TB in aggregate; no case-specific information was collected. In 1985, the system was changed to provide CDC with individual case information, called the "Report of a Verified Case of Tuberculosis" (RVCT). In 1993, the RVCT was expanded to include additional information critical to the changing epidemiology of TB. A software package for data entry, analysis, and transmission of case reports to CDC was implemented as part of the expanded TB surveillance system.

Case Definition of Tuberculosis Disease

The TB case definition for public health surveillance in the United States includes both laboratory and clinical criteria (1) (Table 3.1). According to this definition, a case of TB disease is confirmed by identification of *Mycobacterium tuberculosis* from a clinical specimen or by demonstration of acid-fast bacillus (AFB) in a clinical specimen when a culture has not been or cannot be obtained. In the absence of laboratory confirmation, a case can be confirmed by clini-

C. R. Horsburgh, Jr.: Departments of Epidemiology, Biostatistics, and Medicine, Boston University Schools of Public Health and Medicine; and Department of Medicine, Boston Medical Center, Boston, Massachusetts.

M. Moore: Surveillance Section, Surveillance and Epidemiology Branch, Division of Tuberculosis Elimination, Centers for Disease Control and Prevention,

K. G. Castro: Division of Tuberculosis Elimination, Centers for Disease Control and Prevention, Atlanta, Georgia.

cal criteria. A case may not be counted twice within any consecutive 12-month period. However, patients who had TB verified previously must be reported again if the patients completed therapy and then relapsed. Cases must also be reported again if the patients were lost to supervision for more than 12 months and their disease is verified again. States may also identify and report a case of TB that does not meet the surveillance case definition, and such cases have traditionally also been included in the national database. Case reporting is initiated from several sources (2). Laboratories are required by law in most states to report the isolation of *M. tuberculosis* from a clinical specimen to public health authorities. In addition, health care providers are required to report cases of suspected or confirmed TB to the state. In hospitals, reporting is often done by infection control personnel. Other sources, such as schools, correctional institutions, and nursing homes, also may report cases. For epidemiologic analysis on the national level, yearly incidence is calculated on the basis of the calendar year in which a case report is verified.

Completeness of reporting of TB cases by state health departments to CDC was evaluated in a multisite study during 1993 to 1994, which found reporting to be greater than 95% (3). However, studies using other methodologies have found less complete reporting, and the level likely varies by jurisdiction. In a managed-care setting in Massachusetts, the use of automated pharmacy data found 18% of cases unreported, most of which were clinical cases without laboratory confirmation (4). Other studies using different methodologies have found ranges of completeness of reporting from 40% to 80% (5–9).

In 2000, 83% of adult cases of TB reported to CDC had been confirmed by laboratory isolation of *M. tuberculosis*, 1% had been identified by demonstration of AFB in a clinical specimen, 9% met the clinical definition (Table 3.1), and 7% did not meet the case definition (CDC, unpublished data). Among children, only 26% of reported cases in

TABLE 3.1. TUBERCULOSIS CASE DEFINITION FOR PUBLIC HEALTH SURVEILLANCE

Clinical Description: A chronic bacterial infection caused by *Mycobacterium tuberculosis,* characterized pathologically by the formation of granulomas. The most common site of infection is the lung, but other organs may be involved.

Clinical Case Definition: A case must meet the following criteria:
- Positive tuberculin skin test
- Other signs and symptoms compatible with tuberculosis (e.g., an abnormal, unstable [i.e., worsening or improving] chest radiographs, or clinical evidence of current disease)
- Treatment with two or more antituberculosis medications
- Completed diagnostic evaluation

Laboratory Criteria for Diagnosis
- Isolation of *M. tuberculosis* from a clinical specimen[a] or
- Demonstration of *M. tuberculosis* from a clinical specimen by nucleic acid amplification test,[b] or
- Demonstration of acid-fast bacilli in a clinical specimen when a culture has not been or cannot be obtained.

Case Classification
Confirmed: a case that meets the clinical case definition or is laboratory confirmed

Comment: A case should not be counted twice within any consecutive 12-month period. However, cases in which the patients previously had verified disease should be reported again if the patients were discharged from treatment. Cases also should be reported again if patients were lost to supervision for >12 months and disease can be verified again. Mycobacterial diseases other than those caused by *M. tuberculosis* complex should not be counted in tuberculosis morbidity statistics unless there is concurrent tuberculosis.

[a]Use of rapid identification techniques for *M. tuberculosis* (e.g., DNA probes and mycolic acids, high-pressure liquid chromatography performed on a culture from a clinical specimen) are acceptable under this criterion.
[b]Nucleic acid amplification (NAA) tests must be accompanied by culture for *Mycobacteria* species. However, for surveillance purposes, CDC will accept results obtained from NAA tests approved by the Food and Drug Administration and used according to the approved product labeling on the package insert.
From U.S. Centers for Disease Control and Prevention. Case definitions for infections conditions under public health surveillance. *MMWR Morb Mortal Wkly Rep* 1997;46:40–41, with permission.

2000 were confirmed by isolation of *M. tuberculosis,* whereas 46% of cases met the clinical definition only, and 28% did not meet the case definition. The lower percentage of laboratory-confirmed cases in children occurs because obtaining specimens from children for culture is more difficult and because young children with pulmonary TB are more likely to have low number of mycobacteria in sputum. Some providers do not routinely obtain specimens from children, especially if clinical information on the person who is the source of infection is available.

Temporal Trends

By the late 1940s, TB mortality rates in the United States had dropped by 50% from their levels at the turn of the century (10,11). With the introduction of effective antimicrobial therapy of *M. tuberculosis* in the United States after 1950, a steady decline in the incidence of cases of TB disease was seen. Between 1953 and 1985, the annual number of cases of TB in the United States declined steadily from 84,304 to 22,201, an incidence rate of 53 and 9.3 cases per 100,000 persons, respectively, representing a decrease in the incidence rate of 82% (12) (Fig. 3.1). In 1985, however, the rate and number of cases leveled off and then increased, rising to a peak of 10.5 cases per 100,000 in 1992 (22,201 to 26,673 cases), an increase in rate of 13% (12). When these increases were recognized in the early 1990s, augmented TB control efforts were initiated and federal funding was substantially increased (13). Since 1992, the incidence of TB in the United States has decreased annually, reaching a rate of 5.8 per 100,000 persons in 2000 (16,377 cases).

Several factors were associated with these increased rates. A major factor was increased TB among human immunodeficiency virus (HIV)–infected persons. The increase in TB cases correlated with onset of the acquired immunodeficiency syndrome (AIDS) epidemic; persons aged 25 to 44 had the largest increase in TB cases between 1985 and 1992

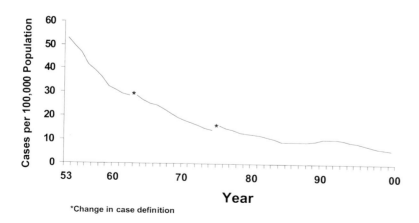

*Change in case definition

FIGURE 3.1. Reported annual incident rates of tuberculosis, United States, 1953–2000.

and were also the age group most heavily affected by AIDS; and the geographic distribution of the two epidemics was similar, with concentration in urban areas and specific states (14). A direct correlation was observed between the percentage of increase in U.S.-born TB patients from 1985 to 1992 and the incidence of AIDS by state (−3.5% per year in states with AIDS incidence of less than 48 per 100,000 to +7.2% in states with more than 100 AIDS cases per 100,000) (14).

Additional evidence about the interaction of the HIV epidemic with TB case rates was obtained indirectly by cross-matching HIV and TB registries. In 1992, the AIDS and TB registries were matched in each state to find AIDS–TB cases for the years 1981 through 1991 (15). Despite the inherent limitation that patients may be reported to only one system even though diagnosed with two separate reportable diseases, approximately 5% of patients were found on both registries, an increase from less than 1% of TB cases in 1981 to nearly 10% by 1990. The estimated proportion of excess TB cases between 1985 and 1990 that could be accounted for by a diagnosis of AIDS was 30%. The impact of HIV infection on the number of TB cases has been estimated to be 57% of excess TB cases in the United States from 1985 to 1991 (16).

Ineffective TB control programs also contributed to the increase in TB cases seen during the period 1985 to 1992. Federal programmatic funding for TB control programs had decreased markedly since the 1970s (13). The overall percentage of patients completing therapy nationwide in the 1980s was poor, with some programs reporting as few as 11% of patients completing therapy (17). Following recognition of this failure to maintain the national infrastructure for TB control, substantial resources were devoted to rebuilding program capacity, and incidence of TB subsequently decreased. In New York City, one of the areas of the United States most heavily affected by the increase in TB, improvement of the TB control infrastructure was associated with a 20% decrease in TB cases between 1992 and 1994; this decrease correlated temporally with an increase in completion of therapy from 50% of patients in 1989 to 90% of patients in 1994 (18). Nationally, after controlling for the effect of HIV infection, decreases in TB cases observed in U.S.-born TB patients between 1991/2 and 1993/4 were associated with improvements in completion of therapy, increases in conversion of sputum culture from positive to negative within 3 months, and increases in the number of contacts per case identified—all indicators of improved program performance (19).

A third factor that was associated with the increases seen between 1985 and 1992 was nosocomial and institutional transmission of *M. tuberculosis*. During this time, CDC and state and local public health departments investigated multiple outbreaks of TB (20–24). Some of the outbreaks were related by overlapping chains of transmission. Nosocomial spread was established by epidemiologic and laboratory evidence in all instances. Common features contributing to these outbreaks included delay in diagnosis, delay in effective therapy, and inadequate isolation procedures. Many patients had severe immunosuppression, with CD4+ lymphocyte counts less than 100 cells/μL, and atypical clinical presentations of TB that made diagnosis more difficult (20–24). In addition, a number of outbreaks were caused by multidrug-resistant organisms that were slow to be recognized and difficult to eradicate.

Nationwide, drug resistance was not a major factor in the increase in TB; high rates of drug resistance, especially multidrug resistance (MDR), mainly occurred in New York City, a primary focus of the increased morbidity. The national TB case report did not include information about drug resistance until 1993, precluding accurate estimates of changes during the period 1985 to 1992. However, in a nationwide survey of the first quarter in 1991, 13 states reported multidrug-resistant TB cases, and more than 60% of these cases were reported in New York City (25). Based on this and a similar survey in 1992, 3.5% of all reported cases involved multidrug-resistant TB at the peak of the resurgence (25,26).

Increased numbers of foreign-born persons in the United States coming from countries with high TB incidence also likely played a role in the increase in TB rates between 1985 and 1992. The foreign-born population increased by more than 20% during the resurgence (27), and the rate of TB among foreign-born persons increased from 28 per 100,000 to 34 per 100,000 during this period. In comparison, the rate of TB among U.S.-born persons remained relatively stable at 8 per 100,000. These changes resulted in an increased proportion of TB cases in the foreign-born and, given the higher intrinsic TB rate of this population, an increase in the overall TB rate.

Demographic Features

Age and Sex

TB case rates by age and sex are shown in Figure 3.2. The age distribution of TB cases reflects the patterns of transmission of *M. tuberculosis* in a community. TB disease in young children indicates recent transmission, since infection is of necessity recently acquired. An increased rate of TB in children often coincides with an increased rate in young adults (i.e., young parents, who are the most common source of infection for children). TB disease in children and TB disease in young adults both usually indicate recent transmission of *M. tuberculosis*. In the elderly, TB disease is more likely due to reactivation of remote infection; incidence in the elderly reflects the prevalence of TB infection when these persons were younger. Males have higher rates of TB disease than females, beginning in the young adult years and persisting throughout life. This predilection has long been observed, and is thought to

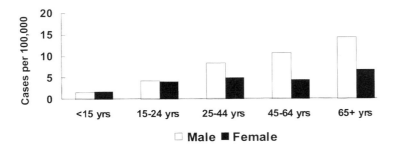

FIGURE 3.2. Incidence rates of tuberculosis by age group and sex, United States, 2000.

reflect increased exposure to *M. tuberculosis* through contacts in the community (28).

Race/Ethnicity

Rates of TB have been consistently higher among racial/ethnic minorities than among whites since national TB surveillance began. While the rates and numbers of cases decreased prior to the mid-1980s, the rate of decline was much slower for nonwhites than for whites (29). In addition, excess cases and increases in numbers of cases were heavily concentrated among racial/ethnic minorities during 1985 to 1992 (14). However, the TB case rates since 1992 have decreased by nearly 50% among non-Hispanic whites, blacks, and Hispanics and by 30% among Asian/Pacific Islanders and Native Americans/Native Alaskans (12). In 2000, racial/ethnic minorities made up 77% of all reported

TB cases; among non-Hispanic whites, the rate was 1.9 per 100,000 persons, whereas it was 15.2 among non-Hispanic blacks, 10.8 among Hispanics, 11.4 among Native Americans/Native Alaskans, and 32.9 among Asian/Pacific Islanders (12). Between 1987 and 1993, TB rates among racial/ethnic minorities were five to ten times higher than those among whites, even after adjusting for age, sex, and country of birth (14). Adjustment for socioeconomic status, however, decreased the rate ratio, especially among U.S.-born blacks, Hispanics, and Native Americans. HIV infection, a risk factor for TB that occurs more frequently among some minority populations, may also explain some of the increased risk for TB among racial/ethnic minorities, but lack of information about prevalence of this factor precluded adjustment for its effect.

The most marked changes in the distribution of TB disease by age are seen in minority populations. As can be seen

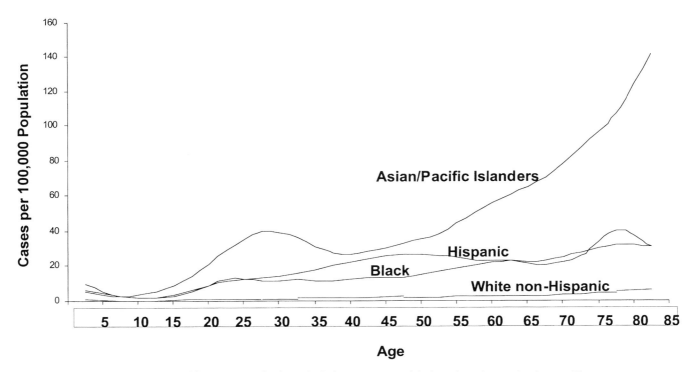

FIGURE 3.3. Incidence rates of tuberculosis by age among blacks, Hispanics, and Asian-Pacific islanders compared with whites, United States, 2000.

in Figure 3.3, TB disease rates for minorities are substantially higher than those for whites in all age groups. Elevated TB disease rates seen among blacks, Hispanics, and Asian/Pacific Islanders in the young adult age group (20 to 45 years of age) suggest TB as a result of recent infection among persons in this age range. In all three groups, the sharp rise after age 65 suggests an additional burden of reactivation disease among minority populations.

Geographic Location

The distribution of TB disease is not uniform across the United States. As shown in Figure 3.4, higher rates are seen in two areas: states with large urban centers and southeastern states. A comparison of TB rates in urban versus rural areas of the United States is shown in Table 3.2. As can be seen, there is a threefold increase in rates from nonurban areas to the largest urban centers, with rates rising from 3.9 per 100,000 to 13.1 per 100,000. Sixty-seven cities in the United States with populations over 250,000 in 2000 reported 38% of the cases in 2000, but these cities represented only 18% of the total U.S. population; the highest TB case rates among these cities occurred in Atlanta, Georgia (30.5 per 100,000), Miami, Florida (27.0 per 100,000), and Newark, New Jersey (26.7 per 100,000) (CDC, unpublished data). The percentage of cases reported from large urban areas (more than 500,000 population) decreased from

35% to 29% between 1992 and 2000, but the percentage of cases reported from nonurban areas (less than 100,000 population) increased slightly from 46% to 49% during the same period. Within urban areas, TB cases frequently cluster in "hot spots"; these have been defined at the zip code or census tract level in several cities (30–32). TB rates as high as 120 per 100,000 have been reported in such areas (30). Higher TB rates in southeastern states appear to partially reflect larger populations of U.S.-born blacks.

Foreign Birth

In 1986, information concerning a patient's place of birth and length of time in the United States was added to the national TB surveillance system. At that time, 22% of TB cases were in persons with foreign birth (27). This percentage has shown a steady increase over time, to 46% of cases in 2000 (12). This reflects a decrease in the number and rate of cases among U.S.-born persons from 19,225 (8.2 per 100,000 population) in 1992 to 8,714 (3.5 per 100,000) in 2000, and an increase in the number of cases but a decrease in rate among foreign-born persons from 7,270 (34.2 per 100,000) in 1992 to 7,554 (25.8 per 100,000) in 2000 (12). Rates of TB disease by age and sex among foreign-born persons in the United States are shown in Figure 3.5.

Seven countries account for the majority of cases of TB in foreign-born persons in the United States: Mexico,

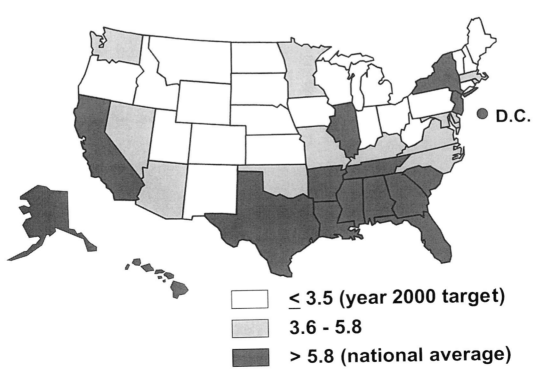

FIGURE 3.4. Incidence rates of tuberculosis by state, United States, 2000. Rate: cases per 100,000.

TABLE 3.2. INCIDENCE RATES OF TUBERCULOSIS IN URBAN AND NONURBAN AREAS, UNITED STATES, 2000

Population of City	Tuberculosis Cases	Case Rate[a]
500,000+	4,704	13.1
250,000–500,000	1,581	11.5
100,000–250,000	2,033	8.0
All other areas	8,059	3.9
United States (overall)	16,377	5.8

[a]Per 100,000 population (total number of cases divided by total population).

Philippines, Vietnam, India, People's Republic of China, Haiti, and Korea (Table 3.3). With the exception of Haiti, these countries also have ranked among the top ten countries of birth of the foreign-born population during the past decade (33). TB case rates among foreign-born persons appear to reflect the level of TB incidence in their birth country or region (27,34) and most likely indicate that a majority of these cases were caused by infection with *M. tuberculosis* in the person's birth country. Among persons from these top countries of birth, rates have been documented to be at least six times that of the U.S.-born population (35). Approximately 50% of foreign-born persons with TB have been in the United States for less than 5 years. The TB case rate among foreign-born persons residing in the United States for 5 years or less is three times higher than that of persons residing in the United States for more than 5 years (27). Within some racial/ethnic populations, the higher TB case rates may be partially explained by the larger proportion of foreign-born persons in that minority group. For example, of Asian/Pacific Islanders who developed TB in 2000, nearly 95% were foreign-born; among Hispanics with TB, over 70% were born outside the United States (12).

Socioeconomic Status

Tuberculosis has traditionally been associated with poverty, but analyses may be confounded by the association between race/ethnicity and economic status. A recent analysis examined the contribution of socioeconomic factors to TB rates among racial/ethnic groups, adjusting for age, sex, and country of birth. There were significant associations between increased risk of TB and increasing levels of crowding, poverty, and decreasing levels of education (36). Utilizing a combined variable including six socioeconomic parameters (i.e., crowding, income, poverty, public assistance, unemployment, and education), TB rate ratios (RRs) were increased with decreasing socioeconomic status among U.S.-born blacks [RR 4.4, 95% confidence interval (CI) 4.3–4.5], Hispanics (RR 2.8, 95% CI 2.7–2.9), Asians (RR 3.5, 95% CI 3.3–3.7), and Native Americans (2.3, 95% CI 2.2–2.4) in comparison with whites of the highest socioeconomic group.

Drug Resistance

Isolates of *M. tuberculosis* that are not susceptible *in vitro* to one or more of the five first-line antituberculosis agents (isoniazid, rifampin, pyrazinamide, ethambutol, and streptomycin) are defined as *drug resistant*. Isolates that are resistant to both isoniazid and rifampin (with or without resistance to other drugs) are termed *multidrug resistant* because these two antibiotics have been shown to be the most potent of the antituberculous drugs and resistance to both greatly complicates the management of patients with active TB. If a patient is infected with a resistant strain, this is termed *primary drug resistance* (PDR), whereas the emergence of drug resistance in a patient on therapy is termed *acquired (secondary) drug resistance* (ADR).

Surveys of selected laboratories in the United States. provide some insight into trends of drug resistance over time. A survey conducted from 1961 to 1968 demonstrated that the rate of PDR to a single drug was 3.5% and to two or more drugs 1% (37). A second survey done from 1975 to 1982 revealed single-drug resistance in 6.9% and resistance to two or more drugs in 2.3% of isolates (38). A third survey done from 1982 to 1986 found single-drug resistance in 9% of isolates, but the increase from 6.9% was thought to be caused by methodologic differences among the studies (39). Within the time span of each study, the rates of resistance were either stable or decreasing, but there were large differences in the rates of resistance between geo-

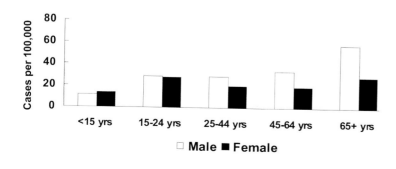

FIGURE 3.5. Incidence rates of tuberculosis by age group and sex among foreign-born persons in the United States, 2000.

TABLE 3.3. TUBERCULOSIS CASES, INCIDENCE RATES, AND DURATION OF UNITED STATES RESIDENCE AMONG FOREIGN-BORN PERSONS BY BIRTH COUNTRY, 2000

Birth Country	No.	Case Rate (%)[a]	Duration U.S. Residence: No. (%)[b]	
			<5 Years	5+ Years
Mexico	1,773	22.0	734 (47)	826 (53)
Philippines	859	69.9	290 (39)	449 (61)
Vietnam	669	81.6	178 (32)	374 (68)
India	562	54.9	305 (64)	169 (36)
China	412	30.6	126 (37)	215 (63)
Haiti	297	92.2	99 (42)	137 (58)
South Korea	208	28.4	56 (35)	103 (65)
Other	2,770	17.6	1,345 (58)	991 (42)
Total[c]	7,550	25.8	3,133 (49)	3,264 (51)

[a]Rates are based on cases per 100,000 persons.
[b]Excludes 1,154 cases with years in United States unknown.
[c]Excludes four cases with unspecified birth country.
Population estimates extrapolated to the April 2000 population from the March 2000 Current Population Survey estimates in the U.S. Census Bureau document, *Profiles of the Foreign-Born Population of the United States: 2000, PPL-145,* Tables 3–2 and 3–4.

graphic areas and among racial/ethnic groups. Also, isolates with drug resistance tended to come from younger persons, indicating that drug-resistant disease was the result of more recent infections. A study examining all culture-positive cases of TB in the United States during the first quarter of 1991 found 14.2% of isolates to be resistant to one or more drugs and 6% to be resistant to two or more drugs (25). Multidrug-resistant TB was found in 3.5% of isolates, and resistance to either rifampin or isoniazid or both was found in 9.5% of isolates. Resistance to rifampin (with or without other drug resistance) was documented in 3.9% of isolates. These increases led to the development of a national plan to combat multidrug-resistant TB (40).

Since 1993, CDC has routinely collected information on drug resistance for all TB cases. Over the period 1993 to 2000, there was a modest decrease in the United States in rates of PDR to isoniazid and in rates of multidrug-resistant TB (Fig. 3.6). Despite these encouraging trends, persons born outside the United States have a markedly increased likelihood of having drug-resistant TB. Between 1993 and 1998, foreign-born persons had rates of PDR for any drug of 17.5% and for MDR of 1.7%, compared to 9.7% and 1.6% among U.S.-born persons; foreign-born persons had rates of ADR for any drug of 30.9% and for MDR of 10.6%, compared to 15.6% and 3.8% among U.S.-born persons (35). Thus, as foreign-born persons continue to account for an increasingly large proportion of the U.S. TB case burden, overall drug resistance rates may increase. In addition, the mobility of the U.S. population can lead to rapid dispersion of drug resistant TB (41,42). During 1993 to 2000, at least one multidrug-resistant TB case was reported from 45 states and from the District of Columbia.

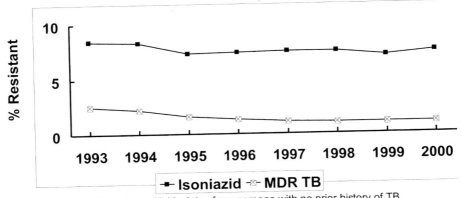

Note: Based on initial isolates from persons with no prior history of TB.
MDR TB defined as resistance to at least isoniazid and rifampin.

FIGURE 3.6. Primary antituberculosis drug resistance, United States, 1993–2000.

Tuberculosis Disease Resulting from Recent Transmission Versus Reactivation Tuberculosis Disease

To optimize TB control strategies, it is useful to know what percentage of TB disease in a community is the result of recent transmission and what percentage is the result of reactivation of latent TB infection. In practice, this means differentiating primary TB disease and reactivation TB disease, but these two types of TB cannot be differentiated by clinical parameters. Molecular clustering of *M. tuberculosis* isolates in a community has been used as a surrogate for disease that results from recent transmission. Using IS6110 typing and other molecular techniques, isolates can be grouped into "clusters" of isolates that are likely to represent chains of TB transmission. One case (the "index" case) is assumed to be the result of reactivation, whereas all others in the cluster are assumed to be the result of spread from that case; isolates that do not cluster are assumed to be the result of reactivation. While such analysis has several limitations (incomplete sampling of cases or failure to sample from neighboring communities will lead to underestimates of clustering, whereas simultaneous reactivations from prior transmission will lead to overestimates), it provides a useful comparative tool.

Cluster analyses from a number of large U.S. cities have concluded that 26% to 50% of their TB cases are the result of recent transmission (42–47). These results are consistent with the rapid decreases in TB seen in New York and San Francisco after improvements in TB control programs, since these improvements were largely targeted at interrupting transmission (18,48). Clustering studies in several cities have suggested that recent transmission is less common among foreign-born patients with TB than among U.S.-born patients (49–52). However, such analyses are less reliable among foreign-born patients because patients whose organism was acquired outside the study area will not be recognized as part of a cluster when the other patients of TB disease with the same organism remain in the country of origin; this may occur when immigrants have recently arrived in the United States or when TB is acquired after a visit abroad (53). Therefore, clustering studies indicating that recent transmission among foreign-born persons is uncommon should be interpreted with caution (54).

DESCRIPTIVE EPIDEMIOLOGY OF TUBERCULOSIS INFECTION

Identification and Reporting of Tuberculosis Infection

Latent tuberculosis infection (LTBI) is an asymptomatic condition. However, because TB infection can reactivate and lead to TB disease, it is important to understand the epidemiology of TB infection. TB infection is diagnosed by the tuberculin skin test (TST). A TST reaction of a predetermined size is indicative of TB infection, but the cutoff for a "positive" test varies depending on the immunologic and epidemiologic status of the individual tested. In the United States, induration of 10 mm or greater is usually considered positive, although in some circumstances, induration of 5 mm is positive. Guidelines for interpreting TST results have recently been updated (55). These guidelines vary the size of the induration required to indicate latent TB infection depending on the epidemiologic risk of infection or the risk of reactivation. Thus, for household contacts or HIV-infected persons a 5-mm induration is positive; for persons with other risk factors for TB, 10 mm is positive; and for persons with no known risk factors for TB, 15 mm is positive. However, in most epidemiologic studies of TB infection, a 10-mm cutoff is used for all subjects.

TB infection is not reportable by law in most parts of the United States. Therefore, epidemiologic information is not systematically collected. Data come largely from TST surveys in specific target populations. These data provide prevalence rates in most cases, although incidence rates have been reported in a few cohorts.

Trends Over Time

Tuberculin skin test trends over time are best understood by examining the results of testing of military recruits. TST surveys were begun among U.S. Navy recruits in 1949 by the United States Public Health Service (USPHS) and have been intermittently performed since that time. These surveys give reliable information about TST rates among largely male recruits aged 18 to 24 years. The 1949 to 1951 survey revealed a prevalence of TB infection of 6.6%, decreasing to 3.2% in surveys done in 1963 to 1964 (28,56). Surveys were then discontinued, but a subsequent survey among Navy recruits performed in 1990 revealed a prevalence of TB infection of 2.5% (57). The decline in TB infection rate is even more notable among those born in the United States; prevalence of TB infection in such recruits fell from 3.9% in the period 1958 to 1969 to 0.6% in 1990 (57). More recent surveys have indicated that the prevalence of a positive TST in the United States has continued to decline (CDC, unpublished observations, 2002). Thus, rates of TB infection have fallen along with the decline in rates of TB disease over the past 50 years.

Demographic Factors

Age and Sex

Several studies have demonstrated that the rate of TB infection increases with age. Surveys performed in Pamlico, North Carolina (1956 to 1960), New York City (1973 to 1974), and Atlanta, Georgia (1994 to 1996) demonstrate a gradual and continuous rise in TB infection prevalence with age, leveling off at 50 to 65 years (58–60). These results are consistent with continued incidence over the lifetime of the individual or a cohort effect (where higher rates among older persons reflect increased incidence at an early age). In the United States, where TB disease rates have been declining over many decades, a cohort effect is the more likely explanation. Among cohorts of elderly persons entering nursing homes in Arkansas, the prevalence of TB infection declined from 20% in 1980 to 1981 to 7% in 1994 to 1995 (61). This decline likely also reflects such a cohort effect, as younger cohorts age and became candidates for nursing home admission.

TB infection rates among children have been studied over the past decade in New York City, Baltimore, and northern California, with reported rates of 0.8% to 2.1% (62–65). Such rates are similar to those reported among children from New Orleans and Chicago in the 1970s (66,67). While TB infection among children necessarily represents more recent infection, these low rates indicate that transmission of *M. tuberculosis* to children in the United States is uncommon. In contrast, among children in Alaska during a time when active TB was common, rates among children reached 90% in 1949 to 1951, declining to roughly 5% by 1969 to 1970 (68).

As with TB disease, TB infection appears to be more common among men than women. Several studies have observed odds ratios of 1.6 to 1.7 among men compared with women (58,60,69). However, other studies have failed to observe differences in TB infection rate by gender (57,59,70).

Race

Tuberculosis infection has long been more common in the United States among racial and ethnic minority populations than among whites. In the USPHS survey among naval recruits performed in 1958 to 1969, rates in blacks were 3.3 times higher than in whites and Hispanics, whereas rates in Asians were 15.8 times higher (56). In the 1990 survey, rates in blacks were 4.1 times higher than in whites and Hispanics, whereas rates in Asians were 22 times higher (57). However, consistent with declines over time, rates in blacks fell from 12.4% in 1958 to 1969 to 4.9% in 1990, whereas rates in Asians fell from 60.2% in 1958 to 1969 to 26.4% in 1990 (57). The increased risk of TB infection in blacks compared with whites is seen in all age groups (58–61). Increased rates of TB infection have also been observed in Hispanics compared with whites and in Native Americans compared with whites (59,69–71).

Geographic Location

In the 1958 to 1969 USPHS surveys, recruits with a lifetime history of living in an urban area had higher rates of TB infection (4.1%) than those with a lifetime history of living in a rural area (2.7%) (28). A similar trend was seen in the 1990 survey (1.8% in areas under 250,000 population versus 6.5% in areas over 500,000), but this difference did not remain statistically significant after controlling for other predictors of TB infection (57).

Foreign Birth

Birth outside the United States is the strongest predictor of TB infection, as it is the strongest predictor of TB disease. In the 1958 to 1969 USPHS survey, persons born in the United States had a TB infection prevalence of 3.9%, whereas persons born outside the United States had a prevalence of 19.2% (56). In the 1990 survey, persons born in the United States. had a prevalence of 0.6%, whereas those born outside the United States had a prevalence of 17.4% (57). In recent surveys, the odds ratio for TB infection among foreign-born persons compared to U.S.-born persons has been reported to be between 2.9 and 25 (60,65,70). Among children, a history of bacille Calmette–Guérin (BCG) vaccination has been shown to account for a portion of this association; among adults the significance of this relationship is less clear (72,73).

Socioeconomic Status

In a survey performed in New York City in 1973 to 1974, lower socioeconomic status (as assessed by a zip code–associated rating of income, occupation, education, and house value) was an independent predictor of TB infection, with a fourfold increase in prevalence between the highest and lowest socioeconomic groups (59).

RISK FACTORS FOR TUBERCULOSIS INFECTION AND DISEASE

Events leading to TB disease follow a progression from exposure to infection to disease, as shown in Figure 3.7. The risk of infection is made up of two components: the risk of exposure, and the risk of infection if exposed. Similarly, risk of disease is composed of the risk of infection plus the risk of primary disease, if infected, and the risk of reactivation, if latent. In areas of the world where exposure is common, there is an additional state, reinfection, that adds to the risk of TB disease; however, in the United States the risk of reinfection is negligible and its contribution to the risk of TB disease will not be further considered.

The term "primary TB disease" is used in its epidemiologic sense, meaning TB disease occurring soon after infection, rather than in its pathologic sense; others have used the term "progressive primary disease" to refer to this stage (74,74).

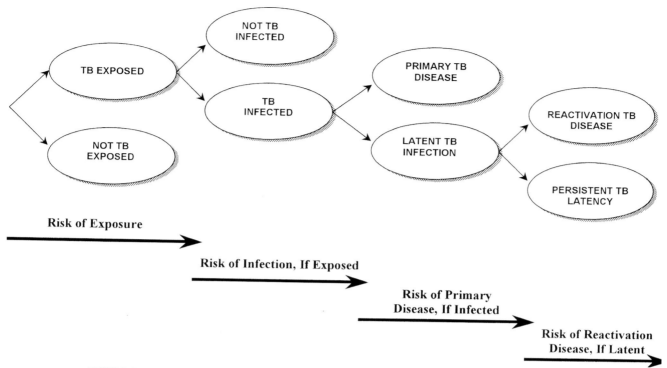

FIGURE 3.7. Time course of events from exposure to disease and definition of transition risks.

Risk of Tuberculosis Infection

Risk of Exposure

Persons in the general U.S. population are presumed to have a very low risk of infection. This has not been directly measured, but the rate among white men is estimated to be between 0.02% and 0.08% per year (76,77). The primary reason for such a low rate is the low likelihood of exposure because TB disease is not common in the United States. In practice, factors that influence the rate of infection among exposed persons, such as intensity and duration of exposure, are rarely measured, and the risk of infection is largely defined by the risk of exposure. Risk of exposure is most directly related to the circumstances that bring a susceptible individual into close contact with an infectious source case.

Persons living or working in congregate settings where risk of exposure to *M. tuberculosis* is often high include employees and residents of hospitals, correctional facilities, nursing homes, and homeless shelters. In hospital employees, prevalence of TB infection has been reported to be as high as 11.3% (78–80). While this prevalence is higher than would be expected for the general population, hospital employees are likely to be demographically distinct from the general population, with substantial numbers of minorities and foreign-born persons, groups that have higher baseline rates of infection. When these factors were controlled for in one study, employees with increased

patient contact had increased risk for TB infection compared with employees with no patient contact, with a relative risk for physicians of 2.35 (1.01 to 5.44) and for housekeepers of 4.33 (1.87 to 9.98) (79). Incidence of TB infection has been reported to be as high as 11.7 per 100 person-years in some hospital employee groups (79,80). It should be noted that these high rates and risks were observed at a time when hospital infection control practices were largely suboptimal. Subsequent changes in administrative and environmental controls have greatly reduced this risk (79,80). Sites of incarceration also provide an environment where risk of exposure to *M. tuberculosis* is high. Prevalence of TB infection among prison populations has been reported to be as high as 27% and to increase with the duration of incarceration (81–84); incidence rates as high as 6.3 infections per 100 person-years have been reported (84). Outbreaks of TB disease among prisoners have been reported (24,85), and prison outbreaks may extend to the surrounding community (85)

Nursing homes, like hospitals, can provide an environment for exposure to *M. tuberculosis*. Nursing home residents have a high prevalence of TB infection, largely reflecting the rate of infection on admission. However, nursing home residents also have substantial incidence of new infection, with reported rates of 3.5% to 5% (86). This increased incidence occurs among persons without infection on admission, and is likely the result of admission to the nursing home of persons with unrecognized active TB (87).

Homeless shelters are another environment where exposure to TB disease may be increased. The prevalence of TB infection among homeless persons has been shown to be between 18% and 70% (60,71,88–90), and a number of outbreaks of TB disease at homeless shelters have been reported (91–95).

Also at high risk for exposure to TB disease are migrant farm workers, intravenous drug users, and persons visiting countries where TB disease is common. No studies of the incidence of TB infection among foreign-born persons while in the United States have been reported, but among children who were born outside the United States or had a parent born outside the United States, the risk of TB infection was increased in association with travel outside the United States [odds ratio (OR) 3.9, 95% CI 1.9–7.9] and having a visitor from outside the United States in the household (OR 2.4, 95% CI 1.0–5.5) (53). Thus, the risk of TB infection related to foreign birth may persist after the foreign-born individual comes to the United States.

Among migrant farm workers in North Carolina, TB infection prevalence was 53% (96). Most farm worker populations have substantial numbers of foreign-born persons, and this may account for much of the TB infection prevalence. In the North Carolina Study, 45% of persons surveyed were foreign-born. Nonetheless, among U.S.-born blacks (representing 88% of the U.S.-born population in this study), 44% were TB infected (96). Risk factors for TB infection included histories of homelessness and incarceration and number of years of farm work. In a prospective study of these farm workers, 14 (30%) of 47 TB-uninfected persons acquired TB infection in a 3-year period, a rate of 10% per year (97). Villarino (98) reported TB infection in 45% of immunocompetent adult farm workers tested at a site in Florida. However, 71% of the population tested was foreign-born, so that the high rates of positive TSTs may have been related to foreign birth and not farm worker status.

Prevalence of TB infection among intravenous drug users has been reported to be 15% to 44% (69,99–103), and incidence has been reported to be 3% to 13% per year (99–101). The degree of risk for TB infection conferred by drug use is difficult to ascertain, as drug users usually have other risk factors for TB infection, including low socioeconomic status, minority race/ethnicity, and history of incarceration. Moreover, HIV prevalence among drug users may be high (30% to 42%) (99,101), and potential anergy among such persons makes identification of TB infection difficult.

Risk of Tuberculosis Infection, If Exposed

While exposure is required for transmission of *M. tuberculosis*, other factors determine whether transmission occurs. These factors include the ability of the infected person to transmit the organism, the biologic capacity of the organism to infect a new host, and the susceptibility of the exposed individual. The ability of the infected host to transmit *M. tuberculosis* has been shown to increase as the concentration of organisms in the sputum increases (104–106); ideally, analysis of risk factors for transmission should control for this factor. In practice, this parameter, as assessed by the number of AFBs seen on sputum smear, is seldom known, since the source case is only identified in contact studies. Persons with laryngeal TB and persons who sing are particularly efficient transmitters (107), but such persons are uncommonly encountered. There is as yet little evidence of wide variability in biologic infectivity between different isolates of *M. tuberculosis*, but such variability occurs in other infectious agents and could contribute to the risk of TB transmission (108).

Several factors can influence the susceptibility of exposed individuals to infection. Persons with enhanced immunity, such as those with prior TB, BCG vaccination, or nontuberculous mycobacterial infection, may have some degree of protection from infection and/or disease (109). However, it is difficult to ascertain the magnitude of this protection because all of these conditions interfere with the assessment of the incidence of TB infection by skin testing.

Persons with immune defects, such as familial immune deficiencies or HIV infection, may have enhanced susceptibility to TB infection when exposed, but convincing evidence that this occurs is lacking. HIV-infected persons have been shown to have increased risk for TB infection in some studies but not in others (24,99,110). Similarly, when exposure is controlled, blacks are seen to be at increased risk for TB infection compared with whites in some studies but not in others (111,112).

Risk of Tuberculosis Disease

Risk of Primary Tuberculosis Disease, If Infected

Persons who become infected with *M. tuberculosis* have a substantial risk of progressing directly to TB disease. In a study of 20,687 household contacts (age 5 years or older), 59% were *M. tuberculosis*–infected when first evaluated. Of these, 598 (4.9%) had TB disease (75). Risk factors for primary TB disease among recently infected persons are shown in Table 3.4.

Risk of Reactivation Tuberculosis Disease, If Latent

The risk of reactivation TB is greatest in recently infected persons. This risk was defined in prospective studies performed by the USPHS between 1950 and 1970 (74,75). Among TB-infected household contacts who were TST positive but had no radiographic evidence of disease, TB disease (pulmonary or extrapulmonary) occurred at a rate of 0.74% per year (0.74 per 100 person-years) in years 1 and 2, 0.31% per year in years 3 through 5, and 0.16%

TABLE 3.4. RISK FACTORS FOR PRIMARY AND REACTIVATION TUBERCULOSIS

Primary Tuberculosis		Reactivation Tuberculosis	
Risk Factor	**Relative Risk (95% CI)**	**Risk Factor**	**Relative Risk (95% CI)**
Age [75][a]		TST size [115]	
0–4	5.51 (4.83–6.28)	5–9 mm	1.0 (Referent)
5+ yr	1.0 (Referent)	10–14 mm	2.30 (1.65–3.21)
		15+ mm	2.86 (1.92–4.27)
HIV Infection [117]		Age [75]	
No	1.0 (Referent)	0–4	4.80 (1.80–12.8)
Yes	8.6 (5.8–13)	5–14	1.0 (Referent)
		15–29	4.99 (2.40–10.4)
		30–44	4.06 (1.84–8.93)
		45+	2.04 (0.83–5.01)
		HIV Infection [116]	
		No	1.0 (Referent)
		Yes	9.5 (3.6–25)
		Weight [113,118]	
		Underweight (≥10%)	1.57 (1.10–2.24)
		Normal Weight	1.0 (Referent)
		Overweight (≥10%)	0.44 (0.26–0.77)
		Abnormal Radiograph [74]	
		No	1.0 (Referent)
		Yes	5.20 (3.35–8.08)

[a]Numbers in brackets indicate source reference.
TST, tuberculin skin test; HIV, human immunodeficiency virus.

per year in years 6 and 7. It is difficult to know with certainty the magnitude of the rate of reactivation TB disease to be expected among persons with latent TB infection, who are identified as having prevalent positive infections without a known date of infection. To the extent that such persons were recently infected, they would contribute excess disease risk. Among young children, persons who are known contacts of a person with TB disease, and persons who are residents of institutions where exposure risk is high, the likelihood that prevalent infections are recent is substantial; for most other groups, the likelihood that such infections in the United States are recent is small. Therefore, rates of reactivation TB can be inferred from studies that have followed prevalent TB-infected persons over time without therapy.

In a study of naval recruits begun in 1949 and followed until 1955, the rate of TB disease among persons with a TST of 10 mm or more at entry was 0.11% (113). Among TB-infected adults in mental health institutions in the United States who were assigned the placebo arm in trials of isoniazid prophylaxis and followed for 10 years, the overall rate of TB was 0.12% per year (74). In a study of children and adolescents with a positive TST at enrollment, the average annual rate of TB disease among persons with a skin test reaction of 11 mm or greater was 0.11% (114). In a study of older adults performed in Georgia and Alabama, the average annual rate of TB disease among persons with a skin test of 10 mm or greater was 0.07% (115). Risk factors for reactivation TB disease among persons with latent TB infection are shown in Table 3.4.

Other Conditions Associated with Tuberculosis Disease

A number of medical conditions, including silicosis, insulin-dependent diabetes mellitus, cancer, renal failure with dialysis, and gastrectomy have been associated with increased risk of TB disease (55). However, the TB infection status of the patients studied is usually not specified; therefore, it is difficult to determine whether the elevated risk observed is due to increased risk of exposure, increased risk of primary disease, or increased risk of reactivation disease.

ACKNOWLEDGMENTS

The authors thank the local and state health department TB staff who collect and submit TB surveillance data to CDC. Special thanks also go to Gloria Kelly for assistance with data analysis and preparation of figures, and to George Comstock and Richard O'Brien for thoughtful review of this chapter.

REFERENCES

1. Centers for Disease Control and Prevention. Case definitions for infectious conditions under public health surveillance. *MMWR Morb Mortal Wkly Rep* 1997;46:40–41.
2. Centers for Disease Control and Prevention. Tuberculosis control laws—United States, 1993. *MMWR Morb Mortal Wkly Rep* 1993;42:3–4.

3. Curtis AB, McCray E, McKenna M, et al. Completeness and timeliness of tuberculosis case reporting: a multistate study. *Am J Prev Med* 2001;20:108–112.

4. Yokoe DS, Subramanyan GS, Nardell E, et al. Supplementing tuberculosis surveillance with automated data from health maintenance organizations. *Emerg Infect Dis* 1999;5:779–787.

5. Compos-Outcalt D, England R, Porter B. Reporting of communicable diseases by university physicians. *Public Health Rep* 1991;106:579–583.

6. Glaser D, Hammersten JE. Pharmacy notification for surveillance and drug utilization review in a metropolitan tuberculosis control program in a low-incidence county. *Maryland Pharm* 1978; July 10.

7. Weinbaum C, Ruggiero D, Schneider, E, et al. TB reporting. *Public Health Rep* 1998;113:288.

8. Trepka MJ, Beyer TO, Proctor ME, et al. An evaluation of the completeness of tuberculosis case reporting using hospital billing and laboratory data—Wisconsin, 1995. *Ann Epidemiol* 1999;9:419–423.

9. Driver CR, Braden CR, Nieves RL, et al. Completeness of tuberculosis case reporting, San Juan and Caguas regions, Puerto Rico, 1992. *Public Health Rep* 1996;111:157–161.

10. Lowell AM, Edwards LB, Palmer CE. *Tuberculosis*. Cambridge: Harvard University Press, 1969:137–138.

11. Rich AR. *The pathogenesis of tuberculosis*. Springfield, IL: Charles C Thomas, 1944:883–892.

12. Centers for Disease Control and Prevention. *Reported tuberculosis in the United States, 2000*. Atlanta, GA:US Department of Health and Human Services, August 2001.

13. Binkin NJ, Vernon AA, Simone PM, et al. Tuberculosis prevention and control activities in the United States: an overview of the organization of tuberculosis services. *Int J Tuberc Lung Dis* 1999;3:663–674.

14. Cantwell MF, Snider DE, Cauthen GM, et al. Epidemiology of tuberculosis in the United States, 1985–1992. *JAMA* 1994; 272:535–539.

15. Burwen DR, Bloch AB, Griffin LD, et al. National trends in the concurrence of tuberculosis and acquired immunodeficiency syndrome. *Arch Intern Med* 1995;155:1281–1286.

16. Bloom BR, Murray CJL. Tuberculosis: commentary on a reemergent killer. *Science* 1992;257:1055–1064.

17. Brudney K, Dobkin J. Resurgent tuberculosis in New York City. *Am Rev Respir Dis* 1991;144:745–749.

18. Frieden TR, Fujiwara PI, Washko RM, et al. Tuberculosis in New York City—turning the tide. *N Engl J Med* 1995;333: 229–233.

19. McKenna MT, McCray E, Jones JL, et al. The fall after the rise: tuberculosis in the United States, 1991 through 1994. *Am J Public Health* 1998;88:1059–1063.

20. Edlin BR, Tokars JI, Grieco MH, et al. An outbreak of multidrug-resistant tuberculosis among hospitalized patients with the acquired immunodeficiency syndrome. *N Engl J Med* 1992; 326:1514–1521.

21. Centers for Disease Control and Prevention. Nosocomial transmission of multidrug-resistant tuberculosis among HIV-infected persons—Florida and New York, 1988–91. *MMWR Morb Mortal Wkly Rep* 1991;40:585–591.

22. Pearson ML, Jereb JA, Frieden TR, et al. Nosocomial transmission of multidrug-resistant *Mycobacterium tuberculosis*: a risk to patients and health care workers. *Ann Intern Med* 1992;117: 191–196.

23. Beck-Sague C, Dooley SW, Hutton MD, et al. Hospital outbreak of multidrug-resistant *Mycobacterium tuberculosis* infections: factors in transmission to staff and HIV-infected patients. *JAMA* 1992;268:1280–1286.

24. Valway SE, Richard SB, Kovacovich J, et al. Outbreak of mul-

tidrug-resistant tuberculosis in a New York State prison, 1991. *Am J Epidemiol* 1994;140:113–122.

25. Bloch AB, Cauthen GM, Onorato IM, et al. Nationwide survey of drug-resistant tuberculosis in the United States. *JAMA* 1994; 271:665–671.

26. Moore M, Onorato IM, McCray E, et al. Trends in drug-resistant tuberculosis in the United States, 1993-1996. *JAMA* 1997; 278:833–837.

27. McKenna MT, McCray E, Onorato I. The epidemiology of tuberculosis among foreign-born persons in the United States, 1986 to 1993. *N Engl J Med* 1995;332:1071–1076.

28. Comstock GW. Epidemiology of tuberculosis. *Am Rev Respir Dis* 1982;125:8–15.

29. Centers for Disease Control and Prevention. Tuberculosis in minorities—United States. *MMWR Morb Mortal Wkly Rep* 1987;36:77–80.

30. Sotir MJ, Parrott P, Metchock B, et al. Tuberculosis in the inner city: impact of a continuing epidemic in the 1990s. *Clin Infect Dis* 1999;29:1138–1144.

31. Acevedo-Garcia, D. Zip code-level risk factors for tuberculosis: neighborhood environment and residential segregation in New Jersey, 1985–1992. *Am J Public Health* 2001;91:734.

32. Barr RG, Diez-Roux AV, Knirsch CA, et al. Neighborhood Poverty and the resurgence of tuberculosis in New York City, 1984–1992. *Am J Public Health* 2001;91:1487–1493.

33. Schmidley DA. *U.S. Census Bureau, Current Population Reports, Series P23-206, Profile of the foreign-born population in the United States, 2000*. Washington, DC: U.S. Government Printing Office, 2001.

34. Zuber PLF, McKenna MT, Binkin NJ, et al. Long-term risk of tuberculosis among foreign-born persons in the United States. *JAMA* 1997;278:304-307.

35. Talbot EA, Moore M, McCray E, et al. Tuberculosis among foreign-born persons in the United States, 1993–1998. *JAMA* 2000;284:2894–2900.

36. Cantwell MF, McKenna MT, McCray E, et al. Tuberculosis and race/ethnicity in the United States: impact of socioeconomic status. *Am J Respir Crit Care Med* 1998;157:1016–1020.

37. Doster B, Caras GJ, Snider DE. A continuing survey of primary drug resistance in tuberculosis, 1961 to 1968. *Am Rev Respir Dis* 1976;113:419–425.

38. Centers for Disease Control and Prevention. Primary resistance to antituberculosis drugs—United States. *MMWR Morb Mortal Wkly Rep* 1983;32:521–522.

39. Snider DE, Cauthen GM, Farer LS, et al. Drug resistant tuberculosis. *Am Rev Respir Dis* 1991;144:732.

40. Centers for Disease Control and Prevention. National action plan to combat multidrug-resistant tuberculosis. *MMWR Morb Mortal Wkly Rep* 1992;41:1–48.

41. Bifani PJ, Plikaytis BB, Kapur V, et al. Origin and interstate spread of a New York City multidrug-resistant *Mycobacterium tuberculosis* clone family. *JAMA* 1996;275:452–457.

42. Agerton TB, Valway SE, Blinkhorn RJ, et al. Spread of strain W, a highly drug-resistant strain of *Mycobacterium tuberculosis*, across the United States. *Clin Infect Dis* 1999;29:85–92.

43. Barnes PF, Yang Z, Pogoda JM, et al. Foci of tuberculosis transmission in central Los Angeles. *Am J Respir Crit Care Med* 1999; 159:1081–1086.

44. Bishai WR, Graham NM, Harrington S, et al. Molecular and geographic patterns of tuberculosis transmission after 15 years of directly observed therapy. *JAMA* 1998;280:1679–1684.

45. Alland D, Kalkut GE, Moss AR, et al. Transmission of tuberculosis in New York City. An analysis by DNA fingerprinting and conventional epidemiologic methods. *N Engl J Med* 1994;330: 1710–1716.

46. Small PM, Hopewell PC, Singh SP, et al. The epidemiology of

tuberculosis in San Francisco. A population-based study using conventional and molecular methods. *N Engl J Med* 1994;330: 1703–1709.

47. Burman WJ, Reves RR, Hawkes AP, et al. DNA fingerprinting with two probes decreases clustering of *Mycobacterium tuberculosis*. *Am J Respir Crit Care Med* 1997;155:1140–1146.

48. Jasmer RM, Hahn JA, Small PM, et al. A molecular epidemiologic analysis of tuberculosis trends in San Francisco, 1991–1997. *Ann Intern Med* 1999;130:971–978.

49. Chin DP, DeRiemer K, Small PM, et al. Differences in contributing factors to tuberculosis incidence in U.S.-born and foreign-born persons. *Am J Respir Crit Care Med* 1998;158: 1797–1803.

50. Tornieporth NG, Ptachewich Y, Poltoratskaia N, et al. Tuberculosis among foreign-born persons in New York City, 1992–1994: implications for tuberculosis control. *Int J Tuberc Lung Dis* 1997;1:528–535.

51. Borgdorff MW, Behr MA, Nagelkerke NJ, et al. Transmission of tuberculosis in San Francisco and its association with immigration and ethnicity. *Int J Tuberc Lung Dis* 2000;4:287–294.

52. Jasmer RM, Ponce de Leon A, Hopewell PC, et al. Tuberculosis in Mexican-born persons in San Francisco: reactivation, acquired infection and transmission. *Int J Tuberc Lung Dis* 1997;1:536–541.

53. Lobato MN, Hopewell PC. *Mycobacterium tuberculosis* infection after travel to or contact with visitors from countries with a high prevalence of tuberculosis. *Am J Respir Crit Care Med* 1998;158:1871–1875.

54. Murray M, Alland D. Methodological problems in the molecular epidemiology of tuberculosis. *Am J Epidemiol* 2001;155: 565–571.

55. Centers for Disease Control and Prevention. Targeted tuberculin testing and treatment of latent tuberculosis infection. *MMWR Morb Mortal Wkly Rep* 2000;49:23–24.

56. Comstock GW, Edwards LB, Livesay VT. Tuberculosis morbidity in the U.S. Navy: its distribution and decline. *Am Rev Respir Dis* 1974;110:572–580.

57. Trump DH, Hyams KC, Cross ER, et al. Tuberculosis infection among young adults entering the US Navy in 1990. *Arch Intern Med* 1993;153:211–216.

58. Edwards LB, Smith DT. Community-wide tuberculin testing study in Pamlico County, North Carolina. *Am Rev Respir Dis* 1965;92:43–54.

59. Reichman LB, O'Day R. Tuberculous infection in a large urban population. *Am Rev Respir Dis* 1978;117:705–712.

60. Bock NN, Metzger BS, Tapia JR, et al. A tuberculin screening and isoniazid preventive therapy program in an inner-city population. *Am J Respir Crit Care Med* 1999;159:295–300.

61. Stead WW. Tuberculosis among elderly persons, as observed among nursing home residents. *Int J Tuberc Lung Dis* 1998;2: S64–S70.

62. Serwint JR, Hall BS, Baldwin RM, et al. Outcomes of annual tuberculosis screening by Mantoux test in children considered to be at high risk: results from one urban clinic. *Pediatrics* 1997; 99:529–533.

63. Froehlich H, Ackerson LM, Morozumi PA. Targeted testing of children for tuberculosis: validation of a risk assessment questionnaire. *Pediatrics* 2001;107:E54.

64. Ozuah PO, Ozuah TP, Stein RE, et al. Evaluation of a risk assessment questionnaire used to target tuberculin skin testing in children. *JAMA* 2001;285:451–453.

65. Scholten JN, Fujiwara PI, Frieden TR. Prevalence and factors associated with tuberculosis infection among new school entrants, New York City, 1991–1993. *Int J Tuberc Lung Dis* 1999;3:31–41.

66. Greenberg HB, Trachtman L, Thompson DH. Finding recent tuberculous infection in New Orleans. Results of tuberculin skin tests on New Orleans children from the inner city and contact investigation program. *JAMA* 1976;235:931–932.

67. Kraut JR, Christoffel KK, Berkelhamer JE, et al. Assessment of tuberculin screening in an urban pediatric clinic. *Pediatrics* 1979;64:856–859.

68. Kaplan G J, Fraser RI, Comstock GW. Tuberculosis in Alaska, 1970. The continued decline of the tuberculosis epidemic. *Am Rev Respir Dis* 1972;105:920–926.

69. Gourevitch MN, Hartel D, Schoenbaum EE, et al. Lack of association of induration size with HIV infection among drug users reacting to tuberculin. *Am J Respir Crit Care Med* 1996; 154:1029–1033.

70. Lifson AR, Halcon LL, Johnston AM, et al. Tuberculin skin testing among economically disadvantaged youth in a federally funded job training program. *Am J Epidemiol* 1999;149:671–679.

71. Zolopa AR, Hahn JA, Gorter R, et al. HIV and tuberculosis infection in San Francisco's homeless adults. Prevalence and risk factors in a representative sample. *JAMA* 1994;272:455–461.

72. Menzies R, Vissandjee B. Effect of bacille Calmette–Guerin vaccination on tuberculin reactivity. *Am Rev Respir Dis* 1992; 145:621–625.

73. Mckay A, Kraut A, Murdzak C, et al. Determinants of tuberculin reactivity among health care workers: interpretation of positivity following BCG vaccination. *Can J Infect Dis* 1999;134–139.

74. Ferebee SH. Controlled chemoprophylaxis trials in tuberculosis. A general review. *Adv Tuberc Res* 1970;17:28–106.

75. Ferebee SH, Mount FW. Tuberculosis morbidity in a controlled trial of the prophylactic use of isoniazid among household contacts. *Am Rev Respir Dis* 1962;85:490–521.

76. Menzies D, Fanning A, Yuan L, et al. Tuberculosis among health care workers. *N Engl J Med* 1995;332:92–98.

77. Daniel TM, Debanne SM. Estimation of the annual risk of tuberculosis infection for white men in the United States. *J Infect Dis* 1997;175:1535–1537.

78. Bailey TC, Fraser VJ, Spitznagel EL, et al. Risk factors for a positive tuberculin skin test among employees of an urban, midwestern teaching hospital. *Ann Intern Med* 1995 122:580–585.

79. Louther J, Rivera P, Feldman J, et al. Risk of tuberculin conversion according to occupation among health care workers at a New York City hospital. *Am J Respir Crit Care Med* 1997;156:201–205.

80. Blumberg HM, Watkins DL, Berschling JD, et al. Preventing the nosocomial transmission of tuberculosis. *Ann Intern Med* 1995;122:658–663.

81. Tulsky JP, White MC, Dawson C, et al. Screening for tuberculosis in jail and clinic follow-up after release. *Am J Public Health* 1998;88:223–226.

82. Hutton MD, Cauthen GM, Bloch AB. Results of a 29-state survey of tuberculosis in nursing homes and correctional communities. *Public Health Rep* 1993;108:305–313.

83. Martin V, Gonzalez P, Cayla JA, et al. Case finding of pulmonary tuberculosis on admission to a penitentiary center. *Tuber Lung Dis* 1994;74:49–53.

84. MacIntyre CR, Kendig N, Kummer L, et al. Impact of tuberculosis control measures and crowding on the incidence of tuberculous infection in Maryland prisons. *Clin Infect Dis* 1997;24:1060–1067.

85. Jones TF, Craig AS, Valway SE, et al. Transmission of tuberculosis in a jail. *Ann Intern Med* 1999;131:557–563.

86. Stead WW, Lofgren JP, Warren E, et al. Tuberculosis as an endemic and nosocomial infection among the elderly in nursing homes. *N Engl J Med* 1985;312:1483–1487.

87. Stead WW, To T. The significance of the tuberculin skin test in elderly persons. *Ann Intern Med* 1987;107:837–842.

88. Barry MA, Wall C, Shirley L, et al. Tuberculosis screening in Boston's homeless shelters. *Public Health Rep* 1986;101:487–494.

89. McAdam JM, Brickner PW, Scharer LL, et al. The spectrum of tuberculosis in a New York City men's shelter clinic (1982–1988). *Chest* 1990;97:798–805.

90. Curtis AB, Ridzon R, Novick LF, et al. Analysis of *Mycobacterium tuberculosis* transmission patterns in a homeless shelter outbreak. *Int J Tuberc Lung Dis* 2000;4:308–313.

91. Schieffelbein CW Jr, Snider DE Jr. Tuberculosis control among homeless populations. *Arch Intern Med* 1988;148:1843–1846.

92. Pablos-Mendez A, Raviglione MC, Batta R, et al. Drug-resistant tuberculosis among the homeless in New York City. *N Y State J Med* 1990;90:351–355.

93. Drug-resistant tuberculosis among the homeless—Boston. *MMWR Morb Mortal Wkly Rep* 1985;34:429–431.

94. Nolan CM, Elarth AM, Barr H, et al. An outbreak of tuberculosis in a shelter for homeless men. *Am Rev Respir Dis* 1991;143:257–261.

95. Nardell E, McInnis B, Thomas B, et al. Exogenous reinfection with tuberculosis in a shelter for the homeless. *N Engl J Med* 1986;315:1570–1575.

96. Ciesielski SD, Seed JR, Esposito DH, et al. The epidemiology of tuberculosis among North Carolina migrant farm workers. *JAMA* 1991;265:1715–1719.

97. Ciesielski S, Esposito D, Protiva J, et al. The incidence of tuberculosis among North Carolina migrant farmworkers, 1991. *Am J Public Health* 1994;84:1836–1838.

98. Villarino ME, Geiter LJ, Schulte JM, et al. Purified protein derivative tuberculin and delayed-type hypersensitivity skin testing in migrant farm workers at risk for tuberculosis and HIV coinfection. *AIDS* 1994;8:477–481.

99. Selwyn PA, Hartel D, Lewis VA, et al. A prospective study of the risk of tuberculosis among intravenous drug users with human immunodeficiency virus infection. *N Engl J Med* 1989;320:545–550.

100. Durante AJ, Selwyn PA, O'Connor PG. Risk factors for and knowledge of *Mycobacterium tuberculosis* infection among drug users in substance abuse treatment. *Addiction* 1998;93:1393–1401.

101. Daley CL, Hahn JA, Moss AR, et al. Incidence of tuberculosis in injection drug users in San Francisco: impact of anergy. *Am J Respir Crit Care Med* 1998;157:19–22.

102. Reichman LB, Felton CP, Edsall JR. Drug dependence, a possible new risk factor for tuberculosis disease. *Arch Intern Med* 1979;139:337–339.

103. Friedman LN, Sullivan GM, Bevilaqua RP, et al. Tuberculosis screening in alcoholics and drug addicts. *Am Rev Respir Dis* 1987;136:1188–1192.

104. Shaw J, Wynn-Williams N. Infectivity of pulmonary tuberculosis in relation to sputum status. *Am Rev Tuberc* 1954;69:724–732.

105. Behr MA, Warren SA, Salamon H, et al. Transmission of *Mycobacterium tuberculosis* from patients smear-negative for acid-fast bacilli. *Lancet* 1999;353:444–449.

106. Reichler MR, Reves R, Bur S, et al. Evaluation of investigations conducted to detect and prevent transmission of tuberculosis. *JAMA* 2002;287:991–995.

107. Loudon RG, Spohn SK. Cough frequency and infectivity in patients with pulmonary tuberculosis. *Am Rev Respir Dis* 1969;99:109–111.

108. Rhee JT, Piatek AS, Small PM, et al. Molecular epidemiologic evaluation of transmissibility and virulence of *Mycobacterium tuberculosis. J Clin Microbiol* 1999;37:1764–1770.

109. Comstock GW, Edwards PQ. An American view of BCG vaccination, illustrated by the results of a controlled trial in Puerto Rico. *Scand J Resp Dis* 1972;53:207–217.

110. Daley CL, Small PM, Schecter GF, et al. An outbreak of tuberculosis with accelerated progression among persons infected with the human immunodeficiency virus. An analysis using restriction-fragment-length polymorphisms. *N Engl J Med* 1992;326:231–235.

111. Stead WW, Senner JW, Reddick WT, et al. Racial differences in susceptibility to infection by *Mycobacterium tuberculosis. N Engl J Med* 1990;322:422–427.

112. Hoge CW, Fisher L, Donnell HD Jr, et al. Risk factors for transmission of *Mycobacterium tuberculosis* in a primary school outbreak: lack of racial difference in susceptibility to infection. *Am J Epidemiol* 1994;139:520–530.

113. Palmer CE, Jablon S, Edwards PQ. Tuberculosis morbidity of young men in relation to tuberculin sensitivity and body build. *Am Rev Tuberc Pulm Dis* 1957;76:517–539.

114. Comstock GW, Palmer CE. Long-term results of BCG vaccination in the southern United States. *Am Rev Respir Dis* 1966;93:171–183.

115. Comstock GW, Livesay VT, Woolpert SF. The prognosis of a positive tuberculin reaction in childhood and adolescence. *Am J Epidemiol* 1974;99:131–138.

116. Moss AR, Hahn JA, Tulsky JP, et al. Tuberculosis in the homeless. A prospective study. *Am J Respir Crit Care Med* 2000;162:460–464.

117. Marks SM, Taylor Z, Qualls NL, et al. Outcomes of contact investigations of infectious tuberculosis patients. *Am J Respir Crit Care Med* 2000;162:2033–2038.

118. Edwards LB, Livesay VT, Acquaviva FA, et al. Height, weight, tuberculous infection and tuberculous disease. *Arch Environ Health* 1971;22:106–112.

4

MOLECULAR EPIDEMIOLOGY OF *MYCOBACTERIUM TUBERCULOSIS*

BARUN MATHEMA
BARRY N. KREISWIRTH

Mycobacterium tuberculosis, the etiologic agent of tuberculosis (TB), has been extensively studied ever since Robert Koch's initial cultivation of the acid-fast rod-shaped tubercle bacillus more than a century ago. Despite the availability of effective antitubercle chemotherapy for more than 50 years and major advances in the biology and epidemiology of *M. tuberculosis*, TB remains the leading cause of adult mortality attributable to a single pathogen, claiming approximately 2 million individuals annually (1,2). It is projected that TB will remain among the ten leading causes of global disease burden even in the year 2020 (3).

The control and prevention of TB in recent years has been further complicated by the interactive and transforming effect of human immunodeficiency virus/acquired immunodeficiency syndrome (HIV/AIDS). Although TB incidence in general has been well controlled in developed nations, the urgency in resource-poor countries is dire as over 90% of all incident and prevalent cases are reported from developing nations where, not surprisingly, the HIV seroprevalence is also high (2–4). Therefore, it is imperative to better understand clinical, epidemiologic, biologic, and socioeconomic parameters associated with this pathogen to aid in the reduction and possible control of worldwide TB morbidity and mortality.

Historically, much of our understanding of TB has stemmed from descriptive epidemiologic and clinical observations as well as from limited animal studies. The results from numerous TB studies, from bacille Calmette–Guérin (BCG) vaccination to isoniazid preventive trials, has been central to formulating a generalized hypothesis regarding all phases of the pathogenesis, from exposure, to successful infection to subsequent disease (5–11). Infection is estab-

lished in approximately one third of individuals exposed to the tubercle bacilli during the course of their lifetime, and among those infected only 10% ever become symptomatic (5,12–14). In addition, disease presentation is quite variable in regard to severity, duration, and therapeutic indices, and the site of pathology, although commonly pulmonary, includes numerous tissues such as the meninges, lymph nodes, and spine (14–16). The variability is multifaceted, and paramount in the disease process is the ongoing interaction between the *M. tuberculosis* strain and the host immune status (17). Environmental factors greatly contribute to the spread of the bacillus, and comorbidity factors, including coinfection with other pathogens and other underlying medical conditions such as diabetes, influence the progression and severity of the disease process.

The *M. tuberculosis* infection route is primarily from aerosolized bacilli being passed on from an infectious, symptomatic individual to another close or casual contact. As a result, the hallmark of TB control has relied on active case finding and effective disease management. This includes contact tracing, Mantoux testing, and prophylaxis of close contacts who may have been exposed to the index patient. TB generally involves a long latency period with symptomatic presentation occurring from 3 months (mainly in the immunocompromised) to a lifetime after the establishment of infection (5,17). As a result, a proportion of incident cases will be due to reactivation or activation of a historical infection, whereas others will be due to a recent event suggesting active transmission (18). Therefore, the distinction between a recent and a historical transmission event is important in assessing the public health implication incident cases bear as well as the overall effectiveness of the local TB control program.

Differentiation or subspeciation of clinical isolates of *M. tuberculosis* is demonstrative in supporting or refuting patient linkages. Techniques for subspeciating *M. tuberculosis* historically have relied on phenotypic characteristics, such as mycobacterial growth rates, colony morphology, bio-

B. Mathema: Public Health Research Institute at the International Center of Public Health, Newark, New Jersey.
B. N. Kreiswirth: Department of Medicine, New York University School of Medicine, New York, New York; and Publich Health Research Institute TB Center, Newark, New Jersey.

chemical assays, phage typing, and susceptibility to selected antibiotics (19). Although useful, these methods have poor discriminatory power, thus limiting the further development of TB epidemiology. This was the case until the late 1980s when molecular biologic techniques were integrated as specific tools of epidemiology (molecular epidemiology).

Molecular epidemiology is largely a hybrid field that integrates epidemiologic methods with the principles and tools of molecular biology to better understand disease causation, spread, and pathogenesis. Over the last decade, molecular epidemiologic studies of *M. tuberculosis* have enhanced our ability to detect and in some instances confirm patient links and identify laboratory cross-contamination (20–24). Prior to the use of molecular tools, understanding the spread of TB was imprecise and was mostly dependent on observational data (25). The difficulty in identifying the links between patients is partly due to TB's latent nature and also because the secondary, tertiary, or quaternary spread often sufficiently obscures the epidemiologic thread needed to understand transmission dynamics.

Among the number of molecular techniques available to subspeciate *M. tuberculosis* isolates, IS (insertion sequence) *6110*-based restriction fragment length polymorphism (RFLP) analysis is the primary DNA fingerprinting method (26). This method has been complemented using a number of secondary genotyping techniques, and together these multiple targets have enhanced the discriminatory power to subspeciate *M. tuberculosis* (27). The increasing use of molecular methods to differentiate clinical isolates of *M. tuberculosis* and the integration of this data with conventional TB epidemiology has made for better characterization of transmission dynamics and in some circumstances has enhanced TB control efforts.

This chapter reviews current genotyping techniques, and their application and utility within the framework of enhancing our understanding of TB epidemiology and control efforts. In addition, we discuss new technologies being tested and future research directions in the study of TB molecular epidemiology.

METHODS OF GENOTYPING *MYCOBACTERIUM TUBERCULOSIS*

Extensive genomic characterization of *M. tuberculosis*, including the complete DNA sequencing of two strains, H37Rv and CDC1551, has revealed remarkable DNA conservation between chromosomes. Sequence comparison of the 275-base pair (bp) internal transcribed spacer region, which separates 16S ribosomal DNA (rDNA) and 23S rDNA, is completely conserved among members of the *M. tuberculosis* complex *(M. tuberculosis, M. bovis, M. africanum, M. canettii, M. microti)*(28). Extending this finding, sequence analysis of 56 structural genes in several hundred geographically and phylogenetically diverse strains

of *M. tuberculosis* complex revealed that allelic polymorphism is extremely rare, occurring in approximately 1 in 10,000 bp (29–31). The remarkably high degree of DNA conservation within this species has led to the suggestion that members of the *M. tuberculosis* complex underwent an evolutionary bottleneck at the time of speciation estimated to have occurred 15,000 to 20,000 years ago (30).

Although the *M. tuberculosis* genome is highly conserved in comparison with other pathogenic bacterial species, there are polymorphic regions that are usually associated with insertion sequences, as well as repetitive elements that are dispersed throughout the chromosome and are used as targets for genotyping.

The first molecular based technique to subspeciate *M. tuberculosis* was a direct gel electrophoresis comparison of restriction digests of genomic DNA as described by Collins and De Lisle (32). However, this method was limited by the complexity of the resulting patterns and the subjective nature of comparing the outcomes from different experiments. The method was improved by using cloned fragments of mycobacterial DNA in a Southern blot format to probe restriction endonuclease–digested chromosomal DNA from *M. tuberculosis* isolates (33). However, the discrimination power was limited. This technique was furthered by the identification of repetitive DNA sequences that are present in variable number and locations and when used as probes yield highly polymorphic hybridization patterns (34,35). This approach forms the bases of modern *M. tuberculosis* genotyping.

Insertion Sequence *6110*

Bacterial insertion sequences (IS), such as IS*6110*, are small (200 to 1,500 bp), mobile, genetic elements that encode their own transposition but, unlike transposons, do not encode a phenotypic marker. Insertion sequence elements are present in variable copy numbers in different species, such as IS*1* in *Escherichia coli* strains, which has a range of 2 to 17 copies and in *Shigella* species from 2 to 40 (36). IS*6110*, a member of the IS*3* family (37), is a 1,355-bp mobile element first described by Thierry et al. that when intact is unique to the *M. tuberculosis* complex (35,38). This insertion sequence has an imperfect 28-bp inverted repeat at its ends, and it generates a 3- to 4-bp target duplication on insertion. Although there are observed "hot spots," IS*6110* insertions are more or less randomly distributed throughout the genome with copy number ranging from rare clones that lack any insertion to those with 26 copies (39,40).

The standardization of IS*6110* Southern blot hybridization initially proposed by van Embden et al. (26) is based on a common restriction enzyme, *Pvu*II, standardized molecular weight markers, and matching software analysis for interlaboratory comparison. The restriction enzyme *Pvu*II was recommended as it cleaves IS*6110* at only one asymmetric site. The DNA probe target was directed against IS*6110* sequences to the right of the *Pvu*II cleavage site; consequently, each hybridizing band corresponds to a single IS*6110* insertion (35). The computer-assisted analysis of the resulting IS*6110* DNA fingerprint patterns (Figs. 4.1 and 4.2 has allowed for large interlaboratory comparison of individual strain patterns as well as the creation of large national and international fingerprint archives (such as those kept at the Centers for Disease Control and Prevention, Atlanta, GA; Public Health Research Institute, Newark, NJ; and National Institute of Public Health and the Environment, Bilthoven, The Netherlands) (41–43).

The observed genetic polymorphism inherent to IS*6110* and the relative stability required of this element to be used as a genetic marker are conflicting and cause for concern regarding the selection of this gauge to study the epidemiology of TB and reliably link related cases. That is, the rate of IS*6110* change must be adequate to distinguish nonepidemiologically related strains yet slow enough to group relevant cases based on identical or similar hybridizing patterns. DNA fingerprints did not change in strains cultured in macrophages over a 4-week period, in a guinea pig model for more than 2 months, or *in vitro* (liquid media) for 6

months (44,45). In addition, two recent studies addressing this point have shown IS*6110* to be stable on the short time scale of months while transposing at an observable rate over longer periods of time. The instability of IS*6110*, taken from sequentially positive cultures with intervals ranging from days to years, determined the half-life or time of IS*6110*-based DNA fingerprint alteration to range between 3 and 4 years (46,47). Although the movement of this insertion element is a replicative process, half-life may vary based on *in vivo* replication rates due to either host–pathogen or site pathologic properties. However, the general stability of IS*6110* within an epidemiologically relevant time frame makes this method applicable for studying transmission dynamics at the local or population level. Noteworthy is a study by Lillebaek et al. (48) that uses IS*6110* genotyping to demonstrate endogenous reactivation of *M. tuberculosis* after 33 years of latency.

The utility of molecular epidemiologic methods in a population analysis relies on sufficient polymorphism within circulating isolates. Defining a clonal type is strengthened when there is adequate background strain diversity. In a population-based study in New Jersey, Bifani et al. (49) reported that approximately one third of the

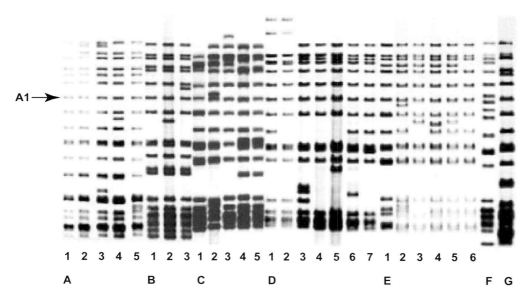

FIGURE 4.1. Insertion sequence *6110* (IS*6110*) Southern blot hybridization DNA fingerprint patterns of W-Beijing family *Mycobacterium tuberculosis* strains isolated from tuberculosis patients in different studies (Public Health Research Institute, Tuberculosis Center collection, B.N.K.). **A:** *lanes 1–5:* Representative members of the W4 strain group from a population-based study, New Jersey (49); **B:** *lanes 1–3:* Representative members of the W14 strain group from a community cluster in New York City (NYC) (72); **C:** lanes *1–5:* Representative members of the W-Beijing family isolated in China (73); **D:** lanes *1–7:* Representative members of the W family strains isolated in the former Soviet Union (145); **E:** *lanes 1–6:* multidrug-resistant strain W and descendants isolated from the NYC outbreak (89); **F:** W family strain W82 identified in nosocomial transmission study, Tennessee (23); **G:** W family strain 210 found in California–Colorado–Texas outbreak (52,142). The *A1 arrow* indicates the IS*6110* insertion (common to all W-Beijing family strains) in *dnaA-dnaN* region of the *M. tuberculosis* chromosome (40). (From Bifani et al. Global dissemination of the *Mycobacterium tuberculosis* W-Beijing family strains. *Trends Microbiol* 2002;10:45–52, with permission.)

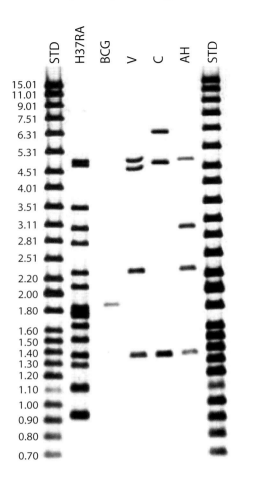

FIGURE 4.2. Southern blot hybridization of *Mycobacterium tuberculosis* isolates, showing *Pvu*II-restricted chromosomal DNA blot hybridized with *Bam*HI – *Sal*I fragment of insertion sequence *6110* (IS*6110*). *Lane 1*, Laboratory strain H37Ra; *lane 2*, *M. bovis* bacille Calmette–Guérin (*BCG*); *lane 3*, common low-copy-number strain in the Public Health Research Institute database; *lane 4*, strain that caused widespread dissemination in the New York City area (123); *lane 5*, strain that caused large outbreak in clothing manufacturing factory (CDC1551) (104). *STD*, molecular weight standards.

1,207 isolates analyzed by IS*6110*-based genotyping were unique to this sample. Another third of the isolates were grouped into 11 major strain groups that included 10 or more patients. In this example, finding a genotype common between patients distinct to the population would strengthen the ability to make inference regarding epidemiologic links. However, defining a DNA fingerprint as unique or uncommon is contingent on the comparison database size and collection method, as there are presumably a finite number of genetic backgrounds within a particular community or group. Nevertheless, the strength of this method is greatly enhanced when genotyping data corroborate with conventional epidemiologic methods of TB control.

IS*6110*-based DNA fingerprinting is not only the most widely used genetic method for subspeciating *M. tuberculosis* with well over 70,000 isolates characterized worldwide, but has since also become a model system to study the molecular epidemiology of a given bacterial species. Although IS*6110*-based DNA fingerprinting has proven to be robust in discriminating strains of *M. tuberculosis*, limitations do exist. One such limitation is the interpretation of genotyping data to draw epidemiologic conclusions. This is especially important in studies in isolated geographic areas where there is low genetic diversity or in regions of high incidence of TB (50–52). Under such conditions, the clustering of patients with common strain genotypes is not always synonymous with recent infection or transmission, as a new infection may involve a number of different transmission pathways. This limitation is somewhat similar to that of conventional field epidemiology involving contact investigations that often fail to identify patterns of transmission, particularly in high incidence areas (25,53).

Another limitation with this genotyping method is the discriminatory power among isolates with six or fewer copies of IS*6110* (low copy number) (27,54–56). That is, isolates with the identical hybridization pattern may not be clonal when six or fewer bands comigrate. An IS*6110* band on a blot only indicates the presence and size of the insertion and does not provide the chromosomal location. Therefore, it is possible to have identical bands that are from different regions of the chromosome. This ambiguity is especially pronounced in low-copy-number isolates as the cumulative probability supporting clonality is decreased given the limited number of independent events (IS*6110* insertions). In contrast, identical or similar patterns in high-copy-number isolates (e.g., more than six IS*6110* insertions) present higher confidence in determining clonality such that the probability of six or more insertions being of similar size but from different chromosomal positions is low. In fact, low-copy-number isolates with the same IS*6110* pattern were shown in a number of studies to be genetically distinct when independent secondary biomarkers were used (54–58). There also exist, though rarely, isolates that do not contain IS*6110* (59,60). Finally, this genotyping tool cannot distinguish among *M. tuberculosis* complex members (61).

Secondary Genotyping Methods

Developed either independently or to overcome the inherent limitations with IS*6110*-based DNA fingerprinting, a number of secondary molecular tools can be used to assess differences in the bacterial genomic organization among clinical specimens. The biologic function, genetic structure, and rate of polymorphism of secondary genetic markers vary greatly, but alone tend to be inferior to the discriminatory ability of IS*6110*-based genotyping. The most commonly used secondary methods include spacer oligonucleotide typing (spoligotyping) and polymorphic GC-rich repetitive sequence (PGRS) typing (56,58,62–65). In general, these techniques are used to augment IS*6110*-based genotypic analysis.

Spoligotyping, first described by Groenen et al. (66), is a polymerase chain reaction (PCR)–based method for differentiating clinical isolates of *M. tuberculosis*. This technique is based on detection of spacer DNA sequences interspersed among 36-bp direct repeats (DRs) in the genomic DR region of *M. tuberculosis* complex strains. The number of repeats and spacer sequences in the DR region vary among *M. tuberculosis* complex strains (67). Forty-three synthetic oligonucleotides based on DNA sequence data of the spacer regions in laboratory strain H37Rv and *M. bovis* BCG vaccine strain P3, have been ordered on a hybridization membrane. Genotyping is performed by first amplifying the DR locus and then by hybridizing the labeled population of synthesized spacers to the membrane. The resulting hybridization to the spotted synthetic oligonucleotide sequences can be detected by chemiluminescence (67). The highly reproducible results are based on a binary (present/absent) system that can be easily interpreted, computerized, and exchanged between laboratories (Fig. 4.3).

There are some clear advantages of using spoligotyping over IS*6110* fingerprinting. Unlike IS*6110* genotyping, which requires approximately 2 µg of bacterial DNA, spoligotyping can be performed using much less DNA and in a fraction of the time. Also, spoligotyping has been shown to provide genotypes on nonviable specimens, on paraffin-embedded material, and on slides of Ziehl–Neelsen stainings (68–70). In addition, this method can distinguish among isolates of the *M. tuberculosis* complex based on specific spacers present in some species of the complex and absent in others (67,71). However, the discriminatory power of spoligotyping alone is less when compared with IS*6110* (27). There have been a number of reports documenting strains with distinct IS*6110* fingerprint patterns sharing the same spoligotype pattern (65,72). As an example, the W-Beijing family of strains defines a large phylogenetic lineage of *M. tuberculosis* strains that comprise hundreds of IS*6110* variations and subtypes, and yet all these strain share a common spoligotype (Fig. 4.3) (73,74). In contrast, spoligotyping has been shown to further subtype IS*6110*-based low-copy-number strains (56,62). It has been shown that spoligotyping, when used in conjunction with IS*6110*-based fingerprinting, creates a robust and discriminatory genotyping system (27).

PGRS typing, first described by Ross et al. (75), is a Southern blot hybridization protocol that uses the restriction enzyme *Alu*I and a consensus PGRS-specific probe. The PGRS probe, designated pTBN12, is a 3.4-kb insert of a PGRS contained in the recombinant plasmid pTBN12. Chaves et al. (58) demonstrated that this technique, like spoligotyping, discriminated isolates clustered by IS*6110* genotyping. This is particularly the case when analyzing IS*6110* low-copy-number strains. This method, like IS*6110*, is labor and time intensive, but in contrast to the IS*6110* system, PGRS hybridization patterns are too complex to computerize for both standardization and analysis.

More recently, PCR and DNA sequence–based methods have been developed that compare variable number tandem repeat elements and single nucleotide polymorphisms (SNPs) to describe the epidemiology of TB. Frothingham and Meeker-O'Connell (76) used PCR to determine the exact number of tandem DNA repeats at each of the five chromosomal loci containing variable number tandem

Spoligotype[a]

CDC	Binary format		Octal Code[c]	PHRI
	1[b]	43		
0001	■■■■■■■■■■■■■■■■■■□□■■■■■■■■■■■■■■■■■□□□□■■■■■■		777777477760771	H37Rv/Ra
0025	■■□■■■■□■■■■□■■■■■■■■■■■■■■■■■■■■■■■■□□□□□		676773777777600	BCG
0075	■■■■■■■■■■■■□■□□□□□□■■■■■■■■■■■■□□□□■■□□□□■		777776407760601	S75 group
0030	■■■□□□□□□□□□□□■□■■■■■■■■■■■■■■■■■□□□□■■■□■■■		700036777760731	C strain
0089	■■■□□□□□□□□□■■■□■■■■□■■■□■■■■■■■■■□□□□■■■■■		700076757760771	CDC1551
0034	□□□□□□□□□□□□□□□□□□□□□□□□□□□□□□□□□□□■■■■■■■■■		000000000003771	W-Beijing strains

[a]Spoligotyping performed at the Wadsworth Center, New York State Department of Health, Albany, New York.

[b]Denotes spacer number.

[c]see Dale *et al.* 2001.

FIGURE 4.3. Binary depiction of spacer oligonucleotide typing (spoligotyping) of *Mycobacterium tuberculosis*. Positive hybridization with 43 different spacers is denoted by *black boxes*; spacer number are indicated at the ends. *Row 1*, H37Rv/Ra, spoligotype 0001 (107); *row 2*, bacillus Calmette–Guérin (*BCG*), spoligotype 0025; *row 3*, S75 group of strains (65); *row 4*, C strain, spoligotype 0030; *row 5*, strain CDC1551 (AH), spoligotype 0089; *row 6*, W-Beijing family strains (74), spoligotype 0034. For octal code[c], see ref. 61. *CDC*, Centers for Disease Control and Prevention; *PHRI*, Public Health Research Institute.

repeat sequences (VNTR loci ETR-A through ETR-E). More recently, Supply et al. (77) reported the use of a mycobacterial interspersed repetitive unit (MIRU) to differentiate clinical *M. tuberculosis* isolates. These VNTR units have been identified around the *M. tuberculosis* genome and located in mammalian-like minisatellite regions. The objective nature of this method and the ability to automate the system may provide an advantage in genotyping large populations.

Given the highly conserved nature of the *M. tuberculosis* genome, genetic alterations at the nucleotide level have given researchers precise targets to assess subtle differences among clinical isolates (29). Both synonymous and nonsynonymous SNPs provide genetic information, but their analyses address different biologic questions (78,79). In general, nonsynonymous changes create an amino acid change, the effect of which on the protein may be subject to environmental selection (80). The nonsynonymous changes in drug resistance gene targets, which are under strong selection pressure, provide a robust method to genotype antibiotic resistance in *M. tuberculosis*. Synonymous changes, which are viewed as functionally neutral, are excellent markers to assess genetic drift and evolutionary relationships among bacterial strains. Recently, Brosch et al. (81) used comparative genomic analysis and identified regions of deletion to infer evolutionary relationships among members of the *M. tuberculosis* complex and other closely related mycobacteria. A similar method was used to differentiate among clinical strains of *M. tuberculosis* and discern lineages of *M. bovis* BCG (82,83).

Sreevatsan et al. (29) used two functionally neutral nonsynonymous SNPs (nsSNPs) located in codon 463 of the catalase-peroxidase-encoding gene *katG* and codon 95 of the A subunit of DNA gyrase gene *gryA* to categorize all modern *M. tuberculosis* strains into three broad genetic groups. More currently, Gutacker et al. (84) used more than 200 synonymous (silent) SNPs (sSNPs), based on the four available *M. tuberculosis* complex genomes, to assess the genetic relationships within *M. tuberculosis* species and to the other members of the complex. The results of this method prove to be robust and rapid in delineating relationships among closely related strains and establishing genetic frameworks to further study biologically relevant properties of the pathogen. Although the use of SNP technology to study transmission dynamics is still in its infancy, with optimization and further studies among molecular epidemiologically characterized strains taking place, this objective method can in theory achieve better resolution than IS*6110*-based fingerprinting.

Perhaps the most direct application of genomic data has been in evaluating alterations in genes that result in reduced susceptibility to antituberculous agents (Table 4.1). Drug resistance in *M. tuberculosis*, in contrast to many other bacterial pathogens, nearly always correlates with a genetic alteration (nonsynonymous point mutations, small deletions or insertions) in the antibiotic-specific resistance–determining region(s) in the chromosome. The molecular genetic basis of resistance has advanced rapidly in recent years, with target genes and specific alterations determined for all first-line (and some second-line) chemotherapeutic agents (85). Assessment of target mutations have aided in determining whether the occurrence of drug resistance in clinical samples is due to primary or secondary (acquired) transmission. That is, whether the isolate was spread as a drug-resistant clone (primary) or whether it developed resistance within the patient (secondary) due to factors such as poor therapeutic compliance, low bioavailability, or drug malabsorption (86–88). In addition, drug resistance markers have been used to elucidate transmission, clonality, and microevolutionary pathways (72,89).

TABLE 4.1. RESISTANCE-DETERMINING GENE LOCI IN *MYCOBACTERIUM TUBERCULOSIS*[a,b]

Antitubercular Agent	Gene	Product	Reported Mutation Frequency Among Resistant Clinical Isolates (%)[a,b]
Streptomycin	*rps* L	Ribrosomal protein S12	~60
	rrs	16S rRNA	<10
Isoniazid	*kat* G	Catalase-peroxidase	60–70
	oxy R–*ahp* C	Alkylhydroreductase	~20
	inh A	Enoyl-ACP reductase	<10
	kasA	β-ketoacyl-ACP synthase	<10
Rifampicin	*rpo* B	β-subunit of RNA polymerase	>95
Ethambutol	*emb* CAB	EmbCAB	~70
Pyrazinamide	*pnc* A	Amidase	70–100
Ethionamide	*inh* A	Enoyl-ACP reductase	<10
Kanamycin	*rrs*	16S rRNA	~65
Fluoroquinolone	*gyr* A	DNA gyrase	>90

[a]For a comprehensive review, see Ramaswamy S, Musser JM. Molecular genetic basis of antimicrobial agent resistance in *Mycobacterium tuberculosis*: 1998 update. *Tuber Lung Dis* 1998;79:3–29.
[b]Mutation frequencies determined by sequencing and polymerase chain reaction/single-strand conformational polymorphism.
ACP, acyl carrier protein.

APPLICATIONS OF MOLECULAR EPIDEMIOLOGIC METHODS IN THE CONTROL AND PREVENTION OF TUBERCULOSIS

Within the past decade, the application of molecular tools has reinforced in some cases, and changed in others, the study of TB transmission dynamics and epidemiology. Although the integration and analysis of *M. tuberculosis* genotyping in the control and prevention of TB is still nascent, genotypic analysis of clinical samples has been extensive, including diverse epidemiologic settings and geographic regions. In general, the increased resolution of molecular methods has provided the opportunity for analysis of both short-term (local epidemiologic) investigations, such as suspected outbreaks or laboratory contamination (23,89–91), and long-term (global epidemiologic) questions, such as understanding spatiotemporal transmission and evolutionary dynamics (29,81,92).

Molecular genotyping of *M. tuberculosis* used in concert with traditional epidemiologic methods has dramatically enhanced our understanding of the patterns of strain transmission. The direct applications to TB control have been wide and diverse. Molecular techniques have been used to estimate the fraction of cases attributable to recent transmission versus reactivation (25,93,94), confirm laboratory cross-contamination (21,91), differentiate recurrent TB into either endogenous reactivation or exogenous reinfection (95–97), identify host-specific risk factors (49,53,98), and study different properties and patterns of drug resistance (99–102). In addition to detecting unsuspected transmission links (49,65), molecular markers are increasingly being used to study transmission patterns within populations (57) and to evaluate host- and strain-specific risk factors and possible genotype-specific differences in phenotypes, such as virulence, tissue tropism, and transmissibility (29,103,104).

The direct applicability and strength of molecular techniques for public health are best shown when carried out to either lead or augment traditional TB control and prevention activities. The following sections present case studies to illustrate the utility of these methods.

Laboratory Cross-Contamination

Laboratory cross-contamination or the identification of a false-positive culture occurs when a clinical sample is mislabeled or contaminated as an error in the handling or processing of primary patient samples being submitted for mycobacterial analyses. This phenomenon occurs at a rate that is quite variable from one clinical laboratory to another. There are several ways in which this can occur, usually involving a growth of bacteria from contaminated instruments (e.g., bronchoscopes), or during laboratory processing (21). In general, sampling needles from

BACTEC (Becton, Dickinson and Company, Franklin Lakes, NJ, U.S.A.) machines are the major source of contamination; however, it has been shown that during conventional decontamination of specimens, there can be splashing and transfer of microbes from the bacterial solution (105). These false-positive results may lead to important clinical errors, as most antituberculous agents require long-term therapy and may pose chemotherapeutic toxicity to the falsely diagnosed patient. Using molecular methods, it has become apparent that this phenomenon occurs more frequently than was previously thought (21,106). Identification of cross-contamination based on molecular types has mainly relied on sufficient strain diversity within the TB population and distinction between clinical versus laboratory strains. That is, given heterogeneous *M. tuberculosis* genotypes in the community, the probability of finding two clinical isolates with identical fingerprints (within a short time period) would be low and warrant an investigation. As most clinical laboratories use a laboratory strain (such as H37Ra/Rv) for identification and drug susceptibility testing, differentiating between patient isolate and control strain is crucial in identifying contamination stemming from the control strain to clinical specimen (107). The latter is especially suspected when there are inconsistencies between clinical findings and microbiologic results (108).

In a study of cross-contamination in a clinical mycobacteriology laboratory, Small et al. (109) suggested that the presentation of two identical fingerprints cultured within 7 days should be investigated. Generally the initial steps in identifying cross-contamination is to determine whether the patient has only a single positive acid-fast stain (out of three smears taken on consecutive days) that grows a positive culture and if the laboratory had processed any other *M. tuberculosis* isolate during the same time period. If the latter is true, then molecular typing can be used to determine the possibility of *in vitro* cross-contamination. In this manner, there have been a number of studies documenting the use of genotyping to prove or refute a potential false-positive classification (20,109–111). Finally, it is crucial to the patient's well-being for the clinical microbiologists and clinicians to maintain close communication to distinguish between pseudo-outbreaks (when a series of false-positive cultures occur) and outbreaks.

Population-Based Studies: Elucidating Transmission Dynamics

M. tuberculosis infection is generally followed by a latency period that can vary from several months (among highly immunocompromised patients) to a lifetime. In fact, about 90% of infected individuals never become symptomatic for TB (5,17). This pathogen's persistence coupled with the reproductive number (number of new infections that one symptomatic case causes annually) makes it extremely difficult to assess the level of transmission at the population level and to determine the thread of epidemiologic links. As mentioned earlier, formerly the assessment of transmission relied solely on the methods of conventional "shoe leather" TB control, which is based on contact investigation. Contact investigation or tracing involves identification of individuals named as close contacts of the index case, which is followed by tuberculin testing (for infection) and, if needed, isoniazid chemoprophylaxis. These methods are useful, especially in low-incident environments or in small or defined situations, and are still an integral part of local TB control government health departments (112). However, conventional approaches are imprecise and often tend to underestimate the level of transmission occurring within the community (25,53). In addition, when there is good case/contact finding and appropriate chemoprophylaxis, a smaller percentage of individuals from the infected pool become symptomatic, and can make case-to-case linkages difficult and seem more sporadic.

The imprecision of contact investigation is further indicated by several recent reports showing that limited or casual contact is adequate for transmission of TB. Population-based molecular epidemiologic studies from San Francisco and Baltimore identified, using extensive contact investigations, only 10% to 25% patient links in molecular-designated clusters (25,53). Moreover, as part of an ongoing population-based study, Yaganehdoost et al. (113) documented complex transmission among a large group of individuals patronizing bars in a specific area in Houston. The Baltimore study by Bishai et al. (53) found that molecularly clustered cases without epidemiologic links shared similar risk profiles, suggesting the importance of casual contact transmission. In support, Valway et al. (104) documented extensive transmission of a clone of *M. tuberculosis* associated with casual contact in a region with a low incidence of TB. These studies have suggested that one of the benefits of conducting population-based molecular epidemiologic studies is the identification of high-risk groups or areas for transmission.

Population-based molecular epidemiologic studies have enabled investigators to uncover outbreaks or epidemic situations not only in defined areas but also in situations when extensive transmission is not suspected. Bifani et al. (49) conducted a population survey of all incident culture-positive TB cases (76% capture) reported in New Jersey between January 1996 to September 1998 and identified 68 members of the W-Beijing family strains that met previously described phylogenetic criteria (74). Using subtle differences in the IS*6110* banding patterns and secondary molecular techniques, the 68 strains were further subdivided into groups A and B (Fig. 4.1, panel A). Unlike group B, group A strains were very closely related based on the molecular data (e.g., IS*6110* motifs), and this was supported by patient demographics such as age, race/ethnicity, HIV serology, birth place, and county of residence.

Although members of group A and B were related phylogenetically, the former represents a clone that has spread and evolved within a defined community and the latter were scattered throughout New Jersey. Group B patients were most probably cases of reactive disease as they were non-U.S.-born and the infecting strains were shown to have diverse IS*6110* patterns within the W-Beijing lineage. Similarly, a study by Mathema et al. (65) identified a recently evolved IS*6110* low-copy-number cluster comprising 56 patients (Fig. 4.4). Here as with the previous study, multiple genotyping methods were employed to confirm clonality of the isolates. Moreover, this study, using clinical, demographic, and contact tracing information, identified 30% case links within the prescribed cluster. There are two significant points from these studies. First, that isolates with similar but not identical fingerprint patterns may be related and part of or an extension of an ongoing outbreak, even in the case of low-copy-number strains. Second, systematic collection of large molecular data sets used in concert with traditional TB surveillance and control activities can make for the identification of previously unrecognized transmission events or outbreaks even in populations with a high background of reported cases (49,65).

Previously, it was assumed that in low-incidence countries, such as the United States, most TB cases were due to endogenous reactivation. Recent population-based studies performed in New York, San Francisco, Denmark, and the Netherlands estimate that on average 35% to 45% of cases were molecularly clustered, suggesting that a good proportion of the incidence is due to recent transmission (25,114–116). The precise contribution of recent transmission to the total number of new cases is quite variable. A number of factors influence transmission dynamics including the size of the infected pool of individuals, population susceptibility (e.g., HIV prevalence), and sampling strategies (117). When population studies take into account the independent parameters and are used with conventional methods, insight into the dynamics of TB transmission can be inferred within specific communities or the general population.

Selected Sample Studies

Perhaps the most common of molecular epidemiologic studies are those involving selected or sometimes convenience sampling. These studies have been carried out in various epidemiologic settings, including congregate areas, health care facilities, and in the community. Three selected studies, described below, illustrate different settings in which these sampling techniques have been used. They include a large multi-institutional outbreak, extensive transmission in a commercial community setting, and widespread dissemination of a drug-susceptible clone among a high-risk group.

W Strain Outbreak

The mid- to late 1980s, coinciding with the emergence of HIV/AIDS and the dismantling of the TB control infrastructure, saw the resurgence of TB in the United States. This was further complicated by the surfacing and spread of drug-resistant organisms and more specifically multidrug-resistant *M. tuberculosis.* Prior to the mid-1980s, outbreaks of multidrug-resistant TB were uncommon in the United States (118).

New York City (NYC), one of the main epicenters of TB, reported more than 3,800 incident cases at the peak of the epidemic (119). During the 43 months spanning 1990 to 1993, 357 cases that were invariably untreatable with isoniazid (INH), rifampin (RIF), ethambutol (EMB), streptomycin (STR), pyrazinamide (PZA), and often kanamycin (KAN) were reported from multiple hospitals and prisons in NYC (112). IS*6110*-based DNA fingerprinting of 253 *M. tuberculosis* isolates cultured from these patients were identical. They each had 18 identical hybridizing bands (Fig. 4.1, panel E1), and this pattern was arbitrarily labeled as strain W (89). These cases were strongly associated with HIV-positive status and poor therapeutic outcomes with mortality rates exceeding 85% (112). Further molecular analysis revealed strain W to harbor a number of unique molecular markers that are summarized in a review article by Bifani et al. (74). Also, DNA sequence analysis of five drug resistance targets among 50 randomly selected W isolates revealed an identical array of mutations strongly suggesting that the spread of this clone was primary in nature (89,120). Since the early 1990s, 11 multidrug-resistant variants have been identified in NYC, with subtle IS*6110* changes and/or with additional (acquired) resistance when compared to the original 18 band strain W (Fig. 4.1, panel E) (74,89). Sequence analysis of the drug resistance target confirmed these variants to be descendants of the outbreak strain. Noteworthy is that fluoroquinolone (120) and capreomycin resistance has been acquired in a subset of W strains and only cycloserine retains activity in some isolates (personal communication, B.N.K., 2002). The distinction of primary spread was crucial in the eventual control of this outbreak and in designing appropriate infrastructure measures for TB prevention and control (121).

CDC1551 Strain Outbreak

Valway et al. (104) in 1995 investigated a large outbreak in a small, rural community with a low incidence of TB. Twenty-one cases were identified of which 15 yielded positive culture results. IS*6110*- and PGRS-based genotyping was performed on 13 of the 15 isolates. IS*6110* analysis identified a four-band hybridization pattern that defines the CDC1551 strain (Fig. 4.4, lane 5), and their identity was confirmed on the basis of an identical PGRS fingerprint (*n* = 13) and spoligotype (Fig. 4.3, unpublished observation,

B.N.K., 2000). Moreover, molecular analysis of 25 isolates from cases residing in surrounding counties was shown to be diverse and different from the four-band CDC1551 strain. Among the 429 close and casual contacts investigated, 72% (311) were skin test positive, including 86 individuals with known skin test conversions. In general, these cases were at minimal risk for TB. The investigators suggested that the extensive transmission occurred due to delayed diagnosis and the extent of disease in the index patient. The fact that the transmission occurred in a clothing manufacturing factory indicates that the environment was a contributory factor in this outbreak.

Given the high skin test conversion, the investigators attempted to assay for particular strain-specific characteristics. The outbreak strain (CDC1551) and virulent laboratory strain Erdman were compared in growth studies in mice. The bacillary load recovered from mice lungs at 10 and 20 days were substantially higher in CDC1551 than the laboratory strain (104). From the animal studies, Valway et al. (104) suggested that extensive transmission was due the outbreak strain's virulence and not only environmental factors. These initial observations led to this strain being selected by the Institute of Genomic Research (www.tigr.org) for complete genomic sequencing. Further analysis by Manca et al. (122), investigating strain-specific host responses, concluded that CDC1551 is not more virulent per se but rather is more immunogenic, that is, eliciting a more rapid and robust host immune response. This result is consistent with the strong PPD reactions observed among the casual exposures. The molecular epidemiology surrounding CDC1551 was important both in distinguishing the outbreak strain and in advancing animal models, immunologic studies, and genomic analysis.

C-Strain Community Spread

During the mutlidrug-resistant strain W outbreak in NYC during the early 1990s, there was also widespread dissemination of a drug-susceptible strain of *M. tuberculosis.* Based on a NYC-wide survey of incident cases, more than 20% were caused by one drug-susceptible isolate. IS*6110*-based fingerprinting resulted in three hybridizing bands; this pattern was arbitrarily labeled strain C (Fig. 4.2, lane 4). To assess the possible epidemiologic and biologic factors associated with this strain, Friedman et al. (123) conducted a case-control investigation of all TB patients consecutively identified in four large NYC hospitals between 1991 and 1994. The four hospitals identified more than 600 cases, 54 with C strain (cases), 69 with non-C clustered (control 1), and 42 with nonclustered pattern (control 2). The clonality of the low-copy-number C strain was confirmed using both 5′ and 3′ IS*6110* DNA fragment probes, PGRS, spoligotype (Fig. 4.3), and double repetitive element PCR (124). The study found that C-strain patients were more likely to have used injecting drugs and less likely to have extrapul-

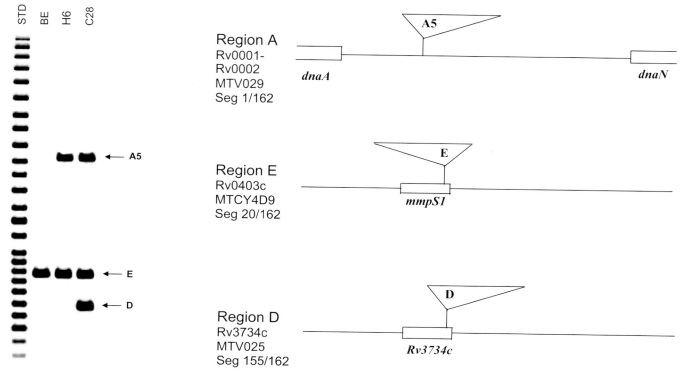

FIGURE 4.4. Southern blot hybridization of *Mycobacterium tuberculosis* strains BE, H6, and C28 (S75 group), a large strain cluster from New Jersey, and results of the insertion sequence (IS*6110*) insertion-site mapping. *Arrows* indicate the hybridization bands corresponding to the IS*6110* insertions in three chromosomal regions. All three strains share the same insertion in E. BE was found to have wild-type sequences in the A and D regions, and H6 had wild-type sequence in region D (compared with H37Rv and CDC1551 genomes). Taken together the authors suggest a stepwise acquisition of IS*6110* from BE to H6 to C28. Triangles schematically demonstrate the position and orientation of IS*6110*. *Seg*, segment; *STD*, molecular weight standards. *Rv* numbers from Cole et al. (144). (From Mathema B, et al. Identification and evolution of an IS*6110* low-copy-number *Mycobacterium tuberculosis* cluster. *J Infect Dis* 2002;185:641–649, with permission.)

monary TB when compared with both control groups. In addition, factors such as being born in the United States, being non-Asian, and living in a shelter for the homeless were positively associated with the C strain cases. Besides injection drug use and extrapulmonary disease, the other factors were also associated with control group 1 or clustered non-C strain cases indicating recent transmission. The initial molecular categories (cases, control 1, and control 2) were crucial in distinguishing strain-specific and recent/reactive transmission. The C strain was also found to be more resistant to reactive nitrogen intermediates (RNIs), which may play a role in the control of tubercle bacillus by human macrophages (125), in comparison with control strains. Although the mechanism and selection of RNI is unclear (126), the investigators speculated that the latter may be due to the fact that repeated injecting drug users have a high level of nitric oxide (NO) and that the prevalence of this clone in such cases results from its capacity to resist NO-mediated clearance (123).

RECURRENT TUBERCULOSIS: SHIFTING DOGMAS

Acquired immunity to TB infection and disease has been heavily debated since the administration of BCG vaccine in the early 1920s (127). The basic premise behind the BCG vaccine, an attenuated form of *M. bovis*, is the induction of the host immune system to recognize specific antigens present in *M. tuberculosis* that protect against uncontrolled replication and dissemination. Although widely used, the efficacy of BCG to prevent individuals from contracting pulmonary TB disease in a number of reports has been inconsistent and in some instances conflicting (11). Although the general belief is that BCG has little to no effect in the control of pulmonary tuberculosis, there is consensus that it does prevent some forms of extrapulmonary TB in children (128). Moreover, the ongoing high incidence of both pulmonary and extrapulmonary forms in regions where BCG has been widely administered supports the near-null effect of the vaccine. The fact that 90% of those infected with *M. tuberculosis* never develop disease supports the thought that the immune response induced by the pathogen is capable of preventing disease in the vast majority of the population. On the basis of several studies, it is accepted that the host's innate T-cell-independent immunity is important in the protection against pulmonary TB (17,129). It remains unclear whether individuals develop disease as a result of their immune response that has been affected by intrinsic host susceptibility or an exogenous event. Furthermore, the extent of immunity against *M. tuberculosis*, from either early exposure or prior disease, is also not well understood despite being a crucial factor in the design of control activities.

Distinguishing episodes of postprimary or recurrent TB into endogenous reactivation or exogenous reinfection has immense implications in the understanding of TB epidemiology and control. A recurrent TB case is defined as a diseased individual with a prior episode of TB that had been cured. Endogenous reactivation is defined as a postprimary episode caused by the initial strain and distinguished from exogenous reinfection, which is caused by a strain different from the primary infection. The longstanding belief was that the majority of recurrent TB is due to endogenous reactivation of the primary *M. tuberculosis* infection. Although debatable, it is thought that successful completion and cure from TB does not always result in bacterial sterilization (130,131). Furthermore, Ziegler et al. (132) using a guinea pig model showed no support for the hypothesis that a second or third exposure to the bacilli leads to an adverse effect on host response to the primary infecting strain. Although there have been limited case reports documenting the occurrence of exogenous reinfection (mainly among immunocompromised individuals), host–pathogen factors influencing this uncommon phenomenon have not been clearly elucidated (133). Distinguishing exogenous from endogenous infection in a given population raises several questions regarding the level of active transmission, dose or infectious burden, environmental factors, and specific host susceptibility. Clinical, epidemiologic, and/or microbiologic data cannot conclusively differentiate recurrent TB caused by reactivation or reinfection. Molecular techniques can, when primary (or historical) and secondary samples are available, help distinguish endogenous from exogenous infection.

A study by van Rie et al. (96) documented the first comprehensive study addressing the contribution of exogenous reinfection among recurrent TB patients in a population-based sample in Cape Town, South Africa. In this study, the investigators sampled and genotyped approximately 700 cases over a 6-year period from an area of high TB incidence (225 cases per 100,000). Forty-eight patients were distinguished on the basis of having antitubercular retreatment following a documented cure. *M. tuberculosis* cultures from both the primary and secondary episodes were captured and genotyped from 16 of the 48 patients. Fifteen of the 16

patients were determined to be HIV seronegative. Comparative analysis of the IS*6110* patterns from the initial versus recurrent isolates revealed that disease in 12 of the 16 (75%) cases was due to an exogenous or a new strain of *M. tuberculosis*. Supporting this finding, Vynnycky and Fine (18) proposed, based on estimates of TB incidence and annual risk of infection, that the fraction of recurrent disease attributable to exogenous reinfection increases proportionally to the regional incidence of disease. Caminero et al. (97) carried out a study in Gran Canaria, Spain, a country of moderate TB burden, that attests to the importance and prevalence of exogenous reinfection. Using genotypic analysis, they found that approximately 44% of recurrent TB was attributable to an exogenous reinfection.

A recent study by Sonnenberg et al. (95) reported on the risk of recurrent disease among HIV-1-infected patients in comparison with HIV-1-negative TB patients in the Gauteng province of South Africa. The study used IS*6110*-based DNA fingerprinting to distinguish endogenous infection (relapse) after cure, from exogenous reinfection. Twenty percent (65 of 326 patients) of the cohort was determined to have recurrent disease (10.3 episodes per 100 person-years). The recurrence rate was almost three times higher among the HIV-1-positive subgroup than the HIV-1 negative group (16.0 versus 6.4 per 100 person-years, respectively). Paired molecular data for 39 of 65 cases were available for comparison. They found 25 relapse and 14 reinfection cases. When patients were stratified by HIV-1 status, the hazard ratio was 18.7 for HIV-1-positive cases in comparison with non-coinfected patients. Being HIV-1 positive in general increased the risk factor for recurrence by 2.4 times. Here the authors concluded that in situations with a high risk of TB infection, HIV-1 significantly increases the rate of recurrence due to high risk of exogenous reinfection.

The use of molecular tools has not only provided direct evidence for the occurrence of exogenous reinfection but also the framework to develop studies aimed at assessing the prevalence and rate at which this phenomenon occurs. More studies are needed to assess recurrent TB in diverse epidemiologic and demographic settings, such as in countries with low incidence, among individuals with different risk factors and comorbidities or different race and/or ethnic groups. There is substantial evidence for racial variation in the susceptibility or level of innate immunity to *M. tuberculosis* infection (134,135); however, more studies on host susceptibility to infection and reinfection are needed that utilize methods and tools of molecular epidemiology.

EVOLUTION AND PATHOGENESIS: MOLECULAR PERSPECTIVE

Genetic determinants and mechanisms of virulence or pathogenesis have been extensively studied in a number of major human pathogenic bacteria. More recently, molecular epidemiologic factors have been used to pose various hypotheses regarding a particular bacterium's pathogenesis. Work done with *Staphylococcus aureus* showed that a clone marked by multilocus enzyme genotyping ET41 commonly harbors the *TSST-1* gene and is responsible for a large proportion of toxic shock syndrome cases (136). Similarly, serotype M18 (M protein) group A *Streptococcus*, a significant human pathogen, was found to be strongly associated with acute rheumatic fever outbreaks (137). With both of these pathogens, defined epidemiologic outcomes were correlated with a specific genetic marker or genotype. Although not commonly practiced among bench scientists, the identification of genetic markers in clinically and epidemiologically relevant strains can aid in elucidating a number of previously unknown virulence properties/factors. This is especially true since the sequencing of clinical *M. tuberculosis* strains CDC1551 (138) and 210 (nearly complete, www.tigr.org), which have become important research strains that are used in both *in vitro* and *in vivo* experimental models.

The pathogenesis studies of *M. tuberculosis* have been extensive; however, only few reports have utilized molecularly well-characterized clinical strains. Given the robust *M. tuberculosis* strain typing data accumulated in the last decade, we are now able to explore the epidemiologic consequences of genetic variability in *M. tuberculosis*. A recent study by Manca et al. (139) sought to evaluate the virulence of various epidemiologically important clinical strains and characterize host–pathogen interaction by establishing a pulmonary infection system in mice. One strain, HN878, was found to be hypervirulent as measured by the exceptionally early death of the infected immunocompetent mice. Furthermore, the investigators suggest that the hypervirulence may be due to the failure of strain HN878 to induce Th1-type immunity. In another study by the same investigators, strain CDC1551 (see "Selected Sample Studies") was thought to be hypervirulent based on growth studies and the high number of contacts infected by the index case (122). However, it was found that infected mice elicit a rapid and vigorous cytokine response when compared to two clinical and two laboratory strains (H37Rv and Erdman). Further studies utilizing genetically well-characterized clinical strains of *M. tuberculosis* may provide insight into strain-specific host susceptibilities, transmissibility, and virulence (as measured by clinical indices) to make for more effective control strategies.

The population structure of *M. tuberculosis* has been difficult to decipher due to the paucity of sequence variation in structural genes, rendering analysis by common population genetics tools, multilocus enzyme electrophoresis (MLEE), or multilocus sequence typing (MLST) poor (27,140,141). However, investigators have used other, nontraditional, methods in suggesting the existence of clonal types (65,72,142). Mathema et al. (65) used multiple molecular markers to confirm relatedness among a group of IS*6110* low-copy number isolates. Sequence analysis of the naked

IS*6110* flanking regions revealed a stepwise acquisition of IS*6110* from one to two to three copies (Fig. 4.4). In two studies by Bifani et al. (49,89), a distinct IS*6110* banding motif, among other molecular markers, was used to suggest clonality (Fig. 4.1, panel A and E). The focus of both studies revolved around strains that are members of a large phylogenetic group known as the W-Beijing family of strains. Kurepina et al. and others have shown that all W-Beijing family members bear specific and distinct IS*6110* insertions (e.g., A1 insertion; Fig. 4.1) (40,143). Furthermore, these strains have been reported to cause extensive disease globally and in some regions account for the majority of all TB cases. In at least one *in vivo* study, the W-Beijing prototype strain (strain 210; Fig. 4.1, panel G) was shown to multiply more rapidly in macrophages than in other clinical and laboratory strains (144). These strains can be distinguished based on a battery of specific molecular markers (74), including 50 structural genes, that are conserved within this well-characterized clonal lineage (29,31). Bifani et al. (in preparation) have further proposed an evolutionary scenario using a group of specific molecular makers to demonstrate unequivocally that this lineage derived from a recent common ancestral cell line. The global success of this lineage is not well understood but may be due to any one or a combination of the following factors: increased transmissibility, more robust replication, stability, and/or distinct gene expression of as-yet-unknown virulence factors.

CONCLUSION

Regardless of whether a natural population is challenged by various anti-TB programs (e.g., vaccination and antitubercular chemotherapy), in general there is observed a low proportion of diseased to infected individuals, which suggests that this is important for the survival of the bacteria. The slow intracellular growth of *M. tuberculosis* and its ability to remain elusive forms the basis for chronicity of infection and disease, which not only complicates the microbiologic diagnosis and necessitates exceptionally long-term chemotherapy, but also hinders accurate description of TB transmission dynamics.

The use of molecular biologic techniques in concert with conventional epidemiologic methods has greatly enhanced the precision and accuracy of describing the epidemiology of TB. Data from both molecular epidemiology and population genetics studies have provided a better understanding of some clinically relevant properties that follow phylogenetic or clonal lines, such as specific virulence factors, tissue tropism, and replication rate (during latency or active disease). Furthermore, strain-specific immunologic studies of successful or prevalent genotypes may yield better understanding of host–pathogen interaction and provide some insight into developing better chemotherapeutic agents or vaccines.

There will soon be three complete *M. tuberculosis* genomes sequenced [H37Rv (145) and CDC1551 (138),

210], and both *M. bovis* and BCG are currently being analyzed. In addition, the advances in gene expression analyses and proteomics will continue to increase our knowledge regarding the genetic basis of diversity and virulence. In turn, these advances will further our understanding of disease causation, spread, and mechanism within the framework of epidemiology and pathogenesis, with the ultimate aim to reduce and control the profound health burden of this human pathogen. Thus, the continual integration of molecular methods with traditional control strategies and development and use of precise markers (e.g., s/nsSNPs and MIRU-VNTR) allows for some optimism in the struggle against this pathogen (146).

ACKNOWLEDGMENTS

We are indebted to W. Eisner, A. Whitelaw, and A. Ravikovitch for their help in editing and with manuscript preparation.

REFERENCES

1. Bloom BR, Murray CJ. Tuberculosis: commentary on a reemergent killer. *Science* 1992;257:1055–1064.
2. Raviglione MC, Snider DE Jr, Kochi A. Global epidemiology of tuberculosis. Morbidity and mortality of a worldwide epidemic. *JAMA* 1995;273:220–226.
3. Murray CJ, Salomon JA. Modeling the impact of global tuberculosis control strategies. *Proc Natl Acad Sci U S A* 1998;95:13881–13886.
4. Murray CJ, Styblo K, Rouillon A. Tuberculosis in developing countries: burden, intervention and cost. *Bull Int Union Tuberc Lung Dis* 1990;65:6–24.
5. Comstock GW. Frost revisited: the modern epidemiology of tuberculosis. *Am J Epidemiol* 1975;101:363–382.
6. Comstock GW, Edwards PQ. An American view of BCG vaccination, illustrated by results of a controlled trial in Puerto Rico. *Scand J Respir Dis* 1972;53:207–217.
7. Comstock GW, Woolpert SF, Livesay VT. Tuberculosis studies in Muscogee County, Georgia. Twenty-year evaluation of a community trial of BCG vaccination. *Public Health Rep* 1976;91:276–280.
8. Ferebee S. Controlled chemoprophylaxis trials in tuberculosis: a general review. *Adv Tuberc Res* 1969;17:29–106.
9. Stead WW. Pathogenesis of the sporadic case of tuberculosis. *N Engl J Med* 1967;277:1008–1012.
10. Stead WW, Slagel WA, Noble J. INH prophylaxis. *N Engl J Med* 1972;286:159–160.
11. Colditz GA, Brewer TF, Berkey CS, et al. Efficacy of BCG vaccine in the prevention of tuberculosis. Meta-analysis of the published literature. *JAMA* 1994;271:698–702.
12. Puffer RR, Steward HC, Gass RS. Tuberculosis in household contacts associates: the influence of age and relationship. *Am Rev Tuberc* 1945;52:89–103.
13. Grzybowski S, Barnett GD, Stylbo K. Contacts of cases of active pulmonary tuberculosis. *Bull Int Union Tuberc* 1975;50:90–106.
14. Jagirdar J, Zagzag D. Pathology and insights into pathogenesis of tuberculosis. In: Rom WN, Garay S, eds. *Tuberculosis*. New York: Little, Brown and Company; 1996:467–482.
15. Klotz SA, Penn RL. Acid-fast staining of urine and gastric contents is an excellent indicator of mycobacterial disease. *Am Rev Respir Dis* 1987;136:1197–1198.
16. Sepkowitz KA, Raffalli J, Riley L, et al. Tuberculosis in the AIDS era. *Clin Microbiol Rev* 1995;8:180–199.
17. Kaufmann SH. How can immunology contribute to the control of tuberculosis? *Nature Rev Immunol* 2001;1:20–30.
18. Vynnycky E, Fine PE. The natural history of tuberculosis: the implications of age-dependent risks of disease and the role of reinfection. *Epidemiol Infect* 1997;119:183–201.
19. Herold CD, Fitzgerald RL, Herold DA. Current techniques in mycobacterial detection and speciation. *Crit Rev Clin Lab Sci* 1996;33:83–138.
20. Bauer J, Thomsen VO, Poulsen S, et al. False-positive results from cultures of *Mycobacterium tuberculosis* due to laboratory cross-contamination confirmed by restriction fragment length polymorphism. *J Clin Microbiol* 1997;35:988–991.
21. Braden CR, Templeton GL, Stead WW, et al. Retrospective detection of laboratory cross-contamination of *Mycobacterium tuberculosis* cultures with use of DNA fingerprint analysis. *Clin Infect Dis* 1997;24:35–40.
22. Edlin BR, Tokars JI, Grieco MH, et al. An outbreak of multidrug-resistant tuberculosis among hospitalized patients with the acquired immunodeficiency syndrome. *N Engl J Med* 1992;326:1514–1521.
23. Haas DW, Milton S, Kreiswirth BN, et al. Nosocomial transmission of a drug-sensitive W-variant *Mycobacterium tuberculosis* strain among patients with acquired immunodeficiency syndrome in Tennessee. *Infect Control Hosp Epidemiol* 1998;19:635–639.
24. HIV-related tuberculosis in a transgender network—Baltimore, Maryland, and New York City area, 1998–2000. *MMWR Morb Mortal Wkly Rep* 2000;49:317–220.
25. Small PM, Hopewell PC, Singh SP, et al. The epidemiology of tuberculosis in San Francisco. A population-based study using conventional and molecular methods. *N Engl J Med* 1994;330:1703–1709.
26. van Embden JD, Cave MD, Crawford JT, et al. Strain identification of *Mycobacterium tuberculosis* by DNA fingerprinting: recommendations for a standardized methodology. *J Clin Microbiol* 1993;31:406–409.
27. Kremer K, van Soolingen D, Frothingham R, et al. Comparison of methods based on different molecular epidemiological markers for typing of *Mycobacterium tuberculosis* complex strains: interlaboratory study of discriminatory power and reproducibility. *J Clin Microbiol* 1999;37:2607–2618.
28. Frothingham R, Wilson KH. Molecular phylogeny of the *Mycobacterium avium* complex demonstrates clinically meaningful divisions. *J Infect Dis* 1994;169:305–312.
29. Sreevatsan S, Pan X, Stockbauer KE, et al. Restricted structural gene polymorphism in the *Mycobacterium tuberculosis* complex indicates evolutionarily recent global dissemination. *Proc Natl Acad Sci U S A* 1997;94:9869–9874.
30. Kapur V, Whittam TS, Musser JM. Is *Mycobacterium tuberculosis* 15,000 years old? *J Infect Dis* 1994;170:1348–1349.
31. Musser JM, Amin A, Ramaswamy S. Negligible genetic diversity of *Mycobacterium tuberculosis* host immune system protein targets: evidence of limited selective pressure. *Genetics* 2000;155:7–16.
32. Collins DM, De Lisle GW. DNA restriction endonuclease analysis of *Mycobacterium tuberculosis* and *Mycobacterium bovis* BCG. *J Gen Microbiol* 1984;130 (Pt 4):1019–1021.
33. Eisenach KD, Crawford JT, Bates JH. Genetic relatedness among strains of the *Mycobacterium tuberculosis* complex. Analysis of restriction fragment heterogeneity using cloned DNA probes. *Am Rev Respir Dis* 1986;133:1065–1068.

34. Zainuddin ZF, Dale JW. Polymorphic repetitive DNA sequences in *Mycobacterium tuberculosis* detected with a gene probe from a Mycobacterium fortuitum plasmid. *J Gen Microbiol* 1989;135 (Pt 9):2347–2355.

35. Hermans PW, van Soolingen D, Dale JW, et al. Insertion element IS986 from *Mycobacterium tuberculosis*: a useful tool for diagnosis and epidemiology of tuberculosis. *J Clin Microbiol* 1990;28:2051–2058.

36. Galas D, Chandler M. Bacterial insertion sequences. In: Berg B, Howe M, eds. *Mobile DNA* Washington, DC: American Society of Microbiology; 1989:109–162.

37. McAdam RA, Hermans PW, van Soolingen D, et al. Characterization of a *Mycobacterium tuberculosis* insertion sequence belonging to the IS3 family. *Mol Microbiol* 1990;4:1607–1613.

38. Thierry D, Cave MD, Eisenach KD, et al. IS*6110*, an IS-like element of *Mycobacterium tuberculosis* complex. *Nucleic Acids Res* 1990;18:188.

39. McHugh TD, Gillespie SH. Nonrandom association of IS*6110* and *Mycobacterium tuberculosis*: implications for molecular epidemiological studies. *J Clin Microbiol* 1998;36:1410–1413.

40. Kurepina NE, Sreevatsan S, Plikaytis BB, et al. Characterization of the phylogenetic distribution and chromosomal insertion sites of five IS*6110* elements in *Mycobacterium tuberculosis*: nonrandom integration in the dnaA-dnaN region. *Tuber Lung Dis* 1998;79:31–42.

41. Van Embden JD, Van Soolingen D, Heersma HF, et al. Establishment of a European network for the surveillance of *Mycobacterium tuberculosis*, MRSA and penicillin-resistant pneumococci. *J Antimicrob Chemother* 1996;38:905–907.

42. Heersma HF, Kremer K, van Embden JD. Computer analysis of IS*6110* RFLP patterns of *Mycobacterium tuberculosis*. *Meth Mol Biol* 1998;101:395–422.

43. Suffys PN, Ivens de Araujo ME, Rossetti ML, et al. Usefulness of IS*6110*–restriction fragment length polymorphism typing of Brazilian strains of *Mycobacterium tuberculosis* and comparison with an international fingerprint database. *Res Microbiol* 2000; 151:343–351.

44. van Soolingen D, Hermans PW, de Haas PE, et al. Occurrence and stability of insertion sequences in *Mycobacterium tuberculosis* complex strains: evaluation of an insertion sequence–dependent DNA polymorphism as a tool in the epidemiology of tuberculosis. *J Clin Microbiol* 1991;29:2578–2586.

45. Cave MD, Eisenach KD, Templeton G, et al. Stability of DNA fingerprint pattern produced with IS*6110* in strains of *Mycobacterium tuberculosis*. *J Clin Microbiol* 1994;32:262–266.

46. de Boer AS, Borgdorff MW, de Haas PE, et al. Analysis of rate of change of IS*6110* RFLP patterns of *Mycobacterium tuberculosis*-based on serial patient isolates. *J Infect Dis* 1999;180:1238–1244.

47. Yeh RW, Ponce de Leon A, Agasino CB, et al. Stability of *Mycobacterium tuberculosis* DNA genotypes. *J Infect Dis* 1998;177: 1107–1111.

48. Lillebaek T, Dirksen A, Baess I, et al. Molecular evidence of endogenous reactivation of *Mycobacterium tuberculosis* after 33 years of latent infection. *J Infect Dis* 2002;185:401–404.

49. Bifani PJ, Mathema B, Liu Z, et al. Identification of a W variant outbreak of *Mycobacterium tuberculosis* via population-based molecular epidemiology. *JAMA* 1999;282:2321–2327.

50. Braden CR, Templeton GL, Cave MD, et al. Interpretation of restriction fragment length polymorphism analysis of *Mycobacterium tuberculosis* isolates from a state with a large rural population. *J Infect Dis* 1997;175:1446–1452.

51. Bifani PJ, Shopsin B, Alcabes P, et al. Molecular epidemiology and tuberculosis control. *JAMA* 2000;284:305–307.

52. Barnes PF, Yang Z, Preston-Martin S, et al. Patterns of tuberculosis transmission in Central Los Angeles. *JAMA* 1997;278: 1159–1163.

53. Bishai WR, Graham NM, Harrington S, et al. Molecular and geographic patterns of tuberculosis transmission after 15 years of directly observed therapy. *JAMA* 1998;280:1679–1684.

54. Yang Z, Chaves F, Barnes PF, et al. Evaluation of method for secondary DNA typing of *Mycobacterium tuberculosis* with pTBN12 in epidemiologic study of tuberculosis. *J Clin Microbiol* 1996;34:3044–3048.

55. Goyal M, Saunders NA, van Embden JD, et al. Differentiation of *Mycobacterium tuberculosis* isolates by spoligotyping and IS*6110* restriction fragment length polymorphism. *J Clin Microbiol* 1997;35:647–651.

56. Bauer J, Andersen AB, Kremer K, et al. Usefulness of spoligotyping to discriminate IS*6110* low-copy-number *Mycobacterium tuberculosis* complex strains cultured in Denmark. *J Clin Microbiol* 1999;37:2602–2606.

57. Rhee JT, Tanaka MM, Behr MA, et al. Use of multiple markers in population-based molecular epidemiologic studies of tuberculosis. *Int J Tuberc Lung Dis* 2000;4:1111–1119.

58. Chaves F, Yang Z, el Hajj H, et al. Usefulness of the secondary probe pTBN12 in DNA fingerprinting of *Mycobacterium tuberculosis*. *J Clin Microbiol* 1996;34:1118–1123.

59. Das S, Paramasivan CN, Lowrie DB, et al. IS*6110* restriction fragment length polymorphism typing of clinical isolates of *Mycobacterium tuberculosis* from patients with pulmonary tuberculosis in Madras, south India. *Tuber Lung Dis* 1995;76:550–554.

60. Sahadevan R, Narayanan S, Paramasivan CN, et al. Restriction fragment length polymorphism typing of clinical isolates of *Mycobacterium tuberculosis* from patients with pulmonary tuberculosis in Madras, India, by use of direct-repeat probe. *J Clin Microbiol* 1995;33:3037–3039.

61. Dale JW, Brittain D, Cataldi AA, et al. Spacer oligonucleotide typing of bacteria of the *Mycobacterium tuberculosis* complex: recommendations for standardised nomenclature. *Int J Tuberc Lung Dis* 2001;5:216–219.

62. Soini H, Pan X, Teeter L, et al. Transmission dynamics and molecular characterization of *Mycobacterium tuberculosis* isolates with low copy numbers of IS*6110*. *J Clin Microbiol* 2001;39:217–221.

63. Burman WJ, Reves RR, Hawkes AP, et al. DNA fingerprinting with two probes decreases clustering of *Mycobacterium tuberculosis*. *Am J Respir Crit Care Med* 1997;155:1140–1146.

64. Sola C, Devallois A, Horgen L, et al. Tuberculosis in the Caribbean: using spacer oligonucleotide typing to understand strain origin and transmission. *Emerg Infect Dis* 1999;5: 404–414.

65. Mathema B, Bifani PJ, Driscoll J, et al. Identification and evolution of an IS*6110* low-copy-number *Mycobacterium tuberculosis* cluster. *J Infect Dis* 2002;185:641–649.

66. Groenen PM, Bunschoten AE, van Soolingen D, et al. Nature of DNA polymorphism in the direct repeat cluster of *Mycobacterium tuberculosis*; application for strain differentiation by a novel typing method. *Mol Microbiol* 1993;10:1057–1065.

67. Kamerbeek J, Schouls L, Kolk A, et al. Simultaneous detection and strain differentiation of *Mycobacterium tuberculosis* for diagnosis and epidemiology. *J Clin Microbiol* 1997;35:907–914.

68. Qian L, Van Embden JDA, Van Der Zanden AGM, et al. Retrospective analysis of the Beijing family of *Mycobacterium tuberculosis* in preserved lung tissues. *J Clin Microbiol* 1999;37: 471–474.

69. van der Zanden AG, Hoentjen AH, Heilmann FG, et al. Simultaneous detection and strain differentiation of *Mycobacterium tuberculosis* complex in paraffin wax embedded tissues and in stained microscopic preparations. *Mol Pathol* 1998;51:209–214.

70. Driscoll JR, McGarry MA, Taber HW. DNA typing of a nonviable culture of *Mycobacterium tuberculosis* in a homeless shelter outbreak. *J Clin Microbiol* 1999;37:274–275.

71. Heyderman RS, Goyal M, Roberts P, et al. Pulmonary tubercu-

losis in Harare, Zimbabwe: analysis by spoligotyping. *Thorax* 1998;53:346–350.

72. Bifani P, Mathema B, Campo M, et al. Molecular identification of streptomycin monoresistant *Mycobacterium tuberculosis* related to multidrug-resistant W strain. *Emerg Infect Dis* 2001;7:842–848.

73. van Soolingen D, Qian L, de Haas PE, et al. Predominance of a single genotype of *Mycobacterium tuberculosis* in countries of east Asia. *J Clin Microbiol* 1995;33:3234–3238.

74. Bifani PJ, Mathema B, Kurepina NE, et al. Global dissemination of the *Mycobacterium tuberculosis* W-Beijing family strains. *Trends Microbiol* 2002;10:45–52.

75. Ross BC, Raios K, Jackson K, et al. Molecular cloning of a highly repeated DNA element from *Mycobacterium tuberculosis* and its use as an epidemiological tool. *J Clin Microbiol* 1992;30:942–946.

76. Frothingham R, Meeker-O'Connell WA. Genetic diversity in the *Mycobacterium tuberculosis* complex based on variable numbers of tandem DNA repeats. *Microbiology* 1998;144(Pt 5): 1189–1196.

77. Supply P, Mazars E, Lesjean S, et al. Variable human minisatellite-like regions in the *Mycobacterium tuberculosis* genome. *Mol Microbiol* 2000;36:762–771.

78. Schork NJ, Fallin D, Lanchbury JS. Single nucleotide polymorphisms and the future of genetic epidemiology. *Clin Genet* 2000;58:250–264.

79. Gut IG. Automation in genotyping of single nucleotide polymorphisms. *Hum Mutat* 2001;17:475–492.

80. Levin BR, Lipsitch M, Bonhoeffer S. Population biology, evolution, and infectious disease: convergence and synthesis. *Science* 1999;283:806–809.

81. Brosch R, Gordon SV, Marmiesse M, et al. A new evolutionary scenario for the *Mycobacterium tuberculosis* complex. *Proc Natl Acad Sci U S A* 2002;99:3684–3689.

82. Behr MA, Wilson MA, Gill WP, et al. Comparative genomics of BCG vaccines by whole-genome DNA microarray. *Science* 1999;284:1520–1523.

83. Kivi M, Liu X, Raychaudhuri S, et al. Determining the genomic locations of repetitive DNA sequences with a whole-genome microarray: IS*6110* in *Mycobacterium tuberculosis. J Clin Microbiol* 2002;40:2192–2198.

84. Gutacker MM, Smoot JC, Migliaccio CA, et al. Genome-wide analysis of synonymous single nucleotide polymorphisms in *Mycobacterium tuberculosis* complex organisms: resolution of genetic relationships among closely related microbial strains. *Genetics* 2002;162:1533–1543.

85. Ramaswamy S, Musser JM. Molecular genetic basis of antimicrobial agent resistance in *Mycobacterium tuberculosis*: 1998 update. *Tuber Lung Dis* 1998;79:3–29.

86. Espinal MA, Kim SJ, Suarez PG, et al. Standard short-course chemotherapy for drug-resistant tuberculosis: treatment outcomes in 6 countries. *JAMA* 2000;283:2537–2545.

87. Peloquin CA, MacPhee AA, Berning SE. Malabsorption of antimycobacterial medications. *N Engl J Med* 1993;329: 1122–1123.

88. Iseman MD, Madsen LA. Drug-resistant tuberculosis. *Clin Chest Med* 1989;10:341–353.

89. Bifani PJ, Plikaytis BB, Kapur V, et al. Origin and interstate spread of a New York City multidrug-resistant *Mycobacterium tuberculosis* clone family. *JAMA*1 996;275:452–457.

90. Edlin BR, Tokars JI, Grieco MH, et al. An outbreak of multidrug-resistant tuberculosis among hospitalized patients with the acquired immunodeficiency syndrome. *N Engl J Med* 1992; 326:1514–1521.

91. Nivin B, Fujiwara PI, Hannifin J, et al. Cross-contamination with *Mycobacterium tuberculosis*: an epidemiological and laboratory investigation. *Infect Control Hosp Epidemiol* 1998;19:500–503.

92. Sola C, Filliol I, Legrand E, et al. *Mycobacterium tuberculosis*-phylogeny reconstruction based on combined numerical analysis with IS1081, IS*6110*, VNTR, and DR-based spoligotyping suggests the existence of two new phylogeographical clades. *J Mol Evol* 2001;53:680–689.

93. Borgdorff MW, Nagelkerke N, van Soolingen D, et al. Analysis of tuberculosis transmission between nationalities in the Netherlands in the period 1993–1995 using DNA fingerprinting. *Am J Epidemiol* 1998;147:187–195.

94. Barnes PF, el-Hajj H, Preston-Martin S, et al. Transmission of tuberculosis among the urban homeless. *JAMA* 1996;275: 305–307.

95. Sonnenberg P, Murray J, Glynn JR, et al. HIV-1 and recurrence, relapse, and reinfection of tuberculosis after cure: a cohort study in South African mineworkers. *Lancet* 2001;358:1687–1693.

96. van Rie A, Warren R, Richardson M, et al. Exogenous reinfection as a cause of recurrent tuberculosis after curative treatment. *N Engl J Med* 1999;341:1174–1179.

97. Caminero JA, Pena MJ, Campos-Herrero MI, et al. Exogenous reinfection with tuberculosis on a European island with a moderate incidence of disease. *Am J Respir Crit Care Med* 2001;163 (Pt 1):717–720.

98. Garcia-Garcia ML, Jimenez-Corona ME, Ponce-de-Leon A, et al. *Mycobacterium tuberculosis* drug resistance in a suburban community in southern Mexico. *Int J Tuberc Lung Dis* 2000;4 (Suppl 2):S168–170.

99. Escalante P, Ramaswamy S, Sanabria H, et al. Genotypic characterization of drug-resistant *Mycobacterium tuberculosis* isolates from Peru. *Tuber Lung Dis* 1998;79:111–118.

100. Lutfey M, Della-Latta P, Kapur V, et al. Independent origin of mono-rifampin-resistant *Mycobacterium tuberculosis* in patients with AIDS. *Am J Respir Crit Care Med* 1996;153:837–840.

101. Marttila HJ, Soini H, Eerola E, et al. A Ser315Thr substitution in KatG is predominant in genetically heterogeneous multidrug-resistant *Mycobacterium tuberculosis* isolates originating from the St. Petersburg area in Russia. *Antimicrob Agents Chemother* 1998;42:2443–2445.

102. van Rie A, Warren RM, Beyers N, et al. Transmission of a multidrug-resistant *Mycobacterium tuberculosis* strain resembling "Strain W" among noninstitutionalized, human immunodeficiency virus–seronegative patients. *J Infect Dis* 1999;180: 1608–1615.

103. Rhee JT, Piatek AS, Small PM, et al. Molecular epidemiologic evaluation of transmissibility and virulence of *Mycobacterium tuberculosis. J Clin Microbiol* 1999;37:1764–1770.

104. Valway SE, Sanchez MP, Shinnick TF, et al. An outbreak involving extensive transmission of a virulent strain of *Mycobacterium tuberculosis. N Engl J Med* 1998;338:633–639.

105. Wurtz R, Demarais P, Trainor W, et al. Specimen contamination in mycobacteriology laboratory detected by pseudo-outbreak of multidrug-resistant tuberculosis: analysis by routine epidemiology and confirmation by molecular technique. *J Clin Microbiol* 1996;34:1017–1019.

106. Bhattacharya M, Dietrich S, Mosher L, et al. Cross-contamination of specimens with *Mycobacterium tuberculosis*: clinical significance, causes, and prevention. *Am J Clin Pathol* 1998;109: 324–330.

107. Bifani P, Moghazeh S, Shopsin B, et al. Molecular characterization of *Mycobacterium tuberculosis* H37Rv/Ra variants: distinguishing the mycobacterial laboratory strain. *J Clin Microbiol* 2000;38:3200–3204.

108. Misdiagnoses of tuberculosis resulting from laboratory cross-contamination of *Mycobacterium tuberculosis* cultures—New Jersey, 1998. *MMWR Morb Mortal Wkly Rep* 2000;49:413–416.

109. Small PM, McClenny NB, Singh SP, et al. Molecular strain typing of *Mycobacterium tuberculosis* to confirm cross-contamina-

tion in the mycobacteriology laboratory and modification of procedures to minimize occurrence of false-positive cultures. *J Clin Microbiol* 1993;31:1677–1682.

110. Nivin B, Driscoll J, Glaser T, et al. Use of spoligotype analysis to detect laboratory cross-contamination. *Infect Control Hosp Epidemiol* 2000;21:525–527.

111. Agerton T, Valway S, Gore B, et al. Transmission of a highly drug-resistant strain (strain W1) of *Mycobacterium tuberculosis.* Community outbreak and nosocomial transmission via a contaminated bronchoscope. *JAMA* 1997;278:1073–1077.

112. Frieden TR, Sherman LF, Maw KL, et al. A multi-institutional outbreak of highly drug-resistant tuberculosis: epidemiology and clinical outcomes. *JAMA* 1996;276:1229–1235.

113. Yaganehdoost A, Graviss EA, Ross MW, et al. Complex transmission dynamics of clonally related virulent *Mycobacterium tuberculosis* associated with barhopping by predominantly human immunodeficiency virus-positive gay men. *J Infect Dis* 1999;180:1245–1251.

114. van Soolingen D, Borgdorff MW, de Haas PE, et al. Molecular epidemiology of tuberculosis in the Netherlands: a nationwide study from 1993 through 1997. *J Infect Dis* 1999;180:726–736.

115. Bauer J, Yang Z, Poulsen S, et al. Results from 5 years of nationwide DNA fingerprinting of *Mycobacterium tuberculosis* complex isolates in a country with a low incidence of *M. tuberculosis* infection. *J Clin Microbiol* 1998;36:305–308.

116. Alland D, Kalkut GE, Moss AR, et al. Transmission of tuberculosis in New York City. An analysis by DNA fingerprinting and conventional epidemiologic methods. *N Engl J Med* 1994;330:1710–1716.

117. Murray M. Determinants of cluster distribution in the molecular epidemiology of tuberculosis. *Proc Natl Acad Sci U S A* 2002;99:1538–1543.

118. Cantwell MF, Snider DE Jr, Cauthen GM, et al. Epidemiology of tuberculosis in the United States, 1985 through 1992. *JAMA* 1994;272:535–539.

119. Frieden TR, Sterling T, Pablos-Mendez A, et al. The emergence of drug-resistant tuberculosis in New York City. *N Engl J Med* 1993;328:521–526.

120. Sullivan EA, Kreiswirth BN, Palumbo L, et al. Emergence of fluoroquinolone-resistant tuberculosis in New York City. *Lancet* 1995;345:1148–1150.

121. Frieden TR, Fujiwara PI, Washko RM, et al. Tuberculosis in New York City—turning the tide. *N Engl J Med* 1995;333:229–233.

122. Manca C, Tsenova L, Barry CE III, et al. *Mycobacterium tuberculosis* CDC1551 induces a more vigorous host response *in vivo* and *in vitro*, but is not more virulent than other clinical isolates. *J Immunol* 1999;162:6740–6746.

123. Friedman CR, Quinn GC, Kreiswirth BN, et al. Widespread dissemination of a drug-susceptible strain of *Mycobacterium tuberculosis.* *J Infect Dis* 1997;176:478–484.

124. Friedman CR, Stoeckle MY, Johnson WD Jr, et al. Double-repetitive-element PCR method for subtyping *Mycobacterium tuberculosis* clinical isolates. *J Clin Microbiol* 1995;33:1383–1384.

125. Nicholson S, Bonecini-Almeida Mda G, Lapa e Silva JR, et al. Inducible nitric oxide synthase in pulmonary alveolar macrophages from patients with tuberculosis. *J Exp Med* 1996;183:2293–2302.

126. Schneemann M, Schoedon G, Linscheid P, et al. Nitrite generation in interleukin-4-treated human macrophage cultures does not involve the nitric oxide synthase pathway. *J Infect Dis* 1997;175:130–135.

127. Behr MA. BCG—different strains, different vaccines? *Lancet* 2002;2:86–92.

128. Colditz GA, Berkey CS, Mosteller F, et al. The efficacy of bacillus Calmette–Guerin vaccination of newborns and infants in the prevention of tuberculosis: meta-analyses of the published literature. *Pediatrics* 1995;96(Pt 1):29–35.

129. van Crevel R, Ottenhoff TH, van der Meer JW. Innate immunity to *Mycobacterium tuberculosis*. *Clin Microbiol Rev* 2002;15:294–309.

130. Stead WW. Pathogenesis of a first episode of chronic pulmonary tuberculosis in man: recrudescence of residuals of the primary infection or exogenous reinfection? *Am Rev Respir Dis* 1967;95:729–745.

131. Manabe YC, Bishai WR. Latent *Mycobacterium tuberculosis*—persistence, patience, and winning by waiting. *Nat Med* 2000;6:1327–1329.

132. Ziegler JE, Edwards ML, Smith DW. Exogenous reinfection in experimental airborne tuberculosis. *Tubercle* 1985;66:121–128.

133. Kaufmann SH. Understanding immunity to tuberculosis: guidelines for rational vaccine development. *Kekkaku* 2001;76:641–645.

134. Stead WW, Senner JW, Reddick WT, et al. Racial differences in susceptibility to infection by *Mycobacterium tuberculosis*. *N Engl J Med* 1990;322:422–427.

135. Crowle AJ, Elkins N. Relative permissiveness of macrophages from black and white people for virulent tubercle bacilli. *Infect Immun* 1990;58:632–638.

136. Musser JM, Schlievert PM, Chow AW, et al. A single clone of *Staphylococcus aureus* causes the majority of cases of toxic shock syndrome. *Proc Natl Acad Sci U S A* 1990;87:225–229.

137. Smoot JC, Barbian KD, Van Gompel JJ, et al. Genome sequence and comparative microarray analysis of serotype M18 group A *Streptococcus* strains associated with acute rheumatic fever outbreaks. *Proc Natl Acad Sci U S A* 2002;99:4668–4673.

138. Fleischmann RD, Alland D, Eisen JA, et al. Whole-genome comparison of *Mycobacterium tuberculosis* clinical and laboratory strains. *J Bacteriol* 2002;184:5479–5490.

139. Manca C, Tsenova L, Bergtold A, et al. Virulence of a *Mycobacterium tuberculosis* clinical isolate in mice is determined by failure to induce Th1 type immunity and is associated with induction of IFN-alpha/beta. *Proc Natl Acad Sci U S A* 2001;98:5752–5757.

140. Maiden MC, Bygraves JA, Feil E, et al. Multilocus sequence typing: a portable approach to the identification of clones within populations of pathogenic microorganisms. *Proc Natl Acad Sci U S A* 1998;95:3140–3145.

141. Feizabadi MM, Robertson ID, Cousins DV, et al. Genomic analysis of *Mycobacterium bovis* and other members of the *Mycobacterium tuberculosis* complex by isoenzyme analysis and pulsed-field gel electrophoresis. *J Clin Microbiol* 1996;34:1136–1142.

142. Le TK, Bach KH, Ho ML, et al. Molecular fingerprinting of *Mycobacterium tuberculosis* strains isolated in Vietnam using IS*6110* as probe. *Tuber Lung Dis* 2000;80:75–83.

143. Beggs ML, Eisenach KD, Cave MD. Mapping of IS*6110* insertion sites in two epidemic strains of *Mycobacterium tuberculosis*. *J Clin Microbiol* 2000;38:2923–2928.

144. Zhang M, Gong J, Yang Z, et al. Enhanced capacity of a widespread strain of *Mycobacterium tuberculosis* to grow in human macrophages. *J Infect Dis* 1999;179:1213–1217.

145. Cole ST, Brosch R, Parkhill J, et al. Deciphering the biology of *Mycobacterium tuberculosis* from the complete genome sequence. *Nature* 1998;393:537–544.

146. Kurepina N. The sequence analysis of the pncA gene determining the PZA-resistance in the predominant *M. tuberculosis*-strains isolated in the Tomsk penitentiary system, Western Siberia, Russia. *Int J Tuberc Lung Dis* 2001;5:S41.

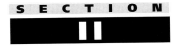

SECTION

II

GENOMICS AND MICROBIOLOGY

5

COMPARATIVE GENOMICS OF THE *MYCOBACTERIUM TUBERCULOSIS* COMPLEX: EVOLUTIONARY INSIGHT AND APPLICATIONS

ROLAND BROSCH
SAYERA BANU
STEWART T. COLE

Genomics, the systematic analysis of the complete genetic material found in an organism by means of DNA sequencing and bioinformatics, is undoubtedly the most powerful tool now available to biological researchers. A massive return can be obtained for a single investment because genomics not only provides the DNA sequence of an organism but also generates complete data sets of its genes, proteins, enzymes, and antigens. Based on this information, the metabolic pathways, physiology, and evolution can be reconstructed *in silico* and rich biological, evolutionary, and medical insight obtained. At the time of writing, four complete genome sequences were available for pathogenic mycobacteria (two strains of *Mycobacterium tuberculosis*, one strain each of *Mycobacterium bovis* and *Mycobacterium leprae*), and several others are at different stages of completion. (For an overview, see http://www.pasteur.fr/unites/recherche/Lgmb/mycogenomics.html/). In this chapter we will briefly describe the various approaches that have been employed, present some selected findings, and show how this information can be used to improve diagnostic procedures.

THE *MYCOBACTERIUM TUBERCULOSIS* COMPLEX

The most predominant human pathogen is *M. tuberculosis*, the etiologic agent of human tuberculosis, that accounts worldwide for 8 million new infections and 2 million deaths per year (1). Together with other highly related bacteria, *M. tuberculosis* forms a tightly knit complex, a single species as defined by DNA/DNA hybridization studies (2), and characterized by a singular lack of genetic diversity (3). The complex includes *M. tuberculosis,* the causative agent in the vast majority of human tuberculosis cases; *Mycobacterium canettii,* a smooth variant that is very rarely encountered; *Mycobacterium africanum,* an agent of human tuberculosis in sub-Saharan Africa; *M. microti,* the agent of tuberculosis in voles; *Mycobacterium bovis,* which infects a wide variety of mammalian species including humans; and bacille Calmette–Guérin (BCG), an attenuated derivative of *M. bovis* that is used as a live vaccine against human tuberculosis.

The Genome Sequence and Biology of *Mycobacterium tuberculosis* H37Rv

For the genome project of the widely used reference strain *M. tuberculosis* H37Rv, a combined strategy consisting of sequencing selected cosmid and bacterial artificial chromosome (BAC) clones, as well as whole-genome shotgun sequencing, was employed. The minimally overlapping set of BAC clones containing large inserts of *M. tuberculosis* H37Rv DNA (4) was of critical importance for the timely completion of the *M. tuberculosis* H37Rv genome sequence, as it allowed the extremely GC-rich areas of the genome, corresponding to the PE-PGRS genes (discussed below), to be obtained as these were underrepresented in the small insert shotgun libraries. The complete genome sequence of *M. tuberculosis* H37Rv comprises 4,411,532 bp and has an average GC content of 65.6%. As the findings of the analysis have been described extensively elsewhere (5–8), only a brief description of selected features

R. Brosch and S. T. Cole: Unité de Génétique Moléculaire Bactérienne, Institut Pasteur, Paris, France.
S. Banu: International Centre for Diarrhoeal Disease Research, Dhaka, Bangladesh.

of the sequence will be presented here. The genome contains approximately 4,000 genes distributed fairly evenly between the two strands. More than 51% of the genes have arisen as a result of gene duplication or domain shuffling events, and 3.4% of the genome is composed of insertion sequences (ISs) and phages (phiRv1, phiRv2). There are 56 copies of IS elements belonging to the well-known IS3, IS5, IS21, IS30, IS110, IS256, and ISL3 families, as well as a new IS family, IS1535, that appears to employ a frameshifting mechanism to produce its transposase (9). IS6110, a member of the IS3 family, is the most abundant element and has played an important role in shaping the genome.

The information deduced from the genome sequence provided new and valuable insight into the biology of the tubercle bacilli, and highlighted the importance of lipid metabolism to its lifestyle as at least 8% of the genome is dedicated to this activity. While *M. tuberculosis* was known to contain a remarkable array of lipids, glycolipids, lipoglycans, and polyketides (10) and the genome sequence revealed many of the genes required for their production, it was surprising to note the presence of numerous genes and proteins that could confer lipolytic functions. Estimates of the concentrations of potential substrates available to a pathogen in host tissues suggest that lipids and sterols are more abundant than carbohydrates. While *M. tuberculosis* has the prototype β-oxidation cycle required for lipid catabolism, catalyzed by the multifunctional FadA/FadB proteins, it also appears to have approximately 100 enzymes potentially involved in alternative lipid oxidation pathways in which exogenous lipids from host cells could be degraded.

One of the major findings of the *M. tuberculosis* genome project was the identification of large gene families that were either unknown previously or poorly understood. Foremost among these were the novel PE and PPE families comprising 100 and 67 members, respectively (5,11). Members of each family share a conserved N-terminal domain of about 110 and 180 amino acid residues, with the characteristic motifs ProGlu (PE in single-letter code), or ProProGlu (PPE) at positions 8–9 or 8–10, respectively. The N-terminal domain is generally followed by a C-terminal extension that is often of highly repetitive sequence; of particular interest are the PE proteins belonging to the PGRS (polymorphic GC-rich sequence) subclass (12) as nearly half of their amino acid content is composed of glycine and this occurs in tandem repetitions of the motif

AsnGlyGlyAlaGlyGlyAla, or variants thereof. As there has been extensive recent progress in the characterization of these proteins, and their genes represent a major source of diversity, they will be discussed in detail in a subsequent section.

The Genome Sequence of *Mycobacterium tuberculosis* CDC1551 and *Mycobacterium bovis* AF2122/97

The CDC1551 strain of *M. tuberculosis* is of interest because it appears to be highly transmissible, causing widespread skin test conversion in a rural area of the United States (13). Contrary to what was first thought, CDC1551 is less virulent in animal models of the disease than the H37Rv strain of *M. tuberculosis*, but it does induce a more rapid and robust immunologic response by the host (14). Its genome sequence was obtained by the whole-genome shotgun method and is nearly identical to that of *M. tuberculosis* H37Rv but is slightly smaller at 4,403,836 bp (Table 5.1A) (14a).

The *M. bovis* strain AF2122/97 was responsible for numerous cases of tuberculosis in cattle in the county of Devon in the United Kingdom in the 1990s, and has also been isolated from diseased badgers, and other wildlife, in the same area (15). No association with human tuberculosis has yet been reported. The genome sequence of *M. bovis* AF2122/97 has also been obtained through a combined approach involving the sequencing of whole-genome shotgun clones and selected BACs. This genome is nearly 70 kb smaller than those of the two *M. tuberculosis* isolates (Table 5.1) and contains about 60 fewer genes. Of particular interest was the presence of a stretch of additional DNA in *M. bovis* AF2122/97, known as TbD1, as this has helped us to understand the evolution of the *M. tuberculosis* complex by providing a valuable diagnostic marker (16). The TbD1 region of *M. bovis* (and all other tubercle bacilli except modern *M. tuberculosis*) contains two genes: *mmpS6* and *mmpL6* (Fig. 5.1) that may be involved in the transport of complex (glyco)lipids by analogy with MmpL7, which is required for the translocation of phthiocerol-dimycocerosate across the cytoplasmic membrane (17,18).

TABLE 5.1A. GENOME STATISTICS

Species	*M. tuberculosis* H37Rv	*M. tuberculosis* CDC1551	*M. bovis* AF2122/97
Genome size (bp)	4,411,532	4,403,836	4,345,492

TABLE 5.1B. GENOME POLYMORPHISMS

Difference	H37Rv × CDC1551	H37Rv × *M. bovis*	CD1551 × *M. bovis*
SNP	1135	2348	2380
Deletions	72	117	114
Insertions	63	108	104

SNP, single nucleotide polymorphism.

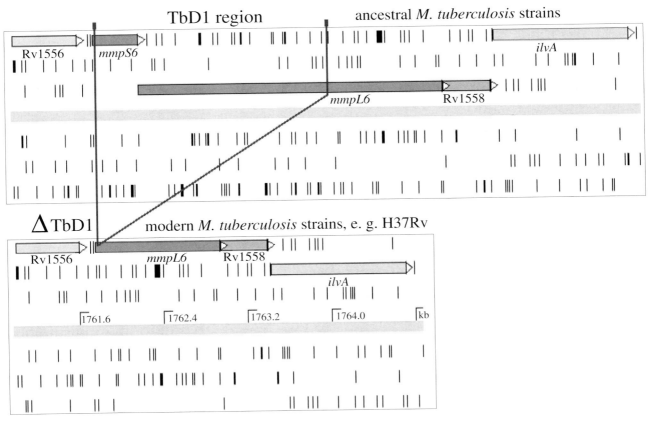

FIGURE 5.1. The lineage of modern *Mycobacterium tuberculosis* strains is characterized by a specific deletion (*TbD1*), resulting in an in-frame gene fusion of *mmpS6'* and *'mmpL6* **(lower portion of the figure)** whereas all other members of the *M. tuberculosis* complex harbor *mmpS6* and *mmpL6* at this locus **(upper portion of the figure)**. All six possible reading frames are shown. *Vertical bars* indicate stop codons.

Initial Comparison of the Three Genome Sequences

The pioneering work of Musser and his colleagues on the diversity and population genetics of the *M. tuberculosis* complex indicated that single nucleotide polymorphisms (SNPs) were unusually rare and that synonymous substitutions occurred infrequently. This led these workers to suggest that the tubercle bacillus may have become a human pathogen as recently as 15,000 years ago and that, having adopted this highly specialized niche, it encountered an evolutionary bottleneck that restricted its divergence (3,19). However, the lack of diversity is somewhat surprising given the absence of the MutL-S mismatch repair system from the proteome (20).

With the availability of three complete genome sequences, finer comparisons of nucleotide sequence divergence can be undertaken than those of Sreevatsan et al. (3), which targeted 26 loci. The initial analysis, presented in Table 5.1B, reveals that SNPs are very uncommon and account for less than 0.02% of the differences between the

M. tuberculosis strains H37Rv and CDC1551, or 0.05% of the differences between *M. bovis* and the two *M. tuberculosis* strains. This confirms and extends the previous findings (3). In contrast, the major source of diversity may be found in the form of insertions or deletions (InDels), ranging in size from 2 bp to 13 kb (Table 5.1). Ten of these result from IS*6110* copy number differences whereas others correspond to some of the well-characterized "regions of difference" (RDs) described further below. On comparison of the two *M. tuberculosis* strains, 55% of these InDels were found to affect genes, especially those encoding PE-PGRS proteins, while the remainder were intergenic. Similar findings and values were obtained when the *M. bovis* genome was examined. Among the intergenic sequences that display variation are the mycobacterial interspersed repetitive units or MIRUs (21,22). There are 41 loci in *M. tuberculosis* H37Rv that contain MIRUs and these often occur as tandem repeats, situated between genes in operons. Variability in MIRU copy number has been observed at certain loci and this has been exploited to develop an epidemiological test to distinguish between strains (23).

OTHER METHODS FOR GENOME-WIDE COMPARISONS

One of the first methods that enabled whole-genome comparisons was pulsed-field gel electrophoresis (PFGE) of macrorestriction fragments of chromosomal DNA. PFGE has been used as a tool for molecular epidemiologic and population genetic studies of the *M. tuberculosis* complex (24,25) and for the construction of integrated genome maps of *M. tuberculosis* H37Rv and *M. bovis* BCG Pasteur (26,27). These maps were of the utmost importance for estimating genome size (about 4.4 Mb) and structure (circular chromosome, absence of plasmids), for establishing ordered cosmid and BAC libraries (4,27), and for guiding and controlling assembly of the *M. tuberculosis* H37Rv genome sequence (5).

Subtractive hybridization, which is based on the hybridization of DNA from two genomes and removal of any common sequences (28), is another powerful technique for whole-genome comparisons and was applied to the genomes of *M. bovis* and *M. bovis* BCG. Three genomic regions of difference (RD1 to RD3) were identified that were absent from *M. bovis* BCG relative to *M. bovis* (29). This initial comparison of the BCG vaccine strain to virulent strains of the *M. tuberculosis* complex has recently been extended by the use of genome hybridization arrays based on a minimal set of BAC clones (4,30), microarrays employing spotted polymerase chain reaction products (31), or oligonucleotide-based GeneChip technology (Affymetrix, Santa Clara, CA, U.S.A.) (32,33). These combined approaches identified 18 RD regions that are absent from *M. bovis* BCG but present in H37Rv and other *M. tuberculosis* strains. Similar array analyses have been applied to clinical isolates and additional variable regions identified, some of which occur on multiple occasions whereas others are confined to a particular strain.

In silico comparison of genome sequences from related mycobacterial species represents an alternative strategy to the various hybridization and array techniques. With the growing number of completed genome sequences, and advances in bioinformatics, more refined comparisons of sequence variation among strains become possible such as those outlined above in which TbD1 was initially identified. More details of the techniques used in comparative mycobacterial genomics may be found in a recent review together with the principal findings (34).

SUMMARY OF GENOMIC VARIABILITY

Genetic variability can arise as a result of mutations involving single-nucleotide changes or from more complex events such as the insertion or deletion of stretches of nucleotides within genes. The transposition of IS elements can also lead to the inactivation or loss of genes depending on the site of insertion or even result in up-regulation if the transposon contains an outward-pointing promoter and inserts upstream of a gene.

Although SNPs occur in the genomes of members of the *M. tuberculosis* complex (Table 5.1B) at the relatively low level for a bacterium (3) of 1 in every 2,000 to 4,000 bp, depending on the species, InDels appear to be a more common means of generating diversity. Most of the insertions result from transposition events, generally involving IS*6110*, or more rarely from gene duplication. There is no evidence in favor of recent horizontal gene transfer, and the closest example of this is provided by RD3 or RD11, the presence or absence of the prophage genomes, phiRv1 or phiRv2, respectively (8). The deletions fall into two groups: ancient and recent. The ancient deletions occurred at different stages in the speciation process and are widespread, whereas the recent deletions have a more restricted distribution. Examples of the latter are the IS*6110*-mediated deletion of the 7-kb locus RvD2 in *M. tuberculosis* H37Rv, still present in the closely related avirulent derivative H37Ra (35), which also undergoes great variability in clinical isolates of *M. tuberculosis* (36). Other IS*6110*-mediated deletions are represented by RvD3-RvD5 that have removed three, two, and four genes from *M. tuberculosis* H37Rv. An example of a recent deletion in BCG Pasteur is the loss of the 8-kb locus RD14, which is still present in all other BCG substrains (31).

In contrast to these deletion events, the absence of regions RD7, RD8, RD9, and RD10 from *M. microti*, *M. bovis*, and BCG seems to be a much older event in evolutionary terms (Fig. 5.2). From close inspection of the sequences that border these RD regions it is apparent that deletions occurred within coding regions. Genes that are present in *M. tuberculosis* in full length were found to be disrupted in BCG, *M. bovis*, and *M. microti* at exactly the same location, whereas these genes are still intact in *M. tuberculosis* and *M. canettii* strains. This observation indicates that these RD regions result from real deletions and not the insertion of genes into *M. tuberculosis* as might be speculated. Based on the presence or absence of such conserved RD regions, a degree of relatedness to the last common ancestor of the *M. tuberculosis* complex was proposed that shows that the lineages of *M. tuberculosis* and *M. bovis* separated before the *M. tuberculosis*-specific deletion TbD1 occurred (Fig. 5.2). This analysis has identified some evolutionarily "old" *M. canettii*, *M. tuberculosis*, and *M. africanum* strains, most of them of African origin, as well as "modern" *M. tuberculosis* strains, the latter including representatives from major epidemic clusters like Beijing, Haarlem, and Africa (16).

Some of these regions, primarily RD9 and TbD1 but also RD1, RD2, RD4, RD7, RD8, RD10, RD12, and RD13, represent very interesting candidates for the development of powerful diagnostic tools for the rapid and

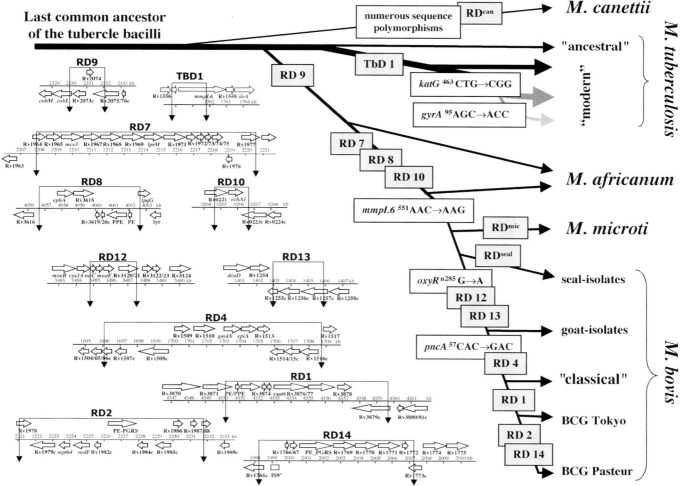

FIGURE 5.2. Scheme of the evolutionary pathway of the tubercle bacilli. *Boxes* indicate deletions *(gray)* and point mutations *(white)* that appeared in the various lineages during the evolution of the tubercle bacilli. (Adapted from Brosch R, Gordon SV, Marmiesse M, et al. A new evolutionary scenario for the *Mycobacterium tuberculosis* complex. *Proc Natl Acad Sci U S A* 2002;99:3684–3689.)

unambiguous identification of members of the *M. tuberculosis* complex (16). Figure 5.2 presents a differential scheme for identifying individual species that relies on the presence of these markers in association with selected SNPs, such as *mmpL6*551 AAC→AAG. This diagnostic strategy offers great promise for the study of the epidemiology and evolutionary biology of the tubercle bacilli. Its application has already shaken one of the tenets of our understanding of the origin of human tuberculosis, namely, that *M. tuberculosis*, the etiologic agent of human tuberculosis disease, evolved from *M. bovis*, the agent of bovine disease. From Figure 5.2 it is clear that this cannot have been the case but instead that *M. canettii* and ancestral *M. tuberculosis* strains appear to be direct descendants of tubercle bacilli that existed before the *M. africanum*→*M. bovis* lineage separated from the *M. tuberculosis* lineage.

VARIABILITY ASSOCIATED WITH THE PE AND PPE MULTIGENE FAMILIES

Genome comparisons and functional genomics have shed new light on the possible roles of the PE and PPE proteins. When the PE genes of *M. tuberculosis* strains H37Rv and CDC1551 were compared *in silico*, it was found that the genes encoding a PE domain or a PE domain followed by a unique protein sequence were identical in both cases (37,38). In contrast, 39 of the 62 common PE-PGRS proteins displayed variability as a result of frameshift mutations or the in-frame insertion or deletion of different Ala,Gly-rich coding sequences in the PGRS component of the gene (Fig. 5.3). Furthermore, consistent with this finding, size variation was also seen on Western blot analysis of protein samples, prepared from different clinical isolates, using PE-PGRS-specific

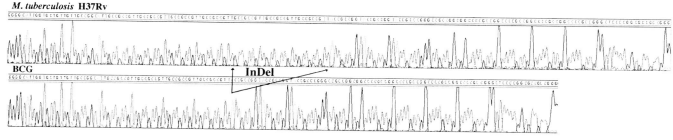

FIGURE 5.3. Example of an in-frame nine-codon deletion in an orthologous PE-PGRS gene in *M. bovis* bacille Calmette–Guérin (*BCG*) corresponding to gene Rv3507 from *M. tuberculosis* H37Rv. The sequence shown originates from the complementary strand.

antibodies. As expected from the conserved repetitive structure, the antibodies cross-reacted with more than one PE-PGRS protein, suggesting that different proteins share common epitopes. An example of this and variability between H37Rv and CDC1551 proteins may be seen in Figure 5.4.

Subcellular fractionation studies and immunogold or fluorescent antibody staining localized many PE-PGRS proteins in the cell wall and cell membrane of *M. tubercu-*

losis (37,39). Disruption of the gene encoding the PE-PGRS protein Rv1818c in *M. tuberculosis* led to greatly reduced bacterial clumping, suggesting that this protein may mediate cell–cell adhesion and altered phagocytosis by macrophages (39). Another PE-PGRS protein, Rv1759c, is capable of binding fibronectin and could thus mediate bacterial attachment to host cells (40,41). In addition, members of the PE-PGRS families have been implicated in the

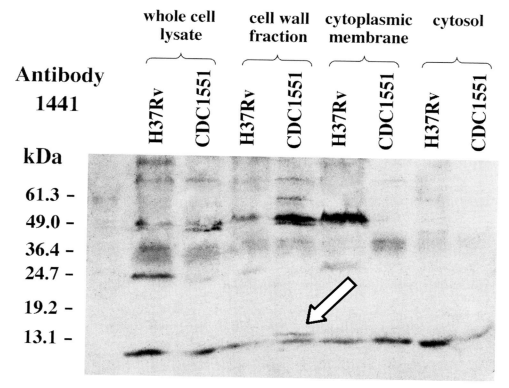

FIGURE 5.4. Subcellular localization of PE-PGRS proteins in two strains of *M. tuberculosis.* Cell wall, cell membrane, and cytosol fractions were prepared and proteins separated by sodium dodecyl sulfate–polyacrylamide gel electrophoresis. After transfer to nylon membranes, antibody 1441c was used to locate the PE-PGRS protein in the cell. The antibody recognized several proteins in each cell fraction. The molecular weight markers (in kilodaltons) are indicated on the left. The *white arrow* indicates size variation of PE proteins that hybridize to antibody 1441 in the two tested *M. tuberculosis* strains.

pathogenesis of *M. marinum* (42), where at least two genes were shown to be strongly up-regulated following phagocytosis of the bacterium.

The immunogenicity of the PE-PGRS protein Rv1818c has been studied in great detail in mice (43) where immunization with the PE domain induced Th1-type responses that were not found when the complete PE-PGRS protein was used. Instead, the PGRS part of the protein elicits antibody production and suppresses the Th1 response induced by the PE domain. The PE-PGRS proteins bear some sequence similarity to EBNA, the Epstein–Barr virus nuclear antigen, that blocks antigen presentation by the major histocompatibility complex (MHC) class I pathway, through its action as a proteasome inhibitor (5). It was speculated that PE-PGRS proteins may also have this activity, and it was recently shown that the PGRS domain, when fused to green fluorescent protein, confers increased resistance to proteosomal attack (44). If these immunologic and adhesive properties are shared among other members of the family, it is conceivable that the extensive variation observed at the gene level could bestow very different phenotypes on the different strains.

The PPE proteins also fall into subfamilies, and by far the most spectacular of these is the major polymorphic tandem repeat (MPTR) subfamily, which contains multiple repetitions of the motif AsnXGlyXGlyAsnXGly. The largest PPE-MPTR protein detected contains 3,300 amino acid residues and, as with the PE-PGRS proteins, these are also associated with polymorphic DNA sequences (11). Extensive sequence variation due to InDels has been reported between the PPE proteins Rv1917c and Rv1753c of *M. tuberculosis* and *M. bovis* (15). There is little evidence concerning their possible function, but Rv1917c was recently shown to be cell wall associated and surface exposed (45).

CLUES FROM THE GENOME FOR IMPROVED BACILLE CALMETTE–GUÉRIN VACCINE DEVELOPMENT

The only tuberculosis vaccine is BCG (46), one of the six components of the expanded program of immunization of the World Health Organization. Since 1921, more than 3 billion doses have been administered worldwide with negligible side effects in immunocompetent individuals. BCG is highly effective against disseminated forms of tuberculosis in children (47), such as miliary disease and meningitis, and also was shown to protect against leprosy in a recent controlled trial (48). However, the protection conferred by BCG vaccination against pulmonary TB in adults, representing the majority of the disease burden, is highly variable and ranges from 0 to 80%, depending on the population, the country, and the BCG strain used (49).

BCG vaccination will probably continue until controlled long-term vaccine trials prove that new vaccines offer better

protection. Consequently, molecular and immunologic characterization of the presently used BCG vaccine strains continues to be an important research topic as it will allow us to identify the genetic basis for the attenuation of BCG and to understand why some BCG substrains offer better protection or cause more scarring than others (50). Encouragingly, it has been found recently that engineering BCG to overproduce a 30-kd major secretory protein, known as antigen 85-B, results in more effective protection against tuberculosis in guinea pigs (51).

By elucidating the genomic differences between the virulent and avirulent members of the *M. tuberculosis* complex, comparative genomics has the potential to define mycobacterial virulence determinants specific for humans and other host range–determining factors that may have important impact on vaccine design. In addition to the many RD regions described above, two large duplications (DU1 and DU2) have been found in BCG strains. Some important potentially protective antigens may have been lost from BCG during the attenuation process. For example, ESAT-6 and CFP10, two strongly immunogenic proteins, are found in early culture filtrates of *M. tuberculosis* but not in BCG (52,53). Interestingly, the ESAT-6 and CFP10 genes are located in the RD1 region of *M. tuberculosis*, a 10-kb genomic region that is absent from all BCG strains. One attractive approach is to use recombinant BCG carrying the missing genes (54) to determine whether better protection can be obtained.

Besides loss of genes, gene duplication undoubtedly played an important role in the differentiation of BCG. Evidence that this phenomenon is still ongoing can be seen in the presence of two large tandem duplications (DU1, DU2) in BCG Pasteur, detected by comparative genomics (55). These duplications of 29 and 36 kb seem to have appeared independently from each other as their presence and/or their size may vary in the different BCG substrains. While DU1 appears to be confined to BCG Pasteur, DU2 has been detected in all BCG substrains tested so far, but this duplication can exhibit size variation (our unpublished observations, 2000). Gene dosage effects may result from these duplications, thereby accounting for some of the differences in immunogenicity displayed by the various BCG vaccine strains.

CONCLUSIONS

Genomic analysis of *M. tuberculosis* has provided us with a rich source of information about the pathogen that is of inestimable value. Application of this new knowledge will surely result in better understanding of the molecular basis of pathogenesis and, hopefully, translate into new drugs, diagnostic tests, and vaccines to combat the disease. Comparative genomics of the *M. tuberculosis* complex has revealed that, on the one hand, the majority of the genome is well conserved in sequence and highly stable, while, on the other hand, extensive variation may occur as a result of a limited range of InDels. Some of these, especially the more numerous deletion events, may affect features such as host range and persistence, whereas others may have more subtle effects. Of particular interest, and some concern, is the finding that the major source of diversity between strains is due to variation in the sequences of the PE and PPE proteins. If these proteins serve as variable surface antigens, as seems increasingly likely, and affect interactions with host cells and phagocytes, development of a more effective vaccine will be most challenging.

ACKNOWLEDGMENTS

We thank T. Garnier and S. V. Gordon for helpful discussions, and B. Saint-Joanis for technical assistance. Parts of this work were supported by grants from the European Union (QLRT-2000-02018), the Institut Pasteur (PTR35), and the Association Française Raoul Follereau.

REFERENCES

1. Dye C, Sheele S, Dolin P, et al. Global burden of tuberculosis: estimated incidence, prevalence, and mortality by country. *JAMA* 1999;282:677–686.
2. Imaeda T. Deoxyribonucleic acid relatedness among selected strains of *Mycobacterium tuberculosis, Mycobacterium bovis, Mycobacterium bovis BCG, Mycobacterium micoti* and *Mycobacterium africanum. Int J Syst Bact* 1985;35:147–150.
3. Sreevatsan S, Pan X, Stockbauer KE, et al. Restricted structural gene polymorphism in the *Mycobacterium tuberculosis* complex indicates evolutionarily recent global dissemination. *Proc Natl Acad Sci U S A* 1997;94:9869–9874.
4. Brosch R, Gordon SV, Billault A, et al. Use of a *Mycobacterium tuberculosis* H37Rv Bacterial Artificial Chromosome (BAC) library for genome mapping, sequencing and comparative genomics. *Infect Immun* 1998;66:2221–2229.
5. Cole ST, Brosch R, Parkhill J, et al. Deciphering the biology of *Mycobacterium tuberculosis* from the complete genome sequence. *Nature* 1998;393:537–544.
6. Cole ST. Learning from the genome sequence of *Mycobacterium tuberculosis* H37Rv. *FEBS Lett* 1999;452:7–10.
7. Tekaia F, Gordon SV, Garnier T, et al. Analysis of the proteome of *Mycobacterium tuberculosis in silico. Tuber Lung Dis* 1999;79:329–342.
8. Brosch R, Gordon SV, Eiglmeier K, et al. Genomics, biology, and evolution of the *Mycobacterium tuberculosis* complex. In: Hatfull GF, Jacobs WR Jr, eds. *Molecular genetics of mycobacteria.* Washington, DC: American Society of Microbiology Press, 2000:19–36.
9. Gordon SV, Heym B, Parkhill J, et al. New insertion sequences and a novel repeated sequence in the genome of *Mycobacterium tuberculosis* H37Rv. *Microbiology* 1999;145:881–892.
10. Daffe M, Draper P. The envelope layers of mycobacteria with reference to their pathogenicity. *Adv Microb Physiol* 1998;39:131–203.
11. Cole ST, Barrell BG. Analysis of the genome of *Mycobacterium tuberculosis* H37Rv. *Genetics and Tuberculosis (Novartis Found Symp 217)* 1998;160–172.
12. Poulet S, Cole ST. Characterisation of the polymorphic GC-rich repetitive sequence (PGRS) present in *Mycobacterium tuberculosis. Arch Microbiol* 1995;163:87–95.
13. Valway SE, Sanchez MP, Shinnick TF, et al. An outbreak involving extensive transmission of a virulent strain of *Mycobacterium tuberculosis. N Engl J Med* 1998;338:633–639.
14. Manca C, Tsenova L, Barry Cr, et al. *Mycobacterium tuberculosis* CDC1551 induces a more vigorous host response *in vivo* and *in vitro*, but is not more virulent than other clinical isolates. *J Immunol* 1999;162:6740–6746.
14a. Fleischmann RD, Alland D, Eisen JA, et al. Whole-genome comparison of *Mycobacterium tuberculosis* clinical and laboratory strains. *J Bacteriol* 2002;184:5479–5490.
15. Gordon SV, Eiglmeier K, Garnier T, et al. Genomics of *Mycobacterium bovis. Tuberculosis (Edinb)* 2001;81:157–163.
16. Brosch R, Gordon SV, Marmiesse M, et al. A new evolutionary scenario for the *Mycobacterium tuberculosis* complex. *Proc Natl Acad Sci U S A* 2002;99:3684–3689.
17. Camacho LR, Ensergueix D, Perez E, et al. Identification of a virulence gene cluster of *Mycobacterium tuberculosis* by signature-tagged transposon mutagenesis. *Mol Microbiol* 1999;34:257–267.
18. Cox JS, Chen B, McNeil M, et al. Complex lipid determines tissue-specific replication of *Mycobacterium tuberculosis* in mice. *Nature* 1999;402:79–83.
19. Kapur V, Whittam TS, Musser J. Is *Mycobacterium tuberculosis* 15,000 years old? *J Infect Dis* 1994;170:1348–1349.
20. Mizrahi V, Andersen SJ. DNA repair in *Mycobacterium tuberculosis.* What have we learnt from the genome sequence? *Mol Microbiol* 1998;29:1331–1339.
21. Supply P, Mazars E, Lesjean S, et al. Variable human minisatellite-like regions in the *Mycobacterium tuberculosis* genome. *Mol Microbiol* 2000;36:762–771,.
22. Supply P, Magdalena J, Himpens S, et al. Identification of novel intergenic repetitive units in a mycobacterial two-component system operon. *Mol Microbiol* 1997;26:991–1003.
23. Mazars E, Lesjean S, Banuls AL, et al. High-resolution minisatellite-based typing as a portable approach to global analysis of *Mycobacterium tuberculosis* molecular epidemiology. *Proc Natl Acad Sci U S A* 2001;13:1901–1906.
24. Singh SP, Salamon H, Lahti CJ, et al. Use of pulsed-field gel electrophoresis for molecular epidemiologic and population genetic studies of *Mycobacterium tuberculosis. J Clin Microbiol* 1999;37:1927–1931.
25. Zhang Y, Wallace RJ, Jr. Genetic differences between BCG substrains. *Tuber Lung Dis* 1995;76:43–50.
26. Philipp WJ, Nair S, Guglielmi G, et al. Physical mapping of *Mycobacterium bovis* BCG Pasteur reveals differences from the genome map of *Mycobacterium tuberculosis H37Rv* and from *Mycobacterium bovis. Microbiology* 1996;142:3135–3145.
27. Philipp WJ, Poulet S, Eiglmeier K, et al. An integrated map of the genome of the tubercle bacillus, *Mycobacterium tuberculosis* H37Rv, and comparison with *Mycobacterium leprae. Proc Natl Acad Sci U S A* 1996;93:3132–3137.
28. Straus D, Ausubel FM. Genomic subtraction for cloning DNA corresponding to deletion mutations. *Proc Natl Acad Sci U S A* 1990;87:1889–1893.
29. Mahairas GG, Sabo PJ, Hickey MJ, et al. Molecular analysis of genetic differences between *Mycobacterium bovis* BCG and virulent *M. bovis. J Bacteriol* 1996;178:1274–1282.
30. Gordon SV, Brosch R, Billault A, et al. Identification of variable regions in the genomes of tubercle bacilli using bacterial artificial chromosome arrays. *Mol Microbiol* 1999;32:643–656.
31. Behr MA, Wilson MA, Gill WP, et al. Comparative genomics of BCG vaccines by whole-genome DNA microarrays. *Science* 1999;284:1520–1523.

32. Salamon H, Kato-Maeda M, Small PM, et al. Detection of deleted genomic DNA using a semiautomated computational analysis of GeneChip data. *Genome Res* 2000;10:2044–2054.

33. Kato-Maeda M, Rhee JT, Gingeras TR, et al. Comparing genomes within the species *Mycobacterium tuberculosis. Genome Res* 2001;11:547–554.

34. Brosch R, Pym AS, Gordon SV, et al. The evolution of mycobacterial pathogenicity: clues from comparative genomics. *Trends Microbiol* 2001;9:452–458.

35. Brosch R, Philipp W, Stavropolous E, et al. Genomic analysis reveals variation between *Mycobacterium tuberculosis* H37Rv and the attenuated *M. tuberculosis* H37Ra. *Infection Immun* 1999;67: 5768–5774.

36. Ho TBL, Robertson BD, Taylor GM, et al. Comparison of *Mycobacterium tuberculosis* genomes reveals frequent deletions in a 20 kb variable region in clinical isolates. *Yeast (Comp Funct Genomics)* 2001;17:272–282.

37. Banu S, Honoré N, Saint-Joanis B, et al. Are the PE-PGRS proteins of *Mycobacterium tuberculosis* variable surface antigens? *Mol Microbiol* 2002;44:9–19.

38. Betts JC, Dodson P, Quan S, et al. Comparison of the proteome of *Mycobacterium tuberculosis* strain H37Rv with clinical isolate CDC 1551. *Microbiology* 2000;146:3205–3216.

39. Brennan MJ, Delogu G, Chen Y, et al. Evidence that mycobacterial PE-PGRS proteins are cell surface constituents that influence interactions with other cells. *Infect Immun* 2001;69: 7326–7333.

40. Espitia C, Laclette JP, Mondragon-Palomino M, et al. The PE-PGRS glycine-rich proteins of *Mycobacterium tuberculosis*: a new family of fibronectin-binding proteins? *Microbiology* 1999;145: 3487–3495.

41. Singh KK, Zhang X, Patibandla AS, et al. Antigens of *Mycobacterium tuberculosis* expressed during preclinical tuberculosis: serological immunodominance of proteins with repetitive amino acid sequences. *Infect Immun* 2001;69:4185–4191.

42. Ramakrishnan L, Federspiel NA, Falkow S. Granuloma-specific expression of mycobacterium virulence proteins from the glycine-rich PE-PGRS family. *Science* 2000;288:1436–1439.

43. Delogu G, Brennan MJ. Comparative immune response to PE and PE-PGRS antigens of *Mycobacterium tuberculosis*. *Infect Immun* 2001;69:5606–5611.

44. Brennan MJ, Delogu G. The PE multigene family: a molecular mantra for mycobacteria. *Trends Microbiol* 2002;10:246–249.

45. Sampson SL, Lukey P, Warren RM, et al. Expression, characterization and subcellular localization of the *Mycobacterium tuberculosis* PPE gene Rv1917c. *Tuberculosis (Edinb)* 2001;81: 305–317.

46. Calmette A. *La vaccination préventive contre la tuberculose.* Paris: Masson, 1927:250.

47. Hart PD, Sutherland I. BCG and vole bacillus vaccines in the prevention of tuberculosis in adolescence and early adult life. *Br Med J* 1977;2 (6082):293–295.

48. Ponnighaus JM, Fine PE, Sterne JA, et al. Efficacy of BCG vaccine against leprosy and tuberculosis in northern Malawi. *Lancet* 1992;339:636–639.

49. Tuberculosis Prevention Trial Madras. Trial of BCG vaccines in south India for tuberculosis prevention. *Indian J Med Res* 1980; 72(Suppl):1–74.

50. Lagranderie MR, Balazuc AM, Deriaud E, et al. Comparison of immune responses of mice immunized with five different *Mycobacterium bovis* BCG vaccine strains. *Infect Immun* 1996;64: 1–9.

51. Horwitz MA, Harth G, Dillon BJ, et al. Recombinant bacillus Calmette–Guérin (BCG) vaccines expressing the *Mycobacterium tuberculosis* 30-kDa major secretory protein induce greater protective immunity against tuberculosis than conventional BCG vaccines in a highly susceptible animal model. *Proc Natl Acad Sci U S A* 2000;97:13853–13858.

52. Brandt L, Oettinger T, Holm A, et al. Key epitopes on the ESAT-6 antigen recognized in mice during the recall of protective immunity to *Mycobacterium tuberculosis*. *J Immunol* 1996;157: 3527–3533.

53. Brandt L, Elhay M, Rosenkrands I, et al. ESAT-6 subunit vaccination against *Mycobacterium tuberculosis*. *Infect Immun* 2000;68: 791–795.

54. Pym AS, Brodin P, Majlessi L, et al. Recombinant BCG exporting ESAT-6 confers enhanced protection against tuberculosis. *Nat Med* 2003;9:533–539.

55. Brosch R, Gordon SV, Buchrieser C, et al. Comparative genomics uncovers tandem chromosomal duplications in some strains of *Mycobacterium bovis* BCG: implications for vaccination. *Comp Funct Genomics (Yeast)* 2000;17:111–123.

GENETIC DIVERSITY OF THE *MYCOBACTERIUM TUBERCULOSIS* COMPLEX

MARCEL A. BEHR

Without a doubt, the most exciting development in tuberculosis (TB) research during the past decade has been the determination of the complete genomic sequence of the causative organism, *Mycobacterium tuberculosis* (1). At the time of writing, the laboratory strain (*M. tuberculosis* H37Rv) (2), a recent clinical isolate (*M. tuberculosis* CDC-1551) (3), and a recent bovine isolate (*Mycobacterium bovis* 2122) (4) have been completely sequenced. These sequences permit genome-wide comparisons across these sequenced isolates, providing insights into the degree and nature of genetic diversity between strains (5). Furthermore, these prototype sequences serve as the cornerstone for genetic comparisons across larger samples of clinical and laboratory isolates. Such comparisons are fueled by a number of pressing questions about the biology of *M. tuberculosis*, including: Why is *M. tuberculosis* virulent? Why are bacille Calmette–Guérin (BCG) vaccines attenuated in virulence? Why do some strains appear to spread more successfully than others? Where did TB come from?

The ready access to sequence information along with the high degree of sequence conservation within the *M. tuberculosis* complex permit one to rapidly design comparative sequencing experiments to attempt to address these and other questions. Such studies can be designed at the level of any selected gene (6) or group of related genes (7) or may be performed on a genome-wide scale, using postgenomic tools such as DNA microarrays (8) and GeneChip (Affymetrix, Santa Clara, CA, U.S.A.) (9). In this chapter, the author will review how these approaches have been used to characterize the genetic diversity of a laboratory strain family (the BCG vaccines) and circulating virulent isolates of the *M. tuberculosis* complex.

DIVERSITY IN ATTENUATED BACILLE CALMETTE–GUÉRIN VACCINES

Mycobacterium bovis BCG refers to a family of closely related vaccine strains that shared a common *M. bovis* ancestor in the early 20th century. Through *in vitro* passage every 2 weeks over 13 years, Calmette and Guérin were able to render this strain attenuated in virulence and first introduced it as a vaccine in 1921 (10). Over the subsequent half century, BCG vaccines were dispersed to a variety of different laboratories where BCG continued to be propagated *in vitro* under a variety of similar conditions. By the 1940s it was first observed that different BCG strains were phenotypically different *in vitro* (11), precipitating efforts to develop standardized lyophilized seed lots. These seed lots currently available for study consist of essentially immortalized forms of BCG strains from the 1960s, which are now about 900 to 1,100 passages removed from the original BCG of 1921 and some 250 to 2,000 passages removed from each other (12).

Phenotypic information from clinical experience and animal models concurs that BCG vaccines are less virulent than circulating strains of *M. tuberculosis*. A nationwide survey in France suggested that BCG disease occurs in perhaps 1 vaccine recipient per 100,000, in contrast to the 1 in 10 often reported to develop TB following infection with *M. tuberculosis* (13). Other phenotypic properties of the BCG family are known from clinical and reference laboratories where BCG strains have a different growth morphology than virulent *M. bovis* and produce a distinct pattern in chromatographic analysis (14). Moreover, beyond there being phenotypic differences between BCG and virulent strains, variability among BCG strains has also been documented. Examples include differences in production of mycolic acids (15) and antigenic proteins (16), as well as less reproducible differences in virulence and protective efficacy (17,18). These differences are certainly encoded in the genomes of the BCG strains. The ability to interrogate the

M. A. Behr: Department of Medicine, McGill University; Department of Medicine, Montreal General Hospital, Montreal, Quebec, Canada.

respective genomes to search for the basis of these properties has provided an interesting opportunity both to study BCG vaccines and to develop an approach that may be applicable for genomic study of other strains of the *M. tuberculosis* complex.

TOOLS FOR GENETIC STUDY OF BACILLE CALMETTE–GUÉRIN STRAINS

Techniques used to interrogate the BCG genome have included targeted analysis of specific BCG genes (6) and whole genomic comparisons by a variety of modalities. For the former, the sequence of the gene can be determined in BCG strains by amplification and standardized sequencing modalities. For genome-wide comparisons, four techniques are used. Subtractive hybridization (with comparison to *M. bovis*) permits the identification of genomic regions absent from BCG in the absence of any *a priori* knowledge of the genomes under study (19). Bacterial artificial chromosome (BAC) libraries permit both the determination of regions missing from BCG strains and also the detection of extra genetic material in BCG strains, either because of deletion from *M. tuberculosis* H37Rv (20) or duplication within BCG (21). Whole-genome spotted DNA microarrays permitted the rapid detection of polygenic deletions of a number of different BCG strains (8). More recent application of the GeneChip has permitted the uncovering of genomic deletions from BCG strains as small as hundreds of base pairs (22). The most intensive study of BCG vaccines will follow from the determination of the complete genome sequence of BCG Pasteur by Cole et al. (23).

BACILLE CALMETTE–GUÉRIN COMPARISONS AT THE LEVEL OF A SINGLE GENE

Because the history of BCG strain dissemination has been largely recorded, it has been possible to determine with relative precision the laboratory site and chronology of genetic differences among BCG strains. As examples, BCG strains obtained from the Pasteur Institute in 1931 or later are unable to synthesize methoxymycolic acid and do not produce the MPB64 antigen. Since strains obtained before 1927 do produce methoxymycolates and MPB64, the responsible mutations can be assigned to the interval between 1927 and 1931 at the Pasteur Institute. From this it is possible to study the relevant genes and determine (a) that a single point mutation at position 293 in the *mmaA3* gene is responsible for the loss of methoxymycolates (6), and (b) that the *mpt64* gene is part of a deleted region, explaining the absence of the

antigenic protein in later BCG strains (19,24). Ongoing studies are now attempting to determine the impact of these mutations on relevant vaccine properties, notably virulence and protective efficacy.

WHOLE-GENOME COMPARISONS OF BACILLE CALMETTE–GUÉRIN VACCINES

Using subtractive hybridization, Mahairas et al. (19) uncovered three regions, called regions of difference (RDs), that were present in *M. bovis* but missing from BCG Connaught. The first of these regions, called RD1, is consistently absent from all BCG strains subsequently studied and thus serves as a diagnostic marker for BCG disease (25). Although the genes encoded in this region have unknown function, two of them encode well-described antigenic proteins (ESAT-6 and CFP-10) (26), suggesting that deletion of this region may alter the antigenicity or virulence of the organism. In the original report, complementation of RD1 did not restore virulence to BCG Brazil (18), suggesting that (a) RD1 is not important for virulence, (b) the complementation did not completely restore function of this region, and/or (c) the strain of BCG used for complementation had undergone further attenuation of virulence. The deletion of this region from *M. tuberculosis* H37Rv has now been accomplished and results in attenuated host pathology and bacterial growth, thus confirming that the deletion of this region likely contributed to the attenuation of BCG (27). Further study is aimed at determining the mechanism of attenuation resulting from the deletion of RD1.

Further genomic analysis of BCG strains has been facilitated by the complete genome sequence of H37Rv, studying differences in genome content via BAC libraries or array/chip platforms. A summary of documented genetic events in the evolution of BCG strains is provided as Figure 6.1. The use of BAC libraries has permitted the demonstration of two duplications in BCG Pasteur, one apparently unique to BCG Pasteur and one also seen in other BCG strains (21). Array- and chip-based platforms have succeeded in uncovering deletions from most BCG strains: as of the summer of 2002, ten genomic deletions have been documented in BCG strains after 1921, and all BCG strains currently in use are separated from the original BCG by at least one genomic deletion (22). Beyond providing unequivocal evidence of the ongoing evolution of BCG strains, the 41 genes represented in BCG deletions provide clues into the nature of evolution of *M. tuberculosis* complex isolates *in vitro* (Table 6.1).

Two classes of genes appear overrepresented in these genetic events: regulatory genes and genes encoding antigenic proteins. Of the genes involved in transcriptional regulation, *M. tuberculosis* H37Rv has 13 σ factors: *sigI* is

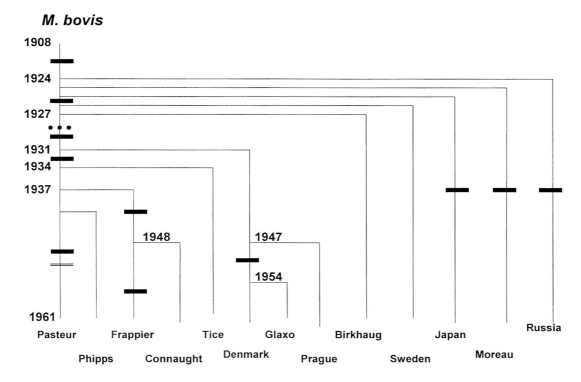

FIGURE 6.1. Genetic events documented to have occurred to bacille Calmette–Guérin (BCG) strains between derivation by Calmette in 1908 and lyophilization of seed lots in the 1960s and 1970s. Deletions are denoted by *solid lines*, the point mutation in *mmaA3* is a *dotted line*, and the duplication (DU1) unique to BCG Pasteur is a *double line*. The second duplication (DU2) is not mapped because its chronology is still under investigation.

TABLE 6.1. PREDICTED FUNCTION OF OPEN READING FRAMES DELETED FROM ONE OR MORE BCG STRAINS ACCORDING TO HIERARCHICAL GENE CLASSIFICATION PROPOSED BY COLE ET AL. (1)

Putative Function	Genes Deleted from BCG Family
Small-molecule metabolism (7 genes)	
Energy metabolism; miscellaneous oxidoreductases and oxygenases	*Rv1771*
Central intermediary metabolism; sugar nucleotides	*Rv3400*
Purines, pyrimidines, nucleosides, and nucleotides; 2′-deoxyribonucleotide metabolism	*Rv1981c*
Broad regulatory functions; repressors/activators	*Rv1773c, Rv1985c, Rv3405c* (twice)
Macromolecule metabolism (9 genes)	
Synthesis and modification of macromolecules; RNA synthesis, RNA modification, DNA transcription	*Rv1189*
Cell envelope; surface polysaccharides, lipopolysaccharides, proteins, and antigens	*Rv1980c, Rv1984c, Rv1987, Rv3874, Rv3875*
Cell envelope; other membrane proteins	*Rv1979c, Rv1986, Rv3402c*
Other (6 genes)	
PE and PPE families; PE family; PE subfamily	*Rv3872*
PE and PPE families; PE family; PE-PGRS subfamily	*Rv1768, Rv1983*
PE and PPE families; PPE family	*Rv3873*
Miscellaneous transferases	*Rv1978, Rv1988*
Conserved hypotheticals (12 genes)	
Conserved hypothetical proteins	*Rv0310c, Rv0312, Rv1190, Rv1191, Rv1766, Rv1767, Rv1770, Rv1982c, Rv3401, Rv3871, Rv3876, Rv3877*
Unknown (8 genes)	
Unknowns	*Rv0309, Rv0311, Rv1769, Rv1772, Rv3403c, Rv3404c, Rv3878, Rv3879c*

BCG, bacille Calmette–Guérin; PE, Pro-Glu; PPE, Pro-Pro-Glu; PGRS, polymorphic GC-rich repetitive sequence.
Note: Although originally annotated as a conserved hypothetical protein, *Rv3874* has since been proposed by Arend et al. (26) to encode for the antigenic protein CFP-10.

deleted from strains after 1934, and *sigH* and *sigM* are seen in the genomic duplications. Outside of σ factors, four different deletions encode a gene predicted to encode a transcriptional regulator (*Rv3405c* is independently deleted on two occasions). The preferential loss of regulatory genes during prolonged *in vitro* growth suggests that in the relatively restricted conditions of the laboratory, genes involved in responding to environmental change are dispensable.

Genes encoding antigenic proteins are also lost during the evolution of BCG strains *in vitro*. The absence of antigenic proteins is predictably a concern for a live attenuated vaccine whose purpose is to elicit an immune response in the host. Two genes known to encode antigens were lost in RD1: *Rv3874* encoding CFP-10 and *Rv3875* encoding ESAT-6. Subsequently, the second deletion, RD2, dated to 1927–1931, encodes three more antigenic proteins: *Rv1980c* (*mpt64*), *Rv1984c* (probable cutinase precursor) and *Rv1987* (chitinase c precursor). Furthermore, two other antigenic proteins that are not deleted (MPB70 and MPB83) are produced in drastically reduced quantities after this interval (28). The loss or shut-off of these antigens from BCG strains suggests that these proteins have a negligible role during *in vitro* growth.

DIVERSITY IN CLINICAL ISOLATES OF THE *MYCOBACTERIUM TUBERCULOSIS* COMPLEX

From early studies on the development of antibiotic resistance, it is known that *M. tuberculosis* is capable of mutation and selection in the face of the relevant selective pressure. Mutations in such isolates demonstrate that diversity is generated not by horizontal gene transfer from other organisms but rather through mutations within the genome, such as single nucleotide polymorphisms, deletions, insertion sequence (IS)–mediated transposition events, and so forth. It therefore follows that isolates circulating in different hosts and environmental conditions will also manifest a number of genetic polymorphisms of the nature described above for BCG strains. Furthermore, if *M. tuberculosis* has been with its host (humans) for more than 10,000 years (29), there would appear to be greater opportunity for genetic diversity in *M. tuberculosis* isolates than has been witnessed in the 50-year history of BCG strains. Indeed, the diversity observed with molecular fingerprinting tools, such as spoligotyping and IS*6110*-based restriction fragment length polymorphism (RFLP), attests to the considerable genetic diversity among clinical isolates. More recently, the application of bacterial genetic tools has shifted from tags used to track organisms in a population to modalities used to discern molecular differences that may impact on bacterial phenotypes. These epi-

demiologically relevant phenotypes include antibiotic resistance (important for treatment), host range (important for rational TB control), antigenic variability (important for design of a new vaccine), and what is broadly described as virulence (important for targeting efforts at particularly problematic strains). For this discussion, the term *virulence* will be replaced with *transmissibility*, defined as the capacity of the organism to spread to other hosts, and *pathogenicity*, defined as the capacity of the infecting organism to cause disease.

HOST RANGE OF *MYCOBACTERIUM TUBERCULOSIS* COMPLEX MEMBERS

Since the early laboratory study of the tubercle bacillus, researchers have distinguished between the bovine forms and the human forms. One of the earliest assays was virulence in an animal model, where both forms were virulent to guinea pigs but only the bovine form caused disease in rabbits (30). From these and later studies have come the different names *M. tuberculosis* and *M. bovis*, as well as the laboratory criteria for these different species and the notion that *M. tuberculosis* is generally a human pathogen whereas *M bovis* has a broad host range. Throughout this period, the definition of these and other subspecies has rested on laboratory phenotypes, and intermediate forms with some of the phenotypic descriptors have eluded simple classification (31). As a result, some of these other forms have been recognized with separates names, such as *M. africanum, M. microti,* and *M. caprae.*

Recent genomic comparisons have uncovered a number of genomic deletions that appear to reliably distinguish between these subspecies. The value of these deletions is twofold. First, because genomic deletions represent unidirectional genetic events, their distribution across isolates of the *M. tuberculosis* complex suggests the evolutionary relationship of these organisms. Second, deletions lend themselves to simple polymerase chain reaction–based assays producing binary results (present/absent) and therefore can be easily exploited in a diagnostic laboratory for robust classification of clinical isolates.

Because of the genetic similarity between *M. tuberculosis* and *M. bovis*, it has long been considered that the human TB epidemic may have begun as a zoonotic infection from cattle. This hypothesis suggested that with domestication, contact of infected animals with humans increased, humans probably drank contaminated milk, and, after a period of host adaptation, a humanized form of *M. bovis* evolved. The existence of forms of the *M. tuberculosis* complex in undomesticated mammals such as seals, voles, dassies, and surikats poses some challenge to this model, suggesting that the spread of this organism is more complex than an interplay between humans and

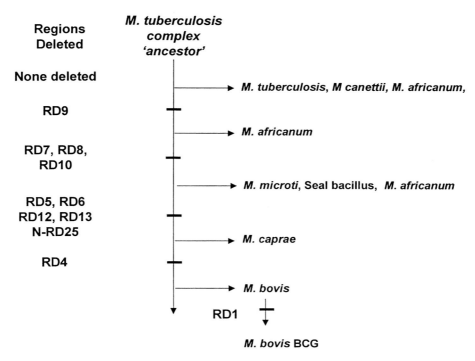

**Regions
Deleted**

None deleted

RD9

**RD7, RD8,
RD10**

**RD5, RD6
RD12, RD13
N-RD25**

RD4

FIGURE 6.2. Distribution of genomic deletions among members of the *Mycobacterium tuberculosis* complex, adapted from ref. 33 with data from refs. 32 and 35. Vertical axis represents time, from ancestor, with genomic deletions represented as *solid lines* crossing the main axis. Deletions represented are those in ref. 33. Isolates called *M. africanum* have been observed to have 0, 1, or 4 deletions. Other members of the *M. tuberculosis* complex to date have been found with a consistent number of regions deleted.

farm stock. Using genomic deletions, two groups have recently evaluated this hypothesis, using independent collections of isolates and somewhat different sets of deletions (32,33). Notable differences in the studies are that the former analysis included the newly described *M. canettii* (34) and that the former study included a larger number of deletions. Despite these differences, the results are remarkably concordant. Isolates with the most conserved genome (fewest genomic deletions) are *M. tuberculosis* and *M. canetii*, whereas increasing numbers of genomic deletions are observed in isolates called *M. africanum*, *M. microti*, the seal bacillus, *M. caprae* followed by *M. bovis* and, finally, *M. bovis* BCG (Fig. 6.2). These results conclusively argue that the precursor of current *M. tuberculosis* was ancestral to contemporary *M. bovis*, thus arguing against a bovine origin of human TB. As *M. canetii* was found near the putative ancestral form of the *M. tuberculosis* complex, a tantalizing alternative hypothesis for the origin of TB is suggested (32). This hypothesis now requires further exploration.

The second valuable application of genomic deletions is in correct classification of clinical isolates. Since the laboratory subspeciation of *M. tuberculosis* complex previously relied on laborious and imperfect phenotypic markers, many laboratories have been content to perform DNA probe–based speciation and simply report presence of *M. tuberculosis* complex. In the absence of a robust method to characterize isolates, the true prevalence of *M. bovis* disease in humans or *M. tuberculosis* disease in cattle may be difficult to ascertain. Recently, Parsons et al. have subjected a large collection of clinical isolates to deletion-based typing and put forth a simple algorithm based on three regions as a first screen and three additional regions where any of the first are negative (35). This approach was validated in 605 consecutive clinical isolates and shown to accurately distinguish *M. tuberculosis*, *M. africanum*, *M. bovis*, and *M. bovis* BCG. The application of this algorithm to other settings, including animal studies, should serve as a first step to determine the host range of members of the *M. tuberculosis* complex.

From this it will then be possible to apply some of the genomic tools described above to further determine the genomic composition of all members of the complex and propose reasons for the observed host specificity.

DIVERSITY IN ANTIBIOTIC RESISTANCE GENES

The resurgence of TB in the 1990s along with the spread of drug-resistant forms spurred on the study of both the molecular targets of antimicrobials (36) and the mutations in these genes that confer resistance (37). Genetic mechanisms responsible for the development of resistance to commonly used anti-TB medications are now established to varying degrees, and their application to both molecular diagnosis and the management of TB are the subject of Chapters 49–52. Polymorphisms in these genes have also served as clonal markers to track the spread of notorious drug-resistant strains of *M. tuberculosis*, most notably the W strain in New York and beyond (38). Two further examples suggest the value of studying genes encoding antibiotic resistance as clonal markers, even in the absence of evident antibiotic pressure.

In a search across 26 genes to determine the degree of genetic polymorphism observed within the *M. tuberculosis* complex, Sreevatsan et al. (39) found a strikingly low frequency of silent nucleotide substitution polymorphisms and two nonsynonymous polymorphisms that occur at high frequency. These latter polymorphisms are nucleotide substitutions in codon 463 of the *katG* gene and codon 95 of the *gyrA* gene, genes respectively encoding catalase-peroxidase and the A subunit of gyrase. Although these polymorphisms do not translate into isoniazid nor quinolone resistance, the observation that genes responsible for antibiotic resistance are naturally polymorphic suggests a role for these beyond that encountered in clinical practice. The use of these polymorphisms in predicting virulence is discussed later.

A second example of polymorphism in an antibiotic resistance gene is the natural occurrence of pyrazinamide-resistant strains. It has long been observed that isolates of *M. bovis* do not have pyrazinamidase activity, necessary to convert pyrazinamide to the active form, owing to a mutation at codon 57 in the *pncA* gene. That this occurs in animals not being treated with antimicrobials suggests that it occurred as part of the natural evolution of this species, at around the same time as the deletion of the RD4 region also missing from *M. bovis* strains (32). Recently, it has been observed that an important proportion of clinical isolates of *M. tuberculosis* from the province of Quebec, Canada manifest monopyrazinamide resistance due to the same 8-bp deletion within the *pncA* gene (40). Further analysis of this phenomenon reveals an epidemiologic pattern inconsistent with recent transmission in a low-incidence setting (less than 3 per 100,000) (41). Moreover, the introduction of pyrazinamide into routine clinical practice in Quebec dates to the 1980s because of low levels of antibiotic resistance, yet most of these patients are elderly persons suspected to be reactivating infections acquired earlier in the 20th century. This anecdote demonstrates that pyrazinamide resistance can occur spontaneously in the absence of drug pressure and does not appear to translate to a significant reduction in fitness. The applicability of this observation to other antibiotic resistance genes requires further study.

DIVERSITY IN GENES ENCODING ANTIGENS

One of the goals of current TB research is the development of a new vaccine, one that not only is protective in a variety of settings but performs equally against all circulating strains of *M. tuberculosis* that may be encountered. Thus, it follows that the antigenic diversity in clinical isolates must be established in order to predict the capacity of novel vaccine candidates to provide consistent protection. To date, the determination of antigenic diversity among clinical isolates is limited to one paper (7).

Calling upon a set of 16 strains selected for their genetic diversity and a random collection of 24 genes known or predicted to encode antigenic proteins, the authors performed targeted sequencing looking for synonymous and nonsynonymous single nucleotide polymorphisms. In contrast to the prominence of antigen-encoding genes in BCG deletions, polymorphisms in clinical isolates were remarkably rare. Specifically, 19 genes were invariant, and only six polymorphisms were detected in the remaining five genes examined. The authors conclude that these data support a recent global dissemination of *M. tuberculosis* and that these results should foster optimism in the development of a new vaccine. If additional studies across larger sample collections confirm these findings, a monovalent anti-TB vaccine could be envisioned.

TOWARD THE MOLECULAR CAUSE OF VIRULENCE

The other important phenotype at issue is bacterial "virulence," that is, the capacity of the strain to spread and cause disease. Since the era of molecular typing, anecdotal reports of strains appearing to be more virulent have proliferated (42–45). The converse phenotype, strains that despite all opportunities for spread are seen only once, has not knowingly been published, but a brief perusal of the San Francisco database provides highly suggestive anecdotes for this occurrence (Small PM, unpublished data, 1997). The evident difficulty with the interpretation of these reports is in accurately and prudently accounting for the many confounders that may cause variable spread (environment), variable attack rate (host immune status), and variable site of disease or infection. (For example, extrapulmonary predominance of *M. bovis* could be due to organism and/or intestinal site of inoculum.) One approach has been to compare responses to this and other isolates of *M. tuberculosis* in experimental settings, using inbred animals and controlled conditions, as was done to evaluate CDC1551 (42). This approach suffers from the major problems plaguing the validity of animal models but also depends on the phenotype under scrutiny. For instance, a strain described in humans to have increased virulence actually had a relatively normal attack rate among those infected but a very high rate of tuberculin conversions in contacts (high transmissibility) (42). The original report noted increased bacterial growth compared to a reference strain, but subsequently others have seen unremarkable growth but a greater induction of inflammatory cytokines (which may explain the high rate of tuberculin conversions) (46). From this example it would appear that using animal models to confirm epidemiologically remarkable strains is a promising avenue because certain properties of the strain are now amenable to controlled study. A further refinement may include subjecting a number of different control strains isolated from the same setting as the outbreak and transferring these different strains in a blinded manner to the same animal model to determine whether one isolate clearly stands apart from the others.

The alternative approach to study virulence has been to categorize the genetic diversity of bacteria within the context of a collection of epidemiologically defined isolates. This approach accepts that given a community of persons and isolates that have been circulating for a number of years, certain strains, or their attributes, may be over- or underrepresented in terms of clinical and epidemiologic variables. The responsible genomic differences then suggest polymorphisms in the genome that are either related to the property of interest or have coevolved with the genetic event that selects for the outcome observed. Typically, epidemiologically important outcomes include the appearance of large clusters of identical RFLP patterns, termed *clusters*, that suggest a chain of ongoing transmission. Clinical outcomes have received less attention and include, for example, the presence of cavitation on chest radiograph. The genetic tools for studying bacterial diversity are the same as described above for BCG, specifically interrogating isolates on arrays/chips for genomic deletions and targeted sequencing of known polymorphic genes.

The polymorphic genes most often studied include two nonsynonymous single nucleotide polymorphisms in katG and gyrA used to divide isolates into three principal genetic groups (39). Group 1, 2, and 3 isolates were not found to differ in terms of IS*6110* copy number, but group 3 isolates appeared less likely to present in an RFLP-defined cluster. This latter suggestion was subsequently tested using epidemiologically defined isolates from San Francisco. Again, isolates were categorized into the three principal genetic groups (47). These groups were compared for the propensity to fall within RFLP-defined clusters, and the proportion of contacts with tuberculous infection or tuberculosis disease. Although the San Francisco study failed to find an association between these outcomes and genetic groups, it did establish the feasibility of such an approach.

A more recent report exploited whole-genome comparisons by GeneChip to look for genomic deletions in clinical isolates collected from San Francisco. This study was driven by important aspects in both the field and the laboratory. The San Francisco molecular epidemiology study has been ongoing since 1992; therefore, it is now possible to exploit natural TB experiments in the field that include characterization not only of the public health scenario but also of the clinical presentation. In the laboratory, the use of GeneChip for genome typing had been previously validated against the H37Rv/CDC 1551 comparison and in detecting previously uncovered genomic deletions from BCG Pasteur (9). Thus, it was possible to assemble a collection of clones, some representing outbreak strains and some representing uniquely observed cases of reactivation disease, and explore the genome content of the responsible bacteria (48).

Among the observations made, isolates with shared RFLP patterns had the same deletion type, providing further evidence that genomic deletions can serve as clonal markers. On average, isolates lacked 2.7 deleted regions, representing 0.3% of the genome. Otherwise stated, in the typical isolate, 99.7% of the reference genome is present. Predictably, genomic regions lost in clinical isolates often encode mobile elements, such as phages and insertion elements (Table 6.2). In contrast, genes encoding information pathways were not deleted in clinical isolates, and only two genes encoding a predicted antigenic protein were among clinical deletions. This study failed to detect an association between the percentage of the genome deleted and either tuberculous infection or active TB in contacts. However, isolates with less genome deleted were more likely to be associated with cavitary disease on the chest radiograph, which may be considered both a marker of more severe pathology in this host and a more contagious form of TB. These findings remain to be confirmed in other settings and/or with larger collections of isolates.

TABLE 6.2. PREDICTED FUNCTION OF OPEN READING FRAMES DELETED FROM ONE OR MORE CIRCULATING CLONES OF *M. TUBERCULOSIS* IN SAN FRANCISCO STUDY BY KATO-MAEDA ET AL. (48), LISTED ACCORDING TO HIERARCHICAL GENE CLASSIFICATION PROPOSED BY COLE ET AL. (1)

Putative Function	Genes Deleted in Clinical Clones
Small-molecule metabolism (10 genes)	
Energy metabolism; TCA cycle	*Rv0794c*
Energy metabolism; miscellaneous oxidoreductases and oxygenases	*Rv0147, Rv3083, Rv3085*
Central intermediary metabolism; sugar nucleotides	*Rv1525*
Amino acid biosynthesis; aspartate family	*Rv2124c*
Polyketide and nonribosomal peptide synthesis	*Rv1527c*
Broad regulatory functions; repressors/activators	*Rv0144, Rv0792c, Rv0377*
Macromolecule metabolism (11 genes)	
Synthesis and modification of macromolecules; nucleoproteins	*Rv0143c*
Degradation of macromolecules; esterases and lipases	*Rv1755c, Rv2349c, Rv2350c, Rv2351c, Rv3084*
Cell envelope; surface polysaccharides, lipopolysaccharides, proteins, and antigens	*Rv1758, Rv1984c*
Cell envelope; other membrane proteins	*Rv3448, Rv3887c, Rv3901c*
Cell processes (1 gene)	
Detoxification	*Rv3617*
Other (43 genes)	
IS elements, repeated sequences, and phage; IS*6110*	*Rv1763, Rv1764, Rv2648, Rv2649, Rv2814c, Rv2815c*
IS elements, repeated sequences, and phage; IS elements; others	*Rv3427c, Rv3428c*
IS elements, repeated sequences, and phage; phage-related functions	*Rv1573, Rv1574, Rv1575, Rv1576c, Rv1577c, Rv1578c, Rv1579c, Rv1580c, Rv1581c, Rv1582c, Rv1583c, Rv1584c, Rv1585c, Rv1586c, Rv2646, Rv2647, Rv2650c, Rv2651c, Rv2652c, Rv2653c, Rv2654c, Rv2655c, Rv2656c, Rv2657c, Rv2658c, Rv2659c*
PE and PPE families; PE-PGRS subfamily	*Rv1983*
PE and PPE families; PPE family	*Rv2352c, Rv3425, Rv3426, Rv3429, Rv2123*
Cytochrome P450 enzymes	*Rv3518c*
Miscellaneous transferases	*Rv1524, Rv1526c*
Conserved hypotheticals (15 genes)	
Conserved hypotheticals	*Rv0146, Rv0145, Rv0376c, Rv0378, Rv0793, Rv1754c, Rv1760, Rv1765c, Rv2314c, Rv2406c, Rv2407, Rv2415c, Rv3767c, Rv3769, Rv3888c*
Unknown (12 genes)	
Unknowns	*Rv1179c, Rv1761c, Rv1762c, Rv2313c, Rv2645c, Rv2660c, Rv3519c, Rv3766c, Rv3768c, Rv3889c, Rv3902c, Rv3903c*

TCA, triarboxylic acid; IS, insertion sequence; PE, Pro-Glu; PPE, Pro-Pro-Glu; PGRS, polymorphic GC-rich repetitive sequence.

LIMITATIONS

In the study of *M. tuberculosis* complex genetic diversity, the limitations may be categorized as technical or biologic. It is the author's contention that the latter will be more formidable.

The current tools to explore genetic diversity are vastly improved from a decade ago when investigators were essentially working in the dark. With the complete genome sequence of H37Rv serving as a scaffold, one can easily design primers to amplify and sequence any gene of interest across whatever collection of isolates is at hand. Moreover, the tools for genomic comparison are becoming increasingly powerful, so while the current GeneChips are capable of screening for genomic deletions of a few hundred base pairs, the technology exists to design newer iterations of such chips to scan for even smaller regions of difference. In theory, one would be delighted to be able to determine the entire genome sequence of all interesting isolates, but there are clearly time and cost issues that limit this approach. Nonetheless, using existing tools, the ability to detect small genetic differences among closely related strains is at hand.

More important than technical issues are the biologic issues regarding samples, biases, and interpretation of genomic information pertaining to these samples. Unlike the study of BCG vaccines, the study of circulating isolates is restricted because of both the host–pathogen biology and potential biases introduced in the laboratory. For instance, the majority of persons infected with *M. tuberculosis* do not develop active tuberculosis, so that only bacteria that cause disease are available for study. Furthermore, it is theoretically possible that a number of different bacteria coexist in the same host (49). Currently, these may be overlooked if one clone outcompetes the others, either to cause disease in the host or during growth in the laboratory (50). While either scenario may theoretically result in a restricted analysis, to date such reports are anecdotal in the face of large molecular epidemiologic studies, suggesting that these are rare occurrences rather than important events.

A more important issue is whether isolates studied come with well-defined phenotypes and sufficient data to measure the impact of potential confounders. Through molecular epidemiologic projects, there are now a number of strain collections that are readily amenable to study. The challenge will be to go beyond describing the genetic variability within these collections to drawing a direct link between genetic variant and a phenotypic outcome, usually a form of disease in the host. Tuberculosis can be envisioned as a dysfunctional interaction of two genomes under the influence of environmental confounders and host modifiers acquired in his or her environment. As promising as the opportunities are, the failure to carefully consider sampling issues in selection of isolates and potential confounders in the analysis of results will likely be the most important stumbling block to understanding the implications and relevance of genetic diversity in *M. tuberculosis*.

CONCLUDING THOUGHTS AND FUTURE DIRECTIONS

With the advent of increasing powerful tools to explore the genome of pathogenic and attenuated strains, it is now possible to better estimate the degree of genetic diversity and begin to explore the impact of these genetic differences on important phenotypes. With this capacity, some major questions still at large can be addressed, including: Why is *M. tuberculosis* virulent and BCG attenuated? Is *M. tuberculosis* antigenically homogeneous? Are certain strains more likely to cause disease, and by inference, better targets for preventive interventions? Are certain strains more likely to cause disease in hosts with specific genetic predispositions? In both BCG vaccines and clinical isolates, the vast majority of the genome is conserved. Despite the numerous deletions incurred by BCG Pasteur over several decades in the laboratory, the current genome can be estimated to present >99% of the *M. bovis* genome from which it was derived. Likewise, clinical isolates have on average 99.7% of the genome conserved. Other sources of genetic polymorphism have now been uncovered, including duplications in BCG vaccines, single nucleotide polymorphisms among *M. tuberculosis* isolates, and genomic rearrangements as documented in the comparison of the completed sequences of H37Rv and CDC 1551. Despite the infrequency of genetic differences, across a genome of 4 million base pairs, there are still sufficient genetic candidates to explore the described phenotypic variations detailed above. From this, it is hoped that a better understanding of how *M. tuberculosis* causes disease will emerge and the necessary tools towards the control of this epidemic can be developed.

ACKNOWLEDGMENTS

Work by the author is funded by the Canadian Institutes for Health Research, of which the author is a New Investigator, and the Sequella Global Tuberculosis Foundation, of which the author is a Core Scientist. The author gratefully acknowledges the considerable assistance of Serge Mostowy and Dao Nguyen for their input in preparing this chapter.

REFERENCES

1. Cole ST, Brosch R, Parkhill J, et al. Deciphering the biology of *Mycobacterium tuberculosis* from the complete genome sequence. *Nature* 1998; 393:537–544.
2. www.sanger.ac.uk/m_tuberculosis.
3. http://www.tigr.org/tigr-scripts/CMR2/GenomePage3. spl? database=gmt.
4. www.sanger.ac.uk/m_bovis.
5. Fraser CM, Eisen J, Fleischmann RD, et al. Comparative genomics and understanding of microbial biology. *Emerg Infect Dis* 2000;6:505–512.
6. Behr MA, Schroeder BG, Brinkman JN, et al. A point mutation in the mma3 gene is responsible for impaired methoxymycolic acid production in *Mycobacterium bovis* BCG strains obtained after 1927. *J Bacteriol* 2000;182:3394–3399.
7. Musser JM, Amin A, Ramaswamy S. Negligible genetic diversity of *Mycobacterium tuberculosis* host immune system protein targets: evidence of limited selective pressure. *Genetics* 2000;155: 7–16.
8. Behr MA, Wilson MA, Gill WP, et al. Comparative genomics of BCG vaccines by whole-genome DNA microarray. *Science* 1999; 284:1520–1523.
9. Salamon H, Kato-Maeda M, Small PM, et al. Detection of deleted genomic DNA using a semiautomated computational analysis of GeneChip data. *Genome Res* 2000;10:2044–2054.
10. Calmette, A. Preventive vaccination against tuberculosis with BCG. *Proc R Soc Med* 1931;24:85–94.
11. Jensen KA. Practice of the Calmette vaccination. *Acta Tuberc Scand* 1946;20:1–45.
12. Behr MA, Small PM. A historical and molecular phylogeny of BCG strains. *Vaccine* 1999;17:915–922.
13. Casanova JL, Blanche S, Emile JF, et al. Idiopathic disseminated bacillus Calmette–Guérin infection: a French national retrospective study. *Pediatrics* 1996;98:774–778.
14. Floyd MM, Silcox VA, Jones WD Jr, et al. Separation of *Mycobacterium bovis* BCG from *Mycobacterium tuberculosis* and *Mycobacterium bovis* by using high-performance liquid chromatography of mycolic acids. *J Clin Microbiol* 1992;30: 1327–1330.
15. Minnikin DE, Parlett JH, Magnusson M, et al. Mycolic acid patterns of representatives of *Mycobacterium bovis* BCG. *J Gen Microbiol* 1984;130:2733–6273.
16. Harboe M, Nagai S, Patarroyo ME, et al. Properties of proteins MPB64, MPB70, and MPB80 of *Mycobacterium bovis* BCG. *Infect Immun* 1986;52:293–302.
17. Dubos RJ, Pierce CH: Differential characteristics *in vitro* and *in vivo* of several substrains of BCG. IV. Immunizing effectiveness. *Am Rev Tuberc Pulm Dis* 1956;74:699–717.
18. Lagranderie MR, Balazuc AM, Deriaud E, et al. Comparison of immune responses of mice immunized with five different *Mycobacterium bovis* BCG vaccine strains. *Infect Immun* 1996;64: 1–9.

19. Mahairas GG, Sabo PJ, Hickey MJ, et al. Molecular analysis of genetic differences between *Mycobacterium bovis* BCG and virulent *M. bovis*. *J Bacteriol* 1996;178:1274–1282.

20. Gordon SV, Brosch R, Billault A, et al. Identification of variable regions in the genomes of tubercle bacilli using bacterial artificial chromosome arrays. *Mol Microbiol* 1999;32:643–655.

21. Brosch R, Gordon SV, Buchrieser C, et al. Comparative genomics uncovers large tandem chromosomal duplications in *Mycobacterium bovis* BCG Pasteur. *Yeast* 2000;17:111–123.

22. Mostowy S, Tsolaki AG, Small PM, et al. Genomic events which define BCG vaccines. 02-GM-A-2480, American Society of Microbiology 102nd General Meeting, May 19–23, 2002, Salt Lake City.

23. http://www.pasteur.fr/recherche/unites/Lgmb/mycogenomics.html

24. Li H, Ulstrup JC, Jonassen TO, et al. Evidence for absence of the MPB64 gene in some substrains of *Mycobacterium bovis* BCG. *Infect Immun* 1993;61:1730–1734.

25. Talbot EA, Williams DL, Frothingham R. PCR identification of *Mycobacterium bovis* BCG. *J Clin Microbiol* 1997;35:566–569.

26. Arend SM, Geluk A, van Meijgaarden KE, et al. Antigenic equivalence of human T-cell responses to *Mycobacterium tuberculosis*–specific RD1-encoded protein antigens ESAT-6 and culture filtrate protein 10 and to mixtures of synthetic peptides. *Infect Immun* 2000;68:3314–3321.

27. Lewis KN, Liao R, Guinn KM, et al. Deletion of RD1 from *M. tuberculosis* mimics bacille Calmette–Guérin attenuation. *J Infect Dis* 2003;187:117–123.

28. Wiker HG, Nagai S, Hewinson RG, et al. Heterogenous expression of the related MPB70 and MPB83 proteins distinguish various substrains of *Mycobacterium bovis* BCG and *Mycobacterium tuberculosis* H37Rv. *Scand J Immunol* 1996;43:374–380.

29. Kapur V, Whittam TS, Musser JM. Is *Mycobacterium tuberculosis* 15,000 years old? *J Infect Dis* 1994;170:1348–1349.

30. Smith T. A comparative study of bovine tubercle bacilli and of human bacilli from sputum. *J Exp Med* 1898 3:451–511.

31. Hoffner SE, Svenson SB, Norberg R, et al. Biochemical heterogeneity of *Mycobacterium tuberculosis* complex isolates in Guinea-Bissau. *J Clin Microbiol* 1993;31:2215–2217.

32. Brosch R, Gordon SV, Marmiesse M, et al. A new evolutionary scenario for the *Mycobacterium tuberculosis* complex. *Proc Natl Acad Sci U S A* 2002;99:3684–3689.

33. Mostowy S, Cousins D, Brinkman J, et al. Genomic deletions suggest a phylogeny for the *Mycobacterium tuberculosis* complex. *J Infect Dis* 2002;186:74–80.

34. Pfyffer GE, Auckenthaler R, van Embden JD, et al. *Mycobacterium canettii*, the smooth variant of *M. tuberculosis*, isolated from a Swiss patient exposed in Africa. *Emerg Infect Dis* 1998;4: 631–634.

35. Parsons LM, Brosch R, Cole ST, et al. Rapid and simple approach for identification of *Mycobacterium tuberculosis* complex isolates by PCR-based genomic deletion analysis. *J Clin Microbiol* 2002;40:2339–2345.

36. Mdluli K, Slayden RA, Zhu Y, et al. Inhibition of a *Mycobacterium tuberculosis* beta-ketoacyl ACP synthase by isoniazid. *Science* 1998;280:1607–1610.

37. Scorpio A, Zhang Y. Mutations in pncA, a gene encoding pyrazinamidase/nicotinamidase, cause resistance to the antituberculous drug pyrazinamide in tubercle bacillus. *Nat Med* 1996;2: 662–667.

38. Bifani PJ, Plikaytis BB, Kapur V, et al. Origin and interstate spread of a New York City multidrug-resistant *Mycobacterium tuberculosis* clone family. *JAMA* 1996;275:452–457.

39. Sreevatsan S, Pan X, Stockbauer KE, et al. Restricted structural gene polymorphism in the *Mycobacterium tuberculosis* complex indicates evolutionarily recent global dissemination. *Proc Natl Acad Sci U S A* 1997;94:9869–9874.

40. Cheng SJ, Thibert L, Sanchez T, et al. pncA mutations as a major mechanism of pyrazinamide resistance in *Mycobacterium tuberculosis*: spread of a monoresistant strain in Quebec, Canada. *Antimicrob Agents Chemother* 2000;44:528–532.

41. Nguyen D, Westley J, Gatewood A, et al. Molecular Characterization Of PZA Resistant M. tuberculosis Strains In Quebec. Abstract LB2, Poster: D21, 98th International Conference of the American Thoracic Society, May 17–22, 2002.

42. Valway SE, Sanchez MP, Shinnick TF, et al. An outbreak involving extensive transmission of a virulent strain of *Mycobacterium tuberculosis*. *N Engl J Med* 1998;338:633–639.

43. Friedman CR, Quinn GC, Kreiswirth BN, et al. Widespread dissemination of a drug-susceptible strain of *Mycobacterium tuberculosis*. *J Infect Dis* 1997;176:478–484.

44. Zhang M, Gong J, Yang Z, et al. Enhanced capacity of a widespread strain of *Mycobacterium tuberculosis* to grow in human macrophages. *J Infect Dis* 1999;179:1213–1217.

45. Caminero JA, Pena MJ, Campos-Herrero MI, et al. Epidemiological evidence of the spread of a *Mycobacterium tuberculosis* strain of the Beijing genotype on Gran Canaria Island. *Am J Respir Crit Care Med* 2001;164:1165–1170.

46. Manca C, Tsenova L, Barry CE III, et al. *Mycobacterium tuberculosis* CDC1551 induces a more vigorous host response *in vivo* and *in vitro*, but is not more virulent than other clinical isolates. *J Immunol* 1999;162:6740–6746.

47. Rhee JT, Piatek AS, Small PM, et al. Molecular epidemiologic evaluation of transmissibility and virulence of *Mycobacterium tuberculosis*. *J Clin Microbiol* 1999;37:1764–1770.

48. Kato-Maeda M, Rhee JT, Gingeras TR, et al. Comparing genomes within the species *Mycobacterium tuberculosis*. *Genome Res* 2001;11:547–554.

49. du Plessis DG, Warren R, Richardson M, et al. Demonstration of reinfection and reactivation in HIV-negative autopsied cases of secondary tuberculosis: multilesional genotyping of *Mycobacterium tuberculosis* utilizing IS*6110* and other repetitive element-based DNA fingerprinting. *Tuberculosis (Edinb)* 2001;81:211–220.

50. Yeh RW, Hopewell PC, Daley CL. Simultaneous infection with two strains of *Mycobacterium tuberculosis* identified by restriction fragment length polymorphism analysis. *Int J Tuberc Lung Dis* 1999;3:537–539.

TUBERCULOSIS LATENCY IN HUMANS

CHARLES L. DALEY

The primary complex may indeed heal completely as such, thereby showing the highest conceivable degree of resistance to the disease. In a large number of cases, however, the healing of the primary complex remains no complete one. Rather, it is incomplete in that it goes over from its active stage only into one of latency.

Anton Ghon, 1923

Mycobacterium tuberculosis possesses the ability to remain quiescent for long periods, "reactivating" years later to produce clinical disease. This property of the tubercle bacillus produces both obstacles and opportunities for tuberculosis control. Because latent tuberculosis infection (LTBI) remains clinically silent, it can only be detected through the use of tuberculin skin testing or the QuantiFERON-TB test (Cellestis Ltd., Carnegie, Victoria, Australia). Screening of large populations is both economically and practically difficult, so that many infected individuals are not identified prior to their developing active tuberculosis disease. However, once identified, these individuals provide an opportunity to halt the progression to disease and thus interrupt the cycle of transmission. As the incidence of tuberculosis declines in the United States and other industrialized nations, identification and treatment of LTBI will become an even more important strategy in our efforts to control and eventually eliminate tuberculosis. This chapter will review the current evidence supporting the concept of clinical latency and the risk factors that are known to result in progression of LTBI to tuberculosis disease.

DEFINITION OF LATENCY

Latency can be viewed as an equilibrium that exists between host and organism. LTBI is a clinical syndrome that occurs after an individual has been exposed to *M. tuberculosis*, the

infection has been established, and an immune response develops to control the pathogen resulting in a quiescent state (1). Whether or not *M. tuberculosis* can develop a state of true latency or dormancy in which no metabolic activity can be detected is still uncertain. However, there are a great deal of pathologic, epidemiologic, and clinical data that demonstrate conclusively that latency does occur clinically. Thus, the term latency, as used in this chapter, will refer to the clinical condition wherein a person with tuberculous infection has no clinical or microbiologic evidence of tuberculosis disease.

EVIDENCE FOR LATENT TUBERCULOSIS

Despite decades of investigation into the pathogenesis of tuberculosis, little is known about the location and state of *M. tuberculosis* in latently infected individuals (1). Nevertheless, in our current model of the pathogenesis of tuberculosis, clinical latency plays a very important role. What follows is a review of the evidence that has accumulated over the past century that supports the concept of latent tuberculosis.

Pathologic Evidence for Latency

Investigations conducted in the early part of the 20th century demonstrated that postmortem tissues from humans who were asymptomatic showed evidence of viable *M. tuberculosis* (2–7). Not long after the identification of the tubercle bacillus by Koch, investigators began to report the isolation of viable *M. tuberculosis* in grossly normal and, in some cases, microscopically normal lymph nodes from apparently nontuberculous patients (2,3). For example, in 1890 Loomis (2) reported that eight of 30 patients who died from nontuberculous causes had evidence of tubercle bacilli by animal inoculation. Most of the studies examined either bronchial, mesenteric, or cervical lymph nodes and noted that approximately 12% of those examined grew *M. tuberculosis* or, in some cases, *M. bovis* (3). Thus, there was evidence that the organism could persist in the granuloma-

C. L. Daley: Department of Medicine, University of California at San Francisco; Chest Clinic, Division of Pulmonary and Critical Care Medicine, San Francisco General Hospital, San Francisco, California.

tous lesion in humans for many years, leading to the phrase, "Once infected, always infected" (4).

Subsequent investigators attempted to determine in which type of pulmonary lesions mycobacteria could be identified. In 1907, Rabinowitsch (6) reported viable tubercle bacilli in nearly one half of calcified lesions and in nearly two thirds of nodules with chalk-like contents. In 1927, Opie and Aronson (7) evaluated healed lesions to see if they contained viable mycobacteria. Material from 169 bodies was examined and found to be culture positive in guinea pig inoculations in 30% of the cases; in 45% of cases mycobacteria could be obtained in "normal" lung tissue. Latent fibrocaseous lesions in the pulmonary apex grew *M. tuberculosis* in most instances examined, and the fibrous scars in the apex grew *M. tuberculosis* in about 25% of the cases, even when there was no gross or histologic evidence of disease. Calcified nodules seldom grew *M. tuberculosis.*

Adding to the mystery of latency was the fact that in some cases acid-fast bacilli could be identified in surgical specimens, but no mycobacteria grew in culture (8,9). Medlar et al. (8) examined surgically removed lung tissue from 72 patients. Acid-fast bacilli were identified in 73% of the specimens but growth of *M. tuberculosis* was detected in only 20%. This finding led to debates about whether or not the organisms were simply dead or perhaps viable but not culturable (persistent). Hobby and associates evaluated 31 necrotic lesions that were surgically resected from 19 patients and demonstrated growth of *M. tuberculosis* in 15 patients using liquid cultures (9). Unlike previous investigators, they held the cultures for a prolonged time and noted that in nine cases it took 63 days of incubation for growth to be detected. Thus, the organisms were present but only in very low numbers or in an altered metabolic state.

Epidemiologic and Clinical Evidence for Latency

Latent tuberculosis infection most often is identified clinically by detection of a delayed-type hypersensitivity reaction to intradermal injection of purified protein derivative (PPD) (10). As proof of latency, persons with a positive tuberculin skin test (TST) should be more likely to progress to tuberculosis than those who are nonreactors. Epidemiologic studies have demonstrated the usefulness of the TST by noting that persons with a positive skin test result are more likely to develop tuberculosis disease than those with a negative skin test reaction. In a study of naval recruits from the 1950s, it was demonstrated that tuberculosis morbidity was five times higher in young men with definitely positive reactions to the 5 tuberculin unit (TU) test compared with nonreactors (11). Morbidity rates were 157 per 100,000 per year for the positive reactors compared with 29 per 100,000 per year for the nonreactors. Similarly, Ferebee and Palmer (12) and Grzybowski (13,14) estimated that the

risk of developing tuberculosis among reactors was three to five times greater than that among nonreactors.

A positive reaction to intradermal PPD injection indicates that a person has an increased probability of being infected with *M. tuberculosis* compared with someone who has a negative skin test reaction. Clinically, the diagnosis of LTBI is defined as the presence of a positive TST reaction in someone who is asymptomatic and who has no microbiologic evidence of tuberculosis. In most cases the chest radiograph is normal, but in some individuals there may be apical fibrotic opacities consistent with old, healed tuberculosis. If viable tubercle bacilli are present in the body of persons with positive tuberculin reactions, then the use of drugs that kill viable bacilli should reduce the subsequent risk of developing tuberculosis. Numerous clinical trials investigating the treatment of latent infection have been conducted, and the evidence is overwhelming that such treatment significantly reduces the subsequent risk of tuberculosis (15).

Although these clinical trials indirectly demonstrated the presence of latent infection, they also raised questions regarding the mechanisms by which *M. tuberculosis* establishes latent infection. How does isoniazid, which kills live replicating extracellular organisms, kill *M. tuberculosis* in the human host? If the organisms are metabolically inactive, how does isoniazid therapy reduce the risk of progression to tuberculosis? Although these questions continue to foster active investigation, to date actual mechanisms of latency are incompletely understood.

PATHOGENESIS OF TUBERCULOSIS

Tuberculosis can develop through progression of recently acquired infection (primary disease), reactivation of latent infection, or exogenous reinfection. After *M. tuberculosis* is inhaled into the lower respiratory tract, ingested by alveolar macrophages, and the patient becomes infected, a series of immunologic events occur. The results of this early immune response dictate whether the infected individual eradicates the infection, becomes latently infected, or develops progressive primary disease. In approximately 3% to 10% of individuals, the primary infection is not contained and the person develops clinically evident primary tuberculosis (16). However, most individuals are able to contain the primary infection (17), which often results in calcified lesions at the initial site of infection called Ghon lesions (18). As noted previously, these lesions typically do not contain viable bacilli (7). In other individuals, parenchymal abnormalities develop in the apices of the lung and are referred to as Simon foci (19). These lesions are more likely to contain viable bacilli than calcified lesions and thus are more likely to lead to postprimary tuberculosis.

After the primary infection is contained, subsequent perturbations in the immune system can result in "reactiva-

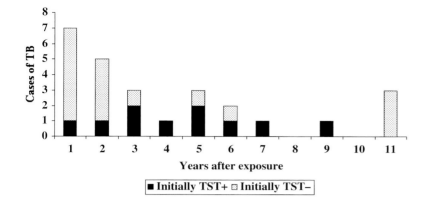

FIGURE 7.1. Time to development of tuberculosis among girls exposed to a teacher with infectious tuberculosis. Girls who were initially tuberculin skin test (*TST*) negative developed tuberculosis soon after the exposure and then the number of cases decreased during the follow-up period. Girls who were initially TST positive developed tuberculosis sporadically throughout the follow-up period (25).

tion" of *M. tuberculosis*, resulting in clinically active disease. For much of the early part of the 20th century, whether tuberculosis resulted from endogenous as opposed to exogenous reinfection was hotly debated (20–22). Stead, in his classic review, argued that endogenous activation of latent infection was the most common pathway to active tuberculosis in adults (23–25). Based on astute observations of previous work, he noted that (a) tuberculosis in tuberculin-negative persons developed in proportion to exposure; (b) among heavily exposed subjects, those with positive TSTs developed less disease than the nonreactors; and (c) among tuberculin reactors, the development of postprimary tuberculosis did not appear to be influenced by reexposure. An outbreak of tuberculosis at a school's girl was used to argue these points (25,26) (Fig. 7.1). As can be seen in the figure, the majority of cases of tuberculosis in the initially tuberculin-negative girls occurred soon after the exposure and then declined over the 12 years of follow-up. However, among the initially tuberculin-positive girls who were exposed, tuberculosis developed sporadically during the ensuing years; not affected by the exposure, the girls were developing tuberculosis as a result of endogenous reactivation of latent infection rather than exogenous infection.

In the recent past it was estimated that approximately 90% of adult cases of tuberculosis were the result of endogenous reactivation of latent infection (27). More recently, with the aid of molecular genotyping, the proportion of reactivated cases is thought to be approximately 60% to 70%, with 30% to 40% of the cases resulting from recent infections (27,28). However, this proportion has been shown to vary significantly depending on the amount of ongoing transmission within a population. Exogenous reinfection has been demonstrated in both human immunodeficiency virus (HIV)–infected (29) and uninfected populations (30,31), but the true frequency with which reinfection causes a first episode of tuberculosis is completely unknown.

The arguments offered by Stead and others for endogenous reinfection were largely circumstantial in nature but convincing nonetheless. Today most authorities believe that

adult forms of tuberculosis are usually the result of reactivation of latent infection acquired previously. Little is known about the signals that cause *M. tuberculosis* to begin to actively replicate, but an understanding of these mechanisms is critical to the understanding of the pathogenesis of tuberculosis. Several factors have been shown to alter the course of tuberculosis, increasing the risk of progression to active disease (10). These factors will be reviewed below.

FACTORS ASSOCIATED WITH PROGRESSION TO TUBERCULOSIS DISEASE

Risk of Primary Tuberculosis Disease After Infection

The risk of developing tuberculosis is greatest soon after infection with *M. tuberculosis*. In studies performed by the U.S. Public Health Service (UHPHS) between 1950 and 1970, the incidence rate of tuberculosis disease among household contacts decreased with time from infection (15,32). Among untreated tuberculosis-infected household contacts, tuberculosis disease occurred at a rate of 0.74% per year in years 1 and 2 after exposure, 0.31% per year in years 3 through 5, and 0.16% per year in years 6 and 7. In two placebo-controlled clinical trials evaluating the use of isoniazid in the United States, 1,472 persons who were allocated to the placebo arm converted their TST during the first year of the study (15). During a 7-year follow-up period, 29 patients developed tuberculosis disease, of which 64% occurred within a year of infection. Twenty-two percent developed tuberculosis disease during the next 3 years and 13% during the last 3 years.

The age at which infection occurs is associated with a differential risk for progression to tuberculosis disease. Among tuberculin reactors in the USPHS household contact study described above, the risk of tuberculosis varied with age. Compared to the risk at ages 5 to 14 (the group with the lowest incidence), the relative risk of primary disease for those aged 0 to 4 years was 4.8 (1.8 to 12.9), whereas for those aged 15 to 29 it was 5.0 (2.4 to 10.4), for those 30 to 44 it was 4.1 (1.8 to 9.0), and for those 45 or older it was 2.0 (0.8 to 5.0) (15,32). The incidence of tuberculosis among tuberculin reactors by age was described in a bacille Calmette–Guérin (BCG) trial from Puerto Rico (33). Among 82,269 tuberculin reactors aged 1 to 18 years who were followed for 18 to 20 years, 1,400 cases of tuberculosis occurred. There were two peaks in the incidence, one among children aged 1 to 4 years and the second during early adolescence and early adulthood. The higher incidence in early childhood and infancy is likely related to the fact that these represent recent infections. The reason for the higher incidence in adolescence is unknown.

The size of the TST has been associated with the risk of progression to primary disease. In a USPHS study, the risk of progression increased with each 5-mm increment in the size of the TST. Compared to the risk with a skin test having 5 to 9 mm induration, the risk increased when skin test size was 10 to 14 mm [(rate ratio (RR) 1.84, 0.78–4.36]; the risk increased further when the skin test was 15 to 19 mm (RR 1.94, 0.76–4.92) and was greatest when the skin test was 20 mm or more (RR 3.87, 1.58–9.48) (15). In the study from Puerto Rico described earlier, children with reactions measuring 16 mm or more in diameter to 1 TU of PPD had a subsequent risk of tuberculosis disease over five times greater than children with reactions of 6 to 10 mm following a test with 10 TU of PPD (33). It is not known if the increasing risk with increasing skin test size is due to an increased risk of progression or a greater likelihood that tuberculosis infection is present. In the latter circumstance, because smaller size reactions may be due to false-positive TST results, it is possible that the larger sizes are more likely to represent true infection.

Most patients who become infected with *M. tuberculosis* are able to control the infection. However, individuals whose immune system is impaired are less likely to be able to control the initial infection and are thus more likely to progress to tuberculosis disease. HIV-infected persons represent one such population, and there are numerous examples of high rates of primary tuberculosis in these patients (34,35). In an outbreak in a residential care facility for persons with HIV infection, 11 of 15 (60%) persons developed tuberculosis within 2 years, compared with none of the staff (34).

Risk of Reactivation (Postprimary) Tuberculosis Disease

The risk of progressing to tuberculosis disease decreases with time from exposure, as noted above. However, the risk of developing tuberculosis persists at a lower level, presumably indefinitely in latently infected individuals. Incidence rates of reactivation disease have been inferred from studies that have followed prevalent infected persons over time. Depending on the design of the study, newly infected per-

sons may be mixed with remotely infected individuals, falsely elevating the risk of progression. Therefore, studies that begin follow-up soon after exposure, such as studies of contacts, make it easier to identify the incidence of tuberculosis later in life. As noted previously, the rate of reactivation disease among household contacts 6 or more years after exposure was 0.16% per year, significantly lower than the rate soon after infection (15). In addition, a population that is screened and followed over time and in which transmission/exposure is limited is also a good population to follow to establish a baseline rate of tuberculosis. In a study of naval recruits who were skin tested upon admission to the service, the rate of tuberculosis disease among persons with skin tests of 10 mm or more at entry was also 0.16% per year (9). The overall rate of tuberculosis disease among patients in a psychiatric hospital who had positive TST and were followed for 10 years was 0.12% per year (15). These studies have helped to determine a baseline incidence of reactivation after the initial high-risk period.

Certain risk factors have been demonstrated to increase the risk of progression to tuberculosis disease above that described previously. These risk factors will be discussed below. It is important to point out that in many studies it is difficult to determine if the populations were more easily infected and/or had a higher risk of progressing to tuberculosis disease. However, it is generally believed that for most

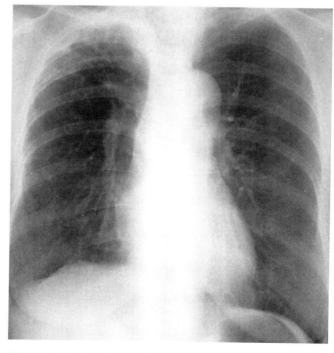

FIGURE 7.2. The chest radiograph demonstrates right upper lobe fibrotic opacities with superior retraction of the right hilum and elevation of the right hemidiaphragm, consistent with volume loss. The patient was asymptomatic and had three negative mycobacterial sputum cultures.

populations the risk of progressing to tuberculosis disease is higher than that in persons without these risk factors. Recent studies have documented that host genetic factors can play an important role in determining who develops tuberculosis, and these factors will be discussed in subsequent chapters.

Fibrotic, Inactive Radiographic Lesions

Individuals who have fibrotic lesions on a chest radiograph consistent with prior healed tuberculosis (Fig. 7.2) have been shown to have an increased risk of progression to tuberculosis disease compared with persons who have normal (or minimally abnormal) chest radiographs. Prior to the availability of isoniazid, it was noted that individuals who developed postprimary tuberculosis as an adult often had apical fibrotic lesions on prior chest radiographs (25). These observations led to both retrospective and prospective studies to determine the risk of developing tuberculosis

in persons with these chest radiographic findings (Table 7.1). In 1969, Horwitz (36) reported that the incidence of tuberculosis in patients whose disease had "arrested" was 130 per 10,000 persons per year, approximately 30-fold higher than in the general population. In a USPHS study in psychiatric hospitals, it was noted that tuberculin-positive persons with fibrotic residua on the chest radiograph developed tuberculosis over a 10-year period at the rate of 36 per 1,000 persons (0.36% per year), compared with 6.9 per 1,000 persons (0.069% per year) in those with normal chest radiographs (including only calcifications) (15) (Fig. 7.3).

In British Columbia, the incidence of tuberculosis in patients with "healed primary complex" was 6.7 per 10,000 per year, which was similar to the rate in patients with abnormalities unrelated to tuberculosis (rate of 2.6 to 8.4 per 10,000 per year) (14). The estimated incidence rate of tuberculosis in tuberculin reactors at the time was around 5.1 per 100,000 per year. On the other hand, the rate of tuberculosis among persons with "apical scarring" was 21.5

TABLE 7.1. INCIDENCE OF TUBERCULOSIS AMONG PERSONS WITH FIBROTIC ABNORMALITIES ON THE CHEST RADIOGRAPH

Study	Population	N	Total Cases of TB	Annual Rate Per 1,000
Natural History Studies				
Gryzbowski, 1971	Inactive TB	10,784		
	"Good chemotherapy"[a]	6,427	76 (53)[b]	2.4 (1.7)[b]
	"Poor chemotherapy"	1,542	86 (61)	11.1 (7.9)
	"No chemotherapy"	2,815	180 (129)	12.8 (9.2)
	Presumed TB, inactive	10,469		
	No previous active disease	5,531	111 (78)	4.0 (2.8)
	"Apical scarring"	4,938	60 (53)	2.4 (2.2)
	Healed primary complex	7,424	26 (25)	0.67 (0.67)
	Old pleurisy	6,413	24 (18)	0.75 (0.56)
	Probably unrelated to TB	13,853	59 (55)	0.85 (0.79)
Nakielna, 1975	Inactive TB	14,552		
	"Good chemotherapy"[a]	8,801	59	2.2
	"Poor chemotherapy"	1,923	45	7.8
	"No chemotherapy"	3,828	77	6.7
Clinical Trials				
Katz, 1965	Inactive TB, placebo group	266		
	Never active	107	10	43.0[c]
	Previously active	159	39	63.0
Ferebee, 1970	Inactive TB, placebo group	1,415		
	Never active	714	49	16.8[c]
	Previously active untreated	286	14	10.5
	Previously active treated	1,060	35	7.1
Falk, 1978	Inactive TB, placebo group	2,314		
	"Good chemotherapy"[a]	944	6	6.4[d]
	"Poor chemotherapy"	598	5	8.3
	"No chemotherapy"	772	15	19.4
IUAT, 1982	Inactive TB, placebo group	6,795		
	<2 cm^2	4,701	53	11.6[d]
	≥2 cm^2	2,094	43	21.3

[a]"Good chemotherapy"—history of >12 mo of at least two drugs, one drug being isoniazid; "poor chemotherapy"—history of <12 mo of two drugs or longer without isoniazid.
[b]Numbers in parentheses are culture confirmed.
[c]Annual rate per 1,000 over 2-year midpoint of study.
[d]Rate per 1,000 over entire study.
IUAT, International Union Against Tuberculosis; TB, tuberculosis.

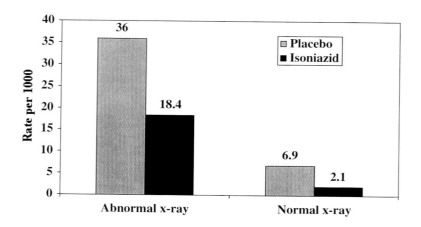

FIGURE 7.3. Ten-year morbidity from tuberculosis among initial tuberculin reactors and converters, classified by radiographic findings on entry into U.S. Public Health Service study in psychiatric hospitals (15,38).

per 10,000 per year; in those classified as inactive tuberculosis with previous active episode, the rate was 28.2 per 10,000; and among patients who had previous active disease but had received no therapy, the rate was 91.7 per 10,000. In a similar study, among 14,552 persons with "inactive tuberculosis" who were followed for 3 years in British Columbia, there were 6.7 cases of tuberculosis per 1,000 persons per year in those individuals who had never been treated (37). This rate was three times higher than that seen in persons who had received adequate chemotherapy in the past (2.2 cases per 1,000 persons per year) and similar to the rate of those who had not received adequate therapy (7.8 cases per 1,000 persons per year).

Although the rates of tuberculosis differed between studies, the incidence among those with evidence of inactive disease on the chest radiograph was higher than in those with normal or minimally abnormal radiographs. These findings led to several randomized clinical trials evaluating the use of isoniazid for preventing the progression to tuberculosis disease in persons with fibrotic, inactive tuberculosis. By evaluating the placebo arm of these studies we can gain further insight into the rates of tuberculosis among persons with fibrotic lesions on the chest radiograph.

Among 1,414 participants with fibrotic radiographic abnormalities in a USPHS clinical trial involving 27 cooperating health departments, the incidence of tuberculosis among persons in the placebo arm was 20 per 1,000 during the treatment year, decreasing to an average of less than 8 per 1,000 in years 4 and 5 of follow-up (15). For the entire 5-year period, the rate was 68.6 per 1,000 for the placebo group and 25.7 per 1,000 for the isoniazid group. The annual rate of tuberculosis among persons who had never had active disease was 10.5 per 1,000 for the midpoint of the study. A placebo-controlled trial of isoniazid given for 2 years in the Hudson River State Hospital noted that the incidence of tuberculosis in the control group was 4.1 per 100 person-years over the 6-year study period (38). The rate decreased from 3.9 per 100 person-years in the first year of

the study (during treatment) to 1.5, 6 years later. Among those who never had active tuberculosis, the rate was 9.3 per 100 persons per year over the 6-year study period (15). At the midpoint of the study, the incidence among persons who had never been diagnosed with active tuberculosis was 43.0 per 1,000 population (Fig. 7.3).

Comstock and Ferebee-Woopert (39) reported the results of a study that provided treatment for latent infection in patients with inactive tuberculosis in an Eskimo population with high rates of tuberculosis. During the first year, 4% of persons in the placebo group developed tuberculosis disease. Over the ensuing 5 years, the average incidence of disease was nearly 1.5% per year, so that the probability of tuberculosis disease by the end of 6 years of follow-up was nearly 12%. A cooperative Veterans Administration double-blind placebo-controlled randomized trial was begun in 1964 when it was noted that 6.3% of 3,200 veterans with inactive disease developed tuberculosis over a 5-year period (40). Among veterans in the placebo arm with "inactive TB," who had never been treated, the rate of tuberculosis disease was 19.4 per 1,000 cases (0.35% per year) (41). Almost all of the patients had documentation of inactive disease for 5 or more years prior to entry into the trial. Thus, in both low- and high-incidence settings, persons with fibrotic abnormalities on the chest radiograph have been shown to have a considerable risk of developing tuberculosis.

The last study to address the efficacy of isoniazid for preventing tuberculosis in persons with fibrotic lesions of the chest radiograph was conducted in several countries in eastern Europe (42). A total of 28,000 individuals with inactive tuberculosis who had fibrotic abnormalities on a chest radiograph were randomized to receive placebo or one of three different isoniazid treatment regimens of varying duration. The incidence of tuberculosis among patients in the placebo arm who had fibrotic parenchymal lesions smaller than 2 cm^2 was 11.6 per 1,000 persons at risk compared with 21.3 per 1,000 persons at risk in those whose radiographic abnormality measured ≥2 cm² (42). This often-quoted study demonstrated that the more extensive the radiographic abnormality, the higher the risk of progression to active tuberculosis.

Human Immunodeficiency Virus Infection

Underlying HIV infection is the most powerful predictor of progression to active disease among latently infected individuals. Rates of progression to tuberculosis have ranged from 4.5 to 16.2 per 100 person-years of observation in several cohort studies (43–53) (Table 7.2). In a prospective study of tuberculosis among HIV-infected injection drug users with tuberculous infection in New York City, active tuberculosis developed in seven of 49 persons (a rate of 7.9% per year); there were no cases in the 62 HIV-negative injection drug users (44). Among HIV-infected injection drug users in San Francisco, the rate of tuberculosis among tuberculin-positive persons was similarly high at 5.0% per year (53), whereas the rate of tuberculosis among HIV-infected homeless persons was almost ten times greater than the rate among HIV-uninfected individuals (54). The variations in the incidence rates among HIV-infected cohorts are likely due to differences in the prevalence of tuberculosis infection in the cohorts, differences in the severity of immunosuppression, and the amount of ongoing transmission that was occurring in the cohorts.

The incidence and predictors of tuberculosis in HIV-infected persons was evaluated in a prospective multicenter study in which 1,130 HIV-seropositive patients without acquired immunodeficiency syndrome (AIDS) were followed for a median of 53 months (52). During the follow-up period, 31 HIV-seropositive patients developed tuberculosis (0.7 case per 100 person-years). The most important demographic risk factor was location. Tuberculosis was four times more likely to occur in sites on the East Coast com-pared with the West Coast and Midwest. Tuberculosis occurred more frequently in persons whose CD4 cell count was less than 200 cells/mm³. The rate was highest in those persons who had a positive TST (4.5 cases per 100 person-years) and those with documented skin test conversions (5.4 cases per 100 person-years) indicating recent infection.

Diabetes Mellitus

Since the time of Avicenna (980–1027 A.D.), diabetes was recognized as a predisposing factor for the development of tuberculosis (55). In the 19th century there were numerous reports describing the common occurrence of tuberculosis in postmortem examinations of patients with diabetes mellitus (55). After the advent of insulin, and with the declining incidence of pulmonary tuberculosis, the incidence of tuberculosis in diabetics was reported to be 1% to 5% (56). Root reported in 1934 that the development of pulmonary tuberculosis in juvenile diabetics was ten times that among nondiabetic Massachusetts grade and high-school children (57). Oscarsson (55) reviewed the chest radiographs of 1,270 diabetics in Kristianstad in 1953. The frequency of pulmonary tuberculosis among diabetics aged 30 years or more was about two to five times higher than in the same age group among the general population. Subsequent reports also described the prevalence of tuberculosis among diabetics to be two to five times higher than that seen in nondiabetics (58,59).

Two recent studies evaluated the rate of tuberculosis in diabetics using large existing databases. Using a database of health insurance claims, investigators in South Korea reported that pulmonary tuberculosis was diagnosed in 170 of 8,015 (2%) diabetics (60). The annual rate of tuberculosis was 1,061 per 100,000 compared with 306 per 100,000 among nondiabetics; the relative risk was 3.5. Pablos-Mendez et al. (61) reported that diabetes mellitus was an

TABLE 7.2. INCIDENCE RATES[a] OF TUBERCULOSIS AMONG COHORTS OF HUMAN IMMUNODEFICIENCY VIRUS-1 SEROPOSITIVE AND SERONEGATIVE INDIVIDUALS

Study Location	Population	HIV +			HIV -	
		All Subjects	PPD +	PPD -	Anergic	PPD +
New York City	IDUs	2.1	7.9	0.3	—	0
New York City	IDUs	—	9.7	—	6.6	1.0
Kigali, Rwanda	Young women	2.5	—	—	—	—
Port-au-Prince, Haiti	General	7.5	10.0	5.7	—	—
Madrid, Spain	84% IDUs	9.1	10.4	5.4	12.4	—
Madrid/Barcelona, Spain	60% IDUs	—	16.2	2.4	2.6	—
Italy, multicenter	72% IDUs	2.3	5.4	0.5	3.0	—
Baltimore, MD	IDUs	1.9	—	—	—	—
U.S.A., multicenter	23% IDUs	0.7	4.5	0.4	0.7	—
San Francisco, CA	IDUs	0.7	5.0	1.0	0	0.4

[a]Rates in 100 person-years for persons who did not take or complete isoniazid preventive therapy.
HIV, human immunodeficiency virus; PPD, purified protein derivative; IDU, injection drug user.

independent risk factor for the development of tuberculosis. In a case-control study involving 5,290 discharges from civilian hospitals in California during 1991 who had tuberculosis and 37,366 controls, the estimated risk of tuberculosis attributable to diabetes (25.2%) was equivalent to that attributable to HIV infection (25.5%).

Few studies have attempted to determine the differential risk of developing tuberculosis among persons with insulin-dependent diabetes (IDDM) versus non–insulin-dependent diabetes (NIDDM). Swai et al. (62) in Tanzania followed 1,250 patients with diabetes and noted that 70 (5.6%) individuals developed tuberculosis. The prevalence of tuberculosis was greatest in the young, in those with low body mass index, and in those with IDDM. Tuberculosis occurred in 24 (8.8%) of the 272 IDDM patients compared with 22 (2.7%) of the 825 patients with NIDDM. Because there was no nondiabetic control group it is not possible to determine if the rate of tuberculosis in the patients with NIDDM was higher than expected. Poor glucose control is thought to confer a higher risk of tuberculosis (61–63), but whether or not the many well-controlled diabetics who have tuberculous infection have a significantly increased risk of progressing to tuberculosis is not known.

End-Stage Renal Disease

Pradham et al. (64) in New York reported five cases of tuberculosis in dialysis patients in 1974 and first suggested that they had an increased incidence of tuberculosis. Subsequently, more reports described elevated incidence rates in comparison with the general population, but there have been few appropriately controlled studies (Table 7.3) (65–74). From 1975 to 1977, 6 of 180 patients undergoing maintenance hemodialysis in Brooklyn, New York developed tuberculosis representing an incidence of approximately 3% per year (66). The mean incidence of tuberculosis from 1973 to 1977 in the adult population of Brooklyn was 2.9 per 1,000 per year (0.29%). Thus, the relative risk of tuberculosis among dialysis patients was 10 times higher than that of the general adult population. In similar studies from San Francisco (65) and Japan (68), the incidence of tuberculosis was six to 16 times that seen in the general

population. Using a dialysis registry and a tuberculosis registry, investigators in British Columbia reported a case rate of 252 per 100,000 compared with an age-matched rate of 10.1 per 100,000, giving a relative risk of 25.3 (70).

Most of the studies have not been population based, do not have a well-matched control group, and do not control for other risk factors such as diabetes as is common in most series. Thus it is difficult to make cross-study comparisons. However, with this in mind, the estimated relative risk from the studies in Table 7.3 ranges from 2 to 25. Whether some of this increased risk is related to new transmission within the dialysis units themselves or other risk factors, such as diabetes mellitus, is not known.

Silicosis

A high incidence of tuberculosis among miners was noted by Georgius Agricola in 1556 in his classic treatise, *De re metallica* (75). Early in the 20th century, 75% of gold miners (who are typically exposed to silica dusts) had evidence of tuberculosis at autopsy (75). During that time in the United States, it was estimated that approximately half of the deaths among lead and zinc miners were due to tuberculosis (76). Although the prevalence of silicosis in the United States has decreased dramatically, the disease continues to be prevalent in some areas of the world, such as the mining areas of Africa.

The rate of tuberculosis among Rhodesian miners with silicosis (1950 to 1959) averaged 30 times that seen in nonsilicotic miners, with an incidence of 3% per year (77). Among 750 hard-coal miners in Pennsylvania studied between 1946 and 1950, 12.6% were diagnosed with tuberculosis (78). Compared with industrial workers of similar age, tuberculosis was eight times more common in men aged 35 to 44 years. In a study from Sweden of 712 cases of silicosis reported during 1959 to 1977, 29 cases of pulmonary tuberculosis occurred compared with one case among 810 nonsilicotic control subjects; thus, there were in excess of 30-fold more cases among the silicotic patients (79).

More recent reports from South Africa document the ongoing problem with tuberculosis and silicosis. Cowie

TABLE 7.3. INCIDENCE OF TUBERCULOSIS AMONG PATIENTS ON LONG-TERM HEMODIALYSIS

Study	Years	Dialysis Cases	TB Cases (%)	TB Rate (%/yr)	General Population Rate (%/yr)[a]	Relative Risk[a]
Lundin, 1979	1975–77	180	6 (3.3)	3.0	0.29	10
Sasaki, 1979	1967–76	367	12 (3.3)	0.33	0.11	3
Andrew, 1980	1967–77	172	10 (5.8)	0.58	0.048	12
Malhotra, 1981	1975–80	150	20 (13.3)	2.7	1.0	3
Garcia-Leoni, 1990	1985–87	108	5 (4.6)	0.85	0.035	24
Chia, 1998	1990–94	886	9 (1.3)	0.25	0.01	25
Shohaib, 1999	1992–97	210	17 (8.1)	1.6	0.063	25

[a]Estimated.

(80), using surveillance data, reported an annual risk of tuberculosis among miners with silicosis of 2,707 per 100,000 compared with 981 per 100,000 among miners without silicosis; the relative risk was approximately 3 [95% confidence interval (CI), 1.9–4.1]. The risk increased with increasing radiographic severity of silicosis. After 7 years follow-up, more than 40% of the patients with the most extensive silicosis developed tuberculosis.

Perhaps one of the best assessments of the incidence of tuberculosis among silicotic patients came from a randomized controlled clinical trial aimed at reducing the risk of tuberculosis among silicotics (81). Twenty-seven percent of silicotic patients in Hong Kong enrolled in the placebo arm of the trial evaluating different treatment regimens for latent infection developed tuberculosis during the 5-year study. The rate of development of tuberculosis in the placebo group was a constant 7% per year over the 5-year period. Based on these studies and others, it appears that the risk of tuberculosis is extremely high in patients with underlying silicosis, ranging from three to 30 times the risk in nonsilicotic individuals.

Concurrent Corticosteroid Therapy

It has been widely reported that treatment with corticosteroids may predispose to active tuberculosis, but the actual excess risk attributed to corticosteroid use is difficult to derive from the literature. Experimental studies demonstrated that glucocorticoid administration in animals was associated with worsening of the disease (82,83), and patients with pulmonary tuberculosis who were given corticosteroids were also reported to do poorly and showed progression of their disease (84–86). Moreover, administration of higher doses of corticosteroids (i.e., more than 15 mg/day for 2 to 4 weeks) is associated with loss of delayed-type hypersensitivity reactions (87). However, many of the earlier clinical reports were anecdotal in nature and included small numbers of patients (88). In a review of the complications of corticosteroids in 2,830 asthmatic patients, only three cases of tuberculosis disease were identified (89). In one study, the prevalence of tuberculosis among asthmatics was one of 550 patients treated with corticosteroids, compared with two of 499 patients with similar disease but not treated with steroids (90). Similarly, in a study of 132 asthmatic patients representing 620 steroid-treated years, of whom 28% had a positive TST, no cases of tuberculosis were identified (91).

Even in high-risk settings, the rate of tuberculosis in corticosteroid-treated individuals appears low. Cowie and King (92) reported that the relative risk of developing tuberculosis was 2.3 for black miners with asthma receiving corticosteroids compared with those who were not. Although the difference was not statistically significant, the CIs were extremely wide and thus the study was likely underpowered to detect a significant difference.

More recently, Kim et al. (93) reviewed the incidence and risk factors for developing tuberculosis among 269 patients with various forms of rheumatologic disease. The mean daily dose of corticosteroids was 18.7 mg prednisolone. Twenty-one patients developed tuberculosis resulting in an incidence rate of 20 per 1,000 patient-years. Risk factors for developing tuberculosis included the mean daily steroid dose during follow-up and for the first year of treatment, and a history of steroid pulse therapy.

The studies described above all suffered from methodologic flaws, so that it is difficult to determine the true excess risk, if any, associated with corticosteroid use. It is important to note that the dose of corticosteroids used, the duration of therapy, other co-risk factors for tuberculosis, and the overall prevalence of tuberculosis in the populations, varied significantly. Based on these data, it appears that chronic corticosteroid use, at least with low to intermediate dosing, represents no more than a modest increased risk for tuberculosis. It is likely that corticosteroids given in sufficient doses for sufficient periods would exert an immunosuppressive effect that would result in an increased risk of tuberculosis. Unfortunately, the dose and duration is not known.

Gastrectomy and Jejunoileostomy

Patients who have undergone gastric resection are considered at increased risk of developing tuberculosis. In 1927, four patients were reported to have developed fulminant tuberculosis following gastric resection, and the authors of this report suggested a causal relationship (94). Subsequently, there have been a number of reports describing a high frequency of tuberculosis among patients who have undergone partial gastrectomy with the prevalence ranging from 1.7 to 12.3 % (95). Although these studies did not have control groups for comparison, the authors noted that the prevalence of gastrectomy among patients with tuberculosis was higher than would have been expected in a suitable control group (95).

Other studies have investigated the incidence of tuberculosis among patients who have undergone partial gastrectomy: the incidence varied from 0.4% to 5.0% with 1 to 16 years of follow-up (95). Thorn et al. (96) followed 749 patients who had undergone partial gastrectomy for peptic ulcer disease and who had normal chest radiographs before surgery. Fourteen of the subjects developed tuberculosis over the next 6.5 years. The authors reported that the rate of tuberculosis was five times higher than in men of the same age and from the same area. Low preoperative weight was predictive of developing disease. Among those whose preoperative weight was less than 85% ideal body weight, the rate of developing tuberculosis was 14 times that of persons of normal weight for height. It is notable that the rate of tuberculosis was not higher if the patient's preoperative chest radiograph and weight were normal. In another study

(97), severe dumping was more common among patients with tuberculosis who had undergone gastrectomy than among those without tuberculosis, suggesting that malnutrition may play a role in the increased risk.

Wills (98) first reported two cases of tuberculous cervical adenitis in patients who had undergone jejunoileostomy for obesity in 1969. This was followed by the report of an additional two cases of tuberculosis among 200 people who underwent jejunoileal bypass surgery (99). Compared with the national rate of tuberculosis, the authors concluded that the rate was excessive. Because both patients developed tuberculosis during the active weight loss phase of the postoperative period, the authors postulated that malnutrition was to blame. Bruce et al. (100) reported four (two culture confirmed) patients who developed tuberculosis from a group of 101 consecutive patients who had undergone jejunoileal bypass for obesity between 1972 and 1975. The rate among these women was at least 60-fold that of the community rate of 12 per 100,000. All four women had developed tuberculosis within 10 months of the bypass coincident with the period of rapid weight loss. The authors reviewed a total of 7 reported cases in the literature and noted that only two of the 11 patients had developed pulmonary tuberculosis.

The lack of good prospective, controlled studies makes it difficult to assign a specific relative risk of tuberculosis following partial gastrectomy or jejunoileal bypass surgery. Other factors associated with the subjects reported could have resulted in the apparent increased risk related to gastrectomy or bypass surgery. It is possible that malnutrition or weight loss was the primary factor causing in increased risk.

Neoplastic Diseases

Neoplastic diseases maintain an important place in the history of the pathogenesis of tuberculosis. Since Sternberg (100a) originally described Hodgkin disease as a peculiar form of tuberculosis in 1898, there has been a great deal of literature speculating on the role of tuberculosis in the etiology of Hodgkin disease and other malignancies (101). Ewing

wrote that "tuberculosis follows Hodgkin's disease like a shadow"; even in the 1940 edition of his textbook, he argued that Hodgkin disease might be caused by tuberculosis (101). In 1928, in the previous edition of his book, Ewing (102) wrote that tuberculosis was the primary cause of bronchogenic carcinoma, although he later retracted this statement. With time this notion that malignancies were caused by tuberculosis lost favor and investigators began to evaluate the possibility that persons with underlying neoplastic disease were at greater risk of developing tuberculosis.

During the early 1930s Parker et al. (103) in Boston reviewed several hundred autopsies to determine the coexistence of tuberculosis among various malignancies. They found active tuberculosis in 20% of the persons who died with Hodgkin disease compared with 10% of those with myelogenous leukemia and 11% in general autopsies. Razis et al. (104) reviewed the medical records of 1,102 patients with Hodgkin disease, 220 patients with leukemia, and 1,269 patients with lymphosarcoma. They noted that patients with Hodgkin disease were significantly more likely to have tuberculosis than those with lymphosarcoma and that, in all cases, tuberculosis followed the diagnosis of Hodgkin disease. In a number of postmortem studies of patients who died with leukemia, no association could be made for an increased risk of tuberculosis (97–108). In fact, Sussman (105) in 1903 thought that the two diseases were "antagonistic." In a review of 213 autopsies in patients with leukemia conducted by the Atomic Bomb Casualty Commission, Hiroshima (1949–1962), the overall frequency of tuberculosis noted at postmortem examination was similar to that of the other 2,135 autopsies performed (108).

Kaplan et al. (109) reviewed 201 cases of tuberculosis between 1950 and 1971 that developed in patients with various underlying malignancies (Table 7.4). Patients with Hodgkin disease, lung cancer, lymphosarcoma, and reticulum cell sarcoma had prevalences of 96, 92, 88, and 78 cases per 10,000 patients, respectively. Patients with head and neck carcinoma, stomach cancer, acute lymphatic leukemia, and acute myelogenous leukemia had a prevalence of 51, 55, 37,

TABLE 7.4. INCIDENCE OF TUBERCULOSIS IN VARIOUS CANCERS

Study	Type of Cancer	Total Cancers	TB Cases	TB Incidence per 1,000
Kaplan, 1973	Hodgkin disease	1,463	14	9.6
	Lung	4,805	44	9.2
	Lymphosarcoma	912	8	8.8
	Stomach	1,646	9	5.5
	Head and neck	8,781	45	5.1
	Bladder (ref.)	2,372	1	0.4
Feld, 1976	Head and neck	1,366	10	7.3
	Lung	1,247	4	3.2
	Leukemias	802	3	1.2
	Lymphomas	1,155	1	0.87
	Total cancers (ref.)	90,022	34	0.38

TB, Tuberculosis.

and 28 per 10,000 patients at risk. During a 5-year study conducted from 1968 to 1973, Feld et al. (110) reported that the incidence of tuberculosis at M. D. Anderson Cancer Center was 65 cases per 100,000 compared with 21 to 29 per 100,000 during the 5-year study period. The highest rate occurred in patients with head and neck carcinoma (7.3 per 1,000), following by lung carcinoma (3.2 per 1,000).

Based on the studies described above (109,110), it is difficult to determine a true relative risk of developing tuberculosis with a specific cell type. The rate of tuberculosis was highest in persons with Hodgkin disease, lung carcinoma, and head and neck carcinoma. If another type of cancer with a low rate of tuberculosis is used as the reference, the relative risk of tuberculosis in the above malignancies was approximately 10 to 20.

Post-Organ Transplantation

There are numerous anecdotal reports of mycobacterial infections in persons who have undergone organ transplantation. Singh and Paterson (111) performed a meta-analysis of the published literature and noted that the incidence of tuberculosis in solid-organ transplantation recipients ranged from 0.35% to 15%. Nonrenal transplantation, rejection within 6 months before the onset of tuberculosis, and type of primary immunosuppressive regimen were all predictors of developing tuberculosis within 12 months of transplantation. Disseminated disease was common, occurring in 33% of patients with tuberculosis.

Most of the published literature deals with tuberculosis post renal transplantation. Based on a review of the literature, Lichtenstein and MacGregor (112) estimated that the rate of tuberculosis among renal transplant recipients was 480 cases per 100,000 versus 13.1 per 100,000 in the general population. Since this review, there have been a number of reports from low- and high-incidence countries (113–118). The incidence in renal transplant recipients varies from 0.35% to 1.2% in the United States to 5% to 15% in India and Pakistan (111). The incidence of tuberculosis in posttransplantation patients at the King Faisal Hospital and Research Center in Riyadh, Saudi Arabia was

reported to be 50 times that of the general population (117). The risk of developing tuberculosis among renal transplantation patients was higher in persons receiving cyclosporine, those with diabetes mellitus, and those with underlying chronic liver disease (118).

In a review of all heart transplantation patients in Germany from 1989 to 1996, 727 orthotopic heart transplantations were identified (119). Tuberculosis was proved in 7 (1%) resulting in a rate of 1,300 per 100,000 per year compared with 17.5 per 100,000 per year in the general population. The incidence of tuberculosis in heart transplant recipients was 20-fold that of the general population in Spain (120). The mean time to the development of tuberculosis after transplantation was 76 days.

There have been few reports of tuberculosis occurring post liver transplantation (121–123). The incidence of tuberculosis among 751 liver transplant candidates and recipients at Stanford was 73.4 per 100,000 person-years (123). Among TST-positive individuals, the rate increased to 800 cases per 100,000 person-years. The incidence among TST-positive persons who had not received treatment for LTBI was 1,585.3 per 100,000 person-years, although the total number of cases was small.

Patients who have undergone organ transplantation must remain immunosuppressed for life, so it is not surprising that they develop tuberculosis once infected with *M. tuberculosis*. In fact, immune impairment in the human host provides some evidence for the concept of clinical latency. For *M. tuberculosis* to remain in a clinically latent state, there must be an equilibrium established; the host immune system must be able to keep the organism's growth in check. When humans are immunosuppressed, this allows for a disequilibrium to occur and the tubercle bacilli are allowed to grow. When tuberculosis develops in relation to the transplant is critical to this argument. Development of tuberculosis soon after transplantation is consistent with endogenous activation of latent infection. The further removed from the transplantation, the more likely new infection or reinfection could occur. Singh and Paterson noted the time of development of tuberculosis post transplantation in solid-organ transplant recipients (111) (Table 7.5). In the

TABLE 7.5. TIMING OF THE ONSET OF TUBERCULOSIS IN SOLID-ORGAN TRANSPLANT RECIPIENTS

Type of Transplant	No. of Patients	No. (%) of Patients with Tuberculosis at Indicated Time of Onset				
		<6 mo	6–12 mo	>1–2 yr	>2–5 yr	> 5 yr
Renal	150	53 (35)	33 (22)	24 (16)	28 (19)	12 (8)
Liver	29	18 (62)	6 (21)	2 (7)	3 (10)	
Heart	11	6 (55)	1 (9)	1 (9)	3 (27)	
Lung	10	8 (80)	1 (10)	1 (10)		
Total	200	85 (43)	41 (20)	28 (14)	34 (17)	12 (6)

From Singh N, Paterson DL. *Mycobacterium tuberculosis* infection in solid-organ transplant recipients: impact and implications for management. *Clin Infect Dis* 1998;27:1266–1277, with permission.

TABLE 7.6. INCIDENCE OF TUBERCULOSIS AMONG VARIOUS TRANSPLANT RECIPIENTS

Study	Design	Dates	Total Patients	TB Cases (%)	Annual Rate per 1,000	General Population per 1,000	RR[a]
Renal transplantation							
Lichtenstein, 1983	Review	1962–72	NA	47	4.8	0.13	37
Qunibi, 1990	Retrospective and review	9 yr	403	14 (3.5)	32.3	0.60	53
John, 2001	Prospective	1986–99	1251	166 (13.3)	35[b]	NA	
Heart transplantation							
Munoz, 1995	Retrospective and review	1989–93	144	3 (2)	13.5	0.30–0.50	27–45
Korner, 1997	Retrospective	1989–96	716	7 (1)	13.0	0.18	72
Liver transplantation							
Meyers, 1994	Retrospective	1988–93	550	4 (0.7)	3.2	0.10	32
Chapparo, 1999	Retrospective	1988–98	751	NA	0.73	NA	NA

[a]RR, estimated relative risk.
[b]Approximate 3-year average at midpoint of study.

studies reviewed, 35% to 80% of the time tuberculosis developed within 6 months of transplantation. In 63% of cases, tuberculosis had developed within a year (Table 7.6).

Physical Habitus

The concept that body build is associated with susceptibility to tuberculosis dates back to the time of Hippocrates when it was noted that patients with tuberculosis were often tall and thin (124). The first scientific evidence came from World War I when Reed and Love (125) reported that Army officers with tall thin physiques were more likely to have tuberculosis, particularly those who were underweight for their height. A similar finding was reported in a study of 3,000 men discharged from the Army after World War II (126). Berry and Nash (124) performed an interesting study in which they measured the skin fold layer from mass miniature radiographs and correlated this with the development of tuberculosis: there was a tendency for lean men to develop tuberculosis. Tuberculin reactivity was not measured in any of the above studies, so it was not possible to determine whether or not the tall thin habitus was related to an increased risk of infection or progression to active disease.

The incidence of active tuberculosis in relation to tuberculin reactivity and body build was studied in 70,000 white men 17 to 21 years of age who were recruited by the Navy from 1949 to 1951 (11). The follow-up period was an average of 4 years. Body build, as measured by height, weight, and height–weight index was shown to be significantly associated with the incidence of tuberculosis. Morbidity rates in persons with a positive TST (≥10 mm) were more than two times higher among those who were 15% or more underweight for their height (2.6 per 1,000 person-years) than in those who were within 5% of standard weight (1.1 per 1,000 person-years). The rate of tuberculosis among men who were 10% or more above standard weight was twice that of standard weight. Body build was not found to

be related to whether or not a man had been infected with tubercle bacilli. Given that these were generally young healthy men, malnutrition is unlikely to be the reason for the increased rate among the men who were underweight for their height.

Although the observations noted above seem to indicate that there is an increased risk of developing tuberculosis in latently infected persons who are underweight for their height, this risk factor is seldom used to determine who should be treated for LTBI.

SIGNIFICANCE OF LATENCY

The World Health Organization estimates that approximately one third of the world's population, or 2 billion people, is infected with *M. tuberculosis*. As industrialized nations move toward elimination of tuberculosis, identification and treatment of latent infection will become a critical component of tuberculosis control efforts. Unfortunately, the largest pool of latently infected individuals resides in endemic countries where the current approach to detecting and treating LTBI is often logistically impractical. The large number of infected individuals presents a major impediment to tuberculosis control worldwide. However, among high-risk individuals such as HIV-infected persons and contacts to infectious cases, an argument can be made to develop models for treatment of LTBI even in resource-poor countries. Early interventions to prevent these high-risk latently infected individuals from developing tuberculosis could have an immediate impact on tuberculosis morbidity and mortality worldwide.

REFERENCES

1. Parrish NM, Dick JD, Bishai WR. Mechanisms of latency in *Mycobacterium tuberculosis*. *Trends Microbiol* 1998;3:107–112.

2. Loomis HP. Some facts in the etiology of tuberculosis, evidenced by thirty autopsies and experiments upon animals. *M Rec* 1890;38:689–698.
3. Wang CY. An experimental study of latent tuberculosis. *Lancet* 1916;2:417–419.
4. Robertson HE. The persistence of tuberculous infections. *Am J Pathol* 1933;9:711–719.
5. Feldman WH, Baggenstoss AH. The residual infectivity of the primary complex of tuberculosis. *Am J Pathol* 1939;5:501–515.
6. Rabinowitsch L. Zur Frage latenter Tuberkelbacillen. *Berl Klin Wchnschr* 1907;44:35–39.
7. Opie EL, Aronson JD. Tubercle bacilli in latent tuberculosis lesions an in lung tissue without tuberculous lesions. *Arch Pathol* 1927;4:1–21.
8. Medlar EM, Bernstein S, Steward DM. A bacteriologic study of resected tuberculosis lesions. *Am Rev Tuberc* 1952;66:36–43.
9. Hobby GL, Auerbach O, Lenert TF, et al. The late emergence of *M. tuberculosis* in liquid cultures of pulmonary lesions resected from humans. *Am Rev Tuberc* 1954;70:191–218.
10. American Thoracic Society/Centers for Disease Control and Prevention. Targeted tuberculin testing and treatment of latent tuberculosis infection. *AJRCCM* 2000;161:5221–5227.
11. Palmer CE, Jablon S, Edwards PQ. Tuberculosis morbidity of young men in relation to tuberculin sensitivity and body build. *Am Rev Tuberc* 1957;76:517–539.
12. Ferebee SH, Palmer CE. The epidemiologic bonus. *Am Rev Respir Dis* 1965;91:104.
13. Grzybowski S. Epidemiology of tuberculosis. *Med Serv J Canada* 1996;22:856–858.
14. Grzybowski S, Fishaut H, Rowe J, et al. Tuberculosis among patients with various radiologic abnormalities followed by the chest clinic service. *Am Rev Respir Dis* 1971;104:605–608.
15. Ferebee SH. Controlled chemoprophylaxis trials in tuberculosis. A general review. *Adv Tuberc Res* 1970;17:28–106.
16. Hopewell PC, Bloom BR. Tuberculosis and other mycobacterial disease. In: Murray JF, Nadel JA, eds. *Textbook of respiratory medicine*, 3rd ed. Philadelphia: WB Saunders, 2000:1043–1105.
17. Meyers JA, Bearman JE, Dixon G. The natural history of tuberculosis in the human body. *Am Rev Respir Dis* 1963;87:354–369.
18. Ghon A. The primary complex in human tuberculosis and its significance. *Am Rev Tuberc* 1923;7:314–317.
19. Simon G. Die Tuberkulose der Lungenspitzen Beitr. *Z Klin Di Tuberck* 1927;67:467–479.
20. Opie EL. Phthisiogenesis and latent tuberculosis infection. *Am Rev Tuberc* 1922;6:525–546.
21. Terplan K. Anatomical contribution to primary and postprimary human pulmonary tuberculosis. *Am Rev Tuberc* 1934;29:77–87.
22. Medlar EM. Incidence of tuberculosis pulmonary cavities in unexpected deaths investigated at necropsy. *Arch Intern Med* 1947;80:403–410.
23. Stead WW. The pathogenesis of pulmonary tuberculosis among older persons. *Am Rev Respir Dis* 1965;91:811–822.
24. Stead WW. Pathogenesis of the sporadic case of tuberculosis. *N Engl J Med* 1967;277:1008–1012.
25. Stead WW. Pathogenesis of a first episode of chronic pulmonary tuberculosis in man: recrudescence of residuals of the primary infection or exogenous reinfection? *Am Rev Respir Dis* 1967;95:729–745.
26. Hyge TV. The efficacy of BCG-vaccination. *Acta Med Scand* 1957;32:7–107.
27. Small PM, Hopewell PC, Singh SP, et al. The contemporary urban epidemiology of tuberculosis: a population-based study using conventional and molecular methods. *N Engl J Med* 1994;330:1703–1709.
28. Geng E, Kreiswirth B, Driver C, et al. Changes in the transmission of tuberculosis in New York City from 1990 to 1999. *N Engl J Med* 2002;346:1453–1458.
29. Small PM, Shafer RW, Hopewell PC, et al. Exogenous reinfection with multidrug-resistant *Mycobacterium tuberculosis* in patients with advanced HIV infection. *N Engl J Med* 1993 22;328:1137–1144.
30. Shafer RW, Singh SP, Larkin C, et al. Exogenous reinfection with multidrug-resistant *Mycobacterium tuberculosis* in an immunocompetent patient. *Tuber Lung Dis* 1995;76:575–577.
31. van Rie A, Warren R, Richardson M, et al. Exogenous reinfection as a cause of recurrent tuberculosis after curative treatment. *N Engl J Med* 1999;341:1174–1179.
32. Ferebee SH, Mount FW. Tuberculosis morbidity in a controlled trial of the prophylactic use of isoniazid among household contacts. *Am Rev Respir Dis* 1962;85:490–521.
33. Comstock GW, Livesay VT, Woolpert SF. The prognosis of a positive tuberculin reaction in childhood and adolescence. *Am J Epidemiol* 1974;99:131–138.
34. Daley CL, Small PM, Schecter GF, et al. Transmission and accelerated progression of tuberculosis in patients infected with the human immunodeficiency virus: characterization of an outbreak using restriction fragment length polymorphism analysis. *N Engl J Med* 1992;326:321–325.
35. DiPerri G, Crucian M, Danzi ML, et al. Nosocomial epidemic of active tuberculosis among HIV-infected patients. *Lancet* 1989;2:1502–1504.
36. Horwitz O. The risk of tuberculosis in different groups of the general population. *Scand J Respir Dis* 1970:72:55–60.
37. Nakiela EM, Cragg R, Grzybowski S. Lifelong follow-up of inactive tuberculosis: its value and limitations. *Am Rev Respir Dis* 1975;112:765–772.
38. Katz J, Kunofsky S, Damijonaitis V, et al. Effect of isoniazid upon the reactivation of inactive tuberculosis. A final report. *Am Rev Respir Dis* 1965;91:345–350.
39. Comstock GW, Ferebee-Woopert S. Preventive treatment of untreated, nonactive tuberculosis in an Eskimo population. *Arch Environ Health* 1972;25:333–337.
40. Fuchs GF. Criteria for prophylaxis in active tuberculosis. *Arch Environ Health* 1965;10:937–941.
41. Falk A, Fuchs GF. Prophlyaxis with isoniazid in inactive tuberculosis. A Veterans Administration Cooperative Study XII. *Chest* 1978:73:44–48.
42. International Union Against Tuberculosis Committee on Prophylaxis. Efficacy of various durations of isoniazid preventive therapy for tuberculosis: five years of follow-up in the IUAT trial. *Bull WHO* 1982;60:555–564.
43. Daley CL. HIV-related tuberculosis. In: Volberding PA, Jacobson MA, eds. *AIDS clinical review 1997/1998*. New York: Marcel Dekker, 1998:289–321.
44. Selwyn PA, Hartel D, Lewis VA, et al. A prospective study of the risk of tuberculosis among intravenous drug users with human immunodeficiency virus infection. *N Engl J Med* 1989;320:545–550.
45. Selwyn P, Skell B, Alcabes P, et al. High risk of active tuberculosis in HIV-infected drug users with cutaneous anergy. *JAMA* 1992;268:504–509.
46. Pape JW, Jean SS, Ho JL, et al. Effect of isoniazid prophylaxis on incidence of active tuberculosis and progression of HIV infection. *Lancet* 1993;342:268.
47. Moreno S, Baraia-Etxaburu J, Bouza E, et al. Risk for developing tuberculosis among anergic patients infected with HIV. *Ann Intern Med* 1993;119:194–198.
48. Guelar A, Gatell J, Verdejo J, et al. A prospective study of the risk of tuberculosis among HIV-infected patients. *AIDS* 1993;7:1345–1349.

49. Antonucci G, Girardi E, Raviglione MC, et al., for the Gruppo Italiano di Studio Tuberculosi e AIDS (GISTA). Risk factors for tuberculosis in HIV-infected persons. A prospective cohort study. *JAMA* 1995;274:143–148.

50. Graham NHM, Galai N, Nelson KE, et al. Effect of isoniazid chemoprophylaxis on HIV-related mycobacterial disease. *Arch Intern Med* 1996;156:889–894.

51. Allen S, Batungwanayo J, Kerlikowske K, et al. Incidence of tuberculosis in HIV-infected and uninfected urban Rwandan women. *Am Rev Respir Dis* 1992;146:1439–1444.

52. Markowitz N, Hansen NI, Hopewell PC, et al. Incidence of tuberculosis in the United States among HIV-infected persons. *Ann Intern Med* 1997;126:123–132.

53. Daley CL, Hahn JA, Moss A, et al. Incidence of tuberculosis in injection drug users in San Francisco. *Am J Respir Crit Care Med* 1998;157:19–22.

54. Moss AR, Hahn JA, Tulsky JP, et al. Tuberculosis in the homeless. A prospective study. *Am J Respir Crit Care Med* 2000;162:460–464.

55. Oscarsson PN, Silwer H. Incidence of pulmonary tuberculosis among diabetics. *Acta Med Scand* 1958;161 (Suppl. 335):23–48.

56. Banyai AL. Diabetes and pulmonary tuberculosis. *Am Rev Tuberc* 1931;24:650–667.

57. Root HF. The association of diabetes and tuberculosis. *N Engl J Med* 1934;210:1–13.

58. Opsahl R, Riddervold HO, Aas TW. Pulmonary tuberculosis in mitral stenosis and diabetes mellitus. *Acta Tuberc Scand* 1961;40:290–296.

59. Turner Warwick M. Pulmonary tuberculosis and diabetes mellitus. *Q J Med* 1957;26:31–42.

60. Kim SJ, Hong YP, Lew WJ, et al. Incidence of pulmonary tuberculosis among diabetics. *Tuber Lung Dis* 1995;76:529–533.

61. Pablos-Mendez A, Blustein J, Knirsch CA. The role of diabetes mellitus in the higher prevalence of tuberculosis among Hispanics. *Am J Public Health* 1997;87:574–579.

62. Swai ABM, Mugusi F, McLarty DG. Tuberculosis in diabetic patients in Tanzania. *Trop Doctor* 1990;20:147–150.

63. Boucot KR, Cooper DA, Dillon ES, et al. Tuberculosis among diabetics. The Philadelphia survey. *Am Rev Tuberc* 1952;65 (Suppl):1–50.

64. Pradhan RP, Katz LA, Nidus BD, et al. Tuberculosis in dialyzed patients. *JAMA* 1974;229:798–800.

65. Andrew OT, Schoenfeld PY, Hopewell PC, et al. Tuberculosis in patients with end-stage renal disease. *Am J Med* 1980;68:59–65.

66. Lundin AP, Adler AJ, Berlyne GM, et al. Tuberculosis in patients undergoing maintenance hemodialysis. *Am J Med* 1979;67:597–602.

67. Malhotra KK, Bhuyan UN, Parashar MK, et al. Tuberculosis in maintenance haemodialysis patients. Study from an endemic area. *Postgrad Med J* 1981;57:492–498.

68. Sasaki S, Akiba T, Suenaga M, et al. Ten year's survey of dialysis-associated tuberculosis. *Nephron* 1979;24:141–145.

69. Cengiz K. Increased incidence of tuberculosis in patients undergoing hemodialysis. *Nephron* 1996;73:421–424.

70. Chia S, Karim M, Elwood RK, et al. Risk of tuberculosis in dialysis patients: a population-based study. *Int J Tuberc Lung Dis* 1998;2:989–991.

71. Shohaib SA, Scrimgeour EM, Shaerya F. Tuberculosis in active dialysis patients in Jeddah. *Nephrology* 1999;19:34–37.

72. Vachharajani A, Abreo K, Phadke A, et al. Diagnosis and treatment of tuberculosis in hemodialysis and renal transplant patients. *Nephrology* 2000;20:273–277.

73. Garcia-Leoni ME, Martin-Scapa C, Rodeno P, et al. High incidence of tuberculosis in renal patients. *Eur J Clin Microbiol Infect Dis* 1990;9:283–285.

74. Kursat S, Ozgur B. Increased incidence of tuberculosis in chronic hemodialysis patients. *Nephrology* 2001;21:490–493.

75. Snider DE Jr. The relationship between tuberculosis and silicosis. *Am Rev Respir Dis* 1978;118:455–460.

76. Lanza AJ, Vane RJ. The prevalence of silicosis in the general population and its effects upon the incidence of tuberculosis. *Am Rev Tuberc* 1934;29:8–16.

77. Paul R. Silicosis in northern Rhodesia copper miners. *Arch Environ Health* 1961;2:96–109.

78. Theodos PA, Gordon B. Tuberculosis in anthracosilicosis. *Am Rev Tuberc* 1952;65:24–46.

79. Westerholm P, Ahlmark A, Maasing R, et al. Silicosis and risk of lung cancer or lung tuberculosis: a cohort study. *Environ Res* 1986;41:339–350.

80. Cowie RL. The epidemiology of tuberculosis in gold miners with silicosis. *Am J Respir Crit Care Med* 1994;159:1460–1462.

81. Hong Kong Chest Service/Tuberculosis Research Center, Madras/British Medical Research Council. A double-blind placebo-controlled clinical trial of three antituberculosis chemoprophylaxis regimens in patients with silicosis in Hong Kong. *Am Rev Respir Dis* 1992;145:36–41.

82. Karlson AG, Gainer JH. The influence of cortisone on experimental tuberculosis of guinea pigs. *Dis Chest* 1951;20:469–481.

83. Spain DM, Molomut N. Effects of cortisone on the development of tuberculous lesions in guinea pigs and on their modification by streptomycin therapy. *Am Rev Tuberc* 1950;62:337–344.

84. Traut EF, Ellman J. Exacerbation of tuberculosis during treatment with cortisone. *JAMA* 1952;149:1214–1218.

85. Capon AW. ACTH, cortisone and tuberculosis. *Cana Med Assoc J* 1952;62:46–48.

86. Deleterious effects of ACTH and cortisone on tuberculosis. *N Engl J Med* 1951;245:662–664.

87. Borvornkitti S, Kangsadai P, Sathirapat P, et al. Reversion and reconversion rate of tuberculin skin test reactions in correlation with use of prednisone. *Dis Chest* 1960;38:51–55.

88. Bateman ED. Is tuberculosis chemoprophylaxis necessary for patients receiving corticosteroids for respiratory disease? *Resp Med* 1993;87:485–487.

89. Leiberman P, Patterson R, Kunske R. Complications of long-term steroid treatment for asthma. *J Allergy Clin Immunol* 1972;49:329.

90. Smyllie HC, Connolly CK. Incidence of serious complications of corticosteroid therapy in respiratory disease. *Thorax* 1968;23:571–581.

91. Schatz M, Patterson R, Kloner R, et al. The prevalence of tuberculosis and positive tuberculin skin tests in a steroid-treated asthmatic population. *Ann Intern Med* 1976;84:261–265.

92. Cowie RL, King LM. Pulmonary tuberculosis in corticosteroid-treated asthmatics. *S Afr Med J* 1987;72:849–850.

93. Kim HA, Yoo CD, Baek HJ, et al. *Mycobacterium tuberculosis* infection in corticosteroid-treated rheumatic disease patient population. *Clin Exp Rheumatol* 1998;16:9–13.

94. Winkelbauer A, Frisch AV. Ulcus pepticum und Lungentuberkulose fur Frage ihrer gegenseitigen Beeinflussung. *Wien Klin Wochenschr* 1927;10:309–313.

95. Snider DE Jr. Tuberculosis and gastrectomy. *Chest* 1985;87:414–415.

96. Thorn PA, Brookes VS, Waterhouse JAH. Peptic ulcer, partial gastrectomy, and pulmonary tuberculosis. *Br Med J* 1956;1:603–608.

97. Hanngren A, Reizenstein P. Studies of dumping syndrome. *Am J Dig Dis* 1969;14:700–710.

98. Wills CE Jr. Jejuno-ileostomy for obesity. *J Med Assoc Ga* 1969; 58:456–461.

99. Pickleman JR, Evans LS, Kane JM, et al. Tuberculosis after jejunoileal bypass for obesity. *JAMA* 1975;234:744.

100. Bruce RM, Wise L. Tuberculosis after jejunoileal bypass for obesity. *Ann Intern Med* 1977;87:574–576.

100a. Sternberg C. Ueber eine eigenartige unter dem Bilde der Pseudoleukämie verlaufende tuberkulose des lymphatischen apparetes. *Ztschr F Heilk* 1898:19,21.

101. Ewing J. *Neoplastic diseases. A treatise on tumors. Lymphoma and lymphosarcoma,* 4th ed. Philadelphia: WB Saunders, 1940:416.

102. Ewing J. *Neoplastic diseases,* 3rd ed. Philadelphia: WB Saunders, 1928:421.

103. Parker F, Jackson H, Bethea JM, et al. Studies of diseases of the lymphoid and myeloid tissues. V. The coexistence of tuberculosis with Hodgkin's disease and other forms of malignant lymphoma. *Am J Med Sci* 1932;184:694–699.

104. Razis DV, Diamond HD, Craver LF. Hodgkin's disease associated with the other malignant tumors and certain non-neoplastic diseases. *Am J Med Sci* 1959;327–335.

105. Sussman WJ. An enquiry into the relationship of leukaemia and tuberculosis. *The Practitioner* 1903;71;536–548.

106. Abbatt JD, Lea AJ. Leukaemia and pulmonary tuberculosis. *Lancet* 1957;2:917–918.

107. Lowther CP. Leukemia and tuberculosis. *Ann Intern Med* 1959;51:52–56.

108. Morrow LB, Anderson RE. Active tuberculosis in leukemia. *Arch Pathol* 1965;79:484–493.

109. Kaplan MH, Armstrong D, Rosen P. Tuberculosis complicating neoplastic disease. A review of 201 cases. *Cancer* 1974;l33:850–858.

110. Feld R, Bodey GP, Groschel D. Mycobacteriosis in patients with malignant disease. *Arch Intern Med* 1976;136:67–70.

111. Singh N, Paterson DL. *Mycobacterium tuberculosis* infection in solid-organ transplant recipients: impact and implications for management. *Clin Infect Dis* 1998;27:1266–1277.

112. Lichtenstein IH, MacGregor RR. Mycobacterial infections in renal transplant recipients: report of five cases and review of the literature. *Rev Infect Dis* 1983;5:216–226.

113. Aslani J, Einollahi B. Prevalence of tuberculosis after renal transplantation in Iran. *Transplant Proc* 2001;33:2804–2805.

114. Niewczas M, Ziolkowski J, Rancewicz Z, et al. Tuberculosis in patients after renal transplantation remains still a clinical problem. *Transplant Proc* 2002;34:677–679.

115. Koseoglu F, Emiroglu R, Karakayali H, et al. Prevalence of mycobacterial infection in solid organ transplant recipients. *Transplant Proc* 2001;33:1782–1784.

116. Hall CM, Willcox PA, Swanepoel CR, et al. Mycobacterial infection in renal transplant recipients. *Chest* 1994;106:435–439.

117. Qunibi WY, Al-Sibai MB, Taher S, et al. Mycobacterial infection after renal transplantation-report of 14 cases and review of the literature. *Q J Med* 1990;282:1039–1060.

118. John GT, Shankar V, Abraham AB, et al. Risk factors for post-transplant tuberculosis. *Kidney Int* 2001;60:1148–1153.

119. Korner MM, Hirata N, Tenderich G, et al. Tuberculosis in heart transplant recipients. *Chest* 1997;111:365–369.

120. Munoz P, Palomo J, Munoz R, et al. Tuberculosis in heart transplant recipients. *Clin Infect Dis* 1995;21:398–402.

121. Meyers BR. Halpern M, Sheiner P, et al. Tuberculosis in liver transplant patients. *Transplantation* 1994;58:301–306.

122. Salizzoni JL, Tiruviluamala P, Reichman LB. Liver transplantation: an unheralded probable risk for tuberculosis. *Tuber Lung Dis* 1992;73:232–238.

123. Chaparro SV, Montoya JG, Keeffe EB, et al. Risk of tuberculosis in tuberculin skin test-positive liver transplant patients. *Clin Infect Dis* 1999;29:207–208.

124. Berry WTC, Nash FA. Studies in the aetiology of pulmonary tuberculosis. *Tubercle* 1955;36:164–174.

125. Reed LJ, Love AG. Biometric studies on U.S. Army officers: somatological norms in disease. *Hum Biol* 1933;5:61.

126. Long ER, Jablon S. *Tuberculosis in the United States Army in World War II. An epidemiological study with an evaluation of X-ray screening.* VA Medical Monograph, May 1, 1955.

8

PERSISTENCE AND DRUG TOLERANCE

JAMES E. GOMEZ
JOHN D. MCKINNEY

"Not only does man lack the power to create life but his ability to destroy it, at least at the microbial level, is sharply limited."

—Walsh McDermott, 1959 (1)

The invention of antimicrobial chemotherapy must be ranked among the most important medical advances of the 20th century. It would be difficult to overstate the medical impact of the miraculous "magic bullets," which demoted to the status of minor and treatable ailments several of the most common and deadly infections that had ravaged the United States and Europe for centuries. Although the first antimicrobials proved ineffective against tuberculosis (TB), the early success in the management of other infectious diseases inspired several groups of biologists and chemists to persevere in their search for a remedy against "The Great White Plague." These efforts culminated, in the mid-1940s, in the discovery of streptomycin by Schatz and Waksman and of paraaminosalicylate (PAS) by Lehmann. When the more effective drugs isoniazid (INH) and pyrazinamide (PZA) were introduced in the early 1950s, TB became a manageable disease in most cases. As predicted by Ehrlich (2), combination therapy with multiple drugs was widely adopted once it was found that "under the influence of two different medicines the danger of rendering the parasites immune, which naturally would be a very great obstacle in connection with further treatment, is apparently greatly minimized." In his optimistically entitled book *The Conquest of Tuberculosis*, Waksman went so far as to predict that "the ancient foe of man, known as consumption, the great white plague, tuberculosis, or by whatever other name, is on the way to being reduced to a minor ailment of man. The future appears bright indeed, and the complete eradication of the disease is in sight" (3).

Forty years later, and despite half a century of anti-TB chemotherapy, the world still sees 8 million to 10 million new cases of active TB each year, and nearly 2 billion individuals are believed to harbor latent TB based on tuberculin skin test (TST) surveys (Fig. 8.1) (4). Why has this manageable bacterial infection failed to yield to modern medicine? While the full answer to this question is certainly complex, one issue seems clear: the features that enable *M. tuberculosis* to persist in the tissues of its host have also allowed TB to remain one of the world's great killers into the 21st century. This problem was anticipated by Ehrlich (2) in 1913, in a historic address at the dawn of the chemotherapy era: "Now that the liability to, and danger of, disease are to a great extent circumscribed . . . the efforts of chemotherapeutics are directed as far as possible to fill up the gaps left in this ring, more especially to bring healing to diseases in which the natural powers of the organism are insufficient." Ninety years later, the ring has not yet been closed in the case of TB, where the "natural powers" of the human immune system are clearly "insufficient" to resolve infection.

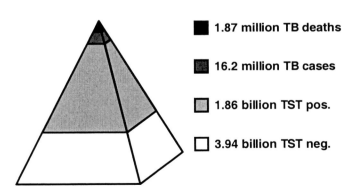

FIGURE 8.1. The "iceberg of pathogenesis." Worldwide, the number of prevalent tuberculosis (*TB*) cases (16.2 million) and annual TB deaths (1.87 million) is dwarfed by the number of latent TB infections (1.86 billion) as indicated by tuberculin skin test (*TST*) surveys. (Data from Dye C, Scheele S, Dolin P, et al. Global burden of tuberculosis: estimated incidence, prevalence, and mortality by country. *JAMA* 1999;282:677–686.)

J. E. Gomez and J. D. McKinney: Laboratory of Infection Biology, The Rockefeller University, New York, New York.

LATENCY, DORMANCY, AND PERSISTENCE

Three terms—*latency, persistence*, and *dormancy*—are commonly used in describing *Mycobacterium tuberculosis* and TB pathogenesis. Because these terms have not always been used consistently, they will be defined here as they will be used in this chapter. *Latency* was defined by Amberson (5) as "the presence of any tuberculous lesion which fails to produce symptoms of its presence." Latency can be achieved through either the early restriction of *M. tuberculosis* growth in the lungs prior to the onset of TB disease or the spontaneous resolution of primary TB. Most people exposed to *M. tuberculosis* mount a vigorous cell-mediated immune response that arrests the progress of the infection, largely limiting it to the initial site of invasion in the lung parenchyma and the local draining lymph nodes [the "Ghon complex" (6)]. The complete elimination of the pathogen, however, is slow and difficult to achieve. Without antibiotic treatment, chronic or latent infection is thought to be the typical outcome of TB infection. Latent TB can reactivate after years or even decades of subclinical persistence, leading to progressive disease and active transmission of the pathogen.

Dormancy has been used to describe both TB disease and the metabolic state of the tubercle bacillus. TB lesions are described as active or dormant, based on whether the associated pathology is progressing or healing, respectively. Active lesions generally contain easily detectable populations of acid-fast, culturable *M. tuberculosis*, but the precise bacteriologic status of dormant lesions remains unclear despite nearly a century of study and debate. The term *dormancy* has also become strongly associated with an *in vitro* model of *M. tuberculosis* growth under limiting oxygen tension, developed by Wayne and Hayes (7). It has been suggested that this model may approximate the state of *M. tuberculosis* surviving in closed, necrotic lesions during clinical latency. It should be emphasized that the model remains speculative because the location and physiologic state of *M. tuberculosis* during latency have not yet been firmly established.

The word *persistence* literally means "continuing steadfastly or obstinately, especially in the face of opposition or adversity." As a pathogen, *M. tuberculosis* manifests its unusual capacity to persist in many ways. On the cellular level, mycobacteria reside within macrophages, which are cells that typically function to eliminate pathogens and other foreign material from the body. At a more systemic level, *M. tuberculosis* is able to avoid elimination from the human host despite the development of vigorous cell-mediated immunity. Another less obvious but profoundly important manifestation of *M. tuberculosis* persistence is the slow rate at which this bacterium is cleared by anti-TB drugs. The 6 months or more of chemotherapy required to cure TB makes the management of this disease an especially formidable challenge to global public health infrastructure, particularly in the developing world.

PERSISTENCE *EX VIVO*

Long before the discovery of streptomycin and other antimicrobials, *M. tuberculosis* was known to be an unusually hardy bacterium, both inside and outside the body. In the early 20th century, researchers subjected *M. tuberculosis* to a barrage of environmental assaults to ascertain which conditions affected the organism's viability and virulence [(8) and references therein]. *Mycobacterium tuberculosis* proved quite adept at withstanding a wide variety of *ex vivo* insults, including desiccation, nutrient deprivation, and osmotic shock, but was found to be highly sensitive to direct exposure to sunlight—an Achilles heel that was later exploited by installation of ultraviolet lights in public spaces such as hospital wards and homeless shelters. It was frequently observed that bacterial samples subjected to environmental affronts retained their virulence for guinea pigs longer that they retained their ability to be subcultured on artificial media. These qualitative observations were probably due in part to the primitive culture media and technology of the time, as well as the exquisite susceptibility of guinea pigs to TB. A more quantitative study of the longevity of tubercle bacilli in culture was carried out by Corper and Cohn (8), who placed several hundred sealed cultures of various human and bovine isolates in a 37°C incubator in 1920 and left them untouched until 1932. Of 56 bottles that were subsequently analyzed, 24 yielded culturable organisms, with an estimated survival of 0.01% in the culturable human samples and approximately 1% survival in the bovine isolates. The viability of the cultures was strongly dependent on the pH of the conditioned medium; samples in which the pH had dropped below 6.1 or risen above pH 7.6 failed to yield viable bacteria. Strains that were known to be virulent prior to their placement in the incubator in 1920 retained their virulence upon subculture in 1932. The authors of this remarkable study speculated that the ability of TB to persist in a closed culture vessel for so many years might be connected to long-term persistence during latency, and drew an analogy between their sealed bottles and the healed human lesions thought to contain persistent *M. tuberculosis*. These observations provided a foundation for the "Wayne model" of TB persistence in oxygen-limited cultures, which has been the focus of renewed interest in recent years (9).

PERSISTENCE AND LATENCY

Prior to the antibiotic era, TB was considered a lifelong infection: "once tuberculous, always tuberculous." This clinical adage was recently given a new twist by a molecular epidemiology study in Denmark, which provided the first compelling molecular evidence for the existence of extraordinarily long periods of latency in untreated humans (10). This study examined the case of a Danish man who first

8: Persistence and Drug Tolerance **103**

developed TB in 1990. When the IS*6110* fingerprint of the _M. tuberculosis_ strain isolated from this patient was compared to fingerprints from the national strain collection, the only match was to an isolate dating from 1958—his father's.

Despite the common feature of persistence, in the preantibiotic era the clinical outcome of infection was clearly variable in different individuals. While some succumbed relatively quickly to a steadily progressive primary infection, others were able to contain the disease. This containment was often temporary, and postprimary TB developing after an extended incubation period was commonplace. The reemergence of TB in those who had previously been diagnosed with TB was generally assumed to be due to reactivation of the earlier infection. The introduction of antibiotic therapy substantially reduced the risk of reactivation, further underscoring the inability of many patients to eliminate _M. tuberculosis_ from the tissues without therapeutic intervention. In the early years of chemotherapy, post-therapy relapse rates hovered around 20%—a substantial improvement from the era when 50% to 80% of TB cases proved fatal within a few years of diagnosis, but still far from ideal. A major step forward was taken in the 1960s with the introduction of short-course combination chemotherapy consisting of INH, rifampin (RIF), and PZA, which further reduced the posttherapy relapse rate to a more acceptable 1% to 2% (11).

Historically, the contribution of exogenous reinfection to the incidence of postprimary TB was largely ignored because it was assumed (on scant evidence) that the first infection would provide substantial protection against secondary infection. Recently, however, it has become clear that exogenous reinfection can be an important source of postprimary TB in high-prevalence areas (11,12). It is currently unclear what proportion of the incident cases of postprimary TB on a global scale is contributed by exogenous reinfection as opposed to endogenous reactivation. As discussed by Styblo (13), the relative importance of these two sources of postprimary TB in a geographically delimited population is probably determined by the local trajectory of the epidemic. Where TB rates are high and rising, as in much of sub-Saharan Africa, reinfection should become increasingly important; where TB rates are low and falling, as in the United States and western Europe, reactivation should predominate.

It is widely assumed that latent TB is due to the incomplete healing of tuberculous lesions, that these smoldering lesions are the site of persistence of dormant tubercle bacilli, and that under certain circumstances the standoff between host and parasite shifts in the bacterium's favor, allowing reactivation. The puzzle is how to reconcile this picture with the fact that the human immune system is clearly capable of mounting a vigorous response against _M. tuberculosis_. Although locally destructive, this necrotizing response can lead to the extensive fibrosis of tuberculous lesions, caseation of infectious foci, and the eventual calci-

fication of the surrounding tissue (14,15). Is it possible that tubercle bacilli are capable of persisting for years within these apparently healed lesions? Or does lymphohematogenous or bronchogenic spread allow the persistence of tubercle bacilli in other regions of the lung? Finally, do other tissues or cell types also harbor viable bacilli during latent infection? Conclusive answers to these questions are not yet available, although numerous investigators have addressed the issues for the better part of a century [reviewed in (16)].

Surgical resection of tuberculous lesions was uncommon in the preantibiotic era, so that early attempts to assess the viability of tubercle bacilli in human lesions were largely limited to necropsy specimens. Lesions obtained from cadavers were frequently shown to contain acid-fast bacilli, sometimes in great numbers. In the mid-1920s, Opie and Aronson (17) collected several hundred necropsy specimens and inoculated this material into guinea pigs. They found that homogenates of fibrocaseous lesions of the apex of the lung typically caused TB in guinea pigs, whereas homogenates of caseous encapsulated or calcified lesions seldom did. Interestingly, nearly half of the samples derived from superficially normal lung tissue were found to be infectious for guinea pigs. In contrast, Feldman and Baggenstoss (18), working at the Mayo Clinic in the late 1930s, found tubercle bacilli in normal lung tissue in only 3 of 51 cases. These authors also observed that the Ghon complex, the calcified primary tubercle and the draining tracheobronchial lymph node, were almost never infectious for guinea pigs (19). Similarly, Sweany et al. (20) were unable to recover viable tubercle bacilli from most lesions and the tissue surrounding them. Together these data suggested that humans are capable of sterilizing primary lesions in the lung and draining lymph nodes, but that tubercle bacilli may persist more effectively in newer secondary lesions, or perhaps even in essentially normal tissue. A new twist was recently added to this story: more than 70 years after Opie and Aronson's original studies were published, the presence of IS*6110* DNA, an insertion element found in multiple copies in the _M. tuberculosis_ chromosome, was demonstrated in the superficially normal lung tissue of Ethiopians and Mexicans who died of causes other than TB (21). _In situ_ polymerase chain reaction revealed that mycobacterial genomic DNA frequently localized to cells other than macrophages, including lung endothelial cells and type II pneumocytes. This intriguing study raises the possibility that invasion of nonprofessional phagocytes lacking major histocompatibility complex class II antigen-presenting molecules may be a novel immune evasion strategy of _M. tuberculosis_; however, the persistence of viable bacilli was not explicitly demonstrated.

PERSISTENCE AND CHEMOTHERAPY

If the fate of bacilli in naturally healed lesions continues to be controversial, the status of tubercle bacilli within patients treated with antimicrobials is even less clear. Following the introduction of TB chemotherapy in the late 1940s, surgical resection of tuberculous lesions became increasingly common and provided material for numerous bacteriologic studies. Several reports published in the mid-1950s showed that large numbers of acid-fast bacilli could be observed by microscopy in tubercles resected months after patients on chemotherapy became sputum negative (22–28). Although *M. tuberculosis* could be cultured from some of these lesions, most failed to yield culturable bacilli; this was especially true of "closed lesions" lacking patent bronchial communication. However, whether these visible but nonculturable bacteria were truly and irreversibly dead or were instead "viable but nonculturable" remained the subject of vigorous debate (24). A proponent of the latter idea, McDermott speculated that these nonculturable bacteria might be not dead, but merely "dormant," and perhaps capable of being resuscitated under the right conditions. Throughout the 1950s and 1960s, McDermott et al. carried out extensive studies in mice to evaluate the fate of *M. tuberculosis* during and after chemotherapy (29–32). These classic studies, which laid the foundation for our current understanding of the efficacy of antituberculous agents used individually and in combination, led to the development of a mouse model of *M. tuberculosis* persistence and reactivation (the "Cornell model") still in use today.

Work by Hobby et al. (25) suggested that inhibitors of mycobacterial growth might be present in resected tissue specimens. By careful washing of samples and extended culture times, Hobby's group was able to substantially increase the rate at which they successfully recovered bacteria from the resected lesions. Although efforts by others to duplicate these findings were not always successful, Vandiviere et al. (27) used extended culturing to obtain even more intriguing results (Fig. 8.2). While their 94% success rate in culturing bacilli from the open lesions of drug-treated patients was somewhat high but not exceptional, their observations regarding closed lesions were striking. By extending the incubation period of their cultures from the standard 8 weeks to 3–10 months, they were able to culture bacilli from nine of 22 closed lesions. Seven of these nine isolates were fully drug sensitive, in contrast to the open cavities, where 37 of 45 isolates were resistant to one or more of the drugs with which the patient was treated. Lack of drug access was presumably not responsible for the survival of *M. tuberculosis* within the closed lesions because INH had been shown previously to penetrate all types of lesions in the human lung (33). To explain their observations, the authors postulated that conditions within closed lesions—such as lowered oxygen tension, long-chain fatty acids, lactic acid, and other bacteriostatic agents—reduced bacterial metabolism and rendered tubercle bacilli refractory to drugs. In this context, it is noteworthy that all of the front-line drugs currently used to manage TB target processes that are involved in cell growth and division, which may explain their poor activity against *in vivo* bacteria and particularly against bacteria in closed lesions. Despite their success in culturing viable bacilli from closed lesions, Vandiviere et al. speculated that "if this state of dormancy lasted long enough, the normal effect of host resistance . . . could, with

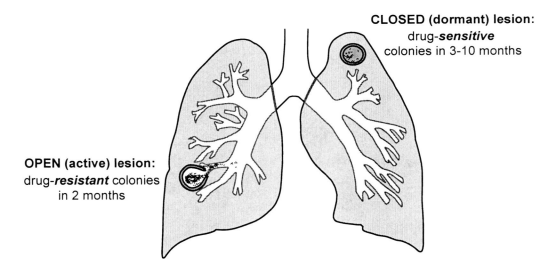

FIGURE 8.2. The death of resurrection of drug-managed *Mycobacterium tuberculosis.* Resected lung lesions were cultured from treated patients. Open/active cavitary lesions, with patent airway connections, typically yielded drug-resistant tubercle bacilli in the normal time frame (2 months or less). Closed/dormant and encapsulated lesions, unconnected to an airway, yielded drug-susceptible tubercle bacilli only after extended incubation (3–10 months). (Data from Loring WE, Vandiviere HM. The treated pulmonary lesion and its tubercle bacillus. I. Pathology and pathogenesis. *Am J Med Sci* 1956;232:20–29.)

sufficient time, reduce the viable units, finally leading to sterilization of the cavity."

In a further attempt to characterize the differences between open and closed lesions, Haapanen et al. (34) obtained gas samples by needling 20 cavities from the lungs of living TB patients and measuring the concentrations of carbon dioxide and oxygen therein. Blocked cavities, where the overall pressure was negative, were enriched for carbon dioxide (10.5% on average versus 3.5% for open cavities) and partially depleted for oxygen (6.3% on average versus 17.8% in open cavities). Like Vandiviere et al., these authors also expressed concern that closure of cavities might slow the metabolism of any viable tubercle bacilli remaining inside, thereby interfering with the bactericidal activity of antitubercular agents such as INH and streptomycin. INH and streptomycin were known to be far more effective against actively replicating *M. tuberculosis* than against nondividing cells, as demonstrated by Hobby and Lenert in 1957 (35). The striking difference in antibiotic susceptibility of actively replicating bacterial cells and nondividing cells has profound implications for the management of TB.

MODELING PERSISTENCE *IN VITRO*

The simplest model of *M. tuberculosis* persistence is the stationary phase culture. The kinetics of replication of *M. tuberculosis* in the lungs of mice are reminiscent of the organism's replication kinetics in culture: an initial period of exponential growth is followed by an extended period during which the number of viable bacilli remains stable. Admittedly, the forces that bring about the cessation of growth *in vitro* (nutrient exhaustion) are not equivalent to those *in vivo* (acquired immunity, although this may play a role in restricting nutrient availability). Still, the stationary phase culture provides a simple, inexpensive, and easily

manipulated system to analyze the long-term survival of nonreplicating cells of *M. tuberculosis*.

Among the more important observations made using axenic stationary phase cultures of *M. tuberculosis* are those relating to drug susceptibility (Fig. 8.3). In one of the earliest studies of its kind, Hobby and Lenert (35) demonstrated that when actively growing *M. tuberculosis* cultures were washed and resuspended in buffered saline (without carbon source), the resulting cessation of bacterial growth was accompanied by the acquisition of refractoriness to killing by INH and PAS. This phenomenon is not unique to the genus *Mycobacterium*; for example, Hobby (36) had previously observed that stationary phase cultures of *Escherichia coli* were refractory to killing by penicillin. The inverse relationship between the bacterial growth rate and the rate of antibiotic-dependent killing is one manifestation of a more general phenomenon known as antibiotic "tolerance," a term coined by Tomasz in 1970 (37). More specifically, slowly replicating bacteria are said to exhibit *phenotypic tolerance* (38); certain mutations can also give rise to *genotypic tolerance*, but there is scant evidence for this form of antibiotic tolerance in *M. tuberculosis* (39). The mechanisms underlying phenotypic tolerance have been studied in both gram-negative and gram-positive bacteria.

Phenotypic antibiotic tolerance is not heritable but instead results from exposure to any of a variety of growth-limiting conditions. Among the conditions that result in phenotypic tolerance in nonmycobacterial species are amino acid starvation and acidic pH, conditions that *M. tuberculosis* may encounter within the host (40). Phenotypic tolerance has been demonstrated to involve the stringent response controlled by the *relA* gene (38). In response to amino acid–deficient conditions, RelA synthesizes tetra- and pentaphosphorylated guanosine (ppGpp and ppGppp, also known as "magic spot"). Association of ppGpp with the β subunit of RNA polymerase results in inhibition of

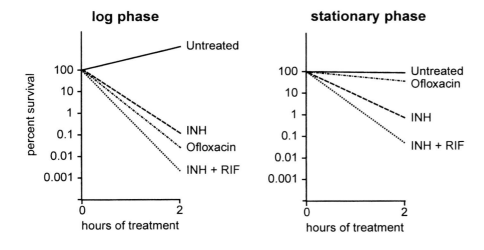

FIGURE 8.3. Differential kill rates of liquid cultures of *Mycobacterium tuberculosis* during exponential and stationary phase growth. All antibiotics have diminished activity against stationary phase bacteria as compared to replicating bacteria. This effect is most pronounced for the fluoroquinolone ofloxacin, a DNA gyrase inhibitor that causes double-stranded DNA breaks during replication of the bacterial genome. *INH*, isoniazid; *RIF*, rifampin. (Adapted from Herbert D, Paramasivan CN, Venkatesan P, et al. Bactericidal action of ofloxacin, sulbactam-ampicillin, rifampin, and isoniazid on logarithmic- and stationary-phase cultures of *Mycobacterium tuberculosis*. *Antimicrob Agents Chemother* 1996;40: 2296–2299.)

transcription. A *relA* mutant of *M. tuberculosis* was recently shown to survive poorly in stationary phase (41), but no data on the antibiotic tolerance or *in vivo* persistence of this mutant have yet been reported.

The early work of Tomasz (37) focused on genotypic tolerance, which is a heritable trait. In a study of *Streptococcus pneumoniae* mutants that were inhibited, but not killed, by penicillin, Tomasz observed that cell death was not a passive event. Mutations in the *lytA* gene, encoding a cell wall autolysin, allowed *S. pneumoniae* cultures to survive penicillin treatment. The penicillin-binding proteins in *lytA* mutants were still inhibited by β-lactams, but breakdown of the cell wall and lysis did not occur; in the presence of antibiotic, bacterial growth was arrested, but *lytA* mutants were not killed. If the drug was removed, bacterial replication resumed. There is but one example of genotypically tolerant *M. tuberculosis* in the literature (39); however, the phenotype of *M. tuberculosis* isolates described in this report was very modest as compared to pneumococcal *lytA* mutants, and the genetic basis of tolerance was not investigated. There are no obvious *lytA* homologs in the *M. tuberculosis* genome (42), but the LytA protein does not appear to be highly conserved throughout the eubacteria. In fact, little is known about the details of antibiotic-induced death in *M. tuberculosis*, although studies to better understand this phenomenon are underway in a number of laboratories.

Recent research on the response of *M. tuberculosis* to antibiotics has focused on transcriptional effects of drug exposure (43–46). Also, a model in which unaerated, 100-day-old stationary phase cultures are treated with RIF (47) has been developed as a way of studying bacteria that are phenotypically RIF tolerant. As more information becomes available on cell wall synthesis and breakdown, the stringent response, cell division, and cell death in *M. tuberculosis*, the mechanisms of tolerance that limit the efficacy of TB chemotherapy can be better evaluated.

An *in vitro* model of dormancy that has received much attention recently was developed by Wayne (9) in the 1970s. The conceptual foundation for this model was laid by Wayne in the 1950s, when the controversy surrounding the viability of *M. tuberculosis* in drug-treated lesions was at its peak. Wayne speculated that difficulties in recovering tubercle bacilli from resected lesions might be related to oxygen availability (48), as bacterial adaptation to the reduced oxygen tension within lesions might render them refractory to culture in well-aerated media. Wayne's attempts to resuscitate bacteria in resected lesions by altering the oxygenation of cultures were unsuccessful (48,49). Later, however, he succeeded in demonstrating that *M. tuberculosis* was capable of survival under anaerobic conditions *in vitro* (50) and that the bacteria that survived anaerobiosis underwent stage-specific cell cycle arrest (51). In Wayne's model, unshaken *M. tuberculosis* cultures were allowed to settle slowly through a self-generated oxygen gra-

dient into the anaerobic conditions present at the bottom of the culture vessel. The gradual transition to a state of anaerobiosis allowed the settling cells to become "dormant" after a transition period that was marked by increased expression of the enzymes isocitrate lyase and glycine dehydrogenase. The latter were proposed to constitute a novel pathway for regeneration of NAD$^+$ in the absence of aerobic respiration (52). The dormant state induced by oxygen deprivation was characterized by a near total shutdown of DNA, RNA, and protein synthesis (47,51) and a concomitant loss of sensitivity to antibiotics such as INH and RIF, along with increased sensitivity to metronidazole, an antibiotic used in the management of anaerobic infections (53). Upon resuscitation of the cultures by oxygenation, the bacteria underwent several rounds of synchronous replication, indicating that cell cycle arrest was stage specific. Although the Wayne model of dormancy is an *in vitro* phenomenon, it has been suggested that some of the phenotypic alterations observed may be relevant to the *in vivo* phenomenon of *M. tuberculosis* latency (54). The relevance of the Wayne model has been questioned because treatment of experimentally infected mice with metronidazole failed to affect *M. tuberculosis* persistence (55,56). However, it can be argued that the mouse model fails to reproduce important forms of tissue pathology, such as caseation necrosis, that have been postulated (but not proven) to influence intralesional oxygen tension and bacterial latency.

MODELING PERSISTENCE IN ANIMALS

The phenomenon of latency has been difficult to reproduce in a small-animal model. Apart from nonhuman primates (57), which are prohibitively expensive and impractical for general use, rabbits provide the closest facsimile of human tuberculosis in terms of tissue pathology and disease progression. Half a century ago, Lurie bred resistant and susceptible strains of rabbits, and demonstrated that the differential outcome of TB infections in these strains was determined by early events prior to the emergence of a specific T cell response, as well as late events involving acquired cell-mediated immunity (58). Both sensitive and resistant rabbits were able to curtail bacterial replication once a specific T cell response was established and to maintain a stable census in the lungs for many months thereafter. The long-term maintenance of a stable bacterial load in the lungs is a common characteristic of animal models of TB, including guinea pigs and mice as well as rabbits. However, the consequences of *M. tuberculosis* persistence are strikingly different in terms of tissue pathology and disease progression. As described by Lurie, the pathology that develops in persistently infected rabbits includes the softening and liquefaction of caseous tubercles leading to cavitation—a hallmark of human tuberculosis that is not reproduced in the guinea pig or mouse models. This makes the rabbit a uniquely valuable small-animal model to study the persistence of *M. tuberculosis* in cavitary lesions. Despite these advantages, the rabbit model is not widely used today. This is due in part to economic and logistic considerations, but also to a long history of research focused on the immunology and chemotherapy of infectious diseases in the mouse.

As mentioned already, infected mice are able to arrest bacterial replication in the lungs within a few weeks of exposure, depending on the dose and the route of inoculation. Low-dose aerosol infection, and moderate doses of *M. tuberculosis* inoculated intravenously, can be used to reproducibly achieve peak bacterial loads in the lungs of mice between 10^4 and 10^7 organisms (59). Resistant strains of mice, such as the C57BL/6 strain (60), are capable of surviving for long periods of time with such loads, during which time they show slowly progressive pathology in the lungs but few signs of overt disease. The early arrest of bacterial replication and the continued stability of the lung census are dependent on intact immunity, which makes this model attractive for the study of host factors needed for controlling infection as well as bacterial genes necessary for persistence within an immune host. In this regard, much has been learned about host immunity through studies in mice. The cytokines interferon-γ (IFN-γ) (61,62) and tumor necrosis factor-α (TNF-α) (63) have been shown to be essential for both the arrest and continued control of *M. tuberculosis* replication. These cytokines are involved in the activation of macrophages and the induction of inducible nitric oxide synthase (iNOS or NOS2), which has been shown to be essential in mice for protection against TB (64). Neutralization of either TNF-α (65) or NOS2 (66) during the persistent phase of infection leads to a resumption of bacterial replication, underscoring their importance in the long-term control of *M. tuberculosis*. Clinical evidence suggests that TNF-α may also be essential for maintenance of TB latency in humans because treatment of latently infected individuals with infliximab, a TNF-α blocker, has been associated with increased risk of reactivation (67). Both CD4+ T cells (68) and CD8+ T cells (69) have been shown to have important roles in the sustained arrest of *M. tuberculosis* in chronically infected mice. The increased risk of reactivation in latently infected individuals who become coinfected with human immunodeficiency virus suggests that CD4+ T cells are also important for maintenance of latency in humans.

While it seems clear that mice are less able than humans to eliminate *M. tuberculosis* from the lungs, their ability to restrict bacterial expansion for an extended duration provides a system in which the standoff between host and pathogen can be dissected. Two models can be proposed to account for this stalemate. In one, a balance between continued bacterial replication and host killing may be achieved at the onset of acquired immunity. This model is supported by evidence that the granulomas found in another TB animal model, *Mycobacterium marinum* infec-

tion of frogs, are dynamic structures that may allow continued *M. marinum* replication (70). Alternately, acquired immunity may drive *M. tuberculosis* into an "*in vivo* stationary phase," a state in which little or no cell division occurs. This model is supported by a classic study by Rees and Hart (71). They hypothesized that continuous bacterial turnover due to balanced growth and death would lead to an accumulation of bacterial bodies, since they and others had shown that the corpses of heat- or drug-killed *M. tuberculosis* were quite stable in mouse lungs. Because they observed stable numbers of acid-fast bacilli in the lungs during persistent infection of mice, they concluded that there was little turnover in the *M. tuberculosis* population. This conclusion was supported by a concomitant study on the heat resistance of *M. tuberculosis* derived from mouse lungs, which demonstrated that *in vivo* bacteria, like stationary phase bacteria grown *in vitro*, were better able to tolerate exposure to 53°C (72). The resistance of *in vivo* bacteria to thermal stress was particularly marked when bacteria were derived from chronically infected rather than acutely infected mice. While direct measurements of *M. tuberculosis* cell division rates in the lungs of mice have not been carried out, the available evidence would seem to indicate that replication rates are slowed or halted in response to acquired immunity.

Another mouse model of TB latency is based on the reduction, but not elimination, of *M. tuberculosis* populations in the organs of mice via antimicrobial therapy. The Cornell model, as it is commonly known, was developed by McDermott et al. at Cornell University in the 1950s. The contemporaneous debate over the viability of microscopically detectable but nonculturable bacilli found in tissues resected from drug-treated patients led the Cornell group to examine the effects of antimicrobials on *M. tuberculosis* in the lungs and spleens of mice. They examined the efficacy of four anti-TB agents, including all of the drugs that were in use clinically, alone and in various combinations (30). As assessed by quantitative analysis of plated lung homogenates, many of the antibiotics studied were severely limited in their capacity to sustain their antimicrobial activity after only a few weeks of administration. The bacterial census in the lungs and spleen dropped during the initial weeks of treatment but tended to stabilize over time, particularly in the spleen. These observations were not the result of the emergence of drug resistant mutants, since the populations of surviving bacteria were typically more than 99% sensitive. Even when the drug dosage was increased or multiple drugs were used in combination, a plateau was typically reached after which no additional killing could be achieved. McDermott (73) coined the term "persisters" to designate the long-term, drug-sensitive survivors of drug therapy and further suggested that "this capacity of drug-susceptible organisms to survive drug attack when subsisting in an animal body may be designated as *microbial persistence.*" He also acknowledged the importance of the problem: "In clinical practice this phenomenon obviously has to do with the post-treatment 'carrier state' and with post-treatment relapse. In short, it is this phenomenon which is responsible for our inability to eradicate an infection from a person or a community by the use of drugs."

The Cornell investigators found that the only drug that would consistently reduce the bacterial load to undetectable levels in both lungs and spleens was PZA, and only when it was given for a minimum of 12 weeks in combination with a companion drug such as INH (29). Later work by a number of investigators demonstrated that RIF also has potent sterilizing power (74). Despite the initial appearance of success, further investigations established that the "sterile state" that was apparently achieved with INH and PZA was problematic. When mice were sacrificed and examined after 12 weeks of INH and PZA, they appeared devoid of viable *M. tuberculosis* organisms (31,32). No bacteria could be cultured from these mice, despite efforts that included plating every organ in its entirety, and then homogenizing the remaining flesh and bones and plating that material. Likewise, it proved impossible to transfer the infection to highly susceptible guinea pigs using extracts from these tissues. Yet it became clear that the drugs had not in fact eradicated infection, but merely rendered it "latent" in the sense that "the presence of the infection cannot be demonstrated by any of the available methods and the fact that it *is* present can only be detected in retrospect by the appearance of relapse" (73). When treated mice were maintained for several months without further intervention, the majority began to show spontaneous bacteriologic relapse (reappearance of culturable bacilli in the tissues). Furthermore, the rate of relapse could be accelerated and increased to 100% of treated animals by administration of high-dose corticosteroids. In keeping with McDermott's definition of "persisters," the bacilli cultured from the relapsing animals remained fully sensitive to INH and PZA, indicating that they were not merely drug-resistant mutants selected during therapy. How had these bacilli "vanished" and then reappeared? And what implications did this phenomenon have for the management of human TB?

One clear implication is the existence of a subpopulation of bacteria *in vivo* that are phenotypically tolerant to the effects of antibiotics. The question that arises is, what are the conditions *in vivo* that trigger the tolerant state? Pathophysiologic studies on human lesions led to the hypothesis that the development of potentially bacteriostatic tissue environments, such as that associated with reduced oxygen tension, nutrient limitation, or acidic pH, could result in the acquisition of drug tolerance by nonreplicating bacteria. However, it is important to point out that the forms of tissue damage proposed to contribute to bacteriostasis in human lung lesions seem to differ in important respects from the pathology of tuberculous lesions in mice. The granulomas that develop in human TB are highly organized structures, containing macrophages and giant cells at their center, surrounded by a rim of lymphocytes at the periphery. The necrotic death of cells at the center of these lesions leads to an accumulation of caseous material that may eventually liquefy and cavitate. In contrast, mouse granulomas comprise a looser accumulation of macrophages, neutrophils, and lymphocytes, and caseation necrosis is less common and occurs more slowly (75). Yet, despite the differences in TB tissue pathology in mice and humans, it is clear that *M. tuberculosis* drug tolerance develops in both host species.

Since tissue pathology does not account for *M. tuberculosis* drug tolerance in the Cornell model, what might? While mycobacterial growth inhibition by acquired immunity appears to reduce the initial rate of drug-induced killing in the mouse, it does not prevent the drugs from working altogether. Nonetheless, the Cornell studies showed that any drug administered alone, or combinations of drugs not including INH and PZA, became less effective with time. At least two alternative explanations can be envisaged. In the first scenario, chemotherapy would rapidly kill all but a small, highly tolerant subpopulation of bacteria ("persisters"), which would still be present and capable of reactivating after 12 weeks of treatment. In the second scenario, the slow killing of a moderately but more uniformly tolerant population of organisms during 12 weeks of INH and PZA therapy would be insufficient to achieve complete sterilization by 12 weeks, leaving a small number of surviving bacteria. In either case, but for very different reasons, the surviving organisms would be in a physiologic state that would render them nonculturable and noninfectious to guinea pigs, although capable of reactivating *in situ*. Either model is consistent with observations of Grosset et al., using fluctuation analysis with genetically marked strains, that the number of organisms reactivating after drug-induced latency is very small, probably less than 10 (76).

The basic distinction between the two scenarios that have been proposed to account for the difficulty of eradicating TB with drugs is whether a "special" subpopulation of highly drug-tolerant bacteria does (first model) or does not (second model) exist *in vivo*. For the better part of a century, many investigators have proposed that alternate forms of *M. tuberculosis* cells (e.g., protoplasts, L forms, or spores) (77) may go undetected *in vivo*, such alternate forms being ill suited for growth in culture or transfer to guinea pigs. As yet, however, no compelling evidence has been adduced for the existence of radically altered forms of tubercle bacilli or for a role of such altered forms in drug tolerance. Indeed, the kinetics of drug-induced killing in the mouse would seem to support the second model, in which the entire bacterial population is relatively, but not completely, refractory to killing. In this regard, it is noteworthy that, in the Cornell studies, prolongation of INH/PZA treatment to 26 weeks apparently resulted in complete sterilization (i.e., the treated animals did not relapse even when severely immune suppressed). This would seem to indicate that the residual bacterial population after 12 weeks of therapy does not consist of nonculturable "alternate forms" that are completely indifferent to drugs. Perhaps the inability to culture organisms from the tissues after prolonged chemotherapy is simply due to accumulated drug-induced damage rendering the organisms too fragile to survive the shock of passage to a new environment.

Since drug tolerance is an *in vivo* phenomenon, it is important to ascertain which aspects of the tissue environment are responsible. Unfortunately, this remains a very murky area of mycobacteriology despite its manifest importance. One important point, at least, is clear: From the very earliest stages of infection, the alterations in bacterial metabolism and physiology that accompany the shift from growth in culture to growth in the lung appear to affect drug activity. This cannot be due solely to alteration of the overall growth rate; during the initial weeks of infection, *M. tuberculosis* replicates as rapidly in the lungs of mice as in artificial medium, yet drug-dependent kill rates in the two conditions are vastly different. For example, exposure to INH and RIF kills 99.9% of the cells in a culture of *M. tuberculosis* within 48 hours, yet comparable killing with these drugs *in vivo* requires 3 to 4 weeks (Fig. 8.4). The concentration of antibiotics achieved in the tissues is not likely to account entirely for the reduced drug sensitivity of *M. tuberculosis in vivo*. Drugs like INH seem to be capable of accumulating to very high levels within TB lesions (33). Thus, it is not surprising that the slow rate of killing *in vivo* cannot be overcome by simply increasing the drug dosage (78). Why, then, are drugs like INH, which are rapidly bactericidal *in vitro*, so poorly effective *in vivo*? A definitive

answer to this question remains elusive, but an improved understanding of the physiology of *M. tuberculosis* while living in the lungs should provide clues.

Recently, the Cornell model has been resurrected as a tool for studying various aspects of *M. tuberculosis* persistence. The original model and its various adaptations are clearly useful for the study of antibiotic effects, particularly their activity against persisters. The late effects of rifapentine (79), metronidazole (56), moxifloxacin (80), and other drugs have been evaluated in various permutations of the Cornell model. The model has also been used to study the immunological control of persistent *M. tuberculosis* infection [(81), reviewed in (82)]. The difficulty in reliably achieving the "sterile state" and consistently reviving the infection, in conjunction with the uncertain relationship between drug-induced latency and the immunity-driven latency seen in humans, implies that experiments using the Cornell model need to be designed and interpreted with care (81).

NEW DEVELOPMENTS

During the past 15 years, the development of molecular genetic tools for the analysis of *M. tuberculosis* has significantly advanced our ability to study the *in vivo* biology of *M. tuberculosis* (83). Genetic and gene expression–based studies have led to the identification of genes that appear to be involved in the adaptation of *M. tuberculosis* to life in the lungs. The mouse continues to be the most frequently used model for studies of *M. tuberculosis* pathogenesis, although there has been a renewal of interest in other models, including guinea pigs, rabbits, and nonhuman primates. Most importantly, new technologies are making it possible, for the first time, to analyze *M. tuberculosis* physiology directly in tissues obtained from infected humans (84).

A growing number of genes appear to have their most important role during the late or chronic phases of infection. The "persistence factors" encoded by these genes may offer particularly attractive targets for drug development, with the possibility of shortening the required treatment time significantly (85). One of the first persistence factors identified affected an unusual behavior of *M. tuberculosis* known as "cording," that is, formation of ropelike tangles of laterally associated bacilli—which has long been thought to be associated with bacterial virulence (86). The cording phenotype was shown to depend on the *pcaA* gene product, an enzyme responsible for the cyclopropanation of α-mycolates, which are long-chain α-alkyl β-hydroxy fatty acids that comprise a major constituent of the mycobacterial cell wall. Disruption of *pcaA* resulted in a slight enhancement of bacterial replication in mice during the acute phase of infection as well as a later defect in persistence. The rather modest reduction in the bacterial load in the lung at late stages of infection was associated with a seemingly disproportion-

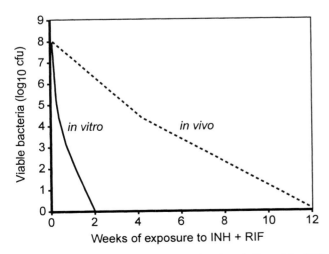

FIGURE 8.4. Drugs such as isoniazid (*INH*) and rifampicin (*RIF*), which are rapidly bactericidal against *Mycobacterium tuberculosis* growing in liquid culture (*in vitro*) are much less effective against *M. tuberculosis* in the lungs of infected mice (*in vivo*). (Drawn from unpublished data, JD McKinney, 2003.)

ate impact on the survival of the infected mice. This may have been attributable to the profoundly altered cellular infiltrate and granuloma organization in mice infected with *pcaA* mutant bacteria lacking proximally cyclopropanated mycolic acids. The role of *M. tuberculosis* cell wall components in modulating host immunity has been studied intensively, and the cell wall–associated molecule phthiocerol dimycocerosate has recently been shown to be important for bacterial replication in mouse lungs at early stages of infection (87). The *pcaA* mutant demonstrates that cell wall components may modulate the host response in a stage-specific manner.

There has recently been a resurgence of interest in the metabolism of *M. tuberculosis* during life in the lung. The first observations that "*in vivo*-grown" bacteria were metabolically distinct from bacteria grown *in vitro* were reported in 1956 by Segal and Bloch. These authors demonstrated that tubercle bacilli isolated from mouse lungs showed a marked enhancement of enzymatic activities related to the breakdown and utilization of fatty acids as a source of carbon and energy (88). Among the pathways required for utilization of fatty acids is the glyoxylate cycle, an anaplerotic pathway that is present in most bacteria but absent in vertebrates. Recently, the *icl1* gene encoding isocitrate lyase, one of the enzymes of the glyoxylate cycle, was shown to be essential for late-stage persistence of *M. tuberculosis* in the mouse model (89). Disruption of the *M. tuberculosis icl1* gene had no effect on bacterial growth *in vitro* or during the acute phase of infection in mice. However, coincident with the onset of cell-mediated immunity, the *icl1* mutant was slowly but progressively eliminated from the lungs. This stage-specific persistence defect resulted in a profound attenuation of virulence (i.e., survival of animals infected with the *icl1* mutant was greatly extended as compared to animals infected with wild-type bacteria). The *icl1* mutant phenotype was largely reversed in mice deficient in IFN-γ, underscoring the key role of the host immune response in driving the dependence of *M. tuberculosis* on this metabolic pathway.

Persistence of *M. tuberculosis in vivo* presumably involves mechanisms for evading the onslaught of the host immune response. A fascinating example of this interplay may be provided by a recent study in which deletion of the *M. tuberculosis hspR* gene, encoding a transcription factor that represses expression of the Hsp70 heat-shock protein, resulted in a delayed defect in bacterial survival (90). The uncontrolled expression of Hsp70 in *M. tuberculosis* had no discernible impact on growth *in vitro* or during the acute phase of infection in mice. However, at later stages of infection, the bacterial load was dramatically reduced in mice infected with the *hspR* mutant bacteria as compared with mice infected with wild-type bacteria. An intriguing possibility is that the uncontrolled expression of the highly immunogenic Hsp70 protein, or a general enhancement of protein (antigen) secretion due to overproduction of this

chaperonin, may have resulted in an enhancement of the host immune response and more effective control of infection. Consistent with this idea, splenocytes from mice infected with *hspR* mutant bacteria contained a twofold higher frequency of Hsp70-specific, IFN-γ-secreting cells as compared with splenocytes derived from mice infected with wild-type bacteria.

The transition from the acute to the chronic phase of infection, accompanied by the shift from exponential bacterial growth to stationary phase persistence, is likely to involve profound alterations in *M. tuberculosis* gene expression. Sequencing of the *M. tuberculosis* genome revealed a large repertoire of putative transcriptional regulatory proteins, including 13 sigma factors, 11 complete two-component regulatory systems, and a multitude of additional uncharacterized transcription factors (42). Emerging evidence suggests that some of these regulatory factors are required for the induction and repression of persistence genes.

Two-component regulatory systems, consisting of a "sensor kinase" and a "response regulator" that binds to promoter regions to regulate transcription, are involved in the responses to a diversity of environmental stimuli in eubacteria. In *M. tuberculosis*, disruption of the Rv0981 gene encoding the MprA response regulator was recently shown to impair persistence in the organs of chronically infected mice, with the deficiency being most pronounced in the spleens (91). Alternative sigma factors bind to the core RNA polymerase ($\alpha_2\beta\beta'$) and direct it to promoters that are not recognized by the polymerase when it is programmed by the "housekeeping" sigma factor (σ^A). In *M. tuberculosis*, a key role for alternative sigma factors in pathogenesis is emerging from studies in a number of laboratories, and there is some evidence that certain of the alternative sigma factors may have their most important role at later stages of infection (92). Intriguingly, disruption of the *M. tuberculosis sigH* gene was shown to result in profound attenuation of virulence in mice while having no discernible impact on the bacterial load in the tissues at any stage of infection (93). Likewise, disruption of the *M. tuberculosis whiB3* gene, encoding a putative transcriptional regulator, led to prolonged survival of infected mice without affecting bacterial numbers (94). In both cases, mice infected with the mutant bacteria (*sigH* or *whiB3*) showed a dramatically altered inflammatory process in the lungs as compared with mice infected with wild-type bacteria. These elegant studies underscore the importance of elucidating the host–pathogen interactions that influence the most important outcome of infection—death or survival—independently of the rather crude metric of bacterial numbers in the tissues. An important goal for future studies will be the identification of the key genes controlled by these and other transcriptional regulators and the elucidation of their specific roles in pathogenesis. This is a very active area of TB research, and it is anticipated that the key regulatory processes and gene networks that control *M. tuberculosis* growth, persistence, and pathogenesis at different stages of infection will soon be revealed.

CONCLUSIONS

During the past decade, there has been a resurgence of interest in the phenomenon of *M. tuberculosis* persistence. In the United States, this has been due in part to the recognition that the demographics of TB are shifting. In 1990, three fourths of all TB cases in the United States were among the U.S.-born; a decade later, the numbers of cases among the U.S.-born and foreign-born were roughly equal (Fig. 8.5). Most significantly, from 1990 to 2000, there was a marked fall in the absolute number of TB cases among the U.S.-born; in contrast, during the same period, the absolute number of cases among the foreign-born actually rose (Fig. 8.5), despite increased investment in TB control during the 1990s. These statistics underscore the unusual difficulty of controlling a persistent infection like TB via conventional public health measures, particularly in the context of an increasingly global society like ours in which the far side of the globe is just a plane ride away. Rising rates of immigration to the United States from high-incidence countries means that more and more persons with latent TB will enter the country in the years to come. Reactivation after arrival will continue to generate new cases of TB and new foci for transmission within the United States. The tools that are currently available to combat this threat to public health—essentially, the TST and isoniazid chemoprophylaxis—are antiquated and woefully inadequate. In recognition of this unmet need, a recent report from the Institute of Medicine warned that "Tuberculosis elimination is not possible with the tools that are currently available. The first priority for research is development of an understanding of latent infection" (95–97).

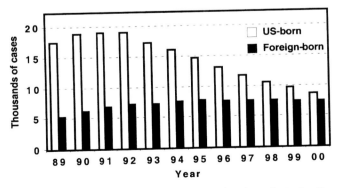

FIGURE 8.5. Changing demographics of tuberculosis in the United States, 1989–2000. (Data from Centers for Disease Control and Prevention. Tuberculosis morbidity among U.S.-born and foreign-born populations—United States, 2000. *MMWR Morb Mortal Wkly Rep* 2002;51:101–104.)

TB control programs in rich and poor countries alike would benefit enormously from four types of new interventions targeting latent TB:

1. *An improved diagnostic test for latent TB infection to replace the TST, which lacks sensitivity and specificity.* In particular, a diagnostic test that can reliably distinguish between latent TB infection and bacille Calmette–Guérin (BCG) vaccination will be essential for use in countries where childhood BCG vaccination is routine; recently, significant progress has been made toward development of such a discriminatory tool (98).

2. *A test to identify individuals with latent TB who are at risk for future reactivation.* Since about 90% of latently infected individuals never develop active TB, it would be very useful if the 10% of individuals who will could be identified before reactivation occurs so that resources (e.g., prophylactic therapy) could be focused on them.

3. *Improved chemoprophylactic therapy for latent TB to prevent reactivation.* The regimen currently recommended by the U.S. Centers for Disease Control and Prevention—9 months of daily INH monotherapy (99)—is impractical for application on a large scale, particularly in resource-limited countries. It is important to note that INH prophylaxis for latent TB infection is not associated with increased risk of acquired INH resistance, implying that the bacterial load must be very small (less than 10^6 organisms). Surely it should be possible to devise new drugs to eliminate such a small population of organisms more effectively and rapidly. An analogous example may be provided by the recent introduction of effective single-dose combination therapy (RIF, ofloxacin, minocycline) for single-lesion paucibacillary leprosy, caused by the related organism *Mycobacterium leprae* (100). A comparable regimen—effective, affordable, and ultrashort course—for the management of latent TB infection would revolutionize global TB control programs.

4. *Perhaps most speculative, an effective postexposure vaccine that could be administered to individuals with latent TB infection to prevent subsequent reactivation.* Although this approach is fraught with conceptual and practical challenges, a recent study suggests that it may be feasible. Using the murine Cornell model of chemotherapy-induced latency, Lowrie et al. demonstrated that post-therapy relapse could be prevented by vaccinating the treated mice with a DNA vaccine encoding the mycobacterial Hsp65 heat-shock protein (101). Remarkably, severe immune suppression failed to reactivate the vaccinated animals, suggesting that the immune boost provided by vaccination allowed the complete eradication of bacteria from the tissues. Although it must be cautioned that DNA vaccination in humans has so far given somewhat disappointing results (102), an important "proof of principle" has been established: that postexposure vaccination, alone or in combination with drug

therapy, could provide a more rapid and effective intervention against latent TB.

Development of new interventions against latent TB infection hinges on an improved understanding of the mechanisms that allow *M. tuberculosis* to persist in the face of host immunity or chemotherapy. It is not yet clear whether these forms of persistence are associated with the same or distinct cellular processes. Recent important advances have been made in identifying *M. tuberculosis* "persistence factors" that promote long-term survival in the mouse model of TB. However, it is not yet clear whether targeting these persistence factors with new drugs will actually promote more rapid killing of bacteria *in vivo*, nor is it clear whether persistence factors that are essential in the mouse model will likewise be important in the context of human infection. The Cornell model has been a useful tool for the study of chemotherapy-induced latency in the mouse, but this form of artificially induced latency may not be relevant to latency in humans, which is typically brought about by the unaided immune response (82). A major challenge for future research will be to take findings from model systems and prove their relevance in humans. With recent spectacular advances in technology opening, for the first time, the possibility of exploring the biology of *M. tuberculosis* in its natural habitat, the human lung, this promises to become an area of vigorous research activity in the near future (84).

REFERENCES

1. McDermott W. Inapparent infection: relation of latent and dormant infection to microbial persistence. *Public Health Rep* 1959;74:485–499.
2. Ehrlich P. Address in pathology on chemotherapeutics: scientific principles, methods, and results. *Lancet* 1913;2:445–451.
3. Waksman SA. *The conquest of tuberculosis.* London: Robert Hale Ltd, 1964.
4. Dye C, Scheele S, Dolin P, et al. Global burden of tuberculosis: estimated incidence, prevalence, and mortality by country. *JAMA* 1999;282:677–686.
5. Amberson JB. The significance of latent forms of tuberculosis. *N Engl J Med* 1938;219:572–576.
6. Ghon A. The primary complex in human tuberculosis and its significance. *Am Rev Tuberc* 1923;7:314–317.
7. Wayne LG, Hayes LG. An *in vitro* model for sequential study of shiftdown of *Mycobacterium tuberculosis* through two stages of nonreplicating persistence. *Infect Immun* 1996;64:2062–2069.
8. Corper HJ, Cohn ML. The viability and virulence of old cultures of tubercle bacilli: studies on twelve-year broth cultures maintained at incubator temperature. *Am Rev Tuberc* 1933;28:856–874.
9. Wayne LG, Sohaskey CD. Nonreplicating persistence of *Mycobacterium tuberculosis*. *Annu Rev Microbiol* 2001;55:139–163.
10. Lillebaek T, Dirksen A, Baess I, et al. Molecular evidence of endogenous reactivation of *Mycobacterium tuberculosis* after 33 years of latent infection. *J Infect Dis* 2002;185:401–404.
11. van Rie A, Warren R, Richardson M, et al. Exogenous reinfec-
tion as a cause of recurrent tuberculosis after curative treatment. *N Engl J Med* 1999;341:1174–1179.
12. Sonnenberg P, Murray J, Glynn JR, et al. HIV-1 and recurrence, relapse, and reinfection of tuberculosis after cure: a cohort study in South African mineworkers. *Lancet* 2001;358:1687–1693.
13. Styblo K. *Epidemiology of tuberculosis*. The Hague: Royal Netherlands Tuberculosis Association, 1991.
14. Rich AR. *The pathogenesis of tuberculosis*. Springfield, IL: Charles C Thomas, 1944.
15. Dannenberg AM Jr. Immunopathogenesis of pulmonary tuberculosis. *Hosp Pract (Off Ed)* 1993;28:51–58.
16. Balasubramanian V, Wiegeshaus EH, Taylor BT, et al. Pathogenesis of tuberculosis: pathway to apical localization. *Tuber Lung Dis* 1994;75:168–78.
17. Opie EL, Aronson JD. Tubercle bacilli in latent tuberculous lesions and in lung tissue without tuberculous lesions. *Arch Pathol* 1927;4:1–21.
18. Feldman WH, Baggenstoss AH. The occurence of virulent tubercle bacilli in presumably non-tuberculous lung tissue. *Am J Pathol* 1939;15:501–515.
19. Feldman WH. The residual infectivity of the primary complex of tuberculosis. *Am J Pathol* 1938;14:473–490.
20. Sweany HC, Levinson SA, Stadnichenko AMS. Tuberculous infection in people dying of causes other than tuberculosis. *Am Rev Tuberc* 1943;47:131–173.
21. Hernandez-Pand R, Jeyanathan M, Mengistu G, et al. Persistence of DNA from *Mycobacterium tuberculosis* in superficially normal lung tissue during latent infection. *Lancet* 2000;356:2133–2138.
22. Beck F, Yegian D. A study of the tubercle bacillus in resected pulmonary lesions. *Am Rev Tuberc* 1952;66:44–50.
23. Medlar EM, Bernstein S, Steward DM. A bacteriologic study of resected tuberculous lesions. *Am Rev Tuberc* 1952;66:36–43.
24. American Trudeau Society. Report of a panel discussion on survival and revival of tubercle bacilli in healed and tuberculous lesions. *Am Rev Tuberc* 1953;68:477–495.
25. Hobby GL, Auerbach O, Lenert TF, et al. The late emergence of *M. tuberculosis* in liquid cultures of pulmonary lesions resected from humans. *Am Rev Tuberc* 1954;70:191–218.
26. Loring WE, Vandiviere HM. The treated pulmonary lesion and its tubercle bacillus. I. Pathology and pathogenesis. *Am J Med Sci* 1956;232:20–29.
27. Vandiviere HM, Loring WE, Melvin I, et al. The treated pulmonary lesion and its tubercle bacillus. II. The death and resurrection. *Am J Med Sci* 1956;232:30–37.
28. Wayne LG. The bacteriology of resected tuberculous pulmonary lesions. I. The effect of interval between reversal of infectiousness and subsequent surgery. *Am Rev Tuberc Pulm Dis* 1956;74:376–387.
29. McCune RM, Tompsett R. Fate of *Mycobacterium tuberculosis* in mouse tissues as determined by the microbial enumeration technique. II. The conversion of tuberculosis infection to the latent state by the administration of tuberculosis and a companion drug. *J Exp Med* 1956;104:763–802.
30. McCune RM, Tompsett R, McDermott W. Fate of *Mycobacterium tuberculosis* in mouse tissues as determined by the microbial enumeration technique. I. The persistence of drug susceptible bacilli in the tissues despite prolonged antimicrobial therapy. *J Exp Med* 1956;104:737–762.
31. McCune RM, Feldman FM, Lambert HP, et al. Microbial persistence. II. Characteristics of the sterile state of tubercle bacilli. *J Exp Med* 1966;123:469–486.
32. McCune RM, Feldman FM, Lambert HP, et al. Microbial persistence. I. The capacity of tubercle bacilli to survive sterilization in mouse tissues. *J Exp Med* 1966;123:445–468.
33. Barclay WR, Ebert RH, Le Roy GV, et al. Distribution and

excretion of radioactive isoniazid in tuberculosis patients. *JAMA* 1953;151:1384–1388.

34. Haapanen JH, Kass I, Gensini G, et al. Studies on the gaseous content of tuberculous cavities. *Am Rev Respir Dis* 1959;80:1–5.

35. Hobby GL, Lenert TF. The *in vitro* action of antituberculous agents against multiplying and non-multiplying microbial cells. *Am Rev Tuberc* 1957;76:1031–1048.

36. Hobby GL, Meyer K, Chaffee E. Observations on the mechanism of action of penicillin. *Proc Soc Exper Biol Med* 1942;50:281–285.

37. Tomasz A, Albino A, Zanati E. Multiple antibiotic resistance in a bacterium with suppressed autolytic system. *Nature* 1970;227:138–140.

38. Tuomanen E. Phenotypic tolerance: the search for beta-lactam antibiotics that kill nongrowing bacteria. *Rev Infect Dis* 1986;8:S279–S291.

39. Wallis RS, Patil S, Cheon SH, et al. Drug tolerance in *Mycobacterium tuberculosis*. *Antimicrob Agents Chemother* 1999;43:2600–2606.

40. Höner zu Bentrup K, Russell DG. Mycobacterial persistence: adaptation to a changing environment. *Trends Microbiol* 2001;9:597–605.

41. Primm TP, Andersen SJ, Mizrahi V, et al. The stringent response of *Mycobacterium tuberculosis* is required for long-term survival. *J Bacteriol* 2000;182:4889–4898.

42. Cole ST, Brosch R, Parkhill J, et al. Deciphering the biology of *Mycobacterium tuberculosis* from the complete genome sequence. *Nature* 1998;393:537–543.

43. Alland D, Kramnik I, Weisbrod TR, et al. Identification of differentially expressed mRNA in prokaryotic organisms by customized amplification libraries (DECAL): the effect of isoniazid on gene expression in *Mycobacterium tuberculosis*. *Proc Natl Acad Sci U S A* 1998;95:13227–13232.

44. Alland D, Steyn AJ, Weisbrod T, et al. Characterization of the *Mycobacterium tuberculosis iniBAC* promoter, a promoter that responds to cell wall biosynthesis inhibition. *J Bacteriol* 2000;182:1802–1811.

45. Michele TM, Ko C, Bishai WR. Exposure to antibiotics induces expression of the *Mycobacterium tuberculosis sigF* gene: implications for chemotherapy against mycobacterial persistors. *Antimicrob Agents Chemother* 1999;43:218–225.

46. Wilson M, DeRisi J, Kristensen HH, et al. Exploring drug-induced alterations in gene expression in *Mycobacterium tuberculosis* by microarray hybridization. *Proc Natl Acad Sci U S A* 1999;96:12833–12838.

47. Hu YM, Butcher PD, Sole K, et al. Protein synthesis is shut down in dormant *Mycobacterium tuberculosis* and is reversed by oxygen or heat shock. *FEMS Microbiol Lett* 1998;158:139–145.

48. Wayne L. Growth of *Mycobacterium tuberculosis* from resected specimens under various atmospheric conditions. *Am Rev Tuberc* 1954;70:910–911.

49. Wayne LG. The bacteriology of resected tuberculous pumonary lesions. II. Observations on bacilli which are stainable but which cannot be cultured. *Am Rev Respir Dis* 1960;82:370–377.

50. Wayne LG. Dynamics of submerged growth of *Mycobacterium tuberculosis* under aerobic and microaerophilic conditions. *Am Rev Respir Dis* 1976;114:807–811.

51. Wayne LG. Synchronized replication of *Mycobacterium tuberculosis*. *Infect Immun* 1977;17:528–530.

52. Wayne LG, Lin KY. Glyoxylate metabolism and adaptation of *Mycobacterium tuberculosis* to survival under anaerobic conditions. *Infect Immun* 1982;37:1042–1049.

53. Wayne LG, Srameck HA. Metronidazole is bactericidal to dormant cells of *Mycobacterium tuberculosis*. *Antimicrob Agents Chemother* 1994;38:2054–2058.

54. Wayne LG. Dormancy of *Mycobacterium tuberculosis* and latency of disease. *Eur J Clin Microbiol Infect Dis* 1994;13:908–914.

55. Brooks JV, Furney SK, Orme IM. Metronidazole therapy in mice infected with tuberculosis. *Antimicrob Agents Chemother* 1999;43:1285–1288.

56. Dhillon J, Allen BW, Hu YM, et al. Metronidazole has no antibacterial effect in Cornell model murine tuberculosis. *Int J Tuberc Lung Dis* 1998;2:736–742.

57. Walsh GP, Tan EV, Dela Cru EC, et al. The Phillipine cynomolgus monkey *(Macaca fasicularis)* provides a new nonhuman primate model of tuberculosis that resembles human disease. *Nat Med* 1996;2:430–436.

58. Lurie M. *Resistance to tuberculosis: experimental studies in native and acquired defensive mechanisms.* Cambridge: Harvard University Press, 1964.

59. Orme IM, Collins FM. Mouse model of tuberculosis. In: Bloom BR, ed. *Tuberculosis: pathogenesis, protection, and control.* Washington, DC: ASM Press, 1994:2003:113–134.

60. Medina E, North RJ. Resistance ranking of some common inbred mouse strains to *Mycobacterium tuberculosis* and relationship to major histocompatibility complex haplotype and *Nramp1* genotype. *Immunology* 1998;93:270–274.

61. Cooper AM, Dalton DK, Stewart TA, et al. Disseminated tuberculosis in interferon gamma gene–disrupted mice. *J Exp Med* 1993;178:2243–2247.

62. Flynn JL, Chan J, Triebold KJ, et al. An essential role for interferon-γ in resistance to *Mycobacterium tuberculosis* infection. *J Exp Med* 1993;178:2249–2254.

63. Flynn JL, Goldstein MM, Chan J, et al. Tumor necrosis factor-α is required in the protective immune response against *Mycobacterium tuberculosis* in mice. *Immunity* 1995;2:561–572.

64. MacMicking JD, North RJ, LaCourse R, et al. Identification of nitric oxide synthase as a protective locus against tuberculosis. *Proc Natl Acad Sci U S A* 1997;94:5243–5348.

65. Mohan VP, Scanga CA, Yu K, et al. Effects of tumor necrosis factor alpha on host immune response in chronic persistent tuberculosis: possible role for limiting pathology. *Infect Immun* 2001;69:1847–1855.

66. Flynn JL, Scanga CA, Tanaka KE, et al. Effects of aminoguanidine on latent murine tuberculosis. *J Immunol* 1998;160:1796–1803.

67. Keane J, Gershon S, Wise RP, et al. Tuberculosis associated with infliximab, a tumor necrosis factor alpha–neutralizing agent. *N Engl J Med* 2001;345:1098–1104.

68. Scanga CA, Mohan VP, Yu K, et al. Depletion of CD4(+) T cells causes reactivation of murine persistent tuberculosis despite continued expression of interferon gamma and nitric oxide synthase 2. *J Exp Med* 2000;192:347–358.

69. van Pinxteren LA, Cassidy JP, Smedegaard BH, et al. Control of latent *Mycobacterium tuberculosis* infection is dependent on CD8 T cells. *Eur J Immunol* 2000;30:3689–3698.

70. Chan K, Knaak T, Satkamp L, et al. Complex pattern of *Mycobacterium marinum* gene expression during long-term granulomatous infection. *Proc Natl Acad Sci U S A* 2002;99:3920–3925.

71. Rees RJW, Hart PD. Analysis of the host–parasite equilibrium in chronic murine tuberculosis by total and viable bacillary counts. *Br J Exp Pathol* 1961;42:83–88.

72. Wallace JG. The heat resistance of tubercle bacilli in the lungs of infected mice. *Am Rev Respir Dis* 1961;83:866–871.

73. McDermott W. Microbial persistence. *Yale J Biol Med* 1958;30:257–291.

74. Grosset J. The sterilizing value of rifampicin and pyrazinamide in experimental short-course chemotherapy. *Bull Int Union Tuberc* 1978;53:5–12.

75. Orme IM. The immunopathogenesis of tuberculosis: a new working hypothesis. *Trends Microbiol* 1998;6:94–97.

76. LeCoeur HF, Lagrange PH, Truffot-Pernot C, et al. Relapses after stopping chemotherapy for experimental tuberculosis in genetically resistant and susceptible strains of mice. *Clin Exp Immunol* 1989;76:458–462.

77. Khomenko AG. The variability of *Mycobacterium tuberculosis* in patients with cavitary pulmonary tuberculosis in the course of chemotherapy. *Tubercle* 1987;68:243–253.

78. McCune R, Lee SH, Deuschle K, et al. Ineffectiveness of isoniazid in modifying the phenomenon of microbial persistence. *Am Rev Tuberc Pulm Dis* 1957;76:1106–1109.

79. Miyazaki E, Chaisson RE, Bishai WR. Analysis of rifapentine for preventive therapy in the Cornell mouse model of latent tuberculosis. *Antimicrob Agents Chemother* 1999;43:2126–2130.

80. Lounis N, Bentoucha A, Truffot-Pernot C, et al. Effectiveness of once-weekly rifapentine and moxifloxacin regimens against *Mycobacterium tuberculosis* in mice. *Antimicrob Agents Chemother* 2001;45:3482–3486.

81. Scanga CA, Mohan VP, Joseph H, et al. Reactivation of latent tuberculosis: variations on the Cornell murine model. *Infect Immun* 1999;67:4531–4538.

82. Flynn JL, Chan J. Tuberculosis: latency and reactivation. *Infect Immun* 2001;69:4195–4201.

83. Glickman MS, Jacobs WR, Jr. Microbial pathogenesis of *Mycobacterium tuberculosis*: dawn of a discipline. *Cell* 2001;104:477–485.

84. Abbott A. Live lung tissue enlisted in fight against tuberculosis. *Nature* 2002;415:823.

85. McKinney JD. *In vivo veritas*: the search for TB drug targets goes live. *Nat Med* 2000;6:1330–1333.

86. Glickman MS, Cox JS, Jacobs WR Jr. A novel mycolic acid cyclopropane synthetase is required for coding, persistence, and virulence of *Mycobacterium tuberculosis*. *Mol Cell* 2000;5:717–727.

87. Cox JS, Chen B, McNeil M, et al. Complex lipid determines tissue-specific replication of *Mycobacterium tuberculosis* in mice. *Nature* 1999;402:79–83.

88. Segal W, Bloch H. Biochemical differentiation of *Mycobacterium tuberculosis* grown *in vivo* and *in vitro*. *J Bacteriol* 1956;72:132–141.

89. McKinney JD, Höner zu Bentrup K, Munoz-Elias EJ, et al. Persistence of *Mycobacterium tuberculosis* in macrophages and mice requires the glyoxylate shunt enzyme isocitrate lyase. *Nature* 2000;406:735–738.

90. Stewart GR, Snewin VA, Walzl G, et al. Overexpression of heat-shock proteins reduces survival of *Mycobacterium tuberculosis* in the chronic phase of infection. *Nat Med* 2001;7:732–737.

91. Zahrt TC, Deretic V. *Mycobacterium tuberculosis* signal transduction system required for persistent infections. *Proc Natl Acad Sci U S A* 2001;98:12706–12711.

92. Mehrotra J, Bishai WR. Regulation of virulence genes in *Mycobacterium tuberculosis*. *Int J Med Microbiol* 2001;291:171–182.

93. Kaushal D, Schroeder BG, Tyagi S, et al. Reduced immunopathology and mortality despite tissue persistence in a *Mycobacterium tuberculosis* mutant lacking alternative sigma factor, SigH. *Proc Natl Acad Sci U S A* 2002;99:8330–8335.

94. Steyn AJC, Collins DM, Hondalus MK, et al. *Mycobacterium tuberculosis* WhiB3 interacts with RpoV to affect host survival but is dispensable for *in vivo* growth. *Proc Natl Acad Sci U S A* 2002;99:3147–3152.

95. Institute of Medicine. *Ending neglect: the elimination of tuberculosis in the United States*. Washington, DC: National Academy Press, 2000.

96. Perlman DC, El-Helou P, Salomon N. Tuberculosis in patients with human immunodeficiency virus infection. *Semin Respir Infect* 1999;14:344–352.

97. World Health Organization. *The world health report 1999: making a difference*. Geneva: WHO, 1999.

98. Andersen P, Munk ME, Pollock JM, et al. Specific immune-based diagnosis of tuberculosis. *Lancet* 2000;356:1099–1104.

99. Centers for Disease Control and Prevention. Tuberculosis morbidity among U.S.-born and foreign-born populations—United States, 2000. *MMWR Morb Mortal Wkly Rep* 2002;51:101–104.

100. World Health Organization. WHO expert committee on leprosy. *WHO Tech Rep Ser* 1998;874:1–43.

101. Lowrie DB, Tascon RE, Bonato VLD, et al. Therapy of tuberculosis in mice by DNA vaccination. *Nature* 1999;400:269–271.

102. Sharma AK, Khuller GK. DNA vaccines: future strategies and relevance to intracellular pathogens. *Immunol Cell Biol* 2001;79:537–546.

9

THE CELL WALL OF *MYCOBACTERIUM TUBERCULOSIS*

DEAN C. CRICK
PATRICK J. BRENNAN
MICHAEL R. MCNEIL

OVERVIEW OF ENTIRE CELL ENVELOPE

The envelope of mycobacteria consists of a plasma membrane, a cell wall, and a capsule-like outermost layer. While considerable information regarding the chemical composition and immunologic properties of the cell envelope of mycobacteria is available, relatively little is known about the manner in which these components are spatially arranged. Electron microscopy using freeze-substitution methods indicates that there are at least four layers that have significantly different properties (1). These include an inner plasma membrane (PM), an electron-dense layer (EDL), an electron transparent zone (ETZ), and an outer electron-dense layer (OL). The PM is a typical bilayer and is approximately 4 to 4.5 nm thick. The EDL is located outside the PM and likely contains the peptidoglycan (PG) layer (1). The ETZ is 9 to 10 nm thick (2) and appears to be hydrophobic due to the inability of water-soluble dyes to penetrate the region. Therefore, it is assumed that the ETZ is primarily composed of mycolic acids (MAs). The OL seems to vary in thickness, electron density, and appearance among species, growth conditions, and preparation methods for microscopy (3–5). The OL from *Mycobacterium tuberculosis* consists of lipids, protein, glucans, mannans, arabinomannans (AMs), and xylan (6), and it has been postulated that lipoarabinomannan (LAM) is also associated with this layer (7) as well as the PM (8,9). In addition, freeze-fracture experiments show that the mycobacteria cell envelope has two planes of weakness—one associated with the PM, as expected, and another associated with the outer part of the envelope (10).

A model of the mycobacterial cell envelope proposed by Minnikin (11) in 1982 was based primarily on the chemical structure of the MAs. In this model, the PM is surrounded by a PG layer, which in turn is surrounded by the polysaccharide arabinogalactan (AG) that covalently tethers the mycolic acids to the PG layer. The MAs are packed in a monolayer, parallel to each other, and oriented perpendicularly to the PM. Minnikin further hypothesized that noncovalently linked lipids would intercalate into the outer portion of the MA layer due to the asymmetry of the two arms of the mycolate. A second model was subsequently proposed (7) that was similar, except that the noncovalently linked lipids were proposed to form a monolayer that did not intercalate with the MAs, thus providing a model that more nearly approximated a cell envelope with two bilayers. The key concept of an MA monolayer in both models was supported by subsequent experiments that showed that the MAs were, in fact, aligned perpendicularly to the cell surface and formed tight crystalline arrays (12). Currently, there are no convincing data to indicate which model is correct, and either model could explain the existence of two freeze-fracture planes in the cell envelope. However, there has been no indication in electron micrographs that a second lipid bilayer exists in the mycobacterial cell envelope (4,5). Therefore, we prefer the earlier, Minnikin model, as one would be likely to see a bilayer structure in electron micrographs if this alternative was correct.

Figure 9.1 is a variation of the original model that is consistent with both the ultrastructure and current chemical structure data. In this figure, the PG and AG layers are proposed to correspond to the EDL seen in electron micrographs. The MA layer corresponds to the ETZ, and the capsule-like (CL) layer corresponds to the OL. As in the Minnikin model, the noncovalently linked or peripheral lipids (PLs) are shown intercalated with the MAs, a configuration that seems consistent with the data and is intuitively satisfying. The glycan chains of the AG and LAM are

D. C. Crick, P. J. Brennan, and M. R. McNeil: Department of Microbiology, Immunology and Pathology, Colorado State University, Fort Collins, Colorado.

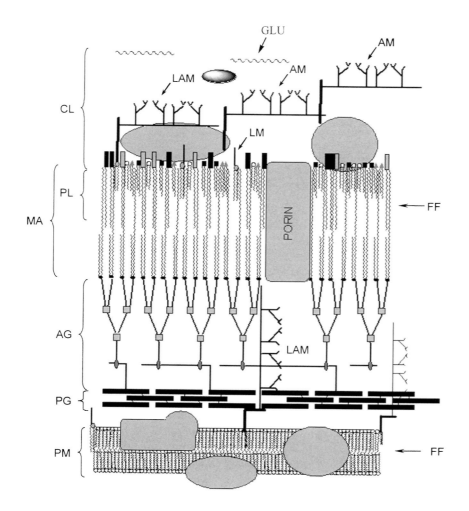

FIGURE 9.1. Schematic model of the mycobacterial cell envelope based on the model first proposed by Minnikin. The plasma membrane (*PM*) is shown at the bottom of the figure and is drawn with anchored lipomannan (*LM*), lipoarabinomannan (*LAM*), and a few representative proteins. For simplicity's sake, many constituents of the PM, such as phosphoinositolmannosides, prenyl phosphates, and other lipids, are not depicted. The cell wall core components [peptidoglycan (*PG*), arabinogalactan (*AG*), and mycolic acids (*MA*)] are shown connected to each other. Peripheral lipids (*PLs*) associated with the mycolate monolayer are shown schematically with a variety of randomly chosen and sized head groups. These PLs are drawn intercalated with the mycolates as in the Minnikin model and include many species, such as diacyl trehalose, sulfolipids, and cord factor. LAM is shown intercalated with both the PM and the capsule-like layer (*CL*). The carbohydrate region of LAM anchored in the PM is depicted as existing between the two lipid layers. The CL is depicted as containing LAM extending from the mycolates, arabinomannan (*AM*), glucan (*GLU*), and proteins. Possible freeze-fracture planes (*FF*) are indicated on the right side of the diagram. Relatively little is known about the proteins associated with the outer cell envelope or their physical arrangement. It is probable that they are associated with all portions of the cell envelope, even though only porins are shown associated with the cell wall core.

drawn in an extended configuration with distinct features. However, since oligosaccharides rarely have a single rigid structure (13) and furanosides are even more flexible than pyranosides (14), this portrayal is likely misleading. The fact that the galactose and arabinose residues are all in the furanose form and connected primarily through 1,5 and 1,6 linkages suggests that the polysaccharides may be optimized for maximal flexibility in order to allow packing of the MAs (15). If this is the case, the thickness of the AG layer (EDL) and the conformation of the AG itself could be dependent on the number of mycolates present and the hydrophobic forces that maintain the mycolate monolayer.

In the previous edition of this book, we presented a model of the cell envelope in which LAM was depicted as extending through the MA layer. This was due primarily to the observations that subcellular fractionation experiments indicated that LAM was associated with the plasma membrane (8,9) and that monoclonal antibodies raised against LAM recognize intact mycobacteria (16). The latter observation indicates that the epitope is accessible to the external milieu. If the saccharide residues are modeled in an extended conformation, it is possible that the molecule

could extend from the PM to the outside of the cell envelope. However, given the inherent flexibility of the structure and the fact that the MA layer presents a formidable permeability barrier (17), it seems unlikely that the carbohydrate could penetrate the MA layer and still maintain the impermeable nature of the cell envelope. Thus, in the current model, LAM is depicted to be anchored in both the PM with the carbohydrate chains between the two lipid layers, and anchored in the MAs themselves with the carbohydrate in the CL, as suggested by Rastogi (7). It seems probable that the LAM anchored in the PM is not exposed to the surface of the cell and that the reactivity of the whole bacterium to monoclonal LAM antibodies is generated by molecules anchored in the MA layer and/or by structurally similar AM molecules (18) located in the CL.

The permeability barrier presented by the mycobacterial cell wall was demonstrated to allow the diffusion of cephalosporin almost three orders of magnitude more slowly than the *Escherichia coli* outer membrane (19). The existence of porins as the main mechanism for diffusion of small hydrophilic molecules through the cell wall of *Mycobacterium chelonae* was reported (20), and subsequently, a gene encoding a porin of the OmpA family was identified in *M. tuberculosis* and expressed (21).

The model described above raises a number of interesting questions. How do the macromolecules found in the CL and secreted molecules pass through a rigid crystalline MA monolayer? How are the PLs transported to the surface of the bacterium and where are they synthesized? Does biosynthesis of macromolecules such as AG take place outside of the PM? Is the AG extruded through the PM, or are precursors assembled inside of the PM, moved outside of the PM, and then assembled? Does the AG/PG layer constitute a space that is analogous to a periplasm? Do the AG and LAM have preferred three-dimensional structures? These and other intriguing questions remain to be investigated. Undoubtedly, the answers obtained will result in extensive revision of the cell envelope model presented here.

STRUCTURE OF THE CELL WALL CORE

The mycobacterial cell wall is made up of the covalently linked molecules known as the cell wall core and the noncovalently associated cell wall extractable lipids (the extractable lipids are discussed later in this chapter). The cell wall core is made up of a cross-linked PG, which is covalently linked to AG chains via phosphoryl-*N*-acetylglu-

cosaminosylrhamnosyl linkage units. The AG is, in turn, esterified to a variety of α-alkyl, β-hydroxy fatty acids known as the mycolic acids. Strictly speaking, lipomannan (LM) and LAM are not part of the cell wall core as they are not part of this covalent network, but are noncovalently attached lipidated polysaccharides. However, due to the structural and biosynthetic similarities of the arabinan portion of LAM to that of AG, discussion of these molecules is included in this section and the cell wall core biosynthesis section.

Peptidoglycan Structure

The PG of the mycobacterial cell wall core is the innermost layer, adjacent to the plasma membrane, and is classified as "chemotype IV" cell wall (22) (Fig. 9.2) or A1γ (23), and is analogous to that found in other bacteria such as *E. coli*. Both Dap-D-Ala and Dap-Dap cross-links are found between the peptide side chains (24). Whether the Dap cross-link goes from a D center to an L center or a D center of the Dap donor apparently has not been established for *M. tuberculosis*, but the cross-link is assumed to be **D-L**, since this has been shown recently for *E. coli* (25). The muramic acids are *N*-glycolylated (MurNGly) rather than *N*-acetylated (26), and carboxylic acids of the peptide are often amidated (27). Recent studies on the biosynthetic

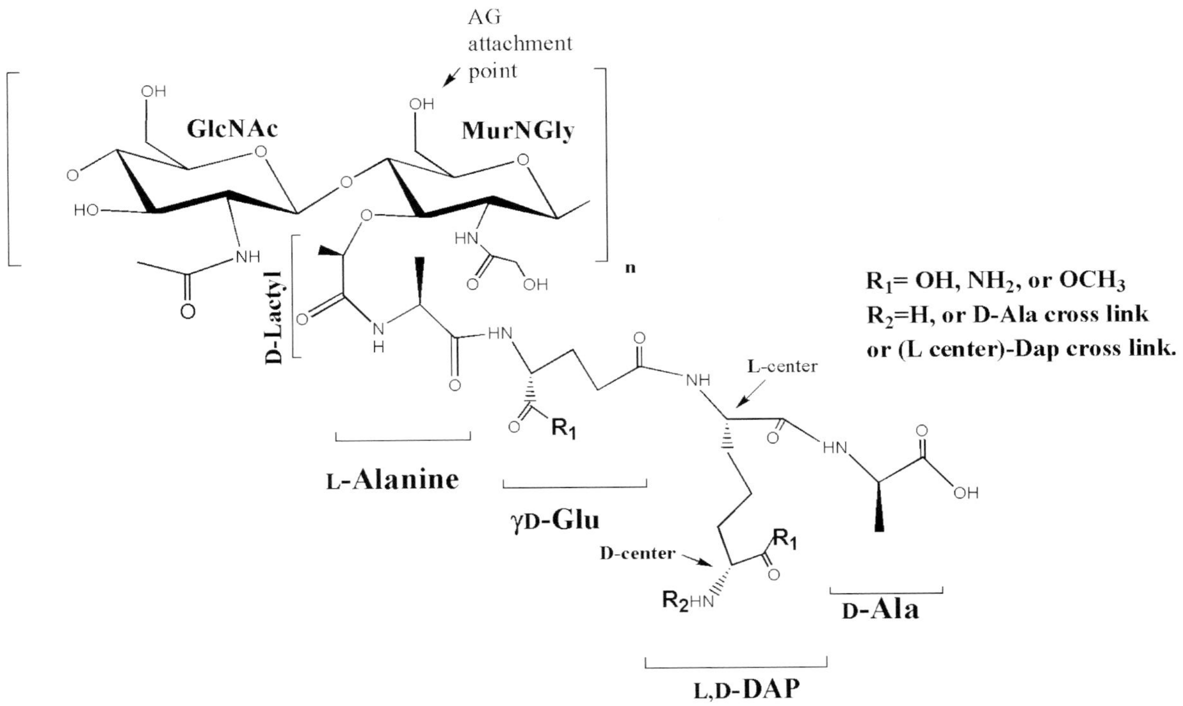

FIGURE 9.2. The peptidoglycan monomeric repeating unit. Note the position of cross-linking at the D center of Dap. Arabinogalactan (*AG*) is attached via a phosphodiester on approximately one of every ten MurNGly units at C-6, as indicated.

intermediates of PG (28) have confirmed the presence of primary amides and shown that methyl esters of the carboxylic acid groups as well as free carboxylates are present on lipid II, a biosynthetic intermediate of PG. As shown in Figure 9.1, the PG is thin in mycobacteria and suspected to be only a few layers thick.

Arabinogalactan Structure

The structure of AG is conveniently divided into three regions as shown in Figure 9.3: the linker region, a D-galactofuran region, and a D-arabinofuran region (29). The linker region consists of the simple disaccharide α-L-rhamnopyranosyl-(1→3)-D-α-N-acetyl-glucosaminosyl-(1→phosphate) (30). This phosphate is esterified to the oxygen at position 6 of a muramic acid (Mur) residue in the PG (Fig. 9.2). The galactofuran is attached to the linker (at O-4 of the L-rhamnosyl residue) and consists of an alternating 1→5, 1→6 β-D-galactofuran (29). Finally the complex D-arabinofuran with both α and β linkages is attached to galactofuran (29,31). Present evidence suggests that three arabinofurans, each with approximately 22 residues (32), are attached at 3 separate points to the 5-position of a 6-linked β-D-galactofuranosyl residue. Furthermore, the available evidence suggests that these branched points are located near the linker region (32). The MAs are esterified to approximately two thirds the nonreducing termini as shown in Figure 9.3 (33). The apparent function of the polymer as a whole is the tethering of the MA layer to the PG; the function of the galactan region beyond where arabinan attaches is unknown, but it might be to produce a viscous hydrophilic region between the PG layer and the MA layer.

Mycolic Acid Structure

The MAs (Fig. 9.3) contain 70 to 90 carbon atoms arranged in an α-branched β-hydroxylated fashion and are attached to arabinosyl residues. They constitute more than 50% by weight of the mass of the cell wall core and apparently interact via powerful hydrophobic interactions (3,12,34,35) to form a lipid shell surrounding the organisms. This property is undoubtedly responsible for the notorious "lipid barrier" and consequent endogenous resistance to many drugs. The structures, functions, and biosyntheses of these complex lipids have recently been reviewed in detail (36)

Lipomannan and Lipoarabinomannan Structure

Phosphatidylinositol mannosides (PIMs) (described later), LM, and LAM appear to be biosynthetically related to each other in that LM appears to be mannosylated PIM, and LAM appears to be arabinosylated LM. Thus, the fully mature molecule LAM is most easily conceptualized as being composed of four regions: a lipidated reducing end (PIM region), the mannan core (LM region), and the arabinofuran with its mannose (Man) caps (Fig. 9.4). The reducing end is well understood, consisting of a phosphatidylinositol (PI) unit (8). The mannan backbone, which is attached to the inositol at C-6, consists of linear 6-linked α-D-Manp units to which are attached t-α-D-Manp side chains on position 2 (37). The arabinan side chains are attached to the mannan backbone at an unknown position. The fact that LM contains an α-1,5-diarabinoside (or α1,5-triarabinoside) attached to the mannan backbone strongly suggests that only a single arabinan chain is present on LAM in contrast to the two or three arabinan side chains present on AG. This fact, along with partial acid hydrolysis experiments (37), linkage analysis (37,38), and enzymatic degradation of LAM (38), suggest that, in contrast to AG, the arabinan of LAM has an arabinan backbone from which side chains of approximately seven arabinosyl residues extend from every fifth backbone residue. These side-chain arabinosides are then capped with mannosyl residues and occasionally arabinosylated with β-D-Araf-(1→2)-α-D-Araf at position 3 of the last 5-linked α-Araf unit, as shown in Figure 9.4. Although it is only a hypothesis, one way to make sense of the complex arabinan structure in LAM is to conceive of it as having a 12-residue repeating unit structure (circled in Fig. 9.4) that is sometimes further elaborated with β-D-Araf-(1→2)-α-D-Araf and Man capping (Fig. 9.4).

BIOSYNTHESIS OF PEPTIDOGLYCAN, ARABINOGALACTAN, AND LIPOARABINOMANNAN

As discussed above, the cell envelope carbohydrate polymers are composed of the sugar monomers, D-GlcNAc, D-MurNGly, L-Rha, D-Galf, and D-Manp. Another precursor to be considered is the carrier molecule, decaprenyl phosphate, which is essential to the biosynthesis of all three polymers. Finally, AG is substituted with MAs. The biosynthesis of these components will be described next, followed by a section on how these monomers are utilized to form the complete polymers.

Synthesis of *N*-Acetylglucosamine and *N*-Acetylmuramic Acid

These molecules are required for PG synthesis with GlcNAc also being required for AG synthesis. GlcNAc, besides being required in its own right, is also the biosynthetic precursor of MurNAc. These two sugars are synthesized in the form of uridine 5′-diphosphate (UDP) nucleotides as shown in Figure 9.5. Although this pathway is common in all eubacteria, it may be of special importance in developing

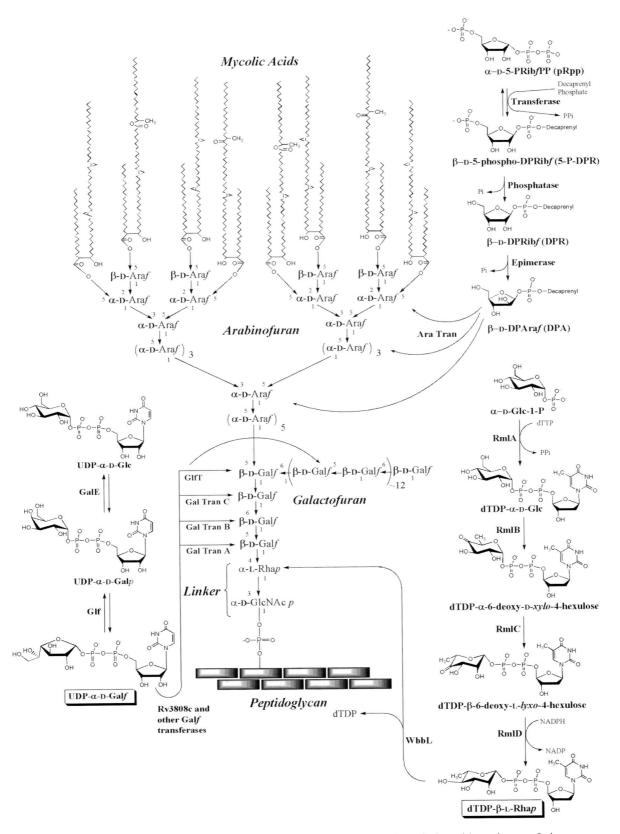

FIGURE 9.3. Structure and biosynthesis of *Mycobacterium tuberculosis* arabinogalactan. Only one arabinan chain is shown; two additional chains are attached near the reducing end of the galactan. The biosynthetic pathways of the formation of the L-rhamnosyl, D-galactofuranosyl, and D-arabinofuranosyl residues are also shown. *UDP,* uridine 5′-diphosphate.

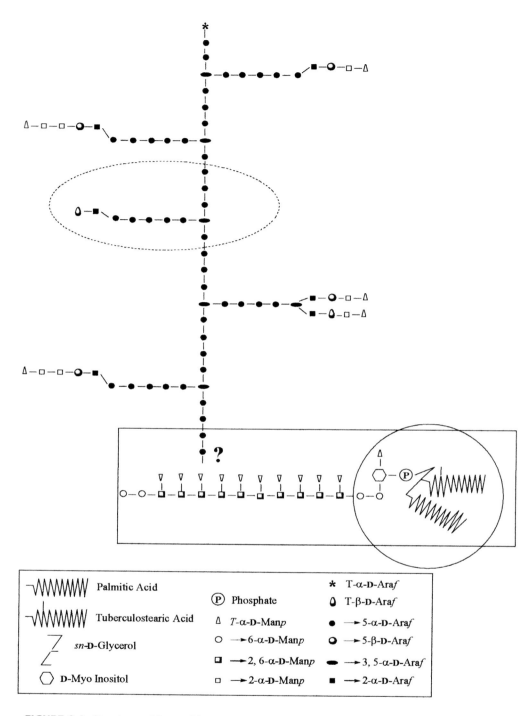

FIGURE 9.4. Structure of lipoarabinomannan. The phosphatidylinositol mannoside (*solid circle*) and lipomannan (*solid square*) components are marked. The arabinan can be considered a 12-arabinosyl repeating unit (*broken ellipse*), forming both the initial side chains (which are further modified) and an arabinan backbone. Although this structure is consistent with the known structural data, other arrangements of the arabinosyl residues are also possible. The reducing end structures are the best understood, and work remains to fully elucidate the interior arabinan regions as well as the attachment site to the mannan.

FIGURE 9.5. Formation of uridine 5′-diphosphate (*UDP*)-GlcNAc and UDP-MurNAc in bacteria. The *Mycobacterium tuberculosis* Rv numbers are assigned by sequence homology, except for Rv1018c and Rv1315, which have been demonstrated to have the assigned function. *NADPH*, nicotinamide adenine dinucleotide phosphate.

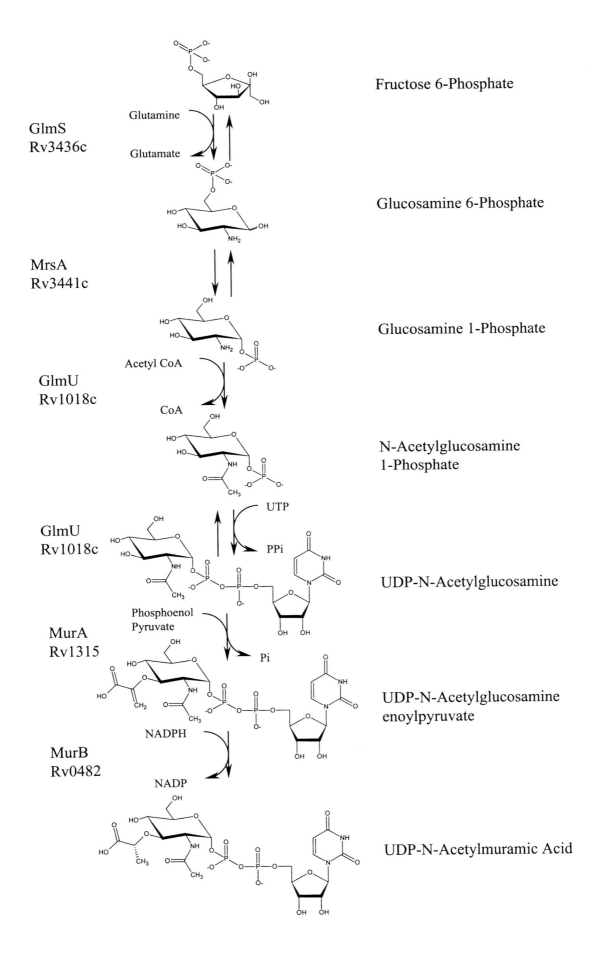

Fructose 6-Phosphate

GlmS
Rv3436c

Glutamine

Glutamate

Glucosamine 6-Phosphate

MrsA
Rv3441c

Glucosamine 1-Phosphate

GlmU
Rv1018c

Acetyl CoA

CoA

N-Acetylglucosamine
1-Phosphate

GlmU
Rv1018c

UTP

PPi

UDP-N-Acetylglucosamine

MurA
Rv1315

Phosphoenol
Pyruvate

Pi

UDP-N-Acetylglucosamine
enoylpyruvate

MurB
Rv0482

NADPH

NADP

UDP-N-Acetylmuramic Acid

new TB drugs. Lack of UDP-GlcNAc has been implicated in cell lysis previously (39), and it is possible that inhibition of formation of any PG precursor, such as UDP-GlcNAc or UDP-MurNAc, might have such an effect.

Synthesis of Deoxythymidine 5′-Diphosphate (dTDP)-Rhamnose and Uridine 5′-Diphosphate–Galactofuranose

The pathways for the formation of these two sugar nucleotides have been delineated in detail and are summarized in Figure 9.3 (40–44). The enzyme forming UDP-Gal*f*, UDP-galactopyranose mutase (Fig. 9.3), has been shown to be essential for mycobacterial viability (45) as has RmlD, one of the enzymes required for dTDP-Rha formation (46). Assays to screen for inhibitors for dTDP-Rha and UDP-Gal*f* formation have been developed and some inhibitors identified (40,47).

Synthesis of Decaprenyl Phosphate

It has been shown that *M. tuberculosis* and *M. smegmatis* utilize prenyl phosphate (Pol-P) molecules in many stages of cell envelope biosynthesis. In *M. smegmatis*, MAs appear to be formed from precursors while attached to a heptaprenyl phosphate molecule (48), although an analogous molecule has not been identified in *M. tuberculosis*. However, decaprenyl phosphorylarabinose is a precursor of the arabinan portions of AG, AM, and LAM (49) in all mycobacteria. Of special importance, a Pol-P molecule has been implicated as the carrier lipid in the assembly of AG (50).

Common Pol-P structures are confined to four main groups: (a) all-*E*, (b) di-*E*, poly-*Z*, (c) tri-*E*, poly-*Z*, and (d) all-*Z* (51). Mycobacteria are not typical in this respect. Most bacteria contain a single predominant Pol-P species, consisting of 11 isoprene units in the di-*E*, poly-*Z* configuration, known as undecaprenyl phosphate or bactoprenyl phosphate. However, *M. smegmatis* contains two dominant forms of Pol-P: a decaprenyl phosphate and a heptaprenyl phosphate (52); these are structurally unusual in that the decaprenyl phosphate (Fig. 9.6) contains one *omega*-, one *E*- and eight *Z*-isoprene units (mono-*E*, poly-*Z*) (53), and the heptaprenyl phosphate consists of four saturated isoprene units on the omega end of the molecule, two *E*- and one *Z*-isoprene units (48) or four saturated and three *Z*-isoprene units (54). *Mycobacterium tuberculosis* appears to be more typical than *M. smegmatis* as a single predominant Pol-P (decaprenyl phosphate) was identified in the tubercle bacillus (55).

Experiments on the biosynthesis of Pol-P in mycobacteria show that *M. tuberculosis* synthesizes decaprenyl diphosphate but not heptaprenyl diphosphate (56), a result that is consistent with the structural data. *M. tuberculosis* open reading frame Rv1086 encodes an *E,Z*-farnesyl pyrophosphate (FPP) synthase (57). This enzyme specifically adds a single isoprene unit to geranyl diphosphate (a ten-carbon molecule) in the *Z* configuration. As of this writing, the enzyme responsible for the synthesis of geranyl diphosphate from dimethylallyl diphosphate and isopentenyl diphosphate has not been identified, although it is now known that *M. tuberculosis* utilizes the nonmevalonate pathway for the synthesis of these five-carbon precursors (58). *Mycobacterium tuberculosis* open reading frame

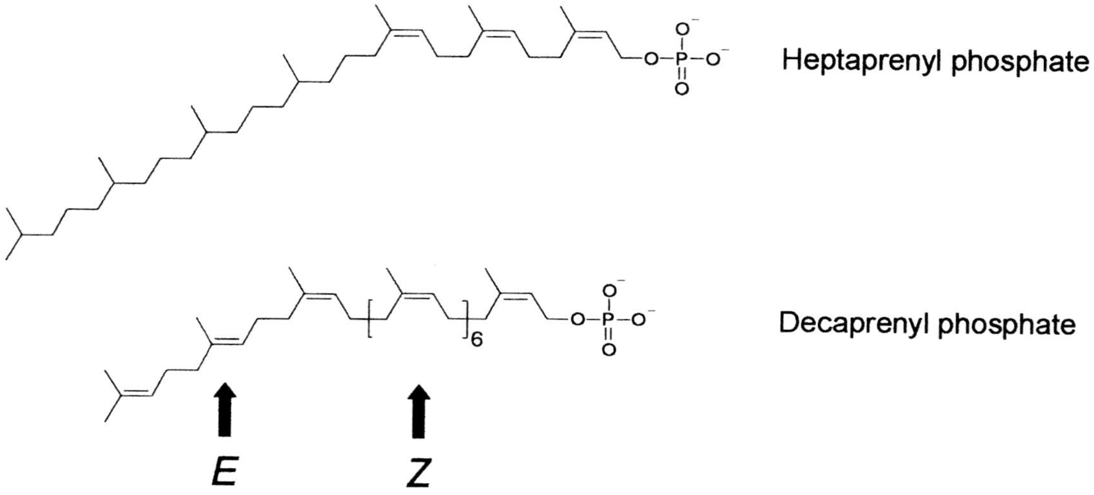

FIGURE 9.6. Structures of prenyl phosphates found in mycobacteria. Heptaprenyl phosphate is drawn with three isoprene units in the *E* configuration. Representative isoprene units having *E* or *Z* stereo configuration are indicated by the arrows.

Rv2361c encodes a decaprenyl diphosphate synthase (59). *E,Z*-FPP, the product of Rv1086, is the substrate for the enzyme encoded by Rv2361c (Kaur D, Crick DC; unpublished observations, 2002); thus, a decaprenyl diphosphate having the mono-*E*, poly-*Z* configuration is the expected product, which is identical to the decaprenyl phosphate found in *M. smegmatis*. Since these enzymes are prenyl diphosphate synthases, further modification is required to generate Pol-P. The enzymatically synthesized prenyl diphosphates must undergo dephosphorylation to form Pol-P prior to entering the various cell envelope synthetic pathways. It is unclear whether this is a simple dephosphorylation or whether both phosphates are removed and the resulting free alcohol is then rephosphorylated by a kinase. A phosphatase/kinase system could be used to regulate the amount of available Pol-P in bacteria. The step(s) necessary to form decaprenyl phosphate from decaprenyl diphosphate have, as yet, not been described for any *Mycobacterium* species.

Synthesis of Decaprenylphosphoryl-D-Arabinose

Decaprenylphosphoryl-D-arabinose is the only donor of D-arabinose known to exist, and it is unusual that this Pol-P-activated sugar is formed directly from the pentose shunt without involvement of a sugar nucleotide (60) (Fig. 9.3). Neither the genes nor the enzymes responsible for this formation have yet been isolated, although this is an active area of research.

Synthesis of Guanosine 5′-Diphosphate–Mannose and Decaprenylphosphoryl-D-Mannose

Guanosine 5′-diphosphate (GDP)–mannose is formed, in both eukaryotes and prokaryotes, from fructose-6-phosphate via an isomerase (ManA) to make Man-6-phosphate, a mutase (ManB) to make Man-1-phosphate, and a guanylyltransferase (ManC) to make GDP-Man. These enzymes have been studied very little in *M. tuberculosis*. Genes that encode enzymes with homology to ManA (Rv3255c) and ManB (Rv3257c) are present in the genome, but their function has not been confirmed. In contrast, Rv3264c, a gene grouped with rhamnose biosynthetic genes, has been shown biochemically to encode ManC (40). Although Rv3264c unequivocally condenses guanosine 5′-triphosphate (GTP) and Man-1-phosphate to make GDP-Man, it is annotated as RmlA2 in the published genome sequence (61), and it was incorrectly labeled as ManB (40) in the report where its function was elucidated.

Although some of the mannosyl residues in LM and LAM arise from GDP-Man, others arise from decaprenylphosphoryl-D-Man, a sugar donor analogous to decaprenylphosphoryl-D-Ara. However, in the case of decaprenylphosphoryl-D-Man, the Man originates from a nucleotide sugar (GDP-Man) (49). The gene encoding this enzymatic activity has been identified as *ppm1* (Rv2051c). Interestingly, the protein has both a catalytic domain sufficient for activity and what appears to be a regulatory domain (62). In other mycobacteria, these two domains are expressed from separate genes (62).

Synthesis of Mycolates

The importance of MAs to bacterial survival and pathogenesis has generated much interest in the enzymes responsible for their biosynthesis. A thorough summary of this work is beyond the scope of this chapter, but a detailed review of this subject was published recently (36). Briefly, MAs are synthesized as a C_{26} units and, separately, as larger (about C_{60}) units, known as the meromycolates, and then these two units are condensed and processed to form the finished MA. The biosynthesis of these precursors requires the interaction of two fatty acids synthase (FAS) systems: the multifunctional polypeptide, FAS I, and the dissociated FAS II system. As in fatty acid synthesis in general, both systems contain the four enzymatic activities necessary for elongation [condensation via β-ketoacyl synthase (KAS), keto reduction via β-ketoacyl reductase, dehydration via β-hydroxyacyl dehydrase, and carbon/carbon double-bond reduction via enoyl reductase]. The fatty acids are thus elongated by repeated cycles using these enzymes; generally the FAS I system is responsible for the shorter chains (up to C_{16} to C_{26}) and the FAS II system for the longer chain lengths found in the meromycolates (36). The genes of the proteins responsible for these various reactions, as well as genes of proteins responsible for shuttling between the two systems, and genes of the proteins involved in covalent modification of the meromycolate, such as those required for formation of cyclopropane rings, are actively being elucidated as described in the Barry review (36) and by others (63,64). In spite of intense effort, the condensation of the meromycolate and the C_{26} straight-chain fatty acids has yet to be shown in mycobacteria, although an analogous condensation reaction has been shown in *Corynebacterium diphtheriae* in which the meromycolate analog and the straight-chain fatty acid are both simple C_{16} precursors (36,65). After condensation, the MA is still presumed to be on a carrier molecule, such as coenzyme A (CoA), and is then transferred to end products such as cord factor (see discussion of cord factor below) and AG (Fig. 9.3).

Since the cessation of MA synthesis is one of the primary effects of isoniazid (INH), a front-line antituberculosis drug (66), fruitful efforts to identify and further exploit the enzyme(s) inhibited by INH and to determine the mechanism of action of INH have been undertaken. First, INH must be activated, and the catalase-peroxidase KatG has been shown to catalyze this activation (67). An enoyl ketoreductase, InhA (68,69), and a β-ketoacyl acyl carrier protein synthase, KasA (70–72), have both been implicated as the actual target(s) of the activated INH. Various other compounds, including ethionamide (73,74), isoxyl (73,75), and thiolactomycin (76), have also been shown to inhibit MA synthesis.

Assembly of Peptidoglycan

The assembly of PG is a well-studied topic in other bacteria (77–80), and the biosynthetic pathway is shown in Figure 9.7. The unique issues for mycobacterial PG formation include the conversion of the *N*-acetyl group on the muramic acid to *N*-glycolyl, the esterification and amidation of the COOH groups of D-Glu and D,L-Dap, and the formation of the Dap-Dap cross-link (Fig. 9.2). Studies in the authors' laboratories suggest that the *N*-glycolyl group is generated after the formation of UDP-MurNAc and before the formation of UDP-Mur-pentapeptide. In addition, it has been shown that some of the carboxylates of lipid II (the PG monomer unit) have undergone methyl esterification and amino amidation (28), as indicated in Figure 9.2.

The penicillin-binding proteins are responsible for both the carbohydrate polymerization (transglycosylase activity) and Dap-Ala cross-linking. The most important of these, PBP1a (PonA, Rv0050) and the closely related PonA′ (Rv 3682), have been identified in the genome by sequence homology and are targets of penicillin. It is generally believed that the combination of active β-lactamases coupled with the permeability barrier of the mycolates results in the lack of susceptibility of *M. tuberculosis* to β-lactams (15). The proteins responsible for Dap-Dap cross-linking have not been identified.

Assembly of Arabinogalactan

Arabinogalactan has been shown to be biosynthesized on the carrier lipid Pol-P (50) and then transferred as a polysaccharide phosphate to PG (Fig. 9.8). The synthesis begins with the transfer of GlcNAc-1-phosphate to Pol-P (50), followed by the attachment of the rhamnosyl residue (50,81). The attachment of galactofuranosyl residues then occurs with branch points occurring early in the galactofuran formation (82,83) presumably because of the addition of short arabinan chains that will be elongated later in the pathway. However, the size of these putative early arabinan side chains is not known. A galactofuranosyltransferase utilizing UDP-Gal*f* has been identified (82,83) and shown to be a bifunctional enzyme capable of adding Gal*f* to either the 5-position or the 6-position of another Gal*f* residue (82). This enzyme is believed to add the bulk of the galactan after the Gal*f* units near the reducing end are added. The identity of the protein(s) that add the Gal*f* units near the rhamnosyl residues is not known.

The EmbA and EmbB proteins are believed to have a key role in arabinosylation of AG, perhaps directly as arabinosyltransferases or perhaps indirectly as a scaffold that directs arabinosylation. These proteins were first identified as the targets of ethambutol (84), which inhibits arabinosylation of AG (85–87) and LAM (88). More recent experiments involving knockouts of *embA*, *embB*, and *embC* in *M. smegmatis* have led to the striking conclusion that EmbA and EmbB are responsible for arabinosylation of AG, and EmbC is responsible for arabinosylation of LAM (89). This sheds light on the profound problem of how the slightly different arabinosylation of galactofuran to form AG and mannan to form LAM are controlled. Thus single gene knockouts of either *embA* or *embB* produced bacteria with

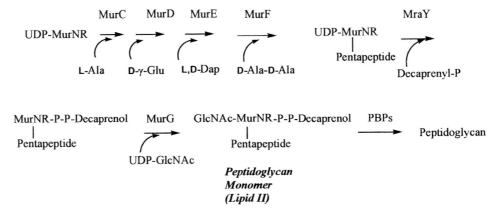

FIGURE 9.7. Biosynthesis of lipid II via MurC-F, MraY, and MurG and its polymerization by penicillin-binding proteins (*PBPs*) to form peptidoglycan. The PBPs polymerize the polysaccharide and cross-link many of the peptides. The structures are shown in detail in Figure 9.2. The R group on Mur begins as acetyl and is enzymatically converted to glycolyl before the transfer to decaprenyl phosphate catalyzed by MraY occurs. *UDP*, uridine 5′-diphosphate.

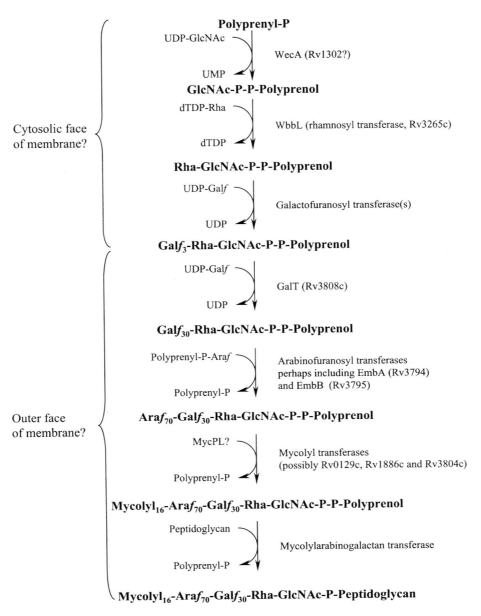

FIGURE 9.8. Biosynthesis of arabinogalactan (AG). The synthesis begins on the carrier lipid, decaprenyl phosphate. There is some evidence to suggest that the early reactions shown in the top bracket occur on the cytosol face of the membrane, whereas the later reactions occur on the outside face of the membrane (*lower bracket*). It is likely that some Ara residues are added before the full complement of Gal*f* residues are present; this is not depicted in the figure. It is not known at what point the AG is transferred from the carrier lipid to the peptidoglycan or at what point the mycolates are transferred to the arabinosyl residues. Although mycolylmannosylphosphorylpolyprenol (*MycPL*) is shown as the mycolate carrier, this role has not been conclusively established. *UDP*, uridine 5'-diphosphate.

a defective AG in which the arabinosylation of the galactofuran was decreased, the size of the galactofuran increased, and the number of terminal β-D-Ara*f*-(1→2)-α-D-Ara*f* units at position 3 of the branched α-Ara*f* (Fig. 9.4) was reduced (89). Presumably EmbA compensates for lack of EmbB and vice versa, which is why these two knockouts were still viable, although the bacteria grew slowly with an altered morphology. In contrast, the *embC* knockout synthesized essentially normal AG but no LAM, although both PIM and LM were formed (89). Thus, EmbA and EmbB are fundamentally involved in arabinosylation of galactofuran, but their exact role has not yet been determined. It is tempting to think that they are part of a multiple protein complex leading to the maturation of galactofuran to AG.

At some point, the mycolates are attached to the terminal arabinosyl residues, although it is not known whether this happens before or after the polymer is attached to PG. Genetic evidence strongly suggests that the fibronectin-binding proteins [FbpA, FbpB, and FbpC (Rv3804c, Rv1886c, and Rv0129c, respectively)], which are also known as antigen 85 proteins, catalyze the transfer of mycolates from a donor molecule such as mannosylphosphorylpolyprenol or trehalose mycolate (90–93). A related protein was found to be inactive (93,94). Importantly, it was noted that all three Fbp isozymes transferred mycolates onto the four sites present in the arabinogalactan nonreducing end hexaarabinoside (93) (Fig. 9.3). These proteins have been shown biochemically to catalyze an exchange reaction between trehalose monomycolate and trehalose (95); crystal structures have been assigned to FbpC (96) and FbpB (97), although *in vitro* biochemical evidence of transfer of mycolate to arabinose is lacking.

Assembly of Lipoarabinomannan

There is intense interest in the role of LAM in tuberculosis. LAM from *M. tuberculosis* has short Man-containing oligosaccharide "caps" (Fig. 9.4) that allow it to bind to the Man receptor on macrophages, unlike the product from *M. smegmatis*, which has no such Man caps. Also, LAM can bind to Toll receptors and can physically insert itself into membranes, inducing signaling events important in the host response in tuberculosis. Thus, understanding the biosynthesis of LAM is a major priority.

Although not strictly proven, it is believed that LAM is synthesized from LM or a very closely related molecule and that LM is biosynthesized from PIM (49). The biosynthesis of PIM is discussed later in this chapter. It has been shown that the α-1,6-Man backbone of LM comes from an elongation of PIM and that the mannosyl donor is decaprenylphosphoryl-D-Man (49). However, from the first reports of *in vitro* synthesis of α-1,6-Man (98) to the more recent studies (49), cell-free enzymatic synthesis of the single mannosyl side chains attached to the 2-position of the 1,6-α-D-mannan has been elusive.

As mentioned above, the arabinosylation of LAM is dependent on the presence of the EmbC protein (89), and decaprenylphosphoryl-D-arabinose is believed to be the sole donor of arabinosyl residues in *M. tuberculosis*. LM contains a di- or tri-α-1,5-D-arabinoside, suggesting that it is elongated by EmbC (and likely supporting proteins) to the mature arabinan of Figure 9.4. However, details of how this arabinan is synthesized are lacking. There are several possibilities, including the addition of one arabinosyl residue at a time to the mannan core. An alternative is the synthesis of oligoarabinan units, perhaps like the one circled in Figure 9.4, which are then polymerized. Given the complexity of the arabinan, the latter hypothesis seems more likely, but as yet no oligoarabinan precursors have been found in mycobacteria.

STRUCTURES OF THE NONCOVALENTLY BOUND CELL ENVELOPE LIPIDS OF MYCOBACTERIA

Our understanding of the chemistry of the free lipids noncovalently associated with the core cell wall of *M. tuberculosis* began in 1937 when the Medical Research Committee of the U.S. National Tuberculosis Association initiated a study under the direction of R. J. Anderson of Yale University on the lipids of acid-fast bacilli. Anderson and colleagues defined most of the biologically relevant cell wall materials that have been the basis of intensive studies in subsequent years: the MAs, the phospholipids, AG, the various "waxes" (a term seldom used nowadays), as well as the single-branched and multibranched fatty acids. Subsequent researchers expanded on this knowledge, notably H. Bloch and H. Noll in their detailed description of "cord factor," and E. Lederer and J. Asselineau, who, with developments in chromatography, nuclear magnetic resonance spectrometry, and mass spectrometry techniques, were able to fully characterize these substances. M. B. Goren was responsible for the full definition of the sulfolipids that are associated with virulent strains of *M. tuberculosis*. C. E. Ballou and E. Lee, following on earlier work by E. Vilkas and E. Lederer, fully defined the PIMs, and P. J. Brennan and S. W. Hunter realized that the LAMs and LMs were based on phosphoinositides.

From early times, it was recognized that many of the chemically novel lipids of the cell wall of *M. tuberculosis* were extractable with various organic solvents. These extracted lipids could be separated into "phosphatide," "acetone-soluble fat," and various "wax fractions." Anderson's group first identified trehalose as a component of the "neutral fats." However, it was many years later that Bloch recognized trehalose as part of the trehalose glycolipids, trehalose-6,6′-dimycolate, or "cord factor" (99) (Fig. 9.9).

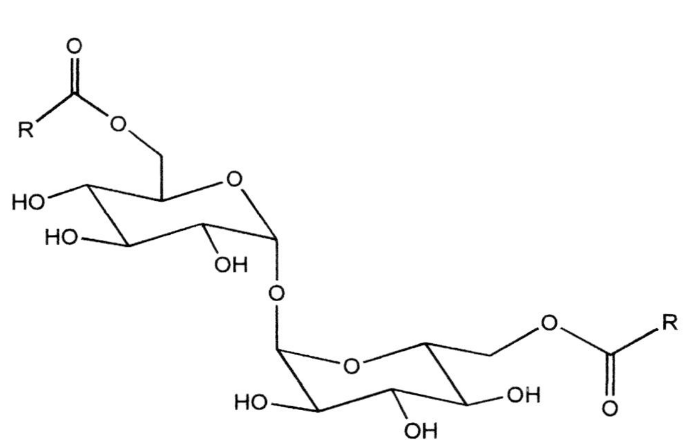

FIGURE 9.9. Structure of trehalose-6,6′-dimycolate, or "cord factor." The R groups correspond to mycolic acids (see Fig. 9.3 for their structure).

The sulfolipids, or sulfatides, of *M. tuberculosis* are another group of trehalose esters. Full structural characterizations, particularly identification of the fatty acid constituents and localization on the trehalose hydroxy functions, has been accomplished (99). It was demonstrated that the structures of the sulfolipid family are based on trehalose 2-sulfate. The fatty acyl functions are members of the methyl-branched fatty acid families, the phthioceranic and hydroxyphthioceranic acids, which are apparently unique to the mycobacterial sulfatides (Fig. 9.10).

Anderson et al. first isolated a methoxyglycol from *M. tuberculosis*, which they called "phthiocerol" (97). The diester of phthiocerol involving the mycocerosic acids is the form in which phthiocerol (and mycocerosic acids) are usually found (99) (Fig. 9.11). The diesters of phthiocerol are variously known as dimycocerosate (DIM) or phthiocerol dimycocerosate. Apparently, dimycocerosate/phthiocerol dimycocerosate is found only in members of the *M. tuberculosis* complex. Clearly, it is found only in mycobacterial species that contain phthiocerol or the phenolphthiocerols, such as mycosides A and B of the *M. tuberculosis* complex or the phenolic glycolipids I to III of *M. leprae*.

Mycocerosic acids are the most prominent of several subgroups of multimethyl-branched fatty acids present in biologically important mycobacterial lipids (Fig. 9.12). They were first isolated from the various waxes of *M. tuberculosis* and identified as C_{30} and C_{31} methyl-branched levorotatory acids (99). Other methyl-branched fatty acids include tuberculostearic acid, apparently exclusively present in the phosphoinositides; the phthienoic acids, which are largely

found as esters of trehalose; and the previously mentioned phthioceranic and hydroxyphthioceranic acids, which are exclusive to the sulfolipids.

Another group of biologically important lipids is the "phosphatides," more specifically the PIMs. These are probably located mostly in the plasma membrane, although there is evidence of their presence in the cell wall proper. In 1938, a "phosphatide" fraction was isolated from *M. tuberculosis*, which, on hydrolysis, yielded glycerol phosphate, Man, and the hexahydric alcohol "inoside" (99). Alkaline saponification of the phosphatides yielded a "phosphorus-containing glycoside," which, on dephosphorylation, produced a mannoinositide containing Man and inositol in the proportions of 2:1. Subsequently, the same approach was used (100) to arrive at the complete structure of the PIMs (Fig. 9.13). Extensive structural studies were conducted on the deacylated glycophospholipids (99). In these studies it was assumed that these glycophospholipids were simple PI derivatives with acyl substituents found only on the glycerol, as is the case with the parent phospholipid, PI. However, Pangborn and McKinney (101) and, later, Brennan and Ballou [as reviewed in (99)] isolated a series of phosphatidylinositol dimannosides (PIM2s) from *M. tuberculosis* containing a total of two, three, and four acyl functions. It is now obvious that multiacyl forms of all of the individual members of the PIM family (PIM$_2$ to PIM$_6$) exist in the cell envelope of *M. tuberculosis*. Subsequently, it was demonstrated that the LMs and LAMs (Fig. 9.4) of mycobacteria are also based on a PI moiety and apparently are modifications of the PIMs, presumably PIM$_3$ (99).

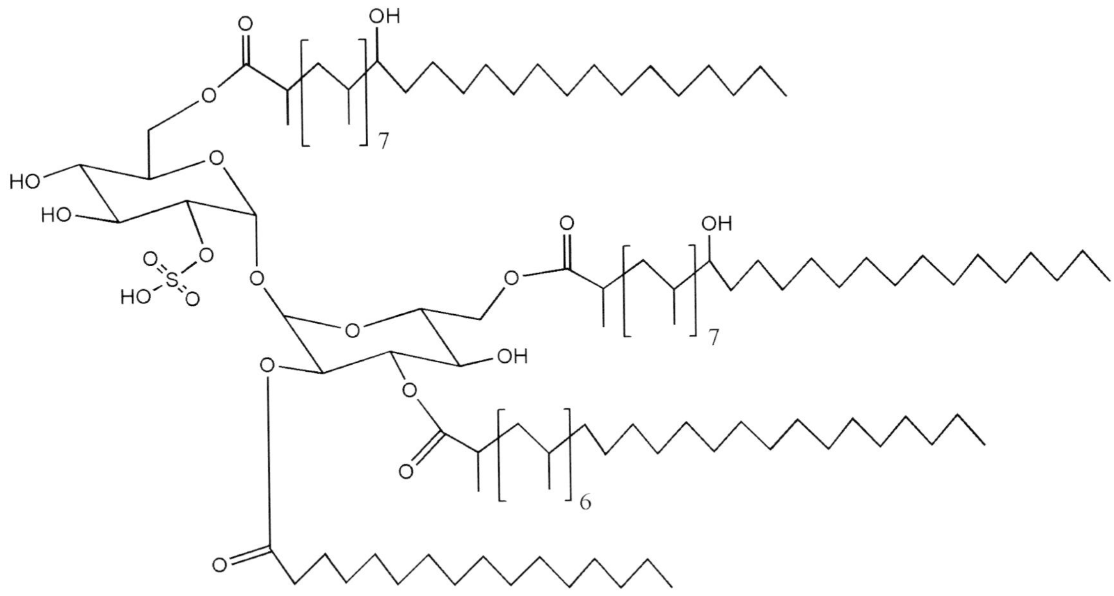

FIGURE 9.10. Structure of sulfolipid-I, one of the sulfatides found in *Mycobacterium tuberculosis.*

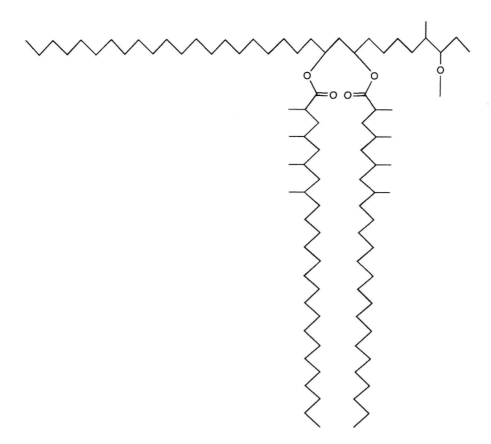

FIGURE 9.11. Structure of phthiocerol dimycocerosate. The phthiocerol moiety (*horizontal structure*) contains two hydroxyl groups to which the mycocerosic acids (*vertical structures*) are esterified.

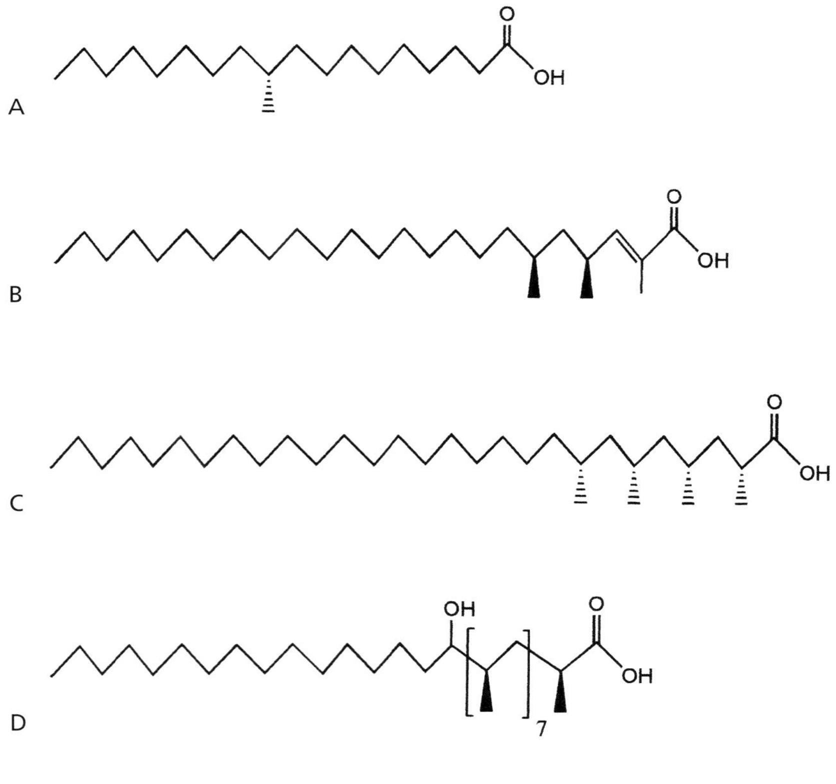

A

B

C

D

FIGURE 9.12. Structures of methyl-branched fatty acids of *Mycobacterium tuberculosis*. **A:** Tuberculostearic acid; **B:** phthienoic acid; **C:** mycocerosic acid; **D:** hydroxyphthioceranic acid.

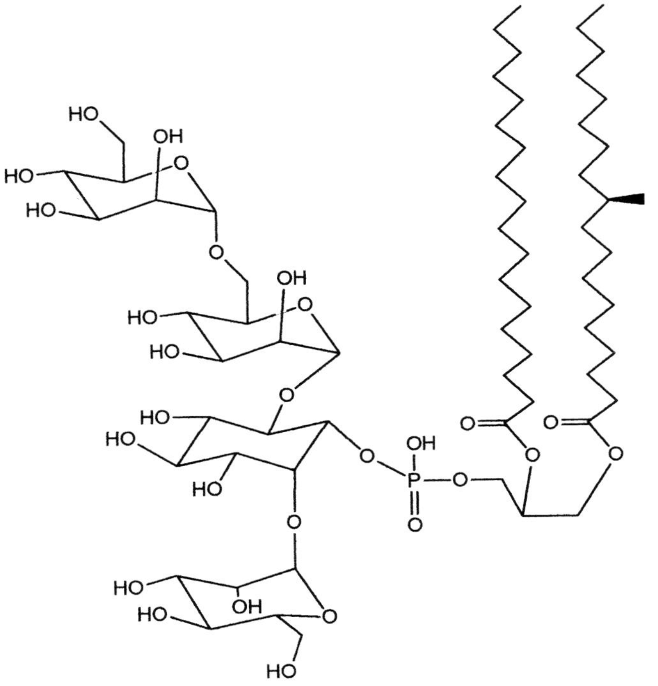

Dimycocerosate and Related Lipids and Methyl-Branched Fatty Acids

Considerable progress has been made on the biosynthesis of both the phthiocerol and mycocerosic acid moieties of DIM (Fig. 9.11). The *M. tuberculosis* genome contains a 50-kB fragment containing a cluster of 13 genes (Fig.9.14) relevant to DIM synthesis. Some of these genes encode proteins with homology to known polyketide synthases. In the midst of this cluster is a gene (*mas*) encoding a large multifunctional enzyme that was shown to be a mycocerosic acid synthase. This enzyme produces mycocerosic acid by extending a fatty acyl CoA using methylmalonyl CoA as the carbon donor (102,103). This suggested that the other

FIGURE 9.13. Structure of phosphatidylinositol mannoside type 3 (PIM₃). It is believed that PIM₃ is further elongated to form PIM₄, PIM₅, and PIM₆ and that it is also elongated to form lipomannan and, ultimately, lipoarabinomannan.

BIOSYNTHESIS OF THE NONCOVALENTLY BOUND CELL ENVELOPE LIPIDS OF MYCOBACTERIA

A major development in our understanding of the cell wall of *M. tuberculosis* was sequencing of the complete genome (61). Elucidation of the genome has allowed identification of gene function by homology search, an advance that has greatly increased the speed with which the understanding of mycobacterial biochemistry has proceeded. An example of this is the cluster of genes responsible for PG synthesis. The *mur* operon is almost identical to that in *E. coli* and other bacteria, telling us that at least the early stages of PG synthesis in *M. tuberculosis* are very similar to those in *E. coli*. Thus, the genome can lead to tentative identification of enzymes by homology searches, but only after cloning and expression of candidate genes followed by demonstration of the appropriate enzymatic activity can identifications be considered valid. This approach is being applied to the genes responsible for the synthesis and subsequent modification of MAs, the genes responsible for the synthesis of the PIMs and LAM, the genes responsible for the synthesis of DIM, and likewise the genes within the so-called cell wall cluster which are responsible for aspects of the synthesis of arabinogalactan.

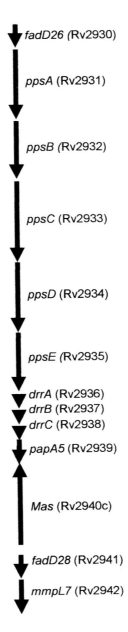

fadD26 (Rv2930)

ppsA (Rv2931)

ppsB (Rv2932)

ppsC (Rv2933)

ppsD (Rv2934)

ppsE (Rv2935)

drrA (Rv2936)
drrB (Rv2937)
drrC (Rv2938)
papA5 (Rv2939)

Mas (Rv2940c)

fadD28 (Rv2941)

mmpL7 (Rv2942)

FIGURE 9.14. Schematic diagram of the organization of the phthiocerol dimycocerosate locus of *Mycobacterium tuberculosis*.

genes of the cluster could be responsible for phthiocerol synthesis, and elegant evidence to this effect has been provided (102,104–106). Recently, it was demonstrated that FadD28 is an acyl CoA synthase-like enzyme that may be responsible for the attachment of mycocerosic acids synthesized by Mas to the phthiocerol (105).

The role of DIM in disease pathogenesis has recently been addressed. Using signature-tagged transposon mutagenesis, mutants with insertions upstream of *fadD26* in the *pps* region and within *fadD28* and *mmpL7* have been isolated (107). Mutants have also been isolated with insertions within *fad26, drrC,* and *mmpL7* (108). The phenotypes were intriguing. No DIM production or production of a related lipid was seen in the upstream *fadD26* (*pps*) mutant or the *fadD28* mutant. However, the *mmpL7* mutant could synthesize DIM but could not excrete DIM into the medium; it and the *drrC* mutant were defective in DIM export/excretion.

Some interesting studies have been done on the biology of the mutants, which are devoid of DIM. They show much higher cell wall permeability (108) and attenuated growth in the mouse lung (107), consistent with early work showing that a DIM-less variant of *M. tuberculosis* H37Rv had attenuated growth in the guinea pig (99).

Reports have also recently come from Kolattukudy's laboratory on the generation of mutants devoid of sulfolipids (106). These researchers have identified a *mas*-like *pks*2 gene responsible for their synthesis and were successful in disrupting this by homologous recombination. In light of the controversial role of sulfolipids in tuberculosis pathogenesis, it will be intriguing to see the phenotype of these mutants.

Biosynthesis of Phosphatidyinositol Mannosides

Based on structures of the PIMs, one would predict that the first biosynthetic event would be synthesis of PI, followed by the addition of Man to give PIM$_2$, PIM$_3$, and so on. However, in the originally published genome sequence, only the genes for phosphatidylserine and phosphatidylethanolamine were clearly annotated. All other genes for phospholipid synthesis, including the one responsible for PI synthesis, could not be distinguished, because the CDP-diacylglycerol binding motif dominated the structures of the genes. Hence, these genes were designated *pgsA, pgsA$_2$, pgsA$_3$*. Each of these genes has been overexpressed in *M. smegmatis,* and the enzyme encoded by *pgsA* was shown to be responsible for the synthesis of PI (109). Rv2612c (*pgsA*) is part of a small operon-like cluster that also contains Rv2609c, Rv2610c, and Rv2611c. It has now been shown that *pimA* (Rv2610c) adds the first Man to PI (110), and Rv2611c potentially adds a fatty acid. The function of Rv2609c is still unclear. Previously, it had been shown that *pimB* (Rv0557), half a chromosome away, encodes the enzyme that adds the second Man (111).

Thus, PgsA catalyzes the formation of PI, and PimA catalyzes the addition of the first Man. PimB adds the second Man, and PimC, which attaches the third Man, has been recently described (112). It is speculated that PIM$_3$, the product of PimC, is the direct precursor of LM and LAM.

STRUCTURE AND BIOSYNTHESIS OF EXTRACELLULAR GLUCAN AND ARABINOMANNAN

The existence of the OL as revealed by electron microscopy (see "Overview of Entire Cell Envelope") has been recognized for a long time but only recently has the chemical composition of this layer (and the related extracellular material) been examined (4,18,113,114). Daffe and colleagues used mechanical means to isolate the OL from *M. tuberculosis,* and it was found to consist of polysaccharide (about 75%) and protein (about 22%) with only traces of lipid (114). Thus, *M. tuberculosis* is now known to have a hydrophilic capsule outside its hydrophobic MA layer. The extracellular glucan represents up to 70% of the surface polysaccharides and is composed of repeating units of five or six 1,4-α-D-Glc*p*, with one of them substituted at position 6 with a single α-D-Glcp residue (18). The structure of the extracellular AM appears to be identical to that of LAM except for the loss of the lipid anchor (18). The ramifications of these polysaccharides in pathology are only beginning to be unraveled. Certainly molecular recognition, perhaps by the Man receptor (115) of AM, might take place and be important in uptake of *M. tuberculosis* into the macrophage. AM may also be involved in immunosuppressive action as well (116). The role of the glucan is less studied, but it may be involved in *M. tuberculosis* evasion of the immune system by molecular mimicry (18).

The proteins in the capsule (OL) were found, in general, to be similar but not identical to the proteins found in the growth medium (114). In particular, 19- and 38-kd lipoproteins as well as the Fpb (antigen 85) proteins were present. A 38-kd protein not found in the growth medium was detected, and a 240-kd protein (MBP/T64) found in the growth medium was not found in the capsule (114).

Very little is known about the biosynthesis of glucan or AM. No studies on the biosynthesis of the extracellular glucan are extant. The structure of AM suggests that it may be formed from LAM by a specific hydrolytic enzyme. However, there is little evidence for this hypothesis.

ACKNOWLEDGMENTS

Research conducted in the authors' laboratories was funded by grants from the National Institutes of Health, National Institute of Allergy and Infectious Diseases: AI-18357, AI-46393, AI-33706, and AI-49151. The authors thank Mr.

Michael Scherman and Dr. Varalakshmi Vissa for assistance in preparing some of the figures and Mrs. Marilyn Hein for assistance in preparing the manuscript.

REFERENCES

1. Paul TR, Beveridge TJ. Reevaluation of envelope profiles and cytoplasmic ultrastructure of mycobacteria processed by conventional embedding and freeze-substitution protocols. *J Bacteriol* 1992;174:6508–6517.
2. Brennan PJ, Draper P. Ultrastructure of *Mycobacterium tuberculosis*. In: Bloom B, ed. *Tuberculosis: pathogenesis, protection, and control.* Washington, DC: ASM Press, 1994:271–284.
3. Brennan PJ, Nikaido H. The envelope of mycobacteria. *Annu Rev Biochem* 1995;64:29-63.
4. Daffe M, Draper P. The envelope layers of mycobacteria with reference to their pathogenicity. *Adv Microb Physiol* 1998;39: 131–203.
5. Draper P. The outer parts of the mycobacterial envelope as a permeability barrier. *Front Biosci* 1998;3:1253-1261.
6. Ortalo-Magne A, Lemassu A, Laneelle MA, et al. Identification of the surface-exposed lipids on the cell envelopes of *Mycobacterium tuberculosis* and other mycobacterial species. *J Bacteriol* 1996;178:456–461.
7. Rastogi N. Recent observations concerning structure and function relationships in the mycobacterial cell envelope: elaboration of a model in terms of mycobacterial pathogenicity, virulence and drug resistance. *Res Microbiol* 1991;142:464–476.
8. Hunter SW, Brennan PJ. Evidence for the presence of a phosphatidylinositol anchor on the lipoarabinomannan of *Mycobacterium tuberculosis. J Biol Chem* 1990;265:9272–9279.
9. Hunter SW, Gaylord H, Brennan PJ. Structure and antigenicity of the phosphorylated lipopolysaccharide antigens from the leprosy and tubercle bacilli. *J Biol Chem* 1986;261:12345–12351.
10. Barksdale L, Kim K-S. *Mycobacterium. Bacteriol Rev* 1977;41: 217–372.
11. Minnikin DE. Lipids: complex lipids, their chemistry, biosynthesis and roles. In: Ratledge C, Stanford JL, eds. *The biology of the mycobacteria,* Vol. 1. London: Academic Press, 1982: 95–184.
12. Nikaido H, Kim SH, Rosenberg EY. Physical organization of lipids in the cell wall of *Mycobacterium chelonae. Mol Microbiol* 1993;8:1025–1030.
13. van Halbeek H. ^{1}H nuclear magnetic resonance spectroscopy of carbohydrate chains of glycoproteins. *Meth Enzymol* 1994;230: 132–168.
14. Bush CA, Martin-Pastor M, Imberty A. Structure and conformation of complex carbohydrates of glycoproteins, glycolipids, and bacterial polysaccharides. *Annu Rev Biophys Biomol Struct* 1999;28:269–293.
15. Jarlier V, Nikaido H. Mycobacterial cell wall: structure and role in natural resistance to antibiotics. *FEMS Microbiol Lett* 1994; 123:11–18.
16. Gaylord H, Brennan PJ, Young D, et al. Most *Mycobacterium leprae* carbohydrate-reactive monoclonal antibodies are directed to lipoarabinomannan. *Infect Immun* 1987;55:2860–2863.
17. Nikaido H. Preventing drug access to target: cell surface permeability barrier and active efflux in bacteria. *Cell Dev Biol* 2001;12:215–223.
18. Lemassu A, Daffe M. Structural features of the exocellular polysaccharides of *Mycobacterium tuberculosis. Biochem J* 1994;297: 351–357.
19. Jarlier V, Nikaido H. Permeability barrier to hydrophilic solutes in *Mycobacterium chelonei. J Bacteriol* 1990;172:1418–1423.
20. Trias J, Jarlier V, Benz R. Porins in the cell wall of mycobacteria. *Science* 1992;258:1479–1481.
21. Senaratne RH, Mobasheri H, Papavinasasundaram KG, et al. Expression of a gene for a porin-like protein of the OmpA family from *Mycobacterium tuberculosis* H37Rv.*J Bacteriol* 1998; 180:3541–3547.
22. Ghuysen JM. Use of bacteriolytic enzymes in determination of wall structure and their role in cell metabolism. *Bacteriol Rev* 1968;32:425–464.
23. Schleifer KH, Kandler O. Peptidoglycan types of bacterial cell walls and their taxonomic implications. *Bacteriol Rev* 1972;36: 407–477.
24. Wietzerbin J, Das BC, Petit JF, et al. Occurrence of D-alanyl-(D)-meso-diaminopimelic acid and meso-diaminopimelyl-meso-diaminopimelic acid interpeptide linkages in the peptidoglycan of mycobacteria. *Biochemistry* 1974;13:3471–3476.
25. Glauner B, Holtje JV, Schwarz U. The composition of the murein of *Escherichia coli. J Biol Chem* 1988;263:10088–10095.
26. Petit JF, Lederer E. The structure of the mycobacterial cell wall. In: Kubica GP, Wayne LG, eds. *The mycobacteria: a sourcebook.* New York: Marcel Dekker, 1984:301–322.
27. Kotani S, Yanagida I, Kato K, et al. Studies on peptides, glycopeptides and antigenic polysaccharide–glycopeptide complexes isolated from an L-11 enzyme lysate of the cell walls of *Mycobacterium tuberculosis* strain H37Rv. *Biken J* 1970;13:249–275.
28. Mahapatra S, Crick DC. Isolation and characterization of TB peptidoglycan biosynthetic intermediates *(in preparation).*
29. Daffe M, Brennan PJ, McNeil M. Predominant structural features of the cell wall arabinogalactan of *Mycobacterium tuberculosis* as revealed through characterization of oligoglycosyl alditol fragments by gas chromatography/mass spectrometry and by ^{1}H and ^{13}C-NMR analyses. *J Biol Chem* 1990;265:6734–6743.
30. McNeil M, Daffe M, Brennan PJ. Evidence for the nature of the link between the arabinogalactan and peptidoglycan components of mycobacterial cell walls. *J Biol Chem* 1990;265:18200–18206.
31. McNeil MR, Robuck KG, Harter M, et al. Enzymatic evidence for the presence of a critical terminal hexaarabinose in the cell walls of *Mycobacterium tuberculosis. Glycobiology* 1994;4:165–174.
32. Besra GS, Khoo K-H, McNeil M, et al. A new interpretation of the structure of the mycolyl-arabinogalactan complex of *Mycobacterium tuberculosis* as revealed through characterization of oligoglycosylalditol fragments by fast-atom bombardment mass spectrometry and ^{1}H nuclear magnetic resonance spectroscopy. *Biochemistry* 1995;34:4257–4266.
33. McNeil M, Daffe M, Brennan PJ. Location of the mycolyl ester substituent in the cell walls of mycobacteria. *J Biol Chem* 1991;266:13217–13223.
34. Liu J, Barry CE, Besra GS, et al. Mycolic acid structure determines the fluidity of the mycobacterial cell wall. *J Biol Chem* 1996;271:29545–29551.
35. Nikaido H, Jarlier V. Permeability of the mycobacterial cell wall. *Res Microbiol* 1991;142:437–443.
36. Barry CE, III, Lee RE, Mdluli K, et al. Mycolic acids: structure, biosynthesis and physiological functions. *Progr Lipid Res* 1998; 37:143–179.
37. Chatterjee D, Hunter SW, McNeil M, et al. Lipoarabinomannan: multiglycosylated form of the mycobacterial mannosylphosphatidylinositols. *J Biol Chem* 1992;267:6228–6233.
38. Khoo KH, Dell A, Morris HR, et al. Inositol phosphate capping of the nonreducing termini of lipoarabinomannan from rapidly growing strains of *Mycobacterium. J Biol Chem* 1995;270: 12380–12389.
39. Fujita K, Tanaka T, Taniguchi M. A bacteriolytic effect of UDP-sugar hydrolase on *Escherichia coli* via its overproduction using a modified ushA gene expression system. *J Ferment Bioeng* 1996;81:68–71.

40. Ma Y, Stern R, Scherman MS, et al. Drug targeting *M. tuberculosis* cell wall synthesis: the genetics of dTDP-rhamnose synthetic enzymes and development of a microtiter plate based screen for inhibitors of the conversion of dTDP-glucose to dTDP-rhamnose. *Antimicrob Agents Chemother* 2001;45:1407–1416.

41. Hoang TT, Ma YF, Stern RJ, et al. Construction and use of low-copy number T7 expression vectors for purification of problem proteins: purification of *Mycobacterium tuberculosis* RmlD and *Pseudomonas aeruginosa* LasI and RhlI proteins, and functional analysis of purified RhlI. *Gene* 1999;237:361–371.

42. Stern RJ, Lee TY, Lee TJ, et al. Conversion of dTDP-4-keto-6-deoxyglucose to free dTDP-4-keto-rhamnose by the*rmlC* gene products of *Escherichia coli* and *Mycobacterium tuberculosis*. *Microbiology* 1999;145:663–671.

43. Weston A, Stern RJ, Lee RE, et al. Biosynthetic origin of mycobacterial cell wall galactofuranosyl residues. *Tuber Lung Dis* 1998;78:123–131.

44. Ma Y, Mills JA, Belisle JT, et al. Drug targeting rhamnose biosynthesis in mycobacteria: determination of the pathway for rhamnose biosynthesis in mycobacteria and cloning, sequencing, expressing and determining the genetic organization of the *Mycobacterium tuberculosis* gene encoding α-D-glucose-1-phosphate thymidylyltransferase. *Microbiology* 1997;143:937–945.

45. Pan F, Jackson M, Ma Y, et al. Determination that cell wall galactofuran synthesis is essential for growth of mycobacteria. *J Bacteriol* 2001;183:3991–3998.

46. Ma Y, Pan F, McNeil MR. Determination that dTDP-rhamnose formation is essential for growth of mycobacteria. *J Bacteriol* 2002;184:3392–3395.

47. Scherman MS, Winans KA, Stern RJ, et al. Drug targeting mycobacterium tuberculosis cell wall synthesis: development of a microtiter plate-based Screen for UDP-galactopyranose mutase and identification of an inhibitor from a uridine-based library. *Antimicrob Agents Chemother* 2003;47:378–382.

48. Besra GS, Sievert T, Lee RE, et al. Identification of the apparent carrier in mycolic acid synthesis. *Proc Natl Acad Sci U S A* 1995;91:12735–12739.

49. Besra GS, Morehouse CB, Rittner CM, et al. Biosynthesis of mycobacterial lipoarabinomannan. *J Biol Chem* 1997;272:18460–18466.

50. Mikusova K, Mikus M, Besra G, et al. Biosynthesis of the linkage region of the mycobacterial cell wall. *J Biol Chem* 1996;271:7820–7828.

51. IUPAC-IUB Joint Commission on Biochemical Nomenclature. Prenol nomenclature. Recommendation 1986. *Eur J Biochem* 2002;167:181–184.

52. Takayama K, Schnoes HK, Semmlier EJ. Characterization of the alkali-stable mannophospholipids of *Mycobacterium smegmatis*. *Biochim Biophys Acta* 1973;136:212–221.

53. Wolucka BA, McNeil MR, de Hoffmann E, et al. Recognition of the lipid intermediate for arabinogalactan/arabinomannan biosynthesis and its relation to the mode of action of ethambutol on mycobacteria. *J Biol Chem* 1994;269:23328–23335.

54. Wolucka BA, de Hoffmann E. Isolation and characterization of the major form of polyprenyl-phospho-mannose from *Mycobacterium smegmatis*. *Glycobiology* 1998;8:955–962.

55. Takayama K, Goldman DS. Enzymatic synthesis of mannosyl-1-phosphoryldecaprenol by a cell-free system of *Mycobacterium tuberculosis*. *J Biol Chem* 1970;245:6251–6257.

56. Crick DC, Schulbach MC, Zink EE, et al. Polyprenyl phosphate biosynthesis in *Mycobacterium tuberculosis* and *Mycobacterium smegmatis*. *J Bacteriol* 2000;182:5771–5778.

57. Schulbach MC, Mahapatra S, Macchia M, et al. Purification, enzymatic characterization, and inhibition of the Z-farnesyl diphosphate synthase from *Mycobacterium tuberculosis*. *J Biol Chem* 2001;276:11624–11630.

58. Bailey AM, Mahapatra S, Brennan PJ, et al. Identification, cloning, purification and enzymatic characterization of *Mycobacterium tuberculosis*1-deoxy-D-xylulose 5-phosphate synthase. *Glycobiology* 2002;12:813–820.

59. Schulbach MC, Brennan PJ, Crick DC. Identification of a short (C-15) chain Z-isoprenyl diphosphate synthase and a homologous long (C-50) chain isoprenyl diphosphate synthase in *Mycobacterium tuberculosis*. *J Biol Chem* 2000;275:22876–22881.

60. Scherman MS, Kalbe-Bournonville L, Bush D, et al. Polyprenylphosphate-pentoses in mycobacteria are synthesized from phosphoribose pyrophosphate. *J Biol Chem* 1996;271:29652–29658.

61. Cole ST, Brosch R, Parkhill J, et al. Deciphering the biology of *Mycobacterium tuberculosis* from the complete genome sequence. *Nature* 1998;393:537–544.

62. Gurcha SS, Baulard AR, Kremer L, et al. Ppm1, a novel polyprenol monophosphomannose synthase from *Mycobacterium tuberculosis*. *Biochem J* 2002;365:441–450.

63. Schaeffer ML, Agnihotri G, Kallender H, et al. Expression, purification, and characterization of the *Mycobacterium tuberculosis* acyl carrier protein, AcpM. *Biochim Biophys Acta Mol Cell Biol Lipids*2001;1532:67–78.

64. Schaeffer ML, Agnihotri G, Volker C, et al. Purification and biochemical characterization of the *Mycobacterium tuberculosis* beta-ketoacyl-acyl carrier protein synthases KasA and KasB. *J Biol Chem* 2001;276:47029–47037.

65. Gastambide-Odier M, Lederer E. Biosynthese de l'acide corynomycolique a partir de deusc molecules d'acide palmitique. *Biochem Zeitschr* 1960;333:285–295.

66. Takayama K, Wang L, David HL. Effect on isoniazid on *in vivo* mycolic acid synthesis, cell growth, and viability of *Mycobacterium tuberculosis*. *Antimicrob Agents Chemother* 1972;2:29–35.

67. Zhang Y, Heym B, Allen B, et al. The catalase-peroxidase gene and isoniazid resistance of *Mycobacterium tuberculosis*. *Nature* 1992;358:591–593.

68. Banerjee A, Dubnau E, Quemard A, et al. InhA, a gene encoding a target for isoniazid and ethionamide in *Mycobacterium tuberculosis*. Science 1994;263:227–230.

69. Dessen A, Quemard A, Blanchard JS, et al. Crystal structure and function of the isoniazid target of *Mycobacterium tuberculosis*. Science 1995;267:1638–1641.

70. Slayden RA, Lee RE, Barry CE. Isoniazid affects multiple components of the type II fatty acid synthase system of *Mycobacterium tuberculosis*. Molecular Microbiology 2000;38:514–525.

71. Mdluli K, Slayden RA, Zhu Y, et al. Inhibition of a *Mycobacterium tuberculosis* beta-ketoacyl ACP synthase by isoniazid. *Science*1998;280:1607–1610.

72. Mdluli K, Sherman DR, Hickey MJ, et al. Biochemical and genetic data suggest that InhA is not the primary target for activated isoniazid in *Mycobacterium tuberculosis*. *J Infect Dis* 1996;174:1085–1090.

73. Winder FG, Collins PB, Whelan D. Effects of ethionamide and isoxyl on mycolic acid synthesis in*Mycobacterium tuberculosis* BCG. *J Gen Microbiol* 1971;66:379-380.

74. Quemard A, Laneelle G, Lacave C. Mycolic acid synthesis: a target for ethionamide in mycobacteria. *Antimicrob Agents Chemother* 1992;36:1316–1321.

75. Phetsuksiri B, Baulard AR, Cooper AM, et al. Antimycobacterial activities of isoxyl and new derivatives through the inhibition

of mycolic acid synthesis. *Antimicrob Agents Chemother* 1999; 43:1042-1051.

76. Slayden RA, Lee RE, Armour JW, et al. Antimycobacterial action of thiolactomycin: an inhibitor of fatty acid and mycolic acid synthesis. *Antimicrob Agents Chemother* 1996;40:2813-2819.

77. Holtje JV, Heidrich C. Enzymology of elongation and constriction of the murein sacculus of *Escherichia coli. Biochimie* 2001; 83:103–108.

78. Holtje JV. From growth to autolysis: the murein hydrolases in *Escherichia coli. Arch Microbiol* 1995;164:243–254.

79. van Heijenoort J. Assembly of the monomer unit of bacterial peptidoglycan. *Cell Mol Life Sci*1998;54:300–304.

80. Heijenoort JV. Biosynthesis of the bacterial peptidoglycan unit. In: Ghuysen JM, Hakenbeck R, eds. *Bacterial cell wall.* New York: Elsevier, 1994:39–54.

81. Mills JA, Motichka K, Jucker M, et al. The cell wall arabino-galactan linker formation enzyme, dTDP-Rha:-α-D-GlcNAc-diphosphoryl polyprenol, α-3-L-rhamnosyl transferase, is essential for mycobacterial viability. Unpublished data, 1998.

82. Kremer L, Dover LG, Morehouse C, et al. Galactan biosynthesis in *Mycobacterium tuberculosis*: identification of a bifunctional UDP-galactofuranosyltransferase. *J Biol Chem* 2001;276: 26430–26440.

83. Mikusova K, Yagi T, Stern R, et al. Biosynthesis of the galactan component of the mycobacterial cell wall. *J Biol Chem* 2000; 275:33890–33897.

84. Belanger AE, Besra GS, Ford ME, et al. Molecular characterization of the target of the antimycobacterial drug ethambutol. *Proc Natl Acad Sci U S A* 1996;93:11919–11924.

85. Takayama K, Kilburn JO. Inhibition of synthesis of arabino-galactan by ethambutol in *Mycobacterium smegmatis. Antimicrob Agents Chemother* 1989;33:1493–1499.

86. Deng L, Mikusova K, Robuck KG, et al. Recognition of multiple effects of ethambutol on metabolism of mycobacterial cell envelope. *Antimicrob Agents Chemother* 1995;39: 694–701.

87. Mikusova K, Slayden RA, Besra GS, et al. Biogenesis of the mycobacterial cell wall and the site of action of ethambutol. *Antimicrob Agents Chemother* 1995;39:2484–2489.

88. Khoo KH, Douglas E, Azadi P, et al. Truncated structural variants of lipoarabinomannan in ethambutol drug-resistant strains of *Mycobacterium smegmatis.* Inhibition of arabinan biosynthesis by ethambutol. *J Biol Chem* 1996;271:28682–28690.

89. Escuyer VE, Lety MA, Torrelles JB, et al. The role of the embA and embB gene products in the biosynthesis of the terminal hexaarabinofuranosyl motif of *Mycobacterium smegmatis* arabinogalactan. *J Biol Chem* 2001;276:48854–48862.

90. Puech V, Bayan N, Salim K, et al. Characterization of the *in vivo* acceptors of the mycoloyl residues transferred by the corynebacterial PS1 and the related mycobacterial antigens 85. *Mol Microbiol* 2000;35:1026–1041.

91. Daffe M. The mycobacterial antigens 85 complex—from structure to function and beyond. *Trends Microbiol* 2000;8: 438–440.

92. Jackson M, Raynaud C, Laneelle MA, et al. Inactivation of the antigen 85C gene profoundly affects the mycolate content and alters the permeability of the *Mycobacterium tuberculosis* cell envelope. *Mol Microbiol* 1999;31:1573–1587.

93. Puech V, Guilhot C, Perez E, et al. Evidence for a partial redundancy of the fibronectin-binding proteins for the transfer of mycoloyl residues onto the cell wall arabinogalactan termini of *Mycobacterium tuberculosis. Mol Microbiol* 2002;44: 1109–1122.

94. Kremer L, Maughan WN, Wilson RA, et al. The *M. tuberculo-*

*sis*antigen 85 complex and mycolyltransferase activity. *Lett Appl Microbiol* 2002;34:233–237.

95. Belisle JT, Vissa VD, Sievert T, et al. Role of the major antigen of *Mycobacterium tuberculosis* in cell wall biogenesis. *Science* 1997;276:1420–1422.

96. Ronning DR, Klabunde T, Besra GS, et al. Crystal structure of the secreted form of antigen 85C reveals potential targets for mycobacterial drugs and vaccines. *Nat Struct Biol* 2000;7: 141–146.

97. Anderson DH, Harth G, Horwitz MA, et al. An interfacial mechanism and a class of inhibitors inferred from two crystal structures of the *Mycobacterium tuberculosis* 30 kDa major secretory protein (antigen 85B), a mycolyl transferase. *J Mol Biol* 2001;307:671–681.

98. Yokoyama K, Ballou CE. Synthesis of alpha 1–6 man-nooligosaccharides in *Mycobacterium smegmatis.* Function of beta-mannosylphosphoryldecaprenol as the mannosyl donor. *J Biol Chem* 1989;264:21621–21628.

99. Goren MB, Brennan PJ. Mycobacterial lipids: chemistry and biological activities. In: Youmans GP, ed. *Tuberculosis.* Philadelphia: WB Saunders, 1979:63–193.

100. Ballou CE, Lee YC. The structure of a myoinositol mannoside from *Mycobacterium tuberculosis* glycolipid. *Biochemistry* 1964; 3:682–685.

101. Pangborn MC, McKinney JA. Purification of serologically active phosphoinositides of *Mycobacterium tuberculosis. J Lipid Res* 1966;7:627–633.

102. Azad AK, Sirakova TD, Fernandes ND, et al. Gene knockout reveals a novel gene cluster for the synthesis of a class of cell wall lipids unique to pathogenic mycobacteria. *J Biol Chem* 1997; 272:16741–16745.

103. Rainwater DL, Kolattukudy PE. Fatty acid biosynthesis in *Mycobacterium tuberculosis* var. *bovis* bacillus Calmette–Guérin. *J Biol Chem* 1985;260:616–623.

104. Fernandes ND, Kolattukudy PE. A newly identified methyl-branched chain fatty acid synthesizing enzyme from *Mycobacterium tuberculosis* var. *bovis* BCG. *J Biol Chem* 1998;273: 2823–2828.

105. Fitzmaurice AM, Kolattukudy PE. An acyl-CoA synthase (acoas) gene adjacent to the mycocerosic acid synthase (mas) locus is necessary for mycocerosyl lipid synthesis in *Mycobacterium tuberculosis* var. *bovis* BCG. *J Biol Chem* 1998;273: 8033–8039.

106. Sirakova TD, Thirumala AK, Dubey VS, et al. The *Mycobacterium tuberculosis* pks2 gene encodes the synthase for the hepta- and octamethyl-branched fatty acids required for sulfolipid synthesis. *J Biol Chem* 2001;276:16833–16839.

107. Cox JS, Chen B, McNeil M, et al. Complex lipid determine tissue specific replication of *Mycobacterium tuberculosis* in mice. *Nature* 1999;402:79–83.

108. Camacho LR, Constant P, Raynaud C, et al. Analysis of the phthiocerol dimycocerosate locus of *Mycobacterium tuberculosis*: evidence that this lipid is involved in the cell wall permeability barrier. *J Biol Chem* 2001;276:19845–19854.

109. Jackson M, Crick DC, Brennan PJ. Phosphatidylinositol is an essential phospholipid of mycobacteria. *J Biol Chem* 2000;275: 30092–30099.

110. Kordulakova J, Gilleron M, Mikusova K, et al. Definition of the first mannosylation step in phosphatidylinositol mannoside synthesis: PimA is essential for growth of mycobacteria. *J Biol Chem* 2002;277:31335–31344.

111. Schaeffer ML, Khoo KH, Besra GS, et al. The *pimB* gene of *Mycobacterium tuberculosis* encodes a mannosyltransferase involved in lipoarabinomannan biosynthesis. *J Biol Chem* 1999; 274:31625–31631.

112. Kremer L, Gurcha SS, Bifani P, et al. Characterization of a putative alpha-mannosyltransferase involved in phosphatidylinositol trimannoside biosynthesis in *Mycobacterium tuberculosis. Biochem J* 2002;363:437–447.
113. Lemassu A, OrtaloMagne A, Bardou F, et al. Extracellular and surface-exposed polysaccharides of non-tuberculous mycobacteria. *Microbiology* 1996;142:1513–1520.
114. Ortalo-Magne A, Dupont MA, Lemassu A, et al. Molecular composition of the outermost capsular material of the tubercle bacillus. *Microbiology* 1995;141:1609–1620.
115. Schlesinger LS. Macrophage phagocytosis of virulent but not attenuated strains of *Mycobacterium tuberculosis* is mediated by mannose receptors in addition to complement receptors. *J Immunol* 1993;150:2920–2925.
116. Ellner JJ, Daniel TM. Immunosuppression by mycobacterial arabinomannan. *Clin Exp Immunol* 1979;35:250–257.

10

MYCOBACTERIUM TUBERCULOSIS VIRULENCE: A GENETIC ANALYSIS

ISSAR SMITH

Tuberculosis (TB), one of the oldest recorded human afflictions, is still one of the biggest killers among infectious diseases, as documented elsewhere in this book. At the same time, the causative agent, *Mycobacterium tuberculosis*, is one of the most difficult bacterial subjects for scientific investigation. As a result of these two related phenomena, most research in nonpathogenic as well pathogenic mycobacteria has the ultimate aim of finding innovative strategies for the prevention and cure of mycobacterial diseases. To rationally develop new approaches, it is essential to study the genetics and physiology of *M. tuberculosis* and related mycobacteria. It is equally important to understand the *M. tuberculosis*–host interaction to learn how these bacteria circumvent host defenses and cause disease. The approaches described in this review have allowed the identification of *M. tuberculosis* genes that are involved or potentially involved in virulence. In the future, some of these genes and the proteins they encode, as well as newly discovered ones, are expected to provide new bacterial targets that can be used for creating vaccines and drugs as well as more selective diagnostic reagents.

DEFINING *MYCOBACTERIUM TUBERCULOSIS* VIRULENCE

What makes *M. tuberculosis* virulent? Unfortunately, there is no simple answer yet, despite the knowledge obtained in the last 100 or more years. *M. tuberculosis* does not have classical virulence factors like those which are the major causes of diseases brought on by other bacterial pathogens, such as toxins produced by *Corynebacterium diphtheriae, Escherichia coli* 0157:H7, *Shigella dysenteriae, Vibrio cholerae*, and so forth. The purpose of much of the research discussed in this chapter has been to help answer this question, that is, defining *M. tuberculosis* virulence by finding those factors that are

important for the progression of TB. While we have only limited knowledge of how the tubercle bacillus causes disease, its virulence can be measured. This quantitative view can then be used to ascertain the effects of modifying the bacterium on the disease process. The standard terms *mortality* and *morbidity* are used for a description of *M. tuberculosis* virulence and can be defined in the following ways. *Mortality* is the percentage of infected animals that die and is also measured as the time it takes for an animal to die after being infected. Another important parameter that is usually associated with virulence is bacterial load or burden, that is, numbers of bacteria found in the infected host after the initial infection. This information allows a comparison of the fitness of different bacterial strains to survive host responses during an infection. In addition, *M. tuberculosis* virulence mutants that have lower bacterial loads during animal infections exhibit different growth curves during this process, and in one publication they have been grouped into various classes: *sgiv* (*severe growth in vivo*), that is, mutants that do not replicate at all. These are cleared rapidly or may persist with no increase in cell numbers; *giv* (*growth in vivo*, that is, mutants that grow initially but at lower rates than the wild type; *per* (*persistence genes*), that is, those growing normally at earlier stages but declining in numbers at the onset of cell-mediated immunity (1). This classification of mutations, especially when more are obtained, will be useful for understanding how the stages of the infectious process are controlled by different *M. tuberculosis* genes. In this chapter, to conform to standard genetic nomenclature, *M. tuberculosis* mutants that show attenuated growth in mice will be classified with the same terminology but as phenotypes (SGIV, GIV, and PER). *Morbidity* in terms of histopathology analyses is important to characterize another class of *M. tuberculosis* mutants affecting virulence, namely, those that do not affect the bacterial load. One example of these is the *M. tuberculosis sigH* mutant that shows normal *M. tuberculosis* survival in macrophages and mice (2,3), but whose histopathology in infected mouse lungs is much less than that caused by wild-type *M. tuberculosis* (3).

I. Smith: Tuberculosis Center, Public Health Research Institute at the International Center for Public Health, Newark, New Jersey.

To better measure morbidity and mortality caused by *M. tuberculosis*, it is important to understand the pathogenesis that is associated with TB. Uncontrolled *M. tuberculosis* growth in its human host, given the usual site of the infection, is associated with extensive lung damage that ultimately causes death by suffocation due to insufficient oxygenation. This anoxia causes the obliteration of lung parenchymal cells involved in oxygen uptake as well as obstruction of bronchiolar passageways by granulomatous growths and by blood that is released by the rupture of liquefied granulomas in adjacent lung tissue (4). Other untreated forms of tuberculosis, such as tubercular meningitis that occurs in the meningeal membranes of the brain, can result in death because of inflammation of brain tissue and resulting hydrocephalus and seizures. Tuberculomas, another form of TB in the brain, are large structures formed by the enlargement of brain granulomas also due to inflammatory responses and they are also associated with seizures (5). Inflammatory responses are also believed to play a role in other extrapulmonary manifestations of TB, such as in bone (6).

Inflammation is a key word here as the growth of the tubercle bacillus elicits inflammatory host responses that are necessary to control infections but that can also cause extensive tissue damage. Among the cellular agents involved in tissue destruction are various proteases like cathepsin D (7) that are also believed to be major factors in the liquefaction of granulomas (8). In addition, *M. tuberculosis* uptake can cause apoptosis of macrophages (9,10), and this could play a role in adjacent tissue damage. A key cytokine in the inflammatory or T_H1 response of the cellular immune system is tumor necrosis factor-α (TNFα). Mice that are unable to produce or respond to it can not form granulomas to restrict bacterial dissemination (11,12). Similarly, TNFα is a major determinant of disease in a rabbit model of TB meningitis, as there is a direct correlation between the extent of disease caused by several *M. bovis* and *M. tuberculosis* strains and levels of this cytokine in the cerebrospinal fluid (13). However, data from analyses of cytokine responses and virulence in mice that are infected with various *M. tuberculosis* strains indicate there are factors additional to TNF-α in TB progression. CDC1551 is a clinical strain that was originally thought to be highly virulent (14), and recently it has been shown that CDC1551 induces levels of cytokines, including TNF-α, in mice that are higher than other *M. tuberculosis* strains. However, it is not more virulent than the other strains, as defined by bacterial load and mortality (15). Also, another study compared the ability of two clinical *M. tuberculosis* strains HN878 and NHN5 to cause disease and to elicit a cytokine response in a mouse model. HN878, the more virulent of the two as determined by mortality measurements, induces lower amounts of the inflammatory cytokines, including TNF-α, than HN5 (16). Interestingly, HN878 induces higher levels of T_H2 cytokines like interleukin-4 (IL-4) and interferon-α

(IFN-α). It has also been reported that the apoptosis that is sometimes observed when *M. tuberculosis* infects macrophages is dependent on TNF-α and that more virulent *M. tuberculosis* cause less apoptosis (17). The above experiments illustrate the complexity of the immune system and its effectors, as their results are not consistent with a simple direct relationship between the levels of one or a few cytokines like TNF-α and the progression of the disease in macrophage and animals. Clearly an optimal balance of these immunomodulators is crucial. Despite the different results in the experiments just discussed that are difficult to interpret, these studies are of value, as they show that some *M. tuberculosis* strains are more virulent than others, using the criteria of mortality and morbidity, in macrophages and animal models (18).

MODELS FOR MEASURING *MYCOBACTERIUM TUBERCULOSIS* VIRULENCE

M. tuberculosis virulence is studied both in tissue culture, using macrophages and more recently dendritic cells, and animal models. Although tissue culture models are easier to work with and give faster and more meaningful results, as discussed in the next section, the animal models are arguably better because all stages of TB can be studied. Significantly, in this regard, certain *M. tuberculosis* mutants do not have an attenuated phenotype in macrophages yet are defective for growth in mice (19,20). Thus, genetic selections or screens for *M. tuberculosis* virulence mutations that use macrophages alone may miss some attenuated *M. tuberculosis* mutants. The choice of animal models is an important one in virulence studies, and the three major models— mice, guinea pigs, and rabbits—each have their advantages and disadvantages. Mice are the most frequently used *in vivo* models because of their well-studied genetics, involving the existence of inbred strains (including some that have mutations in the immune system), the availability of reagents to measure cytokine levels, as well as their low costs of maintenance relative to other animal models (21). Another big advantage to mouse experiments is that there are inbred strains that show widely different levels of resistance to *M. tuberculosis* and other pathogens. This has allowed the development of a set of recombinant congenic mouse strains, made by mating strains A/J and C57/BL6, that is now being used to chromosomally map loci conferring resistance/sensitivity to bacterial infections (22). The progression of TB in mice is unlike that of humans in that the granulomas formed are not as distinct, but the fact that mice are generally not as sensitive to the disease as other animal models and can become chronically infected is more like the human situation. Guinea pigs are very sensitive to *M. tuberculosis* infection, and the stages of the disease, including early stages of granuloma formation, in this animal are similar to those in humans (21). The disadvantages are the lack of inbred strains and reagents as well as the high maintenance costs (21). The rabbit model has one big advantage over the other animal system in that the lung granulomas formed during the disease show the same progression of stages (caseation, liquefaction, and cavitation), as is observed in advanced cases of human TB (8). The disadvantages of rabbits are similar to those of guinea pigs, but their upkeep is even more expensive.

M. tuberculosis is an intracellular pathogen that infects macrophages primarily, and these phagocytic cells are also used to analyze the virulence of *M. tuberculosis* strains and mutants. These *ex vivo* studies serve as a model for the early stages of infection, which involve the phagocytosis of *M. tuberculosis* by resident macrophages in the lung alveoli. Since human alveolar macrophages are difficult to obtain, model macrophage systems are generally used. These can be from either mice or humans and can be primary cultures or immortalized cell lines. Each model has advantages, as primary cells are natural (not immortalized) and are more representative of the actual *in vivo* situation, but they are usually harder to obtain and are more variable, especially macrophages from human donors. Mouse macrophages can be primary, isolated from bone marrow, from lung alveoli by bronchoalveolar lavage, and from peritoneal exudates after injection of thioglycollic acid into the peritoneal cavities of mice. Many mouse macrophage cell lines are available, including the widely used J774 line and MH-S cells, the latter an immortalized alveolar macrophage cell line whose behavior is very similar to that of primary mouse alveolar macrophages (23). Since mice are the most widely used animal model, there are advantages to using macrophages from this mammal, including reagent availability, as discussed above. In addition, the use of primary mouse cells allows the preparation of macrophages from animals with defined mutations so that the effect of specific host factors on interactions with *M. tuberculosis* at the macrophage level can be tested (24). Activation of primary mouse macrophages or macrophages cell lines by the addition of IFN-γ and lipopolysaccharide, which induces the levels of the inducible nitric oxide synthase enzyme to form nitric oxide (NO), is necessary to observe the *M. tuberculosis* killing activity of these cells (25).

Human macrophages are also widely used, and a big advantage in these studies is that the early stages of human disease can be studied. Human macrophages used in these experiments are primary cultures derived from peripheral blood monocytes [monocyte-derived macrophages (MDMs)] that are allowed to differentiate into macrophages as well as the more difficult to obtain alveolar macrophages derived by bronchoalveolar lavage. Transformed monocytic cell lines like THP-1 that can be differentiated into macrophage like phagocytic cells by the addition of phorbol esters (26) are frequently used, as are similar immortalized monocytic cell lines like U-937 (27). Studies have shown that differentiated THP-1 macrophages are quite similar to human MDMs in their response to *M. tuberculosis* infection (28). In addition, many reagents are available to study human host responses to *M. tuberculosis* infection. Human macrophages from TB-negative donors or cell lines do not kill *M. tuberculosis* well, presumably because they do not produce NO (29). This is an advantage if one is testing the survival of bacterial mutants, since the wild-type *M. tuberculosis* cells usually grow well and a mutant growth phenotype can be more accurately quantified than in activated mouse macrophages (30).

GENETICS OF *MYCOBACTERIUM TUBERCULOSIS*

Description of the *Mycobacterium tuberculosis* Genome

Prior to a few years ago, the genetics of *M. tuberculosis* was a neglected subject because of difficulties in working with the organism and lack of suitable tools. A review published as recently as 1994 stated that this field "is still in its infancy" (31), but the study of mycobacterial genetics has blossomed in recent years as demonstrated by an entire book that is dedicated to this area (32). This is due to many innovations, such as the complete DNA sequencing and annotation of the *M. tuberculosis* H37Rv genome (33) and those of related mycobacteria that are currently being completed by the Sanger Center–Pasteur Institute consortium and by the Institute for Genomic Research, as well as the development of many genetic methods, mainly by the Gicquel and Jacobs laboratories (32,34).

The *M. tuberculosis* H37Rv genome consists of approximately 4.5 million base pairs (bp) and contains approximately 4,000 genes (33). Annotation of the *M. tuberculosis* genome shows that *M. tuberculosis* is not remarkable in its content of most groups of genes and their products found in microorganisms. For example, among transcriptional regulatory proteins, *M. tuberculosis* has 13 sigma factors (proteins that confer transcriptional specificity to RNA polymerases), corresponding to 0.3% of the total genes, and 22 other regulatory proteins, including 13 two-component response regulators (usually transcriptional regulators that are activated by and serve to transduce environmental signals), corresponding to 0.6% of the total. These numbers are quite similar to the frequency of genes that encode these regulators in the genomes of *Corynebacterium diphtheriae*, *Bacillus subtilis*, and *Escherichia coli*. This is much lower than the corresponding numbers for the soil-dwelling, spore-forming actinomycete *Streptomyces coelicolor*, which has 55 sigma factor genes (0.7% of the total) and 74 response regulator genes (>2% of the total) (35). It has been postulated that the soil environment in which *Streptomyces* species are found has selected for the ability of these microorganisms to adapt to radically changing conditions.

This would occur by gene duplication and divergent evolution, which would give rise to many transcriptional regulators that would allow appropriate bacterial responses to a changeable environment. In agreement with this idea of environmental selection, the number of predicted transport proteins encoded in the *S. coelicolor* genome is 614, corresponding to 8% of the total genes. The equivalent number in *M. tuberculosis* is 125 annotated genes for transport functions (3% of the total). Circumstantial evidence for this idea of gene duplication is the fact that the *S. coelicolor* genome is more than 8.5 million bp, twice as big as that of *M. tuberculosis* and encoding twice as many proteins (35). There must be additional reasons for these dramatic differences in the *Streptomyces* genome when compared with other eukaryotes. *B. subtilis* is also a spore-forming soil dweller, but its 4-Mb genome has levels of regulatory and transporter proteins that are similar to those of bacteria other than *Streptomyces.*

There are some unique features in the *M. tuberculosis* genome. Two hundred and twenty-five genes are annotated as encoding enzymes for the metabolism of fatty acids, comprising 6% of the total. Among these are approximately 100 that are predicted to function in the β oxidation of fatty acids, whereas *E. coli* has only 50 enzymes involved in fatty acid metabolism. *S. coelicolor* has a total of 115, corresponding to a little more than 1% of the proteins, of which 59 are annotated as being involved in fatty acid degradation. This large number of *M. tuberculosis* enzymes that putatively use fatty acids may be related to the ability of this pathogen to grow in the tissues of the infected host where fatty acids may be the major carbon source. This important aspect of *M. tuberculosis* physiology during infection is described later in this chapter.

Another unusual feature of the *M. tuberculosis* genome is the presence of the unrelated PE and PPE families of acidic, glycine-rich proteins. The names come from the Pro-Glu (PE) and Pro-Pro-Glu (PPE) sequences found in the two conserved N-terminal regions in each of these protein families that are approximately 110 and 180 amino acids long, respectively. The 172 genes, 104 of the PE class and 68 of the PPE variety, comprise more than 4% of the genes in *M. tuberculosis*, and similar levels of abundance are noted in other members of the *M. tuberculosis* complex in which sequence data are available (36). PE and PPE genes are not unique to members of the *M. tuberculosis* complex, as *M. leprae* has 26 genes for these two families. Nineteen of these are pseudogenes, reflecting the extensive physical and genetic downsizing of the *M. leprae* genome by deletion and mutation during the evolution of this obligate parasite (37). *M. marinum,* a pathogenic mycobacterium that infects frogs and fish and causes a TB-like disease, has some PE genes that are involved in virulence (38). These proteins are not restricted to pathogenic mycobacteria as *M. smegmatis* has some proteins of the PE–polymorphic GC-rich sequence (PGRS) family (39). In *M. tuberculosis,* proteins encoded by the 100 PE genes can be further subdivided into three classes: 29 that contain the PE region alone, 8 in which the PE region is followed by unrelated C-terminal sequences, and the largest group of 67 termed the PE-PGRS subfamily. This group of proteins has the conserved PE domain followed by C-terminal extensions with multiple repeats of Gly-Gly-Ala or Gly-Gly-Asn that are in the PGRS domains. The function of these large families of related proteins is unknown, but size variation has been observed in members of the PE-PGRS subfamily in clinical TB strains, and many of these proteins have been localized in the cell wall and cell membrane (39). These data and the fact that these proteins are antigenic has led to the hypothesis that at least some of these proteins may be involved in antigenic variation of *M. tuberculosis* during infection (39). Significantly, many of the PE genes encoding proteins that contain only the 110-amino-acid domain are closely followed by a gene encoding a PPE protein. In one case thus far analyzed, a tandem PE-PPE pair, Rv2431c-Rv2430c, is coexpressed and can form a complex (M. Strong and D. Eisenberg, personal communication, 2002).

Methods of Genetic Analysis in Mycobacteria

The complete sequence and annotation of the *M. tuberculosis* genome has allowed many new genetic approaches to study of the physiology and pathogenicity of this organism, but much important work was done in this area before the genome sequencing project was initiated. These pre-genome approaches largely dealt with developing methods for creating mutations in specific genes. The choice of which genes to explore and ultimately inactivate in the study of virulence was frequently based on the existence of natural mutations occurring in normally virulent strains that affected pathogenicity, such as *katG* and *sigA* (40,41), or predictions as to which genes should be important in some aspect of *M. tuberculosis* virulence and/or physiology by inference from studies of other bacterial pathogens, such as genes encoding sigma factors and iron acquisition regulators (42). The following discussion will address methods used for genetic analysis in mycobacterial species. Their application for the identification and characterization of *M. tuberculosis* genes that play a role in virulence will be discussed later in his chapter. Some methods, such as bacterial conjugation (43) and bacteriophage-mediated transduction (44), have been used for genetic studies in *M. smegmatis* but will not be discussed here as they have not yet been successfully applied to *M. tuberculosis.*

Initial Genetic Studies

Early studies on the creation of mutations in mycobacteria concentrated on the faster growing nonpathogenic species because of the relative ease in working with these bacteria owing to the fact that there is no requirement for BL3 containment facilities, as well as the relative rapidity of the experiments. For example, *M. smegmatis* has a 3-hour generation time whereas that of *M. tuberculosis* is 20 to 24 hours. Several methods were developed to inactivate genes in these bacteria (reviewed in reference 45), and while there was some success in *M. tuberculosis* with these methods, the process remained difficult in this pathogen. In addition to its extremely slow growth rate that makes it time consuming to do the standard types of gene inactivation (it takes 3 weeks for a single *M. tuberculosis* cell to become a visible colony on solid media), this bacterium reportedly had lower rates of homologous recombination and higher rates of illegitimate recombination than other mycobacteria, which would complicate gene disruption by standard gene replacement techniques (45). The original observation that the *M. tuberculosis* RecA protein was synthesized with an intein (protein intron) that had to be spliced out led to speculation that this process contributed to the supposedly low levels of homologous recombination in this species (46). However, later results indicated that the *M. tuberculosis recA* gene is as competent in restoring function to an *M. smegmatis recA* mutant as the *M. smegmatis* inteinless gene, suggesting that the splicing out of inteins does not affect RecA's capability for homologous recombination (47,48). In addition, later experiments have shown that *M. tuberculosis* has rates of homologous recombination that are similar to those of the faster growing nonpathogenic *M. smegmatis* (49).

Current Genetic Methods

Despite the problems mentioned in the previous section, several current techniques have been used with success in inactivating *M. tuberculosis* genes. Gene disruption techniques in mycobacteria, as described below, can be divided into directed and global methods but generally require a selectable phenotype (usually resistance to an antibiotic). The most frequently used antibiotic resistance cassettes used in mycobacteria are those conferring resistance to kanamycin, hygromycin, and streptomycin (50). These antibiotics are also useful for selection in *E. coli*, allowing most cloning procedures to take place in this organism, with appropriate plasmid vectors. Selection for kanamycin resistance (KanR) is favored in many mycobacteria like *M. smegmatis* because of the generally low levels of spontaneous KanR mutations and the high stability and low cost of the antibiotic. However, kanamycin is not a good selective marker in *M. tuberculosis* because there is a high spontaneous mutation rate resulting from the presence of only one ribosomal RNA (*rrn*) cistron in which the 16S rRNA gene can undergo mutations to KanR at a significant level. *M. smegmatis* has two *rrn* cistrons, and mutations to KanR in one of these are masked by the dominance of the second, sensitive *rrn* cistron (51). The high background to KanR in *M. tuberculosis* can be bypassed by introducing a second

resistance marker, such as a streptomycin resistance cassette, into the plasmid construct and doing a double-antibiotic selection for kanamycin and the second antibiotic (e.g., streptomycin) (52); however, this modification requires a more complex cloning strategy. Hygromycin resistance is the preferred antibiotic selection in *M. tuberculosis* in spite of its cost because its frequency of spontaneous mutation to this drug is very low.

Directed Gene Disruption

Directed gene inactivation entails the insertion of an antibiotic resistance cassette in the middle of the gene of interest and transforming this DNA into mycobacteria as a linear or circular molecule, using electroporation. The desired result is allelic replacement of the chromosomal gene by the mutated one. In members of the *M. tuberculosis* complex, directed gene disruptions have been made with long linear molecules, up to 40 kb (53), or shorter ones, in the range of 4 kb (54,55). The use of single-stranded linear DNA increases allelic replacement by homologous recombination in *Streptomyces* (56), and this effect is also observed in gene inactivation experiments in *M. smegmatis* and in the *M. tuberculosis* complex (57). The advantage of the linear DNA method is that cloning is relatively easy, especially when short DNA fragments are used. A disadvantage is that unique restriction enzyme sites are required unless one employs more elaborate manipulation of the DNA sequence of interest, and this problem is magnified as the DNA increases in length. This is true for linear DNAs and plasmid-based systems that are described below. One early way of avoiding this problem was by the use of transposition systems that function in *E. coli* to disrupt genes contained in large segments of mycobacterial DNA cloned into plasmids with *E. coli* replicons. Many transposition insertion events in several genes contained in a 7-kb *M. smegmatis* chromosomal fragment were obtained in *E. coli* using transposon mγδ-200 (58). The desired disruption in the *ideR* gene contained in the *M. smegmatis* DNA fragment, determined by restriction enzyme digestion analyses, was then used to create an *M. smegmatis ideR* mutant gene by homologous recombination, using techniques described in the next paragraph (59). A newer transposon delivery system uses a cell-free approach to disrupt mycobacterial genes. A complex, called the transposome, is made between the transposable element Tn5 containing a selectable antibiotic resistance marker and its transposase, the enzyme responsible for the integration of the transposon into other DNAs. The transposome is commercially available and has been used to make random mutations in cloned mycobacterial DNAs as well as random mutations in mycobacteria after electroporation of the transposome into recipient bacteria (60).

Most directed mutations in mycobacteria are performed with bifunctional or shuttle plasmid vectors that can be maintained in *E. coli* and many are available for this use (50). Circular plasmid integration, using a vector that cannot replicate in the recipient or has a temperature-sensitive (*ts*) replicon (61), is the most widely used method for directed gene disruption by allelic replacement in mycobacteria (45). It usually entails a two-step process in which the plasmid containing the desired gene disrupted with an antibiotic resistance cassette integrates into the genome by a single crossover event (Campbell-type integration) at the region of homology, selecting for the antibiotic resistance cassette. This event forms a direct repeat at one of two positions relative to the antibiotic cassette. In a second crossover event, the plasmid backbone is excised out by means of recombination at the other direct repeat than the one initially used, when the antibiotic selection is maintained, resulting in the desired gene disruption. This technique can be relatively efficient when coupled with a counterselection to facilitate plasmid elimination in the second step. Two methods have been used for counterselection; the first is resistance to streptomycin (StrR), using wild-type *rpsL* in the plasmid vector and a mutated *rpsL* (StrR) allele in the chromosome of the recipient (62). Since the sensitive *rpsL* allele is dominant, resistance to streptomycin is only observed when it is lost along with the plasmid backbone, leaving the unique *rpsl* (StrR) chromosomal gene. The second counterselection is sucrose resistance when *sacB* encoding levansucrase is in the plasmid backbone. This enzyme converts sucrose to levans that are toxic to mycobacteria lacking a functional levanase that coverts levans to fructose and glucose (63). In both cases, the presence of the vector in the bacterial chromosome prevents bacterial growth on selective media (streptomycin or sucrose). Of the two methods, the *sacB* selection is easier because one does not have to make a specific StrR-resistant recipient in which *rpsL*, but not *rrnA*, is mutated. Another advantage to the *sacB* sucrose selection is that it can be used to introduce silent or unmarked mutations into the chromosome of the recipient, dispensing with the need for an antibiotic resistance marker. This method was used in *M. smegmatis* (64) and later in *M. tuberculosis* (49), and is important for the development of live, attenuated *M. tuberculosis* vaccine strains, as discussed later in this chapter. The drawbacks of the two-step procedure are again the necessity of a unique restriction site in the gene of interest coupled with the time required for the process, i.e., approximately 2 to 3 months from the initial transformation to the verification, by DNA analysis, of the gene disruption in survivors of the counterselection. In addition, mutations that inactivate the plasmid-born *rpsl* or *sacB* during the selection and counterselection procedure will be erroneously scored as desired events in which the plasmid has been excised from the chromosome. A way of avoiding these false positives is by introducing another easily screenable marker in the plasmid backbone that should also be eliminated with the vector. An StrR cassette (52) and reporter fusions that give a visible plate phenotype have

been used for this purpose, including fusions with *xylE* (65) and *lacZ* (66).

A simpler and faster one-step variation of single crossover gene inactivation with circular DNA has been employed to inactivate mycobacterial genes. This technique utilizes the property of internal gene fragments carried on a circular plasmid to disrupt the corresponding gene when the DNA integrates into the chromosome by a single Campbell-type event. It has been possible to disrupt the *M. smegmatis sodA* with DNA fragments as short as 180 bp with this method (67). However, these events can be unstable because recombination at the direct repeats in the chromosome formed during the plasmid integration, which is the basis of plasmid elimination in the two-step plasmid procedure, can lead to excision of the plasmid, restoring the intact wild-type gene in the absence of the selecting antibiotic.

The major problem with the above methods is they are for the most part inefficient as the frequency of introducing DNA into mycobacterial species, especially *M. tuberculosis,* by the standard electroporation technique is quite low, even with the utilization of modifications that increase transformation, such as raising the temperature at which the DNA is introduced into *M. tuberculosis* (68). A new method of directed gene inactivation using a *ts* bacteriophage delivery system has been described recently that bypasses these problems and is the current method of choice for directed mutation (69). The gene of interest, disrupted with an antibiotic resistance cassette, is cloned into a plasmid containing a lytic mycobacteriophage genome with a *ts* replicon and also has a bacteriophage λ packaging site. This allows the formation of viable transducing bacteriophage particles by an *in vitro* packaging reaction that can be transduced into *E. coli.* Cosmid DNA is prepared in *E. coli* and is then transformed into *M. smegmatis* at 30°C (the permissive temperature that allows the formation of infectious mycobacteriophage). *M. smegmatis* lysates with the bacteriophage construct are then used to infect *M. tuberculosis* at 30°C (the nonpermissive temperature), with high enough multiplicities to transduce all of the bacteria. Transductants are then selected on antibiotic-containing media for those events in which the *M. tuberculosis* gene has integrated into the chromosome. This technique is very efficient as essentially all of the recipient cells can be transduced and the selection is robust.

Global Gene Inactivation

The principle of global gene inactivation is the insertion of foreign DNA, usually a transposable element, into many sites in the bacterial genome, ideally on a completely random basis. This event requires a selectable phenotype, usually an antibiotic resistance marker carried on the transposable element. Two groups have developed efficient transposition systems that produce integration events in the genomes of mycobacterial species, including *M. tuberculosis*. These systems use transposable elements carried by vectors that cannot replicate above 39°C— in one case a *ts* plasmid carrying Tn 1096 (61), and in the other case a *ts* bacteriophage, similar to the one described in the previous section, that carries Tn 5367 (70). The advantage of these systems is that one can start with a transformed or infected population of cells and easily get many integrative events by passage at the restricting temperature. Both systems have been used to identify *M. tuberculosis* virulence genes using the signature tagged mutagenesis (STM) method developed to clone *Salmonella* genes essential for bacterial survival during mouse infections (71). In this technique, uniquely tagged transposon *M. tuberculosis* mutants were made in broth cultures and were negatively screened by hybridization for those that did not survive during animal infections (72,73). A drawback of these systems in *M. tuberculosis* is that the transposition events are not completely random in that there seem to be "hot spots" of transposition integration, based on the genes found in initial STM mutant screens, as discussed below (72,73). Since the *M. tuberculosis* genome has approximately 4,000 open reading frames (ORFs), many events would be needed to saturate the genome and mutagenize every gene using a nonrandom inactivating system. A transposition system has been developed more recently from the mariner transposable element *Himar-1* that overcomes some of these drawbacks. The mariner element recognition sequence is simply an A-T base pair and is be expected to be truly random in its integration, unlike Tn 1096 and Tn 5367, which recognize much larger integration sites. The *Himar-1* system has been used to introduce transposition events in *M. smegmatis* (74), in *M. bovis* bacillus Calmette–Guérin (BCG) (75), and, more recently, in *M. tuberculosis* H37Rv where 100,000 transposon insertions have been obtained. DNA sequencing and other analyses indicate that more than 2,600 *M. tuberculosis* genes have been thus far inactivated (E. Rubin, personal communication, 2002). STM tagging was not used to make these mariner transposon mutations, so there is no global screening method for virulence genes as there are with the two transposon systems previously described. The transposome complex mentioned previously can also be used to introduce random mutations into mycobacterial genomes, but this system also lacks tagging capability to make screening for mutants with attenuated virulence.

Complementation

Genetic complementation has also been used to identify *M. tuberculosis* virulence genes. These studies use either *M. tuberculosis* strains that were previously known to be avirulent or nonpathogens as recipients for genes that can be selected for a virulence phenotype, using assays that were described earlier in this chapter. It was shown that the random cloning of an *M. tuberculosis* cosmid library into an avirulent *M. bovis* strain localized the attenuating mutation in *sigA*, encoding the major mycobacterial sigma factor, as the wild-type *sigA* restored virulence in a guinea pig morbidity (spleen focus) assay (41). A similar *M. tuberculosis* cosmid library transformed into the avirulent *M. tuberculosis* strain H37Ra permitted isolation of a DNA fragment that increased bacterial survival in mouse spleens but not lungs (76). In another type of complementation experiment, the nonpathogenic *M. smegmatis* was transformed with a cosmid library from *M. bovis* BCG, and a chromosomal fragment conferring increased survival to *M. smegmatis* in mouse peritoneal macrophages and mouse spleens was isolated (77). An *M. tuberculosis* plasmid library was used to identify *eis,* a gene that increases the survival of *M. smegmatis* in the human macrophage-like cell line U-937 (27), and a plasmid library allowed the isolation of *mce1,* a gene that increases the entry of *E. coli* into HeLa cells that are nonphagocytic (78). The ability of specific genes to increase virulence of a nonpathogen has also been tested. The *M. leprae* fused thioredoxin–thioredoxin reductase gene, cloned into a plasmid vector, was capable of increasing the survival of *M. smegmatis* in human MDMs (79).

Antisense Methods

Antisense RNAs are employed to reduce expression of specific genes as they prevent the translation of the mRNAs to which they are complementary. They are especially useful in systems where gene inactivation is difficult as well as when genes are essential as antisense inhibition of translation is rarely, if ever, complete. A general system for conditionally controlling the production of antisense RNA in mycobacteria was developed using the regulatable acetamide/acetamidase system (80). In a demonstration of the usefulness of this method, a prototrophic *M. smegmatis* strain was made into a histidine auxotroph when a *hisD5* antisense RNA was induced by acetamide. Other applications of the antisense method were in *M. bovis* to lower the levels of AhpC (81) and in *M. tuberculosis* H37Rv to reduce the amounts of SodA (82). These are discussed later in this chapter. A related antisense approach, but using phosphorothioate antisense deoxyoligonucleotides, was used to reduce levels of the *M. tuberculosis* glutamine synthetase in growing cells (83).

Other Methods

Gene inactivation, either directed or global, and the subsequent analysis of mutant phenotypes is the most straightforward way to identify and characterize genes and proteins that are involved in a specific process and, in the case of *M. tuberculosis*, its virulence. A major problem with this approach is that some genes may be essential and cannot be disrupted. Thus, methods that do not rely on the absence of a function are also useful, and these "nongenetic" screens usually rely on the differential expression of genes and their products in different environments. As in the genetic methods, they can be used to characterize the expression of individual genes identified by other means or can function in global searches for genes that show the desired pattern of gene expression. The output of these methods can be enzyme activity using reporter genes, levels of RNA or proteins, and in some cases direct selection of genes using a selectable or screenable phenotype.

Reporter Fusions and Promoter Traps

A general method for studying bacterial gene expression is that of reporter gene methodology. This utilizes plasmid vectors that contain a promoterless gene encoding a protein that in most cases catalyzes an easily assayable enzymatic reaction. Specific promoter sequences from known genes or random chromosomal fragments are cloned upstream of the promoterless reporter gene, and this construct is electroporated into the mycobacterial cell so that the activity of the gene in question can be simply measured under different *in vitro* conditions and, in the case of *M. tuberculosis,* during infections. Among the reporter genes used for this purpose in mycobacteria and the proteins they encode are *lacZ* (β-galactosidase), *xylE* (catechol 2,3-dioxygenase), *phoA* (alkaline phosphatase), *lux* (luciferase), *gfp* (green fluorescence protein), and *cat* (chloramphenicol transacetylase), and plasmid vectors with these reporters have been described (reviewed in reference 84). In addition to measuring the levels of individual *M. tuberculosis* genes under different conditions, such as during infection of macrophages (85,86) and iron starvation (87), reporter technology has permitted the selection or screening of mycobacterial genes that are differentially expressed—a technique known as promoter trap cloning. The *cat* gene was used for the cloning of physiologically functional promoters of *M. smegmatis* and *M. tuberculosis* by means of chloramphenicol resistance (88), and *lacZ* screening on solid indicator media allowed the cloning of *M. tuberculosis* H37Rv genes that were induced by NO (86). *M. marinum* genes that are more highly expressed during infection of macrophages were also cloned by differential fluorescence of *gfp* fusions, using fluorescence-activated cell sorting (38,89), and a similar method was used in *M. bovis* BCG (90).

A novel promoter trap system has been recently developed that has allowed the cloning of several *M. tuberculosis* genes that are induced in human macrophages (91). This selection system is similar in principle to In Vitro Expression Technology (IVET) initially developed to identify virulence genes in gram negative pathogens (92, 93). The *M. tuberculosis* system is based on the observation that overexpression of the *inhA* gene in mycobacteria confers resistance to the frontline antitubercular drug isoniazid (INH) (94). This occurs because INH's mode of action, when activated, is to irreversibly bind to and inactivate the essential InhA

protein that is involved in mycolic acid biosynthesis (95). Thus, the drug will be sequestered because it is bound by the high levels of InhA, resulting in phenotypic INH resistance. The promoter trap selection uses a plasmid in which a library of *M. tuberculosis* DNA fragments can be inserted upstream of a promoterless *inhA* gene. *M. tuberculosis* cells containing plasmids with functional promoters are then selected by growth in the presence of INH under different conditions, such as during macrophage infections (91) and in the lungs of *M. tuberculosis*-infected mice (E. Dubnau and I. Smith, unpublished results, 2003).

Hybridization-Based Methods

Several methods that can characterize *M. tuberculosis* mRNA transcripts have been described, and these can be used to quantitate the expression of specific genes or to globally identify and measure many RNA transcripts. Generally these methods utilize production of cDNA from RNA, using specific primers for known genes or random priming for unknown ones, frequently followed by polymerase chain reaction (PCR) amplification. Among these methods used in *M. tuberculosis* to measure individual transcripts are classical reverse transcriptase–polymerase chain reaction (RT-PCR) that was used to examine differences in levels of specific mRNAs in *M. bovis* BCG after heat shock (96) and during human macrophage (97) and animal infections (98). A similar study was carried with several bacterial genes during *M. tuberculosis* H37Rv infection of human macrophages (99).

One of the problems in the standard RT-PCR method when used to measure specific *M. tuberculosis* RNA transcripts during infection is that the products of the PCR amplification step are frequently not unique because of contaminating host RNA. Quantitation of the transcripts is also not always reliable. A variation of RT-PCR has been developed that uses fluorescent molecular beacons to measure the levels of the PCR product in real time with a spectrophotofluorometric thermal cycler (100). Molecular beacons are single-stranded DNA probes that fluoresce only when hybridized to a complementary single-stranded DNA sequence. The hairpin structure of the molecular beacon gives extremely high specificity to its annealing with its target, so that a one-base mismatch will eliminate this interaction (101,102). This highly specific and sensitive assay has been used to measure levels of several sigma factor gene mRNAs when *M. tuberculosis* H37Rv is grown under different stress conditions (103) and to quantitate the mRNAs of various bacterial genes during *M. tuberculosis* infections of human macrophages (91) and mouse lungs (J. Timm et al., unpublished results, 2002; E. Dubnau and I. Smith, unpublished results, 2002).

Amplification-based hybridization techniques have also been used to globally identify *M. tuberculosis* transcripts. An example of these procedures is differential display, which has allowed the identification of several genes that are differentially expressed in *M. tuberculosis* H37Rv grown in broth in comparison with its avirulent descendant, *M. tuberculosis* H37Ra (104). A cDNA method using isolation of differentially expressed mRNAs by customized amplification libraries (DECAL) was developed that eliminated abundant RNAs that could interfere with the specificity of PCR amplification; DECAL also optimized various parameters and was used to identify transcripts that were induced after antibiotic treatment of *M. tuberculosis* growing in broth culture (105). Another method using selective capture of transcribed sequences (SCOTS), utilizing random cDNA synthesis followed by subtractive hybridization and PCR amplification, was used to identify *M. tuberculosis* (106) and *M. avium* genes (107) expressed in human macrophages.

An important benefit of the completion of the *M. tuberculosis* genome and its annotation has been the development of DNA arrays that allow expression profiling of all the *M. tuberculosis* genes. DNA arrays (DNA chips) are dense grids of DNA bound to a solid matrix that can be probed with a complex mixture of labeled cDNAs. The major advantages of microarrays over older technology are the increase in the number of genes being analyzed, the substantial reduction in sample size requirements, and the use of fluorescence detection schemes for high signal to noise. Microarrays can be used for genotyping as well as for expression profiling studies.

There are two major DNA chip platforms currently in use and many more in development. The most widely used method is based on a technique (spotting arrays) invented by Dr. Pat Brown and colleagues at Stanford University (108). It begins with the isolation and placement of individual (500 to 5,000 bp) PCR products (representing individual genes) on a small glass microscope slide in an array format with each gene occupying a unique location. The PCR products are robotically printed and bonded onto the glass slide, denatured, and hybridized to two fluorescently (Cy5 vs. Cy3)-labeled samples representing the expressed mRNAs from two different cell types or conditions. The reference sample is prepared by isolating mRNA from cells growing in one condition and generating a fluorescently labeled probe. A second sample of mRNA is extracted from differently treated cells and used to generate a second probe labeled with the differently colored fluorescent molecule. Labeled cDNAs from the two cell samples are simultaneously applied to a single microarray, where they competitively react with the arrayed cDNA molecules. Each position on the microarray can then be scanned for the two fluorescent colors, using fluorescence detection coupled to microscanning instrumentation. As the fluorescence intensity is proportional to the expression level of a gene in a particular sample, comparing the ratio of the two fluorescent intensities provides a highly accurate and quantitative measurement of differences in the relative levels of gene expression in the two samples. The Brown-type platform has been used in many prokaryotic systems including pathogens and

an open reading frame array of essentially all of the *M. tuberculosis* genes was first made by Dr. Gary Schoolnik's group at Stanford University (109). This and newer *M. tuberculosis* DNA arrays have been used to do a genotyping analysis of the evolutionary relationship between *M. bovis* BCG vaccine strains (110) and to localize insertion sites for the IS*6110* element (111). They have been used for a global gene expression analysis of *M. tuberculosis* exposed to the antitubercular drug INH (112) and to acidic growth conditions (113). These DNA arrays have also been used to study the affects of mutations in *M. tuberculosis* genes encoding transcriptional regulatory proteins on global gene expression. Among the mutations analyzed are some in genes for sigma factors (2,3,30), two-component system response regulators (114) (S. Walters and I. Smith, unpublished results, 2002), and the major *M. tuberculosis* iron flux regulator, IdeR (52).

A second microarray platform, which essentially differs in the manufacturing of the microarray, is exclusively available from Affymetrix. Instead of using PCR products, approximately 15 pairs of overlapping oligonucleotide 25-mers are synthesized for every gene. For each pair, one represents the wild type sequence, and the second contains a single nucleotide mismatch located in the center of the oligonucleotide sequence. Each oligonucleotide is coupled on a unique glass wafer as it is synthesized in parallel using photolithographic methods. An Affymetrix chip for the complete *M. tuberculosis* genome has not been described yet, but one has been developed for genotyping that has DNA sequences corresponding to several alleles of the *M. tuberculosis* rpoB gene and multiple sequences of the 16S rRNA gene of the *M. tuberculosis* rrnA cistron (115).

Proteomics

Proteomic analyses have also provided global information on gene expression by measuring the levels of proteins during different *M. tuberculosis* growth conditions, such as iron starvation (116) and macrophage infections (117). The introduction of two-dimensional gene electrophoresis technology to resolve many of the *M. tuberculosis* proteins, together with mass spectrophotometric determinations that can identify these molecules (118,119), has also been employed to study proteins whose presence is not predicted by the DNA sequence (120), some whose levels are regulated by iron starvation (121) and low levels of oxygen (122), and to identify proteins that are released into the extracellular media when *M. tuberculosis* is grown in broth culture (123). Determination of individual protein levels on a global scale is a very important complementary procedure to DNA array analyses because levels of proteins can frequently be determined by regulation at posttranscriptional steps, such as intein excision of polypeptides from *M. tuberculosis* RecA precursor, as discussed above.

Nevertheless, knowledge of the levels of specific mRNAs and the proteins they encode, obtained from DNA arrays and proteomic determinations, respectively, does not give a complete picture of the levels of functional proteins when *M. tuberculosis* or any cell is exposed to different conditions. The activity of many proteins can also be controlled by various posttranscriptional processes that themselves may be regulated. Among these are protein–protein interaction between certain sigma factors, anti-sigma factors, and anti-anti-sigma factors (reviewed in reference 124) that also occur in *M. tuberculosis* (125; Roderigue et al., unpublished results, 2003). In addition, the activity of proteins can be controlled by covalent modification, such as the phosphorylation of two-component response regulators (126) and the activation of some DNA-binding proteins by the electrostatic binding of divalent metals. The best known example of this is the activation of proteins in the Fur (127) and DtxR families (128) by iron and related metals. IdeR, a mycobacterial protein that regulates iron acquisition and storage (52,129), requires the binding of divalent metal ions such as iron for its interaction with specific DNA sequences (130).

Validation of Results Obtained from Genetic and Gene Expression Technologies

Use of the techniques described in this section has already resulted in identification of many genes that are important for virulence or a particular physiologic property, or are differentially expressed in various conditions, including infection of macrophages or animal models. In many of these studies, the initial results obtained must be considered as preliminary until they are validated by separate experiments.

In the case of the genetic experiments in which a mutated phenotype is obtained when a gene is inactivated, it is essential to secondarily construct a mutant strain that contains a wild-type copy of the gene, ideally integrated into the chromosome in single copy at an ectopic site and under the control of its natural promoter. For this purpose, plasmid vectors that utilize the *att* system of mycobacteriophage L5 for ectopic integration of DNA are widely used (131). The complemented mutant strain should show reversion of all mutant phenotypes to those of the wild-type parent. Only in this way can one be sure that the phenotypes observed after a gene is inactivated are specifically due to the mutation. Since many genes are in polycistronic clusters, it is always possible that the phenotype associated with a mutation is due to a polar effect on a downstream gene. Even if a gene is monocistronic and polarity effects can be ruled out, other events not directly due to the mutation can occur when a gene is disrupted. An example of this occurred during the construction of an *M. tuberculosis* mutant with a disrupted *ideR* gene (52). The mutant had very clear *in vitro* phenotypes with regard to production of siderophores and response to oxidative stress that were completely restored to those of the wild type in a complemented

mutant strain. The poor growth of the mutant in human macrophages was also returned to wild-type levels when the wild-type *ideR* gene was present. However, the mutant's extremely attenuated growth phenotype in mice, manifested by a bacterial load that was 4 log orders lower than the wild type, was not restored in the complemented strain (G. M. Rodriguez and I. Smith, unpublished results, 2002). Other experiments then showed that the mutant and the complemented mutant strains were deficient in the uptake of iron so they could not grow in low-iron-containing media. Evidently, a suppressor mutation that affected the ability of *M. tuberculosis* to acquire iron had occurred during the disruption of *ideR*, which is now believed to be an essential gene. Thus, the initial conclusion that *ideR* was necessary for *M. tuberculosis* growth in mice was wrong and only by using the complemented mutant could the erroneous conclusion be corrected (52). The majority of studies in which *M. tuberculosis* genes are inactivated show that complementation with the wild-type gene restores all phenotypes to the normal situation, but the literature includes some studies in which this was not done. Since many of the *M. tuberculosis* gene inactivation studies concern virulence phenotypes, any conclusion that a gene is important for virulence should be interpreted with caution unless this phenotype can be complemented with the wild-type gene.

Results obtained from gene expression studies, especially those done on a global scale, should be considered preliminary until they are validated using a different technique, in which the levels of individual mRNAs are directly measured by RT-PCR, Northern analysis, or primer extension. In DNA array analyses, since the levels of 4,000 genes are being compared usually as a ratio between two conditions or bacterial strains, many factors, such as background noise (108) and statistical considerations (132,133), may give erroneous results for the values obtained with specific genes. Validation for representative genes is routinely done in most *M. tuberculosis* DNA array papers (2,30,112).

Similarly, results obtained in experiments in which gene expression is studied with multicopy plasmids should be validated. The use of multicopy plasmids for reporter fusions (85) or promoter traps (38,89,91) simplifies cloning, but frequently chromosomal genes are regulated differently when contained on plasmids presumably because DNA conformation is altered. An example of this is the *M. tuberculosis hsp60* gene that is induced after heat shock but is constitutive when present on a multicopy plasmid (134). In work discussed above using a promoter trap carried on a multicopy plasmid during *M. tuberculosis* infection of human macrophages, 43 genes were identified as having been induced during the infection based on their differential resistance to INH. To validate these results, molecular beacon RT-PCR was used to measure the mRNA of a subset of these genes, and it was found that 8 of the 13 tested were induced during infection of macrophages by normal (plasmid-free) *M. tuberculosis* H37Rv (91). This result indicates that the promoter trap was useful in identifying some genes that have the desired gene expression pattern, allowing further investigation on their roles in virulence, but that false positives are also selected.

MYCOBACTERIUM TUBERCULOSIS VIRULENCE FACTORS

As described above, the virulence of *M. tuberculosis* can be measured during the infection of macrophages and animals using several different assays, and various strategies have been developed to make mutations in *M. tuberculosis* genes. Use of a combination of these methodologies has allowed researchers to identify several genes that are important for various aspects of *M. tuberculosis* pathogenicity; this section of the chapter will discuss some of these genes and the cellular components they encode. They are grouped below according to the known or predicted function of the proteins, based on DNA sequence annotation. Some genes have also been identified as being up-regulated during infection. In most cases, their essentiality for virulence has not been established by gene inactivation studies, and some of them will be briefly discussed in the context of related genes that are known to be essential to this process.

Transcriptional Regulators

Sigma Factors

Transcriptional regulators control the transcription of many genes. Therefore, a directed mutational strategy to inactivate regulatory genes could be expected to uncover some that are important for *M. tuberculosis* virulence. This has been demonstrated in other pathogens, such as in the case of *Salmonella typhimurium* virulence factors response regulator PhoP (135,136) and alternative sigma factor RpoS (137).

Sigma A (Rv2703, sigA)

Sigma A is the essential principal mycobacterial sigma factor that is presumably necessary for most mycobacterial housekeeping gene transcription (138,139). Unlike most of the other transcriptional regulator genes that were directly inactivated, it was identified as a virulence factor by complementation of an attenuated *M. bovis* strain (ATCC 35721) with an *M. tuberculosis* cosmid library, using a guinea pig morbidity assay (41). The original mutation in *sigA* that causes attenuation is a partial loss of function that allows sigma A protein to function in general transcription, since the mutant grows normally *in vitro* (broth cultures and solid media), but is presumably unable to transcribe at least one virulence gene. The attenuating mutation is an arginine-to-histidine substitution at amino acid residue 515 (R515H) of the protein and is localized to a C-terminal domain that in other sigma factors interacts with transcrip-

tional activators. A search for a potential activator that interacts with sigma A, utilizing a yeast two-hybrid system, has shown that WhiB3 (Rv3416) interacts with sigma A, and a *whiB3* mutant made in *M. bovis* has a virulence phenotype in guinea pigs similar to that of the original *sigA* R515H mutant (140). Hopefully, DNA array analyses will soon compare the global expression profiles of ATCC 35721 and its complemented derivative strain to see which genes are not transcribed in the mutant strain, as has been done for other *M. tuberculosis* sigma factor mutations. These analyses should allow the identification of genes in the sigma A regulon that require WhiB3 and possibly other activators and should ultimately lead to members of this group that are essential for virulence.

Sigma F (Rv3286c, sigF)

The derived amino acid sequence of the *M. tuberculosis* sigma F is very similar to the sigma F proteins of *S. coelicolor* and *B. subtilis* that are essential for sporulation in these two species as well as the sigma B of *B. subtilis* that controls responses to environmental stress (141). It was speculated that the latency of *M. tuberculosis* in human TB could be similar to bacterial sporulation. To provide evidence for this hypothesis, *sigF* in *M. tuberculosis* CDC1551 was inactivated by allelic replacement using a two-step plasmid method (142). The mutant has no macrophage phenotype and is attenuated for virulence in mice using mortality as a criterion. The mice infected with the mutant all died by 334 days after infection (50% died at 246 days), whereas mice infected with the wild type were all dead by 184 days (50% died at 161 days). It is not known which genes transcribed by RNA polymerase containing sigma F (RNAP–sigma F) are important for this virulence phenotype. Recently, direct transcription assays have identified genes transcribed by RNAP–sigma F, and a promoter sequence has been identified that strongly resembles the *B. subtilis* RNAP–sigma B consensus promoter sequence (125). This information and future DNA array analyses should allow identification of sigma F–dependent *M. tuberculosis* virulence genes. Interestingly, this work also showed that the activity of sigma F is controlled posttranslationally by its binding to an anti-sigma (Rv3287c) that previously had been identified as having sequence similarity to the anti-sigma F and anti-sigma B proteins of *B. subtilis* (143). In turn, the activity of the *M. tuberculosis* anti-sigma F is down-regulated by its binding to two different anti-anti-sigma factors, Rv1356c and Rv3687c, an interaction that allows sigma F to function. Significantly, the function of Rv1356c is regulated by redox potential, while it is proposed that Rv3687c activity is controlled by phosphorylation (125).

Sigma E (Rv1221, sigE)

Sigma E is a member of the extracytoplasmic function (ECF) group of sigma factors that control bacterial response to external stimuli. *sigE* transcripts are induced after exposure of *M. tuberculosis* to various environmental stresses like high temperature and detergent stress (103). Since these stresses might be found during *M. tuberculosis* infections, and a hybridization-based method showed that *sigE* mRNA levels increased during *M. tuberculosis* growth in human macrophages (106), there was a possibility that sigma E would be necessary for virulence. To test this idea, *sigE* was inactivated in *M. tuberculosis* H37Rv by allelic replacement using a two-step plasmid procedure, and its phenotype was analyzed *in vitro* and during infection of mouse and human macrophages (30). The mutant is more sensitive to detergent, high temperature, and oxidative stress than the wild-type parent *M. tuberculosis* H37Rv and grows more poorly than the wild type in both types of macrophages. Preliminary results show that the mutant is attenuated in wild-type mice with a GIV phenotype and kills severe combined immunodeficient (SCID) mice more slowly that the wild type; that is, all mice infected with the mutant were dead by 70 days, whereas *M. tuberculosis* H37Rv killed all mice by 30 days (R. Manganelli et al., unpublished results, 2002). DNA array analyses comparing the *sigE* mutant and the wild-type parent showed that 38 genes required Sigma E for expression during normal growth, whereas 23 other genes in 13 transcription units required this transcription factor for induction after sodium dodecyl sulfate (SDS) stress. Nine of these transcription units had a conserved ECF-like promoter sequence in the region directly upstream of the first gene in each unit. Among the genes requiring sigma E for their expression during unstressed growth are some encoding proteins involved in translation, in transcriptional control, in mycolic acid biosynthesis, in electron transport, and in oxidative stress response. Genes requiring sigma E during SDS stress encode for proteins that are involved in fatty acid degradation, some that are heat-shock proteins (HSPs), and several that are putative transcriptional regulators. *sigB* encoding sigma B, a nonessential sigma factor (M. Gomez and I. Smith, unpublished results, 2001), required sigma E in stressed and unstressed conditions, and recent experiments have shown that RNAP–sigma E can transcribe *sigB* (S. Roderigue et al., unpublished results, 2003). *sigB* mutations do not affect *M. tuberculosis* pathogenicity (M. Gomez and I. Smith, unpublished results, 2001), nor is it known which of the other genes requiring sigma E for their transcription are necessary for virulence. This question is currently being investigated. As is the case with many ECF sigma factors, sigma E activity is down-regulated by an anti-sigma factor, RseA, that is encoded by a gene (Rv1222) adjacent to *sigH* (S. Roderigue et al., unpublished results, 2002). The possible role of RseA in virulence is not known and is also being studied.

Sigma H (Rv3223c, sigH)

Sigma H, like sigma E, is another member of the ECF family of sigma factors and is very similar to the sigma R of *Streptomyces* species. Sigma R responds to certain types of

oxidative stress such as diamide treatment, which involves oxidation of protein SH groups that subsequently form intramolecular disulfide bonds (144). Its promoter recognition activity is blocked by binding of the anti-sigma factor RsrA, which is encoded by a gene adjacent to *sigR*. After oxidative (diamide) stress, key SH groups in RsrA become oxidized and the RsrA binding to sigma R is disrupted (145). Sigma R can then transcribe several genes, such as its own structural gene *sigR* and those encoding thioredoxin and thioredoxin reductase, that can reduce proteins oxidized by diamide treatment. Thioredoxin and its reductase function to return the system to the unstressed state as the newly reduced RsrA can again bind to sigma R (146). The *M. tuberculosis sigH* is induced after various stresses like heat shock and SDS treatment (103) and during macrophage infection (106). Subsequently, this gene was inactivated in three laboratories (2,3,147). The *in vitro* phenotype of the *sigH* mutant is as expected from the *Streptomyces* experiments and the earlier *M. tuberculosis* gene expression experiments, as it is sensitive to SDS, diamide, and heat shock. A combination of DNA array analyses and individual gene expression assays showed there are no genes that require sigma H during unstressed growth (2), but genes similar to those transcribed by the *Streptomyces* RNAP–sigma R, including those encoding thioredoxin and its reductase, are dependent on sigma H for expression after diamide stress (2,3,147). Many of these *M. tuberculosis* genes have promoter sequences that are very similar to those recognized by the *Streptomyces* RNAP–sigma R and the mycobacterial RNAP–sigma E. Transcription assays have shown that some of these genes are transcribed by mycobacterial RNAP–sigma H (147). Among these is *sigB* that is also transcribed by mycobacterial RNAP–sigma E, which uses the same *sigB* promoter as the RNAP–sigma H (S. Roderigue et al., unpublished results, 2003). The virulence phenotype of the *sigH* mutant is subtle in that its growth in macrophages and mice is normal in terms of bacterial load (2,3), but there are differences in lung histopathology, including fewer granulomas and a generally delayed pulmonary inflammatory response (3). As is the case in *Streptomyces*, *M. tuberculosis* has an anti-sigma H factor, RshA (Rv3221A), whose sequence is similar to the *Streptomyces* RsrA, and its structural gene maps near *sigH*. Biochemical experiments have shown that the purified *M. tuberculosis* RshA binds to sigma H, preventing it from functioning in transcription, similar to the *Streptomyces* RsrA–sigma R interaction (S. Roderigue et al., unpublished results, 2003).

Response Regulators

PhoP (Rv0757, Phop)

PhoP is a member of the response regulator class of transcriptional regulators that shows high similarity to the PhoP response regulator of *S. typhimurium* that senses

Mg^{2+} starvation and controls expression of virulence genes (148). On this basis, *phoP* was disrupted in a clinical *M. tuberculosis* isolate strain MT103 by a two-step plasmid procedure and virulence phenotypes were determined (149). The mutant grows poorly in mouse macrophages and is severely attenuated in mice organs where it has an SGIV phenotype. These results have been confirmed and extended as *phoP* has been disrupted in *M. tuberculosis* H37Rv by a two-step plasmid procedure, and this mutant is also attenuated in human and mouse macrophages as well as in mice where it has an SGIV phenotype (S. Walters and I . Smith, unpublished data, 2001). *In vitro* experiments have shown that the *M. tuberculosis* H37Rv *phoP* mutant grows poorly in low Mg^{2+}-containing media, and it is now believed that the *M. tuberculosis* PhoP senses Mg^{2+} starvation as does the *S. typhimurium* PhoP (S. Walters and I. Smith, unpublished observations, 2002). Genes controlled by PhoP, including those important for virulence, are not yet known, and investigations are underway. On the basis of preliminary DNA array data (S. Walters and I. Smith, unpublished data), it appears that the annotated *M. tuberculosis mgtC*, a likely candidate that is discussed later in this section, is not controlled by PhoP.

PrrA (Rv0903c, prrA)

PrrA is one of the 13 annotated response regulators in the *M. tuberculosis* genome. It had been previously shown that this gene was up-regulated during *M. tuberculosis* infection of human macrophages (106), and screening of an ordered transposon mutagenesis library for mutants found one with an insertion near the beginning of the coding sequence for PrrA (150). The growth of the *prrA* mutant in mouse primary macrophages was slightly lower than the wild-type *M. tuberculosis* 103 at 3 and 6 days, reaching wild-type levels at 7 days, and the mutant grew as well as the wild type in mice. In agreement with these observation, green fluorescence protein (GFP) reporter fusions with the *prrA* promoter showed that this gene was transiently induced in macrophages with peak levels of gene expression 4 hours after infection, declining after that time. The significance of PrrA to virulence is not clear, given the very subtle attenuation phenotype.

Rv0981 (Rv0981, mprA)

Rv0981 is another *M. tuberculosis* two-component response regulator, and it was inactivated in *M. tuberculosis* H37Rv by a two-step plasmid procedure (65). The mutant had an unusual phenotype in that it grew better than the wild type in murine macrophages and human MDMs. However, it did not persist in the lungs and livers of infected mice, growing initially and being cleared after 140 days, respectively, showing a delayed PER phenotype. *mprA* is induced when *M. bovis* BCG infects macrophages, using an *mprA*-GFP fusion, but the same *mprA* GFP construct in *M.*

tuberculosis H37Rv does not show induction of *mrpA* in macrophages (65).

Virulence phenotypes of other two component gene mutations have been measured in the response regulator RgX (Rv0491) and in the histidine kinase TrcS (Rv1032c). No macrophage phenotype was observed, and these genes were not induced in macrophages (150). In agreement with these results, 10 of the 13 two-component response regulator genes in *M. tuberculosis* were inactivated, and only the *phoP* mutant, discussed above, had a virulence phenotype in human macrophages and mice (S. Walters and I. Smith, unpublished results, 2001). Included in this group were mutants with disruptions in *regX* and *trcS*. Other two-component systems in *M. tuberculosis* have been studied; MtrA-MtrB (Rv3264c-Rv3245c) is essential for growth, as *mtrA* can not be disrupted (151). Interestingly, GFP reporter fusions with the *mtrA* promoter in *M. bovis* BCG are induced in murine macrophages but not when the fusion is in *M. tuberculosis*, as was observed in gene expression studies with Rv0981 (151). Another response regulator, Rv3133c, controls oxidative stress and low oxygen response, including the expression of the anoxia-induced *hspX* gene as well as its own expression (114). A proteomic analysis of *M. bovis* BCG grown in microaerophilic conditions showed up-regulation of the same genes (152), and *M. smegmatis* genes corresponding to Rv3133c and Rv3132c, encoding the cognate histidine kinase and *hspX* were also induced in anoxic conditions (153). Thus, Rv3133c is important for mycobacterial response to various environmental stresses, but its role in virulence is not clear as a mutation in Rv3133c has no effect on *M. tuberculosis* growth in human macrophages (S. Walters and I. Smith, unpublished results, 2001).

Other Transcriptional Regulators

HspR (Rv0353, hspR)

HspR is a repressor of key heat-shock genes such as *hsp70* where it binds to a specific DNA sequence, the HAIR element (*Hsp*R-*a*ssociated *i*nverted *r*epeat) in the *hsp70* promoter region in *S. coelicolor* (154) and *Helicobacter pylori* (155). The repression occurs at the permissive temperature 37°C and is lifted at 45°C. *M. tuberculosis* also has an ortholog of this ORF (156). The synthesis of *M. tuberculosis* HSPs, some of which are immunodominant antigens (157), is increased after infection (117). Investigations were carried out to see whether the *M. tuberculosis* HspR was a repressor of *hsp70* and whether the regulation of HSPs would be important for virulence (19). Biochemical studies showed that purified *M. tuberculosis* HspR binds to DNA sequences containing the HAIR element, and physiologic experiments indicated that *hspR* mutants in both *M. tuberculosis* and *M. bovis* BCG, constructed by the two-step plasmid technique, are derepressed for Hsp70 synthesis at 37°C, unlike the wild-type strains. The *M. tuberculosis* mutant survives better than the wild type after heat shock, presumably because of the protective effect of the higher level of HSPs. Thus, *M. tuberculosis* HspR functions in the same manner as other bacterial HspRs. While the *M. tuberculosis hspR* mutant has no phenotype in murine macrophages, it is attenuated in mice, with a GIV phenotype. The reason for this attenuation is not currently known, but it was suggested that the higher levels of HSPs in the mutant might cause increased host immunosurveillance, followed by more efficient killing of the pathogen (19).

In addition to potential roles in immunosurveillance, *M. tuberculosis* HSPs may have a more direct role in virulence. GroES is a highly conserved HSP that has chaperonin activity and is also known as cpn10. The *M. tuberculosis* GroES (Rv3418c) is found as a major constituent in the culture filtrate or media in which *M. tuberculosis* grows (123), suggesting that it will be directly exposed to the phagosomal milieu. Recombinant *M. tuberculosis* GroES is a stimulator of bone resorption and induces osteoclast recruitment in bone explant cultures, while also inhibiting the proliferation of an osteoblast bone-forming cell line (6). It has recently been shown that the *M. tuberculosis* GroES binds calcium (158). This suggests a role for GroES in Pott disease, the extrapulmonary form of TB that is marked by the weakening and resorption of spinal vertebrae. This role could be related to the physical depletion of calcium in bones and/or the disruption of calcium signaling in host cells (158).

IdeR (Rv2711, *ideR*)

IdeR is a DNA-binding protein whose ability to interact with a conserved DNA sequence requires the binding of Fe^{2+} or related divalent cations and is a structural and functional homolog of the *C. diphtheriae* DtxR (130,159). IdeR is the major mycobacterial regulator of iron uptake and storage genes, repressing the former and activating the latter (59,87,129). *ideR* is an essential gene that can only be inactivated in the presence of a second site suppressor (52); thus, it has not been possible to directly assess IdeR's role in virulence, as previously discussed in this chapter. However, it is included in this section on virulence factors because of a report that the presence of a mutated DtxR, which exhibits iron-independent repression in other contexts, reduces the growth of *M. tuberculosis* in mice (160). Although not demonstrated directly *in vitro* or during infection, it was postulated that the mutated DtxR is repressing *M. tuberculosis* iron uptake genes during growth of the bacterium in mice. Despite certain caveats, this interesting observation suggests that iron acquisition is essential for *M. tuberculosis* growth in mice as is indicated by other experiments that are discussed below (52) (J. Timm et al., unpublished, 2002).

Enzymes Involved in General Cellular Metabolism

Since many pathogens become starved for certain essential nutrients and cofactors during infection (e.g., amino acids, purines, pyrimidines, and divalent metals such as Mg^{2+} and Fe^{2+}), *M. tuberculosis* researchers have systematically made mutations in genes encoding enzymes in the biosynthetic pathways and acquisition systems for some of these factors. In addition, mutations have been made in genes encoding respiratory enzymes.

Amino Acid and Purine Biosynthetic Genes

LeuD (Rv2987c, *leuD*)

leuD, encoding isopropyl malate isomerase, an enzyme that functions in the biosynthesis of leucine, was inactivated by a two-step plasmid procedure in *M. tuberculosis* H37Rv. The mutant cannot grow in primary murine macrophages, nor can it kill SCID mice (161). The *leuD* auxotroph was also able to protect against virulent *M. tuberculosis* infection of wild-type mice to approximately the same extent as *M. bovis* BCG. *LeuD* mutations were also made earlier in *M. bovis* BCG; in addition, they cannot grow in mice exhibiting an SGIV phenotype (162), nor can they grow in human macrophages (163).

TrpD (Rv2192c, *trpD*)

TrpD is anthranilate phosphoribosyltransferase, in the tryptophan biosynthetic pathway. The *M. tuberculosis* gene was inactivated by a two-step plasmid procedure, but with an initial denaturing DNA step to increase the frequency of homologous recombination (66). The mutant is severely attenuated in murine macrophages, hardly grows in SCID mice (suggesting an SGIV phenotype), and did not kill any of these mice (164).

ProC (Rv0500, *proC*)

ProC is a pyrroline-5-carboxylate reductase involved in proline biosynthesis, and the *M. tuberculosis* gene was inactivated in the same manner as the *trpD* gene, just described. Its virulence phenotype is intermediate between that of the wild-type *M. tuberculosis* H37 parent and the *trpD* mutant (164). It is killed in murine macrophages but not as rapidly as the *trpD* strain, and it kills SCID mice with a median killing time of 130 days, in contrast to the wild-type infection in which all mice were killed by 29 days.

PurC (Rv0780, *purC*)

PurC, which is 1-phosphoribosylaminoimidazole–succinocarboxamide synthase involved in purine biosynthesis, was inactivated in both *M. bovis* BCG and *M. tuberculosis* 103 by a two-step plasmid procedure (165). The growth of both mutants in unactivated murine macrophages is attenuated, with the *M. bovis* BCG mutant showing a large decrease in bacterial numbers, and the *M. tuberculosis* mutant not growing but maintaining the initial numbers of bacteria. Both mutants are severely attenuated in mice with an SGIV phenotype.

Metal Uptake

MgtC (Rv1811, *mgtC*)

The *Salmonella* MgtC is a transporter involved in Mg^{2+} uptake (166). Its presence is essential to the growth of this pathogen in low-Mg^{2+} media and in macrophages, indicating that these environments are limiting for this divalent cation (148). Since there is an *mgtC* ortholog annotated in the *M. tuberculosis* genome, this gene was inactivated in *M. tuberculosis* Erdman, using a linear DNA construct containing the *M. tuberculosis* Erdman *mgtC* disrupted with an antibiotic resistance cassette (167). The mutant grows poorly in low-Mg^{2+} media and in human MDMs, suggesting that the *M. tuberculosis* MgtC has the same function as *Salmonella* PhoP and that the mycobacterial phagosome is also limiting for Mg^{2+}. The mutant is also severely attenuated for growth in mice, exhibiting a SGIV phenotype. However, a similar *mgtC* mutant made in *M. tuberculosis* H37Rv has no attenuated phenotype in THP-1 human macrophages and is able to grow in media containing low Mg^{2+} (S. Walters and I. Smith, unpublished results, 2002). While the *Salmonella mgtC* is positively regulated by PhoP, the main sensor of Mg^{2+} starvation in this bacterium, preliminary DNA array results indicate that this is not the case in *M. tuberculosis* H37Rv. Global expression patterns of *M. tuberculosis* H37Rv grown in different media and compared with its isogenic *PhoP* mutant do not show any induction of *mgtC* in low-Mg^{2+} media or any effect of a *phoP* mutation on *mgtC* expression. The reasons for the discordant results in two laboratories are not known, but different *M. tuberculosis* strains and macrophages were used in the two sets of experiments. The actual role of *mgtC* in *M. tuberculosis* physiology and virulence as well as its regulation awaits further investigation.

MbtB (Rv2383c, *mbtB*)

The *mbt* operon, consisting of *mbtA–J*, encodes enzymes whose function is to synthesize mycobactin and carboxymycobactin (168,169), the major siderophores in *M. tuberculosis* (170). This regulon is repressed by IdeR under high-iron conditions (52,129). MbtB is an enzyme in this pathway that catalyzes formation of an amide bond between salicylate and serine (a step in mycobactin synthesis). Since iron is essential for most life forms but is usually in the form of the largely insoluble ferric salts in the environment, iron uptake systems are required to solubilize these salts and to transport iron into the cell. In bacteria, siderophores usually perform this chelation/solubilization function, and the iron they carry is taken into cells by high-affinity transporters. In addition, pathogens require iron acquisition systems, usually siderophores during infection to obtain iron from host iron-containing proteins like transferrin and lactoferrin. In response to infection, the host frequently sequesters iron to prevent bacterial growth (171). Since mutations in siderophore biosynthetic genes frequently cause attenuation of virulence in bacterial pathogens, the *M. tuberculosis* mycobactin locus was disrupted by inactivation of the *mbtB* gene, using a two-step plasmid procedure (169). The mutant shows wild-type growth in iron-rich media, grows poorly when iron is limiting, and is unable to synthesize the two mycobactin-derived siderophores. It also grows at a slower rate than wild type in human macrophages, as measured by a luminescence assay, indicating that the mycophagosome may be low in iron. This latter hypothesis is supported by experiments showing that levels of *mbtB* and *mbtI* mRNA are increased during *M. tuberculosis* infection of human macrophages (129). As yet, there is no published report on the growth phenotype of the *mbtB* mutant in mice. However, several lines of evidence, all indicating that iron is limiting in the *M. tuberculosis*-infected host, suggest that it will be attenuated. These are as follows: (a) Excess iron exacerbates the progression of TB in humans and animal models (172); (b) Measurements of bacterial mRNA in *M. tuberculosis*-infected mouse lungs show that *mbtB* is highly induced in comparison with its levels when *M. tuberculosis* is grown in broth culture (J. Timm et al., unpublished results, 2002). (c) A mutation in *M. tuberculosis* that prevents growth in low-iron-containing media and is believed to affect a component of the high-affinity iron uptake system (52) also severely attenuates growth in mice because the mutant does not replicate (i.e., has an SGIV phenotype) (G. M. Rodriguez and I. Smith, unpublished results, 2002). The identity of this gene is currently under investigation, but it is expected that the gene will be an important tool for the study of *M. tuberculosis* virulence.

Nitrate Reductase (Rv1161, *narG*)

NarG is a subunit of the prokaryotic respiratory (anaerobic) nitrate reductase that plays a major role in respiration in the absence of oxygen, and anaerobic nitrate reductase activity increases when *M. tuberculosis* becomes microaerophic (173). The *M. tuberculosis* genome has several ORFs with similarity to the subunits of nitrate reductase, including one gene cluster that is annotated as *narGHIJ*, the usual nitrate reductase–encoding genomic structure in prokaryotes (33). The *M. tuberculosis narGHIJ* cluster was shown to have anaerobic nitrate reductase activity (174), and a *narG* mutation was made in *M. bovis* BCG, using a two-step plasmid procedure. The mutant had no anaerobic nitrate reductase activity, but its growth in aerobic or anaerobic conditions was unaffected. When the *M. bovis* BCG *narG* mutant was used to infect mice, a significant virulence phenotype was observed. In SCID mice, the wild-type parent grew well, whereas the mutant showed no replication but was not cleared. In normal mice, the wild-type BCG strain did not replicate, but the mutant was rapidly cleared from lungs, livers, and kidneys, exhibiting an SGIV phenotype (175). These results have not yet been confirmed in *M. tuberculosis*, but they suggest that anaerobic or microaerophilic growth is an important feature of *M. tuberculosis* physiology during infection.

Lipid and Fatty Acid Metabolism

As discussed above, observations made approximately 50 years ago indicated that *M. tuberculosis* shifts from a metabolism that preferentially use carbohydrates when growing *in vitro* to one that utilizes fatty acids when in an infected host (176). These old observations are supported by more recent work, such as the complete sequencing and annotation of the *M. tuberculosis* genome in which more than 200 genes were annotated as being involved in fatty acid degradation (33), and in work discussed directly below.

Icl (Rv0467, *icl* or *aceA*)

Icl, or isocitrate lyase, is an enzyme that converts isocitrate to succinate in the glyoxalate shunt. This allows bacteria and plants to grow on acetate or fatty acids as sole carbon sources and thus provide a source of carbon that can enter the Krebs cycle. Initial observations using an *in vitro* model to study *M. tuberculosis* persistence showed that isocitrate lyase enzyme activity increases dramatically as cells reach stationary phase (177), and its mRNA increases when *M. tuberculosis* infects human macrophages (91,106). The *M. tuberculosis* Erdman *icl* was inactivated by means of allelic replacement using a two-step plasmid system, and the mutant cannot grow on C$_2$ carbon sources. It initially grows normally in mice, but stops growing in lungs and is cleared when cell-mediated immunity is initiated—a PER phenotype (178). The mutant has wild-type growth in IFN-γ knockout mice and in unactivated primary murine macrophages but is killed more rapidly than the wild type when these macrophages are activated with IFN-γ and lipopolysaccharide. Additional evidence indicating the importance of isocitrate lyase is the observation that *icl* mRNA levels increase markedly in the lungs of *M. tuberculosis*-infected mice as the infection progresses (J. Timm et al., unpublished results, 2002).

LipF (Rv3487c, *lipF*)

LipF is annotated as a lipase/esterase that may function in lipid degradation. It was inactivated by the STM procedure in *M. tuberculosis* 103, and when the mutant was individually tested for bacterial load at one time point (3 weeks after infection), it grew approximately 2 log orders less well in mouse lungs than the wild-type strain. In the same experiment, *M. bovis* BCG grew 3 log orders less well than the wild type (72). Other annotated fatty acid metabolic genes have been identified as being induced in human macrophages *fadA4*, *fadA5*, and *echA19* using a promoter trap selection, but only the *fadA4* results were tested and validated by mRNA determinations (91). Similar promoter trap experiments have now identified nine annotated *fad* genes as being induced in the lungs of *M. tuberculosis*-

infected mice, including *fadA4* (E. Dubnau et al., unpublished results, 2002). These mouse results have not yet been validated, nor have mutations been made in any promoter trap–identified genes to determine their virulence phenotypes; however, such experiments are underway.

Phospholipases C (Rv2351c, Rv2350c, Rv2349c, Rv1755c, *plcA, plcB, plcC, plcD*)

The *M. tuberculosis* genome has four ORFs annotated as encoding phospholipase C–type enzymes. Three of these—*plcA, B,* and *C*—are closely linked to each other, but *plcD* is not. This latter gene is missing or disrupted in many *M. tuberculosis* strains, including *H37Rv*, and the *plcABC* cluster is not present in *M. bovis* and its BCG derivatives (179). Disruptions of the *plc* genes were obtained by screening a transposon mutant library made in *M. tuberculosis* 103 that has an intact *plcD*. In addition, some mutations were made by a two-step plasmid procedure (179). Phospholipase C activity was determined in cell extracts of strains that had individual and multiply mutated *plc* genes, and all individual mutants have lower enzyme activity than the wild-type *M. tuberculosis* 103. Triple (*plcABC*) and quadruple (*plcABCD*) mutants have negligible enzyme activity, and strains in which a *plcABC* mutant was the recipient for individual *plc* genes showed that all restore some activity. All of the *plc* genes in *M. tuberculosis* H37 Rv are induced in human (THP-1) macrophages, but the triple and quadruple *plc* mutants grow normally in these cells. However, both of these multiple *plc* mutants are attenuated in mice, showing a GIV phenotype.

Stress Response Proteins

Bacteria and other life forms respond to various oxidative stresses by increasing the activity of enzymes that degrade toxic reactive oxygen intermediates (ROIs). Among these enzymes are catalases and superoxide dismutases. Since phagocytic cells produce ROIs to kill invading bacteria, it would be expected that these enzymes would be important for *M. tuberculosis* virulence.

KatG (Rv1908c, *katG*)

KatG is a catalase-peroxidase that inactivates H$_2$O$_2$ and organic peroxides. It is the only enzyme with catalase activity in *M. tuberculosis* and, in addition to degrading ROIs, it activates the prodrug INH to form a reactive species that inhibits mycolic acid biosynthesis. Spontaneous mutations to INH resistance are usually found in *katG*, and a mutant of this type in *M. bovis* was attenuated in guinea pigs, using a spleen morbidity assay (40). In addition, an *M. tuberculosis* H37R v*katG* mutant, also isolated on the basis of its resistance to INH, was shown to be attenuated in the lungs and spleen of infected mice and was rapidly cleared after initial normal growth, a PER phenotype (180). Another *katG* mutant of *M. tuberculosis* H37Rv showed a similar

PER phenotype in mice, and virulence in guinea pigs was also attenuated by the *M. tuberculosis katG* mutation. Complementation with the wild-type *katG* restored enzyme activity and virulence (181). In *M. smegmatis* (182) and *M. tuberculosis* (183), *katG* is negatively regulated by the FurA protein whose structural gene is directly upstream of *katG*. The role of FurA in virulence is not known.

AhpC (Rv2428, *ahpC*)
AhpC is a subunit of the alkyl hydroperoxide reductase, and enzymes of this type are important in detoxifying organic hydroxyperoxides. Attempts to inactivate this gene in the *M. tuberculosis* complex have been unsuccessful, and an antisense method has been used to phenotypically lower the expression of the *ahpC* gene in *M. bovis* (81). In comparison with the wild type, the resulting phenotypic mutant produced less AhpC and was more sensitive to H_2O_2 and cumene hydroperoxide. The mutant was also much less virulent in a guinea pig model, showing 3 log orders less colony-forming units than the wild type. It has been postulated that AhpC can compensate for the lack of catalase-peroxidase activity in *M. tuberculosis katG* mutants, as there are several reports of increased *ahpC* expression in some *katG* mutants (180,184), However levels of AhpC are not correlated with the virulence of *katG* mutants (180).

SodA (Rv3846, *soda*)
SodA is the iron-factored superoxide dismutase that degrades superoxides that are normal by-products of normal aerobic respiration and are also produced by the phagocytic respiratory burst enzyme. It is therefore important for the survival of intracellular pathogens during infections. SodA is the major enzyme with this activity in *M. tuberculosis*, and attempts to inactivate this gene have not been successful (185). To circumvent this problem, as was done with the *ahpC* gene just discussed, an antisense approach was used to make a phenotypic *sodA* mutation in *M. tuberculosis* H37Rv (82). The phenotypic mutant produced much less SodA protein and was severely attenuated in mice, showing up to 5 log orders less colony-forming units than the wild type in lungs and spleens, and was rapidly cleared demonstrating an SGIV phenotype. Recent results have indicated that the *M. tuberculosis* SodA inhibits redox signaling by macrophages, and it is proposed that this would affect the initiation of the cellular immune response after infection (D. Kernodle, personal communication, 2002).

SodC (Rv342, *sodC*)
SodC is the Cu, Zn-factored superoxide dismutase that is responsible for a small part of total Sod activity in *M. tuberculosis*. Two laboratories have inactivated this gene in *M. tuberculosis* with different virulence results. In one case, *sodC* was inactivated in *M. tuberculosis* Erdman using a linear DNA construct. The resulting mutant was more sensitive to superoxides than the wild type and was killed more

efficiently in activated primary (peritoneal) murine macrophages. It was not affected in unactivated murine macrophages or activated macrophages from respiratory deficient mice (186). In the other case, the *M. tuberculosis* H37Rv *sodC* was inactivated by a two-step plasmid procedure, and while this mutant also showed increased sensitivity to superoxides and H_2O_2, it exhibited wild-type growth in activated primary (bone marrow) murine macrophages and in guinea pigs (185). The reasons for the discrepant results are not known, but different *M. tuberculosis* strains and macrophages were used.

Cell Envelope Function or Secretion

In this category are listed genes encoding proteins that are expected to be exposed to the environment in which *M. tuberculosis* grows, either in culture media or in the context of the mycophagosome. Among these are secreted proteins and enzymes that play a role in the synthesis of various cell surface molecules. The structure of the mycobacterial cell wall/envelope is extremely complex, and a complete discussion of this important and unique barrier that separates *M. tuberculosis* from its external environment is not discussed here for due to space limitations. However, there are some excellent reviews on this subject (187,188).

Culture Filtrate Proteins
M. tuberculosis culture filtrate proteins (CFPs) are those found in the culture medium in which *M. tuberculosis* is grown. They are so defined because mechanisms of secretion are not known for all these proteins, approximately 200 in number (123). In addition, some of these proteins are also associated with cells, so that the definition of CFP is an operational one. CFPs are actively studied by many *M. tuberculosis* researchers because many these are proteins are recognized by the sera of TB patients. It has also been postulated that live, attenuated *M. tuberculosis* vaccines are better than those made from heat-killed cells because during growth in the host *M. tuberculosis* releases CFPs that stimulate host immune mechanisms (189). Interestingly, KatG and SodA, enzymes that degrade ROIs and are important for *M. tuberculosis* survival during infection as discussed above, are found in the culture filtrate. The significance of this localization is not known, but it has been speculated that the location may allow more efficient detoxification of harmful molecules produced by the host in the phagosome (190).

HspX (Rv2031c, *hspX*)
HspX, also known as Acr (the α-crystalline protein homolog or the 14-kd protein), is a major *M. tuberculosis* antigen recognized by the sera of a high proportion of TB patients and is induced under anoxic conditions (191). This gene is also induced in human THP-1 macrophages, and an *M. tuberculosis* mutant in which the *hspX* gene was inacti-

vated was severely attenuated for growth in these macrophages (192). It is postulated that HspX, which has chaperone-like properties, is speculated to be an important controlling element in *M. tuberculosis* latency or persistence, as overexpression of the protein inhibits *M. tuberculosis* growth (193). As discussed above, the induction of *hspX* under anoxic conditions requires the response regulator Rv3133c (114).

Esat6 and CF-10 (Rv3875-Rv3874)

The Esat6 and CF-10 proteins are members of the Esat6 family of related small secreted proteins found in *M. tuberculosis* culture filtrates. Both proteins are immunodominant antigens that are recognized by the sera in a majority of TB patients (194). A mutation that disrupted both closely linked genes in *M. bovis* results in severe attenuation in a guinea pig model of infection, using the criteria of histopathology in several tissues and bacterial load in spleens (195). It is not known which of the two genes is necessary or if both are necessary for the virulence of *M. bovis* in this animal model. Rv3874-Rv3875 is located in the RD1 deletion region that contains the structural genes for nine proteins, Rv3971 to Rv23979. This region is found in all virulent *M. tuberculosis* and *M. bovis* strains but is the only deletion found in all *M. bovis* BCG strains, suggesting that some of the genes in this region are important for virulence (196). The Esat6 and CF-10 genes are cotranscribed in *M. tuberculosis* (197), and when coexpressed in *E. coli*, form a tight 1:1 complex (198). The members of the *M. tuberculosis* Esat6 family are frequently found in the same type of genomic arrangement as many of their genes are found in closely linked pairs in the *M. tuberculosis* genome (33). This suggests that similar 1:1 complexes will also be formed. Another member of the Esat6 family, Rv0288, has been identified as being differentially expressed in mouse lung using a promoter trap screen, and it is also induced in macrophages as determined by RT-PCR analysis (E. Dubnau and I. Smith, unpublished results, 2003). TB10.4, the product of Rv0288, is recognized by sera from 70% of TB patients, and T cells from this cohort show a strong cytokine response (IFN-γ release) when the protein is presented (194). The role of Rv0288 in virulence has not been analyzed yet, but these experiments are in progress. Rv0288 is also found adjacent to another gene, Rv0287, which encodes a member of the Esat6 family, suggesting the existence of a complex.

19-kd Protein (Rv3763, *lpqH*)

The 19-kd glycoprotein is an immunodominant antigen that is recognized by T cells and sera from TB patients. It and other cell surface factors are believed to cause signaling in the macrophage, as it has been shown that the effects of adding the 19-kd protein to macrophages requires the presence of toll-like receptor 2 (TLR2) (199,200), However, as discussed below in this section, these effects are not at all clear. It was

noted that an *M. tuberculosis* strain, I2646, did not produce this protein, and subsequent analyses demonstrated that the I2646 *lpqH* gene was disrupted. The strain was rapidly cleared from the lungs and spleen of infected mice, an SGIV phenotype. Adding back the wild-type *M. tuberculosis* gene to *M. tuberculosis* I2646 allowed growth in lungs that was similar to standard wild-type strains, suggesting that the 19-kd protein was essential for virulence (201). Subsequent experiments were less conclusive as it was shown that the mutations in the gene encoding the 19-kd protein has no effect on *M. intracellulare* virulence (202) and that the addition of genes encoding the 19-kd protein to nonpathogenic mycobacteria actually lowered their efficacy as vaccines (203). In addition, it was found that neither overexpressing the 19-kd protein nor deleting its structural gene in *M. bovis* BCG had any effects on the efficacy of the parent strain as a vaccine in a mouse infection model (204). Thus, the role of this protein in *M. tuberculosis* virulence is not clear. Equally uncertain is the effect the protein has on macrophage responses during *M. tuberculosis* infection of macrophages. It has been reported that addition of the purified 19-kd protein to human MDMs causes up-regulation of the important T_H1 cytokine IL-12 (205). Similarly, addition of the 19-kd protein can activate human neutrophils (206). On the other hand, when the gene for the 19-kd protein was introduced into *M. smegmatis* and the recombinant strain was used to infect human MDMs, IL-12 production is inhibited (207). Another report demonstrated that the addition of the 19-kd protein to murine macrophages causes the inhibition of major histocompatibility complex type II expression and major histocompatibility complex type II antigen processing (200), The reasons for these widely discrepant results are not known. When virulent *M. tuberculosis* infects human MDMs, IL-12 is induced much less than when *E. coli* is used for the infection (208). This suggests that, in a physiologic context, *M. tuberculosis* and its surface components, such as the 19-kd protein, downmodulate the initial cytokine response, including IL-12, in the macrophage.

Cell Surface Components

As discussed above, the mycobacterial cell wall/envelope is a complex structure containing many proteins, lipids, and carbohydrates, many of which are found only in these bacteria. There is a subset of these components that are unique to pathogenic mycobacteria and thus are expected to be excellent targets for further investigations into *M. tuberculosis* virulence.

Erp (Rv 3810, *erp*)

Erp is a surface-located protein that was originally identified by means of a *phoA* fusion strategy to identify secreted *M. tuberculosis* proteins (209). The protein is similar to an exported 28-kd antigen (the PLGTS antigen) in *M. leprae*, but is absent from nonpathogenic mycobacteria. The *M.*

tuberculosis protein has six tandem repeats with the sequence (PA/G)LTS, which is similar to the *M. leprae* protein. The *M. tuberculosis erp* gene was inactivated by a two-step plasmid procedure; the mutant showed attenuation of growth in primary murine macrophages and was also attenuated in the lungs and spleen of infected mice, exhibiting an SGIV phenotype. A similar *erp* mutation was made in *M. bovis* BCG, and this mutant showed a PER attenuation phenotype in mice (210). The function of the protein is unknown as the mutant shows normal growth *in vitro,* but mutant bacteria recovered from infected mice grow much more slowly than the wild-type and complemented mutant strains.

Mas (Rv2940c, *mas*)

mas encodes the mycocerosic acid synthase, an enzyme that catalyzes the synthesis of long-chain, multiple methylated branched fatty acids called mycocerosic acids that are only found in pathogenic mycobacteria. The *mas* gene was disrupted in *M. bovis* BCG using a linear DNA construct and was shown to be deficient in the synthesis of mycocerosic acids and their phthiocerol dimycoserate (PDIM) derivatives (211). No virulence phenotypes of these mutants have been published, but, as discussed in the next paragraphs, inactivation of other genes in the *mas* region results in the attenuation of virulence and the failure of *M. tuberculosis* to produce PDIM. The Kolattukudy group has also made mutations in genes encoding related cell wall components, but their virulence phenotypes have also not been reported (211,212).

FadD26 (Rv2930, *fadD26*)

FadD26 was originally annotated as an acyl coenzyme A synthetase involved in fatty acid degradation. It was identified in the same series of STM experiments in which *lipF* was found, as discussed above (72), and had a similar attenuated phenotype in mice. Similar mouse results were obtained by another group using STM technology in *M. tuberculosis* H37Rv, with the *fadD26* mutant in this study exhibiting a GIV phenotype (73). In the latter case, the transposon inserted in the promoter region of *fadD26* and the disruption also affected the expression of the downstream *ppsA-E* operon (Rv2931-2935) encoding a polyketide synthase required for phthiocerol biosynthesis (211), and one of the mutant phenotypes is the absence of PDIM. It has not yet been shown whether the phenotypes of the *fadD26* mutations are due to a polar effect on the downstream *pps* operon or to a specific role for the FadD26 protein. However, the fact that *fad26* is closely linked to genes for PDIM synthesis, including *mas,* as discussed directly above, suggests that FadD26 may have a synthetic rather than a degradative function, as originally annotated.

FadD28 (Rv2941, *fadD28*)

fadD28 was found in the same STM search that identified *fadD26* (73). Like the latter gene, it was also annotated as a fatty acid coenzyme A synthase, and the *fadD28* mutant has a similar GIV phenotype in mice. *fadD28* is in the *mas* region, and the mutant also does not make PDIM.

MmpL7 (Rv2942, *mmpL7*)

MmpL7 was identified as being important for *M. tuberculosis* virulence in STM transposon searches (72,73). This protein is a member of a large group of related proteins, and one of the phenotypes of the mutant is the failure to transport PDIM (73,213). The mutant is attenuated for growth in mice exhibiting a GIV phenotype. Additional *mmpL* genes, along with several other genes, were identified in one of the transposon searches but will not be discussed here because they have not been studied in great detail (72).

FbpA (*fbpA*, Rv3804c)

Mycobacteria have three mycolyltransferase enzymes, encoded by three genes—*fbpA, fbpB,* and *fbpC*—that transfer long-chain mycolic acids to trehalose derivatives, and the proteins can also bind the cell matrix protein fibronectin (214). Fbp proteins are also found in the culture filtrate and are also known as the antigen 85A, 85B, or 85C complex or the 30- to 32-kd proteins. The three *fbp* genes have been separately inactivated, but only the *M. tuberculosis fbpA* mutant, made with a linear DNA construct, showed severely attenuated growth phenotype in human and murine macrophages (215). The observation that these proteins are immunodominant has led to the creation of a new live vaccine that was made by introducing the *M. tuberculosis fbpB* gene into *M. bovis* BCG. This recombinant strain shows better protection against virulent *M. tuberculosis* infection than the parent BCG strain, using a guinea pig model (216). This vaccine strategy has not been employed with the *M. tuberculosis fbpA* gene, but presumably this will be done, given the reported virulence phenotype of the *fbpA* mutant.

MmaA4 (*mmaA4*, Rv 0642c)

A gene cluster in *M. tuberculosis* has been described that encodes four closely related methyltransferases whose function is to form methoxy and keto derivatives of the meromycolic acid chain that are unique to members of the *M. tuberculosis* complex (217,218). It was postulated that the reaction catalyzed by the methyltransferase encoded by *mmaA4* (methylation of a double bond) is the initial step for all subsequent derivatizations of meromycolic acids (218). To verify this, and to see the effects of this mutation on *M. tuberculosis* virulence, the *M. tuberculosis mmaA4* was inactivated by a two-step plasmid procedure. The mutant grows normally but does not make methoxy- and ketomycolates as originally predicted. In addition, the mutant shows marked cell wall alterations as it is less permeable to various compounds like glycerol and chenodeoxycholate but is more resistant to oxidative stress than the wild-type *M. tuberculosis* H37Rv. The mutant strain was attenuated in mice showing a GIV phenotype (20).

PcaA (Rv0470c, *pcaA*)

PcaA is a methyltransferase that forms cyclopropane residues in mycolic acids. It was originally detected by the unusual colony morphology of an *M. bovis* BCG transposon mutant. Microscopic examination of the mutant showed a corded structure of the clumped bacterial cells. Analysis of the mutated gene showed it was a member of a family of proteins that introduce cyclopropane residues into mycolic acids. To analyze the role of PcaA in *M. tuberculosis* physiology and virulence, the gene was inactivated by a bacteriophage-mediated system (69). The colonial and microscopic phenotype of the mutant was similar to that of the *M. bovis* BCG *pcaA* mutant, and biochemical studies indicated that the role of the enzyme was to synthesize the proximal cyclopropane ring of the α-mycolate chain of mycolic acids. While the BCG mutant was cleared more rapidly from lungs than its parent, the *M. tuberculosis* mutant's growth was essentially similar to that of the wild type. However, the *M. tuberculosis pcaA* mutant was less virulent in a mortality assay, in which five of five mice infected with the wild type all died after 219 days whereas all five of the mice infected with the mutant were alive at this time. Microscopic observations showed much less pathology in the lungs of mice infected with the mutant compared with the wild-type strain.

Lipoarabinomannan

Lipoarabinomannan (LAM) is included in this list of virulence factors because of its importance as an immunomodulator as determined by experiments similar to those described above for the 19-kd protein. LAM, a complex glycolipid that contains repeating arabinose-mannose disaccharide subunits, is a major component of the *M. tuberculosis* cell wall (219). Addition of LAM to murine macrophages depresses IFN-γ, which in turn blocks expression of IFN-γ-induced genes (220). LAM can also scavenge oxygen radicals *in vitro* and inhibits the host phosphokinase, PKC. These multiple phenotypes suggest that LAM functions to down-modulate host responses to *M. tuberculosis* infection, protecting the bacterium from potentially lethal mechanisms such as respiratory burst (220). *M. tuberculosis* mutants that do not make LAM have not been isolated yet, but these should be valuable for the insights they will provide regarding *M. tuberculosis*–host interactions.

FUTURE PROSPECTS AND CONCLUSIONS

As shown in this chapter, much work has been devoted to the search for *M. tuberculosis* virulence factors. Various targets have been identified, such as enzymes involved in the synthesis of unique cell wall structures and secreted proteins. More work has to be performed to ensure that every potential gene is systematically inactivated in the *M. tuber-*

culosis genome so that the virulence of these mutants can be assayed. Ideally, the mariner transposon system (75) can be modified to incorporate signature tagging so that many potential mutants can be tested *in vivo* at the same time. In addition to this global search, more specific approaches can be undertaken. As mentioned previously, the fact that all *M. bovis* BCG strains have one common deletion (RD1) strongly suggests that genes in this region are important for virulence (221). It would seem relatively easy to complement a BCG strain with all or a subset of the genes in the RD1 region to see whether this restores virulence. The use of DNA arrays should be extended so that the global gene expression of *M. tuberculosis*–attenuated mutants can be studied during infections. This is especially important for regulatory mutants (30,140), as those *M. tuberculosis* genes not expressed in the mutant during infections would be good candidates for encoding virulence factors. Another important area to investigate is the host–pathogen interaction with the new technologies that are being developed. The use of DNA arrays to measure host responses to *M. tuberculosis* infection is a new area of research, and two recent publications describing studies in which *M. tuberculosis*-infected murine (24) and human macrophages (208) have provided much useful information. Hopefully, these experiments can be extended in the near future to measure host gene expression in the lungs of infected animals. It will also be interesting to look at the host response when various *M. tuberculosis* mutants are used for infections, such as those that cannot make the 19-kd protein or other immunomodulatory factors. This is attributable to the fact that, as previously discussed, the addition of purified immunomodulators may not give the most meaningful results because the amounts may be nonphysiologic and are not in the context of the intact bacterium. Mutants that are defective in the synthesis of LAM, yet to be made, would be very useful for these experiments.

With the targets already found and the expectation of finding new ones, the next question is what should be done with this information. It is beyond the scope of this chapter to discuss new vaccines and drugs in detail, and these areas have been recently reviewed (222,223). Rather these concluding remarks will list some of the areas that the author thinks could be exploited for better therapies. Live vaccines that are more protective than *M. bovis* BCG are still worth pursuing, even though the problem of giving these to immunocompromised individuals must be addressed. The use of vaccines that have recombinant *M. bovis* BCG containing *M. tuberculosis* genes is a new approach that has great promise (216), and it will be important to use other *M. tuberculosis* genes in this delivery system as well. Another approach to the manufacture of live vaccines is to systematically use attenuated *M. tuberculosis* mutants for protection studies. In this regard, the protection results obtained with a phenotypic *M. tuberculosis sodA* mutant (82) are extremely encouraging. It will be important to use other mutants obtained by standard allelic replacement for protection studies as these will confer less risk of reversion. Subunit vaccines and DNA vaccines are other areas that should be developed as more *M. tuberculosis* virulence factors are identified. The identification of new antitubercular drugs is an important and complex undertaking, and, again, it would seem that unique systems found in *M. tuberculosis* are prime candidates as new targets for rational drug design. One area that should be exploited is the *M. tuberculosis* iron acquisition system as this essential element is limiting for *M. tuberculosis* growth *in vivo*. Since *M. tuberculosis* siderophores, and presumably their receptors, are highly specific, it should be possible to use them to deliver toxic agents directly to *M. tuberculosis*.

The advances in our understanding of *M. tuberculosis* virulence summarized in this chapter are expected to bring many new treatments that should help prevent or control the spread of TB throughout the world. However, it is important to remember René Dubos's cautionary words: "Tuberculosis is a social disease, and presents problems that transcend the conventional medical approach. . . . Its understanding demands that the impact of social and economic factors on the individual be considered as much as the mechanisms by which tubercle bacilli cause damage to the human body" (224). The new vaccines and drugs will work to some extent as *M. bovis* BCG, streptomycin, and INH have worked in the past, but TB will only be eradicated when poverty and inequitable development are ended.

ACKNOWLEDGMENTS

I thank the members of my research group and colleagues at the Tuberculosis Center of the Public Heath Research Institute for helpful discussions. Work from my laboratory that was discussed in this chapter was supported by National Institutes of Health grants RO1 AI44856, RO1 HL 64544, and RO1 HL 68513. The literature survey for this review was completed in September 2002.

REFERENCES

1. Glickman MS, Jacobs WR Jr. Microbial pathogenesis of *Mycobacterium tuberculosis*: dawn of a discipline. *Cell* 2001;104:477–485.
2. Manganelli R, Voskuil MI, Schoolnik GK, et al. Role of the extracytoplasmic-function sigma factor sigma H in *Mycobacterium tuberculosis* global gene expression. *Mol Microbiol* 2002;45:365–374.
3. Kaushal D, Schroeder BG, Tyagi S, et al. Reduced immunopathology and mortality despite tissue persistence in a *Mycobacterium tuberculosis* mutant lacking alternative sigma factor, SigH. *Proc Natl Acad Sci U S A* 2002;99:8330–8335.
4. Garay SM. Pulmonary tuberculosis. In: Rom WN, Garay S, eds. *Tuberculosis*. Boston: Little, Brown and Company, 1996:373–412.
5. Zugar A, Lowy FD. Tuberculosis of the brain, meninges, and the spinal cord. In: Rom WN, Garay S, eds. *Tuberculosis*. Boston: Little, Brown and Company, 1996:541–556.
6. Meghji S, White PA, Nair SP, et al. *Mycobacterium tuberculosis* chaperonin 10 stimulates bone resorption: a potential contributory factor in Pott's disease. *J Exp Med* 1997;186:1241–1246.
7. Munger JS, Chapman HA Jr. Tissue destruction by proteases. In: Rom RN, Garay S, eds. *Tuberculosis*. Boston: Little, Brown and Company, 1996:353–361.
8. Converse PJ, Dannenberg AM Jr, Estep JE, et al. Cavitary tuberculosis produced in rabbits by aerosolized virulent tubercle bacilli. *Infect Immun* 1996;64:4776–4787.
9. Laochumroonvorapong P, Paul S, Elkon KB, et al. H$_2$O$_2$ induces monocyte apoptosis and reduces viability of *Mycobacterium avium–M. intracellulare* within cultured human monocytes. *Infect Immun* 1996;64:452–459.
10. Keane J, Balcewicz-Sablinska MK, Remold HG, et al. Infection by *Mycobacterium tuberculosis* promotes human alveolar macrophage apoptosis. *Infect Immun* 1997;65:298–304.
11. Senaldi G, Yin S, Shaklee CL, et al. *Corynebacterium parvum*- and *Mycobacterium bovis* bacillus Calmette–Guérin–induced granuloma formation is inhibited in TNF receptor I (TNF- RI) knockout mice and by treatment with soluble TNF-RI. *J Immunol* 1996;157:5022–5026.
12. Bekker LG, Haslett P, Maartens G, et al. Thalidomide-induced antigen-specific immune stimulation in patients with human immunodeficiency virus type 1 and tuberculosis. *J Infect Dis* 2000;181:954–965.
13. Tsenova L, Bergtold A, Freedman VH, et al. Tumor necrosis factor alpha is a determinant of pathogenesis and disease progression in mycobacterial infection in the central nervous system. *Proc Natl Acad Sci U S A* 1999;96:5657–5662.
14. Jacobs W, Brennan P, Curlin G, et al. 1996. Comparative sequencing. *Science* 1996;274:17–18.
15. Manca C, Tsenova L, Barry CE III, et al. *Mycobacterium tuberculosis* CDC1551 induces a more vigorous host response *in vivo* and *in vitro*, but is not more virulent than other clinical isolates. *J Immunol* 1999;162:6740–6746.
16. Manca C, Tsenova L, Bergtold A, et al. Virulence of a *Mycobacterium tuberculosis* clinical isolate in mice is determined by failure to induce Th1 type immunity and is associated with induction of IFN-alpha /beta. *Proc Natl Acad Sci U S A* 2001;98:5752–5757.
17. Balcewicz-Sablinska MK, Keane J, Kornfeld H, et al. Pathogenic *Mycobacterium tuberculosis* evades apoptosis of host macrophages by release of TNF-R2, resulting in inactivation of TNF-alpha. *J Immunol* 1998;161:2636–2641.
18. Dunn PL, North RJ. Virulence ranking of some *Mycobacterium tuberculosis* and *Mycobacterium bovis* strains according to their ability to multiply in the lungs, induce lung pathology, and cause mortality in mice. *Infect Immun* 1995;63:3428–3437.
19. Stewart GR, Snewin VA, Walzl G, et al. Overexpression of heat-shock proteins reduces survival of *Mycobacterium tuberculosis* in the chronic phase of infection. *Nat Med* 2001;7:732–737.
20. Dubnau E, Chan J, Raynaud C, et al. Oxygenated mycolic acids are necessary for virulence of *Mycobacterium tuberculosis* in mice. *Mol Microbiol* 2000;36:630–637.
21. Orme IM, McMurray DN. The immune response to tuberculosis in animal models. In: Rom WN, Garay S, eds. *Tuberculosis*. Boston: Little, Brown and Company, 1996:269–280.
22. Fortin A, Diez E, Rochefort D, et al. Recombinant congenic strains derived from A/J and C57BL/6J: a tool for genetic dissection of complex traits. *Genomics* 2001;74:21–35.
23. Melo MD, Stokes RW. Interaction of *Mycobacterium tuberculosis* with MH-S, an immortalized murine alveolar macrophage cell line: a comparison with primary murine macrophages. *Tuber Lung Dis* 2000;80:35–46.
24. Ehrt S, Schnappinger D, Bekiranov S, et al. Reprogramming of the macrophage transcriptome in response to interferon-gamma

and *Mycobacterium tuberculosis*: signaling roles of nitric oxide synthase-2 and phagocyte oxidase. *J Exp Med* 2001;194:1123–1140.

25. Chan J, Xing Y, Magliozzo RS, et al. Killing of virulent *Mycobacterium tuberculosis* by reactive nitrogen intermediates produced by activated murine macrophages. *J Exp Med* 1992; 175:1111–1122.

26. Tsuchiya S, Kobayashi Y, Goto Y, et al. Induction of maturation in cultured human monocytic leukemia cells by a phorbol diester. *Cancer Res* 1982;42:1530–1536.

27. Wei J, Dahl JL, Moulder JW, et al. Identification of a *Mycobacterium tuberculosis* gene that enhances mycobacterial survival in macrophages. *J Bacteriol* 2000;182:377–384.

28. Stokes RW, Doxsee D. The receptor-mediated uptake, survival, replication, and drug sensitivity of *Mycobacterium tuberculosis* within the macrophage-like cell line THP-1: a comparison with human monocyte-derived macrophages. *Cell Immunol* 1999; 197:1–9.

29. Denis M. Human monocytes/macrophages: NO or no NO. *J Leukocyte Biol.* 1994;55:682–684.

30. Manganelli R, Voskuil MI, Schoolnik GK, et al. The *Mycobacterium tuberculosis* ECF sigma factor sigmaE: role in global gene expression and survival in macrophages. *Mol Microbiol* 2001; 41:423–437.

31. Cole ST, Smith DR. Toward mapping and sequencing the genome of *Mycobacterium tuberculosis*. In: Bloom BR, ed. *Tuberculosis: pathogenesis, protection, and control.* Washington, DC: American Society for Microbiology, 1994:227–238.

32. Jacobs WR. *Mycobacterium tuberculosis*: a once genetically intractable organism. In: Hatfall GF, Jacobs WR, eds. *Molecular genetics of mycobacteria.* Washington, DC: American Society for Microbiology, 2000:1–16.

33. Cole ST, Brosch R, Parkhill J, et al. Deciphering the biology of *Mycobacterium tuberculosis* from the complete genome sequence. *Nature* 1998;393:537–544.

34. Collins DM, Gicquel B. Genetics of mycobacterial virulence. In: Hatfall GF, Jacobs WR, eds. *Molecular genetics of mycobacteria.* Washington, DC: American Society for Microbiology, 2000:265–278.

35. Bentley SD, Chater KF, Cerdeno-Tarraga AM, et al. Complete genome sequence of the model actinomycete *Streptomyces coelicolor* A3(2). *Nature* 2000;417:141–147.

36. Brosch R, Gordon SV, Pym A, et al. Comparative genomics of the mycobacteria. *Int J Med Microbiol* 2000;290:143–152.

37. Cole ST, Eiglmeier K, Parkhill J, et al. Massive gene decay in the leprosy bacillus. *Nature* 2001;409:1007–1011.

38. Ramakrishnan L, Federspiel NA, Falkow S. Granuloma-specific expression of *Mycobacterium* virulence proteins from the glycine-rich PE-PGRS family. *Science* 2000;288:1436–1439.

39. Banu S, Honore N, Saint-Joanis B, et al. Are the PE-PGRS proteins of *Mycobacterium tuberculosis* variable surface antigens? *Mol Microbiol* 2002;44:9–19.

40. Wilson TM, Lisle GWD, Collins DM. Effect of *inhA* and *katG* on isoniazid resistance and virulence of *Mycobacterium bovis. Mol Microbiol* 1995;15:1009–1015.

41. Collins DM, Kawakami RP, de Lisle GW, et al. Mutation of the principal sigma factor causes loss of virulence in a strain of the *Mycobacterium tuberculosis* complex. *Proc Natl Acad Sci U S A* 1995;92:8036–8040.

42. Smith I, Dussurget O, Rodriguez GM, et al. Extra- and intracellular expression of *Mycobacterium tuberculosis* genes. *Tuber Lung Dis* 1998;79:91–97.

43. Parsons LM, Jankowski CS, Derbyshire KM. Conjugal transfer of chromosomal DNA in *Mycobacterium smegmatis. Mol Microbiol* 1998;28:571–582.

44. SundarRaj CV, Ramakrishnan T. Transduction in *Mycobacterium smegmatis. Nature* 1970;228:280–281.

45. McFadden J. Recombination in mycobacteria. *Mol Microbiol* 1996;21:205–211.

46. Davis EO, Thangaraj HS, Brooks PC, et al. Evidence of selection for protein introns in the RecAs of pathogenic bacteria. *EMBO J* 1994;13:699–703.

47. Frischkorn K, Sander P, Scholz M, et al. Investigation of mycobacterial *recA* function: protein introns in the RecA of pathogenic mycobacteria do not affect competency for homologous recombination. *Mol Microbiol* 1998;29:1203–1214.

48. Papavinasasundaram KG, Colston MJ, Davis EO. Construction and complementation of a *recA* deletion mutant of *Mycobacterium smegmatis* reveals that the intein in *Mycobacterium tuberculosis recA* does not affect RecA function. *Mol Microbiol* 1998; 30:525–534.

49. Pavelka MS Jr, Jacobs WR Jr. Comparison of the construction of unmarked deletion mutations in *Mycobacterium smegmatis, Mycobacterium bovis* bacillus Calmette–Guérin, and *Mycobacterium tuberculosis* H37Rv by allelic exchange. *J Bacteriol* 1999; 181:4780–4789.

50. Caseli N, Ehrt S. Plasmid vectors. In: Parish T, Stoker NG, eds. Mycobacterium tuberculosis *protocols.* Totowa, NJ: Humana Press, 2001:1–17.

51. Sander P, Prammananan T, Bottger E. Introducing mutations into a chromosomal rRNA gene using a genetically modified eubacterial host with a single rRNA operon. *Mol Microbiol* 1996;22:841–848.

52. Rodriguez GM, Voskuil MI, Gold B, et al. ideR, an essential gene in *Mycobacterium tuberculosis*: role of IdeR in iron-dependent gene expression, iron metabolism, and oxidative stress response. *Infect Immun* 2002;70:3371–3381.

53. Balasubramanian V, Pavelka MS, Bardarov SS, et al. Allelic exchange in *Mycobacterium tuberculosis* with long linear substrates. *J Bacteriol* 1996;178:273–279.

54. Aldovini A, Husson RN, Young RA. The uraA locus and homologous recombination in *Mycobacterium bovis* BCG. *J Bacteriol* 1993; l75:7282–7289.

55. Reyrat JM, Berthet F-X, Gicquel B. The urease gene of *Mycobacterium tuberculosis* and its utilization for the demonstration of allelic exchange in *Mycobacterium bovis* BCG. *Proc Natl Acad Sci U S A* 1995;92:8768–8772.

56. Oh SH, Chater KF. Denaturation of circular or linear DNA facilitates targeted integrative transformation of *Streptomyces coelicolor* A3(2): possible relevance to other organisms. *J Bacteriol* 1997;179:122–127.

57. Hinds J, Mahenthiralingam E, Kempsell KE, et al. Enhanced gene replacement in mycobacteria. *Microbiology* 1999;145:519–527.

58. Fogg GC, Gibson CM, Caparon MG. The identification of *rofA*, a positive acting regulatory component of *prtF* expression: use of an mγδ-based shuttle mutagenesis strategy in *Streptococcus pyogenes. Mol Microbiol* 1994;11:671–684.

59. Dussurget O, Rodriguez GM, Smith I. An *ideR* mutant of *Mycobacterium smegmatis* has a derepressed siderophore production and an altered oxidative-stress response. *Mol Microbiol* 1996;22:535–544.

60. Derbyshire KM, Takacs C, Huang J. Using the EZ:TN Transposome for transposon mutagenesis in *Mycobacterium smegmatis. Epicentre Forum* 2000;7:1–4.

61. Pelicic V, Jackson M, Reyrat JM, et al. Efficient allelic exchange and transposon mutagenesis in *Mycobacterium tuberculosis. Proc Natl Acad Sci U S A* 1997;94:10955–10960.

62. Sander P, Meier A, Bottger EC. *rpsl*+ : a dominant selectable marker for gene replacement in mycobacteria. *Mol Microbiol* 1995;16:991–1000.

63. Pelicic V, Reyrat J-M, Gicquel B. Expression of the *Bacillus subtilis sacB* gene confers sucrose sensitivity on mycobacteria. *J Bacteriol* 1996;178:1197–1199.

64. Pelicic V, Reyrat J-M, Gicquel B. Generation of unmarked directed mutations in mycobacteria, using sucrose counter-selectable suicide vectors. *Mol Microbiol* 1996;20:919–925.

65. Zahrt TC, Deretic V. *Mycobacterium tuberculosis* signal transduction system required for persistent infections. *Proc Natl Acad Sci U S A* 2001;98:12706–12711.

66. Parish T, Gordhan BG, McAdam RA, et al. Production of mutants in amino acid biosynthesis genes of *Mycobacterium tuberculosis* by homologous recombination. *Microbiology* 1999;145:3497–3503.

67. Dussurget O, Rodriguez GM, Smith I. Protective role of the mycobacterial IdeR against reactive oxygen species and isoniazid toxicity. *Tuber Lung Dis* 1998;79:99–106.

68. Wards BJ, Collins DM. Electroporation at elevated temperatures substantially improves transformation frequency of slow-growing mycobacteria. *FEMS Microbiol Lett* 1996;145:101–105.

69. Glickman MS, Cox JS, Jacobs WR Jr. A novel mycolic acid cyclopropane synthetase is required for cording, persistence, and virulence of *Mycobacterium tuberculosis*. *Mol Cell* 2000;5:717–727.

70. Bardarov S, Kriakov J, Carriere C, et al. Conditionally replicating mycobacteriophages: a system for transposon delivery to *Mycobacterium tuberculosis*. *Proc Natl Acad Sci U S A* 1997;94:10961–10966.

71. Hensel M, Shea SJ, Gleeson C, et al. Simultaneous identification of bacterial virulence genes by negative selection. *Science* 1995; 269:400–403.

72. Camacho LR, Ensergueix D, Perez E, et al. Identification of a virulence gene cluster of *Mycobacterium tuberculosis* by signature-tagged transposon mutagenesis. *Mol Microbiol* 1999;34:257–267.

73. Cox JS, Chen B, MacNeil M, et al. Complex lipid determines tissue-specific replication of *Mycobacterium tuberculosis* in mice. *Nature* 1999;402:79–83.

74. Rubin EJ, Akerley BJ, Novik VN, et al. *In vivo* transposition of mariner-based elements in enteric bacteria and mycobacteria. *Proc Natl Acad Sci U S A* 1999;96:1645–1650.

75. Sassetti CM, Boyd DH, Rubin EJ. Comprehensive identification of conditionally essential genes in mycobacteria. *Proc Natl Acad Sci U S A* 2001;98:12712–12717.

76. Pascopella L, Collins FM, Martin JM, et al. Use of *in vivo* complementation in *Mycobacterium tuberculosis* to identify a genomic fragment associated with virulence. *Infect Immun* 1996; 62:1313–1319.

77. Falcone V, Bassey E, Jacobs W Jr, et al. The immunogenicity of recombinant *Mycobacterium smegmatis* bearing BCG genes. *Microbiology* 1995;141:1239–1245.

78. Arruda S, Bomfim G, Knights R, et al. Cloning of an *M. tuberculosis* DNA fragment associated with entry and survival inside cells. *Science* 1993;261:1454–1457.

79. Wieles B, Ottenhoff THM, Steenwijk TM, et al. Increased extracellular survival of *Mycobacterium smegmatis* containing the *Mycobacterium leprae* thioredoxin-thioredoxin reductase gene. *Infect Immun* 1997;65:2537–2541.

80. Parish T, Stoker NG. Development and use of a conditional antisense mutagenesis system in mycobacteria. *FEMS Microbiol Lett* 1997;154:151–157.

81. Wilson T, de Lisle GW, Marcinkeviciene JA, et al. Antisense RNA to ahpC, an oxidative stress defence gene involved in isoniazid resistance, indicates that AhpC of *Mycobacterium bovis* has virulence properties. *Microbiology* 1998;144:2687–2695.

82. Edwards KM, Cynamon MH, Voladri RK, et al. Iron-cofactored superoxide dismutase inhibits host responses to *Mycobacterium tuberculosis*. *Am J Respir Crit Care Med* 2001;164:2213–2219.

83. Harth G, Zamecnik PC, Tang JY, et al. Treatment of *Mycobacterium tuberculosis* with antisense oligonucleotides to glutamine synthetase mRNA inhibits glutamine synthetase activity, formation of the poly-L-glutamate/glutamine cell wall structure, and bacterial replication. *Proc Natl Acad Sci U S A* 2000;97:418–423.

84. Tyagi AK, Gupta SKD, Jain S. Gene expression: reporter technologies. In: Hatfull GF, Jacobs WR, eds. *Molecular genetics of mycobacteria*. Washington, DC: American Society for Microbiology, 2000:131–147.

85. Dellagostin OA, Esposito G, Eales LJ, et al. Activity of mycobacterial promoters during intracellular and extracellular growth. *Microbiology* 1995;141:1785–1792.

86. Hobson RJ, McBride AJ, Kempsell KE, et al. Use of an arrayed promoter-probe library for the identification of macrophage-regulated genes in *Mycobacterium tuberculosis*. *Microbiology* 2002;148:1571–1579.

87. Rodriguez GM, Gold B, Gomez M, et al. Identification and characterization of two divergently transcribed iron regulated genes in *Mycobacterium tuberculosis*. *Tuber Lung Dis* 1999;79:287–298.

88. Das Gupta SK, Bashyam MD, Tyagi AK. Cloning and assessment of mycobacterial promoters by using a plasmid shuttle vector. *J Bacteriol* 1993;175:5186–5192.

89. Barker LP, Brooks DM, Small PL. The identification of *Mycobacterium marinum* genes differentially expressed in macrophage phagosomes using promoter fusions to green fluorescent protein. *Mol Microbiol* 1998;29:1167–1177.

90. Triccas JA, Berthet FX, Pelicic V, et al. Use of fluorescence induction and sucrose counterselection to identify *Mycobacterium tuberculosis* genes expressed within host cells. *Microbiology* 1999;145:2923–2930.

91. Dubnau E, Fontan P, Manganelli R, et al. *Mycobacterium tuberculosis* genes induced during infection of human macrophages. *Infect Immun* 2002;70:2787–2795.

92. Mahan M, Slauch J, Mekalanos JJ. Selection of bacterial virulence genes that are specifically induced in host tissues. *Science* 1993;259:686–688.

93. Mahan MJ, Tobias JW, Slauch JM, et al. Antibiotic-based selection for bacterial genes that are specifically induced during infection of a host. *Proc Natl Acad Sci USA* 1995;92:669–673.

94. Banerjee A, Dubnau E, Quemard A, et al. inhA, a gene encoding a target for isoniazid and ethionamide in *Mycobacterium tuberculosis*. *Science* 1994;263:227–230.

95. Quémard A, Dessen A, Sugantino M, et al. Binding of catalase-peroxidase–activated isoniazid to wild-type and mutant *Mycobacterium tuberculosis* enoyl-ACP reductases. *J Am Chem Soc* 1996;118:1561–1562.

96. Patel BK, Banerjee DK, Butcher PD. Characterization of the heat shock response in *Mycobacterium bovis* BCG. *J Bacteriol* 1991;173:7982–7987.

97. Butcher PD, Mangan JA, Monahan IM. Intracellular gene expression. In: Parish T, Stoker NG, eds. Mycobacterium tuberculosis *protocols*. Totowa, NJ: Humana Press, 1998:285–306.

98. Hu Y, Mangan JA, Dhillon J, et al. Detection of mRNA transcripts and active transcription in persistent *Mycobacterium tuberculosis* induced by exposure to rifampin or pyrazinamide. *J Bacteriol* 2000;182:6358–6365.

99. Mariani F, Cappelli G, Riccardi G, et al. *Mycobacterium tuberculosis* H37Rv comparative gene-expression analysis in synthetic medium and human macrophage. *Gene* 2000;253:281–291.

100. Manganelli R, Tyagi S, Smith I. Real time PCR using molecular beacons: a new tool to identify point mutations and to analyze gene expression in *Mycobacterium tuberculosis*. In: Parish T, Stoker N, eds. *Methods in molecular medicine*: Mycobacterium tuberculosis *protocols*, vol 54. Totowa, NJ: Humana Press, 2001:295–310.

101. Tyagi S, Kramer FR. Molecular beacons: probes that fluoresce upon hybridization. *Nat Biotechnol* 1996;14:303–308.

102. Tyagi S, Bratu DB, Kramer FR. Multicolor molecular beacons for allele discrimination. *Nat Biotechnol* 1998;16:49–53.

103. Manganelli R, Dubnau E, Tyagi S, et al. Differential expression of 10 sigma factor genes in *Mycobacterium tuberculosis*. *Mol Microbiol* 1999;31:715–724.

104. Rivera-Marrero CA, Burroughs MA, Masse RA, et al. Identification of genes differentially expressed in *Mycobacterium tuberculosis* by differential display PCR. *Microb Pathogen* 1998;25:307–316.

105. Alland D, Kramnik I, Weisbrod TR, et al. Identification of differentially expressed mRNA in prokaryotic organisms by customized amplification libraries (DECAL): the effect of isoniazid on gene expression in *Mycobacterium tuberculosis*. *Proc Natl Acad Sci U S A* 1998;95:13227–13232.

106. Graham JE, Clark-Curtiss JE. Identification of *Mycobacterium tuberculosis* RNAs synthesized in response to phagocytosis by human macrophages by selective capture of transcribed sequences (SCOTS). *Proc Natl Acad Sci U S A* 1999;96:11554–11559.

107. Hou JY, Graham JE, Clark-Curtiss JE. *Mycobacterium avium* genes expressed during growth in human macrophages detected by selective capture of transcribed sequences (SCOTS). *Infect Immun* 2002;70:3714–3726.

108. Eisen MB, Brown PO. DNA arrays for analysis of gene expression. *Meth Enzymol* 1999;303:179–205.

109. Schoolnik GK. Microarray analysis of bacterial pathogenicity. *Adv Microb Physiol* 2002;46:1–45.

110. Behr MA, Wilson MA, Gill WP, et al. Comparative genomics of BCG vaccines by whole-genome DNA microarray. *Science* 1999;284:1520–1523.

111. Kivi M, Liu X, Raychaudhuri S, et al. Determining the genomic locations of repetitive DNA sequences with a whole-genome microarray: IS*6110* in *Mycobacterium tuberculosis*. *J Clin Microbiol* 2002;40:2192–2198.

112. Wilson M, DeRisi J, Kristensen HH, et al. Exploring drug-induced alterations in gene expression in *Mycobacterium tuberculosis* by microarray hybridization. *Proc Natl Acad Sci U S A* 1999;96:12833–12838.

113. Fisher MA, Plikaytis BB, Shinnick TM. Microarray analysis of the *Mycobacterium tuberculosis* transcriptional response to the acidic conditions found in phagosomes. *J Bacteriol* 2002;184:4025–4032.

114. Sherman DR, Voskuil M, Schnappinger D, et al. Regulation of the *Mycobacterium tuberculosis* hypoxic response gene encoding a-crystallin. *Proc Natl Acad Sci U S A* 2001;98:7534–7539.

115. Troesch A, Nguyen H, Miyada CG, et al. *Mycobacterium* species identification and rifampin resistance testing with high-density DNA probe arrays. *J Clin Microbiol* 1999;37:49–55.

116. Calder KM, Horwitz MA. Identification of iron-regulated proteins of *Mycobacterium tuberculosis* and cloning of tandem genes encoding a low iron-induced protein and a metal transporting ATPase with similarities to two-component metal transport systems. *Microb Pathogen* 1998;24:133–143.

117. Lee B-Y, Horwitz MA. Identification of macrophage and stress-induced proteins of *Mycobacterium tuberculosis*. *J Clin Invest* 1995;96:245–249.

118. Jungblut PR, Schaible UE, Mollenkopf HJ, et al. Comparative proteome analysis of *Mycobacterium tuberculosis* and *Mycobacterium bovis* BCG strains: towards functional genomics of microbial pathogens. *Mol Microbiol* 1999;33:1103–1117.

119. Mollenkopf HJ, Jungblut PR, Raupach B, et al. A dynamic two-dimensional polyacrylamide gel electrophoresis database: the mycobacterial proteome via Internet. *Electrophoresis* 1999;20:2172–2180.

120. Jungblut PR, Muller EC, Mattow J, et al. Proteomics reveals open reading frames in *Mycobacterium tuberculosis* H37Rv not predicted by genomics. *Infect Immun* 2001;69:5905–5907.

121. Wong DK, Lee BY, Horwitz MA, et al. Identification of Fur, aconitase, and other proteins expressed by *Mycobacterium tuberculosis* under conditions of low and high concentrations of iron by combined two-dimensional gel electrophoresis and mass spectrometry. *Infect Immun* 1999;67:327–336.

122. Rosenkrands I, Slayden RA, Crawford J, et al. Hypoxic response of *Mycobacterium tuberculosis* studied by metabolic labeling and proteome analysis of cellular and extracellular proteins. *J Bacteriol* 2002;184:3485–3491.

123. Sonnenberg MG, Belisle JT. Definition of *Mycobacterium tuberculosis* culture filtrate proteins by two-dimensional polyacrylamide gel electrophoresis, N-terminal amino acid sequencing, and electrospray mass spectrometry. *Infect Immun* 199765:4515–4524.

124. Helmann JD. Anti-sigma factors. *Curr Opin Microbiol* 1999;2:135–141.

125. Beaucher J, Roderigue S, Jacques P-E, et al. Novel *Mycobacterium tuberculosis* anti-s factor antagonists control s^F activity by distinct mechanisms. *Mol Microbiol* 2002;45:1527–1540.

126. Hoch JA, Silhavy TJ, eds. *Two-component signal transduction*. Washington, DC: American Society of Microbiology Press, 1995.

127. Fuangthong M, Herbig AF, Bsat N, et al. Regulation of the *Bacillus subtilis fur* and *perR* genes by PerR: not all members of the PerR regulon are peroxide inducible. *J Bacteriol* 2002;184:3276–3286.

128. Tao X, Schiering N, Zeng HY, et al. Iron, DtxR, and the regulation of diphtheria toxin expression. *Mol Microbiol* 1994;14:191–197.

129. Gold B, Rodriguez GM, Marras SA, et al. The *Mycobacterium tuberculosis* IdeR is a dual functional regulator that controls transcription of genes involved in iron acquisition, iron storage and survival in macrophages. *Mol Microbiol* 2001;42:851–865.

130. Schmitt MP, Predich M, Doukhan L, et al. Characterization of an iron-dependent regulatory protein (IdeR) of *Mycobacterium tuberculosis* as a functional homolog of the diphtheria toxin repressor (DtxR) from *Corynebacterium diphtheriae*. *Infect Immun* 1995;63:4284–4289.

131. Lee MH, Pascopella L, Jacobs WR Jr, et al. Site-specific integration of mycobacteriophage L5: integration-proficient vectors for *Mycobacterium smegmatis, Mycobacterium tuberculosis*, and bacille Calmette–Guérin. *Proc Natl Acad Sci U S A* 1991;88:3111–3115.

132. Hughes TR, Marton MJ, Jones AR, et al. Functional discovery via a compendium of expression profiles. *Cell* 2000;102:109–126.

133. Lee ML, Kuo FC, Whitmore GA, et al. Importance of replication in microarray gene expression studies: statistical methods and evidence from repetitive cDNA hybridizations. *Proc Natl Acad Sci U S A* 2000;97:9834–9839.

134. Stover CK, de la Cruz VF, Fuerst TR, et al. New use of BCG for recombinant vaccines. *Nature* 1991;351:456–460.

135. Fields PI, Groisman EA, Heffron F. A *Salmonella* locus that controls resistance to microbicidal proteins from phagocytic cells. *Science* 1989;243:1059–1062.

136. Miller SI, Kukral AM, Mekalanos JJ. A two-component regulatory system (*phoP phoQ*) controls *Salmonella typhimurium* virulence. *Proc Natl Acad Sci U S A* 1989;86:5054–5058.

137. Fang FC, Libby SJ, Buchmeier NA, et al. The alternative s factor KatF (RpoS) regulates *Salmonella* virulence. *Proc Natl Acad Sci USA* 1992;89:11978–11982.

138. Predich M, Doukhan L, Nair G, et al. Characterization of RNA polymerase and two σ-factor genes from *Mycobacterium smegmatis*. *Mol Microbiol* 1995;15:355–366.

139. Gomez M, Nair G, Doukhan L, et al. *sigA*is an essential gene in*Mycobacterium smegmatis. Mol Microbiol* 1998;29:617–628.

140. Steyn AJ, Collins DM, Hondalus MK, et al. *Mycobacterium tuberculosis* WhiB3 interacts with RpoV to affect host survival but is dispensable for *in vivo* growth. *Proc Natl Acad Sci U S A* 2002;99:3147–3152.

141. DeMaio J, Zhang Y, Ko C, et al. A stationary-phase stress-response sigma factor from *Mycobacterium tuberculosis. Proc Natl Acad Sci U S A* 1996;93:2790–2794.

142. Chen P, Ruiz RE, Li Q, et al. Construction and characterization of a *Mycobacterium tuberculosis* mutant lacking the alternate sigma factor gene, sigF. *Infect Immun* 2000;68:5575–5580.

143. DeMaio J, Zhang Y, Ko C, et al. *Mycobacterium tuberculosis sigF* is part of a gene cluster with similarities to the*Bacillus subtilis sigF* and *sigB* operons. *Tuber Lung Dis* 1997;78:3–12.

144. Paget MSB, Kang J-G, Roe J-H, et al. σR, an RNA polymerase sigma factor that modulates expression of the thioredoxin system in response to oxidative stress in *Streptomyces coelicolor* A3(2). *EMBO J* 1998;17:5776–5782.

145. Kang JG, Paget MS, Seok YJ, et al. RsrA, an anti-sigma factor regulated by redox change. *EMBO J* 1999;18:4292–4298.

146. Paget MS, Molle V, Cohen G, et al. Defining the disulphide stress response in *Streptomyces coelicolor* A3(2): identification of the sigma R regulon. *Mol Microbiol* 2001;42:1007–1020.

147. Raman S, Song T, Puyang X, et al. The alternative sigma factor SigH regulates major components of oxidative and heat stress responses in *Mycobacterium tuberculosis. J Bacteriol* 2001;183:6119–6125.

148. Groisman EA. The pleiotropic two-component regulatory system PhoP-PhoQ. *J Bacteriol* 2001;183:1835–1842.

149. Perez E, Samper S, Bordas Y, et al. An essential role for *phoP* in *Mycobacterium tuberculosis* virulence. *Mol Microbiol* 2001;41:179–187.

150. Ewann F, Jackson M, Pethe K, et al. Transient requirement of the PrrA-PrrB two-component system for early intracellular multiplication of *Mycobacterium tuberculosis. Infect Immun* 2002;70:2256–2263.

151. Zahrt TC, Deretic V. An essential two-component signal transduction system in *Mycobacterium tuberculosis. J Bacteriol* 2000;182:3832–3838.

152. Boon C, Li R, Qi R, et al. Proteins of *Mycobacterium bovis* BCG induced in the Wayne dormancy model. *J Bacteriol* 2001;183:2672–2676.

153. Mayuri, Bagchi G, Das TK, et al. Molecular analysis of the dormancy response in *Mycobacterium smegmatis*: expression analysis of genes encoding the DevR-DevS two component system, Rv3134c and chaperone a-crystalline homologues. *FEMS Microbiol Lett* 2002;211:231–237.

154. Bucca G, Hindle Z, Smith CP. Regulation of the *dnaK* operon of *Streptomyces coelicolor* A3(2) is governed by HspR, an autoregulatory repressor protein. *J Bacteriol* 1997;179:5999–6004.

155. Spohn G, Scarlato V. The autoregulatory HspR repressor protein governs chaperone gene transcription in *Helicobacter pylori. Mol Microbiol* 1999;34:663–674.

156. Gomez, M, Smith, I. Determinants of mycobacterial gene expression. In: Hatfull GF, Jacobs WR, eds. *Molecular genetics of mycobacteria*. Washington, DC: ASM Press, 2000:111–129.

157. Young D, Lathigra R, Hendrix R, et al. Stress proteins are immune targets in leprosy and tuberculosis. *Proc Natl Acad Sci USA* 1988;85:4267–4270.

158. Taneja B, Mande SC. Metal ions modulate the plastic nature of *Mycobacterium tuberculosis* chaperonin-10. *Protein Eng* 2001;14:391–395.

159. Pohl E, Holmes RK, Hol WG. Crystal structure of the iron-dependent regulator (IdeR) from *Mycobacterium tuberculosis* shows both metal binding sites fully occupied. *J Mol Biol* 1999;285:1145–1156.

160. Manabe YC, Saviola BJ, Sun L, et al. Attenuation of virulence in *Mycobacterium tuberculosis* expressing a constitutively active iron repressor. *Proc Natl Acad Sci U S A* 1999;96:12844–12848.

161. Hondalus MK, Bardarov S, Russell R, et al. Attenuation of and protection induced by a leucine auxotroph of *Mycobacterium tuberculosis. Infect Immun* 2000;68:2888–2898.

162. McAdam RA, Weisbrod TR, Martin J, et al. *In vivo* growth characteristics of leucine and methionine auxotrophic mutants of *Mycobacterium bovis* BCG generated by transposon mutagenesis. *Infect Immun* 1995;63:1004–1012.

163. Bange FC, Brown AM, Jacobs WR Jr. Leucine auxotrophy restricts growth of *Mycobacterium bovis* BCG in macrophages. *Infect Immun* 1996;64:1794–1799.

164. Smith DA, Parish T, Stoker NG, et al. Characterization of auxotrophic mutants of *Mycobacterium tuberculosis* and their potential as vaccine candidates. *Infect Immun* 2001;69:1142–1150.

165. Jackson M, Phalen SW, Lagranderie M, et al. Persistence and protective efficacy of a *Mycobacterium tuberculosis* auxotroph vaccine. *Infect Immun* 1999;67:2867–2873.

166. Moncrief MB, Maguire ME. Magnesium and the role of MgtC in growth of *Salmonella typhimurium. Infect Immun* 1998;66:3802–3809.

167. Buchmeier N, Blanc-Potard A, Ehrt S, et al. A parallel intraphagosomal survival strategy shared by *Mycobacterium tuberculosis* and *Salmonella enterica. Mol Microbiol* 2000;35:1375–1382.

168. Quadri LE, Sello J, Keating TA, et al. Identification of a *Mycobacterium tuberculosis* gene cluster encoding the biosynthetic enzymes for assembly of the virulence-conferring siderophore mycobactin. *Chem Biol* 1998;5:631–645.

169. De Voss JJ, Rutter K, Schroeder BG, et al. The salicylate-derived mycobactin siderophores of *Mycobacterium tuberculosis* are essential for growth in macrophages. *Proc Natl Acad Sci U S A* 2000;97:1252–1257.

170. Ratledge C, Ewing M. The occurrence of carboxymycobactin, the siderophore of pathogenic mycobacteria, as a second extracellular siderophore in *Mycobacterium smegmatis. Microbiology* 1996;142:2207–2212.

171. Litwin CM, Calderwood SB. Role of iron in regulation of virulence genes. *Clin Microbiol Rev* 1993;6:137–149.

172. Lounis N, Truffot-Pernot C, Grosset J, et al. Iron and *Mycobacterium tuberculosis* infection. *J Clin Virol* 2001;20:123–126.

173. Wayne LG. Dormancy of *Mycobacterium tuberculosis* and latency of disease. *Eur J Clin Microbiol Infect Dis* 1994;13:908–914.

174. Weber I, Fritz C, Ruttkowski S, et al. Anaerobic nitrate reductase (*narGHJI*) activity of *Mycobacterium bovis* BCG *in vitro* and its contribution to virulence in immunodeficient mice. *Mol Microbiol* 2000;35:1017–1025.

175. Fritz C, Maass S, Kreft A, et al. Dependence of *Mycobacterium bovis* BCG on anaerobic nitrate reductase for persistence is tissue specific. *Infect Immun* 2002;70:286–291.

176. Segal W, Bloch H. 1956. Biochemical differentiation of *Mycobacterium tuberculosis* grown *in vivo* and *in vitro. J Bacteriol* 1956;72:132–141.

177. Wayne LG, Lin KY. Glyoxylate metabolism and adaptation of *Mycobacterium tuberculosis* to survival under anaerobic conditions. *Infect Immun* 1982;37:1042–1049.

178. McKinney JD, Bentrup KHZ, Munoz-Elias EJ, et al. Persistence of *Mycobacterium tuberculosis* in macrophages and mice requires the glyoxalate shunt enzyme isocitrate lyase. *Science* 2000;406:735–738.

179. Raynaud C, Guilhot C, Rauzier J, et al. Phospholipases C are involved in the virulence of *Mycobacterium tuberculosis. Mol Microbiol* 2002;45:203–217.

180. Heym B, Stavropoulos E, Honore N, et al. Effects of overex-

pression of the alkyl hydroperoxide reductase AhpC on the virulence and isoniazid resistance of *Mycobacterium tuberculosis*. *Infect Immun* 1997;65:1395–1401.

181. Li Z, Kelley C, Collins F, et al. Expression of *katG* in *Mycobacterium tuberculosis* is associated with its growth and persistence in mice and guinea pigs. *J Infect Dis* 1998;177:1030–1035.

182. Zahrt TC, Song J, Siple J, et al. Mycobacterial FurA is a negative regulator of catalase-peroxidase gene katG. *Mol Microbiol* 2001;39:1174–1185.

183. Pym AS, Domenech P, Honore N, et al. Regulation of catalase-peroxidase (KatG) expression, isoniazid sensitivity and virulence by furA of *Mycobacterium tuberculosis*. *Mol Microbiol* 2001;40:879–889.

184. Sherman DR, Sabo PJ, Hickey MJ, et al. Disparate responses to oxidative stress in saprophytic and pathogenic mycobacteria. *Proc Natl Acad Sci U S A* 1995;92:6625–6629.

185. Dussurget O, Stewart G, Neyrolles O, et al. Role of *Mycobacterium tuberculosis* copper-zinc superoxide dismutase. *Infect Immun* 2001;69:529–533.

186. Piddington DL, Fang FC, Laessig T, et al. Cu,Zn superoxide dismutase of *Mycobacterium tuberculosis* contributes to survival in activated macrophages that are generating an oxidative burst. *Infect Immun* 2001;69:4980–4987.

187. Brennan PJ, Nikaido H. The envelope of mycobacteria. *Annu Rev Biochem* 1995;64:29–63.

188. Daffe M, Draper P. The envelope layers of mycobacteria with reference to their pathogenicity. *Adv Microb Physiol* 1998;39:131–203.

189. Andersen P. Effective vaccination of mice against *Mycobacterium tuberculosis* infection with a soluble mixture of secreted mycobacterial proteins. *Infect Immun* 1994;62:2536–2544.

190. Braunstein M, Belisle J. Genetics of protein secretion. In: Hatfull GF, Jacobs WR, eds. *Molecular genetics of mycobacteria*. Washington, DC: American Society for Microbiology, 2000: 203–220.

191. Wayne LG, Hayes LG. An *in vitro* model for sequential study of shiftdown of *Mycobacterium tuberculosis* through two stages of nonreplicating persistence. *Infect Immun* 1996;64:2062–2069.

192. Yuan Y, Crane DD, Simpson RM, et al. The 16-kDa a-crystallin (Acr) protein of *Mycobacterium tuberculosis* is required for growth in macrophages. *Proc Natl Acad Sci U S A* 1998;95:9578–9583.

193. Yuan Y, CraneDD, Barry CE III. Stationary phase-associated protein expression in *Mycobacterium tuberculosis*: function of the mycobacterial alpha-crystallin homolog. *J Bacteriol* 1996;178:4484–4492.

194. Skjot RL, Oettinger T, Rosenkrands I, et al. Comparative evaluation of low-molecular-mass proteins from *Mycobacterium tuberculosis* identifies members of the ESAT-6 family as immunodominant T-cell antigens. *Infect Immun* 2000;68:214–220.

195. Wards BJ, de Lisle GW, Collins DM. An esat6 knockout mutant of *Mycobacterium bovis* produced by homologous recombination will contribute to the development of a live tuberculosis vaccine. *Tuber Lung Dis* 2000;80:185–189.

196. Brosch R, Gordon SV, Marmiesse M, et al. A new evolutionary scenario for the *Mycobacterium tuberculosis* complex. *Proc Natl Acad Sci U S A* 2002;99:3684–3689.

197. Berthet FX, Rasmussen PB, Rosenkrands I, et al. A *Mycobacterium tuberculosis* operon encoding ESAT-6 and a novel low-molecular-mass culture filtrate protein (CFP-10). *Microbiology* 1998;144:3195–3203.

198. Renshaw PS, Panagiotidou P, Whelan A, et al. Conclusive evidence that the major T-cell antigens of the *Mycobacterium tuberculosis* complex ESAT-6 and CFP-10 form a tight, 1:1 complex and characterization of the structural properties of ESAT-6, CFP-10, and the ESAT-6*CFP-10 complex. Implications for pathogenesis and virulence. *J Biol Chem* 2002;277:21598–21603.

199. Thoma-Uszynski S, Stenger S, Takeuchi O, et al. Induction of direct antimicrobial activity through mammalian toll-like receptors. *Science* 2001;291:1544–1547.

200. Noss EH, Pai RK, Sellati TJ, et al. Toll-like receptor 2-dependent inhibition of macrophage class II MHC expression and antigen processing by 19-kDa lipoprotein of *Mycobacterium tuberculosis*. *J Immunol* 2001;167:910–918.

201. Lathigra R, Zhang Y, Hill M, et al. Lack of production of the 19-kDa glycolipoprotein in certain strains of *Mycobacterium tuberculosis*. *Res Microbiol* 1996;147:237–249.

202. Mahenthiralingam E, Marklund BI, Brooks LA, et al. Site-directed mutagenesis of the 19-kilodalton lipoprotein antigen reveals no essential role for the protein in the growth and virulence of *Mycobacterium intracellulare*. *Infect Immun* 1998;66:3626–3634.

203. Yeremeev VV, Lyadova IV, Nikonenko BV, et al. The 19-kD antigen and protective immunity in a murine model of tuberculosis. *Clin Exp Immunol* 2000;120:274–279.

204. Yeremeev VV, Stewart GR, Neyrolles O, et al. Deletion of the 19kDa antigen does not alter the protective efficacy of BCG. *Tuber Lung Dis* 2000;80:243–247.

205. Brightbill HD, Libraty DH, Krutzik SR, et al. Host defense mechanisms triggered by microbial lipoproteins through toll-like receptors. *Science* 1999;285:732–736.

206. Neufert C, Pai RK, Noss EH, et al. *Mycobacterium tuberculosis* 19-kDa lipoprotein promotes neutrophil activation. *J Immunol* 2001;167:1542–1549.

207. Post FA, Manca C, Neyrolles O, et al. *Mycobacterium tuberculosis* 19-kilodalton lipoprotein inhibits *Mycobacterium smegmatis*-induced cytokine production by human macrophages *in vitro*. *Infect Immun* 2001;69:1433–1439.

208. Nau GJ, Richmond JF, Schlesinger A, et al. Human macrophage activation programs induced by bacterial pathogens. *Proc Natl Acad Sci U S A* 2002;99:1503–1508.

209. Berthet F, Rauzier J, Lim EM, et al. Characterization of the *Mycobacterium tuberculosis* erp gene encoding a potential cell surface protein with repetitive structures. *Microbiology* 1995;141:2123–2130.

210. Berthet FX, Lagranderie M, Gounon P, et al. Attenuation of virulence by disruption of the *Mycobacterium tuberculosis* erp gene. *Science* 1998;282:759–762.

211. Azad AK, Sirakova TD, Fernandes ND, et al. Gene knockout reveals a novel gene cluster for the synthesis of a class of cell wall lipids unique to pathogenic mycobacteria. *J Biol Chem* 1997;272:16741–16745.

212. Dubey VS, Sirakova TD, Kolattukudy PE. Disruption of msl3 abolishes the synthesis of mycolipanoic and mycolipenic acids required for polyacyltrehalosesynthesis in *Mycobacterium tuberculosis* H37Rv and causes cell aggregation. *Mol Microbiol* 2002;45:1451–1459.

213. Camacho LR, Constant P, Raynaud C, et al. Analysis of the phthiocerol dimycocerosate locus of *Mycobacterium tuberculosis*. Evidence that this lipid is involved in the cell wall permeability barrier. *J Biol Chem* 2001;276:19845–19854.

214. Belisle JT, Vissa VD, Sievert T, et al. Role of the major antigen of *Mycobacterium tuberculosis* in cell wall biogenesis. *Science* 1997; 276:1420–1422.

215. Armitige LY, Jagannath C, Wanger AR, et al. Disruption of the genes encoding antigen 85A and antigen 85B of *Mycobacterium tuberculosis* H37Rv: effect on growth in culture and in macrophages. *Infect Immun* 2000;68:767–778.

216. Horwitz MA, Harth G, Dillon BJ, et al. Recombinant bacillus Calmette–Guérin (BCG) vaccines expressing the *Mycobacterium tuberculosis* 30-kDa major secretory protein induce

greater protective immunity against tuberculosis than conventional BCG vaccines in a highly susceptible animal model. *Proc Natl Acad Sci U S A* 2000;97:13853–13858.

217. Yuan Y, Barry CE III. A common mechanism for the biosynthesis of methoxy and cyclopropyl mycolic acids in *Mycobacterium tyberculosis. Proc Natl Acad Sci U S A* 1996;93: 12828–12833.

218. Dubnau E, Laneelle M-A, Soares S, et al. *Mycobacterium bovis* BCG genes involved in the biosynthesis of cyclopropyl keto- and hydroxy-mycolic acids. *Mol Microbiol* 1997;23: 313–322.

219. Hunter SW, Gaylord H, Brennan PJ. Structure and antigenicity of the phosphorylated lipopolysaccharide antigens from the leprosy and tubercle bacilli. *J Biol Chem* 1986;261: 12345–12351.

220. Chan J, Ran X, Hunter SW, et al. Lipoarabinomannan, a possible virulence factor involved in persistence of *Mycobacterium tuberculosis* within macrophages. *Infect Immun* 1991;59:1755–1761.

221. Gordon SV, Eiglmeier K, Garnier T, et al. Genomics of *Mycobacterium bovis. Tuberculosis* 2001;81:157–163.

222. Barry CE III. Preclinical candidates and targets for tuberculosis therapy. *Curr Opin Invest Drugs* 2001;2:198–201.

223. von Reyn CF, Vuola JM. New vaccines for the prevention of tuberculosis. *Clin Infect Dis* 2002;35:465–474.

224. Dubos R, Dubos J. *The white plague.* Boston: Little, Brown and Company, 1952.

11

LABORATORY DIAGNOSIS

BRUCE A. HANNA

In the first edition of this book, written more than 8 years ago, I began this chapter with the following quote from Riviere's *The Early Diagnosis of Tubercule*, published in 1921: "In the diagnosis of pulmonary tuberculosis examination, and constantly repeated examination, of the sputum must be carried out." (1). At that time, I suggested that despite the great advances in clinical microbiology since that time, this advice on the rigors of detecting *Mycobacterium tuberculosis* in clinical material remained essential. In this update, I try to assess the significant changes in the laboratory detection of mycobacteria and perhaps see whether we can finally improve on the path urged by Riviere.

The insidious increase in the incidence of tuberculosis in the United States during the early 1990s quickly put to rest the notion that tuberculosis was a disease that the developed world need not be concerned about. As can readily be seen in Table 11.1, from a nadir in 1978, the number of cases of tuberculosis in the city of New York dramatically increased, reaching a peak in 1992. If there can be any, albeit oblique, gain from the resurgence in tuberculosis in the developed world, perhaps it is the renewed interest in the development of laboratory methods for the detection and isolation of mycobacteria. As a result, several new techniques and instruments have been developed and marketed that dramatically improve the speed and reliability with which clinical laboratories can isolate and characterize mycobacteria. This chapter reviews these developments, with an emphasis on those current laboratory methods for detecting *M. tuberculosis* in human clinical material.

LABORATORY SERVICE LEVELS

Because mycobacteriology laboratory techniques are very elaborate and require substantial expertise, the full range of services should not be offered by all laboratories. Yet

prompt and economic access to proficient services is essential to manage the individual patient and to safeguard the public health. It has become increasingly popular, therefore, to consolidate such services among laboratories. In 1982, the American Thoracic Society, recognizing the complex nature of mycobacteriology, recommended a level of service approach to laboratory testing (2). More recently, the American Thoracic Society reaffirmed this position and advised that only those laboratories having a sufficient volume of work and assured competence should provide clinical mycobacteriology services (3). Furthermore, those laboratories without the proper facilities to ensure biologic safety should refer all mycobacteriology specimens to an appropriate specialist. Only those laboratories with biologic safety level 3 facilities and an adequate number of specimens to make daily processing feasible should attempt to perform acid-fast smears and culture. Some laboratories may consider using a referral center for more complex procedures, such as species identification and drug testing.

TABLE 11.1. INCIDENCE OF TUBERCULOSIS IN NEW YORK CITY

Year	No. of Cases	Incidence/ 100,000	No. of Cases MDRTB
1978	1,307	17.2	—
1990	3,520	49.8	—
1991	3,673	50.2	366 (10%)
1992	3,811	52	441 (11%)
1993	3,235	44.2	296 (9%)
1994	2,995	40.9	176 (6%)
1995	2,245	33.4	109 (4.3%)
1996	2,053	28	84 (4.1%)
1997	1,730	23.6	56 (3.1%)
1998	1,558	21.3	38 (2.4%)
1999	1,460	19.9	31 (2.1%)
2000	1,332	16.6	25 (1.9%)

MDRTB, multidrug-resistant strains of tuberculosis.
Data from the City of New York Department of Health.

B.A. Hanna: Departments of Pathology and Microbiology, New York University School of Medicine; Department of Pathology, Bellevue Hospital, New York, New York.

LABORATORY SAFETY

A carefully developed and implemented infection control policy and an appreciation of the concept of universal precautions are fundamental for the protection of all laboratory personnel, especially those working in mycobacteriology. Central to such a policy is an annual health assessment for each employee. In the laboratory, mycobacteriology personnel should be required to wear protective garb and perform all tasks with specimens or cultures in a properly functioning biologic safety cabinet under negative pressure to the laboratory or in a centrifuge with containers that are sealed to prevent leakage. These infection control precautions are commonly referred to as biologic safety level 3. It should be intrinsic in all activities to guard against the generation of aerosols that may contain infectious particles. Rigorous attention to the decontamination of work areas and general orderliness of the laboratory and a detailed understanding of mycobacteriology laboratory design and safety are critical to the protection of personnel (4).

SPECIMEN COLLECTION AND TRANSPORT

With the widespread emergence of multidrug resistant strains of *M. tuberculosis* (MDRTB) in the early 1990s, the need to isolate, identify, and characterize isolates recovered from human clinical material became even more important. In general, the principles used to collect specimens examined for other microbes also apply to specimens examined for the presence of mycobacteria. In particular, it is always easiest to recover microorganisms before starting patients on antimicrobial agents. Sterile, leakproof containers without fixative should be used for collection and quickly transported to the laboratory where examination should be performed on the day of receipt. If brief storage is necessary, specimens other than blood should be refrigerated to inhibit the growth of contaminating microorganisms. General guidelines for the collection of various types of specimens are listed in Table 11.2.

Because sputum is the most frequently examined specimen for the detection of acid-fast bacilli, some additional caveats are in order. It is important to evaluate a sufficient number of specimens from each patient to ensure recovery of even low numbers of mycobacteria. From patients with a productive cough, three to six specimens collected on different days are usually adequate. For patients whose smears are negative for acid-fast bacilli, additional samples may be necessary for successful cultivation of the organism. Although sputum may be collected in a sterile, wide-mouth container, a commercially available device that incorporates a 50-mL disposable centrifuge tube (BD Falcon Sputum Collection System, Becton Dickinson Microbiology Systems, Sparks, MD, U.S.A.) provides a secure collection, transport, and processing system in a single unit. For patients who are unable to produce a deep cough sample, sputum induction by the inhalation of sterile saline solution may be necessary. Induced sputum samples should be clearly labeled so that they are not mistaken for saliva. When sputum is unavailable or the findings are consistently negative in patients with convincing clinical evidence of tuberculosis, gastric lavage may be necessary. Such specimens must reach the laboratory promptly, however, because mycobacteria do not survive for extended periods in the acidic gastric washings. If a delay in processing is unavoidable, the specimens should be neutralized with the addition of 10% sodium carbonate.

Although it is common practice to evaluate sputum specimens for quality before bacterial culture, no such standards or conventions have been applied to mycobacteriology. A study of 873 sputum specimens examined and categorized based on the ratio of squamous epithelial cells to neutrophils found that the usual criteria for routine bacterial culture were not helpful in the evaluation of specimen quality for mycobacterial culture (5). Conversely, these investigators reported that when sputum specimens were categorized according to the presence of neutrophils alone,

TABLE 11.2. SPECIMENS FOR EXAMINATION

Specimen	Procedure
Aspirates, fluids	Sterile syringe, container, or direct inoculation to culture media
Blood, bone marrow	Direct inoculation to broth culture media designed for mycobacterial blood cultures or lysis centrifugation system
Bronchial washings	Sterile container
Gastric lavage	50 mL of gastric aspirate in sterile container with 100 mg of sodium carbonate
Sputum	Exudate from lungs by a productive cough (not saliva), sterile container
Stool	Clean container
Tissues, biopsy specimens	Sterile container
Urine	First morning void; do not pool

more than 90% of the positive smears and cultures were found in the group that contained neutrophils.

SPECIMEN PREPARATION

Specimens that are normally expected to be sterile, such as blood, biopsy tissue, bone marrow, and aspirated fluid, may be inoculated directly to culture media. Conversely, specimens that may be contaminated with normal flora microorganisms require digestion and decontamination before inoculation to culture media to prevent the overgrowth of these more rapidly growing microbes. In addition to its normal flora, sputum may also contain mucin and other material that may bind mycobacteria and inhibit their recovery. Because all digestion and decontamination procedures are toxic to microbial cells, including mycobacteria, the goal is to eliminate the normal flora while doing as little harm as possible to the hardier mycobacteria.

Several methods for the digestion and decontamination of specimens are available, and although there is no clear consensus among microbiologists as to which is ideal, some advantages are apparent. The most commonly used and widely preferred reagent is sodium hydroxide (NaOH) usually in combination with *N*-acetyl-L-cysteine or occasionally dithiothreitol. Although NaOH is effective as both a mucolytic and a decontaminating agent, concentrations of as much as 4% are required for maximal efficiency. At this concentration, however, excessive mycobacterial toxicity may develop. By adding as much as 2% of the mucolytic agent *N*-acetyl-L-cysteine, rapid digestion of mucin-rich sputum can be followed by effective decontamination with as little as 2% NaOH. It is important for the laboratory to monitor the overall rate of specimen contamination. The goal is not to reduce this rate to zero because that would indicate that too many mycobacteria are being lost in the decontamination process. Rather, between 2% and 5% of specimens should be found to be overgrown by normal flora. If over time contamination rates are more than 5%, the method used is likely inadequate, whereas if the rate is less than 2%, it is too harsh (4,6). In the mycobacteriology laboratory of Bellevue Hospital Center in New York, we have found the procedure outlined in Table 11.3 results in an acceptable level of contaminants yet is not overly harsh. Other agents that have found acceptance among some laboratories and under some circumstances are Zephiran-trisodium phosphate, oxalic acid, and cetylpyridinium chloride. Complete discussions of these methods are provided in recent technical manuals (4,6). In addition to these methods, sodium dodecyl (lauryl) sulfate in combination with NaOH is occasionally used in Europe (7,8).

After digestion and decontamination, the specimen must be centrifuged to sediment the mycobacteria. The relative centrifugal force (RCF) and time selected for sedimentation of the sample after decontamination will greatly affect the probability of recovery of mycobacteria that may be present. Although there is some disagreement as to the ideal combination of time and RCF, it is clear that both must be monitored closely. It is not enough to measure centrifuge rotor speed [in revolutions per minute (rpm)] alone without knowing the RCF, which is expressed in g units and is a true measure of the sedimenting efficiency. The RCF is unique to each centrifuge because it is a function of the radius and angle of the rotor and may be calculated from the formula $RCF = 1.12 R_{max} (rpm/1,000)^2$, where R_{max} is the radius in millimeters from the center of the rotating head to the bottom of the rotating centrifuge (4). For any given centrifuge and rotor configuration, the number of rpm needed to achieve the desired RCF may be calculated from the following formula (4):

$$rpm = 1,000 \sqrt{RCF/1.12 R_{max}}.$$

In a retrospective study of more than 14,500 specimens, the sensitivity of acid-fast smears and cultures was found to

TABLE 11.3. PROCESSING OF SPUTUM BY METHOD USING *N*-ACETYL-L-CYSTEINE AND SODIUM HYDROXIDE

Per liter of digestant mix:

Reagent A	4% NaOH	500 mL
Reagent B	2.9% sodium citrate dehydrate or 2.6% sodium citrate anhydrous	500 mL
Reagent C	NALC	5 gm

1. Mix reagents A and B, sterilize, and store for later use.
2. Just before use, add reagent C. Use within 24 hr.
3. Transfer 10 mL of sputum or less to a 50-mL plastic screw-capped centrifuge tube. Add an equal volume of the NALC-NaOH solution.
4. Cap the tube tightly and mix it vigorously until the solution is liquified (approximately 5 to 20 seconds on a test tube mixer). Let stand for 15 minutes at room temperature.
5. Add sterile distilled water. Mix by inversion and centrifuge in a safety-shielded rotor (3,000 g for 15 minutes).
6. Pour off supernatant into a splash-proof vessel containing a disinfectant.
7. Disinfect the lip of the tube and resuspend the sediment in 1 to 2 mL of sterile saline solution.
8. Mix gently and inoculate appropriate culture media.

NALC, *N*-acetyl-L-cysteine; NaOH, sodium hydroxide.

improve when the RCF during sedimentation was increased from 1,260 *g* to 3,800 *g* (9). In a more recent study using split samples, an improved sensitivity was noted when the RCF was increased from 2,074 *g* to 3,005 *g*; however, no further increase was found with an RCF as high as 3,895 *g* (10).

Such increased forces, however, raise the concern of excessive heat, especially with prolonged spin cycles, and a refrigerated centrifuge may be necessary. In addition, as speeds increase, one should also be aware of the possible rupture of the centrifuge tubes. Currently, the minimal recommended centrifugation criterion is 3,000 *g* for 15 minutes (6).

ACID-FAST SMEAR

Although less sensitive than culture, the acid-fast smear is an essential and rapid adjunct to the diagnosis of tuberculosis. In one study of paired specimens obtained before treatment from patients with pulmonary tuberculosis, a specimen with a count of 10^4 colony-forming units per milliliter is more likely to result in a positive smear, whereas a negative smear is likely if the count is lower (11). Nonetheless, whether by light or fluorescence microscopy, the acid-fast smear examination is specific, rapid, and simple to perform. Although a single smear of a respiratory specimen has a reported sensitivity of between only 22% and 43%, when multiple specimens are examined, the detection rate improves and as many as 96% of patients with pulmonary tuberculosis may be detected by acid-fast smear examination (6). The sensitivity of smears derived from other specimen sources, however, is

lower (12). It should be pointed out, however, that although in a survey of public health laboratories (13), 29 of respondents preferred the Ziehl–Neelsen or Kinyoun stain, the use of a fluorochrome dye such as auramine O is superior. Because fluorochrome-stained smears are viewed under high dry magnification rather than the oil immersion magnification required by fuchsin-stained smears, they may be examined more rapidly and efficiently. Furthermore, with a fluorochrome dye, mycobacteria seen as staining bright against a dark background are easier to detect; hence, smears examined by this method have been found to have a greater sensitivity than those stained with fuchsin (14). Detailed formulas and procedures for the preparation of the stains and proper performance of the acid-fast smear can be found in standard reference manuals (4,6).

The acid-fast smear remains of enormous value in the primary care setting because, in the hands of a trained microbiologist, it is easy to perform and reliably interpreted. A flow chart for the preparation of Kinyoun- (cold carbolfuchsin), Ziehl–Neelsen-, and fluorochrome-stained smears and a list of suppliers for commercially prepared reagents is provided in Table 11.4.

Regardless of the staining technique used, it is important for the laboratory staff to be vigilant when examining acid-fast smears. The frequency and morphology of acid-fast bacilli found in specimens can be quite variable. If the interpretation of a fluorochrome-stained smear is in doubt, a Ziehl–Neelsen- or Kinyoun-stained smear should be examined for evaluation of microscopic morphology (Figures 11.1–11.4). It is also essential to develop quantitative crite-

TABLE 11.4. PREPARATION OF ACID-FAST SMEARS BY THREE METHODS

Steps	Kinyoun	Ziehl–Neelsen	Fluorochrome
1. Apply specimen	Apply specimen to central area of slide and allow to air dry	Apply specimen to central area of slide and allow to air dry	Apply specimen to central area of slide and allow to air dry
2. For all 3 methods	Fix by immersing in absolute methanol for 1 min	Fix by immersing in absolute methanol for 1 min	Fix by immersing in absolute methanol for 1 min
3. Primary stain	Kinyoun carbolfuchsin, 2 min	Carbolfuchsin, cover with filter paper, heat to steaming, let stand 5 min, remove paper	Auramine O or auramine-rhodamine, 15 min
4. Rinse	Rinse gently with water and drain excess from slide	Rinse gently with water and drain excess from slide	Rinse gently with water and drain excess from slide
5. Decolorize	3% acid-alcohol until color no longer runs from slide	3% acid-alcohol until color no longer runs from slide	0.5% acid-alcohol, 2 min
6. Rinse	Rinse gently with water and drain excess from slide	Rinse gently with water and drain excess from slide	Rinse gently with water and drain excess from slide
7. Counterstain	Methylene blue or brilliant green, 30 sec	Methylene blue or brilliant green, 30 sec	Acridine orange or potassium permanganate, 2 min
8. Rinse	Rinse gently with water and drain excess from slide	Rinse gently with water and drain excess from slide	Rinse gently with water and drain excess from slide
9. Dry	Allow slide to air dry without blotting	Allow slide to air dry without blotting	Allow slide to air dry without blotting
10. Examine thoroughly	1,000×	1,000×	Screen 200–400×, confirm 600–1,000×

Reagents for the acid-fast stains may be obtained from Becton-Dickinson Microbiology Systems, Cockeysville, MD; Difco Laboratories, Detroit, MI; and Remel Laboratories, Lenexa, KS.

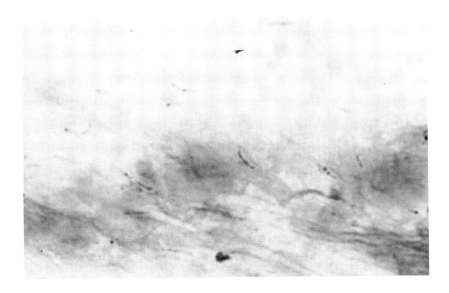

FIGURE 11.1. Kinyoun-stained smear of sputum concentrate, showing numerous acid-fast bacilli displaying the typical beaded appearance of *Mycobacterium tuberculosis* (original magnification, ×1,000).

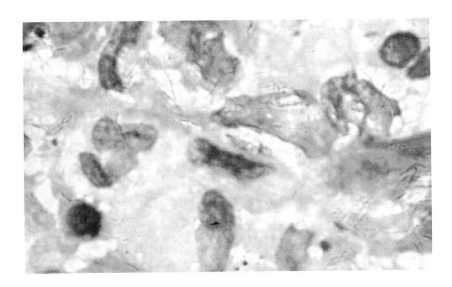

FIGURE 11.2. Kinyoun-stained smear of specimen concentrate, showing numerous acid-fast bacilli. While digestion procedures will disrupt the tendency toward cord formation, the aggregates shown here are suggestive of *Mycobacterium tuberculosis* (original magnification, ×1,000).

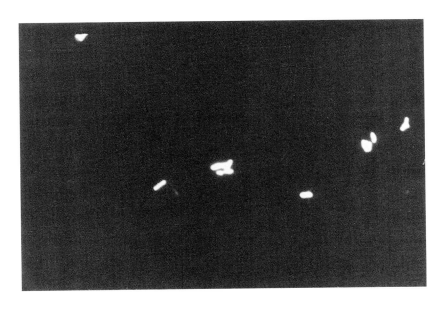

FIGURE 11.3. Auramine O–stained smear of sputum concentrate, showing numerous acid-fast bacilli (original magnification, ×1,000).

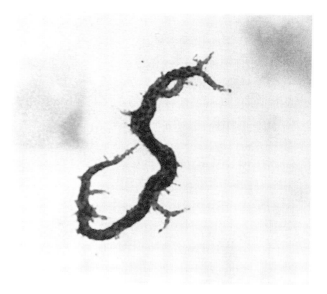

FIGURE 11.4. Kinyoun-stained smear from broth culture of Mycobacterium tuberculosis showing cored formation (original magnification, ×1,000)

ria for reporting smear results. Correlations for fuchsin-stained smears examined at 1,000× versus fluorochrome-stained smears examined at various magnifications are available (4). In the mycobacteriology laboratory of Bellevue Hospital Center, we have found that the interpretive criteria listed in Table 11.5, if carefully applied to rigorously examined smears regardless of the staining method, provide useful clinical information. Although smears remain an important adjunct to the detection of *M. tuberculosis*, they are not an adequate criterion alone and must be followed by culture, both to confirm species identity and drug susceptibility.

LABORATORY CULTIVATION OF *MYCOBACTERIUM TUBERCULOSIS*

Among the great advances in mycobacteriology during the 20th century is the development of solid growth media such as the Middlebrook, Lowenstein–Jensen (LJ), and others. The main advantage of solid media is that they allow the

TABLE 11.5. INTERPRETATION OF ACID-FAST SMEARS

No. of Acid-Fast Bacilli Seen	Result
0	None seen
1–2/slide	Doubtful
3–9/slide	Rare
>10/slide	Few
>1/field	Numerous

determination of characteristic features of colonial morphology, growth rate, and pigment production, which can yield significant preliminary information. Solid media also incorporate malachite green and may be made more selective by the addition of antimicrobial agents, all of which help to suppress the normal contaminating flora. There are proponents for each type of medium, and although not all strains of mycobacteria can be recovered on a single substrate, it is widely recommended and generally accepted that one solid medium substrate should be a part of any primary isolation protocol (6). Among the egg-based media, the most popular in clinical laboratories is LJ, whereas the somewhat more selective Petragnani is preferred in reference and public health laboratories where prolonged transport may lead to specimens more heavily contaminated with normal flora. Among the agar-based media, which are transparent (vs. the opaque LJ), Middlebrook 7H10 and 7H11 formulations provide good performance and may be modified for susceptibility testing and biochemical identification.

Solid media alone, however, are not sufficient for rapid detection of mycobacteria because as long as several weeks of incubation may be necessary for the visible detection of organisms. Substantial improvement in the time to detection and the total number of positive cultures can be realized from using a broth-based growth system. The first broth-based mycobacterial detection system was the BACTEC 460 (BBL; Becton Dickinson Microbiology Systems), which uses a modified Middlebrook broth and a novel radiometric detection scheme. In this system, 4 mL of Middlebrook 7H12 broth containing carbon 14 (^{14}C)–labeled palmitic acid and a supplement of antibiotics (PANTA antibiotic mixture, BBL) is inoculated with 0.5 mL of the processed specimen and the vial incubated in the usual fashion. In this manner, growth can periodically be ascertained by the liberation of $^{14}CO_2$ as metabolized by the mycobacteria and detected by the BACTEC 460 instrument. With the BACTEC system, the average time to the recovery of *M. tuberculosis* from smear-positive specimens is 8 days compared with 18 days for conventional media (15). When culture-positive, smear-negative samples were examined, the mean time to detection with the BACTEC was 14 days compared with 26 days for conventional media (16). For more than 20 years, the BACTEC 460 was the only truly rapid mycobacterial detection system available and even today remains the standard against which others must be compared. However, because sample reading with the BACTEC 460 is not automated, it is a very labor-intensive system, and concern about radioactive waste disposal issues has prompted the development of newer methods.

One of the earlier methods was the ISOLATOR tube (Wampole Laboratories, Princeton, NJ, U.S.A.) that provides a unique approach to the recovery of mycobacteria from blood. Approximately 10 mL of blood is collected into the ISOLATOR tube containing an anticoagulant and saponin, which lyses the red blood cells, releasing any microbes within. After centrifugation, the sediment can be used to inoculate a variety of mycobacterial media. Although the ISOLATOR has been reported to be particularly helpful in recovering *Mycobacterium avium-intracellulare complex* from blood (17), more recent studies indicate the lysis centrifugation fluid may actually inhibit the growth of *M. avium-intracellulare complex* (18).

In the biphasic Septi-Chek AFB (BBL; Becton, Dickinson and Company), broth and solid media are combined into a single device. Septi-Chek AFB contains 20 mL of modified Middlebrook 7H9 broth in a carbon dioxide–enriched culture bottle. After inoculation of the sample, the bottle is capped with a slide containing three solid media: a nonselective Middlebrook 7H11 agar, an egg-based medium, and chocolate agar. Although as sensitive as the BACTEC 460, the time to detection for the Septi-Chek AFB is somewhat longer (19).

The first of the new generation of growth detection systems is the Mycobacteria Growth Indicator Tube (MGIT, BBL; Becton, Dickinson and Company). MGITs contain 4.5 mL of enriched Middlebrook 7H9 broth with an oxygen-sensitive fluorescent sensor to indicate growth in sufficient quantity so that the mycobacteria may be identified by AccuProbe (Gen-Probe, San Diego, CA, U.S.A.) on the day of detection. In general, the sensitivity and time to detection of mycobacteria in the MGIT are comparable with that of the BACTEC 460 (20). Thus, the MGIT offers the advantage of a rapid and reliable detection system without the need for sophisticated equipment. Although not indicated for the recovery of mycobacteria from blood, the MGIT has been shown to provide greatly improved recovery and time to detection over those with solid media (21). A unique observation made during the study of the MGIT was that the time to a culture signal may provide insight into the prognosis for the patient. In one study, a dissociation in the time to detection of mycobacterial growth was observed in patients for whom sequential samples were tested (22). Based on the time to MGIT detection of *M. tuberculosis*, two groups of patients became apparent. In one group whose disease was resolving, a consistent monotonic relationship was observed between the elapsed time from the patient's first specimen and the time to detection of positive growth in the MGIT containing the current specimen. In the second group, in whom clinical improvement was delayed, the time to detection in the MGIT remained brief and constant during the course of the study.

The development of fully automated, continuously monitored incubator-reader systems has significantly improved mycobacteriology laboratory workflow. In a similar fashion to the manual systems, after the sample is processed and inoculated into the growth vial or test tube, it is placed into an incubator-reader module. According to proprietary methods and algorithms, vials are scanned continuously and monitored for growth. When the instrument detects a positive growth signal, the vial is flagged by an instrument display and may be removed for staining and identification in the usual fashion. At present, four such systems are available: the BACTEC 9000 MB and the high-capacity BACTEC MGIT 960 (Becton, Dickinson and Company), the MB/BacT (Organon Teknika Corporation, Durham, NC, U.S.A.), and the ESP II (TREK Diagnostic Systems, Inc., Cleveland, OH, U.S.A.). Although the two BACTEC systems use the same fluorescent technology as the MGIT, the MB/BacT uses a colorimetric CO_2 sensor, whereas the ESP II detects pressure changes in the vial head space. Each of these systems offers significant advantages over manual methods and, with subtle differences, performance characteristics comparable with the BACTEC 460. The reader is urged to review the published reports of the system evaluations for in-depth analyses of each system (23–26). In addition to the routine media used by these systems, a BACTEC MYCO/F lytic medium specifically designed for the BACTEC 9000 instrument has made blood cultures for mycobacteria compatible with commonly available instrumentation (27). These systems have also been developed for drug susceptibility testing, as discussed later.

Despite the advantages of the broth-based cultivation systems, traditional solid media have an important role in the recovery of mycobacteria. In a study of 1,184 respiratory specimens inoculated to both liquid and solid media, no single medium resulted in recovery of all 143 isolates (28). Although the BACTEC 12B provided the highest percentage (93%) of *M. tuberculosis* isolates recovered, the concomitant use of either 7H11 or LJ media increased the recovery of mycobacteria by 4% to 6%.

IDENTIFICATION OF *MYCOBACTERIUM TUBERCULOSIS*

Among the characteristics useful for the species identification are growth rate, colony morphology, and pigmentation. Mycobacteria that form visible colonies on solid media within 1 week are called growers and those that require longer are called slow growers. Mycobacteria that produce a yellow-orange (carotenoid) pigment only when grown in the light but not when grown in the dark are known as photochromogens. Those that produce a carotenoid pigment regardless of whether they are grown in the light or dark are known as scotochromogens, whereas those that do not display a pigment or only a pale yellow-tan hue that does not intensify on exposure to light are nonchromogens. Originally described by Runyon (29), these cultural characteristics can provide a presumptive identification schema for mycobacteria (6).

The conventional or biochemical approach to the identification of mycobacteria is similar to the methods used to identify other microorganisms. By determining the rate of growth, colonial and microscopic morphology, and biochemical characteristics of an isolate and comparing these findings with archetype species descriptions, identification can be accomplished by a consensus of agreement. Although there is a trend toward more sophisticated methods of identification, there are many instances in which conventional methods are sufficient and even preferable. Among the most germane preliminary observations that the laboratory can make of a newly detected isolate are the simplest. For example, a slow-growing, nonpigmented, rough colony with a tendency toward cord formation is quite likely *M. tuberculosis* (30).

Confirmation of *M. tuberculosis* requires that an isolate display positive reactions on the niacin production and nitrate reduction tests. As mycobacteria grow, they produce niacin. Virtually all strains of *M. tuberculosis* and occasional strains of *Mycobacterium chelonae* and *Mycobacterium simiae* are unable to metabolize the niacin produced, and it tends to be secreted into the surrounding growth medium where it can be detected. Although there are several methods of detecting the niacin, all of them require the addition of cyanogen bromide, a compound that requires care in handling. The nitrate reduction test measures the ability of a strain to produce the enzyme nitrate reductase and reduce sodium nitrate to sodium nitrite. Essentially all strains of *M. tuberculosis* are nitrate positive as are *Mycobacterium kansasii* and *Mycobacterium szulgai*. These tests are rapid, easy to perform, and the two most useful biochemical determinants for the rapid identification of *M. tuberculosis*. A strain displaying positive reactions for both the niacin and the nitrate test may be identified as *M. tuberculosis* with a high degree of confidence. In a study by the Centers for Disease Control and Prevention of control *M. tuberculosis* strains, 95% were found to be niacin positive and 97% were nitrate positive (31).

The various catalase tests may be used to provide corroboration. The results of both the semiquantitative catalase test and the test for catalase at 68°C should be negative for *M. tuberculosis*. It should be noted that when the catalase test is performed by the classical method in which a drop of Tween 80–hydrogen peroxide is placed directly on a colony, virtually all mycobacteria display positive reactions, with the notable exception of isoniazid-resistant strains, including those of *M. tuberculosis* (6). Although this is an intriguing observation, its reliability as a predictor of drug resistance has not been tested.

Also useful in the separation of *M. tuberculosis* from another members of the *M. tuberculosis* complex, such as *Mycobacterium bovis*, is the thiophen-2-carboxylic acid hydrazide susceptibility test (32). Strains susceptible to less than 5 µg/mL of thiophen-2-carboxylic acid hydrazide are likely *M. bovis*. In addition, *M. tuberculosis* strains typically display negative reactions for Tween hydrolysis, Tween opacity, tellurite reduction, and arylsulfatase production at 3 and 14 days and will not grow in the presence of 5% NaCl or on MacConkey agar. Conversely, positive reactions for the production of pyrazinamidase and urease are typical

TABLE 11.6. BIOCHEMICAL TESTS USEFUL FOR THE IDENTIFICATION OF *MYCOBACTERIUM TUBERCULOSIS*

Biochemical Test	Reaction of *M. Tuberculosis*
Niacin production	Positive
Nitrate reduction	Positive
Catalase production	
At 68°C	Negative
Semiquantitative	Negative
TCH susceptibility	Resistant
Tween hydrolysis	Negative
Tellurite reduction	Negative
Arylsulfatase production	Negative
Pyrazinamidase production	Positive
Tolerance of 5% sodium chloride	Negative
Growth on MacConkey agar	Negative

TCH, thiophen-2-carboxylic acid hydrazide.

of *M. tuberculosis*. A detailed description of the methods and interpretation for these and other techniques for the identification of clinically important mycobacteria is provided in standard references (4,6). For the convenience of the reader, a brief summary of biochemical tests useful for the conventional identification of *M. tuberculosis* is provided in Table 11.6.

A procedure unique to the BACTEC system for the identification of the *M. tuberculosis* complex is based on the observation that *p*-nitro-α-acetylamino-β-hydroxypropiophenone (NAP) will inhibit organisms belonging to the *M. tuberculosis* complex while having little or no effect on other mycobacteria. A test organism inoculated to a BACTEC NAP vial (BBL) containing a 5-µg NAP disk displaying a significant increase in the growth index over a 5-day incubation period would tend to rule out *M. tuberculosis* complex organisms (33).

A reliable method for identifying mycobacteria is the use of chromatography for analysis of the fatty acids extracted from the mycobacterial cell wall and then methylated to form volatile esters. When analyzed by high-performance liquid chromatography (34), gas-liquid chromatography (35), thin-layer chromatography (36), the resulting fatty acid profiles can be compared with a library of those from known species. Chromatographic techniques are quite accurate and are able to identify many of the mycobacterial species. The commercially available gas-liquid chromatography system that includes hardware and software by Microbial ID, (Newark, DE, U.S.A.) has been reported to perform well (37).

Nucleic Acid Probe Assays

First introduced in 1987, clinical microbiology laboratories have adopted probe assays to speed the identification of *M. tuberculosis*. Early probe kits provided an iodine 125 ([125I])–labeled strand of DNA that was complementary to, and specific for, the ribosomal RNA (rRNA) of the target microbial group. Following a fairly straightforward lysis procedure, the rRNA was released from the test organism and reacted with the ^{125}I DNA probe. The resulting ^{125}I DNA-rRNA hybrid was then detected easily. Because there are many copies of rRNA per cell and a large number of cells was used to perform the assay, these probes were found to have high specificity and sensitivity for the identification of mycobacteria from primary cultures (38). Today, nonradiolabeled DNA probes, especially the synthetic oligonucleotide probes targeting rRNA, have a major role in the identification of medically important microorganisms, not the least of which is *M. tuberculosis*. Probe hybridization analysis offers significant advantages over conventional methods for slow-growing organisms such as mycobacteria for which identification by the methods described above is time-consuming. The acridinium ester–labeled AccuProbe system (Gen-Probe) for identification of the *M. tuberculosis* complex, the *M. avium-intracellulare complex*, *Mycobacterium gordonae*, and *M. kansasii* can identify an isolate within a single working day and have excellent specificity and sensitivity (39).

If there is a single qualification for the use of the AccuProbe, however, it is that the *M. tuberculosis* complex also includes *M. bovis*, *M. bovis* BCG, *Mycobacterium africanum*, and *Mycobacterium microti*; thus, it cannot distinguish between these species (40). More recently, false-positive reactions with *Mycobacterium terrae* also have been reported (41). In addition to direct probe analysis, nucleic acid sequencing can provide significant information, including identification and epidemiologic profiling. By amplifying the 16S rRNA gene and comparing the hypervariable regions with known sequences, the test organism may be identified (42).

SUSCEPTIBILITY TESTING OF *MYCOBACTERIUM TUBERCULOSIS*

The emergence of MDRSTB in the early 1990s emphasized the need for laboratories to perform susceptibility tests on all initial patient isolates. Because *M. tuberculosis* can spontaneously mutate developing resistance to antituberculous drugs, isolates from patients who continue to have positive cultures and from those whose disease has relapsed during or after therapy should also be tested. In addition to the immediate benefit in planning a therapeutic regimen, such information is of value to the public health. In areas that serve patient populations in which drug resistance is prevalent, rapid culture detection followed by dependable susceptibility testing is essential. In some cases, the direct screening of smear-positive sputum for susceptibility to the first-line or primary drugs isoniazid, rifampin, streptomycin, ethambutol, and pyrazinamide (PZA) by a rapid method provides a strategic advantage for the treatment and control of tuberculosis. Several second-line drugs useful in

the treatment of MDRSTB can also be tested by an indirect method after the microorganism has been successfully cultivated in the laboratory.

Rapid, reliable, and comprehensive susceptibility testing of mycobacteria, however, is complex, laborious, and fraught with the potential for error and as such may not be within the expertise of all laboratories. The choice of methods and drugs to be tested requires careful consideration. The cited references in this section should be consulted for the intricacies of these techniques. Clearly, laboratories that do not have a sufficient number of specimens to test or cannot make a commitment to a rigorously controlled protocol for antituberculous drug testing should send newly isolated cultures of *M. tuberculosis* to a reference laboratory.

The principles of *M. tuberculosis* drug testing established four decades ago by Canetti et al. (43,44) have evolved over time. These complex techniques were reviewed elsewhere in detail (45–47) and are summarized here. In brief, random mutants of *M. tuberculosis* occur spontaneously and independently of drug exposure. The definition of resistance is, therefore, founded on the notion that if a proportion of a clinical isolate displays a significantly diminished susceptibility to a critical concentration of a drug, as compared with a wild strain that has not previously been exposed to antituberculous drugs, the clinical response to that drug is tenuous. By convention in the United States, an isolate is considered susceptible if the proportion of resistant cells does not exceed 1% of the total population. The critical concentration of a given drug, however, varies according to the method and growth medium used in the assay, and each requires careful selection.

Although there are many versions of *M. tuberculosis* susceptibility tests, it is useful to distinguish between two inclusive categories: direct and indirect tests, each of which may be performed by either conventional or rapid methods. As the name implies, the inoculum for the direct tests is the processed clinical specimen in which acid-fast bacilli have been observed (i.e., smear-positive sputum). The specimen may be diluted according to the number of acid-fast bacilli seen in the smear and used directly as the inoculum for the susceptibility test. The inoculum for the indirect test, conversely, is the primary isolate culture. There are advantages and limitations to each method. Although direct tests provide results sooner and the inoculum is a true representative of the bacterial population *in situ*, it may be difficult to ensure a uniform distribution of bacilli in the inoculum. For the indirect test, preparation of a uniform inoculum is easier; however, it is essential to avoid selecting a predominant population of resistant or susceptible cells in a subculture. This bias can be minimized by preparing a dilution of the entire growth of the subculture for use as the inoculum.

The conventional methods may be performed as direct or indirect tests by inoculating the microorganisms to a solid medium that contains a known concentration of the test drug. For each of the methods described, test concentrations of drugs may be prepared in the medium by appropriate dilutions of stock solutions of antimicrobial drugs. For the disk modification of these tests, the test concentrations are achieved by incorporating the necessary number of commercially available antimicrobial drug–containing elution disks into the medium.

There are three commonly used conventional methods. The absolute concentration method is one in which a carefully standardized suspension of the isolate is inoculated to a drug-free control and to multiple concentrations of the drugs to be tested. This technique most closely resembles a minimal inhibitory concentration (MIC) test in that the result is expressed in terms of the lowest concentration of drug that inhibits growth of the isolate. In a similar fashion, the resistance ratio method compares the MIC of the test isolate with that of a control strain, usually H37Rv, performed concurrently. Results of the test isolate are expressed as a ratio of MIC of the test isolate to that of the control strain. In general, a ratio of 8 or higher suggests that the isolate is resistant, whereas a ratio of 2 or lower indicates susceptibility.

The most commonly used conventional technique in the United States is the proportion method with its various modifications. Common to all variations, dilutions of the inoculum are made so that growth on control media results in the production of a number of colonies that can be counted (i.e., 50 to 100). The test is performed in a replicate for each dilution of the inoculum. In this manner, the number of colonies that grow on the drug-containing media is counted and compared with the number of organisms calculated to have been in the inoculum. Thus, the proportion of organisms resistant to a drug can be measured and expressed as a percentage of the total population. The Centers for Disease Control and Prevention modification of the proportion method, especially the disk modification of that method performed in quadrant plates of Middlebrook 7H10 agar supplemented with oleic acid, albumin, dextrose, and catalase, has been recommended by the National Committee for Clinical Laboratory Standards as the standard medium for this method (47).

It should be noted that susceptibility tests for PZA can be performed in conventional media only at a reduced pH of approximately 5.5, at which point some strains of *M. tuberculosis* will not grow. It is recommended, therefore, that PZA be tested by the BACTEC 460 method, which is described. Essential to all susceptibility tests, regardless of method, are the critical concentrations of the drugs to be tested. Listed in Table 11.7 are the critical concentrations for several popular methods: the Centers for Disease Control and Prevention version of the proportion method (4), the National Jewish modification of the proportion method (45), and the modified proportion agar dilution test as recommended in the *Manual for Clinical Microbiology* (46). It should be noted that all these methods are performed in Middlebrook 7H10 agar, except for the National Jewish

TABLE 11.7. CRITICAL CONCENTRATIONS (μGML) OF DRUGS TESTED BY THE PROPORTION METHOD

Drug	CDC (4)	National Jewish (45)	ASM (7H10) (46)
Isoniazid	0.2	0.2	0.2, 1
Streptomycin	2	2	2, 10
Ethambutol	5	7.5	5, 10
Rifampin	1	1	1
Pyrazinamide			25, 50
p-Aminosalicylic acid		2.0	2
Ethionamide	5	10	5
Kanamycin	5	6	5
Capreomycin	10	10	10
D-Cycloserine	20	30	30

ASM, American Society for Microbiology; CDC, Centers for Disease Control and Prevention.
Data from Kent PT, Kubica GP. *Public health mycobacteriology:* a guide for the Level III Laboratory. Atlanta: U.S. Department of Health and Human Services, Centers for Disease Control, 1985; Heifets LB, ed. *Drug susceptibility in the chemotherapy of mycobacterial infections.* Boca Raton: CRC Press, 1991; and Inderlied C, Salfinger M. Antimycobacterial agents and susceptibility tests. In: Murray PR, Baron EJ, Phaller MA, et al., eds. *Manual of clinical microbiology, 7th ed.* Washington, DC: American Society for Microbiology, 1999:1601–1623.

version, which specifies 7H11 agar. Critical concentrations for the drugs listed, however, may be different if other growth media are used.

Results for any of the modifications of the proportion method should be read weekly for 3 weeks after inoculation and may be reported as the percentage of the test population observed to be resistant to the test concentration of the drug compared with the control quadrant. If more than 1% of the test population is resistant to the drug being tested, it should be considered that resistance to that drug has developed or is in an advanced stage of development (4). By reporting the interpretation and the percentage of the resistant population, the laboratory may provide an effective guide for a therapeutic regimen.

During the early 1980s, the BACTEC acid-fast bacilli radiometric system for the primary isolation of mycobacteria was adapted to a susceptibility test protocol (48–50). Because the BACTEC method was already well established as a rapid cultivation and detection system, the adaptation to drug testing offered increased speed in the detection of resistant strains. In contrast to the 3 weeks required for the interpretation of results by the conventional methods, BACTEC results are available in as little as 4 to 6 days after inoculation. The BACTEC method can be performed as a direct or an indirect test using the BACTEC 12B vial containing Middlebrook 7H12 broth at the drug test concentrations listed in Table 11.8 (46). In this manner, the BACTEC system provides rapid results with a high correlation with the proportion method. A particular advantage of the BACTEC system is the ability to readily test for susceptibility to PZA. When a modified BACTEC 12B vial

TABLE 11.8. CRITICAL CONCENTRATIONS (µGML) OF DRUGS TESTED BY THE BACTEC 460 METHOD

Drugs	Concentrations
For direct or indirect tests	
Isoniazid	0.1, 0.4
Streptomycin	2, 6
Pyrazinamide	100
Ethambutol	2.5, 7.5
Rifampin	2
For indirect tests only	
p-Aminosalicylic acid	4
Ethionamide	5
Kanamycin	5
Capreomycin	5
D-Cycloserine	50

Data from Kent PT, Kubica GP. *Public health mycobacteriology: a guide for the level III laboratory.* Atlanta: U.S. Department of Health and Human Services, Centers for Disease Control, 1985; and Metchock BG, Nolte FS, Wallace RJ. Mycobacterium. In: Murray PR, Baron EJ, Phaller MA, et al., eds. *Manual of clinical microbiology*, 7th ed. Washington, DC: American Society for Microbiology, 1999:399–437.

adjusted to pH 6.0 is used, results obtained are consistent with those from other methods (51).

Among the developments is a recently reported new agar medium with which to perform PZA susceptibility testing (52). With an acidic pH of 6.0 and the addition of animal serum instead of oleic acid, albumin, dextrose, and catalase, good growth of *M. tuberculosis* using a critical concentration of 900 or 1,200 µg PZA per milliliter made it possible to differentiate between PZA-susceptible and -resistant clinical isolates and determine the actual proportion of resistant bacteria in the isolate.

Arguably, the greatest stimulus to the clinical laboratory has been a result of the increasing incidence of MDRSTB. The search for simpler and quicker drug susceptibility test methods was begun with the MGIT as a screen for susceptibility to isoniazid and rifampin in clinical isolates of *M. tuberculosis* directly from specimens and indirectly from primary culture (53).

The simple and rapid MGIT system, without the need for complex instrumentation, can provide those laboratories, particularly in the developing areas of the world where the incidence of MDRSTB is the highest, access to modern drug susceptibility methods. Several comparative studies of the MGIT drug susceptibility method have recently been published (53–58). Importantly, in these studies, the time to detect resistance with the MGIT method was comparable with that for the BACTEC system.

With the advent of the automated growth and detection systems previously described, the adaptation to drug susceptibility testing was a natural development. Protocols and evaluations for primary drug susceptibility testing of isoniazid, rifampin, streptomycin, and ethambutol using the automated instrument platforms BACTEC MGIT 960, TSP II, and MB/BacT have recently been published (59–65). All these systems, which are commercially avail-

able in the United States and the rest of the world, have similar performance characteristics and are comparable in speed with the BACTEC 460.

A novel method for the detection, identification, and susceptibility testing of *M. tuberculosis*, the luciferase reporter mycobacteriophages (LRPs), has also been reported as a rapid method that may have potential applications in the clinical laboratory (66). In a study of 523 sputum samples cultivated in Middlebrook 7H9, MGIT, and LJ media, 71 mycobacterial isolates were recovered as follows; 76% with the LRPs, 97% with the MGIT 960 method, and 90% with LJ. The median time to detection of bacteria was 7 days with both the LRPs and the MGIT 960 method. In this same study, the accuracy and speed of LRP antibiotic susceptibility testing with rifampin, streptomycin, isoniazid, and ethambutol were compared with those of the BACTEC 460 method. Among 50 *M. tuberculosis* isolates, agreement between the LRP and BACTEC 460 results was 98.5%; however, the LRP susceptibility turnaround time was only 2 days compared with 10.5 days with the BACTEC 460 method.

Laboratory Caveats

It is fitting to conclude this section on the laboratory detection and characterization of *M tuberculosis* with some sobering caveats. Although the preceding techniques have become much more automated than they were just a decade ago, the potential for serious laboratory error during all stages of the processing and examination is great. For example, in a review of all laboratory isolates of *M. tuberculosis* recovered in New York City during in 1 month, 3% of patients had false-positive cultures as a result of laboratory error (67). There is the potential for cross-contamination to occur at many stages during the initial processing of the specimens and during the examination of cultures. Laboratory staff must be vigilant to guard against the generation of aerosols during these stages and be especially mindful of patients from whom multiple samples are examined and are all smear negative but only one sample becomes culture positive. These "smear negative–one positive" patients should be viewed in light of the potential for cross-contamination from either specimens or cultures processed at the same time. It is advisable in such circumstances to seek epidemiologic typing of the isolates in question (68). Several techniques have been reported that use DNA fingerprinting using the IS6110 repetitive insertion sequence and other methods, all of which have been reviewed elsewhere (6).

Characteristics of Various Species of Mycobacteria

As our methods have improved, so have our discoveries, many of which ask as many questions as they answer. For example, at Bellevue Hospital Center, soon after we added a liquid detection system to our solid media, we observed a striking increase in *Mycobacterium xenopi* isolates. Recovery of *M. xenopi* went from 29 isolates from 1975 to 1990, using LJ and Middlebrook, to 12 isolates in 1990 to 1994, using the Septi-Check AFB System, to 381 isolates from 1995 to 1998, using the MGIT. It was not clear, however, whether this represented a true increase in incidence or whether it was a result of the improved culture media. A chart review of all patients with positive cultures for *M. xenopi* revealed in our case that the dramatic surge in *M. xenopi* isolates was predominantly owing to more sensitive laboratory techniques and was not truly the harbinger of an emerging pathogen (69). In a similar fashion, in the period 1990 to 2000, 32 new nontuberculous mycobacterial species have been discovered and characterized, bringing the number of species in the genus to almost 100 (70). All may be cultivated *in vitro* with the exception of *Mycobacterium leprae*, which appears to have undergone reductive evolution and gene decay (71).

REFERENCES

1. Riviere C. *The early diagnosis of tubercle*, 3rd ed. London: Oxford Medical, 1921.
2. Hawkins JE, Good RC, Kubica GP, et al. Levels of laboratory services for mycobacterial diseases: official statement of the American Thoracic Society. *Am Rev Respir Dis* 1982;128:213.
3. The official statement of The American Thoracic Society and The Centers for Disease Control and Prevention. *Am J Respir Crit Care Med* 2000;161:1376–1395.
4. Kent PT, Kubica GP. *Public health mycobacteriology: a guide for the level III laboratory*. Atlanta: U.S. Department of Health and Human Services, Centers for Disease Control, 1985.
5. McCarter YS, Robinson A. Quality evaluation of sputum specimens for mycobacterial culture. *Am J Clin Pathol* 1996;105: 769–773.
6. Metchock BG, Nolte FS, Wallace RJ. Mycobacterium. In: Murray PR, Baron EJ, Phaller MA, et al., eds. *Manual of clinical microbiology*, 7th ed. Washington, DC: American Society for Microbiology, 1999:399–437.
7. Engbaek HC, Vergmann B, Bentzon MW. The sodium lauryl sulphate method in culturing sputum for mycobacteria. *Scand J Respir Dis* 1967;48:268–284.
8. Salfinger M, Kafader FM. Comparison of two pretreatment methods using sodium dodecyl (lauryl) sulfate-sodium hydroxide and *N*-acetyl-L-cysteine-sodium hydroxide for the detection of mycobacteria on BACTEC and Löwenstein slants. *J Microbiol Methods* 1987;6:315–321.
9. Rickman TW, Moyer NP. Increased sensitivity of acid-fast smears. *J Clin Microbiol* 1980;11:618–620.
10. Ratnam S, March SB. Effect of relative centrifugal force and centrifugation time on sedimentation of mycobacteria in clinical specimens. *J Clin Microbiol* 1986;23:582–585.
11. Allen BW, Mitchison DA. Counts of viable tubercle bacilli in sputum related to smear and culture gradings. *Med Lab Sci* 1992; 49:94–98.
12. Lipsky BJ, Gates J, Tenover FC, et al. Factors affecting the clinical value for acid fast bacilli. *Rev Infect Dis* 1984;6:214–222.
13. Huebner RE, Good RC, Tokars JI. Current practices in mycobacteriology: results of a survey of state public health laboratories. *J Clin Microbiol* 1993;31:771–775.
14. Strumpf IJ, Tsang AY, Sayre JW. Reevaluation of sputum staining for the diagnosis of pulmonary tuberculosis. *Am Rev Respir Dis* 1979;119:599–602.
15. Roberts GD, Goodman NL, Heifets L, et al. Evaluation of the BACTEC radiometric method for recovery of mycobacteria and drug susceptibility testing of *Mycobacterium tuberculosis* from acid-fast smear positive specimens. *J Clin Microbiol* 1983;18: 689–696.
16. Morgan MA, Horstmeier CD, DeYoung DR, et al. Comparison of a radiometric method (BACTEC) and conventional culture media for recovery of mycobacteria from smear negative specimens. *J Clin Microbiol* 1983;18:384–388.
17. Gill VE, Park CH, Stock F, et al. Use of lysis centrifugation (Isolator) and radiometric (BACTEC) blood culture systems for the detection of mycobacteria. *J Clin Microbiol* 1985;22:543–546.
18. Wasilauskas BL, Morrell RM. Isolator component responsible for inhibition of *Mycobacterium avium-M. intracellulare* in BACTEC 12B medium. *J Clin Microbiol* 1997;35:588–590.
19. Sewell D, Rashad W, Rourke W, et al. Comparison of the Septi-Chek AFB and BACTEC systems and conventional culture for recovery of mycobacteria. *J Clin Microbiol* 1993;31:2689–2691.
20. Pfyffer GE, Welscher HM, Kissling P, et al. Comparison of the mycobacteria growth indicator tube (MGIT) with radiometric and solid culture for recovery of acid-fast bacilli. *J Clin Microbiol* 1997;35:364–368
21. Hanna BA, Walters SB, Bonk SJ, et al. Recovery of mycobacteria from blood in the MGIT and Lowenstein-Jensen after lysis-centrifugation. *J Clin Microbiol* 1995;33:3315–3316.
22. Epstein MD, Schluger NW, Davidow N, et al. Time to detection of *Mycobacterium tuberculosis* in sputum culture correlates with outcome in patients receiving treatment for pulmonary tuberculosis. *Chest* 1998;113:379–386.
23. Pfyffer GE, Cieslak C, Welscher HM, et al. Rapid detection of mycobacteria in clinical specimens by using the automated BACTEC 9000 MB system and comparison with radiometric and solid-culture systems *J Clin Microbiol* 1997;35:2229–2234.
24. Woods GL, Fish G, Plaunt M, et al. Clinical evaluation of Difco ESP culture system II for growth and detection of mycobacteria *J Clin Microbiol* 1997;35:121–124.
25. Hanna BA, Ebrahimzadeh A, Elliott LB, et al. Multi-center evaluation of the BACTEC® MGIT(tm) 960 for the recovery of mycobacteria. *J Clin Microbiol* 1999;37:748–752.
26. Roggenkamp A, Hornef MW, Masch A, et al. Comparison of MB/BacT and BACTEC 460 TB systems for recovery of mycobacteria in a routine diagnostic laboratory. *J Clin Microbiol* 1999;37:3711–3712.
27. Waite RT, Woods, GL. Evaluation of BACTEC MYCO/F lytic medium for recovery of mycobacteria and fungi from blood. *J Clin Microbiol* 1998;36:1176–1179.
28. Stager CE, Libonati JP, Siddiqi SH, et al. Role of solid media when used in conjunction with the BACTEC system for mycobacterial isolation and identification. *J Clin Microbiol* 1991; 29:154–157.
29. Runyon EH. Identification of mycobacterial pathogens using colony characteristics. *Am J Clin Pathol* 1970;54:578–586.
30. Yagupsky PV, Kaminski DA, Palmer KM, et al. Cord formation in BACTEC 7H12 medium for rapid, presumptive identification of *Mycobacterium tuberculosis* complex. *J Clin Microbiol* 1990;28:1451–1453.
31. Good RC, Silcox VA, Kilburn JO, et al. Identification and drug susceptibility test results for *Mycobacterium* spp. *Clin Microbiol Newslett* 1985;7:133–135.
32. Vestal AL, Kubica GP. Differential identification of mycobacteria III. Use of thiacetazone, thiophen-2-carboxylic acid hydrazide

and triphenyltetrazolium chloride. *Scand J Respir Dis* 1967;48: 142–148.

33. Morgan MA, Doerr KA, Hempel NL, et al. Evaluation of the *p*-nitro-α-acetylamino-β-hydroxypropiophenone differential test for the identification of *Mycobacterium tuberculosis* complex. *J Clin Microbiol* 1985;21:634–635.

34. Glickman SE, Kilburn JO, Butler WR, et al. Rapid identification of mycolic acid patterns of mycobacteria by high-performance liquid chromatography using pattern recognition software and a *Mycobacterium* library. *J Clin Microbiol* 1994;32:740–745.

35. Tisdall PA, DeYoung DR, Roberts GD, et al. Identification of clinical isolates of mycobacteria with gas-liquid chromatography: a 10-month follow-up study. *J Clin Microbiol* 1982;16:400–402.

36. Laszlo A, Papa F, David HL. Thin-layer chromatography systems for the identification of *Mycobacterium tuberculosis, M. bovis* BCG, *M. kansasii, M. gastri* and *M. marinum. Res Microbiol* 1992;143:519–524.

37. Smid I, Salfinger M. Mycobacterial identification by computer-aided gas-liquid chromatography. *Diagn Microbiol Infect Dis* 1994;19:81–88.

38. Gonzalez R, Hanna BA. Identification of *Mycobacterium tuberculosis* and *Mycobacterium avium-intracellulare* by DNA probe. *Diagn Microbiol Infect Dis* 1987;8:69–77.

39. Alcaide F, Benitez MA, Escriba JM, et al. Evaluation of the BACTEC MGIT 960 and the MB/BacT systems for recovery of mycobacteria from clinical specimens and for species identification by DNA AccuProbe. *J Clin Microbiol* 2000;38:398–401.

40. Heifets L. Gen-Probe test should not be considered final in *Mycobacterium tuberculosis* identification. *J Clin Microbiol* 1989; 27:229.

41. Martin C, Levy-Frebault VV, Cattier B, et al. False positive result of *Mycobacterium tuberculosis* complex DNA probe hybridization with a *Mycobacterium terrae* isolate. *Eur J Clin Microbiol Infect Dis* 1993;12:309–310.

42. Kirschner P, Mier A. Bottger EC. Genotypic identification of mycobacteria—facing novel and uncultured pathogens. In: Persing D, Smith TF, Tenover FC, et al., eds. *Diagnostic molecular microbiology.* Washington, DC: American Society for Microbiology, 1993:173–190.

43. Canetti G, Froman S, Grosset J, et al. Mycobacteria: laboratory methods for testing drug sensitivity and resistance. *Bull World Health Organ* 1963;29:565–578.

44. Canetti G, Rist N, Grosset J. Mesure de la sensibilite du bacille tuberculeux aux drogues antibacillaires par la methode des proportions. *Rev Tuberc* 1963;27:217–272.

45. Heifets LB, ed. *Drug susceptibility in the chemotherapy of mycobacterial infections.* Boca Raton, FL: CRC Press, 1991.

46. Inderlied C, Salfinger M. Antimycobacterial agents and susceptibility tests. In: Murray PR, Baron EJ, Phaller MA, et al., eds. *Manual of clinical microbiology,* 7th ed. Washington, DC: American Society for Microbiology, 1999:1601–1623.

47. National Committee for Clinical Laboratory Standards. *M24-T2 susceptibility testing of mycobacteria,* Nocardia *, and other aerobic actinomycetes; tentative standard,* 2nd ed. Villanova, PA: National Committee for Clinical Laboratory Standards, 2001.

48. Snider DE, Good RC, Kilburn JO, et al. Rapid drug susceptibility testing of *Mycobacterium tuberculosis. Am Rev Respir Dis* 1981; 123:402–406.

49. Siddiqi SH, Libonati JP, Middlebrook G. Evaluation of a rapid radiometric method for drug susceptibility testing of *Mycobacterium tuberculosis. J Clin Microbiol* 1981;13:908–912.

50. Roberts GD, Goodman NL, Heifets L, et al. Evaluation of BACTEC radiometric method for recovery of mycobacteria and drug susceptibility testing of *Mycobacterium tuberculosis* from acid-fast smear positive specimens. *J Clin Microbiol* 1983;18: 689–696.

51. Salfinger M, Reller B, Demchuck B, et al. Rapid radiometric method for pyrazinamide susceptibility testing of *Mycobacterium tuberculosis. Res Microbiol* 1989;140:301–309.

52. Heifets L, Sanchez T. New agar medium for testing susceptibility of *Mycobacterium tuberculosis* to pyrazinamide. *J Clin Microbiol* 2000;38:1498–1501.

53. Walters SB, Hanna BA Testing of susceptibility of *Mycobacterium tuberculosis* to isoniazid and rifampin by mycobacterium growth indicator tube method. *J Clin Microbiol* 1996;34: 1565–1567.

54. Rüsch-Gerdes S, Domehl C, Nardi G, et al. Multicenter evaluation of the mycobacteria growth indicator tube for testing susceptibility of *Mycobacterium tuberculosis* to first-line drugs. *J Clin Microbiol* 1999;37:45–48.

55. Goloubeva V, Lecocq M, Lassowsky P, et al. Evaluation of mycobacteria growth indicator tube for direct and indirect drug susceptibility testing of *Mycobacterium tuberculosis* from respiratory specimens in a Siberian prison hospital. *J Clin Microbiol* 2001;39:1501–1505.

56. Palaci M, Ueki SY, Sato DN, et al. Evaluation of mycobacteria growth indicator tube for recovery and drug susceptibility testing of *Mycobacterium tuberculosis* isolates from respiratory specimens. *J Clin Microbiol* 1996;34:762–764.

57. Piersimoni C, Nista D, Bornigia S, et al. Evaluation of a new method for rapid drug susceptibility testing of *Mycobacterium avium* complex isolates by using the mycobacteria growth indicator tube. *J Clin Microbiol* 1998;36:64–67.

58. Bergmann JS, Woods GL. Reliability of mycobacteria growth indicator tube for testing susceptibility of *Mycobacterium tuberculosis* to ethambutol and streptomycin. *J Clin Microbiol* 1997; 35:3325–3327.

59. Bemer P, Palicova F, Rüsch-Gerdes S, et al. Multicenter evaluation of fully automated BACTEC mycobacteria growth indicator tube 960 system for susceptibility testing of *Mycobacterium tuberculosis. J Clin Microbiol* 2002;40:150–154.

60. Tortoli E, Benedetti M, Fontanelli A, et al. Evaluation of automated BACTEC MGIT 960 system for testing susceptibility of *Mycobacterium tuberculosis* to four major antituberculous drugs: comparison with the radiometric BACTEC 460TB method and the agar plate method of proportion. *J Clin Microbiol* 2002;40: 607–610.

61. Ardito A, Posteraro B, Sanguinetti M, et al. Evaluation of BACTEC mycobacteria growth indicator tube (MGIT 960) automated system for drug susceptibility testing of *Mycobacterium tuberculosis. J Clin Microbiol* 2001;39:4440–4444.

62. Bergmann JS, Woods GL. Evaluation of the ESP culture system II for testing susceptibilities of *Mycobacterium tuberculosis* isolates to four primary antituberculous drugs. *J Clin Microbiol* 1998;36: 2940–2943.

63. Ruiz P, Zerolo FJ, Casal MJ. Comparison of susceptibility testing of *Mycobacterium tuberculosis* using the ESP Culture System II with that using the BACTEC method. *J Clin Microbiol* 2000;38: 4663–4664.

64. Díaz-Infantes MS, Ruiz-Serrano MJ, Martínez-Sánchez L, et al. Evaluation of the MB/BacT Mycobacterium Detection System for susceptibility testing of *Mycobacterium tuberculosis. J Clin Microbiol* 2000;38:1988–1989.

65. Brunello F, Fontana R. Reliability of the MB/BacT System for testing susceptibility of *Mycobacterium tuberculosis* complex isolates to antituberculous drugs. *J Clin Microbiol* 2000;38: 872–873.

66. Banaiee N, Bobadilla-del-Valle M, Bardarov S Jr, et al. Luciferase reporter mycobacteriophages for detection, identification, and antibiotic susceptibility testing of *Mycobacterium tuberculosis* in Mexico. *J Clin Microbiol* 2001;39:3883–3888.

67. Frieden T, Woodley CL, Crawford JT, et al. The molecular epi-

demiology of tuberculosis in New York City: the importance of nosocomial transmission and laboratory error. *Tuber Lung Dis* 1996;77:407–413.

68. Dunlap NE, Harris RH, Benjamin WH, et al. Laboratory contamination of *Mycobacterium tuberculosis* cultures. *Am J Respir Crit Care Med* 1995;152:1702–1704.

69. Donabella V, Salazar-Schicchi J, Bonk S, et al. Increasing incidence of *Mycobacterium xenopi* at Bellevue Hospital. *Chest* 2000; 118:1365–1370.

70. Hale YM, Pfyffer G, Salfinger M. Laboratory diagnosis of mycobacterial infections: new tools and lessons learned. *Clin Infect Dis* 2001;33:834–846.

71. Cole ST, Eiglmeir J, Parkhill KD, et al. Massive gene decay in the leprosy bacillus. *Nature* 2001;409:1007–1011.

12

NOVEL APPROACHES TO THE RAPID DIAGNOSIS OF TUBERCULOSIS

NEIL W. SCHLUGER

In most of the world, the approach to diagnostic testing for tuberculosis has changed little in a qualitative sense in the past 100 years. Clinical suspicion, chest radiographs, staining for acid-fast organisms on expectorated sputum samples, and culture for mycobacteria from sputum specimens together form the diagnostic armamentarium available and in use in most of the world. All these tests, in one form or another, have been used throughout the 20th century and are still widely used at the start of the 21st century.

There is a manifest need for new and better diagnostic tests for tuberculosis. The nature of the need differs, however, in resource-poor and resource-rich countries (1). In poor countries, current approaches to diagnosis leave a significant number of cases undetected. Sputum-smear examination will detect only approximately 50% of cases (with a high estimate of perhaps 70%). When resources are extremely limited, as they are in most of the regions where tuberculosis is most common, focusing on smear-positive cases, which are likely to be the most infectious, makes sense from an economic perspective. However, there are certainly costs involved in the underdiagnosis of tuberculosis. For individuals with smear-negative disease, the reliance on smears means that their cases will go undiagnosed for longer periods and may lead to more morbidity, if not more mortality, from tuberculosis. On a population basis, although smear-positive cases in general are highly infectious, smear-negative cases have been shown using molecular epidemiology techniques to contribute significantly to transmission as well (2). Furthermore, and perhaps of greatest significance, many patients with human immunodeficiency virus infection, particularly those with advanced immunosuppression, are more likely to have smear-negative tuberculosis (3). The consequences of delaying diagnosis in such patients may be very high for individual patients. Because substantial numbers of patients with tuberculosis

also have human immunodeficiency virus infection, particularly in regions such as sub-Saharan Africa, this issue is not trivial.

In resource-rich countries such as the United States, it seems less likely that significant numbers of cases are undiagnosed. However, large numbers of patients are essentially overdiagnosed, i.e., admitted to hospital isolation rooms, started on empirical therapy, and subjected to a variety of expensive and invasive diagnostic procedures. The costs of these approaches, in economic terms and in terms of patient inconvenience and discomfort, are substantial (4). Currently, clinical strategies to improve diagnostic accuracy lack sufficient sensitivity or specificity to be of great clinical utility (5–7).

An ideal diagnostic test for active tuberculosis would have the following characteristics: rapid (results available within a day), high sensitivity and specificity, inexpensive, robust (i.e., able to provide reproducible results in a variety of settings), highly automated (or at least not requiring a great deal of sample preparation or highly technically trained personnel), and able to provide drug susceptibility data. At present, no technology currently in use achieves these goals, although several already licensed products or products in late stages of development represent significant improvements over available methods. For the diagnosis of latent tuberculosis infection, a test that can reliably distinguish between *Mycobacterium tuberculosis* and bacille Calmette–Guérin (BCG) vaccination and infection with other mycobacteria would be highly desirable as well. Recent progress has been made in this area, as is discussed in the following sections. Ideally, such a test could also distinguish between persons with latent infection and those with active disease, a more elusive goal.

TESTS FOR LATENT TUBERCULOSIS INFECTION

The tuberculin skin test, which in one form or another has been in use for a century or more, is somewhat limited in

N. W. Schluger: Departments of Medicine and Epidemiology, Columbia University College of Physicians and Surgeons; Department of Medicine, Division of Pulmonary, Allergy, and Critical Care Medicine, Columbia Presbyterian Medical Center, New York, New York.

its utility. The test cannot distinguish between those with latent infection and those with active disease, there is some cross-reactivity with nontuberculous mycobacteria, BCG vaccination can cause a positive result for at least a few years after administration, false-negative results may occur in patients with anergy, and the test requires skilled personnel for both administration and interpretation.

In developing new tests for latent tuberculosis infection, a major hurdle is the lack of a true gold standard against which a novel diagnostic test can be measured. In the absence of this, the best approach might be to apply the new test to a population in a controlled study and observe all patients positive by the novel and reference tests and determine which more accurately predicts the development of active disease. This approach is limited, however, by both ethical and practical considerations. Another approach is to evaluate a novel test in comparison with a reference standard and to collect demographic information about patients that is as detailed as possible to evaluate the test results in the most informed environment. Recently, a test based on the production of interferon gamma (IFN-γ) from T lymphocytes after stimulation with *M. tuberculosis* proteins was developed (8,9). The rationale for the test lies in the fact that a protective immune response to *M. tuberculosis* has as its hallmark the release of the T_H1-type cytokine IFN-γ from circulating lymphocytes. It has been demonstrated that it is technically feasible to measure IFN-γ in whole-blood samples that have been stimulated *in vitro* with mycobacterial proteins. The best and most comprehensive study of the utility of this assay was recently published by Mazurek et al. (10). This study provides evidence that this new assay may indeed be able to distinguish BCG vaccination from true infection with *M. tuberculosis*, and there seemed to be excellent discrimination between *Mycobacterium avium* and *M. tuberculosis* as well. In the study, 1,226 adults underwent standard tuberculin skin testing and testing with the whole-blood IFN-γ release assay (QuantiFERON-TB, Cellestis Ltd., St. Kilda, Australia). In the cohort, 390 persons had a positive skin test and 349 had a positive IFN-γ assay result. Overall agreement between the two tests was 83.1% (κ = 0.60). Most interesting, however, were the results of a multivariate analysis that aimed to elucidate the factors associated with the test results. In this analysis, the odds of having a positive skin test but negative IFN assay were seven times higher in patients who had received BCG vaccination. In addition, the results indicated that in 21.2% of non–BCG-vaccinated persons with positive skin tests and negative IFN-γ assay results, the skin test result was likely owing to exposure to nontuberculous mycobacteria, probably *M. avium*. The results of this study suggest that the IFN-γ release assay might be more discriminating than skin testing for diagnosing latent tuberculosis infection. However, another recent study found poor agreement between the results of the IFN-γ release assay and tuberculin skin testing, even in patients with a known history of culture-proven, active tuberculosis disease (11). In 21 such patients, the IFN-γ assay had a sensitivity of 71% compared with 95% sensitivity for tuberculin skin testing. The specificity was 85% for IFN-γ release assay and 96% for tuberculin skin testing among 52 subjects with no known history of exposure to tuberculosis.

The test has the advantage of not requiring the patient to return for interpretation (although patients will have to return for initiation of therapy, presumably), but it is somewhat more technically complex than skin testing and probably more expensive. Specificity of the IFN-γ release assay can probably be improved by using more *M. tuberculosis*–specific antigens, such as the early secreted antigen ESAT-6, to stimulate blood samples rather than the tuberculin reagent currently used (12–19).

TESTS FOR ACTIVE TUBERCULOSIS

Broth-Based Culture Systems

It is worth noting that broth-based culture systems, such as BACTEC (BBL; Becton, Dickinson and Company, Sparks, MD, U.S.A.), MGIT (a nonradiometric method) (BBL; Becton, Dickinson and Company), MB/BacT (Organon Teknika Corporation, Durham, NC, U.S.A.), Septi-Check(BBL; Becton, Dickinson and Company), and ESP (TREK Diagnostic Systems, Inc., Cleveland, OH, U.S.A.), when combined with DNA probes for rapid species identification, are capable of producing positive results in 2 weeks or less for the majority of sputum smear–positive specimens and within 3 weeks for smear-negative specimens (20–22). The value of culture is currently unsurpassed because it is the only widely available technology that allows drug susceptibility testing.

Nucleic Acid Amplification Assays

There are currently two nucleic acid amplification (NAA) assays available for commercial use in the United States: MTD (GenProbe, San Diego, CA, U.S.A.) and Amplicor (Roche, Basel, Switzerland), and the MTD test has been approved for use in smear-negative cases when the clinical suspicion is high. The MTD assay is an isothermal strategy for DNA amplification, and the Amplicor kit uses the polymerase chain reaction to amplify nucleic acid targets that uniquely identify *M. tuberculosis* in clinical specimens. Despite these different approaches to amplification of target DNA regions of interest, substantial published experience indicates that the tests are roughly equivalent in clinical use (23,24). Each test accurately diagnoses nearly every case of sputum smear–positive pulmonary tuberculosis, and each diagnoses approximately half of the cases of smear-negative, culture-positive pulmonary tuberculosis. Based on these operating characteristics, the U.S. Food and Drug Administration initially approved these tests for the confirmation of a positive sputum smear in a case of possible pulmonary tuberculosis.

An American Thoracic Society workshop recently asked, regarding the role of rapid diagnostic tests for tuberculosis, "What is the appropriate use?" (25). The published experience with currently available NAA assays indicates that they perform well for the indications for which they were approved, i.e., the reliable confirmation that a sputum smear–positive specimen indeed represents *M. tuberculosis*. However, the literature also suggests that the use of these tests might be greatly expanded and allow more accurate diagnosis of pulmonary tuberculosis generally than is now accomplished (23,24). In a recent comparison of both commercially available NAA assays with conventional smear and culture, the specificity of all techniques was extremely high, but the sensitivity varied widely. For smear, sensitivity was an expected 50%, and for culture, it was nearly 100%. For the NAA assays, sensitivity was in the 80% to 84% range, also an expected value given the repeated demonstration that these tests detect all the smear-positive cases of tuberculosis and approximately half of the smear-negative, culture-positive cases. Thus, the overall accuracy of the NAA assays [(true positives + true negatives)/all test results] was much higher than that of smear and not very much lower than that of culture. Newer versions of these tests appear to have a significantly improved ability to detect smear-negative cases as well (26). In other words, if NAA assays are used to ask the question "Does my patient have active pulmonary tuberculosis?", the answer will be correct 92% to 95% of the time compared with 80% of the time if smears are used. (This will be true as long as the patient in question has no history of recently treated tuberculosis, a setting in which NAA assays may be less accurate.) In fact, if the cost of these assays were low enough, they could and should replace sputum smears for the purpose of making a diagnosis of pulmonary tuberculosis in previously untreated patients if the specificity of the NAA assay were equal to or greater than that of the acid-fast bacilli (AFB) smear, which may in fact be the case in some areas. At present, however, given their cost ($50 to $100 per assay in most laboratories), such use of NAA assays would strain laboratory budgets unbearably. However, in some settings, such as centralized laboratories to which a large number of specimens can be quickly and easily referred, these tests may in fact be economically feasible and clinically useful (27). Some analyses also suggest that there are scenarios in which the use of NAA assays, at particular price points, might be cost-effective in resource-poor countries (28).

The Centers for Disease Control and Prevention recently updated its recommendations for the use of NAA assays for the diagnosis of active tuberculosis (29). They now recommend that an AFB smear and an NAA assay be performed on the first sputum smear collected. If the smear and NAA assay results are both positive, tuberculosis is diagnosed with nearly total certainty. If the smear is positive and the

NAA assay result is negative, the statement recommends testing the sputum for inhibitors by spiking the sputum sample with an aliquot of lysed *M. tuberculosis* and repeating the assay. If inhibitors are not detected, the patient can be presumed to have nontuberculous mycobacteria. If the sputum smear result is negative but the NAA assay result is positive, the Centers for Disease Control and Prevention recommend sending additional sputum samples. If positive, the patient can be presumed to have tuberculosis. If both the smear and NAA assay results are negative, an additional specimen should be tested by NAA assay. If the result is negative, the patient can be presumed not to have infectious tuberculosis. The recommendations conclude by noting that clinicians must always rely on clinical judgment and that, ultimately, definitive diagnosis rests on response to therapy and culture results. Although there is a particular logic to them, these recommendations are expensive and, unfortunately, are based on few published data.

In the view of this author, reasonable use of NAA assays for rapid diagnosis of tuberculosis is as follows: NAA assays should be used to confirm that a positive AFB smear does indeed represent *M. tuberculosis*. If smears are negative, but clinical suspicion is high [based on the impression of experienced observers (6)], an NAA assay should be done on a sputum sample, either expectorated or induced. Although as many as 50% of smear-negative, culture-positive cases may not be rapidly diagnosed in this way, the benefit of rapidly diagnosing a sizable proportion of smear-negative cases is obvious. Such uses of the test in smear-negative cases have been approved by the U.S. Food and Drug Administration for the GenProbe MTD-2 assay. An NAA assay should not be done on sputum samples from patients for whom the clinical index of suspicion is low and the AFB smear is negative.

Several questions about the clinical use of NAA assays remained unanswered. Sputum-smear examination is commonly used to gauge both the infectiousness of a patient and the patient's response to therapy. No data are available regarding the utility of NAA assays for these purposes. In addition, the optimal number of sputum samples needed to exclude tuberculosis as a diagnostic possibility remains undefined, although some studies indicate that two negative NAA assay results on different sputum samples make pulmonary tuberculosis quite unlikely. Moreover, the utility of the NAA assay in extrapulmonary forms of tuberculosis is incompletely defined. It appears that NAA assays are more sensitive than smears in these cases, although not sensitive enough to exclude tuberculosis as a diagnostic possibility if negative (30,31). Thus, for example, although a cerebrospinal fluid sample with a positive NAA assay result can be considered presumptively to represent a case of tuberculous meningitis, a negative NAA assay result from the cerebrospinal fluid of a patient in whom the diagnosis is likely considered from a clinical standpoint cannot reliably be used to exclude the diagnosis (32). At present, these tests certainly cannot replace cultures.

RAPID DETECTION OF DRUG RESISTANCE

In parts of the world where multidrug-resistant tuberculosis is a significant problem (Russia, for example), rapid detection of drug resistance would be greatly beneficial to tuberculosis treatment and control efforts. In most instances, detection of rifampin resistance alone would suffice to signal the need for treatment with second-line drugs. Rapid detection of rifampin resistance is technologically feasible by several approaches that examine either genotypic abnormalities (by identifying mutations in the region of the *M. tuberculosis rpoB* gene associated with rifamycin resistance) or actual phenotypic resistance (persistence of the organism in a rifamycin-containing medium) (33). One such approach, the line-probe assay, which detects rifampin resistance–related mutations in the *rpoB* gene of *M. tuberculosis*, is commercially available in Europe (34–36). Such assays may be particularly useful in countries such as Russia, where multidrug-resistant tuberculosis is common, or in situations in which there is a question about acquired drug resistance (e.g., cases of treatment failure or relapse after apparently successful completion of therapy). At present, however, these assays are not in clinical use in the United States, and they are likely to be at least as costly as the available NAA assays.

Luciferase Reporter Gene Assay

In this assay, a sample such as sputum is placed into medium and is then transfected with a lucerifase-containing mycobacterial phage. If viable *M. tuberculosis* is present in the sample, it will take up the phage and the luciferase gene will function, producing visible light when luciferin is added to the assay. Drug susceptibility testing can be obtained by inoculating the clinical sample into antibiotic-containing medium (37).

Although the initial demonstration of this assay was impressive, clinical development of this assay has been slow. The developers of this approach have worked hard to create a technologically simple and inexpensive assay that can be used in countries that have limited financial and personnel resources. The current version of the assay, the "Bronx Box" uses Polaroid film for the readout and has promise as a clinically useful tool. It is a self-contained unit that may be capable of detecting viable *M. tuberculosis* in as few as 2 days (37). Field trials of this assay are underway in the United States and abroad.

Molecular Beacons

An assay for tuberculosis that uses the technology of molecular beacons has also recently been described. Molecular beacons are molecules that emit light when a chemical reaction occurs (38). This reaction will only occur when primers with DNA specificity bind their appropriate target region in polymerase chain reaction amplicons. In this way, rapid and sensitive diagnosis can be established. Recent studies by Piatek et al. (39,40) demonstrated both the sensitivity and specificity of this assay not only in making a diagnosis of tuberculosis but also in rapidly identifying mutations associated with antibiotic resistance. However, as the authors of the study themselves note, "the molecular beacon assay requires expensive equipment that is not yet widely available," although they speculate that this equipment will soon become more widely available as sophisticated polymerase chain reaction assays for a variety of infectious diseases are developed and adopted by clinical laboratories. It seems apparent, however, that the widespread adoption of such sophisticated technology will be limited to wealthy nations.

CONCLUSION

Rapid diagnosis of active tuberculosis and rapid detection of drug resistant *M. tuberculosis* are currently feasible from a technical standpoint using a variety of methods that appear robust and reproducible. The major factor limiting the widespread adoption of these technologies is their cost. Eighty percent of the world's burden of tuberculosis occurs in 22 countries, none of which appears to have the resources to allow routine use of these new approaches. However, cost savings associated with more rapid diagnosis and treatment of active cases, particularly those that are smear negative, might shift the economic calculus more favorably in the direction of newer technologies.

REFERENCES

1. Foulds J, O'Brien R. New tools for the diagnosis of tuberculosis: the perspective of developing countries. *Int J Tuberc Lung Dis* 1998;2:778–783.
2. Behr MA, Warren SA, Salamon H, et al. Transmission of *Mycobacterium tuberculosis* from patients smear-negative for acid-fast bacilli. *Lancet* 1999;353:444–449.
3. Haramati LB, Jenny-Avital ER, Alterman DD. Effect of HIV status on chest radiographic and CT findings in patients with tuberculosis. *Clin Radiol* 1997;52:31–35.
4. Griffiths RI, Hyman CL, McFarlane SI, et al. Medical-resource use for suspected tuberculosis in a New York City hospital . *Infect Control Hosp Epidemiol* 1998;19:747–753.
5. Catanzaro A, Perry S, Clarridge JE, et al. The role of clinical suspicion in evaluating a new diagnostic test for active tuberculosis: results of a multicenter prospective trial. *JAMA* 2000;283:639–645.
6. Divinagracia RM, Harkin TJ, Bonk S, et al. Screening by specialists to reduce unnecessary test ordering in patients evaluated for tuberculosis. *Chest* 1998;114:681–684.
7. Samb B, Henzel D, Daley CL, et al. Methods for diagnosing tuberculosis among in-patients in eastern Africa whose sputum smears are negative. *Int J Tuberc Lung Dis* 1997;1:25–30.
8. Streeton JA, Desem N, Jones SL. Sensitivity and specificity of a gamma interferon blood test for tuberculosis infection. *Int J Tuberc Lung Dis* 1998;2:443–450.
9. Pottumarthy S, Morris AJ, Harrison AC, et al. Evaluation of the

tuberculin gamma interferon assay: potential to replace the Mantoux skin test. *J Clin Microbiol* 1999;37:3229–3232.

10. Mazurek GH, LoBue PA, Daley CL, et al. Comparison of a whole-blood interferon gamma assay with tuberculin skin testing for detecting latent *Mycobacterium tuberculosis* infection. *JAMA* 2001;286:1740–1747.

11. Bellete B, Coberly J, Barnes GL, et al. Evaluation of a whole-blood interferon-gamma release assay for the detection of *Mycobacterium tuberculosis* infection in 2 study populations. *Clin Infect Dis* 2002;34:1449–1456.

12. Arend SM, Engelhard AC, Groot G, et al. Tuberculin skin testing compared with T-cell responses to *Mycobacterium tuberculosis*-specific and nonspecific antigens for detection of latent infection in persons with recent tuberculosis contact. *Clin Diagn Lab Immunol* 2001;8:1089–1096.

13. Pathan AA, Wilkinson KA, Klenerman P, et al. Direct ex vivo analysis of antigen-specific IFN-gamma-secreting CD4 T cells in *Mycobacterium tuberculosis*-infected individuals: associations with clinical disease state and effect of treatment. *J Immunol* 2001;167:5217–5225.

14. Lalvani A, Pathan AA, Durkan H, et al. Enhanced contact tracing and spatial tracking of *Mycobacterium tuberculosis* infection by enumeration of antigen-specific T cells. *Lancet* 2001;357:2017–2021.

15. Lalvani A, Pathan AA, McShane H, et al. Rapid detection of *Mycobacterium tuberculosis* infection by enumeration of antigen-specific T cells. *Am J Respir Crit Care Med* 2001;163:824–828.

16. Lalvani A, Nagvenkar P, Udwadia Z, et al. Enumeration of T cells specific for RD1-encoded antigens suggests a high prevalence of latent *Mycobacterium tuberculosis* infection in healthy urban Indians. *J Infect Dis* 2001;183:469–477.

17. Wu-Hsieh BA, Chen CK, Chang JH, et al. Long-lived immune response to early secretory antigenic target 6 in individuals who had recovered from tuberculosis. *Clin Infect Dis* 2001;33:1336–1340.

18. Vekemans J, Lienhardt C, Sillah JS, et al. Tuberculosis contacts but not patients have higher gamma interferon responses to ESAT-6 than do community controls in The Gambia. *Infect Immun* 2001;69:6554–6557.

19. Brock I, Munk ME, Kok-Jensen A, et al. Performance of whole blood IFN-gamma test for tuberculosis diagnosis based on PPD or the specific antigens ESAT-6 and CFP-10. *Int J Tuberc Lung Dis* 2001;5:462–467.

20. Kanchana MV, Cheke D, Natyshak I, et al. Evaluation of the BACTEC MGIT 960 system for the recovery of mycobacteria. *Diagn Microbiol Infect Dis* 2000;37:31–36.

21. Sharp SE, Lemes M, Sierra SG, et al. Lowenstein-Jensen media. No longer necessary for mycobacterial isolation. *Am J Clin Pathol* 2000;113:770–773.

22. Sharp SE, Lemes M, Erlich SS, et al. A comparison of the Bactec 9000MB system and the Septi-Chek AFB system for the detection of mycobacteria. *Diagn Microbiol Infect Dis* 1997;28:69–74.

23. Dalovisio JR, Montenegro-James S, Kemmerly SA, et al. Comparison of the amplified *Mycobacterium tuberculosis* (MTB) direct test, Amplicor MTB PCR, and IS6110-PCR for detection of MTB in respiratory specimens. *Clin Infect Dis* 1996;23:1099–1106.

24. Della-Latta P, Whittier S. Comprehensive evaluation of performance, laboratory application, and clinical usefulness of two direct amplification technologies for the detection of *Mycobacterium tuberculosis* complex. *Am J Clin Pathol* 1998;110:301–310.

25. Rapid diagnostic tests for tuberculosis: what is the appropriate use? American Thoracic Society Workshop. *Am J Respir Crit Care Med* 1997;155:1804–1814.

26. Bergmann JS, Yuoh G, Fish G, et al. Clinical evaluation of the enhanced Gen-Probe amplified *Mycobacterium tuberculosis* direct test for rapid diagnosis of tuberculosis in prison inmates. *J Clin Microbiol* 1999;37:1419–1425.

27. Chedore P, Jamieson FB. Routine use of the Gen-Probe MTD2 amplification test for detection of *Mycobacterium tuberculosis* in clinical specimens in a large public health mycobacteriology laboratory. *Diagn Microbiol Infect Dis* 1999;35:185–191.

28. Roos BR, van Cleeff MR, Githui WA, et al. Cost-effectiveness of the polymerase chain reaction versus smear examination for the diagnosis of tuberculosis in Kenya: a theoretical model. *Int J Tuberc Lung Dis* 1998;2:235–241.

29. Update: nucleic acid amplification tests for tuberculosis. *MMWR Morb Mortal Wkly Rep* 2000;49:593–594.

30. Piersimoni C, Callegaro A, Scarparo C, et al. Comparative evaluation of the new Gen-Probe *Mycobacterium tuberculosis* amplified direct test and the semiautomated Abbott LCx *Mycobacterium tuberculosis* assay for direct detection of *Mycobacterium tuberculosis* complex in respiratory and extrapulmonary specimens. *J Clin Microbiol* 1998;36:3601–3604.

31. Gamboa F, Fernandez G, Padilla E, et al. Comparative evaluation of initial and new versions of the Gen-Probe amplified *Mycobacterium tuberculosis* direct test for direct detection of *Mycobacterium tuberculosis* in respiratory and nonrespiratory specimens. *J Clin Microbiol* 1998;36:684–689.

32. Lang AM, Feris-Iglesias J, Pena C, et al. Clinical evaluation of the Gen-Probe amplified direct test for detection of *Mycobacterium tuberculosis* complex organisms in cerebrospinal fluid. *J Clin Microbiol* 1998;36:2191–2194.

33. Hellyer TJ, DesJardin LE, Teixeira L, et al. Detection of viable *Mycobacterium tuberculosis* by reverse transcriptase-strand displacement amplification of mRNA. *J Clin Microbiol* 1999;37:518–523.

34. Cooksey RC, Morlock GP, Glickman S, et al. Evaluation of a line probe assay kit for characterization of rpoB mutations in rifampin-resistant *Mycobacterium tuberculosis* isolates from New York City. *J Clin Microbiol* 1997;35:1281–1283.

35. Hirano K, Abe C, Takahashi M. Mutations in the *rpoB* gene of rifampin-resistant *Mycobacterium tuberculosis* strains isolated mostly in Asian countries and their rapid detection by line probe assay. *J Clin Microbiol* 1999;37:2663–2666.

36. Marttila HJ, Soini H, Vyshnevskaya E, et al. Line probe assay in the rapid detection of rifampin-resistant *Mycobacterium tuberculosis* directly from clinical specimens. *Scand J Infect Dis* 1999;31:269–273.

37. Riska PF, Su Y, Bardarov S, et al. Rapid film-based determination of antibiotic susceptibilities of *Mycobacterium tuberculosis* strains by using a luciferase reporter phage and the Bronx Box. *J Clin Microbiol* 1999;37:1144–1149.

38. Leone G, van Schijndel H, van Gemen B, et al. Molecular beacon probes combined with amplification by NASBA enable homogeneous, real-time detection of RNA. *Nucleic Acids Res* 1998;26:2150–2155.

39. Piatek AS, Tyagi S, Pol AC, et al. Molecular beacon sequence analysis for detecting drug resistance in *Mycobacterium tuberculosis*. *Nat Biotechnol* 1998;16:359–363.

40. Piatek AS, Telenti A, Murray MR, et al. Genotypic analysis of *Mycobacterium tuberculosis* in two distinct populations using molecular beacons: implications for rapid susceptibility testing. *Antimicrob Agents Chemother* 2000;44:103–110.

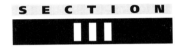

HOST RESPONSE

13

IMMUNODIAGNOSIS

SUMAN LAAL

More than 90% of the cases with active tuberculosis (TB) occur in countries with limited resources, making rapid diagnosis of active TB their major priority (1). The same countries also have a high incidence of latent infection, and the spread of human immunodeficiency virus (HIV) infection in them has created a need for tests that can identify coinfected individuals who are at risk of progressing to TB. In contrast, developed countries have significantly fewer patients and have the resources and infrastructure not only to diagnose and treat relatively early cases of active TB but also to conduct extensive contact investigations and offer preventive therapy to individuals considered at risk of clinical TB. For these reasons, accurate diagnosis of latent *Mycobacterium tuberculosis* infection is the priority in these countries. The different immunodiagnostic tests currently being developed include:

1. Tests for active TB that can identify individuals who have progressed to clinical disease,
2. Tests for detection of incipient, preclinical TB, especially in HIV-infected individuals and other high-risk populations,
3. Tests for latent TB that can distinguish *M. tuberculosis*–infected individuals from bacille Calmette–Guérin (BCG)–vaccinated or nontuberculous mycobacteria (NTM)–sensitized individuals.

The low cost and relative simplicity of immunoassays have encouraged several investigators to attempt to develop serologic tests for active TB. The antigens that have been evaluated in a several different studies include purified protein derivative (PPD), mycobacterial sonicates, mycobacterial glycolipids, 38-kd antigen, 16-kd α-crystallin, 45/47-kd antigen MPT32, Ag 85A, Ag 85B, antigen A60, Kp90, lipoarabinomannan (2,3). The details of sensitivity, specificity, and negative and positive predictive values obtained with these antigens have recently been reviewed and are not

discussed here (3). Of all these, the 38-kd antigen is the most extensively studied protein of *M. tuberculosis* for serodiagnosis (2–5). Although this protein provides very high specificity (>98%), anti–38-kd antibodies are found primarily in patients with advanced and recurrent cavitary TB (4). Studies showed that the sensitivity of anti–38-kd antibody detection varied from approximately 50% in smear-positive patients from Cleveland, Ohio, to approximately 90% in patients from India and China (2,6,7); the sensitivity in smear-negative patients is low (5% to 15%). Despite the correlation with advanced TB, the 38-kd is not well recognized by HIV-infected patients with TB (8). In recent years, several tests based on the 38-kd antigen, alone or in combination with other antigens, have been developed commercially. A recent study compared the reactivity of sera from the same cohort with six different tests (9). The sensitivities and specificities with these tests ranged from 16% to 57% and 62% to 100%, respectively. Clearly, although the 38-kd antigen is a promising candidate, other antigens that can either provide higher sensitivity or enhance the sensitivity obtained with the use of the 38-kd antigen are required for developing immunodiagnosis for active TB.

The genome of *M. tuberculosis* has the ability to express approximately 4,000 proteins (10). The availability of the genome sequence and the ability to clone genes to express large amounts of purified recombinant proteins have made it possible to rapidly evaluate potential candidate antigens for immunodiagnosis of TB. There is also considerable evidence that *M. tuberculosis* regulates its gene expression to survive in different environments *in vitro* and *in vivo* (11–17). The best antigens for devising immunodiagnostic tests to identify active TB would be expected to be those that (a) are recognized by patients with active but not latent infection—the corollary being that the antigens are expressed only by actively replicating *in vivo M. tuberculosis*; (b) elicit immune responses in all or most of the individuals with active disease (i.e., the antigens are expressed by all strains of *M. tuberculosis*); (c) elicit immune responses in patients with different forms of active disease [e.g., in noncavitary, cavitary, HIV-coinfected, and extrapulmonary

S. Laal: Department of Pathology, New York University School of Medicine; VA Medical Center, New York, New York.

TB (EPTB) patients]; and (d) are either specific to *M. tuberculosis* or have serodominant specific epitopes.

Several different approaches have been used in the search for antigens for devising immunodiagnosis for active TB. Our laboratory has focused on the proteins present in culture filtrates of *M. tuberculosis* replicating in minimal bacteriologic media with the expectation that detection of antibodies to antigens released by actively replicating bacteria would be indicative of active disease (16,18,19). Other laboratories have cloned antigens by screening expression libraries of genomic *M. tuberculosis* DNA with sera from rabbits that were hyperimmunized with culture-filtrate proteins of *M. tuberculosis* or monoclonal antibodies or with sera from patients with TB (20–23). Another approach has been to clone proteins encoded by regions of *M. tuberculosis* genome that are absent in BCG (23,24) or to clone some of the secreted proteins of *M. tuberculosis* (25).

Lyaschenko et al. (26,27) evaluated the reactivity of sera from smear-positive and smear-negative patients with TB with 12 *M. tuberculosis* proteins, including ESAT-6, 14-kd protein, MPT63, 19-kd protein, MPT70, MPT64, MPT51, MTC28, Ag 85B, 38-kd protein, MPT32, and KatG. Results showed that, except for the 38-kd antigen that was recognized by approximately 30% of patients with TB, all other antigens tested were recognized by fewer patients (6% to 22%); the additive reactivity with all the antigens provided approximately 77% sensitivity. The same investigators also cloned genes encoded by the RD1 region of *M. tuberculosis*, a region that is missing in *Mycobacterium bovis* BCG, and reported that although ESAT-6 and MTSA 10 were recognized by 13% and 16%, respectively, of the patients with TB, other antigens were recognized only by two to five of the 75 patients tested (24). MTSA10, also called CFP10, was also cloned by Dillon et al. (23) and was shown to be recognized by approximately 10% of the smear-positive patients lacking anti–38-kd antibodies.

Our laboratory has performed two-dimensional mapping of fractionated culture filtrates that are recognized by antibodies from patients with TB classified on the basis of their acid-fast bacilli smear results, radiologic status, and HIV status to delineate candidate antigens for serodiagnosis of TB (16,28). These studies show that:

1. Of the more than 100 proteins present in culture filtrates of *M. tuberculosis* growing in minimal bacteriologic media, only a subset of approximately 12 proteins is well recognized by antibodies from patients with noncavitary TB.
2. Patients with cavitary TB differ from noncavitary patients in that they have antibodies to the same subset of approximately 12 antigens and to an additional subset of approximately 10 antigens, one of which is the 38-kd protein.
3. HIV-coinfected patients with noncavitary TB have antibodies to the same subset of approximately 12 antigens as the non-HIV, noncavitary TB patients.

4. Smear-positive and smear-negative noncavitary patients recognize the same set of antigens, although the titers of antibodies are generally higher in the former group.
5. Despite the fact that different individuals would be infected with different strains, there is a significant homogeneity in the subset of antigens recognized in different individuals.

The antigens from this subset of approximately 12 proteins that are recognized by sera from cavitary, noncavitary, and HIV-coinfected TB patients would be rational choices for developing serodiagnosis for active TB (16,19,29). One antigen of this subset is an 88-kd protein initially identified in our studies (18), which was later reported as antigen Mtb81 (30), and has now been identified to be the 81-kd GlcB protein (10). To avoid confusion, this antigen is referred to as the 88/81-kd (GlcB) in this review. Antibodies to the 88/81-kd (GlcB) are present in approximately 75% of the cavitary TB patients (18,19). Studies show that almost all smear-positive cavitary patients who have anti–38-kd antibodies and that a significant proportion of patients who lack anti–38-kd antibodies possess anti–88/81-kd (GlcB) antibodies. The *M. tuberculosis* GlcB shows strong similarity to the enzyme malate synthase G of *Pseudomonas*, *Corynebacterium*, and *Escherichia coli*, and the high specificities (>95%) obtained with the *M. tuberculosis* antigen indicate the existence of specific serodominant epitopes on the protein (19,30).

Our two-dimensional mapping studies also provide insight into some of the reasons underlying the confusion that arises when the literature on serodiagnosis is analyzed. Most studies of serodiagnosis are based on patients classified by the smear test rather than the radiologic profile, whereas it is the presence and extent of cavitary lesions that affect the antigen profile recognized by antibodies. Moreover, the sensitivity of the smear test itself varies considerably (30% to 70%) in different laboratories (1). Patients in developing countries have poor access to health care and tend to present later and with more advanced TB than patients in developed countries; as a result, smear-positive patients from developing countries are more likely to have cavitary lesions. Thus, cohorts used in different studies are not necessarily comparable, and, thus, the same antigen differs in performance in studies conducted at different sites. Another confounding factor is that often smear-positive HIV patients are noncavitary owing to dysfunctional cellular immune responses, and antigens that are primarily recognized by cavitary patients (such as the 38-kd Ag, 85B) would be expected to be, and are, poorly recognized by HIV-TB patients. In developing countries, the HIV status of patients with TB is not routinely ascertained, and so patients with equivalent smear status would differ in their antibody responses depending on the HIV status. Another important source of confusion is the choice of control individuals; the specificities with the same test vary depending on whether control individuals included are from low prevalence or from endemic countries. For all these reasons, it is difficult to make meaningful comparisons of different tests/antigens evaluated in different regions.

Recent studies show that the sensitivity and specificity obtained with some antigens may differ depending on whether the native or recombinant proteins are studied (19). Studies with native antigens obtained from culture filtrates of *M. tuberculosis* show that the antigen profiles recognized by different patients are quite homogeneous (16). In contrast, results obtained from studies based entirely on recombinant antigens give the impression that responses of patients with TB are heterogeneous and that patients randomly develop antibodies to different mycobacterial antigens (26). The immunogenicity of several (but not all) mycobacterial antigens is affected by posttranslational modifications, especially glycosylation and acylation (16,19). Although the responses obtained with culture filtrate–derived and recombinant 88/81-kd (GlcB) were equivalent when compared in the same patient cohort (Laal S, Singh KK, unpublished data, 2002), when reactivity was evaluated with native and recombinant MPT32 and Ag 85C expressed in *E. coli*, the latter antigens were poorly recognized compared with the native counterparts (19). These differences between native and recombinant proteins are another source of confusion in the literature on serodiagnostics.

The best sensitivity of antibody detection in smear-positive TB patients detected with any antigen or set of antigens is approximately 75% to 80%. It is not clear why approximately 20% of the multibacillary TB patients lack serum antibodies. It has been hypothesized that the antibody-negative patients may have a strong Th1 response and may therefore fail to make antibodies to species-restricted mycobacterial antigens (2). The alternate hypothesis is that circulating antigen may complex with antibodies, thus precluding the detection of free antibody (2). Recent studies determined the presence of antimycobacterial antibodies in paired urine and serum from smear-positive TB patients and found that urine antibodies are often present in the absence of detectable serum antibodies. These results suggest that the inability to detect antibodies in a proportion of TB patients is owing to low titers of antibodies being trapped in immune complexes rather than the absence of antibodies. When paired serum and urine samples were tested, anti–88/81 (GlcB) antibodies were detected in 39 of 43 patients tested (48).

Two glycolipid antigens of *M. tuberculosis*, 2,3-diacyltrehalose (also called sulfolipid IV) and phenolic glycolipid Tb1, have also provided promising results when evaluated for the diagnosis of active TB (31). Antibodies to these two antigens were detected in approximately 75% of the non–HIV-TB smear-positive and smear-negative patients (31). Additional cohorts need to be evaluated, and it would be interesting to determine whether patients lacking antibodies to the protein antigens of *M. tuberculosis* have detectable antiglycolipid antibodies.

A new immunodiagnostic test, a transdermal patch bearing a 24-kd antigen (MBP-64), was recently evaluated in a small cohort of patients and contacts or PPD-positive volunteers and provided high sensitivity (87%) and specificity (100%). The performance of this test in other forms of TB is yet to be evaluated and may be severely limited in high-risk groups with weakened cellular immune responses like the HIV-infected individuals and in individuals on suppressive therapy because it is based on delayed-type hypersensitivity responses (32).

Approximately half of the patients with bacteriologically confirmed pulmonary TB are smear negative. It has been observed with several antigens (19 kd, lipoarabinomannan, Ag 85A, 38 kd) that, compared with smear-positive patients, the sensitivity of antibody detection is lower in smear-negative patients (3). Thus, sensitivities with the 38-kd antigen varied from 16% to 82% in smear-negative patients (3). Recently, six different commercially available tests based on the 38-kd antigen were evaluated, and sensitivities with smear-negative patients ranged from 17% to 50% (9). When the reactivity of the same cohort of noncavitary, smear-negative patients with the culture filtrate–derived 38-kd and 88/81-kd (GlcB) antigens was compared, the former was recognized in approximately 10% and the latter in approximately 35% of the patients (19). Screening of an expression library with sera from patients lacking anti–38-kd antibodies led to the cloning of CFP10 (also called MTSA10) (23). Anti-CFP10 antibodies were present in approximately 25% of the smear-negative patients tested; inclusion of reactivity with the 38-kd antigen increased the sensitivity to approximately 40% (23). Another antigen, MTB48, obtained by the screening of an expression library with sera from patients with EPTB, was recognized by approximately 15% of the smear-negative TB patients; use of both the MTB48 and the 38-kd antigens increased the sensitivity to approximately 30% (22). Because both CFP10 and MTB48 were cloned in the same laboratory, presumably use of the two antigens together did not result in increased sensitivity of antibody detection. Because smear-negative patients have low titers of antibodies, multiple antigens chosen based on their dominance during human infection may be useful to enhance the sensitivity of antibody detection (16).

As the HIV infection spreads in countries that already have a high incidence of TB, the ability of any serodiagnostic test to diagnose TB in coinfected patients assumes increasing importance. The 38-kd antigen, Ag 85B, and lipoarabinomannan are poorly recognized by serum antibodies from HIV-TB patients (8,19,33,34). Studies show that the 88/81-kd (GlcB) is a dominant target of antibody responses in coinfected patients (16,19,29,30). In our cohort of HIV-TB patients from the United States, approximately 65% of the patients had anti–88/81-kd (GlcB) antibodies (19,29). In another cohort of HIV-TB patients from Uganda and South Africa, the sensitivity of anti–88/81-kd (GlcB) antibody detection was 92% (30); in both studies, the specificity was greater than 98%. Other investigators have reported the presence of anti–2,3-diacyl-trehalose and anti–phenolic glycolipid Tb1 antibodies in approximately 74% of HIV-TB patients (31).

Few studies have directly addressed development of a serodiagnostic test for EPTB; generally, antigens tested for pulmonary TB are evaluated in patients with EPTB (2,3,9). In a recent study, anti–38-kd antibodies were reported to be present in 9% to 46% of EPTB patients (9); it is not clear whether sensitivity varied in patients with different subtypes of EPTB (lymphadenitis, miliary, pleural, peritoneal) and how many patients had coincident pulmonary involvement. Moran et al. (25) randomly cloned nine secreted proteins of *M. tuberculosis* and evaluated the reactivity of sera from EPTB patients with these antigens. Fusion proteins of four of these antigens (Sanger IDs MTCY 253.27c, MTCY02B12.02, MTV004.48, and MTCY31.03c) were recognized by antibodies from 35% to 60% of the patients with EPTB; the remaining five were recognized only sporadically. Additive reactivity with all nine proteins provided approximately 70% sensitivity. The reported specificities with these antigens were high, at least with the small number of controls tested. Reactivities of the same antigens with sera from patients with pulmonary TB is not reported nor is the breakdown of different forms of EPTB; therefore, it is not possible to assess whether responses to any of these antigens correlate with any specific site of the disease. As mentioned previously, studies with cavitary and noncavitary TB patients show that the antigens recognized by antibodies are affected by the presence or absence and by the extent of cavitary lesions in patients (16). This suggests that the expression or the accessibility of the antigenic proteins to the immune system is affected by the *in vivo* environment in which the bacteria survive. The pathogenesis of different types of EPTB differs, and in view of the effect of the *in vivo* environment on antigens expressed by the bacteria, it is conceivable that the immunodominant antigens for pulmonary TB and EPTB may show only limited overlap. Although there is sufficient evidence that supports the existence of antibody responses in patients with EPTB, careful studies with well-characterized patients with different forms of EPTB remain to be conducted.

TB in children is difficult to diagnose because they rarely produce bacteriologically positive sputum and have a greater incidence of disseminated disease. For these reasons, immunodiagnosis for TB in children would be very useful. Several studies based on detection of antibodies to PPD, autoclaved suspension of *M. tuberculosis*, and the A60 antigen have been reported (2,3). As observed with adult patients, sensitivities and specificities vary depending on the inclusion criteria used for the cohort, and no conclusive results have been obtained. Although a diagnostic test for pediatric TB would be useful, specific efforts to develop such a test have not been made in recent years.

TESTS FOR INCIPIENT, PRECLINICAL TUBERCULOSIS

The spread of HIV infection to populations that have a high incidence of TB is making an increasing contribution to TB cases worldwide. The immune dysfunction caused by progressive HIV infection leads to a very high rate of reactivation of latent TB, rapid progression of primary infection to clinical disease, and an accelerated course of disease progression. There are no tests currently available that can distinguish between a truly latent, inactive infection and active, incipient, preclinical TB. Cutaneous reactivity to PPD is currently used for detection of *M. tuberculosis* infection, but this test fails to distinguish between latent and active infection and can result in a false-positive result owing to BCG vaccination or exposure to other mycobacteria, and the sensitivity of the test is markedly reduced in HIV-infected individuals. In addition, the time between a positive skin test and the development of clinical TB may range from months to years, and there are no markers to identify individuals who have current, active replication of previously latent bacteria. Several clinical trials with isoniazid monotherapy or with multidrug regimens have provided evidence that preventive therapy significantly decreases the risk of developing active TB in HIV-infected patients (35,36). However, the role of preventive therapy in developing countries is seriously limited by the high rate of PPD positivity, lack of adequate infrastructure and economic resources for procuring drugs, monitoring adherence and potential toxic side effects, and the risks of fostering resistance by treating individuals with undetectable, incipient TB with monotherapy (36). In view of the high rate of reactivation of latent infection in HIV-infected individuals in many parts of the world, tests that can diagnose incipient, preclinical TB would be useful for determining the optimal time and recipients of preventive therapy.

Three groups have provided evidence that antibodies directed against some mycobacterial antigens are present in retrospective sera obtained *before* the development of clinical TB from HIV-TB patients. Antibodies directed against the culture-filtrate proteins of BCG were reported to be present in serial retrospective sera from a patient with acquired immunodeficiency syndrome who initially presented with pleural effusion and was found to be sputum culture positive several months later (37). Sulfolipid IV (2,3-diacyltrehalose)–specific antibodies were reported to be present in retrospective sera from 12 of 13 HIV-TB patients, and these antibodies were detectable 1 to 30 months before the clinical manifestation of TB (38). There was no correlation between positive or negative skin test reactivity and the presence of antibodies. We evaluated the reactivity of 136 retrospective serum samples obtained from 38 culture-confirmed HIV-TB patients with fractionated culture-filtrate proteins of *M. tuberculosis* and found that 88/81-kd (GlcB) antigen was recognized by multiple, serial serum samples from approximately 75% of the patients with HIV who later progressed to TB (29). These antibodies were detectable in the retrospective sera obtained several months to years (3 years) *before* the development of clinical TB (29). Recent studies in our laboratory with serial retrospective sera from two individuals over several months showed that the profile of antigens recognized by antibodies was stable over extended periods. These studies suggest that it should be possible to devise serodiagnostic tests that can identify HIV-infected individuals with incipient, preclinical TB. Prospective studies in which cohorts of HIV-infected patients are monitored for clinical, radiologic, bacteriologic, and serologic criteria for the diagnosis of TB are required to determine the utility of these tests in diagnosing incipient TB. Such studies are clearly warranted in view of the enormity of the HIV-TB problem in developing countries.

Tests for incipient, preclinical TB for other high-risk groups would also be useful. Because clinical material from non-HIV individuals who progressed to clinical TB is unavailable, it has not been possible to conduct specific studies so far. Although the profile of culture-filtrate antigens recognized by noncavitary patients is unaffected by HIV coinfection (16), it remains to be proven that non–HIV-infected individuals also have antimycobacterial antibodies for extended periods before the clinical presentation with TB and that the antigen profile recognized is similar to that recognized by the retrospective, preclinical TB sera from HIV-TB patients. A test for incipient, preclinical TB would also be extremely useful to evaluate new vaccines.

TESTS FOR LATENT TUBERCULOSIS THAT CAN DISTINGUISH *MYCOBACTERIUM TUBERCULOSIS*–INFECTED INDIVIDUALS FROM BACILLE CALMETTE–GUÉRIN– VACCINATED AND NONTUBERCULOUS MYCOBACTERIA–SENSITIZED INDIVIDUALS

TB control in industrialized countries relies not only on rapid diagnosis and monitoring of treatment of patients with active TB but also on identification and screening of contacts of infectious patients. Immigrants from high-prevalence countries constitute a high-risk population because of the high rates of reactivation, and estimates suggest that there are approximately 10 to 15 million individuals in the United States who harbor latent *M. tuberculosis* infection. Close contacts of infectious TB patients are also at a high risk of developing TB because approximately 30% of the contacts get infected, and the risk of progression of latent infection to clinical disease has been estimated to be significantly higher in close contacts compared with the general population (35). Because preventive therapy has been found to reduce the risk of progression of latent *M. tuberculosis* infection to clinical TB by 70%, accurate identification of individuals with latent *M. tuberculosis* infection

is an important component for TB control programs in low-prevalence countries (35).

Currently, the PPD skin test is the only tool available for identification of latent TB. However, the skin test has several drawbacks because PPD is a crude mixture of more than 100 different secreted and somatic proteins, many of which are shared among *M. tuberculosis*, *M. tuberculosis complex*, *M. bovis* BCG, NTM, and environmental mycobacteria. As a result, the PPD test fails to distinguish between BCG vaccination and *M. tuberculosis* infection, and BCG vaccination is routinely given in many countries. Moreover, this test cannot distinguish between exposure to other NTM and *M. tuberculosis* infection. In addition, PPD reactivity gives a false-negative reaction in 20% to 30% of the TB patients with confirmed diagnosis.

Although several antigens have been tested for utility in tests for the identification of latent TB, only results with antigens tested in humans are discussed in this chapter. ESAT-6 and CFP10 are two *M. tuberculosis*–specific proteins that have been investigated extensively as potential candidates for the development of immunodiagnosis for latent *M. tuberculosis* infection (39–42). The genes encoding both these antigens are part of the same operon on the RD1 region of the *M. tuberculosis* genome, a region that has been reported to be absent from all the substrains of *M. bovis* BCG (43). Early studies with small cohorts showed that although PPD induced interferon gamma (IFN-γ) production in a significant proportion of patients with TB and in BCG-vaccinated individuals, ESAT-6 and/or CFP10 elicited the cytokine primarily in a large proportion of patients with TB (39,40). More recently, a whole-blood IFN-γ assay was used to compare the sensitivity and specificity obtained with PPD, ESAT-6, and CFP10 (41). Although almost half the BCG-vaccinated individuals responded by producing IFN-γ in response to PPD, only 10% of the same individuals produced the cytokine in response to ESAT-6 or CFP10; the sensitivity in patients with TB with the two purified antigens was similar to that obtained with PPD (41). Studies in contacts of patients with TB in endemic countries have shown that the prevalence of ESAT-6 responses is high in the contacts of patients with TB compared with community controls (42). Using a sensitive Elispot assay for detection of antigen-specific T cells without *in vitro* stimulation, Lalvani et al. (44) showed that there is a strong positive relationship between the numbers of IFN-γ–producing cells in the peripheral blood mononuclear cells (PBMCs) and the degree of exposure to *M. tuberculosis*. Although more studies are required, the ability of ESAT-6 and CFP10 to distinguish latent *M. tuberculosis* infection from BCG vaccination or sensitization with other mycobacteria will be useful for TB control in industrialized countries where preventive therapy is a viable option.

PBMCs from approximately 80% of the healthy individuals tested in India produced IFN-γ in response to ESAT-6 and CFP10, and the results from sub-Saharan

Africa and other high-prevalence countries are likely to be similar (45). In view of the high prevalence of latent infection with *M. tuberculosis* and the economic constraints that exist, tests that can identify incipient, preclinical TB are likely to be more important for developing countries. Preliminary studies suggest that high levels of ESAT-6–induced IFN-γ in contacts show a strong correlation with progression to clinical TB, but more definite results are awaited. Routine use of any test in resource-poor countries will depend on the test being rapid and inexpensive and requiring minimal laboratory support or infrastructure. Moreover, as an increasing proportion of patients with TB will also have HIV coinfection, the utility of any cellular immune response–based test will have to be assessed in the coinfected individuals.

The other antigen that is a potential candidate for immunodiagnosis of *M. tuberculosis* infection is called DPPD (46,47). This is an approximately 10-kd protein originally selected from fractionated PPD because of its ability to elicit delayed-type hypersensitivity responses in all *M. tuberculosis*–infected guinea pigs tested but not in guinea pigs immunized with several other pathogenic or environmental mycobacteria (46). A recent clinical investigation using DPPD in pulmonary TB patients and healthy subjects suggested that it may be useful for distinguishing between *M. tuberculosis* infection and exposure to other mycobacteria, although it is unlikely to be of use in distinguishing BCG vaccination from *M. tuberculosis* infection.

Much has been achieved in the past few years, and it is obvious that the availability of the genome sequence and the new tools of genomics and proteomics have greatly accelerated pace of development of immunodiagnostic tests for TB. It is also clear that different antigens may be useful for different stages of TB. Preliminary studies suggest that it may be feasible to design immunodiagnosis for incipient, preclinical TB, at least in HIV-infected individuals. Focused studies of development of immunodiagnosis for children and for various forms of EPTB need to done. As more potential candidates are identified, cloned, and characterized, the next challenge will be to develop and optimize technologies related to the use of these antigens in inexpensive, rapid formats that can provide on-the-spot diagnosis.

REFERENCES

1. Foulds J, O'Brien R. New tools for the diagnosis of tuberculosis: the perspective of developing countries. *Int J Tuberc Lung Dis* 1998;2:778–783.
2. Bothamley GH. Serological diagnosis of tuberculosis. *Eur Respir J* 1995;8:676–688.
3. Chan ED, Heifets L, Iseman MD. Immunologic diagnosis of tuberculosis: a review. *Tuber Lung Dis* 2000;80:131–140.
4. Bothamley GH, Rudd R, Festenstein F, et al. Clinical value of the measurement of *Mycobacterium tuberculosis* specific antibody in pulmonary tuberculosis. *Thorax* 1992;47:270–275.
5. Daniels TM. Immunodiagnosis of tuberculosis. In: Rom WR, Garay S, eds. In: *Tuberculosis*. Boston: Little, Brown, 1996: 223–231.
6. Daniel T, Debanne SM, van der Kuyp F. Enzyme-linked immunosorbent assay using *Mycobacterium tuberculosis* antigen 5 and PPD for the serodiagnosis of tuberculosis. *Chest* 1985;88: 388–392.
7. Ma Y, Wang YM, Daniel TM. Enzyme-linked immunoabsorbent assay using *Mycobacterium tuberculosis* antigen 5 for the diagnosis of pulmonary tuberculosis in China. *Am Rev Respir Dis* 1986; 134:1273–1275.
8. McDonough JA, Sada ED, Sippola AA, et al. Microplate and dot immunoassays for the serodiagnosis of tuberculosis. *J Lab Clin Med* 1992;120:318–322.
9. Pottumarthy S, Weels VC, Morris AJ. A comparison of seven tests for serological diagnosis of tuberculosis. *J Clin Microbiol* 2000;38:2227–2231.
10. Cole ST, Brosch R, Parkhill J, et al. Deciphering the biology of *Mycobacterium tuberculosis* from the complete genome sequence. *Nature* 1998;393:537–544.
11. Wong DK, Lee B-Y, Horwitz MA, et al. Identification of fur, aconitase, and other proteins expressed by *Mycobacterium tuberculosis* under conditions of low and high concentrations of iron by combined two-dimensional gel electrophoresis and mass spectrometry. *Infect Immun* 1999;67:327–336.
12. Garbe TR, Hibler NS, Deretic V. Response to reactive nitrogen intermediates in *Mycobacterium tuberculosis*: induction of the 16 kilodalton alpha-crystallin homolog by exposure to nitric oxide donors. *Infect Immun* 1999;67:460–465.
13. Graham JE, Clark-Curtis JE. Identification of *Mycobacterium tuberculosis* RNAs synthesized in response to phagocytosis by human macrophages by selective capture of transcribed sequences (SCOTS). *Proc Natl Acad Sci U S A* 1999;96: 11554–11559.
14. Ramakrishnan L, Federspiel NA, Falkow S. Granuloma-specific expression of *Mycobacterium* virulence proteins from the glycine-rich PE-PGRS family. *Science* 2000;288:1436–1439.
15. Triccas JA, Berthet F-X, Pelicic V, et al. Use of fluorescence induction and sucrose counterselection to identify *Mycobacterium tuberculosis* genes expressed within host cells. *Microbiology* 1999;145:2923–2930.
16. Samanich K, Belisle JT, Laal S. Homogeneity of antibody responses in tuberculosis patients. *Infect Immun* 2001;69: 4600–4609.
17. Dubnau Fontan P, Manganelli R, Soares-Appel S, et al. Identification of *Mycobacterium tuberculosis* genes induced during infection of human macrophages. *Infect Immun* 2002;70:2787–2795.
18. Laal S, Samanich KM, Sonnenberg MG, et al. Human humoral responses to antigens of *Mycobacterium tuberculosis*: immunodominance of high molecular weight antigens. *Clin Diagn Lab Immunol* 1996;4:49–56.
19. Samanich KM, Keen MA, Vissa VD, et al. Serodiagnostic potential of culture filtrate antigens of *Mycobacterium tuberculosis*. *Clin Diagn Lab Immunol* 2000;7:662–668.
20. Manca C, Lyashchenko K, Wiker Harald G, et al. Molecular cloning, purification and serological characterization of MPT63, a novel antigen secreted by *Mycobacterium tuberculosis*. *Infect Immun* 1997;65:16–23.
21. Manca C, Lyashchenko K, Colangeli R, et al. MTC28, a novel 28-kilodalton proline-rich secreted antigen specific for the *Mycobacterium tuberculosis* complex. *Infect Immun* 1997;65: 4951–4957.
22. Lodes MJ, Dillon DC, Mohamath R, et al. Serological expression, cloning and immunological evaluation of MTB48, a novel *Mycobacterium tuberculosis* antigen. *J Clin Microbiol* 2001;39: 2485–2493.

23. Dillon DC, Alderson MR, Day CH, et al. Molecular and immunological characterization of *Mycobacterium tuberculosis* CFP-10, an immunodiagnostic antigen missing in *Mycobacterium bovis* BCG. *J Clin Microbiol* 2000;38:3285–3290.

24. Brusasca PN, Colangeli R, Lyashchenko KP, et al. Immunological characterization of antigens encoded by the RD1 region of the *Mycobacterium tuberculosis* genome. *Scand J Immunol* 2001; 54:448–452.

25. Moran AJ, Treit JD, Whitney JL, et al. Assessment of the serodiagnostic potential of nine novel proteins from *Mycobacterium tuberculosis*. *FEMS Microbiol Lett* 2001;198:31–36.

26. Lyashchenko K, Colangeli R, Houde M, et al. Heterogeneous antibody responses in tuberculosis. *Infect Immun* 1998;66: 3936–3940.

27. Lyashchenko KP, Singh M, Colangeli R, et al. A multi-antigen print immunoassay for the development of serological diagnosis of infectious diseases. *J Immunol Meth* 2000;242:91–100.

28. Samanich KM, Belisle JT, Sonnenberg MG, et al. Delineation of human antibody responses to culture filtrate antigens of *Mycobacterium tuberculosis*. *J Infect Dis* 1998;178:1534–1538.

29. Laal S, Samanich KM, Sonnenberg MG, et al. Surrogate marker of preclinical tuberculosis in human immunodeficiency virus infection: antibodies to an 88 kDa secreted antigen of *Mycobacterium tuberculosis*. *J Infect Dis* 1997;176:133–143.

30. Hendrickson RC, Douglass JF, Reynolds LD, et al. Mass spectrometric identification of Mtb81, a novel serological marker for tuberculosis. *J Clin Microbiol* 2000;38:2354–2361.

31. Simonney N, Molina JM, Molimard M, et al. Analysis of the immunological humoral response to *Mycobacterium tuberculosis* glycolipid antigens (DAT, PGLTb1) for diagnosis of tuberculosis in HIV-seropositive and -seronegative patients. *Eur J Clin Microbiol Infect. Dis* 1995;14:883–891.

32. Nakamura RM, Einck L, Velmonte MA, et al. Detection of active tuberculosis by an MPB-64 transdermal patch: a field study. *Scand J Infect Dis* 2001;33:405–407.

33. Boggian K, Fierz W, Vernazza PL. Infrequent detection of lipoarabinomannan antibodies in human immunodeficiency virus-associated mycobacterial disease. *J Clin Microbiol* 1996;34: 1854–1855.

34. Da Costa CTKA, Khanolkar-Young S, Elliot AM, et al. Immunoglobulin subclass responses to mycobacterial lipoarabinomannan in HIV-infected and non infected patients with tuberculosis. *Clin Exp Immunol* 1993;91:25–29.

35. Binkin NJ, Vernon AA, Simone PM, et al. Tuberculosis prevention and control activities in the United States: an overview of the organization of tuberculosis services. *Int J Tuberc Lung Dis* 1999; 3:663–674.

36. Hawken MP, Muhindi DW. Tuberculosis preventive therapy in HIV-infected persons: feasibility issues in developing countries. *Int J Tuberc Lung Dis* 1999;3:646–650.

37. van Vooren P, Farber CM, Motte S, et al. Assay of specific antibody response to mycobacterial antigen for the diagnosis of a pleural effusion in a patient with AIDS. *Tubercle* 1988;69:303–305.

38. Martin-Casabona N, Fuente TG, Papa F, et al. Time course of anti-SL-IV immunoglobulin G antibodies in patients with tuberculosis and tuberculosis-associated AIDS. *J Clin Microbiol* 1992; 30:1089–1093.

39. van Pinxteren LA, Ravn P, Agger EM, et al. Diagnosis of tuberculosis based on the two specific antigens ESAT-6 and CFP10. *Clin Diagn Lab Immunol* 2000;7:155–160.

40. Arend SM, Andersen P, van Meijgaarden KE, et al. Detection of active tuberculosis infection by T cell responses to early-secreted antigenic target 6-kDa protein and culture filtrate protein 10. *J Infect Dis* 2000;181:1850–1854.

41. Brock I, Munk ME, Kok-Jensen A, et al. Performance of whole blood IFN-gamma test for tuberculosis diagnosis based on PPD or the specific antigens ESAT-6 and CFP-10. *Int J Tuberc Lung Dis* 2001;5:462–467.

42. Vekemans J, Lienhardt C, Sillah JS, et al. Tuberculosis contacts but not patients have higher gamma interferon responses to ESAT-6 than do community controls in The Gambia. *Infect Immun* 2001;69:6554–6557.

43. Skjot RL, Oettinger T, Rosenkrands I, et al. Comparative evaluation of low-molecular-mass proteins from *Mycobacterium tuberculosis* identifies members of the ESAT-6 family as immunodominant T-cell antigens. *Infect Immun* 2000;68:214–220.

44. Lalvani A, Pathan AA, Durkan H, et al. Enhanced contact tracing and spatial tracking of *Mycobacterium tuberculosis* infection by enumeration of antigen-specific T cells. *Lancet* 2001;357: 2017–2021.

45. Lalvani A, Nagvenkar P, Udwadia Z, et al. Enumeration of T cells specific for RD1-encoded antigens suggests a high prevalence of latent *Mycobacterium tuberculosis* infection in healthy urban Indians. *J Infect Dis* 2001;183:469–477.

46. Coler RN, Skeiky YA, Ovendale PJ, et al. Cloning of a *Mycobacterium tuberculosis* gene encoding a purified protein derivative protein that elicits strong tuberculosis-specific delayed-type hypersensitivity. *J Infect Dis* 2000;182:224–233.

47. Campos-Neto A, Rodrigues-Junior V, Pedral-Sampaio DB, et al. Evaluation of DPPD, a single recombinant *Mycobacterium tuberculosis* protein as an alternative antigen for the Mantoux test. *Tuberculosis (Edinb)* 2001;81:353–358.

48. Singh KK, Dong Y, Hinds L, et al. Combined use of serum and urinary antibody for diagnosis of TB. *J Infect Dis* 2003 (in press).

14

THE ROLE OF THE *NRAMP1* GENE IN MYCOBACTERIAL INFECTIONS

ELLEN BUSCHMAN
EMIL SKAMENE
ERWIN SCHURR

In this chapter, we review studies that deal with the genetic component of resistance and susceptibility to tuberculosis. Specifically, we focus on the role of the *Nramp1* (natural resistance–associated macrophage protein 1) gene (formerly *Bcg*) in controlling natural resistance to mycobacteria.

The notion that genetic factors are involved in the development of tuberculosis disease is not entirely new. Historically, physicians in Anglo-Saxon and Northern countries favored a familial (inherited) component in the etiology of tuberculosis disease (1). This view was not shared by physicians in southern European countries where tuberculosis control focused on the contagious nature of the disease (1). After Koch's discovery of *Mycobacterium tuberculosis* as the causative agent of tuberculosis, the idea that genetic factors contributed to tuberculosis susceptibility lost credibility, and it took geneticists more than 30 years to return their attention to the study of tuberculosis. During this time, the genetic hypothesis of tuberculosis susceptibility was kept alive primarily by essentially circumstantial evidence of racial differences in tuberculosis susceptibility during epidemics. For example, at the turn of the century soon after their resettlement in the Qu'Appelle Valley, Canadian Indians experienced a tuberculosis epidemic in which the death rate was 9,000 per 100,000, the highest lethality recorded for any documented tuberculosis outbreak. Black African regiments deployed by the British to Ceylon in the early 19th century were essentially decimated by tuberculosis in 15 years (1). After tuberculosis was introduced to South Africa in the first half of the 19th century, not only were native Africans very susceptible, but the illness took a fulminant, acute course that was more like typhoid than tuberculosis (2), and, thus, it seemed that their increased susceptibility was also associated with a faster progression of the disease.

More circumstantial evidence supporting the role of genetic factors in mycobacterial resistance derives from vaccination trials with live, attenuated *Mycobacterium bovis* BCG (3,4), which, since 1921, has been used to immunize more than 2 billion people against tuberculosis. In several of the major vaccination trial studies (5,6), the protective efficacy of BCG has varied widely, and it has been speculated that this variation may arise from genetic differences between the study populations. A second example involved a tragic accident that occurred in Lübeck, Germany, in 1926 in which 251 children were immunized with a virulent strain of BCG (7). Of these children, 47 showed no detectable disease, 127 developed radiologically detectable lesions that healed, and 77 died of the disease. Although not conclusive, this accident provides good evidence that genetic factors are involved in the control of mycobacterial infection in humans.

In the 1930s, several large genetic studies were conducted of tuberculosis incidence among mono- and dizygotic twins (8). The concordance of tuberculosis reached, on average, 60% among monozygotic twins compared with approximately 20% concordance among dizygotic twins and siblings and less than 10% concordance among spouses. Although the concordance rates in these early studies were possibly inflated owing to ascertainment bias and other shortcomings in the study design, more recent twin studies and their analysis using multivariate statistical methods have confirmed the original results (9). It must be stressed that although the earlier twin studies have been criticized extensively by later investigators, these studies represent an important milestone in the genetic analysis of tuberculosis because they focused the attention of tuberculosis researchers on the importance of genetic factors in the control of tuberculosis susceptibility. Conversely, keeping in mind the experimental and conceptual difficulties encountered, twin studies also brought to light the fact that the

E. Buschman and E. Skamene: McGill Centre for the Study of Host Resistance, McGill University Health Center, Montreal, Quebec, Canada.
E. Schurr: Departments of Medicine and Human Genetics, McGill University; Department of Medicine, McGill University Health Centre, Montreal, Quebec, Canada.

analysis of human tuberculosis by itself would never fully reveal the intricate genetically controlled pathways that give rise to tuberculosis.

EARLY STUDIES ON HOST RESISTANCE TO MYCOBACTERIA

Studies Using Inbred Rabbits

The first conclusive evidence that genetic resistance mechanisms were operative in susceptibility to infection with *M. tuberculosis* H37Rv were provided by Lurie and Dannenberg (10), who initiated a systematic analysis of the genetic component involved in the control of tuberculosis susceptibility in rabbits. Using the number of primary tubercles that developed after controlled inhalation of human virulent *M. tuberculosis* bacilli as the selective trait, four inbred strains of rabbits were developed that expressed differing degrees of tuberculosis susceptibility (11). Resistant strains of rabbits had developed only 5% as many primary tubercles compared with their susceptible counterparts at 5 weeks after infection. Moreover, the number of viable tubercle bacilli contained in the lesions of susceptible animals was significantly lower than those found in lesions from susceptible rabbits. These results demonstrated that genetic factors are of crucial importance for the development of early or natural resistance to *M. tuberculosis* infection in immunologically naive animals. A second equally important observation obtained with this experimental system was that naturally resistant rabbits (i.e., those with low numbers of primary tubercles) were also more resistant to the progression of tuberculosis as evidenced by their increased survival times. Because longevity after inhalation of virulent tubercle bacilli was not used as a selective criterion during the generation of the inbred strains, one can speculate that resistance to attack (natural resistance) and resistance to progression of tuberculosis are different facets of the same underlying principle. Considering that the number of primary tubercles (natural resistance) was found associated with increased macrophage anti–tubercle bacillus activity and that acquired immune responses were shown to control progression of the disease, one can further speculate that macrophage expressed genes control both natural and acquired resistance to tuberculosis in inbred strains of rabbits. A more detailed genetic analysis of natural resistance to tuberculosis provided suggestive evidence for a multigenic control of the trait. Multigenic control of the macrophage-mediated anti–tubercle bacillus activity made it exceedingly difficult to provide formal genetic evidence of a link between natural and acquired resistance to tuberculosis. Nevertheless, the studies of inbred strains of rabbits established the validity of the genetic approach for the analysis of tuberculosis susceptibility and still provide one of the best examples of the contribution of genetic factors to the establishment and pathogenesis of tuberculosis disease.

Strain-Specific Differences in Tuberculosis Susceptibility Among Mouse Strains

The observation that different species of mice differ in their susceptibility to tuberculosis dates back to the work of Koch who noted that field mice (*Arvicola arvalis*) were more susceptible than house mice (*Mus musculus*) (12). This early observation was followed up by others (13,14) who tested inbred strains of mice for their tuberculosis susceptibility. These investigators found significant strain differences in the survival rates after *M. tuberculosis* (Ravenel) infection with the C57BL/6 strain exhibiting the highest resistance. They also established the importance of the route of inoculation, revealing that genetically determined strain differences can be masked by the size of the infectious inoculum. These studies in the mouse model confirmed the results obtained with experimentally infected rabbits and illustrated the importance of the interplay between the genetic constitution of a host and the specific environmental conditions that enhance or obliterate existing genetic differences. It was reasonable to expect that, given the right experimental conditions, the multigenic control of tuberculosis susceptibility detected among selectively bred strains of rabbits might be more readily dissected into individual components in the mouse model.

Detection of the *Bcg/Ity/Lsh* Gene

Studies of tuberculosis susceptibility in the mouse have always been hampered by the high pathogenicity of *M. tuberculosis*, which represents a significant safety hazard to the investigators. Consequently, studies of the relative resistance and susceptibility of different inbred strains of mice to attenuated bacille-Calmette–Guérin (BCG) strain of *M. bovis*, commonly known as BCG, were initiated (15). Susceptibility to BCG infection was measured as a qualitative phenotype (resistance or susceptibility) as the spleen or liver colony-forming unit (CFU) count 3 weeks after intravenous injection with low doses (10^4 CFUs) of dispersed bacilli of the Montreal strain of BCG. In these experiments, published 21 years ago, Forget et al. (15) showed that common inbred strains of mice segregated into two groups, based on nonoverlap of the CFU confidence intervals. It was found that low doses of BCG allowed rapid multiplication in the reticuloendothelial organs of susceptible mice during the first 3 to 4 weeks of infection, whereas no or only marginal multiplication occurred in the spleen and liver of resistant mice. The observation that all inbred strains of mice tested segregated into two sharply separated groups with respect to intracellular multiplication of BCG suggested that the trait of innate resistance to early growth of BCG in mice may be under single gene control. Formal segregation analysis of the trait in F1, F2, and backcross animals generated by crossing resistant A/J with susceptible B10.A progenitor mice confirmed this hypothesis. All

(B10.A × A/J)F1 mice, approximately 50% of the (B10.A × A/J)F1 × B10.A mice, and approximately 75% of the F2 mice were refractory to BCG multiplication (16). These results suggested the presence of a single, dominant BCG resistance locus that was termed *Bcg*.

The chromosomal location of the *Bcg* gene was accomplished through linkage analyses in two panels of recombinant inbred strains, BXD and BXH derived from the BCG-susceptible C57BL/6 progenitor, and the BCG-resistant DBA/2 and C3H/He progenitors, respectively. The strain distribution pattern of *Bcg^r* and *Bcg^s* alleles in BXD and BXH recombinant inbred strains established that the *Bcg* locus was on the proximal part of mouse chromosome 1 between the previously mapped markers *Idh-1* and *Pep-3* (17). The most interesting aspect of this mapping analysis was that the location of *Bcg* (17) matched exactly that of two other pathogen resistance genes, *Salmonella typhimurium* (*Ity*) and *Leishmania donovani* (*Lsh*), which had been discovered some years before (18,19). In 1982, two back-to-back articles published in *Nature* confirmed, by linkage analysis to the three different infections by progeny testing, that the resistance to the three pathogens mapped to the same chromosome 1 locus (17,20). It became quickly obvious that a gene of major importance to intracellular pathogen survival was involved, and several predictions were put forth in these papers. It was proposed that a single gene regulated resistance to the three taxonomically distinct pathogens and that such a gene would likely function by affecting a common biochemical or nutritional growth requirement within the macrophage. It was also hypothesized that the relatively small number of susceptible inbred strains implied that the susceptible allele was a recent mutation. Finally, it was proposed that, at least for *Bcg*, a human homolog would likely play a major role in resistance to tuberculosis and leprosy. Time has proven the accuracy of those early predictions; however, in 1982, the sole task was to find out whether *Bcg/Ity/Lsh* was one or three closely linked genes.

FROM *BCG/ITY/LSH* TO *NRAMP1*

The characterization of the function of *Bcg* was important to human disease because, as Bradley (21) put it in 1980, "only when one finds the biochemical mechanism for natural resistance, can one cross species barriers." Yet, without knowledge of an expressed protein or gene function, this undertaking would entail several complementary approaches and nearly 10 years. The first experiments set out to confirm the macrophage as the cell type expressing the *Bcg* gene and, after that, to identify the functional macrophage property or protein most closely associated with the *Bcg* gene phenotype. Our group showed that the *Bcg* gene was expressed by a radiation-resistant mature cell of the macrophage lineage that was susceptible to prolonged exposure to silica and that susceptibility could be trans-ferred with bone marrow–derived precursors (22). The immune phase of BCG infection and of T and B cells was shown not to be involved with the *Bcg* phenotype. Similar results were obtained with the *S. typhimurium* and *L. donovani* models (23,24). Conclusive proof that macrophages expressed the *Bcg* gene was provided by *in vitro* experiments showing that *Bcg^r* macrophages significantly reduced the growth of BCG (25), *Mycobacterium avium* (26), *Mycobacterium intracellulare* (27), *Mycobacterium smegmatis* (28), *L. donovani* (29), and *S. typhimurium* (30) compared with macrophages from *Bcg^s* congenic mice.

During this time, the *Bcg* congenic strains of mice were developed to provide a model for comparing *Bcg^r* and *Bcg^s* phenotypic activities *in vitro* and *in vivo* (31). Several groups (27,32,33) proceeded to assay various markers of functional and phenotypic parameters of macrophage activation in *Bcg* and *Lsh* congenic strains of mice. Macrophages isolated from resistant mice were generally found to demonstrate a greater magnitude of hexose monophosphate shunt and respiratory burst activity after phagocytosis of BCG (34) or stimulation with interferon gamma (35) compared with macrophages from susceptible mice. Macrophages from resistant animals consistently displayed superior expression of other markers, such as class II Ia antigen (33,36), ACM.1 and 5′ nucleotidase (37), lipopolysaccharide-elicited tumor necrosis factor production (32) and support of antigen specific and nonspecific T cell proliferation (36,38,39). In addition, two cloned macrophage cell lines, B10S(*Bcg^s*) and B10R(*Bcg^r*) were derived by immortalizing bone marrow macrophages from *Bcg*-congenic mouse strains to analyze the molecular characteristics of the *Bcg* gene (40). The B10R resistant cell line constitutively expressed increased bactericidal activity and higher levels of both I-Ab messenger RNA (mRNA) and Ia antigen compared with B10S cells. All these effects, termed the pleiotropic effects of the *Bcg* gene, suggested that macrophages isolated from resistant mice were genetically "switched on" to the state of priming for activation. Unfortunately, none of these parameters could be directly linked to innate resistance to the infectious organisms, and no candidate protein product was ever identified in these assays. There were several scenarios proposed for the *Bcg/Lsh* gene product, including an autocrine interleukin (37) and a DNA-binding protein (29). It has been interesting to view these predictions with the function of the Nramp1 protein, which is now partially known (see later).

Cloning of the *Bcg* (*Nramp1*) Gene

The second approach to identify *Bcg* was by positional cloning or reverse genetics, as it was then called, a procedure by which no mouse gene had ever been identified (41). This was an intense 7-year period of narrowing down the *Bcg* region by production of high-resolution genetic linkage maps with an extensive number of mouse crosses (42,43) and the construction of a physical map (44). A breakthrough occurred in 1992 using the technique of exon amplification reported the previous year (45). This method retrieved competent exons buried within cloned genomic fragments and resulted in the discovery of *Nramp1*, the first mouse gene obtained by positional cloning (46). Within 1 year, the 5′ promoter region of *Nramp1* was characterized (47), the human *NRAMP1* gene was cloned as well as a second mouse *Nramp* gene, *Nramp2* (48,49). Today, it is well established that the Nramp proteins comprise a large, conserved family with members identified in bacteria, yeast, plants, flies, and mammals (50,51).

THE *NRAMP1* GENE

Sequence analysis of the *Nramp1* gene in inbred strains revealed that the susceptibility allele is a single aspartic acid 169 (*Nramp1^{Asp169}*) substitution for glycine 169 in the resistant allele (*Nramp1^{Gly169}*) in predicted transmembrane domain 4 of the protein (44). The susceptibility allele, which was shown to coincide with the absence of Nramp1 protein in macrophages, was determined to arise from a recent mutational event and not as a variant of a polymorphic gene (52). Mice expressing the resistant allele express Nramp1 protein and are resistant to infection. Through the study of *Nramp1* knockouts and transgenics, it was at last indisputable that *Bcg*/*Ity*/*Lsh* were indeed one gene, as had been predicted 10 years earlier (53,54).

Nramp1 Protein and Function

Mouse Nramp1 protein is detected by anti-Nramp1 antibodies as a 90- to 110-kd protein (52) expressed in the late endosomal/lysosomal compartment of macrophages (55,56). At the organ level, Northern blot studies detected strong *Nramp1* mRNA expression in the spleen and liver, with almost no detectable expression in the lung (46,54,57,58). At the cellular level, *Nramp1* mRNA is found in the myeloid cells of the bone marrow and professional phagocytes and can be upregulated by lipopolysaccharide and interferon gamma via the nuclear factor interleukin-6 and interferon response elements in the promoter region of *Nramp1* (57,59). These data help to explain the earlier observations that the phenotypic expression of the *Bcg*/*Ity*/*Lsh* gene is most strong in the spleen and liver, along with the pleiotropic effects of the *Bcg* gene in activated macrophages.

At present, much has been revealed about how Nramp1 restricts the growth of intracellular parasites. Immunochemical analyses performed in macrophages have shown that the Nramp1 protein is expressed in endosomes and becomes actively recruited to the membrane of maturing phagosomes after phagocytosis of *S. typhimurium*, *Leishmania*, and *M. avium* (55,56,58,60,61). These results, together with the knowledge that Nramp1 has the structural features of a membrane transport protein, suggested that Nramp1 may transport a substrate that interferes with microbial growth in the macrophage. Extensive studies by several laboratories have shown that Nramp1 functions as a pH-dependent divalent cation pump at the phagolysosomal membrane. The direction of transport (efflux, influx, or both) and the precise divalent cation(s) (Fe^{2+}, Mn^{2+}, Zn^{2+}, Cu^{2+}) have not yet been resolved unambiguously (56, 62–66). One of the most intriguing properties of Nramp1 is its ability to affect the replication of unrelated pathogens within the macrophage. Intracellular pathogens, such as mycobacteria, actively secrete products that are specifically targeted to interfere with phagosomal function. The Nramp1 protein, through its effect on divalent cation availability, seems to be able to efficiently disrupt the function of these various pathogen mediators and, in so doing, allows the natural process of host microbicidal defense to occur.

HUMAN *NRAMP1*

The complete nucleotide sequence and genomic structure of the human *NRAMP1* gene region on chromosome region 2q35 has been determined (48,67,68). Sequence analysis of human *NRAMP1* revealed extensive (88%) conservation of the primary nucleotide sequence with mouse *Nramp1*. Thus, human *NRAMP1* encodes a predicted polytopic membrane transport protein. The protein sequence homology remains strong evidence that the protein is evolutionarily significant, functionally conserved, and thus a major candidate gene in host defense against mycobacterial infections. In some aspects, however, such as tissue expression, differences have been detected between human and mouse *Nramp1*. First, human *NRAMP1* mRNA studies revealed, in contrast to the mouse, strong expression in the lung compared with the spleen and liver (48,48,69). In addition, *NRAMP1* expression was found most strongly in polymorphonuclear cells, rather than in the fixed tissue macrophages of professional phagocytes found in the mouse. Furthermore, sequencing of homologous regions of human *NRAMP1* did not detect a correlate of the mouse susceptibility mutation (G169D). However, several other polymorphisms in the *NRAMP1* gene have been defined and tested for their linkage with mycobacterial disease, which is discussed in the following sections (68,70,71). It is appears that the pattern of Nramp1 tissue expression, in the background of a highly conserved gene sequence, has evolved differently in mice versus humans.

Relevance of *Nramp1* Knockout Studies to Tuberculosis

One seemingly conflicting result to emerge from the mouse *Nramp1* knockout studies is that *Nramp1* does not affect resistance to the H37Rv (virulent human isolate) strain of

M. tuberculosis, with *Nramp1*-resistant (129sv) and -susceptible (129sv *Nramp*$^{-/-}$) mice displaying an equivalent susceptibility to *M. tuberculosis* in all organs examined (72–74). It is important to remember that these experiments do not show that human *NRAMP1* plays no role in tuberculosis but rather that there are differences between the mouse model of tuberculosis and human tuberculosis. For example, it is not known which aspect of susceptibility in mice is the most appropriate correlate of susceptibility to tuberculosis disease in humans (75). In addition, because 129sv mice are relatively resistant to infection with *M. tuberculosis*, at least using CFU counts and survival times, it is possible that deletion of *Nramp1* may not have a strong effect on the employed measures of susceptibility if absence of Nramp1 makes mice more resistant to disease, as recently suggested (76). Another possibility is that weak expression of mouse *Nramp1* in the lung results in an inability of the Nramp1 protein to strongly influence resistance to a lung-tropic pathogen such as *M. tuberculosis*. More recent genetic analyses of tuberculosis in mice have revealed that susceptibility to *M. tuberculosis* is a complex, multigenic trait best examined through quantitative trait loci and recombinant congenic strain analyses rather than knockout approaches (77,78). Examples for quantitative trait loci mapping in mouse models are several recent scans to map loci influencing tuberculosis severity (77–79). These analyses, conducted on mice of different genetic backgrounds, have identified several significant linkages, on distal portion of chromosome 1, proximal chromosome 7, proximal chromosome 9, and distal chromosome 3. Interestingly, the location of the chromosome 9 linkage exactly overlapped the one found in a quantitative trait loci analysis of cutaneous leishmaniasis (80). Possible epigenetic interactions of those loci with *Nramp1* certainly also deserve more detailed study.

Genetic Analysis of *NRAMP1* in Human Mycobacterial Disease

To commence linkage and association analysis of *NRAMP1* with mycobacterial disease, 11 sequence variants have been identified within *NRAMP1* in a screening panel of 15 unrelated individuals of mixed ethnic origins (68,70,71). The variants include a (CA)$_n$ microsatellite repeat in the immediate 5′ region of the gene, a single nucleotide change in intron 4 (469+14G/C) (INT4), a nonconservative single-base substitution at codon 543 that changes aspartic acid to asparagine (D543N), and a TGTG deletion in the 3′ untranslated region. The allele frequencies of these markers have been measured among white, Asian, black, and Polynesian control individuals (70,71). It has been difficult to estimate and test the possible biologic relevance of these polymorphisms before linkage analysis with tuberculosis disease. The D543N coding region polymorphism is present in allele frequencies greater than 1% (68) and so could

be potentially significant. In the 5′ untranslated region, a repeat polymorphism identified with two predominant alleles is found with approximately 75% to 80% (n = 9) and 20% to 25% (n = 10) frequency (81). It has been shown that the n = 9 allele corresponds to significantly higher levels of *NRAMP1* expression than the n = 10 allele (81). However, it is not expected that a single mutation, such as found in mouse *Nramp1*, will explain human susceptibility to tuberculosis.

NRAMP1 and Mycobacterial Disease

Tuberculosis and leprosy are the two major global mycobacterial diseases. In 2000, there were an estimated 8.4 million new cases of tuberculosis and approximately 2 million deaths (82). In the same year, nearly 700,000 new leprosy cases were reported worldwide (83). Tuberculosis and leprosy are both complex diseases. Forty years ago, Neel (84) explained complex disease as a result of the interactions of pathogen factors, heredity, and environmental factors. The genetic analysis of such complex diseases is a formidable challenge and requires detailed knowledge in each epidemiologic setting of the ethnic background, family structure, clinical phenotypes of the disease, and vaccination status (85). The clinical picture of mycobacterial disease presents a multistep process. In tuberculosis, although almost two-thirds of the world's population is actually infected with *M. tuberculosis*, only an estimated 10% of those infected develop tuberculosis over the course of their lifetime. Considering all these various caveats, one must view the results of the genetic studies discussed in the following sections within a realm of possible genetic effects. One intriguing question is whether *NRAMP1* alleles are involved in susceptibility to one particular infection step, as has been found in the mouse. At present, there appears to be evidence of an impact of *NRAMP1* alleles on infection susceptibility, progression from infection to clinical disease, and acquired host responses (86–88). It is therefore likely that, as the genetic studies of *NRAMP1* accumulate, different mechanisms of *NRAMP1* genetic control will be revealed that act on different forms of tuberculosis. Another intriguing question that emerges as the *NRAMP1* studies accumulate is the counterbalancing force for allele maintenance of different *NRAMP1* alleles in different populations. This subject, like the recent studies of G6PD mutation and malaria endemicity, may lead to important clues about the natural history of tuberculosis susceptibility in world populations. It should be pointed out that although our discussion here is confined exclusively to *NRAMP1* as a candidate gene, several other genes, such as the vitamin D receptor gene, are equally attractive candidates, and the reader is referred to other reviews on this subject (89).

We have been collecting DNA samples from multiplex families with leprosy and tuberculosis worldwide for several years. The strongest evidence to date identifying *NRAMP1* as a major gene linked with tuberculosis susceptibility was detected in a tuberculosis outbreak in a community of aboriginal Canadians (85,87). In this linkage study, the *NRAMP1* gene (or a closely linked gene) seemed to control the progression from infected to affected status. This familial outbreak situation was focused on primary tuberculosis, i.e., manifestation of clinical disease within less than 2 years after infection. Assuming a relative risk of 10 for the susceptibility allele, a major tuberculosis susceptibility locus was mapped to the immediate vicinity of *NRAMP1* with high significance ($p < 10^{-5}$). However, in another linkage study in northern Brazil, 98 multiplex families with tuberculosis comprising more than 700 individuals were studied. Complex segregation analyses provided strong evidence of the presence of major tuberculosis susceptibility gene(s) but no significant evidence that this gene was associated with the *NRAMP1* gene (90). These two analyses, in different populations, different epidemiologic situations, and possibly different strains of *M. tuberculosis*, potentially illustrate that different genetic control mechanisms prevail.

However, *NRAMP1* alleles have been found associated with tuberculosis in four distinct ethnic populations. Evidence for association of *NRAMP1* with tuberculosis susceptibility has been obtained in The Gambia. Using a population-based case-control design, a study in The Gambia investigated the contribution of *NRAMP1* alleles to tuberculosis risk among 410 adult patients with pulmonary tuberculosis and 417 ethnically matched controls (91). Four polymorphisms within *NRAMP1* were analyzed for association with tuberculosis and found associated with tuberculosis. An odds ratio of 1.8 to 1.9 was found, with the rare alleles being significant risk factors for the development of tuberculosis. Similarly, the role of *NRAMP1* alleles as risk factors for tuberculosis was analyzed in studies in Japan, Korea, and Conakry, Guinea. In the Japanese study (92), in agreement with the study in The Gambia study (91), the common promoter repeat allele was found to be a protective factor for tuberculosis ($p = 0.039$) (92). In the Korean study, the *NRAMP1* 1729+55del4 polymorphism was found associated with tuberculosis ($p = 0.02$) (93). Finally, in Conakry, Guinea, the transmission of *NRAMP1* alleles to affected children was assessed in 44 families (94). Of the three polymorphisms analyzed, only the 469+14G/C polymorphism in intron 4 showed significant evidence of association with tuberculosis ($p = 0.036$).

NRAMP1 and Leprosy

Strong evidence of a major role of genetics, possibly *NRAMP1*, in susceptibility to leprosy came from studies in 1995 of families with leprosy in southern Vietnam. In this population, complex segregation analysis revealed that Chinese families showed a strong disposition for a complex genetic-epidemiologic model of susceptibility, whereas Vietnamese families displayed evidence of a major codominant gene with age-dependent penetrance controlling susceptibility to leprosy per se (95). Subsequently, 168 members of 20 multiplex Vietnamese families with were genotyped for *NRAMP1* alleles and four closely linked polymorphic markers. Significant evidence for linkage was observed ($p < 0.005$ to 0.02) and the extent of allele sharing was strong (58%) (71). However, it is unlikely that *NRAMP1* is the major locus detected in the preceding complex segregation analysis. In a second study of *NRAMP1* in leprosy in this same Vietnamese population, significant linkage was observed between *NRAMP1* and the Mitsuda reaction, an *in vivo* diagnostic skin test for lepromatous leprosy that measures specific immunity against lepromin (88). Interestingly, this study indicates that *NRAMP1* somehow influences the development of acquired antimycobacterial immune responses. Such an effect of *NRAMP1* would be in contrast to mouse *Nramp1*, which, in mycobacterial infections, does not seem to affect acquired immune responses. Finally, an association of *NRAMP1* alleles with leprosy type, but not leprosy per se, was detected in Mali (96).

Although the studies above strongly implicate *NRAMP1* as a leprosy susceptibility gene, as in tuberculosis, not all studies have detected association with leprosy and *NRAMP1* (97–100). In addition, a recent genome scan of leprosy susceptibility (101) detected a susceptibility locus on chromosome 10p but failed detect the *NRAMP1*, *VDR*, and *HLA* chromosomal regions detected in other studies (97). In addition, two smaller studies of leprosy, one a case-control study in Calcutta, India, and the other a small analysis of seven families in French Polynesia, failed to detect any association or linkage of *NRAMP1* with leprosy (99,100,102).

A possible contribution of *NRAMP1* to mycobacterial disease susceptibility has now been tested in several studies. Although not absolute, adequate replication has been achieved, particularly in the case of tuberculosis, and it has been firmly established that *NRAMP1* alleles are risk factors for clinical tuberculosis. To pursue this finding, it is necessary to further refine clinical definitions to narrow down the infectious step affected by *NRAMP1* alleles. To fully realize this endeavor, it will be necessary to develop assays of *NRAMP1* function to pinpoint the biologic activity of specific *NRAMP1* alleles in the infectious process.

CONCLUSION

The problems confounding genetic analysis in human populations have been most adequately summarized by Sturtevant (103). "Man," he wrote, "is one of the most unsatisfactory of all organisms for genetic study." The truth of this statement is intuitively known to all of us: the complex breeding pattern of human populations, influenced by social structure and religious and political beliefs as much as by chance, complex gene–gene and gene–environment interactions, and the likely interdependence of these factors all contribute to the problem. The complexities of human genetics are a major reason that investigators have turned to animal models of genetic control of infectious disease. Nevertheless, allele frequencies in human populations and thus the relative importance of distinct loci for multigenic trait expression or the extent of genetic heterogeneity are impossible to predict from studies of experimental species. Likewise, complex traits such as susceptibility to tuberculosis disease are characterized by the presence of incomplete penetrance of susceptibility alleles and the occurrence of phenocopies, i.e., individuals who are affected by the disease (e.g., tuberculosis) for nongenetic reasons. Both complications do not exist in the mouse model. Does this mean that animal models are ineffectual for the genetic analysis of human complex traits such as tuberculosis susceptibility? It certainly does not. The candidate gene approach, as suggested by comparative genome studies, is still valid for many genetic disorders and will remain a cornerstone in deciphering mechanisms of pathogenesis for many years to come. In this context, it has been the great fortune of our group to be involved in both the analysis of experimental species as well as human mycobacterial diseases. The results obtained have proved that the exchange of information between mouse and human geneticists is a profitable and powerful tool to advance the genetic study of human infectious disease, and it is our belief that animal models still hold the key for unraveling important mysteries of susceptibility to medically important infectious diseases.

REFERENCES

1. Dubos R, Dubos J. *The white plague.* New Brunswick/London: Rutgers University Press, 1952:28–43.
2. Stead WW. Genetics and resistance to tuberculosis: could resistance be enhanced by genetic engineering? *Ann Intern Med* 1992;116:937–941.
3. Lotte A, Wasz-Hockert O, Poisson N, et al. BCG complications. Estimates of the risks among vaccinated subjects and statistical analysis of their main characteristics. *Adv Tuberc Res* 1984;21:107–193.
4. Behr MA, Small PM. A historical and molecular phylogeny of BCG strains. *Vaccine* 1999;17:915–922.
5. Chaparas SD. Immunity in tuberculosis. *Bull World Health Organ* 1982;60:447–462.
6. ten Dam HG. Research on BCG vaccination. *Adv Tuberc Res* 1984;21:79–106.
7. McKinney JD, Jacobs JR, Bloom BR. Persisting problems in tuberculosis. In: *Emerging infections.* San Diego, London, Boston: Academic Press, 1998:51–146.
8. Simmonds B. *Tuberculosis in twins.* London: Pitman Medical Publishing, 1963.
9. Comstock GW. Tuberculosis in twins: a re-analysis of the Prophit survey. *Am Rev Respir Dis* 1978;117:621–624.
10. Lurie MB, Dannenberg AM Jr. Macrophage function in infectious disease with inbred rabbits. *Bacteriol Rev* 1965;29:466–476.
11. Lurie MB, Abramson S, Heppleston AG. On the response of genetically resistant and susceptible rabbits: the quantitative inhalation of human-type tubercle bacilli and the nature of resistance to tuberculosis. *J Exp Med* 1952;95:119–134.
12. Donovick R, McKee CM, Jambar WP, et al. Use of the mouse in the standardized test for anti-tuberculous activity of compounds of natural or synthetic origin: choice of mouse strain. *Am Rev Tuberc* 1949;60:109–120.
13. Pierce CR, Dubos J, Middlebrook G. Infection of mice with mammalian tubercle bacilli grown in tween-albumin liquid medium. *J Exp Med* 1947;86:159–165.
14. Youmans GP, Youmans AS. The difference in response of four strains of mice to immunization against tuberculous infection. *Am Rev Respir Dis* 1959;80:753–763.
15. Forget A, Skamene E, Gros P, et al. Differences in response among inbred mouse strains to infection with small doses of *Mycobacterium bovis* BCG. *Infect Immun* 1981;32:42–47.
16. Gros P, Skamene E, Forget A. Genetic control of natural resistance to *Mycobacterium bovis* (BCG) in mice. *J Immunol* 1981;127:2417–2421.
17. Skamene E, Gros P, Forget A, et al. Genetic regulation of resistance to intracellular pathogens. *Nature* 1982;297:506–510.
18. Bradley DJ. Genetic control of natural resistance to *Leishmania donovani. Nature* 1974;250:353–354.
19. Plant J, Glynn AA. Genetics of resistance to infection with *Salmonella typhimurium* in mice. *J Infect Dis* 1976;133:72–78.
20. Plant JE, Blackwell JM, O'Brien AD, et al. Are the *Lsh* and *Ity* disease resistance genes at one locus on mouse chromosome 1? *Nature* 1982;297:510–511.
21. Bradley DJ. In: Skamene E, Kongshavn PAL, Landy M, eds. *Genetic control of natural resistance to infection and malignancy.* New York: Academic Press, 1980.
22. Gros P, Skamene E, Forget A. Cellular mechanisms of genetically controlled host resistance to *Mycobacterium bovis* (BCG). *J Immunol* 1983;131:1966–1972.
23. Crocker PR, Blackwell JM, Bradley DJ. Transfer of innate resistance and susceptibility to *Leishmania donovani* infection in mouse radiation bone marrow chimaeras. *Immunology* 1984;52:417–422.
24. O'Brien AD, Scher I, Formal SB. Effect of silica on the innate resistance of inbred mice to *Salmonella typhimurium* infection. *Infect Immun* 1979;25:513–520.
25. Stach JL, Gros P, Forget A, et al. Phenotypic expression of genetically-controlled natural resistance to *Mycobacterium bovis* (BCG). *J Immunol* 1984;132:888–892.
26. Stokes RW, Orme IM, Collins FM. Role of mononuclear phagocytes in expression of resistance and susceptibility to *Mycobacterium avium* infections in mice. *Infect Immun* 1986;54:811–819.
27. Goto Y, Buschman E, Skamene E. Regulation of host resistance to *Mycobacterium intracellulare in vivo* and *in vitro* by the BCG gene. *Immunogenetics* 1989;30:218–221.
28. Denis M, Forget A, Pelletier M, et al. Killing of *Mycobacterium smegmatis* by macrophages from genetically susceptible and resistant mice. *J Leukoc Biol* 1990;47:25–30.
29. Crocker PR, Davies EV, Blackwell JM. Variable expression of the murine natural resistance gene Lsh in different macrophage populations infected *in vitro* with *Leishmania donovani. Parasite Immunol* 1987;9:705–719.
30. Lissner CR, Swanson RN, O'Brien AD. Genetic control of the innate resistance of mice to *Salmonella typhimurium*: expression of the Ity gene in peritoneal and splenic macrophages isolated *in vitro. J Immunol* 1983;131:3006–3013.
31. Potter M, O'Brien AD, Skamene E, et al. A BALB/c congenic strain of mice that carries a genetic locus (Ityr) controlling resistance to intracellular parasites. *Infect Immun* 1983;40:1234–1235.
32. Blackwell JM, Roach TI, Atkinson SE, et al. Genetic regulation

of macrophage priming/activation: the Lsh gene story. *Immunol Lett* 1991;30:241–248.

33. Zwilling BS, Hilburger ME. Macrophage resistance genes: Bcg/Ity/Lsh. *Immunol Ser* 1994;60:233–245.

34. Denis M, Forget A, Pelletier M, et al. Pleiotropic effects of the Bcg gene: III. Respiratory burst in Bcg-congenic macrophages. *Clin Exp Immunol* 1988;73:370–375.

35. Blackwell JM, Toole S, King M, et al. Analysis of Lsh gene expression in congenic B10.L-Lshr mice. *Curr Top Microbiol Immunol* 1988;137:301–309.

36. Denis M, Buschman E, Forget A, et al. Pleiotropic effects of the Bcg gene. II. Genetic restriction of responses to mitogens and allogeneic targets. *J Immunol* 1988;141:3988–3993.

37. Buschman E, Taniyama T, Nakamura R, et al. Functional expression of the Bcg gene in macrophages. *Res Immunol* 1989; 140:793–797.

38. Buschman E, Skamene E. Immunological consequences of innate resistance and susceptibility to BCG. *Immunol Lett* 1988; 19:199–209.

39. Kaye PM, Blackwell JM. Lsh, antigen presentation and the development of CMI. *Res Immunol* 1989;140:810–815.

40. Radzioch D, Hudson T, Boule M, et al. Genetic resistance/susceptibility to mycobacteria: phenotypic expression in bone marrow derived macrophage lines. *J Leukoc Biol* 1991;50:263–272.

41. Gros P, Malo D. A reverse genetics approach to Bcg/Ity/Lsh gene cloning. *Res Immunol* 1989;140:774–777.

42. Schurr E, Skamene E, Forget A, et al. Linkage analysis of the *Bcg* gene on mouse chromosome 1: identification of a tightly linked marker. *J Immunol* 1989;142:4507–4513.

43. Malo D, Schurr E, Epstein DJ, et al. The host resistance locus Bcg is tightly linked to a group of cytoskeleton-associated protein genes that include villin and desmin. *Genomics* 1991;10: 356–364.

44. Malo D, Vogan K, Vidal S, et al. Haplotype mapping and sequence analysis of the mouse Nramp gene predict susceptibility to infection with intracellular parasites. *Genomics* 1994;23: 51–61.

45. Buckler AJ, Chang DD, Graw SL, et al. Exon amplification: a strategy to isolate mammalian genes based on RNA splicing. *Proc Natl Acad Sci U S A* 1991;88:4005–4009.

46. Vidal SM, Malo D, Vogan K, et al. Natural resistance to infection with intracellular parasites: isolation of a candidate for Bcg. *Cell* 1993;73:469–485.

47. Barton CH, White JK, Roach TI, et al. NH2-terminal sequence of macrophage-expressed natural resistance-associated macrophage protein (Nramp) encodes a proline/serine-rich putative Src homology 3-binding domain. *J Exp Med* 1994;179: 1683–1687.

48. Cellier M, Govoni G, Vidal S, et al. Human natural resistance-associated macrophage protein: cDNA cloning, chromosomal mapping, genomic organization, and tissue-specific expression. *J Exp Med* 1994;180:1741–1752.

49. Gruenheid S, Cellier M, Vidal S, et al. Identification and characterization of a second mouse Nramp gene. *Genomics* 1995;25: 514–525.

50. Cellier M, Prive G, Belouchi A, et al. Nramp defines a family of membrane proteins. *Proc Natl Acad Sci U S A* 1995;92: 10089–10093.

51. Cellier MF, Bergevin I, Boyer E, et al. Polyphyletic origins of bacterial Nramp transporters. *Trends Genet* 2001;17:365–370.

52. Vidal SM, Pinner E, Lepage P, et al. Natural resistance to intracellular infections: Nramp1 encodes a membrane phosphoglycoprotein absent in macrophages from susceptible (Nramp1 D169) mouse strains. *J Immunol* 1996;157:3559–3568.

53. Vidal S, Gros P, Skamene E. Natural resistance to infection with

intracellular parasites: molecular genetics identifies Nramp1 as the Bcg/Ity/Lsh locus. *J Leukoc Biol* 1995;58:382–390.

54. Govoni G, Vidal S, Gauthier S, et al. The Bcg/Ity/Lsh locus: genetic transfer of resistance to infections in C57BL/6J mice transgenic for the *Nramp1 Gly169* allele. *Infect Immun* 1996;64: 2923–2929.

55. Gruenheid S, Pinner E, Desjardins M, et al. Natural resistance to infection with intracellular pathogens: the Nramp1 protein is recruited to the membrane of the phagosome. *J Exp Med* 1997; 185:717–730.

56. Searle S, Bright NA, Roach TI, et al. Localisation of Nramp1 in macrophages: modulation with activation and infection. *J Cell Sci* 1998;111:2855–2866.

57. Govoni G, Vidal S, Cellier M, et al. Genomic structure, promoter sequence, and induction of expression of the mouse Nramp1 gene in macrophages. *Genomics* 1995;27:9–19.

58. Govoni G, Canonne-Hergaux F, Pfeifer CG, et al. Functional expression of Nramp1 in vitro in the murine macrophage line RAW264.7. *Infect Immun* 1999;67:2225–2232.

59. Govoni G, Gauthier S, Billia F, et al. Cell-specific and inducible Nramp1 gene expression in mouse macrophages *in vitro* and *in vivo*. *J Leukoc Biol* 1997;62:277–286.

60. Cuellar-Mata P, Jabado N, Liu J, et al. Nramp1 modifies the fusion of *Salmonella typhimurium*-containing vacuoles with cellular endomembranes in macrophages. *J Biol Chem* 2002;277: 2258–2265.

61. Scott CC, Cuellar-Mata P, Matsuo T, et al. Role of 3-phosphoinositides in the maturation of *Salmonella*-containing vacuoles within host cells. *J Biol Chem* 2002;277:12770–12776.

62. Jabado N, Jankowski A, Dougaparsad S, et al. Natural resistance to intracellular infections: natural resistance- associated macrophage protein 1 (Nramp1) functions as a pH-dependent manganese transporter at the phagosomal membrane. *J Exp Med* 2000;192:1237–1248.

63. Zwilling BS, Kuhn DE, Wikoff L, et al. Role of iron in Nramp1-mediated inhibition of mycobacterial growth. *Infect Immun* 1999;67:1386–1392.

64. Kuhn DE, Lafuse WP, Zwilling BS. Iron transport into mycobacterium avium-containing phagosomes from an Nramp1(Gly169)-transfected RAW264.7 macrophage cell line. *J Leukoc Biol* 2001;69:43–49.

65. Atkinson PG, Barton CH. High level expression of Nramp1G169 in RAW264.7 cell transfectants: analysis of intracellular iron transport. *Immunology* 1999;96:656–662.

66. Goswami T, Bhattacharjee A, Babal P, et al. Natural-resistance-associated macrophage protein 1 is an H+/bivalent cation antiporter. *Biochem J* 2001;354:511–519.

67. Marquet S, Lepage P, Hudson TJ, et al. Complete nucleotide sequence and genomic structure of the human NRAMP1 gene region on chromosome region 2q35. *Mamm Genome* 2000;11: 755–762.

68. Liu J, Fujiwara TM, Buu NT, et al. Identification of polymorphisms and sequence variants in the human homologue of the mouse natural resistance-associated macrophage protein gene. *Am J Hum Genet* 1995;56:845–853.

69. Cellier M, Shustik C, Dalton W, et al. Expression of the human NRAMP1 gene in professional primary phagocytes: studies in blood cells and in HL-60 promyelocytic leukemia. *J Leuk Biol* 1997;61:96–105.

70. Buu NT, Cellier M, Gros P, et al. Identification of a highly polymorphic length variant in the 3′UTR of *NRAMP1*. *Immunogenetics* 1995;42:428–429.

71. Abel L, Sanchez FO, Oberti J, et al. Susceptibility to leprosy is linked to the human *NRAMP1* gene. *J Infect Dis* 1998;177: 133–145.

72. Medina E, Rogerson BJ, North RJ. The Nramp1 antimicrobial resistance gene segregates independently of resistance to virulent *Mycobacterium tuberculosis*. *Immunology* 1996;88:479–481.

73. North RJ, LaCourse R, Ryan L, et al. Consequence of NRAMP1 deletion to *Mycobacterium tuberculosis* infection in mice. *Infect Immun* 1999;67:5811–5814.

74. Medina E, North RJ. Resistance ranking of some common inbred mouse strains to *Mycobacterium tuberculosis* and relationship to major histocompatibility complex haplotype and Nramp1 genotype. *Immunology* 1998;93:270–274.

75. Dannenberg AMJ, Collins FM. Progressive pulmonary tuberculosis is not due to increasing numbers of viable bacilli in rabbits, mice and guinea pigs, but is due to a continuous host response to mycobacterial products. *Tuberculosis* 2001;81:229–242.

76. Caron J, Loredo-Osti JC, Laroche L, et al. Identification of genetic loci controlling bacterial clearance in experimental *Salmonella enteritidis* infection: an unexpected role of Nramp1 (Slc11a1) in the persistence of infection in mice. *Genes Immun* 2002;3:196–204.

77. Lavebratt C, Apt AS, Nikonenko BV, et al. Severity of tuberculosis in mice is linked to distal chromosome 3 and proximal chromosome 9. *J Infect Dis* 1999;180:150–155.

78. Kramnik I, Dietrich WF, Demant P, et al. Genetic control of resistance to experimental infection with virulent *Mycobacterium tuberculosis*. *Proc Natl Acad Sci U S A* 2000;97:8560–8565.

79. Mitsos LM, Cardon LR, Fortin A, et al. Genetic control of susceptibility to infection with *Mycobacterium tuberculosis* in mice. *Genes Immun* 2000;1:467–477.

80. Roberts LJ, Baldwin TM, Curtis JM, et al. Resistance to *Leishmania* major is linked to the H2 region on chromosome 17 and to chromosome 9. *J Exp Med* 1997;185:1705–1710.

81. Searle S, Blackwell JM. Evidence for a functional repeat polymorphism in the promoter of the human NRAMP1 gene that correlates with autoimmune versus infectious disease susceptibility. *J Med Genet* 1999;36:295–299.

82. World Health Organization. *Global tuberculosis control. WHO report. 2001* (WHO/CDS/TB/2001.28). Geneva, Switzerland: World Health Organization, 2001.

83. World Health Organization. Leprosy—global situation. *Wkly Epidemiol Rec* 2000;75:226–231.

84. Neel JV. Diabetes mellitus: a thrifty genotype rendered detrimental by progress? *Am J Hum Genet* 1962;14:353–362.

85. Abel L, Casanova JL. Genetic predisposition to clinical tuberculosis: bridging the gap between simple and complex inheritance. *Am J Hum Genet* 2000;67:274–277.

86. Borgdorff MW. The NRAMP1 gene and susceptibility to tuberculosis. *N Engl J Med* 1998;339:199–200.

87. Greenwood CM, Fujiwara TM, Boothroyd LJ, et al. Linkage of tuberculosis to chromosome 2q35 loci, including NRAMP1, in a large aboriginal Canadian family. *Am J Hum Genet* 2000;67:405–416.

88. Alcais A, Sanchez FO, Thuc NV, et al. Granulomatous reaction to intradermal injection of lepromin (Mitsuda reaction) is linked to the human NRAMP1 gene in Vietnamese leprosy sibships. *J Infect Dis* 2000;181:302–308.

89. Casanova JL, Abel L. Genetic dissection of immunity to mycobacteria: the human model. *Annu Rev Immunol* 2002;20:581–620.

90. Shaw MA, Collins A, Peacock CS, et al. Evidence that genetic susceptibility to *Mycobacterium tuberculosis* in a Brazilian population is under oligogenic control: linkage study of the candidate genes NRAMP1 and TNFA. *Tuber Lung Dis* 1997;78:35–45.

91. Bellamy R, Ruwende C, Corrah T, et al. Variations in the NRAMP1 gene and susceptibility to tuberculosis in West Africans. *N Engl J Med* 1998;338:640–644.

92. Gao PS, Fujishima S, Mao XQ, et al. Genetic variants of NRAMP1 and active tuberculosis in Japanese populations. *Clin Genet* 2000;58:74–76.

93. Ryu S, Park YK, Bai GH, et al. 3′UTR polymorphisms in the NRAMP1 gene are associated with susceptibility to tuberculosis in Koreans. *Int J Tuberc Lung Dis* 2000;4:577–580.

94. Cervino AC, Lakiss S, Sow O, et al. Allelic association between the NRAMP1 gene and susceptibility to tuberculosis in Guinea-Conakry. *Ann Hum Genet* 2000;64:507–512.

95. Abel L, Vu DL, Oberti J, et al. Complex segregation analysis of leprosy in southern Vietnam. *Genet Epidemiol* 1995;12:63–82.

96. Meisner SJ, Mucklow S, Warner G, et al. Association of NRAMP1 polymorphism with leprosy type but not susceptibility to leprosy per se in west Africans. *Am J Trop Med Hyg* 2001;65:733–735.

97. Shaw MA, Atkinson S, Dockrell H, et al. An RFLP map for 2q33-q37 from multicase mycobacterial and leishmanial disease families: no evidence for an Lsh/Ity/Bcg gene homologue influencing susceptibility to leprosy. *Ann Hum Genet* 1993;57:251–271.

98. Blackwell JM, Black GF, Peacock CS, et al. Immunogenetics of leishmanial and mycobacterial infections: the Belem family study. *Philos Trans R Soc Lond B Biol Sci* 1997;352:1331–1345.

99. Levee G, Liu J, Gicquel B, et al. Genetic control of susceptibility to leprosy in French Polynesia; no evidence for linkage with markers on telomeric human chromosome 2. *Int J Lepr Other Mycobact Dis* 1994;62:499–511.

100. Roger M, Levee G, Chanteau S, et al. No evidence for linkage between leprosy susceptibility and the human natural resistance-associated macrophage protein 1 (NRAMP1) gene in French Polynesia. *Int J Lepr Other Mycobact Dis* 1997;65:197–202.

101. Siddiqui MR, Meisner S, Tosh K, et al. A major susceptibility locus for leprosy in India maps to chromosome 10p13. *Nat Genet* 2001;27:439–441.

102. Roy S, Frodsham A, Saha B, et al. Association of vitamin D receptor genotype with leprosy type. *J Infect Dis* 1999;179:187–191.

103. Sturtevant AH. Social implications of the genetics of man. *Science* 1954;120:405–407.

Tuberculosis, Second Edition, edited by William N. Rom and Stuart M. Garay. Lippincott Williams & Wilkins, Philadelphia © 2004

PHAGOCYTOSIS AND TOLL-LIKE RECEPTORS IN TUBERCULOSIS

LARRY S. SCHLESINGER

Mycobacterium tuberculosis is an intracellular pathogen of mononuclear phagocytes that is uniquely adapted to the human host. Its survival during phagocytosis and subsequent multiplication within these professional phagocytes are critical for disease pathogenesis. The molecular determinants for phagocytosis are currently being defined, and recent studies provide evidence of their role in influencing both immediate host cell responses and the fate of the pathogen.

During primary lung infection of the human host, *M. tuberculosis* enters and survives in the alveolar macrophage (AM), a cell with several unique attributes. Subsequently, bacilli disseminate from the lung and are phagocytosed by a heterogeneous group of tissue macrophages and dendritic cells. Thus, *M. tuberculosis* has developed unique strategies to circumvent the normal fate of phagocytosed organisms. This chapter reviews advances in our understanding of the molecular determinants of *M. tuberculosis* phagocytosis by mononuclear phagocytes and immediate host responses generated by a family of important regulators of innate immune cell activation: the Toll-like receptor (TLR) family.

ENTRY OF *MYCOBACTERIUM TUBERCULOSIS* INTO THE MONONUCLEAR PHAGOCYTE

M. tuberculosis enters mononuclear phagocytes by receptor-mediated phagocytosis (1), in which several major host cell receptors play a role. These include complement receptors (CRs), the mannose receptor (MR), and type A scavenger receptors (1–5). The CRs involved are CR1 (CD35) and the leukocyte integrins CR3 (CD11b/CD18) and CR4 (CD11c/CD18) (6). The expression of CRs (particularly CR4) and the MR increases during monocyte differentiation

into macrophages, and CR4 and the MR are highly expressed on AMs (7,8). In the absence of specific antibody, Fcγ receptors do not play a role in phagocytosis (1), an important finding because entry via this receptor would be expected to generate a vigorous host response. The phagocytosis of *M. tuberculosis* is enhanced in the presence of nonimmune serum as a result of complement component C3 opsonization of bacteria. However, phagocytosis of nonopsonized *M. tuberculosis* by CRs also occurs via a direct interaction between bacilli and phagocyte receptors. The levels of phagocytosis in fresh serum of live and heat-killed virulent Erdman strain *M. tuberculosis* by human monocyte-derived macrophages (MDMs) are equivalent (L. S. Schlesinger, unpublished data, 1993). Thus, viability of the bacterium does not appear to be a requirement for the phagocytic process itself, although it plays an important role in the events after phagocytosis.

MYCOBACTERIUM TUBERCULOSIS AND COMPLEMENT PROTEIN C3

Complement activation is pertinent to tuberculosis (TB) pathogenesis as the bacteria encounter complement proteins in the alveolus of the lung (9), during hematogenous spread, and in various tissue sites (10). In these sites, macrophages can secrete complement proteins capable of opsonizing phagocytic particles. The phagocytosis of *M. tuberculosis* by mononuclear phagocytes is enhanced in serum as a result of complement activation that leads to opsonization of bacteria with the C3 activation products C3b and C3bi (11). *M. tuberculosis* cell wall components were shown in early studies to mediate the activation of complement (12,13). The C3 acceptor molecule(s) on the surface of *M. tuberculosis* is(are) beginning to be defined. The *M. tuberculosis* heparin-binding hemagglutinin is one such potential acceptor (14).

Several mechanisms exist for mediating the opsonization of pathogenic mycobacteria with C3 products, raising the possibility that C3 opsonization varies in form and amount between different tissue sites and during different stages of

L. S. Schlesinger: Department of Internal Medicine/Infectious Diseases, Ohio State University; Department of Infectious Diseases, Ohio State University Medical Center, Columbus, Ohio.

infection (e.g., primary TB infection versus reactivation disease). Apart from issues related to complement protein availability, strain-dependent differences in the composition of *M. tuberculosis* outer "capsular" polysaccharides have been shown to affect C3 deposition to some extent (15). Differences in C3 opsonization would affect the relative involvement of different CRs during entry and might influence the fate of the bacterium.

Complement activation and C3 deposition on *M. tuberculosis* occur via the alternative complement pathway in high concentrations of nonimmune human serum (1). Mannose-binding lectin (MBL) and its associated serine proteases can activate both classical and alternative complement pathways (reviewed in reference 16). MBL binds to the surface of mycobacteria (17,18) and may thus mediate activation of complement, resulting in C3 opsonization of bacteria. Finally, there is recent evidence that complement protein 2a in serum can cleave C3 independently of the classical complement components C1 and C4b, leading to C3 product deposition on pathogenic mycobacteria, a pathway postulated to be important in tissue sites of infection (19).

In vitro studies have established that human pulmonary cells have the capacity to produce components of the complement cascade. Complement components such as factor B, C2, C4, C3, and C5 are produced by alveolar type II cells, and C2 and factor B are produced by AMs (9,20). In addition, human C3 gene expression can be induced in the A549 cell line by glucocorticoids (21). Thus, C3 present in the airway could serve as an opsonin for *M. tuberculosis* phagocytosis by AMs, even in the absence of an induced inflammatory response.

COMPLEMENT RECEPTORS

CR3 is the major integrin of phagocytic cells (mononuclear phagocytes and polymorphonuclear leukocytes) and is expressed on natural killer cells and a small set of lymphocytes. In addition to phagocytosis, CR3 mediates stable adhesion of leukocytes to endothelium and the subsequent migration into inflamed organs. These functions are mediated through binding to several physiologic ligands including C3bi (6,22,23). The important but less studied CR4 binds C3bi and serves as a receptor for lipopolysaccharide (LPS) (24–26).

CRs play a major role in the phagocytosis of *M. tuberculosis* by human monocytes and macrophages. CR1 and CR3 on human monocytes mediate phagocytosis of the virulent Erdman strain of *M. tuberculosis* (1). Combinations of two monoclonal antibodies against distinct epitopes on the α chain of CR3 reduce the phagocytosis of *M. tuberculosis* by 80%. Monoclonal antibodies against the C3bi binding

epitope of CR3 and those against other ligand-binding epitopes inhibit phagocytosis. Thus, it is possible that more than one epitope is important in binding *M. tuberculosis* (see later).

The phagocytosis by MDMs of two virulent *M. tuberculosis* strains, Erdman and H37Rv, and the attenuated strain H37Ra is enhanced comparably in fresh nonimmune serum relative to no serum. Ingestion of these strains occurs both in the presence and absence of serum, and the bacteria are found within phagosomes (2). A combination of monoclonal antibodies against CR1, CR3, and CR4 on MDMs inhibits the phagocytosis of all three strains by nearly 80% in the presence of serum. Although studies using MDMs provide detailed information that is applicable to human AMs, direct examination of AMs provides additional insights. Phagocytosis of *M. tuberculosis* by human AMs is greater than that by monocytes, and CR4 plays a particularly important role (5).

There is evidence of the direct interaction between *M. tuberculosis* surface components and CR3 during phagocytosis based on *in vitro* studies using human and murine macrophages and CR3-transfected Chinese hamster ovary cell lines (2,3,15,27). Monoclonal antibodies against CRs significantly inhibit the phagocytosis of bacteria by human macrophages in the absence of serum (2). The binding site for *M. tuberculosis* on CR3 of murine macrophages in the absence of serum was found to be distinct from the C3bi binding site as determined by monoclonal antibody–blocking experiments (3). Both elicited and activated murine macrophages bound mycobacteria poorly despite expressing CR3. Thus, binding of *M. tuberculosis* did not correlate with expression of CR3, a finding that the investigators hypothesized was related to the functional state of the binding site on CR3. *M. tuberculosis* binds in nonopsonic fashion to CR3 expressed on Chinese hamster ovary cells (27), an interaction mediated by bacterial polysaccharides (15). Binding sites on CR3 for the bacterium (I domain, which recognizes C3bi versus lectin sites) are predicted to affect the cellular response [i.e., ligation of lectin sites leads to cellular activation such as the generation of an oxidative burst (28)]. In this respect, the host cell response to mycobacterial adherence may also be influenced by the relative involvement of other macrophage receptors, such as the MR, or other CR3-associated receptors, such as CD14 (29).

A recent *in vivo* study using CR3-deficient mice does not show a difference in bacterial burden or pathology between these animals and their controls (30). However, in this study, intravenous inoculation of bacteria was used rather than the aerosol route, which is the natural route of infection. Because compartmentalization of the immune response is well established and the lung is unique in this respect, the relative role of the C3–CR3 pathway in TB pathogenesis remains unresolved.

MANNOSE RECEPTOR

The macrophage MR is a prototypical pattern recognition receptor that binds with high affinity to mannose and fucose-containing glycoconjugates frequently found on the surface of a variety of microbes referred to as pathogen-associated molecular patterns (reviewed in reference 31). The MR is a member of a family of C-type lectins that is expressed on MDMs, tissue macrophages, and dendritic cells but not monocytes (8,32,33). AMs demonstrate high MR activity (34). The MR can serve as a molecular link between innate and adaptive immune responses (33). For example, the MR mediates loading of lipoarabinomannan (LAM) onto CD1 molecules for LAM presentation to T cells (35).

In contrast to CRs, the macrophage MR mediates phagocytosis of the virulent *M. tuberculosis* Erdman and H37Rv strains but not the attenuated H37Ra strain (2,36,37). The MR also mediates uptake of other mycobacteria (38). The linear α1-2-linked oligomannosyl "caps" of *M. tuberculosis* cell wall LAM serve as ligands for the MR during bacterial phagocytosis (37–39). Subtle differences exist in the ability of LAM from different *M. tuberculosis* strains to bind to the MR, and the inositol phosphate–capped AraLAM (LAM lacking the terminal mannosyl units) from *Mycobacterium smegmatis* does not bind to this receptor (37). The linear array of the terminal mannosyl units of Erdman LAM may be important in enhancing the affinity of this ligand for the MR by clustering several carbohydrate-recognition domains as described for other glycoconjugates (40). There is not a direct correlation between terminal mannosylation of LAM and virulence. Mycobacteria that vary in virulence in animal models, including H37Rv *M. tuberculosis*, the attenuated H37Ra strain, and *M. bovis* bacille Calmette–Guérin, all contain LAM types with mannosyl caps, although the interior structure of these lipoglycans may differ (41–43). The ability of these LAM types to interact with the MR also varies (38). Thus, it appears that the precise array, length, and number of caps may be important in determining the interaction with the host cell. Other *M. tuberculosis* surface molecules accessible to the MR are arabinomannans, mannans, and mannoproteins (44,45). In addition to the LAM–MR interaction, *M. tuberculosis* strains have been found to possess their own lectins, some of which are specific for mannans and may be involved in bacterial binding to host cells (46).

The high MR activity on AMs is noteworthy for TB pathogenesis. MR activity is increased by interleukin (IL)-4, IL-13, and glucocorticoids and inhibited by interferon gamma (IFN-γ). It has been postulated that induction by these mediators and by transforming growth factor β produces an alternative activation state of macrophages with many attributes characteristic of AMs (reviewed in reference 47). The phenotypic and molecular characteristics of these macrophages differ considerably from those of classically activated macrophages. For example, alternatively activated macrophages express high levels of pattern recognition receptors, such as the MR and scavenger receptors, but do not display enhanced killing functions toward microbes (48–50). In this regard, the abundant surfactant protein A (SP-A) produced in the lung interacts with macrophages to enhance MR activity (51). Furthermore, nitric oxide and oxidant production in response to stimuli is reduced in these cells (52,53). Thus, AMs seem best adapted for removal of small airborne particulates with minimal induction of inflammatory immune responses. Although such a cell is suitable for the normal homeostatic needs of the lung, it might also be an ideal cell for an adapted intracellular pathogen such as *M. tuberculosis*.

There is recent evidence of potential involvement of the MR in mycobacterial infection in humans. A major locus for human susceptibility to *Mycobacterium leprae* infection has been mapped to chromosome 10p13 (54), the locus of the MR gene (55), and there is a recent report that newly identified variants of the MR are associated with susceptibility to both leprosy and TB (56).

OTHER RECEPTORS AND LIGANDS FOR *MYCOBACTERIUM TUBERCULOSIS* PHAGOCYTOSIS

Although CRs and the MR are major receptors that mediate phagocytosis on mononuclear phagocytes, it remains possible that other receptors also participate in *M. tuberculosis* phagocytosis, either alone or in conjunction with CRs and/or the MR. CD14 has been found to mediate uptake of nonopsonized *M. tuberculosis* by human microglia, the resident macrophage in the brain (29), and uptake of *M. bovis* by porcine AMs (57). Class A scavenger receptors participate in the uptake of nonopsonized *M. tuberculosis* by MDMs (4). Potential *M. tuberculosis* ligands involved in interactions with mononuclear phagocytes and nonprofessional phagocytes include a mammalian cell entry protein (58), a heparin-binding hemagglutinin (59), glucan (15,60,61), PE-PGRS proteins (62), phosphatidylinositol mannoside (18), and antigen 85, which is reported to bind to CR3 (63).

Thus, *M. tuberculosis*, a highly host-adapted intracellular pathogen, has evolved to use several different major host cell receptors to mediate its entry into professional phagocytes. This strategy affords the bacterium greater flexibility for entry because phagocytes differ in expression and/or function of these receptors depending on the tissue site, the degree of cell differentiation, and the presence of inflammatory mediators. The involvement of multiple receptor classes in phagocytosis raises the possibility that receptors cooperate to modulate host cell signaling pathways that generate early host cell responses (see later).

HOST MOLECULES THAT REGULATE PHAGOCYTOSIS OF *MYCOBACTERIUM TUBERCULOSIS*

Regulation of *M. tuberculosis* occurs by several host proteins that vary in their presence and amount in different tissue sites. SP-A, SP-D, MBL, and complement C1q are members of the collectin family of proteins involved in the innate immune response. SP-A enhances the phagocytosis of *M. tuberculosis* through opsonin and nonopsonin mechanisms (64–66), whereas SP-D has been found to reduce the phagocytosis of pathogenic strains of *M. tuberculosis* by binding to LAM on the bacterial surface, thereby inhibiting bacterial interactions with the MR (67). SP-A has also been found to enhance CR1 function (68). Differences in the relative concentrations of SP-A and SP-D between individuals and known genetic polymorphisms raise the possibility that these proteins may play a role in dictating the relative host susceptibility to infection (69). SP-A may be particularly important in influencing *M. tuberculosis* phagocytosis (as well as phagocytosis of other pathogens) in disease states, such as alveolar proteinosis or human immunodeficiency virus infection, in which SP-A levels are increased (70,71). There are also genetic polymorphisms of MBL that account for significant variability in serum concentrations in different populations (72). Elevated concentrations of MBL in the serum of patients with TB have been reported, and the associated genetic polymorphisms have been found to correlate with susceptibility to mycobacterial infections (73,74).

Other host molecules that potentially regulate *M. tuberculosis* phagocytosis include fibronectin through direct and indirect mechanisms (75,76) and IFN-γ. IFN-γ activation of phagocytes down-regulates the expression and/or function of CRs and the MR (77,78) and has been found to decrease the adherence of mycobacteria (79,80). In one study, IFN-γ activation of macrophages decreased *M. tuberculosis* adherence but led to enhanced intracellular multiplication (81). Inasmuch as several cytokines and inflammatory mediators, such as prostaglandins, influence the surface expression of phagocyte receptors and receptor-mediated phagocytosis, it is likely that these mediators are important in regulating the level of phagocytosis of *M. tuberculosis* and the early host cell response during different stages of disease. In this regard, IL-4 and prostaglandin E_2, two mediators that modulate the host response to mycobacterial infection (reviewed in reference 82), markedly up-regulate CR and/or MR expression and function and down-regulate phagocyte effector functions (48,83,84). Treatment of human monocytes with transforming growth factor β_1 is reported to decrease phagocytosis of H37Ra *M. tuberculosis* but enhance intracellular growth (85).

Natural antibody to several species of mycobacteria has been found in healthy purified protein derivative–negative persons (86). Natural antibody could play a role in disease pathogenesis for mycobacteria by enhancing C3 deposition onto the bacillus and hence greater phagocytosis by mononuclear phagocytes (87). Later in infection with *M. tuberculosis* or during active disease, lysis of bacteria-laden macrophages leads to the phagocytosis of *M. tuberculosis* by neighboring macrophages in the presence of high-titer immune antibody. The role of specific antibody in TB pathogenesis and potentially immune protection is not clear and is likely highly dependent on the nature of the antibody produced. High-titer rabbit antimycobacterial immunoglobulin facilitates the multiplication of bacille Calmette–Guérin in the spleens of mice (88). In an *in vitro* study, rabbit antimycobacterial immunoglobulin had no effect on the phagocytosis of H37Rv *M. tuberculosis* by mouse peritoneal macrophages but enhanced phagosome–lysosome (P–L) fusion (89). In a more recent study, an antibody specific for arabinomannan conferred partial protection on mice after a respiratory challenge with *M. tuberculosis* by enhancing the cellular immune response (90). The role of human immune antibody in influencing receptor-mediated phagocytosis and intracellular survival of *M. tuberculosis* by human cells has not been defined. Of interest, the prevention of disseminated forms of TB in childhood has been found to correlate with the production of antibody to LAM (91).

HOST CELL RESPONSES TO PHAGOCYTOSIS OF *MYCOBACTERIUM TUBERCULOSIS*

The mechanisms underlying phagocytosis are complex, culminating in rearrangement of the actin cytoskeleton to engulf the microbe and generation of a variety of biochemical signals (92). There are substantial differences in cellular responses for almost every phagocytic receptor used, and complex interactions between receptors can be expected because a variety of ligands usually coat any given microbe. The phagocytic process for *M. tuberculosis* is no exception. Recent literature provides indications that the nature of the receptor-ligand interactions for *M. tuberculosis* can regulate the early host cell response and the fate of the bacterium.

Phagocytosis of many pathogens by professional phagocytes is accompanied by the rapid generation of the respiratory burst and P–L fusion (93,94). For *M. tuberculosis*, the extent of P–L fusion and the microbial determinants involved in this process, during and immediately after phagocytosis, are not well characterized. These early events may be particularly important in the outcome of the primary infection in the lung, in which the number of bacteria encountering the phagocyte is thought to be very low.

These events may depend more on *M. tuberculosis* surface molecules (95–99) and the receptors used (95).

The C3–CR entry pathway for *M. tuberculosis* has long been postulated to provide the bacterium safe passage into mononuclear phagocytes. CRs are expressed on all mononuclear phagocytes, ensuring access of the bacterium to its intracellular niche. To the potential advantage of the pathogen, ligation of CR3 does not uniformly trigger toxic host cell responses (100) and has recently been shown to selectively suppress IL-12 production, an important mediator of the cellular immune response to *M. tuberculosis* (101). Our data indicate that there is little or no oxidative response to *M. tuberculosis* by nonactivated human macrophages during phagocytosis (102), a result similar to that obtained with *Mycobacterium kansasii* using a human myeloid cell line (103).

Several of the adhesion functions of CR3 are attributed to the I (or A) domain within the α subunit of CD11b that contains the binding sites for several ligands (104). The binding activity of CR3 is not constitutive but is induced by "inside-out" signaling (in response to a variety of soluble and particulate stimuli) that results in a conformational change facilitating receptor function (105,106). Conversely, CR3, when engaged by some ligands, transduces "outside-in" signaling, resulting in particular kinase-dependent cellular effector responses (107). In addition to the I domain, the α subunit of CD11b contains a cation-independent lectin region that, when ligated, generates more potent host responses. Thus, the binding sites for *M. tuberculosis* on CR3 may have an impact on the host cell response and the fate of the bacterium. The precise nature of the binding sites for *M. tuberculosis* on CR3 is not clear. Phagocytosis of C3-opsonized and nonopsonized *M. tuberculosis* by CR3 on human monocytes and macrophages is inhibited by monoclonal antibodies known to inhibit C3bi particle binding (1,2), but not by soluble β glucan (1). Similarly, competitive soluble carbohydrates did not inhibit the binding of *Mycobacterium kansasii* to CR3 (103). These studies indicate that *M. tuberculosis* binds to the I domain of CR3 potentially via distinct binding sites (108). However, there is also evidence that capsular polysaccharides of *M. tuberculosis* bind to the lectin region of CR3 (15,27).

That there are fundamental differences in the binding interactions to CR3 between C3-opsonized and nonopsonized *M. tuberculosis* is further supported by *in vitro* studies in which the phagocyte membrane is depleted of cholesterol to ascertain the importance of cholesterol-rich microdomains (rafts). Cholesterol depletion, in general, results in a significant reduction in mycobacterial uptake (109). Cholesterol depletion of neutrophils decreased the uptake of nonopsonic mycobacteria but not serum-opsonized organisms, indicating that nonopsonic uptake via CR3 selectively involves a glycosylphosphatidylinositol-anchored protein in membrane rafts (110). Different molecular mechanisms for binding that involve distinct epitopes

on CR3 have been found to transduce different cellular responses depending on the state of bacterial opsonization (111).

Although bacterial viability does not influence the extent of CR3-mediated phagocytosis, it can regulate early host responses during the phagocytic process. Live *M. tuberculosis* organisms but not dead bacteria have been found to interfere with host signaling pathways, inhibiting the increase in cytosolic calcium concentration normally seen after CR3-mediated phagocytosis by human macrophages (112). Treatment of the infected cells with a calcium ionophore causes an increase in intracellular calcium concentration that leads to reduced bacterial viability by enhancing P–L fusion. This activity correlated with increased localization of calmodulin and the activated form of calmodulin-dependent protein kinase II to the phagosome, and inhibitors of either calmodulin or the kinase could suppress the enhanced fusion, leading to increased bacterial survival (113).

Phospholipase D (PLD) activity is stimulated early in activated leukocytes, producing the major signal-transducing molecules phosphatidic acid and diacylglycerol. PLD activity and phosphatidic acid increase markedly during the phagocytosis of *M. tuberculosis* by human MDMs in the presence of nonimmune serum (114). The enhanced PLD activity is inhibited by protein tyrosine kinase inhibitors and by 2,3-diphosphoglycerate, a specific competitive inhibitor of PLD. Concomitantly, these inhibitors significantly reduce *M. tuberculosis* phagocytosis. Activation of this signal transduction pathway may therefore play an important role in regulating the phagocytosis of *M. tuberculosis* and in modulating subsequent macrophage functions. The importance of differential activation of signal transduction pathways by pathogenic and nonpathogenic mycobacteria after phagocytosis has recently been reported (115).

The LAM–MR pathway also appears to be preferable for the intracellular pathogen *M. tuberculosis*. MR-dependent phagocytosis is not coupled to activation of the nicotinamide adenine dinucleotide phosphate (reduced form) oxidase (36,116), and the LAM–MR pathway appears to be important in limiting P–L fusion events (117,118). *M. tuberculosis* LAM is reported to inhibit IL-12 production via the MR by generating a negative signal in the cell (119). Finally, mycobacterial LAM can scavenge toxic oxygen radicals (120,121), providing another mechanism for enhancing the survival of these bacteria during phagocytosis. Thus, like CRs, involvement of LAM and the MR during *M. tuberculosis* phagocytosis may enhance intracellular survival.

Little is known about the biochemical pathways activated by ligation of the MR (33). The transmembrane region and short 45-residue cytoplasmic tail are required for phagocytosis (122,123). The cytoplasmic tail appears to be important in endosomal sorting of the MR to prevent lysosomal degradation (124). Although the relationship between MR ligation and CR activity is unknown, the MR appears to regulate Fcγ receptor activity (125,126).

LAM regulates several macrophage effector functions (127,128), and its ability to suppress or augment host immunologic responses is highly dependent on the mycobacterial species from which it is obtained (129–132). AraLAM resembles LPS in that it is a potent inducer of proinflammatory mediators, chemokines, and inducible nitric oxide synthase activity. It enhances immediate early gene expression, is chemotactic for mononuclear phagocytes, scavenges oxygen radicals, and signals phagocytes through CD14 and TLR2 (121,133–138). In contrast, *M. tuberculosis* LAM induces proinflammatory mediators poorly, stimulates the antiinflammatory cytokine transforming growth factor β (139), and regulates phosphatidylinositol-3-OH kinases (117). Differences in the host cell response to AraLAM and *M. tuberculosis* LAM may relate to the fact that *M. tuberculosis* LAM, but not AraLAM, binds to the MR. MR-dependent cytokine and Ca^{2+} responses to *M. tuberculosis* LAM have been reported (140,141), and *M. tuberculosis* LAM can decrease macrophage signaling responses (142,143). The LAM–MR pathway may also shape the development of the adaptive immune response, as discussed previously (35,144).

Thus, there is increasing evidence that intracellular pathogens such as *M. tuberculosis* alter host cell signaling pathways during and after phagocytosis in such a way to disrupt normal host cell microbicidal activities and/or phagocyte effector functions (reviewed in reference 145).

TOLL-LIKE RECEPTORS IN THE INNATE IMMUNE RESPONSE TO TUBERCULOSIS AND LINKS TO THE ADAPTIVE IMMUNE RESPONSE

The discovery of TLRs has provided new insight into our understanding of the mechanisms by which *M. tuberculosis* triggers the innate immune response. TLRs are a phylogenetically conserved family of mammalian pattern recognition receptors that appear to play a critical role in microbial recognition by macrophages and dendritic cells (146,147). They are transmembrane proteins containing repeated leucine-rich motifs in their extracellular domains.

Mammalian TLR proteins derive their name from the drosophila–Toll protein with which they share sequence similarity. Toll was initially shown to be critical for dorsal ventral patterning in fly embryos and subsequently was found to play an important role in host immunity against fungal infection (148,149). The cytoplasmic domain of Toll was found to be homologous to the signaling domain of the IL-1 receptor and links to IL-1 receptor–associated kinase, a serine kinase that activates transcription factors such as nuclear factor-κB to signal the production of cytokines. The so-called hToll (150) was eventually renamed TLR4.

Today, at least ten TLRs have been identified (reviewed in references 151–153). Agonists have been identified for some TLRs. TLR2 agonists include peptidoglycan and bacterial lipopeptides. TLR4 agonists include gram-negative bacterial LPS, respiratory syncytial virus protein F, and the plant LPS mimetic Taxol. Bacterial flagellin is a TLR5 agonist and bacterial CpG-containing DNA is a TLR9 agonist. The complex signal transduction pathways that accompany TLR ligation are beyond the scope of this review (reviewed in references 147,153). Despite overlapping signal transduction pathways by TLR proteins, it is unlikely that all of these receptors generate identical intracellular signals and cellular responses. Qualitative and quantitative differences in TLR signaling contribute to the diverse responses that accompany development of effective innate and adaptive immunity. Differences also relate to TLR expression. Although the exact expression pattern of each TLR varies, the expression of TLR2 and TLR4 is commonly associated with cells of the innate immune system: monocytes and macrophages, antigen-presenting cells and dendritic cells, endothelial cells and mucosal epithelial cells. Most tissues express at least one TLR with several expressing all (spleen, peripheral blood leukocytes). Professional phagocytes clearly express the highest variety (154).

Studies provide evidence that TLR proteins serve as important regulators of the innate immune response during *M. tuberculosis* infection and may dictate the quality of the subsequent cellular immune response. Through TLRs, *M. tuberculosis* lysate or soluble mycobacterial cell wall–associated lipoproteins induce production of IL-12 (155). Myeloid differentiation protein 88, a common signaling component that links all TLRs to IL-1 receptor–associated kinase, was found to be essential for *M. tuberculosis*–induced macrophage activation (156). A mutation of TLR2 specifically inhibited *M. tuberculosis*–induced tumor necrosis factor-α production; this inhibition was incomplete, thereby suggesting that besides TLR2, other TLRs may be involved.

Using stably transfected Chinese hamster ovary cells, expression of TLR2 and TLR4 confers responsiveness to both virulent and attenuated *M. tuberculosis* strains (157). TLR2 is necessary for signaling of the mycolylarabinogalactan–peptidoglycan complex, a total lipid mixture; AraLAM, a 19-kd *M. tuberculosis* lipoprotein; and a heat-stable, protease-resistant, low molecular weight molecule containing phosphatidylinositol mannoside (155,156,158,159). TLR2-dependent activation of cells by AraLAM was found to be dependent on CD14 (135). Importantly, LAM from *M. tuberculosis* does not appear to be an agonist for TLR2 (157). Thus, although mycobacterial glycolipids can activate cells via CD14 and TLR2, the signaling complex exhibits specificity, enabling it to distinguish between the closely related LAM types. Live *M. tuberculosis* activates cells in both a TLR2- and TLR4-dependent fashion (157,160). The agonist for TLR4 activity is cell associated and heat labile in contrast to phosphatidylinositol mannoside (135,157). In addition to TLR2 and TLR4, other TLRs may be involved in the immune recognition of *M. tuberculosis*: heterodimerization of TLR2 with TLR6 or TLR1 is necessary for signal transduction (161,162).

Different mycobacteria differ in their TLR responses. For example, live *M. avium* does not activate cells in a TLR4-dependent manner (163). Tumor necrosis factor-α, IL-1α, and granulocyte-macrophage colony-stimulating factor, but not IFN-γ, induce TLR2 mRNA in murine macrophages after infection with *M. avium* (164).

Until very recently, a significant amount of the literature regarding *M. tuberculosis* and TLRs focused on transfected cell lines, which do not represent resident macrophages. With an increasing number of tools available, the relative role of TLRs in regulating the biologic activities of CRs, Fcγ receptors, and the MR on primary monocytes and macrophages will become clearer. Some TLR proteins have been shown to use coreceptors that augment TLR-dependent responses. For example, both CD14 and CR3 (165,166) have been shown to augment responsiveness of cells to the TLR4 agonist LPS. CD14 is necessary for the activation of TLR2 by AraLAM (135).

Cellular receptors involved in the phagocytosis of *M. tuberculosis*, such as CRs and the MR, are capable of transducing intracellular signals (122,167); however, these receptors do not appear to be major mediators of *M. tuberculosis*–induced cytokine production in the absence of functional TLRs. TLR2 is recruited to phagosomes during phagocytosis of yeast (168). Cytokine production was eliminated by the expression of a mutant TLR2; however, particle binding and internalization were unaffected. This result suggests that receptors such as the MR signal the cell to enable the particle to undergo internalization and TLRs cooperate to signal the inflammatory response.

More recent studies provide some evidence that TLRs play a role in dictating the fate of *M. tuberculosis* in mammalian cells. The 19-kd lipoprotein of *M. tuberculosis* has been shown to induce nitric oxide–dependent antimicrobial mechanisms in mouse macrophages (169) and can inhibit the growth of *M. tuberculosis* in human monocytes without inducing nitric oxide. In experiments using mice deficient in CD14, TLR2, or TLR4, low-dose aerosol infection with *M. tuberculosis* resulted in no difference in granuloma formation, macrophage activation, and secretion of proinflammatory cytokines, indicating redundant roles for these receptors in initiating protective immune responses (170). However, high-dose aerosol challenge revealed that TLR2- but not TLR4-deficient mice were more susceptible to infection than control mice.

Other effects of TLRs on macrophage microbicidal responses and effector functions that can alter the fate of *M. tuberculosis* include regulation of apoptosis (160,171) and inhibition of MHC class II expression by the mycobacterial 19-kd lipoprotein TLR2 agonist (159). Thus, TLRs appear to mediate both the suppression of antigen presentation and induction of antimicrobial responses by macrophages. The evasion of immune surveillance mediated by TLRs is postulated to allow for chronic infection to occur.

CONCLUSIONS

Monocytes and macrophages serve as the host cell niche for the highly adapted *M. tuberculosis*. Phagocytosis by these cells is complex, involving several major host cell receptors and microbial ligands. Regulation of this process depends in part on the tissue site, the degree of phagocyte differentiation, and the presence of local opsonins and inflammatory mediators. Evidence is accumulating that involvement of specific receptor binding domains, cooperation among different receptors, and involvement of specific microbial determinants are important in defining the early host response and microbial fate during and after phagocytosis. In addition to ligating the receptors that mediate bacterial engulfment, *M. tuberculosis* surface determinants bind to different TLRs that further refine the host response including the production of cytokines and regulation of apoptosis and antigen presentation. Further definition of the molecular determinants of *M. tuberculosis* phagocytosis holds promise for the development of specific antagonists that can augment host responses and consequently bacterial killing.

REFERENCES

1. Schlesinger LS, Bellinger-Kawahara CG, Payne NR, et al. Phagocytosis of *Mycobacterium tuberculosis* is mediated by human monocyte complement receptors and complement component C3. *J Immunol* 1990;144:2771–2780.
2. Schlesinger LS. Macrophage phagocytosis of virulent but not attenuated strains of *Mycobacterium tuberculosis* is mediated by mannose receptors in addition to complement receptors. *J Immunol* 1993;150:2920–2930.
3. Stokes RW, Haidl ID, Jefferies WA, et al. Mycobacteria-macrophage interactions: macrophage phenotype determines the nonopsonic binding of *Mycobacterium tuberculosis* to murine macrophages. *J Immunol* 1993;151:7067–7076.
4. Zimmerli S, Edwards S, Ernst JD. Selective receptor blockade during phagocytosis does not alter the survival and growth of *Mycobacterium tuberculosis* in human macrophages. *Am J Respir Cell Mol Biol* 1996;15:760–770.
5. Hirsch CS, Ellner JJ, Russell DG, et al. Complement receptor-mediated uptake and tumor necrosis factor-alpha-mediated growth inhibition of *Mycobacterium tuberculosis* by human alveolar macrophages. *J Immunol* 1994;152:743–753.
6. Harris ES, McIntyre TM, Prescott SM, et al. The leukocyte integrins. *J Biol Chem* 2000;275:23409–23412.
7. Myones BL, Dalzell JG, Hogg N, et al. Neutrophil and monocyte cell surface p150,955 has iC3b-receptor (CR4) activity resembling CR3. *J Clin Invest* 1988;82:640–651.
8. Speert DP, Silverstein SC. Phagocytosis of unopsonized zymosan by human monocyte-derived macrophages: matura-

tion and inhibition by mannan. *J Leukoc Biol* 1985;38: 655–658.

9. Strunk RC, Eidlen DM, Mason RJ. Pulmonary alveolar type II epithelial cells synthesize and secrete proteins of the classical and alternative complement pathways. *J Clin Invest* 1988;81: 1419–1426.

10. McPhaden AR, Whaley K. Complement biosynthesis by mononuclear phagocytes. *Immunol Res* 1993;12:213–232.

11. Schlesinger LS. *Mycobacterium tuberculosis* and the complement system. *Trends Microbiol* 1998;6:47–49.

12. Ramanathan VD, J Curtis, JL Turk. Activation of the alternative pathway of complement by mycobacteria and cord factor. *Infect Immun* 1980;29:30–35.

13. Rourke FJ, Fan SS, Wilder MS. Anticomplementary activity of tuberculin: relationship to platelet aggregation and lytic response. *Infect Immun* 1979;23:160–167.

14. Mueller-Ortiz SL, Wanger AR, Norris SJ. Mycobacterial protein HbhA binds human complement component C3. *Infect Immun* 2001;69:7501–7511.

15. Cywes C, Hoppe HC, Daffe M, et al. Nonopsonic binding of *Mycobacterium tuberculosis* to complement receptor type 3 is mediated by capsular polysaccharides and is strain dependent. *Infect Immun* 1997;65:4258–4266.

16. Matsushita M. The lectin pathway of the complement system. *Microbiol Immunol* 1996;40:887–893.

17. Polotsky VY, Belisle JT, Mikusova K, et al. Interaction of human mannose-binding protein with *Mycobacterium avium*. *J Infect Dis* 1997;175:1159–1168.

18. Hoppe HC, De Wet JM, Cywes C, et al. Identification of phosphatidylinositol mannoside as a mycobacterial adhesin mediating both direct and opsonic binding to nonphagocytic mammalian cells. *Infect Immun* 1997;65:3896–3905.

19. Schorey JS, Carroll MC, Brown EJ. A macrophage invasion mechanism of pathogenic mycobacteria. *Science* 1997;277: 1091–1093.

20. Cole FS, Matthews WJ Jr, Rossing TH, et al. Complement biosynthesis by human bronchoalveolar macrophages. *Clin Immunol Immunopathol* 1983;27:153–159.

21. Zach TL, Hill LD, Herrman VA, et al. Effect of glucocorticoids on C3 gene expression by the A549 human pulmonary epithelial cell line. *J Immunol* 1992;148:3964–3969.

22. Ueda T, Rieu P, Brayer J, et al. Identification of the complement iC3b binding site in the β2 integrin CR3 (CD11b/CD18). *Proc Natl Acad Sci U S A* 1994;91:10680–10684.

23. Rieu P, Ueda T, Haruta I, et al. The A-domain of β2 integrin CR3 (CD11b/CD18) is a receptor for the hookworm-derived neutrophil adhesion inhibitor NIF. *J Cell Biol* 1994;127: 2081–2091.

24. Blackford J, Reid HW, Pappin DJC, et al. A monoclonal antibody, 3/22, to rabbit CD11c which induces homotypic T cell aggregation: evidence that ICAM-1 is a ligand for CD11c/CD18. *Eur J Immunol* 1996;26:525–531.

25. Ingalls RR, Golenbock DT. CD11c/CD18, a transmembrane signaling receptor for lipopolysaccharide. *J Exp Med* 1995;181: 1473–1479.

26. Loike JD, Sodeik B, Cao L, et al. CD11c/CD18 on neutrophils recognizes a domain at the N terminus of the α chain of fibrinogen. *Proc Natl Acad Sci U S A* 1991;88:1044–1048.

27. Cywes C, Godenir NL, Hoppe HC, et al. Nonopsonic binding of *Mycobacterium tuberculosis* to human complement receptor type 3 expressed in Chinese hamster ovary cells. *Infect Immun* 1996;64:5373–5383.

28. Thornton BP, Vetvicka V, Pitman M, et al. Analysis of the sugar specificity and molecular location of the β-glucan-binding lectin site of complement receptor type 3 (CD11b/CD18). *J Immunol* 1996;156:1235–1246.

29. Peterson PK, Gekker G, Hu S, et al. CD14 receptor-mediated uptake of nonopsonized *Mycobacterium tuberculosis* by human microglia. *Infect Immun* 1995;63:1598–1602.

30. Hu C, Mayadas-Norton T, Tanaka K, et al. *Mycobacterium tuberculosis* infection in complement receptor 3-deficient mice. *J Immunol* 2000;165:2596–2602.

31. Medzhitov R, Janeway C Jr. Innate immunity. *N Engl J Med* 2000;343:338–344.

32. Stahl PD. The macrophage mannose receptor: current status. *Am J Respir Cell Mol Biol* 1990;2:317–318.

33. Stahl PD, Ezekowitz RA. The mannose receptor is a pattern recognition receptor involved in host defense. *Curr Opin Immunol* 1998;10:50–55.

34. Wileman TE, Lennartz MR, Stahl PD. Identification of the macrophage mannose receptor as a 175-kDa membrane protein. *Proc Natl Acad Sci U S A* 1986;83:2501–2505.

35. Prigozy TI, Sieling PA, Clemens D, et al. The mannose receptor delivers lipoglycan antigens to endosomes for presentation to T cells by CD1b molecules. *Immunity* 1997;6:187–197.

36. Schlesinger LS, Kaufman TM, Iyer S, et al. Differences in mannose receptor-mediated uptake of lipoarabinomannan from virulent and attenuated strains of *Mycobacterium tuberculosis* by human macrophages. *J Immunol* 1996;157:4568–4575.

37. Schlesinger LS, Hull SR, Kaufman TM. Binding of the terminal mannosyl units of lipoarabinomannan from a virulent strain of *Mycobacterium tuberculosis* to human macrophages. *J Immunol* 1994;152:4070–4079.

38. Astarie-Dequeker C, N'Diaye EN, Le Cabec V, et al. The mannose receptor mediates uptake of pathogenic and nonpathogenic mycobacteria and bypasses bactericidal responses in human macrophages. *Infect Immun* 1999;67:469–477.

39. Kang BK, Schlesinger LS. Characterization of mannose receptor-dependent phagocytosis mediated by *Mycobacterium tuberculosis* lipoarabinomannan. *Infect Immun* 1998;66:2769–2777.

40. Taylor ME, Bezouska K, Drickamer K. Contribution to ligand binding by multiple carbohydrate-recognition domains in the macrophage mannose receptor. *J Biol Chem* 1992;267: 1719–1726.

41. Prinzis S, Chatterjee D, Brennan PJ. Structure and antigenicity of lipoarabinomannan from *Mycobacterium bovis* BCG. *J Gen Microbiol* 1993;139:2649–2658.

42. Khoo K-H, Dell A, Morris HR, et al. Inositol phosphate capping of the nonreducing termini of lipoarabinomannan from rapidly growing strains of *Mycobacterium*. *J Biol Chem* 1995; 270:12380–12389.

43. Venisse A, Berjeaud J-M, Chaurand P, et al. Structural features of lipoarabinomannan from *Mycobacterium bovis* BCG. Determination of molecular mass by laser desorption mass spectrometry. *J Biol Chem* 1993;268:12401–12411.

44. Ortalo-Magné A, Dupont M-A, Lemassu A, et al. Molecular composition of the outermost capsular material of the tubercle bacillus. *Microbiology* 1995;141:1609–1620.

45. Dobos KM, Khoo KH, Swiderek KM, et al. Definition of the full extent of glycosylation of the 45- kilodalton glycoprotein of *Mycobacterium tuberculosis*. *J Bacteriol* 1996;178:2498–2506.

46. Goswami S, Sarkar S, Basu J, et al. Mycotin: a lectin involved in the adherence of *Mycobacteria* to macrophages. *FEBS Lett* 1994;355:183–186.

47. Goerdt S, Orfanos CE. Other functions, other genes: alternative activation of antigen-presenting cells. *Immunity* 1999;10: 137–142.

48. Stein M, Keshav S, Harris N, et al. Interleukin 4 potently enhances murine macrophage mannose receptor activity: a marker of alternative immunologic macrophage activation. *J Exp Med* 1992;176:287–292.

49. Becker S, Daniel EG. Antagonistic and additive effects of IL-4

and interferon-gamma on human monocytes and macrophages: effects on Fc receptors HLA-D antigens, and superoxide production. *Cell Immunol* 1990;129:351–362.

50. Munder M, Eichmann K, Modolell M. Alternative metabolic states in murine macrophages reflected by the nitric oxide synthase/arginase balance: competitive regulation by CD4+ T cells correlates with Th1/Th2 phenotype. *J Immunol* 1998;160: 5347–5354.

51. Beharka AA, Gaynor CD, Kang BK, et al. Pulmonary surfactant protein A up-regulates activity of the mannose receptor, a pattern recognition receptor expressed on human macrophages. *J Immunol* 2002;169:3565–3573.

52. Fels A, Cohn ZA. The alveolar macrophage. *J Appl Physiol* 1986;60:353–369.

53. Oren R, Farnham AE, Saito K, et al. Metabolic patterns in three types of phagocytizing cells. *J Cell Biol* 1963;17:487–501.

54. Siddiqui MR, Meisner S, Tosh K, et al. A major susceptibility locus for leprosy in India maps to chromosome 10p13. *Nat Genet* 2001;27:439–441.

55. Eichbaum Q, Clerc P, Bruns G, et al. Assignment of the human macrophage mannose receptor gene (MRC1) to 10p13 by *in situ* hybridization and PCR-based somatic cell hybrid mapping. *Genomics* 1994;22:656–658.

56. Hill AVS. Genetic susceptibility to mycobacterial disease. Presented at the American Society for Microbiology General Meeting, 2001.

57. Khanna KV, Choi CS, Gekker G, et al. Differential infection of porcine alveolar macrophage subpopulations by nonopsonized *Mycobacterium bovis* involves CD14 receptors. *J Leukoc Biol* 1996;60:214–220.

58. Arruda S, Bomfim G, Knights R, et al. Cloning of an *M. tuberculosis* DNA fragment associated with entry and survival inside cells. *Science* 1993;261:1454–1457.

59. Menozzi FD, Bischoff R, Fort E, et al. Molecular characterization of the mycobacterial heparin-binding hemagglutinin, a mycobacterial adhesin. *Proc Natl Acad Sci U S A* 1998;95: 12625–12630.

60. Schwebach JR, Glatman-Freeman A, Gunther-Cummins L, et al. Glucan is a component of the *Mycobacterium tuberculosis* surface that is expressed *in vitro* and *in vivo*. *Infect Immun* 2002;70: 2566–2575.

61. Ehlers MRW, Daffe M. Interactions between *Mycobacterium tuberculosis* and host cells: are mycobacterial sugars the key? *Trends Microbiol* 1998;6:328–335.

62. Brennan MJ, Delogu G, Chen Y, et al. Evidence that mycobacterial PE-PGRS proteins are cell surface constituents that influence interactions with other cells. *Infect Immun* 2001;69: 7326–7333.

63. Hetland G, Wiker HG. Antigen 85C on *Mycobacterium bovis*, BCG and *M. tuberculosis* promotes monocyte-CR3-mediated uptake of microbeads coated with mycobacterial products. *Immunology* 1994;82:445–449.

64. Gaynor CD, McCormack FX, Voelker DR, et al. Pulmonary surfactant protein A mediates enhanced phagocytosis of *Mycobacterium tuberculosis* by a direct interaction with human macrophages. *J Immunol* 1995;155:5343–5351.

65. Pasula R, Downing JF, Wright JR, et al. Surfactant protein A (SP-A) mediates attachment of *Mycobacterium tuberculosis* to murine alveolar macrophages. *Am J Respir Cell Mol Biol* 1997; 17:209–217.

66. Downing JF, Pasula R, Wright JR, et al. Surfactant protein A promotes attachment of *Mycobacterium tuberculosis* to alveolar macrophages during infection with human immunodeficiency virus. *Proc Natl Acad Sci U S A* 1995;92:4848–4852.

67. Ferguson JS, Voelker DR, McCormack FX, et al. Surfactant protein D binds to *Mycobacterium tuberculosis* bacilli and

lipoarabinomannan via carbohydrate-lectin interactions resulting in reduced phagocytosis of the bacteria by macrophages. *J Immunol* 1999;163:312–321.

68. Tenner AJ, Robinson SL, Borchelt J, et al. Human pulmonary surfactant protein (SP-A), a protein structurally homologous to C1q, can enhance FcR- and CR1-mediated phagocytosis. *J Biol Chem* 1989;264:13923–13928.

69. Floros J, Lin HM, García A, et al. Surfactant protein genetic marker alleles identify a subgroup of tuberculosis in a Mexican population. *J Infect Dis* 2000;182:1473–1478.

70. Reyes JM, Putong PB. Association of pulmonary alveolar lipoproteinosis with mycobacterial infection. *Am J Clin Pathol* 1980;74:478–485.

71. Phelps DS, Rose RM. Increased recovery of surfactant protein A in AIDS-related pneumonia. *Am Rev Respir Dis* 1991;143: 1072–1075.

72. Lipscombe RJ, Beatty DW, Ganczakowski M, et al. Mutations in the human mannose-binding protein gene: frequencies in several population groups. *Eur J Hum Genet* 1996;4:13–19.

73. Garred P, Richter C, Andersen ÅB, et al. Mannan-binding lectin in the sub-Saharan HIV and tuberculosis epidemics. *Scand J Immunol* 1997;46:204–208.

74. Selvaraj P, Narayannan PR, Reetha AM. Association of functional mutant homozygotes of the mannose binding protein gene with susceptibility to pulmonary tuberculosis in India. *Tuber Lung Dis* 1999;79:221–227.

75. Ratliff TL, McCarthy R, Telle WB, et al. Purification of a mycobacterial adhesion for fibronectin. *Infect Immun* 1993;61: 1889–1894.

76. Abou-Zeid C, Garbe T, Lathigra R, et al. Genetic and immunological analysis of *Mycobacterium tuberculosis* fibronectin-binding proteins. *Infect Immun* 1991;59:2712–2718.

77. Wright SD, Detmers PA, Jong MTC, et al. Interferon-gamma depresses binding of ligand by C3b and C3bi receptors on cultured human monocytes, an effect reversed by fibronectin. *J Exp Med* 1986;163:1245–1259.

78. Mokoena T, Gordon S. Human macrophage activation: modulation of mannosyl, fucosyl receptor activity *in vitro* by lymphokines, gamma and alpha interferons, and dexamethasone. *J Clin Invest* 1987;75:624–631.

79. Schlesinger LS, Horwitz MA. Phagocytosis of *Mycobacterium leprae* by human monocyte-derived macrophages is mediated by complement receptors CR1(CD35), CR3(CD11b/CD18), and CR4(CD11c/CD18) and interferon gamma activation inhibits complement receptor function and phagocytosis of this bacterium. *J Immunol* 1991;147:1983–1994.

80. Toba H, Crowford JT, Ellner JJ. Pathogenicity of *Mycobacterium avium* for human monocytes: absence of macrophage activating factor activity of gamma interferon. *Infect Immun* 1989;57:239–244.

81. Douvas GS, Looker DL, Vatter AE, et al. Gamma interferon activates human macrophages to become tumoricidal and leishmanicidal but enhances replication of macrophage-associated mycobacteria. *Infect Immun* 1985;50:1–8.

82. Barnes PF, Modlin RL, Ellner JJ. T-cell responses and cytokines. In: Bloom BR, ed. *Tuberculosis: pathogenesis, protection, and control.* Washington, DC: ASM Press, 1994:417–435.

83. Schreiber S, Perkins SL, Teitelbaum SL, et al. Regulation of mouse bone marrow macrophage mannose receptor expression and activation by prostaglandin E and IFN-gamma. *J Immunol* 1993;151:4973–4981.

84. Abramson SL, Gallin JI. IL-4 inhibits superoxide production by human mononuclear phagocytes. *J Immunol* 1990;144: 625–630.

85. Hirsch CS, Yoneda T, Averill L, et al. Enhancement of intracellular growth of *Mycobacterium tuberculosis* in human monocytes

by transforming growth factor-b1. *J Infect Dis* 1994;170: 1229–1237.

86. Bardana EJ Jr, McClatchy JK, Farr RS, et al. Universal occurrence of antibodies to tubercle bacilli in sera from non-tuberculous and tuberculous individuals. *Clin Exp Immunol* 1973;13: 65–77.

87. Schlesinger LS, Horwitz MA. A role for natural antibody in the pathogenesis of leprosy: antibody in nonimmune serum mediates C3 fixation to the *Mycobacterium leprae* surface and hence phagocytosis by human mononuclear phagocytes. *Infect Immun* 1994;62:280–289.

88. Forget A, Benoit JC, Turcotte R, et al. Enhanced activity of anti-mycobacterial sera in experimental *Mycobacterium bovis* (BCG) infection in mice. *Infect Immun* 1976;13:1301–1306.

89. Armstrong JA, Hart PD. Phagosome-lysosome interactions in cultured macrophages infected with virulent tubercle bacilli: reversal of the usual nonfusion pattern and observations on bacterial survival. *J Exp Med* 1975;142:1–16.

90. Teitelbaum R, Glatman-Freedman A, Chen B. A mAb recognizing a surface antigen of *Mycobacterium tuberculosis* enhances host survival. *Proc Natl Acad Sci U S A* 1998;95:15688–15693.

91. Costello AM, Kumar A, Narayan V, et al. Does antibody to mycobacterial antigens, including lipoarabinomannan, limit dissemination in childhood tuberculosis. *Trans R Soc Trop Med Hyg* 1992;86:686–692.

92. Aderem A. How to eat something bigger than your head. *Cell* 2002;110:5–8.

93. Pitt A, Mayorga LS, Stahl PD, et al. Alterations in the protein composition of maturing phagosomes. *J Clin Invest* 1992;90: 1978–1983.

94. Berón W, Alvarez-Dominguez C, Mayorga L, et al. Membrane trafficking along the phagocytic pathway. *Trends Cell Biol* 1995; 5:100–104.

95. Bouvier G, Benoliel A-M, Foa C, et al. Relationship between phagosome acidification, phagosome-lysosome fusion, and mechanism of particle ingestion. *J Leukoc Biol* 1994;55:729–734.

96. D'Arcy Hart P, Young MR. Polyanionic agents inhibit phagosome-lysosome fusion in cultured macrophages. *J Leukoc Biol* 1988;43:179–182.

97. Crowe LM, Spargo BJ, Ioneda T, et al. Interaction of cord factor (a,a'-trehalose-6,6'-dimycolate) with phospholipids. *Biochim Biophys Acta Bio-Membr* 1994;1194:53–60.

98. Spargo BJ, Crowe LM, Ioneda T, et al. Cord factor (α,α'-trehalose-6,6'-dimycolate) inhibits fusion between phospholipid vesicles. *Proc Natl Acad Sci U S A* 1991;88:737–740.

99. Goren MB, Hart PD, Young MR, et al. Prevention of phagosome-lysosome fusion in cultured macrophages by sulfatides of *Mycobacterium tuberculosis*. *Proc Natl Acad Sci U S A* 1976;73: 2510–2514.

100. Wilson CB, Tsai V, Remington JS. Failure to trigger the oxidative metabolic burst by normal macrophages: possible mechanism for survival of intracellular pathogens. *J Exp Med* 1980; 151:328–346.

101. Marth T, Kelsall BL. Regulation of interleukin-12 by complement receptor 3 signaling. *J Exp Med* 1997;185:1987–1995.

102. Wayne S, Denning G, Kusner DJ, et al. Phagocytosis of virulent and attenuated strains of *M. tuberculosis* by human macrophages does not generate detectable superoxide anion or hydrogen peroxide. *Clin Res* 1995;43:219A.

103. Le Cabec V, Cols C, Maridonneau-Parini I. Nonopsonic phagocytosis of zymosan and *Mycobacterium kansasii* by CR3 (CD11b/CD18) involves distinct molecular determinants and is or is not coupled with NADPH oxidase activation. *Infect Immun* 2000;68:4736–4745.

104. Graves BJ. Integrin binding revealed. *Nat Struct Biol* 1995;2: 181–183.

105. O'Toole TE, Katagiri Y, Faull RJ, et al. Integrin cytoplasmic domains mediate inside-out signal transduction. *J Cell Biol* 1994;124:1047–1059.

106. Williams MJ, Hughes PE, O'Toole TE, et al. The inner world of cell adhesion: integrin cytoplasmic domains. *Trends Cell Biol* 1994;4:109–112.

107. Loftus JC, Smith JW, Ginsberg MH. Integrin-mediated cell adhesion: the extracellular face. *J Biol Chem* 1994;269: 25235–25238.

108. Schlesinger LS, Frist A, Kaufman T, et al. Evidence for the binding of C3-opsonized and non-opsonized *M. tuberculosis* to the A domain of integrin CR3 (CD11b/CD18). Presented at the Keystone Symposia on Macrophage Biology, 1999.

109. Gatfield J, Pieters J. Essential role for cholesterol in entry of mycobacteria into macrophages. *Science* 2000;288:1647–1650.

110. Peyron P, Bordier C, N'Diaye EN, et al.. Nonopsonic phagocytosis if *Mycobacterium kansasii* by human neutrophils depends on cholesterol and is mediated by CR3 associated with glycosylphosphatidylinositol-anchored proteins. *J Immunol* 2000; 165:5186–5191.

111. Le Cabec V, Carreno S, Moisand A, et al. Complement receptor 3 (CD11b/CD18) mediates type I and type II phagocytosis during nonopsonic and opsonic phagocytosis, respectively. *J Immunol* 2002;169:2003–2009.

112. Malik ZA, Denning GD, Kusner DJ. Inhibition of CA^{2+} signaling by *Mycobacterium tuberculosis* is associated with reduced phagosome-lysosome fusion and increased survival within human macrophages. *J Exp Med* 2000;191:287–302.

113. Malik ZA, Iyer SS, Kusner DJ. *Mycobacterium tuberculosis* phagosomes exhibit altered calmodulin-dependent signal transduction: contribution to inhibition of phagosome-lysosome fusion and intracellular survival in human macrophages. *J Immunol* 2001;166:3392–3401.

114. Kusner DJ, Hall CF, Schlesinger LS. Activation of phospholipase D is tightly coupled to the phagocytosis of *Mycobacterium tuberculosis* or opsonized zymosan by human macrophages. *J Exp Med* 1996;184:585–595.

115. Roach SK, Schorey JS. Differential regulation of the mitogen-activated protein kinases by pathogenic and nonpathogenic mycobacteria. *Infect Immun* 2002;70:3040–3052.

116. Ezekowitz RAB, Sim RB, MacPherson GG, et al. Interaction of human monocytes, macrophages, and polymorphonuclear leukocytes with zymosan *in vitro*. *J Clin Invest* 1985;76: 2368–2376.

117. Fratti RA, Backer JM, Gruenberg J, et al. Role of phosphatidylinositol 3-kinase and Rab5 effectors in phagosomal biogenesis and mycobacterial phagosome maturation arrest. *J Cell Biol* 2001;154:631–644.

118. Kang BK, Schlesinger LS. *M. tuberculosis* lipoarabinomannan is a microbial determinant that reduces phagosome-lysosome fusion following phagocytosis events in human macrophages. Presented at the Keystone Symposia on TB: Molecular Mechanisms and Immunologic Aspects, 1998.

119. Nigou J, Zelle-Rieser C, Gilleron M, et al. Mannosylated liparabinomannans inhibit IL-12 production b human dendritic cells: evidence for a negative signal delivered through the mannose receptor. *J Immunol* 2001;166:7477–7485.

120. Chan J, Fujiwara T, Brennan P, et al. Microbial glycolipids: possible virulence factors that scavenge oxygen radicals. *Proc Natl Acad Sci U S A* 1989;86:2453–2457.

121. Chan J, Fan X, Hunter SW, et al. Lipoarabinomannan, a possible virulence factor involved in persistence of *Mycobacterium tuberculosis* within macrophages. *Infect Immun* 1991;59: 1755–1761.

122. Ezekowitz RAB, Sastry K, Bailly P, et al. Molecular characterization of the human macrophage mannose receptor: demon-

stration of multiple carbohydrate recognition-like domains and phagocytosis of yeasts in Cos-1 cells. *J Exp Med* 1990;72: 1785–1794.

123. Kruskal BA, Sastry K, Warner AB, et al. Phagocytic chimeric receptors require both transmembrane and cytoplasmic domains from the mannose receptor. *J Exp Med* 1992;176: 1673–1680.

124. Schweizer A, Stahl PD, Rohrer J. A di-aromatic motif in the cytosolic tail of the mannose receptor mediates endosomal sorting. *J Biol Chem* 2000;275:29694–29700.

125. Murai M, Aramaki Y, Tsuchiya S. Contribution of mannose receptor to signal transduction in Fcγ receptor-mediated phago-cytosis of mouse peritoneal macrophages induced by liposomes. *J Leukoc Biol* 1995;57:687–691.

126. Murai M, Aramaki Y, Tsuchiya S. α₂-Macroglobulin stimula-tion of protein tyrosine phosphorylation in macrophages via the mannose receptor for Fcγ-receptor- mediated phagocytosis acti-vation. *Immunology* 1996;89:436–441.

127. Brennan PJ, Nikaido H. The envelope of mycobacteria. *Annu Rev Biochem* 1995;64:29–63.

128. Juffermans NP, Verbon A, Belisle JT, et al. Mycobacterial lipoarabinomannan induces an inflammatory response in the mouse lung. A role for interleukin-1. *Am J Respir Crit Care Med* 2000;162:486–489.

129. Chatterjee D, Roberts AD, Lowell K, et al. Structural basis of capacity of lipoarabinomannan to induce secretion of tumor necrosis factor. *Infect Immun* 1992;60:1249–1253.

130. Roach TIA, Barton CH, Chatterjee D, et al. Macrophage acti-vation: lipoarabinomannan from avirulent and virulent strains of *Mycobacterium tuberculosis* differentially induces the early genes c-fos, KC, JE, and tumor necrosis factor-alpha. *J Immunol* 1993;150:1886–1896.

131. Fietta A, Francioli C, Galdroni Grassi G. Mycobacterial lipoara-binomannan affects human polymorphonuclear and mononu-clear phagocyte functions differently. *Haematologica* 2000;85: 11–18.

132. Yoshida A, Koide Y. Arabinofuranosyl-terminated and manno-sylated lipoarabinomannans from *Mycobacterium tuberculosis* induce different levels of interleukin-12 expression in murine macrophages. *Infect Immun* 1997;65:1953–1955.

133. Chan ED, Morris KR, Belisle JT, et al. Induction of inducible nitric oxide synthase-NO· by lipoarabinomannan of *Mycobac-terium tuberculosis* is mediated by MEK1-ERK, MKK7-JNK, and NF-κB signaling pathways. *Infect Immun* 2001;69: 2001–2010.

134. Savedra R Jr, Delude RL, Ingalls RR, et al. Mycobacterial lipoarabinomannan recognition requires a receptor that shares components of the endotoxin signaling system. *J Immunol* 1996;157:2549–2554.

135. Means TK, Lien E, Yoshimura A, et al. The CD14 ligands lipoarabinomannan and lipopolysaccharide differ in their requirement for toll-like receptors. *J Immunol* 1999;163: 6748–6755.

136. Orr SL, Tobias P. LPS and LAM activation of the U373 astro-cytoma cell line: differential requirement for CD14. *J Endo-toxin Res* 2000;6:215–222.

137. Zhang Y, Doerfler M, Lee TC, et al. Mechanisms of stimulation of interleukin-1beta and tumor necrosis factor-alpha by *Mycobacterium tuberculosis* components. *J Clin Invest* 1993;91: 2076–2083.

138. Bernier R, Barbeau B, Olivier M, et al. *Mycobacterium tubercu-losis* mannose-capped lipoarabinomannan can induce NF-κB-dependent activation of human immunodeficiency virus type 1 long terminal repeat in T cells. *J Gen Virol* 1998;79:1353–1361.

139. Dahl KE, Shiratsuchi H, Hamilton BD, et al. Selective induc-tion of transforming growth factor b in human monocytes by

lipoarabinomannan of *Mycobacterium tuberculosis*. *Infect Immun* 1996;64:399–405.

140. Riedel DD, Kaufmann SHE. Differential tolerance induction by lipoarabinomannan and lipopolysaccharide in human macrophages. *Microbes Infect* 2000;2:463–471.

141. Bernardo J, Billingslea AM, Blumenthal RL, et al. Differential responses of human mononuclear phagocytes to mycobacterial lipoarabinomannans: role of CD14 and the mannose receptor. *Infect Immun* 1998;66:28–35.

142. Knutson KL, Hmama Z, Herrera-Velit P, et al. Lipoarabino-mannan of *Mycobacterium tuberculosis* promotes protein tyro-sine dephosphorylation and inhibition of mitogen-activated protein kinase in human mononuclear phagocytes. *J Biol Chem* 1997;273:645–652.

143. Rojas M, Garcia LF, Nigou J, et al. Mannosylated lipoarabino-mannan antagonizes *Mycobacterium tuberculosis*-induced macrophage apoptosis by altering Ca⁺²-dependent cell signal-ing. *J Infect Dis* 2000;182:240–251.

144. Sieling PA, Chatterjee D, Porcelli SA, et al. CD1-restricted T cell recognition of microbial lipoglycan antigens. *Science* 1995;269:227–230.

145. Reiner NE. Altered cell signaling and mononuclear phagocyte deactivation during intracellular infection. *Immunol Today* 1994; 15:374–381.

146. Visintin A, Mazzoni A, Spitzer JH, et al. Regulation of Toll-like receptors in human monocytes and dendritic cells. *J Immunol* 2001;166:249–255.

147. Janeway CA Jr, Medzhitov R. Innate immune recognition. *Annu Rev Immunol* 2002;20:197–216.

148. Stein D, Roth S, Vogelsang E, et al. The polarity of the dorsoventral axis in the *Drosophila* embryo is defined by an extracellular signal. *Cell* 1991;65:725–735.

149. Lemaitre B, Nicolas E, Michaut L, et al. The dorsoventral reg-ulatory gene cassette Spatzle/Toll/cactus controls the potent antifungal response in *Drosophila* adults. *Cell* 1996;86: 973–983.

150. Medzhitov R, Preston-Hurlburt P, Janeway CA Jr. A human homologue of the *Drosophila* Toll protein signals activation of adaptive immunity. *Nature* 1997;388:394–397.

151. Akira S, Takeda K, Kaisho T. Toll-like receptors: critical proteins linking innate and acquired immunity. *Nat Immunol* 2001;2: 675–680.

152. Heldwein KA, Fenton MJ. The role of Toll-like receptors in immunity against mycobacterial infection. *Microbes Infect* 2002; 4:937–944.

153. Imler J-L, Hoffmann JA. Toll receptors in innate immunity. *Trends Cell Biol* 2001;11:304–311.

154. Jefferies C, O'Neill LAJ. Signal transduction pathway activated by Toll-like receptors. *Mod Asp Immunobiol* 2002;2:169–175.

155. Brightbill HD, Libraty DH, Krutzik SR. Host defense mecha-nisms triggered by microbial lipoproteins through Toll-like receptors. *Science* 1999;285:732–736.

156. Underhill DM, Ozinsky A, Smith KD, et al. Toll-like receptor-2 mediates mycobacteria-induced proinflammatory signaling in macrophages. *Proc Natl Acad Sci U S A* 1999;96:14459–14463.

157. Means TK, Wang S, Lien E, et al. Human Toll-like receptors mediate cellular activation by *Mycobacterium tuberculosis*. *J Immunol* 1999;163:3920–3927.

158. Jones BW, Means TK, Heldwein KA, et al. Different Toll-like receptor agonists induce distinct macrophage responses. *J Leukoc Biol* 2001;69:1036–1044.

159. Noss EH, Pai RK, Sellati TJ, et al. Toll-like receptor 2-depen-dent inhibition of macrophage class II MHC expression and antigen processing by 19-kDa lipoprotein of *Mycobacterium tuberculosis*. *J Immunol* 2001;167:910–918.

160. Means TK, Jones BW, Schromm AB, et al. Differential effects of a

Toll-like receptor antagonist on *Mycobacterium tuberculosis–*induced macrophage responses. *J Immunol* 2001;166:4074–4082.

161. Bulut Y, Faure E, Thomas L, et al. Cooperation of Toll-like receptor 2 and 6 for cellular activation by soluble tuberculosis factor and *Borrelia burgdorferi* outer surface protein A lipoprotein: role of Toll-interacting protein and IL-1 receptor signaling molecules in role of Toll-interaction protein and IL-1 receptor signaling molecules in Toll-like receptor 2 signaling. *J Immunol* 2001;167:987–994.

162. Ozinsky A, Underhill DM, Fontenot JD, et al. The repertoire for pattern recognition of pathogens by the innate immune system is defined by cooperation between Toll-like receptors. *Proc Natl Acad Sci U S A* 2000;97:13766–13771.

163. Lien E, Sellati TJ, Yoshimura A, et al. Toll-like receptor 2 functions as a pattern recognition receptor for diverse bacterial products. *J Biol Chem* 1999;574:33419–33425.

164. Wang T, Lafuse WP, Zwilling BS. Regulation of Toll-like receptor 2 expression by macrophages following *Mycobacterium avium* infection. *J Immunol* 2000;165:6308–6313.

165. Fenton MJ, Golenbock DT. LPS-binding proteins and receptors. *J Leukoc Biol* 1998;64:25–32.

166. Perera PY, Mayadas TN, Takeuchi O, et al. CD11b/CD18 acts in concert with CD14 and Toll-like receptor (TLR) 4 to elicit full lipopolysaccharide and Taxol-inducible gene expression. *J Immunol* 2001;166:574–581.

167. Fallman M, Andersson R, Andersson T. Signaling properties of CR3 (CD11b/CD18) and CR1 (CD35) in relation to phagocytosis of complement-opsonized particles. *J Immunol* 1993;151:330–338.

168. Underhill DM, Ozinsky A, Hajjar AM, et al. The Toll-like receptor 2 is recruited to macrophage phagosomes and discriminates between pathogens. *Nature* 1999;401:811–815.

169. Thoma-Uszynski S, Stenger S, Takeuchi O, et al. Induction of direct antimicrobial activity through mammalian Toll-like receptors. *Science* 2001;291:1544–1547.

170. Reiling N, Hölscher C, Fehrenbach A, et al. Cutting edge: Toll-like receptor (TLR)2- and TLR4-mediated pathogen recognition in resistance to airborne infection with *Mycobacterium tuberculosis*. *J Immunol* 2002;169:3480–3484.

171. Aliprantis AO, Yang R-B, Mark MR, et al. Cell activation and apoptosis by bacterial lipoproteins through Toll-like receptor-2. *Science* 1999;285:736–739.

16

NITRIC OXIDE IN TUBERCULOSIS

CARL F. NATHAN
SABINE EHRT

TWO KINDS OF PERSISTENCE: PROLONGED SURVIVAL OF *MYCOBACTERIUM TUBERCULOSIS* AND OUR INABILITY TO EXPLAIN IT

Mycobacterium tuberculosis is among the most successful pathogens of humankind, judging by the infectious dose (one to ten inhaled organisms), proportion of the species infected (approximately one-third), duration of infection (lifelong), incidence of death (the most for any one bacterium), and induction of pathology that promotes dissemination (liquefaction of lung and provocation of cough to generate infectious aerosols). The burden of tuberculosis has been evident throughout medical history. Where sanitation and science accompanied prosperity, tuberculosis transmission rates fell and chemotherapy reduced the case fatality rate from approximately 50% to less than 1%. These triumphs temporarily tucked tuberculosis below the horizon in the very countries best equipped to shed light on its immunobiology. The difficulty of prolonged-course chemotherapy and the consequent rise of drug resistance, the advent of human immunodeficiency virus (HIV)–induced immunosuppression with markedly increased rates of tuberculosis among the infected and decreased rates of cure among the treated, and the unparalleled migration of masses of people across geographic boundaries have combined to convince a now globalized scientific community that tuberculosis is no less a threat to humanity today than it was before the advent of chemotherapy.

More than 120 years have passed since Koch's discovery of *M. tuberculosis*. Given the importance of the information to the survival of our species, it would stand to reason that we would by now have achieved a firm understanding of why the tubercle bacillus so effectively resists elimination by the immune system. Presumably, this would begin with detailed knowledge of how the immune system usually holds the bacillus in check. As it happens, our grasp of these

points is recent and rudimentary. The difficulty that our immune system has in eradicating *M. tuberculosis* and our difficulty in understanding immunity to *M. tuberculosis* are interrelated problems. Reflection on these problems will help set the stage for the topic of this chapter: the evaluation of the production of nitric oxide (NO) as a host defense mechanism that helps to control *M. tuberculosis*.

Persistence of *Mycobacterium tuberculosis* Infection

Fresh evidence continues to support long-standing epidemiologic and pathologic inferences that *M. tuberculosis* persists in the infected host and that avoidance of disease requires an ongoing effort by the immune system. For example, investigators recently sought evidence of cryptic *M. tuberculosis* infection in tissues from 47 HIV-negative Ethiopians and Mexicans who died without a history of tuberculosis and whose purified protein derivative skin test reactivity had been unknown. *In situ* polymerase chain reaction revealed *M. tuberculosis* in the lungs of 32% of these subjects. Macrophages were the most frequently infected cell type (1). Although residence of *M. tuberculosis* in dendritic, epithelial, and other types of cells may contribute to persistence (2), we must still explain bacillary persistence in macrophages, the very cells believed to be responsible for killing mycobacteria.

That the immune system must exert an ongoing effort to prevent persistent *M. tuberculosis* infection from manifesting clinically as tuberculosis was underscored anew by the emergence of active tuberculosis in scores of patients in Europe and the United States who were given antibodies that neutralize tumor necrosis factor (TNF) (3). These agents were administered in an effort to treat rheumatoid arthritis or Crohn disease; the recipients had no clinical signs of tuberculosis before they were given the immunosuppressive agent.

HIV and acquired immunodeficiency syndrome (AIDS) give the most powerful evidence that *M. tuberculosis* is only suppressed by the normal immune system, not eliminated. Although *M. tuberculosis* eventually causes tuberculosis in

C. F. Nathan and S. Ehrt: Department of Microbiology and Immunology, Joan and Sanford I. Weill Medical College of Cornell University, New York, New York.

only approximately 5% to 10% of the infected immuno-competent, latent *M. tuberculosis* infection eventuates in tuberculosis in approximately 50% to 80% of people with supervening HIV infection (4–7). Worldwide, tuberculosis may be the leading cause of death in AIDS (4–7), over and above its indirect contribution to mortality through exacer-bating the growth of HIV (8,9).

The immune system is not alone in usually failing to sterilize *M. tuberculosis* by itself and requiring the aid of drugs. The converse is also true: chemotherapy often fails to sterilize *M. tuberculosis in vivo* without the help of the immune system. This can be inferred from the fact that even when infected with drug-sensitive *M. tuberculosis* and optimally treated, patients with AIDS face a tuberculosis mortality rate of more than 25%, a more than 100-fold increase compared with patients without AIDS.

It is reasonable to judge an immune response as success-ful when it sterilizes the infectious agent and blocks its transmission without irreparable tissue damage to the host. By these criteria, the prevalence and persistence of *M. tuberculosis* infection brand the immune system as a routine failure. At the same time, the fact that 90% or more of immunocompetent people infected with *M. tuberculosis* never develop clinical tuberculosis speaks to the success of immunity by lower standards: prolonged postponement of disease and substantial reduction of transmission. Thus, infection by *M. tuberculosis* usually leads to an ongoing con-test between host and pathogen in which neither can gen-erally claim victory. That the host may occasionally achieve sterilizing immunity is a speculation for which we have scant evidence. That the bacterium occasionally achieves the upper hand is documented millions of times each year.

Thus, *M. tuberculosis* joins many other pathogens that cause persistent infections. There are multiple mechanisms for the persistence of infectious agents in the human host, and more than one mechanism can pertain to a given host–pathogen relationship (Table 16.1). This chapter con-siders just one aspect of persistence: how macrophages kill *M. tuberculosis* and our emerging view of the means by which *M. tuberculosis* avoids being completely eliminated.

Obstacles to Understanding How Macrophages Control *Mycobacterium tuberculosis*

Leaving aside the social forces that shape funding alloca-tions, there are scientific lessons to draw from the very fact that our understanding of effector mechanisms against *M. tuberculosis* has come so late and remains so little. The fore-most impediment was the lack of genetic systems for manip-ulation of mycobacteria, a consequence, in part, of the extra-ordinary glycolipid armor of *M. tuberculosis*. With the discovery of mycobacteriophages (10), it has been possible to knock out *M. tuberculosis* genes efficiently in a targeted or random manner (11,12). Discovery has accelerated with the advent of these techniques, in tandem with the means to sequence genomes, including that of *M. tuberculosis* (13).

A further impediment to insight has been the lack of identification of human genotypes that predispose to tuber-culosis (14). In contrast, mutations have been identified that predispose to life-threatening infections by mycobacte-rial species that rarely cause disease in normal hosts (15). The phenotype of these mutations rarely extends to disease caused by *M. tuberculosis* itself. Perhaps *M. tuberculosis* is so threatening a pathogen that humans have evolved a redun-dancy of defenses; redundancy can rob otherwise informa-tive mutations of their most revealing phenotypes. Alterna-tively, mutations predisposing to exacerbation of tuberculosis may lead to early lethality from primary dissemination. This would leave no time for the endobronchial inflammation and pulmonary cavitation that promote cough and hemoptysis, the signs that propel tuberculosis to the forefront in the physician's differential diagnosis. The same mutations could also predispose to rapid lethality from other prevalent pathogens, including viruses (16). Especially in locales with high infant and child mortality, it would be exceptionally difficult to recognize such a case as an immunodeficiency. The health care systems with the greatest ability to under-take an appropriately focused genetic workup exist in the countries with the lowest rates of *M. tuberculosis* infection. Thus, as rarely as they arise, mutations imparting the sever-

TABLE 16.1. MECHANISMS OF PERSISTENT INFECTION

Antigenic variation (e.g., *Plasmodium falciparum*)
Generalized immunodepletion (e.g., human immunodeficiency virus)
Blockade at specific steps in immune recognition, leading to a deficit in the generation of signals that normally activate effector cells
  (e.g., cytomegalovirus)
Induction of signals that deactivate effector cells (e.g., *Leishmania donovani*)
Dysregulation of signal transduction in host cells (e.g., hepatitis C)
Production of inhibitors of host cell effector enzymes (e.g., *Pseudomonas*)
Deprivation of substrates needed to generate bactericidal molecules (e.g., *Helicobacter pylori* arginase)
Refuge in antimicrobially ineffective host cells (e.g., *Trypanosoma cruzi*)
Interference with vesicular trafficking of effector systems (e.g., *Salmonella typhimurium*[a])
Catabolism of host bactericidal molecules (all microbial pathogens)
Repair of lesions inflicted by host chemistry (all microbial pathogens)

[a]Used in mice to model *Salmonella typhi,* a cause of persistent infections in humans.

est phenotypes may be swept away in the tide of infant and child mortality, out of sight of the few medical geneticists who engage in infectious disease research.

Polymorphisms that exert subtle effects on the incidence of tuberculosis in a given population may be easier to detect, notwithstanding the enormous effort (17,18). The next major breakthroughs in understanding the immunobiology of tuberculosis will likely come from population-based genetic analyses in humans and mice (19), facilitated by the advent of genomics.

A third factor that may have delayed understanding is the power of preconception to restrain progress. Chronic granulomatous disease (CGD) is a life-threatening immunodeficiency caused by inactivating mutations in phagocyte oxidase (phox), an enzyme that produces superoxide (20). Notwithstanding the lesson afforded by CGD, it remained the presumption of many scientists that eukaryotes would not synthesize inorganic reactive radicals for host defense because to do so would be biochemically and biologically implausible and would violate the tenets of specificity by which the immune system was presumed to be bound. On the contrary, it is now clear that evolution has come up with such a solution not just once but twice, independently constructing mutually nonhomologous, multisubunit flavocytochromes to produce superoxide (O_2^-) or NO. Having done so, evolution has conserved both enzyme families throughout the plant and animal kingdoms, where they are integrated into systems for homeostasis through inter- and intracellular signaling and for host defense (21).

MECHANISMS BY WHICH MACROPHAGES MAY CONTROL *MYCOBACTERIUM TUBERCULOSIS*

Importance of Macrophage Antimicrobial Mechanisms in the Control of *Mycobacterium tuberculosis*

As reviewed elsewhere in this book, the established immune response to *M. tuberculosis* depends critically on CD4[+] lymphocytes (22,23) and perhaps also on CD8[+] lymphocytes with cytolytic capacity that recognize formylated mycobacterial peptides presented by infected macrophages (24). These lymphocytes and macrophages themselves release cytokines essential for the control of mycobacterial replication, such as interferon gamma (IFN-γ), interleukin (IL)-12, and TNF. Some of the same cytokines may have deleterious actions as well (25). In part, these cytokines act by orchestrating antigen presentation, cell migration, and tissue remodeling, including granuloma formation (26). They also increase the antimicrobial activity of macrophages that ingest *M. tuberculosis* (27), in part through induction of inducible NO synthase (iNOS) (NOS2) (22), the isoform of NOS that is independent of elevated intracellular calcium ions. However, CD4[+] T cells exert an antituberculous

effect in mice in addition to induction of iNOS (23); the mechanism of this latter effect is undefined. Cytolytic T lymphocytes can kill macrophages containing *M. tuberculosis*, but it is not clear whether this leads to death of the *M. tuberculosis*, and if so, how. Human cytolytic T lymphocytes can discharge a mycobactericidal protein (28), but because a mouse homolog is lacking, the contribution of this mechanism *in vivo* is difficult to judge experimentally.

Most intracellular *M. tuberculosis* organisms reside in macrophages and the closely related but probably much smaller population of myeloid dendritic cells. Macrophages are the major cells with the demonstrated capacity either to sustain the replication or substantially reduce the number of viable *M. tuberculosis* organisms (29) according to their state of differentiation. Thus, mechanisms of macrophage antimicrobial activity against *M. tuberculosis* are of central importance to understanding the pathogenesis of the infection and its persistence.

After hematogenous dissemination, *M. tuberculosis* reactivates more often in lung than elsewhere. From this, it appears that pulmonary macrophages may be less mycobactericidal than those in other organs. We do not know whether this reflects intrinsic differences in the macrophages at disparate locations or something in the lung that equips or stimulates *M. tuberculosis* better to resist macrophages.

Candidate Antimicrobial Mechanisms of Macrophages Besides Production of Reactive Oxygen Intermediates and Reactive Nitrogen Intermediates

Mycobacteria can induce apoptosis via a TNF-α- and caspase-1–dependent pathway (30,31), and avirulent or attenuated mycobacteria induce significantly more apoptosis than virulent *M. tuberculosis* (32). Apoptosis of infected macrophages can lead to death of intracellular *M. tuberculosis*, but we do not understand what kills the bacteria in this scenario nor do we know whether macrophage apoptosis occurs in or is advantageous to the host with tuberculosis. Extracellular adenosine 5′-triphosphate can trigger macrophages to kill mycobacteria *in vitro* by an unknown mechanism associated with phagosome–lysosome fusion (33). We do not know whether this phenomenon operates *in vivo*.

It has been inferred, based on nonspecific phospholipase inhibitors, that macrophage-derived fatty acids may help to restrict the replication of *M. tuberculosis* (34). The enzymatic basis and functional importance of such a pathway have not been established genetically.

Antitoxoplasma activity of macrophage-derived lipoxygenase products was reported (35) but has apparently not been pursued for other microbes.

Phagosome acidification has been credited with killing *M. tuberculosis* in IFN-γ–activated macrophages, but when such macrophages lacked iNOS, they no longer killed (29), although it is presumed that they still acidified their phagosomes. This does not exclude that phagosomal hydrogen ion may play a supportive or redundant role. Conversely, the possibility still needs to be considered that phagosome acidification could potentially favor the intracellular survival of *M. tuberculosis*, as is the case for several other pathogens, such as *Salmonella*, *Coxiella*, *Brucella*, *Candida*, and *Trypanosoma cruzi* (reviewed in reference 36).

Gene disruption studies in mice have demonstrated an antimicrobial role for a family of IFN-γ–induced proteins with homology to GTPases (37). Their mechanism of action appears to be independent of iNOS but is otherwise undefined. Whether these proteins contribute to macrophage antimycobacterial activity is under study.

Macrophages probably achieve antimycobacterial action not just by generating noxious factors but also by withholding beneficial ones, for example, by depleting the phagosome of Mg^{2+} (38) or Fe^{2+} (39). However, the movements of Fe^{2+} in and out of the phagosome remain controversial. Several studies suggest that the *M. tuberculosis*–containing phagosome is Fe^{2+} poor (40–42). Others have argued that a polytopic late endosomal and lysosomal membrane protein termed Nramp1 contributes to early resistance against BCG infection in mice (43) by importing Fe^{2+} into the phagosome, where it participates in generating hydroxyl radicals (44). A contrasting view is that Nramp1 may pump iron out of the phagosome to starve the pathogen of this essential element. The potential of Nramp1 to transport other ions should not be discounted. Nramp1 does not appear to affect resistance of mice to *M. tuberculosis*, in contrast to BCG (45). Nonetheless, Nramp1 polymorphisms appear to be associated with differences in the risk of tuberculosis in human populations (18).

Role of Reactive Oxygen Intermediates in Tuberculosis

The first and perhaps best understood macrophage antimicrobial mechanism is the production of reactive oxygen intermediates (ROIs) by phox (46). Thus, it is important to weigh carefully the available evidence bearing on the contribution of phox. The most clear-cut evidence would be expected to arise from the phenotype of people and mice deficient in the enzyme. Because tuberculosis is common and most people

carrying a known diagnosis of CGD have had access to technologically sophisticated medical attention, one would expect that tuberculosis would eventually occur, be diagnosed, and be reported in some individuals with CGD. Yet, this has happened rarely and without case-control analysis (47,48). Thus, tuberculosis is not generally considered one of the infections to which CGD is a predisposing factor (20).

Treatment of human monocyte-derived macrophages with 1α,25-dihydroxyvitamin D_3 can activate phox. Macrophages treated with the vitamin acquired modest antimycobacterial activity against *M. tuberculosis* (49). It is not clear whether this activity represented mycobacterial killing or merely inhibition of replication, a critical distinction. It amounted to only approximately 0.5 $\log_{10}$ reduction in colony-forming units (CFUs) below the number recovered from untreated macrophages at the same time point. That phox actually mediated the antimycobacterial activity was suggested by studies with ROI scavengers (49). Unfortunately, this point was not proven because CGD monocytes were not tested, and there are no specific chemical inhibitors of phox.

Epidemiologic studies are difficult in a disease as rare as CGD. In contrast, it is relatively straightforward to analyze the role of phox in experimental tuberculosis in mice in which gene disruption is feasible. Bone marrow–derived macrophages from phox-deficient mice killed *M. tuberculosis* normally *in vitro* (Fig. 16.1) (29). Phox-deficient mice showed a defect at restraining the proliferation of *M. tuberculosis*, but only in the lung (50), temporarily (51), and to a small degree (50,51). Most important, *M. tuberculosis* has not been reported to cause phox-deficient mice to die any earlier than wild-type mice. From studies of mice deficient in both iNOS and phox, it emerged that these two pathways can exert mutually redundant protection against commensal organisms, such as *Escherichia coli*. Toward these commensal organisms, no phenotype was evident when either enzyme alone was missing, but only when both were disrupted (52). However, even in these doubly deficient mice, *M. tuberculosis* grew no faster than in mice lacking iNOS alone (K. Hisert and J. McKinney, unpublished data, 2002). Thus, in mice, phox does not appear to be a major nonredundant mechanism of host defense against *M. tuberculosis*.

However, there are sources of ROIs other than phox. Among these is iNOS. When the substrate L-arginine is lim-

FIGURE 16.1. Mouse macrophages require inducible nitric oxide synthase (*iNOS*) but not phagocyte oxidase (*phox*) to kill *Mycobacterium tuberculosis in vitro*. In contrast, their mycobacteriostatic effect is independent of both iNOS and phox. Primary macrophages derived from bone marrow were infected with *M. tuberculosis* strain 1254 at a multiplicity of infection of five bacteria per macrophage and washed. Colony-forming units were determined in the adherent macrophage monolayers at the time points indicated. Mouse genotypes, all on the C57BL/6 background, were as follows: wild type (*wt*) **(A)**; deficient in gp91 component of phox **(B)**; deficient in iNOS **(C)**; deficient in both iNOS and phox **(D)**. (From Ehrt S, Schnappinger D, Bekiranov S, et al. Reprogramming of the macrophage transcriptome in response to interferon-gamma and *Mycobacterium tuberculosis*: signaling roles of nitric oxide synthase-2 and phagocyte oxidase. *J Exp Med* 2001;194:1123–1140, with permission.)

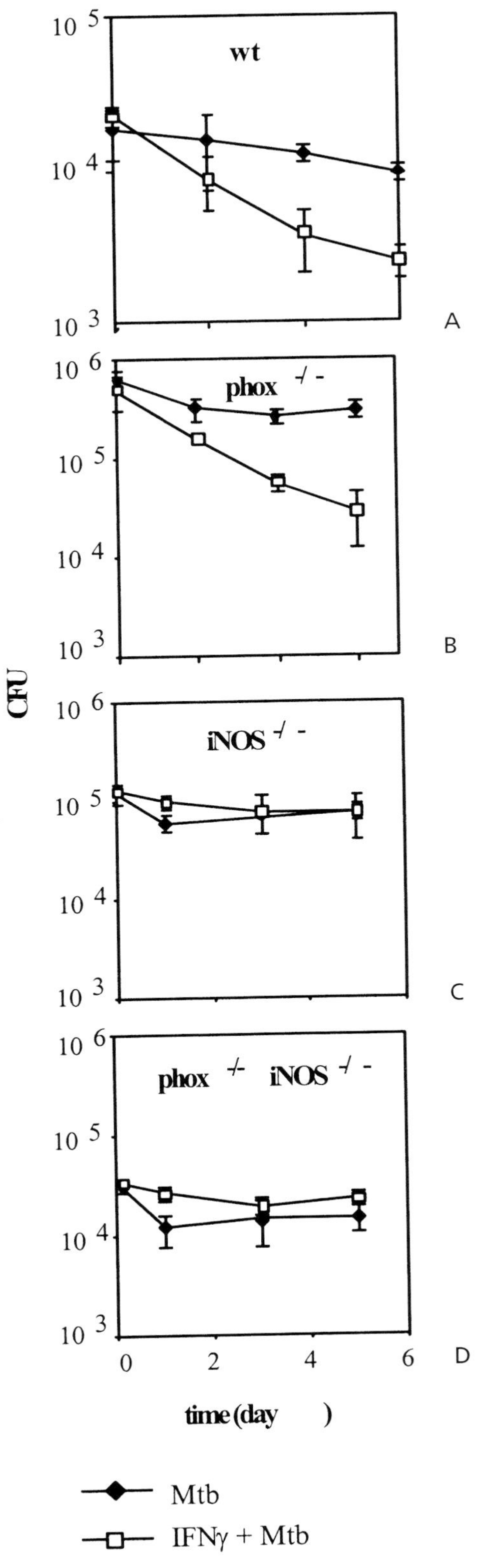

iting, iNOS can produce superoxide (O_2^-) along with or instead of NO. When both are produced together, they combine to generate peroxynitrite ($OONO^-$). ROIs also arise when electrons "leak" from the mitochondrial electron transport chain, generating O_2^-. NO and the $OONO^-$ to which it gives rise both inhibit mitochondrial electron transport and can thus promote the generation of more O_2^-.

One approach to address the role of ROIs apart from the role of phox is to consider the phenotype of mutants in pathways within *M. tuberculosis* that may defend the bacilli against ROIs. Unfortunately, this approach is confounded by two problems: (a) redundancies in defenses of *M. tuberculosis* against ROIs and (b) overlapping roles of defenses against ROIs and RNIs. For example, *M. tuberculosis* encodes multiple superoxide dismutases (SODs), thioredoxins, and peroxiredoxins. Potentially, all these might protect against *both* ROIs and RNIs. SODs, for example, protect against RNIs by decreasing the formation of $OONO^-$ via lowering the concentration of O_2^-, one of its precursors (53). *M. tuberculosis* organisms deficient only in *sodC* (encoding the Cu,Zn SOD) were more susceptible than wild-type *M. tuberculosis* organisms to killing by mouse macrophages *in vitro* (54). However, the *sodC* mutant grew as well as wild-type *M. tuberculosis* in mice, at least over the first 60 days after infection by aerosol (54). This leaves open the possibility that ROI may be important to host defense later on, but if so, such ROIs are not likely to arise from phox because phox deficiency appeared to be inconsequential after day 30 of the infection (51).

Role of Reactive Nitrogen Intermediates in Tuberculosis

At present, there is only one mechanism of macrophage antimicrobial activity about which we can say the following: infected macrophages in the tuberculous host contain a defined enzyme; *in vitro*, a product of that enzyme kills *M. tuberculosis*; when the enzyme is present in macrophages, they can reduce the number of viable *M. tuberculosis* organisms markedly to less than the number initially taken up; when the enzyme is inhibited or deleted, macrophages *in vitro* and the host itself lose control of the infection. That pathway is the generation of NO by iNOS.

Antimicrobial actions of reactive nitrogen intermediates (RNIs) (21,55–58) can be seen as a special case of the widespread role of NO in cell signaling (59). The earliest appreciation of the bactericidal properties of RNI came from the study of mildly acidified nitrite as a food preservative (60,61). Phagosomes are expected to contain nitrite as a spontaneous oxidation product of NO. Phagosomes of activated macrophages are acidic ($pH \geq 4.5$) (62). Mycobacteria can impede acidification of the phagosome (63–65), but immune activation can restore the macrophage's ability to acidify normally (66). Even when acidification is blocked, the pH (approximately 6) remains low enough to promote significant bacterial toxicity from nitrite (61). Mild acidification of nitrite provides HNO_2 (nitrous acid), which dismutates to generate NO, nitrogen dioxide (NO_2), N_2O_3, N_2O_4, and, in biologic media, *S*-nitrosothiols (61). Macrophages secrete glutathione (GSH). Because the intraphagosomal space is topologically equivalent to the extracellular space, phagosomes of activated macrophages are thus expected to contain *S*-nitrosoglutathione (GSNO). GSNO enters *Salmonella typhimurium* (67) and mycobacteria (68) through a peptide permease and once inside exerts bactericidal effects. Targets of RNIs include sulfhydryls in enzymes and Zn-binding transcription factors; Fe, Fe-S clusters, and tyrosyl radicals in enzymes; and nucleic acids (59).

ROIs can enhance the antimicrobial potential of RNIs. For example, H_2O_2 synergizes with NO to cause double-strand DNA breaks, Fe^{2+} release, GSH depletion, and death in *E. coli* (69). Peroxidases can use H_2O_2 to oxidize nitrite to NO_2, itself a potent oxidant (70).

Although O_2^- titrates NO, their product, $OONO^-$, decomposes to more bactericidal species (69,71,72). The importance of $OONO^-$ to bacterial killing by RNIs was suggested by the finding that both nitrite and GSNO could kill *E. coli* in air, but neither could do so under strictly anaerobic conditions (72); that is, O_2 and RNIs exerted a synergistic microbicidal effect. The lethality of RNIs in the presence of O_2 was markedly exacerbated when *E. coli* organisms were rendered selectively deficient in methionine sulfoxide reductase A (MsrA), an enzyme whose function is to reduce oxidized methionine residues (72). Because nitrite and GSNO are not themselves capable of oxidizing methionine, these observations suggested that RNIs become lethal to bacteria when they interact with products of O_2-dependent bacterial metabolism to form a species that oxidizes methionine. O_2^- is a product of aerobic metabolism that gives rise to $OONO^-$ when it encounters NO. $OONO^-$ readily oxidizes methionine. When extracellularly applied, $OONO^-$ is not mycobactericidal (73), most likely because it rapidly dissipates through spontaneous decomposition or reaction with bicarbonate, and hydroxyl radical, its most reactive product, goes on to react with almost any organic molecule that it encounters. In contrast, intracellularly generated peroxynitrite would have access to the inner membrane, cytosol, and chromosome of the pathogen and may be a highly potent mediator of the bactericidal action of externally applied RNIs.

Diverse Sources of Reactive Nitrogen Intermediates in the Tuberculous Lung

Previously, it was noted that there may be important sources of ROIs besides phox. Likewise, there are other sources of RNIs besides iNOS and other cells expressing iNOS besides macrophages. Various cell types in the lung contain NOS1 and NOS3, the two other NOS isoforms. Indeed, sections of lung from patients with tuberculosis stained intensely with an antibody directed against NOS3, particularly in

macrophages in the tuberculous granulomas (74). NOS3 is normally inactive until triggered for a period of minutes by transient elevation of intracellular Ca^{2+} or during phosphorylation by the serine kinase Akt. In macrophages infected with *M. tuberculosis*, it is unknown whether such signals are engendered to activate NOS3, and if so, whether activation is sustained enough to contribute to an antimycobacterial effect. If this were to occur, it would be unprecedented, so the apparent presence of abundant NOS3 in human macrophages in tuberculosis remains a biologic puzzle.

Normal human bronchoalveolar lavage fluid is rich in *S*-nitrosothiols (75). The origin of these RNIs is uncertain, but they may arise from the iNOS that is constitutively expressed by epithelial cells in the large airways (76). Similarly, exhaled human breath contains NO, which arises in part from iNOS in large airway epithelium and from NOS1 in other cells. Thus, even if residing in cells that are iNOS negative, intrapulmonary *M. tuberculosis* organisms will probably encounter some NO and its spontaneous oxidation products, nitrite and nitrate.

Finally, *M. tuberculosis* may make nitrite for itself during anaerobic respiration of nitrate (77). In a low-pH environment, nitrite forms HNO_2. HNO_2 dismutates to produce NO and higher oxides of nitrogen. Thus, when *M. tuberculosis* resides in an acidic environment and respires nitrate, it must deal with the NO generated indirectly as a waste product. To evaluate the likelihood of this scenario, it is necessary to consider whether *M. tuberculosis* will simultaneously encounter (a) a source of nitrate, (b) a deficiency of oxygen, and (c) an abundance of hydrogen ions. In fact, the likelihood seems high. Nitrate is absorbed from the diet and produced by endothelial cell–derived NO (among other sources) when NO reacts with molecular O_2. Nitrate is thus a normal component of blood and body fluids. Granulomas may be the largest nonmineralized tissue structures that exist in the human body without being vascularized. From what is known about tissue PO_2 as a function of distance from a blood vessel, it can be predicted that some of the volume of a granuloma is nearly anoxic. With decreased mitochondrial respiration, increased glycolysis, and decreased removal of metabolic waste, a low pH is to be expected. At the same time, low PO_2 will compromise the ability of iNOS to produce NO (78). Thus, it is conceivable that the closer one comes to the center of a tuberculous granuloma, the less important the macrophage becomes and the more important the tubercle bacillus becomes as the source of NO to which *M. tuberculosis* is exposed.

Evidence Bearing on the Contribution of Inducible Nitric Oxide Synthase to Control of *Mycobacterium tuberculosis In Vitro* and in Mice

Long et al. (79) demonstrated that NO gas kills *M. tuberculosis* in a manner dependent on concentration and time.

A 2-log$_{10}$ reduction in CFUs followed exposure of *M. tuberculosis* to 90 ppm NO over a 48-hour period. Similar concentrations of NO have been inhaled for days or weeks by patients being treated for pulmonary hypertension (80). In an atmosphere of 90 ppm, the maximal NO concentration that could be achieved in the aqueous phase is estimated at approximately 150 nM. Chemotherapeutic agents, such as isoniazid, ethambutol, and pyrazinamide, have minimal inhibitory concentrations toward *M. tuberculosis* of approximately 0.1 μg/mL (0.73 μM), 2 μg/mL (7.2 μM), and 6 μg/mL (40 μM), respectively. NO is the only molecule known to be produced by mammalian cells that can kill tubercle bacilli *in vitro* with a molar potency comparable with that of chemotherapy.

Compared with NO gas, much higher concentrations of nitrite (sub- to low millimolar range) are required for a mycobactericidal effect (81; H. Darwin and C. Nathan, unpublished data, 2002). This makes sense if nitrite works by giving back NO through dismutation of HNO$_2$, considering that such experiments were conducted at pH approximating that in the phagosome, a hydrogen ion concentration orders of magnitude lower than that at the pK_a (3.8) for HNO$_2$. The susceptibility of clinical isolates of *M. tuberculosis* to nitrite correlated inversely with their virulence as assessed in guinea pigs (81). *M. tuberculosis* was also susceptible to killing by NO$_2$ and *S*-nitrosothiols (73).

Only a few studies (29) have reported that macrophages activated *in vitro* can reduce the number of *M. tuberculosis* CFUs to substantially less than the initial number of CFUs taken up. Figure 16.1 demonstrates that the mycobactericidal effect exerted by activated wild-type mouse bone marrow–derived macrophages depended on iNOS. In contrast, nonactivated wild-type macrophages and activated or nonactivated iNOS-deficient macrophages all exerted a mycobacteriostatic rather than mycobactericidal effect. Similarly, an iNOS-independent mycobacteriostatic effect has been reported in human macrophages from healthy donors (82,83).

When wild-type mice were infected with *M. tuberculosis*, their infected macrophages expressed iNOS (Fig. 16.2) (22, 84,85). Expression of iNOS was decreased in mice during protein-calorie malnutrition (86) and in mice that lack IFN-γ, IFN-γ receptor, or TNF receptor 1 (84,87–89). *M. tuberculosis* was much more quickly lethal in these immunodeficient mice than in wild-type mice. When put back on a normal diet, malnourished mice reacquired pulmonary iNOS and control over tuberculosis (86). Conversely, immunization with BCG, which confers partial protection against tuberculosis, induced long-lasting expression of iNOS (90). NOS inhibitors blocked the antimycobacterial activity of mouse macrophages (91–94) and exacerbated acute disease in mice (85,92).

Most important, mice deficient in iNOS died very early of rapid proliferation of *M. tuberculosis* (85) (Fig. 16.3). In one study, iNOS deficiency appeared to be consequential only late after aerosol infection (95), but three other studies con-

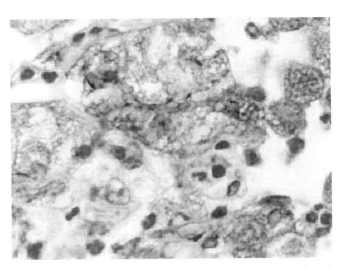

FIGURE 16.2. Expression of inducible nitric oxide synthase (iNOS) in macrophages during infection of mice with *Mycobacterium tuberculosis*. Brown reaction product marks an immunohistochemical reaction for iNOS in the lungs of wild-type mice. Tubercle bacilli (stained red) are contained within iNOS-positive macrophages. (From Mogues T, Goodrich ME, Ryan L, et al. The relative importance of T cell subsets in immunity and immunopathology of airborne *Mycobacterium tuberculosis* infection in mice. *J Exp Med* 2001;193:271–280, with permission.) (See Color Plate 1.)

firmed the importance of iNOS both early and late after infection by recent clinical isolates of *M. tuberculosis* and by laboratory strains, given by both intravenous and inhalational routes (22,96; J. McKinney, personal communication, 2002).

A key role for iNOS was evident not only in acute *M. tuberculosis* infection but also during the chronic phase when wild-type mice appeared clinically well. Administration of a highly specific iNOS inhibitor in the drinking water led to rapid recrudescence of bacillary proliferation and death of the wild-type mice. An enantiomer given as a control compound had no effect (85) (Fig. 16.4). These results were confirmed with another iNOS inhibitor (97).

Finally, McKinney et al. (in preparation) demonstrated that chemotherapy did not cure mice of tuberculosis without the participation of iNOS. Wild-type and iNOS$^{-/-}$ mice were infected with *M. tuberculosis* Erdman strain. From postinfection days 8 through 105, mice received a daily dose of 25 mg/kg isoniazid and 2,000 mg/kg pyrazinamide. On day 108, a cohort of each genotype was killed; undiluted homogenates of their lungs, livers, and spleens yielded no CFUs. From day 106 onward, the remaining mice were maintained without chemotherapy. By 36 weeks, all iNOS$^{-/-}$ mice were dead with massive burdens of *M. tuberculosis*, whereas all the wild-type mice lived to the end of the experiment (52 weeks after infection) and their organs remained free of detectable *M. tuberculosis*. This experiment may help to explain why defective cell-mediated immunity makes it difficult to eradicate mycobacterial infection with chemotherapy. These observations also suggest that chemotherapy might achieve its full potential if

AFB

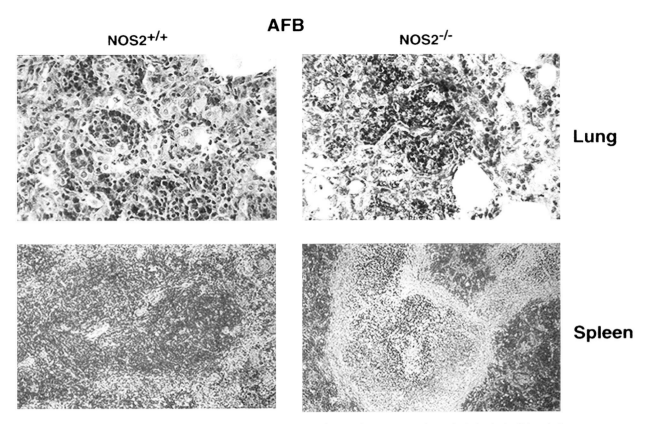

FIGURE 16.3. Much more extensive growth of *Mycobacterium tuberculosis* in inducible nitric oxide synthase (iNOS)–deficient mice than in wild-type mice. Red-stained *M. tuberculosis* (acid-fast bacilli, *AFB*) are observed in much greater numbers in the lung and spleen 30 days after injection of 10^5 *M. tuberculosis* Erdman strain in iNOS-deficient mice (*NOS2^{-/-}*) than in wild-type mice (*NOS2^{+/+}*). (From MacMicking JD, North RJ, La Course R, et al. Identification of nitric oxide synthase as a protective locus against tuberculosis. *Proc Natl Acad Sci U S A* 1997;94:5243–5248, with permission.) (See Color Plate 2.)

decreased expression of iNOS in immunodeficient patients were compensated by making *M. tuberculosis* more sensitive to RNIs.

Evidence Bearing on the Contribution of Inducible Nitric Oxide Synthase in Human Tuberculosis

What does iNOS contribute to the control of tuberculosis in humans? There are two parts to this question. First, is iNOS expressed in human tuberculosis? This question is relatively simple to study, and the answer is "yes." Second, is iNOS functionally important in human tuberculosis? This question is hard to answer without identification of a genetic deficiency of iNOS in humans and given that one would not want to block iNOS pharmacologically in subjects with tuberculosis. This makes it all the more important to judge whether work in the mouse has bearing on the human condition, notwithstanding the differences in the course of the disease in the two species. With respect to iNOS, we are aware of no basis for discounting the potential relevance of murine tuberculosis to human tuberculosis.

Nonetheless, the matter is shrouded in confusion because there are very few studies in which human macrophages *in vitro* have expressed as much iNOS as those *in vivo* in tuberculosis, and there are very few studies in which human macrophages *in vitro* have actually killed *M. tuberculosis* (reduced the numbers to less than those initially present) rather than merely inhibited the growth of *M. tuberculosis*. If one is studying macrophages that do not express iNOS and do not kill *M. tuberculosis*, it is difficult to draw any conclusion about the potential ability of the macrophages to use iNOS to kill *M. tuberculosis*. Because iNOS is abundantly expressed by human macrophages *in vivo*, the lack of expression of substantial amounts of iNOS by human macrophages *in vitro* is most reasonably interpreted as a deficiency of the culture systems, reflecting a lack of knowledge of the variables that control human macrophage differentiation.

The problem stems in part from the fact that iNOS has been intermittently but not consistently inducible in the monocytes of healthy donors. For example, infection with *M. tuberculosis* induced iNOS in normal human monocytes, but only to levels at which product was detected by a

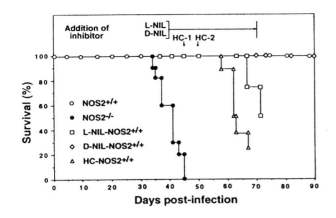

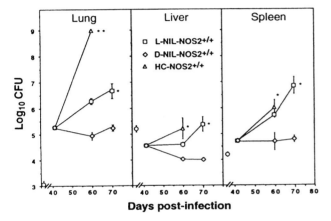

FIGURE 16.4. Survival of *Mycobacterium tuberculosis*–infected wild-type and inducible nitric oxide synthase (iNOS)–deficient mice after intravenous infection with 10^5 *M. tuberculosis* Erdman strain: requirement for iNOS to control acute infection and to maintain clinical well-being during chronic infection. Untreated iNOS-deficient mice died early with large mycobacterial burdens. Wild-type mice appeared clinically well unless immunosuppressed by two injections of hydrocortisone (*HC-1, HC-2*), an agent that inhibits expression of iNOS, or given a highly selective iNOS inhibitor, N^6-(l-iminoethyl)-L-lysine (*L-NIL*), in their drinking water. The latter two groups of mice relapsed and died of florid tuberculosis. As a control, another set of wild-type mice was given the inactive entantiomer N^6-(1-iminoethyl)-D-lysine (*D-NIL*), and these mice continued to suppress the infection. *CFU*, colony-forming unit. (From MacMicking JD, North RJ, La Course R, et al. Identification of nitric oxide synthase as a protective locus against tuberculosis. *Proc Natl Acad Sci U S A* 1997;94: 5243–5248, with permission.)

highly sensitive assay; RNIs were undetectable by the assay used in most other reports (98). Because high-level iNOS can be induced consistently by cytokines and microbial products in mouse tissue macrophages but not human blood monocytes, some workers have concluded that there is a species difference between the human and the mouse such that human macrophages cannot express iNOS, notwithstanding the ready expression of iNOS in many other types of human cells, such as inflamed hepatocytes and keratinocytes. In contrast, others regard monocytes and tissue macrophages as representing distinct states of differ-

entiation and note that human tissue macrophages commonly express abundant iNOS, whereas it is unknown whether normal mouse blood monocytes can be induced to express it.

In contrast to the situation with monocytes from healthy donors, more than 60 reports document expression or induction of iNOS in human monocytes or macrophages that have been studied in or collected from subjects with infectious or inflammatory states (reviewed in references 57, 99). For example, monocytes collected from patients with infectious or inflammatory disorders, such as viral hepatitis and rheumatoid arthritis, are already iNOS positive or are more consistently inducible for iNOS expression *in vitro* than those from normal donors (reviewed in references 57, 99). Likewise, the tissue macrophages from such subjects are iNOS positive as observed *in situ*, as recovered, or after culture with particular stimuli. In the most germane example, studies of human pulmonary alveolar macrophages demonstrated that inflammation provided a first signal and ingestion of mycobacteria a second signal for induction of iNOS (100). Unfortunately, the molecular nature of neither signal was defined. In one study, ingestion of *M. tuberculosis* led to expression of iNOS and production of NO in alveolar macrophages from normal donors, but only after 4 to 7 days (101). This is past the time when most other investigators terminated their experiments.

Focusing on mononuclear phagocytes from subjects with tuberculosis, evidence is compelling for the expression and enzymatic function of iNOS in bronchoalveolar and pulmonary macrophages and its inducibility in peripheral blood monocytes (102). Using an antibody of carefully documented monospecificity, Nicholson et al. (103) detected iNOS in most bronchoalveolar macrophages lavaged from each of 11 patients with tuberculosis, but not in macrophages from normal subjects (Fig. 16.5). Cytochemistry demonstrated that the enzyme was catalytically active but did not permit stoichiometric assessment of product formation. These findings were confirmed and extended to show a 2.5-fold increase in exhaled NO in the breath of patients with tuberculosis compared with healthy controls (104), along with a 370-fold increase in nitrite-releasing capacity of explanted bronchoalveolar macrophages of tuberculosis patients compared with normals (104,105), reaching levels that can be mycobactericidal *in vitro* (81). Those subjects responded best to antituberculous chemotherapy whose bronchoalveolar macrophages made the most nitrite at diagnosis (105) (Table 16.2). Moreover, in surgically resected lungs from eight patients with tuberculosis, iNOS and nitrotyrosine immunoreactivity were abundant in the inflammatory zone of granulomas and throughout the nongranulomatous regions affected by pneumonitis. The cells expressing iNOS and nitrotyrosine were epithelioid macrophages, multinucleated giant cells, alveolar macrophages, and epithelial cells (74) (Fig. 16.6), a picture closely resembling that in mice (Fig. 16.2). Other recent studies have independently con-

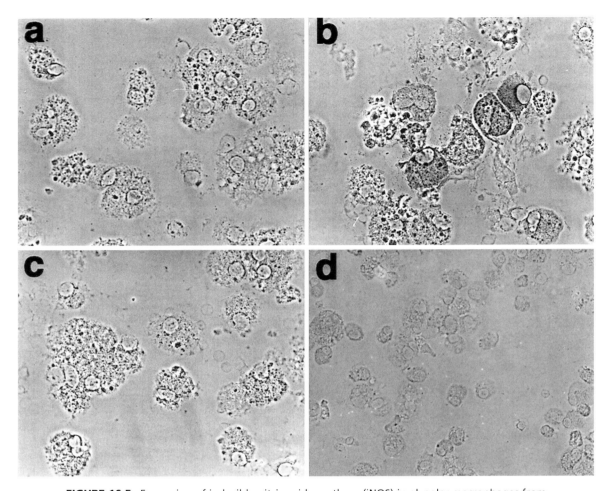

FIGURE 16.5. Expression of inducible nitric oxide synthase (iNOS) in alveolar macrophages from human subjects with tuberculosis. **A–C:** Macrophages lavaged from the lungs of an individual with tuberculosis. **D:** Macrophages from the lungs of a normal subject. Immunocytochemistry was carried out with the following agents: **A,** preimmune serum; **B,D,** antihuman iNOS antipeptide antibody; **C,** as in **B** but with the reaction specifically blocked by the immunizing peptide. Results were similar in each of 11 patients studied. (From Nicholson S, Bonecini-Almeida MdG, Lapa e Silva JR, et al. Inducible nitric oxide synthase in pulmonary alveolar macrophages from patients with tuberculosis. *J Exp Med* 1996;183:2293–2302, with permission.) (See Color Plate 3.)

TABLE 16.2. REACTIVE NITROGEN INTERMEDIATE PRODUCTION BY HUMAN ALVEOLAR MACROPHAGES *EX VIVO*

Study Population (No. of Subjects)	Improvement in Chest X-ray	NO_2^-, μmol/L from 10^6 Cells in 24 Hr (Mean ± SEM)
Normals (8)	—	0.03 ± 0.00
Tuberculosis (8)	Not followed	2.23 ± 1.02
Tuberculosis (10)	>50% in <3 mo	24.97 ± 13.8
Tuberculosis (7)	>50% in 3–6 mo	0.25 ± 0.04
Tuberculosis (5)	<50% in >6 mo	0.16 ± 0.02

Adapted from Wang CH, Kuo HP. Nitric oxide modulates interleukin-1beta and tumour necrosis factor-alpha synthesis, and disease regression by alveolar macrophages in pulmonary tuberculosis. *Respirology* 2001;6:79–84.

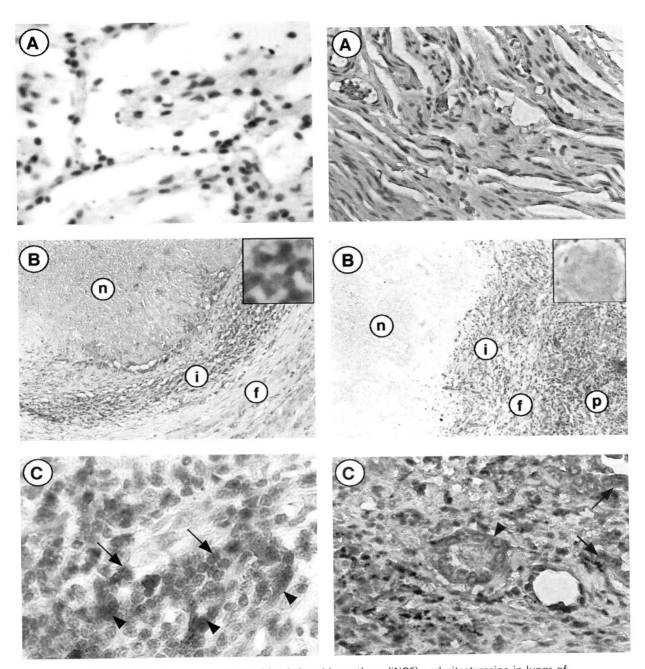

FIGURE 16.6. Expression of inducible nitric oxide synthase (iNOS) and nitrotyrosine in lungs of patients with tuberculosis. Brown reaction product marks an immunohistochemical reaction for iNOS **(left)** or nitrotyrosine **(right)**. Each set of panels shows a field from a normal lung **(A)**, a granuloma from a surgically resected tuberculous lung **(B)**, and a field from an area of pneumonitis in a tuberculous lung **(C)**. In the two panels **B**, the necrotic center (*n*), the inflammatory zone (*i*), the fibrotic capsule (*f*), and the surrounding pneumonitic area (*p*) are shown. The **insets** at higher magnification show iNOS in epithelioid macrophages **(B, left column)** and nitrotyrosine in a multinucleated giant cell **(B, right column)**. Comparison of Figures 16.2, 16.5, and the present figure indicates that tuberculosis in mice models tuberculosis in humans with respect to the expression of iNOS in *M. tuberculosis*–infected macrophages in the tissues. (From Choi HS, Rai PR, Chu HW, et al. Analysis of nitric oxide synthase and nitrotyrosine expression in human pulmonary tuberculosis. *Am J Respir Crit Care Med* 2002;166:178–186, with permission.) (See Color Plate 4.)

firmed that iNOS and nitrotyrosine are coexpressed in human macrophages in tuberculous pulmonary, pleural, and lymph node granulomas (106,106a).

What is the significance of the nitrotyrosine immunoreactivity in tuberculous granulomas? Protein tyrosine residues become nitrosated when OONO⁻ arises in their vicinity from the interaction of NO and O_2^- or when nitrite (arising from NO) is oxidized by hydrogen peroxide (arising from O_2^-) through the agency of myeloperoxidase. Thus, protein tyrosine nitrosation in granulomatous macrophages provides an indication that the local environment sustained sufficient oxidative metabolism to give rise to either NO or O_2^- and most likely both at once. The findings of Choi et al. (74), Schön et al. (106), and Facchetti et al. (106a) suggest that in at least some tuberculous granulomas, there must have been sufficient P_{O_2} to sustain catalysis by iNOS at some point during the evolution of the granuloma.

Human macrophages expressing large amounts of iNOS reduced the number of viable mycobacteria (BCG) by 2.5 logs or more *in vitro*, and this was prevented by an iNOS inhibitor (100). In contrast, human macrophages expressing what appeared to be intermediate or undetectable amounts of iNOS did not kill mycobacteria (*M. tuberculosis* or BCG) (82,83,100,101), although in some cases there was a mycobacteriostatic effect (83), as in the mouse (Fig. 16.1).

Thus, human macrophages can be obtained in various states along a continuum: iNOS negative (as is usually the case from normal donors), iNOS low (as is sometimes seen after infecting normal donors' monocytes or alveolar macrophages with *M. tuberculosis in vitro*) (98), and iNOS high (as is often seen in tissue macrophages from donors with infectious or inflammatory states, including tuberculosis). When human macrophages lack iNOS, they can sometimes exert *mycobacteriostatic* activity by an unknown mechanism. As one would expect, iNOS inhibitors do not affect the mycobacteriostatic activity of iNOS-negative macrophages. When human macrophages express iNOS in small amounts, the macrophages are still only *mycobacteriostatic*, and this activity is sometimes partially reversed by iNOS inhibitors (98). When human macrophages express iNOS in large amounts, they can be *mycobactericidal*, at least toward BCG, and iNOS inhibitors have abolished this activity. In all these respects, close parallels are evident between the human and the mouse. What is lacking and much needed are experiments in which investigators test the course of infection by *M. tuberculosis* itself in human macrophages that express iNOS at the levels expressed by macrophages *in situ* in immunocompetent individuals with tuberculosis.

Some investigators argue that because iNOS is detected in macrophages from individuals with tuberculosis, it must be useless in the control of *M. tuberculosis*. That argument would reject the contribution of every element of the immune system expressed in people with clinically active tuberculosis. As with any infectious disease, active tubercu-

losis reflects a *failure* of the immune system. We need to learn how the normal immune system usually does hold *M. tuberculosis* in check and how *M. tuberculosis* sometimes gets the upper hand in the face of a functional immune system.

In sum, at present, it would be rash to dismiss the potential importance of iNOS in human tuberculosis, given the ability of NO, the primary product of iNOS, to kill *M. tuberculosis*, the proven role of iNOS in tuberculosis in mice, and the presence of iNOS in human tuberculosis.

Signaling Effects of Reactive Nitrogen Intermediates on *Mycobacterium tuberculosis*

The impact of RNIs on *M. tuberculosis* is not limited to growth restriction and death. RNIs are also recognized as signaling molecules by the pathogen. The extensive impact of reagent and macrophage-derived RNIs on gene expression in *M. tuberculosis* became evident with the advent of DNA microarrays that allow global assessment of gene expression. Schoolnik et al. identified more than 70 genes that were induced after treatment of *M. tuberculosis* with low concentrations of RNIs *in vitro* (M.I. Voskuil, et al., submitted) Many of the same genes were also up-regulated in *M. tuberculosis* when the bacilli resided in primary, IFN-γ–activated mouse macrophages. Induction of these genes was abolished when *M. tuberculosis* inhabited IFN-γ–activated macrophages that were iNOS deficient. Thus, *M. tuberculosis* responded to the activation of macrophages by IFN-γ similarly to being exposed to RNIs (D. Schnappinger, et al., submitted).

A subgroup of the RNI response genes was also induced on hypoxia (107). *In vitro*, adaptation of *M. tuberculosis* to a gradual decrease in oxygen concentrations induces a state of nonreplicating persistence (108). The nonreplicating bacteria stay viable for months and can be resuscitated to a replicating state by the introduction of oxygen. The overlap in the genomic response of *M. tuberculosis* to RNIs and hypoxia may suggest that gene regulation occurring in response to RNIs, especially at low RNI concentrations, also leads to nonreplicating persistence. NO can inhibit mycobacterial respiration, which might mimic hypoxia (109).

Treatment with RNIs also induced a group of genes that were otherwise expressed under low iron conditions (110). Restricting the access of bacteria to iron is a host defense mechanism that has been thought to occur mainly by iron sequestration. However, the gene expression profile of RNI-treated *M. tuberculosis* points toward the participation of RNI in functional iron deprivation (D. Schnappinger, et al., submitted). NO destroys Fe-S clusters and may therefore cause a relative deficiency of iron-containing prosthetic groups independently of the pathogen's ability to import iron from its environment. If this leads to activation of the iron scavenging system, perhaps the bacteria would be flooded with iron. Free iron can react with reactive oxygen species through the Fenton reaction, generating DNA-damaging hydroxyl radicals (111).

MECHANISMS OF MYCOBACTERIAL PERSISTENCE IN THE FACE OF INDUCIBLE NITRIC OXIDE SYNTHASE EXPRESSION

There are several scenarios by which *M. tuberculosis* could suppress or deregulate an otherwise protective host immune response, leading to suboptimal expression of iNOS. For example, CD4$^+$ regulatory T cells have been described that secrete both IFN-γ and IL-10 (112). IL-10, by suppressing TNF release (113), can indirectly suppress iNOS induction (114). NO derived from iNOS can nitrosylate the active site cysteine in caspase-1 and thereby inactivate the protease (115). Because caspase-1 processes pro–IL-18, its inactivation might lead to deficient IL-18 production and thus blunt the response of host cells to IL-12 and IFN-γ. *M. tuberculosis* also stimulates host cells to release transforming growth factor β (116). Transforming growth factor β can block iNOS expression by interfering with transcription and translation of iNOS mRNA and shortening the half-life of iNOS protein (117).

Nonetheless, because substantial amounts of iNOS have been detected at sites of *M. tuberculosis* infection in immunocompetent individuals, in both mice and people, it seems necessary to consider what factors may be at work to limit product formation by iNOS, to increase catabolism of the products of iNOS, and to resist or repair their injury.

Limitation of Substrates

Limitation of substrate is a plausible potential explanation for inadequate action of iNOS in tuberculous lesions despite robust expression of the enzyme. To produce NO, iNOS requires three cosubstrates: L-arginine, molecular oxygen, and nicotinamide adenine dinucleotide phosphate (reduced form) (NADPH). L-Arginine might be limiting in a granuloma from a combination of impaired circulatory delivery of L-arginine, which is synthesized mainly in the liver, and the expression by macrophages of L-arginase, an enzyme that breaks down L-arginine to ornithine and urea. It is commonly maintained that Th1 cytokines induce iNOS at the expense of L-arginase, whereas Th2 cytokines induce L-arginase at the expense of iNOS (118). However, when macrophages are exposed to *both* Th1 cytokines and *M. tuberculosis*, L-arginase is synergistically induced (29). As discussed earlier, the avascular nature and large size of some granulomas may make their centers hypoxic. A shortage of O_2 is likely to impair iNOS catalysis (78). There is very little information about NADPH levels in macrophages (119) and none pertaining to macrophages in tuberculous lesions. To summarize, even though macrophages in tuberculous granulomas express iNOS, they may release less NO than

the iNOS-expressing alveolar macrophages from the same patient population.

Interference with Subcellular Trafficking

M. tuberculosis may defend itself against RNIs by blocking the trafficking of organelles or soluble effector enzymes to the phagosome. Virulent *S. typhimurium* uses its type III secretion system to block host cell mobilization of phox to the phagosome (120). The mechanism may involve interference with recruitment of phox-containing vesicles (121). Recent evidence suggests that iNOS, approximately half of which is vesicular (122), may also traffic to bacterial phagosomes in a manner susceptible to interruption by virulent *S. typhimurium* (123). It will be of great interest to learn whether a similar phenomenon takes place during *M. tuberculosis* infection.

However, it is difficult to imagine that iNOS can be converted from bactericidal to inconsequential solely by being held a few microns away from the phagosome. NO diffuses readily from a point source. If altered trafficking does markedly blunt the impact of iNOS, there may be additional events that account for the impact, such as the diversion of iNOS-containing vesicles to fuse with other vesicles containing enzymes that catabolize the products of iNOS.

Microbial Defenses Against Reactive Nitrogen Intermediates and Reactive Oxygen Intermediates: An Overview

There are so many defenses against ROIs and RNIs that it is useful to rationalize their multiplicity. (a) Because oxidants can inactivate some antioxidant defenses, redundancy is a form of defense. (b) Distinct forms of ROIs and RNIs require specific defenses. (c) ROIs and RNIs are particularly dangerous when they interact to produce OONO$^-$, and diverse defenses can protect against OONO$^-$ at each step: prevent formation of OONO$^-$, hasten its catabolism, and reverse its molecular damage.

Thus, SODs protect from NO by blocking formation of OONO$^-$ (53). The downside of SODs is the generation of H_2O_2, which can in turn interact with cuprous or ferrous ions to form hydroxyl radicals that can initiate lipid peroxidation and damage DNA. Thus, expression of SODs is coupled with expression of catalases and organic peroxide peroxidases. GSH also copes with the peroxide output of SODs (124). Synthesis of γ-glutamylcysteine or GSH is confined to halo and purple bacteria (124) and a few gram-positive bacteria (100). GSH contributes to the anti-RNI defense of *Salmonella* (125). GSH peroxidase as a selenoenzyme can detoxify OONO$^-$ (126). Some microbes (125, 127,128) use nonprotein thiols other than GSH, e.g., homocysteine defends *Salmonella* against *S*-nitrosothiols (129). Actinomycetes contain mycothiol, an *N*-acetylcysteine disaccharide (125). Small, Cys-containing enzymes active in redox reactions include as many as three glutaredoxins whose redox cycle involves GSH (130), as many as three thioredoxins (130) that reduce protein disulfides and are cycled by thioredoxin reductase and NADPH, and thioredoxin peroxidases, now called peroxiredoxins (131, 132).

Another way to block OONO⁻ formation, in addition to catabolizing O₂⁻, is to catabolize NO. Bacterial flavohemoglobins serve as NO dioxygenases (133,134), and some bacterial cytochromes can act as NO reductases (135). In *E. coli*, anaerobiosis induces a flavorubredoxin with NO reductase activity (134).

A major action of OONO⁻ is to oxidize protein-bound methionine. This is reversed by MsrA and MsrB in a cycle dependent on thioredoxin, thioredoxin reductase, and NADPH. *E. coli* MsrA increases the cells' resistance to H₂O₂ (136). As noted earlier, MsrA also protects *E. coli* against RNIs (72).

Peroxiredoxins were mentioned previously as thioredoxin peroxidases active against hydrogen peroxide and lipid peroxides. Peroxiredoxins warrant further discussion because it has emerged that they are even more active as peroxynitrite reductases (137). Ames' group first purified alkylhydroperoxide reductase (Ahp) as the enzyme that appeared to be necessary and sufficient to protect enterobacteria from oxidative mutagenesis (138–140). Ahp uses nicotinamide adenine dinucleotide (reduced form) to reduce alkylperoxides to alcohols and provides the primary defense of *E. coli* against endogenous and exogenous H₂O₂ in the micromolar range (141). The enzyme comprises two gene products: a dimer of a 21-kd subunit designated AhpC because the purified protein is *c*olorless and a dimer of a 57-kd protein that is yellow because of its *f*lavin content and hence was designated AhpF. As increasing numbers of AhpC homologs were recognized throughout phylogeny and within individual species, the superfamily was renamed peroxiredoxins (132). Peroxiredoxins are more widely distributed among species than SODs or catalases. Peroxiredoxins can protect against RNIs (142) by serving as peroxynitrite reductases (137).

Defenses of *Mycobacterium tuberculosis* Against Reactive Nitrogen Intermediates and Reactive Oxygen Intermediates

Although the role of RNIs is established in host defense against experimental *M. tuberculosis* and we know that strains or isolates of *M. tuberculosis* vary in their susceptibility to RNIs (81), we have little understanding of how *M. tuberculosis* resists RNIs. This remains an active frontier of research.

Mycobacteria lack GSH (125). Mycothiol seems likely to substitute, but such a function has not been established. *M. tuberculosis* encodes as many as three thioredoxins and one thioredoxin reductase (13), but their role against ROIs

or RNIs is only now being studied via specific knockouts. The *oxyR* regulon of *M. tuberculosis* is nonfunctional (143–145) and the *soxRS* regulon is absent. Nonetheless, some of the genes controlled by these regulons in *E. coli* are expressed in *M. tuberculosis*: catalase-peroxidase (KatG) (144), SOD (54), and AhpC (142,145). As noted earlier, SOD deficiency impairs the growth of *M. tuberculosis* in macrophages but not in mice and guinea pigs (54,146). katG was the only peroxide-inducible protein found in *M. tuberculosis* (147). The effect of selectively engineered and complemented katG deficiency has yet to be reported. Cyclopropanated mycolic acids and phenolic glycolipid (148) may confer resistance to ROIs but have not been tested against RNIs. Exposure to RNIs induces at least eight proteins in *M. tuberculosis* (147), but it is not known whether they have a role in RNI resistance. The *M. tuberculosis* genome encodes two truncated hemoglobins that have been postulated to oxidize NO (149). Knock out of one of these in BCG markedly decreased the rate of NO consumption by the bacillus and rendered its respiration more susceptible to inhibition by NO (109). Tests are awaited of the phenotype of *M. tuberculosis* exposed to RNIs *in vitro* and its survival in macrophages and in mice after the genes encoding one or both of these truncated hemoglobins have been disrupted. MsrA from *M. tuberculosis* protected MsrA-deficient *E. coli* from being killed by hydrogen peroxide, nitrite, or GSNO (72). We are now studying the function of *MsrA* and *MsrB* in *M. tuberculosis*.

Several powerful approaches have been initiated to identify genes in *M. tuberculosis* that may play a nonredundant role in resistance to ROIs and RNIs, such as signature tagged mutagenesis in mice of the appropriate genotypes and saturation transposon mutagenesis with subsequent *in vitro* selection in RNIs. Those studies are in progress.

A less robust approach was launched some years earlier that did not require specialized vectors or containment facilities. This involved expression of *M. tuberculosis* genes in recombinant enterobacteria and selection by survival in RNI stress. In the first such study, *E. coli* organisms containing a library of *M. tuberculosis* genomic DNA were subjected to killing by nitrite (150). An *M. tuberculosis* gene identified in this way, *noxR1*, conferred resistance to nitrite, GSNO, hydrogen peroxide, hypochlorous acid, and hydrogen ion but not to high salt concentrations, heat, detergent, ethanol, or nalidixic acid (150). However, no phenotype was detected when *M. tuberculosis* was rendered selectively *noxR1* deficient and injected into wild-type mice (151). Of course, lack of a phenotype on knock out of a gene in the pathogen may either mean that the gene is inconsequential under the conditions tested or that its function is redundant. Thus, the significance of *noxR1* remains undefined. In the second such search, recombinant *S. typhimurium* pathogens were subjected to killing by GSNO (152). An *M. tuberculosis* gene identified by this approach, *noxR3*, conferred resistance to GSNO, nitrite, hydrogen peroxide and salt but not to acid, heat, detergent, or nalidixic acid (152). Its knockout in *M. tuberculosis* is now being prepared.

AhpC from *M. tuberculosis* protected AhpCF-deficient *S. typhimurium* pathogens from death caused by exposure to nitrite or GSNO (142). On transfection, AhpC from *M. tuberculosis* also protected human cells from death caused by the simultaneous expression of iNOS (142). The mechanism appeared to be related to the ability of AhpC to react rapidly with peroxynitrite (137). In *S. typhimurium*, AhpC interacts with either AhpF or thioredoxin to serve as a peroxynitrite reductase. However, it remained to identify a reducing partner for AhpC in *M. tuberculosis*. *M. tuberculosis* lacks AhpF. In its place in the chromosome appears an unrelated sequence termed AhpD simply to denote by alphabetization that it lies just downstream of AhpC. AhpD had weak peroxidase activity against lipid peroxides (153).

Recent work clarified the physiologic function of AhpD. Purification and crystallization of AhpD allowed its structure to be solved by x-ray diffraction at 2 Å resolution (154). AhpD presents a novel protein fold consisting of a trimer of monomers built up chiefly of seven α-helices. This contrasts with thioredoxins, which display three α helices surrounding five to seven β sheets. However, the C terminus of AhpD's C-terminal α helix can be modeled closely on the active site in thioredoxins. Cysteine 130 and cysteine 133 in AhpD become disulfide bonded when AhpD is oxidized by lipoamide. Thus, AhpD appears to be a lipoamide-sensitive ortholog of thioredoxin.

Armed with this information, Bryk et al. (154) worked out a pathway in *M. tuberculosis* that functions to catabolize hydrogen peroxide, alkyl peroxides, and OONO⁻. The pathway begins when AhpC encounters the oxidant. As the oxidant is reduced to the corresponding alcohol or nitrite, AhpC's conserved N-terminal cysteine is oxidized to the sulfenic acid (137). Further oxidation is prevented by inter-monomeric disulfide bonding. AhpC is reduced by AhpD via its thioredoxin-like cysteine pair. AhpD is then reduced by the lipoamide attached to the enzyme dihydrolipoamide succinyltransferase (SucB). This enzyme is reduced in turn by dihydrolipoamide dehydrogenase (LPD) at the expense of nicotinamide adenine dinucleotide (reduced form). SucB and LPD represent the E2 and E3 components of the α-ketoacid dehydrogenase complexes. Along with a variable representative of E1, these complexes include pyruvate dehydrogenase, α-ketoglutarate dehydrogenase and branched chain ketoacid dehydrogenase. Thus, AhpD helps to connect the enzymes of intermediary metabolism directly to antioxidant defense in *M. tuberculosis* (154). Gene disruption experiments are underway to determine the contribution of AhpC, AhpD, SucB, and LPD to the pathogenesis of *M. tuberculosis* in mice.

Existing literature about the expression of these four proteins deals only with AhpC and is contradictory. KatG-deficient variants of *M. tuberculosis* often harbor compen-

satory mutations in the promoter of *ahpC*, leading to its overexpression (145,155). Aside from *KatG*-deficient mutants, which are often isoniazid resistant, the ability of *M. tuberculosis* to express AhpC was questioned (156). However, expression of AhpC at the protein level has been repeatedly demonstrated, including in *M. tuberculosis* isolates that are KatG replete and both isoniazid sensitive or resistant (142,157–159). AhpC was then said to be repressed during growth of *M. tuberculosis* in mice (158), but our studies by molecular beacon real-time reverse transcription polymerase chain reaction indicate robust expression of *ahpC* within *M. tuberculosis* pathogens recovered from the lungs of infected mice. The *ahpD* gene is cotranscribed with *ahpC*, and transcripts were also detected for *sucB* and *lpd* (S. Shi, S. Ehrt, C. Nathan, unpublished observations, 2002). Knockout of *ahpC* in *M. tuberculosis* led to no growth defect in wild-type mice (158). However, our preliminary experiments indicate a marked phenotype in some mice. AhpC is one of five peroxiredoxins encoded by the *M. tuberculosis* genome (157). One or more of the others may be redundant with AhpC, complicating interpretation. When expression of *ahpC* was blocked in *Mycobacterium bovis*, the mycobacteria lost virulence in the guinea pig (159).

IMPACT ON REACTIVE NITROGEN INTERMEDIATES ON HOST IMMUNE RESPONSES

The host is not indifferent to the large amounts of oxidizing and nitrosating species produced by its own cells during infection and inflammation. In fact, many perturbations of host immunity can be traced back to host-derived ROIs and RNIs. These have been studied at four levels: the organism, cell populations, intercellular signals, and intracellular signals. From this extensive literature, salient findings at the first two levels are noted below in mycobacteria-infected mice and in macrophages that are engaged in killing *M. tuberculosis* pathogens.

Impact of Reactive Nitrogen Intermediates on the Regulation of the Systemic Immune Response to Mycobacteria

The function of RNIs and ROIs in the immune response to microbial infections pertains not only to their bacteriostatic or bactericidal activities; both groups of molecules also participate in shaping the host response. Mice deficient in phagocyte oxidase do not form typical granulomas in response to *Aspergillus fumigatus* (160). This altered granulomatous response was not observed in phox-deficient mice challenged with BCG (161). However, mice deficient in iNOS produced larger and more necrotic granulomas on aerogenic infection with virulent *M. tuberculosis* than did wild-type mice (95). NO has inhibitory effects on the adherence and migration of monocytes and granulocytes, which may contribute to the increased granuloma size in iNOS-deficient mice (162,163). In contrast, iNOS is dispensable for the development of *Mycobacterium avium*–induced pulmonary caseous necrosis (164). However, the mechanisms controlling *M. avium* immunopathology differ from those involved in controlling *M. tuberculosis*. For example, iNOS-deficient mice are more efficient in clearing an *M. avium* infection than are wild-type mice (165).

The functions of NO as modulator of the immune system have been reviewed (166,167). The ability of NO to inhibit T-cell proliferation and leukocyte recruitment may have an impact on an infection with *M. tuberculosis*. In addition, NO modulates the production and function of chemokines and cytokines, such as IL-12, TNF, IL-10, and IFN-γ, whose importance in the pathogenesis of tuberculosis has been documented (84,88,168,169). It has been argued that NO can differentially suppress Th1 responses, perhaps via its interference with signal transduction in response to IL-12 (170).

Despite the signaling activities of NO, the increased susceptibility of the iNOS-deficient mouse toward an *M. tuberculosis* infection is most likely owing to a direct effect on the pathogen and not to a lack of signaling events. IFN-γ levels were preserved in the iNOS$^{-/-}$ mouse and histopathologic responses appeared normal (85). The iNOS$^{-/-}$ phenotype is manifest at the single cell level (29) and products of the enzyme kill *M. tuberculosis in vitro* (79,81).

Regulation of Macrophage Gene Expression

Recent work used a genomic approach to address the impact of RNIs and ROIs on host gene regulation in *M. tuberculosis*–infected macrophages (29). High-density oligonucleotide arrays containing probe sets for approximately 11,000 genes and representing approximately one-third of the mouse genome were used to analyze changes in gene expression of primary mouse macrophages. The macrophages were wild type, iNOS deficient, phox deficient, and deficient in both iNOS and phox. They were cultured with and without IFN-γ followed (or not) by infection with virulent *M. tuberculosis*. Exposure to IFN-γ and/or *M. tuberculosis* resulted in altered gene expression of 25% of the monitored genes. Altered expression of more than half of the regulated genes was dependent on or significantly affected by deficiency of iNOS, phox, or both. Although many of the genes responding to IFN-γ and *M. tuberculosis* were related to immunity and inflammation, the majority of the genes whose expression was affected by iNOS and/or phox were not in this category. This may provide evidence for the existence of regulatory mechanisms to insulate most immunity- and inflammation-related genes

from the influences of iNOS and phox. The study illustrates the considerable impact of RNIs and ROIs on gene regulation and therefore the phenotype of infected macrophages.

POTENTIAL IMPLICATIONS FOR PROPHYLAXIS AND THERAPY

Macrophages have diverse antimicrobial mechanisms. Our knowledge of them ranges from the extensive (e.g., cDNA of enzyme cloned, enzyme purified, catalytic mechanism defined, products shown to be bactericidal, knock out of the gene encoding the enzyme makes mice hypersusceptible to the infection) to the introductory (e.g., antimicrobial effect exists, known mechanisms do not account for it). Two of the antimicrobial pathways of tissue macrophages qualify as extensively defined: production of RNIs via iNOS and production of ROIs via phox (21). Of these, iNOS is critical for the acute and chronic control of experimental tuberculosis and is expressed in human tuberculosis. However, in a biologic setting as complex as tuberculosis, redundancy and synergy can complicate inference (21). Extensive evidence for one pathway is not evidence against another. It can be taken as a given that microbicidal mechanisms other than generation of RNI are also profoundly important to the control of *M. tuberculosis*.

Our understanding of the NO pathway in tuberculosis remains at an early stage. When our grasp of the subject is mature, we will understand why the NO pathway fails to sterilize *M. tuberculosis in vivo* when the products of the same pathway do so *in vitro*. We might have experimental drugs based on that knowledge, such as inhibitors of the RNI-resistance mechanisms of *M. tuberculosis*. By administering such agents, we would be testing whether antituberculous immunity in the normal host can be rendered sterilizing, so that purified protein derivative–positive individuals could become free of the risk of reactivation tuberculosis. We would be asking whether crippling the resistance to host immunity of *M. tuberculosis* could help patients rid themselves more quickly of viable *M. tuberculosis* during chemotherapy, thus reducing the emergence of drug resistance and diminishing the impact of preexistent drug resistance. Finally, we would be asking whether such agents would allow conventional chemotherapy to cure tuberculosis routinely in the HIV-infected host.

ACKNOWLEDGMENT

We thank Drs. R. Bryk, H. Darwin, B. Gold, K. Hisert, D. Schnappinger, and S. Shi for critical comments and Drs. E. Chan, G. Schoolnik, D. Schnappinger, M. Voskuil, and I. Smith for sharing results before publication. Preparation of this article and some of the work herein were supported by National Institutes of Health grants HL61241 to C.N. and

HL68525 to S.E. The Department of Microbiology and Immunology acknowledges the support of the William Randolph Hearst Foundation.

REFERENCES

1. Hernandez-Pando R, Jeyanathan M, Mengistu G, et al. Persistence of DNA from *Mycobacterium tuberculosis* in superficially normal lung tissue during latent infection. *Lancet* 2000;356: 2133–2138.
2. Pethe K, Alonso S, Biet F, et al. The heparin-binding haemagglutinin of *M. tuberculosis* is required for extrapulmonary dissemination. *Nature* 2001;412:190–194.
3. Keane J, Gershon S, Wise RP, et al. Tuberculosis associated with infliximab, a tumor necrosis factor alpha-neutralizing agent. *N Engl J Med* 2001;345:1098–1104.
4. Tuberculosis and AIDS. Statement on AIDS and tuberculosis. Geneva, March 1989. Global Programme on AIDS and Tuberculosis Programme, World Health Organization, in collaboration with the International Union Against Tuberculosis and Lung Disease. *Bull Int Union Tuber Lung Dis* 1989;64:8–11.
5. Bloom BR, Murray CJ. Tuberculosis: commentary on a reemergent killer. *Science* 1992;257:1055–1064.
6. Daley CL, Small PM, Schecter GF, et al. An outbreak of tuberculosis with accelerated progression among persons infected with the human immunodeficiency virus. An analysis using restriction-fragment-length polymorphisms. *N Engl J Med* 1992;326: 231–235.
7. Lienhardt C, Rodrigues LC. Estimation of the impact of the human immunodeficiency virus infection on tuberculosis: tuberculosis risks re-visited? *Int J Tuberc Lung Dis* 1997;1: 196–204.
8. Nakata K, Rom WN, Honda Y, et al. Mycobacterium tuberculosis enhances human immunodeficiency virus-1 replication in the lung. *Am J Respir Crit Care Med* 1997;155:996–1003.
9. Whalen C, Horsburgh CR, Hom D, et al. Accelerated course of human immunodeficiency virus infection after tuberculosis. *Am J Respir Crit Care Med* 1995;151:129–135.
10. Snapper SB, Lugosi L, Jekkel A, et al. Lysogeny and transformation in mycobacteria: stable expression of foreign genes. *Proc Natl Acad Sci U S A* 1988;85:6987–6991.
11. Cox JS, Chen B, McNeil M, et al. Complex lipid determines tissue-specific replication of *Mycobacterium tuberculosis* in mice. *Nature* 1999;402:79–83.
12. Rubin EJ, Akerley BJ, Novik VN, et al. *In vivo* transposition of mariner-based elements in enteric bacteria and mycobacteria. *Proc Natl Acad Sci U S A* 1999;96:1645–1650.
13. Cole ST, Brosch R, Parkhill J, et al. Deciphering the biology of *Mycobacterium tuberculosis* from the complete genome sequence. *Nature* 1998;393:537–544.
14. Sofia M, Maniscalco M, Honore N, et al. Familial outbreak of disseminated multidrug-resistant tuberculosis and meningitis. *Int J Tuberc Lung Dis* 2001;5:551–558.
15. Remus N, Reichenbach J, Picard C, et al. Impaired interferon gamma-mediated immunity and susceptibility to mycobacterial infection in childhood. *Pediatr Res* 2001;50:8–13.
16. Karupiah G, Xie QW, Buller RM, et al. Inhibition of viral replication by interferon-gamma-induced nitric oxide synthase. *Science* 1993;261:1445–1448.
17. Bellamy R, Ruwende C, Corrah T, et al. Variations in the NRAMP1 gene and susceptibility to tuberculosis in West Africans. *N Engl J Med* 1998;338:640–644.
18. Shaw MA, Collins A, Peacock CS, et al. Evidence that genetic susceptibility to *Mycobacterium tuberculosis* in a Brazilian population is under oligogenic control: linkage study of the candidate genes NRAMP1 and TNFA. *Tuber Lung Dis* 1997;78: 35–45.
19. Kramnik I, Dietrich WF, Demant P, et al. Genetic control of resistance to experimental infection with virulent *Mycobacterium tuberculosis*. *Proc Natl Acad Sci U S A* 2000;97: 8560–8565.
20. Winkelstein JA, Marino MC, Johnston RB Jr, et al. Chronic granulomatous disease. Report on a national registry of 368 patients. *Medicine (Baltimore)* 2000;79:155–169.
21. Nathan C, Shiloh MU. Reactive oxygen and nitrogen intermediates in the relationship between mammalian hosts and microbial pathogens. *Proc Natl Acad Sci U S A* 2000;97:8841–8848.
22. Mogues T, Goodrich ME, Ryan L, et al. The relative importance of T cell subsets in immunity and immunopathology of airborne *Mycobacterium tuberculosis* infection in mice. *J Exp Med* 2001;193:271–280.
23. Scanga CA, Mohan VP, Yu K, et al. Depletion of CD4(+) T cells causes reactivation of murine persistent tuberculosis despite continued expression of interferon gamma and nitric oxide synthase 2. *J Exp Med* 2000;192:347–358.
24. Chun T, Serbina NV, Nolt D, et al. Induction of M3-restricted cytotoxic T lymphocyte responses by N-formylated peptides derived from *Mycobacterium tuberculosis*. *J Exp Med* 2001;193: 1213–1220.
25. Engele M, Stossel E, Castiglione K, et al. Induction of TNF in human alveolar macrophages as a potential evasion mechanism of virulent *Mycobacterium tuberculosis*. *J Immunol* 2002;168: 1328–1337.
26. Kindler V, Sappino AP, Grau GE, et al. The inducing role of tumor necrosis factor in the development of bactericidal granulomas during BCG infection. *Cell* 1989;56:731–740.
27. Nathan CF, Murray HW, Wiebe ME, et al. Identification of interferon-gamma as the lymphokine that activates human macrophage oxidative metabolism and antimicrobial activity. *J Exp Med* 1983;158:670–689.
28. Stenger S, Hanson DA, Teitelbaum R, et al. An antimicrobial activity of cytolytic T cells mediated by granulysin. *Science* 1998; 282:121–125.
29. Ehrt S, Schnappinger D, Bekiranov S, et al. Reprogramming of the macrophage transcriptome in response to interferon-gamma and *Mycobacterium tuberculosis*: signaling roles of nitric oxide synthase-2 and phagocyte oxidase. *J Exp Med* 2001;194: 1123–1140.
30. Keane J, Balcewicz-Sablinska MK, Remold HG, et al. Infection by *Mycobacterium tuberculosis* promotes human alveolar macrophage apoptosis. *Infect Immun* 1997;65:298–304.
31. Rojas M, Olivier M, Gros P, et al. TNF-alpha and IL-10 modulate the induction of apoptosis by virulent *Mycobacterium tuberculosis* in murine macrophages. *J Immunol* 1999;162: 6122–6131.
32. Keane J, Remold HG, Kornfeld H. Virulent *Mycobacterium tuberculosis* strains evade apoptosis of infected alveolar macrophages. *J Immunol* 2000;164:2016–2020.
33. Kusner DJ, Barton JA. ATP stimulates human macrophages to kill intracellular virulent *Mycobacterium tuberculosis* via calcium-dependent phagosome-lysosome fusion. *J Immunol* 2001;167: 3308–3315.
34. Akaki T, Tomioka H, Shimizu T, et al. Comparative roles of free fatty acids with reactive nitrogen intermediates and reactive oxygen intermediates in expression of the anti-microbial activity of macrophages against *Mycobacterium tuberculosis*. *Clin Exp Immunol* 2000;121:302–310.
35. Yong EC, Chi EY, Henderson WR Jr. *Toxoplasma gondii* alters eicosanoid release by human mononuclear phagocytes: role of

leukotrienes in interferon gamma-induced antitoxoplasma activity. *J Exp Med* 1994;180:1637–1648.

36. Boschiroli ML, Ouahrani-Bettache S, Foulongne V, et al. The *Brucella* suis virB operon is induced intracellularly in macrophages. *Proc Natl Acad Sci U S A* 2002;99:1544–1549.

37. Collazo CM, Yap GS, Sempowski GD, et al. Inactivation of LRG-47 and IRG-47 reveals a family of interferon gamma-inducible genes with essential, pathogen-specific roles in resistance to infection. *J Exp Med* 2001;194:181–188.

38. Buchmeier N, Blanc-Potard A, Ehrt S, et al. A parallel intraphagosomal survival strategy shared by *Mycobacterium tuberculosis* and *Salmonella enterica*. *Mol Microbiol* 2000;35:1375–1382.

39. Forbes JR, Gros P. Divalent-metal transport by NRAMP proteins at the interface of host-pathogen interactions. *Trends Microbiol* 2001;9:397–403.

40. De Voss JJ, Rutter K, Schroeder BG, et al. Iron acquisition and metabolism by mycobacteria. *J Bacteriol* 1999;181:4443–4451.

41. Gold B, Rodriguez GM, Marras SA, et al. The *Mycobacterium tuberculosis* IdeR is a dual functional regulator that controls transcription of genes involved in iron acquisition, iron storage and survival in macrophages. *Mol Microbiol* 2001;42:851–865.

42. Manabe YC, Saviola BJ, Sun L, et al. Attenuation of virulence in *Mycobacterium tuberculosis* expressing a constitutively active iron repressor. *Proc Natl Acad Sci U S A* 1999;96:12844–12848.

43. Vidal S, Gros P, Skamene E. Natural resistance to infection with intracellular parasites: molecular genetics identifies Nramp1 as the Bcg/Ity/Lsh locus. *J Leukoc Biol* 1995;58:382–390.

44. Cuellar-Mata P, Jabado N, Liu J, et al. Nramp1 modifies the fusion of *Salmonella typhimurium*-containing vacuoles with cellular endomembranes in macrophages. *J Biol Chem* 2002;277:2258–2265.

45. Medina E, North RJ. Evidence inconsistent with a role for the Bcg gene (Nramp1) in resistance of mice to infection with virulent *Mycobacterium tuberculosis*. *J Exp Med* 1996;183:1045–1051.

46. Nathan CF. Mechanisms of macrophage antimicrobial activity. *Trans R Soc Trop Med Hyg* 1983;77:620–630.

47. Lau YL, Chan GC, Ha SY, et al. The role of phagocytic respiratory burst in host defense against *Mycobacterium tuberculosis*. *Clin Infect Dis* 1998;26:226–227.

48. Mouy R, Fischer A, Vilmer E, et al. Incidence, severity, and prevention of infections in chronic granulomatous disease. *J Pediatr* 1989;114:555–560.

49. Sly LM, Lopez M, Nauseef WM, et al. 1alpha,25-Dihydroxyvitamin D3-induced monocyte antimycobacterial activity is regulated by phosphatidylinositol 3-kinase and mediated by the NADPH-dependent phagocyte oxidase. *J Biol Chem* 2001;276:35482–35493.

50. Adams LB, Dinauer MC, Morgenstern DE, et al. Comparison of the roles of reactive oxygen and nitrogen intermediates in the host response to *Mycobacterium tuberculosis* using transgenic mice. *Tuber Lung Dis* 1997;78:237–246.

51. Cooper AM, Segal BH, Frank AA, et al. Transient loss of resistance to pulmonary tuberculosis in p47(phox−/−) mice. *Infect Immun* 2000;68:1231–1234.

52. Shiloh MU, MacMicking JD, Nicholson S, et al. Phenotype of mice and macrophages deficient in both phagocyte oxidase and inducible nitric oxide synthase. *Immunity* 1999;10:29–38.

53. DeGroote MA, Ochsner UA, Shiloh MU, et al. Periplasmic superoxide dismutase protects *Salmonella* from products of phagocyte NADPH-oxidase and nitric oxide synthase. *Proc Natl Acad Sci U S A* 1997;94:13997–14001.

54. Piddington DL, Fang FC, Laessig T, et al. Cu,Zn superoxide dismutase of *Mycobacterium tuberculosis* contributes to survival in activated macrophages that are generating an oxidative burst. *Infect Immun* 2001;69:4980–4987.

55. Butler AR, Flitney FW, Williams DL. NO, nitrosonium ions, nitroxide ions, nitrosothiols and iron-nitrosyls in biology: a chemist's perspective. *Trends Pharmacol Sci* 1995;16:18–22.

56. Fang FC. Perspectives series: host/pathogen interactions. Mechanisms of nitric oxide-related antimicrobial activity. *J Clin Invest* 1997;99:2818–2825.

57. MacMicking J, Xie QW, Nathan C. Nitric oxide and macrophage function. *Annu Rev Immunol* 1997;15:323–350.

58. Nathan C. Natural resistance and nitric oxide. *Cell* 1995;82:873–876.

59. Stamler JS, Lamas S, Fang FC. Nitrosylation. the prototypic redox-based signaling mechanism. *Cell* 2001;106:675–683.

60. Klebanoff SJ. Reactive nitrogen intermediates and antimicrobial activity: role of nitrite. *Free Radic Biol Med* 1993;14:351–360.

61. Stuehr DJ, Nathan CF. Nitric oxide. A macrophage product responsible for cytostasis and respiratory inhibition in tumor target cells. *J Exp Med* 1989;169:1543–1555.

62. Ohkuma S, Poole B. Fluorescence probe measurement of the intralysosomal pH in living cells and the perturbation of pH by various agents. *Proc Natl Acad Sci U S A* 1978;75:3327–3331.

63. Clemens DL, Horwitz MA. Characterization of the *Mycobacterium tuberculosis* phagosome and evidence that phagosomal maturation is inhibited. *J Exp Med* 1995;181:257–270.

64. Sturgill-Koszycki S, Schlesinger PH, Chakraborty P, et al. Lack of acidification in *Mycobacterium* phagosomes produced by exclusion of the vesicular proton-ATPase. *Science* 1994;263:678–681.

65. Xu S, Cooper A, Sturgill-Koszycki S, et al. Intracellular trafficking in *Mycobacterium tuberculosis* and *Mycobacterium avium*-infected macrophages. *J Immunol* 1994;153:2568–2578.

66. Schaible UE, Sturgill-Koszycki S, Schlesinger PH, et al. Cytokine activation leads to acidification and increases maturation of *Mycobacterium avium*-containing phagosomes in murine macrophages. *J Immunol* 1998;160:1290–1296.

67. DeGroote MA, Granger D, Xu Y, et al. Genetic and redox determinants of nitric oxide cytotoxicity in a *Salmonella typhimurium* model. *Proc Natl Acad Sci U S A* 1995;92:6399–6403.

68. Green RM, Seth A, Connell ND. A peptide permease mutant of *Mycobacterium bovis* BCG resistant to the toxic peptides glutathione and S-nitrosoglutathione. *Infect Immun* 2000;68:429–436.

69. Pacelli R, Wink DA, Cook JA, et al. Nitric oxide potentiates hydrogen peroxide-induced killing of *Escherichia coli*. *J Exp Med* 1995;182:1469–1479.

70. Espey MG, Xavier S, Thomas DD, et al. Direct real-time evaluation of nitration with green fluorescent protein in solution and within human cells reveals the impact of nitrogen dioxide vs. peroxynitrite mechanisms. *Proc Natl Acad Sci U S A* 2002;99:3481–3486.

71. Beckman JS, Beckman TW, Chen J, et al. Apparent hydroxyl radical production by peroxynitrite: implications for endothelial injury from nitric oxide and superoxide. *Proc Natl Acad Sci U S A* 1990;87:1620–1624.

72. St John G, Brot N, Ruan J, et al. Peptide methionine sulfoxide reductase from *Escherichia coli* and *Mycobacterium tuberculosis* protects bacteria against oxidative damage from reactive nitrogen intermediates. *Proc Natl Acad Sci U S A* 2001;98:9901–9906.

73. Yu K, Mitchell C, Xing Y, et al. Toxicity of nitrogen oxides and related oxidants on mycobacteria: *M. tuberculosis* is resistant to peroxynitrite anion. *Tuber Lung Dis* 1999;79:191–198.

74. Choi HS, Rai PR, Chu HW, et al. Analysis of nitric oxide synthase and nitrotyrosine expression in human pulmonary tuberculosis. *Am J Respir Crit Care Med* 2002;166:178–186.

75. Moya MP, Gow AJ, McMahon TJ, et al. S-nitrosothiol repletion

by an inhaled gas regulates pulmonary function. *Proc Natl Acad Sci U S A* 2001;98:5792–5797.

76. Guo FH, De Raeve HR, Rice TW, et al. Continuous nitric oxide synthesis by inducible nitric oxide synthase in normal human airway epithelium *in vivo*. *Proc Natl Acad Sci U S A* 1995;92:7809–7813.

77. Weber I, Fritz C, Ruttkowski S, et al. Anaerobic nitrate reductase (narGHJI) activity of *Mycobacterium bovis* BCG *in vitro* and its contribution to virulence in immunodeficient mice. *Mol Microbiol* 2000;35:1017–1025.

78. Dweik RA, Laskowski D, Abu-Soud HM, et al. Nitric oxide synthesis in the lung. Regulation by oxygen through a kinetic mechanism. *J Clin Invest* 1998;101:660–666.

79. Long R, Light B, Talbot JA. Mycobacteriocidal action of exogenous nitric oxide. *Antimicrob Agents Chemother* 1999;43: 403–405.

80. Zapol WM, Hurford WE. Inhaled nitric oxide in the adult respiratory distress syndrome and other lung diseases. *New Horiz* 1993;1:638–650.

81. O'Brien L, Carmichael J, Lowrie DB, et al. Strains of *Mycobacterium tuberculosis* differ in susceptibility to reactive nitrogen intermediates *in vitro*. *Infect Immun* 1994;62:5187–5190.

82. Aston C, Rom WN, Talbot AT, et al. Early inhibition of mycobacterial growth by human alveolar macrophages is not due to nitric oxide. *Am J Respir Crit Care Med* 1998;157: 1943–1950.

83. Thoma-Uszynski S, Stenger S, Takeuchi O, et al. Induction of direct antimicrobial activity through mammalian Toll-like receptors. *Science* 2001;291:1544–1547.

84. Flynn JL, Chan J, Triebold KJ, et al. An essential role for interferon gamma in resistance to *Mycobacterium tuberculosis* infection. *J Exp Med* 1993;178:2249–2254.

85. MacMicking JD, North RJ, La Course R, et al. Identification of nitric oxide synthase as a protective locus against tuberculosis. *Proc Natl Acad Sci U S A* 1997;94:5243–5248.

86. Chan J, Tian Y, Tanaka KE, et al. Effects of protein calorie malnutrition on tuberculosis in mice. *Proc Natl Acad Sci U S A* 1996;93:14857–14861.

87. Dalton DK, Pitts-Meek S, Keshav S, et al. Multiple defects of immune cell function in mice with disrupted interferon-gamma genes. *Science* 1993;259:1739–1742.

88. Flynn JL, Goldstein MM, Chan J, et al. Tumor necrosis factor-alpha is required in the protective immune response against *Mycobacterium tuberculosis* in mice. *Immunity* 1995;2:561–572.

89. Huang S, Hendriks W, Althage A, et al. Immune response in mice that lack the interferon-gamma receptor. *Science* 1993;259:1742–1745.

90. Kahn DA, Archer DC, Gold DP, et al. Adjuvant immunotherapy is dependent on inducible nitric oxide synthase. *J Exp Med* 2001;193:1261–1268.

91. Chan J, Xing Y, Magliozzo RS, et al. Killing of virulent *Mycobacterium tuberculosis* by reactive nitrogen intermediates produced by activated murine macrophages. *J Exp Med* 1992; 175:1111–1122.

92. Chan J, Tanaka K, Carroll D, et al. Effects of nitric oxide synthase inhibitors on murine infection with *Mycobacterium tuberculosis*. *Infect Immun* 1995;63:736–740.

93. Denis M. Interferon-gamma-treated murine macrophages inhibit growth of tubercle bacilli via the generation of reactive nitrogen intermediates. *Cell Immunol* 1991;132:150–157.

94. Flesch IE, Kaufmann SH. Mechanisms involved in mycobacterial growth inhibition by gamma interferon-activated bone marrow macrophages: role of reactive nitrogen intermediates. *Infect Immun* 1991;59:3213–3218.

95. Cooper AM, Pearl JE, Brooks JV, et al. Expression of the nitric oxide synthase 2 gene is not essential for early control of *Mycobacterium tuberculosis* in the murine lung. *Infect Immun* 2000;68:6879–6882.

96. Scanga CA, Mohan VP, Tanaka K, et al. The inducible nitric oxide synthase locus confers protection against aerogenic challenge of both clinical and laboratory strains of *Mycobacterium tuberculosis* in mice. *Infect Immun* 2001;69:7711–7717.

97. Flynn JL, Scanga CA, Tanaka KE, et al. Effects of aminoguanidine on latent murine tuberculosis. *J Immunol* 1998;160: 1796–1803.

98. Jagannath C, Actor JK, Hunter RL Jr. Induction of nitric oxide in human monocytes and monocyte cell lines by *Mycobacterium tuberculosis*. *Nitric Oxide* 1998;2:174–186.

99. Weinberg JB. Human mononuclear phagocyte nitric oxide production and nitric oxide synthase type 2 expression. In: Fang FC, ed. *Nitric oxide and infection*. New York: Kluwer Academic/Plenum Publishers, 1998:95–150.

100. Nozaki Y, Hasegawa Y, Ichiyama S, et al. Mechanism of nitric oxide-dependent killing of *Mycobacterium bovis* BCG in human alveolar macrophages. *Infect Immun* 1997;65:3644–3647.

101. Rich EA, Torres M, Sada E, et al. *Mycobacterium tuberculosis* (MTB)-stimulated production of nitric oxide by human alveolar macrophages and relationship of nitric oxide production to growth inhibition of MTB. *Tuber Lung Dis* 1997;78: 247–255.

102. Wang CH, Lin HC, Liu CY, et al. Upregulation of inducible nitric oxide synthase and cytokine secretion in peripheral blood monocytes from pulmonary tuberculosis patients. *Int J Tuberc Lung Dis* 2001;5:283–291.

103. Nicholson S, Bonecini-Almeida MdG, Lapa e Silva JR, et al. Inducible nitric oxide synthase in pulmonary alveolar macrophages from patients with tuberculosis. *J Exp Med* 1996; 183:2293–2302.

104. Wang CH, Liu CY, Lin HC, et al. Increased exhaled nitric oxide in active pulmonary tuberculosis due to inducible NO synthase upregulation in alveolar macrophages. *Eur Respir J* 1998;11: 809–815.

105. Wang CH, Kuo HP. Nitric oxide modulates interleukin-1beta and tumour necrosis factor-alpha synthesis, and disease regression by alveolar macrophages in pulmonary tuberculosis. *Respirology* 2001;6:79–84.

106. Schön T. Nitric oxide in tuberculosis and leprosy. Dissertation, No. 749, Department of Clinical and Molecular Medicine, Sweden: Linköping University, 2002.

106a. Facchetti F, Vermi W, Fiorentini S, et al. Expression of inducible nitric oxide synthase in human granulomas and histiocytic reactions. *Am J Pathol* 1999;154:145–152.

107. Sherman DR, Voskuil M, Schnappinger D, et al. Regulation of the *Mycobacterium tuberculosis* hypoxic response gene encoding alpha -crystallin. *Proc Natl Acad Sci U S A* 2001;98:7534–7539.

108. Wayne LG. Dynamics of submerged growth of *Mycobacterium tuberculosis* under aerobic and microaerophilic conditions. *Am Rev Respir Dis* 1976;114:807–811.

109. Ouellet H, Ouellet Y, Richard C, et al. Truncated hemoglobin HbN protects *Mycobacterium bovis* from nitric oxide. *Proc Natl Acad Sci U S A* 2002;99:5902–5907.

110. Rodriguez GM, Voskuil MI, Gold B, et al. IdeR, an essential gene in *Mycobacterium tuberculosis*: role of IdeR in iron-dependent gene expression, iron metabolism, and oxidative stress response. *Infect Immun* 2002;70:3371–3381.

111. Imlay JA, Linn S. DNA damage and oxygen radical toxicity. *Science* 1988;240:1302–1309.

112. Trinchieri G. Regulatory role of T cells producing both interferon gamma and interleukin 10 in persistent infection. *J Exp Med* 2001;194:F53–F57.

113. Bogdan C, Vodovotz Y, Nathan C. Macrophage deactivation by interleukin 10. *J Exp Med* 1991;174:1549–1555.

114. Gazzinelli RT, Oswald IP, James SL, et al. IL-10 inhibits parasite killing and nitrogen oxide production by IFN-gamma-activated macrophages. *J Immunol* 1992;148:1792–1796.

115. Kim YM, Talanian RV, Li J, et al. Nitric oxide prevents IL-1beta and IFN-gamma-inducing factor (IL-18) release from macrophages by inhibiting caspase-1 (IL-1beta-converting enzyme). *J Immunol* 1998;161:4122–4128.

116. Dahl KE, Shiratsuchi H, Hamilton BD, et al. Selective induction of transforming growth factor beta in human monocytes by lipoarabinomannan of *Mycobacterium tuberculosis. Infect Immun* 1996;64:399–405.

117. Vodovotz Y, Bogdan C, Paik J, et al. Mechanisms of suppression of macrophage nitric oxide release by transforming growth factor beta. *J Exp Med* 1993;178:605–613.

118. Hesse M, Modolell M, La Flamme AC, et al. Differential regulation of nitric oxide synthase-2 and arginase-1 by type 1/type 2 cytokines *in vivo*: granulomatous pathology is shaped by the pattern of L-arginine metabolism. *J Immunol* 2001;167: 6533–6544.

119. Tsunawaki S, Nathan CF. Enzymatic basis of macrophage activation. Kinetic analysis of superoxide production in lysates of resident and activated mouse peritoneal macrophages and granulocytes. *J Biol Chem* 1984;259:4305–4312.

120. Vazquez-Torres A, Xu Y, Jones-Carson J, et al. *Salmonella* pathogenicity island 2-dependent evasion of the phagocyte NADPH oxidase. *Science* 2000;287:1655–1658.

121. Vazquez-Torres A, Fantuzzi G, Edwards CK 3rd, et al. Defective localization of the NADPH phagocyte oxidase to *Salmonella*-containing phagosomes in tumor necrosis factor p55 receptor-deficient macrophages. *Proc Natl Acad Sci U S A* 2001;98: 2561–2565.

122. Vodovotz Y, Russell D, Xie QW, et al. Vesicle membrane association of nitric oxide synthase in primary mouse macrophages. *J Immunol* 1995;154:2914–2925.

123. Chakravortty D, Hansen-Wester I, Hensel M. *Salmonella* pathogenicity island 2 mediates protection of intracellular *Salmonella* from reactive nitrogen intermediates. *J Exp Med* 2002;195: 1155–1166.

124. Fahey RC, Buschbacher RM, G.L. Newton. The evolution of glutathione metabolism in phototrophic microorganisms. *J Mol Evol* 1987, 25:81–88.

125. Newton GL, Arnold K, Price MS, et al. Disruption of thiols in microorganisms: mycothiol is a major thiol in most actinomycetes. *J. Bacteriol.* 1996;178:1990–1995.

126. Sies H, Sharov VS, Klotz LO, et al. Glutathione peroxidase protects against peroxynitrite-mediated oxidations. A new function for selenoproteins as peroxynitrite reductase. *J Biol Chem* 1997; 272:27812–27817.

127. Spies HS, Steenkamp DJ. Thiols of intracellular pathogens. Identification of ovothiol in Leishmania donovani and structural analysis of a novel thiol from *Mycobacterium bovis. Eur J Biochem* 1994;224:203–213.

128. Tovar J, Fairlamb AH. Extrachromosomal, homologous expression of trypanothione reductase and its complementary mRNA in *Trypanosoma cruzi. Nucleic Acids Res* 1996;24:2942–2949.

129. DeGroote MA, Testerman T, Xu Y, et al. Homocysteine antagonism of nitric oxide-related cytostasis in *Salmonella typhimurium. Science* 1996;272:414–417.

130. Holmgren A. Thioredoxin and glutaredoxin systems. *J Biol Chem* 1989;264:13963–13966.

131. Chae HZ, Chung SJ, Rhee SG. Thioredoxin-dependent peroxide reductase from yeast. *J Biol Chem* 1994;269:27670–27678.

132. Chae HZ, Robison K, Poole LB, et al. Cloning and sequencing of thiol-specific antioxidant from mammalian brain: alkyl hydroperoxide reductase and thiol-specific antioxidant define a

133. Crawford MJ, Goldberg DE. Regulation of the *Salmonella typhimurium* flavohemoglobin gene. A new pathway for bacterial gene expression in response to nitric oxide. *J Biol Chem* 1998;273:34028–34032.

134. Gardner AM, Gardner PR. Flavohemoglobin detoxifies nitric oxide in aerobic, but not anaerobic, *Escherichia coli*. Evidence for a novel inducible anaerobic nitric oxide- scavenging activity. *J Biol Chem* 2002;277:8166–8171.

135. Cross R, Lloyd D, Poole RK, et al. Enzymatic removal of nitric oxide catalyzed by cytochrome c' in *Rhodobacter capsulatus. J Bacteriol* 2001;183:3050–3054.

136. Weissbach H, Etienne F, Hoshi T, et al. Peptide methionine sulfoxide reductase: structure, mechanism of action, and biological function. *Arch Biochem Biophys* 2002;397:172–178.

137. Bryk R, Griffin P, Nathan C. Peroxynitrite reductase activity of bacterial peroxiredoxins. *Nature* 2000;407:211–215.

138. Jacobson FS, Morgan RW, Christman MF, et al. An alkyl hydroperoxide reductase from *Salmonella typhimurium* involved in the defense of DNA against oxidative damage. Purification and properties. *J Biol Chem* 1989;264:1488–1496.

139. Storz G, Jacobson FS, Tartaglia LA, et al. An alkyl hydroperoxide reductase induced by oxidative stress in *Salmonella typhimurium* and *Escherichia coli*: genetic characterization and cloning of ahp. *J Bacteriol* 1989;171:2049–2055.

140. Tartaglia LA, Storz G, Brodsky MH, et al. Alkyl hydroperoxide reductase from *Salmonella typhimurium*. Sequence and homology to thioredoxin reductase and other flavoprotein disulfide oxidoreductases. *J Biol Chem* 1990;265:10535–10540.

141. Costa Seaver L, Imlay JA. Alkyl hydroperoxide reductase is the primary scavenger of endogenous hydrogen peroxide in *Escherichia coli. J Bacteriol* 2001;183:7173–7181.

142. Chen L, Xie QW, Nathan . Alkyl hydroperoxide reductase subunit C (AhpC) protects bacterial and human cells against reactive nitrogen intermediates. *Mol Cell* 1998;1:795–805.

143. Deretic V, Philipp W, Dhandayuthapani S, et al. *Mycobacterium tuberculosis* is a natural mutant with an inactivated oxidative-stress regulatory gene: implications for sensitivity to isoniazide. *Mol Microbiol* 1995;17:889–900.

144. Sherman DR, Sabo PJ, Hickey MJ, et al. Disparate responses to oxidative stress in saprophytic and pathogenic mycobacteria. *Proc Natl Acad Sci U S A* 1995;92:6625–6629.

145. Sherman DR, Mdluli K, Hickey MJ, et al. Compensatory ahpC gene expression in isoniazid-resistant *Mycobacterium tuberculosis. Science* 1996;272:1641–1643.

146. Dussurget O, Stewart G, Neyrolles O, et al. Role of *Mycobacterium tuberculosis* copper-zinc superoxide dismutase. *Infect Immun* 2001;69:529–533.

147. Garbe TR, Hibler NS, Deretic V. Response to reactive nitrogen intermediates in *Mycobacterium tuberculosis*: induction of the 16-kilodalton α-crystallin homolog by exposure to nitric oxide donors. *Infect Immun* 1999;67:460–465.

148. Chan J, Fujiwara T, Brennan P, et al. Microbial glycolipids: possible virulence factors that scavenge oxygen radicals. *Proc Natl Acad Sci U S A* 1989;86:2453–2457.

149. Couture M, Yeh SR, Wittenberg BA, et al. A cooperative oxygen-binding hemoglobin from Mycobacterium tuberculosis. *Proc Natl Acad Sci U S A* 1999;96:11223–11228.

150. Ehrt S, Shiloh MU, Ruan J, et al. A novel antioxidant gene from *Mycobacterium tuberculosis. J Exp Med* 1997;186:1885–1896.

151. Stewart GR, Ehrt S, Riley LW, et al. Deletion of the putative antioxidant noxR1 does not alter the virulence of *Mycobacterium tuberculosis* H37Rv. *Tuber Lung Dis* 2000;80:237–242.

152. Ruan J, St John G, Ehrt S, et al. noxR3, a novel gene from

Mycobacterium tuberculosis, protects *Salmonella typhimurium* from nitrosative and oxidative stress. *Infect Immun* 1999;67: 3276–3283.

153. Hillas PJ, del Alba FS, Oyarzabal J, et al. The AhpC and AhpD antioxidant defense system of *Mycobacterium tuberculosis*. *J Biol Chem* 2000;275:18801–18809.

154. Bryk R, Lima CD, Erdjument-Bromage H, et al. Metabolic enzymes of mycobacteria linked to antioxidant defense by a thioredoxin-like protein. *Science* 2002;295:1073–1077.

155. Wilson TM, Collins DM. ahpC, a gene involved in isoniazid resistance of the *Mycobacterium tuberculosis* complex. *Mol Microbiol* 1996;19:1025–1034.

156. Dhandayuthapani S, Zhang Y, Mudd MH, et al. Oxidative stress response and its role in sensitivity to isoniazid in mycobacteria: characterization and inducibility of ahpC by peroxides in *Mycobacterium smegmatis* and lack of expression in *M. aurum* and *M. tuberculosis*. *J Bacteriol* 1996;178:3641–3649.

157. Domenech P, Honore N, Heym B, et al. Role of OxyS of *Mycobacterium tuberculosis* in oxidative stress: overexpression confers increased sensitivity to organic hydroperoxides. *Microbes Infect* 2001;3:713–721.

158. Springer B, Master S, Sander P, et al. Silencing of oxidative stress response in *Mycobacterium tuberculosis*: expression patterns of ahpC in virulent and avirulent strains and effect of ahpC inactivation. *Infect Immun* 2001;69:5967–5973.

159. Wilson T, de Lisle GW, Marcinkeviciene JA, et al. Antisense RNA to ahpC, an oxidative stress defence gene involved in isoniazid resistance, indicates that AhpC of *Mycobacterium bovis* has virulence properties. *Microbiology* 1998;144:2687–2695.

160. Morgenstern DE, Gifford MA, Li LL, et al. Absence of respiratory burst in X-linked chronic granulomatous disease mice leads to abnormalities in both host defense and inflammatory response to *Aspergillus fumigatus*. *J Exp Med* 1997;185:207–218.

161. Nicholson SC, Grobmyer SR, Shiloh MU, et al. Lethality of endotoxin in mice genetically deficient in the respiratory burst oxidase, inducible nitric oxide synthase, or both. *Shock* 1999; 11:253–258.

162. Cooper A, Adams LB, Dalton DK, et al. IFN-g and NO in mycobacterial disease: new jobs for old hands. *Trends Microbiol* 2002;5:221–226.

163. Grisham MB, Granger DN, Lefer DJ. Modulation of leukocyte-endothelial interactions by reactive metabolites of oxygen and nitrogen: relevance to ischemic heart disease. *Free Radic Biol Med* 1998;25:404–433.

164. Ehlers S, Benini J, Held HD, et al. Alphabeta T cell receptor-positive cells and interferon-gamma, but not inducible nitric oxide synthase, are critical for granuloma necrosis in a mouse model of mycobacteria-induced pulmonary immunopathology. *J Exp Med* 2001;194:1847–1859.

165. Gomes MS, Florido M, Pais TF, et al. Improved clearance of *Mycobacterium avium* upon disruption of the inducible nitric oxide synthase gene. *J Immunol* 1999;162:6734–6739.

166. Bogdan C. Nitric oxide and the immune response. *Nat Immunol* 2001;2:907–916.

167. Dalton TP, Shertzer HG, Puga A. Regulation of gene expression by reactive oxygen. *Annu Rev Pharmacol Toxicol* 1999;39: 67–101.

168. Cooper AM, Dalton DK, Stewart TA, et al. Disseminated tuberculosis in interferon gamma gene-disrupted mice. *J Exp Med* 1993;178:2243–2247.

169. Cooper AM, Roberts AD, Rhoades ER, et al. The role of interleukin-12 in acquired immunity to *Mycobacterium tuberculosis* infection. *Immunology* 1995;84:423–432.

170. Diefenbach A, Schindler H, Rollinghoff M, et al. Requirement for type 2 NO synthase for IL-12 signaling in innate immunity. *Science* 1999;284:951–955.

ANIMAL MODELS OF TUBERCULOSIS

JOANNE L. FLYNN
JOHN CHAN

The study of any disease benefits from the availability of an animal model. Infectious disease research is no exception. The closer the model is to the human disease, the more useful it is in research. Additional considerations for a model include ease of use, availability of animals or reagents, housing, and cost. Animal models are very useful for testing hypotheses regarding pathogenicity of a particular microbe. In fact, fulfilling either Koch's postulates or Falkow's (1) molecular Koch's postulates generally requires an animal model. As an example, a proposed virulence factor can be tested for relevance in disease with an appropriate animal model. Conversely, a less appropriate animal model may suggest that a virulence factor plays no role in disease when, in fact, this very factor is important in human infection. Immune responses to infections are often characterized in animal models. Mice have been particularly useful for immunologic studies because of the vast knowledge of the murine immune system and the availability of unique reagents, such as transgenic and targeted knockout strains. Vaccines and drugs need to be tested initially in animal models rather than the human population for efficacy against an infection.

Success in more than one animal model provides support for the relevance of a virulence factor or the efficacy of a vaccine or drug candidate. This is the case in tuberculosis, for which a wide range of models exists or is in development. Animal models of tuberculosis have contributed immensely to our understanding of pathogenesis, immunology, and treatment of *Mycobacterium tuberculosis* infection. Although much of the research has been performed in mice, classic and current studies in guinea pigs and rabbits have been invaluable in their impact on the field. A major difficulty in the use of animal models in tuberculosis research has been modeling the various stages

of infection, particularly latent infection. In addition, the pathology in the lungs is variable in the models but is very important in human disease. This chapter discusses each model for tuberculosis research currently in use, the advantages and disadvantages of each, similarities to or differences from human infection and disease, and how each model has been and might be used in the study of tuberculosis.

A special consideration for animal models used to study tuberculosis is the need for biosafety level 3 (BSL3) containment. This can be a major obstacle to using animals for this purpose. The exact conditions required for BSL3 containment vary with species and depend on whether the infection can be easily spread by the animal as well as the size and caging requirements of the animals.

MOUSE

The mouse is the most commonly used animal model in the study of tuberculosis. This model has many faces, depending on the strain of mouse or *M. tuberculosis* used, route of infection, and purpose of the study. A great deal of information regarding *M. tuberculosis* pathogenesis, immunology, pathology, and persistence has been gleaned using the mouse model. The advent of immunologic knockouts (mice with specific genetic defects) allowed researchers to determine the contributions of various components of the immune response to control of infection. Further developments in transgenic mice, including inducible knockouts, cells tagged with green fluorescent protein, and human immunodeficiency virus–transgenic mice, will provide new opportunities for studying host–pathogen interactions important in tuberculosis.

Acute Infection

The most commonly studied aspect of tuberculosis in mice is the acute or initial infection. Mice can be infected by a variety of routes, including aerosol, intravenous, intraperitoneal, and intranasal. Infection by aerosol is the most physiologically appropriate route because small numbers of

J. L. Flynn: Department of Molecular Genetics and Biochemistry, University of Pittsburgh School of Medicine, Pittsburgh, Pennsylvania.

J. Chan: Departments of Medicine and Microbiology and Immunology, Albert Einstein College of Medicine; Department of Medicine, Montefiore Medical Center, Bronx, New York.

organisms [10 to 50 colony-forming units (CFUs)] can be delivered accurately and reproducibly to the lungs of mice without infecting other organs first. This does require specific equipment, namely, an aerosol infection machine, of which there are two basic models: whole-body exposure in a chamber or nose-only exposure in individual units. A suspension of *M. tuberculosis* is placed in a nebulizer, and only small aerosolized particles are passed by the mice for a set period. This prevents the problem of clumping of the mycobacteria, which is inherent in other routes of infection and can lead to difficulty in determining and reproducing input dose. On infection of the lungs, the bacilli replicate and within 2 to 3 weeks spread to the spleen, liver, and lymph nodes.

Intravenous infection requires higher numbers of bacteria, and usually 10^4 to 10^6 bacilli are delivered, depending on the strain of *M. tuberculosis* or the purpose of the study. A good rule of thumb is that approximately 1% of the initial intravenous inoculum is delivered to the lungs, with the majority delivered to the spleen and liver (2,3). The mouse can tolerate a much higher intravenous inoculum compared with aerosol inoculum, although the outcome of infection can be different with aerosol versus intravenous infections (4,5). However, in immunocompetent resistant strains of mice, the bacteria replicate in the lungs to similar levels regardless of infection route or dose (as long as it is a sublethal dose) and stabilize at 10^5 to 10^6 CFUs in the lungs by 4 weeks post-infection (Fig. 17.1). The adaptive immune response has established control of the infection by 3 to 4

weeks post-infection and does not generally permit growth beyond this level. In some immunocompromised mice, the adaptive response is not capable of controlling the replication; bacterial load exceeding 5×10^7 CFUs in the lungs is generally fatal to mice.

Various inbred mouse strains are used for studies of *M. tuberculosis*. C57BL/6 mice, which are fairly resistant to the infection, are most commonly used in recent years, but BALB/c and DBA2 mice are also used. There is a differential susceptibility of inbred mouse strains to infection, which persists even after vaccination (6,7). Higher inocula can overcome the resistance of mouse strains and cause fulminant tuberculosis. There is a limited number of *M. tuberculosis* strains used in research, including H37Rv, CDC1551, and Erdman, although other clinical strains are sometimes used as well. The genomes of the first two strains are sequenced. Occasionally, avirulent *M. tuberculosis* strains, such as H37Ra, or other mycobacterial species or strains, such as bacille Calmette–Guérin (BCG), are used to model *M. tuberculosis* infection. Although this strategy may be necessary when BSL3 conditions are not available, the findings need to be verified using virulent *M. tuberculosis*. The use of avirulent or low virulence strains or species can provide results that are not similar to those seen when virulent *M. tuberculosis* is used in similar studies.

Persistent Infection

As in humans, *M. tuberculosis* infection in the mouse is generally controlled but not eliminated. In contrast to latent *M. tuberculosis* infection in humans, the bacterial load in the lungs is still fairly high (Fig. 17.1). The infection persists for the lifetime of the mouse, and, depending on the strain of mouse, the animal can appear clinically well for many months. The chronically infected mouse has been used as a model of latent tuberculosis, although it is more correct to think of this as a persistent rather than truly latent infection. There is evidence that once the immune response establishes control of the infection, the bacilli remaining are in a quiescent or metabolically altered state (8; J. McKinney, personal communication, 2002), although this is still controversial. Nonetheless, the persistent infection is clearly an equilibrium between the host immune response and the pathogen, and interfering with the host immune response can upset the balance and lead to reactivation of the infection. Such intervention as pan-immunosuppression (e.g., steroids), depletion of cell types, and neutralization of cytokines or enzyme activities can cause reactivation of the infection, with increased bacterial growth or pathology in the organs (reviewed in reference 9). This model of persistent infection provides an opportunity for studying the virulence factors that contribute to the ability of *M. tuberculosis* to persist within a host and to evade the immune response. In addition, the host factors involved in containing a persistent infection, as well as the

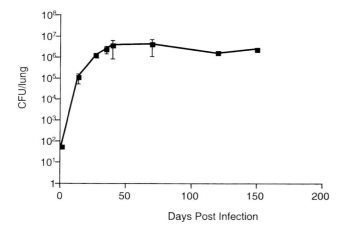

FIGURE 17.1. Course of aerogenic *Mycobacterium tuberculosis* infection in mice. C57BL/6 mice were infected with 50 colony-forming units (*CFUs*) of *M. tuberculosis* Erdman strain in a nose-only aerosolization unit (InTox Products, Albuquerque, NM, U.S.A.). A suspension containing 1×10^7 CFUs in phosphate-buffered saline + 0.05% Tween was placed in the nebulizer; mice were placed in the chambers and exposed to the aerosolized suspension for 20 minutes, followed by 5 minutes of air only. This reproducibly deposits 20 to 70 CFUs into the lungs of the mice. Lungs were obtained from mice at various time points, and bacterial numbers were determined by plating homogenates on 7H10 plates and counting colonies after 21 days.

immune responses that are unique to a chronic infection, can be addressed in this model. For example, the isocitrate lyase gene is believed to be important in long-term survival of *M. tuberculosis* within a host because a strain with a mutant in this gene was less capable of persistent infection in the mouse model (10). Depletion of CD4 T cells, neutralization of tumor necrosis factor (TNF)-α or interferon gamma (IFN-γ), and inhibition of nitric oxide synthase 2 activity affect the ability of a mouse to control a persistent *M. tuberculosis* infection (reviewed in reference 9). This model has also been used to test vaccines to simulate the situation of vaccinating previously infected humans (11). The advantage of this model for studying latent or persistent infection is the natural immunologic control of the pathogen by the host, which mimics the human situation, and the disadvantage is the relatively high bacterial burden in the lungs and spleens of chronically infected mice.

Another mouse model used to study persistent or latent *M. tuberculosis* infection is the Cornell model, so named for the site of the development of this model. Developed by McCune et al. (12–15) in the 1950s, this model involves infecting mice with *M. tuberculosis*, treating the mice with antimycobacterial drugs, and then resting them. Bacterial numbers were usually undetectable in the mice after this treatment. In the original reports, as well as more recent reports, a variable percentage of mice spontaneously reactivated the infection (14,16). Immunosuppression by steroids increased reactivation in the infected and drug-treated mice. The features of this model that make it attractive to researchers interested in studying latent tuberculosis include the low (or undetectable) numbers of organisms in the mouse after drug treatment, the tendency for spontaneous reactivation, and the ability to induce reactivation with immunosuppression. The original Cornell model researchers examined numerous conditions and found vari-

ability in the model with respect to reactivation, spontaneous or induced. This was confirmed in subsequent studies (17). Although this model has many attractive features, the use of this model depends on the conditions used, and the outcome is influenced by initial dose, antibiotic choice, timing for initiation of antibiotic treatment and length of treatment, length of rest period, and choice of immunosuppression for reactivation (17). In addition, clinically latent tuberculosis in humans does not generally depend on antimycobacterial drug treatment, and the treatment interrupts the natural host–pathogen interaction. However, this model has been used by researchers to demonstrate the importance of various immune factors in controlling a persistent infection as well as to test vaccines, drugs, and virulence genes (reviewed in reference 9). It also has potential as a model for bacteria persisting in the drug-treated host, which does parallel the human situation.

Granuloma Formation and Pathology

In response to immunologic signals (cytokines, chemokines) of *M. tuberculosis* infection of the lungs or other organs, lymphocytes and monocytes/macrophages migrate to the site of infection. These cells surround infected macrophages, forming a granuloma. In human infection, the granuloma is composed of a central core of macrophages, including multinucleated giant cells, surrounded by more macrophages and lymphocytes (CD4 and CD8 T cells and B cells) (18). This structure serves to wall off the infection from the lung and provides a localized environment for the immune cells to act against the infection. In the mouse, although the components are similar to the human granuloma, the architecture of the granuloma differs and is better described as a collection of activated and epithelioid macrophages and lymphocytic clusters (Fig. 17.2). This may be a disadvantage of the mouse model because granuloma structure is an important feature

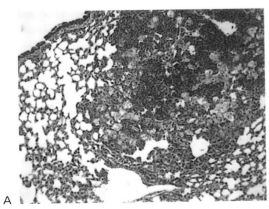
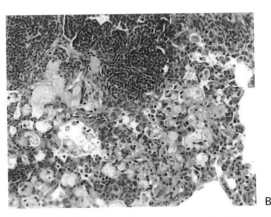

FIGURE 17.2. Granuloma formation in mice infected with *Mycobacterium tuberculosis*. The lungs of infected C57BL/6 mice were fixed in formalin and embedded in paraffin, and sections were stained with hematoxylin and eosin. Granulomas from the lungs are shown demonstrating lymphocytic clusters and activated macrophages as well as unaffected lung tissue. Original magnifications: **A:** original magnification, × 100, **B:** original magnification, × 200.

of the immune response to this infection. The status and structure of the granuloma likely affect localized immune control of the infection, dissemination, pathologic consequences of infection, and drug treatment. Although granuloma structure may be quite different in mice and humans, the function is likely to be similar, i.e., containment of the infection and a localized environment for the immune response to kill organisms. Disruption or inadequate formation of the granuloma owing to immunologic deficiency can have serious consequences with respect to control of the infection and pathology in the lungs (19–21). Caseating granulomas are not observed in immunocompetent mice and rarely seen even in immunocompromised mice. Multinucleated giant cells are also rarely observed in mouse granulomas. Necrosis is observed in murine tuberculous granulomas but is usually owing to increased bacterial numbers.

Genetically Manipulated Mice Used in Tuberculosis Research

A striking advantage of the mouse model is the availability of genetically defined and constructed mice expressing or disrupted in specific genes (transgenic or knockout mice) that can be used to test the contribution of a component of the immune response to *M. tuberculosis*. Before the advent of genetic manipulation of mouse cells and embryos, the only mice deficient in various aspects of the immune system available were the result of natural mutations. Such mice were used in studies, but the ability to specifically target a factor or cell type was a major step forward in our understanding of the host response to infections. Transgenic mice are those that have been engineered to express a specific gene under the control of a particular promoter. The cloned gene is microinjected into the pronucleus of a fertilized egg and implanted in the uterus of a pseudopregnant female mouse. The DNA can be randomly integrated into the genome, and such an egg can give rise to a mouse expressing the gene of interest (the transgene). By backcrossing progeny mice that express the gene, a transgenic line can be established in which some or all of the progeny express the transgene. The promoter can be relatively nonspecific, resulting in gene expression in many cells of the mouse. Alternatively, the promoter can be specific to a cell type, a specific organ, or a developmental stage. These mice can be useful for determining the effects of a gene expressed by certain cells during the course of infection.

Gene knockout mice have been more commonly used to examine the requirement for a particular immune factor in control of infections. A mutation in the gene of interest is made in embryonic stem cell lines by homologous recombination of a mutated copy of the gene and the normal gene in the embryonic stem genome. The embryonic stem cells are injected into mouse blastocysts and then implanted in female mice for development. The resulting progeny can carry a copy of the mutated gene in the genome. Heterozy-

gotes can be screened and are bred to obtain mice with the mutation in both copies of the gene of interest (homozygotes). These mutant mice can be infected with an infectious organism to determine whether the mutated gene is necessary for control of the infection. This technology has been exploited in many fields, and our understanding of the host response to tuberculosis has been dramatically enhanced using knockout mice.

There are other techniques used to address the role of a particular factor or cell type in the control of tuberculosis, such as neutralization or depletion with antibodies. This is useful, particularly when the timing of expression is important. For example, if one wished to test whether a particular cytokine crucial to control of initial infection was also important during chronic infection, neutralization of the cytokine only during chronic infection could be achieved with *in vivo* administration of antibody against that cytokine. In addition, to confirm results with knockout mice, antibody neutralization can be an important tool. There are other types of knockout mice being developed, including inducible knockouts in which the gene of interest can be turned on or off by administration of a drug and mice in which some cells are tagged with green fluorescent protein so that the cells can be tracked during infection.

Immunologic Findings from Genetically Manipulated Mice

The roles of various cell subsets have been explored through the use of knockout mice. Mice with a mutation in a major histocompatibility complex class II gene (22) or in the gene for the CD4 molecule (23) are deficient in CD4 T cells which provided the opportunity to test the requirement for this cell subset in the control of *M. tuberculosis* infection. Both these knockout mice were much more susceptible to *M. tuberculosis* infection and succumbed more quickly than the wild-type control mice (3,24). These data confirmed previous experiments in which CD4 T cells were depleted *in vivo* with antibody (25) and demonstrated conclusively that these cells are essential to control *M. tuberculosis* infection. Immunologic analysis of the CD4 or major histocompatibility complex class II knockout mice indicated that IFN-γ expression in the lungs and macrophage activation were delayed in the absence of CD4 T cells (3). These deficiencies likely contributed to the inability of these mice to control the replication of the bacilli. However, as observed in the knockout or CD4 T cell–depleted mice, there are other roles for CD4 T cells in addition to IFN-γ–mediated macrophage activation (26,27), and additional cell types that produce IFN-γ and activate macrophages (24,28).

A role for CD8 T cells was initially reported using antibody depletion and cell transfer experiments. Mice deficient in β_2-microglobulin, an essential subunit of the class I molecule, were more susceptible than wild-type mice (29,30), which confirmed that CD8 T cells have a role to play in the control of *M. tuberculosis* infection. Although this has been a controversial finding, most studies indicate that mice lacking CD8 T cells are less resistant than control mice (25,29–32). The function of CD8 T cells has also been explored in various knockout mice, including CD4-, perforin-, and granzyme-deficient mice (27,33), but the role of these cells in the control of tuberculosis is not completely clear. However, mice do not have a gene for granulysin or an apparent homolog, a molecule thought to be important in CD8 T cell–mediated killing of intracellular *M. tuberculosis* (34), and thus this role cannot be tested currently in mice.

The requirement for B cells in the control of tuberculosis has been dismissed for many years. Antibodies are believed to be relatively unimportant in the protective response against tuberculosis, although there are a few recent papers that argue that certain antibodies may provide some protection (35,36). B cells are found in fairly large numbers in the granulomas of the lungs (in mice and humans). B-cell knockout mice have been used to examine the role that these cells may play. Although B cell–deficient mice were similar to wild-type mice with respect to control of lung infection, either acute or chronic, lung pathology was clearly affected by the lack of B cells and dissemination of the infection to the spleen was delayed (37,38).

Cytokines believed to be important in the control of *M. tuberculosis* infection have been tested in knockout mouse systems. From these studies, the most important cytokine appears to be IFN-γ. IFN-γ knockout mice are the most susceptible mice of any of the knockouts tested to date, either by intravenous or aerosol infection, and die rapidly with uncontrolled bacterial replication (39,40). Although granulomas form to some extent, they quickly become necrotic owing to overwhelming bacterial replication. These mice have impaired macrophage activation, demonstrating that IFN-γ is the key cytokine for activating macrophages to kill intracellular bacilli (40). Mice lacking interleukin (IL)-12 are also more susceptible than wild-type mice (41), and this is likely related, at least in part, to the subsequent deficiency in IFN-γ because IL-12 is important for the complete induction of IFN-γ production by natural killer and T cells. IL-12 is a heterodimer, consisting of a p40 and a p35 subunit. Mice deficient in the p40 subunit are more susceptible than p35-deficient mice (42). This suggests that both IL-12 and IL-23, another cytokine that uses the p40 subunit, may be involved in control of this infection.

The type I IFNs may also play a role in control of tuberculosis. Knockout mice deficient in the receptor for IFN-α and IFN-β were reported to show a slightly higher bacterial load early, but this was not sustained (43). The IFN regulatory factor-1 knockout mice were quite susceptible to *M. tuberculosis* infection (43), although this may be related to control of IFN-γ signaling. Interestingly, some strains of *M. tuberculosis* that induce more IFN-α are more virulent (44). In addition, intranasal treatment with IFN-α resulted in

increased lung bacillary loads and reduced survival (44). The roles of these IFNs in the protection or pathology of tuberculosis remain to be determined (45).

The roles of TNF-α in tuberculosis are complex. This cytokine is clearly essential for the control of infection, as demonstrated by mice deficient in TNF-α (20), the 55-kd TNF receptor (19), and antibody- or receptor-mediated depletion of TNF-α (19,46). The mice are extremely susceptible to infection and die within 4 weeks of aerosol or intravenous infection. The high bacterial loads observed in mice deficient in TNF-α or TNF-mediated signaling are likely owing, at least in part, to delayed macrophage activation (19). However, there are additional defects in these mice after *M. tuberculosis* infection, which point to an important role for TNF-α in granuloma formation and maintenance (19,20,47). The absence of TNF-α prevents appropriate granuloma formation, apparently by preventing the immune cells from migrating to or within the lungs properly. In chronic infection, when granulomas are already formed and containing the bacteria, neutralizing TNF-α leads to loss of granuloma structure and subsequent aberrant pathology (21). This contributes to the rapid demise of the mice in this model. TNF-α overexpression in the lungs can also lead to pathology (48), suggesting that the level of this cytokine must be tightly controlled during mycobacterial infection to limit pathology and maximize bacterial killing. Thus, mouse models have been used to demonstrate that TNF-α has important roles in macrophage activation, cell migration, bacterial control, granuloma formation, and pathology. This cytokine has recently been implicated as important in preventing reactivation of human latent tuberculosis; a much higher than expected incidence of tuberculosis, and in particular disseminated tuberculosis, was found in patients treated with anti-TNF antibody (infliximab) for rheumatoid arthritis (49). The available animal data on the effects of a reduction in TNF-α in mouse tuberculosis models are consistent with the human results, demonstrating the importance and usefulness of animal models in the study of the immunology of tuberculosis.

IL-10 has also been explored as a regulatory cytokine in the complex immune response to tuberculosis. The chronicity of the infection strongly suggests that inducing and down-regulating the immune response are both necessary components of a successful response to *M. tuberculosis*. Without down-regulatory immune signals, the type 1 T-cell response (producing IFN-γ and activating macrophages) would be induced continually and cause excessive pathology. IL-10 can also deactivate macrophages, which would impair control of bacterial replication. This cytokine is produced in the lungs of mice infected with *M. tuberculosis* (21). However, IL-10 knockout mice were similar to or only slightly more resistant than wild-type mice in the ability to control *M. tuberculosis* infection (50,51; H. Scott, J. Chan, and J. L. Flynn, unpublished data, 2002), although these mice were more susceptible to BCG (52,53). However, mice transgenic for IL-10 (i.e., producing IL-10 constitutively) were more susceptible to BCG infection (54,55). The overproduction of IL-10 may be detrimental to the regulation of the immune response to mycobacterial infection, and, as with TNF-α, the balance of IL-10 levels is likely to be important in the control of tuberculosis. The precise roles of this cytokine in controlling or exacerbating *M. tuberculosis* infection or pathology remain to be determined.

Genetically manipulated mouse models have also been used to investigate the importance or roles of various other cytokines, cell types, chemokines, and effector mechanisms. The models can be useful in determining the contribution of a factor or cell to the protective or pathologic response to *M. tuberculosis*, but caution must also be exercised in interpreting the data obtained in these models.

Although one must interpret data in knockout mice cautiously because a mutation in one gene can have unsuspected effects on other aspects of the immunology or physiology of the mouse, these reagents can provide clues about immune responses important in tuberculosis. This has been exploited by a number of groups and has added to our current understanding of the complex immune response to this pathogen. From these studies, roles for CD4 and CD8 T cells, activation of macrophages, and various cytokines and chemokines have been postulated. The advent of inducible knockouts and mice transgenic for human genes will greatly expand the usefulness of the mouse system for exploring immune responses to *M. tuberculosis*. It should be noted, however, that using bacterial load or survival as the primary measures of the importance of a particular immune component is probably not sufficient because genetic deficiencies that affect the composition of the cellular response or pathology may also be relevant, although the mouse may be able to overcome such deficits and control an infection.

Immune Analysis in Mouse Tissues

It is quite straightforward to analyze immune cell populations, cytokine production, and a variety of immune effector mechanisms in the mouse. Lung and lung-draining lymph node cells can be easily studied and used in a variety of assays. There are many reagents for studying *in vivo* immune responses in the mouse, including a wealth of antibodies for flow cytometry and immunohistochemistry, cytokine assays, gene expression assays (including microarrays), cell proliferation markers, and cell transfer technology for reconstitution of the immune response. For this reason, great strides have been made in understanding the immune response to *M. tuberculosis* using the mouse model.

The mouse is a commonly used model for testing vaccine candidates. Most vaccine candidates are tested as preexposure vaccines, and the most physiologically relevant strategy is to challenge the vaccinated mouse via aerosol with virulent *M. tuberculosis*. The extent of protection can be measured by examining bacterial burden in the organs at various times after infection. The gold standard for vaccines is BCG, although this provides only a modest level of protection (approximately tenfold reduction CFUs in the lungs). Survival of mice can also be used to compare vaccines. As noted previously, the two commonly used long-term infection models have also been used to determine the efficacy of potential vaccines in a postexposure scenario to prevent reactivation of latent infection.

In summary, the advantages of using mice for the study of tuberculosis are numerous. The relatively low cost and ease of containing the animals in a BSL3 environment allow one to use a larger number of animals per experiment. The use of inbred mouse strains increases reproducibility among experiments and researchers. The course of infection is well established, and the parameters of drug treatment, immunization, and so forth are known. A major advantage is the availability of transgenic and knockout mouse strains and immunologic reagents, such as antibodies and cytokines. The disadvantages of the mouse model include the differences from humans in pathology and granuloma formation in the lungs, the relatively high number of organisms persisting in the lungs and spleen, and the lack of a true latency model. It must be said, however, that much of what has been gleaned about tuberculosis from the mouse model has also been found to be true in human tuberculosis, such as the importance of CD4 T cells and TNF-α. Thus, this is likely to remain the easiest, most practical, and most cost-effective model for the study of tuberculosis.

GUINEA PIG

Of all the animal models used for the study of tuberculosis, the guinea pig model is most associated with momentous historical events. Koch (56,57) used guinea pigs to establish the Koch postulates and to identify the tubercle bacillus as the etiologic agent of tuberculosis. In a series of seminal studies, Riley et al. (58) tested and proved the droplet nuclei theory for the respiratory transmission of *M. tuberculosis*, a hypothesis originally put forth by Wells (59) using the guinea pig. Because of the exquisite sensitivity of this species to the tubercle bacillus, classic studies to examine the persistence of *M. tuberculosis* in the human lungs relied substantially on guinea pig inoculation (60). As recent as the 1980s, guinea pig inoculation of patient samples was still practiced in some parts of the world as one of the modalities for diagnosing tuberculous infection (61). Although the latter approach to diagnosing tuberculosis has been replaced by more economic and perhaps more sensitive means (26), the guinea pig model of experimental tuberculosis remains an important tool for the identification of effective antituberculous chemotherapy and vaccines and for the characterization of mycobacterial virulence factors and the host immune response to *M. tuberculosis* (62–66).

Compared with mice, the response of the guinea pig to *M. tuberculosis*, as assessed by the characteristics of tissue pathology, bears a much closer resemblance to that observed in humans (64–66). The tuberculous granuloma in the lungs of guinea pigs infected with virulent *M. tuberculosis*, which consists largely of mononuclear cells, typically undergoes necrosis as the infection progresses. Necrosis, which causes tissue damage, is characteristic of the human tuberculous granuloma. This process, not typically seen in mice infected with the tubercle bacillus, likely plays an important role in the immunopathology of tuberculosis and may be requisite to subsequent liquefaction and cavitation, although these latter pathologic changes, critical to the respiratory transmission of *M. tuberculosis*, do not occur in the guinea pig (see the rabbit and nonhuman primate models). From the practical standpoint of the development of new antituberculous intervention, one of the readouts of vaccine efficacy is the prevention of tissue damage, as represented by necrosis in the lungs of guinea pigs infected with virulent *M. tuberculosis*. Another feature of the guinea pig granuloma is the existence of the poorly characterized Langhans giant cells (Fig. 17.3). This is a characteristic of the human granuloma not generally observed in the mouse. Thus, the guinea pig granuloma exhibits many characteristics typical of the human counterpart. A difference from humans is the inherent susceptibility of guinea pigs, indicating that the immune response that functions so well in humans to contain the infection in most infected persons is deficient to some extent in guinea pigs. An understanding of the exquisite susceptibility of *M. tuberculosis*–infected guinea pigs to progressive disease may provide clues about the more successful immune response of humans.

The guinea pig experimental tuberculosis model has been well characterized (reviewed in reference 63). Based on the classic experiment of Riley et al. (58) and confirmed using

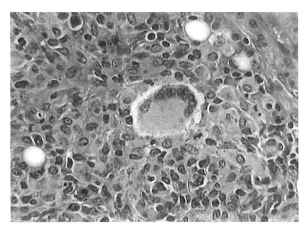

FIGURE 17.3. Granuloma structure in the lung of a guinea pig infected with *Mycobacterium tuberculosis*. Langhans giant cells can be observed in the granuloma. (Original magnification, × 400.) (Courtesy of Lynne Cassone and Todd Lasco, Texas A&M University.)

aerogenic delivery of organisms (63), an effective infective dose of *M. tuberculosis* for the guinea pig amounts to only a few bacilli; this is similar to that estimated for the inoculum required for infecting the human lungs. The procedure used to deliver a low dose of bacilli directly into the lungs has been standardized using a chamber designed by Wiegeshaus et al. (67) and built at the University of Wisconsin in the 1960s. Typically, this small inoculum leads to the establishment of infection randomly in two of the six lobes of the guinea pig lungs. At these sites of primary infection, the bacilli grew exponentially from day 3 to approximately day 21 post-infection. Toward the end of this period of rapid growth, hematogenous spread from the primary foci of infection to other organs and to the lungs occurs. The route of dissemination most likely originates in the lymph nodes draining the primary sites of infection, entering the bloodstream subsequently via the lymphatics. Coinciding with the onset of hematogenous spread, a rigorous delayed-type hypersensitivity response, as assessed by subcutaneous injection of purified protein derivative of *M. tuberculosis*, develops. At this point, the tissue bacterial burden plateaus at approximately 10^5 to 10^6 CFUs. Eventually, all infected animals die of the disease. The invariably fatal course of disease progression affords another reliable parameter by which the efficacy of vaccine and drug candidates can be assessed. It is noteworthy that preexposure BCG vaccination can decrease by 2 to 3 log the peak pulmonic bacterial burden that remains stable for weeks before eventual disease exacerbation (63,66). Compared with the approximately 1-log decrease in peak lung bacillary load achievable by BCG vaccination in the mouse, the 2- to 3-log drop in the guinea pigs provide a substantially wider dynamic range for the assessment of vaccine efficacy.

An interesting and important aspect of the guinea pig tuberculosis model is that it allows differentiation between primary and secondary tuberculous lesions, the latter being the result of hematogenous spread (68,69). It has been observed that secondary lesions do not appear until after 18 to 21 days post-infection. More important, these lesions can be differentiated from primary sites of infection by radiographic examination of the infected lungs. Because it is generally accepted that an important attribute of an effective antituberculous intervention is its ability to prevent secondary dissemination and that *M. tuberculosis* virulence correlates with its propensity to spread hematogenously, the guinea pig tuberculosis model affords a unique system for the evaluation of vaccine and chemotherapeutic candidates as well as the mechanisms involved in disease pathogenesis.

Clearly, the guinea pig is an attractive experimental system for evaluating many aspects of tuberculous infection. The susceptibility of the guinea pig to fatal disease after infection with a few bacilli makes this a rigorous model for testing vaccines because one would hope to be able to protect the most susceptible host with an effective vaccine. The limitations of this model stem mostly from economic and logistic issues. Compared with the expenses incurred by mouse studies, it is substantially more costly to maintain guinea pig colonies in a biocontainment facility. In addition, the availability of immunologic reagents for guinea pig experimentation pales compared with that available for mouse or monkey studies. Still, substantial progress has been made in recent years in the immunology of tuberculosis in the guinea pig (63,64,70). In fact, most recent studies designed to examine the immunologic mechanisms underlying the historical association between malnutrition and tuberculosis have been carried out using the guinea pig (65). Thus, in this important but understudied area of tuberculosis research, the guinea pig reigns.

RABBIT

A classic piece of tuberculosis literature is Lurie's (71) book on tuberculosis in rabbits. This work established the rabbit model and made seminal observations about resistance and susceptibility, the course of infection in the lungs, and pathology. Lurie's work was carried on by others, and some of our current understanding of tuberculosis comes from the classic as well as more modern studies. In recent years, the rabbit has been used to examine granuloma structure, compare virulence of various strains, and for vaccine studies.

The rabbit is much more susceptible to *Mycobacterium bovis* than to *M. tuberculosis* (71). On aerosol infection with *M. bovis*, primary lesions form in the lungs, and the infection can spread to other organs. Cell-mediated immune responses result in granuloma formation with caseous centers. The caseous center can liquefy in the rabbit, and this may lead to large numbers of bacilli within the granuloma (72). Unlike the mouse model, cavity formation is a classic hallmark of tuberculosis in the rabbit, with erosion of granulomas into the bronchus, resulting in bacilli in the airways (73). After *M. tuberculosis* infection, the number of mycobacteria in the granulomas is reduced compared with *M. bovis* infection (71). Rabbits recover from *M. tuberculosis* infection, although it can take many months, but can die of *M. bovis*. The exquisite susceptibility of the rabbit to *M. bovis* limits the use of this for studying human-like tuberculosis; using *M. tuberculosis*, which is less virulent in rabbits, allows the study of resistance and susceptibility, tubercle formation, and vaccine effectiveness. Infection with *M. tuberculosis* (rather than *M. bovis*) may more closely resemble infection of humans with *M. tuberculosis* because most humans control the infection. In fact, *M. tuberculosis* infection resulting in tubercle formation in the lungs can apparently heal without grossly visible lesions or cultivatable bacteria after a number of months (Y. Manabe, personal communication, 2002). It remains to be seen whether this represents latent disease that could be reactivated or actual clearance of the infection; in either case, this aspect is an important feature of the animal model that may lead to a clearer understanding of tuberculosis in humans.

One approach to studying mycobacterial infection in the rabbit is to use the tubercle-count method developed by Lurie (71). The volume of air inhaled by each rabbit to be infected is measured using a whole-body plethysmograph, and the number of viable mycobacteria in an aliquot of air used for aerosol infection is measured using an impinger. These numbers are used to calculate the actual infectious dose for each rabbit. Rabbits are killed 5 weeks after infection, and grossly visible tubercles in the lungs are counted. From this, the number of bacteria required to form one tubercle can be determined. This can be used as a measure of virulence of the organism or as an assessment of the immune response of each rabbit to the infection because survival of the infecting organisms and the resulting tubercle formation are the result of the interaction of host and pathogen. With virulent *M. tuberculosis*, approximately 1,500 to 2,000 inhaled bacilli were required to produce one tubercle (74). In contrast, fewer than ten virulent *M. bovis* bacilli were required to produce one tubercle (75).

The tubercle count method has been used to compare strains of *M. tuberculosis* and *M. bovis* for virulence (74,76), to examine resistance or susceptibility of the host (71), and to compare efficacy of various vaccines (77). For additional testing, bacteria can be cultured and enumerated from the granulomas, and histology and tuberculin skin test responses can be performed. This model is likely to be a useful source of bacteria for studying *in vivo* responses of the pathogen to the host immune response and bacterial gene expression within the granuloma, using a variety of genetic techniques, including genome arrays.

The rabbit has also been used as a model for tuberculous meningitis (78). Meningitis is a serious complication of *M. tuberculosis* infection, particularly in children; it has a high mortality rate, and serious neurologic sequelae occur in many survivors. Using *M. bovis* inoculated directly into the cisterna magna of rabbits, acute mycobacterial meningitis was induced (78). Leukocyte and protein accumulation was observed in the cerebrospinal fluid as well as acid-fast bacilli. Severe clinical signs were also observed 2 to 8 days after infection. A granulomatous meningitis was observed by histology. Antibiotic treatment reduced bacterial numbers, but survival was increased only modestly. This model may be useful for studying mycobacterial meningitis and possible interventions.

Lurie's original observations on rabbits used inbred strains that were either susceptible or resistant (71). Those breeds were lost, and the rabbits available now are outbred. The commercially available rabbits (New Zealand white) are generally resistant to *M. tuberculosis* but are still susceptible to *M. bovis*. The outbred nature of available rabbits results in greater variability in virulence and vaccine testing, and a larger number of animals per group are often needed to obtain statistical significance.

There are advantages to studying tuberculosis in rabbits, including pathology similar to human pathology; the potential for studying different aspects of the disease including meningitis, cavitation (with *M. bovis*), and innate resistance to infection, and a method for comparing virulence or resistance that is more sophisticated than simply enumerating organisms. These factors make the rabbit very attractive for studying aspects of tuberculosis that are not present in the mouse or guinea pig model. This model should be excellent for studying the virulence of strains, efficacy of vaccines and drugs, and virulence factors associated with persistence in human-like granulomas and cavity formation. Disadvantages include the specialized equipment needed for infections (and performing the tubercle count method), cost and space requirements of housing larger animals, and biocontainment of infected rabbits. These factors restrict the ability of most laboratories to develop or use this model. In addition, the paucity of immunologic or other host reagents limits the study of immune responses to the infection or the protective response induced by vaccines.

NONHUMAN PRIMATE

The use of nonhuman primates for the study of tuberculosis dates back many decades. Fifty years ago, the monkey model was more commonly used than it is today. The cost and containment requirements of nonhuman primates preclude the use of this model by most laboratories today. However, the monkey is the closest model of human tuberculosis and is beginning to be used again by a few laboratories. Active tuberculosis can be fatal in monkeys. Nonhuman primate colonies have been addressing the problem of tuberculosis outbreaks for many years. Outbreaks cause substantial damage, in terms of lost research, containment, animal testing and monitoring, and euthanizations. All nonhuman primate colonies have strict control programs to limit introduction of *M. tuberculosis*–infected monkeys, including repeated tuberculin testing during the 31- to 90-day quarantine period. However, tuberculin testing does not identify all infected monkeys, depending on the stage of infection. Aggressive control programs and better husbandry practices have greatly reduced the incidence of tuberculosis outbreaks in research colonies.

In early studies using monkeys for tuberculosis research on vaccines and drugs, the rhesus macaques were used. In some older studies, a very low dose aerosol infection (fewer than 20 CFUs) caused severe and often fatal disease in most animals, reinforcing the belief that monkeys have an innate susceptibility to tuberculosis (79,80). It is generally believed that tuberculosis occurs in monkeys after contact with humans or captive infected monkeys rather than in the wild and that these animals have little resistance to the infection. Recent data suggest that this susceptibility may be overestimated. Clearly, outbreaks occur and can be devastating to a primate colony. In these cases, it is impossible to estimate the infectious dose for the monkeys, and monkeys kept in close proximity can increase the spread of infection. Even in these outbreaks, not all monkeys develop active disease. In accordance with these observations, experimental infection with low doses of *M. tuberculosis* does not necessarily lead to fulminant disease in macaques (81; J. L. Flynn, unpublished data, 2002).

Macaques are commonly used in research. For studies with *M. tuberculosis*, both rhesus (*Macaca mulatta*) and cynomolgus (*Macaca fasicularis*) macaques have been used. Although aerosol infection is possible (79,82), specialized equipment is necessary, and standardizing a dose delivered to the monkeys can be difficult. Delivery of organisms via the trachea or a bronchoscope into the lungs is more commonly performed. In one study, a dose curve was performed using cynomolgus monkeys, with doses ranging from 10 to 10^5 CFUs *M. tuberculosis* (81). All monkeys infected with higher doses (10^3 to 10^5) showed signs of disease and died of tuberculosis between 3 and 29 weeks after inoculation. However, a subset of monkeys infected with 10 to 100 CFUs apparently controlled the infection until the time of euthanasia (6 months) and showed only minimal lung disease on necropsy. This study suggested that low-dose infection could lead to a model that mimicked human infection and suggested the possibility that a latent infection could be achieved in this model.

Our own unpublished data using cynomolgus monkeys indicate that low-dose infection results in a spectrum of disease, including rapid and fulminant tuberculosis, active or chronic disease, and latent infection. The latter is defined as infection in a monkey that does not cause clinical signs of illness for at least 6 to 9 months, with the infection contained in a few small granulomas in the lungs. Approximately 40% of the cynomolgus monkeys that we infected with a low dose of *M. tuberculosis* (fewer than 50 bacilli, Erdman strain) appear to have latent tuberculous infection. There are numerous reports of tuberculosis cases in closed primate colonies, strongly suggesting that natural *M. tuberculosis* or *M. bovis* infections in monkeys can result in latent disease and can reactivate and cause active disease.

Available data regarding *M. tuberculosis* or *M. bovis* outbreaks in nonhuman primate colonies suggested that cynomolgus macaques were less susceptible to tuberculosis than rhesus macaques. A recent study compared these two macaque species with respect to BCG-induced immunity with a *M. tuberculosis* challenge of 3,000 CFUs, a relatively high dose (83). Unimmunized cynomolgus and rhesus macaques both developed progressive tuberculosis, although cynomolgus macaques were somewhat more resistant. However, BCG immunization was much more protective in cynomolgus macaques compared with rhesus macaques. These data suggest that both species will be useful in studying immunology and pathogenesis of tuberculosis and for testing vaccine candidates.

The pathology of tuberculosis in the monkey lungs is strikingly similar to human pathology. The granulomas have a classic structure, with macrophages and multinucleated giant cells surrounded by lymphocytes (Fig. 17.4); granulocytes and fibroblasts are also observed. Caseation of granulomas and granulomas with necrotic centers but healthy tissue otherwise are commonly seen. Caseation is more often observed in more severely affected monkeys. Liquefaction and cavity formation are also found in the lungs of monkeys with advanced disease (83; J. L. Flynn, unpublished observations, 2002). Granulomas can also be fibrotic or solid, and these types of granulomas were observed more commonly in animals with less extensive disease, possibly representing resolving or successful granulomas (J. L. Flynn, unpublished observations, 2002). Disseminated disease can be observed in some monkeys, with visible lesions in the spleen or liver.

Following the course of tuberculosis in monkeys can be challenging. Mammalian tuberculin, rather than purified protein derivative, is generally used for tuberculin skin testing, but the response to this is variable, even in monkeys with active disease. Infected monkeys are not necessarily tuberculin positive, and, in fact, this test seems to be most useful in the early stages of infection, but after 4 to 6 weeks post-infection. The currently available diagnostics are not sufficient for reliable detection of latent or even active infection in monkeys. Chest radiographs can detect pulmonary lesions and provide information about disease severity. However, a surrogate marker of disease or protection does not exist, just as is the case in human tuberculo-

sis. The monkey may be a good model to search for a surrogate marker because the full spectrum of human disease can be recapitulated on experimental infection of the monkey. The immunology of tuberculosis can be studied in the monkey model because the reagents exist already because of cross-reactivity of human reagents and the development of macaque-specific reagents by researchers in the simian immunodeficiency virus field.

Nonhuman primates are also a useful model for testing vaccines that have given promising results in other models, although monkeys are too expensive for the initial screening of vaccine candidates. Although it remains to be proved, it seems reasonable that a vaccine demonstrating protection in rhesus and cynomolgus macaques would have a higher probability of providing protection in humans. The immune responses involved in protection could be investigated more easily in monkeys than in immunized humans, particularly because the peripheral blood, which is the sample most available from humans, may not be the best site to study immunity manifested in the lungs. Nonhuman primates are also a good model for studying antituberculosis drugs. There is a long history of using monkeys for this purpose (84–87). It has been demonstrated that 6 to 12 months of multidrug chemotherapy is effective in monkeys with active disease, although relapse rates over time have not been well studied (88). Monkeys may be useful in studies of new drugs that may reduce therapy duration and relapse rates. This model, with human-like pathology and granulomas and the potential for latent infection, represents an excellent opportunity to test the ability of drugs to penetrate the granulomatous environment or affect bacilli in latent disease.

The advantages of the nonhuman primate model include the similarity to human tuberculosis and, unlike the guinea pig or rabbit model, the abundance of reagents for research. This translates into obtaining results that are more directly applicable to the human situation. The disadvantages are the high cost of nonhuman primate research, biosafety containment, and the outbred nature of the animals. The latter is, however, similar to humans, and although this may cause more variability in experiments, it is a more realistic situation. Cost and biocontainment are serious obstacles to nonhuman primate research in tuberculosis. Monkeys with tuberculosis are contagious to other animals, including monkeys, and to humans, posing a serious risk in an animal facility. Biocontainment is of the utmost importance, and this can be achieved by isolating the animals from other animals and requiring personnel to wear protective gear, including respirators, when in contact with the monkeys. The cost of nonhuman primate research is related to the actual cost of the monkeys, the need for veterinary care and veterinary technicians on a regular basis, and the space needed per animal. Thus, this model, which is quite attractive in many aspects, remains difficult to integrate into many research institutions.

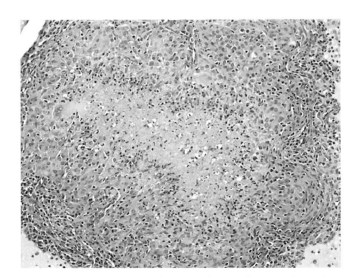

FIGURE 17.4. Granuloma from the lungs of a *Mycobacterium tuberculosis*–infected cynomolgus macaque. The monkey was euthanized at 4 months after infection; a portion of the right lower lobe was fixed in formalin and embedded in paraffin, and sections were stained with hematoxylin and eosin. A granuloma with necrosis in the middle surrounded by macrophages and lymphocytes is shown. Occasional giant cells can be observed. (Original magnification, × 200.)

FROG AND FISH (*MYCOBACTERIUM MARINUM*)

A recent development in modeling tuberculosis has been the use of *M. marinum*, a species that causes a granulomatous disease in fish and frogs and skin granulomas in humans (known as aquarium tank granuloma), as a surrogate for *M. tuberculosis*. *M. marinum* was first isolated from saltwater fish with disseminated tuberculosis in 1926 (89) and is very closely related to *M. tuberculosis*. This mycobacterial species grows at low temperatures (25°C to 35°C) and can cause disease in many species of fish. It is relatively fast growing, genetically tractable, and not a BSL3 pathogen, which makes it quite attractive for the screening of mutants involved in persistence or virulence. Recent studies in using *M. marinum* as a model for tuberculosis have been carried out in goldfish, frogs, and zebra fish.

The pathology of *M. marinum* infection in goldfish is characterized by granuloma formation in numerous organs, including the liver and spleen. The granulomas observed consist mostly of macrophages and some epithelioid macrophages and giant cells, with occasional lymphocytes. The organisms persist within macrophages in the host. Fish are inoculated intraperitoneally and maintained in aquaria. Both acute and chronic infections can be induced in the goldfish, depending on the dose (90). Doses of 10^8 to 10^9 CFUs caused death in less than 10 days, but doses of 10^7 CFUs or less resulted in survival and long-term chronic infection. As few as 600 CFUs caused infection and granuloma formation in goldfish. Bacterial numbers increased over time in the liver and to a lesser extent in the spleen and kidneys. Various granuloma types were observed in this fish model, including necrotizing, nonnecrotizing, and caseous granulomas. This makes the fish an excellent model for studying microbial persistence within a caseous or noncaseous granuloma. Recently, signature-tagged mutagenesis has been performed on *M. marinum* to identify genes expressed in the goldfish. Mutation of some of these genes

caused reduced virulence in the fish (M. Trucksis, personal communication, 2002); such genes are virulence candidates to be tested in *M. tuberculosis*. Early experiments using zebra fish suggest that infection is possible in this species, opening the possibility for studying host genetics in the context of tuberculosis (94).

The leopard frog has also been used as an animal model for *M. marinum*. In the frog, the disease is generally chronic, with low numbers of organisms within granulomas persisting for as long as a year (91). Frogs are inoculated intraperitoneally, and the liver, spleen, kidney, and lungs are colonized by 2 weeks after infection. A dose of 10^4 CFUs is necessary to induce granuloma formation. The granulomas are primarily histiocytic and composed of epithelioid macrophages, with occasional granulomas containing cells that appeared to be lymphocytes. Caseation and giant cells were not observed, in contrast to the goldfish model (92). One interesting aspect of the frog is that treatment with hydrocortisone results in a fulminant, acute infection rather than a subclinical chronic infection (91). Therefore, one can assume that the possibility of reactivation of a latent infection also exists in this model. *M. marinum* genes preferentially expressed in persistent granulomas were identified, and mutants in these genes were deficient in persistence in frogs (93). Thus, both the frog and fish are good models for the identification of potential virulence factors of *M. marinum* that may also contribute to the pathogenesis of *M. tuberculosis*.

SUMMARY

The availability of a variety of animal models is a great asset to research on tuberculosis. Each model has advantages, and a researcher has the opportunity to choose a model depending on which aspect of tuberculosis is of interest for a particular project (Table 17.1). Mice have the advantages of small size, genetically identical, knockouts, and available

TABLE 17.1. HISTOPATHOLOGIC ASPECTS OF THE VARIOUS ANIMAL MODELS OF TUBERCULOSIS

Model	Histopathology				
	Mononuclear Cells	Multinucleated Giant (Langerhans) Cells	Necrosis	Caseation	Liquefaction/ Cavitation
Human	++	++	++	++	++
Mouse	++	−	+/−[a]	−	−
Guinea pig	++	++	++	++	++[b]
Rabbit	++	++	++	++	++
Monkey	++	++	++	++	++
Fish	+[c]	+	++	+	−

[a]More frequent in immunocompromised or susceptible mouse strains.
[b]With *Mycobacterium bovis* or high dose *Mycobacterium tuberculosis*.
[c]Mostly macrophages.
++, present in moderate to high amounts; +, present to a minimal degree; −, not present.

TABLE 17.2. PRACTICAL ASPECTS OF EACH MODEL

Model	Biocontainment	Cost	Immunologic Reagents
Mouse	+	+	+++
Guinea pig	+	++	+/–
Rabbit	++	+++	+/–
Monkey	++++	++++	+++
Frog/fish	–	+/–	–

Biocontainment: +, relatively easy; ++, more difficult and more space needed; +++, very difficult to contain, larger space requirements; –, biosafety Level 3 containment not required.
Cost: +/–, relatively low costs; + to ++++, relative costs.
Immunologic Reagents Availability: +++, very available; +/–, not very available; –, not available.

reagents, whereas guinea pigs display an extreme susceptibility that makes them particularly useful for vaccine research. Rabbits demonstrate human-like pathology, such as caseation and cavity formation. Nonhuman primates also have human-type lesions and recapitulation of the entire spectrum of human tuberculosis, including latent infection. Cost, biocontainment, and reagent availability are disadvantages for some of these models (Table 17.2). The frog or fish model of *M. marinum* does not use *M. tuberculosis* but may be a useful and inexpensive model for testing hypotheses and developing leads for study in virulent *M. tuberculosis* with more conventional animal models. Overall, the wide range of animal models of tuberculosis coupled with the advances in genetics, genomics, and immunology presents unique opportunities to researchers in this field.

ACKNOWLEDGMENT

We are grateful to Drs. Yukari Manabe, Lalita Ramakrishnan, Saverio Capuano III, John McKinney, David McMurray, William Bishai, and Michelle Trucksis for providing useful comments, information, and unpublished data and to the work of many people in the field, past and present. We thank the following for providing photographs for figures: Holly Scott (mouse histology), Dr. David McMurray, Lynne Cassone, and Todd Lasco (guinea pig), and Dr. Edwin Klein (monkey histology). Our work is supported by National Institutes of Health grants AI38411 (J.L.F.), AI37859 (J.L.F.), AI47485 (J.L.F.), AI49157 (J.C. and J.L.F.), and American Lung Association (J.L.F.).

REFERENCES

1. Falkow S. Molecular Koch's postulates applied to microbial pathogenicity. *Rev Infect Dis* 1988;10[Suppl 2]):S274–S276.
2. Orme IM, Collins FM. Mouse model of tuberculosis. In: Bloom BR, ed. *Tuberculosis: pathogenesis, protection, and control.* Washington, DC: American Society for Microbiology Press, 1994.
3. Caruso AM, Serbina N, Klein E, et al. Mice deficient in CD4 T cells have only transiently diminished levels of IFN-γ, yet succumb to tuberculosis. *J Immunol* 1999;162:5407–5416.
4. North RJ. *Mycobacterium tuberculosis* is strikingly more virulent for mice when given via the respiratory than via the intravenous route. *J Infect Dis* 1995;172:1550–1553.
5. Scanga CA, Mohan VP, Tanaka K, et al. The NOS2 locus confers protection in mice against aerogenic challenge of both clinical and laboratory strains of *Mycobacterium tuberculosis*. *Infect Immun* 2001;69:7711–7717.
6. Medina E, North RJ. Resistance ranking of some common inbred mouse strains to *Mycobacterium tuberculosis* and relationship to major histocompatibility complex haplotype and Nramp1 genotype. *Immunology* 1998;93:270–274.
7. Medina E, North RJ. Genetically susceptible mice remain proportionally more susceptible to tuberculosis after vaccination. *Immunology* 1999;96:16–21.
8. Rees RJW, Hart D'A. Analysis of the host-parasite equilibrium in chronic murine tuberculosis by total and viable bacillary counts. *Br J Exp. Pathol* 1961;42:83–88.
9. Flynn JL, Chan J. Tuberculosis: latency and reactivation. *Infect Immun* 2001;69:4195–4201.
10. McKinney JD, zu Bentrup KH, Miczak A, et al. Persistence of *Mycobacterium tuberculosis* in macrophages and mice requires the glyoxylate shunt enzyme isocitrate lyase. *Nature* 2000;406:735–738.
11. Turner J, Rhoades ER, Keen M, et al. Effective preexposure tuberculosis vaccines fail to protect when they are given in an immunotherapeutic mode. *Infect Immun* 2000;68:1706–1709.
12. McCune RM, Tompsett R, McDermott W. The fate of *Mycobacterium tuberculosis* in mouse tissues as determined by the microbial enumeration technique. II. The conversion of tuberculous infection to the latent state by the administration of pyrazinamide and a companion drug. *J Exp Med* 1957;104:763–802.
13. McCune RM, Lee SH, Deuschle K, et al. Ineffectiveness of isoniazid in modifying the phenomenon of microbial persistence. *J Exp Med* 1957;104:1106–1109.
14. McCune RM, Feldmann FM, Lambert HP, et al. Microbial persistence I. The capacity of tubercle bacilli to survive sterilization in mouse tissues. *J Exp Med* 1966;123:445–468.
15. McCune RM, Feldman FM, McDermott W. Microbial persistence. II. Characteristics of the sterile state of tubercle bacilli. *J Exp Med* 1966;123:469–486.
16. Lowrie DB, Tascon RE, Bonato VLD, et al. Therapy of tuberculosis in mice by DNA vaccination. *Nature* 1999;400:269–271.
17. Scanga CA, Mohan VP, Joseph H, et al. Reactivation of latent tuberculosis: variations on the Cornell murine model. *Infect Immun* 1999;67:4531–4538.
18. Randhawa PS. Lymphocyte subsets in granulomas of human tuberculosis: an *in situ* immunofluorescence study using monoclonal antibodies. *Pathology* 1990;22:153–155.
19. Flynn JL, Goldstein MM, Chan J, et al. Tumor necrosis factor-α is required in the protective immune response against *M. tuberculosis* in mice. *Immunity* 1995;2:561–572.
20. Bean AGD, Roach DR, Briscoe H, et al. Structural deficiencies in granuloma formation in TNF gene-targeted mice underlie the heightened susceptibility to aerosol *Mycobacterium tuberculosis* infection, which is not compensated for by lymphotoxin. *J Immunol* 1999;162:3504–3511.
21. Mohan VP, Scanga CA, Yu K, et al. Effects of tumor necrosis factor alpha on host immune response in chronic persistent tuberculosis: possible role for limiting pathology. *Infect Immun* 2001;69:1847–1855.
22. Cosgrove D, Gray D, Dierich A, et al. Mice lacking MHC class II molecules. *Cell* 1991;66:1051–1066.
23. Rahemtulla A, Fung-Leung WP, Schilham MW, et al. Normal development and function of CD8+ cells but markedly decreased helper cell activity in mice lacking CD4. *Nature* 1991;353:180–184.

24. Tascon RE, Stavropoulos E, Lukacs KV, et al. Protection against *Mycobacterium tuberculosis* infection by CD8 T cells requires production of gamma interferon. *Infect Immun* 1998;66:830–834.
25. Muller I, Cobbold S, Waldmann H, et al. Impaired resistance to *Mycobacterium tuberculosis* infection after selective *in vivo* depletion of L3T4+ and Lyt2+ T cells. *Infect Immunol* 1987;55:2037–2041.
26. Scanga CA, Mohan VP, Yu K, et al. Depletion of CD4+ T cells causes reactivation of murine persistent tuberculosis despite continued expression of IFN-γ and NOS2. *J Exp Med* 2000;192:347–358.
27. Serbina NV, Lazarevic V, Flynn JL. CD4+ T cells are required for the development of cytotoxic CD8+ T cells during *Mycobacterium tuberculosis* infection. *J Immunol* 2001;167:6991–7000.
28. Serbina NV, Flynn JL. Early emergence of CD8+ T cells primed for production of type 1 cytokines in the lungs of *Mycobacterium tuberculosis*–infected mice. *Infect Immun* 1999;67:3980–3988.
29. Flynn JL, Goldstein MM, Triebold KJ, et al. Major histocompatibility complex class I-restricted T cells are required for resistance to *Mycobacterium tuberculosis* infection. *Proc Natl Acad Sci U S A* 1992;89:12013–12017.
30. Behar SM, Dascher CC, Grusby MJ, et al. Susceptibility of mice deficient in CD1D or TAP1 to infection with *Mycobacterium tuberculosis*. *J Exp Med* 1999;189:1973–1980.
31. Rolph MS, Raupach B, Kobernick HHC, et al. MHC class Ia-restricted T cells partially account for β2-microglobulin-dependent resistance to *Mycobacterium tuberculosis*. *Eur J Immunol* 2001;31:1944–1949.
32. Mogues T, Goodrich ME, Ryan L, et al. The relative importance of T cell subsets in immunity and immunopathology of airborne *Mycobacterium tuberculosis* infection in mice. *J Exp Med* 2001;193:271–280.
33. Sousa AO, Mazzaccaro RJ, Russell RG, et al. Bloom, Relative contributions of distinct MHC class I-dependent cell populations in protection to tuberculosis infection in mice. *Proc Natl Acad Sci U S A* 1999;97:4204–4208.
34. Stenger S, Hanson DA, Teitelbaum R, et al. An antimicrobial activity of cytotoxic T cells mediated by granulysin. *Science* 1998;282:121–125.
35. Glatman-Freedman A, Casadevall A. Serum therapy for tuberculosis revisited: reappraisal of the role of antibody-mediated immunity against *Mycobacterium tuberculosis*. *Clin Microbiol Rev* 1998;11:514–532.
36. Teitelbaum R, Glatman-Freedman A, Chen B, et al. A mAb recognizing a surface antigen of *Mycobacterium tuberculosis* enhances host survival. *Proc Natl Acad Sci U S A* 1998;95:15688–15693.
37. Bosio CM, Gardner D, Elkins KL. Infection of B cell deficient mice with CDC1551, a clinical isolate of *Mycobacterium tuberculosis*: delay in dissemination and development of lung pathology. *J Immunol* 2000;164:6417–6425.
38. Johnson CM, Cooper AM, Frank AA, et al. *Mycobacterium tuberculosis* aerogenic challenge infections in B cell-deficient mice. *Tuber Lung Dis* 1997;78:257–261.
39. Cooper AM, Dalton DK, Stewart TA, et al. Disseminated tuberculosis in IFN-γ gene-disrupted mice. *J Exp Med* 1993;178:2243–2248.
40. Flynn JL, Chan J, Triebold KJ, et al. An essential role for interferon-γ in resistance to *Mycobacterium tuberculosis* infection. *J Exp Med* 1993;178:2249–2254.
41. Cooper AM, Magram J, Ferrante J, et al. Interleukin 12 (IL-12) is crucial to the development of protective immunity in mice intravenously infected with *Mycobacterium tuberculosis*. *J Exp Med* 1997;186:39–45.
42. Cooper AM, Kipnis A, Turner J, et al. Mice lacking bioactive IL-12 can generate protective, antigen-specific cellular responses to mycobacterial infection only if the Il-12 p40 subunit is present. *J Immunol* 2002;168:1322–1327.
43. Cooper AM, Pearl JE, Brooks JV, et al. Expression of the nitric oxide synthase 2 gene is not essential for early control of *Mycobacterium tuberculosis* in the murine lung. *Infect Immun* 2000;68:6879–6882.
44. Manca C, Tsenova L, Bergtold A, et al. Virulence of a *Mycobacterium tuberculosis* clinical isolate in mice is determined by failure to induce Th1 type immunity and is associated with induction of IFN-alpha/beta. *Proc Natl Acad Sci U S A* 2001;98:5752–5757.
45. Pine R. IRF and tuberculosis. *J Interferon Cytokine Res* 2002;22:15–25.
46. Adams LB, Mason CM, Kolls JK, et al. Exacerbation of acute and chronic murine tuberculosis by administration of a tumor necrosis factor receptor-expressing adenovirus. *J Infect Dis* 1995;171:400–405.
47. Kindler V, Sappino A-P, Grau GE, et al. The inducing role of tumor necrosis factor in the development of bactericidal granulomas during BCG infection. *Cell* 1989;56:731–740.
48. Bekker L-G, Moreira AL, Bergtold A, et al. Immunopathologic effects of tumor necrosis factor alpha in murine mycobacterial infection are dose dependent. *Infect Immun* 2000;68:6954–6961.
49. Keane J, Gershon S, Wise RP, et al. Tuberculosis associated with Infliximab, a tumor necrosis factor a-neutralizing agent. *N Engl J Med* 2001;345:1098–1104.
50. North RJ. Mice incapable of making IL-4 and IL-10 display normal resistance in infection with *Mycobacterium tuberculosis*. *Clin Exp Immunol* 1998;113:55–58.
51. Roach DR, Martin E, Bean AG, et al. Endogenous inhibition of antimycobacterial immunity by IL-10 varies between mycobacterial species. *Scand J Immunol* 2001;54:163–170.
52. Murray PJ, Young RA. Increased antimycobacterial immunity in interleukin-10-deficient. *Infect Immun* 1999;67:3087–3095.
53. Jacobs M, Brown N, Allie N, et al. Increased resistance to mycobacterial infection in the absence of interleukin-10. *Immunology* 2000;100:494–501.
54. Murray PJ, Yang L, Onufryk C, et al. T cell-derived IL-10 antagonizes macrophage function in mycobacteria infection. *J Immunol* 1997;158:315–321.
55. Lang R, Rutschman RL, Greaves D, et al. Autocrine deactivation of macrophages in transgenic mice constitutively overexpressing IL-10 under control of human CD68 promotor. *J Immunol* 2002;168:3402–3411.
56. Koch R. Aeriologie der Tuberculose. *Berlin Klin Wochenschr* 1882;19:221–230.
57. Koch R. Die Aetiologie der Tuberculose. *Am Rev Tuberc* 1932;25:285–323. Pinner B, Pinner M, translators.
58. Riley RL, O'Grady MC, Sultan F, et al. Infectiousness of air from a tuberculosis ward. *Am Rev Respir Dis* 1962;85:511–525.
59. Riley R. How it really happened. What nobody needs to know about airborne infection. *Am J Respir Crit Care Med* 2001;163:7–8.
60. Opie EL, Aronson JD. Tubercle bacilli in latent tuberculous lesions and in lung tissue without tuberculous lesions. *Arch Pathol* 1927;4:1–21.
61. Pallen M. The inoculation of tissue specimens into guinea-pigs in suspected cases of mycobacterial infection—does it aid diagnosis and treatment? *Tubercle* 1987;68:51–57.
62. Smith DW, Balasubramanian V, Wiegeshaus E. A guinea pig model of experimental airborne tuberculosis for evaluation of the response to chemotherapy: the effect on bacilli in the initial phase of treatment. *Tubercle* 1991;72:223–231.
63. McMurray DN. Guinea pig model of tuberculosis. In: Bloom BR, ed. *Tuberculosis: pathogenesis, protection, and control.* Washington, DC: American Society for Microbiology, 1994:135–147.
64. McMurray D. Disease model: pulmonary tuberculosis. *Trends Mol Med* 2001;7:135–137.

65. Dai G, Phalen S, McMurray DN. Nutritional modulation of host responses to mycobacteria. *Front Biosci* 1998;3:E110–E122.

66. Orme IM, McMurray DN, Belisle JT. Tuberculosis vaccine development: recent progress. *Trends Microbiol* 2001;9:115–118.

67. Wiegeshaus E, McMurray DN, Grover AA, et al. Host-parasite relationships in experimental airborne tuberculosis. III. Relevance to microbial enumeration to acquired resistance in guinea pigs. *Am Rev Respir Dis* 1970;102:422–429.

68. Smith DW, McMurray DN, Wiegeshaus EH, et al. Host-parasite relationships in experimental airborne tuberculosis. IV. Early events in the course of infection in vaccinated and nonvaccinated guinea pigs. *Am Rev Respir Dis* 1970;102:937–949.

69. Ho R, Fok JS, Harding GE, et al. Host-parasite relationships in experimental airborne tuberculosis. VII. Fate of *Mycobacterium tuberculosis* in primary lung lesions and in primary lesion-free lung tissue infected as a result of bacillemia. *J Infect Dis* 1978;138:237–241.

70. Jeevan A, Yoshimura T, Foster G, et al. Effect of *Mycobacterium bovis* BCG vaccination on interleukin-1β and RANTES mRNA expression in guinea pig cells exposed to attenuated and virulent mycobacteria. *Infect Immun* 2002;70:1245–1253.

71. Lurie MB. *Resistance to tuberculosis: experimental studies in native and acquired defense mechanisms*. Cambridge, MA: Harvard University Press, 1964.

72. Dannenberg AM. Rabbit model of tuberculosis. In: Bloom BR, ed. *Tuberculosis: pathogenesis, protection, and control*. Washington, DC: American Society for Microbiology, 1994:149–156.

73. Converse PJ, Dannenberg AM, Estep JE, et al. Cavitary tuberculosis produced in rabbits by aerosolized virulent tubercle bacilli. *Infect Immun* 1996;64:4776–4787.

74. Bishai WR, Dannenberg AM, Parrish N, et al. Virulence of *Mycobacterium tuberculosis* CDC1551 and H37Rv in rabbits evaluated by Lurie's pulmonary tubercle count method. *Infect Immun* 1999;67:4931–4934.

75. Dannenberg AMJ. Pathogenesis of pulmonary *Mycobacterium bovis* infection: basic principles established by the rabbit model. *Tuberculosis* 2001;81:87–96.

76. Converse PJ, Dannenberg AM, Shigenaga T, et al. Pulmonary bovine-type tuberculosis in rabbits: bacillary virulence, inhaled dose effects, tuberculin sensitivity, and *Mycobacterium vaccae* immunotherapy. *Clin Diagn Lab Immunol* 1998;5:871–881.

77. Dannenberg AM, Bishai WR, Parrish N, et al. Efficacies of BCG and vole bacillus (*Mycobacterium microti*) vaccines in preventing clinically apparent pulmonary tuberculosis in rabbits: a preliminary report. *Vaccine* 2001;19:796–800.

78. Tsenova L, Sokol K, Freedman VH, et al. A combination of thalidomide plus antibiotics protects rabbits from mycobacterial meningitis-associated death. *J Infect Dis* 1998;177:1563–1572.

79. Barclay WR, Busey WM, Dalgard DW, et al. Protection of mon-

keys against airborne tuberculosis by aerosol vaccination with bacillus Calmette-Guerin. *Am Rev Respir Dis* 1973;107:351–358.

80. Ribi E, Anacker RL, Barclay WR, et al. Efficacy of mycobacterial cell walls as a vaccine against airborne tuberculosis in the rhesus monkey. *J Infect Dis* 1971;123:527–538.

81. Walsh GP, Tan EV, de la Cruz EC, et al. The Philippine cynomolgus monkey (*Macaca fascularis*) provides a new nonhuman primate model of tuberculosis that resembles human disease. *Nat Med* 1996;2:430–436.

82. Shen Y, Zhou D, Qiu L, et al. Adaptive immune response of Vγ2Vδ2+T cells during mycobacterial infections. *Science* 2002;295:2255–2258.

83. Langermans JAM, Andersen P, van Soolingen D, et al. Divergent effect of bacillus Calmette-Guerin (BCG) vaccination on *Mycobacterium tuberculosis* infection in highly related macaque species: implications for primate models in tuberculosis vaccine research. *Proc Natl Acad Sci U S A* 2001;98:11497–11502.

84. Schmidt LH. Studies on the antituberculous activity of ethambutol in monkeys. *Ann N Y Acad Sci* 1966;135:747–758.

85. Schmidt LH. Induced pulmonary tuberculosis in the rhesus monkey: its usefulness in evaluating chemotherapeutic agents. *Trans Conference Chemother Tuberc* 1955;14:226–231.

86. Schmidt LH. Some observations on the utility of simian tuberculosis in defining the therapeutic potentialities of isoniazid. *Annu Rev Tuberc Pulm Dis* 1956;74:138–153.

87. Francis J. Natural and experimental tuberculosis in monkeys with observations on immunization and chemotherapy. *J Comp Pathol* 1956;66:123–135.

88. Wolf RH, Gibson SV, Watson EA, et al. Multidrug chemotherapy of tuberculosis in rhesus monkeys. *Lab Anim Sci* 1988;38:25–33.

89. Aronson JD. Spontaneous tuberculosis in salt water fish. *J Infect Dis* 1926;39:315–320.

90. Talaat AM, Reimschuessel R, Wasserman SS, et al. *Carassius auratus*, a novel animal model for the study of *Mycobacterium marinum* pathogenesis. *Infect Immun* 1998;66:2938–2942.

91. Ramakrishnan L, Valdivia RH, McKerrow JH, et al. *Mycobacterium marinum* causes both long-term subclinical infection and acute disease in the leopard frog (*Rana pipiens*). *Infect Immun* 1997;65:767–773.

92. Bouley DM, Ghori N, Mercer KL, et al. Dynamic nature of host-pathogen interactions in *Mycobacterium marinum* granulomas. *Infect Immun* 2001;69:7820–7831.

93. Ramakrishnan L, Federspeil NA, Falkow S. Granuloma-specific expression of *Mycobacterium* virulence proteins from the glycine-rich PE-PGRS family. *Science* 2000;288:1436–1439.

94. Davis JM, Clay M, Lewis JL, et al. Real-time visualization of mycobacterium-macrophage interactions leading to initiation of granuloma formation in zebrafish embryos. *Immunity* 2002;17:693–702.

CELL-MEDIATED IMMUNE RESPONSE

TIMO ULRICHS
STEFAN H. E. KAUFMANN

Since the groundbreaking discovery of *Mycobacterium tuberculosis* by Robert Koch in 1882 (1), the multifaceted interactions between this pathogen and its host have been in the focus of interest in infection biology. It soon became clear that the host immune system *acquires* protective immunity to infection with *M. tuberculosis*. Koch himself observed that tuberculous guinea pigs reacted in a qualitatively different way to inoculated mycobacteria when compared with naïve ones. Further studies on the host response in infected tissues revealed that immune cells have to be involved in both the effector reaction to the pathogen and the acquisition of resistance to infection. Since then, different cell types were isolated and their roles in the immunity to *M. tuberculosis* were described. In 1893, Borrel and Metchnikoff (2) formulated a basic observation: "La cellule tuberculeuse est toujours une cellule lymphatique" (The tuberculous cell always is a lymphoid cell). They investigated histologic specimens from infected tissue and consistently observed mycobacteria within cells of the lymphoid system, mainly macrophages.

In his original description of the etiology of tuberculosis, Koch (1) had noted the frequent intracellular location of the bacilli in the tuberculous lesion: "Whenever giant cells are present in the tuberculous lesion, the bacilli are preferentially found in these cells. In slowly progressing tuberculous processes, bacilli are exclusively found within these giant cells."

These granulomatous tissue reactions are consistently found at the sites of bacterial implantation. Their chronic nature correlates with bacterial persistence. Skin reactions with some superficial resemblance to these lesions can be induced by local injection of soluble antigen. These reactions, however, are short-lived and less severe, reflecting rapid elimination of the material. This reaction occurs only in infected individuals and has been categorized as delayed-type hypersensitivity (DTH) reaction because of the delayed onset after approximately 48 hours that distinguishes it from acute hypersensitivity reactions that develop within minutes. Koch (3), who was the first to describe this reaction, clearly noted its diagnostic value. He stated "I assume that the material will be a valuable diagnostic measure in the future. It will become possible to diagnose questionable cases of phthisis even in those cases, where bacilli cannot be detected in the sputum." Helmholtz (4) showed that transfer of DTH to tuberculin could be transferred with whole blood (containing the leukocytes) but not with serum. One year later, Bail (5) demonstrated successful transfer with Organ-Brei (spleen and liver cell suspension). These two findings, however, were not appreciated at that time because immunology was focused on antibodies rather than cells as mediators of specific immunity. In 1945, Chase (6), however, demonstrated the adoptive transfer of DTH with tuberculin using peritoneal exudate cells from immune guinea pigs. This experiment was based on previous findings of Landsteiner and Chase (7) that contact sensitivity was transferable with such cells in the absence of serum. Finally, Lawrence (8), in 1949, reported on cellular transfer of DTH against tuberculin in humans by using leukocytes. The lymphocyte nature of the mediators of immunity was first demonstrated by Wesslén (9) in 1952 and later by Coe et al. (10) in 1966. These researchers used lymphocytes from the thoracic duct of immune animals for adaptive transfer of DTH to tuberculin. The T-cell nature of these lymphocytes was demonstrated using thymectomized, X-irradiated, and bone marrow–reconstituted mice lacking functional T cells (11). Soon it became clear that these T cells fail to directly attack *M. tuberculosis*. Instead, it was found that they activate macrophages via soluble mediators, the cytokines. Patterson and Youmans (12) activated normal macrophages, using spleen cells from *M. tuberculosis*–immune mice. The first cytokine to be identified was macrophage inhibitory factor, originally described independently by Bloom and Bennett (13) and by David (14). The concept of macrophage activation was already spelled out by Metchnikoff (15) and elucidated in much detail by Mackaness (16). Lurie (17) demonstrated that macrophages from bacille Calmette–Guérin (BCG)–vaccinated rabbits expressed higher

T. Ulrichs: Department of Immunology, Max-Planck-Institute for Infection Biology; Department of Medical Microbiology and Infection Immunology, Institute for Infection Medicine of Freie Universität Berlin, Berlin, Germany.

S. H. E. Kaufmann: Department of Immunology, Max-Planck-Institute for Infection Biology, Berlin, Germany.

antimycobacterial activity *in vivo*, and Suter (18) went on to reproduce these findings in a defined *in vitro* system.

Today, we know some specific details about the interplay between different immune cells during the course of infection that were not known in the early 20th century; we have even started to investigate global gene expression patterns that specify the host response to *M. tuberculosis* just like a signature identifies an individual. However, all the complex interactions between the pathogen and host are as yet unknown, and we have not yet determined the precise mechanisms that lead to a successful immune response.

This chapter describes the immune cells and molecular mediators that are central to our understanding of the immune response to *M. tuberculosis*. The following sections describe the different cell types and their roles in cellular immunity to tuberculosis in more detail.

PATHOGENESIS OF TUBERCULOSIS IN THE EARLY PHASE OF INFECTION

Tubercle bacilli are transmitted from person to person by inhalation of small droplets containing mycobacteria (Fig. 18.1A). Most individuals clear most droplets already within the bronchi and alveoli of the lung. The percentage of exposed individuals who become infected depends on environmental conditions, the frequency and duration of exposure, and the concentration and size of mycobacteria-containing droplets in the air but is in general considered to be minute. Of those who become infected, more than 90% successfully contain the infection by virtue of an efficient immune response during their lifetime, so that it remains clinically inapparent. A hallmark of infection with *M. tuberculosis* and specific immunity is the positive tuberculin skin reaction. (Graded doses of tuberculin or purified protein derivative are inoculated into the skin, and the induration is measured after 3 to 4 days.) The state of DTH indicates the presence of specific immunity mostly involving antigen-specific T cells. On encountering antigen presented by professional antigen-presenting cells, these T cells produce inflammatory cytokines that attract monocytes to the

site of reaction and activate them. DTH reactions are transient and vanish once the antigen has been eliminated by the activated monocytes. A similar reaction takes place at the site of mycobacterial persistence. However, because mycobacteria persist and are not readily degraded, the antigenic depot sustains a granulomatous reaction at the site of bacterial implantation.

Because the pathogen is inhaled in small droplets, invading mycobacteria first encounter alveolar macrophages residing within lung alveoli that phagocytose the bacilli. T cells are recruited to the site of primary infection where the bacilli are contained and become activated by interactions with T lymphocytes. In an attempt to avoid direct confrontation with host effector mechanisms, *M. tuberculosis* slows down its replication rate within the phagosomes of macrophages and enters a dormant state of low replication and strongly reduced metabolic activity (reviewed in reference 19).

Approximately one-third of the world population (i.e., two billion people) are infected with this pathogen. A balance between the pathogen and the cellular immune response is established so that *M. tuberculosis* is contained at the primary site of infection by the immune cells. Yet the bacilli are not cleared from the host. Rather, *M. tuberculosis* remains dormant until this labile balance between mycobacterial persistence and the immune response becomes disturbed. Once the host response is impaired owing to a variety of reasons including aging, malnutrition, treatment with steroids, or human immunodeficiency virus infection, reactivation of *M. tuberculosis* infection occurs. The balance is tipped in favor of the pathogen, and bacilli are spread to other sites in the lung or other organs. As a result, active tuberculosis develops (Fig. 18.1B).

Phagocytosis of *M. tuberculosis* by alveolar macrophages is mediated by several host cell receptors. They include receptors recognizing distinct patterns expressed on the surface of the pathogen (pattern recognition receptors), like the macrophage mannose receptor and CD14 (reviewed in references 20,21). At least three members of the Toll-like receptor (TLR) family are also involved in interactions between macrophages and mycobacteria. The TLR2 and TLR4 interact with mycobacterial cell wall components, including

FIGURE 18.1. Balance between *Mycobacterium tuberculosis* and the host immune system. **A:** *M. tuberculosis* is inhaled in droplets. After an incubation period of 4 to 12 weeks, infected alveolar macrophages containing the pathogen either destroy their predators [a mechanism that has not yet been shown but probably accounts for a minute proportion **(left)**] or fail to contain the pathogen and die **(right)**. In the first case, infection is abortive; in the second case, the pathogen spreads throughout the body and causes active disease. When the immune response and virulence of *M. tuberculosis* are balanced **(middle)**, intracellular bacteria are contained by the macrophages, and the immune system isolates the primary site of infection by granuloma formation (primary lesion). In this third scenario, the most frequent one, infection without clinical disease develops as long as there is a balance. **B:** *M. tuberculosis* can persist in a dormant state for long periods. Any disturbance of the balance between host and pathogen after weakening of the cellular immune response (immunosuppression) causes endogenous reactivation, which leads to active (postprimary) tuberculosis. Active tuberculosis can also be caused by exogenous reinfection. *HIV*, human immunodeficiency virus. (Adapted from Ulrichs T, Kaufmann SHE. Mycobacterial persistence and immunity. *Front Biosci* 2002;7:458–469.)

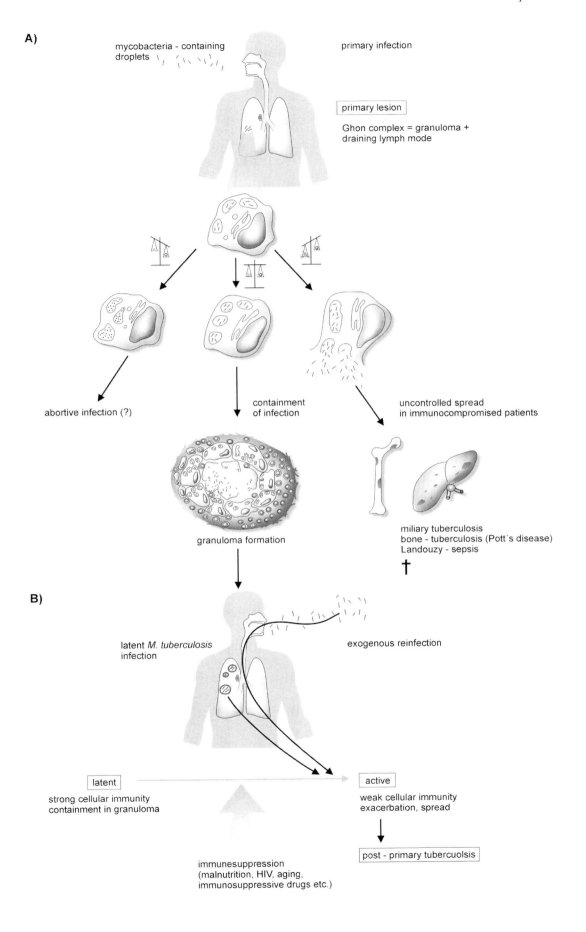

lipoarabinomannan and lipoproteins (22,23), TLR9 interacts with mycobacterial DNA comprising cytosine guanine dinucleotides (CpG) motifs (24,25). Other receptors recognize host molecules, such as surfactant protein, complement proteins, or antibodies from the innate and acquired host response bound to the mycobacterial surface (i.e., surfactant receptors, complement receptors, and Fc receptors) (Fig. 18.2) (25a). The choice of the receptor used to enter the macrophage influences the cellular response: entry of immunoglobulin G–opsonized mycobacteria via Fc receptors results in activation of macrophage antimicrobial systems (26) (see later), whereas internalization via complement receptor 3 fails to activate appropriate effector mechanisms (27). Cholesterol seems to promote docking of mycobacteria to macrophages, and membrane cholesterol is involved in mediating the phagosomal association of tryptophan/aspartate–containing coat protein, which prevents phagosome maturation to the phagolysosome (28). Although the underlying mechanisms are still incompletely understood, arrest of the mycobacterial phagosome at an early stage is a major survival strategy of *M. tuberculosis* to avoid lysosomal degradation. The infected macrophages contain their mycobacterial predators and prevent them from spreading throughout the host organism.

FORMATION OF THE HUMAN TUBERCULOUS GRANULOMA

Restriction of mycobacteria to discrete sites of infection is ensured by the formation of granulomatous reactions at sites of bacterial implantation. Granuloma formation is mediated by a specific immune response and represents a characteristic feature of tuberculosis that lead to its name (granuloma = tubercle, i.e., the anatomic description of a small, distinct

nodule). The granuloma is formed by the recruitment of circulating mononuclear phagocytes and T cells to the site of bacterial replication, with infected macrophages forming the center of the cellular accumulation (Fig. 18.2A). Infected macrophages differentiate into various forms ranging from tissue macrophages to epithelioid and multinucleated giant cells, the latter resulting from fusion of several infected mononuclear cells. Recruited T cells secrete a variety of cytokines that activate infected cells to control their mycobacterial load or activate cytotoxic T cells. A characteristic feature of the tuberculous granulomas is the formation of a caseous center containing necrotic tissue, cell debris, and killed mycobacteria (Fig. 18.2B). Extracellular mycobacteria are found within the zone between the necrotic center and the cellular wall of the granuloma. We are just beginning to understand the strategies used by *M. tuberculosis* to ensure its survival in this hostile environment, e.g., by adapting its metabolism to low oxygen content (29,30) and the switch to lipids as energy source. These lipids are highly abundant components of the caseous center of the granuloma (31). Activation of T cells and macrophages has to be tightly balanced to avoid any disruption of the integrity of the productive granuloma. Excessive cytotoxic activity or apoptosis of infected cells causes liquefaction, allowing dissemination of mycobacteria from the lesion (Fig. 18.2C).

CELL-MEDIATED IMMUNITY AGAINST *MYCOBACTERIUM TUBERCULOSIS*

Cytokines

The majority of immunocompetent human individuals controls mycobacterial infection efficiently. This is mostly owing to an efficient coordination of the immune response by the cytokine network. Leukocyte migration to the site of

FIGURE 18.2. Host response and granuloma formation. **A:** Alveolar macrophages (*MΦ*) phagocytize invading mycobacteria but cannot kill them. T cells and monocytes (*Mo*) are recruited to the site of infection in the lung. **B:** Alveolar macrophages, epithelioid cells (*E*), or Langhans giant cells (generated by fusion of epithelioid cells) harboring intracellular mycobacteria form the center of the productive granuloma. These cells present antigens to T cells and activate them to produce a variety of cytokines and chemokines or to kill the infected cells and intracellular mycobacteria. Chemokines recruit additional cells from the blood circulation to the site of primary infection. Interferon gamma (*IFN-γ*) activates macrophages and other antigen-presenting cells to kill the intracellular bacteria via inducible nitric oxide synthase (iNOS), which generates reactive nitrogen intermediates (*RNI*). CD4+ T cells and macrophages produce tumor necrosis factor-α (*TNF-α*) and lymphotoxin α3 (*LTα3*), which are required for the formation of the wall encapsulating the granuloma. In the center of the granuloma, low oxygen pressure probably forms a hostile environment for released mycobacteria. Activated CD8+ T cells kill mycobacteria in macrophages by means of granulysin and perforin. Killing of infected cells, however, needs to be controlled to retain the integrity of the productive granuloma. **C:** Once the integrity of the granuloma is disturbed in a caseous lesion, mycobacteria can enter blood circulation and surrounding lung tissue and spread throughout the body. Mycobacteria entering the bronchi will be coughed up, spread by aerosols, and infect new individuals. The caseous detritus in the granuloma supports *Mycobacterium tuberculosis* growth, often reaching numbers exceeding 10^9 organisms. With such high bacterial numbers, inadequate chemotherapy leads to the emergence of resistant strains. *NKT*, natural killer T cell; *ROI*, reactive oxygen intermediate; *TGF-β*, transforming growth factor-β. (Adapted from Kaufmann SHE. Immunity to intracellular bacteria. In: Paul WE, ed. *Fundamental immunology*, 5th ed. Philadelphia: Lippincott Williams & Wilkins, 2003:1229–1261.)

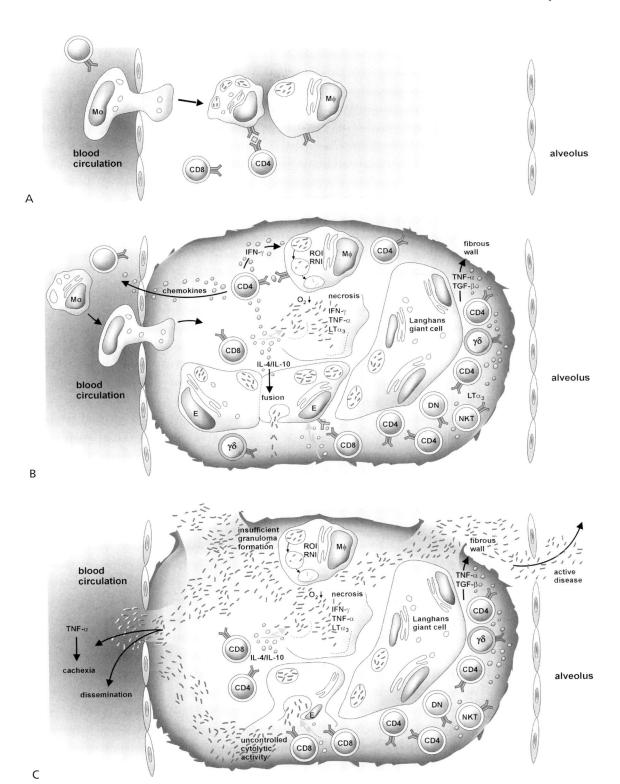

mycobacterial focus and the initiation of the granulomatous lesion are mediated by chemokines and proinflammatory cytokines (Fig. 18.2A). Infected macrophages and dendritic cells produce interleukin-12 (IL-12), the crucial cytokine in controlling early *M. tuberculosis* infection (32,33). IL-12 regulates the immune system toward a T_H1 response with production of interferon gamma (IFN-γ) and down-modulation of IL-10 and IL-4. Patients with genetic defects in IL-12, IL-12 receptor, or IFN-γ are more susceptible to disseminated BCG and *Mycobacterium avium* infections (34,35). Formation and sustaining of the granuloma architecture are supported mainly by tumor necrosis factor-α (TNF-α), IFN-γ, transforming growth factor β, and lymphotoxin $\alpha3$. TNF-α and IFN-γ are also the crucial cytokines responsible for macrophage activation. They activate macrophages to produce inducible nitric oxide synthase (iNOS) and to sustain pathways generating reactive nitrogen intermediates (reviewed in references 36,37). In addition, oxidative effector molecules are generated. Although the oxidative and nitrosative stress reduces mycobacterial growth, it fails to eliminate the pathogen. One reason might be that *M. tuberculosis* resists host effector mechanisms by means of a peroxidase/phosphonitrite reductase system that also participates in its intermediary metabolism (38).

IFN-γ and iNOS (39) are crucial for containing the infection and keeping the balance between persistence of *M. tuberculosis* and immune defense (reviewed in reference 37). Treatment with the iNOS inhibitor aminoguanidine impairs reactive nitrogen intermediate production and reactivates tuberculosis, leading to fatal disease in the mouse model (40). TNF-α synergizes with IFN-γ in the activation of antimycobacterial activities in macrophages (41). More important, TNF-α plays a critical role in the containment of persistent *M. tuberculosis* organisms and in preventing them from spreading to other regions of the lung or to other organs (42,43). Encapsulation of the granuloma and formation of the fibrinous wall are primarily mediated by TNF-α (44), although transforming growth factor-β also seems to be involved in addition (45,46). TNF-α, administered to mice depleted of CD4$^+$ T cells and latently infected with *Mycobacterium bovis* BCG, prevents recrudescence of infection (47,48). In mice, monoclonal antibodies against TNF-α cause reactivation of latent *M. tuberculosis* infection (49), suggesting that TNF-α prevents endogenous spreading of mycobacteria by modulating cytokine levels and limiting histopathology. Mice deficient in lymphotoxin $\alpha3$, also a member of the TNF family, fail to form intact granulomas and have exacerbated tuberculosis (50), suggesting that, together with TNF-α, lymphotoxin $\alpha3$ promotes granuloma formation and its maintenance. Elevated levels of TNF-α, transforming growth factor β, and IL-10 have been detected in sera and pleural fluids of patients with pulmonary tuberculosis (51). In general, the risk of disturbing the delicate balance between pathogen and host seems to increase with decreasing levels of TNF-α. This is illustrated by the fact that reactivation of tuberculosis represents a major side effect of anti–TNF-α antibody therapy of severe rheumatoid arthritis (52,53). TNF-α also regulates the expression of chemokine receptors and the secretion of chemokines. It up-regulates macrophage inflammatory protein (MIP)-1α, MIP-1β, monocyte chemoattractant protein (MCP)-1, and RANTES (the cytokine regulated on activation, normal T cell expressed and secreted), affecting the primary role of chemokines in the immunity to mycobacterial infection, i.e., the recruitment of several immune cells such as monocytes, lymphocytes, and neutrophils (54–58). The induction of MCP-1 and RANTES by lipoarabinomannan can be inhibited by anti–TNF-α antibodies (59). The chemokine receptor CCR5, the receptor for MIP-1α, MIP-1β, and RANTES, is up-regulated on alveolar macrophages isolated from lungs of patients with tuberculosis (60). Mice deficient in CCR2, the receptor for MCP-1, -3, and -5, are highly susceptible to *M. tuberculosis* infection (61), suggesting that chemokines and their receptors play an important role in the formation of the tuberculous granuloma. Mice deficient in CXCR3, the receptor for monokine induced by interferon γ (MIG), interferon-inducible protein 10 (IP-10), and interferon-inducible T-cell α chemokine (I-TAC), have impaired granuloma formation but still are capable of controlling *M. tuberculosis* as controls do. These data not only point to a role of these chemokines in early granuloma formation but also provide evidence of dissociation of granuloma formation and protection in tuberculosis.

CD4$^+$ T Cells

Substantial evidence emphasizes the major role of CD4$^+$ T cells in containing tuberculosis at all stages of disease. CD4$^+$ T cells control persistent mycobacteria contained within the granuloma at least in part in an IFN-γ– and reactive nitrogen intermediate–independent manner (62). Depletion of CD4$^+$ T cells in the mouse model causes rapid reactivation of previously dormant *M. tuberculosis* organisms, resulting in increased bacterial load and exacerbation to rapidly progressing tuberculosis. Major histocompatibility complex (MHC) class II knockout mice are more susceptible to *M. tuberculosis* than mice deficient in CD4$^+$ T cells, probably because some CD4$^-$ T cells can compensate for deficient CD4$^+$ T cells (63). Endogenous reactivation of latent tuberculosis in mice deficient in CD4$^+$ T cells occurs despite normal levels of IFN-γ and iNOS, suggesting that CD4$^+$ T cells regulate the balance between *M. tuberculosis* and activated immune cells. CD4$^+$ and CD8$^+$ T cells are located mainly in the periphery of intact granulomas, and their total numbers correlate with the structural integrity of the granuloma, underlining their key role in containing infection (Fig. 18.2). Patients positive for human immunodeficiency virus with reduced numbers of CD4$^+$ T cells are at increased risk of reactivation of persistent *M. tuberculosis*.

This phenomenon is largely responsible for the recent resurgence of *M. tuberculosis* and the increase of active disease, especially in developing countries with high incidences of human immunodeficiency virus infection.

CD8+ T Cells

In addition to CD4+ T cells, CD8+ T cells also contribute to the successful immune response against *M. tuberculosis* (64) (Fig. 18.2). Experiments with mice deficient in β2-microglobulin, an essential part of MHC class Ia (65), CD1 molecules (66), and CD8α (67,68) as well as with mice deficient in the transporter protein associated with antigen processing (69) revealed that all these animals were more susceptible to *M. tuberculosis* infection than their wild-type counterparts. At first sight, the involvement of antigen-specific CD8+ T cells in the immune response against *M. tuberculosis* is surprising because the pathogen resides within phagosomes (Fig. 18.1) and has no direct contact with the MHC class I antigen-processing machinery. Experiments with antigen model systems suggest that alternative MHC class I pathways permit the processing of phagosomal antigens, thus allowing CD8+ T-cell activation (70). Even active transport of antigen from phagosome to cytosol is conceivable. Finally, *M. tuberculosis* induces apoptosis of host cells and the formation of apoptotic vesicles that can be internalized by bystander dendritic cells and presented to CD8+ T cells.

There are two primary effector functions of CD8+ T cells: production of cytokines, predominantly IFN-γ (as discussed previously), and lysis of infected cells to allow direct bacterial killing. CD8+ T cells lyse target cells via granzymes and perforin or the Fas–FasL interaction (33). Lysed infected macrophages release their mycobacterial load, which can then be taken up and eliminated by activated macrophages or dendritic cells. Recent evidence suggests direct killing of mycobacteria by CD8+ T cells. Killing is facilitated by perforin, which is required to form a pore (71), and executed by granulysin, which has cytotoxic effects on bacteria (72). Perforin-deficient mice, however, are still capable of controlling *M. tuberculosis* infection (67) or die of the infection later (68). Mice do not have a homolog for granulysin. Thus, the contribution of cytolytic CD8+ T cells to protection against tuberculosis is still incompletely understood.

Unconventional T Cells

Presentation of mycobacterial protein antigens via the conventional MHC presentation system is supplemented by the presentation of lipid and glycolipid antigens by CD1 molecules (reviewed in references 73,74) (Fig. 18.3B). The CD1 family consists of antigen-presenting molecules encoded by genes located outside the MHC. The CD1 system is involved in the activation of cell-mediated responses against

mycobacterial infection. Group 1 CD1 molecules (i.e., CD1a, b, and c) are found on professional antigen-presenting cells and present mycobacterial lipid and glycolipid antigens to specific T cells. Group 2 CD1 (i.e., CD1d) is constitutively expressed on a variety of cells and interacts with natural killer T (NKT) cells. In mice, CD1d-restricted NKT cells are activated by mycobacterial cell wall components and are involved in early granuloma formation (75). These NKT cells produce IFN-γ in the early phase after infection of mice with BCG (76). Recently, the first mycobacterial ligand presented by CD1d to T cells was described: isopentenyl-tetra-mannoside. However, it is unclear whether CD1d-restricted T cells play an essential role in the protective immune response to mycobacterial infection because CD1d-deficient mice are not more susceptible to TB (69). Rather, it is likely that CD1d-restricted NKT cells participate in the early regulation of the immune response to tuberculosis.

Several mycobacterial lipid and glycolipid antigens have been identified that elicit a specific group 1 CD1-restricted T-cell response in humans (73). These also include lipoarabinomannan. T cells recognizing CD1-restricted antigens express a broad range of effector mechanisms including cytotoxic activity and IFN-γ secretion. These findings suggest that the CD1 system is involved in cellular immune responses against infection with *M. tuberculosis* in the early and late phases of infection (Fig. 18.3B). However, direct evidence in a suitable animal model is still lacking.

γδ T cells are involved in the rapid, early phase of the immune response to mycobacteria (reviewed in references 77,78) (Fig. 18.4). Human γδ T cells usually recognize pyrophosphate, alkylamine, and nucleotide antigens. The antigen-presenting molecule is still unknown (if it is required at all). Some γδ T cells recognize CD1c on infected cells. In the nonhuman primate model, γδ T cells expand and acquire memory functions after mycobacterial infection (79), suggesting that γδ T cells play a role in the early phase of the immune response after TB infection (80) (Fig. 18.3C).

CONCLUSION

The specific immune response to *M. tuberculosis* infection mainly depends on the activation of various T-cell subsets that produce cytokines that orchestrate appropriate defense mechanisms to keep the pathogen in check. This chapter provides a brief overview of different cell types, cytokines, and chemokines and their specific roles in the balance between the pathogen and the immune response. The intracellular survival of *M. tuberculosis* and its persistence over long periods are major challenges for the immune system. However, the competent immune system is able to cope with mycobacterial infection and indeed does so in more than 90% of all infected humans. Understanding the complex cross talk between the cell-mediated immune response and the pathogen and elucidating the correlates of protection will allow us to develop

A)

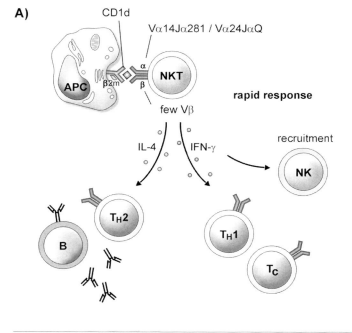

C)

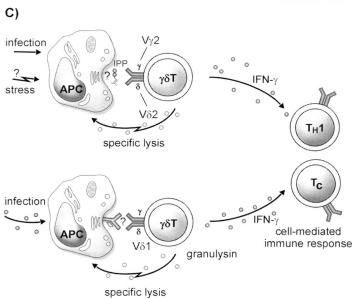

B)

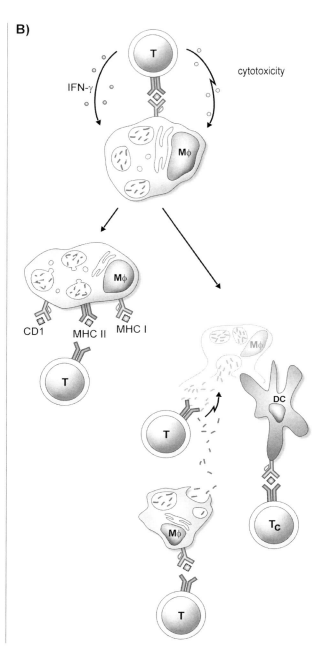

FIGURE 18.3. Unconventional T (*T*) cells involved in immune response to *Mycobacterium tuberculosis*. **A:** Group 2 CD1-restricted natural killer T (*NKT*) cells. NKT cells that recognize lipid antigens presented by CD1d molecules have a variety of different functions. They release high amounts of interferon gamma (*IFN-γ*), directing the immune system to a T$_H$1-type response and recruiting circulating natural killer (*NK*) cells for a rapid immune response before the reaction of activated conventional T cells. The release of interleukin-4 (*IL-4*) induces T$_H$2 cells and causes antibody production by B cells (*B*). After mycobacterial infection, NKT cells become promptly IFN-γ producers (T$_H$1 cells). **B:** Possible roles of group 1 CD1-restricted T cells in the immune response to *M. tuberculosis*. CD1-restricted T cells specific for mycobacterial lipid or glycolipid antigens have several effector functions in the immune response to *M. tuberculosis*: IFN-γ activates antimicrobial activities in mycobacteria-containing macrophages. CD1-restricted T cells also possess cytotoxic activities. The destruction of the mycobacteria-containing macrophages decreases the reservoir of host cells for the pathogen and allows cytotoxic T cells to directly kill mycobacteria. The antigens of the destroyed macrophage can be processed and presented by activated dendritic cells (*DC*), allowing an effective recruitment of additional cytotoxic T cells. **C:** Roles of γδ T cells in early immune responses. γδ T cells expressing Vγ2/Vδ2 recognize pyrophosphate (e.g., isopentenyl-pyrophosphate, *IPP*), alkylamine, and nucleotide antigens derived from microbes. The mechanism of antigen presentation remains unclear. Activated γδ T cells can lyse the antigen-presenting cells (*APC*) and elicit a T$_H$1 immune response. Granulocyte-macrophage colony-stimulating factor derived from activated cells during infection causes the expression of group 1 CD1 molecules on immature dendritic cells. Vδ1$^+$γδ T cells recognize CD1c molecules on the surface of these cells. After activation, Vδ1$^+$γδ T cells release IFN-γ, activating a T$_H$1-type immune response, the release of granulysin, and specific killing of the CD1c$^+$ cell. *MHC I* and *MHC II*, major histocompatibility complex class I and II; *MФ*, macrophages. (Adapted from Ulrichs T, Porcelli S. CD1 proteins: targets of T cell recognition in innate and adaptive immunity. *Rev Immunogenet* 2000;2:416–432.)

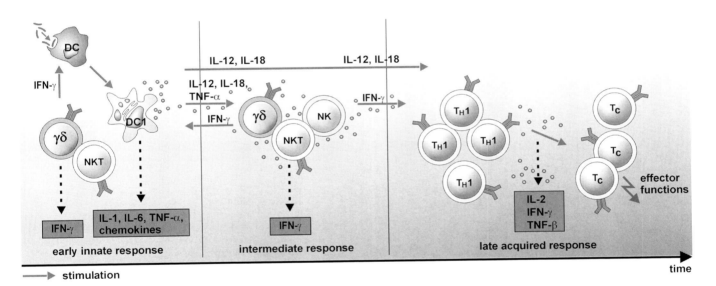

FIGURE 18.4. Overview of phases of infection. Cytokines regulate the immune response toward a T$_H$1-type response. Dendritic cells (*DC*) secrete interleukin (*IL*)-12, IL-18, chemokines, and tumor necrosis factor-α (*TNF-α*), activating natural killer T (*NKT*) cells and γδ T cells. At the same time, these T cells produce interferon gamma (*IFN-γ*), further promoting maturation of DCs. In the intermediary phase, IFN-γ, secreted by activated T cells and natural killer (*NK*) cells activate antigen-presenting cells and secure the maintenance of the T$_H$1 response, resulting in the recruitment of cytolytic T cells. (Adapted from Kaufmann SHE. Immunity to intracellular bacteria. In: Paul WE, ed. *Fundamental immunology*, 5th ed. Philadelphia: Lippincott Williams & Wilkins, 2003:1229–1261.)

both novel therapeutic and prevention strategies to protect the 10% of infected individuals whose immune systems fail to combat tuberculosis on their own (81,82).

ACKNOWLEDGMENT

We thank Lucia Lom-Terborg for proofreading the manuscript and Diane Schad for excellent graphics assistance. S.H.E.K. acknowledges financial support from Bundesministerium für Bildung und Forschung (Joint Project Mykobakterielle Infektionen, Competence Networks Neue Methoden zur Erfassung des Gesamtproteoms von Bakterien, and Genomforschung an Pathogenen Bakterien), E.C. (TB Vaccine Cluster, European Bacterial Proteomics Network, and Structural and Functional Genomics of *M. tuberculosis*), German Science Foundation (SFB 421 and Priority Program Neue Vakzinierungsstrategien), World Health Organization Global Program for Vaccines and Immunization–Vaccine Research and Development (Rational Design of Anti-TB Vaccines), and Fonds der Chemischen Industrie.

REFERENCES

1. Koch R. Die Aetiologie der Tuberculose. *Berl Klin Wochenschr* 1882;19:221–230.
2. Borrel A, Metchnikoff M. Tuberculose pulmonaire expérimentale. *Ann l'Institute Pasteur* 1893;8:594–625.
3. Koch R. Weitere Mittheilungen über ein Heilverfahren gegen Tuberculose. *Dtsch Med Wochenschr* 1890;16:1029–1032.
4. Helmholtz HF. Über passive Übertragung der Tuberkulin-Überempfindlichkeit bei Meerschweinchen. *Z Immunitutsforsch* 1909;3:370.
5. Bail O. Übertragung der Tuberkulinempfindlichkeit, 1. Teil. *Z Immunitatsforsch* 1910;4:470.
6. Chase MW. The cellular transfer of cutaneous hypersensitivity to tuberculin. *Proc Soc Exp Biol* 1945;59:134.
7. Landsteiner K, Chase MW. Experiments on transfer of cutaneous sensitivity to simple chemical compounds. *Proc Soc Exp Biol* 1942;49:688.
8. Lawrence HS. The cellular transfer of cutaneous hypersensitivity to tuberculin in man. *Proc Soc Exp Biol* 1949;71:516.
9. Wesslén T. Passive transfer of tuberculin hypersensitivity by viable lymphocytes from the thoracic duct. *Acta Tuberc Scand* 1952;26:38.
10. Coe JE, Feldmann JD, Lee S. Immunologic competence of thoracic duct cells. I. Delayed hypersensitivity. *J Exp Med* 1966;123:267–281.
11. North RJ. T-cell dependence of macrophage activation and mobilization during infection with *Mycobacterium tuberculosis*. *Infect Immun* 1974;10:66–71.
12. Patterson RJ, Youmans GP. Demonstration in tissue culture of lymphocyte-mediated immunity to tuberculosis. *Infect Immun* 1970;1:600–603.
13. Bloom BR, Bennett B. Mechanism of a reaction *in vitro* associated with delayed-type hypersensitivity. *Science* 1966;153:80–82.
14. David JR. Delayed hypersensitivity *in vitro*: its mediation by cell-free substances formed by lymphoid cell-antigen interaction. *Proc Natl Acad Sci U S A* 1966;56:72–77.
15. Metchnikoff E. *Immunity in infective diseases*. Cambridge: University Press, 1905:591.
16. Mackaness GB. The monocyte in cellular immunity. *Semin Hematol* 1970;7:172–184.
17. Lurie MB. Studies on the mechanism of immunity in tuberculosis. The fate of tubercle bacilli ingested by mononuclear phagocytes derived from normal and immunized animals. *J Exp Med* 1942;75:247–268.
18. Suter E. The multiplication of tubercle bacilli within normal phagocytes in tissue culture. *J Exp Med* 1952;96:137.
19. Ulrichs T, Kaufmann SH. Mycobacterial persistence and immunity. *Front Biosci* 2002;7:D458–D469.
20. Ernst JD. Macrophage receptors for *Mycobacterium tuberculosis*. *Infect Immun* 1998;66:1277–1281.
21. Ehlers MR, Daffe M. Interactions between *Mycobacterium tuberculosis* and host cells: are mycobacterial sugars the key? *Trends Microbiol* 1998;6:328–335.
22. Means TK, Lien E, Yoshimura A, et al. The CD14 ligands lipoarabinomannan and lipopolysaccharide differ in their requirement for Toll-like receptors. *J Immunol* 1999;163:6748–6755.
23. Means TK, Wang S, Lien E, et al. Human toll-like receptors mediate cellular activation by *Mycobacterium tuberculosis*. *J Immunol* 1999;163:3920–3927.
24. Iho S, Yamamoto T, Takahashi T, et al. Oligodeoxynucleotides containing palindrome sequences with internal 5′-CpG-3′ act directly on human NK and activated T cells to induce IFN-gamma production *in vitro*. *J Immunol* 1999;163:3642–3652.
25. Takeshita F, Leifer CA, Gursel I, et al. Cutting edge: role of Toll-like receptor 9 in CpG DNA-induced activation of human cells. *J Immunol* 2001;167:3555–3558.
25a. Kaufmann SHE. Immunity to intracellular bacteria. In: Paul WE, ed. *Fundamental immunology*, 5th ed. Philadelphia: Lippincott Williams & Wilkins, 2003:1229–1261.
26. Armstrong JA, Hart PD. Phagosome-lysosome interactions in cultured macrophages infected with virulent tubercle bacilli. Reversal of the usual nonfusion pattern and observations on bacterial survival. *J Exp Med* 1975;142:1–16.
27. Le CV, Cols C, Maridonneau-Parini I. Nonopsonic phagocytosis of zymosan and *Mycobacterium kansasii* by CR3 (CD11b/CD18) involves distinct molecular determinants and is or is not coupled with NADPH oxidase activation. *Infect Immun* 2000;68:4736–4745.
28. Gatfield J, Pieters J. Essential role for cholesterol in entry of mycobacteria into macrophages. *Science* 2000;288:1647–1650.
29. Tabira Y, Ohara N, Ohara N, et al. The 16-kDa alpha-crystallin-like protein of *Mycobacterium bovis* BCG is produced under conditions of oxygen deficiency and is associated with ribosomes. *Res Microbiol* 1998;149:255–264.
30. Cunningham AF, Spreadbury CL. Mycobacterial stationary phase induced by low oxygen tension: cell wall thickening and localization of the 16-kilodalton alpha-crystallin homolog. *J Bacteriol* 1998;180:801–808.
31. McKinney JD, Honer zu BK, Munoz-Elias EJ, et al. Persistence of *Mycobacterium tuberculosis* in macrophages and mice requires the glyoxylate shunt enzyme isocitrate lyase. *Nature* 2000;406:735–738.
32. Losana G, Rigamonti L, Borghi I, et al. Requirement for both IL-12 and IFN-gamma signaling pathways in optimal IFN-gamma production by human T cells. *Eur J Immunol* 2002;32:693–700.
33. Flynn JL, Chan J. Immunology of tuberculosis. *Annu Rev Immunol* 2001;19:93–129.
34. Altare F, Lammas D, Revy P, et al. Inherited interleukin 12 deficiency in a child with bacille Calmette-Guerin and *Salmonella enteritidis* disseminated infection. *J Clin Invest* 1998;102:2035–2040.

35. Ottenhoff TH, Kumararatne D, Casanova JL. Novel human immunodeficiencies reveal the essential role of type-I cytokines in immunity to intracellular bacteria. *Immunol Today* 1998;19: 491–494.
36. Shiloh MU, Nathan CF. Reactive nitrogen intermediates and the pathogenesis of *Salmonella* and mycobacteria. *Curr Opin Microbiol* 2000;3:35–42.
37. MacMicking J, Xie QW, Nathan C. Nitric oxide and macrophage function. *Annu Rev Immunol* 1997;15:323–350.
38. Bryk R, Lima CD, Erdjument-Bromage H, et al. Metabolic enzymes of mycobacteria linked to antioxidant defense by a thioredoxin-like protein. *Science* 2002;295:1073–1077.
39. MacMicking JD, North RJ, LaCourse R, et al. Identification of nitric oxide synthase as a protective locus against tuberculosis. *Proc Natl Acad Sci U S A* 1997;94:5243–5248.
40. Flynn JL, Scanga CA, Tanaka KE, et al. Effects of aminoguanidine on latent murine tuberculosis. *J Immunol* 1998;160:1796–1803.
41. Flesch IE, Kaufmann SH. Role of cytokines in tuberculosis. *Immunobiology* 1992;189:316–339.
42. Appelberg R. Protective role of interferon gamma, tumor necrosis factor alpha and interleukin-6 in *Mycobacterium tuberculosis* and *M. avium* infections. *Immunobiology* 1994;191:520–525.
43. Ogawa T, Uchida H, Kusumoto Y, et al. Increase in tumor necrosis factor alpha- and interleukin-6-secreting cells in peripheral blood mononuclear cells from subjects infected with *Mycobacterium tuberculosis*. *Infect Immun* 1991;59:3021–3025.
44. Lukacs NW, Chensue SW, Strieter RM, et al. Inflammatory granuloma formation is mediated by TNF-alpha-inducible intercellular adhesion molecule-1. *J Immunol* 1994;152:5883–5889.
45. Aung H, Toossi Z, McKenna SM, et al. Expression of transforming growth factor-beta but not tumor necrosis factor-alpha, interferon-gamma, and interleukin-4 in granulomatous lung lesions in tuberculosis. *Tuber Lung Dis* 2000;80:61–67.
46. Marshall BG, Wangoo A, Cook HT, et al. Increased inflammatory cytokines and new collagen formation in cutaneous tuberculosis and sarcoidosis. *Thorax* 1996;51:1253–1261.
47. Briscoe H, Roach DR, Meadows N, et al. A novel tumor necrosis factor (TNF) mimetic peptide prevents recrudescence of *Mycobacterium bovis* bacillus Calmette-Guerin (BCG) infection in CD4+ T cell-depleted mice. *J Leukoc Biol* 2000;68:538–544.
48. Roach DR, Briscoe H, Baumgart K, et al. Tumor necrosis factor (TNF) and a TNF-mimetic peptide modulate the granulomatous response to *Mycobacterium bovis* BCG infection *in vivo*. *Infect Immun* 1999;67:5473–5476.
49. Mohan VP, Scanga CA, Yu K, et al. Effects of tumor necrosis factor alpha on host immune response in chronic persistent tuberculosis: possible role for limiting pathology. *Infect Immun* 2001; 69:1847–1855.
50. Roach DR, Briscoe H, Saunders B, et al. Secreted lymphotoxin-alpha is essential for the control of an intracellular bacterial infection. *J Exp Med* 2001;193:239–246.
51. Olobo JO, Geletu M, Demissie A, et al. Circulating TNF-alpha, TGF-beta, and IL-10 in tuberculosis patients and healthy contacts. *Scand J Immunol* 2001;53:85–91.
52. Maini R, St Clair EW, Breedveld F, et al. Infliximab (chimeric anti-tumour necrosis factor alpha monoclonal antibody) versus placebo in rheumatoid arthritis patients receiving concomitant methotrexate: a randomised phase III trial. ATTRACT Study Group. *Lancet* 1999;354:1932–1939.
53. Keane J, Gershon S, Wise RP, et al. Tuberculosis associated with infliximab, a tumor necrosis factor alpha-neutralizing agent. *N Engl J Med* 2001;45:1098–1104.
54. Hogaboam CM, Bone-Larson CL, Lipinski S, et al. Differential monocyte chemoattractant protein-1 and chemokine receptor 2 expression by murine lung fibroblasts derived from Th1- and

Th2-type pulmonary granuloma models. *J Immunol* 1999;163: 2193–2201.
55. Warmington KS, Boring L, Ruth JH, et al. Effect of C-C chemokine receptor 2 (CCR2) knockout on type-2 (schistosomal antigen-elicited) pulmonary granuloma formation: analysis of cellular recruitment and cytokine responses. *Am J Pathol* 1999; 154:1407–1416.
56. Boring L, Gosling J, Chensue SW, et al. Impaired monocyte migration and reduced type 1 (Th1) cytokine responses in C-C chemokine receptor 2 knockout mice. *J Clin Invest* 1997;100: 2552–2561.
57. Gao JL, Wynn TA, Chang Y, et al. Impaired host defense, hematopoiesis, granulomatous inflammation and type 1-type 2 cytokine balance in mice lacking CC chemokine receptor 1. *J Exp Med* 1997;185:1959–1968.
58. Chensue SW, Warmington KS, Allenspach EJ, et al. Differential expression and cross-regulatory function of RANTES during mycobacterial (type 1) and schistosomal (type 2) antigen-elicited granulomatous inflammation. *J Immunol* 1999;163:165–173.
59. Juffermans NP, Verbon A, van Deventer SJ, et al. Elevated chemokine concentrations in sera of human immunodeficiency virus (HIV)-seropositive and HIV-seronegative patients with tuberculosis: a possible role for mycobacterial lipoarabinomannan. *Infect Immun* 1999;67:4295–4297.
60. Fraziano M, Cappelli G, Santucci M, et al. Expression of CCR5 is increased in human monocyte-derived macrophages and alveolar macrophages in the course of *in vivo* and *in vitro Mycobacterium tuberculosis* infection. *AIDS Res Hum Retroviruses* 1999;15:869–874.
61. Peters W, Scott HM, Chambers HF, et al. Chemokine receptor 2 serves an early and essential role in resistance to *Mycobacterium tuberculosis*. *Proc Natl Acad Sci U S A* 2001;98:7958–7963.
62. Scanga CA, Mohan VP, Yu K, et al. Depletion of CD4(+) T cells causes reactivation of murine persistent tuberculosis despite continued expression of interferon gamma and nitric oxide synthase 2. *J Exp Med* 2000;192:347–358.
63. Caruso AM, Serbina N, Klein E, et al. Mice deficient in CD4 T cells have only transiently diminished levels of IFN-gamma, yet succumb to tuberculosis. *J Immunol* 1999;162:5407–5416.
64. van Pinxteren LA, Cassidy JP, Smedegaard BH, et al. Control of latent *Mycobacterium tuberculosis* infection is dependent on CD8 T cells. *Eur J Immunol* 2000;30:3689–3698.
65. Rolph MS, Raupach B, Kobernick HH, et al. MHC class Ia-restricted T cells partially account for beta2-microglobulin-dependent resistance to *Mycobacterium tuberculosis*. *Eur J Immunol* 2001;31:1944–1949.
66. Flynn JL, Goldstein MM, Triebold KJ, et al. Major histocompatibility complex class I-restricted T cells are required for resistance to *Mycobacterium tuberculosis* infection. *Proc Natl Acad Sci U S A* 1992;89:12013–12017.
67. Cooper AM, D'Souza C, Frank AA, et al. The course of *Mycobacterium tuberculosis* infection in the lungs of mice lacking expression of either perforin- or granzyme-mediated cytolytic mechanisms. *Infect Immun* 1997;65:1317–1320.
68. Sousa AO, Mazzaccaro RJ, Russell RG, et al. Relative contributions of distinct MHC class I-dependent cell populations in protection to tuberculosis infection in mice. *Proc Natl Acad Sci U S A* 2000;97:4204–4208.
69. Behar SM, Dascher CC, Grusby MJ, et al. Susceptibility of mice deficient in CD1D or TAP1 to infection with *Mycobacterium tuberculosis*. *J Exp Med* 1999;189:1973–1980.
70. Mazzaccaro RJ, Stenger S, Rock KL, et al. Cytotoxic T lymphocytes in resistance to tuberculosis. *Adv Exp Med Biol* 1998;452: 85–101.
71. Serbina NV, Liu CC, Scanga CA, et al. CD8+ CTL from lungs

of *Mycobacterium tuberculosis*-infected mice express perforin *in vivo* and lyse infected macrophages. *J Immunol* 2000;165: 353–363.

72. Stenger S, Mazzaccaro RJ, Uyemura K, et al. Differential effects of cytolytic T cell subsets on intracellular infection. *Science* 1997;276:1684–1687.

73. Ulrichs T, Porcelli SA. CD1 proteins: targets of T cell recognition in innate and adaptive immunity. *Rev Immunogenet* 2000;2: 416–432.

74. Porcelli SA, Modlin RL. The CD1 system: antigen-presenting molecules for T cell recognition of lipids and glycolipids. *Annu Rev Immunol* 1999;17:297–329.

75. Apostolou I, Takahama Y, Belmant C, et al. Murine natural killer T(NKT) cells [correction of natural killer cells] contribute to the granulomatous reaction caused by mycobacterial cell walls. *Proc Natl Acad Sci U S A* 1999;96:5141–5146.

76. Emoto M, Emoto Y, Buchwalow IB, et al. Induction of IFN-gamma-producing CD4+ natural killer T cells by *Mycobacterium bovis* bacillus Calmette Guerin. *Eur J Immunol* 1999;29: 650–659.

77. Morita CT, Mariuzza RA, Brenner MB. Antigen recognition by human gamma delta T cells: pattern recognition by the adaptive immune system. *Springer Semin Immunopathol* 2000;22:191–217.

78. Kaufmann SH. gamma/delta and other unconventional T lymphocytes: what do they see and what do they do? *Proc Natl Acad Sci U S A* 1996;93:2272–2279.

79. Shen Y, Zhou D, Qiu L, et al. Adaptive immune response of Vgamma2Vdelta2+ T cells during mycobacterial infections. *Science* 2002;295:2255–2258.

80. Ladel CH, Blum C, Dreher A, et al. Protective role of gamma/delta T cells and alpha/beta T cells in tuberculosis. *Eur J Immunol* 1995;25:2877–2881.

81. Kaufmann SH. Is the development of a new tuberculosis vaccine possible? *Nat Med* 2000;6:955–960.

82. Kaufmann SH. How can immunology contribute to the control of tuberculosis? *Nat Rev Immunol* 2001;1:20–30.

19

CD1 RESPONSE

PETER A. SIELING
ROBERT L. MODLIN

The CD1 family of proteins presents lipid antigens to T cells in contrast to the major histocompatibility complex (MHC) proteins, which present peptide antigens. This discovery unveiled a new range of potential targets for T cell–mediated immune responses to infection. The mycobacterial cellular envelope is rich with complex lipids that distinguish it from most other common microbial pathogens. Thus, mycobacteria would seem like ideal pathogens with which to investigate the role of CD1 in immunity to infection. In fact, CD1 presentation of microbial antigen was first demonstrated from *Mycobacterium tuberculosis* (1). Much of what is known about human CD1 immunobiology has been established through the investigation of mycobacterial disease and points to the possibility that CD1 presents lipid antigens to T cells to promote protection against infection, in particular, against pathogens rich in lipid content.

CD1 SYSTEM

Similar in structure to the MHC class I molecules, CD1 proteins are heterodimers that consist of an approximately 45-kd α chain that is associated with β$_2$-microglobulin (β2M). Five CD1 genes, CD1A, B, C, D, and E, have been identified in humans. The CD1 isoforms are themselves quite divergent, although the human CD1a, b, and c molecules are more closely related to each other in their nucleic acid and amino acid sequence (and collectively known as group 1 CD1) than to CD1d (group 2 CD1) (2). The murine CD1 locus (two genes) encodes human CD1d homologs (3), whereas murine homologs to human group 1 CD1 genes have not been identified. CD1e is thought to be an intermediate between groups 1 and 2. The structure

P. A. Sieling: Department of Medicine, Division of Dermatology, David Geffen School of Medicine at the University of California at Los Angeles, Los Angeles, California.
R. L. Modlin: Department of Medicine, University of California at Los Angeles; Department of Medicine, Division of Dermatology, University of California at Los Angeles Medical Center, Los Angeles, California.

of mouse CD1 and human CD1b have been solved, and they reveal an antigen-binding groove that is narrower and deeper than MHC class I or II (4). Furthermore, one pocket of the antigen-binding groove of CD1 is made up of entirely hydrophobic residues (4,4a), eliminating the possibility of a hydrogen bonding network that might anchor the NH$_2$ terminus of a bound peptide ligand as MHC class I does (5,6). Together, these data and the conserved sequences of the CD1 family in the antigen-binding groove suggest that the family of CD1 proteins bind highly hydrophobic ligands such as lipids. Evidence suggesting an immunoprotective role for CD1 derives mostly from studies of group 1 CD1 proteins, and evidence of a role of group 2 CD1 proteins in antimycobacterial immunity has been mostly negative (7).

ANTIGENS PRESENTED TO CD1-RESTRICTED T CELLS

Identification of lipid antigens presented through human CD1 presents a major challenge to the paradigm of peptide–MHC–T-cell receptor (TCR) recognition. Previously, only peptide fragments of foreign or self-proteins were thought to bind MHC proteins and activate T cells. Beckman et al. (8) identified protease-resistant and chloroform-soluble mycobacterial antigens presented to T cells via CD1. They reasoned that lipids were prime candidates for CD1 antigens and demonstrated for the first time that *M. tuberculosis*–derived mycolic acid could be presented to T cells. Subsequent findings established a clear pattern that mycobacterial lipids and glycolipids activate T cells through CD1 (9,10) (Table 19.1). The identification of the hydrophobic nature of the antigen-binding pocket (4) and the discovery that CD1 in fact binds lipid (11) refined the model to reflect that lipid attaches to CD1 and the charged/hydrophilic portion of the antigen interacts with T cells. A structural motif for CD1b antigens has been ascribed comprising a hydrophilic or polar head group bound to two fatty acyl chains. A prime example is glucose monomycolate, which contains a glucose (hydrophilic) attached to a mycolic acid with two fatty acyl

TABLE 19.1. MYCOBACTERIAL ANTIGENS PRESENTED BY CD1 ISOFORMS

CD1a	CD1b	CD1c	CD1d
Lipids of unknown structure	Phosphatidyl inositol mannoside, lipoarabinomannan Mycolic acids Glucose monomycolate	Glycosylated phosphoisoprenoids	Unknown

chains (10). Lipid antigens presented by the other group 1 CD1 proteins (CD1a and CD1c) have not been characterized to the extent of CD1b, thus no structural motifs have been ascribed. However, a CD1c antigen from mycobacteria, hexosyl-1-phosphoisoprenoid, is distinct in structure from the CD1b antigens in that it contains only a single fatty acyl chain (12). Identification of the precise lipid structure bound to CD1 awaits crystallization of exogenous antigen inside CD1 or elution of natural lipid from infected cells. Such information should also provide clues to the processing pathway of CD1 antigens.

CD1 ANTIGEN PRESENTATION: ON A COLLISION COURSE WITH MYCOBACTERIA

CD1 proteins are expressed predominantly by hematopoietic cells including thymocytes (CD1a through d), B cells (CD1c, CD1d), monocytes (CD1d), and dendritic cells (CD1a through d). Because monocytes/macrophages are the primary targets for infection by *M. tuberculosis* and dendritic cells are potent antigen-presenting cells for naïve T cells, these two cell types are likely the critical mediators in the immune response to mycobacteria mediated by CD1.

Although structurally similar to MHC class I proteins, the CD1 antigen presentation pathway more closely resembles the MHC class II antigen presentation pathway (Table 19.2). CD1 presents exogenously acquired antigens through pattern recognition receptors such as the macrophage mannose receptor (13). CD1b antigen presentation is inhibited by agents that prevent lysosomal acidification (1,9), suggesting that processing and/or loading of lipid into CD1 requires a low pH environment. Processing of a well-characterized CD1d antigen, α-galactosylceramide, is mediated by

a lysosomal enzyme, α-galactosidase A (14). It is likely that the large, branched carbohydrate structure of lipoarabinomannan (LAM) is also processed in lysosomal compartments by glycosidases and possibly lipases before presentation to T cells.

Several studies indicate that CD1 proteins occupy overlapping but discrete cellular locations, suggesting that the CD1 family of proteins survey distinct intracellular compartments. All CD1 proteins are expressed on the plasma membrane of dendritic cells. Intracellularly, CD1b and CD1d are found predominantly in late endosomes and MHC class II compartment (MIIC) (15,16), a mature endosome-derived vesicle where peptide loading into MHC class II occurs (17). CD1c is not found in MIICs but in early endosomes (18). Endosomal targeting of CD1b, c, and d proteins results from tyrosine-based cytoplasmic tail motifs with the sequence YXXZ, where Y is tyrosine, X is any amino acid, and Z is a bulky hydrophobic amino acid. Deletion of the cytoplasmic tail dramatically reduces intracellular expression and antigen presentation through CD1b (19), although it does not affect CD1c antigen presentation (18). The distinct intracellular trafficking of CD1b and CD1c is thought to be owing to the interaction of the cytoplasmic tails of CD1 with adapters that shuttle proteins within eukaryotic cells. CD1b and CD1d contain amino acid residues at the Y+2 position that mediates interaction with an adapter protein that favors endosome localization over the plasma membrane, similar to the lysosomal protein Lamp-1 (20,21). In contrast, CD1c contains a residue at Y+2 that could lead to an interaction with a distinct adapter protein that favors a default pathway to the plasma membrane and recycling to early endosomes, similar to the transferrin receptor (22,23). Interaction of CD1b with an invariant chain may also regulate intracellular localization, as has

TABLE 19.2. CD1 AND MAJOR HISTOCOMPATIBILITY COMPLEX ANTIGEN-PROCESSING PATHWAYS

Antigen Presentation Pathway	β_2-Microglobulin Required	Antigen Acquisition	Low pH Requirement
CD1	Required	Exogenous	Required
MHC class I	Required	Endogenous	Not required
MHC class II	Not required	Exogenous	Required

MHC, major histocompatibility complex.

been shown for CD1d (24). CD1a, by contrast, lacks an endosomal localization signal altogether and is expressed almost exclusively on the cell surface.

If CD1 proteins function *in vivo* to present antigen to T cells, as indicated by studies of murine CD1 (25–27), they must intersect with mycobacteria inside antigen-presenting cells. *M. tuberculosis* attaches and enters phagocytes via complement receptors and/or a mannose receptor (28,29), migrates to phagolysosomes, and inhibits the lysosomal proton ATPase (30), preventing a low pH environment. Mycobacteria-infected macrophages harbor numerous lipids, including LAM and phosphatidyl inositol mannoside (PIM) in antigen-processing compartments (31,32) normally occupied by CD1 proteins. However, CD1a, b, and c are not expressed on macrophages, raising the question of how mycobacterial antigen gets to CD1⁺ dendritic cells. Although mycobacteria can infect dendritic cells (33), the primary cellular targets *in vivo* are macrophages. One possible explanation is that macrophages apoptose after infection (34), releasing blebs containing mycobacterial antigens that can be phagocytized by dendritic cells. Schaible et al. (32) provided *in vitro* evidence of such a mechanism. Mycobacterial glycolipids including LAM and PIMs were released from infected macrophages and transported from the phagosome into late endosomes/lysosomes and to uninfected bystander cells. CD1a and CD1c were predominantly expressed on the cell surface and in mycobacterial phagosomes of the early endosomal stage. In contrast, CD1b was present in a subset of mycobacterial phagosomes representing mature phagolysosomes. Thus, mycobacterial lipids and CD1 proteins do intersect at sites where the antigens can be loaded into CD1 for presentation at the cell surface to T cells.

Finally, mycobacteria infection can dramatically alter CD1 expression, which can influence antigen presentation by CD1. Direct inhibition of CD1 antigen presentation occurs by down-regulating CD1 expression (33). Indirectly, mycobacteria can induce interleukin-10 secretion, which can prevent the up-regulation of CD1 on dendritic cells (35). Through these regulatory mechanisms, mycobacteria may disrupt presentation and therefore protective immunity against infection (36).

T CELLS THAT RECOGNIZE LIPID ANTIGENS

Initial descriptions of CD1-restricted T cells that recognize mycobacterial antigens were of CD4, CD8, double-negative (DN) T cells, a relatively minor population of circulating T cells (1,8,9). The importance of CD1-restricted T cells was therefore in question. However, CD4 and CD8 single-positive T cells have more recently been shown to recognize mycobacterial antigens in the context of CD1 (37,38), indicating that most T-cell populations recognize antigen in the context of CD1. The role of CD4 and CD8 coreceptors in CD1–T cell interactions is unclear, however,

because neither was required for antigen recognition via CD1 (37,39). These findings also raise the question of how CD1-restricted T cells are educated in the thymus.

The TCRs on CD1-restricted T cells have the same exquisite specificity for antigen as MHC-restricted T cells; for example, changes in the orientation of a single hydroxyl group on glucose monomycolate eliminates TCR recognition (10). Moreover, cloning of TCRs from CD1-restricted T cells into TCR cell lines conferred antigen recognition (39). Sequencing of these CD1-restricted TCRs indicated a positively charged motif in the CDR3 region that could form electrostatic bonds with the negatively charged carboxylic acid of mycolic acids or phosphates of PIM or LAM. Sequencing of TCRs also showed that the TCR α chains for group 1 CD1-restricted T cells are not invariant as are many of the CD1d-restricted T cells (40). Together, these data indicate that the surface receptors of CD1-restricted T cells likely undergo the same rearrangement as MHC-restricted T cells to establish a high degree of antigen specificity.

ROLE OF CD1-RESTRICTED T CELLS IN ANTITUBERCULOSIS IMMUNITY

Addressing the question of *in vivo* protection from mycobacterial infection has been hindered by the lack of group 1 CD1 proteins in rodents. However, mounting evidence suggests that CD1-restricted T cells contribute to a protective role in immunity to tuberculosis. A higher frequency of CD1c antigen-reactive T cells in patients with tuberculosis compared with naïve donors (12) suggests that the antigen has increased the circulating pool of antigen-reactive cells. CD1-restricted T cells have been isolated directly from lesions of patients with mycobacterial infection whose disease is self-limited (9). CD1⁺ dendritic cells are also enriched in the lesions of these patients compared with patients with disseminated infection (36). Finally, CD1-restricted T cells exhibit functions that are associated with protection against *M. tuberculosis* infection, including macrophage-activating Th1 cytokine production (9,38) and cytotoxic T lymphocyte activity (1) that can lyse *M. tuberculosis*–infected cells (41).

Antigen-activated, CD1-restricted T cells can mediate both direct and indirect mechanisms of microbial killing. Both CD4 and CD8 CD1-restricted T cells lyse infected cells and decrease the number of bacteria (41,42) likely mediated by release of cytolytic granule proteins, including granulysin (42,43). CD4, CD8, double-negative T cells, in contrast, lyse infected cells but are unable to directly reduce the bacterial load (41). Presumably, the double-negative T cells allow interferon gamma–activated macrophages to take up the organisms released from lysed cells and kill the bacteria.

Presentation of lipid antigens to T cells via CD1 likely provides the host response with a greater armament against a lipid-rich pathogen such as *M. tuberculosis*. Localization of mycobacterial lipids in CD1-containing, antigen-presenting compartments strengthens the argument that CD1 presents lipids to T cells *in vivo*. The functions of CD1-restricted T cells also support the hypothesis that these T cells contribute to protective immunity to tuberculosis infection. Additional studies should determine whether activation of mycobacteria-reactive, CD1-restricted T cells *in vivo* will have therapeutic value against tuberculosis.

REFERENCES

1. Porcelli S, Morita CT, Brenner MB. CD1b restricts the response of human CD4-8- T lymphocytes to a microbial antigen. *Nature* 1992;360:593–597.
2. Calabi F, Bradbury A. The CD1 system. *Tissue Antigens* 1991;37:1–9.
3. Balk SP, Bleicher PA, Terhorst C. Isolation and expression of cDNA encoding the murine homologues of CD1. *J Immunol* 1991;146:768–774.
4. Zeng Z-H, Castano AR, Segelke B, et al. Crystal structure of mouse CD1: an MHC-like fold with a large hydrophobic binding groove. *Science* 1997;277:339–345.
4a. Gadola SD, Zaccai NR, Harlos K, et al. Structure of human CD1b with bound ligands at 2.3 A, a maze of alkyl chains. *Nat Immunol* 2002;3:721–726.
5. Garrett TP, Saper MA, Bjorkman PJ, et al. Specificity pockets for the side chains of peptide antigens in HLA-Aw68. *Nature* 1989;342:692–696.
6. Bjorkman PJ, Saper MA, Samraoui B, et al. Structure of the human class I histocompatibility antigen, HLA-A2. *Nature.* 1987;329:506–512.
7. Behar SM, Dascher CC, Grusby MJ, et al. Susceptibility of mice deficient in CD1D or TAP1 to infection with *Mycobacterium tuberculosis*. *J Exp Med* 1999;189:1973–1980.
8. Beckman EM, Porcelli SA, Morita CT, et al. Recognition of a lipid antigen by CD1-restricted αβ+ T cells. *Nature* 1994;372:691–694.
9. Sieling PA, Chatterjee D, Porcelli SA, et al. CD1-restricted T cell recognition of microbial lipoglycans. *Science* 1995;269:227–230.
10. Moody DB, Reinhold BB, Guy MR, et al. Structural requirements for glycolipid antigen recognition by CD1b-restricted T cells. *Science* 1997;278:283–286.
11. Ernst WA, Maher J, Cho S, et al. Molecular interaction of CD1b with lipoglycan antigens. *Immunity* 1998;8:331–340.
12. Moody DB, Ulrichs T, Muhlecker W, et al. CD1c-mediated T-cell recognition of isoprenoid glycolipids in *Mycobacterium tuberculosis* infection. *Nature* 2000;404:884–888.
13. Prigozy TI, Sieling PA, Clemens D, et al. The mannose receptor delivers lipoglycan antigens to endosomes for presentation to T cells by CD1b molecules. *Immunity* 1997;6:187–197.
14. Prigozy TI, Naidenko O, Qasba P, et al. Glycolipid antigen processing for presentation by CD1d molecules. *Science* 2001;291:664–667.
15. Sugita M, Jackman RM, van Donselaar E, et al. Cytoplasmic tail-dependent localization of CD1b antigen-presenting molecules to MIICs. *Science* 1996;273:349–352.
16. Chiu YH, Jayawardena J, Weiss A, et al. Distinct subsets of CD1d-restricted T cells recognize self-antigens loaded in different cellular compartments. *J Exp Med* 1999;189:103–110.
17. Rudensky AY, Maric M, Eastman S, et al. Intracellular assembly and transport of endogenous peptide-MHC class II complexes. *Immunity* 1994;1:585–594.
18. Briken V, Jackman RM, Watts GF, et al. Human CD1b and CD1c isoforms survey different intracellular compartments for the presentation of microbial lipid antigens. *J Exp Med* 2000;192:281–288.
19. Jackman RM, Stenger S, Lee A, et al. The tyrosine-containing cytoplasmic tail of CD1b is essential for its efficient presentation of bacterial lipid antigens. *Immunity* 1998;8:341–351.
20. Ohno H, Fournier MC, Poy G, et al. Structural determinants of interaction of tyrosine-based sorting signals with the adaptor medium chains. *J Biol Chem* 1996;271:29009–29015.
21. Boll W, Ohno H, Songyang Z, et al. Sequence requirements for the recognition of tyrosine-based endocytic signals by clathrin AP-2 complexes. *EMBO J* 1996;15:5789–5795.
22. Simpson F, Peden AA, Christopoulou L, et al. Characterization of the adaptor-related protein complex, AP-3. *J Cell Biol* 1997;137:835–845.
23. Dell'Angelica EC, Ohno H, Ooi CE, et al. AP-3: an adaptor-like protein complex with ubiquitous expression. *EMBO J* 1997;16:917–928.
24. Jayawardena-Wolf J, Benlagha K, Chiu YH, et al. CD1d endosomal trafficking is independently regulated by an intrinsic CD1d-encoded tyrosine motif and by the invariant chain. *Immunity* 2001;15:897–908.
25. Chen YH, Chiu NM, Mandal M, et al. Impaired NK1+ T cell development and early IL-4 production in CD1-deficient mice. *Immunity* 1997;6:459–467.
26. Mendiratta SK, Martin WD, Hong S, et al. CD1d1 mutant mice are deficient in natural T cells that promptly produce IL-4. *Immunity* 1997;6:469—477.
27. Kumar H, Belperron A, Barthold SW, et al. Cutting edge: CD1d deficiency impairs murine host defense against the spirochete, *Borrelia burgdorferi*. *J Immunol* 2000;165:4797–4801.
28. Schlesinger LS, Bellinger-Kawahara CG, Payne NR, et al. Phagocytosis of *M. tuberculosis* is mediated by human monocyte complement receptors and complement component C3. *J Immunol* 1990;144:2771–2780.
29. Schlesinger LS, Hull SR, Kaufman TM. Binding of the terminal mannosyl units of lipoarabinomannan from a virulent strain of *Mycobacterium tuberculosis* to human macrophages. *J Immunol* 1994;152:4070–4079.
30. Sturgill-Koszycki S, Schlesinger PH, Chakraborty P, et al. Lack of acidification in *Mycobacterium* phagosomes produced by exclusion of the vesicular proton-ATPase. *Science* 1994;263:678–681.
31. Beatty WL, Rhoades ER, Ullrich HJ, et al. Trafficking and release of mycobacterial lipids from infected macrophages. *Traffic* 2000;1:235–247.
32. Schaible UE, Hagens K, Fischer K, et al. Intersection of group I CD1 molecules and mycobacteria in different intracellular compartments of dendritic cells. *J Immunol* 2000;164:4843–4852.
33. Stenger S, Niazi KR, Modlin RL. Down-regulation of CD1 on antigen-presenting cells by infection with *Mycobacterium tuberculosis*. *J Immunol* 1998;161:3582–3588.
34. Keane J, Balcewicz-Sablinska MK, Remold HG, et al. Infection by *Mycobacterium tuberculosis* promotes human alveolar macrophage apoptosis. *Infect Immun* 1997;65:298–304.
35. Thomssen H, Kahan M, Londei M. Differential effects of interleukin-10 on the expression of HLA class II and CD1 molecules induced by granulocyte/macrophage colony-stimulating factor/interleukin-4. *Eur J Immunol* 1995;25:2465–2470.
36. Sieling PA, Jullien D, Dahlem M, et al. CD1 expression by dendritic cells in human leprosy lesions: correlation with effective host immunity. *J Immunol* 1999;162:1851–1858.

37. Sieling PA, Ochoa MT, Jullien D, et al. Evidence for human CD4+ T cells in the CD1-restricted repertoire: derivation of mycobacteria-reactive T cells from leprosy lesions. *J Immunol* 2000;164:4790–4796.

38. Rosat JP, Grant EP, Beckman EM, et al. CD1-restricted microbial lipid antigen-specific recognition found in the CD8+ αβ T cell pool. *J Immunol* 1999;162:366–371.

39. Grant EP, Degano M, Rosat JP, et al. Molecular recognition of lipid antigens by T cell receptors. *J Exp Med* 1999;189:195–205.

40. Lantz O, Bendelac A. An invariant T cell receptor α chain is used by a unique subset of major histocompatibility complex class I-specific CD4+ and CD4-8- T cells in mice and humans. *J Exp Med* 1994;180:1097–1106.

41. Stenger S, Mazzaccaro RJ, Uyemura K, et al. Differential effects of cytolytic T cell subsets on intracellular infection. *Science* 1997; 276:1684–1687.

42. Ochoa MT, Stenger S, Sieling PA, et al. T-cell release of granulysin contributes to host defense in leprosy. *Nat Med* 2001;7: 174–179.

43. Stenger S, Hanson DA, Teitlebaum R, et al. An antimicrobial activity of cytolytic T cells mediated by granulysin. *Science* 1998; 282:121–125.

20

DENDRITIC CELLS

RALPH M. STEINMAN
THOMAS M. MORAN

Dendritic cells (DCs) function to initiate T cell–mediated immunity and to control its quality and memory. As summarized in chapter 18 and other reviews (1,2), T cell–mediated immunity is at the heart of host resistance to *Mycobacterium tuberculosis*. There has been a recent intensification of research on the properties of DCs in the lung, and now more investigators are studying the interaction of mycobacteria including *M. tuberculosis* with DCs. However, the bulk of this chapter concentrates on the general properties of DCs and their control of T-cell immunity.

T cells have a unique mechanism to recognize and then eliminate infected cells. The requisite antigen receptors on T cells are not engaged by native antigen and extracellular microbes, as is the case with antibodies. Instead, peptide fragments are processed from the infectious agent within cells and then presented at the cell surface. After microbial peptides are processed, the peptides are bound to the peptide binding grooves of major histocompatibility complex (MHC) products usually inside the infected cell. Then the MHC–peptide complexes move to the cell surface for T-cell recognition.

Highly polymorphic MHC products are of two types. MHC class I molecules [human leukocyte antigen (HLA)-A, -B, -C] present peptides derived from cytosolic proteins processed via the multicatalytic proteasome, whereas MHC class II presents peptides processed from proteins within the endocytic system, especially via cathepsins. In this way, T cells recognize MHC molecules presenting foreign peptides as a result of infection within the endocytic system (MHC class II) or in the cytoplasm and nucleus (MHC class I). A more recently recognized mechanism is that glycolipid components of mycobacteria are presented on the CD1 family of MHC class I–related molecules (3–5). Two functional consequences of these types of antigen-presentation mechanisms are that the T cells secrete cytokines, especially

the protective interferon gamma (IFN-γ), and, in some cases, the T cells kill the infected target through perforin-granzyme– and fas ligand–dependent processes.

DCs are one type of antigen-presenting cell. DCs are particularly efficient and specialized in their capacity to capture antigens and to form MHC–peptide and CD1–glycolipid complexes. Nevertheless, all cells that express MHC and CD1 molecules are able to use these molecules to present antigens. Many investigators use the term *antigen-presenting cell* to refer to cells that initiate immunity, but here we use the term in a literal sense, applied to any cell that uses its MHC and CD1 molecules to present peptides and glycolipids. No further terminology seems required other than to refer directly to the specific type of antigen-presenting cell (e.g., DC, macrophage, B cell) and to the type of immune response under consideration.

In addition to being antigen-presenting cells, DCs exert at least three additional sets of controls on T cell–mediated immunity (Fig. 20.1) that enable them to be critical sensors of infection (6,7). DCs are authentic *sentinels* for innate immunity, alerting the host immediately on microbial entry. The innate functions of DCs include transport of antigens to lymphoid organs (where antigen-specific T cells are selected), production of protective cytokines such as interleukin-12 (IL-12) (8) and IFN-α (9,10), and terminal differentiation or maturation. The changes encompassed by the term *DC maturation* control adaptive immunity, as discussed later.

After these innate responses, mature DCs serve as potent *adjuvants* for the adaptive immune response, enhancing its quantity and quality. DCs bind and expand clones of T cells specific for the presented antigens. DCs then control their differentiation into either Th1 or Th2 helper cells. Th1 cells are more protective than Th2 in experimental infections and tumors (11–13). In tuberculosis, Th1 cells will produce IFN-γ to retard mycobacterial growth within macrophages and may kill MHC class II–positive infected macrophages. Th1 cells have additional protective properties, one being their attraction to chemokines produced at many sites of infection. DCs also help to induce high-affinity memory for future antigenic challenge.

R. M. Steinman: Laboratory of Cellular Physiology and Immunology, The Rockefeller University; Rockefeller University Hospital, New York, New York.
T. M. Moran: Department of Microbiology and Immunology, Mt. Sinai School of Medicine, New York, New York.

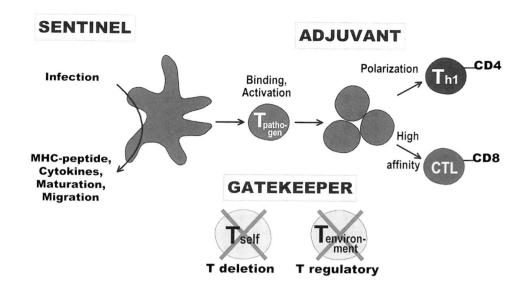

Three broad roles for dendritic cells in controlling immunity.

FIGURE 20.1. Three levels of immune control exerted by dendritic cells. *CTL*, cytolytic T lymphocyte; *MHC*, major histocompatibility complex.

A third level of immune control is that DCs act as *gatekeepers* for immune tolerance, contributing to the vital self–nonself distinction that is essential for immune function. The immune system must defend against tuberculosis and other infections, but it also is important to focus its armamentarium on the pathogen. Ninety percent of individuals resist tuberculosis infection, but when they do, the protective mechanisms are directed against *M. tuberculosis* and not proteins in the airway or self-antigens in lung tissue. This newly recognized gatekeeper function of DCs ensures selective responses against pathogens and not on innocuous targets.

A large part of this chapter reviews DC biology in terms of these three levels of immune control. Then we turn to DCs in the lung, an area that is about to expand given new molecular markers and a new appreciation of their potentially vital role in lung immunology. Finally, we consider the interaction of *M. tuberculosis* with DCs, which also is a topic that is now being approached more vigorously experimentally.

SENTINEL FUNCTIONS OF DENDRITIC CELLS DURING INNATE IMMUNITY

Capture of Antigen for Presentation to T Cells

In the many instances in which it has been tested, DCs prove to be the major cells that successfully capture and present antigens for recognition by T cells. For example, soluble foreign proteins have been injected into animals by many different routes: the airway (14), intestine (15), bloodstream (16), and muscles (17). Then antigen-presenting cells are isolated to test whether they carry the antigen in a form that

stimulates the corresponding antigen-specific T cell. In each case, DCs are the active presenting cells. This efficiency of antigen presentation relative to other cell types relates to DC specializations at the level of antigen uptake (receptors for endocytosis, including receptors for microbial uptake and the uptake of dying infected cells) as well as the machinery for successful processing to MHC–peptide complexes.

DCs express many receptors that have the potential to enhance microbial and antigen uptake. Some known receptors include the macrophage mannose receptor on monocyte-derived DCs (18), the DEC-205 lectin receptor on DCs, especially those in the T-cell areas (19), Langerin on epidermal Langerhans cells and most likely airway epithelium DCs (20), the asialoglycoprotein type 2 receptor on so-called interstitial DCs (21), and Fcγ receptors on most types of DCs (22). Except for DEC-205, the expression of each of these receptors is down-regulated during maturation, as is the capacity to take up substrates by fluid phase pinocytosis and particle phagocytosis. The dampening of endocytic activity has been attributed to an inactivation of Cdc42, a rho family GTPase (23). Nonetheless, the antigens captured by the immature cells are then subject to efficient processing and presentation, as discussed in a separate section.

Cytokine Production and Mobilization of Natural Killer Cells

Cytokines have innate protective functions, and their production can be triggered by infection of DCs. In mice challenged intravenously with particular microorganisms or microbial extracts, the DCs in the T-cell areas of the spleen are the major site for IL-12 production; in contrast, the vast network of macrophages in the marginal sinus and red pulp seems inactive (24,25). Some subsets of DCs also produce IFN-α (9,10,26) and IFN-γ (27) in copious amounts. DCs can directly mobilize natural killer cells (28,29), in part through the production of IL-12 and IFNs. Therefore, on infection, DCs do more than set up the adaptive T-cell response. They quickly contribute valuable innate functions that are considered in other chapters (see Chapters 14–16).

Maturation and Maturation Stimuli for Dendritic Cells

Before infection, i.e., in the steady state, most DCs are at an immature stage of development without potent T-cell stimulatory function. This finding emerged initially from studies of Langerhans cells, the DCs of the epidermis (30,31), but comparable observations have been made with DCs from the spleen (32), lung (33), and various progenitors (34–36). Immature DCs are specialized for antigen capture, whereas mature DCs are specialized for T-cell stimulation (Fig. 20.2). The immature cells express many different receptors for adsorptive uptake as mentioned previously, but most of these are down-regulated during maturation. Reciprocally, maturing DCs dramatically up-regulate several T-cell adhesion and costimulatory molecules, such as B7-2/CD86 (37, 38) (Fig. 20.2). Cytokines and chemokines are also produced, although production ceases approximately 12 hours after the maturation stimulus is applied (39–41).

There are many stimuli for DC maturation, and, importantly, these stimuli are not necessarily the same as the antigens processed for T-cell recognition. In other words, to induce immunity, a microbe must have both antigens and maturation stimuli for DCs. The best understood pathway for DC maturation involves signaling via Toll-like receptors (TLRs) (42,43). Individual TLRs mediate maturation to distinct microbial ligands, e.g., TLR4 is involved in the response to lipopolysaccharide and TLR9 to bacterial DNA and unmethylated CpG (cytosine, guanine) deoxyoligonucleotides. At this time, several distinct mycobacterial products are known to stimulate via TLR2 or TLR4 (44). The tumor necrosis (TNF) receptor family also stimulates DC maturation, particularly CD40L expressed on activated mast cells, platelets, and T cells. It remains to be determined whether different classes of cell surface receptors, such as the TLR, TNF receptor, and hematopoietin receptor families, have different consequences for DC differentiation. Again, for a vaccine or infection to elicit immunity, two sets of events need to take place. There must be capture by immature DCs to provide antigens for processing and presentation on MHC products, but, additionally, microbial products and/or host inflammatory cytokines are required to mature the DCs to become potent stimulators of T-cell immunity.

Dendritic Cells as Specialized Antigen-Processing Cells

The endocytic system of DCs is dedicated to the formation of MHC–peptide complexes and not to full catabolism of antigens and microbial killing, the proviso of macrophages. In the case of MHC class II–peptide complexes, their formation is more than 1,000 times more efficient when DCs capture and process a protein from a dying cell relative to

IMMATURE DC

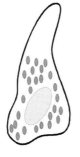

MHC II
lysosome

STIMULI →

Microbial products
(TLRs), TNF family,
NK cells, necrosis,
FcγR, PIR-B, TREM-2

MATURE DC

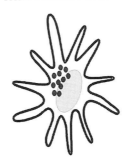

antigen capture

- Adsorptive uptake, eg, DEC-205, FcR
- Macropinocytosis
- Phagocytosis: microbes, dying cells

T cell immunity

- CD40, CD86
- CCR7
- Cytokines, chemokines

Dendritic cell maturation: initiating T cell immunity.

FIGURE 20.2. Dendritic cell (*DC*) maturation, an important control point for immunity and tolerance. *NK*, natural killer; *MHC*, major histocompatibility complex; *TLRs*, toll-like receptors; *TNF*, tumor necrosis factor.

DCs that are fed the preprocessed peptide (45). The formation of MHC–peptide complexes or T-cell receptor (TCR) ligands has been directly visualized within MHC II–rich compartments (46). Immature DCs have numerous MHC II–rich endocytic vesicles that also contain HLA-DM and intact invariant chain (Fig. 20.2). During maturation, proteolysis is stimulated in the endocytic system, including catabolism of the invariant chain especially via cathepsin S (47). One mechanism is that the protease inhibitor cystatin C within the MHC II compartments is removed (47). With the ensuing cathepsin S activation, the invariant chain is "clipped" to produce the CLIP degradation product, and the latter is exchanged via HLA-DM for high-affinity antigenic peptides. The immature DC also is unusual in that it can retain endocytosed proteins for days for subsequent presentation (48). When it finally receives a maturation stimulus, there is active formation and transport of MHC II peptide to the cell surface (Fig. 20.2) in association with CD86 molecules (46,48). In this way, the maturing DC displays aggregates of MHC II peptide and CD86 (the so-called *signal one* and *signal two*, respectively), an ideal situation for setting up the immunologic synapse for effective triggering antigen-specific T cells.

The MHC class I pathway is also regulated in DCs and has some known specializations. The "classic" MHC class I pathway captures endogenous or newly synthesized peptides in the cytosol (49). Peptides produced within the proteasome [the multicatalytic protease that seems to focus on defective ribosomal initiation products (50)] are transported into the lumen of the rough endoplasmic reticulum by the MHC-encoded transporters for antigenic peptides (TAPs). Under the aegis of tapasin, the peptides are loaded onto the newly synthesized MHC class I and transported as to the cell surface.

In DCs, however, nonviable endocytosed proteins can also be presented on MHC class I, and the process is often TAP-dependent. This exogenous pathway is so termed because the peptides are not synthesized initially in the antigen-presenting cell. When intact cells are the source of antigen in the exogenous pathway, the latter is called cross-presentation because after uptake by DCs, peptides cross from the cell of synthesis to the MHC products of the DC. DCs are unusually efficient at the exogenous pathway for protein antigens. Uptake can begin via DEC-205 (51) and FcγR (22), as well as infected cells (52,53) including *M. tuberculosis*-infected macrophages (54). Furthermore, when DCs are induced to mature, they begin to accumulate large aggregates of polyubiquinated proteins (55). Although it may be possible that these are destined for proteosomal digestion and presentation, the function of these aggregates that seem unique to DCs is not yet known.

Ostensibly, the exogenous pathway violates the beauty of MHC-restricted T-cell recognition of infected cells. We outlined previously how antigen presentation allows T cells to focus on infected cells because peptides produced during infection are displayed as MHC–peptide complexes at the cell surface. The exogenous pathway would allow cells that are not actively infected to present peptides to T cells. However, it would be valuable if the exogenous pathway is primarily restricted to DCs. For one thing, DCs would not have to be productively infected to efficiently present peptides on MHC classes I and II. For example, macrophages dying as a result of infection with *Salmonella* pathogens are known to be captured and presented by DCs (53). Another role for the exogenous pathway is to allow DCs to act as gatekeepers (see later) to induce peripheral tolerance in the steady state by cross-presenting self-tissues undergoing cell death and turnover as well as environmental proteins (56).

ADJUVANT ROLES OF DENDRITIC CELLS IN ADAPTIVE IMMUNITY
Priming T-Cell Immunity *In Vitro*

All cells are able to use their MHC products to present peptides, but most cell types are weak *immunogens* or *immune stimulators* with respect to T-cell priming. Instead, immunity best develops when DCs process and present the antigen. Once activated by DCs, T cells carry out the effector limb of immunity by recognizing peptides presented on many antigen-presenting cell types. To summarize, all cells with MHC products can present antigens, which is essential because most cells are subject to infection by one microbe or another. DCs are designed to prime T cells and control many qualitative features of the T-cell response, allowing the activated T cells to act on other infected antigen-presenting cells.

Some of the experimental evidence of the immune adjuvant role of DCs in tissue culture is as follows. Different types of antigen-presenting cells are exposed ("pulsed") to antigens *ex vivo* and then assessed for their capacity to stimulate unprimed or resting T cells (57). In some cases, the stimuli that have been tested do not require that the antigen-presenting cell capture and process antigen, e.g., superantigens that bind directly to MHC class II products (58), mitogens that are directly presented at the cell surface (59,60), or even allogeneic MHC–peptide complexes in the mixed leukocyte reaction (61). In each instance, DCs prove to be potent stimulators of immunity, whereas other antigen-presenting cells are weak and sometimes inactive.

A starting point to understand the potency of DCs is the efficient binding of antigen-specific T cells in culture (57,62) and *in vivo* (63,64). These multicellular DC–T cell aggregates then serve as a microenvironment for triggering T-cell growth and differentiation. In culture, the DCs are observed to continually extend sheetlike processes ("veils") as if it is looking for the appropriate T cell to embrace. Indeed, antigen-reactive CD4+ and CD8+ T cells are gathered in, e.g., in the case of T cells reactive to mycobacterial antigens, and DCs can capture most antigen-specific CD4$^+$ T cells in a day in culture (65). A stable microenvironment thereby develops (but a dynamic one if observed directly because the DC processes continue to move in a vibrant fashion), in which the T cells begin to grow and differentiate while bound to the DC. With time, activated T blasts leave their nests of DCs and are now fully able to respond vigorously to antigens presented on other cells, such as macrophages and B cells (57,62). In other words, a primary immune response takes place in culture in two stages: first, DCs activate vigorous T-cell growth and differentiation (production of lymphokines, such as IL-2 and IFN-γ, and cytolysins, such as perforin) in what is termed the afferent limb; then activated T cells interact with other antigen-presenting cells, such as microbicidal macrophages and antibody-producing B cells, in the efferent or effector limb.

The efficient clonal selection of specific T cells might begin via a recently identified C-type lectin called DC-SIGN [DC-specific, intercellular adhesion molecule (ICAM)-3 grabbing nonintegrin]. This DC lectin interacts with ICAM-3/CD50, a molecule selectively expressed by resting T cells (66). The hypothesis is that the loose binding of T cells via DC-SIGN provides a chance for the T-cell antigen receptor to scan the DC for MHC peptide. Getting an antigen-presenting DC together with the appropriate specific T cell is no small matter. The MHC peptide need only be present in small amounts on DCs [although as mentioned previously, the MHC peptide is coclustered with CD86 costimulatory molecules (48)], so DC-SIGN–mediated "scanning" would allow low-affinity, membrane-bound, antigen receptor on T cells to be selected by DCs.

Although DC-SIGN is the one known DC-restricted adhesion molecule, DCs also express other molecules for T-cell binding and stimulation. Some of these are CD54/ICAM-1, which binds CD11a/LFA-1, and CD48 and CD58/LFA-3, which bind to CD2. The costimulatory molecules include several B7 family members (e.g., CD80, CD86) and the newer family members, such as ICOS-L, B7-H1, and B7-DC. The levels of these molecules can be high on DCs, although levels of expression during different DC maturational states need to be examined further.

DC-derived cytokines also have a stimulatory role for T cells. In the case of IL-12 and IL-18, cytokines that polarize T cells toward Th1-type responses, production by DCs is abundant and peculiarly rapid after microbial stimulation (24,39–41). In humans, IFN-α from plasmacytoid DCs can influence Th1 development as well (67,68). DCs also are able to produce the T-cell growth factor IL-2 early after receiving a maturation stimulus; the IL-2 can then contribute to the subsequent T-cell proliferative response in culture (69). Beyond cytokines, DCs may produce small molecular growth enhancers [cysteine (70)] and inhibitors [produced by indolamine 2,3-dioxygenase (71,72)]. In sum, DCs have a number of mechanisms that help to explain their potency in controlling immunity,

although many of these have only been explored in tissue culture to date.

Dendritic Cells as Adjuvants for Expanding T-Cell Immunity *In Vivo* in Rodents and Humans

One way to establish and characterize the T-cell priming role of DCs *in vivo* is to pulse the cells *ex vivo* with antigens and then reinfuse the antigen-pulsed DCs into syngeneic animals. When this is done, the DCs prime T cells in the draining lymphoid organs. The priming is direct because the T cells only recognize antigens presented on the MHC products of the injected DCs (15,32). To prove this, one primes T cells in an MHC A × MHC B F1 animal. Individual clones can either recognize antigens presented on MHC A or MHC B. If one injects antigen-bearing, MHC A DCs, only the MHC A–restricted T-cell clones are primed, whereas F1 DCs would prime both MHC A– and MHC B–restricted T cells. T-cell priming via DCs leads to protective antimicrobial immunity (73,74). Similar findings can be made with tumor antigens and in humans in whom autologous DCs have been reinfused to expand immunity. As a result, a new field of immunotherapy has begun in which DCs are pulsed *ex vivo* with tumor antigens and then reinfused to actively immunize patients against cancer (75–77) and eventually other diseases (e.g., those caused by chronic infections).

Migration and Homing of Dendritic Cells to Peripheral Lymphoid Organs

An important specialization of DCs is their capacity to migrate and home to the T-cell areas of lymphoid tissues *in vivo* where they encounter resting T cells (Fig. 20.3). DCs move from tissues into the afferent lymph, which takes them to the lymph nodes. This movement to the T-cell areas is valuable for priming because the pool of naïve T cells recirculates through these regions.

The manner in which DCs control their positioning and homing *in vivo* is being unraveled at the level of specific chemokines and chemokine receptors. Macrophage inflammatory protein (MIP)-3α and CCL20 are chemokines expressed in inflamed epithelia, including the antigen-transporting epithelia of mucosa-associated lymphoid tissues and the airway epithelium (78,79). CCL20 may help to recruit DCs expressing the chemokine receptor CCR6 to body surfaces. Immature monocyte-derived DCs express CCR1 and CCR5 (80) and therefore are recruited to the interstitial spaces during inflammation by MIP-1α, MIP-1β, and RANTES (regulated on activation, normal T cell expressed and secreted) (CCL3, 4, 5). CCR2, recognizing the monocyte chemoattractant protein chemokine (CCL2) (81), and CCR7, specific for CCL19 and 21, help move DCs out of the periphery into lymphatics and then the

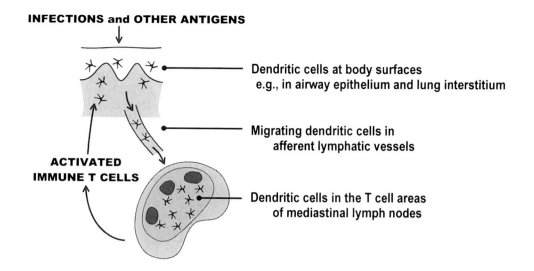

The dendritic cell system: nature's adjuvant.

FIGURE 20.3. Location of dendritic cells in the lung airway epithelium, interstitial spaces, and draining lymph nodes.

lymph node T-cell areas (82,83). Interestingly, DCs express different multidrug resistance receptors (MDR-1, MRP-1) that pump out cysteinyl leukotrienes. The latter in turn enhances responsiveness of CCR7 to the CCL19 chemokine MIP-3β. This is just a sampling of the current work being done to try to understand the remarkable capacity of DCs and their precursors to migrate from blood to tissues and then to peripheral lymphoid organs.

In the lymphoid organs, naïve and central (resting) memory T cells continually leave the blood through high endothelial venules and begin their journey through a network of DC processes. Expression of CD62L (L selectin) allows the T cell in the blood to start rolling on the venular endothelium, while expression of CCR7 provides for activation and chemotaxis to chemokines (CCL19 and 21) present on the endothelium or in the surrounding stroma. Because DCs extend a vast network of processes in the T-cell area, they are perfectly positioned to select T-cell clones specific for the presented antigens. The formation of DC–T cell clusters *in situ* has been visualized in recent years (63, 64). T-cell activation then takes place in the T-cell areas. The activated lymphocytes leave the lymphoid organ, usually via efferent lymphatics, to return to the inflammatory site because of changes in their homing receptors. On activation, T cells lose the L selectin and CCR7 chemokine receptors used originally to home to the T-cell areas, but they gain ligands such as P selectin glycoprotein ligand, active integrins, and higher levels of CD44 needed to recognize inflamed blood vessels and extracellular matrices. These changes in homing receptors help the activated T cell to leave its site of development in the lymph node and home to the peripheral site of infection.

The dynamic anatomy of DCs and T cells in lymphoid tissues parallels in design what one observes in tissue culture. Potent DCs control the afferent limb, picking up antigens and migrating to lymphoid tissues to find and activate rare clones of antigen-specific T cells. Then activated T cells take over for the efferent limb. Activated T cells are modified to seek out the site of infection and inflammation and carry out effector functions in concert with other antigen-presenting cells.

Dendritic Cells Control Polarization of T Cells to the Th1 or Th2 Types

T cells differentiate during an immune response to yield progeny that produce different sets of cytokines and express different repertoires of chemokine receptors. Th1 cells produce IFN-γ for activating macrophages, whereas Th2 cells produce IL-4 and IL-5 for antibody production and eosinophil recruitment.

DCs can rapidly polarize the $CD4^+$ T-cell response toward Th1. For example, DCs from healthy adult volunteers have been pulsed *ex vivo* with antigen, either keyhole limpet hemocyanin protein or MHC class II binding melanoma peptides, and then reinfused. Within a week, antigen-specific $CD4^+$ T cells are primed to secrete IFN-γ but not IL-4 (84,85). DCs can produce Th1 polarizing cytokines such as IL-12, IL-18, and IL-23 (39–41). IFN-α, which is produced in large amounts by the plasmacytoid DC subset during viral infection (9,10,67,68), also can serve to polarize T cells toward the Th1 type.

However, DCs also can contribute to Th2-type responses. If IL-4 or IL-13 is present during T-cell priming, the DCs can polarize toward Th2 (86). Mast cells and phagocytes are sources of IL-4 and IL-13. The microbe itself may influence the outcome, with some microbes causing DCs to produce IL-12 and polarize to Th1 (24) and others, such as yeasts, causing DCs to polarize toward Th2 (87). A fascinating new finding further implicates DCs in the control of Th2 polarization (88). A subset of CD11c-positive but CD14-negative DCs in the blood, often termed myeloid DCs, have receptors for a cytokine called thymic stromal lymphopoietin. This cytokine is abundant in the crypts of the tonsils, mucosa-associated lymphoid tissues that are active in antibody formation, and in the skin of patients with atopic dermatitis (88). The DC subset has thymic stromal lymphopoietin receptors, which includes the IL-7R α chain. When engaged, the DCs polarize T cells to an inflammatory type of Th2 cell, one that produces large amounts TNF-α, but not IL-10, as well as the prototype Th2 cytokine IL-4. In sum, specific microbial products and cytokines work on cells in the environment and through DCs to control the quality of T-cell differentiation.

Dendritic Cells Influence the Development of T-Cell Memory

DCs also can improve the quality of T-cell memory, something that has been tested for CD8+ T cells in humans (89). By quality, we mean the capacity of the T cells to make responses with even lower doses of peptide ligand, also termed improved *functional affinity*. Conceivably, this reflects an improved real TCR affinity for complexes of MHC and microbial peptides. When DCs are pulsed with an MHC class I binding peptide and then reinfused to boost T-cell memory, the selected T cells respond to much lower doses of peptide, i.e., they have a higher functional avidity. An interesting mechanism involves the finding that MHC–peptide complexes can transfer from antigen-presenting cells to T cells (90). MHC–peptide complexes can be abundant on DCs (45,46,91), so despite this apparent "shedding," the DCs will maintain low but sufficient TCR ligand to stimulate T cells. The higher affinity T cells then will be the ones to successfully compete for ligand on DCs, which thereby select a memory repertoire of higher affinity cells. *A priori*, memory cells will be more effective if they are able to respond to lower doses of antigen, especially small amounts of peptide within an infected target.

The presence of a Th1-type CD4+ T-cell response improves the development of memory CD8+ cytolytic T lymphocytes. One relevant mechanism may be that CD4+ T cells help DCs to produce IL-15 (92), which in turn maintains memory CD8+ T cells (93).

A fascinating new path to memory has recently been described in the context of allergic responses in the lung. There, on antigen inhalation, both DCs and Th2-type memory T cells accumulate in the lung, including the bronchoalveolar lavage (94). Importantly, the lung DCs can

continue to present the inhaled antigen for long periods, at least a month.

The capacity of DCs to improve the quality of T cell–mediated immunity will now be pursued in human disease settings. DCs from patients are being pulsed *ex vivo* and then reinfused to induce active immunity, especially against cancer antigens. Many variables need to be worked out in such protocols (95,96). Nonetheless, given the new and improved assays for quantifying cell-mediated immunity, investigators can now use DCs to better manipulate human T-cell immunity to pathogens.

NEW GATEKEEPER ROLES OF DENDRITIC CELLS IN TOLERANCE

Importance of Peripheral Tolerance

One of the central challenges for the immune system is to avoid autoreactivity and additionally, in the case of an organ such as the lung, reactivity to environmental proteins in the airway. A key mechanism for controlling autoreactivity to self is that exposure to antigen during development leads to the deletion of self-reactive T and B cells. Nonetheless, central tolerance is clearly incomplete, both for T and B cells (97). Consider, in addition, that many self-antigens may never access the thymus or may only be expressed after the thymus has populated the periphery with T cells. Furthermore, many environmental proteins enter the body postnatally after the T-cell repertoire has been formed and are constantly being captured by DCs (see previously).

DC biology dramatizes the need for peripheral tolerance and the challenge of "horror autotoxicus," Paul Ehrlich's term for the destruction that the immune system would inflict if it were to react to self. When DCs are exposed to an infectious agent, they must mature to energize immunity. Simultaneously, however, the same DCs are also exposed to self and environmental proteins. Influenza illustrates this. DCs phagocytose and present dying, influenza-infected, epithelial cells (52,98), the hallmark of this infection, and, as mentioned previously, airway DCs are always picking up airway proteins. Yet, after recovery from influenza, one does not exhibit chronic T-cell reactions against the airway or against airway proteins.

These considerations are stimulating research on the capacity of DCs to induce peripheral tolerance (99). An alternative would be that other cells, especially epithelial and connective tissue cells, would induce tolerance, but this would have limited potential. Epithelial and mesenchymal cells are notoriously inefficient in antigen capture and processing, most notably for particulates and for presentation on MHC class II products, which are often lacking. In contrast, DCs in the steady state can carry out several activities basic to the induction of tolerance, including the presentation of antigens on both MHC classes I and II, often by receptor-mediated uptake mechanisms.

Antigen Capture and Migration of Dendritic Cells in the Steady State

In the steady state, DCs continuously sample self and environmental proteins and migrate into lymph and lymphoid tissues. For example, DCs are found in the airway epithelium and in the interstitial spaces of many organs, such as the parenchyma of the lung (14,100). Lung DCs rapidly pick up ovalbumin or fluorescein isothiocyanate–dextran aerosolized into the airways of rodents (14,101), whereas proteins placed into the intestinal lumen are picked up by DCs in mesenteric lymphatics (15). Although these epithelia must serve an overall barrier function, DCs are nonetheless able to capture antigens in the steady state. Capture can be further enhanced by infection because mature DCs can express epithelial junctional proteins and thereby seem able to insert processes between epithelial cells to capture organisms (102). Importantly, the animals are not immunized in the steady state in the absence of infection or inflammation.

Likewise, DCs are able to capture cellular self-constituents, most likely through phagocytosis of cells dying during normal turnover. Epidermal DCs can capture melanin from dying keratinocytes most likely and take it to the lymph node (103). Intestinal DCs can capture and transport intestinal epithelial cells (104). Splenic DCs can capture dying splenocytes (105). Therefore, DCs are the principal known cell type that ferries antigens to the naïve repertoire of lymphocytes circulating through T-cell areas.

DCs continually traffic through peripheral tissues, the turnover being short with half-lives of 1 to 2 days in a tissue such as the lung (106). Then DCs move into afferent lymphatics to gain access to the T-cell areas and the naïve pool of recirculating T cells. The mechanisms that underlie this traffic of DCs through tissues and back into lymph in the steady state are not yet identified. This traffic is occurring at all times, which is likely vital for their gatekeeper role in maintaining tolerance to self and environmental proteins.

Deletional and Regulatory Forms of Peripheral Tolerance

To assess the role of DCs in tolerance, the most direct *in vivo* experiment has been to target an antigen to DCs in lymphoid tissues in the steady state. This experiment has been carried out in two ways: by using an antibody to an endocytosis receptor that targets antigens to DCs in otherwise unstimulated mice (51,107) or by injecting dying antigen-bearing leukocytes that are selectively captured by DCs *in vivo* (108). Then one follows the response of TCR transgenic T cells specific for the antigens that have been delivered to DCs *in vivo*. The antigen-reactive CD4+ and CD8+ cells efficiently recognize the antigen and begin to proliferate actively, but then the T cells are deleted. In contrast, if a DC maturation stimulus is simultaneously administered, the T cells are immunized. Therefore, one pathway to peripheral tolerance is that antigens picked up by DCs in

lymphoid tissues in the steady state delete T cells specific for the innocuous MHC–peptide complexes.

An alternative route to tolerance is the generation of specific suppressor T cells. These T cells can silence antigen-specific immunity, even the response of polarized Th1 cells to mature DCs. The thymus is able to generate antigen-specific CD4+CD25+ suppressor T cells that regulate some types of autoimmunity (109; reviewed in reference 110). It is not clear yet how these suppressor cells are maintained and expanded in the periphery. Conceivably, DCs are playing a role, e.g., they have the capacity to make the IL-2 needed to trigger CD25+, i.e., IL-2 receptor–positive T cells.

DCs may also expand regulatory T cells *de novo* in the periphery, and these T cells perhaps are different from the CD25+ suppressor T cells made in the thymus, although they have a comparable suppressive effect (111). If immature or nonimmunogenic DCs are used to present antigen in humans, IL-10–producing T cells can develop that regulate or dampen responses by Th1-type helpers. In the lung, it is proposed that DCs in the steady state also produce IL-10, which in turn dampens the immune response (112).

For the time being, it is important to introduce this new aspect of DC physiology to mediate peripheral T-cell tolerance. This is likely to be a critical day-to-day function of DCs in an organ such as the lung. In general, the gatekeeper role of DCs is able to control the immune repertoire so that reactivity to self or to nonpathogenic environmental antigens is either deleted or regulated in an antigen-specific fashion. Then when the infection arises, the immune response can focus on the microbe (56). The unknown, as discussed elsewhere, relates to chronic infection (99). If microbial products during chronic infection are captured under circumstances that resemble the steady state, might the DCs induce tolerance rather than immunity?

IDENTIFICATION AND FUNCTION OF DENDRITIC CELLS IN THE LUNG

Identification of a Dendritic Cell Network in Airway Epithelium and Interstitial Spaces

DCs are distributed widely in the mouse (113,114), rat (115–119), and human respiratory tract (113,120). In histologic specimens, the DCs are identified by their dendritic shape, failure to stain with macrophage or B-cell markers, and expression of MHC II and other DC-restricted products (see later). In the upper airway epithelium, the DCs can be visualized *en face* in the epithelium where they have the appearance of a network similar to that of the Langerhans cells of the epidermis. The system begins at the nasal turbinates and extends down the trachea and bronchiolar epithelium (115,117,119,121). In perpendicular sections through the epithelium, airway DCs intercalate their processes between the epithelial cells (117). However, in light of recent findings demonstrating that intestinal tract DCs may be able to penetrate and maintain the integrity of the epithelial tight junctions (102), it is possible that DCs send dendrites into the airway space. In the lower respiratory tract, DCs are found in alveolar septal walls, on the alveolar surfaces, and in the lung parenchyma (106,115, 117). The density of airway DCs ranges from 600 to 800 per square millimeter in the upper airway to approximately 75 per square millimeter in the peripheral lung (119,122, 123).

The ontogeny of DCs in the respiratory tract has been described, primarily in the rat (118,124). MHC class–bearing DCs are not seen until 2 to 3 days after birth if the animals are kept in dust-free conditions. MHC class II–negative precursors carrying the OX62 marker expressed primarily on rat DCs can be observed immediately after birth, but they do not become MHC class II positive for 2 to 3 days, and adult levels are not reached until 21 days in rats (118,125) and as long as a year in humans (126). The MHC class II–positive cells that appear before weaning seem refractory to cytokine stimulation and present antigen poorly (127). This observation has been suggested as one explanation for the increased susceptibility to respiratory infection in neonates (118,127). Class II–positive DCs are first observed in the nasal epithelium, implying that maturation is induced by inflammatory stimuli (124). This is supported by the demonstration that systemic IFN-γ or bacterial infection speeds up the conversion to class II–positive DCs in the trachea, whereas steroids slow it down (118,124). Postmortem studies in children younger than a year of age have confirmed a lack of MHC class II–positive DCs, whereas children who die of respiratory infection have class II–positive DCs in the tracheal mucosa (126).

The turnover of DCs in the tracheal epithelium in the steady state of rodents is rapid, with the half-life being only 1.5 days and the DCs being derived from precursors in the bone marrow (106,121). The presence of allergens or bacterial or viral pathogens accelerates the influx of precursors (128). The turnover in the parenchyma is much slower (10 to 12 days), suggesting some degree of heterogeneity among respiratory tract DCs (106,121,129). It is likely that DCs do not die in the lung, but instead their death occurs after traffic to the lymph node because large numbers of DCs seem to move from the airway to lymph node in the steady state (101).

New Markers for Dendritic Cells in the Lung

The respiratory tract is a major portal for interaction of a host with environmental macromolecules and pathogens. The rapid influx of DCs into the lungs after exposure to inflammatory stimuli ensures that a significant number of immature DCs is always present (130). It is also evident

that turnover rates differ greatly between upper and lower respiratory tracts (106,121). These observations suggest a heterogeneity that might arise from distinct DC subsets or maturational states. Several new DC markers are found in the lung, although more studies are needed to determine their role in monitoring DC numbers, origin, and function.

Langerin, CD207, is a type II, C-type lectin that was first identified in the Birbeck granules of epidermal DCs or Langerhans cells (20). Langerin likely serves as an endocytic receptor to deliver ligands to the Birbeck granules. Although these granules have not been seen in the lung, CD207-positive cells are clearly numerous (20).

DC-SIGN, CD209, like Langerin, is a type II transmembrane protein with a single external C-type lectin domain. It is expressed on monocyte-derived DCs (66), but it has yet to be found on Langerhans cells. CD209 also has an endocytic function (131) but has other significant roles. DC-SIGN binds to ICAM-3 on resting T cells, where it is thought to mediate a loose interaction between DCs and T cells before antigen recognition (66). DC-SIGN also captures the human immunodeficiency virus-1 envelope and is important in transmitting virus to T cells (132). The mRNA for mouse DC-SIGN is present in the lung (133).

DEC-205, CD205, is a type I membrane protein that has ten external, contiguous C-type lectin domains (19). It has been found on some mouse lung DCs (114) but is also detected on alveolar macrophages and the airway epithelium (134). In DCs, DEC-205 is an adsorptive endocytic receptor, mediating rapid uptake of anti–DEC-205 antibodies via coated pits. DEC-205 appears to be additionally specialized for antigen presentation that is beyond uptake. This receptor recycles through late endosomal MHC class II–positive compartments, greatly enhancing presentation of bound ligands (135). DEC-205 greatly enhances the efficiency of presentation *in situ* (107) and mediates the exogenous pathway of presentation on MHC class I (51).

M1204 is a 50-kd mouse DC–restricted protein with sequences homologous to 2′,5′ oligoadenylate synthetase and ubiquitin (136). These sequence homologies raise the possibility that it functions to inhibit virus replication or virus-induced apoptosis. At this time, the only publication on M1204 indicates expression by DCs isolated from the spleen and DCs generated from bone marrow precursors as well as antibody staining of presumptive DCs surrounding the bronchioles (136).

Traffic of Dendritic Cells and Environmental Proteins to the Lung

The movement of DCs from the lungs to the draining pulmonary lymph nodes has been shown by injection of DCs of different origins. Splenic DCs injected into the trachea rapidly migrate to the lymph nodes (137). Bone marrow DCs, charged *ex vivo* with a peptide, rapidly transport antigen to the draining lymph nodes and directly present it to specific T cells (138). Studies using direct inoculation of macromolecules have also suggested DC traffic from lung to lymph nodes and have provided information on kinetics. When fluorescein isothiocyanate–modified dextrans are administered into the trachea, fluorescent MHC class II–positive cells with the CD11c integrin are found in the draining nodes (101). The cells start arriving in the node 6 hours after instillation and peak by 24 hours. They also present the antigen efficiently to TCR transgenic T cells specific for the injected macromolecule (101). Likewise, after intratracheal inoculation of hen egg lysozyme, DCs capable of stimulating hen egg lysozyme–specific T cells are found in draining pulmonary lymph nodes for as long as 7 days (139).

In addition to what appears to be a steady-state migration of DCs from the lung to the draining lymph node, there is also a rapid recruitment of DCs into the airway after exposure to inflammatory stimuli (140). Within 30 minutes of exposure to heat-killed bacteria, an influx of MHC class II–bearing DCs is evident in tracheal tissue. Peak influx is 2 hours after exposure and reaches levels three to four times higher than steady-state numbers. Over the next 2 days, there is an exodus of DCs to the nodes, restoring DC numbers to the steady state by 72 hours. This recruitment can be initiated by bacteria, virus, or soluble protein antigens with slightly different kinetics (130,141). The immigration of DCs seems to be mediated by a number of chemotactic stimuli to which these cells are responsive including chemokines, complement cleavage products, and bacterial f-met-leu-phe (128,130).

Spectrum of Potential Immune Responses via Pulmonary Dendritic Cells

The respiratory epithelium is exposed to many antigenic substances, most of which are handled by such innate defenses as the mucociliary escalator and phagocytosis. Both nonpathogenic and pathogenic substances, however, evade these innate clearance mechanisms. Therefore, the respiratory tract must be capable of coordinating the type of response based on the nature of the inhaled substance. DCs probably play an essential role in this coordination (125, 142).

One type of response is that an environmental protein is simply ignored. Another possibility is that inhaled antigens elicit a Th2-type response, as evident in rodents (143,144) and humans (145). This response is characterized by the induction of immunoglobulin E antibodies and the production of Th2 cytokines (IL-4 and IL-5) in regional lymph nodes (146). Repeated exposure to an antigen can lead to suppression by CD8$^+$ T cells with $\gamma\delta$ TCRs (147–149). A role of $\gamma\delta$ CD8$^+$ cells in suppression has not been found by others (112,150,151). These latter studies have demonstrated that after respiratory exposure to antigens, IL-10–expressing DCs migrate to draining lymph nodes and stimulate the development of CD4$^+$ regulatory T cells that render the mice hyporesponsive to antigen.

The maturation state of the DC influences the type of response that is generated (142). Freshly collected rat lung DCs express an immature phenotype characterized by low expression of MHC class II and costimulatory molecules, poor stimulatory activity in the mixed leukocyte reaction, high endocytic activity, and production of IL-10 (142). After incubation with ovalbumin and injection *in vivo*, these cells only stimulate a weak Th2 response. Such a weak response may represent a prelude or obligatory step toward the generation of T regulatory cells (112). In contrast, after overnight incubation with granulocyte-macrophage colony-stimulating factor, respiratory tract DCs curtail IL-10 production and endocytosis but express high levels of MHC class II and CD86. The cells then stimulate a robust MLR and elicit strong mixed Th1/Th2 responses to protein antigens on injection *in vivo*. Further stimulation of the DCs with TNF, CD40L, or an infectious agent seems necessary to elicit production of IL-12 p70 (142).

In contrast to the response to the previously discussed nonpathogenic aerosol antigens, the response to influenza virus infection is profoundly Th1 in nature, characterized by the production of IFN-γ but not IL-4, strong generation of cytotoxic T cells, and production of complement-fixing antibodies (152–154). Together, these results suggest that *in vivo*, lung DCs are in an immature state, producing IL-10 and priming either Th2 or T regulatory responses. Manipulations that lead to DC maturation gives rise to more protective Th1-type responses (125).

Allergic sensitization seems to require the generation and maintenance of a stable and strong Th2 response (155–157). This may require DCs (158). It is unclear why Th2 responses develop in some individuals but not others. It has been speculated that precocious maturation of lung DCs is involved in chronic asthma (121,129). This is supported by findings in transgenic mice overexpressing granulocyte-macrophage colony-stimulating factor; they show enhanced responsiveness to environmental antigens (159) that is inhibited by IL-10 (160). Moreover, the airway epithelium of atopic individuals has increased numbers of DCs that are reduced after corticosteroid treatment (161). Furthermore, these DCs demonstrate high levels of CD23, an indicator of DC activation (162). A fascinating new perspective is that thymic stromal lymphopoietin is able to differentiate a subset of myeloid DCs to induce an inflammatory type of Th2 immunity with high production of both IL-4 and TNF-α (88).

Thus, the respiratory tract seems capable of inducing tolerance or Th2 or Th1 immunity. The polarity of the response is at least partially determined by the nature of the antigen, the environment of the lungs at the time of exposure, and the subset and maturation state of DCs.

INTERACTION OF DENDRITIC CELLS WITH MYCOBACTERIA

Uptake and Fate of Mycobacteria in Dendritic Cells

Mycobacteria like bacille Calmette–Guérin (BCG) (74,163) and *M. tuberculosis* (8,164) are internalized by cultured DCs. The addition of IFN-γ and lipopolysaccharide allows mouse DCs to resist the growth of *M. tuberculosis*, but the organisms persist nonetheless (165). Likewise, *in vivo*, BCG can be captured by DCs in mouse spleen, and then the organisms seem to persist rather than grow (166). The addition of IL-10 to immature human cultures can convert immature DCs to a more resistant macrophage type of cell (164). Thus, *M. tuberculosis* can be captured by immature DCs, and there is a possibility that these organisms can persist within these cells.

Antigen Presentation via Infected Dendritic Cells

DCs that have taken up BCG have been used to immunize mice via the subcutaneous and intratracheal routes. Strong T-cell priming to purified protein derivative was induced by the subcutaneous route (163), whereas intratracheal priming led rapidly to Th1 immunity and significant protection against aerosol *M. tuberculosis* infection (167,168).

Protection against *M. tuberculosis* refers to the ability of the immune system to prevent reactivation after a primary exposure (2) rather than sterile immunity. Protection depends on cellular immunity leading to the production of a Th1 response and the cytokine IFN-γ (2,169). After their interaction with BCG or *M. tuberculosis*, DCs respond in several ways to enhance antigen presentation. IL-12 production is induced (8,166,167), as are other inflammatory cytokines, such as IL-1 and TNF (170). The DCs also mature, expressing higher levels of antigen-presenting and T-cell costimulatory molecules (167). This up-regulation can be achieved with a cell wall fraction from mycobacteria, which then signals the DCs via either TLR2 or TLR4 (171) (reviewed in reference 44), although activation is better with live organisms (8). DC maturation in response to *M. tuberculosis* is at least partially a result of autocrine stimulation by TNF-α because maturation is greatly reduced in the presence of neutralizing antibodies to TNF-α (170).

Cytotoxic CD8+ T cells are generated during a mycobacterial infection. Because the organisms and their products have only been detected in phagosomes to date, the mechanism whereby cytolytic T lymphocytes are generated has been unclear (1). A newly recognized mechanism is that DCs capture fragments of apoptotic macrophages containing mycobacterial antigens (1). DCs are known to process antigens from apoptotic material onto MHC class I molecules, the exogenous or cross-presentation pathway.

DCs are also able to present mycobacterial antigens using the non–MHC-encoded but class I–like CD1 molecules (5,172–175). Interaction of mycobacterial components with CD1 molecules can occur in early or late endosome/phagosome compartments (174). The epitopes presented by CD1 are primarily lipids or glycolipids (5,173). T cells with specificity for *M. tuberculosis* lipids can be found in the blood of subjects infected with *M. tuberculosis*, but not in uninfected individuals (5). In response to *Mycobacterium leprae*, CD1-restricted CD4+ (175), CD8+ (176), and double-negative (177) T cells have been identified that secrete IFN-γ. The expression of CD1 on DCs correlates with effective immunity because it is up-regulated in mild forms of leprosy but not more severe types of disease (178).

Evolving Field of *Mycobacterium tuberculosis*–Dendritic Cell Interactions

What are some of the themes that are likely to be unraveled by this new interest in the *M. tuberculosis*–DC interaction? A critical part of the experiments should involve the distinction between live and dead mycobacteria. For example, a macrophage infected with BCG is unable to present antigens from the living mycobacteria, but the same cells seem to be able to present the soluble antigens within preparations of purified protein derivative (179). Therefore, different responses to DCs presenting dead versus live mycobacteria may take place in culture or *in vivo*.

To summarize at the level of the three broad functions of DCs outlined in Figure 20.1, beginning with their *sentinel* functions, there is much to be learned concerning mycobacterial uptake and processing pathways. Conceivably, many of the endocytic receptors on DCs bind mycobacteria, but which ones are expressed in the lung? It is likely that mycobacteria will be able to mature DCs, but are there different consequences depending on the maturation receptor that is used, e.g., Toll-like and non–Toll-like? Cytokines can be produced in abundance by DCs, but which ones are made by DCs responding to dead versus live mycobacteria, and are these immunoenhancing versus immunosuppressive, inflammatory versus noninflammatory? With regard to their *adjuvant* roles, DCs are likely to be potent in eliciting adaptive immunity, but which forms of adaptive immunity resist infection and which resist reactivation of infection in macrophages harboring latent mycobacteria? Do DCs allow the immune system to generate *in vivo* multiple types of mycobacterial reactive T cells, including MHC- and CD1-restricted cells, CD4 and CD8, and others? With respect to the new *gatekeeper* function of DCs, does the immunology of tolerance (deletion, suppression) interface with host resistance to mycobacteria, particularly mycobacteria persisting over long periods? Might suppressor mechanisms be generated if mycobacteria exploit the gatekeeper roles of DCs?

REFERENCES

1. Kaufmann SH. How can immunology contribute to the control of tuberculosis? *Nat Rev Immunol* 2001;1:20–30.
2. Flynn JL, Chan J. Immunology of tuberculosis. *Annu Rev Immunol* 2001;19:93–129.
3. Porcelli SA. The CD1 family: a third lineage of antigen-presenting molecules. *Adv Immunol* 1995;59:1–98.
4. Sugita M, Grant EP, van Donselaar E, et al. Separate pathways for antigen presentation by CD1 molecules. *Immunity* 1999;11:743–752.
5. Moody DB, Ulrichs T, Muhlecker W, et al. CD1c-mediated T-cell recognition of isoprenoid glycolipids in *Mycobacterium tuberculosis* infection. *Nature* 2000;404:884–888.
6. Reis e Sousa C. Dendritic cells as sensors of infection. *Immunity* 2001;14:495–498.
7. Rescigno M, Borrow P. The host-pathogen interaction: new themes from dendritic cell biology. *Cell* 2001;106:267–270.
8. Henderson RA, Watkins SC, Flynn JL. Activation of human dendritic cells following infection with *Mycobacterium tuberculosis*. *J Immunol* 1997;159:635–643.
9. Siegal FP, Kadowaki N, Shodell M, et al. The nature of the principal type 1 interferon-producing cells in human blood. *Science* 1999;284:1835–1837.
10. Cella M, Jarrossay D, Facchetti F, et al. Plasmacytoid monocytes migrate to inflamed lymph nodes and produce large amounts of type I interferon. *Nat Med* 1999;5:919–923.
11. Maloy KJ, Burkhart C, Junt TM, et al. CD4(+) T cell subsets during virus infection. Protective capacity depends on effector cytokine secretion and on migratory capability. *J Exp Med* 2000;191:2159–2170.
12. Nishimura T, Iwakabe K, Sekimoto M, et al. Distinct roles of antigen-specific T helper type 1 (Th1) and Th2 cells in tumor eradication *in vivo*. *J Exp Med* 1999;190:617–628.
13. Christensen JP, Cardin RD, Branum KC, et al. CD4(+) T cell-mediated control of a γ-herpesvirus in B cell-deficient mice is mediated by IFN-γ. *Proc Natl Acad Sci U S A* 1999;96:5135–5140.
14. Holt PG, Oliver J, Bilyk N, et al. Downregulation of the antigen presenting cell function[s] of pulmonary dendritic cells *in vivo* by resident alveolar macrophages. *J Exp Med* 1993;177:397–407.
15. Liu LM, MacPherson GG. Antigen acquisition by dendritic cells: intestinal dendritic cells acquire antigen administered orally and can prime naive T cells *in vivo*. *J Exp Med* 1993;177:1299–1307.
16. Crowley M, Inaba K, Steinman RM. Dendritic cells are the principal cells in mouse spleen bearing immunogenic fragments of foreign proteins. *J Exp Med* 1990;172:383–386.
17. Bujdoso R, Hopkins J, Dutia BM, et al. Characterization of sheep afferent lymph dendritic cells and their role in antigen carriage. *J Exp Med* 1989;170:1285–1302.
18. Sallusto F, Cella M, Danieli C, et al. Dendritic cells use macropinocytosis and the mannose receptor to concentrate antigen in the major histocompatibility class II compartment. Downregulation by cytokines and bacterial products. *J Exp Med* 1995;182:389–400.
19. Jiang W, Swiggard WJ, Heufler C, et al. The receptor DEC-205 expressed by dendritic cells and thymic epithelial cells is involved in antigen processing. *Nature* 1995;375:151–155.
20. Valladeau J, Ravel O, Dezutter-Dambuyant C, et al. Langerin, a novel C-type lectin specific to Langerhans cells, is an endocytic receptor that induces the formation of Birbeck granules. *Immunity* 2000;12:71–81.
21. Valladeau J, Duvert-Frances V, Pin J-J, et al. Immature human dendritic cells express asialoglycoprotein receptor isoforms for efficient receptor-mediated endocytosis. *J Immunol* 2001;167:5767–5774.
22. Regnault A, Lankar D, Lacabanne V, et al. Fcg receptor-mediated induction of dendritic cell maturation and major histocompatibility complex class I-restricted antigen presentation after immune complex internalization. *J Exp Med* 1999;189:371–380.
23. Garrett WS, Chen LM, Kroschewski R, et al. Developmental control of endocytosis in dendritic cells by Cdc42. *Cell* 2000;102:325–334.
24. Reis e Sousa C, Hieny S, Scharton-Kersten T, et al. In vivo microbial stimulation induces rapid CD40L-independent production of IL-12 by dendritic cells and their re-distribution to T cell areas. *J Exp Med* 1997;186:1819–1829.
25. Huang LY, Reis e Sousa C, Itoh Y, et al. IL-12 induction by a TH1-inducing adjuvant in vivo: dendritic cell subsets and regulation by IL-10. *J Immunol* 2001;167:1423–1430.
26. Gerosa F, Baldani-Guerra B, Nisii C, et al. Reciprocal activating interaction between natural killer cells and dendritic cells. *J Exp Med* 2002;195:327–333.
27. Ohteki T, Fukao T, Suzue K, et al. Interleukin 12-dependent interferon γ production by CD8α+ lymphoid dendritic cells. *J Exp Med* 1999;189:1981–1986.
28. Piccioli D, Sbrana S, Melazndri E, et al. Contact-dependent stimulation and inhibition of dendritic cells by NK cells. *J Exp Med* 2002;195:335–341.
29. Ferlazzo G, Tsang ML, Moretta L, et al. Human dendritic cells activate resting NK cells and are recognized via the NKp30 receptor by activated NK cells. *J Exp Med* 2002;195:343–351.
30. Schuler G, Steinman RM. Murine epidermal Langerhans cells mature into potent immunostimulatory dendritic cells *in vitro*. *J Exp Med* 1985;161:526–546.
31. Inaba K, Schuler G, Witmer MD, et al. The immunologic properties of purified Langerhans cells: distinct requirements for the stimulation of unprimed and sensitized T lymphocytes. *J Exp Med* 1986;164:605–613.
32. Inaba K, Metlay JP, Crowley MT, et al. Dendritic cells pulsed with protein antigens in vitro can prime antigen-specific, MHC-restricted T cells *in situ*. *J Exp Med* 1990;172:631–640.
33. Bilyk N, Holt PG. Inhibition of the immunosuppressive activity of resident pulmonary alveolar macrophages by granulocyte/macrophage colony-stimulating factor. *J Exp Med* 1993;177:1773–1777.
34. Inaba K, Inaba M, Romani N, et al. Generation of large numbers of dendritic cells from mouse bone marrow cultures supplemented with granulocyte/macrophage colony-stimulating factor. *J Exp Med* 1992;176:1693–1702.
35. Bender A, Sapp M, Schuler G, et al. Improved methods for the generation of dendritic cells from nonproliferating progenitors in human blood. *J Immunol Methods* 1996;196:121–135.
36. Romani N, Reider D, Heuer M, et al. Generation of mature dendritic cells from human blood: an improved method with special regard to clinical applicability. *J Immunol Methods* 1996;196:137–151.
37. Inaba K, Witmer-Pack M, Inaba M, et al. The tissue distribution of the B7-2 costimulator in mice: abundant expression on dendritic cells in situ and during maturation *in vitro*. *J Exp Med* 1994;180:1849–1860.
38. Caux C, Vanbervliet B, Massacrier C, et al. B70/B7-2 is identical to CD86 and is the major functional ligand for CD28 expressed on human dendritic cells. *J Exp Med* 1994;180:1841–1847.
39. Ebner S, Ratzinger G, Krosbacher B, et al. Production of interleukin-12 by human monocyte-derived dendritic cells is optimal when the stimulus is given at the onset of maturation, and is further enhanced by interleukin-4. *J Immunol* 2001;166:633–641.

40. Kalinski P, Schuitemaker JH, Hilkens CM, et al. Final maturation of dendritic cells is associated with impaired responsiveness to IFN-γ and to bacterial IL-12 inducers: decreased ability of mature dendritic cells to produce IL-12 during the interaction with Th cells. *J Immunol* 1999;162:3231–3236.

41. Langenkamp A, Messi M, Lanzavecchia A, et al. Kinetics of dendritic cell activation: impact on priming of Th1, Th2 and nonpolarized T cells. *Nat Immunol* 2000;1:311–316.

42. Kaisho T, Akira S. Dendritic-cell function in Toll-like receptor- and MyD88-knockout mice. *Trends Immunol* 2001;22: 78–83.

43. Horng T, Barton GM, Medzhitov R. TIRAP: an adapter molecule in the Toll signaling pathway. *Nat Immunol* 2001;2: 835–841.

44. Stenger S, Modlin RL. Control of *Mycobacterium tuberculosis* through mammalian Toll-like receptors. *Curr Opin Immunol* 2002;14:452–457.

45. Inaba K, Turley S, Yamaide F, et al. Efficient presentation of phagocytosed cellular fragments on the MHC class II products of dendritic cells. *J Exp Med* 1998;188:2163–2173.

46. Inaba K, Turley S, Iyoda T, et al. The formation of immunogenic MHC class II- peptide ligands in lysosomal compartments of dendritic cells is regulated by inflammatory stimuli. *J Exp Med* 2000;191:927–936.

47. Pierre P, Mellman I. Developmental regulation of invariant chain proteolysis controls MHC class II trafficking in mouse dendritic cells. *Cell* 1998;93:1135–1145.

48. Turley SJ, Inaba K, Garrett WS, et al. Transport of peptide-MHC class II complexes in developing dendritic cells. *Science* 2000;288:522–527.

49. Townsend ARM, Rothbard J, Gotch FM, et al. The epitopes of influenza nucleoprotein recognized by cytotoxic T lymphocytes can be defined with short synthetic peptides. *Cell* 1986;44: 959–968.

50. Schubert U, Anton LC, Gibbs J, et al. Rapid degradation of a large fraction of newly synthesized proteins by proteasomes. *Nature* 2000;404:770–774.

51. Bonifaz L, Bonnyay D, Mahnke K, et al. Efficient targeting of protein antigens to the dendritic cell receptor DEC-205 in the steady state leads to antigen presentation on MHC class I products and peripheral CD8$^+$ T cell tolerance. *J Exp Med* 2002;196: 1627–1638.

52. Albert ML, Pearce SFA, Francisco LM, et al. Immature dendritic cells phagocytose apoptotic cells via $\alpha_v\beta_5$ and CD36, and cross-present antigens to cytotoxic T lymphocytes. *J Exp Med* 1998;188:1359–1368.

53. Yrlid U, Wick MJ. *Salmonella*-induced apoptosis of infected macrophages results in presentation of a bacteria-encoded antigen after uptake by bystander dendritic cells. *J Exp Med* 2000; 191:613–623.

54. Schaible UE, Winau F, Fischer K, et al. Apoptosis facilitates antigen recognition by MHC-1 and CD-1 restricted T-lymphocytes in tuberculosis. 2003 *(submitted)*.

55. Lelouard H, Gatti E, Capello F, et al. Transient aggregation of ubiquinated proteins during dendritic cell maturation. *Nature* 2002;417:177–182.

56. Steinman RM, Turley S, Mellman I, et al. The induction of tolerance by dendritic cells that have captured apoptotic cells. *J Exp Med* 2000;191:411–416.

57. Inaba K, Steinman RM. Protein-specific helper T lymphocyte formation initiated by dendritic cells. *Science* 1985;229: 475–479.

58. Bhardwaj N, Young JW, Nisanian AJ, et al. Small amounts of superantigen, when presented on dendritic cells, are sufficient to initiate T cell responses. *J Exp Med* 1993;178:633–642.

59. Klinkert WEF, Labadie JH, Bowers WE. Accessory and stimu-

60. Austyn JM, Steinman RM, Weinstein DE, et al. Dendritic cells initiate a two-stage mechanism for T lymphocyte proliferation. *J Exp Med* 1983;157:1101–1115.

61. Steinman RM, Witmer MD. Lymphoid dendritic cells are potent stimulators of the primary mixed leukocyte reaction in mice. *Proc Natl Acad Sci U S A* 1978;75:5132–5136.

62. Inaba K, Steinman RM. Resting and sensitized T lymphocytes exhibit distinct stimulatory [antigen-presenting cell] requirements for growth and lymphokine release. *J Exp Med* 1984;160: 1717–1735.

63. Ingulli E, Mondino A, Khoruts A, et al. *In vivo* detection of dendritic cell antigen presentation to CD4+ T cells. *J Exp Med* 1997;185:2133–2141.

64. Matsuno K, Ezaki T, Kudo S, et al. A life stage of particle-laden rat dendritic cells in vivo: their terminal division, active phagocytosis and translocation from the liver to hepatic lymph. *J Exp Med* 1996;183:1865–1878.

65. Pancholi P, Steinman RM, Bhardwaj N. Dendritic cells efficiently immunoselect mycobacterial-reactive T cells in human blood, including clonable antigen-reactive precursors. *Immunology* 1992;76:217–224.

66. Geijtenbeek TBH, Torensma R, van Vliet SJ, et al. Identification of DC-SIGN, a novel dendritic cell-specific ICAM-3 receptor that supports primary immune responses. *Cell* 2000; 100:575–585.

67. Kadowaki N, Antoneko S, Lau JY-N, et al. Natural interferon-α/β-producing cells link innate and adaptive immunity. *J Exp Med* 2000;192:219–226.

68. Cella M, Facchetti F, Lanzavecchia A, et al. Plasmacytoid dendritic cells activated by influenza virus and CD40L drive a potent Th1 polarization. *Nat Immunol* 2000;1:305–310.

69. Granucci F, Vizzardelli C, Pavelka N, et al. Inducible IL-2 production by dendritic cells revealed by global gene expression analysis. *Nat Immunol* 2001;2:882–888.

70. Angelini G, Gardella S, Ardy M, et al. Antigen-presenting dendritic cells provide the reducing extracellular microenvironment required for T lymphocyte activation. *Proc Natl Acad Sci U S A* 2002;99:1491–1496.

71. Fallarino F, Vacca C, Orabona C, et al. Functional expression of indoleamine 2,3-dioxygenase by murine CD8α$^{(+)}$ dendritic cells. *Int Immunol* 2002;14:65–68.

72. Hwu P, Du MX, Lapointe R, et al. Indoleamine 2,3-dioxygenase production by human dendritic cells results in the inhibition of T cell proliferation. *J Immunol* 2000;164:3596–3599.

73. Ludewig B, Ehl S, Karrer U, et al. Dendritic cells efficiently induce protective antiviral immunity. *J Virol* 1998;272: 3812–3818.

74. Demangel C, Bean AG, Martin E, et al. Protection against aerosol Mycobacterium tuberculosis infection using *Mycobacterium bovis* bacillus Calmette Guerin-infected dendritic cells. *Eur J Immunol* 1999;29:1972–1979.

75. Thurner B, Haendle I, Röder C, et al. Vaccination with Mage-3A1 peptide-pulsed mature, monocyte-derived dendritic cells expands specific cytotoxic T cells and induces regression of some metastases in advanced stage IV melanoma. *J Exp Med* 1999;190:1669–1678.

76. Banchereau J, Palucka AK, Dhodapkar M, et al. Immune and clinical responses in patients with metastatic melanoma to CD34(+) progenitor-derived dendritic cell vaccine. *Cancer Res* 2001;61:6451–6458.

77. Fong L, Hou Y, Rivas A, et al. Altered peptide ligand vaccination with Flt3 ligand expanded dendritic cells for tumor immunotherapy. *Proc Natl Acad Sci U S A* 2001;98:8809–8814.

78. Dieu-Nosjean MC, Massacrier C, Homey B, et al. Macrophage

inflammatory protein 3α is expressed at inflamed epithelial surfaces and is the most potent chemokine known in attracting Langerhans cell precursors. *J Exp Med* 2000;192:705–718.

79. Cook DN, Prosser DM, Forster R, et al. CCR6 mediates dendritic cell localization, lymphocyte homeostasis, and immune responses in mucosal tissue. *Immunity* 2000;12:495–503.

80. Sallusto F, Palermo B, Lenig D, et al. Distinct patterns and kinetics of chemokine production regulate dendritic cell function. *Eur J Immunol* 1999;29:1617–1625.

81. Sato N, Ahuja SK, Quinones M, et al. CC chemokine receptor (CCR)2 is required for Langerhans cell migration and localization of T helper cell type 1 (Th1)-inducing dendritic cells. Absence of CCR2 shifts the *Leishmania major*-resistant phenotype to a susceptible state dominated by Th2 cytokines, B cell outgrowth, and sustained neutrophilic inflammation. *J Exp Med* 2000;192:205–218.

82. Forster R, Schubel A, Breitfeld D, et al. CCR7 coordinates the primary immune response by establishing functional microenvironments in secondary lymphoid organs. *Cell* 1999;99:23–33.

83. Robbiani DF, Finch RA, Jaeger D, et al. The leukotriene C4 transporter MRP1 regulates CCL19 (MIP-3β, ELC)-dependent mobilization of dendritic cells to lymph nodes. *Cell* 2000;103:757–768.

84. Dhodapkar MV, Steinman RM, Krasovsky J, et al. Antigen specific inhibition of effector T cell function in humans after injection of immature dendritic cells. *J Exp Med* 2001;193:233–238.

85. Schuler-Thurner B, Schultz ES, Berger TG, et al. Rapid induction of tumor-specific type 1 T helper cells in metastatic melanoma patients by vaccination with mature, cryopreserved, peptide-loaded monocyte-derived dendritic cells. *J Exp Med* 2002;195:1279–1288.

86. Seder RA, Paul WE, Davis MM, et al. The presence of interleukin 4 during *in vitro* priming determines the lymphokine-producing potential of CD4+ T cells from T cell receptor transgenic mice. *J Exp Med* 1992;176:1091–1098.

87. d'Ostiani CF, Del Sero G, Bacci A, et al. Dendritic cells discriminate between yeasts and hyphae of the fungus *Candida albicans*. Implications for initiation of T helper cell immunity *in vitro* and *in vivo*. *J Exp Med* 2000;191:1661–1674.

88. Soumelis V, Reche PA, Kanzler H, et al. Human epithelial cells trigger dendritic cell-mediated allergic inflammation by producing TSLP. *Nat Immunol* 2002;3:673–680.

89. Dhodapkar MV, Krasovsky J, Steinman RM, et al. Mature dendritic cells boost functionally superior T cells in humans without foreign helper epitopes. *J Clin Invest* 2000;105:R9–R14.

90. Kedl RM, Schaefer BC, Kappler JW, et al. T cells down-modulate peptide-MHC complexes on APCs *in vivo*. *Nat Immunol* 2002;3:27–32.

91. Inaba K, Pack M, Inaba M, et al. High levels of a major histocompatibility complex II–self peptide complex on dendritic cells from lymph node. *J Exp Med* 1997;186:665–672.

92. Mattei F, Schiavoni G, Belardelli F, et al. IL-15 is expressed by dendritic cells in response to type I IFN, double-stranded RNA, or lipopolysaccharide and promotes dendritic cell activation. *J Immunol* 2001;167:1179–1187.

93. Ku CC, Murakami M, Sakamoto A, et al. Control of homeostasis of CD8+ memory T cells by opposing cytokines. *Science* 2000;288:675–678.

94. Julia V, Hessel EM, Malherbe L, et al. A restricted subset of dendritic cells captures airborne antigens and remains able to activate specific T cells long after antigen exposure. *Immunity* 2002;16:271–283.

95. Steinman RM, Dhodapkar M. Active immunization against cancer with dendritic cells: the near future. *Int J Cancer* 2001;94:459–473.

96. Nestle FO, Banchereau J, Hart D. Dendritic cells: on the move from bench to bedside. *Nat Med* 2001;7:761–765.

97. Bouneaud C, Kourilsky P, Bousso P. Impact of negative selection on the T cell repertoire reactive to a self-peptide: a large fraction of T cell clones escapes clonal detection. *Immunity* 2000;13:829–840.

98. Albert ML, Sauter B, Bhardwaj N. Dendritic cells acquire antigen from apoptotic cells and induce class I-restricted CTLs. *Nature* 1998;392:86–89.

99. Steinman RM, Nussenzweig MC. Avoiding horror autotoxicus: the importance of dendritic cells in peripheral T cell tolerance. *Proc Natl Acad Sci U S A* 2002;99:351–358.

100. Holt PG, Schon-Hegrad MA, Oliver J, et al. A contiguous network of dendritic antigen presenting cells within the respiratory epithelium. *Int Arch Allergy Appl Immunol* 1990;91:155–159.

101. Vermaelen KY, Carro-Muino I, Lambrecht BN, et al. Specific migratory dendritic cells rapidly transport antigen from the airways to the thoracic lymph nodes. *J Exp Med* 2001;193:51–60.

102. Rescigno M, Urbano M, Valzasina B, et al. Dendritic cells express tight junction proteins and penetrate gut epithelial monolayers to sample bacteria. *Nat Immunol* 2001;2:361–367.

103. Hemmi H, Yoshino M, Yamazaki H, et al. Skin antigens in the steady state are trafficked to regional lymph nodes by transforming growth factor-β1-dependent cells. *Int Immunol* 2001;13:695–704.

104. Huang F-P, Platt N, Wykes M, et al. A discrete subpopulation of dendritic cells transports apoptotic intestinal epithelial cells to T cell areas of mesenteric lymph nodes. *J Exp Med* 2000;191:435–442.

105. Iyoda T, Shimoyama S, Liu K, et al. The CD8+ dendritic cell subset selectively endocytoses dying cells in culture and *in vivo*. *J Exp Med* 2002;195:1289–1302.

106. Holt PG, Haining S, Nelson DJ, et al. Origin and steady-state turnover of class II MHC-bearing dendritic cells in the epithelium of the conducting airways. *J Immunol* 1994;153:256–261.

107. Hawiger D, Inaba K, Dorsett Y, et al. Dendritic cells induce peripheral T cell unresponsiveness under steady state conditions *in vivo*. *J Exp Med* 2001;194:769–780.

108. Liu K, Iyoda T, Saternus M, et al. Immune tolerance after delivery of dying cells to dendritic cells in situ. *J Exp Med* 2002;196:1091–1097.

109. Jordan MS, Boesteanu A, Reed AJ, et al. Thymic selection of CD4+CD25+ regulatory T cells induced by an agonist self-peptide. *Nat Immunol* 2001;2:301–306.

110. Sakaguchi S. Regulatory T cells: key controllers of immunologic self-tolerance. *Cell* 2000;101:455–458.

111. Jonuleit H, Schmitt E, Schuler G, et al. Induction of human IL-10-producing, non-proliferating CD4+ T cells with regulatory properties by repetitive stimulation with allogeneic immature dendritic cells. *J Exp Med* 2000;192:1213–1222.

112. Akbari O, DeKruyff RH, Umetsu DT. Pulmonary dendritic cells producing IL-10 mediate tolerance induced by respiratory exposure to antigen. *Nat Immunol* 2001;2:725–731.

113. Sertl K, Takemura T, Tschachler E, et al. Dendritic cells with antigen-presenting capability reside in airway epithelium, lung parenchyma, and visceral pleura. *J Exp Med* 1986;163:436–451.

114. Pollard AM, Lipscomb MF. Characterization of murine lung dendritic cells: similarities to Langerhans cells and thymic dendritic cells. *J Exp Med* 1990;172:159–168.

115. Holt PG, Schon-Hegrad MA, Oliver J. MHC class II antigen-bearing dendritic cells in pulmonary tissues of the rat. Regulation of antigen presentation activity by endogenous macrophage populations. *J Exp Med* 1987;167:262–274.

116. Rochester CL, Goodell EM, Stoltenborg JK, et al. Dendritic

cells from rat lung are potent accessory cells. *Am Rev Respir Dis* 1988;138:121–128.

117. Gong JL, McCarthy KM, Telford J, et al. Intraepithelial airway dendritic cells: a distinct subset of pulmonary dendritic cells obtained by microdissection. *J Exp Med* 1992;175:797–807.

118. Nelson DJ, McMenamin CM, McWilliam AS, et al. Development of the airway intraepithelial dendritic cell network in the rat from class II major histocompatibility [Ia]-negative precursors: differential regulation of Ia expression at different levels of the respiratory tract. *J Exp Med* 1994;179:203–212.

119. Schon-Hegrad MA, Oliver J, McMenamin PG, et al. Studies on the density, distribution, and surface phenotype of intraepithelial class II major histocompatability complex antigen [Ia]-bearing dendritic cells [DC] in the conducting airways. *J Exp Med* 1991;173:1345–1356.

120. Nicod LP, Lipscomb MF, Weissler JC, et al. Mononuclear cells in human lung parenchyma: characterization of a potent accessory cell not obtained by bronchoalveolar lavage. *Am Rev Respir Dis* 1987;136:818–823.

121. Holt PG, Stumbles PA, McWilliam AS. Functional studies on dendritic cells in the respiratory tract and related mucosal tissues. *J Leukoc Biol* 1999;66:272–275.

122. Holt PG, Schon-Hegrad MA, Phillips MJ, et al. Ia-positive dendritic cells form a tightly meshed network within the human airway epithelium. *Clin Exp Allergy* 1989;19:597–601.

123. Holt PG, Schon-Hegrad MA, McMenamin PG. Dendritic cells in the respiratory tract. *Int Rev Immunol* 1990;6:139–149.

124. McWilliam AS, Nelson DJ, Holt PG. The biology of airway dendritic cells. *Immunol Cell Biol* 1995;73:405–413.

125. Holt PG. Antigen presentation in the lung. *Am J Respir Crit Care Med* 2000;162:S151–S156.

126. Tschernig T, Debertin AS, Paulsen F, et al. Dendritic cells in the mucosa of the human trachea are not regularly found in the first year of life. *Thorax* 2001;56:427–431.

127. Nelson DJ, Holt PG. Defective regional immunity in the respiratory tract of neonates is attributable to hyporesponsiveness of local dendritic cells to activation signals. *J Immunol* 1995;155:3517–3524.

128. Stumbles PA, Strickland DH, Pimm CL, et al. Regulation of dendritic cell recruitment into resting and inflamed airway epithelium: use of alternative chemokine receptors as a function of inducing stimulus. *J Immunol* 2001;167:228–234.

129. Holt PG. Dendritic cell ontogeny as an aetiological factor in respiratory tract diseases in early life. *Thorax* 2001;56:419–420.

130. McWilliam AS, Napoli S, Marsh AM, et al. Dendritic cells are recruited into the airway epithelium during the inflammatory response to a broad spectrum of stimuli. *J Exp Med* 1996;184:2429–2432.

131. Engering A, Geijtenbeek TB, van Vliet SJ, et al. The dendritic cell-specific adhesion receptor DC-SIGN internalizes antigen for presentation to T cells. *J Immunol* 2002;168:2118–2126.

132. Geijtenbeek TBH, Kwon DS, Torensma R, et al. DC-SIGN, a dendritic cell specific HIV-1 binding protein that enhances TRANS-infection of T cells. *Cell* 2000;100:587–597.

133. Park CG, Takahara K, Umemoto E, et al. Five mouse homologues of the human dendritic cell C-type lectin, DC-SIGN. *Int Immunol* 2001;13:1283–1290.

134. Witmer-Pack MD, Swiggard WJ, Mirza A, et al. Tissue distribution of the DEC-205 protein that is detected by the monoclonal antibody NLDC-145. II. Expression *in situ* in lymphoid and nonlymphoid tissues. *Cell Immunol* 1995;163:157–162.

135. Mahnke K, Guo M, Lee S, et al. The dendritic cell receptor for endocytosis, DEC-205, can recycle and enhance antigen presentation via MHC II+, lysosomal compartments. *J Cell Biol* 2000;151:673–683.

136. Tiefenthaler M, Marksteiner R, Neyer S, et al. M1204, a novel 2′,5′ oligoadenylate synthetase with a ubiquitin-like extension, is induced during maturation of murine dendritic cells. *J Immunol* 1999;163:760–765.

137. Havenith CEG, van Miert PPMC, Breedijk AJ, et al. Migration of dendritic cells into the draining lymph nodes of the lung after intratracheal instillation. *Am J Respir Cell Mol Biol* 1993;9:484–488.

138. Lambrecht BN, Pauwels RA, Fazekas De St Groth B. Induction of rapid T cell activation, division, and recirculation by intra-tracheal injection of dendritic cells in a TCR transgenic model. *J Immunol* 2000;164:2937–2946.

139. Xia W, Pinto CE, Kradin RL. The antigen-presenting activities of Ia+ dendritic cells shift dynamically from lung to lymph node after an airway challenge with soluble antigen. *J Exp Med* 1995;181:1275–1283.

140. McWilliam AS, Nelson D, Thomas JA, et al. Rapid dendritic cell recruitment is a hallmark of the acute inflammatory response at mucosal surfaces. *J Exp Med* 1994;179:1331–1336.

141. McWilliam AS, Marsh AM, Holt PG. Inflammatory infiltration of the upper airway epithelium during Sendai virus infection: involvement of epithelial dendritic cells. *J Virol* 1997;71:226–236.

142. Stumbles PA, Thomas JA, Pimm CL, et al. Resting respiratory tract dendritic cells preferentially stimulate T helper cell type 2 (Th2) responses and require obligatory cytokine signals for induction of Th1 immunity. *J Exp Med* 1998;188:2019–2031.

143. Hoyne GF, Tan K, Corsin-Jimenez M, et al. Immunological tolerance to inhaled antigen. *Am J Respir Crit Care Med* 2000;162:S169–S174.

144. Lambrecht BN, De Veerman M, Coyle AJ, et al. Myeloid dendritic cells induce Th2 responses to inhaled antigen, leading to eosinophilic airway inflammation. *J Clin Invest* 2000;106:551–559.

145. Yabuhara A, Macaubas C, Prescott SL, et al. TH2-polarized immunological memory to inhalant allergens in atopics is established during infancy and early childhood. *Clin Exp Allergy* 1997;27:1261–1269.

146. Hoyne GF, Askonas BA, Hetzel C, et al. Regulation of house dust mite responses by intranasally administered peptide: transient activation of CD4+ T cells precedes the development of tolerance *in vivo*. *Int Immunol* 1996;8:335–342.

147. McMenamin C, Holt PG. The natural immune response to inhaled soluble protein antigens involves major histocompatibility complex (MHC) class I-restricted CD8₊ T cell-mediated but MHC class II-restricted CD4₊ T cell-dependent immune deviation resulting in selective suppression of immunoglobulin E production. *J Exp Med* 1993;178:889–899.

148. McMenamin C, Oliver J, Girn B, et al. Regulation of T-cell sensitization at epithelial surfaces in the respiratory tract: suppression of IgE responses to inhaled antigens by CD3+ TCRα-/β-lymphocytes (putative γ/δ T cells). *Immunology* 1991;74:234–239.

149. McMenamin C, Pimm C, McKersey M, et al. Regulation of IgE responses to inhaled antigen in mice by antigen-specific γδ T cells. *Science* 1994;265:1869–1871.

150. Tsitoura DC, DeKruyff RH, Lamb JR, et al. Intranasal exposure to protein antigen induces immunological tolerance mediated by functionally disabled CD4+ T cells. *J Immunol* 1999;163:2592–2600.

151. Tsitoura DC, Kim S, Dabbagh K, et al. Respiratory infection with influenza A virus interferes with the induction of tolerance to aeroallergens. *J Immunol* 2000;165:3484–3491.

152. Moran TM, Isobe H, Fernandez-Sesma A, et al. Interleukin-4 causes delayed virus clearance in influenza virus-infected mice. *J Virol* 1996;70:5230–5235.

153. Moran TM, Park H, Fernandez-Sesma A, et al. Th2 responses to inactivated influenza virus can be converted to Th1 responses and facilitate recovery from heterosubtypic virus infection. *J Infect Dis* 1999;180:579–585.

154. Lopez CB, Fernandez-Sesma A, Czelusniak SM, et al. A mouse model for immunization with *ex vivo* virus-infected dendritic cells. *Cell Immunol* 2000;206:107–115.

155. Lambrecht BN, Carro-Muino I, Vermaelen K, et al. Allergen-induced changes in bone-marrow progenitor and airway dendritic cells in sensitized rats. *Am J Respir Cell Mol Biol* 1999;20: 1165–1174.

156. Drazen JM, Arm JP, Austen KF. Sorting out the cytokines of asthma. *J Exp Med* 1996;183:1–5.

157. van Rijt LS, Lambrecht BN. Role of dendritic cells and Th2 lymphocytes in asthma: lessons from eosinophilic airway inflammation in the mouse. *Microsc Res Tech* 2001;53:256–272.

158. Lambrecht BN, Salomon B, Klatzmann D, et al. Dendritic cells are required for the development of chronic eosinophilic airway inflammation in response to inhaled antigen in sensitized mice. *J Immunol* 1998;160:4090–4097.

159. Stampfli MR, Wiley RE, Neigh GS, et al. GM-CSF transgene expression in the airway allows aerosolized ovalbumin to induce allergic sensitization in mice. *J Clin Invest* 1998;102: 1704–1714.

160. Stampfli MR, Cwiartka M, Gajewska BU, et al. Interleukin-10 gene transfer to the airway regulates allergic mucosal sensitization in mice. *Am J Respir Cell Mol Biol* 1999;21:586–596.

161. Moller GM, Overbeek SE, Van Helden-Meeuwsen CG, et al. Increased numbers of dendritic cells in the bronchial mucosa of atopic asthmatic patients: downregulation by inhaled corticosteroids. *Clin Exp Allergy* 1996;26:517–524.

162. Tunon-De-Lara JM, Redington AE, Bradding P, et al. Dendritic cells in normal and asthmatic airways: expression of the alpha subunit of the high affinity immunoglobulin E receptor (FcεRIα). *Clin Exp Allergy* 1996;26:648–655.

163. Inaba K, Inaba M, Naito M, et al. Dendritic cell progenitors phagocytose particulates, including bacillus Calmette-Guerin organisms, and sensitize mice to mycobacterial antigens *in vivo*. *J Exp Med* 1993;178:479–488.

164. Fortsch D, Rollinghoff M, Stenger S. IL-10 converts human dendritic cells into macrophage-like cells with increased antibacterial activity against virulent *Mycobacterium tuberculosis*. *J Immunol* 2000;165:978–987.

165. Bodnar KA, Serbina NV, Flynn JL. Fate of *Mycobacterium tuberculosis* within murine dendritic cells. *Infect Immun* 2001; 69:800–809.

166. Jiao X, Lo-man R, Guermonprez P, et al. Dendritic cells are host cells for mycobacteria *in vivo* that trigger innate acquired immunity. *J Immunol* 2002;168:1294–1301.

167. Hodge JW, McLaughlin JP, Kantor JA, et al. Diversified prime and boost protocols using recombinant vaccinia virus and recombinant non-replicating avian pox virus to enhance T-cell immunity and antitumor responses. *Vaccine* 1997;15:759–768.

168. Tascon RE, Soares CS, Ragno S, et al. *Mycobacterium tuberculosis*-activated dendritic cells induce protective immunity in mice. *Immunology* 2000;99:473–480.

169. Scanga CA, Mohan VP, Yu K, et al. Depletion of CD4(+) T cells causes reactivation of murine persistent tuberculosis despite continued expression of interferon gamma and nitric oxide synthase 2. *J Exp Med* 2000;192:347–358.

170. Thurnher M, Ramoner R, Gastl G, et al. Bacillus Calmette-Guerin mycobacteria stimulate human blood dendritic cells. *Int J Cancer* 1997;70:128–134.

171. Tsuji S, Matsumoto M, Takeuchi O, et al. Maturation of human dendritic cells by cell wall skeleton of *Mycobacterium bovis* bacillus Calmette-Guerin: involvement of Toll-like receptors. *Infect Immun* 2000;68:6883–6890.

172. Moody DB, Guy MR, Grant E, et al. CD1b-mediated T cell recognition of a glycolipid antigen generated from mycobacterial lipid and host carbohydrate during infection. *J Exp Med* 2000;192:965–976.

173. Porcelli SA, Modlin RL. The CD1 system: antigen-presenting molecules for T cell recognition of lipids and glycolipids. *Annu Rev Immunol* 1999;17:297–329.

174. Schaible UE, Hagens K, Fischer K, et al. Intersection of group I CD1 molecules and mycobacteria in different intracellular compartments of dendritic cells. *J Immunol* 2000;164: 4843–4852.

175. Sieling PA, Ochoa MT, Jullien D, et al. Evidence for human CD4+ T cells in the CD1-restricted repertoire: derivation of mycobacteria-reactive T cells from leprosy lesions. *J Immunol* 2000;164:4790–4796.

176. Rosat JP, Grant EP, Beckman EM, et al. CD1-restricted microbial lipid antigen-specific recognition found in the CD8+ αβ T cell pool. *J Immunol* 1999;162:366–371.

177. Porcelli S, Morita CT, Brenner MB. CD1b restricts the response of human CD4-8-T lymphocytes to a microbial antigen. *Nature* 1992;360:593–597.

178. Sieling PA, Jullien D, Dahlem M, et al. CD1 expression by dendritic cells in human leprosy lesions: correlation with effective host immunity. *J Immunol* 1999;162:1851–1858.

179. Pancholi P, Mirza A, Bhardwaj N, et al. Sequestration from immune CD4+ T cells of mycobacteria growing in human macrophages. *Science* 1993;260:984–986.

CYTOKINE RESPONSE IN TUBERCULOSIS

RANY CONDOS
WILLIAM N. ROM

Despite recent successful efforts at tuberculosis (TB) control in the United States, the worldwide epidemic continues to be fueled by many factors, including lack of resources and the human immunodeficiency virus (HIV) epidemic (1). This latter factor may be the most significant in developing countries where HIV and TB infections are highly prevalent. The increased susceptibility to TB infection and disease among HIV-infected patients is directly related to impaired host immunity and has focused attention on host immunity as a strong determinant of disease (2).

Not all patients with TB infection develop active disease, and before effective therapy was available, some patients recovered without specific treatment (3–5). Although it is possible that virulence differences among various strains of *Mycobacterium tuberculosis* may play a role in outcome, it is generally believed that the clinical presentation of disease is tied to the state of the immune system. A better understanding of this host response at a basic level is likely to result in novel approaches to TB infection. The past decade witnessed an explosion of information on soluble proteins (cytokines) secreted by immunoregulatory cells, which modulate the immune response to intracellular pathogens, including mycobacteria. This chapter summarizes our current understanding of the role played by cytokines in the immune response to *M. tuberculosis* (Table 21.1).

CYTOKINES

Interleukin-1

Macrophages are capable of producing interleukin (IL)-1α, IL-1β, and IL-1Rα, a specific receptor antagonist of IL-1 (6). IL-1 is produced on stimulation with *M. tuberculosis*,

R. Condos: Department of Medicine, Division of Pulmonary and Critical Care Medicine, New York University Medical Center, New York, New York.

W. N. Rom: Department of Medicine, Division of Pulmonary and Critical Care Medicine, New York University Medical Center; Bellevue Chest Service, New York, New York.

and specific mycobacterial components, including lipoarabinomannan, a complex heteropolysaccharide embedded in the mycobacterial cell membrane (7,8). IL-1 induces macrophages to produce the proinflammatory cytokines IL-6 and tumor necrosis factor (TNF)-α and stimulates T-cell proliferation by up-regulating T-cell expression of IL-2 receptors and IL-2 production (9). IL-1 is an endogenous pyrogen and probably contributes to the fever of TB (10).

Studies on knockout mice lacking IL-1β showed defective granuloma formation after infection with *M. tuberculosis* (11). In patients with TB, the production of reactive nitrogen intermediaries by infected alveolar macrophages amplifies the synthesis of IL-1β and TNF-α, probably through nuclear factor κB (NK-κB) activation (12). Binding of IL-1 to its receptor leads to activation of the signal transduction pathway, which includes NF-κB, mitogen-activated protein kinases p38, p42/44, and c-Jun N-terminal kinase (JNK). IL-1 receptor I is part of an IL-1R/Toll-like receptor (TLR) superfamily, an evolutionarily conserved signaling system with a conserved cytosolic region of the receptor (13). Microbial ligands, such as lipopolysaccharides and lipoproteins, activate the TLRs on macrophages. A recent report shows that alveolar macrophages internalize and destroy *M. tuberculosis* at the site of infection in a TLR2-dependent manner (14). This report also showed that activating the macrophages with an antigen derived from *M. tuberculosis* or another infectious agent further reduced the viability of intracellular *M. tuberculosis* by a mechanism involving TLR2. Further research will provide an insight into role of these receptors and the cytokines that they induce in the control of intracellular bacteria.

IL-1β is expressed at the site of disease both in cavitary pulmonary disease and in tuberculous pleural effusions (15–17). Circulating levels of IL-1β have been correlated with disease activity and fever in infected patients. In a study of purified protein derivative (PPD)–positive healthy controls compared with patients with active TB, polymorphisms at the IL-1 locus affected cytokine responses. Patients with tuberculous pleural disease had increased IL-

TABLE 21.1. CYTOKINES PRODUCED BY MACROPHAGES AND TH1 AND TH2 CELLS

Cytokine	Macrophage	Th1	Th2
IL-1	+	−	−
Tumor necrosis factor	+	+	+
IL-6	+	−	+
IL-10	+	−[a]	+
IL-12	+	−	−
Transforming growth factor β	+	−	−
Interferon gamma	−	+	−
IL-2	−	+	−
IL-4	−	−	+
IL-5	−	−	+

[a]Interleukin-10 is produced by human but not murine Th1 cells.
IL, interleukin; +, identified in; −, not identified in.

1β levels reflecting a proinflammatory haplotype associated with self-limited disease (18,19).

Tumor Necrosis Factor-α

Human mononuclear cells and alveolar macrophages produce large quantities of TNF-α in response to *M. tuberculosis* and its components (20,21). TNF-α activates both neutrophils and macrophages, leading to protease release, stimulation of respiratory burst, and induction of vascular adhesion molecule expression essential for cell recruitment at sites of inflammation (22). Clinical and experimental data on animals and humans suggest that TNF contributes both to protection against TB and to immunopathology. In favor of a protective role, granuloma formation in mice infected with *Mycobacterium bovis* bacille Calmette–Guérin (BCG) coincides with local TNF synthesis, and injection of anti-TNF antibodies interferes with the development of granulomas and the elimination of mycobacteria (23). Furthermore, TNF-α messenger RNA (mRNA) and protein are concentrated at the site of disease in patients with tuberculous pleuritis who mount a resistant immune response to infection (24).

TNF-α plays a role in the immunopathology of TB. Administration of TNF-α to animals results in fever and wasting (25). Serum levels of TNF-α are significantly higher in patients with lepromatous leprosy with an ineffective immune response than in patients with tuberculoid leprosy with relative immunologic resistance (26). In addition, peripheral blood mononuclear cells (PBMCs) from patients with TB with cachexia and high-grade fever produce more TNF than do PBMCs from patients with TB without these findings (27,28).

Because TNF can exhibit both protective and pathologic effects in *M. tuberculosis* infection, it is intriguing to speculate that production of physiologic concentrations of TNF is important to antimycobacterial immune defenses and that local release of TNF at the site of disease contributes to granuloma formation, control of infection, and mycobacte-

rial elimination. Excessive local production of TNF may cause marked tissue necrosis that is characteristic of progressive TB and may result in TNF release into the circulation, contributing to systemic manifestations of TB such as fever and cachexia. These observations have prompted interest in TNF-α blocking agents as immunomodulators in the treatment of TB.

Thalidomide, a synthetic derivative of glutamic acid, was shown to alleviate the symptoms of erythema nodosum leprosum by inhibiting production of TNF-α by PBMCs (29). Its use in TB has been associated with reduced TNF-α production and accelerated weight gain even in those who were HIV infected (30). In addition, antigen-specific immune responses *in vitro* and in patients with HIV/TB were enhanced (31). In contrast, infliximab, a humanized antibody against TNF-α used in the treatment of Crohn disease and rheumatoid arthritis, has been associated with the development of active TB (32). There were 70 reported cases of TB after treatment with infliximab, for a median of 12 weeks and active TB developed soon after the initiation of treatment. The complexity of the TNF-α response induced by mycobacterial infection is underscored by these differences.

TNF-α is a member of an emerging family of soluble molecules with several complex immunoregulatory properties that interact with specific receptors. Signals from these receptors mediate apoptosis and the activation of NF-κB, which can influence the production of many other cytokines and the expression of adhesion molecules (33). The TNF receptors (TNF-R1 and TNF-R2) are the sole mediators of TNF signaling. The soluble form of TNF-α binds to TNF-R1 and TNF-R2 binds membrane-associated TNF-α. Signaling occurs when a TNF trimer binds two or three receptors in an extracellular complex, which permits aggregation and activation of the cytoplasmic domains (34). Infliximab binds both soluble and membrane-bound TNF-α, thereby preventing induction of the signaling cascade. Thalidomide simply inhibits production TNF-α by PBMCs.

Clinically, levels of TNF-α in both the peripheral blood and the lung [bronchoalveolar lavage (BAL)] have been correlated with both disease activity and immunopathology (35–37). Finally, TNF-α gene polymorphism has been studied in pulmonary TB and found not to be an independent determinant of susceptibility to disease (38). However, polymorphisms were found to be associated with protection against disease in combination with the human leukocyte antigen genes.

Interleukin-6

IL-6 is a potent B-cell growth and differentiation factor that induces immunoglobulin production by activated B cells and is thought to mediate polyclonal B-cell expansion in infectious and neoplastic diseases (39). IL-6 may therefore mediate the hyperglobulinemia that is characteristic of TB. Limited experimental evidence suggests that IL-6 does not enhance mycobacterial clearance but reduces binding of TNF to murine macrophages and antagonizes the antimycobacterial activity of TNF in macrophages infected with *Mycobacterium avium* (40). In IL-6 knockout mice, the absence of IL-6 led to an early increase in bacterial load with a concurrent delay in the induction of interferon gamma (IFN-γ) (41). However, mice were able to contain and control bacterial growth and developed a protective memory response to secondary infection. This demonstrates that although IL-6 is involved in stimulating early IFN-γ production, it is not essential for the development of protective immunity against *M. tuberculosis*. Addition of IL-6 to human monocytes also enhances intracellular and extracellular mycobacterial growth and can inhibit the production of IL-1β and TNF-α (42). Pleural fluid from patients with TB was shown to have high levels of IL-6 (43). In BAL cells, especially activated alveolar macrophages, spontaneously release increased quantities of IL-1β, IL-6, and TNF-α (15). These cytokines are likely to be involved in directing granuloma formation and control of *M. tuberculosis* infection.

CCAAT/Enhancer Binding Protein-β

The nuclear transcription factor CCAAT/enhancer binding protein (C/EBP)-β (nuclear factor-IL-6) is a 37-kd transcription factor found on the IL-6, IL-1β, IL-1α, IL-8, and TNF-α genes, thus serving as a common pathway for expression of macrophage cytokines (44,45). C/EBP-β and NF-κB are expressed in macrophages and induced by stimulation with lipopolysaccharide (LPS) and *M. tuberculosis* (46). Macrophage differentiation up-regulates C/EBP-β and C/EBP-β is responsible for regulating gene expression in mature macrophages (47). *M. tuberculosis* stimulates production of macrophage cytokines IL-1β, IL-6, and TNF-α, and C/EBP binding sites are involved in the transcriptional regulation of these genes (48).

Cloning of the cytokine gene IL-1β and deletion mutant analysis revealed that a fragment −131/+15 contained the promoter activity in response to lipoarabinomannan and LPS (44,49). There is a C/EBP-β motif 5′ to a NF-κB motif on the IL-6 gene, and both respond to lipoarabinomannan stimulation independently of each other. The C/EBP-β and NF-κB sites have been referred to as mycobacterial response elements, defining a common pathway for *M. tuberculosis* to stimulate cytokine genes (e.g., TNF-α, IL-8) (46). C/EBP-β knockout mice infected with *M. tuberculosis* showed poor granuloma formation and impaired generation of reactive oxygen intermediates from neutrophils despite normal mRNA expression of IFN-γ, TNF-α, and IL-12 (50). By activating C/EBP and NF-κB, macrophage ingestion of *M. tuberculosis* can trigger a cascade of cytokines that can then attract inflammatory and immune effector cells, stimulating cell–cell adhesion and differentiating macrophages into the epithelioid and Langerhans giant cells typical of tuberculous granuloma.

Interleukin-10

IL-10 is an antiinflammatory cytokine that is produced by human and murine macrophages exposed to *M. tuberculosis in vitro* (51,52). IL-10 inhibits cytokine synthesis by monocytes and inhibits the microbicidal activity of murine macrophages (53–55). IL-10 also suppresses antigen-specific T-cell proliferation by down-regulation of macrophage class II major histocompatibility complex (MHC) expression and IL-12 synthesis by antigen-presenting cells, which results in suppression of IFN-γ secretion (56). The production of IL-10 by macrophages and CD8+ cells is induced by LPS and TNF-α. Infection of mice with *M avium* induces IL-10 production and neutralizing anti–IL-10 antibodies reduce the bacterial burden by 2 to 3 log units (57). IL-10 also reverses the mycobactericidal effects of TNF (58). In human TB, IL-10 production is higher in anergic patients, both before and after successful TB treatment (59). These results suggest that IL-10 may play a role in inhibiting the immune response to *M. tuberculosis* and may contribute to the anergy and failure of lymphocytes to proliferate in response to *M. tuberculosis*.

Interleukin-12

IL-12 is a disulfide-linked heterodimeric cytokine composed of two subunits of 40-kd (p40) and 35-kd (p35), both of which are required for bioactivity (60,61). IL-12 mRNA and protein are concentrated at the site of disease in patients with tuberculous pleuritis, and IL-12 is produced by pleural fluid cells in response to *M. tuberculosis* (62). IL-12 favors the development of precursor T cells into Th1 cells, which are thought to mediate resistance against mycobacteria (63,64). IL-12 may also enhance cytotoxicity and augment proliferation by antigen-specific cytolytic T cells and natural killer (NK) cells (60,65). An intriguing property of IL-12 is its capacity to induce proliferation by cytolytic T cells only on costimulation of the T-cell receptor with antigen or anti-CD3 (66). In contrast, cytokines such as IL-2 and IL-7 cause proliferation in the absence or presence of antigen (67).

Functional IL-12 receptors are expressed primarily on activated T and NK cells (68). Two IL-12 receptor subunits, IL-12R1 and IL-12R2, have been cloned from human and mouse T cells, and coexpression of these two subunits is required for high-affinity binding of IL-12 (60,69,70). Expression of IL-12R2 is tightly controlled and may be an important mechanism for regulation of IL-12 responsiveness. IL-12 may also contribute to lymphocyte recognition of *M. tuberculosis* antigens because anti–IL-12 antibodies inhibit *M. tuberculosis*–induced lymphocyte proliferation (71).

Patients with severe mycobacterial disease and autosomal recessive mutations in the genes encoding IL-12 p40 or IL-12R1 have been described, and in each case, the mutation precluded protein expression (72–74). Each patient had severe infection with either nontuberculous mycobacterium or vaccine-associated BCG, and most had severe *Salmonella* infections. However, in most instances, infection was effectively treated with antibiotics. In several patients, administration of adjunctive IFN along with antibiotics was associated with substantial clinical improvement. Well-organized, mature, tuberculoid granulomas were observed on histopathologic examination of affected tissues from IL-12R1–deficient patients, suggesting that IL-12–dependent IFN induction is not required for mature granuloma formation. Despite this, immunohistochemical analysis of mature granulomas in normal patients with TB shows abundant IL-12p40 and IFN-γ (75). Tuberculin-specific delayed-type hypersensitivity testing was normal in IL-12R1–deficient patients with BCG infection, implying that, like IFN, IL-12 is not required for development of delayed-type hypersensitivity (74,76). *In vitro*, activated T lymphocytes and NK cells from patients had markedly diminished but not absent IFN production. This residual IL-12–independent IFN production in IL-12p40– and IL-12R1–deficient patients may account for their milder clinical phenotype compared with patients with complete IFN receptor deficiency. Findings in IL-12p40– and IL-12R1–deficient patients further support that IFN is critical in the control of mycobacterial and *Salmonella* infections and that a principal role of IL-12 in control of these infections is to stimulate IFN production. IL-12 is a regulatory cytokine that connects the innate and adoptive host response to mycobacteria mostly through its induction of IFN-γ.

Transforming Growth Factor β

A macrophage deactivator important in human host defense may be transforming growth factor (TGF) β. This cytokine is widely distributed and produced mainly by monocytes and macrophages (77). Although it has some proinflammatory effects such as enhancement of monocyte chemotaxis and augmented expression of Fc receptors, TGF-β also has important antiinflammatory effects, including deactivation of macrophage production of reactive oxygen and nitrogen intermediates, inhibition of T-cell proliferation, interference with natural killer and cytotoxic T lymphocyte (CTL) function, and down-regulation of IFN-γ, TNF-α, and IL-1 release (78). A series of experiments elucidated a role for TGF-β in growth inhibition of *M. tuberculosis* by macrophages (79–81). When TGF-β is added to cocultures of mononuclear phagocytes and *M. tuberculosis*, both phagocytosis and growth inhibition were inhibited in a dose-dependent manner. TGF-β also blocked the effect of TNF-α on growth inhibition. Tuberculin (PPD) induces TGF-β production by monocytes from healthy individuals, and TGF-β production is increased in PBMCs and lung granulomas from patients with pulmonary TB. Production of IFN-γ after stimulation with PPD by circulating T lymphocytes taken from patients with TB increases in the presence of natural inhibitors of TGF-β.

TGF-β is a product of activated monocytes, and of the five known isoforms, TBFb1 is the predominant one produced by human mononuclear cells. TGF-β is synthesized as a precursor with the N-terminal domain, also termed *latency-associated peptide*, noncovalently associated with the C-terminal bioactive dimer, thereby preventing the binding of TGF-β to its specific cell surface receptor (82). The mature TGF-β protein can be released from the inactive complex by the action of proteases, such as plasmin, or the action of binding proteins, such as thrombospondin (83). TGF-β modulates cell proliferation, differentiation, apoptosis, adhesion, and migration of various cell types. Most cell types, including immature hematopoietic cells, activated T and B cells, macrophages, neutrophils, and dendritic cells, produce TGF-β and/or are sensitive to its effects (84,85). TGF-β inhibits IL-2–dependent T-cell proliferation and IL-2R expression (86). It also down-regulates the expression of human leukocyte antigen–DR and decreases monocyte production of TNF-α and IL-1β (87,88). TGF-β inhibits expression of IFN-γ and activation of macrophages by inhibiting reactive oxygen and nitrogen intermediaries (89). This macrophage deactivating effect has important implications for phagocytic function.

In TB, TGF-β is constitutively overproduced by monocytes from patients (80). Langerhans giant cells and epithelioid cells in tuberculous granulomas also express mRNA for TGF-β, suggesting that local production of TGF-β may result in deactivation of macrophages and immunopathology (90). In human macrophages infected with *M. avium*, production of TGF-β is highest in those infected with the most virulent strains, and addition of recombinant TGF-β inhibits the antimycobacterial effects of TNF (91). In TB, TGF-β increases the intracellular growth of *M. tuberculosis*, whereas neutralizing antibodies to TGF-β reduce intracellular growth (92). Furthermore, IFN-γ enhances antimycobacterial activity of macrophages only in the presence of neutralizing antibodies to TGF-β. These results indicate that TGF-β inhibits antimycobacterial immune defenses and facilitates mycobacterial survival. Excessive production of TGF-β in response to *M. tuberculosis* along with TNF-α induces tissue damage and extensive fibrosis. By stimulating expression of TGF-β, *M. tuberculosis* can lead to T-cell suppression, macrophage deactivation, and tissue destruction. Finally, Th3 CD4+ cells primarily secrete TGF-β, providing help for immunoglobulins and suppression for Th1 and Th2 cells (93).

CYTOKINES PRODUCED BY CD4+ T CELLS

Although T lymphocytes (including a/b CD4+ and CD8+ cells, CTLs, and g/d T lymphocytes) play a role in host defense, the bulk of experimental and clinical data favors a dominant role for CD4+ cells in immune defenses against TB (93). CD4+ T cells are involved in recognition of antigens, including mycobacterial cell wall products, such as lipoarabinomannan, that have been processed in phagosomes and presented in the context of MHC class II molecules on the surface of antigen-presenting cells, such as monocytes, macrophages, and dendritic cells (94).

The importance of CD4+ T cells in human TB is well supported by clinical data. CD4+ T cells are selectively expanded at the site of disease in patients with tuberculous pleuritis and a resistant immune response (95). In HIV infection, depletion of CD4+ cells is most likely responsible for the increased risk of mycobacteremia, extrapulmonary TB, and positive acid-fast bacilli sputum smears (96). For example, the frequency of mycobacteremia increases from 4% in patients with more than 200 CD4 cells per microliter to 49% in those with 100 or fewer CD4 cells per microliter. In addition, there is an inverse correlation between the number of mycobacteria counted in pulmonary granulomas and the peripheral CD4+ count suggesting a protective role for these cells (97). Finally, patients with acquired immunodeficiency syndrome (AIDS) with pulmonary TB are unable to mount the CD4+ lymphocytic alveolitis normally observed during TB (98).

T helper cells can be separated into at least two phenotypic classes, Th1 and Th2 cells, based on murine models of disease (99,100). These cells derive from so-called Th0 or null cells, and their differentiation from precursor cells is under the control of cytokines such as IL-12. Th1 cells are defined by their ability to produce the cytokines IFN-γ and IL-2, whereas Th2 cells produce cytokines such as IL-4, IL-5, IL-10, and IL-13. Functionally, Th1 cells can enhance microbicidal activity of macrophages and augment delayed-type hypersensitivity responses (Table 21.1). Th2 cells can support B-cell growth and differentiation and augment humoral immune responses. Both Th1 and Th2 cells produce IL-3, granulocyte-macrophage colony-stimulating fac-

tor, and TNF. IL-1 is an important growth factor for Th2 but not Th1 cells, and macrophages are optimal antigen-presenting cells for Th1 cells, whereas B cells are optimal for Th2 cells (101,102). In the course of an immune response to a specific pathogen, Th1 and Th2 cells exert cross-regulatory influences that favor the predominance of one subpopulation. IFN-γ produced by Th1 cells inhibits proliferation by Th2 cells, IL-10 produced by Th2 cells inhibits cytokine synthesis by Th1 cells, and IL-4 inhibits generation of Th1 cells (103).

In murine models, the type of T-cell response elicited by the intracellular pathogen can influence disease manifestation. For example, in leishmaniasis, Th1 cells mediate immunologic resistance to infection through production of IFN-γ, whereas Th2 cells exacerbate disease through production of IL-4 (104,105). In *M bovis* infection, resistant mice produce high concentrations of IFN-γ and IL-2 but low levels of IL-4, whereas susceptible mice produce high levels of IL-4 and low levels of IFN-γ and IL-2 (106). In addition, production of IFN-γ but not IL-4 is a functional marker of murine T cells that confer adoptive immunity against *M. tuberculosis* (107).

Human T cells can exhibit dichotomous patterns of cytokine production similar to those of murine Th1 and Th2 cells. However, unlike in mice, IL-10 is produced by both human Th1 and Th2 cells and inhibits proliferation and cytokine production by both subpopulations (108, 109). In humans, IL-4 may be the main Th2 cytokine that inhibits growth of Th1 cells through deactivation of macrophages, perhaps selectively inhibiting antigen presentation to Th1 cells (104). The Th1/Th2 dichotomy has been demonstrated in skin biopsy lesions from patients with leprosy (110). Lepromatous leprosy lesions are characterized clinically by extensive cutaneous involvement with poorly defined lesions, which infiltrate the dermis diffusely. In contrast, tuberculoid lesions are sharply demarcated and are single or few in number on the skin. Yamamura determined that lepromatous leprosy lesions (those that are less able to control bacterial growth) contained cells expressing the genes from IL-4, IL-5, and IL-10, whereas resistant tuberculoid lesions contained cells expressing the cytokine genes IFN-γ and IL-2 (111). The pattern of cytokine gene expression by T helper cells seems to be associated with different manifestations of disease in humans, and the Th1/Th2 paradigm seems tenable in human disease. Asthma, Crohn disease, and organ transplantation are further examples of disease states whose clinical manifestations seem, at least in part, to be related to the Th phenotype present at the site of disease (112,113).

CD4+ Cell Phenotypes in Tuberculosis

Published data on cytokine production by human T cells in response to *M. tuberculosis* are conflicting. Some authors noted that most CD4+ *M. tuberculosis*–reactive T cells propagated *in vitro* are Th1-like, producing high concentrations of IFN-γ but low concentrations of IL-4 and IL-5, and others found that mRNA for Th1 cytokines predominates over that for Th2 cytokines at the site of tuberculin skin tests (114–116). In contrast, one study demonstrated that most *M. tuberculosis*–reactive T-cell clones secrete IFN-γ and IL-4, and another report indicated that most *M. tuberculosis*–reactive T-cell clones produce both Th1 and Th2 cytokines, including IFN-γ, IL-2, IL-4, IL-5, and IL-10 (117). Because these disparate results may reflect selection of T-cell subpopulations by culture conditions *in vitro* and may not reflect events *in vivo*, it is critical to evaluate the cytokine response at the site of mycobacterial disease.

In patients with tuberculous pleuritis, expression of mRNA for the Th1 cytokines IFN-γ and IL-2 is greater in pleural fluid than in blood, and concentrations of IFN-γ are 15-fold higher than those in serum (118,119). In contrast, expression of mRNA for the Th2 cytokine IL-4 is lower in pleural fluid than in blood. Pleural fluid lymphocytes stimulated with *M. tuberculosis* produce more IFN-γ and IL-2 than do peripheral blood lymphocytes. These results provide strong evidence of selective concentration of Th1-like cells at the site of disease in persons with a resistant immune response and suggest that Th1 cells play an important role in human antimycobacterial defenses.

Various studies have attempted to characterize the T-lymphocyte responses associated with TB, although few have studied lymphocytes produced in the lung itself in patients with pulmonary TB. Surcel et al. (120) studied proliferative responses and cytokine production in PBMCs taken from patients with TB and normal controls in response to stimulation with mycobacterial antigens *in vitro*. They found that patients with TB had increased proliferation of cells secreting IL-4 but not IFN-γ in response to stimulation and compared with cells from healthy subjects. Sanchez et al. (121) studied 45 patients with pulmonary TB and 16 tuberculin skin test–positive controls and found that patients had less IFN-γ than controls and more IL-4 production. They concluded that patients with TB had a Th2-type response in their peripheral blood, whereas tuberculin-positive patients had a Th1-type response.

Robinson et al. (122) used *in situ* hybridization to detect cytokine gene expression in BAL cells from nine patients with active pulmonary TB (and compared with healthy controls) and found that increased levels of IFN-γ mRNA localized mainly to T cells with no difference in IL-4/IL-5. Schwander et al. (123) studied a similar group of patients and found that the majority of lymphocytes in the lungs of patients with TB were activated T cells displaying the a/b receptor. In HIV-infected patients, the absolute number and immune activation state of CD4⁺-lymphocytes may be reduced. Sodhi et al. (124) demonstrated that low levels of circulating IFNγ in peripheral blood are associated with severe clinical TB (radiographically far advanced disease). Our group has shown that patients with clinically and radi-

ographically limited TB (negative sputum smears, no cavitation on chest radiographs) have an alveolar lymphocytosis in infected regions of the lung; these lymphocytes produce high levels of IFNγ (37). In patients with far advanced or cavitary disease, no Th1-type lymphocytosis is present. These studies provide some evidence that the local cellular immune response in pulmonary TB is composed, at least in part, of Th1-type CD4⁺ lymphocytes.

In addition to inducing activation of macrophages by secreted cytokines, there is recent evidence that lymphocytes can kill mycobacteria directly through CTL activity (125,126). Lymphocytes taken from the lungs of normal volunteers had the ability to lyse mycobacterial antigen-pulsed alveolar macrophages and peripheral monocytes. The ability to lyse monocytes exceeded the ability to lyse macrophages. CTLs were activated with PPD primarily through MHC class II, whereas when lymphocytes were expanded with both PPD and IL-2, CTLs were both class I and class II expanded. Although the general assumption has been that CD4⁺ T lymphocytes are by far the most important components of cell-mediated immunity in TB, this study also demonstrated significant ability of CD8⁺ T lymphocytes to carry out CTL activity as well. These experiments establish a direct role for CTL in host defense against TB that complements their role as stimulators of macrophage function (127).

Interferon Gamma

Although many cytokines are involved in the host response against TB, IFN-γ plays a key role in modulating the effects of T lymphocytes on alveolar macrophages. The essential role of IFN-γ in combating *M. tuberculosis* has been demonstrated in mice with a targeted disruption of the IFN-gene [IFN-γ (−/−) mice] in which *M. tuberculosis* administered intravenously or aerogenically results in the premature demise of the animal (128,129). These mice can develop granulomas and delayed-type hypersensitivity responses but have progressive, widespread tissue destruction, necrosis, and proliferation of acid-fast bacilli. Similarly, mice with targeted disruption of the IFN-γ receptor gene also died within 7 to 9 weeks after inoculation with BCG.

An intact type II IFN system is critical for effective response to mycobacterial infections in humans. Patients with genetic defects in IFN-γ receptor function have infections with usually nonpathogenic mycobacteria (72). These patient and others with nontuberculous mycobacterial disease treated with exogenous IFN-γ had asymptomatic improvement. Mutations or gene deletions in the IFN-γ signaling pathway may lead to chronic or uncontrolled mycobacterial infection. Recently, it has been reported that patients heterozygous for a point mutation in STAT-1 were susceptible to mycobacterial infection but had normal resistance to viral infections owing to dominant effects on production of STAT-1 homodimers and recessive effects on formation of interferon-stimulated gene factor 3 (130). A point mutation of the IFN-γ receptor gene precluding expression of the receptor on cell surfaces led to dissemination of *M. bovis* BCG after vaccination, which led to death in an infant despite treatment (72). The uncontrolled growth within macrophages in this child was probably owing to impaired activation of bactericidal mechanisms through IFN regulatory factor 1 and inducible nitric oxide synthase. This child had a strongly positive test for delayed-type hypersensitivity to tuberculin, reflecting a normal Th1 response. Patients with persistent disseminated non-TB mycobacterial infections or idiopathic CD4+ lymphocytopenia have responded to recombinant IFN-γ subcutaneously twice weekly with marked clinical improvement, abatement of fever, clearing of lesions, and radiographic improvement (131). Patients with active TB have been described to have reduced PBMCs and BAL induction of IFN-γ (132,133). We have demonstrated clinical improvement after treatment with aerosol IFN-γ in five patients with multidrug–resistant TB who were failing TB therapy (134). In all patients, the only intervention was the addition of aerosol IFN-γ to a failing regimen.

AIDS patients with TB are unable to produce the high levels of IFN-γ mRNA normally seen in the lung during pulmonary TB (98). The failure to increase IFN-γ during TB likely contributes to susceptibility of AIDS patients to infection with *M. tuberculosis*. The increased susceptibility to TB infection and disease among HIV-infected patients is directly related to impaired host immunity. In addition, TB switches the pulmonary microenvironment from one that suppresses HIV-1 replication to one that stimulates it (135,136). The high levels of virus produced during infections such as TB and the increased viral mutation produced by enhanced viral replication may contribute to the accelerated course of AIDS after opportunistic infection.

Interleukin-2

IL-2 is a critical T-cell growth factor that expands populations of antigen-reactive T cells and is likely to increase the local concentration of macrophage-activating factors secreted by T cells. IL-2 induces IFN-γ production, thereby activating macrophages and cytotoxic T cells specific for *M. tuberculosis* antigens. Administration of recombinant IL-2 limits the replication of *M. bovis* BCG in mice and reduces the bacillary burden in lepromatous leprosy (137,138). In TB, PBMCs demonstrated few IL-2–responsive cells when compared with controls. However, soluble IL-2Rα levels have been shown to be increased in the sera of patients with TB and to respond to therapy (139). In addition, IL-2Rα expression was increased in the involved lung of patients with TB. This increase was induced by IFN-γ and regulated by NF-κB binding of the IL-2Rα promoter (140). In HIV-infected patients with TB, IL-2 expression is impaired with low levels of circulating IL-2Rα, and IL-2 when compared with non–HIV-infected TB patients (141).

Studies in leprosy with subcutaneously administered IL-2 showed up-regulation of markers associated with endothelial cell activation, influx of circulating lymphocytes and monocytes, and a decrease in bacillary burden (138). IL-2 administration in patients with multidrug-resistant TB was associated with increased T cells, sputum conversion, and improvement in chest radiographs (142). The immune activation associated with IL-2 treatment was owing to induction of IFN-γ and up-regulation of genes responsible for the development of an antimycobacterial response (143).

Interleukin-4

In contrast to the effects of Th1 cytokines, IL-4 deactivates macrophages and blocks T-cell proliferation by down-regulation of IL-2 receptor expression and inhibition of transcription of the IL-2 gene (144–147). IL-4, therefore, has the capacity to inhibit the immune response to *M. tuberculosis*. In humans, granulomas can express both IL-4 and IFN-γ, and severe pulmonary TB disease has been associated with high production of IL-4 (148). Others have not detected increased IL-4 in patients with TB (149). The ability of the human immune response to simultaneously express T1 and Th2 cytokines underscores the complexity of trying to conform human host responses to murine models of infection. Further studies are needed to determine whether excessive production of IL-4 contributes to suppression of the immune response in patients with TB or simply reflects disease activity.

Chemokines

Chemokines are a recently discovered category of chemotactic cytokines that play a central role in the recruitment and interaction of inflammatory cells at the site of infection (150) (Table 21.2). They are 8- to 10-kd proteins with 20% to 70% homology in amino acid sequences and have been classified according to the characteristic sequence of four cysteines: CXC or α, CC or β, C or γ, and CX3C or δ chemokines (151). CXC (or α) chemokines are chemoattractant for neutrophils, T and B cells, whereas CC (or β) chemokines mediate interactions of monocytes, basophils, eosinophils, and T, dendritic, and NK cells (152). The signaling pathway involves binding to their receptors (seven transmembrane receptors coupled to pertussis toxin–sensitive G1 proteins) and a series of intracellular events including generation of inositol triphosphate, release of intracellular calcium, and activation of protein kinase C (153). Receptor expression can be modified by inflammatory cytokines and down-regulated by their own ligands, with the exception of CCR7 (not down-regulated). CCR1, CXCR3, and CCR5 are expressed by Th1 lymphocytes, whereas CCR3, CCR4, and CCR8 are present on Th2 cells (154).

Via a multistep sequence of events involving selectins and integrins, chemokines lead to extravasation of leuko-

TABLE 21.2. CHEMOKINES INVOLVED IN TUBERCULOSIS IMMUNE RESPONSE

Chemokine	Cell of Production	Receptors	Target Cells
RANTES	Macrophage-monocyte-THP1	CCR1, CCR3, CCR5	Eosinophils, basophils, monocytes, activated T cells, dendritic cells, natural killer cells
MIP-1α	Macrophage-monocyte-THP1-mesothelial cells	CCR1, CCR5	Activated T cells, monocytes, dendritic cells, natural killer cells
MIP-1β	Macrophages, monocytes, THP1	CCR5	Activated T cells, monocytes, dendritic cells, natural killer cells
MCP-1	Macrophage-monocyte-THP1-mesothelial cells	CCR2	Activated T cells, monocytes, dendritic cells, basophils
MCP-2	THP-1	CCR2	Activated T cells, monocytes, dendritic cells, basophils
MCP-3	Monocytes	CCR2	Activated T cells, monocytes, dendritic cells, basophils
MPIF-1	THP-1	CCR1	Monocytes, dendritic cells, inhibitor of myeloid precursors
GRO-α	THP-1, neutrophils	CXCR2	Neutrophils
GRO-β	THP-1	CXCR2	Neutrophils
GRO-γ	THP-1	CXCR2	Neutrophils
MIP-3α	THP-1	CCR6	Dendritic cells
PARC	THP-1	?	Resting T cells, activated T cells
I-309	THP-1	CCR8	Monocytes
Eotaxin	THP-1	CCR3	Eosinophils, basophils, dendritic cells
IP-10	Monocytes, whole blood, epithelial cells	CXCR3	Activated T cells, natural killer cells
MIG	Epithelial cells	CXCR3	Activated T cells, natural killer cells
I-TAC	Epithelial cells	CXCR3	Activated T cells, natural killer cells
Fractalkine	Endothelial cells	CX3CR1	Activated T cells, natural killer cells, monocytes

GRO, growth-related oncogene; IP-10, interferon-inducible protein 10; I-TAC, interferon-inducible T-cell alpha chemoattractant; MCP, monocyte chemoattractant protein (–1, –2, –3); MIG, monokine induced by interferon γ; MIP, macrophage inflammatory protein; PARC, pulmonary and activation-regulated chemokine; RANTES, regulated on activation, normal T expressed and secreted; THP, myelomonocytoma cells.

cytes to areas of infection. The heat shock protein 65 of *M. tuberculosis* increases expression of E selectin and intercellular adhesion molecule-1 (ICAM-1) *in vitro* in human endothelial cells (155). Increased expression of ICAM-1 in human alveolar macrophages from patients with pulmonary TB followed by a decrease later in the disease has been reported (156,157). ICAM-1 is also expressed in pleural mesothelium and thought to be responsible for recruitment of monocytes during tuberculous pleurisy (158).

An effective immune response against *M. tuberculosis* involves interaction of Th1 lymphocytes, effector cells, dendritic cells, and macrophages, leading to granuloma formation and killing (or at least inhibition of the growth) of mycobacteria at the site of disease (158–160). RANTES (the cytokine regulated on activation, normal T cell expressed and secreted) and osteopontin (also called early T-lymphocyte activation protein 1 or Eta-1) have been demonstrated by *in situ* hybridization and immunohistochemistry in TB granulomas from human lymph nodes and pulmonary samples of active TB patients (161). Macrophages in lymph nodes from patients with TB have also been shown to produce monocyte chemoattractant protein 1 (MCP-1) (162). Fractalkine (or CX3CL1) has been demonstrated on the surface endothelial cells in granulomatous lesions of TB lymph nodes. Its receptor, CX3CR1, has been found on surface of NK cells and

Th1 cells, suggesting a role for these molecules in the amplification circuit of polarized Th1 responses in TB (163).

A series of patients with TB with prevalent CD4⁺ lymphocyte pattern in the BAL demonstrated high levels of MCP-1 and RANTES in the BAL in the acute phase of the disease compared with the convalescent phases (164,165). In contrast, IL-8 levels remained elevated during all phases of the disease. The concentration of RANTES correlated with the absolute number of CD4⁺ cells in the involved lobes, suggesting that these chemokines could be implicated in the effective response against *M. tuberculosis*.

The CCR5 receptor binds RANTES and macrophage inflammatory protein (MIP)-α and -1β and is a coreceptor for HIV-1 to enter macrophages (166). It is up-regulated in macrophages in BAL of patients with TB and plays a role in the interaction of HIV and TB (167). Expression of CCR5 was reported to be increased on PBMCs from HIV-1 infected patients during TB disease. Chemokine levels are elevated in both HIV-1 infected and non–HIV-infected TB patients when compared with controls. Interferon-inducible protein 10 (IP-10) and MCP-1 levels are higher in HIV-1–infected patients than in HIV-negative patients, suggesting a possible role for these chemokines in the complex interaction between the two diseases (168). IP-10 serum levels have been correlated also with fever and anorexia in patients.

Studies on pleural effusions from patients with TB demonstrated higher levels of MCP-1 and MIP-1α compared with effusions from congestive heart failure and pneumonia, whereas IL-8 levels were higher in parapneumonic effusions, suggesting a role for these factors in a different mechanism of recruitment of phagocytic cells in infections from different agents (169,170). In addition, *in vitro* studies demonstrated the ability of mesothelial cells to produce MIP-1α and MCP-1 and to express ICAM-1 on their surface, suggesting a leading role for these cells in the pathogenesis of tuberculous pleurisy.

Most of the studies on induction of chemokines have been performed on monocyte-derived macrophages and monocytes after infection by *M. tuberculosis* or challenge with mycobacterial components. MCP-1 spontaneous production is slightly higher in CD4+ cells from patients with TB compared with healthy donors, whereas no significant differences were found after challenge with *M. tuberculosis* (162). Production of IL-8, MCP-1, and MIP-1β but not IP-10 has been reported after stimulation of whole blood from healthy donors with lipoarabinomannan (168).

Dendritic cells are considered the main antigen-presenting cells in the development of an effective immune response against mycobacteria (171). Immature human lung dendritic cells express CCR1 and CCR5 as well as high levels of MHC II (172). Maturation of dendritic cells was demonstrated after challenge with 19-kd lipoprotein from *M. tuberculosis* with a subsequent increased capacity of these cells to stimulate T cells (173). These cells expressed MHC II and other cell surface markers but not chemokines and their receptors. Another elegant study demonstrated cooperation of dendritic and NK cells during challenge with heat-killed *M. tuberculosis*: both cell types matured, resulting in higher killing activity for NK cells and in a greater capacity of dendritic cells to stimulate NK and T-naive cells (174). CCR7 was up-regulated during the maturation process of antigen-presenting cells.

All these findings suggest the existence of a complex network of chemotactic factors and receptors that can influence the immune response against *M. tuberculosis* from the very early phases of the infection to granuloma formation and the killing of bacteria by specialized cells. The exact function of these molecules during the immune response *in vivo* and the pathogenetic mechanisms that *M. tuberculosis* is able to use to avoid an effective response and to cause disease have only begun to be elucidated.

Interleukin-8

IL-8 was one of the first described chemokines and, for this reason, has long been classified as a cytokine. It functions as a chemotactic factor for neutrophils, T lymphocytes, and basophils (175). IL-8 has been demonstrated to be angiogenic, similar to fibroblast growth factor, thus potentially contributing to the high vascularity observed in the healing process at the margins of tuberculous cavities (176).

IL-8 is a member of the CXC chemokine subfamily and binds to either of the two receptors, CXCR-1 (IL-8RA) or CXCR-2 (IL-8RB). Exaggerated release of IL-8 may lead to the increased neutrophils observed in tuberculous infiltrates and may contribute to the necrotic destruction of lung tissue (177). Agonists for IL-8 production include LPSs, TNF-α, IL-1, and phorbol myristate acetate. IL-1, TNF-α, and phorbol myristate acetate activate the IL-8 gene rapidly and directly in the absence of new protein synthesis, probably by a common serine kinase. The 5′ flanking region of the IL-8 gene contains several potential binding sites for known NFs including AP-1, NF-κB-β, C/EBP-β, octomer motif, and interferon regulatory factor 1 (178).

Expression of IL-8 is increased in lymph nodes and granulomas from patients with TB and correlate with the neutrophil infiltration (179). BAL studies have shown a significant increase of IL-8 levels in patients with TB (165,180). Levels of the chemokine have been found to correlate with radiographic findings and with the levels of defensins (181,182). A decrease in the IL-8 production was reported for miliary forms. Virulence of strains of *M. tuberculosis* was reported to be inversely correlated with IL-8 production from monocyte-derived macrophages, highlighting its role in the early phases of infection (183).

Several studies demonstrated the presence of IL-8 in the sera of patients affected by TB. PBMCs from HIV-negative patients with TB expressed mRNA for IL-8 (184). Patients who died of TB had higher basal concentration and a decrease in *in vitro* production of IL-8 (177). A protective role is suggested by the finding that levels of IL-8 in the sera of patients with TB increased with cure. In HIV-infected patients, Juffermans et al. (168) reported that the levels of IL-8 were significantly increased in patients and in close contacts compared with control but not different between HIV-infected and HIV-negative patients. Meddows-Taylor et al. (185) found higher levels of IL-8 in sera from HIV-infected patients and HIV-infected TB patients compared with HIV-negative TB patients. The same study showed that the spontaneous release of IL-8 by PBMCs was enhanced in patients despite a significantly decreased response to phytohemagglutinin compared with normal patients, suggesting again a role in the development of an effective immune response.

Defensins in Human Tuberculosis

Defensins, or human neutrophil peptides, are cationic proteins with antimicrobial activity against gram-positive and -negative bacteria (186). Rich in arginine and cysteine residues, these proteins are 29 to 34 amino acids long and have a molecular weight of 3.5 kd. Constituents of the azurophil granules of neutrophils, they are synthesized as precursors and then activated by the cleavage of a signal peptide (187). Defensins were demonstrated to have high killing activity for *M. tuberculosis* in an *in vitro* assay, causing defects to the tuberculous cell wall and binding to the genomic DNA as the intracellular target (188). Human macrophages do not express defensins, but transfection of mRNA for these molecules enhances the killing capacity of these cells *in vitro*, highlighting the possible utility of these proteins in the treatment of TB (189). No evidence of a protective role of defensins against *M. tuberculosis in vivo* exists. However, levels of defensins in BAL were found to be significantly increased in patients with pulmonary TB compared with healthy controls. Higher levels were detected in patients with cavitary TB and an inverse relationship between plasma levels at the beginning of the treatment and forced expiratory volume/forced vital capacity before and after the treatment were reported, suggesting the role of these molecules as useful markers of severity of disease and deterioration of pulmonary function (182).

Immunotherapeutics

Although chemotherapy will remain the mainstay of anti-TB treatment, the use of adjunctive immunotherapeutic modalities is attractive, particularly in the growing percentage of persons with drug-resistant TB. One approach to immunotherapy is to administer vaccine preparations that stimulate a predominance of Th1 cytokines. Such vaccines could include purified or recombinant mycobacterial antigens or live vaccine vector organisms that secrete specific mycobacterial proteins.

An alternative immunotherapeutic strategy is to directly administer cytokines that enhance bacillary elimination, such as IFN-γ, IL-2, and IL-12. Administration of IL-2 intradermally to patients with TB led to immune activation and decreases in bacillary burden (142). IFN-γ has been successfully used to treat disseminated nontuberculous mycobacteria with clinical improvement (131). We have used aerosol IFN-γ to treat failing multidrug-resistant TB patients (134). The treatment was well tolerated, and patients responded with conversion of sputum smears, decreased cavitary size, and increased time to a positive culture. Clinical improvement was accompanied by IFN-γ signaling in BAL cells and induction of IP-10. Therapeutic uses of cytokines may be limited by high cost and toxicity of large parenteral doses that may be required to attain effective tissue levels. Use of aerosolized cytokine for pulmonary TB may maximize local therapeutic effects while minimizing adverse reactions.

REFERENCES

 1. Raviglione MC, Snider DE Jr, Kochi A. Global epidemiology of tuberculosis. Morbidity and mortality of a worldwide epidemic. *JAMA* 1995;273:220–226.

 2. Jones BE, Young SMM, Antoniskis D, et al. Relationship of the manifestations of tuberculosis to DC4 cell counts in patients with human immunodeficiency virus infection. *Am Rev Respir Dis* 1993;148:1292–1297.

 3. Weisner D. Sanitorium follow-up studies. *Am Rev Tuberc* 1922; 6:320–326.

 4. Mitchell R. Mortality and relapse of uncomplicated advanced pulmonary tuberculosis before chemotherapy: 1,504 consecutive admissions followed for fifteen to twenty-five years. *Am Rev Tuberc* 1955;72:487–512.

 5. Stephens M. Follow-up of 1,041 tuberculosis patients. *Am Rev Tuberc* 1941;44:451–462.

 6. Denis M. Interleukin-1 (IL-1) is an important cytokine in granulomatous alveolitis. *Cell Immunol* 1994;157:70–80.

 7. Barnes PF, Chatterjee D, Abrams JS, et al. Cytokine production induced by *Mycobacterium tuberculosis* lipoarabinomannan. Relationship to chemical structure. *J Immunol* 1992;149:541–547.

 8. Wallis RS, Amir-Tahmasseb M, Ellner JJ. Induction of interleukin 1 and tumor necrosis factor by mycobacterial proteins: the monocyte Western blot. *Proc Natl Acad Sci U S A* 1990;87: 3348–3352.

 9. Toossi Z, Sedor JR, Lapurge JP, et al. Expression of functional interleukin 2 receptors by peripheral blood monocytes from patients with active pulmonary tuberculosis. *J Clin Invest* 1990; 85:1777–1784.

10. Dinarello C. Interleukin-1 and the pathogenesis of the acute-phase response. *N Engl J Med* 1984;311:1413–1418.

11. Fantuzzi C, Dinarelllo CA. The inflammatory response in interleukin-1 beta-deficient mice: comparison with other cytokine-related knock-out mice. *J Leukoc Biol* 1996;59:489–493.

12. Kuo HP, Wang CH, Huang KS, et al. Nitric oxide modulates interleukin-1beta and tumor necrosis factor alpha synthesis by alveolar macrophages in pulmonary tuberculosis. *Am J Respir Crit Care Med* 2000;161:192–199.

13. O'Neill LA. The interleukin-1 receptor/Toll-like receptor superfamily: signal transduction during inflammation and host defense (review). *Sci STKE* 2000 Aug 8;2000(44):RE1.

14. Means TK, Jones BW, Schromm AB, et al. Differential effects of a Toll-like receptor antagonist on *Mycobacterium tuberculosis*-induced macrophage responses. *J Immunol* 2001;166: 4074–4082.

15. Tsao TC, Hong J, Huang C, et al. Increased TNF-alpha, IL-1beta and IL-6 levels in the bronchoalveolar lavage fluid with the upregulation of their mRNA in the macrophages lavaged from patients with active pulmonary tuberculosis. *Tuber Lung Dis* 1999;79:279–285.

16. Tsao TC, Hong J, Li LF, et al. Imbalances between tumor necrosis factor-alpha and its soluble receptor forms, and interleukin-1beta and interleukin-1 receptor antagonist in BAL fluid of cavitary pulmonary tuberculosis. *Chest* 2000;117:103–109.

17. Xirouchaki N, Tzanakis N, Bouros D, et al. Diagnostic value of interleukin-1alpha, interleukin-6, and tumor necrosis factor in pleural effusions. *Chest* 2002;121:815–820.

18. Wilkinson RJ, Patel P, Llewelyn M, et al. Influence of polymorphism in the genes for the interleukin (IL)-1 receptor antagonist and IL-1beta on tuberculosis. *J Exp Med* 1999;189:1863–1874.

19. Bellamy R, Ruwende C, Corrah T, et al. Assessment of the interleukin 1 gene cluster and other candidate gene polymorphisms in host susceptibility to tuberculosis. *Tuberc Lung Dis* 1998;79:83–89.

20. Zhang Y, Doerfler M, Lee TC, et al. Mechanisms of stimulation of interleukin-1β and tumor necrosis factor-α by *Mycobacterium tuberculosis* components. *J Clin Invest* 1993;91:2076–2083.

21. Rom WN, Schluger N, Law K, et al. Human host response to *Mycobacterium tuberculosis*. *Schweiz Med Wochenschr* 1995;125: 2178–2185.

22. Semenzato G, Adami F, Maschio N, et al. Immune mechanisms in interstitial lung diseases. *Allergy* 2000;55:1103–1120.
23. Kindler V, Sappino AP, Grau GE, et al. The inducing role of tumor necrosis factor in the development of bactericidal granulomas during BCG infection. *Cell* 1989;56:731–740.
24. Barnes PF, Fong S-J, Brennan PJ, et al. Local production of tumor necrosis factor and interferon-γ in tuberculosis pleuritis. *J Immunol* 1990;145:149–154.
25. Flynn JL, Goldstein MM, Chan J, et al. Tumor necrosis factor-alpha is required in the protective immune response against *Mycobacterium tuberculosis* in mice. *Immunity* 1995;2:561–572.
26. Pisa P, Gennene M, Soder O, et al. Serum tumor necrosis factor levels and disease dissemination in leprosy and leishmaniasis. *J Infect Dis* 1990;161:988–991.
27. Takashima T, Ueta C, Tsuyuguchi I, et al. Production of tumor necrosis factor alpha by monocytes from patients with pulmonary tuberculosis. *Infect Immun* 1990;58:3286–3292.
28. Cadranel J, Philippe C, Perez J, et al. *In vitro* production of tumour necrosis factor and prostaglandin E₂ by peripheral blood mononuclear cells from tuberculosis patients. *Clin Exp Immunol* 1990;81:319–324.
29. Sampaio EP, Hernandez MO, Carvalho DS, et al. Management of erythema nodosum leprosum by thalidomide: thalidomide analogues inhibit *M. leprae*-induced TNF-alpha production *in vitro*. *Biomed Pharmacother* 2002;56:13–19.
30. Tramontana JM, Utaipat U, Molloy A, et al. Thalidomide treatment reduces tumor necrosis factor alpha production and enhances weight gain in patients with pulmonary tuberculosis. *Mol Med* 1995;1:384–397.
31. Bekker GL, Haslett P, Maartens G, et al. Thalidomide-induced antigen-specific immune stimulation in patients with human immunodeficiency virus type 1 and tuberculosis. *J Infect Dis* 2000;181:954–965.
32. Keane J, Gershon S, Wise PR, et al. Tuberculosis associated with infliximab, a tumor necrosis factor α-neutralizing agent. *N Engl J Med* 2001;345:1098–1104.
33. Agostini C, Zambello R, Sancetta R, et al. Expression of tumor necrosis factor-receptor superfamily members in lung T lymphocytes in interstitial lung disease. *Am J Respir Crit Care Med* 1996;153:1359–1367.
34. Schluter D, Deckert M. The divergent role of tumor necrosis factors in infectious diseases. *Microbes Infect* 2000;1:285–292.
35. Olobo JO, Geletu M, Demissie A, et al. Circulating TNF-alpha, TGF-beta, and IL-10 in tuberculosis patients and healthy contacts. *Scand J Immunol* 2001;53:85–91.
36. Saltini C, Colizzi V. Soluble immunological markers of disease activity in tuberculosis. *Eur Respir J* 1999;149:485–486.
37. Condos R, Liu Y, Rom W, et al. Local immune responses correlate with presentation and outcome in tuberculosis. *Am J Respir Crit Care Med* 1998;57:729–735.
38. Selvaraj P, Sriram U, Mathan Kurian S, et al. Tumour necrosis factor alpha (-238 and -308) and beta gene polymorphisms in pulmonary tuberculosis: haplotype analysis with HLA-A, B and DR genes. *Tuberculosis* 2001;81:335–341.
39. Hirano T, Akira S, Taga T, et al. Biological and clinical aspects of interleukin 6. *Immunol Today* 1990;11:443–449.
40. Bermudez LE, Wu M, Petrofsky M, et al. Interleukin-6 antagonizers tumor necrosis factor-mediated mycobacteriostatic and mycobactericidal activities in macrophages. *Infect Immun* 1992;60:4245–4552.
41. Saunders BM, Frank AA, Orme IM, et al. Interleukin-6 induces early gamma interferon production in the infected lung but is not required for generation of specific immunity to *Mycobacterium tuberculosis* infection. *Infect Immun* 2000;68:3322–3326.
42. Denis M, Gregg EO. Recombinant interleukin-6 increases the

43. Xirouchaki N, Tzanakis N, Bouros D, et al. Diagnostic value of interleukin-1alpha, interleukin-6, and tumor necrosis factor in pleural effusions. *Chest* 2002;121:815–820.
44. Zhang Y, Rom WN. Regulation of the interleukin-1β (IL-1β) gene by mycobacterial components and lipopolysaccharide is mediated by two nuclear factor-IL6 motifs. *Mol Cell Biol* 1993; 13:3831–3837.
45. Akira S, Isshiki H, Sugita T, et al. A nuclear factor for IL-6 expression (NF-IL6) is a member of a C/EBP family. *EMBO J* 1990;9:1897–1906.
46. Zhang Y, Broser M, Rom WN. Activation of the interleukin-6 gene by *Mycobacterium tuberculosis* or lipopolysaccharide is mediated by NF-IL6 and NF-κB. *Proc Natl Acad Sci U S A* 1994;91:2225–2229.
47. Weiden M, Tanaka N, Qiao Y, et al. Differentiation of monocytes to macrophages switches the *Mycobacterium tuberculosis* effect on HIV-1 replication from stimulation to inhibition: modulation of interferon response and CCAAT/enhancer binding protein B expression. *J Immunol* 2000;165:2028–2039.
48. Merola M, Blanchard B, Tovey MG. The kappa B enhancer of the human interleukin-6 promoter is necessary and sufficient to confer an IL-1 beta and TNF-alpha response in transfected human cell lines: requirement for members of the C/EBP family for activity. *J Interferon Cytokine Res* 1996;16:783–789.
49. Hoshino Y, Hoshino S, Nakata K, et al. Maximal HIV-1 replication in alveolar macrophages during tuberculosis requires both lymphocyte contact and cytokines. *J Exp Med* 2002;195: 495–525.
50. Sugawara I, Mizuno S, Yamada H, et al. Disruption of nuclear factor-interleukin-6, a transcription factor, results in severe mycobacterial infection. *Am J Pathol* 2001;158:361–366.
51. Orme IM, Roberts AD, Griffin JP, et al. Cytokine secretion by CD4 T lymphocytes acquired in response to *Mycobacterium tuberculosis* infection. *J Immunol* 1993;151:518–525.
52. Fiorentino DF, Zlotnik A, Mosmann TR, et al. IL-10 inhibits cytokine production by activated macrophages. *J Immunol* 1991;147:3815–3822.
53. de Waal Malefyt R, Abrams J, Bennett B, et al. IL-10 inhibits cytokine synthesis by human monocytes: an autoregulatory role of IL-10 produced by monocytes. *J Exp Med* 1991;174: 1209–1220.
54. Bogdan C, Vodovotz Y, Nathan C. Macrophage deactivation by interleukin 10. *J Exp Med* 1991;174:1549–1555.
55. Oswald IP, Gazzinelli RT, Sher A, et al. IL-10 synergizes with IL-4 and transforming growth factor-β to inhibit macrophage cytotoxic activity. *J Immunol* 1992;148:3578–3582.
56. de Waal Malefyt R, Haanen J, Spits H, et al. Interleukin-10 (IL-10) and viral IL-10 strongly reduce antigen-specific human T cell proliferation by diminishing the antigen-presenting capacity of monocytes via downregulation of class II major histocompatibility complex expression. *J Exp Med* 1991;174:915–924.
57. Bermudez LE, Champsi J. Infection with *Mycobacterium avium* induces production of interleukin-10 (IL-10), and administration of anti-IL-10 antibody is associated with enhanced resistance to infection in mice. *Infect Immun* 1993;61:3093–3097.
58. Redpath S, Ghazal P, Gascoigne NRJ. Hijacking and exploitation of IL-10 by intracellular pathogens. *Trends Microbiol* 2001; 9:86–92.
59. Boussiotis AV, Tsai EY, Yunis EJ, et al. IL-10-producing T cells suppress immune responses in anergic tuberculosis patients. *J Clin Invest* 2000;105:1317–1325.
60. Bertagnolli MM, Lin B-Y, Young D, et al. IL-12 augments antigen-dependent proliferation of activated T lymphocytes. *J Immunol* 1992;149:3778–3783.

61. Gubler U, Chua AO, Schoenhaut DS, et al. Coexpression of two distinct genes is required to generate secreted bioactive cytotoxic lymphocyte maturation factor. *Proc Natl Acad Sci U S A* 1991; 88:4143–4147.

62. Zhang M, Gately MK, Wang E, et al. Interleukin 12 at the site of disease in tuberculosis. *J Clin Invest* 1994;93:1733–1739.

63. Munk ME, Mayer P, Anding P, et al. Increased numbers of IL-12 producing cells in human tuberculosis. *Infect Immun* 1996; 64:1078–1080.

64. Rogge L, Papi A, Presky DH, et al. Antibodies to the IL-12 receptor beta chain mark human Th1 but not Th2 cells *in vitro* and *in vivo*. *J Immunol* 1999;162:3926–3932.

65. Cooper AM, Roberts AD, Rhoades ER, et al. The role of interleukin-12 in acquired immunity to *Mycobacterium tuberculosis* infection. *Immunology* 1995;84:423–432.

66. Bertagnolli M, Herrmann S. IL-7 supports the generation of cytotoxic T lymphocytes from thymocytes. Multiple lymphokines required for proliferation and cytotoxicity. *J Immunol* 1990;145:1706–1712.

67. Gately MK, Renzetti LM, Magram J, et al. The interleukin-12/interleukin-12-receptor system: role in normal and pathologic immune responses. *Annu Rev Immunol* 1998;16:495–521.

68. Zhang M, Gong J, Presky DH, et al. Expression of the IL-12 receptor beta 1 and beta 2 subunits in human tuberculosis. *J Immunol* 1999;162:2441–2447.

69. Sakai T, Matsuoka M, Aoki M, et al. Missense mutation of the interleukin-12 receptor beta1 chain-encoding gene is associated with impaired immunity against *Mycobacterium avium* complex infection. *Blood* 2001;97:2688–2694.

70. Wu C, Wang X, Gadina M, et al. IL-12 receptor beta 2 (IL-12R beta 2)-deficient mice are defective in IL-12-mediated signaling despite the presence of high affinity IL-12 binding sites. *J Immunol* 2000;165:6221–6228.

71. Denis M. Interleukin-12 (IL-12) augments cytolytic activity of natural killer cells towards *Mycobacterium tuberculosis* infected human monocytes. *Cell Immunol* 1994;156:529–536.

72. Dorman SE, Holland SM. Interferon-gamma and interleukin-12 pathway defects and human disease. *Cytokine Growth Factor Rev* 2000;11:321–333.

73. de Jong R, Altare F, Haagen IA, et al. Severe mycobacterial and *Salmonella* infections in interleukin-12 receptor-deficient patients. *Science* 1998;280:1435–1438.

74. Altare F, Durandy A, Lammas D, et al. Impairment of mycobacterial immunity in human interleukin-12 receptor deficiency. *Science* 1998;280:1432–1435.

75. Fenhalls G, Stevens L, Bezuidenhout J, et al. Distribution of IFN-gamma, IL-4 and TNF-alpha protein and CD8 T cells producing IL-12p40 mRNA in human lung tuberculous granulomas. *Immunology* 2002;105:325–335.

76. Verhagen CE, deBoer T, Smits HH, et al. Residual type 1 immunity in patient genetically deficient for interleukin 12 receptor 1 (IL-12R1): evidence for an IL-12R 1independent pathway of IL-12 responsiveness in human T cells. *J Exp Med* 2000;192:5172–5178.

77. Toossi Z, Ellner JJ. The role of TGF beta in the pathogenesis of human tuberculosis. *Clin Immunol Immunopathol* 1998;87: 107–114.

78. Kehrl JH, Wakefield LM, Roberts AB, et al. Production of transforming growth factor-β by human T lymphocytes and its potential role in the regulation of T cell growth. *J Exp Med* 1986;163:1037–1050.

79. Hirsch CS, Yoneda T, Averill L, et al. Enhancement of intracellular growth of *Mycobacterium tuberculosis* in human monocytes by transforming growth factor-beta 1. *J Infect Dis* 1994;170: 1229–1237

80. Toossi Z, Young TG, Averill LE, et al. Induction of transforming growth factor beta 1 by purified protein derivative of *Mycobacterium tuberculosis*. *Infect Immun* 1995;63:224–228.

81. Dahl KE, Shiratsuchi H, Hamilton BD, et al. Selective induction of transforming growth factor beta in human monocytes by lipoarabinomannan of *Mycobacterium tuberculosis*. *Infect Immun* 1996;64:399–405.

82. Koli K, Saharinen J, Hyytiainen M, et al. Latency, activation, and binding proteins of TGF-beta. *Microsc Res Tech* 2001;52: 354–362.

83. Murphy-Ullrich JE, Poczatek M. Activation of latent TGF-beta by thrombospondin-1: mechanisms and physiology. *Cytokine Growth Factor Rev* 2000;11:59–69.

84. Lebman DA, Edmiston JS. The role of TGF-beta in growth, differentiation, and maturation of B lymphocytes. *Microbes Infect* 1999;1:1297–1304.

85. Kapp A, Zeck-Kapp G. Activation of the oxidative metabolism in human polymorphonuclear neutrophilic granulocytes: the role of immuno-modulating cytokines. *J Invest Dermatol* 1990;95:94S–99S.

86. Boom WH, Toossi Z, Wolf SF, et al. The modulation by IL-2, NKSF (IL-12/CLMF) and TGF-β of CD4⁺ T cell mediated cytotoxicity for macrophages. In: *Proceedings of the Twenty-Seventh Joint Conference on Tuberculous Leprosy*, 1992:163–167(abst).

87. Luttmann W, Franz P, Schmidt S, et al. Inhibition of HLA-DR expression on activated human blood eosinophils by transforming growth factor-beta1. *Scand J Immunol* 1998;48:667–671.

88. Bogdan C, Paik J, Vodovotz Y, et al. Contrasting mechanisms for suppression of macrophage cytokine release by transforming growth factor-β and IL-10. *J Biol Chem* 1992;267:23301–23306.

89. Ding A, Nathan C, Srimal S. Macrophage deactivating factor and TGF-β inhibit nitrogen oxide synthesis by IFN γ. *J Immunol* 1990;145:940–945.

90. Toossi Z, Gogate P, Shiratsuchi H, et al. Enhanced production of TGF-beta by blood monocytes from patients with active tuberculosis and presence of TGF-beta in tuberculous granulomatous lung lesions. *J Immunol* 1995;154:465–473.

91. Bermudez LE. Production of transforming growth factor-beta by *Mycobacterium avium*-infected human macrophages is associated with unresponsiveness to IFN-gamma. *J Immunol* 1993; 150:1838–1845.

92. Hirsch CS, Yoneda T, Averill L, et al. Enhancement of growth factor-beta 1. *J Infect Dis* 1994;170:1229–1237.

93. Weiner HL. Oral tolerance: immune mechanisms and the generation of Th3-type TGF-beta-secreting regulatory cells. *Microbes Infect* 2001;3:947–954.

94. Muller I, Cobbold SP, Waldmann H, et al. Impaired resistance to *Mycobacterium tuberculosis* infection after selective *in vivo* depletion of L3T4⁺ and Lyt–2⁺ cells. *Infect Immun* 1987;55: 2037–2041.

95. Barnes PF, Mistry SD, Cooper CL, et al. Compartmentalization of a CD4+ T lymphocyte subpopulation in tuberculous pleuritis. *J Immunol* 1989;142:1114–1119.

96. Barnes PF, Bloch AB, Davidson PT, et al. Tuberculosis in patients with human immunodeficiency virus infection. *N Engl J Med* 1991;324:1644–1650.

97. North RJ, Izzo AA. Granuloma formation in severe combined immunodeficient (SCID) mice in response to progressive BCG infection. Tendency not to form granulomas in the lung is associated with faster bacterial growth in this organ. *Am J Pathol* 1993;142:1959–1966.

98. Law KF, Jagirdar J, Weiden MD, et al. Tuberculosis in HIV-positive patients: cellular response and immune activation in the lung. *Am J Respir Crit Care Med* 1996;153:1377–1384.

99. Delespesse G, Demeure CE, Yang LP, et al. *In vitro* maturation

of naive human CD4+ T lymphocytes into Th1, Th2 effectors. *Int Arch Allergy Immunol* 1997;113:157–159.

100. Romagnani S. The Th1/Th2 paradigm. *Immunol Today* 1997;18:263–267.

101. Greenbaum LA, Horowitz JB, Woods A, et al. Autocrine growth of CD4+ T cells. Differential effects of IL-1 on helper and inflammatory T cells. *J Immunol* 1988;140:1555–1560.

102. Gajewski TF, Pinnas M, Wong T, et al. Murine Th1 and Th2 clones proliferate optimally in response to distinct antigen-presenting cell populations. *J Immunol* 1991;146:1750–1758.

103. Fiorentino DF, Bond MW, Mosmann TR. Two types of mouse T helper cell. IV. Th2 clones secrete a factor that inhibits cytokine production by Th1 clones. *J Exp Med* 1989;170:2081–2095.

104. Salgame P, Abrams JS, Clayberger C, et al. Differing lymphokine profiles of functional subsets of human CD4 and CD8 T cell clones. *Science* 1991;254:279–282.

105. Maggi E, Parronchi P, Manetti R, et al. Reciprocal regulatory effects of IFN-γ and IL-4 on the *in vitro* development of human Th1 and Th2 clones. *J Immunol* 1992;148:2142–2147.

106. Huygen K, Abramowicz D, Vandenbussche P, et al. Spleen cell cytokine secretion in *Mycobacterium bovis* BCG-infected mice. *Infect Immun* 1992;60:2880–2886.

107. Heinzel FP, Sadick MD, Holaday BJ, et al. Reciprocal expression of interferon-γ or interleukin 4 during the resolution or progression of murine leishmaniasis. Evidence for expansion of distinct helper T cell subsets. *J Exp Med* 1989;169:59–72.

108. Yssel H, De Waal Malefyt R, Roncarolo MG, et al. IL-10 is produced by subsets of human CD4 T cell clones and peripheral blood T cells. *J Immunol* 1992;149:2378–2384.

109. Del Prete G, De Carli M, Almerigogna F, et al. Human IL-10 is produced by both type 1 helper (Th1) and type 2 helper (Th2) T cell clones and inhibits their antigen-specific proliferation and cytokine production. *J Immunol* 1993;150:353–360.

110. Sieling PA, Modlin RL. Cytokine patterns at the site of mycobacterial infection. *Immunobiology* 1994;191:378–387.

111. Yamamura M, Uyemura K, Deans RJ, et al. Defining protective responses to pathogens: cytokine profiles in leprosy lesions. *Science* 1991;254:277–279.

112. Parronchi P, Romagnani P, Annunziato F, et al. Type 1 T-helper cell predominance and interleukin-12 expression in the gut of patients with Crohn's disease. *Am J Pathol* 1997;150:823–832.

113. Piccotti JR, Chan SY, VanBuskirk AM, et al. Are Th2 helper T lymphocytes beneficial, deleterious, or irrelevant in promoting allograft survival? *Transplantation* 1997;63:619–624.

114. Del Prete GF, De Carli M, Mastromauro C, et al. Purified protein derivative of *Mycobacterium tuberculosis* and excretory-secretory antigen(s) of *Toxocara canis* expand *in vitro* human T cells with stable and opposite (type 1 T helper or type 2 T helper) profile of cytokine production. *J Clin Invest* 1991;88:346–350.

115. Haanen JBAG, de Waal Malefijt R, Res PCM, et al. Selection of a human T helper type 1-like T cell subset by mycobacteria. *J Exp Med* 1991;174:583–592.

116. Tsicopoulos A, Hamid Q, Varney V, et al. Preferential messenger RNA expression of Th1-type cells (IFN-γ+, IL-2+) in classical delayed-type (tuberculin) hypersensitivity reactions in human skin. *J Immunol* 1992;148:2058–2061.

117. Boom WH, Wallis RS, Chervenak KA. Human *Mycobacterium tuberculosis*–reactive CD4+ T-cell clones: heterogeneity in antigen recognition, cytokine production, and cytotoxicity for mononuclear phagocytes. *Infect Immun* 1991;59:2737–2743.

118. Barnes PF, Abrams JS, Lu S, et al. Patterns of cytokine production by mycobacteria-reactive human T cell clones. *Infect Immun* 1993;61:197–203.

119. Barnes PF, Lu S, Abrams JS, et al. Cytokine production at the site of disease in human tuberculosis. *Infect Immun* 1993;61:3482–3489.

120. Surcel H-M, Troye-Blomberg M, Paulie S, et al. Th1/Th2 profiles in tuberculosis, based on the proliferation and cytokine responses of blood lymphocytes to mycobacterial antigens. *Immunology* 1994;81:171–176.

121. Sanchez FO, Rodriguez JI, Agudelo G, et al. Immune responsiveness and lymphokine production in patients with tuberculosis and healthy controls. *Infect Immun* 1994;62:5673–5678.

122. Robinson DS, Ying S, Taylor IK, et al. Evidence for a Th1-like bronchoalveolar T-cell subset and predominance of interferon-gamma gene activation in pulmonary tuberculosis. *Am J Respir Crit Care Med* 1994;149:989–993.

123. Schwander SK, Sada E, Torres M, et al. T lymphocytic and immature macrophage alveolitis in active pulmonary tuberculosis. *J Infect Dis* 1996;173:1267–1272.

124. Sodhi A, Gong J, Silva C, et al. Clinical correlates of interferon gamma production in patients with tuberculosis. *Clin Infect Dis* 1997;25:617–620.

125. Tan JS, Canaday DH, Boom WH, et al. Human alveolar T lymphocyte responses to *Mycobacterium tuberculosis* antigens: role for CD4+ and CD8+ cytotoxic T cells and relative resistance of alveolar macrophages to lysis. *J Immunol* 1997;159:290–297.

126. Flynn JL, Goldstein MM, Triebold KJ, et al. Major histocompatibility complex class I-restricted T cells are required for resistance to *Mycobacterium tuberculosis* infection. *Proc Natl Acad Sci U S A* 1992;89:12013–12017.

127. Flynn JL, Goldstein MM, Triebold KJ, et al. Major histocompatibility complex class I-restricted T cells are necessary for protection against *M. tuberculosis* in mice. *Infect Agents Dis* 1993;2:259–262.

128. Dalton DK, Pitts-Meek S, Keshav S, et al. Multiple defects of immune cell function in mice with disrupted interferon-γ genes. *Science* 1993;259:1739–1742.

129. Kamijo R, Le J, Shapiro D, et al. Mice that lack the interferon-γ receptor have profoundly altered responses to infection with bacillus Calmette-Guérin and subsequent challenge with lipopolysaccharide. *J Exp Med* 1993;178:1435–1440.

130. Dupuis S, Dargemont C, Fieschi C, et al. Impairment of mycobacterial but not viral immunity by a germline human STAT1 mutation. *Science* 2001;13;293:300–303.

131. Holland SM, Eisenstein EM, Kuhns DB, et al. Treatment of refractory disseminated nontuberculous mycobacterial infection with interferon gamma. A preliminary report. *N Engl J Med* 1994;330:1348–1355.

132. Vilcek J, Klion A, Henriksen-DeStefano D, et al. Defective gamma-interferon production in peripheral blood leukocytes of patients with acute tuberculosis. *J Clin Immunol* 1986;6:146–151.

133. Somoskovi A, Zissel G, Zipfel PF, et al. Different cytokine patterns correlate with the extension of disease in pulmonary tuberculosis. *Eur Cytokine Netw* 1999;10:135–142.

134. Condos R, Rom WN, Schluger NW. Treatment of multidrug-resistant pulmonary tuberculosis with interferon-gamma via aerosol. *Lancet* 1997;349:1513–1515.

135. Zhang Y, Nakata K, Weiden M, et al. *Mycobacterium tuberculosis* enhances HIV-1 replication by transcriptional activation at the long terminal repeat. *J Clin Invest* 1995;95:2324–2331.

136. Condos R, Rom WN, Weiden M. Lung-specific immune response in tuberculosis. *Int J Tuberc Lung Dis* 2000;4:S11–S17.

137. Jeevan A, Asherton GL. Recombinant interleukin-2 limits the replication of *Mycobacterium lepraemurium* and *Mycobacterium bovis* BCG in mice. *Infect Immun* 1988;56:660–664.

138. Kaplan G, Britton WJ, Hancock GE, et al. The systemic influ-

ence of recombinant interleukin 2 on the manifestations of lepromatous leprosy. *J Exp Med* 1991;173:993–1006.

139. Takahashi S, Setoguchi Y, Nukiwa T. Soluble interleukin-2 receptor in sera of patients with pulmonary tuberculosis. *Chest* 1991;99:310–314.

140. Tchou-Wong KM, Tanabe O, Chi C, et al. Activation of NFκB in *Mycobacterium tuberculosis*-induced interleukin-2 receptor expression in mononuclear phagocytes. *Am J Respir Crit Care Med* 1999;159:1323–1329.

141. Lawn SD, Rudolph D, Ackah A, et al. Lack of induction of interleukin-2-receptor-alpha in patients with tuberculosis and human immunodeficiency virus co-infection: implications for pathogenesis. *Trans R Soc Trop Med Hyg* 2001;95:449–445.

142. Johnson BJ, Bekker LG, Rickman R, et al. rhuIL-2 adjunctive therapy in multidrug resistant tuberculosis: a comparison of two treatment regimens and placebo. *Tuber Lung Dis* 1997;78:195–203.

143. Johnson B, Bekker LG, Ress S, et al. Recombinant interleukin 2 adjunctive therapy in multidrug-resistant tuberculosis *Novartis Found Symp* 1998;217:99–106.

144. Lehn M, Weiser WY, Engelhorn S, et al. IL-4 inhibits H_2O_2 production and antileishmanial capacity of human cultured monocytes mediated by IFN-γ. *J Immunol* 1989;143:3020–3024.

145. Ho JL, He SH, Rios MJC, et al. Interleukin-4 inhibits human macrophage activation by tumor necrosis factor, granulocyte-monocyte colony-stimulating factor, and interleukin-3 for antileishmanial activity and oxidative burst capacity. *J Infect Dis* 1992;165:344–351.

146. Martinez OM, Gibbons RS, Garovoy MR, et al. IL-4 inhibits IL-2 receptor expression and IL-2-dependent proliferation of human T cells. *J Immunol* 1990;144:2211–2215.

147. Schwarz EM, Salgame P, Bloom BR. Molecular regulation of human interleukin 2 and T-cell function by interleukin 4. *Proc Natl Acad Sci USA* 1993;90:7734–7738.

148. Fenhalls G, Wong A, Bezuidenhout J, et al. *In situ* production of gamma interferon, interleukin-4, and tumor necrosis factor alpha mRNA in human lung tuberculous granulomas. *Infect Immun* 2000;68:2827–2836.

149. Seah GT, Scott GM, Rook GA. Type 2 cytokine gene activation and its relationship to extent of disease in patients with tuberculosis. *J Infect Dis* 2000;181:385–389.

150. Sallusto F, Mackay CR, Lanzavecchia A. The role of chemokine receptors in primary, effector, and memory immune responses. *Annu Rev Immunol* 2000;18:593–620.

151. Kelner GS, Kennedy J, Bacon KB, et al. Lymphotactin: a cytokine that represents a new class of chemokine. *Science* 1994;266:1395–1399.

152. Mantovani A. The chemokine system: redundancy for robust outputs. *Immunol Today* 1999;20:254–257.

153. Rossi D, Zlotnik A. The biology of chemokines and their receptors. *Annu Rev Immunol* 2000;18:217–242.

154. D'Ambrosio D, Mariani M, Panina-Bordignon P, et al. Chemokines and their receptors guiding T lymphocyte recruitment in lung inflammation. *Am J Respir Crit Care Med* 2001;164:1266–1275.

155. Verdegaal ME, Zegveld ST, van Furth R. Heat shock protein 65 induces CD62e, CD106, and CD54 on cultured human endothelial cells and increases their adhesiveness for monocytes and granulocytes. *J Immunol* 1996;157:369–376.

156. Somoskovi A, Zissel G, Ziegenhagen MW, et al. Accessory function and costimulatory molecule expression of alveolar macrophages in patients with pulmonary tuberculosis. *Immunobiology* 2000;201:450–460.

157. Lopez-Ramirez GM, Rom WN, Bonk SJ, et al. *Mycobacterium tuberculosis* alters expression of adhesion molecules on monocytic cells. *Infect Immun* 1994;62:2515–2520.

158. Nasreen N, Mohammed KA, Ward MJ, et al. Mycobacterium-induced transmesothelial migration of monocytes into pleural space: role of intercellular adhesion molecule-1 in tuberculous pleurisy. *J Infect Dis* 1999;180:1616–1623

159. Orme IM, Cooper AM. Cytokine/chemokine cascades in immunity to tuberculosis. *Immunol Today* 1999;20:307–312.

160. Schluger NW, Rom WN. The host immune response to tuberculosis. *Am J Respir Crit Care Med* 1998;157:679–691.

161. Nau GJ, Guilfoile P, Chupp GL, et al. A chemoattractant cytokine associated with granulomas in tuberculosis and silicosis. *Proc Natl Acad Sci U S A* 1997;94:6414–6419.

162. Lin Y, Gong J, Zhang M, et al. Production of monocyte chemoattractant protein 1 in tuberculosis patients. *Infect Immun* 1998;66:2319–2322.

163. Fraticelli P, Sironi M, Bianchi G, et al. Fractalkine (CX3CL1) as an amplification circuit of polarized Th1 responses. *J Clin Invest* 2001;107:1173–1181.

164. Sadek MI, Sada E, Toossi Z, et al. Chemokines induced by infection of mononuclear phagocytes with mycobacteria and present in lung alveoli during active pulmonary tuberculosis. *Am J Respir Cell Mol Biol* 1998;19:513–521.

165. Kurashima K, Mukaida N, Fujimura M, et al. Elevated chemokine levels in bronchoalveolar lavage fluid of tuberculosis patients. *Am J Respir Crit Care Med* 1997;155:1474–1477.

166. Deng H, Liu R, Ellmeier W, et al. Identification of a major co-receptor for primary isolates of HIV-1. *Nature* 1996;381:661–666.

167. Fraziano M, Cappelli G, Santucci M, et al. Expression of CCR5 is increased in human monocyte-derived macrophages and alveolar macrophages in the course of *in vivo* and *in vitro Mycobacterium tuberculosis* infection. *AIDS Res Hum Retroviruses* 1999;15:869–874.

168. Juffermans NP, Verbon A, van Deventer SJ, et al. Elevated chemokine concentrations in sera of human immunodeficiency virus (HIV)-seropositive and HIV-seronegative patients with tuberculosis: a possible role for mycobacterial lipoarabinomannan. *Infect Immun* 1999;67:4295–4297.

169. Mohammed KA, Nasreen N, Ward MJ, et al. Mycobacterium-mediated chemokine expression in pleural mesothelial cells: role of C-C chemokines in tuberculous pleurisy. *J Infect Dis* 1998;178:1450–1456.

170. Antony VB, Godbey SW, Kunkel SL, et al. Recruitment of inflammatory cells to the pleural space. Chemotactic cytokines, IL-8, and monocyte chemotactic peptide-1 in human pleural fluids. *J Immunol* 1993;151:7216–7223.

171. Demangel C, Britton WJ. Interaction of dendritic cells with mycobacteria: where the action starts. *Immunol Cell Biol* 2000;78:318–324.

172. Cochand L, Isler P, Songeon F, et al. Human lung dendritic cells have an immature phenotype with efficient mannose receptors. *Am J Respir Cell Mol Biol* 1999;21:547–554.

173. Hertz CJ, Kiertscher SM, Godowski PJ, et al. Microbial lipopeptides stimulate dendritic cell maturation via Toll-like receptor 2. *J Immunol* 2001;166:2444–2450.

174. Gerosa F, Baldani-Guerra B, Nisii C, et al. Reciprocal activating interaction between natural killer cells and dendritic cells. *J Exp Med* 2002;195:327–333.

175. Matsushima K, Baldwin ET, Mukaida N. Interleukin-8 and MCAF: novel leukocyte recruitment and activating cytokines. *Chem Immunol* 1992;51:236–265.

176. Koch AE, Polverini PJ, Kunkel SL, et al. Interleukin-8 as a macrophage-derived mediator of angiogenesis. *Science* 1992;258:1798–1801.

177. Friedland JS, Remick DG, Shattock R, et al. Secretion of interleukin-8 following phagocytosis of *Mycobacterium tuberculosis* by human monocyte cell lines. *Eur J Immunol* 1992;22:1373–1378.

178. Mukaida N, Shiroo M, Matsushima K. Genomic structure of the human monocyte-derived neutrophil chemotactic factor IL-8. *J Immunol* 1989;143:1366–1377.

179. Bergeron A, Bonay M, Kambouchner M, et al. Cytokine patterns in tuberculous and sarcoid granulomas: correlations with histopathologic features of the granulomatous response. *J Immunol* 1997;159:3034–3043.

180. Zhang Y, Broser M, Cohen H, et al. Enhanced interleukin-8 release and gene expression in macrophages after exposure to *Mycobacterium tuberculosis* and its components. *J Clin Invest* 1995;95:586–592.

181. Casarini M, Ameglio F, Alemanno L, et al. Cytokine levels correlate with a radiologic score in active pulmonary tuberculosis. *Am J Respir Crit Care Med* 1999;159:143–148.

182. Ashitani J, Mukae H, Hiratsuka T, et al. Elevated levels of alpha-defensins in plasma and BAL fluid of patients with active pulmonary tuberculosis. *Chest* 2002;121:519–526.

183. Fietta A, Meloni F, Francioli C, et al. Virulence of *Mycobacterium tuberculosis* affects interleukin-8, monocyte chemoattractant protein-1 and interleukin-10 production by human mononuclear phagocytes. *Int J Tissue React* 2001;23:113–125.

184. Schauf V, Rom WN, Smith KA, et al. Cytokine gene activation and modified responsiveness to interleukin-2 in the blood of tuberculosis patients. *J Infect Dis* 1993;168:1056–1059.

185. Meddows-Taylor S, Martin DJ, Tiemessen CT. Dysregulated production of interleukin-8 in individuals infected with human immunodeficiency virus type 1 and *Mycobacterium tuberculosis*. *Infect Immun* 1999;67:1251–1260.

186. Ashitani J, Mukae H, Nakazato M, et al. Elevated pleural fluid levels of defensins in patients with empyema. *Chest* 1998;113:788–794.

187. Yount NY, Yuan J, Tarver A, et al. Cloning and expression of bovine neutrophil beta-defensins. Biosynthetic profile during neutrophilic maturation and localization of mature peptide to novel cytoplasmic dense granules. *J Biol Chem* 1999;274:26249–26258.

188. Miyakawa Y, Ratnakar P, Rao AG, et al. *In vitro* activity of the antimicrobial peptides human and rabbit defensins and porcine leukocyte protegrin against *Mycobacterium tuberculosis*. *Infect Immun* 1996;64:926–932.

189. Kisich KO, Heifets L, Higgins M, et al. Antimycobacterial agent based on mRNA encoding human beta-defensin 2 enables primary macrophages to restrict growth of *Mycobacterium tuberculosis*. *Infect Immun* 2001;69:2692–2699.

22

MOLECULAR MECHANISMS OF HUMAN IMMUNODEFICIENCY VIRUS/TUBERCULOSIS INTERACTION IN THE LUNG

YOSHIHIKO HOSHINO
BINDU RAJU
MICHAEL WEIDEN

Patients with human immunodeficiency virus (HIV) and tuberculosis (TB) coinfection present a unique series of problems in both the developed and developing world. HIV infection markedly reduces the resistance to active TB. Unlike many other opportunistic infections, HIV-infected patients with high CD4 lymphocyte counts are at much greater risk for TB than patients without HIV infection. An example of this is latent TB infection. HIV-1-positive injection drug users who are also purified protein derivative (PPD) positive have a 10% annual rate of progression to active disease as compared with a 10% lifetime risk of progression to active disease in PPD-positive HIV-1-negative patients (1). There is also evidence that HIV-1 infection enhances transmission of TB. In hospital outbreaks a large number of acquired immune deficiency syndrome (AIDS) patients progress to active TB disease shortly after exposure (2). Finally, the virulence of *M. bacterium* is markedly increased by HIV infection. HIV-1-positive patients with multidrug-resistant TB have nearly 70% one-year mortality as compared with a 50% lifetime mortality in HIV-uninfected patients with multidrug-resistant infection (3).

The marked immunocompromise produced by HIV-1 necessitates great vigilance to prevent an epidemic of TB in HIV-1-infected patients. This is especially true because a negative PPD has no utility in excluding latent TB infection in HIV-infected patients. An excellent example of the disastrous interaction between infection with HIV and TB

Y. Hoshino: Department of Medicine, Division of Pulmonary and Critical Care Medicine, New York University School of Medicine, New York, New York.
B. Raju: Department of Medicine, Division of Pulmonary and Critical Care Medicine, New York University School of Medicine; Department of Chest Medicine, Bellevue Hospital Center, New York, New York.
M. Weiden: Department of Medicine, Division of Pulmonary and Critical Care Medicine, New York University School of Medicine; Department of Pulmonary Medicine, Bellevue Hospital, New York, New York.

is found in New York City during the last decade. The confluence of the HIV epidemic and dismantling of the infrastructure for TB control produced a spike of TB in the early 1990s. The nadir of the incidence of active TB occurred in late 1970s with approximately 1,200 cases of TB reported to the New York City Department of Health. The peak of the TB epidemic occurred in 1992 when 3,811 cases of TB were reported in the city. Seroprevalence studies documented that HIV-1 infection contributed significantly to the TB epidemic. In 1992, 34% of TB patients were known to be HIV-1 infected and only 16% of TB patients were known to be HIV-1 uninfected. Men aged 25 to 54 had the peak incidence of TB. This was also the group with the highest HIV infection rates, providing further evidence that HIV-1 infection was driving the TB epidemic.

The United States government responded to the epidemic by investing more than $2 billion in TB control in New York City over the next decade. The hallmarks of this effort were accessible and convenient directly observed therapy; a high index of suspicion for the possibility of TB in the hospital setting leading to isolation of patients with cough and infiltrates on chest radiograph while TB was ruled out; and creation of public health laws mandating treatment and isolation of rare recalcitrant patients while they present an infection risk. By 1997 the effectiveness of this program was clear, with only 1,730 cases of TB reported.

Control of TB markedly improved even though the incidence of HIV-1 infection increased during this period and highly active antiretroviral therapy had not yet been widely introduced. In 1997 only 26% of TB patients were HIV-1 seropositive, while 48% of TB patients were found to be seronegative. The New York City experience demonstrates that, despite their expense, currently available strategies for TB control are effective even in the face of an ongoing HIV epidemic. This has important implications for the developing world where a vast majority of patients infected with TB and HIV are located. It has been estimated that more than 500,000 deaths occurred in coinfected patients in the year 2000 (4). Understanding the interaction of these two pathogens is clinically important given the high prevalence of patients coinfected with HIV-1 and *Mycobacterium tuberculosis* in both the developed and developing world.

EFFECTS OF TUBERCULOSIS ON THE COURSE OF ACQUIRED IMMUNE DEFICIENCY SYNDROME

Tuberculosis accelerates the course of AIDS. In addition to the convincing evidence that HIV-1 infection worsens the risk and course of TB, there is increasing clinical evidence that coinfection with *M. tuberculosis* accelerates progression of disease caused by HIV-1 infection. In a case-control study of AIDS patients matched for CD4 counts, patients with HIV/TB coinfection had higher mortality than patients without TB (5). This increased mortality was not due to TB but rather to an increased rate of other lethal opportunistic infections. A prospective cohort study conducted in Uganda confirmed these findings, with an acceleration of AIDS observed in high CD4 count patients after TB (6). It is possible that *M. tuberculosis* infects patients with a more aggressive form of HIV infection and thereby identifies a subgroup of patients predisposed to rapid progression. Alternatively, TB may alter the viral infection in a way that changes viral load or viral pathogenicity.

Recent investigation strongly supports the notion that TB increases viral replication. Bronchoscopy with bronchoalveolar lavage (BAL) has been an extremely useful tool to document the effect of TB on HIV-1 replication. In the absence of opportunistic infection there is little or no viral replication in the lung, and fewer than 1 in 10,000 alveolar macrophages is provirally infected (7). Lung segments involved with TB have a 10- to 1,000-fold increase in HIV-1 viral particles in comparison with uninvolved lung segments of the same patient lavaged at the same time (8). The BAL viral load is higher than that found in plasma, indicating that the lung is supporting high levels of local viral replication (Fig. 22.1). This conclusion is supported by sequence analysis results demonstrating that lung-derived virus is distinct from plasma-derived virus. Similar effects of TB have also been observed by others who have studied viral dynamics in the pleural space and blood during HIV/TB coinfection (9).

The immune response to pulmonary TB is characterized by delayed hypersensitivity with granuloma formation, recruitment of CD4+ lymphocytes to the lung, and the elaboration of a large number of cytokines, including tumor necrosis factor-α (TNF-α), interferon-γ (IFN-γ), interleukin-1β (IL-1β), interleukin-6 (IL-6), and inter-

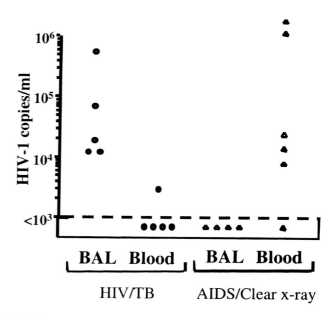

FIGURE 22.1. Viral load in blood and bronchoalveolar lavage (*BAL*) fluid of human immunodeficiency virus/tuberculosis (*HIV/TB*)–coinfected patients and autoimmune deficiency syndrome (*AIDS*) patients with clear chest radiographs.

leukin-8 (IL-8) by bronchoalveolar cells (10). HIV-1 coinfection impairs granuloma formation and CD4+ lymphocytosis (11,12). *M. tuberculosis* and its cell wall component lipoarabinomannan (LAM) increase release of TNF-α, IL-1β, and IL-6 by mononuclear phagocytes at the level of transcription by activation of promoters through increased activity of DNA-binding proteins such as nuclear factor κB (NF-κB) and CCAAT/enhancer-binding protein-β (C/EBP-β) (13,14). The HIV-1 long terminal repeat (LTR), like the promoters of many cytokine genes, contains NF-κB and C/EBP binding sequences. TNF-α increases HIV-1 production in mononuclear phagocytes through transcriptional activation of the LTR promoter by NF-κB (15), although the effect depends in part on the state of cellular differentiation (16,17). Similarly, *M. tuberculosis* and its cell wall component LAM increases HIV-1 promoter activity, increases binding of NF-κB to LTR sequences, and enhances HIV-1 replication. *In vivo* the amount of HIV-1 correlated very well ($R^2 > 0.95$, $p < 0.001$) with TNF-α and IL-6 levels in the BAL fluid of AIDS patients with TB (8). Two possible explanations of this correlation are that (a) inflammatory cytokines stimulate HIV-1 production *in vivo* and (b) the inflammation produced in pulmonary TB increases both HIV-1 replication and cytokine production.

Sequence analysis reveals that virus from involved lung segments has much greater diversity than virus from uninvolved lung segments. The predicted amino acid sequences of viruses obtained from the involved segment suggest that they are more pathogenic than virus from uninvolved lung segments (8). Little or no virus is found in the lymphocytes drawn to the site of TB. This may be due to the short life span of a CD4 lymphocyte in the setting of immune activation. A majority of the lymphocytes at the site of TB in HIV-1-infected patients are CD8 cells. The alveolar macrophage is the predominant source viral replication in the lung during HIV-1 replication (18). Defining the molecular mechanisms suppressing HIV-1 replication in resting macrophages and the switch to high levels of HIV-1 replication seen in activated macrophages in TB is essential to understanding AIDS pathophysiology. This is especially true because macrophages are long-lived cells and latently infected macrophages may be a reservoir for viral reactivation after prolonged highly active antiretroviral therapy (19).

DIFFERENCES BETWEEN TYPE I AND TYPE II INTERFERONS

Type I IFN is essential for innate antiviral immunity, whereas type II IFN is essential for cellular immunity. The IFNs are cytokines that mediate both antigen-independent and antigen-dependent antiviral immunity. Type-I IFNs constitute an essential early arm of the innate immune response (20), which is activated in the first few hours after viral infection (21). Type I IFNs are expressed at low levels in normal tissues. Immunoreactive IFN-α is expressed in tissue macrophages throughout the body (22). Innate immunity is activated by invariant characteristics of the pathogen and provides protection from pathogens in the time window before antigen-specific immunity can occur (23).

In the case of viruses, the IFN response is activated by the presence of double-stranded RNA, which is a common feature of many viruses, including HIV-1. A double-stranded RNA-dependent protein kinase (PKR) is expressed in IFN-treated monocytes and is likely a sensor of viral infection (24). Knockout mice deficient in PKR fail to induce type I IFNs after stimulation with double-stranded RNA and are more susceptible to early death from viral infection than mice with intact PKR (25). Once activated by viral infection, PKR phosphorylates inhibitory κB (I-κB), activating the NF-κB system (26), and phosphorylates translation initiation factors, which shut down protein synthesis. The transactivating region of the HIV-1 genome produces an RNA stem structure that is sensed by a PKR (27). The type I IFN system, once induced, provides early protection against a broad range of viruses. Knockout mice deficient in receptors for type I IFNs are highly prone to early death after viral infection (28). The type I IFN system is strongly activated by HIV-1 infection *in vitro* and *in vivo,* but HIV-1 escapes from the inhibitory effects of the innate immune system in part because IFN receptors are down-regulated (29).

IFN-γ, the only cytokine in the type I IFN response, is essential for control of intracellular pathogens such as *M. tuberculosis.* Produced during the cellular immune response by antigen-specific lymphocytes, IFN-γ serves to activate macrophages. Knockout mice deficient in multiple steps along the type II IFN pathway are extremely prone to death caused by intracellular pathogens (30). AIDS patients who show depletion of CD4+ lymphocytes are unable to produce the high levels of IFN-γ normally seen in the lung during pulmonary TB (Fig.22.2). This may contribute to susceptibility of AIDS patients to infection with *M. tuberculosis.* Knockout mice deficient in Stat-1 manifest a specific dysfunction of type I and type II IFN–mediated immunity (31). Signal transduction by IFN-γ is mediated by a different receptor pair which, when activated, induces Stat-1 homodimer formation (32). The Stat-1 homodimer and ISGF-3, the transcription factor complex that mediates type II IFN, have different sequence specificity. Type I and type II IFNs activate different but overlapping sets of genes that collectively mediate the antiviral, immunomodulatory, and developmental effects of the IFNs.

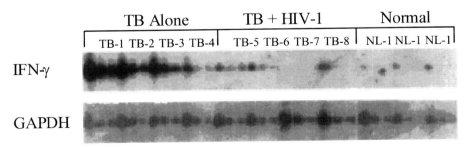

FIGURE 22.2. Interferon-γ (*IFN-γ*) mRNA in bronchoalveolar lavage cells measured by reverse transcriptase–polymerase chain reaction of serial dilutions of input cDNA. Four immunocompetent tuberculosis patients produced high levels of IFN-γ mRNA, whereas four human immunodeficiency virus type 1 (*HIV-1*)–coinfected patients had significantly reduced IFN-γ mRNA. Parallel reactions with glyceraldehyde-3-phosphate dehydrogenase (*GAPDH*) primers were used to ensure equal loading. *NL,* normal control; *TB,* tuberculosis.

VIRAL REPLICATION IN MACROPHAGES AND MONOCYTES

Type I IFN suppresses viral replication in macrophages but not monocytes after proinflammatory stimuli. Surprisingly, proinflammatory stimuli, such as TNF-α and lipopolysaccharide (LPS), suppress viral replication in macrophages (33). The suppression of HIV-1 replication seen after LPS stimulation closely resembles the suppression seen after addition of IFNs (34). The negative regulatory element (NRE) is the DNA element responsible for suppressing the HIV-1 LTR after LPS stimulation (16). The type I IFN system is activated by infection with *M. tuberculosis.* The mycobacterial cell wall component LAM interacts with the Toll-like receptor 4 (TLR-4) with the CD14 adapter molecule. Once TLR-4 is activated type I interferon is induced (35). This may explain the paradox that *in vitro M. tuberculosis* infection inhibits HIV-1 replication. Clearly coinfection of cells in isolation does not reproduce the activation of HIV-1 replication *in vivo.*

Opposite results were observed when monocytes were treated with TNF-α or LPS. Undifferentiated monocytic cell lines or blood monocytes up-regulate HIV-1 LTR promoter activity and HIV-1 replication in response to LPS and other proinflammatory stimuli, such as TNF-α (36,37) or coinfection with many different pathogens (38). This is in part due to NF-κB activation. Interestingly, IFN-β mRNA is equally well induced in monocytes and macrophages after LPS stimulation (33), suggesting that during differentiation macrophages gain the ability to respond to IFN. This is due to induction of IRF-9, a critical component of ISGF-3 and type I IFN signaling (17).

CCAAT/ENHANCER-BINDING PROTEIN

C/EBP-β has 37-kd stimulatory and 16-kd inhibitory isoforms. The C/EBP-β gene (also called NF-IL-6, LAP/LIP, and NF-M) has no introns, but two different proteins are produced from the same mRNA. The model proposed to explain these observations is translation start-site selection. Stimulatory forms (approximately 30 and 37 kd, termed LAP for liver activation protein) are produced when the ribosome starts translation at the first or second AUG codon. The large forms contain DNA binding domains, dimerization domains, and transcriptional activation domains. A small (about 16 to 20 kd) isoform described in rat liver (termed LIP for liver-induced inhibitory protein) functions as an inhibitory transcription factor (39,40). This form is likely produced when the ribosome selects an internal ribosome entry site (IRES) in the C/EBP-β mRNA. The inhibitory form of the protein contains only a DNA binding and dimerization domain but no activation domain, and it can form heterodimers with the stimulatory C/EBP-β (Fig. 22.3). The mechanism that regulates start-site selection is poorly understood.

Importantly, the 16-kd C/EBP-β(LIP) isoform is a dominant negative transcription factor *in vitro,* since heterodimers of the inhibitory and stimulatory C/EBP-β isoforms suppress transcription and bind to C/EBP sites in the DNA with higher affinity than homodimers of the stimulatory 37-kd C/EBP-β isoform (Fig. 22.3). LIP inhibits transcription if present at 20% the level of LAP (39). C/EBP-β knockout mice have a lymphoproliferative disorder similar to Castleman disease, which is associated with elevated levels of IL-6 (41,42). Double-mutant mice deficient in both IL-6 and C/EBP-β do not develop the lymphoproliferative disorder (43). These findings demonstrate that C/EBP-β participates in down-regulation of cytokine production *in vivo* and suggest that the inhibitory C/EBP-β has an important role in maintaining cytokine homeostasis. The HIV-1 LTR NRE has three C/EBP binding domains that bind C/EBP-β (44). The C/EBP binding site closest to the transcription start site is 1 bp from an NF-κB site (Fig. 22.4). Mutation of the C/EBP binding sites produces a virus that is unable to replicate in monocytes but is still able to replicate in lymphocytes (45). The effect on replication is transcriptionally mediated because C/EBP mutation produces marked loss of promoter function in monocytes (46). These data suggest that transcription factors that bind to C/EBP sites in the LTR are important stimulators of HIV-1 replication in monocytes but not in lymphocytes. C/EBP-binding elements can either repress or stimulate transcription, depending on which isoform of C/EBP-β is expressed (47). C/EBP transcription factors are also important regulators of promoter function in adenoviruses (48). Thus, the C/EBP transcription factor family is a good candidate for regulating viral expression in macrophages.

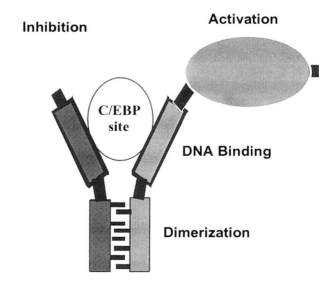

FIGURE 22.3. A 16-kd CCAAT/enhancer-binding protein-β (*C/EBP-β*) is a dominant negative transcription factor because heterodimers of the 37-kd isoform and the 16-kd isoform repress transcription and bind to C/EBP sites in DNA with high affinity.

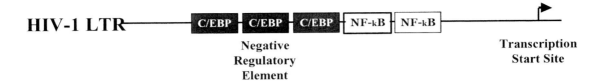

FIGURE 22.4. The human immunodeficiency virus type 1 long terminal repeat (*HIV-1 LTR*) has three CCAAT/enhancer-binding protein (*C/EBP*) binding domains that are required for replication in macrophages but not lymphocytes. *NF-κB*, nuclear factor κB.

EXPRESSION OF CCAAT/ENHANCER-BINDING PROTEIN

Inhibitory C/EBP-β is strongly expressed in alveolar macrophages from lung segments with low viral replication and is down-regulated in inflamed lung segments with high viral replication. Overexpression of the inhibitory 16-kd isoform in transformed monocytes leads to inhibition of HIV-1

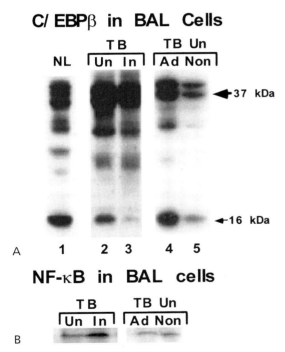

A

FIGURE 22.5. Transcription factor expression in bronchoalveolar lavage (*BAL*) cells from a normal control and a patient with human immunodeficiency virus type 1 infection and pulmonary tuberculosis (*TB*). **A:** *Lane 1,* a normal control (*NL*). *Lanes 2 and 3,* inhibitory 16-kd CCAAT/enhancer-binding protein-β (*C/EBP-β*) was strongly expressed in BAL cells from uninflamed lung and was down-regulated in pulmonary tuberculosis. *Lane 4,* adherent BAL cells (*Ad*) from an uninvolved lobe of an autoimmune deficiency syndrome patient with tuberculosis. Adherent BAL cells contained more than 95% alveolar macrophages. *Lane 5,* nonadherent cells (*Non*), which were 80% to 90% lymphocytes. **B:** Nuclear factor κB (*NF-κB*) expression is up-regulated in BAL cells of involved lung segments in tuberculosis. These immunoblots are from the same patients shown in panel A.

replication and LTR promoter function (46). C/EBP binding sites and NF-κB binding sites also occur in the TNF-α promoter, and overexpression of inhibitory C/EBP-β represses TNF-α transcription (49). C/EBP and NF-κB sites also occur in IL-1 and IL-6 promoters, suggesting that the HIV-1 LTR and proinflammatory cytokine genes undergo similar regulation in monocytes and macrophages (13,14,50). Changes in LTR activity may be regulated by systems that normally regulate inflammatory cytokine promoters. The inhibitory short form C/EBP-β is strongly expressed in alveolar macrophages from normal lung and in the uninvolved lobes of patients with TB (Fig. 22.5). Expression of this dominant negative transcription factor maintains the alveolar macrophage in its baseline quiescent state and may be important for preventing an excessive inflammatory response to a brief inflammatory stimulus. The inhibitory form is lost in the involved lung segments, thus supporting the hypothesis that C/EBP-β is a mediator of the switch from repression of HIV-1 LTR in uninflamed lung to its activation in pulmonary TB (51). It is therefore possible that a two-step process is required to maximally stimulate proinflammatory cytokine and HIV-1 replication: loss of an inhibitor to derepress C/EBP binding promoters and activation of NF-κB to stimulate the promoters.

MACROPHAGE/LYMPHOCYTE CONTACT

Macrophage/lymphocyte contact and cytokines are required to maximally activate HIV-1 replication. In vitro infection of macrophages with *M. tuberculosis* or stimulation with other bacterial products fails to reproduce loss of the inhibitory 16-kd C/EBP-β isoform or the increase in HIV-1 replication observed in involved lungs of AIDS patients with TB (17). Since cell-mediated immunity is central to the control of TB, it is likely that cell interaction between lymphocytes and macrophages is required to reproduce the state of immune activation found in TB. Support for this notion comes from the observation that allogeneic lymphocytes are capable of increasing HIV-1 replication in macrophages (52). Furthermore, isolated membranes from activated lymphocytes enhance HIV-1 replication in macrophages (53). This suggested that contact between lymphocytes and macrophages is essential to produce the type of immune activation produced during TB.

The addition of activated lymphocytes to macrophages reproduces the state of activation found in TB; inhibitory C/EBP-β is lost, NF-κB is activated, and HIV-1 replication is enhanced. If lymphocytes are separated from the macrophages by a membrane that prevents direct cell contact but allows cytokines to move from lymphocytes to macrophages, NF-κB is activated but expression of the inhibitory transcription factor is maintained. Lymphocyte-derived cytokines do not maximally stimulate the HIV-1 LTR in macrophages. Expression of the inhibitory C/EBP-β is abolished by antibodies that cross-linked macrophage-expressed costimulatory molecules B-7, vascular cell adhesion molecules (VCAM), and CD40. All three costimulatory molecules must be activated to abolish inhibitory transcription factor expression, suggesting that lympho-

cyte/macrophage contact derepresses whereas soluble factors activate the HIV-1 LTR and other proinflammatory promoters (Fig. 22.6).

SUMMARY

There exists a devastating reverberation between HIV-1 infection and TB. HIV infection markedly increases the transmission, progression, and severity of TB. Tuberculosis exacerbates AIDS by producing a burst of viral replication and mutation. Preventing TB in the HIV-infected individual is one strategy to slow the progression of AIDS even in the absence of effective antiviral chemotherapy.

The study of HIV/TB interaction has also unveiled important regulatory pathways that influence HIV infection and control production of inflammatory mediators. C/EBP-

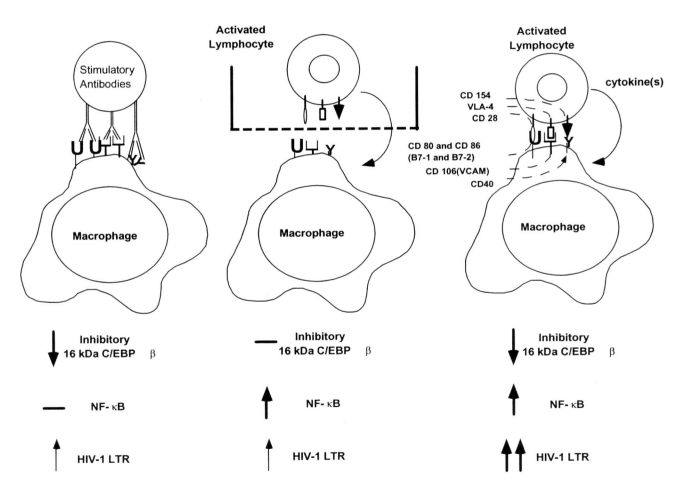

FIGURE 22.6 Two-step signaling achieves high levels of human immunodeficiency virus type 1 long terminal repeat (*HIV-1 LTR*) activation during cellular immunity. Contact between lymphocytes and macrophages down-regulates inhibitory CCAAT/enhancer-binding protein-β (*C/EBPβ*) derepressing the HIV-1 LTR (**left**), whereas soluble factors activate nuclear factor κB (*NF-κB*) enhancing the HIV-1 LTR (**middle**). Both contact and soluble factors are required for maximal stimulation (**right**).

β is a transcription factor that binds the HIV-1 LTR as well as many proinflammatory cytokine promoters in macrophages. Inhibition of these may be important for maintaining lung homeostasis in the absence of infection. Activation of the HIV-1 LTR and proinflammatory cytokines requires a two-step process including contact-mediated derepression and cytokine-mediated activation. One advantage of the requirement for lymphocyte/macrophage contact is that granulomatous inflammation is limited to areas where lymphocytes are activated by the presence of antigen stimulation. This limits the destruction of lung architecture to areas where TB antigens are present to activate lymphocytes.

REFERENCES

1. Selwyn PA, Hartel D, Lewis VA, et al. A prospective study of the risk of tuberculosis among intravenous drug users with human immunodeficiency virus infection. *N Engl J Med* 1989;320: 545–550.
2. Fischl MA, Uttamchandani RE, Daiko GL. An outbreak of tuberculosis caused by multiple-drug-resistant tubercle bacilli among patients with HIV infection. *Ann Intern Med* 1992;117: 177–183.
3. Park MM, Davis A, Schluger N, et al. Outcome of MDR-TB patients, 1983–1993: prolonged survival with appropriate therapy. *Am J Respir Crit Care Med* 1996;153:317–324.
4. WHO Report on the TB epidemic. *WHOTB* 1994;94:177.
5. Whalen C, Horsburgh CR, Hom D, et al. Accelerated course of human immunodeficiency virus infection after tuberculosis. *Am J Respir Crit Care Med* 1995;151:129–135.
6. Toossi Z, Mayanja-Kizza H, Hirsch CS, et al. Impact of tuberculosis (TB) on HIV-1 activity in dually infected patients. *Clin Exp Immunol* 2000;123:233–238.
7. Nakata K, Weiden M, Harkin T, et al. Low copy number and limited variability of proviral DNA in alveolar macrophages from HIV-1 infected patients: evidence for genetic differences in HIV-1 between lung and blood macrophage populations. *Mol Med* 1995;1:744–757.
8. Nakata K, Rom W, Honda Y, et al. *M. tuberculosis* enhances human immunodeficiency virus-1 replication in the lung. *Am J Respir Crit Care Med* 1997;155:996–1003.
9. Toossi Z, Johnson J, Kanost R, et al. Increased replication of HIV-1 at sites of *Mycobacterium tuberculosis* infection: potential mechanisms of viral activation. *J Acq Immun Defic Syndr* 2001;28:1–8.
10. Law KF, Weiden M, Harkin T, et al. Increased release of IL-1β, IL-6, and TNF-α by bronchoalveolar cells lavaged from involved sites in pulmonary tuberculosis. *Am J Respir Crit Care Med* 1996; 153:799–804.
11. Israel-Biet D, Cadranel J, Beldjord K, et al. 1991. Tumor necrosis factor production in HIV-seropositive subjects: relationship with lung opportunistic infections and HIV expression in alveolar macrophages. *J Immunol* 1991;147:490–494.
12. Law KF, Jagirdar J, Weiden M, et al. Tuberculosis in HIV-positive patients: cellular response and immune activation in the lung. *Am J Respir Crit Care Med* 1996;153:1377–1384.
13. Zhang Y, Broser M, Rom WN. Activation of the interleukin-6 gene by *Mycobacterium tuberculosis* or lipopolysaccharide is mediated by NF-IL6 and NF-κB. *Proc Natl Acad Sci U S A* 1994; 91:2225–2229.
14. Zhang Y, Rom WN. Regulation of the interleukin-1β gene by mycobacterial components and lipopolysaccharide is mediated by two NF-IL6-like motifs. *Mol Cell Biol* 1993;13:3831–3837.
15. Duh E, Maury W, Folks T, et al. Tumor necrosis factor α activates human immunodeficiency virus type 1 through induction of nuclear factor binding to the NF-κB sites in the long terminal repeat. *Proc Natl Acad Sci U S A* 1989;86:5974–5978.
16. Bernstein MS, Tong-Starksen SE, Locksley RM. Activation of human monocyte-derived macrophages with lipopolysaccharide decreases human immunodeficiency virus replication at the level of gene expression. *J Clin Invest* 1991;88:540–545.
17. Weiden M, Tanaka N, Qiao Y, et al. Differentiation of monocytes to macrophages switches the *Mycobacterium tuberculosis* effect on HIV-1 replication from stimulation to inhibition: modulation of interferon response and C/EBPβ expression. *J Immunol* 2000;165:2028–2039.
18. Orenstein JM, Fox C, Whal SM. Macrophages as a source of HIV during opportunistic infections. *Science* 1997;276:1857.
19. Finzi D, Hermankova M, Pierson T, et al. Identification of a reservoir for HIV-1 in patients on highly active antiretroviral therapy. *Science* 1997;278:1295–1300.
20. van der Broek M, Muller U, Huang S, et al. Immune defense in mice lacking type I and/or type II interferon receptors. *Immunol Rev* 1995;148:5–18.
21. Eloranta M, Sandberg K, Alm G. The interferon-α/β responses of mice to herpes simplex virus studied at the blood and tissue level *in vitro* and *in vivo*. *Scand J Immunol* 1996;43:355–360.
22. Khan N, Pulford A, Farquharson M, et al. The distribution of immunoreactive interferon-alpha in normal human tissues. *Immunology* 1989;66:201–206.
23. Medzhitov R, Janeway C Jr. Innate immunity: the virtues of a nonclonal system of recognition. *Cell* 1997;91:295–298.
24. Der S, Lau A. Involvement of the double-stranded-RNA-dependent kinase PKR in interferon expression and interferon-mediated antiviral activity. *Proc Natl Acad Sci U S A* 1995;92: 8841–8845.
25. Yaang Y, Reis L, Pavlovic J, et al. Deficient signaling in mice devoid of double-stranded RNA-dependent protein kinase. *EMBO J* 1995;14:6095–6106.
26. Stancovski I, Baltimore D. NF-κB activation: the IκB kinase revealed? *Cell* 1997;91:299–302.
27. Edery I, Petryshyn R, Sonenberg N. Activation of double-stranded RNA-dependent kinase (dsI) by the TAR region of HIV-1 mRNA: a novel translational control mechanism. *Cell* 1989;56:303–312.
28. Muller U, Steinhoff U, Reis L, et al. Functional role of type I and type II interferons in antiviral defense. *Science* 1994;264: 1918–1921.
29. Lau A, Read S, Williams B. Downregulation of interferon α but not γ receptor expression *in vivo* in the acquired immunodeficiency syndrome. *J Clin Invest* 1988;82:1415–1421.
30. Durbin J, Hackenmiller R, Simon M, et al. Targeted disruption of the mouse Stat-1 gene results in compromised innate immunity to viral disease. *Cell* 1996;84:443–450.
31. Maraz M., White J, Sheehan K, et al. Targeted disruption of the Stat-1 gene in mice reveals unexpected physiologic specificity in the JAK-STAT signaling pathway. *Cell* 1996;84:431–442.
32. Bluyssen H., Durbin J, Levy D. ISGF3γ p48, a specificity switch for interferon activated transcription factors. *Cytokine Growth Factor Rev* 1996;7:11–17.
33. Gessani S, Testa U, Varano B, et al. Enhanced production of LPS-induced cytokines during differentiation of human monocytes to macrophages: role of LPS receptors. *J Immunol* 1993; 151:3758–3766.
34. Kornbluth RS, Oh PS, Munis JR, et al. IFNs and bacterial lipopolysaccharide protect macrophages from productive infection by human immunodeficiency virus *in vitro*. *J Exp Med* 1989; 169:1137–1151.
35. Toshchakov V, Jones BW, Perera PY, et al. TLR4, but not TLR2,

mediates IFN-beta-induced STAT1 alpha/beta-dependent gene expression in macrophages. *Nat Immunol* 2002:3:392–398.

36. Tadmori W, Mondal D, Tadmori I, et al. Transactivation of human immunodeficiency virus type 1 long terminal repeats by cell surface tumor necrosis factor α. *J Virol* 1991;65:6425–6429

37. Pomeranz R, Feinberg M, Trono D, et al. Lipopolysacaride is a potent monocyte/macrophage-specific stimulator of human immunodeficient virus type-1 expression. *J Exp Med* 1990;172:253–261.

38. Peterson PK, Gekker G, Chao CC, et al. Human cytomegalovirus-stimulated peripheral blood mononuclear cells induce HIV-1 replication via a tumor necrosis factor-α-mediated mechanism. *J Clin Invest* 1992;89:574–580.

39. Descombes P, Schibler U. A liver-enriched transcriptional activator protein, LAP, and a transcriptional inhibitory protein, LIP, are translated from the same mRNA. *Cell* 1991;67:569–579.

40. Ossipow V, Descombes P, Schibler U. CCAAT/enhancer-binding protein mRNA is translated into multiple proteins with different transcription activation potentials. *Proc Natl Acad Sci U S A* 1993;90:8219–8223.

41. Tanaka T, Akira S. Targeted disruption of the NF-IL6 gene dicloses its essential role in bacterial killing and tumor cytotoxicity by macrophages. *Cell* 1995;80:353–361.

42. Screpanti I., Romani L, Muisiani P., et al. Lymphoproliperative disorder and imbalanced T-helper response in C/EBP-β-deficient mice. *EMBO J* 1995;14:1932–1941.

43. Screpanti I., Muisiani P, Bellavia D, et al. Inactivation of the IL-6 gene prevents development of multicentric Castleman's disease in C/EBPβ-deficient mice. *J Exp Med* 1996;186:1561–1566.

44. Tesmer VM, Rajadhyaksha A, Babin J, et al. NF IL-6-mediated transcriptional activation of the long terminal repeat of the human immunodeficiency virus type 1. *Proc Natl Acad Sci U S A* 1993;90:7298–7303.

45. Henderson AJ, Calame KL. CCAAT/enhancer binding protein (C/EBP) sites are required for HIV-1 replication in primary macrophages but not CD4+ T cells. *Proc Natl Acad Sci U S A* 1997;94:8714–8719.

46. Henderson AJ, Zou X, Calame K. C/EBP proteins activate transcription from human immunodeficiency virus type 1 long terminal repeat in macrophages/monocytes. *J Virol* 1995:69:5337–5344.

47. Sears R, Sealy L. Multiple forms of C/EBP-β bind the EFII enhancer sequence in Rous sarcoma virus long terminal repeat. *Mol Cell Biol* 1994;14:4855–4871.

48. Spergel J, Hsu W, Akira S, et al. NF-IL6, a member of the C/EBP family, regulates E1A-responsive promotors in the absence of E1A. *J Virol* 1992;66:1021–1030.

49. Pope RM, Lentz A, Ness SA. C/EBPβ regulation of the tumor necrosis factor α gene. *J Clin Invest* 1995;94:1449–1455.

50. Zhang Y, Doerfler M, Lee TC, et al. Mechanisms of stimulation of interleukin-1β and tumor necrosis factor-α by *Mycobacterium tuberculosis* and its components. *J Clin Invest* 1993;91:2076–2083.

51. Honda Y, Rogers L, Nakata K, et al. Type I interferon induces inhibitory 16 kDa C/EBP-β repressing the HIV-1 LTR in macrophages: pulmonary tuberculosis alters C/EBP expression enhancing HIV-1 replication. *J Exp Med* 1998;188:1255–1265.

52. Hoshino Y, Nakata K, Hoshino S, et al. Maximal HIV-1 replication in alveolar macrophages during tuberculosis requires both lymphocyte contact and cytokines. *J Exp Med* 2002;195:495–505.

53. Mikovits J, Lohrey N, Schulof R, et al. Activation of infectious virus from latent human-immunodeficiency-virus infection of monocytes *in vivo*. *J Clin Invest* 1992;90:1486–1491.

PROGRAMMED CELL DEATH IN TUBERCULOSIS

JOSEPH KEANE
HARDY KORNFELD

Programmed cell death, also called apoptosis, is a regulated process of cellular self-deconstruction (1,2). Cells undergoing apoptosis shrink in volume as their nuclear and cytoplasmic contents are systematically condensed and degraded (Fig. 23.1). The cells form blebs and fragment into membrane-bound particles called apoptotic bodies that contain the intracellular contents, preventing their release into the extracellular environment. The alternative mode of cell death is necrosis, which is characterized by cellular swelling and catastrophic disruption of the cell and mitochondrial membranes with leakage of cytoplasmic contents into the extracellular space.

The biochemical machinery of apoptosis is constitutively expressed in most eukaryotic cells, and includes a family of cytoplasmic cysteine proteases called caspases that are critical components for the initiation and execution of programmed cell death (3). Caspases are produced as zymogens that are activated by cleavage at aspartate residues in sequence motifs similar to their own target substrates. Activated caspases may cleave other caspases to activate them, and they cleave diverse nuclear and cytoplasmic substrates in the execution phase of apoptosis. Among the latter is caspase-activated DNase, which cleaves genomic DNA between nucleosomes. This results in the characteristic banding pattern of genomic DNA isolated from apoptotic cells. In contrast, DNA isolated from necrotic cells appears as a smear.

Apoptosis is a fundamental mechanism in development where the elimination of unnecessary cells contributes to tissue patterning. In mature organisms, apoptosis maintains structural homeostasis by balancing the production of new cells with the elimination of senescent or redundant cells. The immune system makes extensive use of apoptosis to eliminate autoreactive lymphocytes, to regulate the expan-

sion and persistence of activated leukocytes during inflammation, and as a mechanism to kill infected cells (4,5).

MECHANISMS OF APOPTOSIS

Death signals are initiated by specific cell surface receptors, or by agents of cell injury such as ionizing radiation acting directly within the cell. Receptor-mediated death signaling is reviewed here as it is most pertinent to the pathobiology of tuberculosis. Members of the tumor necrosis factor receptor (TNFR) family link extracellular signals to the machinery of programmed cell death (6). Among these receptors, TNFR1 and Fas (CD95) are the best characterized and dominant members. Their cognate ligands TNF-α and Fas ligand (FasL) are members of the TNF family. Both TNF-α and FasL are expressed as transmembrane proteins that can bind to TNFR1 or Fas expressed on other cells. Cleavage by a membrane metalloproteinase liberates soluble TNF-α and FasL, which are also capable of activating their receptors on target cells independent of cell-to-cell contact (7,8). The extracellular domains of the surface receptors can also be cleaved yielding soluble TNFR1 and Fas that may act as receptor antagonists, adding an additional layer of regulation to the initiation of death signaling.

Trimers of TNF-α or FasL cross-link TNFR1 and Fas, respectively. This promotes the recruitment of signaling adapter complexes that associate with the intracytoplasmic tails of the death receptors through protein interaction motifs called death domains (DDs) and death effector domains (DEDs). Both TNFR1 and Fas have DD sequences that interact with the DD of adaptor proteins. The DD of Fas recruits the death-signaling adapter Fas-associated death domain protein (FADD), whereas the DD of TNFR1 associates with the DD of TNF receptor-1–associated death domain protein (TRADD), which in turn recruits FADD to the receptor. Once associated with either Fas or TNFR1, FADD then recruits procaspase-8 (or procaspase-10) through DED interactions. Activated procaspase-8 (or procaspase-10)

J. Keane: Dublin Molecular Medicine Center, Trinity College Dublin, St. James's Hospital, Dublin, Ireland.
H. Kornfeld: Department of Medicine, University of Massachusetts Medical School, Worcester, Massachusetts.

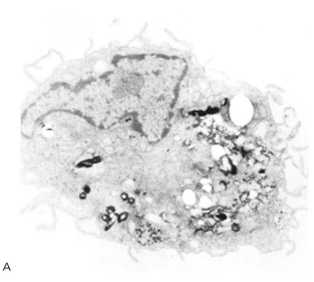
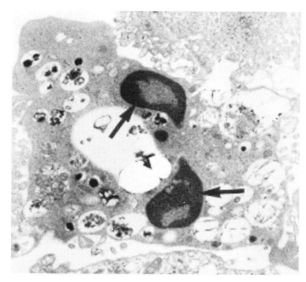

A   B

FIGURE 23.1. Morphology of apoptosis. Electron micrographs of uninfected alveolar macrophages (**A**) or macrophages infected with *Mycobacterium tuberculosis* H37Ra (**B**) were prepared after 2 days in culture. Nuclear fragmentation and condensation (*arrows*) were seen in cells from the H37Ra-infected group. Original magnification ×7,056 in both photomicrographs. (From Keane J, Balcewicz-Sablinska K, Remold HG, et al. Infection by *Mycobacterium tuberculosis* promotes human alveolar macrophage apoptosis. *Infect Immun* 1997;65:298–304, with permission.)

initiates a cascade that culminates in the activation of effector caspases (3, 6, and 7). TNFR1 can also transmit signals that inhibit apoptosis when a different complex of adaptor proteins are recruited to the intracytoplasmic tail. When TNF receptor–associated protein 2 (TRAF2) and receptor-interacting protein (RIP) are bound to TNFR1, signal pathways leading to activation of the c-Jun N-terminal kinase pathway, or signals resulting in the nuclear translocation of the transcription factor nuclear factor κB (NF-κB), are enabled (9). The latter augments the expression of genes that inhibit TNF-α-induced apoptosis (10–12). A second TNF receptor, TNFR2, lacks an intracytoplasmic DD motif and does not bind TRADD. This implies that TNFR2 is not involved in TNF death signaling, although there is evidence that TNFR2 provides cooperative signals that augment TNFR1-mediated death signals (13). The death signaling pathways potentially involved in *Mycobacterium tuberculosis*–induced macrophage apoptosis are depicted in Figure 23.2.

Mitochondrial Regulation of Apoptosis

Death signals can also originate from the mitochondria. Increased mitochondrial permeability results in the release of cytochrome *c*, which, in conjunction with the cytosolic protein Apaf-1, activates procaspase-9 leading to effector caspase activation (14). The precise role of mitochondrial death signals in the overall regulation of cell fate is a matter of debate, with some authorities holding that mitochondria are essential regulators of cell death and others positing that death signals initiated from cell surface receptors may be fully independent of mitochondria (15,16). Whatever the

final outcome of this debate, it is established that a family of important apoptosis-regulating proteins are linked to this organelle (2,17). Members of the Bcl-2 family, including Bax, Bak, and Bok, form pores in the mitochondrial membrane, promoting apoptosis. Countervailing antiapoptotic members of this family include Bcl-2, Bcl-X$_L$, and Bcl-w. It is believed that the initiation or inhibition of mitochondrial death signals depends on the local balance between the proapoptotic and antiapoptotic Bcl-2 family proteins.

Several other families of death signal regulatory proteins have been described in what is coming to be understood as an increasingly complex network. In trying to understand the emerging literature in this area, it is important to recognize that the dominant death signaling pathways in any system vary in a cell- and stimulus-specific manner.

Antiapoptotic Signals

The complexity of apoptosis-regulating factors is increasing as research progresses, and a complete description is beyond the scope of this discussion. In addition to the proapoptotic caspases, and the Bcl-2 family proteins that include both pro- and antiapoptotic members, there are other important apoptosis inhibitors. The inhibitor of apoptosis (IAP) family of antiapoptotic genes counteract programmed cell death by direct inhibition of caspases and probably also by channeling TNF-α signaling to NF-κB activation through interactions with TRAF2 in the TNFR complex (18). The IAP genes were first recognized by the discovery of viral homologs that are expressed by the pathogens to counteract the apoptosis response of infected host cells (19). There are

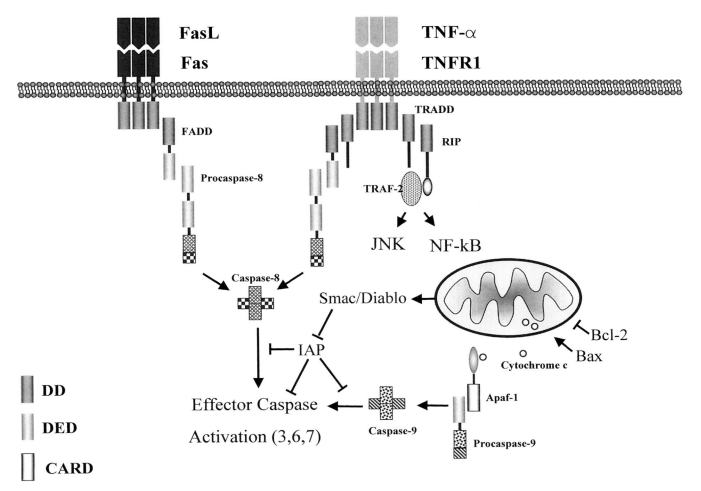

FIGURE 23.2. Death signaling pathways. This simplified schema depicts cell death receptor and mitochondrial signal pathways that may operate in *Mycobacterium tuberculosis*-infected macrophages. Ligation of Fas or tumor necrosis factor receptor-1 (*TNFR1*) can initiate a cascade of caspase activation leading to cell death. Depending on the adaptor proteins recruited to TNFR1, this receptor can also activate the c-Jun N-terminal kinase pathway or signals leading to the nuclear translocation of nuclear factor κB. The latter is known to induce the expression of genes that oppose apoptosis. Not shown in this figure is a potential direct connection between TNFR1 and mitochondrial death signals mediated by the Bcl-2 family member BID. *CARD*, caspase recruitment domain; *DD*, death domain; *DED*, death effector domain; *IAP*, inhibitor of apoptosis.

at least seven IAP homologs expressed in humans. These are characterized by functionally important sequence motifs called baculovirus IAP repeat (BIR) domains, and a C-terminal zinc finger RING motif. Apoptosis induction requires repression of the caspase-inhibiting activity of IAPs. This is mediated by release of an apoptosis-promoting mitochondrial factor called Smac/DIABLO (20).

Fate of Apoptotic Cells

The cellular corpses resulting from programmed cell death are called apoptotic bodies. These membrane-bound remnants contain a portion of the degraded cytoplasmic contents of the cell. Apoptotic bodies display unique cell surface fea-

tures that mark them for clearance by neighboring cells, particularly professional phagocytes including macrophages and neutrophils. One such surface feature is phosphatidylserine, which is normally exposed only on the cytoplasmic surface of the plasma membrane in viable cells. Phosphatidylserine flips to the extracellular surface of the plasma membrane in apoptotic cells (permitting the convenient identification of apoptotic cells by its interaction with annexin V). A specific phosphatidylserine receptor is one means for the recognition of apoptotic cells by phagocytes (21), but additional tethering and phagocytic receptors may also be involved in a phagocyte- and target-specific manner, including $\alpha_v\beta_3$ and $\alpha_v\beta_5$ integrins, CD36, and CD14 (22,23). It has recently been appreciated that the low-density lipoprotein–related protein receptor (CD91) is also involved in the engulfment of apoptotic cells (24). This is of particular interest because CD91 appears to convey extracellular antigens to the class I major histocompatibility complex (MHC) pathway (25).

Apoptosis prevents the release of potentially harmful cell contents and further suppresses inflammation as a result of signals imparted to phagocytes engulfing apoptotic bodies. Contact with apoptotic bodies triggers the release of antiinflammatory factors, including transforming growth factor β (26). In contrast, necrosis can provoke inflammation by allowing bioactive molecules to be discharged into the extracellular environment. This distinction might not be absolute as it recognized that apoptosis of leukocytes can lead to the release of cytokines cleaved from their precursors by caspase activity. These cytokines include the precursors of interleukin-1β (IL-1β) and IL-18 that are cleaved by caspase-1, and IL-16 whose precursor is a substrate for caspase-3 (27–29).

APOPTOSIS AND INFECTION

Immune responses to infection are regulated by apoptosis, but hosts and microbial pathogens also appear to use the induction or inhibition of apoptosis in particular target cells to their respective advantage (30). This paradigm is best understood in the context of infection by viruses (31). Viruses are intracellular parasites that convert host cell resources to the production of new viruses. One mechanism for host cells to control the spread of viral infection is to undergo apoptosis, thereby limiting viral replication. In parallel with the evolution of apoptosis as an innate defense response, many viruses have acquired genes such cowpox virus *crm A*, baculovirus *p35*, and various viral IAP homologs that suppress host cell apoptosis. Preventing host cell apoptosis enables viruses to replicate optimally and to disperse when the burst size is attained. The fate of virus-infected cells depends in some cases on the outcome of a regulatory conflict between host proapoptotic and viral antiapoptotic signals.

A role for apoptosis in bacterial and protozoal infections is increasingly being appreciated (32,33). Bacterial mediators of apoptosis include pore-forming toxins (e.g., listeriolysin O), protein synthesis inhibitors (e.g., *Pseudomonas aeruginosa* Exo-A), and proteins delivered via the type 3 secretion apparatus (e.g., the IpaB antigen of *Shigella*). Bacterial superantigens also induce apoptosis, namely, activation-induced cell death (AICD) of T lymphocytes. AICD normally operates as a regulatory mechanism that limits the expansion of activated T lymphocytes through Fas/FasL signaling (4). A given pathogen might exploit apoptosis to eliminate host defense cells or to penetrate an epithelial barrier. As an example, an apoptosis-inducing exotoxin of *P. aeruginosa* is postulated to facilitate persistent infection by eliminating neutrophils (34).

Similarly, induction of macrophage apoptosis by the group B *Streptococcus* β-hemolysin may be a strategy to overcome host defenses (35). Some gastrointestinal pathogens are known to cause apoptosis of gut epithelial cells. How this contributes to pathogenesis is unclear, but in the case of *Helicobacter pylori* virulence determinants in the cag pathogenicity island confer apoptosis-inducing activity against gastric mucosal cells to the bacterial lipopolysaccharide (36).

In contrast, the host might exploit apoptosis to deny intracellular pathogens a preferred growth niche. As is known to be the case with virus infections, a bacterial or protozoal pathogen faced with this defense strategy might express antiapoptotic activities to maintain a growth advantage. This scenario is suggested by evidence that the intracellular pathogens *Leishmania donovani* and *Chlamydia* inhibit the spontaneous apoptosis of host cells (37,38).

APOPTOSIS OF MACROPHAGES IN TUBERCULOSIS

Evidence is accumulating that apoptosis of macrophages and lymphocytes has a role in the host–pathogen interaction in tuberculosis. In the context of protective immunity, antigen-specific T lymphocytes are regulated by AICD, and cytotoxic T lymphocytes (CTLs) will kill *M. tuberculosis*-infected targets by mechanisms involving apoptosis. Considerable attention has also been paid to the potential role of macrophage apoptosis occurring as a direct consequence of intracellular parasitism by *M. tuberculosis*.

The success of *M. tuberculosis* as a human pathogen, and a characteristic that distinguishes it from nonpathogenic mycobacteria, is its ability to survive within macrophages. Inhaled bacilli commandeer the alveolar macrophage as a niche for efficient replication, at least partially protected from an effective immune response of the host. To achieve this end, tubercle bacilli have evolved mechanisms to control maturation of the phagosome in which they reside after engulfment by lung macrophages. Precisely how this is achieved is unclear, but it has been demonstrated that mycobacterial phagosomes have reduced incorporation of the vesicular adenosine triphosphate (ATP)–dependent proton pump that otherwise acidifies this compartment (39). Mycobacterial phagosomes are also impeded in their ability to fuse with lysosomes, protecting bacilli from toxic antimicrobial effectors including lysosomal hydrolases and free radicals (40,41). As characterized by immunoelectron microscopy, mycobacterial phagosomes most closely resemble early endosomes. In common with several other intracellular macrophage pathogens, *M. tuberculosis* appears to defeat cellular microbicidal mechanisms and establish a environment that favors bacterial survival and replication. In this context, apoptosis of infected macrophages could be a host strategy for innate defense.

Apoptosis of *Mycobacterium tuberculosis*-Infected Macrophages in the Absence of T Lymphocytes

Apoptosis of purified macrophages infected *in vitro* with pathogenic mycobacteria has been reported by several laboratories. Infection-induced apoptosis has been observed both in primary human alveolar macrophages and in monocyte-derived macrophages following exposure to various strains of *M. tuberculosis* and other pathogenic mycobacterial species (42–45). Infection-induced apoptosis has also been observed using primary cells of murine origin and in cell lines of human and murine origin (46,47). The data of Placido and Keane indicate that macrophage apoptosis requires challenge with live mycobacteria; heat-killed organisms had no effect on macrophage viability (43,45). This suggests that the signal that primes macrophage for apoptosis is generated from within the cell as a consequence of bacterial metabolism, rather than resulting from activation of cell surface receptors engaged by bacterial surface components.

Certain strains of *Mycobacterium avium* also induce human macrophage apoptosis, which can be blocked by the addition of anti-TNF antibodies, anti-Fas antibodies, or a caspase inhibitor (48). *M. avium* sonicate was found to induce apoptosis of the human monocyte-derived cell line THP-1 and human monocytes (49). This result contrasts with work with alveolar macrophages, where only viable mycobacteria were found to influence apoptosis (45).

The relative induction of macrophage apoptosis by pathogenic mycobacteria is influenced by several variables. When a number of different mycobacterial strains were tested by infection of human alveolar macrophages, the avirulent strains (H37Ra, *Mycobacterium bovis* BCG) were found to induce abundant apoptosis. In contrast, virulent strains (including H37Rv, *M. bovis* wild type, and clinical *M. tuberculosis* isolates) established productive infection without triggering an alveolar macrophage cell death response (50). The differential expression of apoptosis is best observed when the infecting dose is ten bacilli per macrophage or less.

The occurrence and timing of macrophage apoptosis after infection with *M. tuberculosis* appears to depend on the multiplicity of infection used (51,52), the virulence of the bacillus, the growth phase of the bacilli in culture before addition to macrophages *in vitro*, and the maturity of cell being infected (monocyte versus macrophage). With very high multiplicities of infection even virulent bacilli are cytotoxic, with both apoptosis and necrosis occurring *in vitro* more rapidly than is seen with low-dose infection.

Regarding the differentiation state of monocytic cells, it is known that monocytes are growth factor dependent and undergo spontaneous apoptosis in culture without growth factor support. In contrast, terminally differentiated human alveolar macrophages can be cultured for weeks *in vitro* with minimal spontaneous apoptosis. Monocytes can be rescued from spontaneous apoptosis by infection with the virulent *M. tuberculosis* strain H37Rv (53) or *M. bovis* BCG (54).

Role of Tumor Necrosis Factor

Apoptosis following mycobacterial infection of purified human alveolar macrophages has been shown to depend on macrophage-derived TNF activity. Naive macrophages are insensitive to the cytotoxic effects of TNF, indicating that the TNFR1 signaling complex in resting cells is not assembled to activate procaspase-8. However, when macrophages are infected with certain strains of *M. tuberculosis* they become primed to undergo autocrine and/or paracrine TNF-mediated apoptosis. Inhibiting endogenous TNF by neutralizing monoclonal antibody or by treatment with pentoxifylline completely blocks apoptosis of human alveolar macrophages infected with *M. tuberculosis* H37Ra (45). While a variety of death signaling pathways may be triggered *in vivo*, endogenous TNF alone is both necessary and sufficient for infection-induced macrophage apoptosis *in vitro*. This finding has implications for understanding the mechanism whereby infected macrophages become primed to undergo apoptosis as well as how virulent mycobacterial strains evade this response.

Experiments reported by Balcewicz-Sablinska et al. (55) suggest that evasion of apoptosis by at least one virulent *M. tuberculosis* strain (H37Rv) involves the inhibition of TNF signaling. Infection of primary human macrophages with virulent H37Rv was shown to induce greater production of IL-10 than infection with the isogenic attenuated strain H37Ra. Enhanced expression of IL-10 was linked to the shedding of TNFR2 from the macrophage surface after infection. Complexes of soluble TNFR2 and TNF were identified in supernatant fluid, and it was shown that this neutralized the biologic activity of TNF in the H37Rv-infected macrophage cultures despite equivalent production of TNF by macrophages infected with either strain. The vital importance of TNF in host defense against tuberculosis is amply supported by both human and murine studies (56–58). The postulated role for soluble TNFR antagonism as a mycobacterial virulence mechanism is novel, but it might not apply to all virulent bacterial strains (50).

It has also been suggested that differential expression of TNF by macrophages infected with virulent or attenuated *M. tuberculosis* strains provides a growth advantage for H37Rv. Engele et al. (59) reported that H37Rv induced more TNF production by human alveolar macrophages than H37Ra and that TNF in this setting promoted the growth of H37Rv. While differences in TNF production by alveolar or monocyte-derived macrophages infected with diverse *M. tuberculosis* strains have not been observed in some other published studies, the concept that TNF might stimulate the growth of virulent strains is novel and worthy of further study. Mycobacterial infection might alter TNFR signaling in a manner that favors bacterial replication and host cell survival (via NF-κB). A precedent is suggested by the finding that *M. tuberculosis* alters interferon-γ (IFN-γ) signaling (60).

Fas and Purinergic Receptors

Activation of cell death pathways other than those triggered by TNF have also been identified in macrophages infected with *M. tuberculosis*. Oddo et al. (61) reported that monocyte-derived macrophages constitutively express Fas and the addition of soluble FasL triggers apoptosis. Infection with H37Rv or H37Ra reduces surface expression of Fas but the infected cells remain sensitive to Fas death signals. This *in vitro* study used purified macrophages, and apoptosis induction required exogenous FasL. It is likely that infected macrophages would encounter cell-associated or soluble FasL from a variety of sources *in vivo* (62).

Purinergic receptors expressed on macrophages are also capable of transducing death signals (63). Death signaling is initiated by the ATP-gated purinoreceptor that is widely expressed on immunocytes, including macrophages. Apoptosis and killing of intracellular bacilli following ATP stimulation has been reported (64,65), but it is possible that these two phenomena are not linked or at least that alternative mechanisms exist for the antimicrobial activities activated through P2X (66). Stimulation of the P2X receptor by ATP was shown to promote phagosome–lysosome fusion, enhancing bacillary killing without reducing macrophage viability (67).

Regulation of Death Signaling in Macrophages Infected by *Mycobacterium tuberculosis*

The bacillary and host genetic basis of the macrophage apoptosis response to bacillary infection deserves close attention. Using differential display, Rango et al.(68) investigated mouse macrophage gene expression after infection with H37Rv. They noticed marked down-regulation of murine cytochrome *c* oxidase subunit VIIc (COX VIIc), an enzyme postulated to play a role in apoptosis. Klingler et al. (44) reported that the antiapoptotic gene *bcl-2* is down-regulated and apoptosis is increased in macrophages after infection with *M. bovis* BCG. The Bcl-2 family member *A1*is also reported to be regulated by mycobacterial infection of monocytes (54). It is likely that many more cases of differentially regulated apoptosis genes in *M. tuberculosis*-infected macrophages will be revealed by future studies. Unraveling of the genetic basis of this response is greatly expedited through the use of DNA microarrays (69,70).

Microbicidal Effects of Apoptosis

In addition to simply excluding pathogenic mycobacteria from a preferred growth niche, macrophage apoptosis has been linked by several investigators to reduced bacterial viability. Molloy et al. (64) reported that bacillary cell death occurs when infected host cells are rendered apoptotic by the exogenous administration of ATP. This effect appeared to be specifically linked to apoptosis, as bacterial viability was not impaired when host cells were subjected to H_2O_2-induced necrosis. In a similar vein, Oddo et al. (61) found that Fas-mediated macrophage apoptosis was linked to killing intracellular bacilli, whereas this was not seen with complement-mediated lysis of infected cells. Given the downstream similarities of death signaling initiated by TNF or Fas receptors, it would be expected that the induction of macrophage apoptosis by TNFR1 signaling would also cause a reduction in the viability of infected bacilli. Keane et al. (50) reported that infection of alveolar macrophages with attenuated mycobacteria strains that induced high rates of apoptosis was associated with mycobacterial killing. Alveolar macrophages infected *in vitro* with virulent mycobacterial strains remained viable and supported intracellular bacillary replication.

An antimycobacterial effect of apoptosis has also been observed using mouse macrophages. In these cells, apoptosis (and the associated reduction in bacterial viability) is dependent on TNF and independent of IFN-γ (51). Picolinic acid interferes with tryptophan metabolism and causes apoptosis of infected mouse macrophages with a concomitant reduction in the viability of *M. avium*, especially in the presence of IFN-γ (71).

A microbicidal effect of apoptosis, but not necrosis, for macrophages infected with mycobacteria has thus been confirmed by several laboratories. The mechanism whereby macrophage apoptosis promotes the killing of intracellular bacilli remains to be elucidated, but the preponderance of evidence suggests that key determinants lie in the execution phase of apoptosis since a variety of different initiating signals lead to the same outcome. Duan et al. (72) reported that macrophage apoptosis and arachidonic acid production in macrophages infected by *M. tuberculosis* is dependent on the activity of group IV cytosolic phospholipase A_2 and that these factors are linked to killing of bacilli.

Not all laboratories report increased bacillary killing with apoptosis. Santucci et al. (52) infected monocyte-derived macrophages with the virulent H37Rv strain, finding no bacillary killing when apoptosis was induced by high multiplicity of infection. Of interest, they did not see the bacillary growth typical of virulent *M. tuberculosis* strains such as H37Rv in the absence of apoptosis. The cytotoxic effects of high-dose infection are expressed rapidly *in vitro* and might outpace the induction of a putative microbicidal mechanism in this setting, particularly if necrosis is also induced or if secondary necrosis of apoptotic cells occurs rapidly in the cultures.

Fate of Apoptotic Macrophages After *Mycobacterium Tuberculosis* Infection

The consequence of macrophage apoptosis is the production of apoptotic corpses. Apoptotic cells are cleared with high efficiency *in vivo*, a phenomenon that depends on the expression of unique surface markers that indicate the apoptotic state of the cell for recognition by phagocytes. When macrophages infected with *M. tuberculosis* undergo apoptosis, intracellular bacilli may be retained within the apoptotic bodies. When this occurs *in vivo* it is highly likely that bacilli packaged in apoptotic bodies will therefore be quickly ingested by naive macrophages or neutrophils. These considerations prompted investigators to examine the fate of mycobacteria when fresh macrophages are added to cultures of previously infected macrophages undergoing apoptosis. Fratazzi et al. (73) reported that the addition of naive macrophages to infected apoptotic macrophages prevents the spread of mycobacterial infection in culture and enhances bacterial killing. No such effect was seen when the infected target macrophages were made necrotic by sonication. These studies suggest that bacilli associated with apoptotic bodies suffer a different fate after phagocytosis than occurs when naked bacilli are taken up through complement (or other) receptor–mediated phagocytosis. It is possible that bacilli contained within apoptotic bodies are more efficiently delivered to mature phagolysosomes. This model is far from established, and Bermudez et al. (74) reported that uptake of *M. avium* from apoptotic macrophages facilitates growth of bacilli in naive macrophages.

Macrophage Apoptosis and Host Susceptibility to Tuberculosis

The genetics of tuberculosis susceptibility has been studied in mice as an approach to understanding differences in human susceptibility to infection and disease. Rojas et al. (46) derived macrophage cell lines from congenic mice that differed in the *bcgNramp1* susceptibility allele. By comparing the response to *M. tuberculosis* infection of cell lines from the tuberculosis-resistant or susceptible mice (B10R and B10S), they noted that apoptosis correlated with increased nitric oxide production (NO$^-$) by B10R cells. Infection-induced apoptosis of these cells is differentially regulated by TNF and IL-10, while NO$^-$ and caspase-1 activity are required for its expression (75). They found that the balance of TNF and IL-10 was influenced by the *bcgNramp1* gene, an observation supporting the notion that apoptosis is beneficial to the host, since macrophages of the resistant *bcg* genotype were more prone to undergo apoptosis than those from the *bcg*-susceptible genotype. The relationship between genetic tuberculosis susceptibility factors of mice and humans is not yet resolved, and there is no conclusive evidence that *Nramp1* is a major determinant of

human susceptibility to tuberculosis. In this regard, inhibiting the activity of inducible NO synthase did not alter the apoptosis response of human alveolar macrophages to *M. tuberculosis* infection (45).

Tuberculosis susceptibility is likely to be multigenic and conceivably includes genes governing the macrophage apoptosis response. The common inbred mouse strain BALB/c is inherently resistant to tuberculosis. Peritoneal macrophages from BALB/c mice were found to undergo apoptosis in response to *M. tuberculosis* H37RA, similar to human macrophages. However, infection of macrophages from inherently susceptible C3H/HeJ mice failed to trigger apoptosis (47). The role of genetic factors influencing the apoptotic response of macrophages and the potential relationship to disease susceptibility deserves further attention.

Apoptosis of *Mycobacterium Tuberculosis*-Infected Macrophages in the Presence of T Lymphocytes

In addition to apoptotic pathways triggered as a direct result of mycobacterial infection, infected macrophages also become targets for killing by CTLs. Although *M. tuberculosis* bacilli are contained within phagosomes, mycobacterial antigens are accessible to the MHC class I pathway. It has been proposed that mycobacterial phagosomes are "leaky," allowing the bacteria access to cytoplasmic nutrients but also providing a pathway for antigenic molecules to reach the cytoplasm (76). The engulfment and processing of *M. tuberculosis* from apoptotic macrophages by dendritic cells could also contribute to the eventual cross-presentation of mycobacterial antigens to CD8$^+$ CTL (23).

The CTL response in tuberculosis is covered in depth in Chapter 18, but it should be noted here that the induction of programmed cell death is a predominant mechanism of target cell elimination. Surface expression of FasL particularly on CD4$^+$ CTL triggers Fas-mediated apoptosis in target cells expressing this receptor (77). Based on *in vitro* studies of *M. tuberculosis*-infected macrophages treated with soluble FasL, this CTL function would be expected to reduce the viability of mycobacteria within target macrophages (61). At odds with this model, Stenger et al. (78) reported that the direct antimicrobial effect of a CD8$^+$ T cell–derived protein called granulysin, but not Fas signaling, was responsible for killing intracellular *M. tuberculosis*.

CTLs produce two additional molecules that function cooperatively to kill target cells. The first is perforin, which causes pore formation in the cell membrane. The resulting pores allow both granulysin and another cytotoxic granule protein called granzyme to enter the cell. While nonapoptotic killing mechanisms may be initiated by cytotoxic granule proteins, both granzyme and granulysin have been shown to initiate programmed cell death. Granzyme can activate caspases directly, whereas granulysin disrupts the mitochondrial transmembrane potential causing the release of cytochrome *c* (79,80). Even if Fas- or granzyme-mediated apoptosis does not exert a direct antimicrobial effect, the resulting apoptotic bodies containing *M. tuberculosis* may be engulfed by newly recruited phagocytes possibly resulting in bacillary killing.

ROLE OF MACROPHAGE APOPTOSIS IN HOST DEFENSE AND TUBERCULOSIS DISEASE

While apoptosis is a well-established innate defensive response to viral infection, its participation in resistance to tuberculosis is a novel concept that has not yet been fully validated. The occurrence of infection-induced apoptosis is well supported by *in vitro* data. *In vivo* correlates have not yet been investigated in depth, but apoptosis of alveolar macrophages in the course of human pulmonary tuberculosis has been demonstrated (43,44). There are several obstacles to studying the occurrence and effects of macrophage apoptosis *in vivo*, not the least of which is the myriad mechanisms that may potentially contribute to apoptosis of inflammatory cells at foci of *M. tuberculosis* infection in tissues. However, *in vivo* alveolar macrophages lavaged from *M. tuberculosis* involved lung segments demonstrated fivefold more apoptosis than alveolar macrophages lavaged from normal volunteer controls (44).

Eviction

If alveolar macrophages comprise an essential niche for *M. tuberculosis* growth, then it is reasonable to predict that depletion of these cells would reduce susceptibility to infection. Although it is counterintuitive to posit that loss of the lung's primary host defense cell would protect against infection, this has been demonstrated experimentally. Leemans et al. (81) depleted alveolar macrophages in mice using bisphosphonate-loaded liposomes, finding that this treatment protected mice from lethal *M. tuberculosis* infection and reduced bacterial load in the lung and liver. This result supports the hypothesis that alveolar macrophages provide a necessary environment for bacillary growth following aerosol infection. In this context, programmed cell death of the infected alveolar macrophages could function as an innate immune defense strategy to deprive the bacillus of its optimal habitat. Even if the uptake of apoptotic corpses containing *M. tuberculosis* provides a mechanism for invasion of naive macrophages rather than augmenting bacterial elimination, the necessity for bacilli to reestablish a niche in the new host cell would be expected to restrict their replication kinetics. Furthermore, the process would be repeated sequentially when the new host cells initiate their own programmed cell death. Neutrophils are also recruited to foci

of *M. tuberculosis* infection in the lung and have a role in protection, although this effect has not conclusively been linked to their phagocytic and antimicrobial functions (82,83). Neutrophils avidly engulf apoptotic corpses and would certainly be suboptimal hosts for any viable mycobacteria taken up from apoptotic macrophages. Finally, by containing bacilli in apoptotic bodies, programmed cell death of infected macrophages would limit the extracellular growth of *M. tuberculosis*, which is an important facet of the disease process.

Bacillary Killing

The typical growth curves for *M. tuberculosis* in the lungs, as modeled in mice and other laboratory animals, is characterized by an initial phase of logarithmic expansion followed by plateau phase that occurs after 2 to 4 weeks. The eventual control of bacterial growth is attributed to the expression of an effective adaptive immune response, while the logarithmic phase is taken as evidence that innate defense mechanisms are relatively ineffective. However, most authorities agree that innate defense mechanisms are activated in tuberculosis and contribute to the optimal induction of adaptive immunity. Consistent with this idea is the finding that attenuated strains of pathogenic mycobacteria grow more slowly in the lungs of infected animals than their virulent counterparts during the early phase of logarithmic growth (84). Bacterial burden in the lung at the time when adaptive immunity is expressed may therefore be significantly lower after infection by attenuated strains. By limiting the bacterial burden achieved prior to the expression of adaptive immunity, an effective innate response would limit manifestations of tuberculosis disease that result from delayed-type hypersensitivity. The susceptibility of attenuated mycobacteria to infection-induced apoptosis potentially represents an important part of host protection afforded by TNF.

Granuloma Homeostasis

The hallmark of a successful immune response to tuberculosis is the granuloma. Cree et al. (85) have shown by microscopy that apoptosis is a feature of the granulomatous response in several diseases, including sarcoidosis, leprosy, and tuberculosis. Using more sensitive techniques to identify apoptotic cells, others have confirmed that apoptosis is a prominent feature of granulomas in tuberculosis, involving both macrophages and T lymphocytes (44,45,86). It appears that macrophage apoptosis has an active role in maintaining granuloma integrity, thereby compartmentalizing the infection and limiting the size of the inflammatory lesion. In mice with targeted mutation of TNFR1, granulomas undergo necrosis during mycobacterial infection, whereas granulomas in wild-type mice remain intact (56,87). Necrosis in this setting is associated with death of the mice. The dynamic regulation of granulomas may be an ongoing requirement for the maintenance of latent tuberculosis infection in humans, and TNF is a critical factor. Patients treated with TNF-inhibiting drugs are known to have high rates of tuberculosis reactivation, possibly due to altered control of macrophage apoptosis in granulomas (51,58). It is likely that death signaling is a major mechanism whereby TNF contributes to the regulation of granuloma structure and function.

APOPTOSIS OF LYMPHOCYTES IN TUBERCULOSIS

Several investigators have demonstrated T-cell apoptosis in the setting of mycobacterial infection *in vitro* and *in vivo*. T lymphocytes have a key role in the adaptive immune response to tuberculosis, and they are regulated at least in part by apoptosis in the context of AICD. However, T-cell apoptosis potentially contributes to the immunosuppression that is sometimes a feature of this disease. The challenge to understanding the role of T-cell apoptosis in tuberculosis disease is discriminating between normal and presumably beneficial regulation of T-cell responses by AICD, as opposed to the potential for maladaptive apoptotic T-cell depletion that might impair protective immunity.

Mycobacterial antigens have been shown to induce apoptosis of human T lymphocytes. Soruri et al. (88) generated purified protein derivative (PPD)–specific helper T lymphocytes *in vitro*, finding that a subsequent restimulation with PPD resulted in concentration-dependent hyporesponsiveness resulting from apoptosis of $\alpha\beta$ and $\gamma\delta$ T lymphocytes. This response was mediated by Fas and ascribed to AICD. Similarly, Das et al. (89) found evidence for selective apoptosis of T_H1 cells following *ex vivo* stimulation of T lymphocytes from *M. tuberculosis*-infected mice with anti-CD3 monoclonal antibody and phorbol ester. Since T_H1 responses are associated with protection and T_H2 responses with susceptibility to tuberculosis disease, a preferential loss of T_H1 cells would have unfavorable consequences for the host. Mechanisms other than AICD might also contribute to lymphocyte apoptosis in tuberculosis. In this regard, IL-4 was reported to sensitize *M. tuberculosis*-reactive T lymphocytes to TNF-mediated apoptosis (90). Yet another mechanism for T-cell apoptosis was suggested by evidence that FasL expression may be induced in macrophages in murine tuberculous granulomas (91). Apoptosis was seen at the interface between macrophage and lymphoid aggregates, and it was concluded that *M. tuberculosis* might employ FasL expression by host macrophages for protection against attack by CTLs.

Whatever the mechanisms involved, T-cell apoptosis may be associated with weakened immunity in tuberculosis. Under some circumstances, patients with active tuber-

culosis disease fail to respond to tuberculin skin testing (92), and circulating T lymphocytes may have reduced IFN-γ production on culture with mycobacterial antigens (93,94). Hirsch et al. (95) have shown that T-cell apoptosis is increased in patients with active tuberculosis, and this vulnerability of T lymphocytes to undergo apoptosis improves during successful chemotherapy of disease. Gilbertson et al. (96) model this process in mice infected with *M. avium*. They demonstrated increasing apoptosis of both CD4$^+$ and CD8$^+$ T lymphocytes that correlated with increasing bacterial load and decreasing IFN-γ production. These events are followed by increasing morbidity and mortality.

It is the perspective of many investigators that T-cell apoptosis is associated with disease progression and unhelpful to the immune response to infection. A contrasting view was offered by Watson et al. (62) who suggested that a lack of appropriate T-cell apoptosis after infection with *M. tuberculosis* may contribute to inefficient elimination of lymphocytes, contributing to pulmonary tuberculosis pathology.

SUMMARY

Programmed cell death is a fundamental biologic process whose participation in the pathogenesis of tuberculosis is now being appreciated. The discovery that macrophages may undergo apoptosis in response to *M. tuberculosis* infection, and that evasion of apoptosis is a virulence-associated phenotype of *M. tuberculosis*, suggests that this process might be employed as an innate defense against intracellular parasitism by pathogenic mycobacteria. In the earliest phases of primary infection, prior to the acquisition and expression of adaptive immunity, apoptosis of infected macrophages might constitute one component of innate defense that limits the rate of bacterial growth and extrapulmonary dissemination. As the more effective cell-mediated and delayed-type hypersensitivity responses evolve, the situation becomes much more complex with multiple death signaling pathways acting on a variety of different cell types. With the expression of adaptive immunity, both lymphocytes and macrophages are seen to undergo apoptosis by a variety of intrinsic and cooperative pathways, including TNF, Fas, AICD, and the effector functions of CTLs. In addition to regulating the extent of inflammation, and possibly contributing to the killing of intracellular bacilli, apoptosis must play a key role in the homeostatic maintenance of granulomas. These various processes have implications for controlling the extent of tissue necrosis and for the control of latent tuberculosis infection. As new therapeutic drugs that influence apoptosis enter clinical practice, their potential to suppress or exacerbate manifestations of tuberculosis disease must also be considered.

REFERENCES

1. Steller H. Mechanisms and genes of cellular suicide. *Science* 1995, 267:1445–1449.
2. Zimmermann KC, Bonzon C, Green DR. The machinery of programmed cell death. *Pharmacol Ther* 2001;92:57–70.
3. Thornberry NA, Lazebnik Y. Caspases: enemies within. *Science* 1998;281:1312–1316.
4. Ju ST, Matsui K, Ozdemirli M. Molecular and cellular mechanisms regulating T and B cell apoptosis through Fas/FasL interaction. *Int Rev Immunol* 1999;18:485–513.
5. Savill J. Apoptosis in resolution of inflammation. *J Leuk Biol* 1997;61:375–380.
6. Locksley RM, Killeen N, Lenardo MJ. The TNF and TNF receptor superfamilies: integrating mammalian biology. *Cell* 2001;104:487–501.
7. Gearing AJ, Beckett P, Christodoulou M, et al. Processing of tumour necrosis factor-alpha precursor by metalloproteinases. *Nature* 1994;370:555–557.
8. Kayagaki N, Kawasaki A, Ebata T, et al. Metalloproteinase-mediated release of human Fas ligand. *J Exp Med* 1995;182:1777–1783.
9. Liu Z, Hsu H, Goeddel DV, et al. Dissection of TNF receptor 1 effector functions: JNK activation is not linked to apoptosis while NF-κB activation prevents cell death. *Cell* 1996;87:565–576.
10. Beg AA, Baltimore D. An essential role for NF-κB in preventing TNF-α-induced cell death. *Science* 1996;274:782–784.
11. Chu ZL, McKinsey TA, Liu L, et al. Suppression of tumor necrosis factor–induced cell death by inhibitor of apoptosis c-IAP2 is under NF-κB control. *Proc Natl Acad Sci USA* 1997;94:10057–10062.
12. Wu MX, Ao Z, Prassad KVS, et al. *IEX*-1L, an apoptosis inhibitor involved in NF-κB-mediated cell survival. *Science* 1998;281:998–1001.
13. Li X, Yang Y, Ashwell JD. TNF-RII and c-IAP1 mediate ubiquitination and degradation of TRAF2. *Nature* 2002;416:345–347.
14. Green DR, Reed JC. Mitochondria and apoptosis. *Science* 1998;281:1309–1312.
15. Kroemer G, Dallaporta B, Resche-Rigon M. The mitochondrial death/life regulator in apoptosis and necrosis. *Annu Rev Physiol* 1998;60:619–642.
16. Scaffidi C, Fulda S, Srinivasan A, et al. Two CD95 (APO-1/Fas) signaling pathways. *EMBO J* 1998;17:1675–1687.
17. Pellegrini M, Strasser A. A portrait of the Bcl-2 protein family: life, death, and the whole picture. *J Clin Immunol* 1999;19:365–377.
18. Goyal L. Cell death inhibition: keeping caspases in check. *Cell* 2001;104:805–808.
19. Clem RJ, Fechheimer M, Miller LK. Prevention of apoptosis by a baculovirus gene during infection of insect cells. *Science* 1991;254:1388–1390.
20. Green DR. Apoptotic pathways: paper wraps stone blunts scissors. *Cell* 2000;102:1–4.
21. Fadok VA, Bratton DL, Rose DM, et al. A receptor for phosphatidylserine-specific clearance of apoptotic cells. *Nature* 2000;405:85–90.
22. Fadok VA, Chimini G. The phagocytosis of apoptotic cells. *Semin Immunol* 2001;13:365–372.
23. Albert ML, Pearce SF, Francisco LM, et al. Immature dendritic cells phagocytose apoptotic cells via alphavbeta5 and CD36, and cross-present antigens to cytotoxic T lymphocytes. *J Exp Med* 1998;188:1359–1368.
24. Ogden CA, deCathelineau A, Hoffmann PR, et al. C1q and mannose binding lectin engagement of cell surface calreticulin and CD91 initiates macropinocytosis and uptake of apoptotic cells. *J Exp Med* 2001;194:781–795.
25. Srivastave P. Roles of heat-shock proteins in innate and adaptive immunity. *Nat Rev Immunol* 2002;2:185–194.
26. Huynh ML, Fadok VA, Henson PM. Phosphatidylserine-dependent ingestion of apoptotic cells promotes TGF-beta1 secretion and the resolution of inflammation. *J Clin Invest* 2002;109:41–50.
27. Howard AD, Kostura MJ, Thornberry N, et al. IL-1-converting enzyme requires aspartic acid residues for processing of the IL-1 beta precursor at two distinct sites and does not cleave 31- kDa IL-1 alpha. *J Immunol* 1991;147:2964–2969.
28. Ghayur T, Banerjee S, Hugunin M, et al. Caspase-1 processes IFN-gamma-inducing factor and regulates LPS-induced IFN-gamma production. *Nature* 1997;386:619–623.
29. Zhang Y, Center DM, Wu DM, et al. Processing and activation of pro-interleukin-16 by caspase-3. *J Biol Chem* 1998;273:1144–1149.
30. Zychlinsky A. Programmed cell death in infectious diseases. *Trends Microbiol* 1993;1:114–117.
31. Barber GN. Host defense, viruses and apoptosis. *Cell Death Differ* 2001;8:113–126.
32. Weinrauch Y, Zychlinsky A. The induction of apoptosis by bacterial pathogens. *Annu Rev Microbiol* 1999;53:155–187.
33. Luder CG, Gross U, Lopes MF. Intracellular protozoan parasites and apoptosis: diverse strategies to modulate parasite–host interactions. *Trends Parasitol* 2001;17:480–486.
34. Usher LR, Lawson RA, Geary I, et al. Induction of neutrophil apoptosis by the *Pseudomonas aeruginosa* exotoxin pyocyanin: a potential mechanism of persistent infection. *J Immunol* 2002;168:1861–1868.
35. Fettucciari K, Rosati E, Scaringi L, et al. Group B *Streptococcus* induces apoptosis in macrophages. *J Immunol* 2000;165:3923–3933.
36. Kawahara T, Kuwano Y, Teshima-Kondo S, et al. *Helicobacter pylori* lipopolysaccharide from type I, but not type II strains, stimulates apoptosis of cultured gastric mucosal cells. *J Med Invest* 2001;48:167–174.
37. Moore KJ, Matlashewski G. Intracellular infection by *Leishmania donovani* inhibits macrophage apoptosis. *J Immunol* 1994;152:2930–2937.
38. Fan T, Lu H, Hu H, et al. Inhibition of apoptosis in chlamydia-infected cells: blockade of mitochondrial cytochrome *c* release and caspase activation. *J Exp Med* 1998;187:487–496.
39. Sturgill-Koszycki S, Schlesinger PH, Chakraborty P, et al. Lack of acidification in *Mycobacterium* phagosomes produced by exclusion of the vesicular proton-ATPase. *Science* 1994;263:678–680.
40. de Chastellier C, Thilo L. Phagosome maturation and fusion with lysosomes in relation to surface property and size of the phagocytic particle. *Eur J Cell Biol* 1997;74:49–62.
41. Xu S, Cooper A, Sturgill-Koszycki S, et al. Intracellular trafficking in *Mycobacterium tuberculosis* and *Mycobacterium avium*-infected macrophages. *Cell* 1994;153:2568–2577.
42. Gan H, Newman GW, Remold HG. Plasminogen activator inhibitor type 2 prevents programmed cell death of human macrophages infected with *Mycobacterium avium*, serovar 4. *J Immunol* 1995;155:1304–1315.
43. Placido R, Mancino G, Amendola A, et al. Apoptosis of human monocytes/macrophages in *Mycobacterium tuberculosis* infection. *J Pathol* 1997;181:31–38.
44. Klingler K, Tchou-Wong K-M, Brandli O, et al. Effects of mycobacteria on regulation of apoptosis in mononuclear phagocytes. *Infect Immun* 1997;65:5272–5278.
45. Keane J, Balcewicz-Sablinska K, Remold HG, et al. Infection by *Mycobacterium tuberculosis* promotes human alveolar macrophage apoptosis. *Infect Immun* 1997;65:298–304.

46. Rojas M, Barrera LF, Puzo G, et al. Differential induction of apoptosis by virulent *Mycobacterium tuberculosis* in resistant and susceptible murine macrophages: role of nitric oxide and mycobacterial products. *J Immunol* 1997;159:1352–1361.

47. Keane J, Shurtleff BA, Kornfeld H. TNF-dependent BALB/c murine macrophage apoptosis following *Mycobacterium tuberculosis* infection inhibits bacillary growth in an IFN-γ independent manner. *Tuberculosis (Edinb)* 2002;82:55–61.

48. Bermudez LE, Parker A, Petrofsky M. Apoptosis of *Mycobacterium avium*-infected macrophages is mediated by both tumour necrosis factor (TNF) and Fas, and involves the activation of caspases. *Clin Exp Immunol* 1999;116:94–99.

49. Hayashi T, Catanzaro A, Rao SP. Apoptosis of human monocytes and macrophages by *Mycobacterium avium* sonicate. *Infect Immun* 1997;65:5262–5271.

50. Keane JM, Remold HG, Kornfeld H. Virulent strains of *Mycobacterium tuberculosis* evade apoptosis of infected alveolar macrophages. *J Immunol* 2000;164:2016–2020.

51. Keane J, Gershon SK, Braun MM. Tuberculosis and treatment with infliximab. *N Engl J Med* 2002;346:623–626.

52. Santucci MB, Amicosante M, Cicconi R, et al. *Mycobacterium tuberculosis*–induced apoptosis in monocytes/macrophages: early membrane modifications and intracellular mycobacterial viability. *J Infect Dis* 2000;181:1506–1509.

53. Durrbaum-Landmann I, Gercken J, Flad H-D, et al. Effect of *in vitro* infection of human monocytes with low numbers of *Mycobacterium tuberculosis* bacteria on monocyte apoptosis. *Infect Immun* 1996;64:5384–5389.

54. Kremer L, Estaquier J, Brandt E, et al. *Mycobacterium bovis* bacillus Calmette Guérin infection prevents apoptosis of resting human monocytes. *Eur J Immunol* 1997;27:2450–2456.

55. Balcewicz-Sablinska K, Keane J, Kornfeld H, et al. *Mycobacterium tuberculosis* evades apoptosis of host macrophages by release of TNF-R2 resulting in inactivation of TNF-α. *J Immunol* 1998;161: 2636–2641.

56. Flynn JL, Goldstein MM, Chan J, et al. Tumor necrosis factor-α is required in the protective immune response against *Mycobacterium tuberculosis* in mice. *Immunity* 1995;2:561–572.

57. Garcia I, Yoshitaka M, Marchal G, et al. High sensitivity of transgenic mice expressing soluble TNFR1 fusion protein to mycobacterial infections: synergistic action of TNF and IFN-γ in the differentiation of protective granulomas. *Eur J Immunol* 1997;27:3182–3190.

58. Keane J, Gershon S, Wise RP, et al. Tuberculosis associated with infliximab, a tumor necrosis factor alpha–neutralizing agent. *N Engl J Med* 2001;345:1098–1104.

59. Engele M, Stossel E, Castiglione K, et al. Induction of TNF in human alveolar macrophages as a potential evasion mechanism of virulent *Mycobacterium tuberculosis*. *J Immunol* 2002;168: 1328–1337.

60. Ting LM, Kim AC, Cattamanchi A, et al. *Mycobacterium tuberculosis* inhibits IFN-gamma transcriptional responses without inhibiting activation of STAT1. *J Immunol* 1999;163:3898–3906.

61. Oddo M, Renno T, Attinger A, et al. Fas ligand–induced apoptosis of infected human alveolar macrophages reduces the viability of intracellular *Mycobacterium tuberculosis*. *J Immunol* 1998; 160:5448–5454.

62. Watson VE, Hill LL, Owen-Schaub LB, et al. Apoptosis in *Mycobacterium tuberculosis* infection in mice exhibiting varied immunopathology. *J Pathol* 2000;190:211–220.

63. Kornfeld H, Mancino G, Colizzi V. The role of macrophage cell death in tuberculosis. *Cell Death Differ* 2000;6:71–78.

64. Molloy A, Laochumroonvorapong P, Kaplan G. Apoptosis, but not necrosis, of infected monocytes is coupled with killing of intracellular bacillus Calmette–Guérin. *J Exp Med* 1994;180: 1499–1509.

65. Smith RA, Alvarez AJ, Estes DM. The P2X7 purinergic receptor on bovine macrophages mediates mycobacterial death. *Vet Immunol Immunopathol* 2001;78:249–262.

66. Lammas DA, Stober C, Harvey CJ, et al. ATP-induced killing of mycobacteria by human macrophages is mediated by purinergic P2Z(P2X7) receptors. *Immunity* 1997;7:433–444.

67. Stober CB, Lammas DA, Li CM, et al. ATP-mediated killing of *Mycobacterium bovis* bacille Calmette–Guérin within human macrophages is calcium dependent and associated with the acidification of mycobacteria-containing phagosomes. *J Immunol* 2001;166:6276–6286.

68. Ragno S, Estrada-Garcia I, Butler R, et al. Regulation of macrophage gene expression by *Mycobacterium tuberculosis*: down-regulation of mitochondrial cytochrome *c* oxidase. *Infect Immun* 1998;66:3952–3958.

69. Ragno S, Romano M, Howell S, et al. Changes in gene expression in macrophages infected with *Mycobacterium tuberculosis*: a combined transcriptomic and proteomic approach. *Immunology* 2001;104:99–108.

70. Nau GJ, Richmond JF, Schlesinger A, et al. Human macrophage activation programs induced by bacterial pathogens. *Proc Natl Acad Sci U S A* 2002;99:1503–1508.

71. Pais TF, Appelberg R. Macrophage control of mycobacterial growth induced by picolinic acid is dependent on host cell apoptosis. *J Immunol* 2000;164:389–397.

72. Duan L, Gan H, Arm J, et al. Cytosolic phospholipase A2 participates with TNF-alpha in the induction of apoptosis of human macrophages infected with *Mycobacterium tuberculosis* H37Ra. *J Immunol* 2001;166:7469–7476.

73. Fratazzi C, Arbeit RD, Carini C, et al. Programmed cell death of *Mycobacterium avium* serovar 4-infected human macrophages prevents mycobacteria from spreading and induces mycobacterial growth inhibition by freshly added, uninfected macrophages. *J Immunol* 1997;158:4320–4327.

74. Bermudez LE, Parker A, Goodman JR. Growth within macrophages increases the efficiency of *Mycobacterium avium* in invading other macrophages by a complement receptor-independent pathway. *Infect Immun* 1997;65:1916–1925.

75. Rojas M, Olivier M, Gros P, et al. TNF-alpha and IL-10 modulate the induction of apoptosis by virulent *Mycobacterium tuberculosis* in murine macrophages. *J Immunol* 1999;162:6122–6131.

76. Flynn JL, Chan J. Immunology of tuberculosis. *Annu Rev Immunol* 2001;19:93–129.

77. Lewinsohn DM, Bement TT, Xu J, et al. Human purified protein derivative-specific CD4+ T cells use both CD95-dependent and CD95-independent cytolytic mechanisms. *J Immunol* 1998; 160:2374–2379.

78. Stenger S, Mazzaccaro RJ, Uyemura K, et al. Differential effects of cytolytic T cell subsets on intracellular infection. *Science* 1997; 276:1684–1687.

79. Sharif-Askari E, Alam A, Rheaume E, et al. Direct cleavage of the human DNA fragmentation factor-45 by granzyme B induces caspase-activated DNase release and DNA fragmentation. *EMBO J* 2001;20:3101–3113.

80. Kaspar AA, Okada S, Kumar J, et al. A distinct pathway of cell-mediated apoptosis initiated by granulysin. *J Immunol* 2001;167: 350–356.

81. Leemans JC, Juffermans NP, Florquin S, et al. Depletion of alveolar macrophages exerts protective effects in pulmonary tuberculosis in mice. *J Immunol* 2001;166:4604–4611.

82. Pedrosa J, Saunders BM, Appelberg R, et al. Neutrophils play a protective nonphagocytic role in systemic *Mycobacterium tuberculosis* infection of mice. *Infect Immun* 2000;68:577–583.

83. May ME, Spagnuolo PJ. Evidence for activation of a respiratory burst in the interaction of human neutrophils with *Mycobacterium tuberculosis*. *Infect Immun* 1987;55:2304–2307.

84. North RJ, Izzo AA. Mycobacterial virulence. Virulent strains of *Mycobacterium tuberculosis* have faster *in vivo* doubling times and are better equipped to resist growth-inhibiting functions of macrophages in the presence of specific immunity. *J Exp Med* 1993;177:1723–1733.

85. Cree IA, Nurbhai S, Milne G, et al. Cell death in granulomata: the role of apoptosis. *J Clin Pathol* 1995;40:1314–1319.

86. Fayyazi A, Eichmeyer B, Soruri A, et al. Apoptosis of macrophages and T cells in tuberculosis associated caseous necrosis. *J Pathol* 2000;191:417–425.

87. Ehlers S, Kutsch S, Ehlers EM, et al. Lethal granuloma disintegration in mycobacteria-infected TNFRp55–/– mice is dependent on T cells and IL-12. *J Immunol* 2000;165:483–492.

88. Soruri A, Schweyer S, Radzun HJ, et al. Mycobacterial antigens induce apoptosis in human purified protein derivative-specific alphabeta T lymphocytes in a concentration-dependent manner. *Immunology* 2002;105:222–230.

89. Das G, Vohra H, Saha B, et al. Apoptosis of Th1-like cells in experimental tuberculosis (TB). *Clin Exp Immunol* 1999;115:324–328.

90. Seah GT, Rook GA. Il-4 influences apoptosis of *Mycobacterium*-reactive lymphocytes in the presence of TNF-alpha. J *Immunol* 2001;167:1230–1237.

91. Mustafa T, Phyu S, Nilsen R, et al. Increased expression of Fas ligand on *Mycobacterium tuberculosis* infected macrophages: a potential novel mechanism of immune evasion by *Mycobacterium tuberculosis*? *Inflammation* 1999;23:507–521.

92. Vanham G, Toossi Z, Hirsch CS, et al. Examining a paradox in the pathogenesis of human pulmonary tuberculosis: immune activation and suppression/anergy. *Tuber Lung Dis* 1997;78:145–158.

93. Zhang M, Lin Y, Iyer DV, et al. T-cell cytokine responses in human infection with *Mycobacterium tuberculosis*. *Infect Immun* 1995;63:3231–3234.

94. Sodhi A, Gong J, Silva C, et al. Clinical correlates of interferon gamma production in patients with tuberculosis. *Clin Infect Dis* 1997;25:617–620.

95. Hirsch CS, Toossi Z, Vanham G, et al. Apoptosis and T cell hyporesponsiveness in pulmonary tuberculosis. *J Infect Dis* 1999;179:945–953.

96. Gilbertson B, Zhong J, Cheers C. Anergy, IFN-gamma production, and apoptosis in terminal infection of mice with *Mycobacterium avium*. *J Immunol* 1999;163:2073–2080.

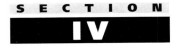

SECTION

IV

CLINICAL ASPECTS

PATHOLOGY AND INSIGHTS INTO PATHOGENESIS OF TUBERCULOSIS

JAISHREE JAGIRDAR
DAVID ZAGZAG

PRIMARY PULMONARY TUBERCULOSIS: THE GHON COMPLEX

Primary pulmonary infection by the tubercle bacillus results in a small patch of caseous bronchopneumonia that is surpassed in size by a similar lesion appearing in the draining hilar lymph nodes. The primary lesions occur predominantly in the middle and lower lung fields in a subpleural location. Their gross appearance was first described by Laennec (1) as a wet/semidry chalky paste. The term *caseation* was applied to describe this pasty chalk and was not originally intended to refer to the microscopic appearance of necrosis (Fig. 24.1) The primary lesion together with the draining lymphatics and affected lymph nodes constitutes the *Ghon complex*. Although Anton Ghon was not the first to describe the primary pulmonary lesions, his was the first detailed autopsy report on 747 consecutive predominantly pediatric autopsies. He found active pulmonary tuberculosis (TB) in 28.6% of the autopsied subjects, and the majority of them had the primary lesion (2).

Among 326 autopsies reviewed at Bellevue Hospital Center between 1989 and 1993, 50 subjects with either active or inactive TB (15.3%) were identified. No primary complexes were recorded although 40% of the autopsied subjects were in the pediatric age group. The incidence of mycobacterial infection was low in the pediatric subjects: There were two *Mycobacterium avium-intracellulare* (MAC) infections and one healed treated *Mycobacterium tuberculosis* infection. Lucas and Nelson (3) made a similar observation in their pediatric autopsy series.

J. Jagirdar: Department of Pathology, University of Texas Health Science Center; Department of Pathology, University Hospital, University of Texas Health Science Center, San Antonio, Texas.

D. Zagzag: Departments of Pathology and Neurosurgery, New York University School of Medicine; Department of Pathology, New York University Medical Center, New York, New York.

AUTOPSY DIAGNOSIS OF TUBERCULOSIS: CURRENT IMPLICATION TO HUMAN IMMUNODEFICIENCY VIRUS–POSITIVE SUBJECTS

In our recent Bellevue autopsy study of 326 cases (Table 24.1), 64% of the decedents were infected with human immunodeficiency virus (HIV), and most were plagued by homelessness, imprisonment, or alcoholism. Of the 50 patients with TB, 39 (78%) had active TB with necrotizing lesions. Eight (2.4% of 326 autopsy cases) had active cavitary TB not diagnosed during life, posing a health hazard not only for the community but also for hospital workers and autopsy personnel. Medlar (4) conducted an autopsy study between 1935 and 1944 and reported for New York City a 1% incidence of active cavitary TB undetected during life, as compared with 2.4% in our current Bellevue study. In an autopsy study from Poland (5), active TB was found in 7.9% of autopsied subjects. TB was not diagnosed during life in one third of their subjects. A similar study done in Hong Kong showed a 3% incidence of clinical nondetection (6). The racial distribution was as expected in our autopsy series and consisted of 60% African American, 21% Hispanic, 16% white, and 2% Asian. A higher prevalence of disseminated mycobacterial infection was noted in the HIV-positive subjects than the HIV-negative ones (Table 24.1), with the common sites of dissemination being the spleen, lymph nodes, kidney, liver, intestines, and bone marrow in descending order. The rate of lung involvement in the HIV-positive subjects was lower than that in the HIV-negative subjects. However, when treated subjects with healed mycobacterial infection were included, the rate of lung involvement rose to 56% in the HIV-positive subjects. Furthermore, patients who had low CD4 cell counts with biopsy-proved *M. tuberculosis* responded to their therapy, with no evidence of disease at autopsy. In

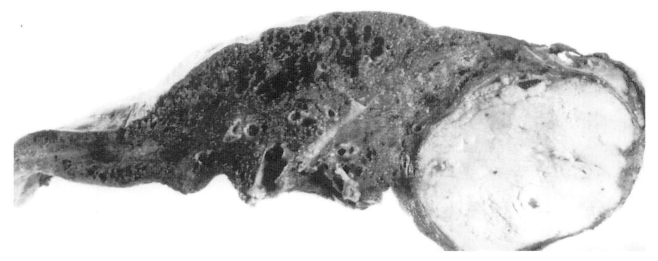

FIGURE 24.1. Gross appearance of a large area of caseous necrosis.

TABLE 24.1. AUTOPSY DIAGNOSIS OF TUBERCULOSIS[a]

Site of Lesions	HIV Positive (%)	HIV Negative (%)
Disseminated	44	10
Lungs	31	7
Lungs only	22[b]	32
All lymph nodes	31	4
Pulmonary hilar lymph nodes	6	7
Pleura only	3	0
Liver	21	4
Spleen	37	7
Kidney	25	0
Intestines	6	4
Adrenal	9	7
Bone marrow	6[c]	4
Skin	3	0
Pericardium	6	0
Omentum and diaphragm	0	7
Pancreas and esophagus	6	0

[a]Total no. of subjects: HIV positive = 32; HIV negative = 28.
[b]Fifty-six percent if subjects with treated healed infections included.
[c]This number may be lower than expected because marrow is not extensively examined at autopsy.
HIV, human immunodeficiency virus.

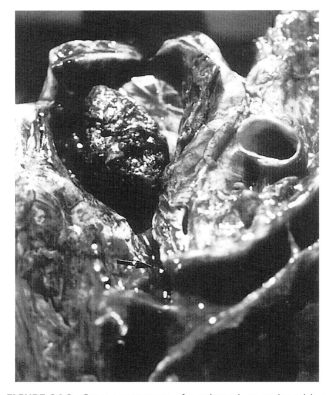

FIGURE 24.2. Gross appearance of a tuberculous cavity with a fungus ball. Note that the cavity communicates with a bronchus (*arrow*). This patient died of massive hemoptysis.

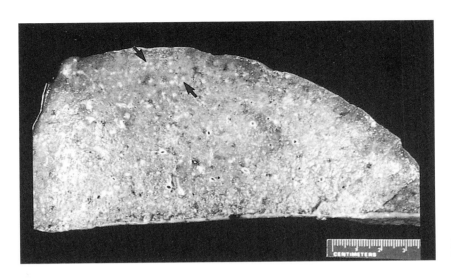

FIGURE 24.3. Gross picture of miliary lesions in the lung parenchyma. (See Color Plate 5.)

the HIV-positive subjects the cause of death was usually not TB but opportunistic infections such as *Pneumocystis carinii* pneumonia, disseminated cytomegalovirus disease, or cryptococcosis. Two subjects with aspergillosis, one colonizing a cavity (Fig. 24.2) and the other invasive, were identified in this group.

PROGRESSIVE PRIMARY COMPLEX

If healing does not occur in the primary phase, the infection progresses to the progressive primary complex, occurring predominantly in the pediatric age group. In this type of infection, enlarging areas of necrosis without encapsulation develop. The draining lymph nodes undergo extensive necrosis.

MILIARY TUBERCULOSIS

Miliary TB is so named because the small lesions resemble 2-mm millet seeds (Fig. 24.3) and occur after hematogenous dissemination. This dissemination can occur in the primary form and can remain dormant, as evidenced by small calcified nodules in the spleen or the liver at autopsy. However, the term miliary TB is most often used to describe the form that occurs in adults with an acute progressive course. Diffuse alveolar damage and rapidly evolving infiltrates may be present. However, symptoms vary greatly and some cases are not diagnosed until autopsy. In our autopsy study, we found 17 cases of miliary TB, with 3 occurring in HIV-negative patients. Microscopically the miliary lesions appear as small foci of necrotizing granulomatous inflammation filling four to five alveolar spaces (Fig. 24.4). With healing they shrink and become hyalin-

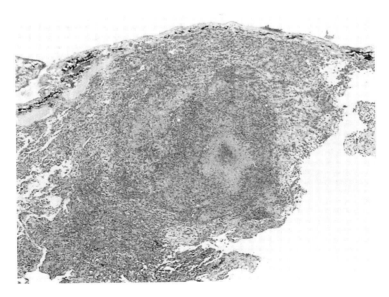

FIGURE 24.4. Microscopic appearance of a miliary lesion on a hemotoxylin–phloxine–saffranin stain. Note the central area of necrosis (original magnification ×20). (See Color Plate 6.)

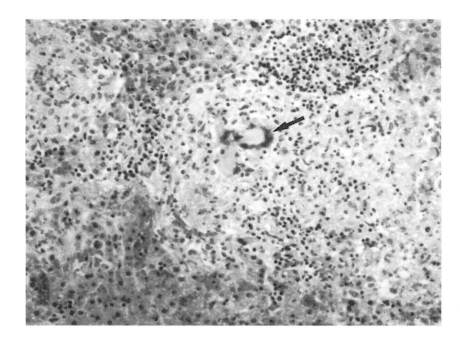

FIGURE 24.5. Microscopic appearance of a miliary lesion in the liver. Note the Langhans giant cell (*arrow*) (hematoxylin–eosin, original magnification ×400).

ized. The sites most frequently involved are the spleen (100%), liver (70%) (Fig. 24.5), lungs (86%), and bone marrow (77%), with lesser involvement of other organs such as skin, kidney, pancreas (Fig. 24.6), and joints. The rate of disseminated organ involvement in our autopsy study was doubtless lowered as a result of many patients being treated during life. In HIV-positive patients with miliary disease there is a paucity of granulomatous response with areas of necrosis containing numerous acid-fast bacilli,

compared with the non–HIV-positive patients (7). Grossly visible miliary lesions in the lung are not pathognomonic for TB; they may occur with histoplasmosis, cytomegalovirus infection (8), and *Legionella pneumophila* infections. Furthermore, similar lesions may be seen in anaplastic Ki-1 lymphoma (9), a recently described entity characterized by large pleomorphic cells, a sinus growth pattern, and expression of Ki-1 (CD30) antigen. Lymphangiectatic spread of carcinoma can produce a miliary appearance in the lung.

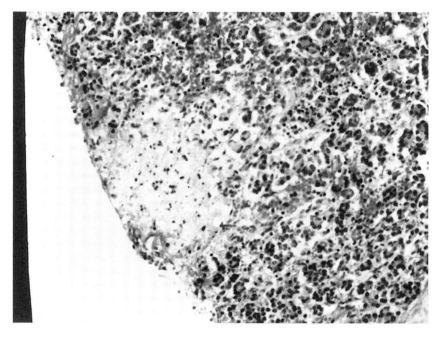

FIGURE 24.6. Microscopic appearance of a miliary lesion in the pancreas. Note the area of necrosis with a lack of giant cells (hematoxylin–eosin, original magnification × 200).

ADULT PULMONARY TUBERCULOSIS

The term *chronic pulmonary TB* is preferred to the terms *postprimary reactivation* and *reinfection TB* because there is controversy as to whether the lesion follows reactivation of an old Ghon focus or represents a reinfection. Stead (10–12) and others (13,14) have reviewed the mode of infection in adults. It is generally believed that reactivation following the primary lesion is the preferred pathogenic mechanism of most adult TB infections. Supporting this hypothesis is the fact that tubercle bacilli have grown in 40% of subapical nodules and 5% of Ghon foci (14,15). However, reinfection can occur as well.

Grossly, adult TB presents as an acute necrotizing pneumonic process in either or both upper-lung fields (Fig. 24.7). There may be liquefaction and bronchial involvement, with rapid intrabronchial spread to adjacent lobes of the lung resulting in "galloping consumption."

Cavitation occurs, with the average size of the cavity being 3 to 10 cm, and is usually located in the upper lobes. The wall is composed of granulation tissue encircled by an outer layer of fibrous tissue. Chronic cavities have

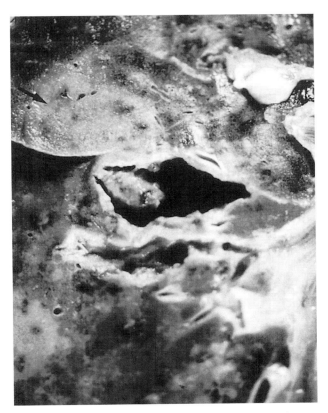

FIGURE 24.7. Gross appearance of a cavitary lesion with pneumonic consolidation (*arrow*).

thicker walls than expanding recent ones. Obliterated pulmonary aneurysmal arteries are seen traversing the cavity (Rasmussen arteries). The exact source of bleeding in these cavities is not clear, but it may be due to oozing of blood from capillaries in the exuberant granulation tissue or from larger vessels caught in the necrotizing process. When aspergillomas are present in these cavities, it is speculated that hemoptysis could be caused by mechanical friction of the mycetoma or by release of endotoxins with hemolytic properties (16). Medlar (4) stated that the morphology of necrotic lesions does not seem to be altered following chemotherapy and, in addition, the latter does not prevent a continuation of liquefaction. He stated that the number of acid-fast bacilli found in cavitary or necrotic lesions is unpredictable, similar to our observations, although cavities are known to support exuberant mycobacterial growth (17).

PULMONARY TUBERCULOMA

Tuberculomas are the most common solitary pulmonary nodules (17) (Fig. 24.8). The term *granuloma* was originally given to a chronic inflammatory mass resembling tumor and may be most appropriate in this instance. Tuberculomas occur more commonly in the elderly and are often resected because carcinoma is suspected half the time, owing to the absence of calcification. Others are resected because they keep growing despite antituberculous therapy. In approximately half of these lesions, which are often cavitating, acid-fast bacillus (AFB) can be identified either by smear or culture (17). In the rest of the lesions a diagnosis of mycobacterial infection is suspected because of the typical microscopic appearance in the absence of other organisms such as *Histoplasma*. In a Japanese study of 36 patients whose tuberculomas were excised, short-term antituberculous therapy following excision (18) was considered to be adequate. *Mycobac-*

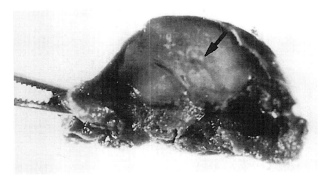

FIGURE 24.8. Gross appearance of a wedge resection specimen with tuberculoma. Note the tiny areas of necrosis within the lesion (*arrow*).

terium gordonae also has been isolated from such an excised nodule (19).

DRUG RESISTANCE AND MORPHOLOGY

The granulomatous inflammation in drug-resistant TB does not differ from that in the non–drug-resistant end-stage lungs for which lobectomy is the treatment of choice (Fig. 24.9). Interestingly, fewer AFBs are observed than expected considering the drug resistance. Guy et al. (20) recently showed that when pan-drug-resistant strains were injected into rabbits, fewer organs grew bacilli on culture as compared with a drug-sensitive strain. These authors suggested that perhaps this was due to lower pathogenicity of the resistant strains. It may be due to slower doubling time; an alternative explanation is that these mycobacteria become non–acid fast due to alteration in their cell walls. Studies are underway to evaluate both of these hypotheses. Chandrasekhar and Ratnam (21) showed that the drug-resistant mycobacteria are converted to their ametabolically inactive "granular" form in the presence of host defenses or antituberculous drug therapy. In addition, these bacilli do not cause disease or tuberculin sensitivity in the normal host but do so in the

immunocompromised host. Due to their deficient cell wall, they are less immunogenic, are non–acid fast, and remain dormant in macrophages.

SURGICAL PATHOLOGY OF TUBERCULOSIS: NEW YORK UNIVERSITY EXPERIENCE

One hundred twenty-five patients with granulomatous inflammation were identified over a 1-year period at New York University Medical Center; 40 had documented mycobacterial infections (Table 24.2). Patients who had positive cultures or AFB in granulomas were selected. The ages ranged from 31 to 72, with a mean of 42 years. The male/female ratio was 7:1. Twenty-five patients were HIV positive. Four more had HIV risk factors. In 11 patients the HIV status was suspect or negative. Since the biopsy was a primary mode of diagnosis, it can be assumed that patients were not on therapy at the time of biopsy. Frequently biopsied sites, in descending order, were lung; lymph nodes (Fig. 24.10), particularly superficial lymph nodes; bone marrow; pleura; liver; and skin. There were 12 MAC- and 15 *M. tuberculosis*-positive cultures, with 2 patients having both. The significance of MAC in these 2 patients is unclear. In our series only half of the patients with MAC-positive cultures had a lower absolute CD4+ count, below 100 cells/mm^3. Interestingly, in 11 patients (27.5%), cultures were positive, with no bacilli in tissue in those with the higher CD4+ counts. In 9 patients (22%) the biopsy specimens contained AFB but the cultures were negative. These observations emphasize the value of a biopsy in making a primary diagnosis of TB. Comparison of morphology in the MAC- and *M. tuberculosis*-positive patients did not show any striking differences in terms of number of giant cells or epithelioid cells, as was suggested by some (22), except that necrosis was more common in *M. tuberculosis* than MAC-positive patients and was statistically significant (13 of 17 vs. 4 of 14 patients, respectively ($R^2 = 0.27$, $p < 0.001$)). Marchevsky et al. (23), in their study of mycobacterial infections other than *M. tuberculosis* in non–HIV-infected patients, found that the most common tissue response was necrotizing granulomatous inflammation, as in *M. tuberculosis* infection. Clinically their patients presented with solitary pulmonary nodules, diffuse interstitial infiltrates, or multiple discrete infiltrates on chest x-ray studies. Moreover, in our study the morphology varied with the organ of involvement, with the bone marrow showing far fewer necrotizing granulomas and variable numbers of AFBs regardless of the CD4+ count. This could be due to the fact that different cytokines were released from the hematopoietic precursors. In miliary disease occurring in non–HIV- and HIV-positive individuals, a wide variety of morphology rang-

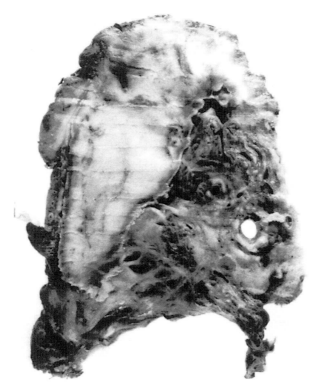

FIGURE 24.9. Gross appearance of end-stage multidrug-resistant lung.

TABLE 24.2. SURGICAL PATHOLOGY OF TUBERCULOSIS

Patient No.	Age (yr)	Sex	HIV Status	Organ Site	Culture	CD4+ Count (cells/mm³) in PBL	No. of Bacilli in Granuloma	Necrosis in Granuloma	Cytotoxic T Cells in Tissue		
									Normal	Granuloma	Necrosis
1	36	M	ND	Bone marrow	MAI, blood	1	Moderate	No	ND	ND	ND
2	31	F	HIV+	LN, TBNA	Treated, none	2	Moderate	Yes	ND	ND	ND
3	52	M	ND	Bone marrow	MAI, blood	2	Numerous	No	1+	ND	ND
4	34	M	HIV+	Lung	BAL-MAI	3	Numerous	Yes	0	ND	ND
5	37	M	HIV+	LN, TBNA	MAI	4	Numerous	No	ND	1+	2+
6	36	M	HIV+	Pleura	Negative	5	Rare	Yes	ND	2+	3+
7	44	M	HIV+	R submandibular LN	MTB	5	Numerous	Yes	ND	2+	ND
8	34	F	HIV+	RUL lung	ND	6	Numerous	Yes	ND	ND	2+
9	ND	M	HIV?	Pleura	ND	9	Moderate	Yes	1+	2+	ND
10	ND	M	HIV?	Lung	On medication	11	Moderate	Yes	ND	ND	ND
11	35	M	HIV+	Bone marrow	BLD MTB	16	Rare	Yes	ND	2+	2+
12	ND	M	ND	Mediastinal LN	MTB	20	Numerous	Yes	ND	ND	ND
13	ND	M	HIV+	Lung, LN	MTB	26	Numerous	No	ND	ND	ND
14	56	M	HIV+	Liver	MAI	28	Rare	Yes	ND	2+	ND
15	51	M	HIV+	RUL lung	MTB	33	Rare	No	ND	ND	ND
16	38	M	HIV+	Lung	MTB	35	None	No	ND	ND	ND
17	41	M	ND	Bone marrow	ND	40	Numerous	Yes	ND	2+	2+
18	ND	M	HIV+	Lung needle aspirate	MAI	48	Moderate	Yes	ND	0	ND
19	ND	M	HIV+	Lung	MTB	51	Moderate	No	0	ND	ND
20	50	M	HIV+	Bone marrow	MTB	61	Rare	No	ND	1+, m2+	ND
21	37	M	HIV+	R thigh skin	MAI	71	Numerous	No	ND	1+	ND
22	ND	M	HIV+	Pleura	MTB	103	Numerous	No	ND	1+, m2+	3+
23	36	M	HIV+	R axillary LN	MTB	104	Numerous	Yes	ND	2+	ND
24	ND	M	HIV+?	LN	Negative	105	Numerous	Yes	ND	ND	ND
25	36	F	HIV+	Lung	Negative	106	Numerous	No	ND	2+, m3+	3+
26	62	M	HIV+	Mediastinal mass	ND	115	Moderate	Yes	ND	3+	ND
27	69	M	HIV+	RLL lung	MAI	128	None	No	ND	ND	ND
28	40	M	HIV+	Bone marrow	MAI	135	Numerous	No	ND	1+, m1+	ND
29	72	F	ND	LLL lung	MAI	152	None	No	ND	ND	ND
30	29	M	HIV+	Lung	MTB	167	None	Yes	ND	ND	ND
31	ND	M	HIV+	Lung	MAI	201	None	Yes	ND	ND	ND
32	40	M	HIV+	L axillary LN	ND	230	Rare	No	ND	2+	3+
33	56	M	ND	Lung	MAI	331	Rare	Yes	ND	ND	ND
34	ND	M	HIV?	Pleura	MTB	386	None	Yes	ND	ND	ND
35	ND	M	ND	ND	MTB	420	None	Yes	1+	ND	ND
36	46	M	ND	RUL lung	BAL-MTB	579	None	Yes	1+	m1+	2+
37	24	M	ND	RLL lung	MAI, MTB	624	None	No	ND	1+	ND
38	ND	M	HIV+	Lung	MTB	801	None	Yes	ND	ND	ND
39	32	M	ND	Lung	MAI, MTB	840	None	Yes	ND	1+, m2+	ND
40	26	F	ND	Left lung	Negative	1179	Rare	Yes	ND	1+	3+

LN, lymph node; m, macrophage; ND, no data; CD4, no. of cells/μ1; none, 0; moderate, mean of 10; TBNA, transbronchial needle aspirate; rare, mean of 2; numerous, mean of 50; 1+, few; 2+, some; 3+, many; PBL, peripheral blood lymphocytes; RUL, right upper lobe; MTB, *Mycobacterium tuberculosis*; BLD, blood; BAL, bronchoalveolar lavage.

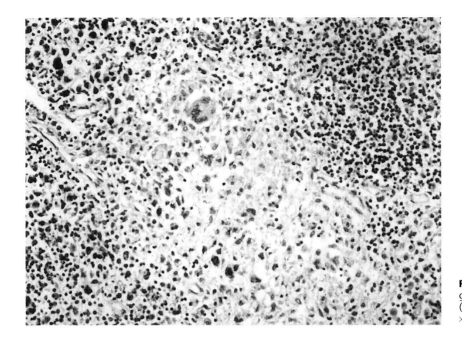

FIGURE 24.10. Microscopic appearance of a granuloma with a giant cell in a lymph node (hematoxylin–eosin, original magnification ×400).

ing from well-formed granulomas with giant cells (Figs. 24.11 and 24.12) to suppurative necrosis with foam cells (Fig. 24.13) was observed in involved organs. While it is true that the suppurative response is associated with numerous AFBs at one end of the spectrum with loss of immune function, and the well-formed granulomas with fewer AFBs at the other end of the spectrum with intact immune function, there is an overlap. Different morphologies coexist so that one cannot assume a direct correlation with immune status, as was suggested by some (24).

STAINING CHARACTERISTICS OF MYCOBACTERIA

The Ziehl–Neelsen stain (Figs. 24.14 and 24.15) or the Kinyoun modification is the stain of choice. Owing to their waxy cell wall components, the mycobacteria are acid fast; that is, they retain the red dye carbol fuchsin after rinsing with acid solvents. When an AFB is detected in the granulomatous area, it is highly specific and indicative of mycobacterial infection. However, between 10^5 and 10^6 bacteria per milliliter of tissue is required before they can be

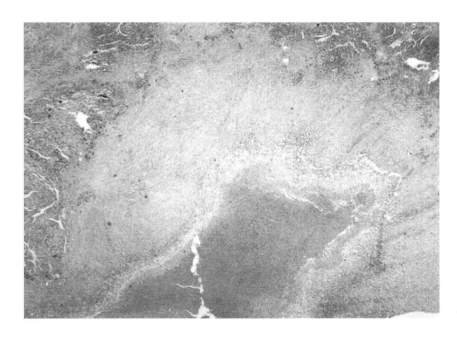

FIGURE 24.11. Microscopic appearance of a large typical necrotizing granuloma (hematoxylin–eosin, original magnification ×20).

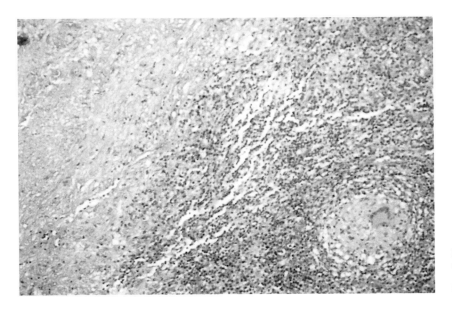

FIGURE 24.12. Microscopic appearance of a granuloma with nonnecrotizing and necrotizing granuloma (hematoxylin–eosin, original magnification ×200).

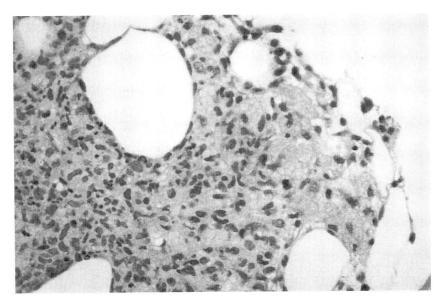

FIGURE 24.13. Microscopic appearance of a suppurative lesion with foamy macrophages in a *Mycobacterium avium* complex infection of the skin (hematoxylin–eosin, original magnification ×400).

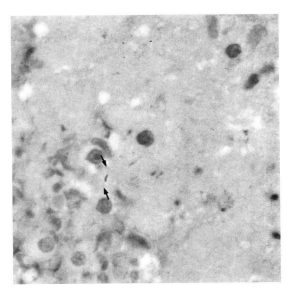

FIGURE 24.14. Rare acid-fast bacillus (Ziehl–Neelsen, original magnification ×1,000). (See Color Plate 7.)

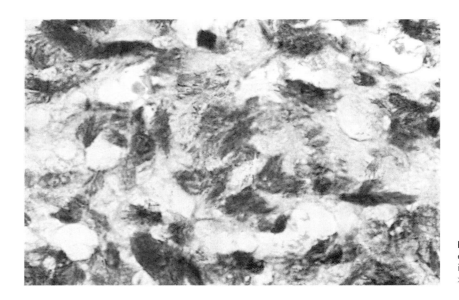

FIGURE 24.15. Numerous acid-fast bacilli in a case of *Mycobacterium avium-intracellulare* infection (Ziehl–Neelsen, original magnification ×1,000). (See Color Plate 8.)

visualized in a light microscope. Staining of mycobacteria is inconsistent with Gram stain. The mycobacteria are stained by Gomori methenamine silver stain and the periodic acid–Schiff stain (25). Other stains that are useful and more sensitive but perhaps not as specific are auramine O (Fig. 24.16) and rhodamine (26).

IMMUNOHISTOCHEMICAL STAINING OF MYCOBACTERIA

With the availability of antibodies to mycobacteria, it is possible to detect mycobacteria immunohistochemically in tissue. Humphrey and Weiner (27) found a slightly improved detection rate of mycobacteria in caseous lesions by using rabbit polyclonal antibodies rather than the traditional Ziehl–Neelsen stain. Their antibody cross-reacted weakly with atypical mycobacteria and was found to be highly specific for mycobacterial infections. Other authors using monoclonal antibodies against different mycobacterial antigens (28, 35, and 65 kd) were able to improve on the false-negative results obtained by traditional staining methods. In addition, the antibody to 35-kd antigen appeared to be specific for *M. tuberculosis* (28). More work is needed to establish the value of immunohistochemical staining over conventional staining techniques and its ability to speciate mycobacteria reliably.

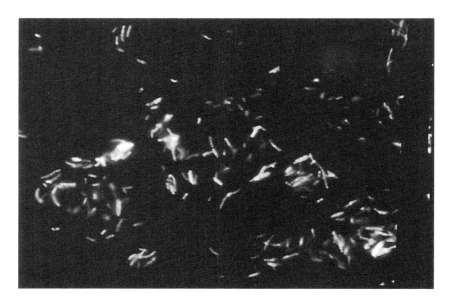

FIGURE 24.16. Numerous mycobacteria on an auramine O stain (original magnification ×1,000). (See Color Plate 9.)

COMPLICATIONS OF PULMONARY TUBERCULOSIS

Several complications of cavities can occur. Erosion of a pulmonary artery with aneurysm can occur with fatal bleeding (Fig. 24.2). Another complication is a bronchopleural fistula due to loss of subpleural tissue with empyema. Colonization of *Aspergillus* with aspergilloma formation in a cavity can occur. A remote association of TB is carcinoma. Dacosta and Kinare (29) found 29 cases of TB associated with 220 cases of lung carcinoma (13% incidence). There were seven "scar cancers" in their group, with two arising in scars associated with TB. The term *scar cancer* is restricted to well-documented previous scarring followed several years later by carcinoma at the same site. This occurs at sites of bullet wounds and with scars caused by grenade splinters or knife blades (30). The stroma in genuine scar cancers is composed of type I, IV, and V collagen, whereas the collagen in most carcinomas with fibrosis is young, type III, and is produced by the tumor or tumor-stimulated stroma (31). Poor clearance of carcinogens in scarred areas could contribute to pulmonary carcinogenesis (32).

CYTOLOGIC DIAGNOSIS OF MYCOBACTERIAL INFECTIONS

Fine-needle aspiration (FNA) in patients with suspected mycobacterial infection is valuable as a screening procedure, particularly in superficial easily accessible locations such as cervical and submandibular regions. Numerous articles have been written on FNA of lymph nodes in these locations (33–35). Three different patterns are observed: epithelioid granulomas without necrosis, epithelioid granulomas with necrosis, and necrosis alone. AFBs are seen most readily in 77% of patients with the necrotic pattern alone. In a study performed at Bellevue Hospital, Finfer et al. (35) found that when caseous or grossly purulent material was aspirated in the proper clinical setting, it was highly specific. Lau et al. (34) reported that FNA has a specificity of 93% and a sensitivity of 77%. The chance of detecting AFBs in these specimens on an average is between 40% and 56%.

Radhika et al. (36) successfully carried out deep abdominal aspiration of ileocecal, colonic, and jejunal regions. In their patients, a clinical diagnosis of TB was made 60% of the time. A pattern of reaction similar to that in lymph nodes was observed, with an AFB yield of 45%.

Maygarden and Flanders (37) reported cytologic findings from three patients with acquired immunodeficiency syndrome (AIDS) in whom mycobacteria were detected as negative images on a Wright-stained slide. In aspirate obtained by FNA of a lymph node we found numerous negative images of AFBs in macrophages on a slide stained with Diff-Quik (Dade Behring AG, Düdingen, Germany) (Fig. 24.17).

Transbronchial needle aspiration is another approach to making a diagnosis of mycobacterial infections. This method originally was used to stage lung carcinomas but is increasingly used to diagnose other conditions at Bellevue Hospital. In 2 patients in our series of 40 patients (Table 24.2), definitive diagnosis of mycobacterial infection was made by transbronchial needle aspiration.

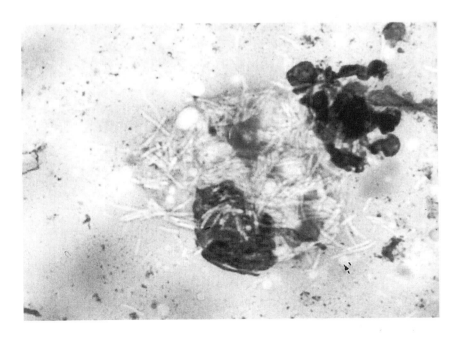

FIGURE 24.17. Negatively stained images of mycobacteria in aspirate (Diff-Quik, original magnification ×1,000). (Courtesy of Dr. Jerry Minkowitz.)

ELECTRON MICROSCOPY

With the electron microscope, epithelioid cells show highly ruffled interdigitating cell membranes, well-developed endoplasmic reticulum, and abundant mycobacteria and large Golgi complexes. Large vesicles may be seen with no lysosomal granules, implying that they are equipped with a secretory function rather than a phagocytic function. Numerous thick-walled mycobacteria can be identified in the cytoplasm, particularly in material from patients with MAC infection (Fig. 24.18). In the latter patients the lesions may resemble dermatofibromas histologically and on electron microscopy the spindled cells have a fibroblastic appearance (38) (Fig. 24.18).

CORRELATION OF CD4 COUNTS WITH MORPHOLOGY AND NUMBER OF BACILLI

Cellular immunity is an integral part of the immune response against mycobacterial infections, with resultant necrotizing or nonnecrotizing granulomatous inflammation. There is convincing evidence that the T_H1 subset of the helper T cells (CD4+) that secrete interferon-γ (IFN-γ) and interleukin-2 (IL-2) confer protective immunity (39). As of yet, no direct phenotypic marker is available to study

the T_H1 subset. However, *in situ* hybridization for IFN-γ and IL-2 cytokines and CD4+ subset analysis at the site of granulomatous inflammation and peripheral blood, when examined in conjunction with the number of AFBs in the tissue, can give insights into bacterial killing. We evaluated 40 patients (Table 24.2) from our surgical pathology files. The CD4+ counts in peripheral blood ranged from 1 to 1,179/mm³. Importantly, 19 of 25 patients with CD4+ counts of 106 cells/mm³ or lower had moderate to numerous bacilli in granulomas, versus 2 of 15 with CD4+ counts higher than 106 cells/mm³, corroborating the need for CD4+ cells in granulomatous mycobacterial killing. The correlation between the number of bacilli and CD4+ cell count was significant ($R^2 = 0.17$, $p < 0.01$). Our finding is not surprising. However, no large studies have shown this correlation *in vivo* in biopsy material. Lucas and Nelson (3), in their study of cadavers in Abidjan, made similar observations. In another study, Jones et al. (40) found an increasing incidence of mycobacteremia with declining CD4+ counts, further supporting our findings and suggesting a key role for the CD4+ cells in limiting the severity of TB. We were unable to find any correlation with the CD4/CD8 ratio or the total number of CD8+ cells, as were Jones et al. (40). Once we established this direct protective correlation between CD4+ cell counts and AFB in tissue, it was possible to dissect out which of the morphologic changes were

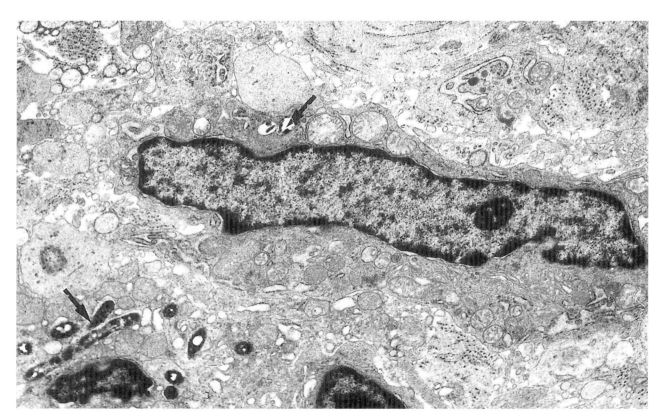

FIGURE 24.18. Electron micrograph of a fibroblastic cell with mycobacteria (*arrows*).

"protective" and occurred with the higher CD4+ counts and low number of bacilli, and vice versa. The rationale for this evaluation was to enable us to define, manage, and eliminate potentially harmful nonprotective immunologic tissue responses. The morphologic changes we evaluated for this purpose were granuloma formation, giant cells, and necrosis. Granuloma formation has been equated with an intact or preserved cellular immunity. We found necrotizing granulomas with low CD4+ counts of 100 cells/mm³ and below. In addition, two sarcoidosis patients in this study were found to have well-formed sarcoidosis granulomas. This is in agreement with other observers (40–42). Consequently, one needs to postulate that granuloma formation is not at least directly influenced by the CD4+ cells and therefore is not protective.

We have shown that intercellular adhesion molecule (ICAM) has an important role in granuloma formation and that its up-regulation is dependent on tumor necrosis factor-α (TNF-α), which is plentiful in HIV-positive patients, the source being the macrophages for TNF-α (43). According to Lucas and Helson (3), Langhans-type giant cell formation (not to be confused with Langerhans cells, which are antigen-presenting cells) correlated with CD4+ counts. However, we were unable to replicate this correlation. We would suggest that giant cell formation is linked with expression of ICAM (see section "Intracellular Adhesion Molecule in Mycobacterial Infection"), which in turn is up-regulated by TNF-α.

In our series, necrosis was seen regardless of the CD4+ count (Table 24.2). Furthermore, tuberculin itself is non-toxic and does not evoke necrosis in skin tests in bacille Calmette–Guérin (BCG) recipients, and necrosis is not seen in tuberculoid leprosy patients. This implies that necrosis is not an inevitable component of a positive cell-mediated immune response to mycobacterial antigen (44). Complementing this observation is the fact that sarcoid patients for the most part do well, perhaps due to the absence of necrosis in the majority of them. However, cavity formation requires intact cell-mediated immunity (45). A factor that may be responsible for necrosis in mycobacterial infections is sustained production of TNF-α and increased end-organ sensitivity (endothelial cells) to TNF-α produced by macrophages stimulated by mycobacteria (44). Abrogation of the end-organ sensitivity to TNF-α or blocking it may have therapeutic implications. In summary, we have observed that most features of the tuberculous granuloma (i.e., giant cells, epithelioid clusters, and necrosis) are not CD4+ dependent and hence should not be affected in AIDS unless there is a total loss or malfunction of the necessary cytokines and adhesion molecules for their formation, such as ICAM-1 and its up-regulators, TNF-α, IL-1, and IFN-γ (46). All of these cytokines are elevated in AIDS patients (42) and can be demonstrated in lymph nodes of AIDS patients by *in situ* hybridization (46). In this context, an additional variable—that the T cells have defective function long before their actual reduction in numbers (47)—must be considered. The granulomatous features may be divorced from mycobacterial numbers and hence from the killing that appears to be a CD4+-dependent phenomenon. However, low CD4+ counts do not affect the effectiveness of antituberculous drug therapy, as suggested by other authors (48) and our autopsy study. The HIV-positive patients are more likely to develop adverse reactions to drugs than are HIV-negative patients.

LYMPHOCYTE SUBSETS IN GRANULOMATOUS INFLAMMATION

There is a preponderance of CD4+ cells (Fig. 24.19) over CD8+ cells (Fig. 24.20) at the site of granulomatous inflammation, in the tissue as well as the pleural (49) and bron-

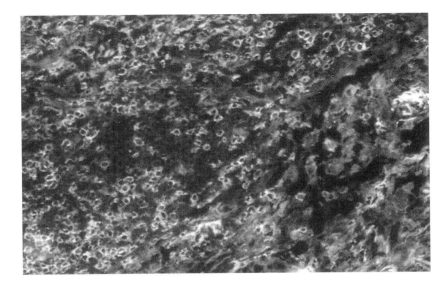

FIGURE 24.19. Numerous CD4+ cells around centrally placed epithelioid cells (negatively stained area, avidin–biotin immunofluorescence, original magnification ×100).

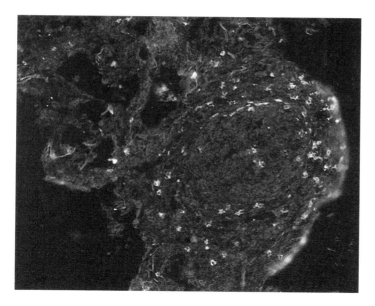

FIGURE 24.20. Few CD8⁺ cells forming a ring around the granuloma (same technique as Fig. 24.19).

choalveolar lavage (BAL) fluids (50). The lymphocytes are distributed in tight cuffs around centrally placed activated epithelioid cells. The markers used to detect activation were human leukocyte antigen (HLA)–DR (51–53) and CD71, a transferrin receptor. In the six TB patients we studied (all HIV negative), the CD4/CD8 ratio in the tissue approximated more than 5:1, while there was a similar increase in CD4/CD8 ratio in BAL fluid from the involved segments (50). However, with disease progression, in patients with suppurative lesions and in AIDS patients there may be increased CD8⁺ cells. Several authors working with granulomatous inflammation of different causes made similar observations (51–54). This correlates well with the finding of Ainslie et al. (55) who demonstrated increased numbers of CD8⁺ cells in the BAL fluid from patients with miliary TB as compared with those with localized pulmonary TB. They believed that

these cells could be of the suppressor phenotype, with resultant suppression of activated macrophages and poor mycobacterial killing. Few γδ T cells and natural killer (NK) cells were detected, suggesting that these cells had a minimal local immunologic contribution in granulomatous inflammation. Approximately 10% to 15% of the cells were proliferating *in situ* as delineated by the MIB-1 immunohistochemical staining, compared with less than 1% in the noninflamed lung (Fig. 24.21). Double staining with CD29, β₁-integrin, a marker for the memory phenotype, and CD4 and CD8 shows that large numbers of cells in the granuloma are of the memory phenotype. Barnes al. (49) showed similar findings of CD4⁺CDw29⁺ T lymphocytes in tuberculous pleuritis. CD4⁺CDw29⁺ but not the CD4⁺CDw29⁻ produced high levels of IFN-γ when stimulated by purified protein derivative (PPD) *in vitro* and were selectively depleted in

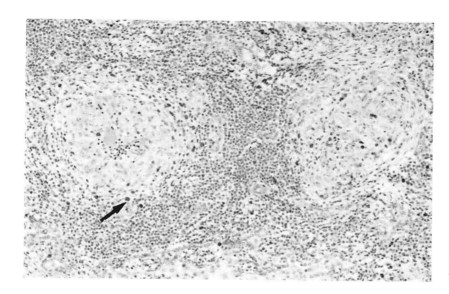

FIGURE 24.21. Immunoperoxidase staining for proliferation marker MIB-1 in granulomas. Note few cells are positive (*arrow*) (original magnification ×20).

AIDS patients, according to Van Noesel et al. (56). This results in an imbalance of naive and memory T cells, with resultant poor responsiveness to antigen in the context of autologous major histocompatibility molecules.

INTERCELLULAR ADHESION MOLECULE IN MYCOBACTERIAL INFECTION

ICAM-1 (CD54) is a chain polypeptide that is heavily glycosylated (M_r 76 to 114,000). It is expressed on both hematopoietic and nonhematopoietic cells and serves as a counterreceptor to integrins, leukocyte function–associated antigen (LFA)–1 (CD11a/CD18), and Mac-1 (CD11b/CD18) (57). Previously, our group (58) showed *in vitro* that *M. tuberculosis* (H37Ra) enhances the expression of ICAM-1 in monocytic cells. It is also found in sarcoid granulomas (59) and in epidermal keratinocytes in tuberculoid leprosy but not in lepromatous leprosy (60). ICAM-1/LFA-1 interactions are also critical for conjugate formation between antigen-presenting cells and T cells as well as activation of the latter. We evaluated 50 biopsy specimens to look at the participation of ICAM-1, *in vivo*, in the generation of mycobacterial granulomas (61). For comparison, granulomatous inflammation, both infectious and noninfectious, from diverse causes was used. ICAM-1 was detected by the biotin–streptavidin complex technique. In the normal tissue, ICAM-1 was identified on type II pneumocytes, large-vessel endothelium, and, rarely, bronchial epithelium. In the granulomas from diverse causes, including sarcoidosis, leishmaniasis, and histoplasmosis, membranous staining was identified on giant cells, epithelioid cells, and degenerate cellular membranes in areas of necrosis. The finding of strong membranous staining of giant cells (Fig. 24.22) is well supported by an *in vitro* study showing that ICAM-1 and its ligand are impor-

tant in the formation of rat macrophage aggregates and giant cells, which can be blocked with the corresponding antibodies (62). In addition, other *in vitro* studies using human peripheral blood monocytes showed the importance of IFN-γ-induced enhanced expression of LFA-1 to the generation of multinucleated giant cells (63). The giant cell formation was completely blocked by anti-ICAM antibodies (63). In the alveolar macrophages away from the granuloma, weak or no expression of ICAM-1 was seen, suggesting that ICAM-1 expression was granuloma specific. In the ill-defined granulomas of MAC infection, ICAM-1 was not expressed (Fig. 24.23). These observations suggest a critical role for ICAM-1 in the development of well-formed granulomas of diverse causes. This was further corroborated recently in ICAM-1 knockout mice given dextran beads. These animals were unable to produce well-formed granulomas (64). It will be interesting to do a similar study using BCG or *M. tuberculosis*. ICAM-1 also may be important for mediating recruitment of the inflammatory cells to the periphery of the granuloma and mediating T-cell cytolysis and necrosis. Recently, it was shown in a mouse ICAM-1 knockout model that ICAM-1 might play an important role in T-cell activation by providing a costimulatory signal (65). Why some granulomas with ICAM-1 expression undergo necrosis and others do not may have to do with the sustained expression of TNF-α and end-organ sensitivity to it (see section "Correlation of CD4 Counts with Morphology and Number of Bacilli"). Our observation of ICAM having a critical role in granuloma formation has been further confirmed by gene disruption of the ICAM-1 molecule. The Mac-1 binding site of ICAM-1 was confirmationally changed so that monocytes could no longer bind. The lymphocyte function–associated antigen (LFA) binding site was intact. When these mice were exposed to low-dose *M. tuberculosis* they developed normal T-cell responses but no delayed

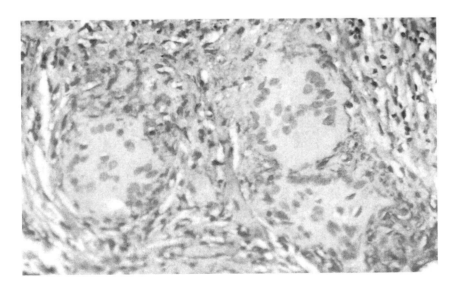

FIGURE 24.22. Immunoperoxidase staining for intercellular adhesion molecule-1 in tuberculous granuloma with giant cells. Note fine membranous staining on the surface of the giant cells (original magnification, ×400).

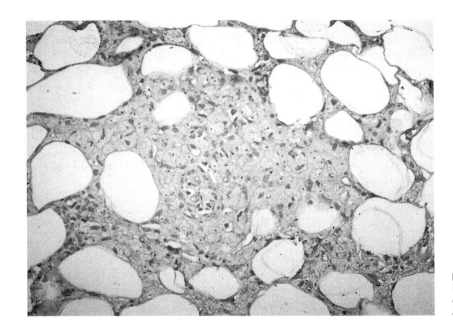

FIGURE 24.23. Immunoperoxidase staining for intercellular adhesion molecule-1 in ill-defined granuloma with foam cells in *Mycobacterium avium* complex. Note that there is no staining.

type hypersensitivity response and no appreciable granuloma formation during the first 90 days. Thus, granuloma formation was not required for the initial containment of infection. However, the animals began to die, with marked inflammation and necrosis at the site of infection. Therefore, according to this study, granuloma formation may serve to wall of the infection and ICAM-1 is necessary for granuloma formation. As infected macrophages die there are other macrophages in the granuloma to phagocytose the released mycobacteria, thus stopping their spread. This study provides strong support for the concept that the granuloma is not merely an overresponsive delayed-type hypersensitivity but rather that it has a crucial role in protective immunity (66).

The presence of IL-1β (Fig. 24.24) in granulomas is consistent with its role in modulating ICAM-1 expression together with TNF-α and IFN-γ (45,67). IL-1β previously was observed in tuberculous and sarcoid granulomas (68) but not in MAC granulomas or foreign-body granulomas. This finding is consistent with our finding of less ICAM-1 expression in MAC with foam cells, perhaps due to the fact that less IL-1 is present to up-regulate it. The IL-1 antagonist, IL-1 receptor antagonist protein (IRAP), was detected in reactive lymph nodes and in these granulomas (69). There have been significant contributions in our understanding of the role of IFN-γ, IL-12, CD4, CD8, and chemokines in granuloma formation in the last 5 years as shown in Tables 24.3 and 24.4 (66,70–82).

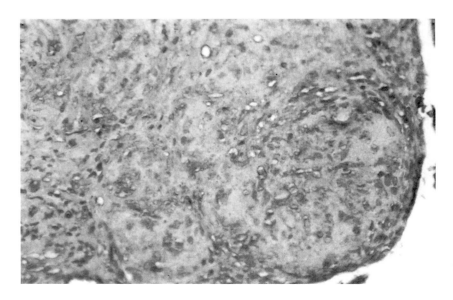

FIGURE 24.24. Immunoperoxidase staining for interleukin-1 in tuberculous granuloma. Note positive brown staining in the cytoplasm in the form of vacuoles and membranous staining (original magnification ×200).

TABLE 24.3. EFFECT OF INTERFERON-γ PRODUCTION OR T-CELL DELETION ON GRANULOMA FORMATION

Gene Knockout	IFN-γ Production	Survival	Granuloma Formation	Ref.
IFN-γ	No IFN-γ	40 d	Granulocyte accumulation, some lymphocytes and macrophages progressing to necrosis.	70
IL-12	No IFN-γ	50 d	Macrophages accumulate in the absence of lymphocytes; increased neutrophils and necrosis.	71
CD4	Reduced	120 d	Delayed inflammation; macrophages/neutrophils, few lymphocytes.	72
CD8	Reduced	180–200 d	Increased lymphocytes early, but loss of control and necrosis prior to death.[a]	
β2m	Reduced early	>200 d	Aerosol infection; increased macrophage with lymphocytes limited to perivascular cuffs.	73
	Reduced	28 d	Intravenous infection; increased granuloma formation, high level of necrotic granulomas.	74
γδ	Normal INF-γ	Normal	Increased numbers of neutrophils within the granuloma.	

[a]Turner J, personal communication, 2000.
IFN-γ, interferon-γ; IL-12, interleukin-12; β2m, β2-microglobulin.

TABLE 24.4. CHEMOKINE RESPONSE DETECTED DURING *MYCOBACTERIUM TUBERCULOSIS* INFECTION

Chemokine	Cell Type(s)	Responses	Ref.
MCP-1	PBMC and alveolar macrophages	Increased expression when stimulated with viable M. TB	76–78
	BALF	Increased expression in patients with acute TB infection	79
	Knockout mice	No effect on bacterial growth *in vivo*, no information on granuloma formation	
CCR2 (MCP-1 receptor)	Knockout mice stimulated *in vivo* with PPD-coated latex beads	Reduced recruitment of monocytes, macrophages; reduced granuloma formation	80
RANTES	BALF	Decreased production of IFN-γ	
	Human MNs and AMs	Increased expression in patients with acute TB infection; both H37Rv and H37Ra infections induce RANTES production	77 78
MIP-1α	Human MNs and AMs	M. TB infection induces rapid expression of MIP-1	76
	Human neutrophils	Increased expression	78
	Murine BMM	Infecting macrophages with M. TB induces rapid expression detectable by day 1	
MIP-1β	Aerosol infection with M. TB	mRNA detectable by 40 d postinfection	81
	Murine BMM	Infecting macrophages with M. TB induces rapid expression detectable by day 1	81
MIP-2	Aerosol infection with M. TB	mRNA detectable by 40 d postinfection	
	Murine BMM	Infecting macrophages with M. TB induces rapid expression detectable by day 1	81
IL-8	Aerosol infection with M. TB	mRNA detectable by 40 d	
	Human alveolar epithelial cells or cell line	M. TB infection induces production of IL-8 and MCP-1 independent of virulence of mycobacterial strain	82
	PBMC, alveolar macrophages	H37Rv and H37Ra infection induces release of IL-8	76
	BALF	Increased expression in patients with acute M. TB infection	77

AM, alveolar macrophages; BALF, bronchoalveolar lavage fluid; BMM, bone marrow–derived macrophages; IFN-γ, interferon-γ; IL, interleukin; MCP, monocyte chemotactic protein; MIP, macrophage inflammatory protein; MN, monocytes; M. TB, *Mycobacterium tuberculosis*; PBMC, peripheral blood mononuclear cell; PPD, purified protein derivative; RANTES, regulated on activation, normal T cell expressed and secreted; TB, tuberculosis.

ROLE OF CYTOTOXIC T CELLS IN GRANULOMATOUS INFLAMMATION

While the role of CD4$^+$ T$_H$1 cells in conferring protective immunity in mycobacterial infections is becoming clear, the role of CD8$^+$ cells, more specifically cytotoxic T cells, is not. Transgenic knockout mice lacking the β$_2$-microglobulin gene infected with *M. tuberculosis* succumb within 3 weeks, defining a murine role for CD8$^+$ cells (83). In tissue immunofluorescence studies (50), we showed that CD8$^+$ cells form a thin cuff around epithelioid cells in granulomas, as did other authors who speculated that these CD8$^+$ cells are probably cytotoxic and responsible for necrosis (53). Furthermore, Pitchie et al. (84) observed that lymphokine-activated macrophages are unable to achieve complete bacteriostasis *in vitro*, creating a need to look for alternative mechanisms. We evaluated cytotoxic T cells using a panantibody that detects all cytotoxic cells including NK, γδ, CD8$^+$, and CD4$^+$ cells. This antibody detects RNA-binding nucleolysin protein in the cytotoxic granules and Golgi apparatus in both activated and inactivated T cells. Since we demonstrated, both in the BAL fluid and in the tissue, that a minority of the cells were NK or γδ, we assumed that a substantial proportion of the cytotoxic cells as defined by the TIA-1 antibody were either CD8$^+$ or CD4$^+$. We evaluated 22 surgical specimens of mycobacterial infection (Table 24.2). Normal tissue from unrelated patients and adjacent to granulomas showed rare scattered cytotoxic T cells (1+). Small granulomas had consistently fewer cells than larger ones. However, more cytotoxic T cells were associated with granulomas than the normal areas, implying a specific role for these cells in granulomas. In the lymph nodes this association was not as obvious, perhaps due to the presence of indigent lymphocytes. Other infections that require cell-mediated immunity, such as leishmaniasis and leprosy, had similar responses. In sarcoidosis granulomas (six patients), fewer cells were identified than in the infectious granulomas. There were many more cytotoxic T cells in the areas of necrosis than in other areas without necrosis, implying a cause-and-effect relationship (Fig. 24.25). Therefore, the mere presence of cytotoxic cells does not inevitably lead to necrosis. The numbers of these cells and mononuclear phagocytes or epithelioid cells capable of releasing cytokines, such as TNF-α and proteases including interstitial collagenase and gelatinase, are important jointly in causing the necrosis characteristic of mycobacterial infections. Interestingly, in hypersensitivity pneumonitis (in which necrosis is uncommon), many cytotoxic T cells were noted. The number of cytotoxic T cells did not correlate with either CD4$^+$ counts or the number of bacilli, suggesting that cytotoxic T cells do not confer any protective immunity. These findings seem to be in agreement with the notion that cell-mediated immunity can be more deleterious to the individual than the mycobacteria. Supporting our observation, Pitchie et al. (84) found CD4 cytolytic T cells capable of specifically lysing autologous antigen-presenting macrophages, particularly in cavitary lesions. They concluded that this cytotoxic response contributes to tissue damage rather than protective immunity to the host. However, they believe that this may help disease localization because there is a reduced capacity to generate mycobacterial antigen–specific cytolytic activity in miliary disease. Additional studies are needed to confirm this finding.

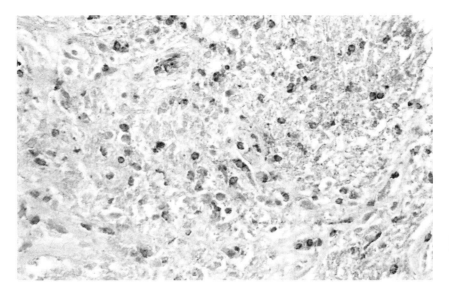

FIGURE 24.25. Immunoperoxidase staining for T-cytotoxic cells using monoclonal antibody TIA-1. Note numerous cytotoxic cells in the area of necrosis in a tuberculous granuloma.

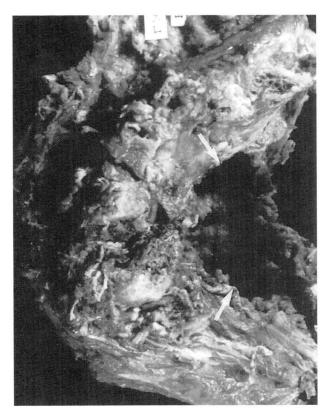

FIGURE 24.26. Gibbus deformity. Note the bony defect (*arrows*) that resulted from a surgical attempt to decompress the underlying spinal cord.

TUBERCULOSIS OF THE CENTRAL NERVOUS SYSTEM

Tuberculosis of the central nervous system (CNS) occurs in patients with preserved immunity and those with immunodeficiency. The bacilli enter through the respiratory system by inhalation, and following bacteremia, small tuberculous foci (Rich foci) develop in the brain, spinal cord, and meninges.

The infection can affect the CNS in several ways. Tuberculous meningitis is the most common manifestation and has accounted for about 10% of all forms of bacterial meningitis in all age groups. It is generally encountered during the first three decades of life and is usually, but not always, associated with active systemic disease. The leptomeninges show characteristic changes. They are diffusely thickened and green–gray, and are more severely affected in the basal cisterns of the brain. The spinal leptomeninges also may be involved. On sectioning, the brain usually shows hydrocephalus and edema. Histologically, the extent of cellular exudate and caseation varies from patient to patient. Central necrotic cores are surrounded by epithelioid histiocytes, lymphocytes, and Langhans giant cells. The leptomeningeal vessels at the base of the brain are frequently affected and show inflammatory infiltrate in the wall or an endarteritis obliterans. AFBs may be abundant or scanty. Tuberculomas may form and require surgical excision (85).

Tuberculous spondylitis most commonly affects the thoracic region of the vertebral column and can involve several levels (86). A paravertebral soft-tissue abscess may develop. In Pott disease, paraparesis or even paraplegia results from compression of the spinal cord secondary to the spinal column deformity (87) (Fig. 24.26).

The presentation, clinical manifestations, cerebrospinal fluid formula, and mortality of tuberculous meningitis are generally similar in patients with and those without HIV infection (88).

Tuberculous abscesses and tuberculomas in the brain parenchyma are well-established causes of brain mass lesions in patients with AIDS (89). The incidence of tuberculomas is approximately 10% of all cases of TB diagnosed in AIDS patients (90). Computed tomography reveals ring-enhancing or hypodense lesions. TB of the CNS can occur in association with other infectious agents commonly encountered with AIDS, such as *Toxoplasma gondii*, *Cryptococcus neoformans*, and cytomegalovirus (89). In HIV-infected patients the lesions are usually necrotic (Fig. 24.27) with abundant histio-

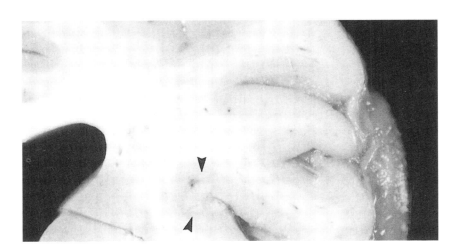

FIGURE 24.27. Intraparenchymal necrotic lesion in the cerebral cortex of a human immunodeficiency virus–positive patient (*arrowheads*). (See Color Plate 10.)

cytes containing numerous acid-fast mycobacteria. The organisms are found around blood vessels or within necrotizing lesions. The etiologic agents are identical to those responsible for systemic disease (*M. tuberculosis* or *M. avium-intracellulare*).

REFERENCES

1. Laennec RTH. *Deflauscultation mediate.* Paris: Brosson, 1918.
2. Ober WB. Ghon but not forgotten: Anton Ghon and his complex. *Pathol Annu* 1983;18:79–85.
3. Lucas S, Nelson AM. Pathogenesis of tuberculosis in human immunodeficiency virus–infected people. In: Bloom BR, ed. *Tuberculosis: pathogenesis, protection, and control.* Washington, DC: American Society for Microbiology, 1994:503–514.
4. Medlar EM. *The behavior of pulmonary tuberculous lesions: a pathological study.* Monograph, 1955.
5. Szopinski J, Remiszewski P, Szymanska D, et al. Tuberculosis found in autopsies done in the Institute of Tuberculosis and Lung Diseases 1972–1991. *Pneumonol Alergol Pol* 1993;61:275–279.
6. Lee JK, Ng TH. Undiagnosed tuberculosis in hospitalized patients—an autopsy survey. *J R Soc Health* 1990;110:141–143.
7. Hill AR, Premkumar S, Burstein S, et al. Disseminated tuberculosis in the acquired immunodeficiency syndrome era. *Am Rev Respir Dis* 1991;144:1164–1170.
8. McGuinness G, Naidich DP, Jagirdar J, et al. High resolution CT finding in miliary lung disease. *J Comput Assist Tomogr* 1992;16:384–390.
9. Close PM, Macrae MB, Hammond JM, et al. Anaplastic large-cell Ki-1 lymphoma. Pulmonary presentation mimicking miliary tuberculosis. *Am J Clin Pathol* 1993;99:631–636.
10. Stead WW. Pathogenesis of a first episode of chronic pulmonary tuberculosis in man: recrudescence of residuals of the primary infection or exogenous reinfection? *Am Rev Respir Dis* 1967;95:729–745.
11. Stead WW. The pathogenesis of pulmonary tuberculosis among older persons. *Am Rev Respir Dis* 1965;91:811–822.
12. Stead WW. Pathogenesis of the sporadic cases of tuberculosis. *N Engl J Med* 1967;277:1008–1012.
13. Heimbeck J. Incidence of tuberculosis in young adult women with special reference to employment. *Br J Tuberc* 1938;32:154–166.
14. Daniels M, Ridehaligh F, Springett VH, et al. *Tuberculosis in young adults: report of the Prophit Tuberculosis Survey 1935–1944.* London: Lewis, 1948.
15. Mankiewicz E. Bacteriophage types of mycobacteria. *Can J Public Health* 1972;63:111:307–312.
16. Pennington JE. Aspergillus lung disease. *Med Clin North Am* 1980;64:475–490.
17. Dannenberg AM Jr. Pathogenesis of tuberculosis. In: Fishman AP, ed. *Pulmonary disease and disorder.* New York: McGraw-Hill, 1980:1264–1281.
18. Ishida T, Yokoyama H, Kaneko S, et al. Pulmonary tuberculoma and indications for surgery: radiographic and clinicopathological analysis. *Respir Med* 1992;86:431–436.
19. Coolop NA. A solitary pulmonary nodule due to *M. gordonae. Respiration* 1990;57:351–352.
20. Guy E, Rocha MP, Faith R, et al. Pathogenicity of multi-drug resistant *M. tuberculosis* in the guinea pig. *Am Rev Respir Dis* 1994;149:A614.
21. Chandrasekhar S, Ratnam S. Studies on cell-wall deficient non-acid fast variants of *M. tuberculosis. Tuber Lung Dis* 1992;73:273–279.
22. Yee HT, Doniguian E, Della-Latta, et al. Mycobacterial infections (MI): a correlative study of culture and tissue diagnosis. *Lab Invest* 1994;70:129A.
23. Marchevsky A, Damsker B, Gribitz A, et al. The spectrum of pathology of nontuberculous mycobacterial infections in open-lung biopsy specimens. *Am J Clin Pathol* 1982;78:695–700.
24. Yang GC, Schinella RA. The histopathology of tuberculosis in the acquired immunodeficiency syndrome: a study of 9 cases. In: Rotterdam H, et al., eds. *Progress in AIDS pathology II.* New York: Field and Wood, 1990:103–110.
25. Wear DJ, Hadfield TL, Connor DH, et al. Letter to the editor. *Arch Pathol Lab Med* 1985;109:701–702.
26. Kommareddi S, Abramowsky C, Swinehart GL, et al. Nontuberculous mycobacterial infections: comparison of the fluorescent auramine-O and Ziehl–Neelsen techniques in tissue diagnosis. *Hum Pathol* 1984;15:1085–1089.
27. Humphrey DM, Weiner MH. Mycobacterial antigen detection by immunohistochemistry in pulmonary tuberculosis. *Hum Pathol* 1987;18:701–708.
28. Barbolini G, Biseti A, Colizzi V, et al. Immunohistologic analysis of mycobacterial antigens by monoclonal antibodies in tuberculosis and mycobacteriosis. *Hum Pathol* 1989;20:1078–1083.
29. Dacosta NA, Kinare SG. Association of lung carcinoma and tuberculosis. *J Postgrad Med* 1991;37:185–189.
30. Chauduri MR. Primary pulmonary scar carcinomas. *Indian J Med Res* 1973;61:858–869.
31. Madri JA, Carter D. Scar cancers of the lung; origin and significance. *Hum Pathol* 1984;15:625–631.
32. Flance IJ. Scar cancer of the lung. *JAMA* 1991;266:2003–2004.
33. Arora B, Arora DR. Fine needle aspiration cytology in diagnosis of tuberculous lymphadenitis. *Indian J Med Res* 1990;91:189–192.
34. Lau SK, Wei WI, Hsu C, et al. Efficacy of fine needle aspiration cytology in the diagnosis of tuberculous cervical lymphadenopathy. *J Laryngol Otol* 1990;104:24–27.
35. Finfer M, Perchick A, Burstein DE. Fine needle aspiration biopsy diagnosis of tuberculous lymphadenitis in patients with and without the acquired immune deficiency syndrome. *Acta Cytol* 1991;35:325–332.
36. Radhika S, Rajwanshi A, Kochhar R, et al. Abdominal tuberculosis. Diagnosis by fine needle aspiration cytology. *Acta Cytol* 1993;37:673–678.
37. Savage RA. Correspondence re: S. J. Maygarden and E. L. Flanders. Mycobacteria can be seen as "negative images" in cytology smears from patients with acquired immunodeficiency syndrome. *Mod Pathol* 1989;2:239.
38. Brandwein M, Choi HS, Strauchen J, et al. Spindle cell reaction to nontuberculous mycobacteriosis in AIDS mimicking a spindle cell neoplasm. *Virchows Arch A Pathol Anat Histopathol* 1990;416:281–286.
39. Del Prete G, Maggi E, Romagnani S. Human Th1 and Th2 cells: functional properties, mechanisms of regulation, and role in disease. *Lab Invest* 1994;70:299–306.
40. Jones BE, Summer M, Young M, et al. Relationship of the manifestations of tuberculosis to CD4 cell counts in patients with human immunodeficiency virus infection. *Am Rev Respir Dis* 1993;148:1292–1297.
41. Sunderam G, McDonald RJ, Maniatis T, et al. Tuberculosis as a manifestation of the acquired immunodeficiency syndrome (AIDS). *JAMA* 1986;256:362–366.
42. Fauci AS. Multifactorial nature of human immunodeficiency virus disease: implications for therapy. *Science* 1993;262:1011–1018.
43. Rook GAW, Al Attiyah R. Cytokines and the Koch phenomenon. *Tubercle* 1991;72:13–20.
44. Theuer CP, Hopewell PC, Elias D, et al. Human immunodefi-

ciency virus infection in tuberculosis patients. *J Infect Dis* 1990; 162:8–12.

45. Webb DS, Mostowski HS, Gerard TL, et al. Cytokine-induced enhancement of ICAM-1 expression results in increased vulnerability of tumor cells to monocyte-mediated lysis. *J Immunol* 1991;146:2682–2686.

46. Emilie D, Peuchmaur M, Maillot M, et al. Production of interleukins in human immunodeficiency virus-1–replicating lymph nodes. *J Clin Invest* 1990;86:148–159.

47. Staal FJT, Anderson MT, Staal GE, et al. Redox regulation of signal transduction: tyrosine phosphorylation and calcium influx. *Immunology* 1994;91:3619–3622.

48. Chaisson RE, Schecter GF, Theur CP, et al. Tuberculosis in patients with the acquired immunodeficiency syndrome. *Am Rev Respir Dis* 1987;136:570–574.

49. Barnes PF, Mistry SD, Cooper CL, et al. Compartmentalization of a CD4⁺ T lymphocyte subpopulation in tuberculous pleuritis. *J Immunol* 1989;142:1114–1119.

50. Law KF, Jagirdar J, Weiden MD, et al. Lymphocyte characteristics in BAL and blood of patients with active pulmonary tuberculosis. *Am Rev Respir Dis* 1994;146:A614.

51. Jagirdar J, Chang JC, Lesser M, et al. In situ analysis of lymphocyte subsets in rat lung granulomas induced by complete Freund's adjuvant using monoclonal antibodies. *Lab Invest* 1983;46: 41A.

52. Van Den Oord JJ, Dewolf-Peeters C, Facchetti F, et al. Cellular composition of hypersensitivity-type granulomas: immunohistochemical analysis of tuberculous and sarcoidal lymphadenitis. *Hum Pathol* 1984;15:559–565.

53. Van Den Oord JJ, Dewolf-Peeters C, Desmet VJ. Cellular composition of suppurative granulomas: an immunohistochemical study of suppurative granulomatous lymphadenitis. *Hum Pathol* 1985;16:1009–1014.

54. Van Voorhis WC, Kaplan G, Sarno EN, et al. The cutaneous infiltrates of leprosy: cellular characteristics and the predominant T-cell phenotypes. *N Engl J Med* 1982;307:1593.

55. Ainslie GM, Solomon JA, Bateman ED. Lymphocyte and lymphocyte subset numbers in blood and in bronchoalveolar lavage and pleural fluid in various forms of human pulmonary tuberculosis at presentation and during recovery. *Thorax* 1992;47: 513–518.

56. Van Noesel CJ, Gruters RA, Terpstra FG, et al. Functional and phenotypic evidence for a selective loss of memory T cells in asymptomatic human immunodeficiency virus-infected men. *J Clin Invest* 1990;86:293–299.

57. Dustin ML, Rothlien R, Bhan AK, et al. Induction by IL 1 and interferon-γ: tissue distribution, biochemistry and function of a natural adherence molecule (ICAM-1). *J Immunol* 1986;137: 245–254.

58. Lopez-Ramirez GM, Bonk SJ, Cronstein BN, et al. *Mycobacterium tuberculosis* alters expression of adhesion molecules on monocytic cells. *Infect Immun* 1994;62:2515–2520.

59. Van Dinther-Janssen ACHM, Van-Maarsseveen TCM, Eckert H, et al. Identical expression of ELAM-1, VCAM-1, and ICAM-1 in sarcoidosis and usual interstitial pneumonitis. *J Pathol* 1993; 170:157–164.

60. Sullivan L, Sano S, Pirmez C, et al. Expression of adhesion molecules in leprosy lesions. *Infect Immun* 1991;59:4154–4160.

61. Lopez-Ramirez GM, Reibman J, Rom WN, et al. The role of intercellular adhesion molecule-1 (ICAM-1) in the modulation of granulomatous response to *Mycobacterium tuberculosis*. *Am J Respir Crit Care Med* 1994;149:A611.

62. Smith KM, Doyle NA, Doerschuk CM. Role of CD11/CD18 and ICAM-1 in the aggregation and fusion of rat alveolar macrophages in response to interferon-γ. *Am Rev Respir Dis* 1994;149:A1098.

63. Most J, Neumayer HP, Dierich MP. Cytokine-induced generation of multinucleated giant cells *in vitro* requires interferon-γ and expression of LFA-1. *Eur J Immunol* 1990;20:1661–1667.

64. Smith KM, Doyle NA, Quinlan WM, et al. Granulomatous inflammation induced by intravenous dextran beads in ICAM-1 deficient mice. *Am J Respir Crit Care Med* 1994;149:A83.

65. Sligh JE, Ballantyne CM, Rich SS, et al. Inflammatory responses are impaired in mice deficient in intracellular adhesion molecule-1. *Proc Natl Acad Sci USA* 1993;90:8529–8533.

66. Bernadette MS, Cooper AM. Restraining mycobacteria: role of granuloma in mycobacterial infections. *Immunol Cell Biol* 2000; 78:334-341

67. Mulligan MS, Vaprociyan AA, Miyasaka M, et al. Tumor necrosis factor α regulates *in vivo* intrapulmonary expression of ICAM-1. *Am J Pathol* 1993;142:1739–1749.

68. Devergne O, Emilie D, Peuchmaur M, et al. Production of cytokines in sarcoid lymph nodes: preferential expression of interleukin-1β and interferon-γ genes. *Hum Pathol* 1992;23: 317–323.

69. Chensue SW, Warmington KS, Berger AN, et al. Immunohistochemical demonstration of interleukin-1 receptor antagonist protein and interleukin-1 in human lymphoid tissue and granulomas. *Am J Pathol* 1992;140:269–275.

70. Flynn JL, Chan J, Triebold KJ, et al. An essential role for interferon gamma in resistance to *Mycobacterium tuberculosis* infection. *J Exp Med* 1993; 178: 2249-54.

71. Cooper AM, Magram J, Ferrante J, et al. Interleukin 12 (IL-12) is crucial to the development of protective immunity in mice intravenously infected with *Mycobacterium tuberculosis*. *J Exp Med* 1997;186:39–45.

72. Caruso AM, Serbina N, Klein E, et al. Mice deficient in CD4 T cells have only transiently diminished levels of IFN-gamma, yet succumb to tuberculosis. *J Immunol* 1999; 162:5407–5416.

73. D'Souza CD, Cooper AM, Frank AA, et al. A novel non-classical β2-microglobulin-restricted mechanism influencing early lymphocyte accumulation and subsequent resistance to tuberculosis in the lung. *Am J Respir Cell Mol Biol* 2000;23:188–193.

74. Flynn JL, Goldstein MM, Triebold KJ, et al. Major histocompatibility complex class I-restricted T cells are required for resistance to *Mycobacterium tuberculosis* infection. *Proc Natl Acad Sci U S A* 1992; 89:12013–12017.

75. D'Souza CD, Cooper AM, Frank AA, et al. An anti-inflammatory role for gamma delta T lymphocytes in acquired immunity to *Mycobacterium tuberculosis*. *J Immunol* 1997;158: 1217–1221.

76. Kasahara K, Tobe T, Tomita M, et al. Selective expression of monocyte chemotactic and activating factor/monocyte chemoattractant protein 1 in human blood monocytes by *Mycobacterium tuberculosis*. *J Infect Dis* 1994;170:1238–1247.

77. Kurashima K, Mukaida N, Fujimura M, et al. Elevated chemokine levels in bronchoalveolar lavage fluid of tuberculosis patients. *Am J Respir Crit Care Med* 1997;155:1474–1477.

78. Sadek MI, Sada E, Toossi Z, et al. Chemokines induced by infection of mononuclear phagocytes with mycobacteria and present in lung alveoli during active pulmonary tuberculosis. *Am J Respir Cell Mol Biol* 1998;19:513–521.

79. Lu B, Rutledge BJ, Gu L, et al. Abnormalities in monocyte recruitment and cytokine expression in monocyte chemoattractant protein 1–deficient mice. *J Exp Med* 1998;187:601–608.

80. Boring L, Gosling J, Chensue SW, et al. Impaired monocyte migration and reduced type 1 (Th1) cytokine responses in C-C chemokine receptor 2 knockout mice. *J Clin Invest* 1997;100: 2552–2261.

81. Rhoades ER, Cooper AM, Orme IM. Chemokine response in mice infected with *Mycobacterium tuberculosis*. *Infect Immun* 1995;63:3871–3877.

82. Lin YG, Zhang M, Barnes PF. Chemokine production by a human alveolar epithelial cell line in response to *Mycobacterium tuberculosis*. *Infect Immun* 1998;66:1121–1126.

83. Flynn JL, Goldstein MM, Triebold KJ, et al. Major histocompatibility complex class I-restricted T cells are required for resistance to *M. tuberculosis* infection. *Proc Natl Acad Sci U S A* 1992;89:12013–12017.

84. Pitchie AD, Rahelu M, Kumararatne DS et al. Generation of cytolytic T cells in individuals infected by *M. tuberculosis* and vaccinated with BCG. *Thorax* 1992;47:695–701.

85. Arseni C. Two hundred and one cases of intracranial tuberculoma treated surgically. *J Neurol Neurosurg Psychiatry* 1958;21: 308–311.

86. Cleveland M, Bosworth DM. The pathology of tuberculosis of the spine. *J Bone Joint Surg* 1942;24:527–546.

87. Martin NS. Pott's paraplegia: a report on 120 cases *Br J Bone Joint Surg* 1971;53:596–608.

88. Berenguer J, Moreno S, Luguna F. Tuberculosis meningitis in patients infected with the human immunodeficiency virus. *N Engl J Med* 1992;326:668–672.

89. Fischl MA, Pitchenik AE, Spira TJ. Tuberculous brain abscess and *Toxoplasma* encephalitis in a patient with the acquired immunodeficiency syndrome. *JAMA* 1985;253:3428–3430.

90. Bishburg E. Central nervous system tuberculosis with the acquired immunodeficiency syndrome and its related complex. *Ann Intern Med* 1986;105:210–213.

Tuberculosis, Second Edition, edited by William N. Rom and Stuart M. Garay. Lippincott Williams & Wilkins, Philadelphia © 2004

PULMONARY TUBERCULOSIS

STUART M. GARAY

Throughout history, tuberculosis (TB) has been identified by its most prominent constitutional symptom—wasting (i.e., "phthisis" or consumption). Although the formation of tubercles in the lungs with resulting symptoms has been recorded since ancient times, the nature and relationship of these lesions to the disease entity of TB became evident only in the 17th and 18th centuries through the works of Sylvius, Morton, Willis, Morgagni, and Laennec. Current clinical experience with TB reveals that 80% to 90% of all cases in patients not infected by human immunodeficiency virus (HIV) involve the lungs.

Failure to diagnose pulmonary TB before a patient dies and delay in diagnosis have persisted as significant problems. In the 1940s, before chemotherapy was available, Farber and Clark recognized the problem of unsuspected TB in hospitalized patients but suggested that this could be solved by routine chest radiographs of all admitted patients (1). Unfortunately, this did not occur. In the post-sanatoria era of the 1970s, failure to diagnose TB was ascribed to the fact that fewer physicians were knowledgeable about diagnosing and managing TB. In addition, physicians had a decreased index of suspicion for TB because of the declining incidence of the disease in the United States (2–9). Greenbaum et al. (9) found that 50% of patients with TB admitted to a teaching hospital during the early 1970s were initially misdiagnosed (9). During that period, as disclosed by a study of nine New England medical schools during the mid-1970s (10), the topic of TB had been eliminated from most curricula. Indeed, in 1977, Byrd et al. (11) found that nonpulmonary physicians administered inappropriate treatment in more than 60% of TB cases. The problem was not restricted to the United States; reports from other developed countries revealed similar findings (12–14). Studies from the mid-1980s found a significant number of unsuspected cases and delays in diagnosis in both inner-city teaching hospitals and suburban community hospitals—even as the number of reported TB cases began to increase in the United States (15,16). In the first decade of the 21st century, delays in diagnosis and management of TB continue to be a problem in the United States and abroad, in community hospitals as well as in university teaching hospitals, attributed to private practitioners as well as academic professors (17–21). This is especially disappointing despite major efforts for an intensive national educational campaign designed to improve the knowledge base of clinicians likely to be challenged by patients with TB (22). This is alarming because delays in diagnosis have led to significant delays in treatment in both HIV and non-HIV patients (23,24). In addition, such delays have led to nosocomial TB infections with sensitive as well as multidrug resistant TB, unnecessary exposure of hospital personnel, treatment failure, and more extensive disease (24–28).

A number of specific patient features have been identified as responsible for the misdiagnosis of TB: lack of pulmonary symptoms (6,16); atypical radiographic findings (16); inconsistent laboratory data, including negative tuberculin skin tests (29); advanced age (15,16); and associated diseases that alter cell-mediated immunity (29,30). In addition to these patient-related issues, physician error has contributed in such ways as misinterpretation of chest radiographs, disregard of radiographic reports suggesting the presence of TB (8), omission of tuberculin skin tests (8), and failure to obtain an adequate number of sputum samples in both HIV and non-HIV patients (6,7,30). In addition, failure to include TB in the differential diagnosis of nonresolving pneumonia (especially in the elderly or immunosuppressed) and the willingness to accept diagnosis of malignancy without tissue confirmation (especially in the elderly) have contributed to the lack of diagnosis of pulmonary TB (6,10,16). Socioeconomic factors, such as homelessness, poor access to health care, and language incompetence, have also contributed to diagnostic and therapeutic delays (23,31).

Thus, varied and "atypical" clinical and radiographic presentations, physician error, and lack of knowledge have all caused difficulties in the diagnosis of pulmonary TB. In light of the resurgence of TB, this chapter attempts to bridge the gap in knowledge for many of today's physicians who have neither diagnosed nor managed TB.

PATHOGENESIS

Understanding the clinical presentation of pulmonary TB requires consideration of its pathogenesis (see Chapter 24

S. M. Garay: Division of Pulmonary and Critical Care Medicine, New York University School of Medicine, New York, New York.

for greater detail) (32). Droplet nuclei of 5 μm or less in diameter are generated by individuals with TB (e.g., by speaking or coughing) and are subsequently inhaled by a susceptible, nonimmunized person (33). The number of bacilli in a 5-μm droplet nucleus is estimated at one to ten. In his classic work, *The Pathogenesis of Tuberculosis,* Rich (34) quoted the results of German investigators who found that the numbers of tubercle bacilli in droplets ranged from 1 to more than 400 organisms per millimeter. A single organism has the potential to cause disease, but usually 5 to 200 inhaled bacilli are needed to cause human infection (32).

Inhaled tubercle bacilli become lodged in a distal respiratory bronchiole or alveolus, located subpleurally. The primary complex is usually located in the lower lobes because of better ventilation to that area. Ghon (35) found that the primary focus was almost equally distributed between upper and lower lobes, with slightly more in the right lung. Frostad (36) observed focal infiltrations "equally distributed all over the lung areas below the clavicles, with a maximum in the infraclavicular region." Medlar (37) determined the location of the primary complex from autopsy analysis of 105 persons; 85% of the lesions were within 1 cm of the pleural surface, 66% were in the lower half of the lungs, and 12% were supraclavicular. Medlar believed that the location of the calcified primary lesions followed "a chance distribution of an airborne infection." In a clinical prospective study regarding the fate of tuberculin reactors, Poulsen (38) followed the radiographic presentation in 133 individuals (62 children and 71 adults). The radiographic changes were almost all unilateral, with 57% occurring on the right side. Perihilar infiltrates (i.e., in the mid-lung field) occurred in 54% of adults and 71% of children. Upper lobe infiltrates occurred in 14% of adults and 19% of children, whereas lower lobe infiltrates occurred in 31% of adults and 10% of children. In a similar prospective study of 76 tuberculin converters who subsequently developed radiographic abnormalities consistent with primary TB, Gedde-Dahl (39) also found a right-sided predominance (62%) with evidence of mid-lung field disease in 50% of patients, lower lobe disease in 37%, and upper lobe disease in only 13%.

Once deposited within the alveolar space, bacilli are ingested by nonactivated alveolar macrophages at the site of implantation and are subsequently transported to hilar and mediastinal nodes. The bacilli either are destroyed or multiply, depending on innate "cidal" capabilities of the macrophages. Intracellular multiplication of bacilli over the course of several days leads to macrophage death. Infected macrophages release chemotactic factors that attract circulating monocytes. The logarithmic multiplication of tubercle bacilli is followed by the onset of cell-mediated immunity in about 3 to 4 weeks (32).

Activated alveolar macrophages and lymphokine-activated T lymphocytes have enhanced capability to destroy intracellular bacilli. The resulting inflammatory process is pathologically recognized as a tubercle or granuloma (i.e., a collection of modified histiocytes surrounded by lymphocytes and cap-

illaries) (see Chapter 24). The granuloma has central necrosis with caseum that inhibits both macrophage function and bacillary growth, and results in a loss of cellular structures. Radiographically, the resulting lesion is referred to as a *Ghon focus* (40). Tubercle bacilli, free or within macrophages, drain along regional peribronchial lymphatic channels to the tracheobronchial lymph nodes, which results in caseating granulomas within the hila. During acute infection, hilar nodes enlarge. Subsequently, these primary lesions shrink with fibrosis and calcification, and (rarely) ossification. The small parenchymal Ghon focus and the associated calcified lymph node compose the Ranke complex (40).

During the first several weeks after infection, tubercle bacilli multiply and enter the bloodstream through lymphatic channels and the smaller pulmonary veins within the inflammatory exudate (41,42). Hematogenous seeding occurs most frequently to sites in which oxygen tension is highest: the brain, epiphyses of long bones, kidneys, vertebral bodies, lymph nodes, and the apical-posterior areas of the lungs. This may explain the high frequency of apical involvement in reactivation TB; higher PO_2 levels favor growth (43). Dock suggested an additional mechanism accounting for the apical-posterior location of reactivated disease: deficiency in lymph production and decreased drainage that impede removal of bacilli from these areas, resulting in organism accumulation and subsequent inflammation of tissue (44,45).

The original focus of disease is usually eradicated within weeks or several months. Tubercle bacilli located in the apex of the lungs and organisms disseminated elsewhere are usually walled off by granulomatous inflammation and destroyed (32). Sometimes the primary focus is eradicated, but disseminated bacilli remain viable within the granulomas. These viable organisms lie dormant until some future event or illness results in loss of cellular immunity and reactivation of TB disease. Occasionally, the primary infection progresses and TB occurs at that site as well as wherever it has disseminated; this is called *progressive primary TB.* The ultimate progression occurs in the host with little or no host response; this is called *disseminated TB* or *miliary TB* (see Chapter 27).

Exposure to a patient with active TB results in infection in approximately one third of those who do not have HIV (46). Of that third, 3% to 5% develop TB within a year. After a year, an additional 3% to 5% develop TB during the remainder of their lifetime. Stead provided convincing evidence that TB in most adults occurs from reactivation of organisms that were seeded during primary infection (47). Nonetheless, reinfection with tubercle bacilli rarely occurs and progresses to clinical disease in both HIV-infected individuals and those without HIV, as demonstrated by identification of different phage types within the same individual as well as analysis by restriction fragment length polymorphisms (48–52). Two studies—one from San Francisco, the other from New York City—estimated that one third of all TB cases were caused by recent infection rather than reactivation of old infection

(53,54). Among HIV-related cases, nearly two thirds of patients were infected within a period of a few months.

PRIMARY TUBERCULOSIS

Epidemiology

Traditionally, primary pulmonary TB has been a disease of childhood. However, between 1952, the year when isoniazid (INH) was introduced clinically, and 1981, the onset of the acquired immunodeficiency syndrome (AIDS) epidemic, the epidemiology of TB in the United States changed dramatically. There was a significant decrease in the prevalence of TB in children; a person's first encounter with TB was often as an adult. As early as 1968, Stead predicted that primary TB infection would occur with increasing frequency in young adults because of the change in epidemiology, and that reactivation disease (postprimary TB) would shift from adolescents and young adults to patients older than 40 years (55). Confirmation of this prediction among certain racial and socioeconomic groups is seen in data collected by Trump et al. (56): tuberculin skin positivity was found in only 0.8% of young white adult males entering the U.S. Navy in 1990. As noted above, even before the onset of AIDS, primary TB was observed with increased frequency in the adult population, including the elderly (57). This explains the many studies claiming "atypical" or "unusual" radiographic findings in the late 1970s (58–63). Most series suggested an incidence of primary TB of 10% to 34% in adults (58–60,64). Only Hadlock et al. (61) failed to find a significant increase in primary TB in adults. The latter investigators believed that higher percentages were found in other series because of patient selection, that is, ordinary cases of TB were not referred to tertiary medical centers, which left a greater percentage of "unusual" cases for the latter. This may have been true to some extent, but most investigators believe that a real shift in the age group contracting TB occurred.

Clinical Presentation

Case 1: A 39-year-old African-American woman was referred to the Bellevue Chest Clinic (New York, NY, U.S.A.) for a tuberculin skin test. She had been told 2 months earlier that she had sarcoidosis because of an abnormal chest radiograph and erythema nodosum on her lower extremities. At the time, she had fever (101°F) and right-sided chest discomfort. She was given a prescription for prednisone but did not fill it and sought a second opinion. She was a nurse who cared for patients with TB. Her purified protein derivative (PPD) skin test was 12 mm but had been negative 1 year earlier. She was asymptomatic and had a dark macular rash on her left lower leg. Her physical examination was otherwise unremarkable. Her sputum smear was acid-fast bacillus (AFB) negative. Pulmonary function tests were normal. A chest radiograph revealed right hilar adenopathy without parenchymal infiltrates (Fig. 25.1). Sputum culture by the Bactec system (Becton, Dickinson and Company; Sparks, MD, U.S.A.) showed

positive results 3 weeks later, and she was treated with INH, rifampin, pyrazinamide, and ethambutol. The organisms proved pansensitive, and after 2 months only INH and rifampin were continued. After 4 months of therapy there was a significant reduction of the hilar adenopathy. She completed a 6-month (total) course of combination chemotherapy.

The most detailed description of the clinical presentation of primary TB comes from the work of Scandinavian inves-

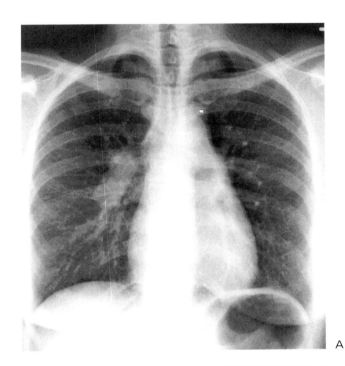

A

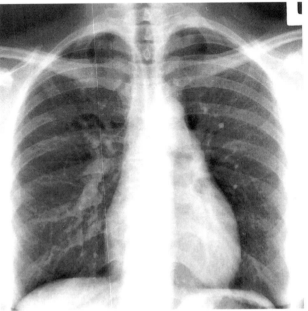

B

FIGURE 25.1. A: Right hilar adenopathy without parenchymal infiltrates. **B:** Resolution of the adenopathy after antituberculous therapy.

tigators before the advent of chemotherapy (36,38,39). Poulsen (38) followed the outcome of 517 new tuberculin converters derived from data collected from the Tuberculosis Centre on the Faroe Islands (off the coast of Norway) from 1932 to 1946. After their conversion had been documented, patients were observed for more than 5 years. The study included 186 children and 331 adults. Initial fever occurred in about 70% of 232 nonselected converters; in the remaining 285 converters, fever was a criterion for enrollment. Most adults had fever as high as 39°C, with an average duration of 2 to 3 weeks. In 23% of patients fever lasted longer than 1 month; however, it had ceased in 98% of patients by 10 weeks. In addition to fever, approximately 25% had subjective symptoms such as retrosternal and interscapular pain, presumably correlated anatomically with the area of the primary infection. Retrosternal pain coincided with the onset of fever and lasted 1 to 2 weeks. In most cases, the pain was described as oppressive, often exacerbated by swallowing, accompanied by tenderness to pressure over the lower sternum, and was thought to be secondary to enlarged bronchial lymph nodes. A second type of pain, occurring in the side of the chest and described as "pricking," was pleuritic in nature; this pain was noted in 39 patients. Pleural effusion was observed in 20 of these patients. Rare symptoms included cough (seven patients), joint pain (four patients), sore throat (two patients), and fatigue (11 patients).

Bradycardia was observed in adults during the first half of the febrile period. Erythema nodosum was striking, usually presenting as blue–red tender nodules in the lower extremities, mostly on the shins (the arms were involved in only five patients), and occurred predominantly in women. The erythema occurred simultaneously with the tuberculin conversion and was usually associated with fever.

Radiographic findings were observed at a very early stage, in most patients during the initial fever. Of the 517 converters, 333 (64%) had hilar adenopathy (78% of 186 children and 56% of 331 adults). Among the 232 nonselected patients (those enrolled solely because of their tuberculin conversion), hilar changes were observed in 55%. Among the 285 selected converters (i.e., patients who presented with fever at the time of conversion) hilar changes were observed in 72%. Nearly half the hilar changes occurred in the right lung and one-third in the left lung. Bilateral changes occurred in 16% of patients. In all cases, radiographic findings occurred within 2 months of tuberculin conversion, although hilar adenopathy was detected within the first week in 41 patients. Hilar enlargement subsided slowly, often as long as 1 to 2 years, and left an accentuated hilum with calcification.

Pleural effusions occurred within the first year, usually 3 to 4 months after tuberculin conversion. Poulsen found 151 (29%) of 517 converters developed pleural effusions. Adults were more apt to develop pleural effusions than children (33% versus 23%), with equal frequency in males and females. Interestingly, adult converters who presented with initial fever, erythema nodosum, or both, demonstrated a

greater frequency of effusions than those who did not (34% and 36%, respectively, versus 26% for those without fever or erythema). In addition, the presence of a pulmonary infiltrate was associated with pleural effusion in 43% of adult cases. Of the 151 cases of pleural effusion, the time of conversion was accurately known for 147, which allowed calculation of the interval between conversion and the onset of pleurisy. A total of 88 patients (60%) were observed within 4 months of conversion, and 80% presented within 6 months. Among the 151 cases of pleurisy, 108 were unilateral: 53% right-sided, 41% left-sided, and 6% bilateral.

Pulmonary infiltrates appeared soon after infection. Poulsen found 139 (27%) of 517 converters with pulmonary infiltrates. Within the first month, 44% had been diagnosed; by the end of 3 months, 78% had been diagnosed. The parenchymal abnormalities were almost always unilateral and associated with ipsilateral hilar enlargement; in addition, many had contralateral hilar changes. Right-sided infiltrates were slightly more common (57%), and bilateral infiltrates occurred in only three patients (2%). The central perihilar areas were most commonly involved (62% in all patients; 54% in adults and 71% in children). Lower lobe infiltrates were observed in 33% of adults and 10% of children. Only 13% of adults had upper lobe infiltrates. The infiltrates were polymorphous, ranging from homogeneous wide bands to mottled or streaky infiltrates. Most infiltrates regressed over months to years. However, in 20 patients (15%) the infiltrates progressed within the first year after conversion (progressive primary TB).

Progressive primary pulmonary TB results when the primary parenchymal disease progresses either at its original site or in other parts of the lung. Poulsen found 20 such cases. He noted continued progression of the infiltrate at the original site (i.e., the Ghon focus) in six patients, regression and then progression of the infiltrate at the original site in eight patients, and cavitation in four patients. In five cases, progression was diffuse without any clear relation to the original focus.

During the late 1970s through mid-1980s, several reviews of radiographic findings in primary pulmonary TB appeared. Unlike Poulsen's longitudinal prospective study, these studies were retrospective and institution based (58–63). In the largest series (103 patients) by Choyke et al. (62), 85% of patients had pulmonary infiltrates, 54% of which occurred in the lower lobes (62). Pleural effusions occurred in 29 of 103 (28%) patients in Choyke's series, but only in about 7% of combined series (58–63). Four to 13% of patients presented with lymphadenopathy, and 3% to 4% demonstrated a normal chest radiograph.

More recently, Krysl et al. (64) prospectively studied all culture-proven cases of TB in British Columbia from 1989 through 1991 (188 cases) to determine patterns of presentation in primary and reactivation TB. Thirty patients (18% of the total) were classified as having primary TB. Similar to Poulsen's findings, lymphadenopathy was observed in 20 (67%) of the 30 patients and was the most common radiographic abnormality in this group. Lymphadenopathy was unilateral and hilar (nine cases) with or without concomitant involvement of the mediastinum. Bilateral hilar and isolated mediastinal lymphadenopathies were rare (one case each). Pulmonary parenchymal involvement was observed in 19 (63%) patients classified as having primary disease, a far greater percentage than that observed by Poulsen. This percentage is reasonable because the basis for enrollment in the Krysl study was an abnormal chest radiograph whereas in the Poulsen study it was tuberculin conversion. The findings consisted of airspace consolidation primarily in the upper lobes. Two patients had radiographic evidence of cavitation. Endo-

bronchial spread was detected in two patients. Similar to the Poulsen study, pleural effusions were present in 33% (10 patients). This was the sole radiographic abnormality in seven patients and occurred most often in the right lung. Isolated lymphadenopathy was not observed.

Case 2: A 25-year-old HIV-negative individual presented to the Bellevue Chest Clinic complaining of cough; sputum, fever, night sweats, and weight loss over 2 months. A previous PPD had been negative. A repeat PPD on admission revealed 15 mm of induration. Physical examination was unremarkable. Posteroanterior (PA) and lateral chest radiographs revealed marked hilar and mediastinal adenopathy (Fig. 25.2A,

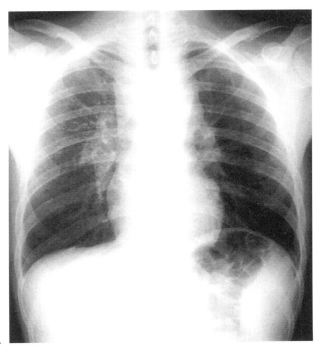

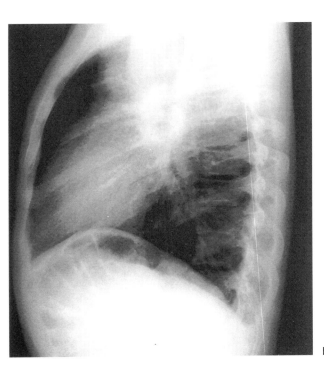

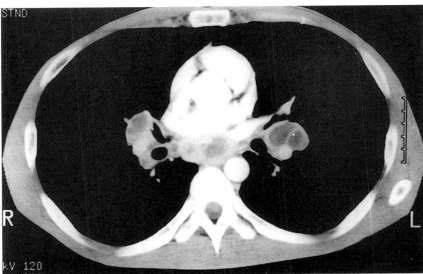

FIGURE 25.2. A, B: Posteroanterior and lateral views reveal marked bilateral hilar and mediastinal adenopathy. **B, C:** Chest computed tomography scan with contrast revealed mediastinal and hilar adenopathy with peripheral ring enhancement and central necrosis.

B) A computed tomography (CT) scan with contrast revealed mediastinal adenopathy with central caseation and peripheral ring enhancement consistent with *Mycobacterium tuberculosis* (Fig. 25.2C). Three sputum smears were AFB negative. The patient underwent fiberoptic bronchoscopy. Bronchoalveolar lavage (BAL) yielded 380×10^3 cells/mL with 89% macrophages, 7% lymphocytes, 3% neutrophils, and 1% eosinophils. Transbronchial needle aspiration resulted in recovery of numerous AFBs on smear.

Intrathoracic lymphadenopathy secondary to TB has been considered an uncommon radiographic finding in adults without HIV, occurring in 0.4% to 13% of all cases of adult pulmonary TB (58–60,62,64–67). Isolated lymphadenopathy is observed more frequently in children with primary TB (68,69). Dhand et al. (70), in a study of 33 adults with lymphadenopathy, found superior mediastinal widening as a result of paratracheal node enlargement to be most common in adults with primary TB. A combination of paratracheal and hilar node enlargement was found in almost 50% of cases. Bilateral hilar adenopathy was found in only 15% of cases, which confirmed its relative infrequency, as noted also by others (71,72).

An unusual phenomenon in primary TB is obstruction of the bronchus, referred to as *epituberculosis* (73). Rarely, enlarging lymph nodes may compress the bronchi, resulting in atelectasis. If the obstruction is not relieved within several weeks, parenchymal destruction and bronchiectasis distal to the obstruction may occur. Epituberculosis may occur despite adequate chemotherapy, especially if therapy is initiated late in the clinical course (see sections "Endobronchial Tuberculosis" and "Complications of Tuberculosis").

LOWER LUNG FIELD TUBERCULOSIS

Case 3: A 45-year-old man with insulin-controlled diabetes mellitus presented complaining of fever, a productive cough, and dyspnea of 4 weeks duration. Physical examination revealed a temperature of 101°F with respirations of 20 per minute. Chest examination revealed egophony at the base. A chest radiograph revealed right lower lobe consolidation (Fig. 25.3) and right hilar prominence. Examination of three expectorated sputa failed to reveal AFB organisms. Fiberoptic bronchoscopy revealed right lower lobe bronchostenosis. AFB smear and culture of the bronchoalveolar washings were positive.

In 1886, Kidd (74) was the first to report lower lung field TB, which is defined as "tuberculous disease found below an imaginary line traced across the hila and including the parahilar regions on a standard posterior-anterior chest roentgenogram" (75). Disease of the lower lobes, middle lobe, and lingula usually arises from bronchogenic spread from an upper lobe cavity. However, isolated disease may be the result of ulceration of a bronchus by a tuberculous lymph node with spillage into the bronchus. Lower lung field TB often masquerades as pneumonia, carcinoma, or bronchiectasis and may be misdiagnosed for a prolonged time. Pathogenic, clinical, and radiologic features differ from that of upper lobe disease. Although some have classified lower lung field TB as a manifestation of primary disease in adults, others have demonstrated its occurrence as reactivated disease (67,76,77). The incidence of lower lung field TB has ranged from 1% to 7%, depending on the

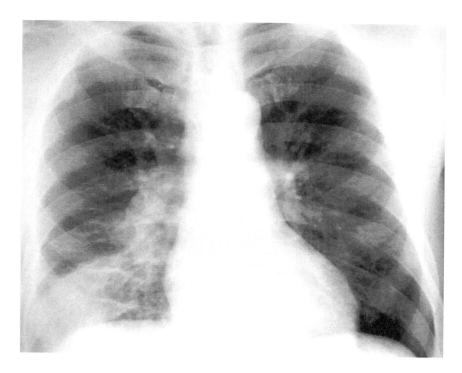

FIGURE 25.3. Diabetic with right lower lobe infiltrate and mild right hilar adenopathy. Smears and cultures of patient's bronchoalveolar lavage fluid were positive for acid-fast bacillus.

patient population studied (75,79). Studies from TB sanatoria report a lower percentage (75,78,79) than those from general hospitals (58,76,77). A recent prospective population-based study found lower lobe TB in 2 (1%) of 158 patients with reactivation TB (64). Older studies have found predominance in females and patients younger than 40 years. Segarra et al. (75) reported these characteristics for 89% of cases, and Berger (76) reported the same for 59% of cases. However, Chang et al. (77) recently reported a series of 85 patients whose mean age was 44 years; 37 were older than 40 years. Lower lung field TB appears to be more common in patients with advanced age, steroid therapy, hepatic or renal disease, diabetes (see "Diabetes Mellitus"), pregnancy, silicosis, and kyphoscoliosis (75–81). Some patients have no underlying conditions (76,77).

The duration of symptoms may be as little as 2 weeks, although the mean is 12 weeks (77). Most series report symptoms for less than 6 months (75–78). Cough with variable amounts of sputum is the most common symptom. Fever, chills, hemoptysis, chest discomfort, dyspnea, and weight loss also occur. Radiographic findings often suggest bacterial or viral pneumonia. Consolidation is more confluent and extensive (homogeneous) than that found in upper lobe TB. Cavities are usually single and may be isolated or lie within an area of consolidation (75,76). Cavities may be large (3 to 4 cm diameter) and tension cavities (thin walled with fluid) may develop (78,82–87).

Tubercle bacilli may be difficult to demonstrate on sputum smear and culture (76,77,84,86,88). Chang et al. (77) reported smear positivity in 57% of patients and an additional 6% with positive cultures. Bronchoscopic examination was highly specific, yielding a positive diagnosis in 32 (76%) of 42 patients. Bronchoscopy was performed in 33 sputum smear–negative patients and in nine patients in whom sputum smears were positive and for whom there was a suspicion of coexistent bronchogenic carcinoma (four patients) or endobronchial lesions (five patients) (77). TB endobronchial involvement was found in 76% of patients who underwent bronchoscopy. Abnormal bronchoscopic findings included ulcerative granuloma in 12 patients, fibrostenosis in nine patients, submucosal infiltration in seven patients, and mucosal swelling and erythema in four patients (see "Endobronchial Tuberculosis").

REACTIVATION TUBERCULOSIS

Multiple terms have been given to this stage of TB: chronic TB postprimary disease, reinfection or recrudescent TB, adult-type progressive TB, endogenous reinfection, and reactivation TB. However, regardless of nomenclature, this form of TB occurs in 90% of adult non-HIV cases. It results from reactivation of a previously dormant organism implanted years before by a primary infection that seeded—usually but not always—to the apical-posterior segments (32,43,45). The original site of spread may leave a small scar radiographically distinguishable as a Simon focus (40).

Clinical Presentation

Case 4: A 56-year-old Chinese woman presented to Bellevue Hospital Center complaining of fever, chills, night sweats, cough, and thick white sputum. This condition had persisted for 1 month. She had immigrated to the United States 3 years earlier. Her chest radiograph revealed bilateral nodular infiltrates with a cavitary density in the right upper lung field (Fig. 25.4A, B). CT scan revealed extensive endobronchial spread with dilatation of bronchi and thick-walled cavity formation (Fig. 25.4C, D). Her sputum smear was positive and grew pansensitive *M. tuberculosis*. Treatment with INH, rifampin, pyrazinamide, and ethambutol cleared her sputum of organisms within 2 months. She continued INH and rifampin for an additional 4 months.

The presence of vague, nonspecific symptoms is common in individuals with TB. Various patterns of presentation are seen, from insidious onset with mild constitutional symptoms of anorexia, weight loss, fatigue, and low-grade temperature to acute onset with fever, night sweats, and productive cough. Often a predominantly "catarrhal" pattern with cough and purulent sputum is seen. Less frequently, patients present with hemoptysis. TB accounts for 7% to 16% of all cases of hemoptysis (89,90). Before chemotherapy was available, TB was one of the leading causes of massive hemoptysis (91) (see "Hemoptysis"). A distinguishing feature of TB is its frequent asymptomatic presentation. Some patients with advanced, bilateral, cavitary, multilobed disease deny all symptoms. When symptoms are acknowledged, however, clinical presentation reveals the destructive and inflammatory process within the lung parenchyma.

Several recent studies have assessed the frequency of symptoms. Barnes et al. (92) prospectively studied 188 patients admitted to a large municipal hospital with culture-proven TB. Cough (78%) and weight loss (74%) occurred most frequently, whereas fatigue (68%), fever (60%), and night sweats (55%) occurred less frequently. Hemoptysis was present in only 37%. Mathur et al. (16) suggested that elderly patients present with fewer symptoms. However, a recent prospective study by Korzeniewska-Kosela et al. (93) of 218 consecutive patients from Canada compared presentations in 142 young adults and 76 elderly patients. The young adults had a mean age of 41 years and the elderly of 75 years. In culture-proven disease, hemoptysis, fever, and cough were slightly more common in young adults (p = 0.03, 0.02, and 0.01, respectively). There was no difference in duration of symptoms (see "Tuberculosis and the Elderly"). Cohen et al. (94) correlated the presence of cough, sputum, and weight loss with smear-positive TB. The absence of these symptoms and the

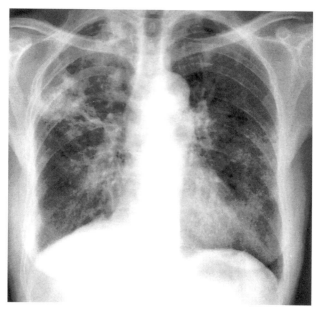

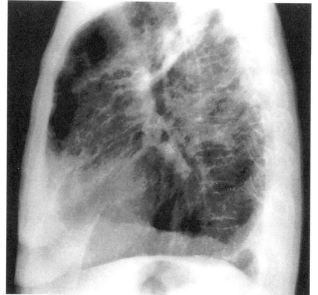

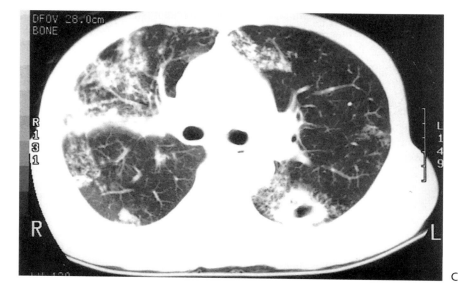

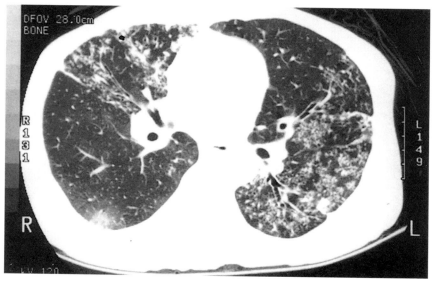

FIGURE 25.4. A: Bilateral fibronodular infiltrates with a right upper lobe cavitary infiltrate. **B:** Lateral chest film reveals the cavitary infiltrate in the posterior segment of the right upper lobe. **C, D:** High-resolution computed tomography scan reveals extensive endobronchial spread with dilatation of the bronchi and thick-walled cavity formation not apparent on the plain films.

lack of a typical chest radiograph were strong negative predictors for pulmonary TB (94).

Finally, chronic symptoms may not always be present. In a large population-based study analyzing symptoms in 254 patients with pulmonary TB (a subset of 526 TB cases diagnosed in Los Angeles County over a 6-month period), Miller et al. (95) found the following symptoms to be present: cough (76%), fever (51%), fatigue (59%), weight loss (43%), sweats (48%), and hemoptysis (24%). Of note, the percentage of patients who had prolonged (2 weeks) symptoms of cough and fever decreased significantly to 48% and 29%, respectively.

Cough is one of the earliest symptoms. Initially, it may be nonproductive. As tissue necrosis occurs, sputum is produced. Cough may be mild and occur only in the morning because secretions accumulate during the night and are expectorated when the person arises. As the disease progresses cough becomes deeper and more continuous throughout the day and at night. Endobronchial TB resulting in ulcerations of the bronchial mucosa is often associated with a harsh, barking cough.

Sputum may be scanty and mucoid initially, but subsequently it becomes yellow or yellow–green. It is rarely foul smelling but often blood streaked. Frank hemoptysis is rarely the initial presenting symptom because it usually results from more extensive disease and causes excavation and ulceration of blood vessels within the cavitary wall. Occasionally, however, hemoptysis is massive because of rupture of a dilated vessel within the cavitary wall, often referred to as a *Rasmussen aneurysm* (see "Hemoptysis") (96,97). In light of the destructive pathologic changes within the lung parenchyma, it is surprising that hemoptysis is not a more frequent occurrence. Vascular thrombosis often precedes destruction of tissue, and causes obliteration of the pulmonary vessels within the areas of necrosis, which prevents gross bleeding. Dyspnea is a late symptom and signifies extensive parenchymal involvement. Alternatively, it may suggest the presence of a complicating process such as a pneumothorax or pleural effusion. Chest pain is unusual but signifies localized pleural inflammation. It is exacerbated by the usual factors associated with pleuritic pain, and may be relieved by changes in body position. Rarely, a dull pain unrelated to respiratory motion is found. Spontaneous pneumothorax may result in severe pleuritic pain and dyspnea.

Although fever usually accompanies TB, as many as 50% of patients may fail to present with this finding initially (98). Often fever does not appear until the disease process is more extensive and largely exudative. Thus, febrile patients are more often symptomatic and have a higher incidence of cavitation and AFB organisms on sputum smears. Febrile patients tend to be younger and have a higher incidence of lymphopenia and hypoalbuminemia (98). The fever has a diurnal variation. It is usually low or normal in the morning and gradually rises during the day, peaking in the late afternoon or evening. At night, the temperature falls and is accompanied by diaphoresis (night sweats). Fever may be intermittent or regular and increase in elevation as the disease progresses.

Hoarseness is unusual in patients presenting with pulmonary TB as opposed to laryngeal TB (see Chapter 30) (99). Hoarseness is usually secondary to bacillary spread to the larynx leading to inflammation of the vocal cords, ventricular folds, or cricoarytenoid joint. Vocal cord paralysis secondary to recurrent nerve palsy is much less common (100,101). In the latter instance, the nerve is compressed on its passage through or adjacent to inflamed tuberculous nodes (102), or is stretched toward the lung apex by retraction of the left upper lobe bronchus due to cicatrization atelectasis (102).

Other constitutional symptoms, such as weight loss and anorexia, are found in advanced disease. When they occur with less advanced pulmonary disease, extrapulmonary TB (e.g., tuberculous enteritis) should be suspected. Alternatively, a concomitant lung carcinoma may be present (see "Relation Between Tuberculosis and Bronchogenic Carcinoma").

Physical examination is often not helpful in establishing or eliminating the diagnosis of TB. A major limitation is the failure to detect mild or even moderate illness, despite apparent radiographic disease. As the disease progresses, posttussive crackles may be heard over areas of tuberculous infiltration. More than 60 years ago, Amberson (103), former chief of the Bellevue Chest Service, related the following:

> In advanced cases these [crackles] may be heard on quiet breathing, but ordinarily only after the cough. In order to secure the proper cooperation of the patient it is of value to illustrate just what is meant, and the physician may go through the procedure, breathing out quietly but fully, giving a short cough at the end of the expiratory effort, and then breathing in quickly. Occasionally it is possible to elicit rales only after a series of three or four sharp successive coughs without intervening inspirations . . . It is just at the end of the expiratory cough or the beginning of the following inspiration that rales are most likely to be heard.

Coarse, bubbling crackles may be heard in the presence of secretions lodged in cavities or larger bronchi. In cases of endobronchial disease, localized wheezing may be heard, even when there is no radiographic evidence of atelectasis or collapse. The wheezing may be accentuated by forced expiration when the patient assumes different positions. As the disease process becomes more advanced, with extensive parenchymal inflammation and the formation of cavities, bronchial breath sounds may be heard over areas of consolidation, and cavernous breathing is occasionally detected.

Extrapulmonary physical findings may be present, especially when TB involves the lymph nodes, liver, spleen, or joints (see Chapters 31, 34, 35, and 38). Other unusual findings include phlyctenular conjunctivitis (Chapter 29), meningeal signs (Chapter 28), changes in pigmentation (due to adrenal insufficiency) (Chapter 39), and clubbing or hypertrophic osteoarthropathy. The latter finding is of interest, because it is not widely recognized that TB may be a cause of clubbing or hypertrophic osteoarthropathy (104,105). Some have doubted its association (106) despite Locke's initial description in 1915 (104). Before the advent of chemotherapy, its reported incidence was 16 to 28% (107). More recently, McFarlane et al. (108) reported that 21% of TB patients admitted to a Nigerian hospital had clubbing. Those with clubbing had more severe disease, including larger cavities and greater mortality.

Radiographic Appearance

Two large studies have documented the apical-posterior predilection of reactivation TB (109,110). Poppius and Thomander (109) reviewed plain films and standard tomograms in 500 patients with cavernous pulmonary disease. Disease was found in the apical and posterior segments of the upper lobe in 84.5% of the patients. Similarly, Adler (110) reviewed radiographic presentations in 423 patients with localized TB; confirmation of localization was often made by comparing the results with those from surgical segmentectomy. Adler found an almost identical percentage to that of Poppius and Thomander: dominant lesions occurred in the apical and posterior segments in 85% of cases. An additional 10% of cases occurred in the superior segments of the lower lobes. Although the remaining segments were not often the site of dominant TB lesions, 3% occurred in the anterior segment of the upper lobes. The anterior segment was involved secondarily in 36% of cases. Recent studies confirm the apical-posterior predominance for reactivation. In a retrospective analysis of 51 patients, Farman et al. (111) found that 44 had involvement of apical, posterior, or both segments, with cavitation or infiltration. A more recent prospective study by Barnes et al. (92) similarly found 137 (90%) of 152 patients with TB had disease localized to these segments.

Reactivation disease that is predominantly in the anterior segment of the upper lobe is rare (110,112). Spencer et al. (113) found nine (6%) of 142 TB patients with this presentation. Disease restricted to the anterior segment was noted in four patients, representing 7% (four of 56) of patients with isolated upper lobe disease, 3% (four of 142) of all patients. Minimal adjacent disease of one other upper lobe segment occurred in the remaining five patients. The incidence of both isolated and predominant anterior segment disease was 16% of patients who had only upper lobe involvement (nine of 56). Five of the nine had reactivation disease, which confirms that anterior disease is not always a manifestation of primary disease. Although the incidence of alcohol abuse, advanced age, concurrent neoplasm, steroid use, and diabetes was higher in these patients, only diabetes was statistically significant (113).

Typical findings of reactivation disease are still found in most adults with TB (see Chapter 26). In the prospective study by Barnes et al. (92), 152 of 188 patients (87%) had "typical" radiographic patterns demonstrating upper lobe infiltrates and or cavitation. More recently, Wilcke et al. (114) found that 92% of 548 patients with pulmonary TB had a "usual" radiographic pattern of reactivation TB. Eight percent had "unusual" patterns, including isolated lower lobe infiltrates (3%), hilar adenopathy (2%), miliary TB (1%), tuberculoma (0.4%), and normal chest radiograph (0.5%).

Cavitation results from liquefaction of the caseous material within the granuloma with dissection into a bronchus (115). When a tuberculous lesion extends into a bronchus, the caseous material softens and flows out, which allows air to take its place and causes a cavity. Dissemination of disease occurs via the bronchi. The rigid, fibrous wall of the original caseous lesion persists as the wall of the cavity. Both the fibrous wall and the elastic tension of the surrounding pulmonary parenchyma are responsible for persistence of the cavity. Occasionally, a "tension cavity" is formed by a valvelike mechanism at the bronchial communication, allowing air to enter but not escape. Tuberculous cavities appear in 19% to 50% of all patients (59,60,64). The wall may be thick or thin, and smooth or nodular internally.

Christensen et al. (116) retrospectively reviewed the radiographic features of 188 patients with TB and compared them with those observed in patients with *Mycobacterium kansasii* and *Mycobacterium intracellulare*. Cavitary disease occurred in 87% of patients, almost exclusively in the posterior portions of the upper lobes. Most patients with *M. tuberculosis* had multiple cavities of varying sizes. Solitary, thin-walled cavities occurred in 4% of *M. tuberculosis* patients compared with 10% of patients with nontuberculous mycobacteria. However, because the incidence of *M. tuberculosis* is far greater than that of *M. kansasii* or *M. intracellulare*, a thin-walled cavity is more likely due to *M. tuberculosis*. Although some investigators have failed to find air-fluid levels in cavities (117), others have observed them in 4% to 20% of patients (59,118,119). Even though the presence of an air-fluid level within a cavity is compatible with TB, superinfection with anaerobic or gram-negative organisms should also be considered. Less common etiologies include intracavitary bleeding, cavitary carcinoma, and infected bullae. A solitary cavity without surrounding reaction should raise the question of possible bronchogenic carcinoma.

Similarly, in a prospective study by Krysl et al. (64) involving 158 patients with reactivation TB, upper lobe infiltrates and cavitation were the most common findings. Pulmonary infiltrates were present in 126 patients (80%), 104 (69%) of which were limited to the upper lobes. The infiltrates were exudative (demonstrating airspace or acinar consolidation) in 87 (55%) and fibroproductive (demonstrating fibronodular areas) in 38 (24%) of the patients.

Cavitation was present in 30 patients (19%); six (41%) had air-fluid levels. Most cavities heal by obliteration, leaving a small scar that can be seen radiographically. Occasionally, there is "open healing" in which the caseous material, epithelioid cell zone, and granulation tissue gradually disappear, leaving the remaining cavity space lined by the scar tissue from the capsule. It has been suggested that open healing is a result of chemotherapy. However, Auerbach (120) demonstrated that this process also occurred before chemotherapy was used.

Endobronchial spread may be observed in 10% to 21% of patients (59–61). Subsequent formation of multiple small, acinar shadows in the lower lobes is highly suggestive of bronchogenic spread. Confluent airspace pneumonia may develop. Bronchogenic spread can occur in the ipsilateral or contralateral lung. Typically, there is a large cavity in the upper lobe with ipsilateral spread to the lower lobe and a small patchy area of focal spread to the superior segment of the contralateral lower lobe (Fig. 25.4).

Other observable radiographic patterns are marked fibrotic responses resulting in lobar atelectasis, hilar retraction, and tracheal deviation (59). Rarely (1% to 10% of the time), patients may have active pulmonary TB with normal chest radiographs (121–123). The presence of calcification in an infiltrate does not signify inactive disease. Furthermore, the activity of disease should never be deduced from the appearance of an isolated plain film.

Recent studies utilizing restriction fragment length polymorphism analysis have suggested that radiographic patterns of primary and reactivation TB may not differ based on recent (within a year) versus remote (more than a year) infection (124). Rather, radiographic patterns such as mediastinal adenopathy (suggesting recent infection) and upper lobe infiltrates (suggesting remote infection) reflect the integrity of an individual's immune response, not the timing of the TB infection (124). Thus, mediastinal adenopathy and pleural effusion are present more often in patients with ineffective immunity (both HIV- and non–HIV-infected patients) (125–127). Furthermore, immunologic status based on CD4 lymphocyte counts have been correlated with high-resolution computed tomography (HRCT) pattern; the lower the CD4 levels, the more atypical patterns have been observed in both HIV- and non–HIV-infected patients (127,128).

Finally, during the past decade CT and HRCT analysis have been used as more precise imaging techniques for evaluating activity (129–132) (see Chapter 26). Moon et al. (130) studied 49 consecutive patients with mediastinal tuberculous lymphadenitis correlating CT findings, biopsy, and culture results. CT findings of nodes with central low attenuation and peripheral rim enhancement suggested active disease, while homogeneous and calcified nodes suggested inactive disease. Low-attenuation areas within the nodes had pathologic correspondence to areas of caseation necrosis and may be a reliable indicator for disease activity.

Various CT findings, such as centrilobular lesions, nodules, branching linear structures 2 to 4 mm in diameter giving a "tree-in-bud" appearance, have been described suggesting activity of disease. Lee et al. (132) prospectively analyzed the utility of HRCT scans in the diagnosis and management of 146 non–HIV-infected patients with confirmed TB. With HRCT, TB was correctly diagnosed in 133 of 146 patients (91%), whereas 32 of 42 patients without TB were correctly excluded. Active (71 of 89; 80%) and inactive (51 of 57; 89%) state of disease could be correctly differentiated by CT. The most common CT patterns of active disease were areas of centrilobular branching linear structures and nodules (see Chapter 26). Similar findings were observed by Im et al. (129). However, these findings are not specific for active TB and can be observed with stable TB. Nonetheless, when CT reveals centrilobular nodules or branching linear structures associated with bronchial dilatation, acinar nodules, lobular or segmental consolidation, and cavitation, the diagnosis of active pulmonary TB is strongly suggested (131).

Case 5: A 55-year-old man, who had smoked two packs of cigarettes per day for 30 years, presented with a routine chest radiograph revealing a right upper lobe nodule. The patient had served in the army during the Vietnam War. Subsequently, he worked in construction for less than a year and had "mild" exposure to asbestos. He denied the presence of symptoms. His physical examination was unremarkable. His PPD was negative but he was not anergic (positive mumps skin test). Chest radiograph revealed a right upper lobe, noncalcified, circumscribed nodule of 2.0 cm (Fig. 25.5). A chest radiograph taken 3 years previously had not revealed the lesion. A chest CT performed with a "phantom technique" to assess density revealed a 2-cm, well marginated, slightly spiculated nodule with no calcification. There were bilateral pleural plaques. Sputum was negative for AFB. Bronchoscopy revealed abundant alveolar macrophages with focal interstitial fibrosis and bronchiolar metaplasia. Cytologic analysis and AFB stains of the BAL fluid were negative. A percutaneous needle aspirate with CT guidance revealed atypical cells with necrotic debris but no granulomas. AFB smear of the aspirate was negative. A thoracotomy was performed. The pathologic specimen revealed multiple caseating granulomas but AFB smear was negative. Culture of the excised lung tissue revealed pansensitive tuberculous organisms.

Isolated nodular masses or tuberculomas are found in less than 10% of patients (64). Tuberculomas range from 0.5 to 4 cm in diameter and are smooth and sharply defined (133–141). A tuberculoma is a tumorlike granuloma caused by the tubercle bacillus; it is encapsulated by connective tissue without evidence of surrounding inflammation. It may arise from a primary infection or reactivation, though the majority of tuberculomas are probably primary infections in which healing has progressed to a localized focus but has stopped at that stage without further resolution. Pathologically, a tuberculoma is a multilayered lesion with continual necrosis around an encapsulated focus.

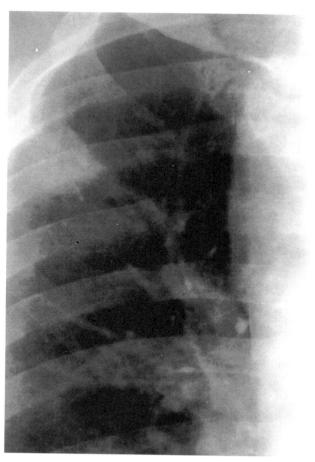

A

FIGURE 25.5. **A:** Posteroanterior chest radiograph reveals a 2-cm nodule. **B:** Chest computed tomography scan reveals a well-marginated, slightly spiculated nodule without calcification.

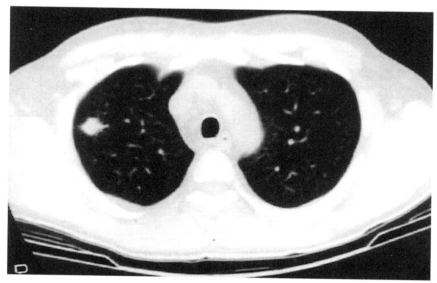

B

Tuberculomas are usually well-circumscribed nodules located in the periphery of the upper lobes. When found in the lower lobes, they are usually located in the superior segment. Hillerdal found cavitation in 49 of 192 tuberculomas (133). Satellite lesions in the vicinity of the tuberculoma suggest its tuberculous origin. Sochocky (136) found that 50% of tuberculomas contained calcification distributed centrally, peripherally, or throughout the entire lesion. Many tuberculomas are incidental findings on the chest radiograph. The patient is in good health and a solitary nodule is found (as in Case 5). The differential diagnosis of a solitary, noncalcified lung nodule includes carcinoma.

Although lymphadenopathy is seldom associated with a tuberculoma, calcified granulomas may occasionally be found either in the hilum or in small satellite lesions. The patient's tuberculin skin test is usually positive. Unfortunately, in some patients there is a negative tuberculin skin test reaction and no calcified granulomas are found. From plain films and conventional tomography, Ishida et al. (137) suspected lung cancer in 21 (58%) of 36 patients who ultimately proved to have benign tuberculomas on surgical resection. Misleading radiographic signs included an ill-defined margin, pleural indentation, and spicular radiation. Chest CT scans did not distinguish benign from malignant disease in nine (41%) of 22 cases; however, densitometry analysis utilizing a reference phantom was not performed (138). Tateishi et al. (140) have shown that contrast-enhanced dynamic CT may help in the noninvasive diagnosis of active versus inactive tuberculomas; peripheral rim enhancement is found most often in active tuberculomas. On pathologic examination this radiographic pattern corresponds to nodal central necrosis with a highly vascular, inflammatory, capsular reaction. Unfortunately, this radiographic pattern is nonspecific and may be seen in lymphoma, carcinoma, and atypical mycobacterial infection. Therefore, culture or pathologic confirmation may be necessary. Nested polymerase chain reaction (PCR) of transthoracic fine-needle aspirate specimens has recently been used as a minimally invasive diagnostic technique in patients with solitary nodules (141). Seven of eight (87.5%) aspirates from proven tuberculous nodules demonstrated positive results on nested PCR, when sputum, bronchial washing, as well as transthoracic needle aspirates were AFB stain negative. Nested PCR appears to have greater sensitivity in specimens with small numbers of *M. tuberculosis* organisms. The rate of recovery of tubercle bacilli organisms from excised tuberculomas varies from 15% to 73% (135,136). Although the majority of these lesions remain stable for a prolonged period, occasionally the capsule in some tuberculomas breaks down leading to active disease (135).

ENDOBRONCHIAL TUBERCULOSIS

Before the advent of chemotherapy, the natural history of endobronchial TB was well described in large clinical and pathologic series (142–147). Endobronchial disease in children is usually a complication of primary TB. Lincoln et al. (147) described a group of 156 children with bronchoscopic evidence of endobronchial TB. Disease occurred more frequently in the right lung. Radiographic evidence of obstruction was observed in 90% of the patients with segmental atelectasis, occurring most frequently in the right middle lobe and the anterior segment of the right upper lobe (147,148). Endobronchial disease in children is caused by encroachment of enlarged nodes on the bronchi. The

nodes become fixed to the bronchial walls as a result of inflammatory changes and the infection progresses through the walls of the bronchi to the mucosal lining, ultimately creating ulceration or granulation tissue. A node may erode through the bronchial wall with extrusion of caseous material (147,149).

In adults, endobronchial disease may occur in primary or reactivation TB. Salkin et al. (143) presented data from 125 consecutive autopsies and 622 consecutive admissions to Hopemont Sanitorium in West Virginia. Every patient underwent an initial rigid bronchoscopy within a few days of admission. Serial bronchoscopies were performed every 3 to 6 months, as well as before operative procedures or when the patient developed new symptoms. The entire group underwent 2,000 bronchoscopies during an average observation period of 32 months. Tuberculous lesions in the tracheobronchial tree were observed in 50 (40%) of the autopsied patients and 97 (15.5%) of the patients undergoing bronchoscopy. Patients with positive sputum and a cavity demonstrated endobronchial lesions more frequently than those without these characteristics. More patients with endobronchial TB had lower lobe disease than upper lobe disease, probably because of pooling of AFB secretions in the lower lobes. Bronchial ulceration progressed to polyp formation and stenosis in these patients within 3 to 6 months. Endobronchial healing correlated with cavity resolution.

Smart (150) suggested five potential mechanisms for endobronchial infection: (a) direct extension from adjacent parenchymal infection (i.e., a cavity), (b) implantation of organisms from infected sputum, (c) hematogenous dissemination, (d) lymph node erosion into a bronchus, and (e) lymphatic drainage from the parenchyma to the peribronchial region.

In a review of 1,000 consecutive autopsies on patients with TB, Auerbach found that 421 (42%) had evidence of tracheobronchial disease (146). Most of the tuberculous ulcers were present in the posterior wall of the tracheobronchial tree. The presence of extensive ulceration was associated with extensive and progressive TB; cavities were always present in the 222 patients with grossly evident ulcers. Auerbach (146), who endorsed the implantation theory of endobronchial disease, stated that endobronchial disease was "the result of infected material passing over the mucous membrane. The pouring out of numerous virulent tubercle bacilli must be considered an important factor . . ." This may be the mechanism for patients with cavitary disease and a large organism load, but endobronchial disease may also develop as a result of lymphatic spread.

Myerson (151) suggested an alternative mechanism of retrograde passage of tubercle bacilli through lymphatics from bronchioles and subsegmental bronchi to the main bronchus. Perforation of tuberculous lymph nodes into the bronchi has been considered uncommon in adults. Before chemotherapy was available, Froste (152) bronchoscopically examined 420 tuberculous patients, of whom 21 were referred because of suspected lymph node perforation (152). Only five (1.2%) had nodal perforation. In contrast, Schwartz (153) found a much higher percentage of perforations—25% of 700 tuberculous patients at autopsy. Arnstein (154) found bronchial perforation in 51 of 135 elderly patients whose lymph nodes demonstrated tuberculous and pneumoconiotic changes. More recently, Chang et al. (67) suggested bronchial perforation as a possible mechanism in some patients.

The clinical and bronchoscopic features of endobronchial TB have also been described during the chemotherapy era of the past 25 years (155–175). The clinical presentation is variable. Endobronchial TB may have an insidious onset, simulating lung carcinoma (159), or may have an acute onset, mimicking asthma (169), foreign body aspiration (170), or pneumonia (156,158,160). It may even appear after completion of therapy (158). Endobronchial TB occurs more commonly in young women (156), but Van den Brande et al. (162) described a significant geriatric population, 11 (15%) of 73 elderly TB patients with endobronchial disease. A barking cough with sputum is found in almost two thirds of patients with endobronchial TB (156,158). The barking cough is not always responsive to antitussive medication, but has been reported to respond to steroids along with antituberculous chemotherapy (156). Sputum production is variable; rarely, bronchorrhea (>500 cm^3/day) has been reported (171). Hemoptysis may occur but is seldom massive (156,161). With lymph node rupture, chest pain may be sharp or dull in the sternal or parasternal region. Dyspnea is often associated with atelectasis. Physical examination may reveal diminished breath sounds, a localized wheeze, or rhonchi (142,160,174). The wheeze is low pitched, constantly present, and heard over the same area on the chest wall (142,160). From 25% to 35% of patients have evidence of collapse on chest radiograph, and 35% to 60% have evidence of consolidation (156,158,162,174). Interestingly, 10% to 20% have normal chest radiographs (156,158). Thus, a clear chest radiograph does not preclude the diagnosis of endobronchial TB (160).

Surprisingly, most recent studies have found a low yield on sputum AFB smears (15% to 20%) (156,158,162,174). In contrast, Chung and Lee (175) found a 53% yield. The explanation given for poor yield on sputum AFB smears is that expectoration of sputum is difficult because of mucus entrapment by proximal bronchial granulation tissue. As a result, bronchoscopic samplings have been key to the diagnosis, producing more than 90% yield on smear as well as culture (156,158,175). The typical bronchoscopic finding is the presence of white, gelatinous granulation tissue. The mucosa is nodular, red, vascular, and sometimes ulcerated; it may simulate bronchogenic carcinoma (156,159,175). Smith et al. (157) confirmed earlier findings regarding the evolution of bronchial ulcers. Hyperplastic inflammatory

polyps developed in areas of previous ulcers and ultimately progressed to fibrostenosis. Bronchostenosis developed despite effective therapy. This complication develops in 60% to 95% of cases and may even involve the main bronchi (156,158,161–168,174,175). Ip et al. (158) performed repeat bronchoscopy in 12 of 20 patients 8 to 49 months after the patients had completed antituberculosis chemotherapy. Eight of 12 patients were asymptomatic, including one with a pinhole stenosis of the left main bronchus. Four patients had severe pinhole stenosis of the trachea or the main bronchus; six patients had mild to moderate narrowing of the main or lobar bronchus. Only one patient had no residual bronchostenosis.

Chung and Lee (175) have recently published a prospective bronchoscopic study of endobronchial TB. During a 6-year period, 114 of 1,938 patients with pulmonary TB proved to have endobronchial TB. The peak incidence occurred in the third decade with an overwhelming female predominance. Sputum smear was positive in 57 of 107 patients (53%), whereas sputum culture was positive in 67 of 91 patients (74%). Endobronchial TB was classified in seven subtypes based upon bronchoscopic findings: actively caseating (43%), edematous-hyperemic (14%), fibrostenosis (10.5%), tumorous (10.5%), granular (11%), nonspecific bronchitic (8%), and ulcerative (3%). Subsequent to diagnosis, 81 patients underwent serial bronchoscopies to analyze subsequent endobronchial changes during treatment. It is noteworthy that antituberculous therapy did not prevent bronchostenosis in 69% of treated patients. Bronchostenosis was related to the extent of disease progression and closely related to formation of granulation tissue.

Chung and Lee (175) relate their classification of endobronchial TB with the extent of disease progression. Pathologically, the initial lesion presents as simple erythema and edema of the mucosa. This is followed by submucosal tubercle formation resulting in erythema and granularity observed at bronchoscopy. Partial bronchial stenosis results from significant mucosal congestion edema. Development of caseous necrosis with TB granuloma formation can be found at the mucosal surface, resulting in active caseating endobronchial TB. When the inflammation erupts through the mucosa, an ulcer is formed that may be covered by caseous material. Finally, the mucosal ulcer evolves into hyperplastic polyps and the endobronchial lesion heals by fibrostenosis (156,157). Tumorous endobronchial TB can also develop by intrathoracic TB lymph nodes eroding into the bronchus (157).

Whether steroid therapy is beneficial in reversing bronchostenosis is unclear. Nemir et al. (176) found that steroid therapy did not reduce the incidence of residual fibrosis in a double-blinded children's study. More recently, Ip (158) concurred with this finding, but Lee et al. (156) claimed benefit with corticosteroids. Chan et al. (177) treated eight patients with endobronchial TB with adjunctive corticosteroids. Only two patients definitely improved. These investigators concluded that the effect of corticosteroids is difficult to predict when the mechanism of airway narrowing includes fibrosis and inflammation. Only the inflammation may respond to steroid therapy. Stenotic lesions may be managed with repeated dilatations (162,174). Aggressive therapeutic modalities, such as stent insertion or laser therapy (178–180), should be considered prior to further development of fibrosis or complete bronchial obstruction.

DIAGNOSIS

Tuberculin Skin Test

The tuberculin skin test is used as an indicator of infection with *M. tuberculosis*; it tests a cell-mediated immune response (see Chapter 55). In most situations, the absence of skin reactivity to tuberculin makes the possibility of TB unlikely. Wier and Schless (181) studied the tuberculin skin test reaction in 530 consecutive tuberculous patients admitted to Fitzsimmons Army Hospital in Denver, Colorado. There were six nonreactors initially, but three reacted positively upon repeat testing. In a World Health Organization study of 3,600 TB patients, less than 4% of patients had reactions to PPD of less than 10 mm to intermediate strength (182). Kent and Schwartz (183) reviewed records at the U.S. Naval Hospital in St. Albans, New York between 1955 and 1964: 12 patients with TB had negative tuberculin skin reactions not only to five tuberculin units (TU) but also to 250 TU. Six patients were asymptomatic but were hospitalized because of an abnormal chest radiograph; six had mild symptoms. In six patients, repeated sputum cultures were negative and the diagnosis was made by open-lung biopsy. Thus, some patients with TB fail to react to tuberculin. Some patients may have generalized anergy secondary to an underlying disease, which affects cellular immunity. However, even when there is no apparent cause of immunosuppression, only 80% to 85% of hospitalized patients with proven TB have a positive reaction to intermediate-strength tuberculin (5 TU) (184).

Rooney et al. (185) tested 100 patients with active TB; 21% failed to react. The nonreactors were identified as patients who were seriously ill with malnutrition that had led to protein depletion with subsequent impaired lymphocyte function. Patients were restudied 2 weeks after institution of a high-protein, high-calorie diet and antituberculous chemotherapy; most became reactive. Similarly, Nash and Douglas (186) found that 49 of 200 patients (25%) with active TB failed to respond to intermediate-strength PPD. Significant factors that determined a negative response included lower serum protein, decreased immunoglobulin G level, and increased age (see "Tuberculosis and the Elderly"). Nonresponders demonstrated a diminished response to *in vitro* transformation of peripheral blood lymphocytes when PPD was added to the culture (186). Ellner et al. (187)

described a population of circulating adherent mononuclear cells (not T lymphocytes) that inhibit transformation of sensitized lymphocytes to PPD but not phytohemagglutinin in patients with a diminished tuberculin response. Other potential mechanisms for false-negative tuberculin response in patients with TB include the presence of serum inhibitors (188), a defect in lymphokine production that prevents the necessary assemblage of leukocytes at the site of the intradermal PPD injection (189), and compartmentalization of sensitized lymphocytes within lymph nodes (190). Compromised immune function in patients with localized pulmonary TB improves with treatment (191,192).

One common cause of lack of response to tuberculin is anergy due to an underlying disease such as sarcoidosis and malignancy, especially lymphoma. Other causes of a negative or diminished response to tuberculin skin testing include acute viral infections, vaccination with live virus, corticosteroids, immunosuppressive drugs, overwhelming infection of any kind, and malnutrition (see Chapter 55).

Microbiologic Examination

> In the future it will not be difficult to decide what is tuberculosis and what is not. . . . The demonstration of tubercle bacilli . . . will settle the question.
>
> *Robert Koch*

Sputum Analysis

A definitive diagnosis of TB requires the recovery of *M. tuberculosis* organisms from a patient's secretions, body fluids, or tissues. Ease of performance and low cost coupled with a reasonable diagnostic yield has made microscopic examination of sputum a key test for pulmonary TB. In the past, controversy developed regarding the predictive value of this test, since a wide range of results regarding AFB smears had been reported. Unfortunately, collection of sputum is often conducted with little supervision. In the hospital, the physician instructs the nurse who, in turn, instructs an aide to collect sputum. In the office or clinic, the patient is given a "sputum cup" and told to return with several samples. In neither setting is there adequate supervision regarding proper technique.

Sputum collection is best accomplished in the morning shortly after a patient awakens. A minimum of three but not more than six specimens should be collected on separate days. A single specimen is not sufficient because bacterial contamination may prevent mycobacterial growth. In a study of 261 patients, Krasnow and Wayne (193) found that only 30% of patients yielded positive sputum on the first collection. They found little advantage in collecting more than five specimens. In fact, the incremental yield between three and five specimens was minimal. Blair et al. (194) related the positivity of AFB smears and cultures with the number of collected specimens in 270 patients. With a single specimen, smears were positive in 47% and cultures in 74%. With three specimens the positive percentage increased to 58% and 90%, respectively. Six daily specimens improved the yield further to 62% and 96%, respectively. There was no significant advantage to more than six specimens.

The need for more than two sputum specimens for diagnostic AFB smear and culture has recently been challenged (195–200). Nelson et al. (195) retrospectively reviewed the smear and culture results for sputum culture–proven cases of TB in 246 patients. Of the patients from whom at least three specimens were collected, only 47% had at least one smear-positive specimen. The third or later specimen was the first smear-positive specimen for 13% and was the first culture-positive specimen for only 7%. Furthermore, of the smear-negative patients only 5% had a third or subsequent specimen submitted that was the first from which AFB was recovered on culture.

Similarly, Van Deun et al. (197) found that a third specimen yielded only a 2.7% increment in positive AFB smears. Furthermore, they found that reading 100 fields per smear was as effective in terms of accuracy as reading 300 fields (i.e., observing 10 AFBs per 100 fields) for making a positive diagnosis by smear. Examination of more than one sputum is necessary to maximize the sensitivity of culture for *M. tuberculosis*. The diagnostic value of the second specimen is significant, increasing the sensitivity of the reading by 30% (195). Despite the low yield from a third sputum specimen, some investigators believe a third reading is still necessary, with public health benefits outweighing demands on laboratory services, even in resource-poor nations (198).

Kestle and Kubica (201) compared 183 pairs of single morning sputum specimens with 24- to 72-hour pooled sputum specimens for the same tuberculous patient. The specimens were mailed for processing and culture. There was no significant difference between the two methods: 64% were positive for single specimens versus 60% for pooled specimens. However, bacterial contamination was observed in 15% of the pooled specimens versus 2% of the single specimens. In contrast, when specimens were processed at the same institution in which they were collected, Krasnow and Wayne (193) recovered significantly more positive cultures from pooled specimens. Earlier mycobacterial growth was observed from single specimens. Although an early-morning specimen collected for overnight processing or a pooled 24-hour collection is preferable, some situations require an immediate specimen. Andrews and Radhakrishna (202) compared the results of cultures from patients presenting to an outpatient chest clinic: two "spot specimens" and two overnight specimens were collected from 348 patients with culture-positive TB. A single spot specimen revealed a positive AFB smear in 66% of patients and a positive culture in 91%. Smear positivity increased to 76% with two spot specimens and to 83% with two overnight specimens. Most of these patients had extensive cavitary disease. When data were analyzed in a subgroup of 48 patients with noncavitary disease, the yield from spot and overnight specimens was much less. In these noncavitary cases, smear positivity was 30% and 46% in spot and overnight specimens, respectively, and culture results were 64% and 80%, respectively.

Various techniques may be used to help patients expectorate sputum spontaneously. One such technique requires the patient to take several deep breaths before expectoration: two breaths are held for several seconds and subsequently exhaled, and the third breath is forcibly exhaled; after the fourth breath, the patient coughs. Warren et al. (203) found that sputum smear sensitivity improved to 92% of specimens, when a minimum of 5.0 mL of sputum was obtained. Approximately 5 to 10 mL of sputum is sufficient. Saliva is not acceptable.

If the patient cannot spontaneously produce sputum, induction by inhalation of aerosolized, warm distilled water, or normal or hypertonic saline may be used. Older as well as more recent studies have documented the high yield from induced sputum (204–211). Microbiologic confirmation of TB ranged from 70% to 90% and compared favorably with results from bronchoscopy (208,209). Indeed, multiple induced sputum specimens increased the cumulative yield for AFB smear and culture from 64% and 70%, respectively, for one specimen to 81% and 91% for two, and 91% and 99% for three induced samples (207). Results may depend on sputum induction technique. Induction with 3 to 5 mL of hypertonic saline will result in an adequate specimen in only 16% of patients. However, the yield increases to 84% following the administration of 30 mL of hypertonic saline with an ultrasonic nebulizer and 95% after 60 to 90 mL is used (209,210). Attractive features for sputum induction are its low cost compared with bronchoscopy, lower risk of occupational exposure to the health care workers compared with bronchoscopy (211), excellent acceptability even in children (212), and safety with minimal if any adverse events occurring. Sputum induction must be conducted in a properly isolated area with adequate ventilation to prevent exposure to personnel (213,214). Sputum produced by induction is watery and resembles saliva; it should be designated as induced sputum to prevent its being discarded by the laboratory (215).

Several techniques are utilized to stain tubercle bacilli (see Chapter 11). The standard method is Neelsen's modification in 1883 of Ziehl's method published in 1882. The Ziehl–Neelsen method requires application of heat for optimal staining; the Kinyoun cold-staining technique does not. Basic fuchsin (magenta) stains AFBs red against a contrasting green, blue, or yellow background. The fluorochrome technique uses the dye auramine alone or in combination with rhodamine and requires a fluorescence microscope. When stained with auramine alone, tubercle bacilli appear white to yellow–green; when the auramine-rhodamine combination is used, AFB appear pink or orange. This technique allows rapid screening for AFB. Fluorochrome-positive specimens should be confirmed by traditional techniques.

The chances of finding tubercle bacilli on a smear increase with their concentration in sputum. Most authorities state that for stains to reliably identify organisms, at least 1×10^4 organisms per milliliter of sputum must be present. This number is based on work by Yeager et al. (216) and Hobby et al. (217). Yeager's group (216) found that the mean sputum bacillary population at the time a smear became negative (after initiation of chemotherapy) on microscopy was 9.5×10^3 organisms per milliliter. Hobby et al. (217) found that the minimal number of organisms per milliliter of sputum detectable was 7.8×10^3. Rouillon et al. (218) stated that at least 5×10^3 bacilli per milliliter of sputum must be present to be identified by microscopy. David estimated that the probability of a positive smear is 50% when there are from 5 to 10×10^3 organisms per milliliter of sputum but falls to a probability of less than 10% at a concentration of 1×10^3 per milliliter (219).

Two studies published in 1975 reported that tubercle bacilli were found on fluorescent smear in less than 25% of specimens from which mycobacteria were cultured (220,221). Furthermore, these studies found that more than 50% of specimens demonstrating AFB on smear proved to be culture negative. These investigators suggested that these findings were supported by application of the Bayes theorem: as the prevalence of a disease in the population decreases, a larger fraction of positive diagnostic test results is falsely positive. Thus, sputum specimens for AFB staining should be submitted only when it is likely that TB is present, thereby increasing the chance to find TB in the population being tested and reducing the false-positive rate.

Subsequent studies have had better positive rates for AFB smears (222–232). Strumpf et al. (228) evaluated the use of the fluorochrome auramine-rhodamine stain. In 81 proven cases, the true-positive rate was 86%. Specificity was greater than 99%, and sensitivity was 66%. Lipsky et al. (229) analyzed smear and culture results of 3,207 clinical specimens submitted for mycobacterial smear and culture. A total of 95 grew *M. tuberculosis*; 65% had positive AFB smears. Furthermore, 96% of patients with TB from whom more than one specimen was processed had at least one positive AFB smear. Gordin and Slutkin (230) examined the validity of AFB smears during two periods: 1975–1978 and 1979–1982. The smear sensitivity ranged from 46% to 55% during the different periods. Of 47 positive smears during the first period, only one was false positive. None of the 96 positive smears during the second period was false positive. The positive predictive values for AFB microscopy were 97.9% and 100% for the two periods. Levy et al. (231) reported the sensitivity and specificity for sputum smears of 53% and 99.8%, respectively, with a positive predictive value of 98.5%. They also studied the significance of "scanty-positive" (four or fewer) AFBs on smear microscopy

from 75 smears obtained from 42 patients with pulmonary TB. Five specimens from four patients were actually false positive. The positive predictive value of scanty-positive smears was 93%. In those patients with positive smears, AFBs were found in the first four specimens. Similarly, four was the optimal number of specimens submitted for culture, with a cumulative positive percentage of 96.3%. As noted previously, recent studies suggest only a minimal (7% to 8%) improvement in yield with three culture specimens and even less with additional specimens (195,207).

Several studies suggest that clinical presentation may affect yield on smear. In a large study of 977 patients with culture-proven TB, Kim et al. (232) found positive smears in 20% to 40% of patients with minimal disease, in 60% to 70% of patients with moderately severe disease, and in 90% to 95% of patients with advanced cavitary disease. Greenbaum et al. (9) found that AFB smears were positive in 43% of the stained specimens from 32 patients with pulmonary TB. Patients with cavitary disease had a greater percentage of positive smears and cultures (57% and 96%, respectively) than those with noncavitary disease (32% and 70%, respectively). *M. tuberculosis* was observed on the first AFB smear in 78% of the patients who had at least one positive AFB smear; it was recovered on culture in the first submitted specimen from 96% of patients. Recently, Barnes et al. (92) found positive smears in 155 (82%) of 188 patients with expectorated sputum. Positive smears were found more often in patients with radiographic findings "typical of reactivation" (90%) than those with "atypical" findings (50%); for cavitary disease, 98% of patients had AFB present on sputum smear compared with 70% of patients with noncavitary disease.

It should not be surprising that negative smears may be found in patients with noncavitary closed lesions because the concentration of tubercle bacilli in sputum is closely related to the character and extent of the underlying pulmonary lesion. Canetti (233) demonstrated that in untreated patients a 2-cm tuberculous nodule contains from 1×10^2 to 1×10^4 organisms, but a cavity of similar size may contain from 10^7 to 10^9 organisms. As noted previously, at least 5×10^3 to 1×10^4 organisms per milliliter of sputum must be present to be observed on microscopic examination of smears. Acid-fast smears are often reported by the microbiology laboratory using a semiquantitative scale (234). A rough estimate of the number of AFB detected per field translates into a semiquantitative report (Table 25.1). The scheme is stain dependent.

Diagnosis of pulmonary TB is ultimately confirmed by positive sputum cultures. The yield for cultures is significantly greater than that of sputum microscopy. As with AFB smears, AFB cultures on solid culture media can be quantified. A widely used scale for semiquantitating growth on agar plates is found in Table 25.2 (234). Note that growth in liquid culture systems cannot be similarly quantitated (see Chapter 11). Levy et al. (231) reported sensitiv-

TABLE 25.1. SEMIQUANTITATIVE SCALE FOR ACID-FAST BACILLUS SMEARS

Fuchsin (10³)	Fluorochrome (×250)	Quantity
No AFB/300 fields	No AFB/30 fields	No AFB seen
1–2 AFB/300 fields	1–2 AFB/30 fields	Doubtful AFB
1–2 AFB/100 fields	1–9 AFB/10 fields	Rare (1+)
1–9 AFB/10 fields	1–9 AFB/field	Few (2+)
1–9 AFB/field	10–90 AFB/field	Moderate (3+)
>9 AFB/field	>90 AFB/field	Numerous (4+)

AFB, acid-fast bacillus.

ity and specificity for sputum cultures of 81.5% and 98.4%, respectively, in a study of 435 specimens from 107 patients with pulmonary TB. Culture yield, like microscopic examination, is also affected by the clinical status of the patients. Greenbaum et al. (9) found that 96% of patients with cavitary disease had positive cultures in contrast to 70% who had focal infiltrates.

True false-positive AFB smears (i.e., positive smears with negative cultures) are uncommon in a well-supervised laboratory and should occur in less than 1% of specimens (229). Adequate quality control of laboratory procedures reduces the incidence of false-positive smears. Numerous technical errors, such as failure to filter reagents properly or transfer of organisms from a specimen that contains AFB to one that does not, have been reported (229,235–237). Narain et al. (238) found that most patients with false-positive smears did not develop TB within 3 years of follow-up. MacGregor et al. (235) studied the significance of isolated low numbers of *M. tuberculosis* in the culture of sputum specimens. Low-colony isolates were defined as comprising less than five colonies. During an 18-month period, 31 patients had 35 low-colony isolates and were easily separated into two groups—those that had TB by clinical criteria and those who appeared to be uninfected. All patients in the "TB unlikely" group were culture negative when reevaluated 2 to 4 months after their first culture. They had no evidence of TB on chest radiograph, despite having received no antituberculosis medication. Epidemiologic evidence suggested cross-contamination of the cultures with those of smear-positive patients.

TABLE 25.2. QUANTITATIVE SCALE FOR ACID-FAST BACILLUS GROWTH ON AGAR PLATES

No. Colonies Observed	Reported Quantity
None	Negative
<50	Actual no.
50–100	1+
100–200	2+
200–500	3+
>500 (confluent)	4+

Recently, a number of investigators utilizing DNA fingerprinting techniques have identified false-positive TB due to cross-contamination (239–244). In two reports the source of cross-contamination appeared to be a laboratory control strain, H37Ra, that is used routinely for routine drug susceptibility testing as well as part of proficiency testing (240,242). As a result of these laboratory errors, the National Tuberculosis Genotyping and Surveillance Network (NTGN) of the Centers for Disease Control and Prevention has established criteria for suspected laboratory cross-contamination of TB (242), which may include at least one of the following: (a) the patient's clinical course is inconsistent with TB; (b) there is a single positive *M. tuberculosis* culture with no AFB seen in any specimen; (c) a culture-positive specimen from a different patient processed or handled on the same day has an identical DNA fingerprint, and no epidemiologic connection exists between patients; (d) a laboratory control strain has an identical fingerprint; (e) time to growth detection is greater than 30 days.

Sputum Smear–Negative, Culture-Positive Tuberculosis

The problem of smear-negative TB is significant in both industrial and underdeveloped countries (245–250). Murray et al. (251) found that in the pre-AIDS era there were 1.22 cases of smear-negative pulmonary and extrapulmonary TB for every case of smear positive pulmonary TB. More recently, a study from western Canada by Long et al. (252) found that for every smear-positive respiratory case there were 2.52 smear-negative respiratory or extrapulmonary cases. The association of AFB-negative smears with lower bacillary numbers and minimal, noncavitary radiographic patterns might imply that smear-negative patients are less infectious. However, a recent DNA fingerprinting study from San Francisco attributed 17% of TB transmission to patients with smear-negative, culture-positive TB (253).

Thus, more rapid, sensitive, and specific diagnostic techniques are necessary to detect smear-negative AFB. The diagnostic approach that has elicited the most excitement in this regard has been the use of nucleic acid amplification (NAA) techniques to identify *M. tuberculosis* organisms (see Chapter 12). Eisenach et al. (254) first demonstrated extremely high sensitivity and specificity (both greater than 90%) utilizing PCR on consecutive sputum samples. However, their results with PCR were no better than those using sputum smears. Schluger et al. (255) demonstrated that PCR might fail to distinguish between active and previous disease.

Currently, there are two NAA assays for commercial use in the United States: MTD (GenProbe, San Diego, CA, U.S.A.) and Amplicor (Roche, Basel, Switzerland). The MTD assay is an isothermal strategy for DNA amplification, and the Amplicor kit utilizes the PCR to amplify specific nucleic acid targets that uniquely identify *M. tuberculosis* in clinical specimens. Despite these different approaches to amplification of target DNA regions of interest, the yields from these tests appear equivalent (256–260). Both tests diagnose nearly every case of sputum smear–positive pulmonary TB and each will diagnose approximately 50% of smear-negative culture-positive pulmonary TB. An "enhanced" NAA test has been approved by the Food and Drug Administration for use on both smear-positive and smear-negative sputa of individuals clinically suspected of having TB. This was based on a multicenter study by Catanzaro et al. (261) in which the suspicion of TB was quantified. When there was an intermediate or high suspicion of TB, the sensitivity of the "enhanced" NAA test was 75% to 88% and the specificity was 100%.

Cohen et al. (262) recently evaluated the efficacy of PCR testing in "front-line" clinical practice. They prospectively studied 85 patients suspected of having TB of whom 27 had culture proven TB. PCR testing of two sputum samples obtained within 24 hours of the patient's arrival at the hospital proved diagnostic in all patients who were smear-positive and 53% to 73% of those who were smear-negative, depending on PCR technique (Amplicor versus an in-house assay, respectively). PCR testing on two specimens allowed detection of 95% to 100% of all patients excluding those with paucibacillary disease; in the latter instance, the detection rate dropped to 74% to 85% for the two PCR assays. Additional studies with large numbers of patients will be required before this PCR assay approach can be adopted in clinical practice (262) (see Chapter 12). Feasibility and costs remain an issue in both wealthy and resource-limited countries (263). An American Thoracic Society workshop has addressed some of these issues (260).

Bronchoscopy

Empirical therapy may be justified in some instances, such as a rapid clinical deterioration, or in some developing countries with limited resources. However, whenever possible, a definitive diagnosis should be pursued. When NAA testing of sputum is not available or is negative and suspicion remains high, the next diagnostic step for a smear-negative patient suspected of having pulmonary TB is fiberoptic bronchoscopy. The diagnostic role of bronchoscopy in patients suspected of having TB has been controversial. Before 1970, multiple studies described the diagnostic utility of rigid bronchoscopy (144,145,152,264–266). With the advent of fiberoptic bronchoscopy, however, studies began to report both its usefulness and its inefficacy (267,268).

Most of the controversy has been resolved, though some persists. The practice of sending all bronchoscopy washings routinely for mycobacterial culture should be discouraged in populations in which the prevalence of TB is low. Kvale et al. (267) found positive AFB cultures in only 2.1% of 859 bronchoscopies, and an exclusively positive rate was observed in only 0.9%. Jett et al. (269) reviewed their experience with mycobacterial culture of bronchoscopic washings in 4,120 patients (60% of total patient bronchoscopies) during a 5-year period. A total of 209 patients had culture-proven TB; 34 of these patients (16%) underwent bronchoscopy. Cultures yielded *M. tuberculosis* in 32 of 34 patients (94%); in 10 patients it provided the only source for the diagnosis. Russell et al. (270) reviewed their 10-year experience with mycobacterial culture of bronchoscopic washings in 1,399 patients (270). Only 25 (1.8%) had positive cultures for *M. tuberculosis*. Bronchoscopic washings had a positive rate of 96% (24 of 25) and were exclusively positive in 10 (40%) of 25 patients. In contrast, Ip et al. (271) reported the results of routine mycobacterial culture of bronchoscopic washings in 1,734 procedures from Hong Kong, an area of high TB prevalence. TB was found in 144 cases (8%). Of these cases, a positive culture of bronchoscopic washings was obtained in 119 cases (83%) and was the exclusive means of diagnosis in 64 (44%).

An important question regarding the role of bronchoscopy concerns the yield in patients with sputum smear–negative TB with respect to immediate diagnosis, definitive diagnosis, and exclusive diagnosis. In addition, which bronchoscopic procedure should be used and whether the yield correlates with chest radiographic findings are other questions to be answered. Danek and Bower (272) reviewed bronchoscopic findings in 41 patients with sputum smear–negative, culture-positive TB. AFB smear of bronchoscopic washings was positive in 14 (34%) of 41 patients. Cultures of bronchoscopic specimens were positive in 39 (95%) of 41 patients and were exclusively positive in 19 (46%) of 41 patients. Postbronchoscopy sputum specimens were culture positive in five patients in whom all other specimens were negative. Brush biopsy was never the sole diagnostic test. Although lung biopsy did not prove to be the exclusive source for diagnosing TB, it revealed bronchogenic carcinoma in four patients.

Most subsequent reports have confirmed the utility of bronchoscopic procedures for diagnosing TB (273–296). An immediate diagnosis can be obtained in 28% to 73% of cases. Only Chan et al. (284) claimed a very low yield of 14%. When data from the 13 largest series were combined, an immediate diagnosis was obtained in 220 (45%) of 494 patients (271–275,278–284,292). A definitive diagnosis of TB was obtained by bronchoscopy in 73% to 93% of cases. When the numbers of patients from all of the previously cited series were totaled, a definitive diagnosis of TB was found in 376 (88%) of 426 patients (271–275,278–284, 292). Bronchoscopic specimens were the exclusive source of diagnosis in up to 44% of cases (271). The diagnosis was made exclusively by transbronchial biopsy in 9% to 37% of cases (273,275,276,281,282,284); by culture of bronchial washings in 12% to 44% (271,272,275); by BAL culture in 9% to 41% (277,280,281,284); and by brush biopsy smears in 20% (283).

A small retrospective study by Stenson et al. (286) found that culture of the transbronchial biopsy was not reliable for diagnosing TB, since it was positive in only two of 12 cases. These investigators obtained their highest yield (75%) by culture of prebronchoscopy sputum. Prebronchoscopy sputum culture proved to be more sensitive than bronchoscopic culture (67% versus 44%), although the latter was occasionally the only positive culture. In a study by de Gracia et al. (277), the yields from BAL cultures, bronchial washings, and postbronchoscopy sputum were compared. This study found BAL positive in 15 (88%) of 17 cases, bronchoscopic washings positive in 9 (53%) of 17 cases, and postbronchoscopy sputum positive in 6 (46%) of 13 cases. Similarly, Baughman et al. (291) found BAL smears and culture positive in 68% and 92% of patients, respectively—a significantly greater yield than for sputum smears and cultures, which were 34% and 51%, respectively. Although Kennedy et al. (281) found a similar yield for BAL cultures, it was not significantly greater than postbronchoscopic sputum cultures (63% from sputum and 66% from BAL). Moreover, they noted a greater yield from prebronchoscopy sputum (93%) and attributed the decreased culture positivity in BAL fluid secondary to growth inhibition by lidocaine (297–299).

Several recent studies have combined BAL with PCR to help diagnose smear-negative TB (293–296). Chen et al. (296) prospectively lavaged 26 smear-positive, 54 smear-negative (TB suspected), and 22 nontuberculous (lung cancer) patients. The sensitivity for smear-positive patients was 96%; the specificity for the non-TB patients was 100%. Of the 54 suspected smear-negative patients, 14 were ultimately diagnosed with TB. The sensitivity and specificity in this group was 36% and 96%, respectively. The combination of BAL smear and PCR was 43%, which was the same as BAL culture alone.

BAL has been used to characterize the inflammatory response in various pulmonary processes. Several investigators have demonstrated an increase in neutrophils and lymphocytes in the BAL fluid of TB patients (300,301). Ozaki et al. (301) demonstrated that BAL fluid obtained simultaneously from TB-affected and nonaffected regions of the lungs yields a normal distribution of cells in the nonaffected regions.

The latest addition to the bronchoscopic procedure includes transbronchial needle aspiration (TBNA), which has been used to diagnose tuberculous mediastinal lymphadenopathy in both HIV and non-HIV patients (302,303). Harkin et al. (303) performed TBNA utilizing a large-caliber (19-gauge) needle to obtain histologic samples from mediastinal and hilar nodes. TBNA provided the diagnosis in 20 (87%) of 23 patients with mycobacterial disease (*M. tuberculosis*, 11; *M. avium-intracellulare*, 7; combined *M. tuberculosis* and *M. avium-intracellulare*, 1; and *M. fortuitum*, 1). In these patients, positive TBNA specimens included smears of aspirated material for AFB in 11 (63%),

mycobacterial culture in 14 (61%), and histology in 15 (65%). An immediate diagnosis was made in 17 (74%) of 23 patients. TBNA provided the only diagnostic specimen in 11 patients (48%): five (33%) of 15 patients with *M. tuberculosis* and six (75%) of eight with nontuberculous mycobacteria.

Wilcox et al. (304) reported the results of fiberoptic bronchoscopy in 41 patients with sputum-negative miliary TB. A definitive diagnosis was obtained in 34 patients. Bronchial brushings yielded *M. tuberculosis* in 24 of 42 bronchoscopies (57%), 13 from direct smear and 11 from culture only. Transbronchial biopsies were diagnostic in 30 (73%) of 41 procedures, 38 from histology, one from direct smear, and one from culture only. A rapid diagnosis was established in 27 of 34 patients by histologic examination only (14 patients), by direct smear of brushings and transbronchial biopsy specimen (five patients), or by both smear of brushings and transbronchial biopsy specimen (eight patients). Similar results were obtained by Pant et al. (305). The diagnosis of miliary TB is discussed in detail in Chapter 27.

Complications related to fiberoptic bronchoscopy are few but include bleeding and pneumothorax. The incidence of fever ranges from 1.2% to 17% (306,307). BAL does not appear to increase the incidence of fever. Rimmer et al. (308) reported two cases in which fever developed rapidly after bronchoscopy and persisted for several weeks. In addition, there was extension of the tuberculous infiltrates due to spillage of infected bronchial secretions, insertion of the bronchoscope into a previously unaffected area, or both. Transmission of AFB from one patient to another by a bronchoscope has also been reported (309,310), as has contamination of bronchoscopies by mycobacteria (311,312). Proper disinfection of the bronchoscopes is necessary to prevent such transmission (313,314). Shim et al. (315) recently demonstrated that adequately washed bronchoscopes do not induce false-positive PCR results on bronchial aspirates.

Alternative approaches for diagnosing TB in the highly suspected smear-negative patient may be pursued, especially in children as well as adults who may be at risk to undergo bronchoscopy. In the past, gastric aspirates were a useful diagnostic technique because bronchial secretions are constantly being swallowed (215,316–324). Gastric AFB smear positivity is dependent on a high bacillary burden within the lungs. Although gastric fluid has a lower diagnostic yield than induced sputum or bronchoscopic washings, it may be used in selected patients, especially children (322–324). The procedure is best performed in-hospital utilizing a standard technique (322). Approximately 50 mL of gastric fluid should be aspirated in the morning after an 8-hour sleep, as soon as the patient awakens and is still fasting. Two gastric aspirate specimens are usually adequate (321,322). Aspirates should be processed within 4 hours because mycobacteria die in gastric washings (215). When delay is necessary, neutralization of the gastric acid should be performed by the addition of buffer tablets. The yield from gastric aspirate cultures varies from 18% to 71% (316,318). Gastric smears are extremely unreliable; sensitivity is only 59% and the false-positive rate is 33% (318).

Alternative Diagnostic Techniques

Other approaches utilizing transtracheal aspiration and transthoracic fine-needle aspiration (TFNA) have also been advocated (325–334). Transtracheal aspiration was popular in the 1970s but is rarely used today. Thadepalli et al. (325) used this technique to diagnose TB in 31 of 35 patients with sputum smears negative for AFB. Several studies have described the yield of TFNA in the detection of TB (327–333). The smear has certain distinct cytomorphologic features suggestive of granulomatous disease (330). In addition, it can be stained for AFB. Qadri et al. (329) found positive smears in 23% and positive cultures in 53% of their patients. Gomes et al. (328) utilized TFNA in 25 patients with smear-negative TB. A positive diagnosis was obtained in eight patients (smear positive, culture positive, or both), and a suggestive diagnosis of TB, on the basis of granulomatous inflammatory changes, was obtained in 10 (40%). The yield from TFNA varied with the extent of the radiographic abnormality: its reliability was greater when lesions were smaller than 4 cm. Yew et al. (331,332) diagnosed TB in 67 patients by percutaneous TFNA. Two thirds of the patients had solitary nodules with or without surrounding parenchymal infiltrates, and one third had consolidation with or without collapse or loculated hydro- or pyothorax. A total of 45 (67%) of 67 patients demonstrated histologic features diagnostic of TB (granulomas with or without caseation plus stainable AFB); 14 (21%) of 67 demonstrated granulomatous inflammation without stainable AFB (331). Matched with sputum culture and bronchial aspirate culture, TNFA was the exclusive method of diagnosis in 28 (42%) patients. Pneumothoraces were observed in 10 (15%) of patients; only one patient required chest tube drainage. Most recently, Kang et al. (333) utilized PCR to enhance the diagnostic yield for TB from percutaneous TFNA. PCR detected TB in 11 of 17 patients (65% sensitivity), compared with only four positive sputum (24% sensitivity). Finally, Khan et al. (334) reported 12 patients with mediastinal lymph node TB in whom CT-guided fine needle aspiration was performed; a positive diagnosis was obtained in eight (66%) patients. Only one patient developed an insignificant pneumothorax following aspiration.

PULMONARY FUNCTION

Before chemotherapy was available, pulmonary function was frequently assessed in patients with pulmonary TB. In 1846, Hutchinson (335) studied vital capacity in 31 patients and 31 control subjects. He found reduced vital capacity in patients with TB and suggested that the degree of reduction was indicative of the extent of the disease and that subsequent change indicated progression or improvement. Today we know that there is no characteristic pulmonary function pattern in patients with pulmonary TB. Indeed, in most patients with minimal or even moderate radiographic abnormalities, there is seldom any permanent physiologic abnormality after completion of therapy for TB—especially if it is administered early.

Abnormalities generally parallel the extent of parenchymal disease (336–338). In widespread fibrotic disease, there is a restrictive pattern with a decrease in lung volume and diffusing capacity (338,339). Several investigators have found that TB may result in airflow limitation (340,341). Skoogh (342,343) utilized plethysmographic measurements measuring airway conductance to demonstrate the existence of airflow limitation in pulmonary TB and demonstrated only a weak response to inhaled β-adrenergic agents. Airflow limitation may be caused by extensive fibrotic disease or endobronchial TB (338,340,341). However, frequently it is secondary to coexisting chronic obstructive pulmonary disease in TB patients who are cigarette smokers (339). Gas exchange abnormalities are uncommon unless there is extensive pulmonary parenchymal disease. The destructive process uniformly affects alveoli and pulmonary vasculature resulting in matched reduction of ventilation and perfusion. Mild hypoxemia with an increased alveolar–arterial O_2 gradient may be present. However, hypercapnia is unusual unless there is extensive parenchymal damage resulting in increased deadspace ventilation.

LABORATORY ABNORMALITIES

Hematologic abnormalities have been associated with pulmonary TB for almost 100 years (344,345). Some studies found anemia in only 16% to 22% of patients (345–348), whereas others have found 60% to 76% of patients to be anemic (349–351). Case selection may account for these discrepancies. However, many patients with pulmonary TB have minimal or no anemia. The sedimentation rate is elevated in more than 75% of patients with moderate to very advanced pulmonary TB (345).

Although nonanemic pulmonary TB patients have elevated sedimentation rates and C-reactive protein levels, the levels in anemic patients are significantly higher (350). The serum iron and total iron binding capacity are lower in anemic patients than in nonanemic patients with pulmonary TB, and the marrow nonheme iron is greater (350). These observations suggest that most patients with pulmonary TB have anemia caused by decreased marrow iron store release and suppression of erythropoiesis by inflammatory mediators.

Macrocytic anemia is rarely associated with pulmonary TB. Anemia attributable to folate or vitamin B_{12} deficiency is infrequently identified, although decreases in serum folic acid levels are documented in as much as 30% of patients with pulmonary TB (345,346,349,351,352). Patients with more advanced disease have a greater incidence of leukocytosis than those with minimal pulmonary TB (345). A relative or absolute neutrophilia may be documented in 29% to 57% of patients (345,346,349).

Mild leukopenia is rarely found in patients with pulmonary TB. About 1.5% to 4% of patients may have a white blood cell count of 4,000 or less (345,346,349,351). Reversible mild thrombocytosis occurs in about 52% of patients with severe pulmonary TB (349,353).

Absolute or relative decreases in peripheral lymphocyte counts have been documented in patients with pulmonary TB (345,354,355). Seventeen to 40% of patients may demonstrate absolute lymphocyte counts of 1,500 or less. Peripheral lymphocyte percentages of 20% or less are found in 21%, 32%, and 47% of patients with minimal, moderate, and far-advanced disease, respectively (345). Decreases in $CD4^+$ counts have also been described (356,357).

A mild absolute or relative monocytosis is found in 29% to 60% of patients (345,349,358). Thrombocytopenia and pancytopenia rarely occur in patients with pulmonary TB (349). The identification of thrombocytopenia or pancytopenia in association with pulmonary TB suggests possible drug toxicity or another underlying process (343,359).

COMPLICATIONS OF TUBERCULOSIS

Pneumothorax

Before the advent of chemotherapy, spontaneous pneumothorax complicating cavitary TB was an important and dangerous complication of pulmonary TB. In 1932, a report by Berry (360) from the Bellevue Chest Service found 55% mortality in 75 patients who developed this complication. Subsequently, in 1941, the mortality rate had fallen to 30% (361). By 1956, Reemtsama et al. (362) reported that there had been no deaths in 20 such patients seen by the Bellevue Chest Service from 1950 to 1954. Since chemotherapy has been used, pneumothorax associated with TB has occurred in only 0.6% to 1.0% of hospitalized TB patients (363,364). Pneumothorax may also occur in patients with miliary TB (365,366). Most recently, Yagi et al. (367) reported on 46 cases of pneumothorax diagnosed in 3,611 patients with TB during a 10-year period (1987 to 1997). Cavitary TB was observed in 41 of 46 patients. Pneumothorax was present on admission in 50% and developed during therapy in the remaining 50%. Twenty-four patients underwent tube drainage, while 7 required surgical intervention. A total of 15 patients died, 13 secondary to respiratory failure.

Auerbach and Lipstein (368) described the pathogenesis of TB-associated pneumothorax. They reviewed 1,000 consecutive autopsies of chronic TB patients and found bronchopleural fistulas in 78 cases (7.8%). Only 19 occurred in

cases of TB in which artificial collapse of the lungs had never been attempted.

Two types of perforation occur in TB-associated pneumothorax—frank rupture of a peripheral cavity into the pleural space or rupture into the pleural space of a subpleural caseous focus that underwent liquefaction with subsequent extension involving the pleura (368). In both instances, a pneumothorax results. An inflammatory response begins at the site of the initial rupture. The bronchopleural fistula may persist or seal off. Occasionally, the seal is permanent and the lung reexpands. More often, intercostal tube drainage is needed, which is usually successful (369,370).

The most important factor affecting the outcome of tube thoracostomy is the size of the bronchopleural fistula, which is influenced by the extent of the underlying parenchymal process of TB. Patients with extensive disease and those whose symptoms are poorly controlled by chemotherapy have large fistulas. A peel develops over the lung that prevents reexpansion despite intercostal tube drainage. In addition, some patients with large bronchopleural fistulas develop a mixed empyema, which complicates the reexpansion process. Ihm et al. (364) noted that in 17 of 28 patients with successful chest tube therapy, the interval between the development of a pneumothorax and chest tube insertion was 24 hours or less. In only two patients was chest tube insertion a failure. However, a long interval did not preclude successful reexpansion; this occurred in six of 28 patients when the chest tube was inserted at intervals of 16 to 75 days. In some patients the airleak may not close until after 6 weeks of chest tube drainage and antituberculous chemotherapy.

A bronchopleural fistula may be seen in patients with "old, healed" TB (369,371), especially in those with old pleural disease who were treated for pneumothorax before chemotherapy was introduced. Diagnosis of a bronchopleural fistula should be considered in patients who have increasing sputum production, air in the pleural space, and a changing air-fluid level. Chest tube drainage along with chemotherapy should be instituted. Subsequently, definitive surgical treatment to fill the pleural space should be undertaken. Some investigators have suggested an association between previous pulmonary TB and subsequent "spontaneous" pneumothorax (372). However, there is little evidence to support this contention.

Hemoptysis

> . . . The spitting of pus follows the spitting of blood . . . Consumption follows the spitting of blood . . . Consumption follows the spitting of this and death follows Consumption.
>
> *Hippocrates*

Tuberculosis is responsible for 7% to 16% of all cases of hemoptysis in the United States (89,90); historically, the percentages have ranged from 13% to 40% (91,373–376). Elsewhere, TB accounts for hemoptysis in 1% to 16% of all cases (377,378). Hemoptysis may occur during active TB or after chemotherapy for TB. During acute TB, bleeding is usually streaky. Most patients are smear positive and have cavitary disease. However, the absence of cavities does not preclude the diagnosis of TB. Furthermore, the presence of a cavity does not assure that it is the source of the bleeding. Until the advent of chemotherapy, 4% to 7% of deaths that occurred in TB sanatoria were caused by massive hemoptysis (96,97).

In 1841, Fern (379) described the rupture of an aneurysm within a tuberculous cavity in a patient who died of multiple recurrent pulmonary hemorrhages. Subsequently, Rasmussen (380, 381) described in detail his experience with cases of massive hemoptysis associated with TB: in each of his patients a pulmonary vessel passed tangentially to the wall of a tuberculous cavity with an aneurysmic dilatation of this vessel into the cavity. The aneurysm ruptured, causing massive hemoptysis. Autopsy studies by Auerbach (96) as well as Plessinger and Jolly (97) confirmed these observations when they found hemoptysis in patients with chronic TB. Extension of TB into the adventitia and media of the vessel wall causes herniation into the lumen of the cavity and the formation of an aneurysm. Continued inflammation of the wall from TB causes rupture of the aneurysm into the cavity, resulting in massive hemoptysis. Cudkowicz (382) confirmed that enlarged bronchial arteries are present in tuberculous lungs and the walls of tuberculous cavities have only a bronchial arterial blood supply. Dilatation of bronchial arterioles was observed near miliary tubercles. Despite the previously supportive data regarding the etiology of massive hemoptysis in TB patients, Thompson et al. (383) questioned the importance of Rasmussen aneurysms. In a retrospective review of 80 autopsied patients with massive hemoptysis, only six had Rasmussen aneurysms. No specific vessel could be identified in 61 patients. Of the remaining 19 cases, the bleeding source was either the pulmonary artery with no aneurysm (eight patients) or the bronchial artery (five patients). Thompson argued that a branch of the pulmonary artery was the most likely source of bleeding at any point in the lung, distal to the secondary bronchi. Most cases of hemoptysis were due to an erosion of a branch of the pulmonary artery without a significant aneurysmal dilatation.

Hemoptysis may also be found in the patient who has completed chemotherapy for TB. In this situation, hemoptysis may be due to residual bronchiectasis, an aspergilloma invading an open healed cavity, a scar carcinoma, a ruptured broncholith or cavernolith, or recurrence of TB. Many patients complete therapy and have only minimal residual fibrotic scarring. However, some patients with extensive disease have significant destruction of the lung, resulting in bronchiectasis (see below). The parenchyma is hypervascularized with a dilated and tortuous bronchial cir-culation. Anastomoses develop between the bronchial and pulmonary circulation (384). Superinfection in these areas of bronchiectasis may result in inflammation and rupture of the vessels, which leads to hemoptysis (385).

Other patients are left with open, healed cavities that become colonized by saprophytic fungi such as *Aspergillus*, resulting in mycetomas. The wall of an aspergilloma cavity is fibrous with highly vascularized granulation tissue. The blood vessels lining the cavity are of bronchial origin. A prospective study by the British Thoracic and Tuberculosis Association demonstrated that of 544 patients with residual tuberculous cavities after chemotherapy, 34% had *Aspergillus* precipitins and 17% developed aspergillomas (386). Characteristically, the fungus ball only partially fills the cavity giving an air-crescent sign on chest radiography. Massive hemoptysis occurs in 5% to 25% of patients (387–391).

Healed, calcified mediastinal or hilar lymph nodes may impinge on bronchi and, occasionally, erode through bronchial arteries into the bronchial lumen (392–396). Such broncholiths may be extruded and expectorated (lithoptysis). Hemoptysis occurs in more than 50% of such cases (392–394). Rarely, massive hemoptysis occurs as a result of erosion through bronchial arteries. This leads to high-pressure hemorrhage that may necessitate surgical intervention to stop the bleeding. Chest CT is effective in detecting broncholiths (397), which may then be visualized directly by bronchoscopy.

Middleton et al. (398) stressed that patients hospitalized with TB-related hemoptysis of any amount, with or without an obvious cavity, should undergo a rapid diagnostic workup to define the site of bleeding and allow rapid surgical intervention if needed. This group described five patients with noncavitary TB with hemoptysis on admission. In each case hemoptysis subsided and then suddenly recurred, causing death by asphyxiation. Yeoh et al. (399) reviewed experience with massive hemoptysis at the Bellevue Chest Service from 1959 through 1966. Forty-three patients were managed conservatively; of these, 10 died from asphyxiation. Surgical resection was performed on 13 patients; two of these patients died. Thus, mortality waas 23% in the nonsurgical patients but only 15% in the surgically treated patients.

In most instances sedation, bed rest, and antituberculous medications control bleeding (400,401). However, if bleeding becomes massive (>600 mL/24 hours) or severe (>200 mL/24 hours) and repetitive, resection of the site of bleeding is indicated (402–404). Alternatively, bronchial artery embolization may be used as a temporizing measure to prepare the patient for surgery or utilized in the patient who is not an operative candidate (see Chapter 43) (405–409). Muthuswamy et al. (405) emphasized that bleeding occurred not only from bronchial or pulmonary arterial systems or both, but also from intercostal arteries and other vessels supplying the lung. Indeed, patients who undergo bronchial arterial embolization only may continue to bleed from pulmonary arterial sources. Uflaker et al. (406) reported a series of 75 patients who underwent bronchial artery embolization; 68 patients had a tuberculous etiology of their life-threatening hemoptysis. Immediate control of bleeding occurred in 83%. By combining bronchial arterial embolization, antituberculosis chemotherapy, and surgical management, long-term control of bleeding was achieved in 95% of their patients. More recently, Ramakantan et al. (408) documented almost complete control of massive hemoptysis in 102 of 140 patients utilizing bronchial artery embolization. Similarly, Wong et al. (409) were able to control life-threatening hemoptysis in posttuberculous bronchiectasis with or without associated mycetomas.

Residual Parenchymal Damage

Bronchiectasis

Bronchiectasis may develop after primary or reactivation TB (410–414). After primary TB, extrinsic compression of a bronchus from enlarged tuberculous nodes may lead to bronchial distention distal to the obstruction and is often associated with secondary infection (411). There may be no evidence of parenchymal TB (413). In reactivation TB, bronchiectasis develops by destruction and fibrosis of lung parenchyma, resulting in retraction and irreversible bronchial dilatation (413,414). Alternatively, localized tuberculous endobronchial infection results in cicatricial bronchostenosis, which leads to postobstructive pneumonia and distal bronchiectasis (412,414). Since reactivation usually occurs in the apical and posterior segments of the upper lobe, bronchiectasis is usually found in these areas. Because of adequate bronchial drainage in these sites, bronchiectasis may produce minimal symptoms (*dry bronchiectasis*). Bronchiectasis may present as a late manifestation of previous TB (415,416). As noted earlier, bronchiectasis is a significant cause of hemoptysis (90). Radiographic documentation of bronchiectasis is obtained by high-resolution chest CT scans (90, 415–418). Bronchography is rarely indicated.

Right Middle Lobe Syndrome

Brock demonstrated that the right middle lobe bronchus is more densely surrounded by lymph nodes than other bronchi (412). This bronchus is particularly vulnerable to nodal compression with subsequent lobar atelectasis (419, 420). In addition, the right middle lobe bronchus has a relatively long length with a small internal caliber and a sharp angle where it branches. Both of these characteristics contribute to the collapsibility of the right middle lobe. Ineffective collateral ventilation has been suggested as a major factor in the pathophysiology of the right middle lobe syndrome (421).

Destroyed Lung

Rarely, TB causes massive destruction in one or both lungs. Palmer notes that this process may occur after either primary or reactivation TB (422). After primary TB, destruction is usually unilateral and involves the upper lobes. It is a result of bronchial obstruction by tuberculous lymph nodes with subsequent distal necrosis, atelectasis, and secondary pyogenic infection. Ultimately, a fibrotic, contracted lobe or lung is left. Frequently, there is an overlying residual pleural effusion or pleural thickening confined to the upper lobe.

When destruction occurs in reactivation TB, evidence of TB in the contralateral upper lobe is usually present (422). There may be striking mediastinal shift to the fibrotic lung. Marked hilar elevation can also occur with compensatory lower lobe emphysema. Ultimately, bronchiectasis and marked fibrosis coexist. Although active TB may be present, it is often difficult to ascertain because sputa may be negative. More often, the TB is quiescent but active superinfection by pyogenic organisms or fungi such as *Aspergillus* occurs. A diagnostic dilemma is to rule out associated malignancy.

Bobrowitz (423) reported 18 patients with "destroyed lung"; of these, eight died. These patients developed excavation of an entire lung or of all the lobes on one side of a lung. The duration from the diagnosis of TB to the first evidence of destroyed lung was 7 to 10 years; in one third of the patients the time was slightly less than 3 years. The interval was influenced by the patients' lack of adequate or continuously effective therapy. Of the eight patients who died, three had fulminant, fatal hemoptysis and two had active TB disease. Three patients died of nontuberculous bacterial lung infections. Hemoptysis occurred in seven other patients. Most patients demonstrated hyperinflation of the lung with overdistention of the contralateral lung. Radiographically, there was a huge cavitary complex with a few strands of tissue extending across it. There was retraction of the lung with the presence of an air-fluid level at the base of the destroyed lung. Lung scans revealed absence of perfusion in the destroyed lung.

A more acute destructive process results from pulmonary gangrene due to TB. Kahn et al. (424) reported four such patients—three of whom died. The radiographic features of pulmonary gangrene show one or more lobes with an initially homogeneous infiltrate that progresses to dense consolidation. Air-filled cysts appear in the area of previous consolidation. Coalescence of these radiolucent areas leads to formation of a thick-walled cavity. The necrotic tissue may remain attached to the wall. Alternatively, there may be a freely mobile, intracavitary mass that looks like an intracavitary clot, fungus ball, or Rasmussen aneurysm. However, the rapidity of onset distinguishes gangrene from these other processes. CT scan may be diagnostic (425). Widespread vascular thrombosis and arteritis of the infected lung causes obliteration of the vascular supply to that particular part of the lung with ensuing necrosis. The gangrenous part of the lung detaches from the surrounding pulmonary parenchyma and drops into the cavity as a freely floating mass. Resolution may occur with prompt institution of antituberculous therapy (426) but occurs less often (425).

Occasionally, pneumonectomy can provide symptomatic relief and physiologic improvement in the appropriately selected patient with parenchymal destruction. Such was the case in a patient reported by Simons et al. (427). Forty years before, the patient had undergone repeated pneumothoraces and a phrenic crush resulting in a unilateral fibrothorax and paralyzed hemidiaphragm for cavitary TB. She developed the onset of respiratory insufficiency with hypoxemia, hypercapnia, pulmonary hypertension, and cor pulmonale. After pneumonectomy, the resultant gas exchange normalized and pulmonary vascular resistance decreased by 25%. Park et al. (428) reported that patients with destroyed lung might progress to respiratory failure.

Respiratory Failure

Although not widely recognized, TB may be a primary cause of acute respiratory failure (ARF) (429). Acute respiratory failure may also occur in patients with destroyed lung (see above) and concomitant lung diseases (such as chronic obstructive pulmonary disease and asthma) or bacterial superinfection (428). Finally, ventilatory failure may develop after an interval of many years in patients with severe thoracic kyphosis due to childhood tuberculous osteomyelitis of the thoracic spine (430).

Tuberculous pneumonia as well as miliary TB may result in ARF and progress to the adult respiratory distress syndrome (ARDS), requiring mechanical ventilation (429,431, 432). During a 10-year period, Penner et al. (429) found that 19% (seven of 37) of patients with miliary TB presented with ARF requiring mechanical ventilation, in contrast to 0.8% (six of 722) of patients with tuberculous pneumonia. Choi et al. (433) found retrospectively that 1.7% (17 of 1,010) of patients with newly diagnosed pulmonary TB presented with ARF.

Prior to 1995, fewer than 75 cases of TB-related ARF had been reported (430–457). In 1969, Goldfine et al. (434) reported a patient with miliary TB who developed ARDS requiring mechanical ventilation. Subsequently, Agarwal et al. (435) reported 16 patients with respiratory failure (defined as PaO$_2$ < 50 mm Hg on room air), 10 of whom required mechanical ventilation. More recently, several studies have reviewed the clinical and radiographic presentation of patients with respiratory failure and TB (429,433,457). Delays in diagnosis and initiation of therapy have contributed to significant mortality, ranging from 47% to 69% (457). Heffner et al. (436) found that TB was not considered as a diagnostic possibility on admission in patients with hypoxic respiratory failure (defined as arterial

PO$_2$/alveolar PO$_2$ < 0.5). The prolonged time from admission to consideration of TB was (mean) 4.7 ± 1.0 days, whereas the time to diagnosis was 7.2 ± 1.7 days. This was significantly greater than that in patients with TB without ARF. Furthermore, delay in diagnosis (symptoms present >1 month prior to admission to the intensive care unit) was a poor prognostic indicator. Even when TB is suspected in this setting, establishing a definitive diagnosis can be difficult and often cannot be accomplished prior to autopsy (6,458).

The presence of risk factors such as alcoholism, diabetes, immunosuppression, malignancy, and HIV infection may distinguish TB from other causes of ARDS. In contrast to non–TB-related ARDS, most (almost 90%) of TB patients had symptoms for more than a week before admission (431,457). These symptoms were often nonrespiratory, including constitutional symptoms such as weight loss, lethargy, and generalized malaise. A protracted prodrome may be the most reliable distinguishing historical feature in patients with TB-related ARF (431). Physical examination is nondiagnostic with fever, tachypnea, and tachycardia often present. Laboratory findings are variable and nonspecific. Hypoalbuminemia is often dismissed, but suggests chronicity of symptoms and when present is a poor prognostic indicator (457). Anemia is often present while most patients have a normal white blood cell count with a left shift. Disseminated intravascular coagulation (DIC) has been observed in almost half of the reported cases. Its incidence in TB-related ARDS is higher than in ARDS of other etiologies (452). DIC occurs more often in miliary TB–associated respiratory failure than in ARF secondary to tuberculous pneumonia (429). DIC may contribute to the pathophysiology of respiratory failure by causing embolization of fibrin and platelet aggregates in the lungs. Thrombotic thrombocytopenic purpura has rarely been reported in association with TB and respiratory failure (459,460).

Hypotension and, in particular, septic shock progressing to respiratory failure is unusual in TB. In the early 1950s, "sepsis tuberculosis gravissima" was defined as an acute, usually fatal infection associated with hematologic abnormalities, altered mental status, renal insufficiency, and disseminated TB (461). More recently, a few cases of sepsis secondary to TB have been reported in some HIV-infected patients (462–466) as well as non–HIV-infected patients (457). However, such cases are extremely rare.

Because the diagnosis of TB is not often considered initially, timely examination of sputum for AFB may not occur. Even then, initial smears may prove negative with repeat examination necessary. Sputum smears provide a definite diagnosis in less than 50% of cases. Thus, specimens obtained by endotracheal suctioning as well as bronchoscopic specimens may prove more valuable.

Unfortunately, the radiographic findings in TB-associated ARDS are rarely classic and may not strongly suggest TB. It is unusual to find focal infiltrates (15%); when present, the focal infiltrates are often in the lower lobes (429,433,457). Cavitary lesions and hilar adenopathy also occur less frequently (10% to 15%). Not surprisingly, the most common radiographic pattern consists of diffuse alveolar/interstitial infiltrates (433), which may often be misdiagnosed as pulmonary edema (433,436,457). Almost as common is a diffuse bilateral micronodular pattern, associated with consolidation and/or "ground glass" opacification (433). HRCT scans may reveal a miliary pattern of nodules or disseminated centrilobular micronodules and a tree-in-bud appearance with background areas of ground-glass attenuation (433,456). This corresponds to the fact that the majority of patients with respiratory failure and TB have miliary disease.

Bacterial pneumonia with subsequent respiratory failure is the most common misdiagnosis. When present, cavitary lesions are often incorrectly attributed to a necrotizing bacterial process (436). Thus, failure of a presumed pneumonia to respond to standard therapy should prompt efforts to diagnose TB (436,457).

As noted above, the prognosis for patients with TB-related respiratory failure is poor. Penner et al. (429) found that multiorgan system failure contributed significantly to mortality, presented in two thirds of the patients dying with TB-related respiratory failure. Similarly, Zahar et al. (457) found that increasing number of organ failures (utilizing the Knaus scale) resulted in an increased 30-day mortality. Despite adequate TB chemotherapy, TB-associated respiratory failure often progresses. Therapy may be inadequate in part due to gut malfunction resulting in malabsorption of medications. Recently, this problem was found in some HIV-infected patients with TB (467).

CLINICAL RESPONSE TO THERAPY

Fever

The resolution of fever after the initiation of therapy has been specifically addressed by three studies performed during different time periods after chemotherapy was introduced (468–470). Berger and Rosenbaum (468) treated 44 patients with INH and paraaminosalicylic acid (PAS), with or without streptomycin, and found that 13 (30%) patients had fever for 21 days or longer and 31 (70%) had fever for less than 21 days. Analysis of patient data at the 2-week interval revealed 34% with persistent fever versus 64% with defervescence. Six (14%) patients had fever lasting longer than 2 months. Patients with prolonged fever had either miliary disease or far-advanced pulmonary disease.

Kiblawi et al. (469) found resolution of fever in 64% of 59 patients after 2 weeks of therapy, which most often consisted of INH, ethambutol, and streptomycin. The mean duration of fever in these patients was 16 days and the median was 10 days, with the range 1 to 109 days. Far-advanced disease and high temperature (>38.8°C) on admission were more frequently observed in the group with fever lasting longer than 2 weeks.

Barnes et al. (470) reported strikingly different results in 161 patients; 89% of their patients defervesced within a week and 93% after 2 weeks of therapy. All but one patient received INH and rifampin, and most also received pyrazinamide. This therapeutic regimen is more potent than those prescribed in the previous studies and most likely accounts for the rapid defervescence in this study. These investigators found that alcoholism and advanced disease (as indicated by anemia, hyponatremia, and hypoalbuminemia) were markers of delayed defervescence. Salomon et al. (471) found that in patients receiving a four-drug regimen, defervescence occurred within 2 weeks in 9% of patients with multidrug-resistant mycobacteria compared with 78% of those with drug-susceptible organisms.

When fever is prolonged, especially lasting 3 to 4 weeks or longer after the initiation of therapy, alternative explanations must be considered, such as coexisting infection or neoplasm, drug hypersensitivity, drug resistance, and poor compliance. Only after these complicating factors have been ruled out and antipyretics have proved ineffective should one consider symptomatic relief of the fever with corticosteroids. Cytokines like tumor necrosis factor-($TNF-\alpha$), interleukin-1 (IL-1), and other interleukins might be responsible for the persistent fever that occurs in some patients (472). The use of corticosteroids in conjunction with antituberculous drugs in this setting has recently been reviewed (473,474). The duration of such therapy to control fever is 4 to 10 weeks.

Cough

Not only is cough a significant symptom of TB, but cough frequency correlates with the degree of infectiousness of the disease. Loudon and Roberts (475) demonstrated that the mean number of droplet particles expelled by coughing was 465 per cough. A bout of coughing may produce up to 3,500 droplet particles; almost half the droplets remain suspended in air as droplet nuclei for at least 30 minutes and are capable of infecting other individuals (475). Loudon and Spohn (476) used a tape recorder placed in the rooms of newly diagnosed TB patients to monitor cough frequency over an 8-hour interval from 11 p.m. to 7 a.m. They followed a group of 20 patients with mild to moderate disease undergoing chemotherapy. Before therapy, the patients' mean number of coughs per 8-hour night was 109. By the end of the second week of therapy, the patients' average cough count had fallen to 38 coughs per night, one third of the original cough count.

Chest Radiograph

Obtaining serial chest radiographs is not a sensitive or efficient method of monitoring response. Radiographic resolution is slow and lags behind patient well-being as well as sputum smear and culture conversion. The chest radiograph begins to show improvement 1 to 3 months after initiation of therapy and should indicate resolution or stability (90% of cases) at 6 months. At the completion of therapy a chest radiograph should document resolution or stabilization.

Bobrowitz reported seven patients who developed progressive pulmonary infiltrates during initial therapy for TB (477). These new areas developed within 3 to 5 weeks after initiation of therapy. At the time of their appearance, there was evidence of clinical improvement. With continuation of therapy, sputum conversion occurred and the areas of progression and the original radiographic abnormalities resolved. Onwubalili et al. (478) and Akira and Sakatani (456) reported progressive respiratory failure following the administration of anti-TB therapy. The former speculated that hypersensitivity to tuberculoproteins released from dying mycobacteria might be responsible for this paradoxical phenomenon.

In patients who have been treated presumptively on the basis of chest radiographs (smear negative and/or culture negative), the major indicator for response to therapy is the chest radiograph. Gordin et al. (479) reported 139 non-HIV patients with negative AFB smears who were treated for a presumptive diagnosis of pulmonary TB on the basis of radiographic abnormalities. They found 66 (48%) of the 139 patients to have TB. In these 66 patients, only 16 (11.5%) eventually had positive cultures, and 50 (36%) had clinical (seven patients) or radiographic (43 patients) improvement with antituberculous chemotherapy.

The intervals at which chest films are obtained depend on the clinical circumstances. Failure of the radiograph to show improvement in the patient after 3 months of therapy suggests that the abnormality seen on the radiograph does not represent active TB or that the patient's treatment regimen is inadequate. Routine chest radiographs do not indicate treatment failures. Rather, persistently positive cultures or the reappearance of positive cultures are more reliable for detecting this problem (480).

Bacteriologic Response

The best measure of treatment response is eradication of tubercle bacilli from a patient's sputum. Jones et al. (481) were among the first to report the effect of chemotherapy in 78 first-time and 52 chronic-disease patients by daily examination of sputum smears and cultures. Patients with sensitive organisms had a rapid decrease (a semilogarithmic response) in the number of AFB during the first 2 weeks. Patients had complete eradication of tubercle bacilli during the first month or had significantly reduced numbers for several weeks longer.

Yeager et al. (216) monitored bacilli counts in sputa of patients with pulmonary TB who were treated with INH

and PAS; some also took streptomycin. Their initial bacilli counts ranged from 10^6 to 10^7 organisms per milliliter. There was great variability in the rate of decline of organisms in the sputa of individual patients. Sputum cultures were negative at a mean of 76 days with a range of 8 to 142 days. Several years later, Hobby et al. (217) analyzed 269 sputum specimens from 28 patients before and after chemotherapy. There was a reduction in the number of tubercle bacilli per milliliter of sputum from 10^6 to 10^4 (≥2 logs) after an average of 16 days of chemotherapy.

Various factors influence the time to sputum conversion among patients with smear-positive pulmonary TB. These include underlying immune status, compliance with therapy, bioavailability of medications, drug susceptibility, and burden of infection. Sputum smear conversion in patients receiving first-line therapy occurs in 75% to 85% of patients after 2 months and in 96% after 6 months (482–484). Culture conversion occurs in 50% by one month and in 95% by 3 months after initiation of therapy (483). Telzak et al. (485) found that cavitary disease, numerous AFB on initial smear, and no prior history of TB were factors associated with an increased number of days for both smear and culture conversion. HIV status was not a significant factor.

It should be noted that a small percentage of patients have persistent positive AFB smears even at the completion of therapy (232,486–488). Vidal et al. (486) that found 10 (2.2%) of 453 patients had positive AFB smears at the completion of their treatment regimen: five patients had only one positive smear, whereas five patients had more than one. Of these ten cases, sputum culture was negative in eight, consistent with these patients having nonviable bacilli in their sputum. In two patients, nontuberculous mycobacteria were found on culture. Previously, Warring (487) reported that these nonviable bacilli—either dead bacilli or those unable to reproduce—originated from necrotic tuberculous lesions. Al-Moamary et al. (488) found that the presence of AFB on smear after conversion to negative cultures was observed at some point during therapy in 18% of 428 patients treated for TB. Only 30% of a subset of 30 patients with persistently positive smear results beyond 20 weeks represented treatment failure. Lack of clinical improvement and worsening chest radiographs were useful indicators of treatment failure. Radiographic improvement on treatment with persistently positive smear results should suggest that the smear result is due to nonviable organisms. Kim et al. (232) observed that persistently positive AFB smears were more common in far-advanced cavitary disease.

In patients with positive pretherapy sputum smears, repeat sputum samples should be obtained at 2- to 4-week intervals until the results of at least two successive examinations are negative. Sputum cultures should be obtained until there is bacteriologic conversion. In patients receiving multidrug therapy containing both INH and rifampin, sputum cultures should become negative for more than 50% of patients at 1 month, for 85% at the end of 2 months, and for more than 90% at the end of 3 months of therapy (483,484). Patients whose sputum cultures have not converted after 2 to 3 months should be evaluated for possible drug resistance or poor compliance.

PREDICTING THERAPEUTIC RESPONSE

As discussed above, early prediction of therapeutic outcome is currently based on clinical status, radiographic resolution, and clearing of AFB organisms from sputum. Several studies have suggested that earlier measures of response to therapy might help to predict possible treatment failure (489–493). Epstein et al. (489) found that treatment failure can be identified after 4 to 6 weeks of therapy by measuring time to detection (TTD) in Mycobacteria Growth Indicator Tube (MGIT; Becton, Dickinson) cultures. The MGIT contains Middlebrook and Cohn 7 Hg broth with various supplements to enhance growth. An indicator at the bottom of the tube fluoresces as the oxygen level decreases, signaling growth. A positive result is verified by AFB smear and subsequent PCR testing. The TTD in serial samples increased in most successfully treated patients. In those in whom TTD did not increase, there was a poor response to therapy. The presence of HIV infection, intravenous drug use, multidrug resistance, treatment with "second-line" agents, extensive radiographic involvement, and cavitary disease were associated with a delayed increase in TTD.

Another novel approach has been reported by Wallis et al. (490,491). Relapse of TB may be predicted by measuring *M. tuberculosis* antigen 85 in sputum after 2 weeks of therapy. These investigators subsequently developed a multivariate model to predict response to therapy in a prospective cohort of 42 HIV-negative patients with drug-sensitive TB. Measurement of sputum *M. tuberculosis* antigen 85 concentration on day 14 of therapy and days-to-positive in Bactec on day 30 were helpful in predicting delayed clearance of bacilli.

Other research techniques including monitoring sputum cytokine levels and sputum messenger RNA have been used to assess early response to chemotherapy (492,493). The rapid disappearance of *M. tuberculosis* in RNA from sputum as well as reduction in interferon-γ correlated with successful anti-TB therapy. Additional large trials will be required to determine the clinical usefulness of these new, sophisticated monitoring tools as predictors of therapeutic success.

IMMUNOSUPPRESSION AND TUBERCULOSIS

Immunosuppressive Therapy

Immunosuppression may result from therapy or disease. As discussed at the beginning of this chapter, intact cellular immunity is crucial for the prevention of TB. Drugs that depress cellular immunity, such as corticosteroids and cytotoxic agents, predispose patients to TB infection. In addition, some disease entities, such as malignancies, renal failure, transplantation, and collagen vascular diseases, may alter immunity and predispose to TB (494). Until the AIDS epidemic, mycobacterial disease in the immunocompromised host was considered uncommon, occurring in less than 5% of patients (495). In contrast, in countries in which TB was endemic, it was seen in up to 19% of immunocompromised patients (496).

Corticosteroids

The occurrence of TB in patients receiving corticosteroids was documented soon after the American debut of corticosteroid therapy in the early 1950s (497–502). However, in two of these reports there was no bacteriologic confirmation of TB (497,502). Subsequent reports confirmed the development of TB in steroid-treated patients (503–507).

The clinical presentation of TB in steroid-treated patients is confusing and may lead to a delay in diagnosis (504,506,507). Dautzenberg et al. (506) found a mean delay between the first symptom of TB and the diagnosis of 48 days. Indeed, the symptoms of TB may mimic those caused by the underlying disease and lead to a delay in diagnosis and an increase in immunosuppressive therapy. Skogsberg et al. (507) found this delay to be the cause of death in six of 13 immunosuppressed patients.

The actual risk of TB in steroid-treated patients is unknown. In pharmacologic doses, steroids suppress inflammation, resulting in lymphocytopenia and monocytopenia. The direct effect of steroids on lymphocyte function is not clear, but adverse effects on monocyte–macrophage function have been reported (508). Daily administration of prednisone suppresses the delayed hypersensitivity skin test and causes anergy in approximately 2 weeks (509). In contrast, alternate-day therapy does not suppress delayed hypersensitivity (510).

Sahn et al. (503) reviewed 14 episodes of reactivation TB in 13 patients. The most common presenting symptoms were productive cough and malaise. Fever and night sweats were rarely observed. Millar and Horne (504) noted similar suppression of symptoms. They found cough, dyspnea, and weight loss to occur, but not to be invariably present, in a group of 11 patients. In contrast, Dautzenberg et al. (506) found high fever to be the most common symptom in their study of 30 immunosuppressed patients; in 21 patients it was the major symptom.

There are few data regarding the utility of tuberculin testing, but Sahn and Lakshminarayan (503) found nine of 12 patients to be PPD positive. They found that eight of 14 episodes occurred during steroid therapy; TB was diagnosed in six patients 3 to 12 months (mean 5.5 months) after discontinuation of therapy. The daily dose of prednisone ranged from 10 mg to 80 mg. Millar and Horne noted a minimum of 10 mg of prednisolone in their patients (504).

In the series by Sahn and Lakshminarayan, the duration of corticosteroid administration before the diagnosis of active TB ranged from 2 months to 7 years. Five of eight episodes occurred during 2 to 8 months of therapy. In four of eight patients, additional immunosuppressive agents such as azathioprine and chlorambucil were used.

The radiographic pattern may reveal typical upper lobe disease suggesting reactivation. Some series confirm the presence of cavitary disease (503); others found that it did not occur frequently (507). Skosberg et al. (507) found that in steroid-treated patients TB was more frequently disseminated (40% vs. 12%; $p < 0.001$); lung infiltrates were more often miliary (44% vs. 13%; $p < 0.001$); and sputum smears were less often positive (30% vs. 62%; $p < 0.05$). In contrast, Sahn and Lakshminarayan (503) as well as Millar and Horne (504) found positive AFB smears in most patients. In steroid-treated patients, TB responds to standard chemotherapy (506), and there is no significant delay in sputum conversion time (503). Interestingly, in the series by Sahn and Lakshminarayan, three of the 11 patients who developed TB while being treated with steroids were also receiving prophylaxis; one patient was noncompliant and the other two patients developed INH-resistant organisms.

In contrast to these series, several large studies of corticosteroid-treated asthmatics revealed a very low incidence of TB in populations with high prevalence of TB as well as low prevalence of TB (511–514). These studies concluded that corticosteroid therapy should not be withheld for fear of inducing TB. Furthermore, it was not necessary to prescribe routine INH prophylaxis to asthmatic patients requiring long-term steroid therapy. Schatz et al. (513) failed to detect TB in 132 steroid-treated asthmatic patients. However, only 28% of their patients had positive tuberculin skin tests. Similarly, in two large British studies, only one case of TB developed in 786 steroid-treated patients, but most patients received 10 mg or less of prednisolone daily or 20 mg or less on alternate days (511,512).

Malignancy

TB in cancer patients occurs at a higher frequency than in the general population. It can occur at any point during the course of the malignancy. Several older series have documented these findings and have shown that TB occurred most frequently in the presence of lung, head and neck, and hematologic malignancies (515–517). More recently, Libshitz et al. (518) retrospectively reviewed the records of 56 cancer patients who developed TB between January 1989 and December 1994. Approximately 50% of the patients developed TB during or within 18 months of therapy, while in another 30% TB was discovered synchronously with the diagnosis of carcinoma. Distant cases of TB (21%) developed 18 months or more after completion of therapy. It is

unclear how many patients in the last group had their immune status altered by the therapy predisposing them to TB as opposed to how many developed TB unrelated to the malignancy or chemotherapy. In comparison with earlier series, TB occurred less frequently in lung, head, and neck carcinomas than in hematologic malignancies. The increase in the latter occurred most significantly in patients with acute leukemia. This is thought to reflect the more vigorous chemotherapy for leukemia during the past 15 years as well as improved antibiotic therapy compared with 25 to 40 years ago. Libshitz et al. (518) found that 50 (89%) of 56 patients had intrathoracic TB. The radiographic findings were consistent with primary TB in 9 (18%) cases, postprimary TB in 31 (62%) cases, and nonspecific in nine (18%) cases. One patient (2%) had a normal chest radiograph.

Kim et al. (519) reviewed their experience with patients with myelodysplastic syndrome (MDS). They found that 12 of 195 consecutive patients with MDS were diagnosed with TB. Six of these 12 patients were initially diagnosed with TB but subsequently were found to have myelodysplastic syndrome. The radiographic pattern was often consistent with primary TB; extrapulmonary involvement was common.

RELATION BETWEEN TUBERCULOSIS AND BRONCHOGENIC CARCINOMA

Pulmonary TB and bronchogenic carcinoma have been confused for centuries (520). Before the 19th century, the word *tubercle* was used to describe both cancer and TB (520). TB may mimic lung cancer and may even lead to thoracotomy (521,522). Such cases usually present atypically with lack of symptoms and confusing chest radiographic findings (521). Equally troubling is that pulmonary TB and bronchogenic carcinoma may coexist in the same patient (523–529). This led to considerable speculation regarding a pathogenetic link between the two diseases (530–532). Shah-Mirany et al. (529) conducted a controlled study comparing 54 patients with both diseases and 41 patients with only bronchogenic carcinoma, and found no significant relation between the two diseases. Similar conclusions were found in larger, retrospective studies (526,528,530,533).

When active TB is dominant, particularly if the patient's sputum is positive, coexistent carcinoma may be overlooked. Tunell et al. (534) found an average delay of 16.3 weeks in the diagnosis of carcinoma in the presence of TB in contrast to an average duration of 3.4 weeks for a control group of patients with lung carcinoma alone. Cytologic analysis of repeated sputum samples improved the yield in diagnosing coexisting carcinoma (527,535,536). When patients with proven TB who are receiving therapy develop progressive abnormalities, or when there is radiographic resolution in one area with persistence or enlargement in another area, there is reason to suspect coexistent disease. Snider and Placik (537) matched 124 patients with coexisting bronchogenic carcinoma and TB according to race, sex, and age. They could not find local mechanisms linking TB with carcinoma, but they found that carcinoma could reactivate TB by eroding encapsulated caseous foci. They also postulated that the cachectic state sometimes associated with a bronchogenic carcinoma might reactivate underlying TB.

Renal Disease

Impaired cellular immunity due to end-stage renal disease may predispose patients to TB (538). More than 20 years ago various investigators noted a high incidence of TB in patients with chronic renal failure undergoing dialysis (539–544). Most patients were maintained on dialysis on average for approximately 1 year. Fever and weight loss were common symptoms. However, the diagnosis was often delayed because symptoms were nonspecific and attributed to uremia. The tuberculin skin test was positive in 50% to 60% of patients (540,541). Chest radiographic patterns were atypical and included diffuse interstitial infiltrates, lower lobe infiltrates, pleural effusions, and normal radiographic appearance (541). Extrapulmonary TB was observed more frequently than expected, including kidneys, liver, meninges, and peritoneum. Despite difficulties in diagnosis, most patients were treated successfully (541).

Approximately 10 years after these initial reports, TB continued to occur in patients on maintenance dialysis in both endemic and nonendemic populations (545–550). Most recently, Quantrill et al. (551,552) found a high incidence of TB in patients with chronic renal failure who presented to the Manchester Royal Infirmary dialysis unit. During a 13-year interval (1986–1999), 24 cases of TB were diagnosed (8 prior to dialysis and 16 in individuals undergoing regular dialysis). Of the 16 dialysis patients, 14 were receiving continuous ambulatory peritoneal dialysis (CAPD). All of the TB cases in the dialysis group were extrapulmonary. Peritoneal TB occurred in eight (57%) of the 14 patients receiving CAPD. The other significant extrapulmonary presentation was TB lymphadenitis. Chest radiographs were nondiagnostic. In most cases the chest radiograph was normal or revealed small pleural effusions, which are common in chronic renal failure patients undergoing dialysis.

In contrast, Kursat and Ozgur (553) reviewed their 3-year experience with 157 chronic hemodialysis patients in Manisa, Turkey. Nine patients were diagnosed with TB (four with pulmonary, four with lymphadenitis, and one with skin). All but one patient were treated successfully. Finally, Smirnoff et al. (554) analyzed the utility of tuberculin and anergy skin testing in patients receiving long-term dialysis: 40% were anergic whereas 19% were tuberculin positive. Despite the high rate of anergy, testing may be useful in identifying anergic patients who require further clin-

ical assessment, chest radiography, and consideration for prophylaxis in high-risk cases (552,555).

Transplantation

The prevalence of TB in renal transplant recipients varies from 0.5% to 11.5%, depending on the country from which data are gathered (556–560). The 11.5% prevalence comes from India, a country with a high TB prevalence in the general population (558). Hall et al. (559) reported 21 cases of *M. tuberculosis* in 487 renal transplantation patients. The median time from transplantation to diagnosis was 14 months (range 2 to 74). Initially, all patients received corticosteroids, with either a combination of cyclosporine and azathioprine or with cyclosporine/azathioprine separately. In seven patients (32%) immunosuppression was intensified with pulsed intravenous corticosteroids for a rejection episode within 3 months of the diagnosis of TB. Most patients presented with cough (73%) and fever (55%). Other symptoms occurred less frequently. Pulmonary infiltrates were observed in 14 patients (67%). The distribution was in the upper lobes in ten patients (48%), middle lobes in seven patients (33%), and lower lobes in four patients (19%). A miliary pattern was seen in four patients (19%), pleural effusion in three (14%), tuberculoma in two (10%), apical cavitary infiltrates in two (10%), and hilar adenopathy in one patient (5%). Diagnosis of TB was made by sputum smears in 40% of patients and by fiberoptic bronchoscopy in almost 50% (eight patients by brushings and three by transbronchial biopsy). Extrapulmonary TB occurred in only 23% of patients, which is significantly less than that reported by Qunibi et al. (557). Not only can TB develop in transplanted patients as a result of immunosuppression, but transplanted organs may also transmit TB to their recipients. Mourad et al. (560) described two cadaver kidney recipients who received allografts procured from the same donor. Both subsequently developed disseminated TB (one with a miliary pattern on chest radiograph) 2 and 6 months after transplantation, respectively.

TB rarely occurs in other types of organ transplantation. Several large series reviewing infections in bone marrow transplant recipients reported the incidence of TB ranging from 0.1% to 2.2% (561–565). There were 10 cases of TB among 5,193 bone marrow transplant recipients, yielding an overall incidence of 0.19%. In contrast, Ip et al. (566) found 10 cases of TB in 183 consecutive bone marrow transplant recipients (5.5% incidence) in a transplant center in Hong Kong. The authors attribute this higher incidence of TB to Hong Kong's having a higher incidence of TB in the general population. The median time for onset of symptoms was 150 days, the main symptoms being fever and cough. Chest radiograph infiltrates were consistent with reactivation. Treatment with standard antituberculosis drugs for a longer duration (1 year) was highly effective.

Risk factors for developing TB included total-body irradiation and chronic graft versus host disease. The latter disrupted reconstitution of immune defenses against TB (566).

The incidence of pulmonary TB after lung transplantation is extremely low (567–573), ranging from 1% to 2%. Two recent series found nontuberculous mycobacteria to be more common (572,573). In most cases TB appears to have been transmitted from the donor lung (567,569–571), although reactivation of endogenous infection has also been reported (568,571). The time from lung transplantation to onset of TB ranges from 2 to 5 months (571). Most cases of TB occurred following the augmentation of corticosteroids (571). TB in transplanted lungs has no characteristic radiographic pattern, ranging from subtle bronchial narrowing and small pleural effusions to cavitary infiltrates. Patients usually respond well to a four-drug treatment regimen (INH, ethambutol, streptomycin, and pyrazinamide). Most series report the avoidance of rifampin as part of the standard therapy because of its capacity to increase the metabolism of cyclosporine via induction of the hepatic cytochrome P-450. Low cyclosporine levels may cause lung rejection. Some investigators have utilized rifampin, carefully monitoring cyclosporine levels (573). Development of TB in liver transplant recipients is discussed in Chapter 35.

Collagen Vascular Disease

Tuberculosis is an important cause of morbidity and mortality in patients with certain rheumatic diseases (574–579). Its incidence in patients with collagen vascular disease is a function of the degree of immunosuppression in these patients (due to the underlying disease or the effect of medication) as well as the prevalence of TB in the general population of a specific country. Thus, TB occurs more frequently in patients with systemic lupus erythematosus (SLE) than in those with rheumatoid arthritis (RA) (574,578–580). In patients with SLE this higher incidence of TB has been attributed to an intrinsic defect in cell-mediated immunity (581–583) as well as the effect of corticosteroid administration (584).

Some studies have revealed that the mean daily dosage of corticosteroids was higher in SLE patients who developed TB (574,579). In contrast to SLE, TB was not observed more frequently in patients with RA who were maintained on cytotoxic agents or low doses of corticosteroids (prednisone less than 15 mg/day or its equivalent) (574,579). Patients with RA may have impaired immunity (581,585,586), which may predispose them to TB but to a lesser extent (579). Several groups of investigators have found that SLE patients more frequently present with extrapulmonary involvement (576–579). Patients with SLE had chest radiographic findings consistent with miliary dissemination, diffuse consolidation, or primary TB (576–579,588). In contrast, patients with RA had radiographic findings consistent with reactivation (579,587).

Recently, Keane et al. (589) reported the development of TB in RA patients treated with infliximab. Infliximab is a humanized antibody against tumor necrosis factor (TNF-α). The role of TNF-α in the human immune response to TB awaits further clarification (see Chapter 21). Antibodies to TNF-α in the mouse model cause reactivation of latent infection (590,591). Most patients developed TB within 12 weeks of initiation of therapy and most had been receiving other immunosuppressive therapy. The majority of patients developed extrapulmonary disease, whereas almost 25% had disseminated disease (589,592). Interestingly, another agent that neutralizes TNF-α, ethanercept, has not been associated with increased TB. This may relate to different ways in which infliximab and ethanercept neutralize TNF-α (589).

Diabetes Mellitus

An association between diabetes and tuberculosis has been implied for centuries. In the late 16th century Morton (593) recognized a link between diabetes and TB. Approximately 100 years ago, diabetic patients often died from diabetic coma or TB (594). In 1927, Sosman and Steidl (595) reported that 9% of 182 hospitalized diabetic patients had evidence of pulmonary TB on routine chest radiograph. All but three patients were older than 45 years. Root obtained chest radiographs of consecutive diabetic patients who attended the Joslin Clinic (Boston, MA, U.S.A.) between 1927 and 1930 (596). He found the incidence rate of TB to be 2.8% among 1,373 hospitalized diabetics, 2.45% among 10,000 diabetics in the Joslin series, and 1.6% in 750 juvenile diabetics. Banyai (597) reported composite data from 1927 through 1931 and found the incidence of TB among diabetics to be 2.6%—three times greater than the estimated incidence of TB in the United States during that time period. In 1946, Boucot et al. (598) conducted a large-scale survey of diabetics in Philadelphia. They found that TB recurred almost twice as frequently in diabetics: the incidence of TB was 8.4% among the city's 3,106 diabetics compared with 4.3% in a nondiabetic control group of 71,767 industrial workers. In 1954, Silwer and Oscarsson (599) published the results of a Swedish survey that documented TB in 3.8% of diabetics; in their survey, the prevalence of TB among diabetics was fourfold that of the population.

More recently, data from the Danish Tuberculosis Index suggested a threefold risk for TB in diabetic patients (600). Similarly, Kim et al. (601) found that Korean diabetic patients have a risk for TB 3.4 times greater than that for nondiabetic patients. A greater risk was observed in those aged 36 to 49 than in those older than 50. Most recently, a case-control study of 5,290 California hospital discharges of diabetic patients found diabetes to be a significant risk factor for TB among Hispanics (602). Mexican Americans predominated in this Hispanic group. Among Hispanics aged 25 to 54, the estimated risk of TB attributable to diabetes (25.2%) was equivalent to that attributed to HIV infection (25.5%).

Boucot et al. (598) found significant factors favoring development of TB in diabetics: age of the patient, duration and severity of diabetes, and weight less than normal (598). Only 5% of diabetic patients under age 40 who had diabetes for less than 10 years had active TB, in contrast to 17% of diabetics under age 40 who had diabetes for more than 10 years. Severity of diabetes also predisposed to TB: 5.3% of diabetics requiring more than 40 units of insulin daily had active TB. The prevalence of TB in diabetics was twice as high in those whose weight was below normal compared with those whose weight was above normal. Holden and Hiltz (603) found a higher proportion of far-advanced cases of TB among diabetics with severe disease compared with those with mild diabetes. Cavitation was greatest among those with more severe disease, that is, those requiring 40 units of insulin or more daily.

The clinical presentation of TB in diabetic patients is similar to that in nondiabetic patients (604). The radiographic findings have been described as both typical and atypical. Some studies suggest an increased frequency of lower lobe TB (595,605,606,610,611) as well as a greater predisposition to cavitary disease (607–611). Other studies have argued against these "unusual" findings (80,604). In a retrospective study by Perez-Guzman et al. (610) of 192 diabetic TB patients matched to a control group, almost two thirds of the diabetic group had both upper and lower lobe involvement in comparison with one third in the controls. Furthermore, predominant upper lobe involvement had a decreased frequency (17% vs. 56%) and lower lobe involvement an increased frequency (19% vs. 7%). More diabetic patients developed cavitations (82% vs. 59%), more often in the lower lobes. Bacakoglu et al. (611) found that cavitary disease occurred more frequently in persons with type I diabetes. Ikezoe et al. (608) reviewed CT patterns of TB in diabetic patients (608). They found no predilection for atypical location (lower lobe, anterior segment of the upper lobes, or right middle lobe). However, they found a higher prevalence of multiple cavities within any given lesion as well as nonsegmental distribution of the TB.

The mechanism predisposing diabetic patients to TB is unclear. Alterations in cellular immunity have been suggested but specifics remain to be defined. Hyperglycemia may predispose to impaired monocyte–macrophage function (612–614). Hyperglycemia is common in patients with TB. Bloom reported 47 men admitted to the San Diego Naval Hospital with newly diagnosed pulmonary TB; one third had an abnormal glucose tolerance test result (615). More recently, Mugasi et al. (616) found that 82 (16%) of 506 consecutive patients admitted with active pulmonary TB had impaired glucose tolerance test results. This was in addition to the 25 who were found to be diabetic (615). Impaired glucose tolerance resolved with appropriate antituberculous therapy (616,617).

Before the introduction of antituberculous chemotherapy, TB caused significant mortality in diabetics. The average annual mortality rate for diabetic patients with TB was 20% (619). Kessler found 21 deaths from TB among 21,477 diabetic patients followed at the Joslin Clinic between 1930 and 1956, which was 1.5 times greater than expected (620). From 1914 to 1922, TB was responsible for 4.9% of total deaths (621). This had fallen to 1.7% between 1944 and 1949, and there were no deaths from TB between 1969 and 1979. However, among 1,043 diabetic patients who underwent autopsy between 1964 and 1980, two cases of TB were found.

With effective chemotherapy, diabetics with TB fare as well as nondiabetics. Holden and Hiltz (603) reported on tuberculous diabetics admitted to Nova Scotia Sanatorium from 1931 through 1961. They found that of 34 patients treated before chemotherapy, 50% were dead within 2 years of discharge. In contrast, only four (17%) of 23 treated patients died. Luntz (622), Banyai (623), and Ross (619) reported larger series of successfully treated tuberculous diabetics with death and relapse rates similar to those of nondiabetic populations. Although therapy has significantly improved overall prognosis, poorly controlled diabetes may still predispose to reactivation TB. Edsall et al. (624) found that diabetes occurred concurrently in 8% of 145 cases, second only to concurrence of TB with severe alcoholism (26%).

Finally, Bashar et al. (625) reported a significant association between multidrug-resistant TB and diabetes. They found 18 (36%) of 50 patients with diabetes and TB had multidrug-resistant TB compared to only 10% in a control group. Both groups had predominantly upper lobe cystic or cavitary disease. This study coincided with large multidrug-resistant TB outbreaks in several hospitals in New York City. These patients may have developed multidrug-resistant TB through undetected nosocomial spread rather than having their diabetes predispose them to multidrug-resistant organisms (626).

Gastrectomy

Patients who have undergone gastrectomy are considered at increased risk of developing TB. In 1927, Winkelbauer and Frisch reported four patients who developed fulminant TB after gastrectomy (627). In a subsequent Swedish study, Forsgren found that the risk of developing TB after partial gastrectomy was ten times greater than the risk of developing TB in the general population (627). According to Snider, the prevalence of gastrectomy among TB patients varied from 1.7% to 2.5%, and the incidence of TB among patients who underwent gastrectomy ranged from 0.4% to 5.0%. However, none of these studies had matched controls.

Thorn et al. (628) reviewed the case histories of 955 patients who underwent partial gastrectomy for peptic ulcer disease. They found that gastric ulcer and preoperative weight loss predisposed to active TB after surgery. Of 955 patients, 809 had chest radiographs before surgery. In 60 there were abnormalities consistent with TB: in eight of these patients, tubercle bacilli were found in sputa before or within a month of surgery. Nine of 45 men patients and five of seven women patients with abnormal radiographs developed TB after surgery. There were 616 men and 133 women who had normal chest radiographs before surgery. None of the women developed postoperative TB. Fourteen men developed TB during a follow-up period of 1.5 to 6.5 years. The annual incidence of TB was five times that of men of the same age. Men with low preoperative weight (less than 85% of ideal body weight before gastrectomy) had a 14-fold greater likelihood of developing TB than men with normal body weight.

Hanngren and Reizenstein (629) studied 38 patients who developed TB after gastrectomy. Because of increased malabsorption, there were increased numbers of AFB in the patients' sputum. They found that severe dumping syndrome was more common among these patients, suggesting that malnutrition secondary to intestinal malabsorption may predispose to TB. Interestingly, Welsh (630) reported a case of drug-resistant TB after gastrectomy. Presumably, subtherapeutic levels of antituberculosis chemotherapy secondary to malabsorption resulted in selection of organisms that were drug resistant.

A related group of patients are those with jejunoileal bypass. In various series, 3% to 4% of patients developed TB (631). Nonpulmonary TB accounted for more than 80% of cases after bypass. The increased risk may have been related to alterations in cellular immunity induced by malnutrition (632). In addition to the increased incidence of TB, abnormal drug metabolism resulting in reduced serum concentrations of rifampin and ethambutol occurred (632). Similar problems were seen in gastrectomy patients (630).

SILICOSIS-RELATED TUBERCULOSIS

In 1556, Agricola (633) was the first to recognize the association between silicosis and TB. Individuals with silicosis have a greater risk of developing pulmonary TB than nonsilicotic individuals in the same population (634). The frequency of coexisting TB is higher among patients with more advanced forms of silicosis (635,636). Studies on South African gold miners and Danish foundry workers demonstrated that the risk of TB was threefold higher among silicotic workers (634,636). Multiple studies have found that pulmonary TB occurs in as many as 20% to 25% of all silicotic patients during their lifetime (636–638). Furthermore, the relative risk of death from TB is three to five times greater than that of the general population.

Cowie (636) showed that the annual incidence of TB increased with the degree of profusion of silicosis as detected by chest radiograph. Recently, Chang et al. (639) found that the size of the small opacities and the presence

of progressive massive fibrosis (PMF) are more important than profusion in determining the risk of TB. Hnizdo and Murray (638) found that the severity of silicosis found at autopsy was associated with an increased risk for developing pulmonary TB. These investigators showed that cumulative dust exposure was a risk factor for TB in gold miners. Finally, Corbett et al. (640) demonstrated that the risks of silicosis and HIV infection are multiplicative with respect to TB. Thus, HIV-positive silicotic individuals have considerably higher TB incidence rates than those reported from other HIV-positive miners.

Inhaled silica particles that reach the lungs are phagocytosed by alveolar macrophages. In turn, silica particles damage cell membranes, which eventually leads to death and lysis of alveolar macrophages. Both humoral and cell-mediated immune abnormalities may be present in silicosis (641). Furthermore, macrophage destruction may not be necessary to increase TB susceptibility (642). Allison et al. (643) demonstrated that sublethal doses of silica enhance the growth of *M. tuberculosis* in macrophage cultures. Previous experiments in guinea pigs demonstrated that inhalation of quartz reactivated TB lesions that were healing (644).

The clinical presentation of pulmonary TB in silicotic patients may be insidious. It is usually a result of reactivation and occurs more often in patients with PMF (645,646). Conversely, at least 50% of patients with PMF develop TB. Symptoms may be nonspecific and mostly constitutional, including fever, night sweats, fatigue, and generalized malaise (645,647). While increased cough may be present, progressive dyspnea and hemoptysis are not common. Chest radiographs may be difficult to interpret in patients with silicosis. Poorly demarcated infiltrates predominantly in the apices favors the diagnosis of TB. These infiltrates may surround preexisting silicotic nodules or conglomerates. Cavity formation may be present in TB but is very unusual in silicotic nodules in the absence of TB (645). Chest CT scans may help clarify these radiologic dilemmas. Ultimately, bacteriologic confirmation is necessary but may prove difficult to obtain in silicotic patients (647). The diagnosis of TB in silicotic patients requires a high index of suspicion, since it is frequently found only as a postmortem finding (646–648). Extrapulmonary TB is rare in silicotic patients (645). When present, it has usually involved the pleura.

While a discussion about management of TB is beyond the scope of this chapter (see Chapter 47), several general points should be made. Early literature suggested a poorer success rate for management of TB in silicotic patients (649,650). It was believed that the intense fibrotic reaction and vascular destruction in the lung parenchyma prevented antituberculous medications from reaching their intended sites. However, most of these studies were conducted prior to modern TB therapy. More recent studies from South Africa and Hong Kong have demonstrated excellent success rates utilizing four-drug regimens that included INH, rifampin, pyrazinamide, and streptomycin (635,651,652).

RELATION BETWEEN TUBERCULOSIS AND SARCOIDOSIS

Various investigators have found an increased incidence of TB in patients with proven sarcoidosis (653–657). As early as 1950, Riley (653) reported the experience of the Bellevue Chest Service in finding TB in 13 of 52 cases of sarcoidosis. Two years before, Ustvedt (654) published an autopsy study reviewing 59 patients with sarcoidosis: TB was the cause of death in 11 of these patients. Subsequently, Scadding (655) found TB in 29 (13%) of 230 cases. In five cases, the clinical picture changed from sarcoidosis to TB; in 18 cases, tubercle bacilli were found without a change in the clinical picture of sarcoidosis; and in six cases, tubercle bacilli were isolated before the clinical appearance of sarcoidosis. Similarly, Haroutunian et al. (656) reported 14 patients in whom both TB and sarcoidosis were present. In the mid-1960s, Mankiewicz (657,658) claimed that sarcoidosis represented an unusual manifestation of pulmonary TB modified by uninhibited mycobacteriophages; sarcoidosis resulted from unrestrained lytic activity against mycobacteria. Chapman and Speight (659) reported the increased incidence of serum mycobacterial antibodies in patients with sarcoidosis. In contrast, Sutherland et al. (660) reviewed the British Medical Research Council's clinical trial of bacille Calmette–Guérin in more than 54,000 young people and found no link between TB and sarcoidosis. In 1970, Vanek and Schwartz (661) demonstrated acid-fast bacilli in tissue from sarcoidosis patients without evidence of TB.

The discussion regarding the association between TB and sarcoidosis faded away until recently, when the application of sophisticated molecular biologic techniques resurrected the previous debate. Saboor et al. (662) utilized PCR to detect mycobacterial DNA in patients with sarcoidosis. *M. tuberculosis* DNA was found in half of the patients with sarcoidosis on the basis of a PCR assay of BAL samples, bronchial washings, and tissue specimens. Nontuberculous mycobacterial DNA was found in an additional 20%. Subsequently, using PCR, some investigators have detected mycobacterial DNA in samples of affected tissue from patients with sarcoidosis (663–665), but others have not (666–669). As of this writing (2003), the controversy still exists. Utilizing PCR, Drake et al. (670) found *Mycobacterium* species DNA in patients with sarcoidosis, whereas Eishi et al. (671) in a large international study did not.

TUBERCULOSIS AND THE ELDERLY

> …The consumption of young men, that are in the Flower of their Age, when the heat of the Blood is yet brisk, and therefore more disposed to a Feverish Fermentation, is for the most part Acute. But in Old Men, where the Natural Heat is decayed, it is more Chronical…
>
> *Richard Morton, 1698* (672)

The geriatric population in both industrial and nonindustrial countries represents a large reservoir of TB infection (673,674). Elderly patients represent a particular problem because mortality of TB in this age group is higher (675). In the past, the diagnosis of TB in the elderly was frequently delayed or found at autopsy (6,9,12,14–16,29, 676–678). The delay in diagnosis had been attributed to atypical clinical and radiologic presentations (679–687). Age-related diminution in immune function, altered mucociliary clearance, and decreased pulmonary function in conjunction with malnutrition and associated diseases (such as diabetes, gastrectomy, malignancy, and alcoholism) may render the elderly more susceptible to TB. Indeed, Morris (686) suggested that the pattern of TB in the elderly was so characteristic that it deserved a separate classification. During the past decade numerous publications have reported on studies about the differences between younger and elderly TB patients; the results have been confusing and contradictory (93,680–696). In 1999, Perez-Guzman et al. (696) performed a meta-analysis on 12 published studies (which included references 93,680,683–685,687,689–691 as well as several other non–English language studies) to help resolve this issue. They defined "older" patients as those over the age of 60 years. The meta-analysis failed to corroborate that there was a significant delay in diagnosis in the elderly; that is, the time elapsed from the beginning of symptoms to the establishment of a TB diagnosis was similar in older and younger patients. More recently, Van den Brande et al. (695) in a retrospective analysis of 251 patients with pulmonary TB (113 patients were older than 70 years) found no difference between elderly and younger patients with respect to "suspicion interval" (time from first complaints to first consideration of TB) or "recognition interval" (time from first consideration of TB to actual diagnosis). In their meta-analysis, Perez-Guzman et al. (696) found no differences between older and younger TB patients with respect to prevalence of cough, sputum production, weight loss, fatigue/malaise, upper lobe radiographic abnormalities, positive sputum AFB, anemia, and serum aminotransferase levels. In the elderly there was a lower prevalence of fever, night sweats, hemoptysis, cavitary lung disease, positive tuberculin test, as well as lower levels of serum albumin and blood leukocytes. Dyspnea was more common in the elderly, perhaps secondary to pulmonary function loss associated with aging. The higher prevalence of hemoptysis in the younger patients was related to the higher frequency of cavitation.

Most elderly patients develop TB from reactivation of infection that occurred 50 to 60 years previously (41,47). Although 80-90% of cases of TB in the elderly occur among individuals living at home, there is a higher incidence of TB among nursing home residents (697,698); the Centers for Disease Control and Prevention reported twice the age-adjusted risk of developing TB (699). Stead et al. (697) reported their experience in a nursing home outbreak in which 30% of previously tuberculin-negative residents became infected and 17% developed progressive primary TB. These investigators also found a lower than expected prevalence of positive tuberculin tests in new admissions to 223 Arkansas nursing homes (700). These data suggested that fewer elderly had been infected with TB, and these elderly nursing home residents represented a potentially large susceptible population that could develop TB (701). Restriction fragment length polymorphism analysis may help determine what proportion of disease in the elderly is due to recent infection as opposed to reactivation of infection.

The most important factor for diagnosing TB in the elderly is to maintain a high index of suspicion. While all patients should undergo tuberculin skin testing, interpretation of results may be confusing because tuberculin reactivity declines with age secondary to a decline in delayed hypersensitivity (702–707). When rechallenged 1 to 5 weeks later, the tuberculin may turn positive due to the "booster phenomenon" (708–711).

Ultimately, the diagnosis of TB depends on demonstration of positive AFB in sputum smears and cultures. Most studies have found no difference in yield between younger and older patients (696). However, elderly patients may not be able to provide adequate sputum, so that induced sputum and even gastric aspirates have been suggested as alternative diagnostic tools. In recent years, fiberoptic bronchoscopy has proven more useful than other methods. Patel et al. (712) found that the diagnosis of TB would have been missed in almost 20% of elderly patients with TB without the aid of bronchoscopy.

Most elderly patients are treated successfully for pulmonary TB. Although some studies have found significant age-related mortality (677,683,693,695), others have not (684,685,687). The principles of therapy for the elderly are the same as those for younger groups (see Chapter 47). However, there is a higher incidence of drug toxicity in the elderly, perhaps due to a greater number of concurrent medical conditions and therapies (694,714–716). Mackay and Cole (677) retrospectively analyzed therapy in 116 patients between 1979 and 1980; major drug toxicity resulting in alteration of therapy increased with age, occurring in 40% of all patients over 65 years of age. Most of the toxicity was related to rifampin. Unfortunately, all regimens include multiple hepatotoxic drugs. In the U.S. Public Health Service hepatitis surveillance study in the early 1970s, 5% of the 13,838 INH-treated patients were older than 64 years (713). The case rate for INH-induced hepatitis was only 8 per 1,000 but might have been as high as 18 per 1,000 if all possible cases had been included. Stead et al. (701) observed INH hepatitis in 4.5% of approximately 2,000 elderly patients. Although older patients appear to be at risk for hepatotoxicity, some studies have not found this problem. Both the study by Korzeniewska-Kosela et al. (93) and the one by Umeki (684) found the risk of hepatotoxic-

ity in the elderly and younger adults to be equal (14.5% vs. 10.1% and 17% vs. 22%, respectively; *p* not significant in both studies). Nonhepatic side effects may also be a problem in the elderly. Umeki reported that 23% of elderly patients developed drug-related neutropenia (684). In addition, drug interactions may be a significant problem for the elderly who are often taking multiple medications for various other ailments.

Rifampin is notorious for producing drug interactions (717). It is a potent inducer of microsomal liver enzymes and enhances the metabolism of various drugs resulting in rapid elimination of drugs metabolized in the liver. Some of these interactions may be found commonly in the elderly and include a diminished anticoagulant affect with coumadin; inadequate control of diabetes in patients taking chlorpropamide, tolbutamide, and other sulfonylureas; as well as inadequate seizure control in patients maintained on phenytoin. Additional drugs that may be affected and require dosage adjustment include cardiac glycosides, β-blockers such as propranolol, calcium channel blockers such as verapamil, corticosteroids, theophylline, thyroxine, and cimetidine.

REFERENCES

1. Farber JE, Clark WT. Unrecognized tuberculosis in a general hospital. *Am Rev Tuberc* 1943;47:129–134.
2. Jacob S, Greenberg HB. Diagnosis and treatment of 20 tuberculous patients who entered a community hospital. *Am Rev Respir Dis* 1972;105:528–531.
3. Ashba JK, Boyce JM. Undiagnosed tuberculosis in a general hospital. *Chest* 1972;61:447–451.
4. MacGregor RR. A year's experience with tuberculosis in a private urban teaching hospital in the post-sanatorium era. *Am J Med* 1975;58:221–228.
5. Furey WW, Stefancie MF. Tuberculosis in a community hospital: a 5 year review. *JAMA* 1976;235:168–176.
6. Bobrowitz ID. Active tuberculosis undiagnosed until autopsy. *Am J Med* 1982;72:650–658.
7. Page MI, Lunn JS. Experience with tuberculosis in a public teaching hospital. *Am J Med* 1984;77:667–670.
8. Craven RB, Wenzel RP, Atuk NO. Minimizing tuberculosis risk to hospital personnel and students to unsuspected disease. *Ann Intern Med* 1975;82:628–632.
9. Greenbaum M, Beyt BE, Murray PR. The accuracy of diagnosing pulmonary tuberculosis at a teaching hospital. *Am Rev Respir Dis* 1980;21:447–481.
10. Huber GL, Miller RD. Training of undergraduate medical school students in pulmonary disease: a regional analysis of New England medical schools. *Chest* 1976;70:267–273.
11. Byrd RB, Horn BR, Solomon DA, et al. Treatment of tuberculosis by the nonpulmonary physician. *Ann Intern Med* 1977; 86:799–802.
12. Rosenthal T, Pitlik S, Michaeli D. Fatal undiagnosed tuberculosis in hospitalized patients. *J Infect Dis* 1975;131(Suppl):51–56.
13. Edlin GP. Active tuberculosis unrecognized until necropsy. *Lancet* 1978;1:650–652.
14. Enarson DA, Gryzbowski S, Dorken E. Failure of diagnosis as a factor in tuberculosis mortality. *Can Med Assoc J* 1978;118: 1520–1522.

15. Counsell SR, Tan JS, Dittus RS. Unsuspected pulmonary tuberculosis in a community teaching hospital. *Arch Intern Med* 1989;149:1274–1278.

16. Mathur P, Auten G, Sall R, et al. Delayed diagnosis of pulmonary tuberculosis in city hospitals. *Arch Intern Med* 1994; 154:306–310.

17. Rao VK, Iadermarco EP, Fraser VJ, et al. Delays in the suspicion and treatment of tuberculosis among hospitalized patients. *Ann Intern Med* 1999;130:404–411.

18. Liam CK, Tang CK. Delay in the diagnosis and treatment of pulmonary tuberculosis in patients attending a university teaching hospital. *Int J Tuberc Lung Dis* 1977;4:326–332.

19. Moran GJ, McCabe F, Morgan MT, et al. Delayed recognition and infection control for tuberculosis patients in the emergency department. *Ann Emerg Med* 1995;26:290–295.

20. Greenway C, Menzies D, Fanning A, et al. Delay in diagnosis among hospitalized patients with active tuberculosis predictors and outcome. *Am J Respir Crit Care Med* 2002;165:927–933.

21. Yilmaz A, Boga S, Sulu E, et al. Delays in the diagnosis and treatment of hospitalized patients with smear-positive pulmonary tuberculosis. *Respir Med* 2001;95:802–805.

22. The American Lung Association Conference on Re-establishing Control of Tuberculosis in the United States. *Am J Respir Crit Care Med* 1996;154:251–262.

23. Sherman LF, Rujiwara PI, Cook SV, et al. Patient and health care system delays in the diagnosis and treatment of tuberculosis. *Int J Tuberc Lung Dis* 1999;3:1088–1095.

24. Bennett CL, Schwartz DN, Parada JP, et al. Delays in tuberculosis isolation and suspicion among persons hospitalized with HIV-related pneumonia. *Chest* 2000;117:110–116.

25. Fischl MA, Uttamehandani RB, Dalkos GL, et al. An outbreak of tuberculosis caused by multiple drug resistant tubercle bacilli among patients with HIV infection. *Ann Intern Med* 1992; 117:177–183.

26. Pearson ML, Jereb JA, Frieden TR, et al. Nosocomial transmission of multi-drug resistant *Mycobacerium tuberculosis*: a risk to patients and health care workers. *Ann Intern Med* 1992;117: 191–196.

27. Menzies RI, Fanning A, Yuan L. Tuberculosis among health care workers. *N Engl J Med* 1995;332:92-98.

28. Centers for Disease Control and Prevention. Recommendations and reports. Guidelines for preventing transmission of *Mycobacterium tuberculosis* in healthcare facilities. *MMWR Morb Mortal Wkly Rep* 1994;43(RR123):1–32.

29. Katz I, Rosenthal T, Michaeli D. Undiagnosed tuberculosis in hospitalized patients. *Chest* 1985;87:770–774.

30. Kramer F, Modilevsky T, Waliany AR, et al. Delayed diagnosis of tuberculosis in patients with human immunodeficiency virus infection. *Am J Med* 1990;89:451–456.

31. Asch S, Leake B, Anderson, Gelberg L. Why do symptomatic patients delay obtaining care for tuberculosis? *Am J Respir Crit Care* 1998;157:1244–1248.

32. Dannenberg AM Jr. Immune mechanisms in the pathogenesis of pulmonary tuberculosis. *Rev Infect Dis*(Suppl 2);1989:11: 369–378.

33. Riley RL, Mills CC, Nyka W, et al. Aerial dissemination of pulmonary tuberculosis. *Am J Hyg* 1959;70:185–196.

34. Rich AR. *The pathogenesis of tuberculosis*, 2nd ed. Springfield, IL: Charles C Thomas, 1951:664.

35. Ghon A, King, DB Trans. *The primary lung focus of tuberculosis in children* (English ed). London: J & A Churchill, 1916:83.

36. Frostad S. Tuberculosis incipiens. *Acta Tuberc Scand* 1944;13 (Suppl):1–294.

37. Medlar EM. The pathogenesis of minimal pulmonary tuberculosis: a study of 1225 necropsies in cases of sudden and unexpected death. *Am Rev Tuberc* 1948;58:583–611.

38. Poulsen A. Some clinical features of tuberculosis. 2. Initial fever. 3. Erythema nodosum. 4. Tuberculosis of lungs and pleura in primary infection. *Acta Tuberc Scand* 1951;33:37–92.

39. Gedde-Dahl T. Tuberculous infection in the light of tuberculin matriculation. *Am J Hyg* 1952;56:139–214.

40. Fraser RG, Pare JAP, Pare PD, et al., eds. *Diagnoses of diseases of the chest*, 3rd ed. Philadelphia: WB Saunders, 1989:890.

41. Rich AR. *The pathogenesis of tuberculosis*, 2nd ed. Springfield, IL: Charles C Thomas, 1951:797, 827.

42. Stead WW, Bates JH. Evidence of a "silent" bacillemia in primary tuberculosis. *Ann Intern Med* 1971;74:559–561.

43. Riley RL. Apical localization of pulmonary tuberculosis. *Bull Johns Hopkins Hosp* 1960;106:232–239.

44. Dock W. Apical localization of phthisis. *Am Rev Tuberc* 1942; 71:345–357.

45. Goodwin RA, DesPrez RM. Apical localization of pulmonary tuberculosis, chronic pulmonary histoplasmosis and progressive massive fibrosis of the lung. *Chest* 1983;83:801–805.

46. Grzybowski S, Barnett GD, Stylbo K. Contacts of cases of active pulmonary tuberculosis. *Bull Int Union Tuberc* 1975;50: 90–106.

47. Stead WW. Pathogenesis of a first episode of chronic pulmonary tuberculosis in man: recrudescence of residuals of primary infection or the exogenous reinfection? *Am Rev Respir Dis* 1967; 95:729–745.

48. Lepeuple A, Thibier R, Vivien JN. A case of transmission of *M. tuberculosis* from one patient with active tuberculosis to a person with healed pulmonary tuberculosis. *Rev Tuberc (Paris)* 1960;24:1312–1321.

49. Raleigh JW, Weichelhausen R. Exogenous reinfection with *Mycobacterium tuberculosis* confirmed by phage typing. *Am Rev Respir Dis* 1973;108:639–642.

50. Nardell E, McInnis B, Thomas B, et al. Exogenous reinfection with tuberculosis in a shelter for the homeless. *N Engl J Med* 1986;315:1570–1575.

51. Daley CL, Small PM, Schecter GF, et al. An outbreak of tuberculosis with accelerated progression among persons infected with the human immunodeficiency virus: an analysis using restriction-fragment-length polymorphisms. *N Engl J Med* 1992;326:231–235.

52. Small PM, Shafer RW, Hopewell PC, et al. Exogenous reinfection with multidrug-resistant *Mycobacterium tuberculosis* in patients with advanced HIV infection. *N Engl J Med* 1993;328: 1137–1144.

53. Small PM, Hopewell PC, Singh SP, et al. The epidemiology of tuberculosis in San Francisco. *N Engl J Med* 1994;330: 1703–1709.

54. Alland D, Kalkut GE, Moss AR, et al. Transmission of tuberculosis in New York City. *N Engl J Med* 1994;330:1710–1716.

55. Stead WW, Kerby GR, Schlueter DP, et al. The clinical spectrum of primary tuberculosis in adults. Confusion with reinfection in the pathogenesis of chronic tuberculosis. *Ann Intern Med* 1968;68:731–744.

56. Trump DH, Hyams KC, et al. Tuberculosis infection among young adults entering the US Navy in 1990. *Arch Intern Med* 1993;153:211–216.

57. Alexander WJ, Avent CK, Baily WC. Simple primary tuberculosis in an elderly woman. *J Am Geriatr Soc* 1979;27:123–125.

58. Kahn MA, Kovnat DM, Bachus B, et al. Clinical and roentgenographic spectrum of pulmonary tuberculosis in the adult. *Am J Med* 1977;62:31–38.

59. Miller WT, MacGregor RR. Tuberculosis: frequency of unusual radiographic findings. *AJR Am J Roentgenol* 1978;130:867–875

60. Woodring JH, Vandiviere HM, Fried AM, et al. Update: the radiographic features of pulmonary tuberculosis. *AJR Am J Roentgenol* 1986;146:497–506.

61. Hadlock FP, Park SK, Awe RJ, et al. Unusual findings in adult pulmonary tuberculosis. *AJR Am J Roentgenol* 1980; 1015–1018.
62. Choyke PL, Sostman HD, Curtis AM, et al. Adult onset of pulmonary tuberculosis. *Radiology* 1983;148:357–362.
63. Tytle TL, Johnson TH. Changing patterns in pulmonary tuberculosis. *S Med J* 1984;77:1223–1227.
64. Krysl J, Korzeniewska-Kosela M, Muller N, et al. Radiologic features of pulmonary tuberculosis: an assessment of 188 cases. *Can Assoc Radiol J* 1994;45:101–107.
65. Lyons HA, Calvy GL, Sammons BP. The diagnosis and classification of mediastinal masses: a study of 782 cases. *Ann Intern Med* 1959;51:897–932.
66. Kent DC, Elliot RC. Hilar adenopathy and tuberculosis. *Am Rev Respir Dis* 1967;96:439–450.
67. Chang S-C, Lee P-Y, Perng R-P. Clinical role of bronchoscopy in adults with intrathoracic tuberculous lymphadenopathy. *Chest* 1988;93:314–317.
68. Weber AL, Bird KT, Janower ML. Primary tuberculosis in childhood with emphasis on changes affecting the tracheobronchial tree. *AJR Am J Roentgenol* 1968;103:123–132.
69. Leung AN, Muller NL, Pineda PR, et al. Primary tuberculosis in childhood: radiographic manifestations. *Radiology* 1992;182: 87–91.
70. Dhand S, Fisher M, Fewell JW. Intrathoracic lymphadenopathy in adults. *JAMA* 1979;241:505–507.
71. Winterbauer RH, Belic N, Moores KD. A clinical interpretation of bilateral hilar adenopathy. *Ann Intern Med* 1973;78:65–71.
72. Sackowitz AJ, Sackowitz GH. Bilateral hilar lymphadenopathy: an uncommon manifestation of adult tuberculosis. *Chest* 1977; 71:421–423.
73. Jones EM, Rafferty TN, Willis HS. Primary tuberculosis complicated by bronchial tuberculosis with atelectasis (epituberculosis). *Am Rev Respir Dis* 1942;476:392.
74. Kidd P. Basic tuberculous phthysis. *Lancet* 1886;2:616.
75. Segarra F, Sherman DS, Rodriguez-Aguero J. Lower lung field tuberculosis. *Am Rev Respir Dis* 1963;87:37–40.
76. Berger HW, Granada MG. Lower lung field tuberculosis. *Chest* 1974;65:522–526.
77. Chang S-C, Pui-Yuen L, Perng R-P. Lower lung field tuberculosis. *Chest* 1987;91:230–232.
78. Parmar MS. Lower lung field tuberculosis. *Am Rev Respir Dis* 1967;96:310–313.
79. Fernandez MZ, Nedwicki EG. Lower lung field tuberculosis. *Mich Med* 1969;68:31–35.
80. Morris JT, Seaworth BJ, McAllister CK. Pulmonary tuberculosis in diabetics. *Chest* 1992;102:539–541.
81. Reisner D. Pulmonary tuberculosis of the lower lobe. *Arch Intern Med* 1935;56:258–280.
82. Chambers JS, Jr. Tuberculous cavities of the lower lobe: results of treatment in 103 patients. *Am Rev Tuberc* 1951;63:625–643.
83. Sokoloff MJ. Lower lobe tuberculosis. *Radiology* 1940;34: 589–594.
84. Pratt-Johnson JH. Observations on lower lobe tuberculosis. *Br J Dis Chest* 1959;53:385–389.
85. Vivas JR, Laubach CA, Jr. Observations on lower lobe disease in pulmonary tuberculosis. *Am Rev Tuberc* 1949;60:15–24.
86. Weidman WH, Campbell HB. Lower lobe tuberculosis. *Am Rev Tuberc* 1937;36:525–541.
87. Hamilton CE, Fredd H. Lower lobe tuberculosis: a review. *JAMA* 1935;105:427–430.
88. Gordon BL, Charr R, Sokoloff MJ. Basal pulmonary tuberculosis: results of treatment. *Am Rev Tuberc* 1944;49:432–436.
89. Johnston H, Reisz G. Changing spectrum of hemoptysis: underlying causes in 148 patients undergoing diagnostic flexible bronchoscopy. *Arch Intern Med* 1989;149:1666–1668.
90. McGuinness G, Beacher JR, Harkin TJ, et al. Hemoptysis: prospective high-resolution CT/bronchoscopic resolution. *Chest* 1994;105:1155–1162.
91. Pursel SE, Lindskag GE. Hemoptysis. A clinical evaluation of 105 patients examined consecutively on a thoracic surgical service. *Am Rev Respir Dis* 1961;84:329–336.
92. Barnes PF, Verdegem TD, Vachon LA, et al. Chest roentgenogram in pulmonary tuberculosis. New data on an old test. *Chest* 1988;94:316–320.
93. Korzeniewska-Kosela M, Krysl J, Muller N, et al. Tuberculosis in young adults and the elderly. *Chest* 1994;106:28–32.
94. Cohen R, Muzaffar S, Capellan J, et al. The validity of classic symptoms and chest radiographic configuration in predicting pulmonary tuberculosis. *Chest* 1996;109:420–423.
95. Miller LG, Asch SM, Yu EI, et al. A population-based survey of tuberculosis symptoms: how atypical are atypical presentations? *Clin Infect Dis* 2000;30:293–299.
96. Auerbach O. Pathology and pathogenesis of pulmonary arterial aneurysm in tuberculosis cavities. *Am Rev Tuberc* 1939;39: 99–115.
97. Plessinger VA, Jolly PN. Rasmussen's aneurysms and fatal hemorrhage in pulmonary tuberculosis. *Am Rev Tuberc* 1949;60: 589–603.
98. Feingold AO. Tuberculosis without fever. *S Med J* 1975;68: 751–753.
99. Yew WW, Chau CH, Lee J, et al. Hoarseness due to recurrent laryngeal nerve palsy from intrathoracic mycobacteriosis (letter). *Int J Tuberc Lung Dis* 2001;11:1074–1075.
100. Vyravanthan S. Hoarseness in tuberculosis. *J Laryngol Otol* 1983;97:523–525.
101. Gupta SK. The syndrome of spontaneous laryngeal palsy in pulmonary tuberculosis. *J Laryngol Otol* 1960;74:106–113.
102. Radner DB, Snider GL. Recurrent laryngeal nerve paralysis as a complication of pulmonary tuberculosis. *Am Rev Tuberc* 1952; 65:93–99.
103. Amberson JB, Jr. *Tuberculosis*. New York: Oxford University Press, 1940:282.
104. Locke EA. Secondary hypertrophic osteoarthropathy and its relation to simple club fingers. *Arch Intern Med* 1915;15: 659–713.
105. Webb JG, Thomas P. Hypertrophic osteoarthropathy and pulmonary tuberculosis. *Tubercle* 1986;67:225–228.
106. Skorneck AB, Ginsberg LB. Pulmonary hypertrophic osteoarthropathy (periostitis) its absence in pulmonary tuberculosis. *N Engl J Med* 1958;258:1079–1082.
107. Kaplan RM, Munson I. Clubbed fingers in pulmonary tuberculosis. *Am Rev Tuberc* 1941;44:439–450.
108. Macfarlane JT, Ibrahim M, Tor-Agbidye S. The importance of finger clubbing in pulmonary tuberculosis. *Tubercle* 1979;60: 45–48.
109. Poppius H, Thomander K. Segmentary distribution of cavities: a radiologic study of 500 consecutive cases of cavernous pulmonary tuberculosis. *Ann Med Int Fenn* 1957;46:113–119.
110. Adler H. Phthisiogenetic studies by means of tomography in cases of localized pulmonary tuberculosis in adults. *Acta Tuberc Scand* 1959;47(Suppl);13–26.
111. Farman DP, Speir WA Jr. Initial roentgenographic manifestations of bacteriologically proven *Mycobacterium tuberculosis*–typical or atypical. *Chest* 1986;89:75–77.
112. Lentino W, Jacobson HG, Poppel M. Segmental localization of upper lobe tuberculosis: the rarity of anterior involvement. *AJR Am J Roentgenol* 1957;77:1042–1047.
113. Spencer D, Ragan R, Blinkhorn R, et al. Anterior segment upper lobe tuberculosis in the adult: occurrence in primary and reactivation disease. *Chest* 1990;97:384–388.
114. Wilcke JT, Askgaard DS, Nybo Jensen B, et al. Radiographic

spectrum of adult pulmonary tuberculosis in a developed country. *Respir Med* 1998;92:493–497.

115. Sutinen S. Evaluation of activity in tuberculous cavities of the lungs. *Scand J Respir Dis* 1968;67(Suppl):5–78.

116. Christensen EE, Dietz GW, Dietz GW, et al. Initial roentgenographic manifestations of pulmonary *Mycobacterium tuberculosis, M. kansasii,* and *M. intracellularis* infections. *Chest* 1981;80: 132–136.

117. Israel RH, Poe RH, Greenblatt DW, et al. Differentiation of tuberculous from nontuberculous cavitary lung disease. *Respiration* 1985;47:151–157.

118. Cohen JR, Amorosa JK, Smith PR. The air fluid level in cavitary tuberculosis. *Radiology* 1978;127:315–316.

119. Makanjvola D. Fluid levels in pulmonary tuberculosis cavities in a rural population in Nigeria. *AJR Am J Roentgenol* 1983; 141:519–520.

120. Auerbach O. The syndrome of persistent cavitation and noninfectious sputum during chemotherapy and its relation to open healing of cavities. *Am Rev Tuberc* 1957;75:242–258.

121. Schmidel NH, Hardy MA. Pulmonary tuberculosis with normal chest radiographs: report of eight cases. *Can Med Assoc J* 1967;97:178–180.

122. Husen L, Fulkerson LL, Del Vecchio E, et al. Pulmonary tuberculosis with negative findings on chest x-ray films: a study of 40 cases. *Chest* 1971;60:540–542.

123. Marciniuk DD, McNab BD, Martin WT, et al. Detection of pulmonary tuberculosis in patients with a normal chest radiograph. *Chest* 1999;115:445–452.

124. Jones BE, Ryu R, Yang Z, et al. Chest radiographic findings in patients with tuberculosis with recent or remote infection. *Am J Respir Crit Care Med* 1997;155:1270–1273.

125. Post FA, Wood R, Pillay GF. Pulmonary tuberculosis in HIV infection: radiographic appearance is related to CD4+ T-lymphocyte count. *Tuber Lung Dis* 1995;76:518–521.

126. Keiper MD, Beumont M, Eistami A, et al. CD4 T lymphocyte count and the radiographic presentation of pulmonary tuberculosis: a study of the relationship between these factors in patients with human immunodeficiency virus. *Chest* 1995;107: 74–80.

127. Laissy JP, Cadi M, Boudiaf ZE, et al. Pulmonary tuberculosis: computed tomography and high resolution computed tomography patterns in patients who are either HIV-negative or HIV-seropositive. *J Thorac Imaging* 1998;13:58–64.

128. Yabuuchi H, Murayama S, Murakami J, et al. Correlation of immunologic status with high-resolution CT and distribution of pulmonary tuberculosis. *Acta Radiol* 2002;43:44–47.

129. Im J-G, Itoh H, Young-Soo S, et al. Pulmonary tuberculosis: CT findings—early active disease and sequential change with antituberculous therapy. *Radiology* 1993; 186:653–660.

130. Moon MK, Im JG, Yean KM, et al. Mediastinal tuberculous lymphadenitis: CT findings of active and inactive disease. *AJR Am J Roentgenol* 1998;170;715–718.

131. Lee KS, Hwang JW, Chung MP, et al. Utility of CT in the evaluation of pulmonary tuberculosis in patients without AIDS. *Chest* 1996;110:977–984.

132. Lee JY, Lee KS, Jung KS, et al. Pulmonary tuberculosis: CT and pathologic correlation. *J Comput Assist Tomogr* 2000;24: 691–698.

133. Hillerdal O. Tuberculoma of the lung. *Acta Tuberc Scand* 1954;34(Suppl):1–191.

134. Culver GJ, Concannon JP, McManus JF. Pulmonary tuberculomas: pathogenesis, diagnosis, and management. *J Thorac Surg* 1950;20:798–822.

135. Bleyer JM, Marks JH. Tuberculoma and hamartomas of the lung: comparative study of 66 proved cases. *AJR Am J Roentgenol* 1957;77:1013–1022.

136. Sochocky S. Tuberculoma of the lung. *Am Rev Tuberc* 1958;78: 403–410.

137. Ishida T, Yokoyama S, Kaneko S, et al. Pulmonary tuberculoma and indications for surgery. *Respir Med* 1992;86:431–436.

138. Zerhouni EA, Stitik FP, Siegelman SS, et al. CT of the pulmonary nodule: a cooperative study. *Radiology* 1986;160: 319–327.

139. Nurayama S, Murakami J, Hashimoto S, et al. Noncalcified pulmonary tuberculomas: CT enhancement patterns with histological correlation. *J Thorac Imaging* 1995;10:91–95.

140. Tateishi U, Kusumoto M, Akiyama Y, et al. Role of contrast-enhanced dynamic CT in the diagnosis of active tuberculoma. *Chest* 2002;122:1280–1284.

141. Shim JJ, Cheong HJ, Kang E-Y, et al. Nested polymerase chain reaction for detection of *Mycobacterium tuberculosis* in solitary pulmonary nodules. *Chest* 1998;113:20–24.

142. Cohen AG, Wessler H. Clinical recognition of tuberculosis of major bronchi. *Arch Intern Med* 1939;63:1132–1157.

143. Salkin D, Cadden AV, Edson RC. The natural history of tuberculous tracheobronchitis. *Am Rev Tuberc* 1943;47:351–369.

144. Wilson NJ. Bronchoscopic observations in tuberculosis tracheobronchitis: clinical and pathological correlations. *Dis Chest* 1945;11:36–59.

145. McRae DM, Hiltz JE, Quinlan JJ. Bronchoscopy in a sanatorium. *Am Rev Tuberc* 1950;61:355–368.

146. Auerbach O. Tuberculosis of trachea and major bronchi. *Am Rev Tuberc* 1949;60:604–620.

147. Lincoln EM, Harris LC, Bovornkitti S, et al. The course and prognosis of endobronchial tuberculosis in children. *Am Rev Tuberc* 1955;71:246–256.

148. Frostad S. Segmental atelectasis in children with primary tuberculosis. *Am Rev Respir Dis* 1959;79:597–605.

149. Frostad S. Lymph nodes perforation through the bronchial tree in children with primary tuberculosis. *Acta Tuberc Scand* 1959;47(Suppl):104–124.

150. Smart J. Endobronchial tuberculosis. *Br J Dis Chest* 1951;45: 61–68.

151. Myerson MC. *Tuberculosis of the trachea and bronchus.* Springfield, IL: Charles C Thomas, 1944:250–275.

152. Froste N. Bronchoscopy in pulmonary tuberculosis. *Acta Tubercl Scand* 1950;23(Suppl):1–119.

153. Schwartz P. The role of the lymphatics in the development of bronchogenic tuberculosis. *Am Rev Tuberc* 1953;67:440–452.

154. Arnstein A. Non-industrial pneumoconiosis, pneumoconiotuberculosis and tuberculosis of the mediastinal and bronchial lymph glands in old people. *Tubercle* 1941;22:281–295.

155. Jokinen K, Pavla T. Nuutinen J. Bronchial findings in pulmonary tuberculosis. *Clin Otolaryngol* 1977;2:139–148.

156. Lee JH, Park SS, Lee DH, et al. Endobronchial tuberculosis. Clinical and bronchoscopic features in 121 cases. *Chest* 1992; 102:990–994.

157. Smith LS, Schillaci RF, Sarlin RF. Endobronchial tuberculosis. Serial fiberoptic bronchoscopy and natural history. *Chest* 1987; 91:644–647.

158. Ip MSM, So SY, Lam WK, et al. Endobronchial tuberculosis revisted. *Chest* 1986;89:727–730.

159. Matthews JI, Matarese SL, Carpenter JL. Endobronchial tuberculosis simulating lung cancer. *Chest* 1984;86:642–644.

160. Seiden HS, Thomas P. Endobronchial tuberculosis and its sequelae. *CAN MED ASSOC J* 1981;124:165–169.

161. Volckaert A, Roels P, Van der Niepen P, et al. Endobronchial tuberculosis: report of three cases. *Eur J Respir Dis* 1987;70: 99–101.

162. Van den Brande PM, Van de Mierop T, Verben K, et al. Clinical spectrum of endobronchial tuberculosis in elderly patients. *Arch Intern Med* 1990;150:2105–2108.

163. Pierson DJ, Lakshminarayan S, Petty TL. Endobronchial tuberculosis. *Chest* 1973;64:537–539.
164. Albert RK, Petty TL. Endobronchial tuberculosis progressing to bronchial stenosis. *Chest* 1976;70:537–539.
165. Caligiuri A, Banner AS, Jensik RJ. Tuberculosis mainstem bronchial stenosis treated with sleeve resection. *Arch Intern Med* 1984;144:1302–1303.
166. Tse CY, Natkunam. Serious sequelae of delayed diagnosis of endobronchial tuberculosis. *Tubercle* 1988;69:213–216.
167. Mellem H, Boye NP, Armkvaern R, et al. Stenotic tuberculous tracheitis treated with resection and anastomosis. *Eur J Respir Dis* 1986;68:224–225.
168. Natkunam R, Ong BH, Tse CY, et al. Carinal resection for stenotic tuberculous tracheitis. *Thorax* 1988;43:491–493.
169. Williams DJ, York EL, Norbert EJ, et al. Endobronchial tuberculosis presenting as asthma. *Chest* 1988;93:836–838.
170. Caglayan S, Coteli I, Acar U, et al. Endobronchial tuberculosis simulating foreign body aspiration. *Chest* 1989;95:1164.
171. So SY, Lam WK, Sham MK. Bronchorrhea—a presenting feature of active endobronchial tuberculosis. *Chest* 1983;84:635–636.
172. Lynch JP, Ravikrishan KP. Endobronchial mass caused by tuberculosis. *Arch Intern Med* 1980;140:1090–1091.
173. Yee A, Wasef E. Pigmented polypoid obstructive endobronchial tuberculosis (letter). *Chest* 1985;87:702–703.
174. Hoheisel G, Chan BK, Chan CH, et al. Endobronchial tuberculosis: diagnostic features and therapeutic outcome. *Respir Med* 1994;88:593–597.
175. Chung HS, Lee JH. Bronchoscopic assessment of the evolution of endobronchial tuberculosis. *Chest* 2000;117:385–392.
176. Nemir RL, Cardonna J, Lacoius A, et al. Prednisone therapy as an adjunct in the treatment of lymph node bronchial tuberculosis in childhood. *Am Rev Tuberc* 1963;74:189–198.
177. Chan HS, Sun A, Hoheisel GB. Endobronchial tuberculosis: is corticosteroid treatment useful?—a report of 8 cases and review of the literature. *Postgrad Med J* 1990;66:822–826.
178. Sawada S, Fujinara Y, Furui S, et al. Treatment of tuberculous bronchial stenosis with expandible metallic stents. *Acta Radiol* 1993;9:153-160.
179. Slonim SM, Razavi M, Kee S, et al. Transbronchial Palmaz stent placement for tracheobronchial stenosis. *J Vasc Interv Radiol* 1993;9:153-160.
180. Wan IYP, Lee TW, Lam HCK, et al. Tracheobronchial stenting for tuberculous airway stenosis. *Chest* 2002;122:370–374.
181. Wier J, Schless J. The tuberculin reaction in 530 patients admitted to the Tuberculosis Service, Fitzsimons Army Hospital. *Am Rev Respir Dis* 1959;80:569–574.
182. Edwards LB, Palmer CE, Edwards PQ. Further studies of geographic variation in naturally acquired tuberculin sensitivity. *Bull WHO* 1955;12:63–83.
183. Kent DC, Schwartz R. Active tuberculosis with negative skin reactions. *Am Rev Respir Dis* 1967;95:411–418.
184. Holden M, Dubin MR, Diamond PH. Frequency of negative intermediate-strength tuberculin sensitivity in patients with active tuberculosis. *N Engl J Med* 1971;285:1506–1509.
185. Rooney JJ, Crocco JA, Kramer S, et al. Further observations on tuberculin reactions in active tuberculosis. *Ann Intern Med* 1968;731:744.
186. Nash DR, Douglas JE. Anergy in active pulmonary tuberculosis. *Chest* 1980;77:32–37.
187. Ellner JJ. Suppressor adherent cells in human tuberculosis. *J Immunol* 1978;121:2573–2579.
188. Wieczorek Z, Szibinski G, Zwolinski J. Characterization of lymphocyte E rosette inhibitory factor in sera from tuberculosis patients. *Arch Immunol Ther Exp (Warsz)* 1977;25:63–68.
189. Waxmar J, Lochskin M. *In vitro* and *in vivo* cellular immunity

190. Rook GAW, Carswell JW, Stanford JL. Preliminary evidence for trapping of antigen-specific lymphocytes in the lymphoid tissue of "anergic" tuberculosis patients. *Clin Exp Immunol* 1976;26:129–132.
191. McMurray DN, Echeverri A. Cell-mediated immunity in anergic patients with pulmonary tuberculosis. *Am Rev Respir Dis* 1978;118:827–834.
192. Maher J, Kelly P, Hughes P, et al. Skin anergy and tuberculosis. *Respir Med* 1992;86:481–484.
193. Krasnow I, Wayne LG. Comparison of methods for tuberculosis bacteriology. *Appl Microbiol* 1969;18:915–917.
194. Blair EB, Brown GL, Tull AW. Computer files and analyses of laboratory data from tuberculosis patients. II. Analyses of six years data on sputum specimens. *Am Rev Respir Dis* 1976;113:427–432.
195. Nelson SM, Deike MA, Cartwright CP. Value of examining multiple sputum specimens in the diagnosis of pulmonary tuberculosis. *J Clin Microbiol* 1998;36:467–489.
196. Stone BL, Burman WJ, Hidred MV, et al. The diagnostic yield of acid-fast-bacillus smear-positive sputum specimens. *J Clin Microbiol* 1997;35:1030–1031.
197. Van Deun A, Salim AH, Cooreman E, et al. Optimal tuberculosis case detection by direct sputum smear microscopy: how much better is more? *Int J Tuberc Lung Dis* 2002;6:222–230.
198. Harries AD, Kamenya A, Subramanayan VR, et al. Sputum smears for diagnosis of smear positive pulmonary tuberculosis. *Lancet* 1996;347:834–835.
199. Walker D, McNerhey R, Kimankinda-Mwembo M, et al. An incremental cost-effectiveness analysis of the first, second and third sputum examination in the diagnosis of pulmonary tuberculosis. *Int J Tuberc Lung Dis* 2000;4:1086–1087.
200. Wu ZL, Wang QL. Diagnostic yield repeated smear microscopy examinations among patients suspected of pulmonary TB in Shandong province of China. *Int J Tuberc Lung Dis* 2000;4:1086–1087.
201. Kestle DG, Kubica GP. Sputum collection for cultivation of mycobacteria. An early morning specimen or the 24- to 72-hour pool? *Am J Clin Pathol* 1967;48:347–349.
202. Andrews RH, Radhakrishna S. A comparison of two methods of sputum collection in the diagnosis of pulmonary tuberculosis. *Tubercle* 1959;40:155–162.
203. Warren JR, Bhattacharya M, DeAlmeida KNF, et al. A minimum of 5.0 mL of sputum improves the sensitivity of acid-fast smear for *Mycobacterium tuberculosis*. *Am J Respir Crit Care Med* 2000;161:1559–1562.
204. Hensler NM, Spivey CG, Dees TM. The use of hypertonic aerosol in production of sputum for diagnosis of tuberculosis. Comparison with gastric specimens. *Dis Chest* 1961;40:639–642.
205. Elliott RC, Reichel J. The efficacy of sputum specimens obtained by nebulization versus gastric aspirates in the bacteriologic diagnosis of pulmonary tuberculosis. *Am Rev Respir Dis* 1963;88:223–227.
206. Jones FL Jr. The relative efficacy of spontaneous sputa, aerosol-induced sputa and gastric aspirates in the bacteriologic diagnosis of pulmonary tuberculosis. *Dis Chest* 1966;50:403–408.
207. Zahrani K, Jahdali H, Loirer L, et al. Yield of smear, culture and amplification tests from repeated sputum induction for the diagnosis of pulmonary tuberculosis. *Int J Tuberc Lung Dis* 2001;9:855–860.
208. Conde MB, Soares SLM, Mello FC, et al. Comparison of sputum induction with fiberoptic bronchoscopy in the diagnosis of tuberculosis. *Am J Respir Crit Care Med* 2000;162:2238–2240.
209. Anderson C, Inhaber N, Menzies D. Comparison of sputum

induction with fiberoptic bronchoscopy in the diagnosis of tuberculosis. *Am J Respir Crit Care* 1955;152:1570–1574.

210. Merrick ST, Sepkowitz KA, Walsh J, et al. Comparison of induced versus expectorated sputum for diagnosis of pulmonary tuberculosis by acid-fast smear. *Am J Infect Control* 1997;25:463–466.

211. Malasky C, Jordan T, Potulski F, et al. Occupational tuberculosis infections among pulmonary physicians in training. *Am Rev Respir Dis* 1990;142:505–507.

212. Shata AMA, Coulter JBS, Parry CM, et al. Sputum induction for the diagnosis of tuberculosis. *Arch Dis Child* 1996;74:535–537.

213. Centers for Disease Control and Prevention. Guidelines for preventing the transmission of *Mycobacterium tuberculosis* in health-care facilities, 1994. *MMWR Morb Mortal Wkly Rep* 1994;43:RR-13.

214. World Health Organization. *Guidelines for prevention of tuberculosis in health care facilities in resource-limiting settings.* 1999;269:1–51.

215. Kubica GP, Gross WM, Hawkins JE, et al. Laboratory services for mycobacterial diseases. *Am Rev Respir Dis* 1975;112:773–787.

216. Yeager H Jr, Lacy J, Smith LR, et al. Quantitative studies of mycobacterial populations in sputum and saliva. *Am Rev Respir Dis* 1966;95:998–1004.

217. Hobby GL, Holman AP, Iseman MC, et al. Enumeration of tubercle bacilli in sputum of patients with pulmonary tuberculosis. *Antimicrobiol Agents Chemother* 1973;4:94–104.

218. Rouillon A, Perdrizet S, Parrot R. Transmission of tubercle bacilli: the effects of chemotherapy. *Tubercle* 1976;56:275–299.

219. David HL. *Bacteriology of mycobacterioses.* Atlanta: Centers for Disease Control and Prevention, 1976:153.

220. Boyd JC, Marr JJ. Decreasing reliability of acid-fast smear techniques for detection of tuberculosis. *Ann Intern Med* 1975;82:489–492.

221. Marraro RV, Rodgers EM, Roberts TH. The acid-fast smear: fact or fiction? *J Am Med Technol* 1975;37:277–279.

222. Stottmeier KD. Acid-fast smears and tuberculosis (letter). *Ann Intern Med* 1975;83:429–430.

223. Fierer J, Merino R. Acid-fast smears and tuberculosis (letter). *Ann Intern Med* 1975;83:430–431.

224. Burdash NM, Manos JP, Ross D, et al. Evaluation of the acid-fast smear. *J Clin Microbiol* 1976;4:190–191.

225. Pollock HM, Wieman EJ. Smear results in the diagnosis of mycobacterioses using blue light fluorescence microscopy. *J Clin Microbiol* 1977;5:329–331.

226. Murray PR, Elmore C, Krogstad J. The acid-fast stain: a specific and predictive test for mycobacterial disease. *Ann Intern Med* 1980;92:512–513.

227. Rickman TW, Moyer NP. Increased sensitivity of acid-fast smears. *J Clin Microbiol* 1980;11:618–620.

228. Strumpf IJ, Tsang AV, Sayre JW. Re-evaluation of sputum staining for the diagnosis of pulmonary tuberculosis. *Am Rev Respir Dis* 1979;119: 599–602.

229. Lipsky BA, Gates J, Tenover FC, et al. Factors affecting the clinical value of microscopy for acid-fast bacilli. *Rev Infect Dis* 1984;6:214–222.

230. Gordin F, Slutkin G. The validity of acid-fast smears in the diagnosis of pulmonary tuberculosis. *Arch Pathol Lab Med* 1990;114:1025–1027.

231. Levy H, Feldman C, Sacho H, et al. A re-evaluation of sputum microscopy and culture in the diagnosis of pulmonary tuberculosis. *Chest* 1989;95:1193–1197.

232. Kim TC, Blackman RS, Heatwole KM, et al. Acid-fast bacilli in sputum smears of patients with tuberculosis: prevalence and significance of negative smears pretreatment and positive smears post-treatment. *Am Rev Respir Dis* 1984;129:264–268.

233. Canetti G. Present aspects of bacterial resistance in tuberculosis. *Am Rev Respir Dis* 1965;92:687–703.

234. Dunlap NE, Bass J, Fujiwara P, et al. American Thoracic Society Statement. Diagnostic Standards and Classification of Tuberculosis in Adults and Children. *Am J Respir Crit Care Med* 2000;161:1376–1395.

235. MacGregor RR, Clark LW, Bass F. The significance of isolating low numbers of *Mycobacterium tuberculosis* in culture of sputum specimens. *Chest* 1975;68:518–523.

236. Aber VR, Allen BW, Mitchison DA, et al. Quality control in tuberculosis bacteriology. 1. Laboratory studies on isolated positive cultures and the efficiency of direct smear examination. *Tubercle* 1980;61:123.

237. Mitchison DA, Keyes AB, Edwards EA, et al. Quality control in tuberculosis bacteriology. 2. The origin of isolated positive cultures from sputum of patients in four studies of short course chemotherapy in Africa. *Tubercle* 1980;67:135–144.

238. Narain R, Rao MS, Chandrasekhar P, et al. Microscopy positive and microscopy negative cases of pulmonary tuberculosis. *Am Rev Respir Dis* 1971;103:761–773.

239. Dunlap WE, Harris RH, Benjamin WH Jr, et al. Laboratory contamination of *Mycobacterium tuberculosis* cultures. *Am J Respir Crit Care Med* 1995;152:1702–1704.

240. Burman WJ, Stone BL, Reves RR, et al. The incidence of false-positive cultures for *Mycobacterium tuberculosis*. *Am J Respir Crit Care Med* 1997;155:321–326.

241. Braden C, Templeton G, Stead W, et al. Retrospective detection of laboratory cross contamination of *Mycobacterium tuberculosis* cultures with the use of DNA fingerprint analysis. *Clin Infect Dis* 1997;24:35–46.

242. Shilkret K, Liu Z, Santos F, et al. Misdiagnoses of tuberculosis resulting from laboratory cross-contamination of *Mycobacterium tuberculosis* cultures. New Jersey, 1998. *MMWR Morb Mortal Wkly Rep* 2000;49:413–416.

243. Chang CL, Kim HH, Son HC, et al. False-positive growth of *Mycobacterium tuberculosis* attributable to laboratory contamination confirmed by restriction fragment length polymorphism analysis. *Int J Tuberc Lung Dis* 2001;9:861–867.

244. Heifets L. False diagnosis of tuberculosis. *Int J Tuberc Lung Dis* 2001;9:789–790.

245. Long R. Smear-negative pulmonary tuberculosis in industrialized countries. *Chest* 2001;120:330–341.

246. Kanaya A, Glidden DV, Chambers HF. Identifying pulmonary tuberculosis in patients with negative sputum smear results. *Chest* 2001;120:349–355.

247. Colebunders R, Bastian. A review of the diagnosis and treatment of smear-negative pulmonary tuberculosis. *Int J Tuberc Lung Dis* 2000;4:97–107.

248. Harries AD, Maher D, Nunn P. An approach to the problems of diagnosing and treating adult smear-negative pulmonary tuberculosis in high HIV-prevalence settings in sub-Saharan Africa. *Bull World Health Organ* 1998;76:651–662.

249. Samb B, Sow PS, Kony S, et al. Risk factors for negative sputum acid-fast bacilli smears in pulmonary tuberculosis: results from Dakar, Senegal, a city with low HIV seroprevalance. *Int J Tuberc Lung Dis* 1999;4:330–336.

250. Hargreaves NJ, Kadzakumanja O, Phiri O, et al. What causes smear negative pulmonary tuberculosis in Malawi, an area of high HIV seroprevalence. *Int J Tuberc Lung Dis* 2001;5:113–122.

251. Murray CJL, Styblo K, Rouillon A. Tuberculosis in developing countries: burden intervention and cost. *Bull Int Union Tuberc Lung Dis* 1990;65:6–24.

252. Long R, Chui L, Kakulphimp J, et al. Postsanitorium pattern of antituberculous drug resistance in western Canada: effect of outpatient care and immigration. *Am J Epidemiol* 2001;153:903–911.

253. Behr MA, Warren SA, Salamon H, et al. Transmission of *Mycobacterium tuberculosis* from patients smear-negative for acid-fast bacilli. *Lancet* 1999;353:444–449 (published erratum apers in Lancet 1999;353:1714).

254. Eisenach KO, Sifford MD, Cave MD, et al. Detection of *Mycobacterium tuberculosis* in sputum samples using a polymerase chain reaction. *Am Rev Respir Dis* 1991;144:1160–1163.

255. Schluger NW, Kinney D, Harkin TJ, et al. Clinical utility of the polymerase chain reaction in the diagnosis of infections due to *Mycobacterium tuberculosis*. *Chest* 1994;105:1116–1121.

256. Schluger NW. Changing approaches to the diagnosis of tuberculosis. *Am J Respir Crit Care Med* 2001;164:2020–2024.

257. Dalovisio JR, Montenegro-James S, Kemmerly SA, et al. Comparison of the amplified *Mycobacterium tuberculosis* (MTB) direct test, Amplicor MTB PCR, and IS 6110-PCR for detection of MTB in respiratory specimens. *Clin Infect Dis* 1996;23:1099–1106.

258. Della-Latta P, Whittier S. Comprehensive evaluation of performance, laboratory application, and clinical usefulness of two direct amplification technologies for the detection of *Mycobacterium tuberculosis* complex. *Am J Clin Pathol* 1998;110:301–310.

259. Cheodore P, Jamieson FB. Routine use of the Gen-Probe MTD2 amplification test for detection of *Mycobacterium tuberculosis* in clinical specimens in a large public health mycobacteriology laboratory. *Diagn Microbiol Infect Dis* 1999;35:185–191.

260. Catanzaro A, Davidson BL, Fujiwara PI, et al. Rapid diagnostic tests for tuberculosis. What is the appropriate use? Proceedings of the American Thoracic Society Workshop. *Am J Respir Crit Care Med* 1997;155:1804–1814.

261. Catanzaro A, Perry S, Clarridge JF, et al. The role of clinical suspicion in evaluating a new diagnostic test for active tuberculosis: results of a multi-center prospective trial. *JAMA* 2000;283:639–645.

262. Cohen RA, Muzaffar S, Schwartz D, et al. Diagnosis of pulmonary tuberculosis using PCR assays on sputum collected within 24 hours of hospital admission. *Am J Respir Crit Care Med* 1998;157:156–161.

263. Roos BR, van Cleeff MR, Githui WA, et al. Cost-effectiveness of the polymerase chain reaction versus smear examination for the diagnosis of tuberculosis in Kenya: a theoretical model. *Int J Tuberc Lung Dis* 1998;2:235–241.

264. Shipman SJ. Diagnostic bronchoscopy in occult tuberculosis. *Am Rev Tuberc* 1939;39:629–632.

265. McIndoe RB, Steele JD, Samson PC, et al. Routine bronchoscopy in patients with active pulmonary tuberculosis. *Am Rev Tuberc* 1939;39:617–628.

266. Pecora DV, Yegia D. Bronchoscopy in the diagnosis and localization of bacteriologically positive tuberculosis lesions. *Am Rev Tuberc* 1956;73:586–588.

267. Kvale PA, Johnson MC, Wroblewski DA. Diagnosis of tuberculosis: routine cultures of bronchial washings are not indicated. *Chest* 1979;76:140–142.

268. Neff TA. Bronchoscopy and Bactec for the diagnosis of tuberculosis: state of the art, or a brief dissertation on the efficient search for the tubercle bacillus? *Am Rev Respir Dis* 1986;133:962.

269. Jett JR, Cortese DA, Dines DE. The value of bronchoscopy in the diagnosis of mycobacterial disease. *Chest* 1981;80:575–578.

270. Russell MD, Torrington KG, Tenholder MF. A ten-year experience with fiberoptic bronchoscopy for mycobacterial isolation. *Am Rev Respir Dis* 1986;133:1069–1071.

271. Ip M, Chan PY, So SY, et al. The value of routine bronchial aspirate culture at fibreoptic bronchoscopy for the diagnosis of tuberculosis. *Tubercle* 1989;70:281–285.

272. Danek SJ, Bower JS. Diagnosis of pulmonary tuberculosis by flexible fiberoptic bronchoscopy. *Am Rev Respir Dis* 1979;119:677–679.

273. Wallace JM, Deutsch AL, Harrel JH, et al. Bronchoscopy and transbronchial biopsy in evaluation of patients with suspected active tuberculosis. *Am J Med* 1981;70:1189–1194.

274. Sarkar SK, Sharma GS, Gupta PR, et al. Fiberoptic bronchoscopy in the diagnosis of pulmonary tuberculosis. *Tubercle* 1980;61:97–99.

275. So SY, Lam WK, Yu DYC. Rapid diagnosis of suspected pulmonary tuberculosis by fiberoptic bronchoscopy. *Tubercle* 1982;63:195–200.

276. Wilcox PA, Benatar SR, Potgieter PD. Use of the flexible fibreoptic bronchoscope in diagnosis of sputum-negative pulmonary tuberculosis. *Thorax* 1982;37:598–601.

277. de Gracia J, Curull V, Vidal R, et al. Diagnostic value of bronchoalveolar lavage in suspected pulmonary tuberculosis. *Chest* 1988;93:329–332.

278. Khoo KK, Meadway J. Fiberoptic bronchoscopy in rapid diagnosis of sputum smear negative pulmonary tuberculosis. *Respir Med* 1989;83:335–338.

279. Mehta J, Krish G, Berro E, et al. Fiberoptic bronchoscopy in the diagnosis of pulmonary tuberculosis. *S Med J* 1990;83:753–755.

280. Al-Kassimi FA, Azhar M, Al-Majed, et al. Diagnostic role of fibreoptic bronchoscopy in tuberculosis in the presence of typical x-ray pictures and adequate sputum. *Tubercle* 1991;72:145–148.

281. Kennedy DJ, Lewis WP, Barnes PF. Yield of bronchoscopy for the diagnosis of tuberculosis in patients with human immunodeficiency virus infection. *Chest* 1992;102:1040–1044.

282. Chan CHS, Chan RCY, Arnold M, et al. Bronchoscopy and tuberculostearic acid assay in the diagnosis of sputum smear–negative pulmonary tuberculosis: a prospective study with the addition of transbronchial biopsy. *Q J Med* 1992;297:15–23.

283. Chawla R, Pant K, Jaggi OP, et al. Fiberoptic bronchoscopy in smear-negative pulmonary tuberculosis. *Eur Respir J* 1988;1:804–806.

284. Chan WS, Sun AJM, Woheisel GB. Bronchoscopic aspiration and bronchoalveolar lavage in the diagnosis of sputum smear-negative pulmonary tuberculosis. *Lung* 1990;168:215–220.

285. Levy H, Feldman C, Kallenbach JM. The diagnostic yield of prebronchoscopy sputa and bronchial washings in patients with biopsy-proven pulmonary tuberculosis. *S Afr Med J* 1989;78:527–528.

286. Stensen W, Aranda C, Bevelaqua FA. Transbronchial biopsy culture in pulmonary tuberculosis. *Chest* 1983;83:883–884.

287. Funahashi A, Lohaus GH, Politis J, et al. Role of fiberoptic bronchoscopy in the diagnosis of mycobacterial diseases. *Thorax* 1983;38:267–270.

288. Fujii H, Fukaura A, Kashima N, et al. Early diagnosis of tuberculosis by fibreoptic bronchoscopy. *Tuberc Lung* 1992;73:167–169.

289. Tevola K. Bronchial aspiration in the diagnosis of pulmonary tuberculosis. *Scand J Resp Dis* 1974;89(Supp):151–154.

290. Norrman E, Keistinen T, Uddenfeldt M, et al. Bronchoalveolar lavage is better than gastric lavage in the diagnosis of pulmonary tuberculosis. *Scand J Infect Dis* 1988;20:77–88.

291. Baughman RP, Dohn MN, Loudon RG, et al. Bronchoscopy with bronchoalveolar lavage in tuberculosis and fungal infections. *Chest* 1991;99:92–97.

292. Charoenratanakul S, Dejsomritrutai W, Chaiprasert A. Diagnostic role of fibreoptic bronchoscopy in suspected smear negative pulmonary tuberculosis. *Respir Med* 1995;89:621–623.

293. Wong CF, Yew WW, Chan CY, et al. Rapid diagnosis of smear-positive pulmonary tuberculosis via fiberoptic bronchoscopy:

utility of polymerase chain reaction in bronchial aspirates as an adjunct to transbronchial biopsies. *Respir Med* 1998;92: 815–819.

294. Lai R-S, Lee S-J, Ting H-C, et al. Diagnostic value of transbronchial lung biopsy under fluoroscopic guidance in solitary pulmonary nodule in an endemic area of tuberculosis. *Respir Med* 1996;90:139–143.

295. Salajka F, Mezensky L, Pokorny A. Commercial polymerase chain reaction test (Amplicor set) in the diagnosis of smear-negative pulmonary tuberculosis from sputum and bronchoalveolar lavage. *Monaldi Arch Chest Dis* 2000;55:9–12.

296. Chen NH, Liu YC, Tsao TC, et al. Combined bronchoalveolar lavage and polymerase chain reaction in the diagnosis of pulmonary tuberculosis in smear-negative patients. *Int J Tuberc Lung Dis* 2002;4:350–355.

297. Conte BA, Laforet EG. The role of the topical anesthetic agent in modifying bacteriologic data by bronchoscopy. *N Engl J Med* 1962;267:957–960.

298. Erlich H. Bacteriologic studies and effects of anesthetic solutions on bronchial secretions during bronchoscopy. *Am Rev Respir Dis* 1961;84:414–421.

299. Schmidt RM, Rosenkranz HS. Antimicrobial activity of local anesthetics: lidocaine and procaine. *J Infect Dis* 1970;121: 597–607.

300. Dhand R, De A, Ganguly NK, et al. Factors influencing the cellular response in bronchoalveolar lavage and peripheral blood of patients with pulmonary tuberculosis. *Tubercle* 1989;69: 161–173.

301. Ozaki T, Nakahira S, Tani K, et al. Differential cell analysis in bronchoalveolar lavage fluid from pulmonary lesions of patients with tuberculosis. *Chest* 1992;102:54–59.

302. Baron KM, Aranda CP. Diagnosis of mediastinal mycobacterial lymphadenopathy by transbronchial needle aspiration. *Chest* 1991;100:1723–1724.

303. Harkin TJ, Ciotoli C, Adrizzo-Harris DJ, et al. Transbronchial needle aspiration (TBNA) in patients infected with HIV. *Am Rev Respir Crit Care Med* 1998;157:1913-1918.

304. Wilcox PA, Potgieter PD, Bateman ED, et al. Rapid diagnosis of sputum negative miliary tuberculosis using the flexible fibreoptic bronchoscope. *Thorax* 1986;41:681–684.

305. Pant K, Chawla R, Mann PS, et al. Fiberoptic bronchoscopy in smear-negative miliary tuberculosis. *Chest* 1989;95:1151–1152.

306. Pereira W, Kovnat DM, Snider GL. Fever and pneumonia following fiberoptic bronchoscopy. *Am Rev Respir Dis* 1975;112: 59–64.

307. Pereira W Jr, Kovnat DM, Snider GL. A prospective study of complications following flexible fiberoptic bronchoscopy. *Chest* 1978;73:813–816.

308. Rimmer J, Gibson P, Bryant DH. Extension of pulmonary tuberculosis after fibreoptic bronchoscopy. *Tubercle* 1988;69: 57–61.

309. Nelson E, Larson PA, Schraufnagel DE, et al. Transmission of tuberculosis by flexible fiberbronchoscopes. *Am Rev Respir Dis* 1983;127:97–100.

310. Michele TM, Cronin WA, Graham MH, et al. Transmission of *Mycobacterium tuberculosis* by a fiberoptic bronchoscope. *JAMA* 1997;278:1093–1095.

311. Dawson DJ, Armstrong JG, Blacklock ZM. Mycobacterial cross-contamination of bronchoscopy specimens. *Am Rev Respir Dis* 1982;126:1095–1097.

312. Jackson J, Leggett JE, Wilson D, et al. Mycobacterium gordonae in fiberoptic bronchoscopes. *Am J Infect Control* 1996; 24:19-23.

313. Best M, Sattar SA, Springthorpe VS, et al. Efficacies of selected disinfectants against *Mycobacterium tuberculosis*. *J Clin Microbiol* 1990;28:2234–2239.

314. Martin MA, Reichelderfer M. APIC guideline for infection prevention and control in flexible endoscopy. *Am J Infect Control* 1994;22:19–23.

315. Shim TS, Chi JS, Lee DS, et al. Adequately washed bronchoscope does not induce false-positive amplification tests on bronchial aspirates in the diagnosis of pulmonary tuberculosis. *Chest* 2002;121:774–781.

316. Hsing CT, Ma YT. A comparative study of the efficacy of laryngeal swab, bronchial lavage, gastric lavage, and direct sputum examination methods in detecting tubercle bacilli in a series of 1,320 patients. *Am Rev Respir Dis* 1962;86:16–20.

317. Lees AW, Miller TJR, Roberts GBS. Bronchial lavage for recovery of the tubercle bacillus. Comparison with gastric lavage and laryngeal swabbing. *Lancet* 1955;269:800–801.

318. Strumpf IJ, Tsang AY, Schork MA, et al. The reliability of gastric smears by auramine-rhodamine staining technique for the diagnosis of tuberculosis. *Am Rev Respir Dis* 1976;114: 971–976.

319. John GT, Juneja R, Mukundan U, et al. Gastric aspiration for diagnosis of pulmonary tuberculosis in adult renal allograft recipients. *Transplantation* 1996;61:972–973.

320. Bahammam A, Choudhri S, Long R. The validity of acid-fast smears of gastric aspirates as an indicator of pulmonary tuberculosis. *Int J Tuberc Lung Dis* 1999;3:62–67.

321. Rizvi N, Rao NA, Houssain M. Yield of gastric lavage and bronchial wash in pulmonary tuberculosis. *Int J Tuberc Lung Dis* 2000;4:147–151.

322. Pomputius WF, Rost J, Dennehy PH, et al. Standardization of gastric aspirate technique improves yield in the diagnosis of tuberculosis in children. *Pediatr Infect Dis J.* 1997;16:222–226.

323. Abadco DL, Steiner P. Gastric lavage is better than bronchoalveolar lavage for isolation of *Mycobacterium tuberculosis* in childhood tuberculosis. *Pediatr Infect Dis J.* 1992;11:735–738.

324. Somy NS, Swaminathan G, Paramasvian D, et al. Value of bronchoalveolar lavage and gastric lavage in the diagnosis of pulmonary tuberculosis in children. *Tuber Lung Dis* 1995;78: 295–299.

325. Thadepalli H, Rambhatia K, Niden AH. Transtracheal aspiration in diagnosis of sputum-smear-negative tuberculosis. *JAMA* 1977;238:1037.

326. Schmerber-Vereerstraeten J, Schoutens E, Lempereur L, et al. Usefulness of transtracheal puncture and aspiration in the bacteriological diagnosis of pulmonary tuberculosis. *Infection* 1977; 5:132–136.

327. Sinner WN. Fine needle biopsy of tuberculomas (letter). *Chest* 1984;85:836.

328. Gomes I, Trindade E, Vidal O, et al. Diagnosis of sputum smear-negative forms of pulmonary tuberculosis by transthoracic fine-needle aspiration. *Tubercle* 1991;72:210–213.

329. Qadri SMH, Akhtar M, Ali MA. Sensitivity of fine needle aspiration biopsy in the detection of mycobacterial infections. *Diagn Cytopathol* 1991;7:142–146.

330. Baily TM, Akhtar M, Ali MA. Fine needle aspiration biopsy in the diagnosis of tuberculosis. *Acta Cytol* 1985;29:732–735.

331. Yew WW, Kwan SYL, Wong PC, et al. Percutaneous transthoracic needle biopsies in the rapid diagnosis of pulmonary tuberculosis. *Lung* 1991;169:285–289.

332. Yew WW, Wong PC, Lee J, et al. Rapid diagnosis of smear-negative pulmonary tuberculosis (letter). *Chest* 1994;106:327–328.

333. Kang EY, Choi JA, Seo BK, et al. Utility of polymerase chain reaction for detecting *Mycobacterium tuberculosis* in specimens from percutaneous transthoracic needle aspiration. *Radiology* 2002;225:205–209.

334. Khan J, Akhtar M, von Sinner WN, et al. CT-guided fine needle aspiration biopsy in the diagnosis of mediastinal tuberculosis. *Chest* 1994;106:1329–1332.

335. Hutchinson J. On the capacity of the lungs, and on the respiratory functions, with a view to establishing a precise and easy method of detecting disease by the spirometer. *Trans Med-Chir Soc London* 1846;29:137–252.

336. Anno H, Tomashefski JF. Studies on the impairment of respiratory function in pulmonary tuberculosis. *Am Rev Tuberc* 1955; 71:333–348.

337. Simpson DG, Kuschner M, McClement J. Respiratory function in pulmonary tuberculosis. *Am Rev Respir Dis* 1963;87:1–16.

338. Lopez-Majano V. Ventilation and transfer of gases in pulmonary tuberculosis. *Respiration* 1973;30:48–63.

339. Skoogh BE. Lung mechanics in pulmonary tuberculosis. I. Static lung volumes. *Scand J Respir Dis* 1973;54:148–156.

340. Lancaster JF, Tomashefski JF. Tuberculosis—a cause of emphysema. *Am Rev Respir Dis* 1963;87:435–437.

341. Snider GL, Doctor L, Demas TA, et al. Obstructive airway disease in patients with treated pulmonary tuberculosis. *Am Rev Respir Dis* 1971;103:625–640.

342. Skoogh BE. Lung mechanics in pulmonary tuberculosis. II. Airways conductance at different lung volumes. *Scand J Respir Dis* 1973;54:369–378.

343. Skoogh BE. Lung mechanics in pulmonary tuberculosis. III. Bronchial reactivity. *Scand J Respir Dis* 1973;54:379–387.

344. Cameron SJ. Tuberculosis and the blood-a special relationship? *Tubercle* 1974;55:55–72.

345. Muller GL. *Clinical significance of blood in tuberculosis.* New York: Commonwealth Fund, 1943.

346. Corr WP, Kyle RA, Bowie EJ. Hematologic changes in tuberculosis. *Am J Med Sci* 1964;122:709–714.

347. Klipstein FA, Berlinger FG, Reed LJ. Folate deficiency associated with drug therapy for tuberculosis. *Blood* 1967;29: 697–712.

348. Roberts PD, Hoffbrand AV, Mollin VL. Iron and folate metabolism in tuberculosis. *BMJ* 1966;2:198–202.

349. Morris CD, Bird AR, Nell H. The hematological and biochemical changes in severe tuberculosis. *Q J Med* 1989;73: 1151–1159.

350. Baynes RD, Flax H, Bothwell TH, et al. Hematological and iron-related measurements in active pulmonary tuberculosis. *Scand J Haematol* 1986;36:280–287.

351. Cameron SJ, Horne NW. The effect of tuberculosis and its treatment on erythropoiesis and folate activity. *Tubercle* 1971;52:37–48.

352. Markkanen T, Lavantoe A, Fallinen G, et al. Folic acid and vitamin B$_{12}$ in tuberculosis. *Scand J Haematol* 1969;4:283–291.

353. Baynes RD, Bothwell TH, Flax H, et al. Reactive thrombocytosis in pulmonary tuberculosis. *J Clin Pathol* 1987;40: 676–679.

354. Beck JS, Potts RC, Kardjito T, et al. T4 lymphopenia in patients with active pulmonary tuberculosis. *Clin Exp Immunol* 1985; 60:49–54.

355. Onwubalili JK, Edwards AJ, Palmer L. T4 lymphopenia in human tuberculosis. *Tubercle* 1987;68:195–200.

356. Bhatnagar R, Nalaviya AN, Narayanan S, et al. Spectrum of immune response abnormalities in different clinical forms of tuberculosis. *Am Rev Respir Dis* 1977;115:207–212.

357. Beck JS, Potts RC, Kardjito T, et al. T4 lymphopenia in patients with active pulmonary tuberculosis. *Clin Exp Immunol* 1985; 60:49–54.

358. Schmitt, Neuert G, Stix L. Monocyte recruitment in tuberculosis and sarcoidosis. *Br J Haematol* 1977;35:11–17.

359. Holdiness MR. A review of blood dyscrasias induced by the antituberculosis drugs. *Tubercle* 1987;68:301–309.

360. Berry FB. Tuberculous pyopneumothorax with pyogenic infection. *J Thorac Surg* 1932;2:139–153.

361. Eglee EP, Wylie RH. Empyema and the unexpanded lung following artificial pneumothorax for tuberculosis. *J Thorac Surg* 1941;10:603–616.

362. Reemtsama, Clauss RH, Wylie RH. The management of spontaneous pneumothorax complicating pulmonary tuberculosis. *Am Rev Tuberc* 1956;74:351–357.

363. Wilder RJ, Beacham EG, Ravitch MM. Spontaneous pneumothorax complicating cavitary tuberculosis. *J Thorac Cardiovasc Surg* 1962;43:561–573.

364. Ihm HJ, Hankins JR, Miller JE, et al. Pneumothorax associated with pulmonary tuberculosis. *J Thorac Cardiovasc Surg* 1972;64: 211–219.

365. Peiken AS, Lamberta F, Seriff NS. Bilateral recurrent pneumothoraces: a rare complication of miliary tuberculosis. *Am Rev Respir Dis* 1974;110:512–517.

366. Narang RK, Kumar S, Gupta A. Pneumothorax and pneumomediastinum complicating acute miliary tuberculosis. *Tubercle* 1977;58:79–82.

367. Yagi T, Yamagishi F, Sasaki Y, et al. Clinical review of pneumothorax cases complicated with active pulmonary tuberculosis (Japanese). *Kekkaku* 2002;77:395–399.

368. Auerbach O, Lipstein S. Bronchopleural fistulas complicating pulmonary tuberculosis. *J Thorac Surg* 1939;8:384–411.

369. Johnson TM, McCann W, Davey WN. Tuberculous bronchopleural fistula. *Am Rev Respir Dis* 1973;107:30–41.

370. Belmonte R, Crowe HM. Pneumothorax in patients with pulmonary tuberculosis (letter). *Clin Infect Dis* 1995;20:1565.

371. Donath J, Kahn FA. Tuberculous and posttuberculous bronchopleural fistula. *Chest* 1984;86:697–703.

372. Lambert HP. Spontaneous pneumothorax and pulmonary tuberculosis. *Tubercle* 1956;37:207–209.

373. Heller R. The significance of haemoptysis. *Tubercle* 1946;26: 70–74.

374. Abbott OA. The clinical significance of pulmonary hemorrhage: a study of 1316 patients with chest disease. *Dis Chest* 1948;14:824–839.

375. Levitt N. Clinical significance of hemoptysis. *J Mich State Med Soc* 1951;50:606–610.

376. Crocco JA, Rooney JJ, Fankushen DS, et al. Massive hemoptysis. *Arch Intern Med* 1968;121:495–498.

377. Hirshberg B, Biran I, Glazer M, et al. Hemoptysis: etiology, evaluation, and outcome in a tertiary referral hospital. *Chest* 1997;112:440–444.

378. Fidan A, Ozdogan S, Salepci B, et al. Hemoptysis: a retrospective analysis of 108 cases. *Respir Med* 2002;96:677–680.

379. Fern SW. Aneurysm of the pulmonary artery (letter). *Lancet* 1840–1841;1:679.

380. Rasmussen V, WD Moore (trans). *On hemoptysis, especially when fatal in its anatomical and clinical aspects.* (Reprinted from *Hospitals-Tilende*, 11th ed., No. 9-13, 1868.) *Edinburgh Med J* 1868;14:384, 486–503.

381. Rasmussen V, Moore WD (trans). Continued observations on hemoptysis. *Edinburgh Med J* 1869;15:97–104.

382. Cudkowicz L. The blood supply of the lung in pulmonary tuberculosis. *Thorax* 1952;7:270–276.

383. Thompson JR. Mechanisms of fatal pulmonary hemorrhage in tuberculosis. *Am J Surg* 1955;89:637–644.

384. Liebow AA, Hales MR, Lindskog GE. Enlargement of the bronchial arteries and their anastomoses with the pulmonary arteries in bronchiectasis. *Am J Pathol* 1949;25:211–233.

385. Stinghe RV, Mangivlea VG. Hemoptysis of bronchial origin occurring in patients with arrested tuberculosis. *Am Rev Respir Dis* 1970;101:84–89.

386. British Thoracic and Tuberculosis Association Research Committee. Aspergilloma and residual tuberculous cavities—the results of a survey. *Tubercle* 1970;51:227–245.

387. Conlan AA, Abramor E, Moyes DG. Pulmonary aspergil-

loma—indications for surgical intervention. An analysis of 22 cases. *S Afr Med J* 1987;71:285–288.

388. Varkey B, Rose HD. Pulmonary aspergilloma. A rational approach to treatment. *Am J Med* 1976;61:626–631.

389. Jewkes J, et al. Pulmonary aspergilloma: analysis of prognosis in relation to haemoptysis and survey of treatment. *Thorax* 1983;38:572–578.

390. Butz RO, Zvetina JR, Leininger BJ. Ten year experience with mycetomas in patients with pulmonary tuberculosis. *Chest* 1985;87:356–358.

391. Tomlinson JR, Sahn SA. Aspergilloma in sarcoid and tuberculosis. *Chest* 1987;92:505–508.

392. Schmidt HW, Clagett OT, McDonald JR. Broncholithiasis. *J Thorac Cardiovasc Surg* 1950;19:226–245.

393. Groves LK, Effler DB. Broncholithiasis. *Am Rev Tuberc* 1956;73:19–30.

394. Dixon GE, Donnerberg RL, Schonfeld SA, et al. Advances in the diagnosis and treatment of broncholithiasis. *Am Rev Respir Dis* 1984;129:1028–1030.

395. Cooley DA. The clinical significance of cavernoliths. *J Thorac Cardiovasc Surg* 1953;25:240–255.

396. Goldermans D, Verhaert J, Van Meerbeeck H, et al. Broncholithiasis: present clinical spectrum. *Respir Med* 1990;84:155–156.

397. Conces DJ, Tarver RD, Vix VA. Broncholithiasis: CT features in 15 patients. *AJR Am J Roentgenol* 1991;157:249–253.

398. Middleton JR, Sen P, Lange M, et al. Death-producing hemoptysis in tuberculosis. *Chest* 1977;72:601–604.

399. Yeoh CB, Hubaytar RT, Ford JM, et al. Treatment of massive hemorrhage in pulmonary tuberculosis. *J Thorac Cardiovasc Surg* 1967;54:503–510.

400. Bobrowitz ID, Ramakrishna S, Shim Y-S. Comparison of medical vs surgical treatment of major hemoptysis. *Arch Intern Med* 1983;143:1343–1346.

401. Corey R, Hla KM. Major and massive hemoptysis: reassessment of conservative management. *Am J Med Sci* 1987;294:301–309.

402. Amirana M, Frater R, Tirschwell P, et al. An aggressive surgical approach to significant hemoptysis in patients with pulmonary tuberculosis. *Am Rev Respir Dis* 1968;97:187–192.

403. Garzon AA, Cerruti MM, Goldring ME. Exsanguinating hemoptysis. *J Thorac Cardiovasc Surg* 1982;84:829–833.

404. Conlan AA, Hurwitz SS, Krige L, et al. Massive hemoptysis: review of 123 cases. *J Thorac Cardiovasc Surg* 1983;85:120–124.

405. Muthuswamy PP, Akbik F, Franklin C, et al. Management of major or massive hemoptysis in active pulmonary tuberculosis by bronchial arterial embolization. *Chest* 1987;92:77–82.

406. Uflacker R, Kaemmerer A, Picon P, et al. Bronchial artery embolization in the management of hemoptysis: technical aspects and long-term results. *Radiology* 1985;157:637–644.

407. Santelli ED, Katz DG, Goldschmidt AM, et al. Embolization of multiple Rasmussen aneurysms as a treatment of hemoptysis. *Radiology* 1994;193:396–398.

408. Ramakantan R, Bandekar VG, Gandhi MS, et al. Massive hemoptysis due to pulmonary tuberculosis: control with bronchial artery embolization. *Radiology* 1996;200:691–694.

409. Wong ML, Szkup P, Hopley MJ. Percutaneous embolotherapy for life-threatening hemoptysis. *Chest* 2002;121:95–102.

410. Rilance AB, Gerstl B. Bronchiectasis secondary to pulmonary tuberculosis. *Am Rev Tuberc* 1943;48:8–24.

411. Roberts JC, Blair LG. Bronchiectasis in primary tuberculosis. *Lancet* 1950;1:386–388.

412. Brock RC. Post-tuberculous broncho-stenosis and bronchiectasis of the middle lobe. *Thorax* 1950;5:5–39.

413. Rosenzweig DY, Stead WW. The role of tuberculosis and other forms of bronchopulmonary necrosis in the pathogenesis of bronchiectasis. *Am Rev Respir Dis* 1966;93:769–785.

414. Curtis JK. The significance of bronchiectasis associated with pulmonary tuberculosis. *Am J Med* 1957;22:894–903.

415. Hatipoglu ON, Osma E, Manisali M, et al. High resolution computed tomographic findings in pulmonary tuberculosis. *Thorax* 1996;51:397–402.

416. Cartier Y, Cavanagh PV, Johkoh T, et al. Bronchiectasis: accuracy of high-resolution CT in differentiation of specific diseases. *Am J Roentgenol* 1999;173:47–52.

417. McGuinness G, Naidich DP. Bronchiectasis: CT/clinical correlations. *Semin Ultrasound Comput Tomogr Magnet Reson Imaging* 1995;16:395–419.

418. McGuinness G, Naidich DP, Leitman BS, et al. Bronchiectasis: CT evaluation. *AJR Am J Roentgenol* 1993;160:253–259.

419. Cohen AG. Atelectasis of the right middle lobe resulting from perforation of tuberculous lymph nodes into bronchi in adults. *Ann Intern Med* 1951;35:820–835.

420. Lindskog GE, Spear HC. Middle lobe syndrome. *N Engl J Med* 1955;253:489–495.

421. Inners CR, Terry PB, Traystman RJ, et al. Collateral ventilation and the middle lobe syndrome. *Am Rev Respir Dis* 1978;118:305–310.

422. Palmer PES. Pulmonary tuberculosis—usual and unusual radiographic presentations. *Sem Roentgenol* 1979;14:28–67.

423. Bobrowitz FD, Rodescu D, Marcus H, et al. The destroyed tuberculous lung. *Scand J Respir Dis* 1974;55:82–88.

424. Khan FA, Rehman M, Marcus P, et al. Pulmonary gangrene occurring as a complication of pulmonary tuberculosis. *Chest* 1980;77:76–80.

425. Lopez-Contreras J, Ris J, Domingo P, et al. Tuberculous pulmonary gangrene. *Clin Infect Dis* 1994;18:243–245.

426. Lorenz R, Kraman SS. Intracavitary mass in a patient with far-advanced tuberculosis. *Chest* 1982;82:91–92.

427. Simons J, Friedman J, Theodore J, et al. Pneumonectomy for unilateral lung disease associated with respiratory failure. *Am Rev Respir Dis* 1973;108:652–655.

428. Park JH, Na Jo, Kim EK et al. The prognosis of respiratory failure in patients with tuberculous destroyed lung. *Int J Tuberc Lung Dis* 2001;5:963–967.

429. Penner C, Roberts D, Kunimoto D, et al. Tuberculosis as a primary cause of respiratory failure requiring mechanical ventilation. *Am J Respir Crit Care Med* 1995;151:867–872.

430. Smith IE, Laroche CM, Jamieson SA, et al. Kyphoscoliosis secondary to tuberculosis osteomyelitis as a cause of ventilatory failure. *Chest* 1996;110:1105–1110.

431. Frame RN, Johnson MC, Eichenhorn MS, et al. Active tuberculosis in the medical intensive care unit: a 15-year retrospective analysis. *Crit Care Med* 1987;15:1012–1014.

432. Levy H, Kallenbach JM, Feldman C, et al. Acute respiratory failure in active tuberculosis. *Crit Care Med* 1987;15:221–225.

433. Choi D, Lee KS, Suh GY, et al. Pulmonary tuberculosis presenting as acute respiratory failure: radiologic findings. *J Comput Assist Tomogr* 1999;23:107–113.

434. Goldfine ID, Schachter H, Barclay WR, et al. Consumption coagulopathy in miliary tuberculosis. *Ann Intern Med* 1969;71:775–777.

435. Agarwal MK, Muthuswamy PP, Banner AS, et al. Respiratory failure in pulmonary tuberculosis. *Chest* 1977;72:605–609.

436. Heffner JE, Strange C, Sahn SA. The impact of respiratory failure on the diagnosis of tuberculosis. *Arch Intern Med* 1988;148:1103–1108.

437. Homan W, Harman E, Braun NM, et al. MIliary tuberculosis presenting as acute respiratory failure: treatment by membrane oxygenator and ventricle pump. *Chest* 1975;67:366-369.

438. Huseby JS, Hudson LD. Miliary tuberculosis and adult respiratory distress syndrome. *Ann Intern Med* 1976;85:609–611.

439. Murray HW, Tuazon CU, Kirmani N,et al. The adult respira-

tory distress syndrome associated with miliary tuberculosis. *Chest* 1978;73:37–43.

440. DeSilva A, Gibson J, Gilbert DN. Miliary tuberculosis and adult respiratory distress syndrome. *Ann Intern Med* 1977;86:659.

441. Hus JT, Padula JP, Ryan SF. Miliary tuberculosis and adult respiratory distress syndrome. *Ann Intern Med* 1978;89:140–141.

442. Raimondi AC, Olmedo G, Roncoroni AJ. Acute miliary tuberculosis presenting as acute respiratory failure. *Intensive Care Med* 1978;4:207–209.

443. Zimmerman HM, Wertheimer DE, Rosner F. Miliary tuberculosis and adult respiratory distress syndrome. *NY State J Med* 1981;81(5):787–789.

444. So SY, Yu D. The adult respiratory distress syndrome associated with miliary tuberculosis. *Tuber Lung Dis* 1981;62:49–53.

445. Vaz AJ. Miliary tuberculosis and the adult respiratory distress syndrome in a renal transplant recipient. *Chest* 1979;75:412.

446. Krauss JS, Walker DH. Miliary tuberculosis and consumption of clotting factors by multifocal vasculopathic coagulation. *South Med J* 1979;72:1479–1481.

447. Fieber SS, Cohn JD, Jacobs FM. Adult respiratory distress syndrome secondary to activated miliary tuberculosis following surgery. *J Med Soc NJ* 1979;76:357–360.

448. Dee P, Teja K, Korzeniowski O, Suratt PM. Miliary tuberculosis resulting in adult respiratory distress syndrome: a surviving case. *AJR Am J Roentgenol* 1980;569–572.

449. Pasculle AW, Kapadia SB, Ho M. Tuberculous bacillemia, hyperexia and rapid death. *Arch Intern Med* 1980;426–427.

450. Hurwitz SS, Marinopoulos G, Conlan AA, et al. Adult respiratory distress syndrome associated with miliary tuberculosis. *S Afr Med J* 1984;65:27–28.

451. Dyer RA, Chappell WA, Potgieter PD. Adult respiratory distress syndrome associated with miliary tuberculosis. *Crit Care Med* 1985;13:12–15.

452. Piqueras AR, Marruecos L, Artigas A, et al. Miliary tuberculosis and adult respiratory distress syndrome. *Intensive Care Med* 1987;13:174–182.

453. Lintin SN, Isaac PA. Miliary tuberculosis presenting as adult respiratory distress syndrome. *Intensive Care Med* 1988;14:672–674.

454. Heap MJ, Bion JF, Hunter KR. Miliary tuberculosis and the adult respiratory distress syndrome. *Respir Med* 1989;83:153–156.

455. Gachot B, Wolff M, Clair B, et al. Severe tuberculosis in patients with human immunodeficiency virus infection. *Intensive Care Med* 1990;16:491–493.

456. Akira M, Sakatani M. Clinical and high-resolution computed tomographic findings in five patients with pulmonary tuberculosis who developed respiratory failure following chemotherapy. *Clin Radiol* 2001;56:550–555.

457. Zahar JR, Azoulay E, DeLassence A, et al. Delayed treatment contributes to mortality in ICU patients with severe active pulmonary tuberculosis and acute respiratory failure. *Intensive Care Med* 2001;27:513–520.

458. Sacks LV, Pendle S. Factors related to in-hospital deaths in patients with tuberculosis. *Arch Intern Med* 1998;158:1916–1922.

459. Toscano V, Bontadini A, Falson G, et al. Thrombotic thrombocytopenic purpura associated with primary tuberculosis. *Infection* 1995;23:58–59.

460. Pene F, Papo T, Brudy-Gulphe L, et al. Septic shock and thrombotic microangiopathy nonimmunocompromised patient (letter). *Arch Intern Med* 2001;161:1347–1348.

461. Pagel W. The evolution of tuberculosis in man. In: Pagel W, Simmonds EAJ, Norman M, eds. *Pulmonary tuberculosis*, 4th ed. New York: Oxford University Press, 1964:147–161.

462. Ahuja SS, Ahuja SK, Phelps KR, et al. Hemodynamic confirmation of septic shock in disseminated tuberculosis. *Crit Care Med* 1992;20:901–903.

463. Vadillo M, Corbella X, Carratala J. AIDS presenting as septic shock caused by *Mycobacterium tuberculosis*. *Scand J Infect Dis* 1994;26:105–106.

464. George S, Papa L, Sheils L, et al. Septic shock due to disseminated tuberculosis. *Clin Infect Dis* 1996;22:188–189.

465. Clark TM, Burman WJ, Cohn DL, et al. Septic shock from *Mycobacterium tuberculosis* after therapy for *Pneumocystis carinii*. *Arch Intern Med* 1998;158:1033–1035.

466. Angoulvant D, Mohammedi I, Duperret S, et al. Septic shock caused by *Mycobacterium tuberculosis* in a non-HIV patient (letter). *Intensive Care Med* 1999;25:238.

467. Morehead RS. Delayed death from pulmonary tuberculosis: unsuspected subtherapeutic drug levels. *S Med J* 2000;93:507–510.

468. Berger HW, Rosenbaum I. Prolonged fever in patients treated for tuberculosis. *Am Rev Respir Dis* 1968;87:140–143.

469. Kiblawi SSO, Jay SJ. Stonehill RB, et al. Fever response of patients on therapy for pulmonary tuberculosis. *Am Rev Respir Dis* 1981;123:20–24.

470. Barnes PF, Chan LS, Wong SF. The course of fever during treatment of pulmonary tuberculosis. *Tubercle* 1987;68:255–260.

471. Saloman N, Perlman DC, Friedman P, et al. Predictors and outcome of multidrug-resistant tuberculosis. *Clin Infect Dis* 1995;21:1245–1252.

472. Barnes PF, Lu S, Abrams JS. Cytokine production at the site of disease in tuberculosis. *Infect Immun* 1993;62:3482–3489.

473. Muthuswamy P, Hu T-C, Carasso B. Prednisone as adjunctive therapy in the management of pulmonary tuberculosis: report of 12 cases and review of the literature. *Chest* 1995;107:1621–1630.

474. Alzeer AH, FitzGerald JM. Corticosteroids and tuberculosis: risks and use as adjunct therapy. *Tuber Lung Dis* 1993;74:6–11.

475. Loudon RG, Roberts RM. Droplet expulsion from the respiratory tract. *Am Rev Respir Dis* 1967;95:435–442.

476. Loudon RG, Spohn SK. Cough frequency and infectivity in patients with pulmonary tuberculosis. *Am Rev Respir Dis* 1969;99:109–111.

477. Bobrowitz ID. Reversible roentgenographic progression in the initial treatment of pulmonary tuberculosis. *Am Rev Respir Dis* 1980;121:735–742.

478. Onwubalili JK, Scatt GM, Smith H. Acute respiratory distress related to chemotherapy of advanced pulmonary tuberculosis: a study of two cases and review of the literature. *Q J Med* 1986;230:599–610.

479. Gordin FEM, Slutkin G, Schecter G, et al. Presumptive diagnosis and treatment of pulmonary tuberculosis based on radiographic findings. *Am Rev Respir Dis* 1989;139:1090–1093.

480. Albert RK, Iseman M, Sbarbaro JA, et al. Monitoring patients with tuberculosis for failure during and after treatment. *Am Rev Respir Dis* 1976;114:1051–1060.

481. Jones JM, McClement JH, Garfield JW. Series counts of tubercle bacilli in the sputum of patients under treatment for tuberculosis. *Transactions of the 25th Research Conference in Pulmonary Diseases*. VA–Armed Forces, Jan 23–27, 1966:17–18.

482. American Thoracic Society/Centers for Disease Control and Prevention/Infectious Diseases Society of America. Treatment of tuberculosis. *Am J Respir Crit Care Med* 2003;167:603–662.

483. Combs DB, O'Brien RJ, Geiter LJ. USPHS tuberculosis short-course chemotherapy trial 21: effectiveness, toxicity, and acceptability. *Ann Intern Med* 1990;112:397–406.

484. American Thoracic Society. Treatment of tuberculosis and tuberculosis infection in adults and children. *Am J Respir Crit Care Med* 1994;149:1359–1374.

485. Telzak EE, Fazal BA, Pollard CL, et al. Factors influencing time

to sputum conversion among patients with smear-positive tuberculosis. *Clin Infect Dis* 1997;25:666–670.

486. Vidal R, Martin-Casabona N, Juan A, et al. Incidence and significance of acid-fast bacilli in sputum smears at the end of antituberculous treatment. *Chest* 1996;109:1562–1565.

487. Warring FC, Sutramongkole U. Nonculturable acid-fast forms in the sputum of patients with tuberculosis and chronic respiratory disease. *Am Rev Respir Dis* 1979;102:714–724.

488. Al-Moamary MS, Black W, Bessuille E, et al. The significance of the persistent presence of acid-fast bacilli in sputum smears in pulmonary tuberculosis. *Chest* 1999;116:726–731.

489. Epstein MD, Schluger NW, Davidow AL, et al. Time to detection of *Mycobacterium tuberculosis* in sputum culture correlates with outcome in patients receiving treatment for pulmonary tuberculosis. *Chest* 1998;113:379–386.

490. Wallis RS, Perkins M, Phillips M, et al. Induction of the antigen 85 complex of *M. tuberculosis* in sputum: a determinant of outcome in pulmonary tuberculosis. *J Infect Dis* 1998;178:1115–1121.

491. Wallis RS, Perkins MD, Phillips M, et al. Predicting the outcome of therapy for pulmonary tuberculosis. *Am J Respir Crit Care Med* 2000;161:1076–1080.

492. Ribeiro-Rodrigues R, Co TR, Johnson JL, et al. Sputum cytokine levels in patients with pulmonary tuberculosis as early markers of mycobacterial clearance. *Clin Diagn Lab Immun* 2002;9:818–823.

493. Desjardin LE, Perkins MD, Wolski K, et al. Measurement of sputum *Mycobacterium tuberculosis* messenger RNA as a surrogate for response to chemotherapy. *Am J Respir Crit Care Med* 1999;160:203–210.

494. Oursler KK, Moore RD, Bishai WR, et al. Survival of patients with pulmonary tuberculosis: clinical and molecular epidemiologic factors. *Clin Infect Dis* 2002;34:752–759.

495. Rosenow E III, Wilson WR, Cockerill FR III. Pulmonary disease in the immunocompromised host. *Mayo Clin Proc* 1985;60:473, 610–631.

496. Chan JC, Shun-Yang S, Lam WK, et al. High incidence of pulmonary tuberculosis in the non-HIV infected immunocompromised patients in Hong Kong. *Chest* 1989;96:835–839.

497. King EQ, Johnson JB, Batten GJ, et al. Tuberculosis following cortisone therapy. *JAMA* 1951;147:238–241.

498. Popp CG, Ottosen P, Brasher CA. Cortisone and tuberculosis. *JAMA* 1951;147:241–242.

499. Fred L, Levin MH, Barrett TF. Development of active pulmonary tuberculosis. *JAMA* 1951;147:241–242.

500. Kleinschmidt RF, Johnston JM. Miliary tuberculosis in a cortisone treated patient: case report with autopsy. *Ann Intern Med* 1951;35:694–702.

501. Doerner AA, Naegele CF, Regan FD, et al. The development of tuberculous meningitis following cortisone therapy. *Am Rev Tuberc* 1951;64:564–571.

502. Walker B. Miliary tuberculosis in a case of acute disseminated lupus erythematosus treated with ACTH. *BMJ* 1952;2:1076–1078.

503. Sahn SA, Lakshminarayan S. Tuberculosis after corticosteroid therapy. *Br J Dis Chest* 1976;70:195–205.

504. Millar JW, Horne NW. Tuberculosis in immunosuppressed patients. *Lancet* 1979;1:1176–1178.

505. Abbott MR, Smith DD. Mycobacterial infections in immunosuppressed patients. *Med J Aust* 1981;1:351–353.

506. Dautzenberg B, Grosset J, Fechner J, et al. The management of thirty immunocompromised patients with tuberculosis. *Am Rev Respir Dis* 1984;129:494–496.

507. Skogberg K, Ruutu P, Tukiainen P, et al. Effect of immunosuppressive therapy on the clinical presentation and outcome of tuberculosis. *Clin Infect Dis* 1993;17:1012–1017.

508. Fauci AS, Dale DC, Balow JE. Glucocorticosteroid therapy: mechanisms of action and clinical considerations. *Ann Intern Med* 1976;84:304.

509. Bovornkitti S, Kangsadal P, Sathirapat, et al. Reversion and reconversion rate of tuberculin skin reactions in correlation with the use of prednisone. *Dis Chest* 1960;38:51.

510. MacGregor RR, Sheagren JN, Lipsett MB, et al. Alternate-day prednisone therapy. *N Engl J Med* 1969;280:1427–1439.

511. Walsh SD, Grant WB. Corticosteroids in treatment of chronic asthma. *BMJ* 1966;2:796–802.

512. Smyllie HC, Connolly CK. Incidence of serious complications of corticosteroid therapy in respiratory disease. *Thorax* 1968;23:571–581.

513. Schatz M, Patterson R, Kloner R, et al. The prevalence of tuberculosis and positive tuberculin skin tests in a steroid-treated asthmatic population. *Ann Intern Med* 1976;84:261–265.

514. Cowie RL, King LM. Pulmonary tuberculosis in corticosteroid-treated asthmatics. *S Afr Med J* 1987;72:849–850.

515. Kaplan MH, Armstrong D, Rosen P. Tuberculosis complicating neoplastic disease. *Cancer* 1974;33:850–858.

516. Feld R, Bodey GP, Groschel D. Mycobacteriosis in patients with malignant disease. *Arch Intern Med* 1976;136:67–70.

517. Ortals DW, Marr JJ. A comparative study of tuberculous and other mycobacterial infections and their associations with malignancy. *Am Rev Respir Dis* 1978;117:39–45.

518. Libshitz HI, Pannu HK, Elting LS, et al. Tuberculosis in cancer patients: an update. *J Thor Imag* 1997;12:41-46.

519. Kim HC, Goo JM, Kim HB, et al. Tuberculosis in patients with myelodysplastic syndromes. *Clin Radiol* 2002;57:408–414.

520. Onuigbo WI. Some nineteenth century ideas on links between tuberculosis and cancerous diseases of the lung. *Br J Dis Chest* 1975;69:207–210.

521. Pitlik SD, Fainstein V, Bodey GP. Tuberculosis mimicking cancer—a reminder. *Am J Med* 1984;76:822–825.

522. Prytz S, Hansen JL. A follow up examination of patients with pulmonary tuberculosis resected on suspicion of tumor. *Scand J Respir Dis* 1976;57:239–246.

523. Helm WH, Moon AJ. The diagnosis and treatment of bronchial carcinoma in the presence of active pulmonary tuberculosis. *Br J Tuberc Dis Chest* 1952;46:87–94.

524. White FC, Beck F, Pecora DV. Coexisting primary lung carcinoma and pulmonary tuberculosis. A report of fifteen cases discovered through a chest clinic and a hospital. *Am Rev Tuberc* 1959;79:134–141.

525. Mody KM, Poole G. Coexistent lung carcinoma and tuberculosis. *Br J Dis Chest* 1963;57:200–203.

526. Gopalakrishnan P, Miller JE, McLaughlin JS. Pulmonary tuberculosis and coexisting carcinoma. *Am J Surg* 1975;41:405–408.

527. Ting YM, Church WR, Ravikrishnan KP. Lung carcinoma superimposed on pulmonary tuberculosis. *Radiology* 1976;119:307–312.

528. Mok CK, Nandi P, Ong GB. Coexistent bronchogenic carcinoma and active pulmonary tuberculosis. *J Thorac Cardiovasc Surg* 1978;76:469–472.

529. Shah-Mirany J, Reimann AF, Adams WE. Coexisting bronchogenic carcinoma and tuberculosis. *Dis Chest* 1966;50:258–264.

530. Meyer EC, Scatliff JH, Lindskog GE. The relationship of antecedent tuberculosis to bronchogenic carcinoma. *J Thorac Cardiovasc Surg* 1959;38:384–397.

531. Berkheiser SW. Atypical bronchiolar proliferation and metaplasia associated with tuberculosis. *Dis Chest* 1964;45:522–527.

532. Chaudhuri MR. Primary pulmonary scar carcinomas. *Indian J Med Res* 1973;61:858–863.

533. Carey JM, Geer AE. Bronchogenic carcinoma complicating

pulmonary tuberculosis: a report of eight cases and a review of 140 cases since 1932. *Ann Intern Med* 1958;49:161–180.

534. Tunell WP, Koh Y-C, Adkins PC. The dilemma of coincidental active pulmonary tuberculosis and carcinoma of the lung. *J Thorac Cardiovasc Surg* 1971;62:563–567.

535. McQuarrie DG, Nicoloff DM, Van Nostrand D, et al. Tuberculosis and carcinoma of the lung. *Chest* 1968;54:427–432.

536. Holden HM, Quinlan JJ, Hiltz JE. Coexisting pulmonary tuberculosis and bronchogenic carcinoma. A report of 15 cases. *CAN MED ASSOC J* 1965;93:1306–1310.

537. Snider GL, Placik B. The relationship between pulmonary tuberculosis and bronchogenic carcinoma. *Am Rev Respir Dis* 1969;99:229–236.

538. Newberry WM, Sanford JP. Defective cellular immunity in renal failure: depression of reactivity of lymphocytes to phytohemagglutinin by renal failure serum. *J Clin Invest* 1971;50:1262–1271.

539. Lundin AP, Adler AJ, Berlyne GM, et al. Tuberculosis in patients undergoing maintenance hemodialysis. *Am J Med* 1979;67:587–602.

540. Pradhan RP, Katz LA, Nidus BD, et al. Tuberculosis in dialyzed patients. *JAMA* 1974;229:798–800.

541. Andrew OT, Schoenfeld PY, Hopewell PC, et al. Tuberculosis in patients with end-stage renal disease. *Am J Med* 1980;68:59–65.

542. Belcon MC, Smith EK, Kahana LM, et al. Tuberculosis in dialysis patients. *Clin Neprol* 1982;17:14–18.

543. Rutsky EA, Rostand SG. Mycobacteriosis in patients with chronic renal failure. *Arch Intern Med* 1980;140:57–61.

544. Malhotra KK, Parashar MK, Sharma RK, et al. Tuberculosis in maintenance dialysis patients: study from an endemic area. *Postgrad Med J* 1981;57:492–498.

545. Cuss FMC, Carmichael DJS, Linington A, et al. Tuberculosis in renal failure: a high incidence in patients burn in the third world. *Clin Nephrol* 1986;25:129–133.

546. Hussein MM, Bakir N, Roujouleh H. Tuberculosis in patients undergoing maintenance dialysis. *Nephrol Dial Transplant* 1990;5:584–587.

547. Mitwalli A. Tuberculosis in dialysis patients on maintenance dialysis. *Am J Kidney Dis* 1991;18:579–582.

548. Garcia-Leoni ME, Martin-Scapa C, Rodeno P, et al. High incidence of tuberculosis in rehab patients. *Eur J Clin Microbiol Infect Dis* 1990;9:283–285.

549. Kwan JTC, Hart PD, Raftery MJ, et al. Mycobacterial infection is an important infective complication in British dialysis patients. *J Hosp Infect* 1991;19:249–255.

550. Cengiz K. Increased incidence of tuberculosis in patients undergoing haemodialysis. *Nephron* 1996;73:421–424.

551. Quantrill SJ, Woodhead MA, Bell CE, et al. Peritoneal tuberculosis in patients receiving continuous ambulatory peritoneal dialysis. *Nephrol Dial Transplant* 2001;16:1024–1027.

552. Quantrill SJ, Woodhead MA, Bell CE, et al. Side-effects of antituberculosis drug treatment in patients with chronic renal failure. *Eur Respir J* 2002;20:440–443.

553. Kursat S, Ozgur B. Increased incidence of tuberculosis in chronic hemodialysis patients. *Am J Nephrol* 2001;21:490–493.

554. Smirnoff M, Patt C, Secker B, Adler JJ. Tuberculin and anergy skin testing of patients receiving long-term hemodialysis. *Chest* 1998;113:25–27.

555. Korzets A, Gafter U. Tuberculosis prophylaxis for the chronically dialysed patient—yes or no? *Nephrol Dial Transplant* 1999; 14:2857–2859.

556. Lichtenstein IH, Macgregor RR. Mycobacterial infections in renal transplant recipients: report of five cases and review of the literature. *Rev Infect Dis* 1983;5:216–226.

557. Qunibi WY, Al-Sibai MB, Taher S, et al. Mycobacterial infection after renal transplantation—report of 14 cases and review of the literature. *Q J Med* 1990;77:1039–1060.

558. Malhotra KK, Dash SC, Dhawan IK, et al. Tuberculosis and renal transplantation—observations from an endemic area of tuberculosis. *Postgrad Med J* 1986;62:359–362.

559. Hall CH, Wilcox PA, Swanepoel CR, et al. Mycobacterial infections in renal transplant recipients. *Chest* 1994;106:435–439.

560. Mourad G, Soulillou JP, Chong-G, et al. Transmission of *Mycobacterium tuberculosis* with renal allografts. *Nephron* 1985; 41:82–85.

561. Kurzrock R, Zander A, Vellekoop L, et al. Mycobacterial pulmonary infections after allogenic bone marrow transplantation. *Am J Med* 1984;77:35–40.

562. Navari RM, Sullivan KM, Springmeyer SC, et al. Mycobacterial infections in marrow transplant patients. *Transplantation* 1983;36:509–513.

563. Hoyle C, Goldman JM. Life-threatening infections occurring more than 3 months after BMT. *Bone Marrow Transplant* 1994; 14:247–252.

564. Roy V, Weisdorf D. Mycobacterial infections following bone marrow transplant (BMT): a retrospective review of 20 year experience. *Blood* 1995;86(Suppl 1):861A.

565. Martino R, Martinez C, Brunet S, et al. Tuberculosis in bone marrow transplant recipients: report of two cases and review of the literature. *Bone Marrow Transplant* 1996;18:809–812.

566. Ip MSM, Yuen KY, Woo PCY. Risk factors for pulmonary tuberculosis in bone marrow transplant recipients. *Am J Respir Crit Care Med* 1998;158:1173–1177.

567. Carlse S, Bergin C. Reactivation of tuberculosis in a donor lung after transplantation. *AJR Am J Roentgenol* 1990;154:495–497.

568. Dromer C, Nashef S, Velly J, et al. Tuberculosis in transplanted lungs. *J Heart Lung Transplant* 1993;12:924–927.

569. Miller RA, Louis LA, Kline JN, et al. *Mycobacterium tuberculosis* in lung transplant recipients. *Am J Respir Crit Care Med* 1995;152:374–376.

570. Ridgeway AL, Warner GS, Phillips P, et al. Transmission of *Mycobacterium tuberculosis* to recipients of single lung transplants from the same donor. *Am J Respir Crit Care Med* 1996; 153:1166–1168.

571. Schulman LL, Scully B, McGregor CC, et al. Pulmonary tuberculosis after lung transplantation. *Chest* 1997;111:1459–1462.

572. Kesten S, Chaparro C. Mycobacterial infections in lung transplant recipients. *Chest* 1999;115:741–745.

573. Malouf MA, Glanville AR. The spectrum of mycobacterial infection after lung transplantation. *Am J Respir Crit Care Med* 1999;160:1611–1616.

574. Kim HA, Yoo CD, Baek HJ, et al. *Mycobacterium tuberculosis* infection in a corticosteroid-treated rheumatic disease patient population. *Clin Exp Rheumatol* 1998;16:9–13.

575. Feng PH, Tan TH. Tuberculosis in patients with systemic lupus erythematous. *Ann Rheum Dis* 1981;41:11–14.

576. Rovensky J, Kovancik M, Kistufek P, et al. Contribution to the problem of tuberculosis in patients with systemic lupus erythematosus. *Rheumatology* 1996;55:180–187.

577. Victorio-Navarra STG, Dy EER, Arroyo CG, et al. Tuberculosis among Filipino patients with systemic lupus erythematosus. *Semin Arthritis Rheum* 1996;26:628–634.

578. Hernandez-Cruz B, Sifuentes-Osornio J, Ponce-deLeon Rosales S, et al. *Mycobacterium tuberculosis* infection in patients with systemic rheumatic diseases. A case series. Clin Exp Rheumatol 1999;17:289–296.

579. Yun J-E, Lee S-W, Kim J-B, et al. The incidence and clinical characteristics of *Mycobacterium tuberculosis* infection among systemic lupus erythematosus and rheumatoid arthritis patients in Korea. *Clin Exp Rheumatol* 2002;20:127–132.

580. Wolfe F, Flowers N, Anderson JJ, et al. Tuberculosis infection in patients with rheumatoid arthritis (abstract). *Arthritis Rheum* 2001;44:S105.

581. Toh BH, Roberts-Thompson JC, Mathews SD, et al. Depression of cell-mediated immunity in old age and the immunopathic diseases, lupus erythematosus, chronic hepatitis and rheumatoid arthritis. *Clin Exp Immunol* 1973;14:193–202.

582. Riccard PJ, Hausman PB, Raff HV. The autologous mixed lymphocyte reaction in systemic lupus erythematosus. *Arthritis Rheum* 1982;25:820–823.

583. Stohl W. Impaired polyclonal T cell cytolytic activity: a possible risk factor for systemic lupus erythematosus. *Arthritis Rheum* 1995;38:505–516.

584. Rosenthal CJ, Franklin EC. Deficiency of cell-mediated immunity in active SLE: changing patterns after steroid therapy. *Arthritis Rheum* 1975;18:207–217.

585. Andriankos AA, Sharp JT, Person DA, et al. Cell-mediated immunity in rheumatoid arthritis. *Ann Rheum Dis* 1977;36:13–20.

586. Paimela I, Johansson-Stephansson EA, Koskimies S, et al. Depressed cutaneous cell-mediated immunity in early rheumatoid arthritis. *Clin Exp Rheumatol* 1990;8:433–437.

587. Durson AB, Kalac N, Ozkan B, et al. Pulmonary tuberculosis in patients with rheumatoid arthritis (four case reports). *Rheumatol Int* 2002;21:153–157.

588. Kim HY, Im J-G, Goo JM, et al. Pulmonary tuberculosis in patients with systemic lupus erythematosus. *AJR Am J Roentgenol* 1999;173:1639–1642.

589. Keane J, Gershon S, Wise R, et al. Tuberculosis associated with infliximab, a tumor necrosis factor–-neutralizing agent. *N Engl J Med* 2001;345:1098–1104.

590. Mohan VP, Scanga CA, Yu K, et al. Effects of tumor necrosis factor alpha on host immune response in chronic persistent tuberculosis: possible role for limiting pathology. *Infect Immun* 2001;69:1847–1855.

591. Garcia I, Miyazaki Y, Marchal G, Lesslauer W, et al. High sensitivity of transgenic mice expressing soluble TNFR1 fusion protein to mycobacterial infections: synergistic action of TNF and IFN-gamma in the differentiation of protective granulomas. *Eur J Immunol* 1997;27:3182–3190.

592. Mayordomo L, Marenco JL, Gomez-Matcos J, et al. Pulmonary miliary tuberculosis in a patient with anti-TNF-alpha treatment. *Scand J Rheumatol* 2002;31:44–45.

593. Morton R. *Phthisiologia*. London, England. Smith and Welford; 1694:360.

594. Fitz R. The problem of pulmonary tuberculosis in patients with diabetes. *Am J Med Sci* 1930;180:192–200.

595. Sosman MC, Steidl JH. Diabetic tuberculosis. *AJR Am J Roentgenol* 1927;17:625–629.

596. Root HF. The association of diabetes and tuberculosis. *N Engl J Med* 1934;210:1–13.

597. Banyai AL. Diabetes and pulmonary tuberculosis. *Am Rev Tuberc* 1931;24:650–667.

598. Boucot K, Dillon E, Cooper D, et al. Tuberculosis and diabetics. *Am Rev Tuberc* 1952;65(Suppl 1):1–50.

599. Silwer H, Oscarrson P. Incidence and coincidence of diabetes mellitus and pulmonary tuberculosis in a Swedish county. *Acta Med Scand* 1958;161(Suppl 335):1–48.

600. Horowitz O. The risk of tuberculosis in different groups of the general population. *Scand J Respir Dis* 1970;72(Suppl):55–60.

601. Kim JJ, Hong YP, Lew WJ, et al. Incidence of pulmonary tuberculosis among diabetics. *Tuberc Lung Disease* 1995;76:529–533.

602. Pablos-Mendez A, Blustein J, Knirsch CA. The role of diabetes mellitus in the higher prevalence of tuberculosis among Hispanics. *Am J Pub Health* 1997;87:574–579.

603. Holden HH, Hiltz JE. The tuberculous diabetic. *Can Med Assoc J* 1962;87:797–801.

604. Al-Wabel AH, Teklu B, Mahfouz AA, et al. Symptomatology and chest roentgenographic changes of pulmonary tuberculosis among diabetics. *East Afr Med J* 1997;74:62–64.

605. Weaver R. Unusual radiographic presentation of pulmonary tuberculosis in diabetic patients. *Am Rev Respir Dis* 1974;109:162–163.

606. Marais RM. Diabetes mellitus in black and colored tuberculosis patients. *S Afr Med J* 1980;57:483–484.

607. Umut S, Tosun GA, Yildirim. Radiographic location of pulmonary tuberculosis (letter). *Chest* 1994;106:326.

608. Ikezoe J, Takeuchi N, Johkoh T, et al. CT appearance of pulmonary tuberculosis in diabetic and immunosuppressed patients. Comparison with patients who have no underlying disease. *AJR Am J Roentgenol* 1992;159:1175–1179.

609. Hendy M, Stableforth D. The effect of established diabetes mellitus on the presentation of infiltrative pulmonary tuberculosis in the immigrant Asian community of an inner city area of the United Kingdom. *Br J Dis Chest* 1983;77:87–90.

610. Perez-Guzman, Torres-Cruz A, Villarreal-Velarde H, et al. Atypical radiological images of pulmonary tuberculosis in 192 diabetic patients: a comparative study. *Int J Tuberc Lung* 2001;5:455–461.

611. Bacakoglu F, Basoglu OK, Cok G, et al. Pulmonary Tuberculosis in patients with diabetes mellitus. *Resputation* 2001;68:595–600.

612. Koziel H, Koziel MJ. Pulmonary complications of diabetes mellitus. *Infect Dis Clin North Am* 1995;9:65–96.

613. Geisler G, Almdal T, Bennedsen J, et al. Monocyte functions in diabetes mellitus. *Acta Pathol Microbiol Immunol Scand* 1982;90:33–37.

614. Glass EJ, Stewart J, Matthews DM, et al. Impairment of monocyte "lect-n-like" receptor activity in type I (insulin dependent) diabetic patients. *Diabetologica* 1987;30:228–231.

615. Bloom JD. Glucose intolerance in pulmonary tuberculosis. *Am Rev Respir Dis* 1969;100:38–41.

616. Mugasi F, Swai ABM, Alberti KGMM, et al. Increased prevalence of diabetes mellitus in patients with pulmonary tuberculosis in Tanzania. *Tubercle* 1990;71:271–276.

617. Gulbas Z, Erdogan Y, Balci S. Impaired glucose tolerance in pulmonary tuberculosis. *Eur J Respir Dis* 1987;71:345–347.

618. Oluboyo PO, Erasmus RT. The significance of glucose intolerance in pulmonary tuberculosis. *Tubercle* 1990;71:135–138.

619. Ross JD. Progress of tuberculous diabetics coming under supervision during the years 1953–65 up to July 1972. *Tubercle* 1973;54:130–140.

620. Kessler I. Mortality experience of diabetic patients: a twenty-six year follow-up study. *Am J Med* 1971;51:715–724.

621. Cooppan R. Infection and diabetes. In: Marble A, et al., eds. *Joslin's Diabetes mellitus*, 12th ed. Philadelphia: Lea & Febiger, 1985:737–747.

622. Luntz GRWN. Management of the tuberculous diabetic. Follow-up of 84 cases for one year. *BMJ* 1957;1:1082–1086.

623. Banyai AL. Diabetes and tuberculosis. *Dis Chest* 1959;36:238–242.

624. Edsall J, Collins JG, Gran JAC. The reactivation of tuberculosis in New York City in 1967. *Am Rev Respir Dis* 1970;102:725–736.

625. Bashar M, Alcabes P, Rom WN, et al. Increased incidence of multidrug-resistant tuberculosis in diabetic patients on the Bellevue Chest Service, 1987 to 1997. *Chest* 2001;120:1514–1519.

626. Villarino ME, Clairy M. Tuberculosis due to environment, biology, or both? *Chest* 2001;120:1435–1437.

627. Snider DE, Jr. Tuberculosis and gastrectomy (editorial). *Chest* 1985;87:414–415.

628. Thorn PA, Brookes VS, Waterhouse JAH. Peptic ulcer, partial

gastrectomy, and pulmonary tuberculosis. *BMJ* 1956;1: 603–608.

629. Hanngren A, Reizenstein P. Studies of dumping syndrome. *Am J Dig Dis* 1969;14:700–710.

630. Welsh CH. Drug-resistant tuberculosis after gastrectomy. *Chest* 1991;99:246–247.

631. Snider DE, Jr. Jejunoileal bypass for obesity. A risk factor for tuberculosis. (editorial). *Chest* 1982;81:531–532.

632. Bruce RM, Wise L. Tuberculosis after jejunoileal bypass for obesity. *Ann Intern Med* 1977;87:574–576.

633. Agricola G. De Re Metallica. Basel, 1556. (translated by HC Hoover and LH Hoover), New York: Dover, 1950.

634. Sherson D, Lander F. Morbidity of pulmonary tuberculosis among silicotic and nonsilicotic foundry workers in Denmark. *J Occup Med* 1990;32:110–113.

635. Cowie RL, Langton ME, Becklake MR. Pulmonary tuberculosis in South African gold miners. *Am Rev Respir Dis* 1989; 139:1086–1089.

636. Cowie RL. The epidemiology of tuberculosis in gold miners with silicosis. *Am J Respir Crit Care Med* 1994;150:1400–1402.

637. Steen TW, Gy-KM, Gabosianelwe T, et al. Prevalence of occupational lung disease among Botswana men formerly employed in the South African mining industry. *Occup Environ Med* 1997;54:19–26.

638. Hnizdo E, Murray J. Risk of pulmonary tuberculosis relative to silicosit and exposure to silica dust in South African gold miners. *Occup Environ Med* 1998;55:496–502.

639. Chang KC, Leung CC, Tam CM. Tuberculosis risk factors in a silicotic cohort in Hong Kong. *Int J Tuberc Lung Dis* 2001; 5:177–184.

640. Corbett EL, Churchyard GJ, Clayton TC, et al. HIV infection and silicosis: the impact of two potent risk factors on the incidence of mycobacterial disease in South African miners. *AIDS* 2000;14:2759–2768.

641. Uber CL, McReynolds RA. Immunotoxicology of silica. *CRC Crit Rev Toxicol* 1982;10:303–319.

642. Lowrie DB. What goes wrong with the macrophage in silicosis? *Eur J Respir Dis* 1982;63:180–182.

643. Allison AC, Hart PD. Potentiation by silica of the growth of *Mycobacterium tuberculosis* in macrophage cultures. *Br J Exp Pathol* 1968;49:465–476.

644. Gardner LU. Studies on experimental pneumoconiosis-the reactivation of healing primary tubercles in the lung by the inhalation of quartz, granite and carborundum dusts. *Am Rev Tuberc* 1929;20:833–875.

645. Snider DE. The relationship between tuberculosis and silicosis (editorial): *Am Rev Respir Dis* 1978;118:455–460.

646. Chatgidakis CB. Silicosis in South African white gold miners: a comparative study of the disease in its different stages. *Med Proc* 1963;9:383–392.

647. Schepers GWH. Silicosis and tuberculosis. *Ind Med Surg* 1964; 33:381–399.

648. Rivers D, James WRL, Davies DG, et al. The prevalence of tuberculosis at necropsy in progressive massive fibrosis of coal workers. *Br J Ind Med* 1957;14:39–42.

649. Morrow CS. The results of chemotherapy in silicotuberculosis. *Am Rev Respir Dis* 1960;82:831–834.

650. Medical Research Council/Miners' Chest Diseases Treatment Center. Chemotherapy for pulmonary tuberculosis with pneumoconiosis. *Tubercle* 1967;48:1–10.

651. Cowie RL. Silicotuberculosis: long term outcome after short course chemotherapy. *Tuberc Lung Dis* 1995;76:39–42.

652. Lin TP, Suo J, Lee CN, et al. Short-course chemotherapy for pulmonary tuberculosis in pneumoconiotic patients. *Am Rev Respir Dis* 1987;136:808–810.

653. Riley EA. Boeck's sarcoid. *Am Rev Tuberc* 1950;62:231–285.

654. Ustvedt HJ. Autopsy findings in Boeck's sarcoid. *Tubercle* 1948; 29:107–111.

655. Scadding JG. *Mycobacterium tuberculosis* in the aetiology of sarcoidosis. *BMJ* 1960;2:1617–1623.

656. Haroutunian LM, Fisher AM, Smith EW. Tuberculosis and sarcoidosis. *Bull Johns Hopkins Hosp* 1964;115:1–28.

657. Mankiewicz E, Beland J. The role of mycobacteriophages and of cortisone in experimental tuberculosis and sarcoidosis. *Am Rev Respir Dis* 1964;89:707–720.

658. Mankiewicz E. The relationship of sarcoidosis to anonymous bacteria. Proceedings of the 3rd International Conference on Sarcoidosis, Stockholm, September 11–14, 1963. *Acta Med Scand* 1964;425(Suppl):68–73.

659. Chapman JS, Speight M. Further studies of mycobacterial antibodies in the sera of sarcoidosis patients. In: Proceedings of the 3rd International Conference on Sarcoidosis, Stockholm, September 11–14, 1963. *Acta Med Scand* 1964;425(Suppl):61–67.

660. Sutherland I, Mitchell DN, D'Arey, et al. Incidence of intrathoracic sarcoidosis among young adults participating in a trial of tuberculosis vaccines. *BMJ* 1965;2:497–503.

661. Vanek J, Schwarz J. Demonstration of acid-fast rods in sarcoidosis. *Am Rev Respir Dis* 1970;101:395–400.

662. Saboor SA, Johnson NM, McFadden J. Detection of mycobacterial DNA in sarcoidosis and tuberculosis with polymerase chain reaction. *Lancet* 1992;339:1012–1015.

663. Mitchell IC, Turk JL, Mitchell DN. Detection of mycobacterial rRNA in sarcoidosis with liquid-phase hybridization. *Lancet* 1992;339:1015–1017.

664. Fidler HM, Rook GA, Johnson NM, et al. *Mycobacterium tuberculosis* DNA in tissue affected by sarcoidosis. *BMJ* 1993; 306:546–549.

665. Popper HH, Winter E, Hoffer G. DNA *Mycobacterium tuberculosis* in formalin-fixed paraffin-embedded tissue in tuberculosis and sarcoidosis detected by polymerase chain reaction. *Am J Clin Pathol* 1994;101:738–741.

666. Bocart D, Lecossiet D, DeLassence A, et al. A search for mycobacterial DNA in granulomatous tissues from patients with sarcoidosis using the polymerase chain reaction. *Am Rev Respir Dis* 1992;145:1142–1148.

667. Richter E, Greinert V, Kirsten D, et al. Assessment of mycobacterial DNA in cells and tissues of mycobacterial and sarcoid lesions. *Am J Respir Crit Care Med* 1996;153:375–380.

668. Vokurka M, Lecossier D, du Bois RM, et al. Absence of DNA from mycobacteria of the *M. tuberculosis* complex in sarcoidosis. *Am J Respir Crit Care Med* 1997;155:1000–1003.

669. Wilsher ML, Menzies RE, Croxson MC. *Mycobacterium tuberculosis* DNA in tissues affected by sarcoidosis. *Thorax* 1998;53: 871–874.

670. Drake WP, Pei Z, Pride DT, et al. Molecular analysis of sarcoidosis tissues for *Mycobacterium* species DNA. *Emerg Infect Dis* 2002;8:1334–1341.

671. Eishi Y, Suga M, Ishige I, et al. Quantitative analysis of mycobacterial and propioni bacterial DNA in lymph nodes of Japanese and European patients with sarcoidosis. *J Clin Microbiol* 2002;40:198–204.

672. Morton R. Phthisiologia: or a treatise of consumption. In: Major R, ed. *Classic descriptions of disease*, 3rd ed. Springfield, IL: Charles C Thomas, 1945:63.

673. Tocque K, Bellis MA, Tam CM, et al. Long-term trends in tuberculosis. Comparison of age-cohort data between Hong Kong and England and Wales. *Am J Respir Crit Care Med* 1998; 158:484–488.

674. World Health Organization. The World health report. Making a difference. Geneva, Switzerland. *WHO*; 1999;3:310–320.

675. Borgadorff MW, Veen J, Kalisvaart NA, et al. Mortality among tuberculosis patients in the Netherlands in the period 1993–1995. *Eur Respir J* 1998;11:816–820.

676. Fullerton JM, Dyer L. Unsuspected tuberculosis in the aged. *Tubercle* 1965;46:193–198.

677. Mackay AD, Cole RB. The problems of tuberculosis in the elderly. *Q J Med* 1984;212:497–510.

678. King D, Davies PD. Disseminated tuberculosis in the elderly: still a diagnosis overlooked. *J R Soc Med* 1992;85:48–50.

679. Morris CDW. The radiography, hematology and biochemistry of pulmonary tuberculosis in the aged. *Q J Med* 1989;71: 529–535.

680. Teale C, Goldman JM, Pearson SB. The association of age with the presentation and outcome of tuberculosis. *Age Ageing* 1993; 22:289–293.

681. Nagami P, Yoshikawa TT. Tuberculosis in the geriatric patient. *J Am Geriatr Soc* 1983;31:356–363.

682. Yoshikawa TT. Tuberculosis in aging adults. *J Am Geriatr Soc* 1992;40:178–187.

683. Alvarez S, Shell C, Berk SL. Pulmonary tuberculosis in elderly men. *Am J Med* 1987;82:602–606.

684. Umeki S. Comparison of younger and elderly patients with pulmonary tuberculosis. *Respiration* 1989;55:75–83.

685. Katz PR, Reichman W, Dube D, et al. Clinical features of pulmonary tuberculosis in young and old veterans. *J Am Geriatr Soc* 1987;35:512–515.

686. Morris CDW. Pulmonary tuberculosis in the elderly: a different disease? (editorial). *Thorax* 1990;45:912–913.

687. Van den Brande P, Vijgen J, Demedts M. Clinical spectrum of pulmonary tuberculosis in older patients: comparison with younger patients. *J Gerontol* 1991;46:M204–M209.

688. Van den Brande P, Lambrechts M, Tack J, et al. Endobronchial tuberculosis mimicking lung cancer in elderly patients. *Respir Med* 1991;85:107–109.

689. Chan CHS, Woo J, Or KKH, et al. The effect of age on the presentation of patients with tuberculosis. *Tuber Lung Dis* 1995; 76:290–294.

690. Liaw YS, Yang PC, Yu CJ, et al. Clinical spectrum of tuberculosis in older patients. *J Am Geriatr Soc* 1995;43:256–260.

691. Rocha M, Pereira S, Barros H, et al. Does pulmonary tuberculosis change with ageing? *Int J Tuberc Lung Dis* 1997;1: 147–151.

692. Perez-Guzman C, Torres-Cruz A, Villareal-Velardee H, et al. Progressive age-related changes in pulmonary tuberculosis images and the effect of diabetes. *Am J Respir Crit Care Med* 2000;162:1738–1740.

693. Chan-Yeung M, Noertjojo K, Tan J, et al. Tuberculosis in the elderly in Hong Kong. *Int J Tuberc Lung Dis* 2002;6: 771–779.

694. Leung CC, Yew WW, Chan CK. Tuberculosis in older people: a retrospective and comparative study from Hong Kong. *J Am Geriatr Soc* 2002;50:1219–1226.

695. Van den Brande P, Berniest T, Vewwerft J, et al. Impact of age and radiographic presentation on the presumptive diagnosis of pulmonary tuberculosis. *Respir Med* 2002;96:979–983.

696. Perez-Guzman, Vargas MH, Torres-Cruz A, et al. Does aging modify pulmonary tuberculosis? *Chest* 1999;116:961–967.

697. Stead WW. Tuberculosis among elderly persons: an outbreak in a nursing home. *Ann Intern Med* 1981;94:606–610.

698. Stead WW, Lofgren JP, Warren E, et al. Tuberculosis as an endemic and nosocomial infection among the elderly in nursing homes. *N Engl J Med* 1985;312:1483–1487.

699. Centers for Disease Control and Prevention. Prevention and control of tuberculosis in facilities providing long-term care to the elderly. Recommendations of the Advisory Committee for the Elimination of Tuberculosis. *MMWR Morb Mortal Wkly Rep* 1990;39:7–20.

700. Stead WW, To T. The significance of tuberculin skin testing in elderly persons. *Ann Intern Med* 1987;107:837–842.

701. Stead WW, To T, Harrison RW, et al. Benefit–risk considerations in preventive treatment for tuberculosis in elderly patients. *Ann Intern Med* 1987;107:843–845.

702. Battershill JH. Cutaneous testing in the elderly patient. *Chest* 1980;77:188–189.

703. Dorken E, Grzybowski S, Allen EA. Significance of the tuberculin test in the elderly. *Chest* 1987;92:237–240.

704. Creditor MC, Smith EC, Gallai JB, et al. Tuberculosis, tuberculin reactivity, and delayed cutaneous hypersensitivity in nursing home residents. *J Gerontol* 1988;43:M97–M100.

705. Welty C, Burstin S, Muspratt S, et al. Epidemiology of tuberculous infection in a chronic care population. *Am Rev Respir Dis* 1985;132:133–136.

706. Ben-Yehuda A, Weksler ME. Host resistance and the immune system. *Clin Geriatric Med* 1994;8:701–711.

707. Francesco FF, Vescovini R, Passeri G, et al. Shortage of circulating naive CD8+ T cells provides new insight on immunodeficiency and ageing. *Blood* 2000;95:2860–2868.

708. Thompson NJ, Glassroth JL, Snider DE Jr, et al. The booster phenomenon in serial tuberculin testing. *Am Rev Respir Dis* 1979;119:587–597.

709. Gordin FM, Perez-Stable EJ, Flaherty D, et al. Evaluation of a third sequential tuberculin skin test in a chronic care population. *Am Rev Respir Dis* 1988;137:153–157.

710. Perez-Stable EJ, Flaherty D, Schecter G, et al. Conversion and reversion of tuberculin reactions in nursing home residents. *Am Rev Respir Dis* 1988;137:801–804.

711. Van den Brande P, Demedts M. Four stage tuberculin testing in elderly subjects induces age-dependent progressive boosting. *Chest* 1992;101:447–450.

712. Patel YR, Mehta JB, Harvill L, et al. Flexible bronchoscopy as a diagnostic tool in the evaluation of pulmonary tuberculosis in an elderly population. *J Am Geriatr Soc* 1993;41:629–632.

713. Kopanoff DE, Snider DE, Caras GJ. Isoniazid-related hepatitis: a US Public Health Service Cooperative Surveillance Study. *Am Rev Respir Dis* 1978;117:991–1001.

714. Pande JN, Singh SP, Khilnans GC, et al. Risk factors for hepatotoxicity from antituberculosis drugs: a case control study. *Thorax* 1996;51:132–136.

715. Chan CH, Or KK, Cheung W, et al. Adverse drug reactions and outcome of elderly patients on antituberculosis chemotherapy with and without rifampin. *J Med* 1995;26:43–52.

716. Sharma SK, Balamurugan A, Saha PK, et al. Evaluation of clinical and immunogenetic risk factors for the development of hepatotoxicity during antituberculosis treatment. *Am J Respir Crit Care Med* 2002;166:916–919.

717. Finch CK, Chrisma CR, Baciewicz AM, et al. Rifampin and rifabutin drug interactions. An update. *Arch Intern Med* 2002; 162:985–992.

Tuberculosis, Second Edition, edited by William N. Rom and Stuart M. Garay. Lippincott Williams & Wilkins, Philadelphia © 2004

IMAGING OF THORACIC TUBERCULOUS INFECTIONS

GEORGEANN MCGUINNESS
AMI N. RUBINOWITZ

In the United States the dramatic decline of tuberculosis (TB) in the past several decades has resulted in a generation of physicians with limited experience in the management of TB. This, as well as the shift of care from specialized institutions to the general medical community, has increased the responsibility of the radiologist to promptly recognize this infection (1). Shifts in epidemiology, impaired immune status of risk groups, and changes in the mycobacterial organism itself have furthered the role of chest radiography in the detection, diagnosis, and management of TB (1,2). In economically developed countries, such as the United States, the majority of TB cases still arise as a result of endogenous reactivation of remote infection. Because of this TB is overall more prevalent in the elderly (3), except in locales where there is a high rate of TB in immigrants from endemic countries. In less industrially developed countries, the majority of TB cases represent recent infection, and therefore 80% of cases occur in persons during their productive years (3). The potential of the radiograph to immediately suggest active disease at a time when other test results are negative, delayed, or equivocal should be recognized. Chest radiographs may also give the first evidence of unsuspected disease or disease reactivation, or suggest the correct diagnosis when TB is an obscure diagnostic possibility.

This chapter discusses optimal utilization of imaging in the detection and management of TB. Traditional uses of radiology in tuberculosis are presented and common presentations of the disease are reviewed. Atypical manifestations of TB are also presented. Finally, the contribution of newer modalities, particularly high-resolution computed tomography (HRCT), is emphasized.

G. McGuinness and **A. N. Rubinowitz:** Department of Radiology, New York University Medical Center, New York, New York.

THE CHEST RADIOGRAPH AND PULMONARY TUBERCULOSIS

The chest radiograph has historically been a major tool in the armamentarium against TB. The chest radiograph is used in concert with the tuberculin skin test as a means of detecting disease. Stability of radiographic findings is a primary component in the assessment of disease activity, as defined by the American Thoracic Society (4). TB is considered active until such time as (a) all bacteriologic tests for the organism are negative for 6 months or longer and (b) serial chest radiographs obtained at intervals of 6 months or less are stable for 6 months or longer.

Tuberculin skin testing remains extremely important for determining infection by mycobacteria. In particular, as the prevalence of TB has declined in recent decades, a positive purified protein derivative (PPD) result is increasingly likely to indicate recent infection rather than response to remote infection. However, tuberculin skin testing has specific limitations that are particularly important to some groups at heightened risk for infection. Tuberculin skin testing has proved unreliable in immunocompromised patients (5); there is also a delay of up to 3 days in interpretation of results. Accordingly, the chest radiograph has become increasingly important in disease detection, particularly for cases in which patient reliability is not assured, in contained populations in which a delay in diagnosis of even a few days could have clinical impact, in human immunodeficiency virus (HIV)–positive patients, and in patients previously treated with bacille Calmette–Guérin (BCG).

Radiographic manifestations of parenchymal disease in the lungs are divided into primary, latent, and postprimary or reactivation phases, corresponding to the clinical stage of disease.

Primary Tuberculosis

Primary TB typically involves the lower lungs, consequent to the physical principles of aerosol deposition. The tubercle bacillus is inhaled into the lungs in the form of a droplet nucleus and is deposited deep in the lungs where it may replicate, having avoided the mucociliary clearance mechanisms of the central airways proximal to the respiratory bronchioles. Normal pulmonary airflow favors the lower lungs. It is important to remember, however, that the infiltrates of primary TB may occur in any lobe. Of the 17 patients with primary TB and lung infiltrates studied by Woodring et al. (6), 50% of the infiltrates occurred in the upper lobes. In some series, upper lobe involvement is seen more frequently in primary infection than is lower lobe involvement (7).

In 90% to 95% of people, the organism may replicate for a few weeks with little host response as cell-mediated immunity to the tuberculous antigen develops. In most cases, cell-mediated immunity effectively acts against the infection within 2 to 6 weeks and prompts a granulomatous response that either contains or eradicates the organism. Discrete granulomata in the lungs, known as *Ghon foci*, may result with or without calcium deposition. When associated with ipsilateral calcifications in hilar lymph nodes, these lesions may be referred to as *Ranke complexes* (Fig. 26.1).

In approximately 5% of cases, if cell-mediated immunity fails to contain or eradicate the infection, primary infection results in clinical pneumonia. Classically, this is seen as a lobar or segmental infiltrate, usually associated with ipsilateral hilar adenopathy. Multiple lobes may be involved, with mediastinal

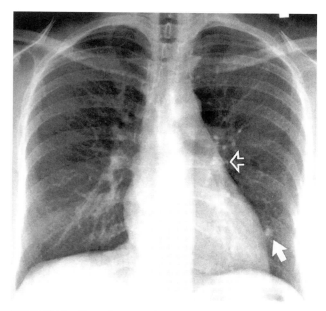

FIGURE 26.1. Ghon focus and Ranke complex in a 44-year-old woman without a history of tuberculosis. Chest radiograph demonstrates a calcified granuloma, known as a Ghon focus, in the left lower lobe (*closed arrow*), indicative of previous exposure to tuberculosis. A Ghon focus coupled with calcified nodes in the ipsilateral hilum (*open arrow*) is referred to as a Ranke complex.

adenopathy or a pleural effusion (Fig. 26.2). This appearance in the past been referred to as the *pediatric pattern* because it has historically been more typical of pediatric tuberculosis (8). This erroneous moniker dates from the time when primary TB was the usual disease manifestation in the pediatric population and was unusual in adults. This term should be discouraged, as it may contribute to a failure to recognize and consider primary TB as a diagnosis in an adult. Interestingly, in primary TB adenopathy is relatively more common in pediatric patients than lung consolidation, whereas the opposite applies to primary TB in adults (8). Areas of consolidation in primary tuberculosis may undergo cavitation, sometimes referred to as *progressive primary disease* (Fig. 26.2).

The incidence of tuberculous lymphadenitis, both in association with pleuroparenchymal disease and as a solitary manifestation of infection, is increasing. This is due to the prevalence of exuberant adenopathy typical of TB in patients with the acquired immunodeficiency syndrome (AIDS) and to the fact that more primary disease is occurring in unexposed adults. In a recent large series, lymphadenopathy was detected radiographically in 67% of adults with primary TB (7), an unexpectedly high number attributed to the increasing number of adults at risk for "childhood tuberculosis." It is important to emphasize that as an unexposed generation reaches adulthood, "pediatric pattern" is being seen with increasing frequency in adults presenting with primary TB. In general, however, the prevalence of lymphadenopathy decreases with age (8). This is reflected in the fact that postobstructive atelectasis and/or hyperinflation resulting from extrinsic airway compression due to enlarged nodes is more common in children, with smaller airways and relatively more adenitis, than in adults, who generally have larger airways and less relative adenitis (3).

Inflammation and consequent fibrotic traction from adenitis can secondarily affect other mediastinal organs. There may be distortion and displacement of major airways, including the trachea. Fistula formation, occurring between the airways and the mediastinum, pleura, or esophagus, is a dreaded complication (Fig. 26.3).

Pleural effusions alone or in combination with adenopathy are also a common manifestation of primary TB (Fig. 26.4). Despite the fact that tuberculous effusions are more common in adults, they are generally recognized as consistent with TB in the pediatric population, but not in adults with such presentations. The appearance of bilateral hilar adenopathy, mediastinal adenopathy, or both in the absence of parenchymal disease in the adult is especially apt to be attributed erroneously to sarcoidosis or lymphoma rather that to TB (Fig. 26.5).

Failure to recognize atypical appearances of TB, particularly in the adult, is one of the most common causes of misdiagnosis. Radiographic diagnosis of TB was initially correct in only 34% of 30 patients with primary TB studied by Woodring et al. (6). Patterns most commonly associated with a misdiagnosis included hilar and mediastinal adenopathy in an adult, atelectasis, pleural effusion, and a normal chest radiograph.

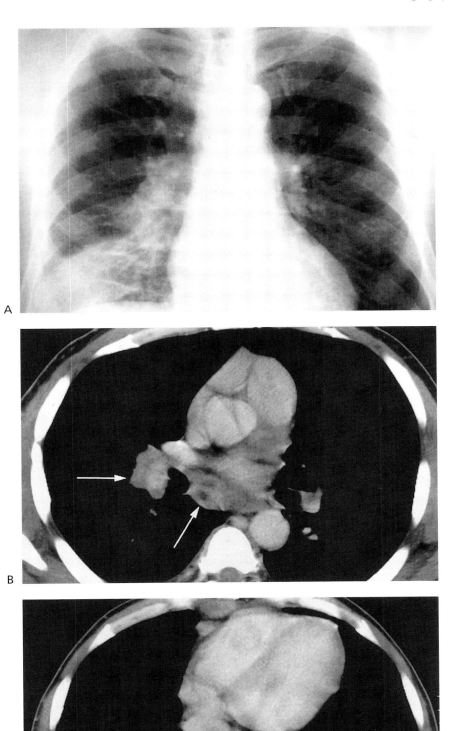

A

B

C

FIGURE 26.2. Radiographic pattern of adult primary tuberculosis in a 45-year-old man presenting with cough and fever. **A:** Chest radiograph demonstrates consolidation in the right lower lobe and ipsilateral hilar lymphadenopathy. **B:** Axial contrast-enhanced computed tomography (CT) scan though the subcarinal space confirms typical enlarged, low-density subcarinal and right hilar lymph nodes (*arrows*). **C:** CT scan through the right lung base demonstrates low-density regions in the infiltrate (*arrows*) indicative of necrosis or early abscess formation.

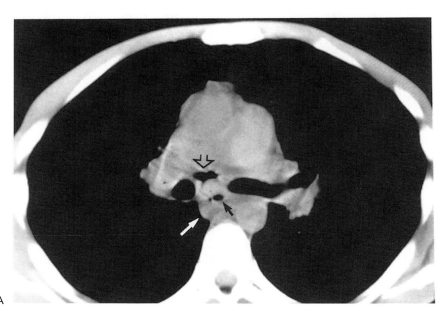

A

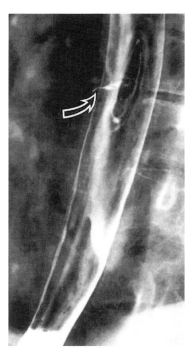

B

FIGURE 26.3. Esophageal perforation secondary to tuberculosis adenitis in a 36-year-old woman. **A:** Axial computed tomography scan through the subcarinal region. Enlarged nodes are noted in the subcarinal region, extending into the azygoesophageal recess (*white arrow*). The esophageal lumen is air filled (*black arrow*), and there is an abnormal collection of mediastinal air (*open arrow*). **B:** Gastrograffin swallow confirms presence of a fistula with extravasation of contrast (*arrow*), due to biopsy-proven tuberculosis adenitis.

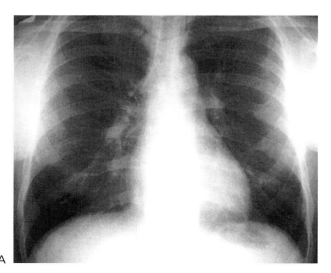

A

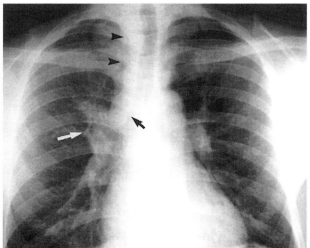

B

FIGURE 26.4. Primary tuberculosis presenting as adenopathy and pleural effusion. **A:** Baseline normal chest radiograph in a 27-year-old woman 1 year before illness. **B:** Chest radiograph at presentation with fevers and night sweats demonstrates extensive mediastinal adenopathy, including paratracheal (*arrowheads*), azygous complex (*black arrow*), and right hilar (*white arrow*) nodes. Note the absence of infiltrate.

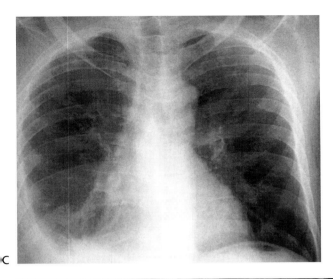

C

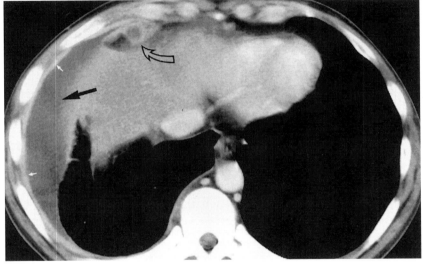

D

FIGURE 26.4. *Continued.* **C:** Chest radiograph in a 42-year-old man presenting with cough, fever, and night sweats of 2 weeks duration reveals a right pleural effusion with little focal consolidation. **D:** Computed tomography demonstrates a homogeneous pleural fluid collection (*black arrow*) as well as uniform thickening and enhancement of the parietal pleura (*white arrows*) following intravenous contrast enhancement. A low-density cardiophrenic angle lymph node (*curved open arrow*) can also be identified. This constellation of findings is highly suggestive of tuberculous effusions.

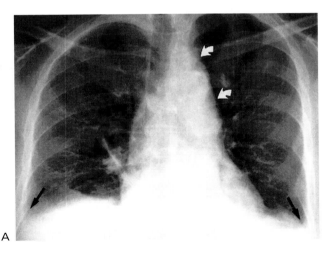

A

FIGURE 26.5. Tuberculous adenopathy misdiagnosed in an adult. **A:** Chest radiograph in a 67-year-old woman presenting with a gastric ulcer demonstrates abundant mediastinal adenopathy (*curved white arrows*) and small bilateral pleural effusions (*black arrows*). *Continued on next page.*

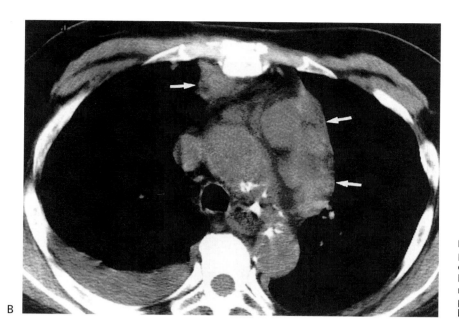

B

FIGURE 26.5. *Continued.* Tuberculous adenopathy misdiagnosed in an adult. **B:** Noncontrast computed tomography image obtained just below the aortic arch shows extensive anterior mediastinal adenopathy (*arrows*). Initially interpreted as most likely neoplastic, subsequent biopsy documented mycobacterial infection.

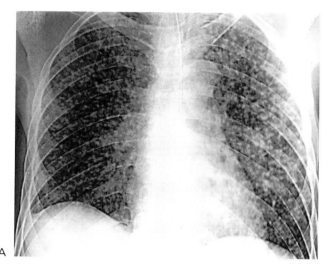

A

FIGURE 26.6. Lymphohematogenous dissemination. **A:** Chest radiograph demonstrates innumerable small parenchymal nodules. **B:** A 1.5-mm high-resolution computed tomography image confirms the presence of sharply defined diffuse nodules (in the range of 3 to 6 mm) randomly scattered throughout the parenchyma without evidence of cavitation. This appearance is distinct from miliary disease, in which, by definition, the nodules are 1 to 3 mm in diameter, and the endobronchial diseases, in which there are indirect centrilobular nodules.

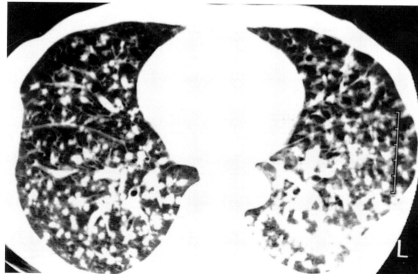

B

It is important to recognize that primary infection is associated with diffuse, early dissemination of organisms to both pulmonary and extrapulmonary sites. In most cases, these foci also succumb to the cell-mediated immune response. However, in situations of less vigorous immune response, some organisms in these isolated foci may remain viable, though contained, serving as potential sources for reactivation disease in the future. Lymphohematogenous dissemination of primary disease may result in a miliary pattern of tiny nodules ranging in size from 1 to 3 mm. This is seen in 3% to 6% of cases (6,9). Hematogenous dissemination may result in diffuse nodules that range in size from 4 to 6 mm (Fig. 26.6). A patient with active TB may present with a normal chest radiograph in up to 15% of cases (6).

Secondary Tuberculosis

When the quiescent residua of primary TB reactivate, the areas of involved lung are typically the apices and superior segments of the lower lobes. The predilection of TB for these areas has been attributed to favorable local environmental conditions in these areas. There is a relatively low level of lymph production and flow in the lung apices and the superior segments of the lower lobes, as compared with the rest of the lungs. Clearance of tubercle bacilli from these regions, after diffuse dissemination during the lymphohematogenous phase of primary infection, is therefore impeded. In addition, the relatively hyperoxic environment of these sites suits the high oxygen demands of the organism, allowing sustained dormancy of the organism, known as latent TB, and subsequent reactivation.

The well-recognized sequelae of primary infection are nodules (with and without calcification), fibrotic bands, and scarring identified in the lung apices. These are sometimes called *fibronodular changes* or *fibroproductive changes* (Fig. 26.7). Apical nodules are sometimes referred to as Simon foci. Radiographic signs indicating reactivation disease include new infiltrates and acinar nodules, new cavities, and changing

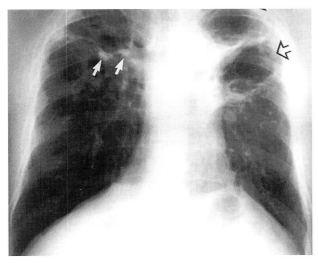

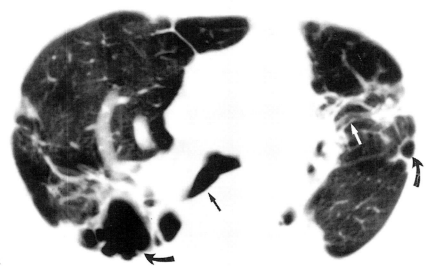

FIGURE 26.7. Upper lobe fibronodular and cavitary changes in a 48-year-old man. **A:** Chest radiograph demonstrates typical lung nodules (*white arrows*), fibrotic bands, and cavities (*black open arrow*) in the upper lobes. Volume loss in the upper lobes has resulted in upward retraction of hilar structures and compensatory hyperexpansion of the lower lobes. **B:** Computed tomography through the upper lobes confirms volume loss and cicatricial distortion of the lung architecture. The right upper lobe bronchus is displaced superiorly and posteriorly (*black straight arrow*). Note the presence of unsuspected bronchiectasis (*white arrow*) associated with bilateral cavities (*curved arrows*).

pleural disease (Fig. 26.8). It must be stressed that recrudescent active disease may lack detectable radiographic changes, albeit rarely. Even a series of stable radiographs demonstrating fibronodular disease cannot assure inactive disease. In select cases, HRCT may identify indicators of active disease not seen on chest radiographs (Fig. 26.9).

Often typical fibroproductive nodular changes in the upper lobes seen radiographically are dismissed as indicative of healed TB when based on a single examination. In many cases this will be true; however, unless stability of the lesions can be documented, the possibility of active disease cannot be excluded. Even the presence of calcification within an infiltrate does not signify inactive disease. On a single examination any abnormality must be considered as representing indeterminate disease activity. In the recent series by Krysl et al. (7), 5% of patients with proven active postprimary TB presented with calcified fibroproductive disease as the only radiographic parenchymal abnormality. Woodring et al. (6) found this to be one of the most common reasons for misdiagnosis of active TB in their series.

Atypical appearances of postprimary tuberculosis are becoming increasingly common. Lower lobe infiltrates, adenopathy, upper lobe masses (tuberculomas), and pleural disease should all be recognized as potentially representing reactivation TB.

In the series by Woodring et al. (6), 56 patients with documented active, postprimary TB were studied. The radiographic diagnosis of active disease was initially correct in 59% of these cases. Common causes of misinterpretation included overlooking fibroproductive changes or interpreting them as inactive, considering involvement of anterior segments of the upper lobes or lung bases as evidence against the diagnosis of TB, and interpreting mass lesions as likely neoplasms. The clinical diagnosis in this series was initially correct in only 55% of cases (6).

Pleural Disease

Pleural effusion is a common manifestation of primary TB occurring after cell-mediated immunity has had time to develop, usually 3 to 6 months after infection (3). The pleuritis that develops is caused by the release of tuberculoprotein into the pleural space, with the consequent hypersensitivity response. Thoracentesis usually yields sterile fluid, with positive cultures seen in only about 20% to 40% of cases (3). Pleural biopsy may yield bacilli and prove culture positive in approximately 65% to 70% of cases (3). The presumed parenchymal focus of disease is not always radiographically apparent. Computed tomography (CT) may be useful in demonstrating the parenchymal infiltrate as well as typical features of tuberculous lymphadenitis, and therefore may suggest the correct diagnosis (10) (Fig. 26.4C, D). Pleural effusions may also be seen in postprimary disease, but slightly less frequently. Pleural effusions secondary to TB are usually unilateral, initially mobile, layer dependently in the hemithorax, and are homogeneous in density. (Fig. 26.10B).

The natural course for most effusions caused by TB is resorption, leaving little residua. In a small percentage of cases, effusion progresses to frank empyema, at which point

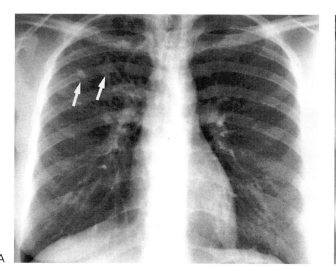
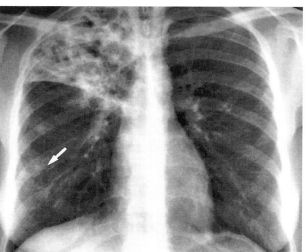

FIGURE 26.8. Reactivation (postprimary) tuberculosis. **A:** Chest radiograph in a patient who had been treated for tuberculosis reveals residual linear and nodular densities (*arrows*) in the right upper lobe. **B:** Follow-up chest radiograph obtained 1 year later because of cough, fever, and weight loss shows patchy consolidation in the right upper lobe consistent with reactivation disease. Sublobar infiltrate in the lower lung is noted (*arrow*). Sputum was positive for acid-fast bacillus.

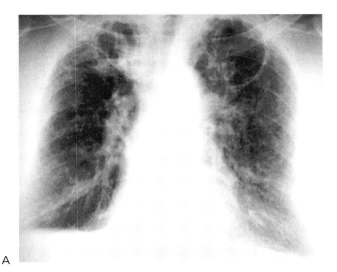

A

FIGURE 26.9. Reactivation disease detected only by high-resolution computed tomography (HRCT). **A:** Chest radiograph in a 47-year-old asymptomatic man with a history of previously documented tuberculosis. Diffuse fibrosis, nodular and linear densities, upper lobe cystic changes, and volume loss are evident. **B:** HRCT through the upper lungs reveals extensive bronchiectasis (*white arrows*), fibrosis, and cavities. **C:** HRCT through the lung bases demonstrates relative absence of disease.

(continued on next page)

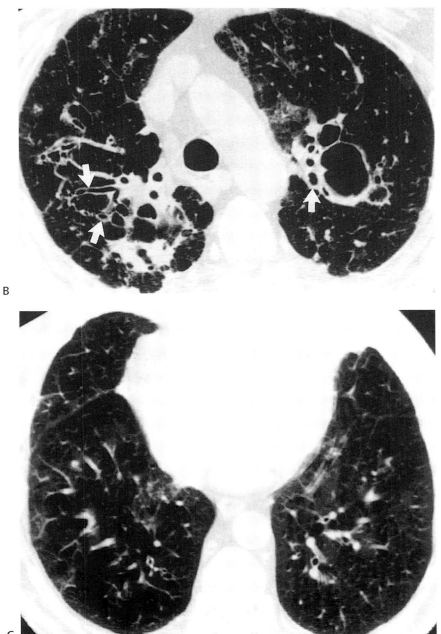

B

C

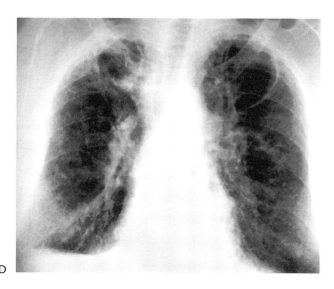

D

FIGURE 26.9. *Continued.* **D:** Follow-up radiograph obtained 3 months later shows no change. **E:** HRCT scan obtained due to suspicion of active disease shows small, centrilobular densities (*arrowheads*), some of which form a "tree-in-bud" appearance (*curved arrow*). These findings are characteristic of endobronchial spread of disease. Although sputum smears were negative, therapy was initiated on the basis of the CT findings. Cultures subsequently proved positive for tuberculosis.

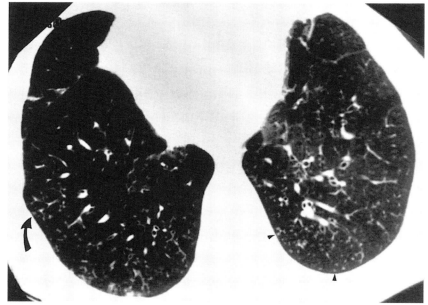

E

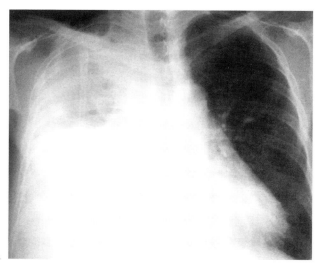

A

FIGURE 26.10. Tuberculous empyema in a 46-year-old man. **A:** Chest radiograph shows a large right and tiny left pleural effusion.

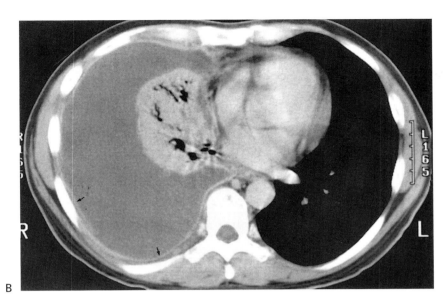

B

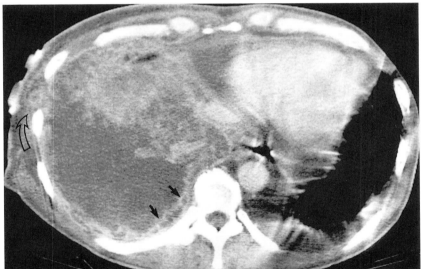

C

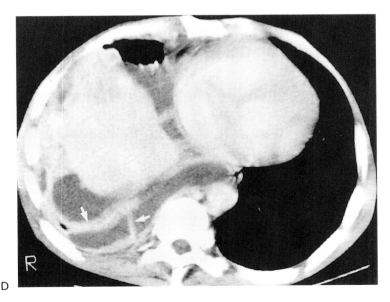

D

FIGURE 26.10. *Continued.* **B:** Initial computed tomography scan demonstrates a homogeneous, low-density, right pleural fluid collection. The parietal pleural surfaces are thin and smooth (*arrows*). **C:** One month later there are innumerable tiny isolated fluid collections between multiple septations within the pleural space (*arrows*). Note extension of disease into the chest wall (*curved arrow*) with resultant cutaneous fistula, despite therapy. **D:** In another patient with tuberculous empyema, the septations are thicker (*arrows*) resulting in larger pleural fluid loculations. These loculations may harbor viable bacilli, despite adequate therapy, and may serve as a source of recurrent disease.

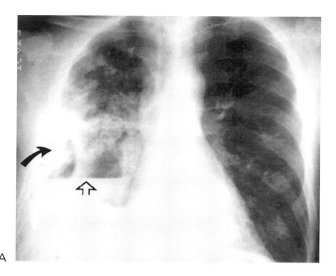

A

FIGURE 26.11. Chronic tuberculosis empyema with bronchopleural fistula evaluated with computed tomography (CT). **A:** Chest radiograph in 62-year-old man with a long history of tuberculous empyema previously treated. At presentation, an air-fluid collection can be identified in the right pleural space (*open arrow*). Pleural calcium can be seen (*curved arrow*), seemingly displaced from the chest wall. **B:** CT scan through the lower lungs confirms the presence of diffuse calcification of the pleural surfaces (*white arrows*), which confirms chronicity. As seen on the scan, extrapleural fibrofatty proliferation (*open arrow*) and thickening of the ribs are characteristic sequelae of chronic tuberculous inflammation. Note that calcium is actually floating within the pleural space (*black arrow*). **C:** CT performed with lung windows at approximately the same level illustrates the presence of a fistulous communication with air dissecting behind the pleura, within the extrapleural space (*arrow*).

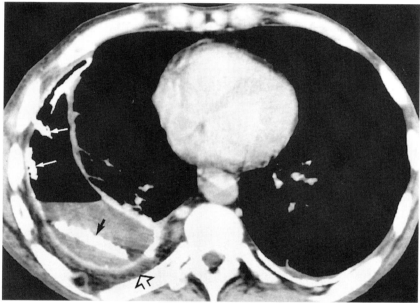

B

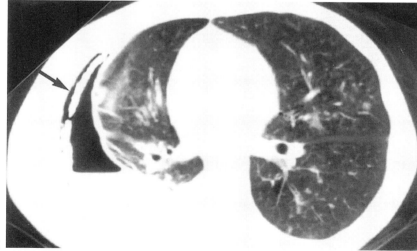

C

loculated pockets, density variations, and strandlike septations can be seen on CT scan (Fig. 26.10). These collections are usually both smear and culture positive (3).

Untreated or inadequately managed TB empyemas may continue as chronic empyemas. On chest radiography these are seen as chronically thickened pleural rinds, sometimes with resultant volume loss of the affected hemithorax. Calcifications and underlying parenchymal changes may be identified. CT is valuable in defining the typical extrapleural fibrofatty proliferation associated with these chronic infections, as well as the typical proliferative changes to subjacent ribs as a result of chronic inflammation (Fig. 26.11). Apical pleural thickening (sometimes designated the "apical cap") commonly seen on chest radiographs in patients with TB is often a source of consternation because of typical asymmetry and, therefore, an overlap in appearance with Pancoast tumors. This appearance in clarified by CT as secondary to extrapleural fat interspersed with vessels (11), thus differentiating it from tumor. Calcifications of the visceral and parietal pleural surfaces are more sensitively detected by CT than by radiography, as is identification of chronic pleural fluid collections that are usually hidden by the thickened pleural rind at plain film radiography (Fig. 26.10). Identification of chronic pleural collections is extremely important because they often harbor numerous tubercle bacilli and are dangerous sources for potential recrudescent disease. In the Hulnick et al. (10) study of ten patients with chronic tuberculous pleural disease, pleural fluid collections were identified in six; in all cases active infection was documented (Fig. 26.11).

If a tuberculous empyema is inadequately managed, encapsulated empyema may erode through the parietal pleura and discharge infectious material into the body wall or mediastinum (Fig. 26.12). The result is empyema necessitatis, suspected clinically in many cases as a chest wall mass. On CT, a low-density body wall collection, often with an enhancing rim after intravenous contrast, is seen in association with a thick-walled pleural collection (Fig. 26.12). Communication between the pleural and chest wall collection is rarely demonstrated (12). Empyema necessitatis has rarely been reported as a manifestation of reactivation disease (13).

Chest wall abscesses may develop in the absence of pleuroparenchymal disease, presumably caused by hematogenous dissemination of organisms (14). Often such abscesses accompany destructive changes of osseous or cartilaginous structures. CT characterizes these "cold abscesses" as low-density collections, often with enhancing rims and occasional calcifications, that cross tissue plains and may cause osseous destruction (Fig. 26.13).

Tuberculosis in the Human Immunodeficiency Virus–Positive Patient

The AIDS epidemic and the current resurgence in tuberculosis are more than temporally linked. The susceptibility of the AIDS population to this infection has contributed significantly to the spread of TB, and TB has become a major complication of HIV/AIDS. This is reflected in the inclusion of pulmonary TB in patients with CD4 cell counts below $200/mm^3$ in the revised list of index infections for the surveillance definition of AIDS (14a). The strongest risk factor for both immediate and delayed progression from infection to active TB is the coexistence of HIV infection. The risk of progression to disease in HIV-positive patients with TB infection is 5% to 10% per year, as opposed to a 5% to 10% lifetime risk in the general population (3). The subset of AIDS patients who are intravenous drug abusers, homeless, or institutionalized are at particular risk for mycobacterial infection.

Health care workers must maintain a very high index of suspicion for TB because its incidence in the AIDS population is estimated at 50 to 200 times that of the general population (15). It is imperative to remember that TB is not only one of the most curable diseases to afflict AIDS patients, it is also one of the most contagious, both to others with AIDS and to the immune-intact population. Moreover, there are data to support the assertion that active TB infection actually accelerates the progression of AIDS (16).

Because of the relative virulence of *Mycobacterium tuberculosis* in comparison with that of other opportunistic infections, TB is a common AIDS-defining illness in HIV-positive patients. A delay in the diagnosis of TB in this setting is common. Multifactorial reasons include the failure to consider this diagnosis in the face of well-known opportunistic infections, unfamiliarity with the spectrum of radiologic changes in this disease, the high incidence of concomitant processes both infectious and noninfectious, and chronic changes in scarred lungs that may mask acute or evolving disease. Factors that may complicate the radiologic follow-up during the treatment period for TB in AIDS are also important to consider and are therefore discussed below.

The radiologist may be the first to suggest tuberculosis as a diagnostic consideration, so familiarity with the spectrum of unique imaging findings associated with this infection in AIDS/HIV is important. In comparison with the general population, the AIDS patient is more likely to present with adenopathy, bronchogenic spread of infection, miliary disease, extrapulmonary disease, and a normal chest radiograph (8,15–18). Recognizing that there may be a broad spectrum of findings in TB increases the likelihood of making a timely diagnosis (19). In a recent series by Kramer et al. (20) of 52 AIDS patients, the diagnosis of tuberculosis was delayed in 48%. Forty-five percent of those in whom the diagnosis was delayed died of TB, as compared with 19% of those in whom a rapid diagnosis was made. These investigators, therefore, supported empiric therapy for TB in all HIV-positive patients with chest radiographic findings suggestive of TB and not explained by other causes.

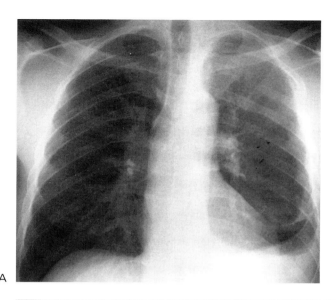

A

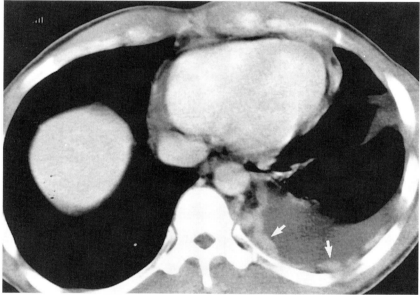

B

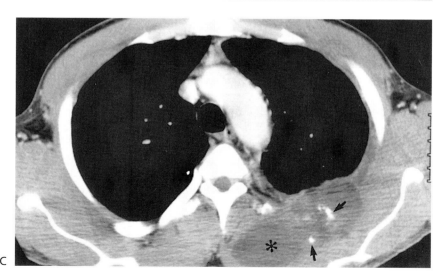

C

FIGURE 26.12. Empyema necessitatis in a 42-year-old man. **A:** Chest radiograph shows left pleural effusion and relative absence of parenchymal consolidation. **B:** Computed tomography (CT) scan through the lung bases demonstrates loculated pleural fluid collection with marked thickening and nodular irregularity of the parietal pleura (*arrows*). **C:** CT scan obtained at the level of the aortic arch shows erosion of the ribs (*arrows*) with extension of fluid into the chest wall (*asterisk*). This constellation of findings strongly suggests empyema necessitatis, which was subsequently confirmed.

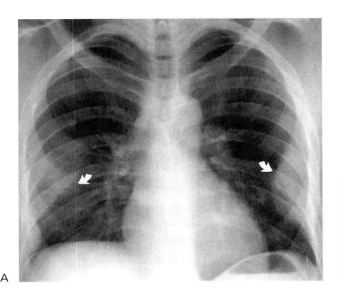

A

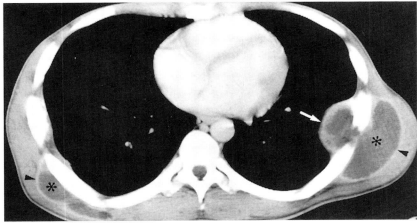

B

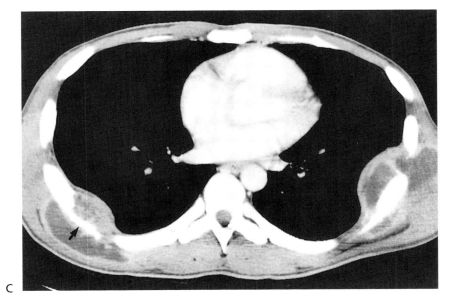

C

FIGURE 26.13. Chest wall abscesses in a 27-year-old male prisoner who noted subcutaneous masses while playing basketball. **A:** Chest radiograph shows smooth, extrapleural densities bilaterally (*arrows*) in the absence of pleural effusions. **B:** Computed tomography (CT) scan demonstrates multiple low-density fluid collections in the chest wall (*asterisks*) and the extrapleural space (*arrow*). The margins of these collections are enhanced (*arrowheads*) after intravenous contrast administration. **C:** CT scan obtained at a lower level shows destruction of adjacent ribs (*arrow*) by "cold abscesses."

The radiographic manifestations of TB in the HIV-positive patient reflect the level of immune compromise. When the immune system is relatively intact (more than 200 CD4 cells/mm³) the most typical radiographic finding is that of reactivation TB. Frequently, these patients still have reactive tuberculin skin tests. The radiographic findings include upper lobe cavities, infiltrates, and nodules. Pleural effusions, consequent to hypersensitivity pleuritis, are seen more commonly in patients with CD4 levels above 200/mm³ (21). Some series report a relatively lower incidence of cavitary disease and more frequent mid- and lower lung infiltrates in AIDS patients as compared with those who have reactivation TB in the immunocompetent population (22). Some of these patients with relatively well-preserved immune function may not have had previous exposure to *Mycobacterium*, and the appearance will then be typical of primary TB.

In contrast, in more severely immunocompromised patients with CD4 counts less than 200 cells per mm³, the most common presentation of TB is the primary TB pattern of adenopathy, consolidation, and miliary disease. In the series by Long et al. (22), the primary pattern of disease was seen on the chest radiograph in 80% of the HIV-positive patients with clinical AIDS and TB, as compared with 30% of the HIV-positive non-AIDS patients and 11% of the HIV-negative patients. Strikingly prominent mediastinal and hilar adenopathy was commonly seen. The prominence of adenopathy inversely correlated with compromised immunity (21). In the study of 128 HIV-positive patients by Pearlman et al. (23), a significantly higher prevalence ($p = 0.01$) of adenopathy and a lower prevalence ($p = 0.08$) of cavitation was identified in 98 patients with CD4 cell counts less than 200/mm³, when compared with 30 patients with CD4 cell counts greater than 200/mm³. Such adenopathy is not only seen in primary disease but may also be a feature of reactivation TB in AIDS patients (22).

Adenitis from TB has been further characterized by CT. The TB adenitis in HIV-positive patients is typically of low density centrally, a feature that may be of diagnostic value.

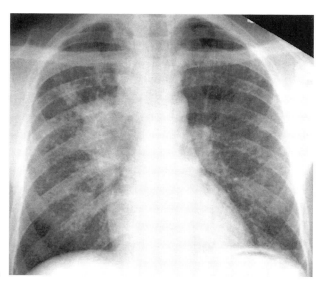

A

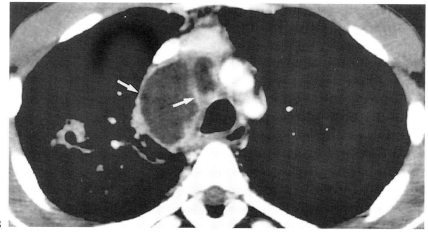

B

FIGURE 26.14. Low-density adenopathy in a 29-year-old man with acquired immune deficiency syndrome and tuberculosis. **A:** Chest radiograph demonstrates extensive right paratracheal and hilar adenopathy. There is associated right perihilar infiltrate. **B:** Contrast-enhanced computed tomography scan obtained just above the aortic arch confirms marked low-density paratracheal adenopathy with striking peripheral rim enhancement (*arrows*).

In a retrospective review of 25 HIV-positive patients with documented TB adenitis evaluated by CT, the most characteristic CT finding was the presence of low-density mediastinal and hilar lymph nodes in 80% of the patients (24). When intravenous contrast was administered, there was marked rim enhancement (Fig. 26.14). These authors concluded that recognition of low-density mediastinal and hilar nodes on CT was sufficiently characteristic of TB to warrant empiric therapy, pending results of culture.

A remarkable feature of TB in patients with HIV infection is the high incidence of extrapulmonary involvement. Since 1987, extrapulmonary TB has been an AIDS-defining condition in HIV-positive patients (25). Extrapul-

monary TB is more common in advanced AIDS and correlates with diminishing CD4 cells counts. In the series by Jones et al. (21), extrathoracic TB was present in 70% of HIV-positive patients with TB and CD4 cell counts less than 100/mm³, as compared with 50% and 44%, respectively, for patients with CD4 levels less than 200 or 300/mm³. Chest roentgenographic features may be consistent with either the primary or secondary pattern of disease, with a miliary pattern occurring in about half of the cases (5). Extrathoracic disease most frequently manifests as lymphadenitis or disseminated multiorgan disease (Fig. 26.15). Bone marrow, genitourinary, central nervous system, and spinal disease are common.

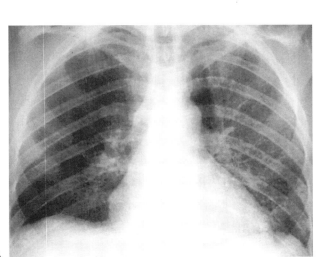

A

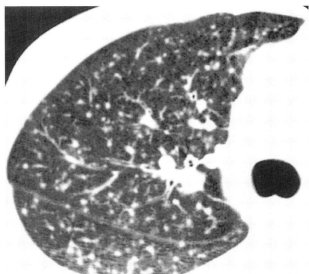

B

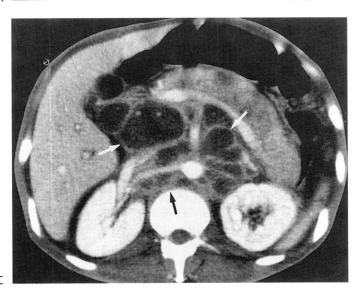

C

FIGURE 26.15. Thoracic and extrathoracic tuberculosis in a 33-year-old male acquired immune deficiency syndrome patient. **A:** Chest radiograph shows subtly increased markings in the left lower lung. **B:** High-resolution, targeted, reconstructed image through the right upper lobe reveals numerous tiny nodules of 1 to 3 mm consistent with miliary disease. On biopsy this proved to be tuberculosis. Sputums were negative. **C:** Computed tomography scanning through the abdomen results in demonstration of extensive, enlarged, low-density lymph nodes (*arrows*), consistent with retroperitoneal and mesenteric tuberculous lymphadenitis.

Radiographic Follow-up in Human Immunodeficiency Virus/Acquired Immune Deficiency Syndrome Patients with Tuberculosis: Paradoxical Worsening and Partial Immune Restoration

Serial chest radiographs to monitor response to therapy should be routinely utilized. If there is radiographic evidence of worsening disease while treatment is ongoing, considerations should include various complicating factors, including the administration of highly active antiretroviral therapy (HAART) with consequent immune restoration disease, the acquisition of multidrug-resistant tuberculosis, failure to comply with therapy, drug reaction, or the development of concomitant thoracic complications of HIV (26–28). In the setting of AIDS the possibility of unrelated pulmonary processes arising during the treatment period must be considered. Twenty-seven percent of the patients with AIDS and TB developed new HIV-related lung disease during the follow-up period of 3 to 6 months in the series by Small et al. (27). A high index of suspicion for other HIV-associated diseases in this setting must be maintained.

Since approximately 1996, the potent combination of protease inhibitors and antiretroviral therapy (HAART), usually consisting of two nucleoside reverse transcriptase inhibitors, has become the cornerstone in the management of HIV-related disease (29,30). This regime is now allowing partial immune restoration (PIR) in AIDS patients, evidenced by declining HIV viral loads, increasing CD4 cell counts, and partial restoration of cell-mediated immunity (29,30). The clinical consequences of such therapeutic advances are reductions in the progression of HIV infection to clinical AIDS, reductions in the incidence of new opportunistic infections, reduction in the need for prophylactic therapy after PIR, and

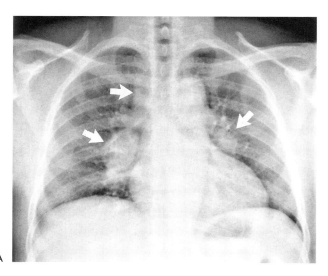

A

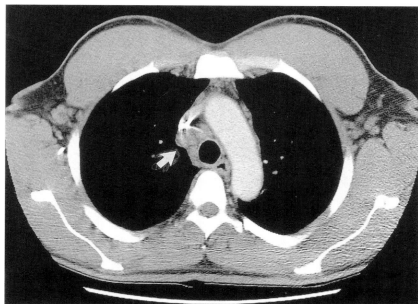

B

FIGURE 26.16. Paradoxical worsening of tuberculous adenitis in a 47-year-old man with acquired immune deficiency syndrome and tuberculosis, occurring after initiation of highly active antiviral therapy (HAART). **A:** Chest radiograph demonstrates abundant mediastinal and hilar adenopathy (*arrows*). **B:** Computed tomography (CT) scan obtained at the level of the aortic arch demonstrates enlarged right paratracheal and retrocaval/pretracheal lymph nodes (*arrow*).

a reduction in mortality from HIV infection (29). With these benefits came recognition of a new clinical and radiographic entity, partial immune restoration disease, mediated by the newly heightened immune response. This paradoxical response occurs most frequently in patients with CD4 cell counts below 100/mm³ before initiation of HAART and represents a restoration of cell-mediated immunity.

Paradoxical clinical and radiographic worsening in patients undergoing treatment for tuberculosis has been described since the 1960s and has been attributed to an inflammatory response consequent to improved host immunity after initiation of antituberculosis therapy. These findings are thought to largely reflect improved cell-mediated immune function, including strengthened delayed hypersensitivity and decreased suppressor mechanisms occurring in the weeks following initiation of therapy (28). In patients coinfected with HIV and TB a similar phenomenon has been

described after institution of HAART, seen in approximately 35% of cases (31). This may occur even if the patient has been undergoing anti-TB therapy for some time, and even after clinical and radiographic improvement has been attained on anti-TB therapy alone. HAART therapy heightens the granulomatous response to the organism by increasing the number and improving the function of the T-helper type 1 cells, a major effector cell in cell-mediated immunity in TB. The cytokines produced by these cells (interferon-γ and interleukin-2) enhance the ability to clear the organisms but also incite the inflammation (32). Soon after HAART is begun, usually within a few days to weeks, restored antimycobacterial cell-mediated immunity may result in new or worsening lymph node enlargement, parenchymal disease, and/or pleural effusions (28) (Fig. 26.16). Clinically fever is common (33). In the series of Fishman et al. (28), paradoxical radiographic worsening occurred in 45% of the AIDS

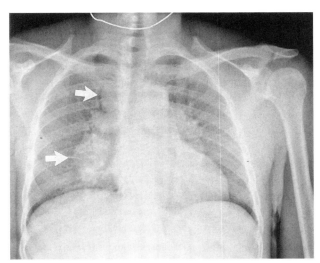

C

FIGURE 26.16. C: Repeat chest radiograph approximately 3 weeks after initiation of HAART shows worsening of lymph node enlargement (*arrows*). **D:** CT scan obtained at the level of the aortic arch a few days later also demonstrates marked worsening in paratracheal and retrocaval adenopathy.

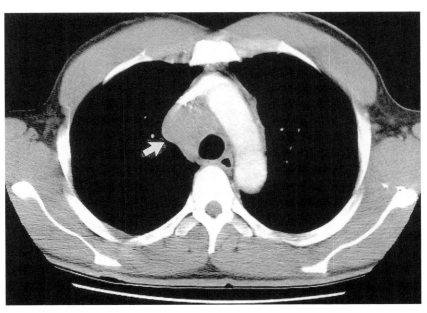

D

patients on HAART, as compared with 20% of HIV-positive patients not on HAART or HIV-negative TB patients. Parenchymal disease was the finding most likely to worsen. Severe worsening occurred in the group with most severe immune suppression initially; all patients in this group had CD4 cell counts less than 100/mm^3.

It is important to appreciate that the worsening clinical and radiographic features of this process do not represent an increase in the replication of mycobacteria. In fact, once PIR disease is established as the cause of worsening clinical and radiographic findings, and other etiologic factors have been excluded, some investigators feel that patients may benefit from steroid therapy (33). However, others have reported an increase in TB relapse (positive culture or histopathologic findings after treatment and documented negative culture findings) in patients with

paradoxical worsening of TB after HAART (34). These data suggest persistent infection as the cause of relapse, and initiation of steroid therapy should be approached with caution. However, in this report by Wendel et al. (34), the paradoxical worsening of TB occurred with the same frequency in AIDS patients both receiving and not receiving HAART.

MULTIDRUG-RESISTANT TUBERCULOSIS

When drug resistance develops during an inadequately managed episode of mycobacterial infection (primary resistance) or when the infecting bacillus is already antibiotic resistant at the time of infection (secondary resistance), the radiographic manifestations of the disease are characterized by the same

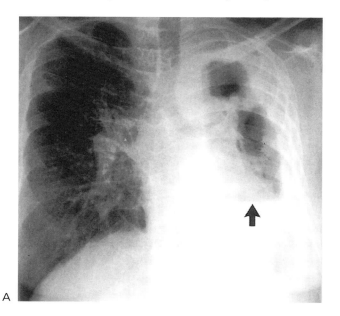

A

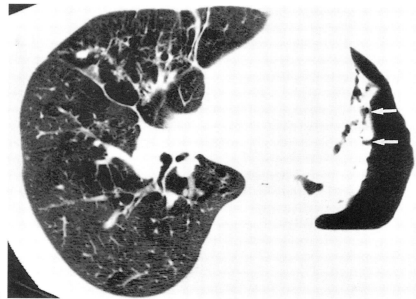

B

FIGURE 26.17. Multidrug-resistant tuberculosis resulting in bronchopleural fistula in a 43-year-old immune-intact woman. **A:** Chest radiograph after 1 year of therapy for multidrug-resistant tuberculosis demonstrates an air-fluid level in the left pleural space (*arrow*), consistent with bronchopleural fistula. The collapsed left lung is densely consolidated. **B:** Computed tomography scanning through the midlungs confirms dense consolidation of the left lung, with areas of cavitation clearly communicating with the pleural space (*arrows*).

processes. However, the disease is usually relentlessly progressive, often is disseminated, demonstrates little response to therapy, and is highly likely to be associated with secondary complications such as bronchopleural fistula (Fig. 26.17). The overall incidence of drug-resistant TB in the United States is under 2%, but in New York City it has been reported to be as high as 38% (35), reflecting the combined risk factors of foreign country of birth and coinfection with HIV.

These changes are magnified when resistant organisms infect the immunocompromised patient. In a comparison of drug-resistant and susceptible tuberculous infections in HIV-positive patients, Fischl et al. (36) found the presence of infiltrates and cavities on chest radiographs more common in the multidrug-resistant TB group than in the susceptible group. Those patients who received three or more drugs effective against their particular organism had a significantly longer survival period than those who received fewer than three effective drugs.

NONTUBERCULOUS MYCOBACTERIAL INFECTION

The presentation of nontuberculous or atypical mycobacterial infections, particularly *Mycobacterium avium* complex (MAC), may be indistinguishable from *M. tuberculosis* in patients with chronic pulmonary diseases, such as chronic obstructive pulmonary disease. The radiographic appearance is often suggestive of postprimary TB. There is also an association between atypical myobacterial infections and bronchiectasis. This subset of patients is often elderly women. The areas of lung involvement in these cases are frequently the lower lobes (37), specifically the middle lobe and lingua (38). Although chest radiographic findings are frequently nonspecific, recognition of CT findings that include nodular or alveolar infiltrates, cavities, and bronchiectasis often suggests this diagnosis (39,40) (Fig. 26.18A). In particular, the presence of bronchiectasis may be more sensitively detected at HRCT. A

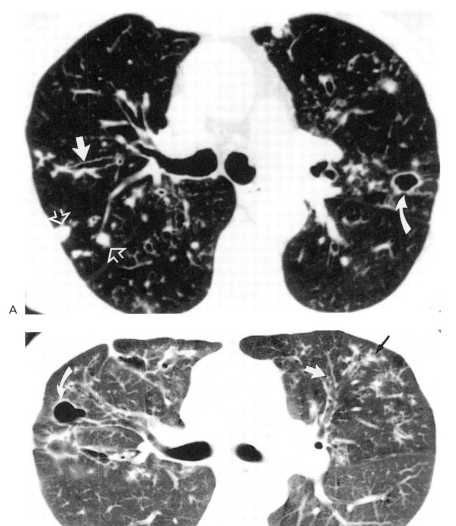

FIGURE 26.18. *Mycobacterium avium* complex (MAC) infection. **A:** High-resolution computed tomography (CT) scan obtained at the level of the carina in a 75-year-old woman demonstrates scattered nodules (*open arrows*), bronchiectasis (*white arrow*), and a small cavity (*curved arrow*). This constellation of findings, especially in elderly women, is suggestive of MAC disease, subsequently confirmed in this case. **B:** CT scan in a 33-year-old acquired immune deficiency syndrome patient presenting with hemoptysis shows similar findings. Note prominent bronchiectasis (*white arrow*), nodular densities (*black arrow*), and small cavity (*curved arrow*), as compared with **A.** Subsequent bronchoalveolar lavage and multiple sputum samples confirmed MAC infection in the absence of other granulomatous or fungal organisms.

study evaluating serial CT findings in these patients reported evidence of developing or progressing bronchiectasis, which suggested that the bronchiectasis, rather than predisposing to the infection, resulted from the infection (40).

The second group at heightened risk for atypical mycobacterial infection is the immunocompromised, particularly AIDS patients. For these patients the portal of entry for the organism is usually the gastrointestinal tract and, accordingly, the disease is disseminated by the time it affects the lungs. Unlike *M. tuberculosis*, MAC is rarely an AIDS-defining illness. Radiographic findings include adenopathy, diffuse patchy infiltrates, cavities (Fig. 26.18B), and frequently a normal radiograph, seen in up to 21% of HIV-positive patients with documented pulmonary MAC (41). The nonspecific chest radiographic findings may not be helpful in making a specific diagnosis of MAC. By comparing the roentgenographic findings in HIV-positive patients with MAC with those of patients with *M. tuberculosis*, Modilevsky et al. (41) were able to prospectively predict the correct diagnosis in 83% of the patients with TB, as opposed to 25% of those with MAC infections.

IMAGING SURGICALLY MANAGED DISEASE

Surgical techniques to control mycobacterial infections in the lung have declined since the introduction of effective antibiotic therapy. Before chemotherapeutic management, either affected lobes with recalcitrant infections were resected surgically or the infection was eradicated by obliterating the oxygen supply necessary for growth of the organism. This was achieved through collapse therapy; therapeutic atelectasis of the affected lobe was created, often through surgical musculoskeletal collapse or by filling the pleural space with a volume-occupying substance (lipid material or artificial plastic spheres) in a process called *plombage therapy* (Fig. 26.19).

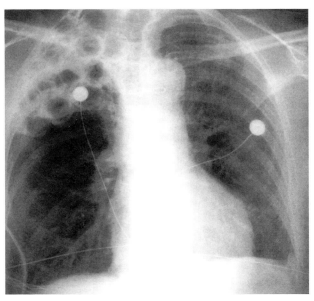

A

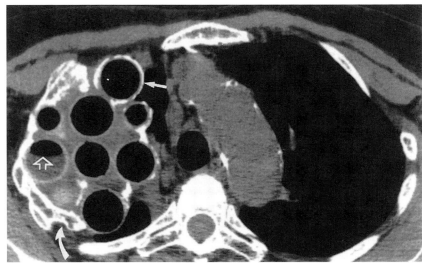

B

FIGURE 26.19. Plombage therapy in a 64-year-old man. **A:** Chest radiograph depicts filling of the right upper hemithorax by plastic spheres. **B:** Computed tomography scan obtained at the level of the aortic arch demonstrates that some of the spheres have calcified (*white arrow*) and fluid has accumulated in others (*open arrow*). Healed fractured ribs are noted (*curved arrow*).

Surgical management techniques are again gaining acceptance for patients failing medical therapy. Typical settings include infection with multidrug-resistant mycobacterial organisms or infection by nontuberculous mycobacteria with limited response to antibiotic therapy. These patients have a high rate of surgical and postsurgical complications, including tissue breakdown at the resection site and consequent bronchopleural fistula. In the series of 80 patients studied by Pomerantz et al. (42), 16% developed bronchopleural fistulas or persistent air leaks postoperatively. These investigators advocated liberal use of mobilized muscle flaps to seal resection sites, particularly in cases in which preoperative sputum tests were positive, in which a postlobectomy space was anticipated, or in which a bronchopleural fistula existed preoperatively (Fig. 26.20).

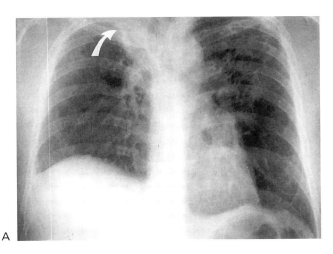

A

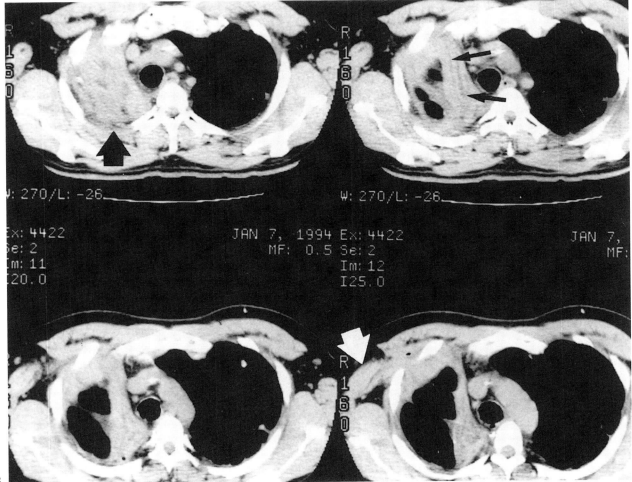

B

FIGURE 26.20. Muscle flap interposition after right upper lobectomy for tuberculosis in a 37-year-old man. **A:** Chest radiograph obtained after right upper lobectomy for multidrug-resistant tuberculosis demonstrates volume loss in the right hemithorax after lobectomy. Note right apical density (*curved arrow*). **B:** Sequential computed tomography images obtained through the right apex and right upper hemithorax depicts a vascularized muscle pedicle traversing the right axillary space (*right lower image, white arrow*) and the muscle flap filling the right apex (*left upper image, black arrow*). Low-density streaks (*right upper image, small arrows*) within the muscle flap are secondary to fatty atrophy.

NONMYCOBACTERIAL SEQUELAE OF TUBERCULOSIS

Despite successful suppression or obliteration of infection, residua of TB infection in the lung parenchyma may remain, including fibrosis, scarring, nodules, cavities, and volume loss (43). Less apparent on chest radiographs, but often clinically important, are the residual effects on the airways, such as bronchiectasis, which may be focal or diffuse (43). Hemoptysis may be the presenting symptom of the patient with postinflammatory bronchiectasis. In a series utilizing CT in the evaluation of patients presenting with hemoptysis, airway bleeding was caused by bronchiectasis in 25%, exclusive of the 16% in whom hemoptysis was directly attributed to TB (44). Postinflammatory bronchial stenosis, classically affecting the middle lobe, may result in a chronically atelectatic, con-solidated lobe. When this involves the middle lobe, it is known as *chronic middle lobe syndrome*. Calcified mediastinal or hilar nodes that erode into airways are referred to as *broncholiths* (45). This may cause airway obstruction or hemoptysis (Fig. 26.21).

Cystic bronchiectasis, or residual cavities, are susceptible to superinfection, particularly by fungi such as *Aspergillus*, and often form discrete mycetomas. Serial radiographs demonstrate internal filling of a known cavity by soft-tissue density material that may be loosely formed initially but becomes tightly formed with time. A characteristic exuberant pleural reaction may be noted adjacent to the affected lobe, corresponding to the time of superinfection. Mycetomas are generally mobile within the cavity and will layer dependently upon changes in positioning (Fig. 26.22).

Bronchogenic carcinoma occurs in the scarred lungs of posttuberculous patients more commonly than it does in

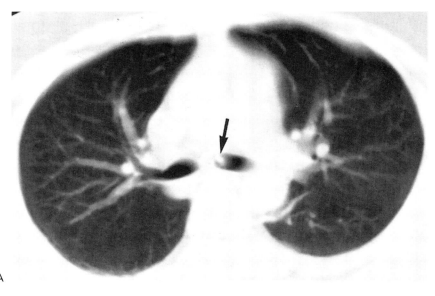

A

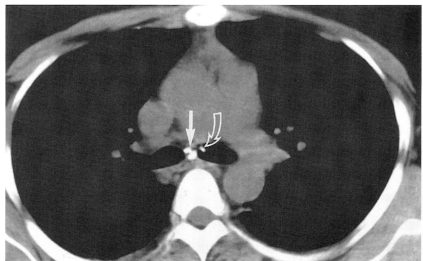

B

FIGURE 26.21. Posttuberculous broncholith in a 44-year-old woman presenting with hemoptysis. **A:** Computed tomography (CT) scan with lung windows obtained at the level of the carina. An endobronchial filling defect is identified within the left main bronchus (*arrow*). **B:** CT scan obtained with mediastinal windows at the same level reveals calcified lymph nodes in the subcarinal region (*arrow*), one of which has eroded into the left main bronchus (*curved arrow*). At bronchoscopy, a calcified node was identified partially eroding through the bronchial wall. Patient had no known history of tuberculosis.

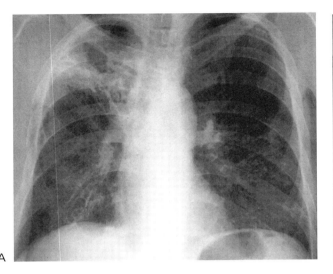
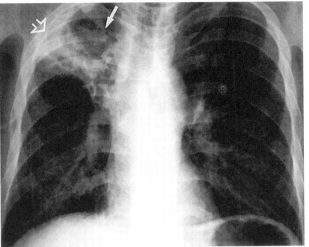

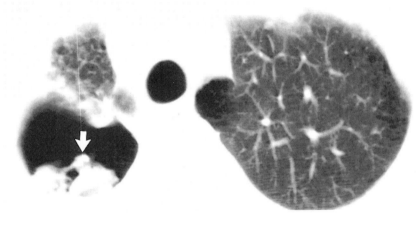

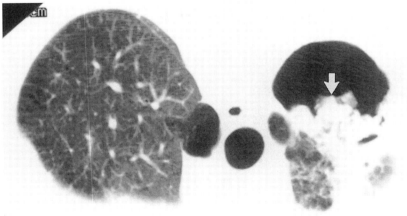

FIGURE 26.22. Mycetoma in a posttuberculous cavity in a 44-year-old man. **A:** Chest radiograph after management of tuberculosis demonstrates volume loss and cavitation in the right upper lobe. **B:** Chest radiograph obtained 3 months later reveals new irregular filling defect within the cavity (*arrow*), as well as adjacent pleural thickening, typical of fungal superinfection (*open arrow*). **C, D:** Computed tomography scanning of the lung apices when the patient is supine (**C**) and prone (**D**), respectively, results in demonstration of mobile dependent material consistent with aspergilloma in the right upper lobe cavity (*arrow*).

the general population. Such cancers are referred to as *scar carcinomas*, although the precise causal relationship of the infection to the malignancy is unclear. What is apparent, however, is that radiographic detection of such cancers is hindered by postinflammatory changes to the chest. Current radiographs must be compared not only with the most recent previous examination, in which interval changes may be subtle or masked, but also with remote examinations in the hope that subtle changes will become conspicuous (Fig. 26.23). A growing mass might represent reactivation disease; however, the possibility of superimposed malignancy should not be ruled out.

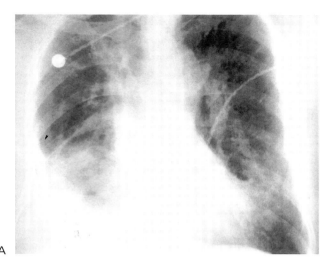

A

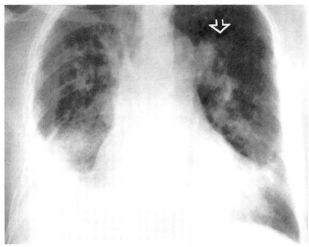

B

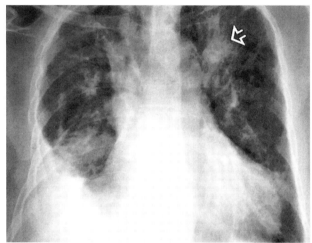

C

FIGURE 26.23. Scar carcinoma in a 64-year-old man with a history of tuberculosis. **A:** Baseline chest radiograph demonstrates increased linear and nodular markings, architectural distortion, and pleural thickening, consistent with history of tuberculosis. **B:** Follow-up radiograph obtained 14 months later was interpreted as unchanged. In retrospect, there is a soft-tissue density in the left suprahilar region (*arrow*). **C:** Chest radiograph obtained 8 months later. The left suprahilar mass is now obvious. **D:** Computed tomography scanning at the level of the aortic arch results in confirmation of a mass in the left upper lobe (*arrow*). Biopsy confirmed the presence of non–small cell lung cancer.

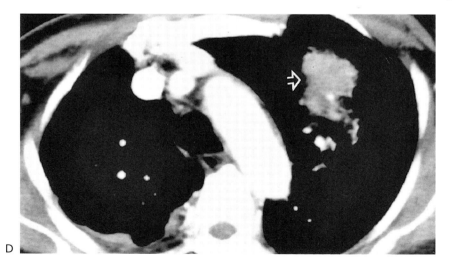

D

ROLE OF COMPUTED TOMOGRAPHY IN THE TUBERCULOSIS PATIENT

CT can provide valuable information in certain complex cases of TB. Current indications for utilization of CT in this setting include (a) detection of occult disease; (b) precise definition of the extent of disease, including evaluation of the mediastinum, pleura, and chest wall; and (c) characterization of disease, including determination of disease activity.

CT is more sensitive than chest radiography in the detection of subtle or occult parenchymal disease (46). In cases in which there is strong clinical suspicion of disease but normal or equivocal radiographic findings, the increased sensitivity of CT may allow prompt diagnosis, even when mycobacteriology results are pending (24). Chest radiographic findings in miliary disease may be subtle and are often missed. HRCT findings in miliary disease have been well described (17). HRCT markedly increases the probability of disease detection (Fig. 26.24) as compared with

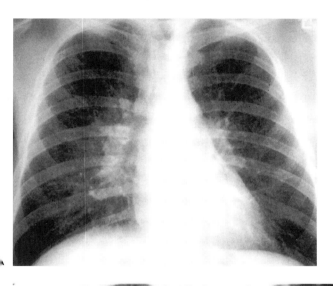

FIGURE 26.24. Miliary tuberculosis in a 36-year-old man. **A:** Chest radiograph demonstrates obvious right hilar adenopathy. Diffuse miliary nodules were missed on initial interpretation. **B:** A 10-mm-thick collimated computed tomography (CT) image (conventional resolution) obtained from the upper lungs. Miliary nodules are subtle and could be missed. **C:** A 1.5-mm high-resolution CT image obtained from the upper lungs. Diffuse nodules, ranging from 1 to 3 mm, are diagnostic of miliary disease. Many of the nodules are subpleural, resulting in an irregular pleural surface (*small arrow*). These findings are characteristic of miliary tuberculosis.

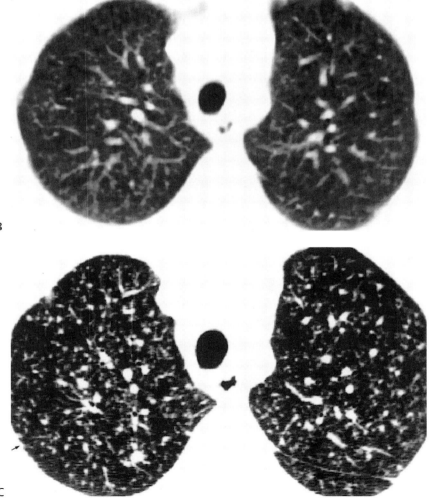

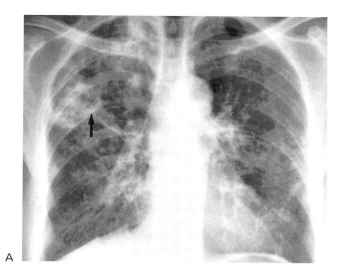

A

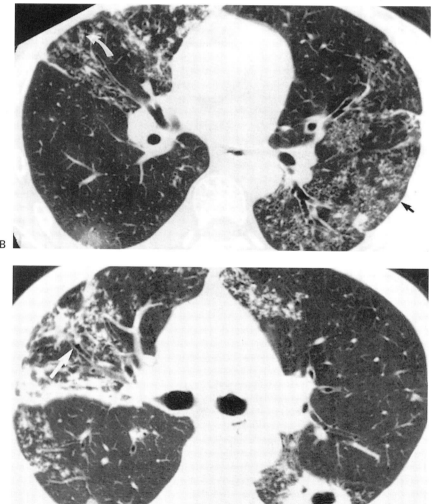

B

C

FIGURE 26.25. Endobronchial tuberculosis in a 56-year-old man. **A:** Chest radiograph shows right upper lobe cavity (*arrow*), patchy infiltrates, and a suggestion of fine nodularity in the left mid-lung. **B:** High-resolution computed tomography (HRCT) through the mid-lungs produced an image showing a myriad of tiny, centrilobular nodules (*arrow*). These represent caseous material filling bronchioles, alveolar ducts, and marginal alveoli. Clustering of these nodules about the branching airway has been termed the "tree-in-bud" appearance (*curved arrow*). **C:** HRCT image obtained at the level of the carina shows a cavity in the superior segment of the left lower lobe (*black arrowhead*) not suspected from the radiograph. Bronchiectasis in the right upper lobe (*white arrow*) was also not predicted from the radiograph. Scattered foci of centrilobular nodules are the result of endobronchial dissemination of infectious material.

conventional CT. CT also may demonstrate subtle adenopathy or early infiltrates before they are detectable radiographically. In addition, HRCT is of proven value in the detection of occult bronchiectasis (47–49).

By eliminating superimposition of structures, CT allows accurate evaluation of the extent of disease. Parenchymal abnormalities, including occult abscesses and cavities as well as unsuspected complications such as fungal superinfection, are clearly depicted (Fig. 26.22). CT is also of proven value in identifying central airway pathology such as bronchial stenoses and broncholiths (Fig. 26.21). As a consequence, in select cases CT may be of value before bronchoscopy as a useful guide to direct the bronchoscopist to optimal sites for transbronchial biopsy or bronchoalveolar lavage.

In addition to identifying and characterizing mediastinal and parenchymal abnormalities, CT is also of value in assessing pleural disease, both acute and chronic. CT identification of parenchymal foci of disease hidden radiographically by a large pleural effusion may be of considerable value in suggesting the correct etiology of an acute effusion. More important, chronic pleural changes, such as loculated fluid collections, are readily detected with CT, even when they are radiographically occult. CT is of particular value in assessing complications such as empyema necessitatis and bronchopleural fistula (Figs. 26.10 through 26.13). The location of the fistulous connection between small peripheral airways and the pleural space may also be identified with HRCT.

Less commonly, CT may have a role in assessing the pericardium. Tuberculous pericarditis is an uncommon complication of TB, causing potentially treatable cardiac compromise. Although rarely seen on plain radiographs, pericardial thickening is easily recognized with CT. In the series by Suchet and Horwitz (50), the constellation of pericardial thickening greater than 3 mm combined with impaired diagnostic filling at cardiac catheterization suggested the diagnosis of tuberculous pericarditis in 157 of 186 patients with such findings.

Of still greater potential value, recent studies have suggested a possible role for CT in assessing disease activity. HRCT findings in active TB have been correlated with pathologic findings (9). As documented by Im et al., 97% of patients with active primary TB had evidence of bronchogenic spread of disease on HRCT. The characteristic HRCT appearance of active endobronchial disease includes poorly defined centrilobular nodules of 5 to 8 mm in diameter, centrilobular branching structures, and the "tree-in-bud" appearance (Fig. 26.25). These lesions represent caseous material filling the bronchioles, alveolar ducts, and peribronchial alveoli as well as peribronchiolar granulomata. These findings are seen in a limited number of entities; in the setting of acute infectious disease, they are characteristic of active TB (9,51,52).

CT may also prove useful in the detection or confirmation of reactivation disease that is suspected radiographically or clinically, but is obscured by chronic fibrotic and postinflammatory pleural or parenchymal changes. New infiltrates, acinar or centrilobular nodules, cavities, effusions, and adenopathy all suggest recrudescent disease (Fig. 26.9). Evidence of bronchogenic spread of tuberculosis was seen in only 20% of cases with postprimary TB radiographically but was identified in up to 95% of cases at CT (53,54). In the appropriate clinical setting, typical HRCT appearances may warrant initiation of therapy before confirmatory microbiology.

CONCLUSION

As we enter a new era in the fight against TB, the role of imaging has moved to the forefront. The historical tool of the physician, the chest radiograph, must be interpreted with a new understanding of the changing and varied presentations of this old disease. Studies must be interpreted with a high index of suspicion for TB, particularly in the new and growing risk groups. The ability of newer modalities such as CT to detect subtle disease, characterize typical changes suggesting this specific diagnosis, and clarify processes masked by complex radiographs should be appreciated and appropriately utilized.

REFERENCES

1. Buckner CB, Leithiser RE, Walker CW, et al. The changing epidemiology of tuberculosis and other mycobacterial infections in the United States: implications for the radiologist. *AJR Am J Roentgenol* 1991;156: 255–264.
2. Brudney K, Dobkin J. Resurgent tuberculosis in New York City. Human immunodeficiency virus, homelessness, and the decline of tuberculosis control programs. *Am Rev Respir Dis* 1991;144: 475–479.
3. Leung AN. Pulmonary tuberculosis: the essentials. *Radiology* 1999;210:307–322.
4. Diagnostic Standards and Classification of Tuberculosis in Adults and Children. This official statement of the American Thoracic Society (ATS) and the Centers for Disease Control and Prevention was adopted by the ATS Board of Directors, July 1999. This statement was endorsed by the Council of the Infectious Disease Society of America, September 1999. *Am J Respir Crit Care Med* 2000;161(4 Pt 1).
5. Hill AR, Premkumar S, Brustein S, et al. Disseminated tuberculosis in the acquired immunodeficiency syndrome era. *Am Rev Respir Dis* 1991;144:1164–1170.
6. Woodring JH, Vandiviere HM, Fried AM, et al. Update: the radiographic features of pulmonary tuberculosis. *AJR Am J Roentgenol* 1986;146:497–506.
7. Krysl J, Korzeniewska-Kosela M, Muller NL, et al. Radiologic features of pulmonary tuberculosis: an assessment of 188 cases. *Can Assoc Radiol J* 1994;45:101–107.
8. Leung AN, Muller NL, Pineda PR, et al. Primary tuberculosis in

childhood: radiographic manifestations. *Radiology* 1992;182: 87–91.

9. Im JG, Itoh H, Shim YS, et al. Pulmonary tuberculosis: CT findings—early active disease and sequential change with antituberculous therapy. *Radiology* 1993;186:653–660.

10. Hulnick DH, Naidich DP, McCauley DI. Pleural tuberculosis evaluated by computed tomography. *Radiology* 1983;149: 759–765.

11. Im JG, Webb WR, Han MC, et al. Apical opacity associated with pulmonary tuberculosis: high-resolution CT findings. *Radiology* 1991;178:727–731.

12. Glicklich M, Mendelson DS, Gendal ES, et al. Tuberculous empyema necessitatis. Computed tomography findings. *Clin Imaging* 1990;14:23–25.

13. Bhatt GM, Austin HM. CT demonstration of empyema necessitatis. *J Comput Assist Tomogr* 1985;9:1108–1109.

14. Adler BD, Padley SP, Muller NL. Tuberculosis of the chest wall: CT findings. *J Comput Assist Tomogr* 1993;17:271–273.

14a. Centers for Disease Control and Prevention. 1993 revised classification system for HIV infection and expanded surveillance for AIDS among adolescents and adults. *MORB MORTAL WKLY REP* 1993;41(RR-13):1–19.

15. Markowitz N, Hansen NI, Hopewell PC, et al. Incidence of tuberculosis in the United States among HIV-infected persons. The Pulmonary Complications of HIV Infection Study Group. *Ann Intern Med* 1997;126:123–132.

16. Havlir DV, Barnes PF. Tuberculosis in patients with human immunodeficiency virus infection. *N Engl J Med* 1999;340: 367–373.

17. McGuinness G, Naidich DP, Jagirdar J, et al. High resolution CT findings in miliary lung disease. *J Comput Assist Tomogr* 1992;16: 384–390.

18. Greenberg SD, Frager D, Suster B, et al. Active pulmonary tuberculosis in patients with AIDS: spectrum of radiographic findings (including a normal appearance). *Radiology* 1994;193:115–119.

19. Barnes PF, Bloch AB, Davidson PT, et al. Tuberculosis in patients with human immunodeficiency virus infection. *N Engl J Med* 1991;324:1644–1650.

20. Kramer F, Modilevsky T, Waliany AR, et al. Delayed diagnosis of tuberculosis in patients with human immunodeficiency virus infection. *Am J Med* 1990;89:451–456.

21. Jones BE, Young SM, Antoniskis D, et al. Relationship of the manifestations of tuberculosis to CD4 cell counts in patients with human immunodeficiency virus infection. *Am Rev Respir Dis* 1993;148:1292–1296.

22. Long R, Maycher B, Scalcini M, et al. The chest roentgenogram in pulmonary tuberculosis patients seropositive for human immunodeficiency virus type 1. *Chest* 1991;99:123–127.

23. Perlman DC, el-Sadr WM, Nelson ET, et al. Variation of chest radiographic patterns in pulmonary tuberculosis by degree of human immunodeficiency virus-related immunosuppression. The Terry Beirn Community Programs for Clinical Research on AIDS (CPCRA). The AIDS Clinical Trials Group (ACTG). *Clin Infect Dis* 1997;25:242–246.

24. Pastores SM, Naidich DP, Aranda CP, et al. Intrathoracic adenopathy associated with pulmonary tuberculosis in patients with human immunodeficiency virus infection. *Chest* 1993;103: 1433–1437.

25. Revision of the CDC surveillance case definition for acquired immunodeficiency syndrome. Council of State and Territorial Epidemiologists; AIDS Program, Center for Infectious Diseases. *MMWR Morb Mortal Wkly Rep* 1987;36 Suppl 1:1S–15S.

26. Fishman JE, Sais GJ, Schwartz DS, et al. Radiographic findings and patterns in multidrug-resistant tuberculosis. *J Thorac Imaging* 1998;13:65–71.

27. Small PM, Hopewell PC, Schecter GF, et al. Evolution of chest radiographs in treated patients with pulmonary tuberculosis and HIV infection. *J Thorac Imaging* 1994;9:74–77.

28. Fishman JE, Saraf-Lavi E, Narita M, et al. Pulmonary tuberculosis in AIDS patients: transient chest radiographic worsening after initiation of antiretroviral therapy. *AJR Am J Roentgenol* 2000; 174:43–49.

29. Powderly WG, Landay A, Lederman MM. Recovery of the immune system with antiretroviral therapy: the end of opportunism? *JAMA* 1998;280:72–77.

30. Lederman MM, Valdez H. Immune restoration with antiretroviral therapies: implications for clinical management. *JAMA* 2000; 284:223–228.

31. Navas E, Martin-Davila P, Moreno L, et al. Paradoxical reactions of tuberculosis in patients with the acquired immunodeficiency syndrome who are treated with highly active antiretroviral therapy. *Arch Intern Med* 2002;162:97–99.

32. Schluger NW, Perez D, Liu YM. Reconstitution of immune responses to tuberculosis in patients with HIV infection who receive antiretroviral therapy. *Chest* 2002;122:597–602.

33. Saurborn DP, Fishman JE, Boiselle PM. The imaging spectrum of pulmonary tuberculosis in AIDS. *J Thorac Imaging* 2002;17: 28–33.

34. Wendel KA, Alwood KS, Gachuhi R, et al. Paradoxical worsening of tuberculosis in HIV-infected persons. *Chest* 2001;120: 193–197.

35. Moore M, Onorato IM, McCray E, et al. Trends in drug-resistant tuberculosis in the United States, 1993-1996. *JAMA* 1997;278: 833–837.

36. Fischl MA, Daikos GL, Uttamchandani RB, et al. Clinical presentation and outcome of patients with HIV infection and tuberculosis caused by multiple-drug-resistant bacilli. *Ann Intern Med* 1992;117:184–190.

37. Miller WT Jr. Spectrum of pulmonary nontuberculous mycobacterial infection. *Radiology* 1994;191:343–350.

38. Wittram C, Weisbrod GL. *Mycobacterium avium* complex lung disease in immunocompetent patients: radiography–CT correlation. *Br J Radiol* 2002;75:340–344.

39. Hartman TE, Swensen SJ, Williams DE. *Mycobacterium avium-intracellulare* complex: evaluation with CT. *Radiology* 1993;187: 23–26.

40. Moore EH. Atypical mycobacterial infection in the lung: CT appearance. *Radiology* 1993;187:777–782.

41. Modilevsky T, Sattler FR, Barnes PF. Mycobacterial disease in patients with human immunodeficiency virus infection. *Arch Intern Med* 1989;149:2201–2205.

42. Pomerantz M, Madsen L, Goble M, et al. Surgical management of resistant mycobacterial tuberculosis and other mycobacterial pulmonary infections. *Ann Thorac Surg* 1991;52:1108–1111; discussion 1112.

43. Kim HY, Song KS, Goo JM, et al. Thoracic sequelae and complications of tuberculosis. *Radiographics* 2001;21:839–858; discussion 859–860.

44. McGuinness G, Beacher JR, Harkin TJ, et al. Hemoptysis: prospective high-resolution CT/bronchoscopic correlation. *Chest* 1994;105:1155–1162.

45. Conces DJ, Jr., Tarver RD, Vix VA. Broncholithiasis: CT features in 15 patients. *AJR Am J Roentgenol* 1991;157:249–253.

46. Webb WR, Müller NL, Naidich DP. Clinical utility of high-resolution computed tomography. In: *High-resolution CT of the lung*, 3rd ed. Philadelphia: Lippincott Williams & Wilkins, 2001:569–597.

47. Grenier P, Maurice F, Musset D, et al. Bronchiectasis: assessment by thin-section CT. *Radiology* 1986;161:95–99.

48. Muller NL, Bergin CJ, Ostrow DN, et al. Role of computed

tomography in the recognition of bronchiectasis. *AJR Am J Roentgenol* 1984;143:971–976.

49. Naidich DP, McCauley DI, Khouri NF, et al. Computed tomography of bronchiectasis. *J Comput Assist Tomogr* 1982;6:437–444.

50. Suchet IB, Horwitz TA. CT in tuberculous constrictive pericarditis. *J Comput Assist Tomogr* 1992;16:391–400.

51. Gruden JF, Webb WR, Warnock M. Centrilobular opacities in the lung on high-resolution CT: diagnostic considerations and pathologic correlation. *AJR Am J Roentgenol* 1994;162:569–574.

52. Lee KS, Song KS, Lim TH, et al. Adult-onset pulmonary tuberculosis: findings on chest radiographs and CT scans. *AJR Am J Roentgenol* 1993;160:753–758.

53. Im JG, Itoh H, Han MC. CT of pulmonary tuberculosis. *Semin Ultrasound Comput Tomogr Magnet Reson Imaging* 1995;16:420–434.

54. Hatipoglu ON, Osma E, Manisali M, et al. High resolution computed tomographic findings in pulmonary tuberculosis. *Thorax* 1996;51:397–402.

MILIARY TUBERCULOSIS

STEPHEN K. BAKER
JEFFREY GLASSROTH

Miliary tuberculosis (TB) represents the unchecked hematogenous dissemination of *Mycobacterium tuberculosis* organisms. Although usually thought of as a radiologic concept in the present era, the notion of miliary disease originated as a pathologic description. In 1679, Theophilus Bonetus (1), in his catalogue of postmortem examinations, *Sepulchretum sive anatomia practica*, described a patient:

> " . . . whom doctors had been treating daily as if asthmatic; but no thick or tenacious humor was found within the airways, but rather throughout the whole substance of the parenchyma, minute but crumbly small stones were found, most similar to a kind of very old cheese."

John Jacobus Manget (2), in republishing Bonetus's work in 1700, added his own observations, and first likened the gross pathologic appearance to that of innumerable millet seeds (hence *miliary*):

> "The whole surface, in front and behind, as well as within the interstitium of the major lobes, was covered with firm small white corpuscles, of the size of millet seeds. . . ."

The relation of miliary TB to caseating or cavitary pulmonary TB remained unsettled for centuries, despite Bonetus's instincts in grouping his case with pulmonary cavitations. Laennec clearly established the connection in 1810 (3), but as late as 1865 no less an authority than Virchow maintained that miliary TB and caseating pulmonary TB were different diseases (4,5). It was ultimately the collective work of von Buhl (1857), who asserted that miliary TB was an infectious disease caused by "tuberculous poison" from caseous foci spreading via the blood (4); of Villemin (1865), who reproduced disseminated TB in rabbits by injection of caseous material and pus from patients; and of Koch (1882), who discovered the tubercle bacillus that proved miliary and pulmonary TB to be variants of one disease.

S. K. Baker (Deceased): Department of Medicine, Northwestern University Medical School, Chicago, Illinois.

J. Glassroth: Department of Medicine, University of Wisconsin School of Medicine; Department of Medicine, University of Wisconsin Hospitals and Clinics, Madison, Wisconsin.

EPIDEMIOLOGY

Data from the Centers for Disease Control and Prevention (CDC) reveal that in 1969 to 1973 (6), 1975 (7), and 1985 to 1988 (8), a remarkably consistent 1.3 % of reported cases of TB were classified as miliary. However, in urban areas especially, the incidence of miliary TB is now increasing, both in absolute numbers and as a percentage of total cases of TB (9), because of the joint emergence of the human immunodeficiency virus (HIV) and multidrug-resistant strains of *M. tuberculosis*. In areas endemic for HIV infection, particularly where effective antiretroviral therapy is not available, the incidence of disseminated TB as a percentage of total TB cases is approaching that of the preantibiotic era. At Boston City Hospital in the preantibiotic era, 20% of all autopsied patients with TB had miliary spread (10); in the late 1970s, this incidence had decreased to 0.7% (11). Similarly, at Johns Hopkins, disseminated TB accounted for 0.7% of all deaths in the preantibiotic era, and by the 1950s this figure had fallen by more than 50% (12). With the emergence of the HIV pandemic in the 1980s, disseminated TB accounted for 8% of all TB cases from 1984 to 1987 in one endemic area, with at least 10% of patients with TB who were coinfected with HIV having clinically recognizable dissemination (13). The incidence of disseminated disease in patients with advanced HIV infection is much higher (14).

Men are more often affected than women in most series (11, 15–17), perhaps reflecting the greater prevalence of TB in general among men (8). Whether blacks are more likely to develop disseminated disease is unclear. Some series reported a higher incidence in blacks, although socioeconomic differences were not controlled for (15,16). Between 1969 and 1973, the CDC found that disseminated disease was present in 2.9% of all cases of TB reported for blacks, whereas less than half that incidence (1.2%) was seen among cases reported for whites (6). The relative contributions of living conditions, access to medical care, nutrition, and comorbidity were not assessed in these older studies, although a more recent analysis suggests that socioeconomic conditions may be a significant factor in explaining apparent disparities between races with respect to tuberculosis in the United States (18). In a study that did not include white participants, Al-Arif et al. (19) reported that a particular human leukocyte antigen (HLA) phenotype (Bw15) appeared to be a marker for advanced tuberculous disease, including disseminated disease, in black persons. The authors did not comment on the relative frequency of this haplotype in blacks as compared with whites.

The age of peak prevalence of miliary TB continues to change. Typically, it is most manifest in population subgroups with the least developed or most impaired cellular immunity. In the preantibiotic era, young children (<3 years) were most affected; in the post-isoniazid era, as the overall prevalence of TB declined, miliary disease became more common in relative terms among the elderly. The rise of the HIV and the increased use of immunosuppressive therapies for other diseases have created a new subset of relatively young adults such that the prevalence curve of miliary TB is becoming biphasic, with peaks in early adulthood and later in life (20).

PATHOGENESIS

Unchecked dissemination can occur during primary infection or after reactivation of a latent focus. During primary infection, small numbers of tubercle bacilli usually gain access to the circulation via the lymphatics and embolize to the capillary beds of most organ systems, with a statistical and perhaps trophic predilection for those most vascular and therefore most reliably oxygenated, such as liver, spleen, marrow, and brain. Almost always these metastatic foci heal by granulomatous encapsulation, sometimes with calcification, and with little tissue necrosis. Reactivation later in life may lead to pulmonary or localized extrapulmonary TB (12). Acute miliary TB occurs when these foci fail to heal and are able to progress (12,21). This is the form most often seen in previously uninfected hosts with impaired cellular immunity, and it usually occurs within 6 months of the primary infection. Alternatively, reactivation of a latent focus of infection, with subsequent caseation and erosion into adjoining blood vessels or large lymphatics, allows hematogenous embolization of large numbers of bacilli (3,10). Synchronous granuloma formation in the affected viscera results in the striking gross pathologic appearance first noted by the 17th century pathologists. Less commonly, caseous necrosis of a mediastinal node, with drainage into the thoracic duct, may lead to miliary TB largely confined to the lungs. Caseation into a pulmonary vein, with prompt systemic spread, or caseation of an extrapulmonary focus drained by the portal circulation (spleen, mesenteric nodes), with initial hepatic involvement, may lead to prominent nonpulmonary symptoms and signs before typical lung involvement becomes clinically or radiologically obvious.

Most cases of disseminated TB in HIV-infected persons in this country have been thought on epidemiologic grounds to be the result of reactivation, although dissemination soon after primary infection or exogenous reinfection has been demonstrated by restriction fragment length polymorphism (RFLP) analysis (23,24).

Determinants of successful dissemination include the state of host cellular immune defenses (nonspecific and specific), mycobacterial virulence factors, and the number of organisms gaining lymphohematogenous access (bacterial load). Prior to the onset of specific cell-mediated immunity, macrophages, natural killer (NK) cells and γ/δ T-lymphocytes participate in a nonspecific response to localize tubercle bacilli (25). Defects in these elements could be a factor in early dissemination. Indeed, disseminated TB has been associated with impaired expansion of γ/δ T cells (26), a CD4$^-$ CD8$^-$ NK subset that may be involved in generating a rapid response to common antigens, such as bacterial or host heat-shock proteins. As noted previously, certain class I major histocompatibility complex (MHC) alleles have also been associated with a higher rate of dissemination. In that study, 9 of 12 black patients with pulmonary TB and the *HLABw15* allele also had evidence of dissemination (19). Failure to generate adequate specific cell-mediated immunity also presumably could to lead to dissemination (27). CD4$^+$ T lymphocytes, by generating activated blood-borne macrophages via interferon-γ (IFN-γ), interleukin-2 (IL-2), and other lymphokines, appear to have a central role in the rapid containment of infection at distant sites, as well as in affecting tuberculin reactivity (25,28). In animal models, tumor necrosis factor-α (TNF-α) has a central role in the host response against tuberculoisis, including granuloma formation and containment of disease (29), and it has been reported that disseminated tuberculosis occurs soon after the initiation of therapy with infliximab, a monoclonal antibody against TNF-α used in the management of rheumatoid arthritis and inflammatory bowel disease (30). MHC class II–restricted target cell lysis is impaired *in vitro* in patients with disseminated disease but not in those with cavitary disease (31). Disseminated infection and impaired tuberculin reactivity are commonly associated with advanced HIV infection and increase in incidence as the CD4$^+$ lymphocyte count falls (14). The role of other infections often seen with advanced HIV disease, such as cytomegalovirus infection, in dissemination of mycobacterial infection is not known. Mycobacteremia is common (32), and suggests defective mycobacteria-containing target cell lysis or macrophage microbicidal activity, or both. Other viral infections, particularly measles and pertussis, may predispose to disseminated TB in early childhood (11); they also transiently reduce CD4 counts.

Kaufmann (28) made the point that certain aspects of the normal cell-mediated immune response may facilitate dissemination. Clonal expansion of CD8$^+$ cytolytic T-cell populations that are able to lyse target cells presenting mycobacterial antigens and MHC type I proteins is known to occur in the course of tuberculous infection. Overexuberant lysis of target cell macrophages, by the release of intracellular proteases, oxidants, and viable organisms, may contribute to tissue necrosis and facilitate extracellular spread of organisms. Dannenberg (33) argued that liquefaction necrosis—probably a manifestation of a vigorous delayed-type hypersensitivity response—is the most important mechanism facilitating dissemination as well as disease transmission.

Virulence factors for *M. tuberculosis* remain poorly characterized. Most work has involved mycobacterial cell surface glycolipids (e.g., trehalose dimycolate, cord factor) and sulfolipids, which may interfere with phagosome-lysome fusion, or disrupt the phagosome membrane (34). Virulent strains of *Mycobacterium tuberculosis* in mice (H37RV, *M. tuberculosis* Erdman) have more rapid doubling times *in vivo*, and a similar situation has been reported in human tuberculosis (35); whether this is the cause of or an effect of their virulence is unknown. Ethanol consumption, which is cited as a risk factor for dissemination in most series (11,15,36,37), has been shown to activate virulence factors analogous to heat-shock proteins in intracellular *Mycobacterium avium* (38). Whether similar mechanisms exist for *M. tuberculosis* is unknown. Evidence exists that certain drug resistance mechanisms may be associated with differences in virulence. Some isoniazid-resistant strains lacking catalase activity are less able to disseminate in guinea pigs, whereas isoniazid-resistant strains that still possess catalase activity are as virulent as sensitive strains (39). In humans, isoniazid- or streptomycin-resistant strains appeared in one study to behave similarly to drug-susceptible strains in terms of infectivity for household contacts (40). Fischl et al. (41) found that 32% of HIV-infected patients in an outbreak of multidrug-resistant TB had disseminated disease at presentation, compared with 16% of an HIV-infected control cohort with single-drug–resistant or susceptible TB. CD4 counts and CD4/CD8 ratios were not significantly different between cohorts.

Sheer number of organisms gaining access to the blood stream after necrosis of a caseous focus was thought to be a factor in dissemination in the preantibiotic era. Fifty years ago most autopsy series could demonstrate a macroscopically apparent portal of entry (12). This likely represents the natural history of untreated localized disease; in the antibiotic era, macroscopic caseous foci are difficult to find (12).

Iatrogenic disseminated TB, the direct result of a medical procedure, occurs rarely, but has been reported to occur after extracorporeal shock wave lithotripsy (42,43), renal allograft placement (44), ureteral catheterization (45), and cardiac valve homograft placement (46). Disseminated bacille Calmette–Guérin (BCG) infection has occurred after intravesicular BCG installation as part of chemotherapy for bladder malignancies (47,48).

Thus, a complex set of interactions between T lymphocytes, macrophages, and the organism, modulated by both exogenous factors (coinfection, nutritional state, medications, toxic exposure) and genetic factors (on the part of the organism as well as the host), seems to determine the likelihood of miliary dissemination.

CLINICAL MANIFESTATIONS

The clinical manifestations of miliary TB are protean. A variety of syndromes have been ascribed to miliary TB, including the adult respiratory distress syndrome (49–51); shock (52) possibly with thrombotic microangiopathy (53); multisystem organ failure (54) or lesser dysfunction of one or two organ systems (55,56); immune hemolytic anemia (57); dermal involvement (58); fever of unknown origin (59); and "failure to thrive" without fever (60). Beyond the obvious contributions of host immune response and comorbidity, these presentations reflect the fact that hematogenous dissemination can range from a massive single bacillary bolus to episodic bursts of relatively low-grade bacillemia, as well as the fact that the site of dissemination may originate in the pulmonary, portal, or systemic circulation. In the mid-1980s in the United States, almost 20% of reported cases of miliary TB were not diagnosed until after death (8).

In the classic syndrome, occurring after sudden massive caseation into the blood stream ("acute generalized miliary tuberculosis") (10) in an apparently immunocompetent host, miliary dissemination is usually identified radiographically at presentation or shortly thereafter. At the other end of the clinical and pathologic spectrum (e.g., in the setting of impaired specific host cell-mediated immunity), miliary disease may be associated with a normal-appearing chest radiograph and only minor constitutional symptoms, and has been compared with lepromatous leprosy, another mycobacterial disease with a limited host response (61). Some refer to this latter presentation as *cryptic* (60).

The typical patient presents with a febrile wasting illness of 2 to 4 months duration; in North America and western Europe, such an individual often has known underlying chronic illness (Fig. 27.1). Symptoms and signs are often nonspecific and limited to fever, mild tachypnea, and ination (Figs. 27.2 and 27.3). Cough and dyspnea are relatively common, occurring in about half of reported cases. Rigors, generally thought to be relatively specific for gram-negative or gram-positive bacteremias, have been associated with miliary TB as well (62). Organomegaly is variable, and more common in children (63). Uveal involvement in the form of choroidal tubercles is said to be a specific finding for miliary TB (64), although such tubercles may be found in patients with localized pulmonary TB when looked for (65). They are rarely noted in most adult series, although mydriatic agents were not routinely used; an autopsy series found choroidal tubercles in 50% of eyes examined (12). Choroidal tubercles, which are found more frequently in

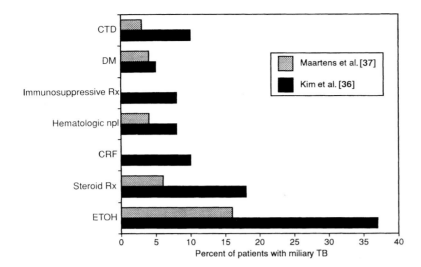

FIGURE 27.1. Frequency with which predisposing conditions are found in patients with miliary tuberculosis. Data are from a U.S. series (*n* = 38) (36) (*shaded bar*) and from an area of high prevalence (South Africa) (*n* = 109) (37) (*black bar*). Human immunodeficiency virus–infected persons were not included in either series. *CTD*, connective tissue disease; *DM*, diabetes mellitus; *nprl*, neoplasm; *CRF*, chronic renal failure; *ETOH*, alcohol.

children (64), are not associated with meningeal involvement but result from hematogenous spread (65). Choroidal hemorrhages have also been reported (66).

Skin involvement in the form of disseminated 3- to 10-mm erythematous macules and papules on thighs, buttocks, genitalia, and extremities (tuberculosis cutis miliaris disseminata) occurs rarely (67,68); most recent reports concerned HIV-infected patients (69,70).

Signs of hepatic involvement are often present but usually are limited to hepatomegaly and elevation of the alkaline phosphatase level. Rarely, a picture of cholestatic jaundice dominates (56,71). Urinary tract involvement occurs in the form of pyuria, proteinuria, or microscopic hematuria. Overt renal insufficiency due to miliary TB is rare, although three cases of renal failure due to extensive granulomatous destruction of the renal interstitium (72) and one case of immune complex glomerulonephritis resolving with antituberculous therapy and corticosteroids (73) have been reported.

Miliary TB on occasion presents as acute hypoxemic respiratory failure and noncardiogenic pulmonary edema, which may cause a delay or failure in correct diagnosis (74). A history of a subacute prodromal illness lasting at least several weeks; a history of TB, alcohol or drug abuse, known HIV infection, or other causes of immune impairment; coupled with a failure to identify other causes of acute lung

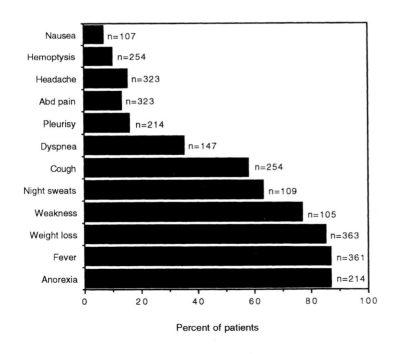

FIGURE 27.2. Frequency of symptoms noted at presentation in patients with miliary tuberculosis. Data are pooled from five clinical series (15,17,36,37,60). The number indicated for each category refers to the number of patients for whom the presence or absence of the symptom was specifically reported. *Abd*, abdominal.

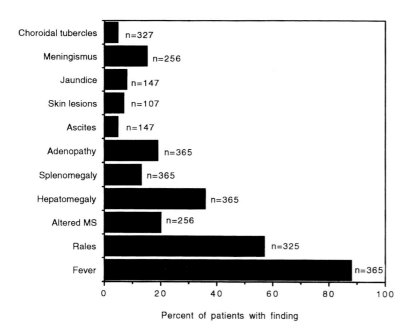

FIGURE 27.3. Frequency of physical findings noted at presentation in patients with miliary tuberculosis. Data are pooled from five clinical series (15,17,36, 37,60). The number indicated for each category refers to the number of patients in whom the physical finding was sought. *MS,* mental status.

injury should suggest the possibility of underlying TB. Disseminated TB should be excluded in HIV-infected patients with diffuse alveolar infiltrates and hypoxemia, especially if corticosteroid therapy—without concomitant antituberculous therapy—is to be given as part of treatment for *Pneumocystis carinii* pneumonia. In one study of 11 HIV-infected patients who died with undiagnosed disseminated TB, nine were treated solely for presumed *P. carinii* pneumonia (75). The purified protein derivative (PPD) test is often nonreactive in patients reported with adult respiratory distress syndrome due to miliary TB (52). Sputum smears are positive less than half the time. Shock can occur (52). Mortality rates in reported series range from 57% to 89% (49).

Central nervous system (CNS) involvement in the form of meningitis or tuberculomas is recognized clinically in 16% to 30% of patients (12,15,17,37), although meningeal involvement can be found postmortem in 29% (17) to 54% (12) of cases. Disseminated cerebral tuberculomas may be clinically silent and may be underappreciated in clinical series; magnetic resonance imaging with gadolinium enhancement allows their noninvasive detection (76,77). Several authors (15,36) noted the specificity of headache for CNS involvement. The cerebrospinal fluid (CSF) can be clear or cloudy, with a usual lymphocytic pleocytosis, ranging from 10 to 1,000 cells/mm³; protein concentrations are usually above 50 mg/dL, and glucose is less than 50 mg/dL in about 70% of patients (17,64). Acid-fast bacillus (AFB) smears are rarely positive (36,37), while the range of positive cultures has been 0% in a recent U.S. series (36) to 60% in a South African report (37). Disseminated TB in HIV-infected patients was associated with a

21% rate of CSF culture positivity in one series (13), although the CSF protein level and cell counts were normal in two of these patients.

Clinically significant cardiac involvement is especially unusual; most autopsy series of miliary TB report an incidence of about 10%, almost always asymptomatic (10,12). Pericarditis occurs rarely (36,37). One patient with miliary TB presenting with sudden cardiac death due to apparent myocardial involvement has been reported (78). Endocardial involvement is rarely recognized antemortem (79), and valvular endocarditis is generally thought to be a result of, rather than a cause of, dissemination (80). Two reports of aortic valve vegetations and insufficiency recognized during life, and occurring during therapy for disseminated TB, have been published (80,81); in one case, valve replacement was required (81). Tuberculous vegetations on a prosthetic mitral valve with multiorgan dissemination have been found postmortem (79). As noted, miliary TB following valve replacement with contaminated valve homografts has occurred (46).

Miliary TB can present with a mycotic aneurysm of the ascending or descending aorta (82). Caseous foci, such as lymph nodes or vertebral (Pott) abscesses, are often found adjacent to the aneurysm, suggesting spread by erosion into the aorta with subsequent miliary dissemination (82). Embolization to aortic wall vasa vasorum during hematogenous spread from a distant focus may be a less common mechanism. It is important to note that antimycobacterial therapy has been associated with aneurysm rupture (82).

Overt adrenal insufficiency at presentation or during therapy for disseminated TB appears to be very unusual (83), occurring in approximately 1% of most series (37,84), although granulomatous involvement of the adrenals is found in up to 42% (15) of postmortem examinations. In a prospective study of adrenal responsiveness before and during therapy for various forms of TB, only 1 of 30 patients with miliary TB had a subnormal response to exogenous corticotropin administration, and had no clinical signs of hypoadrenalism; 60% of those patients had supranormal basal serum cortisol levels (85). Chemical hyperthyroidism, which normalized with antituberculous therapy and which was associated with granulomatous infiltration of the thyroid gland in the setting of postprimary miliary TB, has also been reported (86).

Nongranulomatous vasculitis attributed to disseminated tuberculous infection has been reported; in both instances, host cellular immunity was severely compromised (13,87).

Clearly, almost all of these clinical presentations are entirely nonspecific and require a high index of suspicion for the diagnosis of disseminated TB.

LABORATORY FINDINGS

Imaging

The chest roentgenogram shows a miliary pattern at presentation in more than half of the patients reported in most series (Fig. 27.4). It is important to note that even if not present initially, miliary patterns often become apparent days to weeks later (16,17). In a classic paper, Felson (88) stated that miliary tubercles do not become radiographically apparent until at least 2 to 3 weeks after hematogenous seeding. Miliary patterns may be subtle and are often initially overlooked; for example, 10 of 12 "normal" readings were reared as showing a miliary pattern in one study (89).

Like millet, a small round grain about 1 to 3 mm in diameter with remarkable size consistency (Fig. 27.5), miliary radiologic patterns consist of multiple 1- to 3-mm well-defined nodules that typically are distributed uniformly throughout all lung fields, although a basilar predominance or larger upper-lung zone nodules may be perceived (88) (Figs. 27.6 and 27.7). The miliary pattern is usually described as reflecting a nodular interstitial process, although Felson (90) pointed out that by the time miliary tubercles become large enough to be seen on a chest film, they have almost invariably involved the adjacent alveoli. Conversely, processes that involve the distal airspaces, such as pulmonary alveolar proteinosis, inhalational diseases, alveolar hemorrhage syndromes, or the various causes of pulmonary edema, can appear nodular. These "acinar nodules" are usually larger (5 to 10 mm), less well defined, and more heterogeneous in size than classic hematogenously generated miliary patterns (91), but in many clinical circumstances it can be difficult to make the distinction with certainty. Published differential diagnoses of a miliary pattern on chest roentgenogram have therefore been large (88,92), but the addition of a single piece of clinical information to the interpretation of the film—the presence of fever—narrows the list considerably (Table 27.1). Most miliary nodules seen radiographically are probably summated densities of those tubercles most perfectly aligned in the plane of the film, thus generating sufficiently opaque images (93). Summation of imperfectly aligned nodules may create curvilinear opacities, resulting in a perceived reticulonodularity (93). Bright-light examination, close attention to intercostal spaces, and slight underpenetration of the film increase diagnostic sensitivity. A diffuse interstitial pattern, presumably occurring because of lymphatic obstruction or infiltration (lymphangitis tuberculosa reticu-

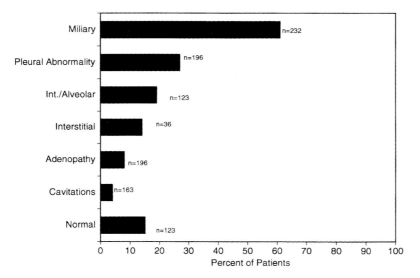

FIGURE 27.4. Frequency of chest radiographic patterns seen at presentation in patients with miliary tuberculosis. A miliary pattern is found slightly more than half the time. Data are pooled from four series (11,17,36,37). The number indicated in each category refers to the number of patients for whom the presence or absence of the finding was specifically reported.

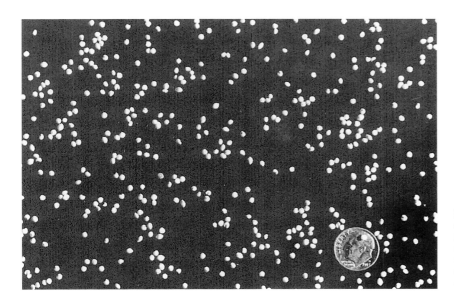

FIGURE 27.5. Millet is compared to a U.S. 10-cent piece (diameter, 15 mm). Note the uniformity of size and shape of the seeds. This same uniformity of size, "roundness" of the individual lesions, and even distribution are hallmarks of miliary tuberculosis seen on chest radiographs.

laris) (94), is seen less frequently. A chronic tuberculous pulmonary focus is seen in approximately 25% to 30% of patients. The radiologic findings of disseminated TB associated with HIV infection are similar to those seen in HIV-seronegative patients. Adenopathy including mediastinal involvement, lower-lobe infiltrates, or clear lung fields is more common when advanced HIV coinfection is present (95–97). Computed tomography is also invaluable for imaging adenopathy and visceral lesions in the setting of extrapulmonary dissemination.

High-resolution computed tomography (HRCT) of the chest can confirm the chest radiographic findings (98,99) and, perhaps, contribute to the differential diagnosis (100). Innumerable 1- to 3-mm nodules, both sharply and poorly defined, are seen, most often uniformly distributed throughout the lung (Fig. 27.8). Diffuse as well as localized

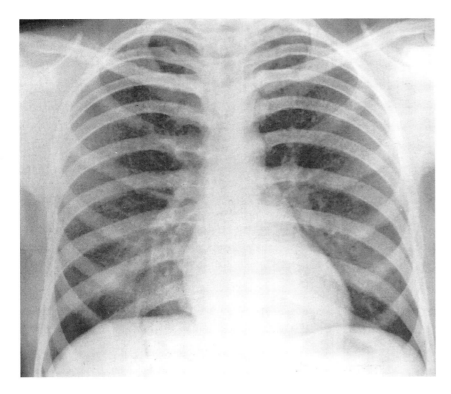

FIGURE 27.6. Posteroanterior chest radiograph of miliary tuberculosis. Note the even distribution of lesions through all lung fields.

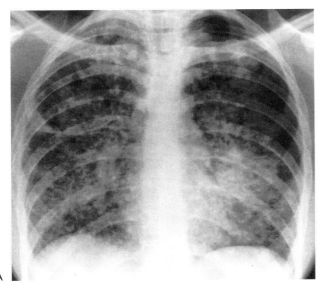
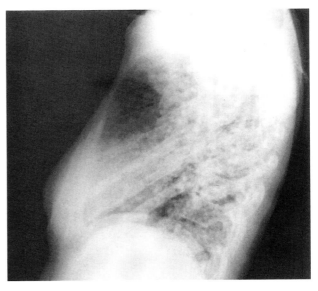

FIGURE 27.7. Posteroanterior (**A**) and lateral (**B**) chest radiographs of somewhat more advanced miliary tuberculosis. Note the coalescence of miliary lesions into larger areas of infiltration. A pneumothorax is present on the left.

TABLE 27.1. MILIARY INFILTRATES WITH FEVER: DIFFERENTIAL DIAGNOSIS

I. Infectious diseases
  A. Mycobacterial
    1. *M. tuberculosis* infection[a]
    2. Atypical mycobacteria in immunocompromised hosts (157)
  B. Fungal
    1. Histoplasmosis[a] (158)
    2. Coccidioidomycosis[a] (159)
    3. Blastomycosis[a] (160)
    4. Cryptococcosis (161)
  C. Viral
    1. Varicella[a] (162)
    2. Influenza[a]
    3. Measles[a] (93)
    4. Cytomegalovirus infection (163)
  D. Bacterial
    1. *Mycoplasma* infection (164)
    2. Nocardiosis (165)
    3. *Legionella micdadei* infection (166)
    4. Brucellosis (167)
    5. *Staphylococcus aureus* infection (168)
    6. Melioidosis (169)
    7. Psittacosis (170)
    8. Tularemia (171)
  E. Parasitic
    1. Schistosomiasis (172)
    2. Toxoplasmosis (173)
    3. Strongyloidiasis (174)
II. Neoplastic diseases
  A. Lymphoma (175)
III. Inflammatory diseases
  A. Hypersensitivity pneumonitis[a]
  B. Sarcoidosis
  C. Goodpasture syndrome (176)
  D. Other alveolar hemorrhage syndromes (177)

[a]More common causes.

septal thickening usually accompanies the nodules (98). Some investigators indicate that HRCT findings do not discriminate miliary TB from other miliary lung diseases; in one study, blinded interpretation of HRCT scans was no more accurate than blinded interpretation of the chest radiograph in suggesting a specific diagnosis of miliary TB (101). Others propose that the presence of multiple small cystlike lesions in addition to the small nodules is suggestive of miliary TB or metastatic cancer (100). At a minimum, HRCT is useful in demonstrating a miliary pattern when the chest radiograph appears atypical (i.e., predominantly linear opacities) (99) or even normal (98).

Because gallium is concentrated by viable mycobacteria as well as by leukocytes (102), gallium scanning can show diffuse pulmonary and extrapulmonary uptake in miliary disease (102–104), but is not specific. In one series, gallium scanning was normal in 3 (19%) of 16 patients with miliary TB, 2 of whom had miliary patterns on chest radiographs (104). It should be remembered that in patients with coexistent illnesses associated with disseminated TB, gallium uptake may reflect the underlying disease. Once a diagnosis of disseminated TB is entertained, concentrating diagnostic efforts on areas of gallium positivity may facilitate evaluation. Progressive diminution of gallium uptake can be used to assess response to theory at extrapulmonary foci (105), but is not cost effective and is rarely indicated for that purpose.

Finally, ultrasonography of the liver can show a "bright" echogenic pattern also seen in cirrhosis, fatty infiltration, congestive heart failure, and lymphoma. The diagnostic utility may be increased when fever is present (106).

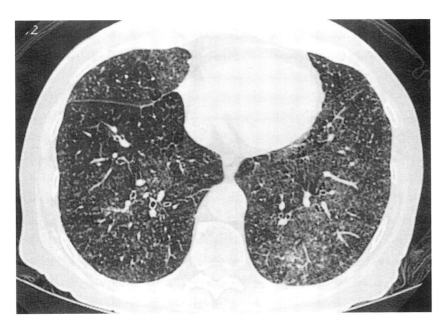

FIGURE 27.8. High-resolution computed tomography of miliary tuberculosis. Numerous punctate 1- to 2-mm nodules are seen evenly distributed through the lung parenchyma. Septal thickening is evident. An area of alveolar infiltration is noted in the left lower lobe. (Film courtesy of Dr. Robert Pugatch, University of Maryland, Baltimore.)

Blood Abnormalities

The complete blood cell count reveals a mild normochromic normocytic anemia in approximately half of patients (15,37). A normal white blood cell count is the rule in miliary TB, but many nonspecific abnormalities have been reported. Neutrophilia can be seen and is more common than lymphocytosis or monocytosis. A left shift with an increased number of band forms may be present and may mislead the clinician to suspect a bacterial rather than mycobacterial process (107). Leukemoid reactions occur (108). Pancytopenia, which is rare, is considered by Hunt et al. (109) to be usually the result of an underlying hematologic disorder rather than of tuberculous marrow infiltration. Although said to be a poor prognostic sign in the context of miliary TB, Maartens et al. (37) reported hematologic recovery in three of six patients with pancytopenia in their series, although follow-up bone marrow examinations were not performed. T cell–mediated inhibition of granulopoiesis *in vitro*, resolving with therapy, has been reported in a man with miliary TB and pancytopenia (110). Several cases of the histiocytic hemophagocytotic syndrome have been reported (111–113), one resolving with antituberculous therapy, etoposide, and corticosteroids (114). Concomitant viral infections, which have the best-described association with this entity, were not rigidly excluded. Disseminated intravascular coagulation occurs in overwhelming and usually fatal disease (37,53). Immune hemolytic anemia responding to antituberculosis therapy has recently been reported (57). The erythrocyte sedimentation rate is usually elevated in miliary TB, as are other acute-phase reactants such as C-reactive protein (115), intercellular adhesion molecule-1 (ICAM-1) (116), and the polyclonal gamma globulins. Hyponatremia is very common, presumably because of the same antidiuretic hormone dysregulation seen in many pulmonary inflammatory processes; there is no correlation with CNS involvement (36) or with adrenal insufficiency. Hypercalcemia can occur, as in other granulomatous processes, but is quite rare (117). Arterial blood gases typically reveal a widened alveolar–arterial (A-a) gradient and a mild respiratory alkalosis. In one report, 40% of patients had an arterial partial oxygen pressure (PaO_2) of less than 60 mm Hg (36). The alkaline phosphatase level is often elevated; transaminase levels are usually normal or mildly elevated.

Other Laboratory Abnormalities

Sterile pyuria was found in 32% of patients in the series of Kim et al. (36) but did not correlate with positive mycobacterial culture. Conversely, Gelb et al. (17) found positive urine cultures in 11 patients who had normal urinary sediment. Pulmonary function testing can reveal a mild restrictive defect (118). Bronchoalveolar lavage (BAL) fluid from patients with miliary TB reveals a predominant lymphocytosis (118,119), with a depressed CD4$^+$ subpopulation in untreated patients (119). After treatment has begun, BAL fluid demonstrates a predominance of CD4$^+$ lymphocytes (118,119). Pulmonary artery pressures were normal at rest in a study of six patients with miliary TB (120); response to exercise was normal in four; in two, pulmonary vascular resistance was increased (120).

Diagnosis

Along with presentation late in the clinical course and insufficient clinical suspicion, the frequent inability to achieve a rapid diagnosis of miliary TB remains the major stumbling block to lowering mortality. A diagnosis of miliary TB should be entertained in any patient with unexplained fever or wasting. A history of TB or exposure should be pursued; evidence of HIV infection should also be sought. Fundi should be examined carefully after use of a mydriatic agent. An initial nonmiliary radiographic pattern does not exclude miliary disease, and films should be obtained at frequent intervals, in addition to considering HRCT of the chest, if suspicion remains high (90). All accessible secretions and body fluids should be examined microscopically and cultured once the diagnosis is suspected (Fig. 27.9); even acid-fast staining of middle ear discharge was reported to have been instrumental in making a diagnosis of miliary TB (121). In HIV-infected patients, acid-fast stains of sputum are positive with a frequency similar to that seen in non–HIV-infected patients with disseminated TB (25% in one series) (9). Culture of urine, blood, or CSF is typically of higher yield in HIV-seropositive than in HIV-seronegative persons with miliary TB (9). Mycobacterial blood cultures, preferably involving lysis centrifugation techniques, should be obtained, especially in HIV-infected patients. Lysis centrifugation blood cultures are positive in as many as 59% of HIV-infected patients with clinically apparent dissemination (13). In one study, positive blood cultures were the initial means of diagnosis in 33% of HIV-infected patients with disseminated TB (32). Although *M. tuberculosis* has been detected by acid-fast stain of the buffy coat of peripheral blood (122), most positive acid-fast smears of the buffy coat are due to *Mycobacterium avium-intracellulare* (123). The tuberculin skin test

result, reported in older studies to be positive in 60% to 73% of patients (15,17), was most often negative in more recent series (36,37), probably reflecting the epidemiologic shift of the disease (Fig. 27.10).

Histopathologic demonstration of granulomas in tissue continues to have a central role in the rapid diagnosis of miliary TB. Acid-fast stains of tissue are neither sensitive (124) nor, in HIV-infected patients, specific (125). Lung, liver, and bone marrow are the three organs in which granulomas are most likely to be found; easily accessible lymph nodes and serosal surfaces, when evidence of their involvement is clinically or radiologically apparent, also have a high yield (Fig. 27.11). The presence of liver granulomas is not specific for disseminated TB; they may be found in 25% of patients with pulmonary TB (124,126). It is also of note that the majority of hepatic granulomas with acid-fast organisms in HIV-infected patients are due to *M. avium-intracellulare* (125,127). The presence of lymphopenia increases the yield of bone marrow biopsy (128).

Two studies examined the utility of fiberoptic bronchoscopy with bronchial washing, brushing, and transbronchial biopsy in smear-negative miliary TB (129,130). An immediate diagnosis (positive smear or histopathology) was made in 65% of patients in both series, and culture results raised the overall diagnostic yield to 79% (Fig. 27.12). As both series were from areas of high prevalence for TB, the negative predictive value of bronchoscopy for miliary TB will be less in areas of lower prevalence. No comparable studies exist in the United States, although Kim et al. (36) found that bronchoscopy added little utility to other diagnostic maneuvers in 11 patients with miliary TB,

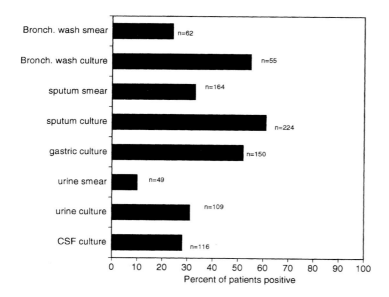

FIGURE 27.9. Pooled data from four series (15,17,36,37) showing the frequency with which a positive smear or culture from common sources occurs in patients with miliary tuberculosis. Note that smears from all sources are relatively insensitive; cultures are more sensitive but do not provide a rapid diagnosis.

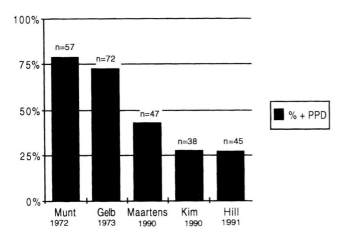

FIGURE 27.10. Frequency of positive tuberculin skin test responses [purified protein derivative (*PPD*), 5-TU (tuberculin units), and/or second-strength PPD] in recent reported series of disseminated tuberculosis (13,15,17,36,37). The frequency of negative or anergic responses has increased significantly in recent years probably reflecting human immunodeficiency virus coinfection.

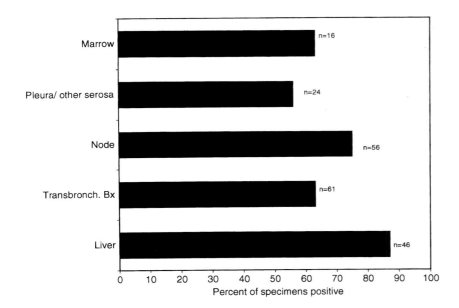

FIGURE 27.11. Frequency with which granulomas are found in biopsy specimens of selected sites in patients with miliary tuberculosis. The number indicated for each site refers to the total number of patients who had biopsies performed at that site. Data are pooled from three sources (17,36,37).

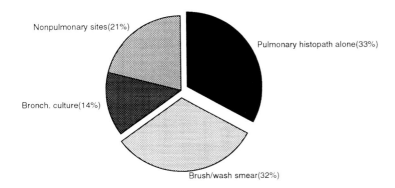

FIGURE 27.12. Frequency with which the diagnosis in patients with sputum smear–negative miliary tuberculosis was confirmed by various bronchoscopically obtained specimens. Data are pooled from two series (126,127). A rapid diagnosis (by smear of brushings and/or washings, or by pathologic appearance of transbronchial biopsy specimens) could be made in 41 (65%) of 63 patients. The diagnosis could not be made by bronchoscopy in 21% of patients and was made on the basis of nonpulmonary specimens.

providing rapid diagnosis in only two patients. The utility of bronchoscopy with biopsy in HIV-infected patients with disseminated TB is likely similar to the yield in HIV-seronegative individuals. In one series, a rapid broncho-scopic diagnosis was made in only two of seven patients (9). In series of HIV-infected patients with all forms of TB, the bronchoscopic yield was lower than (24,131) or equivalent to (132) that in HIV-seronegative patients. Cultures of washings were found to be of low yield by some groups (36,133) although not by others (134), perhaps because certain topical anesthetic agents may have inhibitory effects on mycobacterial growth (133).

In recent years, the more rapid detection of *M. tuberculosis* has been facilitated by the development of several broth-based radiometric and nonradiometric systems (e.g., Bactec, Becton Dickinson Diagnostic Systems, Sparks, MD, U.S.A.; and Mycobacteria Growth Indicator Tube, Becton Dickinson, Franklin Lakes, NJ, U.S.A., respectively) and by nucleic acid probes and amplification systems. More rapid drug susceptibility testing is also possible using these systems (135). Thus, in a study comparing AFB staining, conventional culture, and the Amplicor (Roche, Basel, Switzerland) polymerase chain reaction (PCR)–based testing of respiratory specimens, the positivity rate for the culture and PCR was virtually identical and much greater than for the AFB staining technique The PCR test allowed detection of *M. tuberculosis* at 6 hours following specimen decontamination (136). PCR analysis of sputum cannot yet replace mycobacterial culture but does provide a rapid diagnosis in a significant proportion of patients for whom diagnosis might have been delayed. It can now be applied to a variety of specimen types.

Serologic diagnosis of miliary TB by enzyme-linked immunosorbent assay (ELISA) using antibodies directed against purified secreted antigens or cell wall components continues to be of research interest. In patients with miliary TB, various serologic assays continue to be troubled by low sensitivity (137) or specificity (138), and their role in the diagnosis of miliary disease remains to be defined. Recently, an interferon release assay (QuantiFERON-TB, Cellestis Ltd., Carnegie, Victoria, Australia) has been compared with the tuberculin skin test (PPD) for purposes of identifying latent TB infection (LTBI). In limited testing it has shown some advantages in identifying infected PPD-negative (anergic) individuals (135). The ultimate usefulness of such an assay for identifying latent or active TB infection remains to be defined.

THERAPY

Therapeutic recommendations for disseminated TB are the same as for pulmonary TB (139). A three-drug regimen—isoniazid, rifampin, and pyrazinamide (supplemented by

ethambutol if the local prevalence of primary drug resistance is 4% or more or unknown)—should be started until drug sensitivity information is available. If the organism is fully sensitive, ethambutol may be dropped and isoniazid, rifampin, and pyrazinamide continued. Pyrazinamide is deleted after 2 months, and isoniazid and rifampin are continued for a total of 6 months. Directly observed therapy is desirable for most patients in the continuation phase of treatment to ensure adherence to treatment. If drug resistance is found, regimens need to be appropriately tailored to the organism's susceptibility pattern. In children and in HIV-infected patients, therapy is frequently extended to at least 9 months (139), with 6 months of therapy provided after culture conversion, if that can be documented. Interaction between drugs used to manage TB and those given as antiretroviral therapy may require modification of one or another regimen (97). Dissemination with bone or joint involvement, or extensive lymphadenitis, may require longer therapy (139). Since meningeal involvement remains a major risk factor for morbidity and mortality in miliary TB, drugs that readily penetrate the meninges should theoretically be used. Isoniazid and pyrazinamide achieve the highest CSF levels (140). Falk (141) attributed the dramatic reduction in mortality of miliary TB when isoniazid became available to its ability to easily penetrate the meninges. The role of the fluoroquinolones, which demonstrate excellent penetration of almost all tissues, including the meninges, remains to be defined in miliary TB, although a recent study of drug-resistant tuberculosis suggests that this class of drugs may have some utility particularly when other agents cannot be used (142,143).

The adjunctive use of corticosteroids to modulate the deleterious effects of the inflammatory response has not been prospectively investigated in disseminated TB. Evidence exists that corticosteroids are of benefit in selected patients with meningeal (144) or pericardial (145) inflammation, or when rare and clearly aberrant immunologic phenomena appear, such as immune complex nephritis (75) and histiocytic hemophagocytosis (114). When deterioration of organ function (particularly gas exchange) continues despite adequate antituberculous therapy, some clinicians would add corticosteroids, although the prevalence of multidrug-resistant strains now complicates this decision. Also, in severely immunocompromised patients, other inapparent opportunistic infections may coexist that if not therapeutically addressed may progress during corticosteroid therapy. Replacement doses of corticosteroids should be used if adrenal insufficiency is suspected, with the knowledge that rifampin increases exogenous corticosteroid catabolism (146). A retrospective evaluation of corticosteroid use in miliary TB found no difference in mortality in 43 children given steroids as compared with 51 not given steroids (65). Another retrospective report (147) suggested a reduction in mortality and faster subjective improvement in the steroid-treated cohort, although cohorts were not matched and statistical significance was not demonstrated. It is not clear that the power of either study was sufficient to resolve an effect of corticosteroids within the overwhelmingly beneficial context of antimycobacterial therapy. Reported complications arising during the therapy of miliary TB, excluding those related to any severe prolonged illness for which medication is given, have emphasized perforation of structures at the site of granulomatous involvement: pneumothorax (148), small bowel (149), or mycotic aortic aneurysm (83). Expansion of intracranial tuberculomas (150), hydrocephalus (37), cutaneous abscesses, and tenosynovitis (151) have also been reported to occur well into therapy.

Response to therapy is followed by defervescence, recovery of appetite, and sense of well-being, which usually becomes apparent 7 to 14 days after therapy is initiated (15) but may be delayed by weeks in some patients. The mean time to radiologic clearing ranges from 10 to 19 weeks in most series (16,37,90,119) and is usually complete. The time to radiologic resolution was inversely correlated with the degree of BAL fluid lymphocytosis, particularly the number of CD8[+] lymphocytes, in one series (119), and directly correlated with age in another series (16). Old reports of residual miliary calcifications had poor documentation of mycobacterial infection, and probably represented healed viral (varicella) or fungal lesions.

PREVENTION

Miliary disease, like all forms of TB, can be prevented by the use of isoniazid or other agents to manage LTBI in persons at greatest risk for disease (152). HIV-seropositive patients in particular should be screened for infection; a high priority for screening and management of LTBI should be given to HIV-infected persons (152).

The BCG vaccine appears to reduce the incidence of miliary spread, particularly in children. A meta-analysis of the BCG vaccine literature found three suitable case-control studies pertinent to miliary TB that demonstrated a combined 78% protective effect against disseminated disease (153). The duration of the protective effect could not be assessed. BCG is not effective in patients already infected by *M. tuberculosis*. Moreover, the vaccine should not be given to immunocompromised hosts (including those infected with HIV) because of the risk of disseminated BCG infection (154). Finally, because BCG vaccination may produce skin test conversion, it limits the usefulness of isoniazid prophylaxis. BCG vaccination is therefore best reserved for persons with continuing exposure to *M. tuberculosis* who cannot or will not use isoniazid preventive therapy. When immunosuppressive therapy including corticosteroid therapy at a dosage higher than 15 mg/day of prednisone, or an equivalent, is contemplated, tuberculin reactivity should be assessed and prophylaxis given to reactors with 5 mm or more induration, since disseminated disease may be more likely in the setting of such treatment (152).

PROGNOSIS

Prognosis is related to comorbidity (age, underlying chronic organ dysfunction) (17,107) and to those factors contributing to a delay in diagnosis (lack of fever, lack of respiratory symptoms, negative PPD test result, etc.) (107). Most studies found meningeal or other CNS involvement to be an independent predictor of mortality even in the post-isoniazid era (17,36,141), although others did not (15,37). Pancytopenia, which may reflect an underlying hematologic disorder or overwhelming marrow involvement, is inconsistently associated with increased mortality (37,109). Nonreactivity to tuberculin is not associated with increased mortality in those who are treated (15,37), but was a significant factor in undiagnosed miliary TB subjects coming to autopsy (59,155). Race is not a consistent factor in mortality; excesses of mortality in both whites (141) and blacks (15,36) have been reported.

HIV-infected patients respond to therapy in a fashion similar to those without HIV infection (13,97), although TB has been reported as a significant contributing cause of death in 45% of patients with CD4 counts less than 200 cells/mm^3 (14). Management of HIV infection with combination antiretroviral therapy along with management of tuberculosis has the potential to substantially improve outcome in these patients (156). In general, failure to improve or continued deterioration—assuming multidrug resistance has been excluded—should prompt a search for coexistent infection in the HIV-seropositive patient. Adverse drug reactions and drug interactions (rash, hepatitis, thrombocytopenia) occur more frequently in HIV-infected patients (24,156).

The overall mortality rate stands at approximately 20% and has not changed for 25 years (Fig. 27.13), suggesting that the last major therapeutic impact on the disease was isoniazid; the mortality rate has not changed in the rifampin era (36,37), or with rapid advances in diagnostic and supportive technology. As noted previously, almost 20% of cases of miliary TB reported to the CDC in the mid-1980s were diagnosed after death (8). The emergence of multidrug-resistant strains, progressing hand in hand with the HIV epidemic, makes any immediate progress doubtful. Delay in or failure of diagnosis remains the largest single correctable factor contributing to mortality. A consistently high clinical suspicion, coupled with application of new rapid microbiologic diagnostic techniques, will be important in coming years.

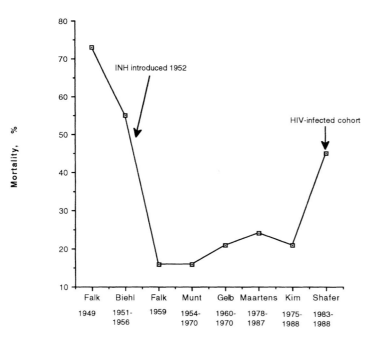

FIGURE 27.13. Reported mortality from selected clinical series of miliary tuberculosis (9,16,17,36,37,141). Mortality remained at approximately 20% during the 30 years after the introduction of isoniazid. Concomitant human immunodeficiency virus infection increases mortality attributable to disseminated tuberculosis.

REFERENCES

1. Bonetus T. *Sepulchretum sive anatomia practica*, Vol .1, Observatio XLVI. Geneva, 1679.
2. Manget JJ. *Sepulchretum sive anatomia practica*, Vol. 1, Observatio XLVII (3 vols). London: Cramer and Perachon, 1700.
3. Auerbach O. Acute generalized miliary tuberculosis. *Am J Pathol* 1944;20:121–136.
4. Keers RY. *Pulmonary tuberculosis: a journey down the centuries.* London: Balliere Tindall, 1978.
5. Mettler CC. *History of medicine.* Philadelphia: Blakiston, 1947.
6. Centers for Disease Control and Prevention. *Extrapulmonary tuberculosis in the United States 1969–1973.* DHEW Publication CDC 78-8260. Atlanta: Department of Health, Education, and Welfare, 1978.
7. Centers for Disease Control and Prevention. *Tuberculosis statistics.* DHEW Publication CDC 77-8249. Atlanta: Department of Health, Education, and Welfare, 1977.
8. Rieder HL, Kelly GD, Bloch AB, et al. Tuberculosis diagnosed at death in the United States. *Chest* 1991;100:678–681.
9. Shafer RW, Kim DS, Weiss JP, et al. Extrapulmonary tuberculosis in patients with human immunodeficiency virus infection. *Medicine* 1991;70:384–397.
10. Chapman CB, Wharton CM. Acute generalized miliary tuberculosis in adults. *N Engl J Med* 1946;235:239–248.
11. Alvarez S, McCabe W. Extrapulmonary tuberculosis revisited: a review of experience at Boston City and other hospitals. *Medicine* 1984;63:25–55.
12. Slavin RE, Walsh TJ, Pollack AD. Late generalized tuberculosis: a clinical pathologic analysis and comparison of 100 cases in the preantibiotic and antibiotic eras. *Medicine* 1980;59:352–366.
13. Hill AR, Premkumar S, Brustein S, et al. Disseminated tuberculosis in the acquired immunodeficiency syndrome era. *Am Rev Respir Dis* 1991;144:1164–1170.
14. Jones BE, Young SMM, Antoniskis D, et al. Relationship of the manifestations of tuberculosis to CD4 cell counts in patients with human immunodeficiency virus infection. *Am Rev Respir Dis* 1993;148: 1292–1297.
15. Munt PW. Miliary tuberculosis in the chemotherapy era: with a clinical review in 69 American adults. *Medicine* 1972;51: 139–155.
16. Biehl JP. Miliary tuberculosis. A review of sixty-eight adult patients admitted to a municipal general hospital. *Am Rev Tuberc* 1958;77:605–622.
17. Gelb AF, Leffler C, Brewin A, et al. Miliary tuberculosis. *Am Rev Respir Dis* 1973;108:1327–1333.
18. Cantwell MF, McKenna MT, McCray E, et al. Tuberculosis and race/ethnicity in the United States: impact of socioeconomic status. *Am J Respir Crit Care Med* 1998;157:1016–1020.
19. Al-Arif LI, Goldstein RA, Affronti LF, et al. HLA-Bw15 and tuberculosis in a North American black population. *Am Rev Respir Dis* 1979;120:1275–1278.
20. Braun MM, Cote TR, Rabkin CS. Trends in death with tuberculosis during the AIDS era. *JAMA* 1993;269:2865–2868.
21. Stead WW. Pathogenesis of tuberculosis: clinical and epidemiologic perspective. *Rev Infect Dis* 1989 11:S366–S368.
22. Selwyn PA, Hartel D, Lewis VA, et al. A prospective study of the risk of tuberculosis among intravenous drug users with human immunodeficiency virus infection. *N Engl J Med* 1989; 320:545–550.
23. Edlin BR, Tokars JI, Grieco MH, et al. An outbreak of multidrug-resistant tuberculosis among hospitalized patients with the acquired immunodeficiency syndrome. *N Engl J Med* 1992;326:1514–1521.
24. Daley CL, Small PM, Schecter GF, et al. An outbreak of tuberculosis with accelerated progression among persons infected with the human immunodeficiency virus: an analysis using restriction fragment-length polymorphisms. *N Engl J Med* 1992;326:231–235.
25. Flynn JL, Chan J. Immunology of tuberculosis. *Annu Rev Immunol* 2001; 19:93–129.

26. Barnes PF, Grisso CL, Abrams JS, et al. T lymphocytes in human tuberculosis. *J Infect Dis* 1992;165:506–512.

27. Ellner JJ. Review: the immune response to human tuberculosis—implications for tuberculosis control. *J Infect Dis* 1997; 176:1351–1359.

28. Kaufmann SHE. *In vitro* analysis of the cellular mechanisms involved in immunity to tuberculosis. *Rev Infect Dis* 1989;11: S448–S454.

29. Flynn JL, Goldstein MM, Chan J, et al. Tumor necrosis factor-alpha is required in the protective immune response against *Mycobacterium tuberculosis* in mice. *Immunity* 1995;2:561–572.

30. Keane J, Gershon S, Wise RP, et al. Tuberculosis associated with infliximab, a tumor necrosis factor alpha-neutralizing agent. *N Engl J Med* 2001;345:1098–1104.

31. Kumararatne DS, Pithie AS, Drysdale P, et al. Specific lysis of mycobacterial antigen-bearing macrophages by class II MHC–restricted polyclonal T-cell lines in healthy donors or patients with tuberculosis. *Clin Exp Immunol* 1990;80: 314–323.

32. Bouza E, Diaz-Lopez MD, Moreno S, et al. *Mycobacterium tuberculosis* bacteremia in patients with and without human immunodeficiency virus infection. *Arch Intern Med* 1993;153: 496–500.

33. Dannenberg AM. Immune mechanisms in the pathogenesis of pulmonary tuberculosis. *Rev Infect Dis* 1989;11:S369–S378.

34. Myrvik QN, Leake ES, Goren MB. Mechanisms of toxicity of tubercle bacilli for macrophages. In: Bendinelli M, Friedman H, eds. *Mycobacterium tuberculosis: interactions with the immune system.* New York: Plenum Press, 1988:303–325.

35. Valway SE, Sanchez MP, Shinnick TF, et al. An outbreak involving extensive transmission of a virulent strain of Mycobacterium tuberculosis. *N Engl J Med* 1998; 338:633–639.

36. Kim JH, Langston AA, Gallis HA. Miliary tuberculosis: epidemiology, clinical manifestations, diagnosis, and outcome. *Rev Infect Dis* 1990;12:583–590.

37. Maartens G, Willcox PA, Benatar SR. Miliary tuberculosis: rapid diagnosis, hematologic abnormalities, and outcome in 109 treated adults. *Am J Med* 1990;89:291–296.

38. Bermudez LE, Young LS, Martinelli J, et al. Exposure to ethanol up-regulates the expression of *Mycobacterium avium* complex proteins associated with bacterial virulence. *J Infect Dis* 1993;168:961–968.

39. Cohn ML, Davis CL. Infectivity and pathogenicity of drug-resistant strains of tubercle bacilli studied by aerogenic infection of guinea pigs. *Am Rev Respir Dis* 1970;102:97–100.

40. Snider DE Jr, Kelly GD, Cauthen GM, et al. Infection and disease among contacts of tuberculosis cases with drug-resistant and drug-susceptible bacilli. *Am Rev Respir Dis* 1985;132: 125–132.

41. Fischl MA, Daikos GL, Uttamchandani RB, et al. Clinical presentation and outcome of patients with HIV infection and tuberculosis caused by multiple-drug-resistant bacilli. *Ann Intern Med* 1992;117:184–190.

42. Amado LEM, Barciela LA, Fernandez AR, et al. Extracorporeal shock wave lithotripsy complicated with miliary tuberculosis. *J Urol* 1993;149:1532–1534.

43. Federmann M, Kley HK. Miliary tuberculosis after extracorporeal shock-wave lithotripsy. *N Engl J Med* 1990;323:1212.

44. Lenk S, Oesterwitz H, Scholz D. Tuberculosis in cadaveric renal allograft recipients: report of 4 cases and review of the literature. *Eur Urol* 1988;14:484–486.

45. Yekanath H, Gross PA, Vitenson JH. Miliary tuberculosis following ureteral catheterization. *Urology* 1980;16:197–198.

46. Anyanwu CH, Nassau E, Yacoub M. Miliary tuberculosis following homograft valve replacement. *Thorax* 1976;31: 101–106.

47. Rabe J, Neff KW, Lehmann KJ, et al. Miliary tuberculosis after intravesical bacille Calmette–Guérin immunotherapy of carcinoma of the bladder. *AJR Am J Roentgenol* 1999;172:748–750.

48. Palayew M, Briedis D, Libman M, et al. Disseminated infection after intravesical BCG immunotherapy. Detection of organisms in pulmonary tissue. *Chest* 1993;104:307–309.

49. Piqueras A, Marruecos R, Artigas A, et al. Miliary tuberculosis and the adult respiratory distress syndrome. *Intensive Care Med* 1987;13:175–182.

50. Lintin SN, Isaac PA. Miliary tuberculosis presenting as the adult respiratory distress syndrome. *Intensive Care Med* 1988; 14:672–674.

51. Heap MJ, Bion JF, Hunter KR. Miliary tuberculosis and the adult respiratory distress syndrome. *Respir Med* 1989;83: 153–156.

52. Ahuja SS, Ahuja SK, Phelps KR, et al. Hemodynamic confirmation of septic shock in disseminated tuberculosis. *Crit Care Med* 1992;20:901–903.

53. Pene F, Papo T, Brudy-Gulphe L, et al. Septic shock and thrombotic microangiopathy due to *Mycobacterium tuberculosis* in a nonimmunocompromised patient. *Arch Intern Med* 2001;161: 1347–1348.

54. Sydow M, Schauer A, Crozier TA, et al. Multiple organ failure in generalized disseminated tuberculosis. *Respir Med* 1992;86: 517–519.

55. Godwin JE, Coleman AA, Sahn SA. Miliary tuberculosis presenting as hepatic and renal failure. *Chest* 1991;99:752–754.

56. Asada Y, Hayashi T, Sumiyoshi A, et al. Miliary tuberculosis presenting as fever and jaundice with hepatic failure. *Hum Pathol* 1991;22:92–94.

57. Kuo P-H, Yang P-C, Kuo S-S, et al. Severe immune hemolytic anemia in disseminated tuberculosis with response to antituberculosis therapy. *Chest* 2001;119:1961–1963.

58. Lowry KJ, Stephan KT, Davis CE. Miliary tuberculosis presenting with rigors and developing unusual cutaneous manifestations. *Cutis* 1999;64:23–27.

59. Bobrowitz ID. Active tuberculosis undiagnosed until autopsy. *Am J Med* 1982;72:650–658.

60. Proudfoot AT, Akhtar AJ, Douglas AC, et al. Miliary tuberculosis in adults. *BMJ* 1969;2:273–276.

61. Lenzini L, Rottoli P, Rottoli L. The spectrum of human tuberculosis. *Clin Exp Immunol* 1977;27:230–237.

62. Harvey C, Eykyn S, Davidson C. Rigors in tuberculosis. *Postgrad Med J* 1993;69:724–725.

63. Hussey G, Chisolm T, Kibel M. Miliary tuberculosis in children: a review of 94 cases. *Pediatr Infect Dis J* 1991;10:832–836.

64. Sahn S, Neff TA. Miliary tuberculosis. *Am J Med* 1974;56: 495–505.

65. Massaro D, Katz S, Sachs M. Choroidal tubercles. A clue to hematogenous tuberculosis. *Ann Intern Med* 1964;60:231–241.

66. Shono T, Abe S, Horiuchi T. A case of miliary tuberculosis with disseminated choroidal hemorrhages. *Br J Ophthalmol* 1990;74: 317–319.

67. Fisher JR. Miliary tuberculosis with unusual cutaneous manifestations. *JAMA* 1977;238:241–242.

68. Rietbroek RC, Dahlmans RPM, Smedts F, et al. Tuberculosis cutis miliaris disseminata as a manifestation of miliary tuberculosis: literature review and report of a case of recurrent skin lesions. *Rev Infect Dis* 1991;13:265–269.

69. Stack RJ, Bickley LK, Coppel IG. Miliary tuberculosis presenting as skin lesions in a patient with acquired immunodeficiency syndrome. *J Am Acad Dermatol* 1990;23:1031–1035.

70. Joly P, Picard-Dahan C, Bamberger N, et al. Acute pustular eruption: an unusual clinical feature of disseminated mycobacterial infection in patients with acquired immunodeficiency syndrome. *J Am Acad Dermatol* 1993;28:264–266.

71. Schaaf HS, Nel ED. Tuberculosis presenting as cholestatic jaundice in early infancy. *J Pediatr Gastroenterol Nutr* 1992;15:437–439.

72. Mallinson WW, Fuller RW, Levison DA, et al. Diffuse interstitial renal tuberculosis—an unusual cause of renal failure. *Q J Med* 1981;198:137–148.

73. Shribman JH, Eastwood JB, Uff J. Immune complex nephritis complicating miliary tuberculosis. *BMJ* 1983;287:1593–1594.

74. Heffner JE, Strange C, Sahn S. The impact of respiratory failure on the diagnosis of tuberculosis. *Arch Intern Med* 1988;148:1103–1108.

75. Flora GS, Modilevsky T, Antoniskis D, et al. Undiagnosed tuberculosis in patients with human immunodeficiency virus infection. *Chest* 1990;98:1056–1059.

76. Eide FF, Gean AD, So YT. Clinical and radiographic findings in disseminated tuberculosis of the brain. *Neurology* 1993;43:1427–1429.

77. Gupta RK, Kohli A, Gaur V, et al. MRI of the brain in patients with miliary pulmonary tuberculosis without symptoms or signs of central nervous system involvement. *Neuroradiology* 1997;9:699-704.

78. Wallis PJW, Branfoot AC, Emerson PA. Sudden death due to myocardial tuberculosis. *Thorax* 1984;39:155–156.

79. Wainwright J. Tuberculous endocarditis—a report of two cases. *S Afr Med J* 1979;56:731–733.

80. Cope AP, Heber M, Wilkins EGL. Valvular tuberculous endocarditis: a case report and review of the literature. *J Infect* 1990;21:293–296.

81. Soyer R, Brunet A, Chevalier B, et al. Tuberculous aortic insufficiency—report of a case with successful surgical management. *J Thorac Cardiovasc Surg* 1981;82:254–256.

82. Felson B, Akers PV, Hall GS, et al. Mycotic tuberculous aneurysm of the thoracic aorta. *JAMA* 1977;237:1104–1108.

83. Braidy J, Pothel C, Amra S. Miliary tuberculosis presenting as adrenal failure. *J Can Med Assoc* 1981;124:748–751.

84. Weir MR, Thornton GF. Extrapulmonary tuberculosis. Experience of a community hospital and review of the literature. *Am J Med* 1985;79:467–478.

85. Barnes DJ, Naraqi S, Temu P, et al. Adrenal function in patients with active tuberculosis. *Thorax* 1989;44:422–424.

86. Nieuwland Y, Tan KY, Elte JWF. Miliary tuberculosis presenting with thyrotoxicosis. *Postgrad Med J* 1992;68:677–679.

87. Lipper S, Watkins DL, Kahn IR. Nongranulomatous septic vasculitis due to miliary tuberculosis. A pitfall in diagnosis for the pathologist. *Am J Dermatopathol* 1980;2:71–74.

88. Felson B. Acute miliary diseases of the lung. *Radiology* 1952;59:32–48.

89. Berger HW, Samortin TG. Miliary tuberculosis: diagnostic methods with emphasis on the chest roentgenogram. *Chest* 1970;58:586–589.

90. Felson B. A new look at pattern recognition of diffuse pulmonary disease. *AJR* 1979;133:183–189.

91. Felson B. The roentgen diagnosis of disseminated pulmonary alveolar diseases. *Semin Roentgenol* 1967;2:3–21.

92. Beuchner HA. The differential diagnosis of miliary diseases of the lungs. *Med Clin N Am* 1959;43:89–112.

93. Genereux GP. Pattern recognition in diffuse lung disease. A review of theory and practice. *Med Radiogr Photogr* 1985;61:2–31.

94. Price M. Lymphangitis reticularis tuberculosa. *Tubercle* 1968;49:377–384.

95. Pitchenik AE, Rubinson HA. The radiographic appearance of tuberculosis in patients with the acquired immunodeficiency syndrome (AIDS) and pre-AIDS. *Am Rev Respir Dis* 1985;131:393–396.

96. Barnes PF, Bloch AB, Davidson PT, et al. Tuberculosis in patients with human immunodeficiency virus infection. *N Engl J Med* 1991;324:1644–1650.

97. Havlir DV, Barnes PF. Tuberculosis in patients with human immunodeficiency virus infection. *N Engl J Med* 1999;340:367–373.

98. McGuinness G, Naidich DP, Jagirdar J, et al. High resolution CT findings in miliary lung disease. *J Comp Assist Tomogr* 1992;16:384–390.

99. Optican RJ, Ost A, Ravin CE. High-resolution computed tomography in the diagnosis of miliary tuberculosis. *Chest* 1992;102:941–943.

100. Voloudaki AE, Tritou IN, Magkanas EG, et al. HRCT in miliary lung disese. *Acta Radiologica* 1999;40:451–456.

101. Nishimura K, Izumi T, Kitaichi M, et al. The diagnostic accuracy of high-resolution computed tomography in diffuse infiltrative lung diseases. *Chest* 1993;104:1149–1155.

102. Moody EB, Delbeke D. Nuclear medicine case of the day. Miliary tuberculosis. *AJR Am J Roentgenol* 1992;158:1382.

103. Winzelberg GG. Radionuclide evaluation of miliary tuberculosis. *Clin Nucl Med* 1981;6:330–331.

104. Kao C-H, Wang S-J, Liao S-Q, et al. Usefulness of gallium-67-citrate scans in patients with acute disseminated tuberculosis and comparison with chest x-rays. *J Nucl Med* 1993;34:1918–1921.

105. Sarkar SD, Ravikrishnan KP, Woodbury DH, et al. Gallium-67 citrate scanning: a new adjunct in the detection and follow-up of extrapulmonary tuberculosis—concise communication. *J Nucl Med* 1979;20:833.

106. Andrew WK, Thomas RG, Gollach BL. Miliary tuberculosis of the liver—another cause of the "bright liver" on ultrasound examination. *S Afr Med J* 1982;62:808–809.

107. Grieco MH, Chmel H. Acute disseminated tuberculosis as a diagnostic problem. A clinical study based on twenty-eight cases. *Am Rev Respir Dis* 1974;109:554–560.

108. Sprung DJ. Miliary tuberculosis, with adult respiratory distress syndrome and a leukemoid reaction. *N Carolina Med J* 1981;42:709–710.

109. Hunt BJ, Andrews V, Pettingale KW. The significance of pancytopenia in miliary tuberculosis. *Postgrad Med J* 1987;63:801–804.

110. Bagby GC, Gilbert DN. Suppression of granulopoiesis by T-lymphocytes in two patients with disseminated mycobacterial infection. *Ann Intern Med* 1981;94:478–481.

111. Cassim KM, Gathiram V, Jogessar VB. Pancytopenia associated with disseminated tuberculosis, reactive histiocytic haemophagocytic syndrome and tuberculous hypersplenism. *Tuber Lung Dis* 1993;74:208–210.

112. Weintraub M, Siegman-Igra Y, Josiphov J, et al. Histiocytic hemophagocytosis in miliary tuberculosis. *Arch Intern Med* 1984;144:2055–2056.

113. Campo E, Condom E, Miro M-J, et al. Tuberculosis-associated hemophagocytic syndrome. *Cancer* 1986;58:2640–2645.

114. Monier BM, Fauroux B, Chevalier JY, et al. Miliary tuberculosis with acute respiratory failure and histiocytic hemophagocytosis. Successful treatment with extracorporeal lung support and epipodophyllotoxin VP 16-213. *Acta Paediatr* 1992;81:725–727.

115. De Beer FC, Nel AE, Gie RP, et al. Serum amyloid A protein and C-reactive protein levels in pulmonary tuberculosis: relationship to amyloidosis. *Thorax* 1984;39:196–200.

116. Shijubo N, Imai K, Nakanishi F, et al. Elevated concentrations of circulating ICAM-1 in far advanced and miliary tuberculosis. *Am Rev Respir Dis* 1993;148:1298–1301.

117. Isaacs RD, Nicholson GI, Holdaway IM. Miliary tuberculosis with hypercalcemia and raised vitamin D concentrations. *Thorax* 1987;42:555–556.

118. Sharma SK, Pande JN, Singh YN, et al. Pulmonary function and immunologic abnormalities in miliary tuberculosis. *Am Rev Respir Dis* 1992;145:1167–1171.
119. Ainslie GM, Solomon JA, Bateman ED. Lymphocyte and lymphocyte subset numbers in blood and in bronchoalveolar lavage and pleural fluid in various forms of human pulmonary tuberculosis at presentation and during recovery. *Thorax* 1992;47:513–518.
120. Sandoval J, Cicero R, Seoane M, et al. Behavior of the pulmonary circulation at rest and during exercise in miliary tuberculosis. *Chest* 1991;99:152–154.
121. Vomero E, Ratner SJ. Diagnosis of miliary tuberculosis by examination of middle ear discharge. *Arch Otolaryngol Head Neck Surg* 1988;114:1029–1030.
122. Biron F, Reveil JC, Penalba C, et al. Direct visualization of *Mycobacterium tuberculosis* in a blood sample from an AIDS patient (letter). *AIDS* 1990;4:259.
123. Eng RH, et al. Diagnosis of *Mycobacterium* bacteremia in patients with acquired immunodeficiency syndrome by direct examination of blood films. *J Clin Microbiol* 1989;27:764–769.
124. Klatskin G. Hepatic granulomata: problems in interpretation. *Ann NY Acad Sci* 1976;278:427–432.
125. Orenstein MS, Tavitian A, Yonk B, et al. Granulomatous involvement of the liver in patients with AIDS. *Gut* 1985;26:1220–1225.
126. Buckingham WB, Turner GC, Knapp WB, et al. Liver biopsy in a tuberculosis hospital. *Dis Chest* 1956;29:675.
127. Kahn SA, Saltzman BR, Klein RS, et al. Hepatic disorders in the acquired immune deficiency syndrome: a clinical and pathological study. *Am J Gastroenterol* 1986;81:1145–1148.
128. Lombard EH, Mansvelt EP. Haematological changes associated with miliary tuberculosis of the bone marrow. *Tuber Lung Dis* 1993;74:131–135.
129. Willcox PA, Potgieter PD, Bateman ED, et al. Rapid diagnosis of sputum negative miliary tuberculosis using the flexible fiberoptic bronchoscope. *Thorax* 1986;41:681–684.
130. Pant K, Chawla R, Mann PS, et al. Fiberbronchoscopy in smear-negative miliary tuberculosis. *Chest* 1989;95:1151–1152.
131. Modilevsky T, Sattler FR, Barnes PF. Mycobacterial disease in patients with human immunodeficiency virus infection. *Arch Intern Med* 1989;149:2201–2205.
132. Salzman SH, Schindel ML, Aranda CP, et al. The role of bronchoscopy in the diagnosis of pulmonary tuberculosis in patients at risk for HIV infection. *Chest* 1992;102:143–146.
133. Wallace JM, Deutsch AL, Harrell JH, et al. Bronchoscopy and transbronchial biopsy in evaluation of patients with suspected active tuberculosis. *Am J Med* 1981;70:1189–1194.
134. Miro AM, Gibilara E, Powell S, et al. The role of fiberoptic bronchoscopy for diagnosis of pulmonary tuberculosis in patients at risk for AIDS. *Chest* 1992;101:1211–1214.
135. Schluger NM. Changing approaches to the diagnosis of tuberculosis. *Am J Respir Crit Care Med* 2001;164:2020–2024.
136. Chin DP, Yajko DM, Hadley WK, et al. Clinical utility of a commercial test based on the polymerase chain reaction for detecting *Mycobacterium tuberculosis* in respiratory specimens. *Am J Respir Crit Care Med* 1995; 151:1872-1877.
137. Sada E, Ferguson LE, Daniel T. An ELISA for the serodiagnosis of tuberculosis using a 30,000-Da native antigen of *Mycobacterium tuberculosis*. *J Infect Dis* 1990;162:928–931.
138. Sada E, Brennan PJ, Herrera T, et al. Evaluation of lipoarabinomannan for the serological diagnosis of tuberculosis. *J Clin Microbiol* 1990;28:2587–2590.
139. American Thoracic Society. Treatment of tuberculosis and tuberculosis infection in adults and children. *Am J Respir Crit Care Med* 1994;149:1359–1374.
140. Ellard GA, Humphries MJ, Allen BW. Cerebrospinal fluid drug concentrations and the treatment of tuberculous meningitis. *Am Rev Respir Dis* 1993;148:650–655.
141. Falk A. U.S. Veterans Administration–Armed Forces Cooperative Study on the chemotherapy of tuberculosis. *Am Rev Respir Dis* 1965;91:6–12.
142. Alegre J, Fernandez de Sevilla T, Falco V, et al. Ofloxacin in miliary tuberculosis. *Eur Respir J* 1990;3:238–239.
143. Tahaoglu K, Torun T, Sevim T, et al. The treatment of multidrug resistant tuberculosis in Turkey. *N Engl J Med* 2001;345:170–174.
144. Girgis NI, Farid Z, Kilpatrick ME, et al. Dexamethasone adjunctive treatment for tuberculous meningitis. *Pediatr Infect Dis J* 1991;10:179–183.
145. Strang JG, Kakaza HHS, Gibson DG, et al. Controlled clinical trial of prednisolone as adjuvant in treatment of tuberculous constrictive pericarditis in Transkei. *Lancet* 1987;2:1418–1422.
146. McAllister WAC, Thompson PJ, Al-Habet SM, et al. Rifampicin reduces effectiveness and bioavailability of prednisolone. *BMJ* 1983;286:923–925.
147. Tongnian S, Jiayu Y, Liye Z et al. Chemotherapy and its combination with corticosteroids in acute miliary tuberculosis in adolescents and adults. Analysis of 55 cases. *Chin Med J (Beijing)* 1981;94:309–314.
148. Chandra KS, Prasad AS, Prasad CE, et al. Recurrent pneumothoraces in miliary tuberculosis. *Trop Geogr Med* 1988;40:347–349.
149. Seabra J, Coelho H, Barros H, et al. Acute tuberculous perforation of the small bowel during antituberculous therapy. *J Clin Gastroenterol* 1993;16:320–322.
150. Lees AJ, Macleod AF, Marshall J. Cerebral tuberculomas developing during treatment of tuberculous meningitis. *Lancet* 1980;1:1208–1211.
151. Corbella X, Carratala J, Rufi G, et al. Unusual manifestations of miliary tuberculosis: cutaneous lesions, phalanx osteomyelitis, and paradoxical expansion of tenosynovitis. *Clin Infect Dis* 1993;16:179–180.
152. American Thoracic Society/Centers for Disease Control Statement. Targeted tuberculin testing and treatment of latent tuberculosis infection. *Am J Respir Crit Care* 2000;161:S221–S247.
153. Colditz GA, Brewer TF, Berkey CS, et al. Efficacy of BCG vaccine in the prevention of tuberculosis. Meta-analysis of the published literature. *JAMA* 1994;271:698–702.
154. Quinn TC. Interactions of the human immunodeficiency virus and tuberculosis and the implications of BCG vaccination. *Rev Infect Dis* 1989;11 Suppl 2:S379–S384.
155. Katz I, Rosenthal T, Michaeli D. Undiagnosed tuberculosis in hospitalized patients. *Chest* 1985;87:770–774.
156. Burman WJ, Jones BE. Treatment of HIV-related tuberculosis in the era of effective antiretroviral therapy. *Am J Respir Crit Care Med* 2001;164:7–12.
157. Peters EJ, Morice R. Miliary pulmonary infection caused by *Mycobacterium terrae* in an autologous bone marrow transplant patient. *Chest* 1991;100:1449–1450.
158. Tong P, Tan WC, Pang M. Sporadic disseminated histoplasmosis simulating miliary tuberculosis. *BMJ* 1983;287:822–823.
159. Randle HW. Miliary coccidiomycosis. *Arizona Med* 1975;32:408–410.
160. Frean J, et al. Disseminated blastomycosis masquerading as tuberculosis. *J Infect* 1993;31:776–782.
161. Douketis JD, Kesten S. Miliary pulmonary cryptococcosis in a patient with the acquired immunodeficiency syndrome. *Thorax* 1993;48:402–403.
162. Meyer B, Stalder H, Wegman W. Persistent pulmonary granulomas after recovery from varicella pneumonia. *Chest* 1986;89:457–459.
163. Beschorner WE, Hutchins GM, Burns WH, et al. Cytomeg-

alovirus pneumonia in bone marrow transplant recipients: miliary and diffuse patterns. *Am Rev Respir Dis* 1990;122: 107–114.

164. Finnegan OC, Fowles SJ, White RJ. Radiologic appearance of *Mycoplasma* pneumonia. *Thorax* 1981;36:469–472.

165. Kim OH, Yang HR, Bahk YU. Pulmonary nocardiosis manifested as miliary nodules in a neonate—a case report. *Pediatr Radiol* 1992;22:229–230.

166. Cluroe AD. Legionnaire's disease mimicking pulmonary miliary tuberculosis in the immunocompromised. *Histopathology* 1993; 22:73–75.

167. Patel PJ, Al-Suhaibani AK, Al-Aska AK, et al. The chest radiograph in brucellosis. *Clin Radiol* 1988;39:39–41.

168. Flores JA. Miliary pattern in neonatal pneumonia. *Pediatr Radiol* 1988;18:355–356.

169. Goetz MD, Finegold SM. Pyogenic bacterial pneumonia, lung abscess, and empyema. In: Murray JF, Nadel JA, eds. *Textbook of respiratory medicine. Third Edition.* Philadelphia: WB Saunders, 2000:985–1041.

170. Cornog JLJ, Hanson CW. Psittacosis as a cause of miliary infiltrates of the lung and hepatic granulomas. *Am Rev Respir Dis* 1968;98:1033–1036.

171. Rubin SA. Radiographic spectrum of pleuropulmonary tularemia. *AJR Am J Roentgenol* 1978;131:277–281.

172. Schaberg T, Rahn W, Racz P, et al. Pulmonary schistosomiasis resembling acute pulmonary tuberculosis. *Eur Respir J* 1991;4: 1023–1026.

173. Prosmanne O, Chalaoui J, Sylvestre J, et al. Small nodular pattern in the lungs due to opportunistic toxoplasmosis. *J Can Assoc Radiol* 1984;35:186–188.

174. Krysl J, Muller N, Miller RR, et al. Patient with miliary nodules and diarrhea. *Can Assoc Radiol J* 1991;42:363–366.

175. Close PM, Macrae MB, Hammond JM, et al. Anaplastic large-cell Ki-1 lymphoma. Pulmonary presentation mimicking miliary tuberculosis. *Am J Clin Pathol* 1993;99:631–636.

176. Curull V, Morell F, Fort J, et al. Dyspnea, fever, and a miliary pattern. *Chest* 1985;88:285–286.

177. Leatherman JW, Davies SF, Hoidal JR. Alveolar hemorrhage syndromes: diffuse microvascular lung hemorrhage in immune and idiopathic disorders. *Medicine* 1984;63:343–361.

28

TUBERCULOSIS OF THE BRAIN, MENINGES, AND SPINAL CORD

MICHAEL HENRY
ROBERT S. HOLZMAN

Tuberculosis of the central nervous system remains among the most serious of all forms of human tuberculosis and is uniformly fatal without treatment. Even now, half a century after the introduction of streptomycin, it can be difficult to diagnose and may respond poorly to treatment. This chapter discusses tuberculosis of the brain, meninges, and spinal cord, with special reference to the impact of newer diagnostic techniques and therapeutic regimens on the management of these forms of the disease.

HISTORY, EPIDEMIOLOGY, AND RISK FACTORS

Tuberculosis of the central nervous system was a recognized disease long before modern understanding of it evolved: a Vedic hymn dated approximately two millennia B.C. invokes a treatment ritual for "consumption seated in thy head. . ." (1). Sir Robert Whytt, an 18th century Scottish physician and scholar of childhood hydrocephalus, provided the first systematic clinical description of the disease (2). The term *tubercular meningitis* was coined by P. H. Green, who published a study of the disease in *The Lancet* in 1836, a half-century before Koch discovered the tubercle bacillus (3).

The epidemiology of central nervous system tuberculosis parallels that of tuberculosis as a whole. In recent large-scale epidemiologic studies, central nervous system involvement accounted for approximately 5% to 10% of cases of clinical tuberculosis in the United States (4).

Central nervous system tuberculosis is both more frequent and more virulent in children (5). Twenty to 60% of children dying of active tuberculosis have brain or meningeal involvement at autopsy, in contrast to 5% or less for adults (6–8). In the 1940s, Elizabeth Lincoln, an expert and distinguished clinician, suggested that, based on her experience, children with antecedent viral infection, head trauma, surgery, or tuberculin positivity were at special risk for tuberculous meningitis (TBM) (9).

PATHOGENESIS

The pathogenesis of TBM is analogous to that of other forms of tuberculosis. Nineteenth and early twentieth century pathologists were puzzled when intracarotid injection of experimental animals with mycobacteria, even in massive numbers, failed to produce TBM. Only rare tubercles were produced, scattered through the brain substance and meninges. In contrast, much of the clinical syndrome of TBM in experimental animals could be easily recreated with intracranial injections of tuberculoprotein in the absence of any infection (10).

In 1933, McCordock and Rich (11) extrapolated from these observations the pathogenetic theory of TBM that is still accepted today. Dissecting tubercular brains with meticulous technique, they observed cases in which submeningeal or intrameningeal tubercles could be seen discharging bacilli into the subarachnoid spaces. They deduced that these bacteria were the progeny of those which had seeded the meninges weeks, months, or years earlier as a part of the primary tuberculous infection. The mycobacteria in these "Rich foci" could erupt from the tubercle with enough antigenic force to cause all of the manifestations of TBM. Thus, the pathogenesis of central nervous system tuberculosis is a two-step process: first, a hematogenous seeding of the meninges; then a quiescent phase of weeks, months, or decades until a stimulus, immune or traumatic, causes organisms and antigen contained in tubercles to be released into the subarachnoid spaces, causing disease. The entire sequence may evolve over

M. Henry: Department of Internal Medicine, New York University Medical Center, New York, New York.
R. S. Holzman: Department of Medicine, New York University School of Medicine; Department of Medicine, Bellevue Hospital, New York, New York.

a span of weeks as part of an overwhelming primary infection in an infant or immunocompromised adult, or it may span many decades if tuberculous infection acquired in childhood reactivates in the waning immunity of old age.

PATHOLOGY

Tuberculous meningitis produces characteristic changes in the meninges, the blood vessels of the brain, and the brain parenchyma itself. In the meninges, a granular, gelatinous exudate lies typically in the subarachnoid space at the base of the brain, most prominent near the optic chiasm and extending into the sylvian fissures. Should a similar exudate cover the ependyma and choroid plexus of the lateral ventricles it may induce a communicating hydrocephalus. Microscopically, the exudate is composed of fibrin and inflammatory cells: neutrophils in early cases and mononuclear cells in later ones. Foci of caseation necrosis surrounded by epithelioid cells and giant cells stud the substance of the exudate. Mycobacteria are present in variable numbers (11,12). Antituberculous treatment induces further caseation of the exudate. With successful treatment, much of the exudate may resolve, leaving residual tubercles, foci of caseation, and fibrosis (13,14).

Atrophy of gray and white matter may be induced by chronic hydrocephalus. In addition, the portion of the brain parenchyma immediately adjacent to the meningeal and ependymal exudates may develop a "border-zone reaction" of edema, perivasculitis, and gliosis. Occasional instances of diffuse cerebral edema, demyelination, and hemorrhagic leukoencephalopathy accompanying TBM have been identified (15,16).

In addition to the exudative inflammation and hydrocephalus, occlusive vascular disease may develop. TBM may produce a vasculitis that involves arteries and veins of all sizes in the vicinity of the meningeal exudate. In the arterial system, the terminal portion of the internal carotid artery and the proximal middle cerebral artery in the sylvian fissure are most often affected. Inflammatory cells infiltrate all layers of the vessels, and tubercles form, first in the adventitia and later in the media and the intima. As the disease progresses, the medial layer of the vessels fibroses, the intima thickens, and the vessel lumen shrinks in a necrotizing vasculitis reminiscent of periarteritis nodosa. With treatment, fibrotic endarteritis persists (17). Thus, TBM may produce ischemic damage to the brain parenchyma.

CLINICAL MANIFESTATIONS

The clinical manifestations of TBM are protean, and many case reports document unusual presentations (18). Some disparities among newer and older clinical series, and among series from different countries, can be explained by the fact that patient age is a most important determinant of presentation. Headache, fever, and stiff neck (meningismus) are common presenting complaints in adults, though they are by no means present in all cases (19–21). Among children, headache is far less common, and nausea and other abdominal complaints often predominate (9,22,23). Behavioral abnormalities ranging from lethargy to agitated paranoia are identified in 30% to 70% of patients of all ages (9,18,24–26). In children, symptoms are typically present for hours to weeks before medical attention is sought. Among adult patients, duration of symptoms is generally somewhat longer, and adult cases with symptoms lasting for years have been reported (21,27). A history of tuberculosis can be elicited in about 50% of pediatric patients and about 10% of adult patients (21,27,28).

Illustrative Case

A 42-year-old man was brought to the emergency room by the police. He was unable to give a medical history, but his wife described a 2-week history of worsening headaches, with fever, blurred vision, cough, and weight loss. One week before admission she had taken him to another hospital because of agitation and confusion. There he received a dose of intramuscular haloperidol and was discharged to psychiatric follow-up. Four days before admission he disappeared from his home. The police found him in a public park and brought him to a hospital.

Previously in apparent good health, he was an intravenous drug user who had recently been incarcerated in a state penitentiary. He was reportedly purified protein derivative (PPD) negative, and his status with respect to human immunodeficiency virus (HIV) infection was unknown.

On admission he was awake and restless. His neck was rigid. Neurologically he was unable to follow simple commands and there was a palsy of the left sixth cranial nerve. The remainder of the physical examination was within normal limits. His white blood cell (WBC) count was 11,100/mm^3 with 23% bands. Lumbar puncture revealed clear, colorless cerebrospinal spinal fluid (CSF) at an opening pressure of 350 mm H_2O. CSF protein was 454 mg %, glucose 13 mg %, WBC 31/mm^3, red blood cell (RBC) count 134/mm^3. A test for CSF cryptococcal antigen was negative. His serum sodium was 121 mEq/L and liver function tests were normal. A computed tomography (CT) scan performed with contrast demonstrated basal meningeal enhancement, enlarged ventricles, and a round, uniformly enhancing lesion in the left parietal area.

Initial therapy was directed against bacterial meningitis, but a second lumbar puncture after 24 hours of therapy was unchanged, and Gram stain, acid-fast bacillus (AFB) stain, and bacterial cultures of both specimens of CSF were negative. Antibacterial therapy was discontinued and isoniazid, rifampin, pyrazinamide, and streptomycin were given. He remained febrile and delirious, and prednisone (60 mg/day) was added to his regimen. Repeat CT scanning 5 days later demonstrated further enlargement of the ventricles due to persistent communicating hydrocephalus. A ventriculostomy was inserted. CSF from the drain showed rare mycobacteria in both fluorochrome and AFB stains. A culture of the fluid grew *Mycobacterium tuberculosis*, sensitive to all agents tested.

Streptomycin and prednisone were stopped after 2 months and isoniazid, rifampin, and pyrazinamide were continued. The patient's neurologic status slowly improved, although after 6 months' therapy his memory and affect were still significantly impaired.

Staging Based on Neurologic Status

Prognosis is still gauged best with a staging system based on neurologic findings that was introduced in 1947 to systematize early treatment trials (29) (Table 28.1). In stage I, there are no neurologic abnormalities. In stage II disease there is some combination of meningismus, lethargy, and/or cranial nerve palsies. Such palsies may be unilateral or bilateral and most often involve the sixth nerve, followed in frequency by the third, fourth, and seventh. Involvement of other cranial nerves is less common (22,27). Cranial nerve palsies are ascribed to the pressure of the thick basilar inflammatory exudate on the cranial nerves, compounded in some cases by the presence of hydrocephalus.

Stage III is characterized by neurologic changes beyond those defining stage II, such as coma, seizures, abnormal movements such as choreoathetosis, and paresis or paralysis of one or more extremities. Paresis most commonly reflects ischemic infarction from tuberculous vasculitis, although it also may be induced or exacerbated by hydrocephalus. In some reports, paresis has been noted in 40% or more of patients, occurring most commonly in the anterior cerebral circulation, in the territory of one or both lenticulostriate, medial striate, thalamotuberal, and thalamoperforating arteries (29,30).

TABLE 28.1. STAGES OF TUBERCULOUS MENINGITIS

Stage	Clinical Signs and Symptoms
I (early)	Nonspecific symptoms Few or no clinical signs of meningitis Fully conscious and alert
II (intermediate)	Signs of meningitis Drowsiness or lethargy Cranial nerve palsies
III (advanced)	Stupor or coma Systemic toxicity Gross paresis or paralysis

Modified from British Medical Research Council. Streptomycin treatment of tuberculous meningitis. *Lancet* 1948;1:582–596.

Ophthalmic examination may reveal papilledema due to increased intracranial pressure. In some cases choroid tubercles may be seen by fundoscopic examination (31). Internuclear ophthalmoplegia has been reported as a complication (32).

DIAGNOSTIC TESTS

Routine laboratory tests are seldom striking in TBM. The absolute WBC counts may be high, normal, or low, and the differential may be normal or show a left shift. Occasional concurrent disseminated tuberculosis may produce a myelophthisic differential, with metamyelocytes and nucleated red cells present. The sedimentation rate may be normal or elevated. Hyponatremia reflecting the inappropriate secretion of antidiuretic hormone has been reported in a substantial number of patients in some series (33,34). Chest x-ray shows evidence of tuberculosis, either active or healed, in as many as 50% of adults and 90% of children (19,22,35,36). PPD tuberculin testing has been reported as negative in 10% to 15% of children and approximately 50% of adults (9,19,24,37).

Cerebrospinal Fluid

Cerebrospinal fluid abnormalities in TBM are not pathognomonic. The most characteristic picture is that of a moderate lymphocytic pleocytosis, moderately elevated spinal fluid protein and moderate hypoglycorrhachia (38,39). These findings are similar to those accompanying a variety of meningeal processes, such as partially managed bacterial meningitis, fungal meningitis, syphilitic meningitis, carcinomatous meningitis, and collagen vascular diseases of the central nervous system. Any or all of these findings may be exaggerated or absent in TBM; in rare cases, the disease has been definitively diagnosed despite a totally normal CSF examination (18). A polymorphonuclear predominance may sometimes be seen. A normal spinal fluid glucose on initial presentation may become lower on repeat sampling, although it is said never to fall to the extremely low or undetectable levels seen in bacterial or carcinomatous meningitis (22,40). An elevated CSF protein, usually in the range of 150 mg % to 200 mg %, is the most reliably present abnormality. Extreme protein elevations are seen almost exclusively in association with spinal block (see below).

Microbiology

Demonstrating *M. tuberculosis* in the CSF of patients with TBM remains difficult, undoubtedly reflecting the very small number of organisms required to provoke even fulminate disease. Smears of spinal fluid are rarely positive; in some series, more than 90% are negative (24,41). Many techniques for enhancing the yield of AFB staining CSF have been reported. Staining the pellicle—the fibrinaceous clot that may form in standing CSF—is one of the more venerable of these techniques (42), and layering the sediment of centrifuged spinal fluid onto a single slide is another (43). In 1979, Kennedy and Fallon (23) convincingly demonstrated the utility of staining multiple specimens of CSF and raised their yield of positive smears to 86% after processing four specimens for each case.

CSF culturing for mycobacteria also lacks sensitivity, and culture-negative cases actually comprise the majority of some series where inclusion was based on other convincing diagnostic criteria (21,24,27,44). Yield of cultures may be enhanced by processing of large volumes or multiple specimens of spinal fluid. A recent study indicates that both cisternal and ventricular CSF are more likely to be culture positive than fluid obtained from the lumbar region (45). Cultures of blood, urine, sputum, or other body fluids may be useful supplements to spinal fluid culture in the presence of extraneural disease.

Despite its disadvantages, a positive mycobacterial culture remains by default the gold standard of diagnosis in TBM. Its lack of sensitivity and the long interval before the result is finalized are particularly frustrating in the context of a disease in which rapid and precise diagnosis is a therapeutic necessity. The ideal diagnostic technique for TBM would combine acceptable sensitivity and specificity with speed, low expense, and ease of execution in the clinical laboratories of developing countries in which the bulk of TBM now occurs. To date, despite many candidates, no single test has met all of these qualifications.

Radiology

Older radiologic techniques are relatively unrevealing in cases of central nervous system tuberculosis. Radiographs of the skull can identify separation of the cranial sutures in infants with hydrocephalus and occasionally distinguish the meningeal calcification of healed disease (46). Radioisotope brain scans may reveal meningeal inflammation if it is extensive and severe (47). A triad of angiographic findings has been reported, comprising ventricular dilatation, narrowing of the vessels at the base of the brain, and cerebral arteritis (48). Because the author noted an association between angiography and subsequent clinical deterioration, he cautioned against its use for routine diagnosis. A more recent study found that findings on digital subtraction angiogram did not predict the development of infarcts or clinical outcome, again leading the authors to discourage the routine use of angiography for diagnosis of TBM (49). However, angiography is useful is differentiating tumor from tuberculoma (50) by the absence of "tumor vascularity."

The introduction of computed tomography (CT) and magnetic resonance imaging (MRI) has revolutionized the role of neuroimaging in the diagnosis and management of

TBM. CT examination with contrast commonly reveals meningeal enhancement of the basal cistern, hydrocephalus, granulomatous lesions, and cerebral infarctions (Figs. 28.1 and 28.2). Less common findings include meningeal enhancement of the cerebral and cerebellar hemispheres, ependymitis (50–53). CT is highly sensitive; in one survey of 289 patients (mostly children), only 35 (12%) had normal CT studies on admission (54). In another study of 64 adults, only 14% had normal CT scans (55).

There are several limitations to the use of CT for diagnosis. Early in TBM the typical findings may be absent, although they may progress with time even in the presence of antituberculous treatment (54). In addition, none of these findings are specific (50). The differential diagnosis includes bacterial or fungal meningitis, carcinomatosis, Wegener's granulomatosis, neurosarcoidosis, and chronic meningitis secondary to actinomycosis or nocardia (56).

MRI has proven to be more sensitive than CT in the radiologic detection of TBM (57), although, like CT, its specificity is limited. MR angiograms demonstrate findings similar to those found in conventional angiography (58). The comparison of magnetic transfer ratios has helped to differentiate meningeal inflammation secondary to tuber-

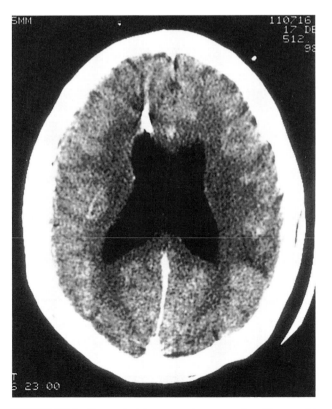

FIGURE 28.1. Computed tomography scan of a 42-year-old man with tuberculous meningitis demonstrates the symmetrically enlarged ventricles seen with communicating hydrocephalus.

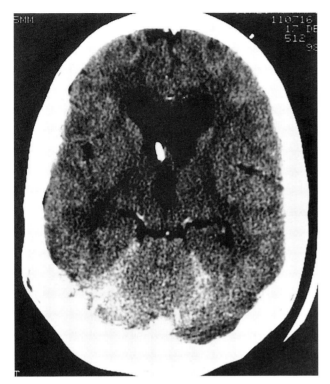

FIGURE 28.2. Dramatic enhancement of the basal meninges on a computed tomography scan with intravenous contrast in a patient with tuberculous meningitis.

culous infection from other etiologies (59). Pui et al. (60) were able to detect small enhancing nodules in tuberculous, bacterial, and fungal meningitis, but not in viral meningitis. By using the criteria of the presence of a solid rim or sizes under 2 cm in diameter, they were able to identify TBM with 86% sensitivity, 90% specificity, and 88% accuracy. MRI may also demonstrate the extent of cerebral disease during miliary spread of tuberculosis (61), even in the absence of frank meningitis (62).

The correlation of CT and MRI findings with clinical disease is not strong, and it has been difficult to assign precise prognostic value to initial CT or MRI findings. Several studies have noted that the presence or degree of meningeal enhancement does not correlate with the severity of disease (54,55,63). Similarly, ventricular size on CT imaging does not correlate well with monitored intracranial pressure (64).

With effective therapy, resolution of the pathologic findings on CT or MRI is the general rule, although the pattern and evolution differs from patient to patient and even from lesion to lesion in same patient (50). Meningeal enhancement can initially worsen on treatment, prior to showing signs of resolution (54).

While CT and MRI scans may eventual return to normal, permanent encephalomalacia in the areas of cerebral infarcts, as well as meningeal granulomas may persist. Some of the granulomas may calcify (65).

Antibody Detection

Antibodies against a variety of mycobacterial antigen preparations may be detected in the CSF of patients with TBM. These assays are inherently more sensitive than they are specific because they are compromised by the presence of low-level, circulating, cross-reactive antibodies (66).

An early study in India demonstrated the pitfalls. Antibodies to a soluble mycobacteria extract were detected in the CSF of 68% of patients with tuberculous but also in 37% of patients with pyogenic meningitis (67). None of the 37% had any known history of tuberculosis in the past. Negative controls from India had an 18% false-positive rate whereas similar negative controls from the United Kingdom had no false positives, underscoring the role of previous exposure and possibly latent infection in persistent antibody production.

More recently, antibodies to a variety of purified antigens, including bacille Calmette–Guérin (BCG), PPD, antigen 5, 14kD antigen, and lipoarabinomannan (LAM) (68–72) have been detected by ELISA and dot-immunobinding assays (73). Some of these studies have demonstrated sensitivities well exceeding those of culture, reaching 85% for some assays (72). Specificities approaching 100% have been reported as well (70–72).

However, other investigators have not been able to consistently replicate these findings. The sensitivity of detecting CSF anti-BCG was only 24% in one study (74), and anti-LAM, previously reported to be 85% sensitive (72), was detected only 42% of the time in a second study (69). A survey of reactivity to various purified antigens found antibody to 38kD (the major constituent of antigen 5) to be positive in only 12% of TBM patients, whereas anti-LAM was detected in 53%. The false-positive rate for anti-LAM was 21% (75). The sensitivity of these assays in this study was notably worse in culture-positive cases, leading the authors to postulate that in those with high numbers of tubercle bacilli in the CSF, excess antigen was absorbing the antibody, rendering it undetectable. In support of their hypothesis, 67% of the culture-positive cases had detectable IgG immune complexes.

Assays to detect CSF cells secreting antimycobacterial antibodies have been promising, although more technically demanding and less clinically useful. One study used an immunoblot assay to detect cells secreting anti-BCG antibodies in 96% of TBM cases, with an 8% false-positive rate (76). A second study, using a cell–ELISA technique, detected CSF-derived B cells producing anti-PPD antibodies in 90% of TBM patients, with no false positives in the control group (77).

Antigen Detection

A variety of techniques have been used to search for mycobacterial antigens or antigen–antibody complexes directly in the spinal fluid. The assays studied include latex agglutination (78), radioimmunoassay (79), ELISA (74,80), inhibition ELISA (81), immunoblotting (82), and reverse passive hemagglutination assays (83,84). The reported sensitivities of these assays have been uniformly better than culture, with specificities of 90% to 100% (85,86). Direct staining of macrophages isolated from CSF with a polyvalent rabbit IgG to *M. bacterium* tuberculosis was 72% sensitive, with no false positive in the control group (87). To further improve the accuracy of a serologic diagnosis, some investigators have combined assays for antibody and antigen (74), antibody and immune complex (88), or simply tested for a series of antibodies (89). Despite these generally robust reported results, none of these tests have been validated in large-scale, multicenter trials. The optimal algorithm for a serologic diagnosis has yet to be determined.

Nucleotide Amplification and Detection

Nucleic acid amplification techniques have been used to assay CSF for mycobacterial DNA and RNA (90–92). A nested amplification technique (93) and use of improved primers (94) was shown to improve both sensitivity and specificity. In a small-scale trial, a nucleic acid amplification kit that has been marketed for detection of *M. tuberculosis* in respiratory specimens (Gen-Probe Amplified *Mycobacterium tuberculosis* Direct Test; Gen-Probe, Inc., San Diego, CA, U.S.A.) was tested for its ability to detect the organism in CSF (95). This study was small, and some of the subjects had tuberculomas, not meningitis. Twenty-nine samples were processed in parallel by both polymerase chain reaction (PCR) and culture. Five of the 29 had TBM and four had tuberculomas without meningitis. All five meningitis patients had both positive cultures and PCR tests. All four tuberculoma patients had negative results on both tests, as did the 20 patients with diagnoses other than tuberculosis. In contrast to these results, in another study the result of PCR was positive in only six of eight patients with culture-proven TBM and in only 40% of a group of culture-negative patients with strong suspicion of disease (96). The role of PCR in diagnosis remains to be determined.

Other Diagnostic Techniques

The bromine partition test, first devised in the 1920s, is based on the observation that TBM tends to disrupt the blood–brain barrier more than other meningitides do (97). Not widely used in the United States, the test requires the intravenous injection of radiolabeled isotopes, either bromine-82 or technetium-99, and CSF assay for radioactivity 48 hours later (98–100). The use of technetium allows both the substance of the brain and CSF flow patterns to be imaged during the course of the test (101).

Adenosine deaminase, an enzyme elaborated by activated T lymphocytes, has been found in significantly ele-

vated concentrations in the CSF of some patients with TBM (102). Conflicting reports on the utility of this assay have appeared. Some have described excellent sensitivity and specificity (102–104), including one series of patients with HIV-associated TBM (105). Others observed low sensitivity and specificity or excess overlap of levels between cases of tuberculous, bacterial, or viral meningitis (106,107) or noted that it added little information to more readily available tests (108,109).

Tuberculostearic acid, a component of the cell wall of *M. tuberculosis*, has been detected in CSF with the use of gas–liquid chromatography (110,111). This molecule has been found to be a fairly sensitive and specific indicator of TBM in several studies, but the need for expensive equipment and experienced operators prevents its widespread use.

MASS LESIONS OF THE CENTRAL NERVOUS SYSTEM

Tuberculoma

A tuberculoma results when intracranial tubercles enlarge without rupturing into the subarachnoid space. Walled off from the brain parenchyma by a thick fibrous capsule, these structures may reach considerable size before symptoms result (112). Tuberculomas usually occur in the absence of TBM but may be present concomitantly (113). In a large autopsy series from the early 20th century, tuberculomas were roughly four times less common than TBM (112); however, such studies may not provide accurate estimates of relative incidence in the general population.

In a series of 39 consecutive patients with central nervous system tuberculosis seen in one Saudi Arabian hospital during a 4-year period, 28 (72%) had brain or spinal cord tuberculomas, but only 11 (28%) had TBM (114).

Tuberculomas may enlarge during management of TBM and cause symptoms of an intracranial mass lesion (115–117). The enlargement may not reflect failure of therapy but is believed to result from the reconstitution, during treatment, of immune inflammatory responses to mycobacterial antigens. No age, gender, racial, or other factor has been identified to predict whether dissemination of *M. tuberculosis* to the central nervous system will subsequently manifest itself as meningitis or as a mass lesion.

Most patients have single lesions, although as many as 12 have been identified within a single cranium (118). They may be found in the cerebral hemispheres, basal ganglia, brainstem, and cerebellum, as well as (rarely) in the substance of the spinal cord (119,120). Tuberculomas are among the most common intracranial mass lesions in developing countries but are now thought to be rare in the Western world (121,122). However, the increased availability of MRI and CT has undoubtedly resulted in greater recognition of these lesions in all contexts.

In the absence of concomitant meningitis, the symptoms of tuberculomas are those of inflamed or enlarging intracranial masses. Symptoms are often limited to seizures; fever and systemic toxicity are rare (123,124). The protein content of the CSF may be elevated, but other abnormalities are not usually reported (113).

The diagnosis is suggested by the radiologic appearance but can only be confirmed by pathologic examination. Angiographically, a tuberculoma appears as an avascular mass, sometimes with a faint tumor blush. CT scanning typically shows either uniform contrast enhancement or a thick rind of enhancement surrounding a punctate area of central clearing representing the caseous center of the lesion (Fig 28.3) (125,126). MRI with enhancement depicts similar findings and appears to be more sensitive than CT in the detection of these lesions (127,128).

The gold standard of diagnosis is the demonstration of caseating granulomata on pathologic examination. AFB smears and stains of tissue specimens are positive in only about 60% of cases; a similar proportion of specimens grow mycobacteria in culture. Surgical resection beyond that required for diagnostic examination is rarely required (129,130), and patients treated with medical therapy alone have achieved better functional recovery than those whose lesions were surgically removed (124,131).

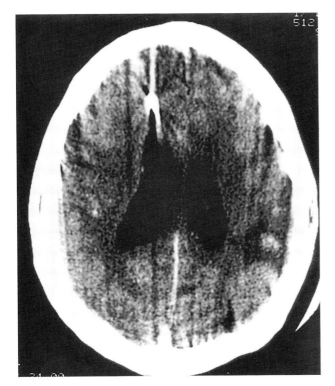

FIGURE 28.3. A small, left parietal tuberculoma in a patient with tuberculous meningitis appears as a round uniformly enhancing lesion on computed tomography scan.

Tuberculous Brain Abscess

Rarely, the caseous center of a tuberculoma liquefies and a tuberculous brain abscess results. Unlike other forms of intracranial tuberculosis, tuberculous abscesses teem with mycobacteria. They may occur as single or multiple lesions, with or without concomitant meningitis (132,133). Patients with abscesses show considerably more toxemia than those with tuberculomas; headache, fever, delirium, and focal neurologic signs occur commonly. Tuberculous abscesses seldom respond adequately to antituberculous drugs alone, and surgical drainage is usually required (134).

Tuberculosis Of The Spinal Cord

All of the varieties of intracranial tuberculosis may occur within the spinal cord and its membranes, including arachnoiditis, vasculitis, and intraparenchymal mass lesions. Disease may be localized to the spinal cord but more often accompanies intracranial disease. The pathogenesis of tuberculous arachnoiditis is similar to that of TBM: the rupture of a submeningeal tubercle into the spinal subarachnoid space (135–138).

Clinically, these events may result in the acute onset of spinal block, in a subacute transverse myelitis-like syndrome, or in a slow, ascending paralysis that develops over months to years (139,140). In rare cases of arachnoiditis ossificans, symptoms do not manifest until years after the active infection has resolved (141). Fever and systemic toxicity are mild or absent in most patients with spinal cord tuberculosis. Their CSF often becomes so proteinaceous and tenacious that it is impossible to obtain. When available, protein content of the fluid may exceed several grams per 100 mL. Hypoglycorrhachia and lymphocytic pleocytosis are seen in 30% to 50% of cases. Myelography demonstrates filling defects that may extend over the length of the cord. An enhancing subarachnoid exudate may be demonstrated on CT or MRI (142).

Definitive surgical therapy of spinal arachnoiditis is not often attempted because of the extent of the exudate and the tenacious network of adhesions that may develop. However, partial neurologic recovery after surgery has been reported (143). Steroids and antituberculous drugs have also led to symptomatic improvement in a few reported cases (137, 144).

Intramedullary and epidural tuberculomas have both been reported within the spinal cord. As in the brain, these tuberculomas are well encapsulated and may mimic spinal cord tumors in virtually all respects. In contrast to the management of intracranial tuberculomas, complete surgical excision of the spinal mass has been the treatment of choice in most reported cases, although some have responded to partial excision and prolonged antimycobacterial treatment (145, 146, 147).

TREATMENT AND PROGNOSIS

Despite major advances in our understanding of the treatment of pulmonary tuberculosis, the optimal regimen and dosing duration of anti-tuberculous therapy for TBM has not been established. Its relative rarity, high early mortality in advanced cases, and difficulty in early diagnosis make it difficult to conduct definitive clinical trials. As a result, current treatment regimens for central nervous system tuberculosis have evolved with the addition of each new antituberculous agent and are based on expert opinion, informed by an amalgam of small clinical trials, descriptive studies of large series, and extrapolations from studies on pulmonary tuberculosis.

Like pulmonary tuberculosis, central nervous system disease is managed with combination chemotherapy to prevent the development of resistant isolates. While the infectious load in typical cases of central nervous system tuberculosis is far less than that of pulmonary, treatment of central nervous system disease is complicated by the need for need for drugs to adequately penetrate the blood–brain barrier and the limited tolerance of the central nervous system to internal inflammation (Table 28.2a–c).

In 1947, the clinician Edith Lincoln (9) voiced concern over the impending availability of drugs to manage TBM. She warned, "Cases [will have to be] recognized early if we are to cure the disease without leaving a damaged brain." Fifty years of treatment studies have amply justified her concern. Although treatment and cure are now routine, morbidity and mortality rates still remain extraordinarily high if the disease is not diagnosed and managed promptly. "The lesson of TBM, to be repeatedly taught, is that treatment should be started as swiftly as possible on clinical grounds. Delay through bewilderment or procrastination through uncertainty is dangerous and often leads to a worse prognosis" (148).

Current Recommendations

As of the writing of this chapter the most recent joint recommendations of the American Thoracic Society, Centers for Disease Control and Prevention, and American Academy of Pediatrics were published in 1994. They suggest that for adults TBM be managed "according to the principles and with the drug regimens outlined for pulmonary tuberculosis," whereas children "should receive at least 12 months of therapy" (149). Children were singled out for more prolonged therapy because the data may have been inadequate to assure the adequacy of a briefer course. The British Thoracic Society recommends a 12-month course in all patients with TBM (150).

Patients have been successfully treated with courses ranging from 6 months (151) to 2 years, and beyond. A recent review of treatment considered trials published between 1978 and 1999 and providing at least 12 months of post-treatment observation. Four studies evaluating a 6-month regimen and seven studies evaluating longer treatment regimens were identified (152). All four studies evaluating a 6-month course were prospective, nonrandomized studies, the largest of which reported 95 children undergoing a 6-month regimen of isoniazid, rifampin, pyrazinamid, and ethambutol. Mortality was 16%, with one patient experiencing a relapse (153). The review concluded that the 6-month courses, which included isoniazid, rifampin, and pyrazinamide, had comparable outcomes to the longer ones, but cautioned that the total number of patients receiving a 6-month course was only 197, and nearly 75% of subjects were younger than 16 years.

Regimens of less than 12 months, supported as they are by several studies (154–156), seem reasonable for at least those patients with sensitive isolates who respond well to therapy and have uncomplicated courses. For those with slow improvement or severe disease, many clinicians give more prolonged therapy. As of 1992, an experienced group of clinicians in Hong Kong was treating patients with TBM who presented in stage I or stage II for 9 to 12 months, whereas patients with stage III disease were treated for 12 to 18 months, and patients with tuberculoma for 18 to 24 months (157).

Evolution of Treatment Regimens

Streptomycin and Paraaminosalicylic Acid

Streptomycin, the first antituberculous agent developed, had an clear and substantial impact on the outcome of TBM, reducing mortality rates from virtually 100% to 50% to 60% (158,159). However, treatment failures were quickly noticed, anticipating later pharmacokinetic studies that would show only modest penetration of streptomycin into the CSF, and almost none in the absence of meningeal inflammation (160). The introduction of paraaminosalicylic acid, when combined with streptomycin, led to even better outcomes in early trials (161), but subsequent studies showed that paraaminosalicylic acid also achieved relatively low levels in the CSF, in part due to an active efflux mechanism (162).

Isoniazid

Isoniazid, first used in 1952, revolutionized the management of all forms of tuberculosis. A small, unbound molecule that penetrates the spinal fluid even in the absence of meningeal inflammation, isoniazid achieves levels well above those necessary for effective management of TBM. Its introduction for the management of TBM was associated with additional reductions in mortality with reported rates from 17% to 30% (Fig. 28.4) (163,164). For the two decades following the introduction of isoniazid, management of central nervous system tuberculosis centered on the

TABLE 28.2A. CEREBROSPINAL FLUID PENETRATION BY ANTITUBERCULOUS DRUGS

Drug	MIC (mg/mL)	Dose	No. of Pts.	Time After Dosing (hr)	Serum	CSF	Cit.
Isoniazid	0.025–0.05	9 mg/kg	19	2	4.4	1.9	160
			8	4	2.6	3.2	160
			8	6	1.0	1.8	160
		10 mg/kg	25	2	4.5	4.6	291
		20 mg/kg	40	4	11.2	11.6	291
Rifampin	0.005–0.20	11 mg/kg	19	2	11.5	0.39	160
			8	4	10.6	0.38	160
			8	6	4.7	0.47	160
		600 mg	5	3	6.85	0.27	292
		600 mg	14	2	10.9	0.19	173
			11	6	8.3	0.28	173
Pyrazinamide	12.5	30 mg/kg	18	2	43.0	26.0	173
			13	6	35.8	42.7	173
		40 mg/kg	13	2		28.5	174
			13	4		30.6	174
		1500 mg or 30 mg/kg	13	3	32.2	33.6	175
Ethambutol	1.0	25 mg/kg	7	3	3.9	0.98	166
		25 mg/kg	5	4	5.2	0.38	167
		25 mg/kg	8	3	5.5	1.39	168
Streptomycin	0.4–10	13 mg/kg	10	2	30.0	2.1	160
			6	4	16.4	1.6	160
			6	6	10.6	2.2	160
Ethionamide	0.6–2.5	250 mg q12h	6	2	1.6	0.85	293
				3	1.0	1.2	293
				4	0.9	0.85	293
		15 mg/kg	18	2		1.71	294
						2.17	294

Drug Level (μg/mL) (Average) spans Serum, CSF, Cit.

TABLE 28.2B. CASE REPORT OF A 21-MONTH-OLD GIRL

Drug	MIC (μg/mL)	Dose	Time After Dosing (hr)	Serum	Inflamed	Uninflamed
Ciprofloxacin	0.25–2.0	250 mg p.o. bid	2.5	3.37		Trace
			9.0	0.29		0.14
			11.0	0.22	Trace	
Cycloserine	10–20	250 mg b.i.d.	2.5	24.4		7.7
			9.0	23.9		22.5
			13.0	16.5	11.5	
Rifabutin	0.125–1.0	300 q.d.	2.5	0.43		0.1
			9	0.43		0.1

Drug Levels (μg/mL); Meninges spans Inflamed, Uninflamed.

b.i.d., twice per day; p.o., orally; q.d., every day.
Adapted from DeVincenzo JP, Berning SE, Peloquin CA, et al. Multidrug-resistant tuberculosis meningitis: clinical problems and concentrations of second-line antituberculous medications. *Ann Pharmacother* 1999;33:1184–1188.

TABLE 28.2C. CASE REPORT OF A 25-YEAR-OLD MAN

Drug	MIC (μg/mL)	Dose	Time After Dosing (hr)	CSF Drug Level (μg/mL)
Levaquin	0.25	750 mg i.v.	0.5	1.05
			4.5	1.88
Amikacin	16	22 mg/kg	2.0	9.8
			6.0	10.1

i.v., intravenous; MIC, minimal inhibitory concentration; CSF, cerebrospinal fluid.
Adapted from Berning SE, Cherry TA, Iseman MD. Novel treatment of meningitis caused by multidrug-resistant *Mycobacterium tuberculosis* with intrathecal levofloxacin and amikacin: case report. *Clin Infect Dis* 2001;32:643–646.

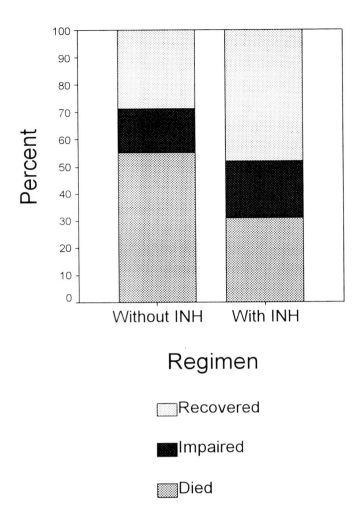

FIGURE 28.4. The impact of isoniazid on the prognosis of tuberculous meningitis. The *bar on the left* represents the results of a study in which patients were treated with streptomycin alone (158). The *bar on the right* represents the weighted average outcomes for eight studies that used various regimens, all of which contained isoniazid (23,33,180,181,185,255,289,290). Averages were weighted by study size.

use of isoniazid, paraaminosalicylic acid, and streptomycin, although with little standardization of dosages or duration of therapy. Despite anecdotal reports of successful treatment courses of less than 9 months (165), most clinicians of the time employed treatment courses of 18 to 36 months.

Ethambutol

Introduced in as an antitubercular agent in 1961, ethambutol penetrates the blood–brain barrier to achieve therapeutic doses, but only in the setting of meningeal inflammation (166,167). Ethambutol is effective in the management of TBM (168); however, a comparison of paraaminosalicylic acid with ethambutol in patients also receiving isoniazid

and streptomycin for TBM showed to no difference in outcome (169)

Pyrazinamide

Pyrazinamide readily passes through the blood–brain barrier, even in the setting of uninflamed meninges (170–175) and has been adapted into the first line of treatment for those with TBM (see below). However, while there is some evidence that pyrazinamide may permit a reduction in treatment duration (176–178), it has not been shown to improve outcome. One prospective trial in 1986 found no difference in outcome when pyrazinamide was added to a then-standard course of isoniazid, rifampin, and streptomycin (179). In addition, a retrospective review of 101 cases between the years 1985 and 1996 found no difference in mortality or morbidity rates between pyrazinamide- and ethambutol-containing regimens, when each was given with isoniazid, streptomycin, and rifampin (180). A retrospective analysis of 199 children treated over the years 1961 to 1984 found no change in outcome with any regimen, in spite of the introduction of rifampin and pyrazinamide during these years (181).

Pyrazinamide has been shown to be more active in an acidic environment, such as that characteristic of necrotic tissue (182). The more neutral pH of the spinal fluid may lessen the activity of pyrazinamide, explaining why improved outcomes have not been demonstrated despite the achievement of supratherapeutic CSF levels (183).

Rifampin

The introduction of rifampin in the early 1970s and the reintroduction of pyrazinamide, both powerful sterilizing agents, changed the management of pulmonary tuberculosis by permitting shorter, more intense courses of therapy. While these regimens have also shortened the management of most cases of TBM, an improvement in the survival of patients has been difficult to establish. Although one group experienced a marked reduction in mortality among children receiving isoniazid (20 mg/kg) and rifampin (15 mg/kg) in comparison with historical controls (184,185), a retrospective study of 143 patients treated between 1967 and 1980 found no improvement in outcome in those patients receiving a rifampin-containing regimen (186). Nor have more contemporary randomized controlled trials demonstrated improved outcomes with rifampin-containing regimens. One study was a controlled trial of 41 children in which rifampin was compared with paraaminosalicylic acid in children receiving 18 months of treatment with isoniazid, streptomycin, and the test drug (187). Two additional randomized controlled trials compared rifampin with ethambutol in patients receiving isoniazid and streptomycin (188,189). None of the three trials demonstrated mortality advantages for rifampin. Thus, mortality rates for TBM remain much as they have since the introduction of isoniazid.

Other Agents

The management of multidrug-resistant *M. tuberculosis* requires the use of antituberculous agents, which, because of toxicity, poor efficacy, or limited clinical experience, have generally been relegated to the second line of therapy. Of these, ethionamide has been the agent studied most for the management of meningitis. It penetrates well into the spinal fluid, regardless of inflammation (190). Cycloserine also enters the spinal fluid in the absence of meningeal inflammation (191). The newer aminoglycosides and capreomycin are similar to streptomycin in their poor ability to cross uninflamed meninges.

Fluoroquinolones have found a role in the management of multidrug-resistant pulmonary tuberculosis, although published data are limited. Their role in the management of TBM is uncertain. Although they are able to enter the spinal fluid, even in the absence of inflammation, levels achieved with fluoroquinolones in the CSF are lower than that found in the serum and in brain parenchyma. Two studies have reported *in vivo* measurements made in patients undergoing treatment for TBM; only one reported fluoroquinolone levels exceeding the minimal inhibitory concentration for *M. tuberculosis* (192,193). In a third study, spinal fluid ciprofloxacin levels were only 9% of the serum levels and 15% of serum levels in bacterial meningitis (194).

Linezolid is a potentially effective agent for the management of *M. tuberculosis*. While linezolid has been used successfully to manage gram-positive bacterial meningitis (195), its efficacy in TBM is unknown at this time.

Dosage and Route of Administration

The dosages of medications used for TBM are generally similar to those used in other forms of tuberculosis. Increasing dosages to overcome the difficulties in penetrating the blood–brain barrier, although a logical intervention, has not been shown to be more effective and will increase the frequency of side effects (196).

In the setting of treatment failure despite drug susceptibility, intrathecal or intraventricular administration of antituberculous agents has been tried. Intrathecal streptomycin was used by some clinicians on a routine basis, especially prior to the availability of rifampin and pyrazinamide (197,198) When used as monotherapy, intrathecal streptomycin combined with systemic administration resulted in better outcomes than systemic streptomycin alone (199). The only controlled study comparing intrathecal to parenteral streptomycin in the setting of modern chemotherapy was too small to demonstrate any difference in outcome (200). Side effects were not reported; however, others have

advised against its use, reporting frequent meningeal irritation from intrathecal injection (201). Intraventricular rifampin has been reported to improve clinical outcome in several cases reports (202,203). Intrathecal levaquin combined with intrathecal amikacin has been used successfully to treat one patient with multidrug-resistant disease (204).

Steroids

The utility of steroid therapy in cases of impending or established spinal block is now virtually unchallenged (205, 206), and steroids should be regarded as standard therapy.

Steroids are also used to ameliorate the inflammatory response that is responsible for so much of the pathology of TBM. In 1992, a subcommittee of the Infectious Disease Society of America concluded that moderate evidence favored the routine use of corticosteroids in cases of TBM (207)—an opinion echoed in current treatment guidelines for tuberculosis (149).

However, despite more than six decades of therapeutic use, the debate continues as to whether steroids have a net beneficial or detrimental effect. Early reports of steroid use consist mostly of case series, uncontrolled trials, and anecdotal accounts, with some reporting benefit (208–210) and others harm or inactivity (211–214). A 1997 review of the literature covering all forms of tuberculosis concluded that steroid therapy ameliorated disease symptoms and signs and did not interfere with the efficacy of chemotherapy. In analyzing the reports of steroid use in TBM, regimens longer than 4 weeks were noted to have better results than those reporting shorter courses of steroid use (215). Other reviews have generally found moderate evidence to recommend the routine use of corticosteroids but noted the general lack of comparable data (216) and likely publication bias (217). In a recent Cochrane metaanalysis, steroid use was found to be associated with fewer deaths (rate ratio 0.79; 95% confidence interval 0.65 to 0.97), but the favorable effect was seen only in children (rate ratio 0.77 for children, 0.96 for adults) (217). This metaanalysis also found that the magnitude of the steroid effect was similar when stage I and II patients were pooled and compared with stage III patients. Pooling was needed because most randomized trials of steroid use include few stage I patients. Likewise, HIV-positive patients have not been included in controlled studies.

The optimal dose and duration of corticosteroid treatment are even less clear. Most experts recommend dexamethasone, 0.2 mg/kg of body weight per day, or prednisone, 1 mg/kg per day (60 mg/day for adults) orally or intravenously gradually tapered over 4 to 6 weeks, depending on the patient's clinical response. Despite the often-cited concern that steroid-induced suppression of meningeal inflammation may impede central nervous system penetration by antituberculous drugs, a recent study indicates no difference in actual CSF levels of isoniazid, rifampin, pyrazinamide, and streptomycin with and without concomitant steroids (218).

Regardless of their role in improving outcomes, corticosteroids have reproducible clinical effects on patients, often muting fever, headache, malaise, and delirium. Steroids allow for a faster resolution of symptoms and more rapid resolution of abnormal CSF parameters. Clinical and laboratory parameters may rebound when steroids are discontinued, even when the dose has been carefully tapered (218,219). Corticosteroids have also been postulated to reduce intracranial pressure and decrease the incidence of cerebral infarction. However, a recent study by Schoeman et al. (220) found no evidence that children treated with steroids experienced either of these benefits.

Surgery

Neurosurgical intervention to relieve hydrocephalus can dramatically improve function, especially in children (221–223). Not every patient requires a mechanical shunt, however, and different protocols have been proposed for the selection of appropriate surgical candidates. In one, stage I and stage II patients receive immediate ventriculoatrial or ventriculoperitoneal shunting, if management of hydrocephalus is indicated; stage III patients undergo internal shunt placement only if neurologic improvement follows external ventricular drainage (224). A less surgically aggressive approach employs a trial of one or more medical modalities for relieving communicating hydrocephalus, such as corticosteroids, furosemide, acetazolamide, intrathecal hyaluronidase, and daily lumbar punctures to avoid the need for surgery in many patients (225–227). Which of these alternative strategies is optimal has not been established by comparative trial, and the course selected may well depend on the locale of practice and the availability and skill of neurosurgical services.

Immunomodulators Other Than Steroids

In addition to corticosteroids, many other agents have been employed in an attempt to decrease the damage inflicted by inflammatory response associated with TBM. Most of these are only of historical interest.

Shortly after the introduction of antituberculous antimicrobials, clinicians experimented with intrathecal streptokinase, streptodornase, and heparin (228,229). These therapies were not beneficial and were abandoned.

The intrathecal administration of PPD, first used in the early 20th century (230), was strongly advocated by some investigators during the 1950s and 1960s. Administration of intrathecal PPD exacerbates meningeal symptoms and increases intracranial pressure, but was thought to hasten the resolution of the basal exudate (231). While numerous case series touting success were reported (232), no controlled trials were conducted. The rationale for intrathecal PPD administration is in direct opposition to that for administration of steroids, and as experience with the latter therapy increased interest in the former waned.

Hyaluronidase is an enzyme that facilitates the breakdown of hyaluronic acid, a mucopolysaccharide that forms a gelatinous material is tissue spaces. In the early 1980s, intrathecal hyaluronidase was evaluated in several small nonrandomized studies as a potential medical therapy for managing communicating hydrocephalus associated with TBM. The hope was that such treatment would allow ventricular shunting to be avoided. Side effects of intrathecal hyaluronidase were minimal but the results of these uncontrolled studies were not consistent, with one finding an advantage over ventriculoperitoneal shunting (233), and the other leading to the opposite conclusion (234). A more recent randomized controlled trial compared three medical regimens, one of which was the use of intrathecal hyaluronidase, to immediate ventriuloperitoneal shunting. There was no difference in outcome among any of the four arms (235). In this study, intrathecal hyaluronidase was shown to decrease intracranial pressure when compared with patients receiving only antibiotics, but the difference was not significant.

The most recent immunomodulatory treatment to be investigated is the administration of thalidomide, an inhibitor of the production of tumor necrosis factor-α (TNF-α). This cytokine has multiple effects. It has a role in containing mycobacterial infections and producing granulomatous reactions, and has also been found to produce increased permeability of the blood–brain barrier in cases of bacterial meningitis (236,237). Also, in bacterial meningitis, increased levels of TNF-α predict a worse outcome (238).

In rabbits with experimental *Mycobacterium bovis* meningitis, administration of thalidomide with antimicrobial therapy lowered TNF-α levels, reduced brain pathology, and reduced mortality from 50% with antimicrobials alone to zero (239). Open-label studies hinted that thalidomide might be useful in humans as well (240,241). However, a randomized controlled trial of thalidomide in children with stage II or stage III TBM was halted secondary to a interim analysis that identified an increased number of adverse outcomes and death in the treatment group (242). At present, the use of thalidomide must be regarded as investigational and of unproven value.

PROGNOSIS AND SEQUELAE

TBM often responds quite slowly to a successful course of treatment. Clinical symptoms and CSF parameters may worsen briefly after the first doses of antibiotics in a Herxheimer-like reaction to released antigen (243,244). Subsequently, weight gain and increased sense of well-being may be the first clinical signs of response. Fever and CSF abnor-

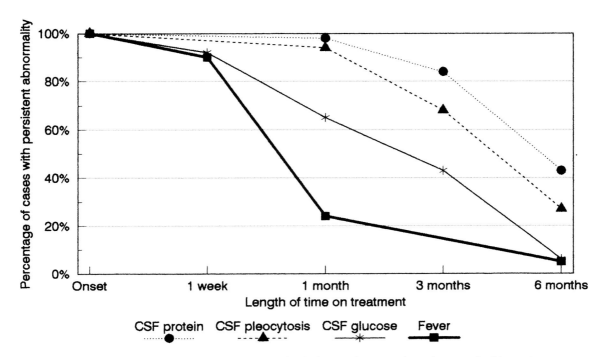

FIGURE 28.5. Fever and cerebrospinal fluid (*CSF*) abnormalities in tuberculous meningitis resolve in a characteristic pattern after treatment is initiated. CSF glucose generally normalizes by 3 to 6 months of therapy, but pleocytosis is slower to resolve and CSF protein may remain elevated for an even longer period. (Data from Lepper MH, Spies HW. The present status of the management of tuberculosis of the central nervous system. *Ann NY Acad Sci* 1963;106:106–123.)

malities may persist for weeks to months in many patients, resolving sequentially in a characteristic pattern (Fig 28.5) (21,212). The *de novo* appearance of brain tuberculomas during a successful treatment course for meningitis has been repeatedly reported (115–117).

One large series from Egypt evaluating more than 1,500 patients with TBM or encephalitis showed a mortality rate of 55%, substantially higher than that of pneumococcal, *Haemophilus influenzae*, or meningococcal meningitis (245). Mortality in other recent series of treated patients is 10% to 30% (24,33,246,247). Investigators seeking prognostic factors for death, despite treatment, have examined variables such as duration of symptoms before presentation, initial CSF parameters, and CSF microbiology. Disease at younger ages (among children) and advanced stage of illness at the start of treatment repeatedly emerge as reliable, independent prognosticators (158,248–251). Pregnant women suffer worse outcomes than other adults (252–254). Among the individual antituberculous agents, only use of isoniazid as a component of the regimen has been a marker of reduced mortality (158,255).

The risk of permanent neurologic impairment is also a direct correlate of the stage of illness at presentation (Fig. 28.5). Neurologic disabilities ranging from mild to severe are reported in as many as 50% of adults and children who survive the infection. These include mental retardation and

behavioral problems in children, organic brain syndrome in adults, ataxia, hemiparesis, persisting seizure disorders, and persistent cranial nerve palsies, including optic nerve atrophy (246,256–261). The development of syringomyelia after an otherwise successful course of treatment has been ascribed to vasculitis of the spinal arteries leading to ischemic myelomalacia (142,262). Similarly, vasculitis or calcification of the hypothalamic–pituitary axis may result in delayed or precocious sexual development, diabetes insipidus, chronic hypothermia, and gonadotropin or growth hormone deficiency many years after treatment (263–265).

CENTRAL NERVOUS SYSTEM TUBERCULOSIS AND THE ACQUIRED IMMUNODEFICIENCY SYNDROME

A pathogen with opportunistic capabilities, *M. tuberculosis* infects patients with HIV infection early in the course of HIV-related immunosuppression. Approximately half of untreated HIV-infected patients with pulmonary tuberculosis develop active disease before the occurrence of an acquired immunodeficiency disease (AIDS)–defining illness (266).

Central nervous system tuberculosis is frequently seen in patients with HIV infection, and in some parts of the world

M. tuberculosis has become the most common central nervous system pathogen encountered in HIV-infected persons (267,268). Whether HIV infection increases the likelihood of central nervous system disease in patients with tuberculosis infection is still debated (267,269). Several retrospective series have shown no differences in presentation, CSF parameters, responses to treatment, or mortality rates in patients with and without HIV infection (267,270–272).

However, some atypical features have been repeatedly encountered in HIV-infected patients. Patients with HIV infection are more likely to have TBM despite the presence of acellular spinal fluid (273). They may also have a higher incidence of intracranial mass lesions (270,274). TBM or encephalitis may occur concomitantly with more opportunistic pathogens such as *Cryptococcus neoformans* and *Toxoplasma gondii* (275,276).

Nontuberculous mycobacteria, such as *Mycobacterium avium-intracellulare* and *Mycobacterium fortuitum*, may also cause meningitis (277,278). Administration of BCG vaccine to an HIV-infected newborn child has resulted in disseminated infection due to the vaccine strain of *M. bovis* (279). The organism was recovered from the spinal fluid.

PREVENTION AND CONTROL

The BCG vaccine does not prevent tuberculosis; rather, it reduces the ability of the bacilli to replicate and disseminate hematogenously. The ability of BCG to prevent cases of TBM in children is widely accepted, and several case-control studies have estimated the vaccine's efficacy for the prevention of TBM to be 75% to 85% (280–283), with unvaccinated children about five times more likely to develop TBM. A metaanalysis in 1993 arrived at a similar conclusion, finding the protective effect to be 86% in randomized controlled trials and 75% in case-control studies (284).

Determining the effectiveness of this vaccine poses several challenges, as there are many other factors related to the incidence of TBM. Some investigators have commented that confounding variables, such as nutritional status, were admittedly difficult to control for (285). A case-control analysis of children in India, controlling for age and vaccination status, concluded that the level of protection from BCG is limited. Cases and controls were similar when compared for vaccination rates. However, a significantly higher proportion of patients were older than 5 years, leading the investigators to conclude that vaccination actually delays the development of TBM rather than preventing it (286). The prevalence of TBM did not rise in a county in China after BCG vaccinations at birth were discontinued, suggesting that other factors may have been responsible for the previously observed decrease in TBM rates (287). When TBM occurs in a vaccinated child, the presentation and radiographic findings do not appear to be altered (288).

REFERENCES

1. *Rig Veda* X(i) 63:1–6. Quoted in Tandon PN, Bhatia R, Baraga S. Tuberculous meningitis. In: Harris AA, ed. *Handbook of clinical neurology*, Vol. 8. New York: Elsevier, 1988:195.
2. Whytt R. *Observations on the dropsy in the brain*. Edinburgh: J. Balfour, 1768.
3. Green PH. Tubercular meningitis. *Lancet* 1836;2:232-235.
4. Rieder HL, Snider DE, Cauthen GM. Extrapulmonary tuberculosis in the United States. *Am Rev Respir Dis* 1990;141:347–351.
5. Farer LS, Lowell AM, Meador MP. Extrapulmonary tuberculosis in the United States. *Am J Epidemiol* 1979;109:205–217.
6. Riggs HE, Rupp C, Ray H. Clinicopathologic study of tuberculous meningitis in adults. *Am Rev Tuberc* 1956;74:830–834.
7. Udani PM, Dastur DK. Tuberculous encephalopathy with and without meningitis: clinical features and pathological correlations. *J Neurol Sci* 1970;10:541–561.
8. Auerbach O. Tuberculous meningitis: correlation of therapeutic results with the pathogenesis and pathologic changes; part I. *Am Rev Tuberc* 1951;64:408–418.
9. Lincoln EM. Tuberculous meningitis in children with special reference to serous meningitis. Part I. *Am Rev Tuberc* 1947;56:75–94.
10. Burn CG, Finley KH. The role of hypersensitivity in the production of experimental meningitis: I. Experimental meningitis in tuberculous animals. *J Exp Med* 1932;56:203–221.
11. Rich AR, McCordock HA. The pathogenesis of tuberculous meningitis. *Bull Johns Hopkins Hosp* 1933;52:5–37.
12. Dastur DK, Lalitha VS. The many facets of neurotuberculosis: an epitome of neuropathology. In: Zimmerman HM, ed. *Progress in neuropathology*, Vol. 2. New York: Grune and Stratton, 1973:351–408.
13. Rich AR. *The pathogenesis of tuberculosis*. Springfield, IL: Charles C Thomas, 1946.
14. Auerbach O. Tuberculous meningitis: correlation of therapeutic results with the pathogenesis and pathologic changes. Part II: Pathologic changes in untreated and treated cases. *Am Rev Tuberc* 1951;64:419–429.
15. Dastur DK, Udani PM. Pathology and pathogenesis of tuberculous encephalopathy. *Acta Neuropathol* 1966;6:311.
16. Udani PM, Dastur DK. Tuberculous encephalopathy with and without meningitis: clinical features and pathological correlations. *J Neurol Sci* 1970;10:541–561.
17. Winkelman NW, Moore MT. Meningeal blood vessels in tuberculous meningitis. *Am Rev Tuberc* 1940;42:315–333.
18. Daif A, Obeid T, Yaqub B, et al. Unusual presentations of tuberculous meningitis. *Clin Neurol Neurosurg* 1992;94:1–5
19. Klein NC, Damsker B, Hirschman SZ. Mycobacterial meningitis: retrospective analysis from 1970–1983. *Am J Med* 1985;79:29–34.
20. Haas EJ, Madhavan T, Quinn EL, et al. Tuberculous meningitis in an urban general hospital. *Arch Intern Med* 1977;137:1518.
21. Barrett-Connor E. Tuberculous meningitis in adults. *S Med J* 1967;60:1061–1067.
22. Lincoln EM, Sordillo SVR, Davies PA. Tuberculous meningitis in children. A review of 167 untreated and 74 treated patients with special reference to early diagnosis. *J Pediatr* 1960;57:807–823.
23. Kennedy DH, Fallon RJ. Tuberculous meningitis. *JAMA* 1979;241:264–268.
24. Ogawa SK, Smith MA, Brennessel DJ, Lowy FD. Tuberculous meningitis in an urban medical center. *Medicine* 1987;66:317–326.

25. Delage G, Dusseault M. Tuberculous meningitis in children: a retrospective study of 79 patients, with an analysis of prognostic factors. *Can Med Assoc J* 1979;120:305–309.

26. Idriss ZH, Sinno AA, Kronfol NM. Tuberculous meningitis in childhood. *Am J Dis Child* 1976;130:364–367.

27. Traub M, Colchester ACF, Kingsley DPE, et al. Tuberculosis of the central nervous system. *Q J Med* 1984;53:81–100.

28. Alvarez S, McCabe WR. Extrapulmonary tuberculosis revisited: a review of experience at Boston City and other hospitals. *Medicine* 1984;63:25–54.

29. Leiguarda R, Berthier M, Starkstein S, et al. Ischemic infarction in 25 children with tuberculous meningitis. *Stroke* 1988;19:200–204.

30. Hsieh FY, Chia LG, Shen WC. Locations of cerebral infarctions in tuberculous meningitis. *Neuroradiology* 1992;34:197–199.

31. Illingsworth RS, Lorber J. Tubercles of the choroid. *Arch Dis Child* 1956;31:467–469.

32. Teoh R, Humphries MJ, Chan JC, et al. Internuclear ophthalmoplegia in tuberculous meningitis. *Tubercle* 1989;70:61.

33. Kent SJ, Crowe SM, Yung A, et al. Tuberculous meningitis: a 30-year review. *Clin Infec Dis* 1993;17:987–994.

34. Smith J, Godwin-Austen R. Hypersecretion of anti-diuretic hormone due to tuberculous meningitis. *Postgrad Med* 1980;56:41–44.

35. Hinman AR. Tuberculous meningitis at Cleveland Metropolitan General Hospital. *Am Rev Respir Dis* 1967;95:670–673.

36. Bateman DE, Newman PK, Foster JB. A retrospective survey of proven cases of tuberculous meningitis in the northern region, 1970–1980. *J R Coll Phys London* 1983;17:106–110.

37. Steiner P, Portugaleza C. Tuberculous meningitis in children. *Am Rev Respir Dis* 1973;107:22–29.

38. Reinitz E, Hubbard D, Grayzel AI. Central nervous system systemic lupus erythematosus versus central nervous system infection: low cerebral spinal fluid glucose and pleocytosis in a patient with a prolonged course. *Arth Rheum* 1982;25:583–587.

39. Jeren T, Beus I. Characteristics of cerebrospinal fluid in tuberculous meningitis. *Acta Cytol* 1982;26:678.

40. Weinstein L. Bacterial meningitis. *Med Clin North Am* 1985;69:219–229.

41. Clark WC, Metcalf JC, Muhlbauer MS, et al. *Mycobacterium tuberculosis* meningitis: a report of twelve cases and a literature review. *Neurosurgery* 1986;18:604–610.

42. Holt LE, Howland J. *The diseases of infancy and childhood*, 9th ed. New York: Appleton, 1926:618.

43. Stewart SM. The bacteriologic diagnosis of tuberculous meningitis. *J Clin Pathol* 1953;6:241–242.

44. Sumaya CV, Simek M, Smith MHD, et al. Tuberculous meningitis in children during the isoniazid era. *J Pediatr* 1975;87:43–49.

45. Radhakrishnan VV, Mathai A, Thomas M. Correlation between culture of *Mycobacterium tuberculosis* and antimycobacterial antibody in lumbar, ventricular and cisternal cerebrospinal fluids of patients with tuberculous meningitis. *Indian J Exp Biol* 1991;29:845–848.

46. Chambers AA, Lukin RR, Tomsick TA. Cranial and intracranial tuberculosis. *Semin Roentgenol* 1979;14:319–324.

47. Maroon JC, Jones R, Mishkin FS. Tuberculous meningitis diagnosed by brain scan. *Radiology* 1972;104:333–335.

48. Lehrer H. The angiographic triad of tuberculous meningitis: a radiographic and clinicopathologic correlation. *Radiology* 1966;87:829–835.

49. Rojas-Echeverri LA, Soto-Hernandez JL, et al. Predictive value of digital subtraction angiography in patients with tuberculous meningitis. *Neuroradiology* 1996;38:20–24.

50. Jinkins JR. Computed tomography of intracranial tuberculosis. *Neuroradiology* 1991;33:126–135.

51. Chu NS. Tuberculous meningitis. Computerized tomographic manifestations. *Arch Neurol* 1980;37:458–460.

52. Shah GV. Central nervous system tuberculosis: imaging manifestations. *Neuroimaging Clin North Am* 2000;10:355–374.

53. de Castro CC, de Barros NG, Campos ZM, et al. CT scans of cranial tuberculosis. *Radiol Clin North Am* 1995;33:753–769.

54. Ozates M, Kemaloglu S, Gurkan F, et al. CT of the brain in tuberculous meningitis. A review of 289 patients. *Acta Radiol* 2000;41:13–17.

55. Teoh R, Humphries MJ, Hoare RD, et al. Clinical correlation of CT changes in 64 Chinese patients with tuberculous meningitis. *J Neurol* 1989;236:48–51.

56. Viallard JF, Blanco P. Images in clinical medicine. Tuberculous meningitis. *N Engl J Med* 1999;341:1197.

57. Chang KH, Han MH, Roh JK, et al. Gd-DTPA-enhanced MR imaging of the brain in patients with meningitis: comparison with CT. *Am J Neuroradiol* 1990;11:69–76.

58. Gupta RK, Gupta S, Singh D, et al. MR imaging and angiography in tuberculous meningitis. *Neuroradiology* 1994;36(2):87–92.

59. Gupta RK, Kathuria MK, Pradhan S. Magnetization transfer MR imaging in CNS tuberculosis. *Am J Neuroradiol* 1999;20;52:867–875.

60. Pui MH, Memon WA. Magnetic resonance imaging findings in tuberculous mengingoencephalitis. *Can Assoc Radiol J* 2001;52:43–49.

61. Eide FF, Gean AD, So YT. Clinical and radiographic findings in disseminated tuberculosis of the brain. *Neurology* 1993;43:1427–1429.

62. Gupta RK, Kohli A, Gaur V, et al. MRI of the brain in patients with miliary pulmonary tuberculosis without symptoms or signs of central nervous system involvement. *Neuroradiology* 1997;39:699–704.

63. Kingsley DP, Hendrickse WA, Kendall BE, et al. Tuberculous meningitis: role of CT in management and prognosis. *J Neurol Neurosurg Psychiatry* 1987;50:30–36.

64. Schoeman JF, Laubscher JA, Donald PR. Serial lumbar CSF presure measurements and cranial computed tomographic findings in childhood tuberculous meningitis. *Childs Nerv Syst* 2000;16:203–208

65. Jinkins JR, Gupta R, Chang KH, et al. MR imaging of central nervous system tuberculosis. *Radiol Clin North Am* 1995;33:771–786.

66. Daniel TM, Debanne SM. The serodiagnosis of tuberculosis and other mycobacterial diseases by enzyme-linked immunosorbent assay. *Am Rev Respir Dis* 1987;135:1137–1151.

67. Chandramuki A, Allen PR, Keen M, et al. Detection of mycobacterial antigen and antibodies in the cerebrospinal fluid of patients with tuberculous meningitis. *J Med Microbiol* 1985;20:239–247.

68. Hernandez, R., Munoz, O., Guiscfre, H Sensitive enzyme immunoassay for early diagnosis of tuberculous meningitis. *J Clin Microbiol* 1984;20:533–535.

69. Chandramuki A, Bothamley GH, Brennan PJ, Ivanyi J. Levels of antibody to defined antigens of *Mycobacterium tuberculosis* in tuberculous meningitis. *J Clin Microbiol* 1989;27:821–825.

70. Radhakrishnan VV, Mathai A, Sehgal S. Correlation between culture of *Mycobacterium tuberculosis* and IgG antibody to *Mycobacterium tuberculosis* antigen-5 in the cerebrospinal fluid of patients with tuberculous meningitis. *J Infect* 1990;21:271–277.

71. Mathai A, Radhakrishnan VV, Mohan PK, et al. ELISA of IgG antibody to *M. tuberculosis* antigen-5, PPD in CSF in tuberculous meningitis patients. *Indian J Med Res* 1990;91:5–30.

72. Park SC, Lee BI, Cho SN, et al. Diagnosis of tuberculous meningitis by detection of immunoglobulin G antibodies to purified protein derivative and lipoarabinomannan antigen in cerebrospinal fluid. *Tuber Lung Dis* 1993;74:317–322.

73. Sumi MG, Annamma M, Sarada C, et al. Rapid diagnosis of tuberculous meningitis by a dot-immunobinding assay. *Acta Neurol Scand* 2000;101:61–64.

74. Watt G, Zaraspe G, Bautista S, et al. Rapid diagnosis of tuberculous meningitis by using an enzyme-linked immunosorbent assay to detect mycobacterial antigen and antibody in cerebrospinal fluid. *J Infect Dis* 1988;158:681–686.

75. Miorner H, Sjobring U, Nayak P, et al. Diagnosis of tuberculous meningitis: a comparative analysis of 3 immunoassays, an immune complex assay and the polymerase chain reaction. *Tuber Lung Dis* 1995;76:381–386.

76. Lu CZ, Quao J, Shen T, et al. Early diagnosis of tuberculous meningitis by detection of anti-BCG secreting cells in cerebrospinal fluid. *Lancet* 1990;336:10–13.

77. Baig SM. Anti-purified protein derivative cell-enzyme-linked immunosorbent assay, a sensitive method for early diagnosis of tuberculous meningitis. *J Clin Microbiol* 1995;33(11): 3040–3041.

78. Krambovitis E, McIllmurray MB, Lock PE, et al. Rapid diagnosis of tuberculous meningitis by latex particle agglutination. *Lancet* 1984;2:1229–1231.

79. Kadival GV, Samuel AM, Mazarelo TBMS, et al. Radioimmunoassay for detecting *Mycobacterium tuberculosis* antigen in cerebrospinal fluids of patients with tuberculous meningitis. *J Infir Dis* 1987;155:608–611.

80. Radhakrishnan VV, Sehgal S, Mathai A. Correlation between culture of *Mycobacterium tuberculosis* and detection of mycobacterial antigens in cerebrospinal fluid of patients with tuberculous meningitis. *J Med Microbiol* 1990;33:223–226.

81. Radhakrishnan VV, Mathai A. Detection of *Mycobacterium tuberculosis* antigen 5 in cerebrospinal fluid by inhibition ELISA and its diagnostic potential in tuberculous meningitis. *J Infect Dis* 1991;163:650–652.

82. Sumi MG, Mathai A, Reuben S, et al. Immunocytochemical method for early laboratory diagnosis of tuberculous meningitis. *Clin Diagn Lab Immunol* 2002;9:344–347.

83. Chandramuki A, Allen PR, Keen M, Ivanyi J. Detection of mycobacterial antigen and antibodies in the cerebrospinal fluid of patients with tuberculous meningitis. *J Med Microbiol* 1985; 20:239–247.

84. Katti MK. Immunodiagnosis of tuberculous meningitis: rapid detection of mycobacterial antigens in cerebrospinal fluid by reverse passive hemag glutination assay and their characterization by Western blotting. *FEMS Immunol Med Microbiol* 2001; 31:59–64.

85. Mathai A, Radhakrishnan VV, George SM, et al. A newer approach for the laboratory diagnosis of tuberculous meningitis. *Diagn Microbiol Infect Dis* 2001;39:225–228.

86. Radhakrishnan VV, Mathai A, Sehgal S. Correlation between culture of *Mycobacterium tuberculosis* and IgG antibody to *Mycobacterium tuberculosis* antigen-5 in the cerebrospinal fluid of patients with tuberculous meningitis. *J Infect* 1990;21: 271–277.

87. Sumi MG, Mathai A, Reuben S, et al. Immunocytochemical method for early laboratory diagnosis of tuberculous meningitis. *Diagn Lab Immunol* 2002;9:344–347.

88. Patil SA, Gourie-Devi M, Anand AR, et al. Significance of mycobacterial immune complexes (IgG) in the diagnosis of tuberculous meningitis. *Tuber Lung Dis* 1996;77:164–167.

89. Chandramuki A, Bothamley GH, Brennan PJ, et al. Levels of antibody to defined antigens of *Mycobacterium tuberculosis* in tuberculous meningitis. *J Clin Microbiol* 1989;27:821–825.

90. Kaneko K, Onodera O, Miyatake T, et al. Rapid diagnosis of tuberculous meningitis by polymerase chain reaction. *Neurology* 1990;40:1617–1618.

91. Brisson-Noel A, Aznar C, Chureau C, et al. Diagnosis of tuberculosis by DNA amplification in clinical practice evaluation. *Lancet* 1991;338:364–366.

92. Shankar P, Manjunath N, Mohan KK, et al. Rapid diagnosis of tuberculous meningitis by polymerase chain reaction. *Lancet* 1991;337:5–7.

93. Narita M, Matsuzono Y, Shibata M, et al. Nested amplification protocol for the detection of *Mycobacterium tuberculosis*. *Acta Paediatr* 1992;81:997–1001.

94. Narayanan S, Parandaman V, Narayanan PR, et al. Evaluation of PCR using TRC(4) and IS6110 primers in detection of tuberculous meningitis. *J Clin Microbiol* 2001;39:2006–2008.

95. Baker CA, Cartwright CP, Williams DN, et al. Early detection of central nervous system tuberculosis with the gen-probe nucleic acid amplification assay: utility in an inner city hospital. *Clin Infect Dis* 2002;35:339–342.

96. Sumi MG, Mathai A, Reuben S, et al. A comparative evaluation of dot immunobinding assay (Dot-Iba) and polymerase chain reaction (PCR) for the laboratory diagnosis of tuberculous meningitis. *Diagn Microbiol Infect Dis* 2002;42:35–38.

97. Smith HV, Taylor LM, Hunter G. The blood–cerebrospinal fluid barrier in tuberculous meningitis and allied conditions. *J Neurol Neurosurg Psychiatry* 1955;18:237–249.

98. Mandal BK, Evans DIK, Ironside AG, et al. Radioactive bromide partition test in differential diagnosis of tuberculous meningitis. *BMJ* 1972;4:413–415.

99. Wiggelinkhuizen M, Mann M. The radioactive bromide partition test in the diagnosis of tuberculous meningitis in children. *J Pediatr* 1980;97:843–847.

100. Mann MD, Macfarlane CM, Verburg CJ, et al. The bromide partition test and CSF adenosine deaminase activity in the diagnosis of tuberculous meningitis in children. *S Afr Med J* 1982; 62:431–433.

101. Von Wenzel KS, Klopper JF, Wasserman HJ. the technetium-99m DTPA partition test in the diagnosis of tuberculous meningitis. *S Afr Med J* 1989;75:488–489.

102. Ribera E, Martinez-Vazquez JM, Ocana I, et al. Activity of adenosine deaminase in cerebrospinal fluid for the diagnosis and follow-up of tuberculous meningitis in adults. *J Infect Dis* 1987;155:603-607.

103. Mishra OP, Loiwal V, Ali Z, et al. Cerebrospinal fluid adenosine deaminase activity for the diagnosis of tuberculous meningitis in children. *J Trop Pediatr* 1996;42:129–132.

104. Choi SH, Kim YS, Bae IG, et al. The possible role of cerebrospinal fluid adenosine deaminase activity in the diagnosis of tuberculous meningitis in adults. *Clin Neurol Neurosurg* 2002; 104:10–15.

105. Ena J, Crespo MJ, Valls V, et al. Adenosine deaminase activity in cerebrospinal fluid: a useful test for meningeal tuberculosis, even in patients with AIDS. *J Infect Dis* 1988;158:896.

106. Coovadia YM, Dawood A, Ellis ME, et al. Evaluation of adenosine deaminase activity and antibody to *Mycobacterium tuberculosis* antigen 5 in cerebrospinal fluid and the radioactive bromide partition test for the early diagnosis of tuberculous meningitis. *Arch Dis Child* 1986;61:42.

107. Chawla RK, Seth RK, Raj B, et al. Adenosine deaminase levels in cerebrospinal fluid in tuberculosis and bacterial meningitis. *Tubercle* 1991;72:190–192.

108. Donald PR, Malan C, Schoeman JF. Adenosine deaminase activity as a diagnostic aid in tuberculous meningitis. *J Infect Dis* 1987;156:1040–1041.

109. Donald PR, Malan C, van der Walt A, et al. The simultaneous determination of cerebrospinal fluid and plasma adenosine

deaminase activity as a diagnostic aid in tuberculous meningitis. *S Afr Med J* 1986;69:505–507.

110. French GL, Teoh R, Chan CY, et al. Diagnosis of tuberculous meningitis by detection of tuberculostearic acid in cerebrospinal fluid. *Lancet* 1987;2:117–119.

111. Brooks JB, Daneshvar MI, Haberberger RL, et al. Rapid diagnosis of tuberculous meningitis by frequency-pulsed electron-capture gas-liquid chromatography detection of carboxylic acids in cerebrospinal fluid. *J Clin Microbiol* 1990;28:989–997.

112. Dastur HM, Desai AD. A comparative study of brain tuberculomas and gliomas based upon 107 case records of each. *Brain* 1965;88:375–386.

113. Sibley WA, O'Brien JL. Intracranial tuberculomas: a review of clinical features and treatment. *Neurology* 1956;6:157–165.

114. Bahemuka M, Murungi JH. Tuberculosis of the nervous system: a clinical, radiological and pathological study of 39 consecutive cases in Riyadh, Saudi Arabia. *J Neurol Sci* 1989;90:67–76.

115. Teoh R, Humphries MJ, O'Mahony G. Symptomatic intracranial tuberculoma developing during treatment of tuberculosis: a report of 10 patients and review of the literature. *Q J Med* 1987;63:449–460.

116. Lees AJ, MacLeod AF, Marshall J. Cerebral tuberculomas developing during treatment of tuberculous meningitis. *Lancet* 1980;1:1208–1211.

117. Shepard WE, Field ML, James DH. Transient appearance of intracranial tuberculoma during treatment of tuberculous meningitis. *Pediatr Infect Dis* 1986;5:599–601.

118. Garland HG, Armitage G. Intracranial tuberculoma. *J Pathol Bacteriol* 1933;37:461–471.

119. Arseni C. Two hundred and one cases of intracranial tuberculoma treated surgically. *J Neurol Neurosurg Psychiatry* 1958;21:308–311.

120. Asenjo A, Valladares H, Fierro J. Tuberculomas of the brain: report of one hundred and fifty-nine cases. *Arch Neurol Psychiatry* 1951;65:146–160.

121. Ramamurthi B. Intracranial tumors in India: incidence and variations. *Int Surg* 1973;58:542–547.

122. DeAngelis LM. Intracranial tuberculoma: case report and review of the literature. *Neurology* 1981;31:1133–1136.

123. Harder E, Al-Kawi MZ, Carney P. Intracranial tuberculoma: conservative management. *Am J Med* 1983;74:570–576.

124. Bagga A, Kaira V, Ghai OP. Intracranial tuberculoma: evaluation and treatment. *Clin Pediatr* 1988;27:487–490.

125. Ramamurthi B, Varadarajan MG. Diagnosis of tuberculomas of the brain: clinical and radiologic correlation. *J Neurosurg* 1961;18:1–7.

126. Whelan MA, Stern J. Intracranial tuberculoma. *Radiology* 1981;138:75–81.

127. Offenbacher H, Fazekas F, Schmidt R, et al. MRI in tuberculous meningoencephalitis: Report of four cases and review of the neuroimaging literature. *J Neurol* 1991;238:340–344.

128. O'Brien NC, van Eys J, Baram TZ, et al. Intracranial tuberculoma in children: a new look at an old problem. *S Med J* 1988;81:1239–1244.

129. Tandon PN, Bhargava S. Effect of medical treatment on intracranial tuberculoma: a CT study. *Tubercle* 1985;66:85–97.

130. Mayers MM, Kaufman DM, Miller MH. Recent cases of intracranial tuberculomas. *Neurology* 1978;28:256–260.

131. Armstrong FB, Edwards AM. Intracranial tuberculoma in native races of Canada: with special reference to symptomatic epilepsy and neurologic features. *Can Med Assoc J* 1963;89:56–65.

132. Whitener DR. Tuberculous brain abscess: report of a case and review of the literature. *Arch Neurol* 1978;35:148–155.

133. Reichentral E, Cohen ML, Schujman E, et al. Tuberculous brain abscess and its appearance on computerized tomography. *J Neurosurg* 1982;56:597–600.

134. Jain VK, Chandramuckh A, Venkataramana NK, et al. The far cry of a TB brain. *Clin Neurol Neurosurg* 1989;91:171–176.

135. Ransome GA, Montiero ES. A rare form of tuberculous meningitis. *BMJ* 1947;1:413–414.

136. Brooks WDW, Fletcher AP, Wilson RR. Spinal cord complications of tuberculous meningitis. *Q J Med* 1954;23:275–290.

137. Kocen RS, Parsons M. Neurological complications of tuberculosis: some unusual manifestations. *Q J Med* 1970;39:17–30.

138. Hernandez-Albujar S, Arribas JR, Royo A, et al. Tuberculous radiculomyelitis complicating tuberculous meningitis: case report and review. *Clin Infect Dis* 2000;30:915–921.

139. Wadia NH, Dastur DK. Spinal meningitides with radiculomyelopathy. Part 1. *J Neurol Sci* 1969;8:239–260.

140. Dastur DK, Wadia NH. Spinal meningitides with radiculomyelopathy: Part 2. Pathology and pathogenesis. *J Neurol Sci* 1969;8:261–293.

141. Van Paesschen W, Van Den Kerchove M, Appel B, et al. Arachnoiditis ossificans with arachnoid cyst after cranial tuberculous meningitis. *Neurology* 1990;40:714–716.

142. Fehlings MG, Bernstein M. Syringomyelia as a complication of tuberculous meningitis. *Can J Neurol Sci* 1992;19:84–87.

143. Naidoo DP, Desai D, Kranidiotis L. Tuberculous meningiomyeloradiculitis—a report of two cases. *Tubercle* 1991;72:65–69.

144. Frelich D, Swash M. Diagnosis and management of tuberculous paraplegia with special reference to tuberculous radiculomyelitis. *J Neurol Neurosurg Psychiatry* 1979;42:12–18.

145. Lin, TH. Intramedullary tuberculoma of the spinal cord. *J Neurosurg* 1960;17:497–499.

146. Rhoton EL, Ballinger WE, Quisling R, et al. Intramedullary spinal tuberculoma. *Neurosurgery* 1988;22:733–736.

147. Gokalp HZ, Ozkal E. Intradural tuberculomas of the spinal cord. *J Neurosurg* 1981;55:289–292.

148. Kennedy DM. Tuberculous meningitis. *Lancet* 1981;2:261.

149. American Thoracic Society. Treatment of tuberculosis and tuberculosis infection in adults and children. *Am J Respir Crit Care Med* 1994;149:1359–1374.

150. British Thoracic Society. Chemotherapy and management of tuberculosis in the United Kingdom: recommendations 1998. Joint Tuberculosis Committee of the British Thoracic Society. *Thorax* 1998;53:536–548.

151. Kendig EL Jr. Evolution of short-course antimicrobial treatment of tuberculosis in children, 1951–1984. *Pediatrics* 1985;75:684–686.

152. van Loenhout-Rooyackers JH, Keyser A, Laheij RJ, et al. Tuberculous meningitis: is a 6-month treatment regimen sufficient? *Int J Tuberc Lung Dis* 2001;5:1028–1035.

153. Donald PR, Schoeman JF, Van Zyl LE, et al. Intensive short course chemotherapy in the management of tuberculous meningitis. *Int J Tuberc Lung Dis* 1998;2:704–711.

154. Dutt AK, Moers D, Stead WW. Short-course chemotherapy for extrapulmonary tuberculosis. *Ann Intern Med* 1986;104:7–12.

155. Visudhiphan P, Chiemchanya S. Tuberculous meningitis in children: treatment with isoniazid and rifampicin for twelve months. *J Pediatr* 1989;114:875–879.

156. Alarcon F, Escalante L, Perez Y, et al. Tuberculous meningitis: short course of chemotherapy. *Arch Neurol* 1990;47:1313–1317.

157. Humphries M. The management of tuberculous meningitis. *Thorax* 1992;47:577–581.

158. Lorber J. The results of treatment of 549 cases of tuberculous meningitis. *Am Rev Tuberc* 1954;69:13–25.

159. Choremis K, Zervos N, Constantinides V, et al. Streptomycin therapy of tuberculous meningitis. *Lancet* 1948;2:595–599.

160. Ellard GA, Humphries MJ, Allen BW.Cerebrospinal fluid drug concentrations and the treatment of tuberculous meningitis. *Am Rev Respir Dis* 1993 Sep;148(3):650–655.

161. Lorber J. Treatment of tuberculous meningitis. *BMJ* 1960;1:1309–1312.

162. Spector R, Lorenzo AV. The active transport of para-aminosalicylic acid from the cerebrospinal fluid. *J Pharmacol Exp Ther* 1973;185:642–648.

163. Lorber J. Treatment of tuberculous meningitis. *BMJ* 1960;1:1309–1312.

164. Falk A. U.S. Veterans Administration–Armed Forces cooperative study on the chemotherapy of tuberculosis. XIII. Tuberculous meningitis in adults, with special reference to survival, neurologic residual, and work status. *Am Rev Respir Dis* 1965;91:823–883.

165. Kendig EL Jr, Burch C. Short-term antimicrobial therapy of tuberculous. *Am Rev Respir Dis* 1960;82:672–681.

166. Place VA, Pyle MM, de la Huerga J. Ethambutol in tuberculous meningitis. *Am Rev Respir Dis* 1969;99:783–785.

167. Pilheu JA, Maglio F, Cetrangolo R, et al. Concentrations of ethambutol in the cerebrospinal fluid after oral administration. *Tubercle* 1971;52:117–122.

168. Bobrowitz ED. Ethambutol in tuberculous meningitis. *Chest* 1972;61:629–632.

169. Girgis NI, Yassin MW, Sippel JE, et al. The value of ethambutol in the treatment of tuberculous meningitis. *J Trop Med Hyg* 1976;79:14–17.

170. Forgan-Smith R, Ellard GA, Newton D, et al. Pyrazinamide and other drugs in tuberculous meningitis. *Lancet* 1973;2:374.

171. Ellard GA, Humphries MJ, Allen BW. Cerebrospinal fluid drug concentrations and the treatment of tuberculous meningitis. *Am Rev Respir Dis* 1993;148:650–655.

172. Ellard GA, Humphries MJ, Gabriel M, et al. Penetration of pyrazinamide into the cerebrospinal fluid in tuberculous meningitis. *BMJ* 1987;294:284–285.

173. Woo J, Humphries M, Chan K, et al. Cerebrospinal fluid and serum levels of pyrazinamide and rifampicin in patients with tuberculous meningitis. *Curr Ther Res* 1987;42:235–242.

174. Donald PR, Seifart H. Cerebrospinal fluid pyrazinamide concentrations in children with tuberculous meningitis. *Pediatr Infect Dis* 1988;7:469–471.

175. Phuapradit P, Sumonchai K, Kaojarern S, et al. The blood/cerebrospinal fluid partitioning of pyrazinamide: a study during the course of treatment of tuberculosis meningitis. *J Neurol Neurosurg Psychiatry* 1990;53:81-82.

176. Alarcon F, Escalante L, Perez Y, et al. Tuberculous meningitis. Short course of chemotherapy. *Arch Neurol* 1990;47:1313–1317.

177. Phuapradit P, Vejjajiva A. Treatment of tuberculous meningitis: role of short-course chemotherapy. *Q J Med* 1987;62:249–258.

178. Jacobs RF, Sunakorn P, Chotpitayasunonah T, et al. Intensive short course chemotherapy for tuberculous meningitis. *Pediatr Infect Dis J* 1992;11:194–198.

179. Ramachandran P, Duraipandian M, Nagarajan M, et al. Three chemotherapy studies of tuberculous meningitis in children. *Tubercle* 1986;67:17–29.

180. Hosoglu S, Ayaz C, Geyik MF, et al. Tuberculous meningitis in adults: an eleven-year review. *Int J Tuberc Lung Dis* 1998;2:553–557.

181. Humphries MJ, Teoh R, Lau J, et al. Factors of prognostic significance in Chinese children with tuberculous meningitis. *Tubercle* 1990;71:161–168

182. Heifets L. Antimycobacterial agents: pyrazinamide. In: Yu V, Merigan T, Barriere S, eds. *Antimicrobial therapy and vaccines*. Baltimore: Williams & Wilkins, 1999:670–671.

183. Berning SE, Cherry TA, Iseman MD. Novel treatment of meningitis caused by multidrug-resistant *Mycobacterium tuberculosis* with intrathecal levofloxacin and amikacin: case report. *Clin Infect Dis* 2001;32:643–646.

184. Visudhiphan P, Chiemchanya S. Evaluation of rifampicin in the treatment of tuberculous meningitis in children. *J Pediatr* 1975;87(6 Pt 1):983–986.

185. Visudhiphan P, Chiemchanya S. Tuberculous meningitis in children: treatment with isoniazid and rifampicin for twelve months. *Pediatrics* 1989;114:875–879.

186. Latorre P, Gallofre M, Laporte JR, et al. Rifampicin in tuberculous meningitis: a retrospective assessment. *Eur J Clin Pharmacol* 1984;26:583–586.

187. Rahajoe NN, Rahajoe N, Boediman I, et al. The treatment of tuberculous meningitis in children with a combination of isoniazid, rifampicin and streptomycin—preliminary report. *Tubercle* 1979;60:245–250.

188. Girgis NI, Yassin MW, Laughlin LW, et al. Rifampicin in the treatment of tuberculous meningitis. *J Trop Med Hyg* 1978;81:246–247.

189. Doganay M, Bakir M, Dokmetas I. Treatment of tuberculous meningitis in adults with a combination of isoniazid, rifampicin and streptomycin: a prospective study. *Scand J Infect Dis* 1989;21:81–85.

190. Holdiness MR. Cerebrospinal fluid pharmacokinetics of the antituberculosis drugs. *Clin Pharmacokinet* 1985;10:532–534.

191. DeVincenzo JP, Berning SE, Peloquin CA, et al. Multidrug-resistant tuberculosis meningitis: clinical problems and concentrations of second-line antituberculous medications. *Ann Pharmacother* 1999;33:1184–1188.

192. Berning SE, Cherry TA, Iseman MD. Novel treatment of meningitis caused by multidrug-resistant *Mycobacterium tuberculosis* with intrathecal levofloxacin and amikacin: case report. *Clin Infect Dis* 2001;32:643–646.

193. DeVincenzo JP, Berning SE, Peloquin CA, et al. Multidrug-resistant tuberculosis meningitis: clinical problems and concentrations of second-line antituberculous medications. *Ann Pharmacother* 1999;33:1184–1188.

194. Barsic B, Himbele J, Beus I, et al. Entry of ciprofloxacin into cerebrospinal fluid during bacterial, viral and tuberculous meningitis. *Neurol Croat* 1991;40:111–116.

195. Zeana C, Kubin CJ, Della-Latta P, et al. Vancomycin-resistant *Enterococcus faecium* meningitis successfully managed with linezolid: case report and review of the literature. *Clin Infect Dis* 2001;33:477–482.

196. Iseman MD. Extrapulmonary tuberculosis in adults. In: *A clinician's guide to tuberculosis*. Philadelphia: Lippincott Williams & Wilkins, 2000:145–197.

197. Wasz-Höckert O, Donner M. Results of the treatment of 191 children with tuberculosis in the years 1949–54. *Acta Paediatr* 1963;51(Suppl 141):7–25.

198. Lorber J. The treatment of tuberculous meningitis. *BMJ* 1960;1309–1312.

199. British Medical Research Council. Streptomycin treatment of tuberculous meningitis. *Lancet* 1948;1:582–596.

200. Freiman I, Geefhuysen J. Evaluation of intrathecal therapy with streptomycin and hydrocortisone in tuberculous meningitis. *J Pediatr* 1970;76:895–901.

201. Choremis K, Zerevos N, Constantinides V, et al. Streptomycin therapy of tuberculous meningitis in children. *Lancet* 1948;ii:595–599.

202. Dajez P, Vincken W, Lambelin D, et al. Intraventricular administration of rifampin for tuberculous meningitis. *J Neurol* 1981;225:153–156.

203. Vincken W, Meysman M, Verbeelen D, et al. Intraventricular rifampicin in severe tuberculous meningo-encephalitis. *Eur Respir J* 1992;5:891–893.

204. Berning SE, Cherry TA, Iseman MD. Novel treatment of meningitis caused by multidrug-resistant *Mycobacterium tuberculosis* with intrathecal levofloxacin and amikacin: case report. *Clin Infect Dis* 2001;32:643–646.

205. Parsons M. The treatment of tuberculous meningitis. *Tubercle* 1989;70:79–82.

206. Molavi A, LeFrock JL. Tuberculous meningitis. *Med Clin North Am* 1985;69:315–331.

207. McGowan JE Jr, Chesney PJ, Crossley KB, et al. Guidelines for the use of systemic glucocorticosteroids in the management of selected infections. *J Infect Dis* 1992;165:1–13.

208. Kendig EL, Choy SH, Johnson WH. Observations on the effect of cortisone in the treatment of tuberculous meningitis. *Am Rev Tuberc* 1956;73:99–109.

209. Johnson JR, Furstenberg NE, Patterson R, et al. Corticotropin and adrenal steroids as adjuncts to the treatment of tuberculous meningitis. *Ann Intern Med* 1957;46:316–331.

210. Ashby M, Grant H. Tuberculous meningitis treated with cortisone. *Lancet* 1955;1:65–66.

211. Parsons M. *Tuberculous meningitis: a handbook for clinicians.* New York: Oxford University Press, 1979;39.

212. Lepper MH, Spies HW. The present status of the treatment of tuberculosis of the central nervous system. *Ann NY Acad Sci* 1963;106:106–123.

213. Weiss W, Flippin HF. The prognosis of tuberculous meningitis in the isoniazid era. *Am J Med Sci* 1961;242:423–430.

214. Weiss W, Flippin HF. The changing incidence and prognosis of tuberculous meningitis. *Am J Med Sci* 1965;250:46–59.

215. Dooley DP, Carpenter JL, Rademacher S. Adjunctive corticosteroid therapy for tuberculosis: a critical reappraisal of the literature. *Clin Infect Dis* 1997;25:872–887.

216. Coyle PK. Glucocorticoids in central nervous system bacterial infection. *Arch Neurol* 1999;56:796–801.

217. Prasad K, Volmink J, Menon GR. Steroids for treating tuberculous meningitis. (Systematic Review) Cochrane Infectious Diseases Group Cochrane Database of Systematic Reviews. Issue 3, 2002.

218. Kaojarern S, Supmonchai K, Phuapradit P, et al. Effect of steroids on cerebrospinal fluid penetration of antituberculous drugs in tuberculous meningitis. *Clin Pharmacol Ther* 1991; 49:6–12.

219. Johnson JR, Furstenberg NE, Patterson R, et al. Corticotropin and adrenal steroids as adjuncts to the treatment of tuberculous meningitis. *Ann Intern Med* 1957;46:316–331.

220. Schoeman JF, Van Zyl LE, Laubscher JA, et al. Effect of corticosteroids on intracranial pressure, computed tomographic findings, and clinical outcome in young children with tuberculous meningitis. *Pediatrics* 1997;99:226–231.

221. Bhagwati SN. Ventriculoatrial shunt in tuberculous meningitis with hydrocephalus. *J Neurosurg* 1971;35:309–313.

222. Chitale VR, Kasaliwal GT. Our experience of ventriculoatrial shunt using Upadhyaya valve in cases of hydrocephalus associated with tuberculous meningitis. *Prog Pediatr Surg* 1982;15: 223–236.

223. Chan KH, Mann KS. Prolonged therapeutic external ventricular drainage: a prospective study. *Neurosurgery* 1988;23: 436–438.

224. Palur R, Rahshekhar V, Chandy MJ, et al. Shunt surgery for hydrocephalus in tuberculous meningitis: a long-term follow-up study. *J Neurosurg* 1991;74:64–69.

225. Schoeman J, Conald P, van Zyl L, et al. Tuberculous hydrocephalus: comparison of different treatments with regard to ICP, ventricular size and clinical outcome. *Dev Med Child Neurol* 1991;33:396–405.

226. Visudhiphan P, Chiemchanya S. Hydrocephalus in tuberculous meningitis in children: treatment with acetazolamide and repeated lumbar puncture. *J Pediatr* 1979;95:657–660.

227. Singhal BS, Bhagwati SN, Syed AH, et al. Raised intracranial pressure in tuberculous meningitis. *Neurology (India)* 1975;23: 32–39.

228. Cathie IAB, McFarlane JCW. Adjuvants to streptomycin in treating tuberculous meningitis in children. *Lancet* 1950;1: 1360–1362.

229. Lorber J. Fibrinolytic agents in the treatment of tuberculous meningitis. *J Clin Pathol* 1964;17:353–354.

230. Don A. Case of tuberculous meningitis in boy treated with tuberculin: recovery, recurrence and death. *BMJ* 1907;1: 1360–1362.

231. Smith H. Tuberculous meningitis. *Int J Neurol* 1964;4: 134–157.

232. Fitzsimons JM, Smith HV. Tuberculous meningitis: special features of treatment. *Tubercle* 1963;44:103–111.

233. Gourie-Devi M, Satish P. Hyaluronidase as an adjuvant in the treatment of cranial arachnoiditis (hydrocephalus and optochiasmatic arachnoiditis) complicating tuberculous meningitis. *Acta Neurol Scand* 1980;62:368–381.

234. Bhagwati SN, George K. Use of intrathecal hyaluronidase in the management of tuberculous meningitis with hydrocephalus. *Childs Nerv Syst* 1986;2:20–25.

235. Schoeman J, Donald P, van Zyl L, et al. Tuberculous hydrocephalus: comparison of different treatments with regard to ICP, ventricular size and clinical outcome. *Dev Med Child Neurol* 1991;33:396–405.

236. Mustafa MM, Lebel MH, Ramilo O, et al. Correlation of interleukin-1 beta and cachectin concentrations in cerebrospinal fluid and outcome from bacterial meningitis. *J Pediatr* 1989; 115:208–213.

237. Saukkonen K, Sande S, Cioffe C, et al. The role of cytokines in the generation of inflammation and tissue damage in experimental gram-positive meningitis. *J Exp Med* 1990;171: 439–448.

238. Sharief MK, Ciardi M, Thompson EJ. Blood–brain barrier damage in patients with bacterial meningitis: association with tumor necrosis factor-alpha but not interleukin-1 beta. *J Infect Dis* 1992;166:350–358.

239. Tsenova L, Soklo K, Freddman VH, et al. A combination of thalidomide plus antibiotics protects rabbits from mycobacterial meningitis–associated death. *J Infect Dis* 1998;177: 1563–1572.

240. Schoeman JF, Springer P, Ravenscroft A, et al. Adjunctive thalidomide therapy of childhood tuberculous meningitis: possible anti-inflammatory role. *J Child Neurol* 2000;15:497–503.

241. Schoeman JF, Ravenscroft A, Hartzenberg HB. Possible role of adjunctive thalidomide therapy in the resolution of a massive intracranial tuberculous abscess. *Childs Nerv Syst* 2001;17: 370–372.

242. Schoeman JF. Thalidomide therapy in childhood tuberculous menigitis. *J Child Neurol* 2000;15:838.

243. Parsons M. *Tuberculous meningitis: a handbook for clinicians.* New York: Oxford University Press, 1979.

244. Bhagwati SN. Ventriculoatrial shunt in tuberculous meningitis with hydrocephalus. *J Neurosurg* 1971;35:309–313.

245. Girgis NI, Sippel JE, Kilpatrick ME, et al. Meningitis and encephalitis at the Abbassia Fever Hospital, Cairo, Egypt, from 1966 to 1989. *Am J Trop Med Hyg* 1993;48:97–107.

246. Falk A. U.S. Veterans Administration–Armed Forces cooperative study on the chemotherapy of tuberculosis. 13. Tuberculous meningitis in adults, with special reference to survival, neurologic residuals, and work status. *Am Rev Respir Dis* 1962;91:823–831.

247. Ramachandran P, Duraipandian M, Reetha AM, et al. Longterm status of children treated for tuberculous meningitis in South India. *Tubercle* 1989;70:235–239.

248. British Medical Research Council. Streptomycin treatment of tuberculous meningitis. *Lancet* 1948;1:582–596.

249. Weiss W, Flippin HF. The prognosis of tuberculous meningitis in the isoniazid era. *Am J Med Sci* 1961;242:423–430.

250. Weiss W, Flippin HF. The changing incidence and prognosis of tuberculous meningitis. *Am J Med Sci* 1965;250:46–59.

251. Humphries MJ, Teon R, Lau J, et al. Factors of prognostic significance in Chinese children with tuberculous meningitis. *Tubercle* 1990;71:161–168.

252. D'Cruz IA, Dandekar AC. Tuberculous meningitis in pregnant and puerperal women. *Obstet Gynecol* 1968;31:775–778.

253. Stephanopoulos C. The development of tuberculous meningitis during pregnancy. *Am Rev Tuberc* 1957;76:1079–1087.

254. Kingdom JC, Kennedy DH. Tuberculous meningitis in pregnancy. *Br J Obstet Gyn* 1989;96:233–235.

255. Ramachandran P, Duraipandian M, Nagarajan M, et al. Three chemotherapy studies of tuberculous meningitis in children. *Tubercle* 1986;67:17–29.

256. Lorber J. Long-term follow-up of 100 children who recovered from tuberculous meningitis. *Pediatrics* 1961;28:778–791.

257. Todd RM, Neville JG. The sequelae of tuberculous meningitis. *Arch Dis Child* 1964;39:213–225.

258. Donner M, Wasz-Hockert O. Late neurologic sequelae of tuberculous meningitis. *Acta Paediatr* (Suppl) 1962;141:34–42.

259. Pentti R, Donner M, Valanne E, et al. Late psychological and psychiatric sequelae of tuberculous meningitis. *Acta Paediatr* (Suppl) 1962;141:65–77.

260. Mooney AJ. Some ocular sequelae of tuberculous meningitis. *Am J Ophthalmol* 1956;41:753–768.

261. Miettinen P, Wasz-Hockert O. Late ophthalmological sequelae of tuberculous meningitis. *Acta Paediatr* (Suppl) 1962;141:43–49.

262. Schon F, Bowler JV. Syringomyelia and syringobulbia following tuberculous meningitis. *J Neurol* 1990;237:122–123.

263. Lorber J. Diabetes insipidus following tuberculous meningitis. *Arch Dis Child* 1958;33:315–319.

264. Dick DJ, Sanders GL, Saunders M, et al. Chronic hypothermia following tuberculous meningitis. *J Neurol Neurosurg Psychiatry* 1981;44:255–257.

265. Lam KS, Sham MM, Tam SC, et al. Hypopituitarism after tuberculous meningitis in childhood. *Ann Intern Med* 1993;118:701–706.

266. Louie E, Rice LB, Holzman RS. Tuberculosis in non-Haitian patients with acquired immune deficiency syndrome. *Chest* 1986;90:542–545.

267. Berenguer J, Moreno S, Laguna F, et al. Tuberculous meningitis in patients infected with the human immunodeficiency virus. *N Engl J Med* 1992;326:668–672.

268. Bergemann A, Karstaedt AS. The spectrum of meningitis in a population with high prevalence of HIV disease. *Q J Med* 1996;89:499–504.

269. Taelman H, Batungwanayo J, Clerinx J, et al. Tuberculous meningitis in patients infected with the human immunodeficiency virus (letter). *N Engl J Med* 1992;327:1171.

270. Dube MP, Holtom PD, Larsen RA. Tuberculous meningitis in patients with and without human immunodeficiency virus infection. *Am J Med* 1992;93:520–524.

271. Porkert MT, Sotir M, Parrott-Moore P, Blumberg HM. Tuberculous meningitis at a large inner-city medical center. *Am J Med Sci* 1997;313:325–331.

272. Yechoor VK, Shandera WX, Rodriguez P, et al. Tuberculous meningitis among adults with and without HIV infection. Experience in an urban public hospital. *Arch Intern Med* 1996;156:1710–1716.

273. Laguna F, Adrados M, Ortega A, et al. Tuberculous meningitis with acellular cerebrospinal fluid in AIDS. *AIDS* 1992;6:1165–1167.

274. Bishburg E, Sunderam G, Reichman LB, et al. Central nervous system tuberculosis with the acquired immunodeficiency syndrome. *Ann Intern Med* 1986;105:210–213.

275. Gomez-Aranda F, Lopez-Dominguez JM, Malaga AM, et al. Meningitis simultaneously due to *Cryptococcus neoformans* and *Mycobacterium tuberculosis*. *Clin Infect Dis* 1993;16:588.

276. Fischl MA, Pitchenik AE, Spira TJ. Tuberculous brain abscess and *Toxoplasma* encephalitis in a patient with the acquired immunodeficiency syndrome. *JAMA* 1985;253:3428–3430.

277. Jacob CN, Henein SS, Heurich AE, et al. Nontuberculous mycobacterial infection of the central nervous system in patient with AIDS. *S Med J* 1993;86:638–640.

278. Hawkins CC, Gold JWN, Whimbey E, et al. *Mycobacterium avium* complex infections in patients with the acquired immunodeficiency syndrome. *Ann Intern Med* 1986;105:184–188.

279. Ninane J, Grymonprez A, Burtonboy G, et al. Disseminated BCG in HIV infection. *Arch Dis Child* 1988;63:1268–1269.

280. Miceli I, de Kantor IN, Colaiacovo D, et al. Evaluation of the effectiveness of BCG vaccination using the case-control method in Buenos Aires, Argentina. *Int J Epidemiol* 1988;17:629–634.

281. Filho VW, de Castilho EA, Rodrigues LC, et al. Effectiveness of BCG vaccination against tuberculosis meningitis: a case-control study in Sao Paulo, Brazil. *Bull WHO* 1990;68:69–74.

282. Camargos PAM, Guimaraes MDC, Antunes CMF. Risk assessment for acquiring meningitis tuberculosis among children not vaccinated with BCG: a case-control study. *Int J Epidemiol* 1988;17:193–197.

283. Thilothammal N, Krishnamurthy PV, et al. Does BCG vaccine prevent tuberculous meningitis? *Arch Dis Child* 1996;74:144–147.

284. Rodrigues LC, Diwan VK, Wheeler JG. Protective effect of BCG against tuberculous meningitis and miliary tuberculosis: a meta-analysis. *Int J Epidemiol* 1993;22:1154–1158.

285. Awasthi S, Moin S. Effectiveness of BCG vaccination against tuberculous meningitis. *Indian Pediatr* 1999;36(5):455–460.

286. Mittal SK, Aggarwal V, Rastogi A, et al. Does B.C.G. vaccination prevent or postpone the occurrence of tuberculous meningitis? *Indian J Pediatr* 1996;63:659–664.

287. Zhang LX, Tu DH, He GX, et al. Risk of tuberculosis infection and tuberculous meningitis after discontinuation of bacillus Calmette–Guérin in Beijing. *Am J Respir Crit Care Med* 2000;162(4 Pt 1):1314–1317.

288. Guler N, Ones U, Somer A, et al. The effect of prior BCG vaccination on the clinical and radiographic presentation of tuberculosis meningitis in children in Istanbul, Turkey. *Int J Tuberc Lung Dis* 1998;2:885–890.

289. Girgis NI, Sultan Y, Farid Z, et al. Tuberculosis meningitis, Abbassia Fever Hospital–Naval Medical Research Unit No. 3, Cairo, Egypt, from 1976 to 1996. *Am J Trop Med Hyg* 1998;58:28–34.

290. Yaramis A, Gurkan F, Elevli M, et al. Central nervous system tuberculosis in children: a review of 214 cases. *Pediatrics* 1998;102:E49.

291. Donald PR, Gent WL, Seifart HI, et al. Cerebrospinal fluid isoniazid concentrations in children with tuberculous meningitis: the influence of dosage and acetylation status. *Pediatrics* 1992;89:247–250.

292. Sippel JE, Mikhail IA, Girgis NI. Rifampin concentrations in cerebrospinal fluid of patients with tuberculous meningitis. *Am Rev Respir Dis* 1974;109:579–580.

293. Hughes IE, Smith H, Kane PO. Ethionamide: its passage into the cerebrospinal fluid in man. *Lancet* 1962;1:616–617.

294. Donald PR, Seifart HI. Cerebrospinal fluid concentrations of ethionamide in children with tuberculous meningitis. *J Pediatr* 1989;115:483–486.

OCULAR COMPLICATIONS

DOROTHY NAHM FRIEDBERG
MONICA LORENZO-LATKANY

I found, on approaching the Zenith of my ambition, the Great Lake in question nothing but mist and glare before my eyes. From the summit of the eastern horn the lovely Tanganyika Lake could be seen in all its glory by everybody but myself.

Captain John H. Speke (1827–1864)

[Captain Speke, discoverer of the source of the Nile River, had ocular tuberculosis diagnosed in 1859 by Sir William Bowman (1).]

In 1711, Maitre-Jan reported the first instance of ocular tuberculosis. Cohnheim, in 1867, described miliary tuberculosis of the choroid as a metastatic phenomenon and part of the systemic infection; he proved that choroidal nodules were identical to tubercles elsewhere in the body. In 1882, Koch discovered the tubercle bacillus, and in 1883, Julius von Michael identified the organism in the eye (2).

Tuberculosis affects all areas of the visual system, from the eyelids to the optic nerve. The current resurgence of tuberculosis makes it imperative that the ophthalmologist and the patient's general physician be aware of the diversity of the presentations of tuberculosis in the eye and ocular adnexa. As in other diseases with protean manifestations, considering the possibility of tuberculosis is often the most difficult part of making the correct diagnosis. Discovery of a tuberculous etiology for a particular ocular condition, especially in a patient without known active infection elsewhere, requires prompt collaboration between the ophthalmologist and internist. A close partnership is also necessary to select therapy, particularly in light of the emergence of multidrug-resistant strains and the difficulty of treating human immunodeficiency virus (HIV)–positive patients in whom tuberculosis is often only one of a multitude of concurrent infections. Several of the mainstay

D. N. Friedberg: Department of Ophthalmology, New York University School of Medicine; Department of Ophthalmology, New York Eye and Ear Infirmary, New York, New York.

M. Lorenzo-Latkany: Department of Ophthalmology, New York University School of Medicine, New York, New York.

drugs, as well as some of the newer antituberculous medications, have known ocular side effects; thus, careful ophthalmic monitoring is important to prevent serious drug toxicities.

Ocular tuberculosis usually requires systemic therapy. Optimal treatments change rapidly and depend on the patient's immune status, history, and probability of drug resistance. This chapter recommends therapies only if they are particular to the ocular form of the disease.

EYELIDS

Lupus vulgaris is a progressive tuberculous infection of the skin. It is a slowly progressive disease with subepithelial nodules that have an "apple jelly" appearance. Lupus vulgaris can affect the eyelids and may result in the development of tuberculous conjunctivitis (3,4). In scrofuloderma, the skin is affected secondarily to involvement of underlying tissues such as the orbital bones or lacrimal sac. The skin can develop a purplish swelling that may ulcerate (4). Tuberculous tarsitis can produce lesions simulating chalazia (4,5). A tuberculous granuloma can present as a firm lid mass (6) and an acute lid abscess (7).

Lacrimal System

Both tuberculous dacryoadenitis, the involvement of the lacrimal gland, and tuberculous dacryocystitis, involvement of the lacrimal sac, have been described in patients without evidence of active tuberculosis. Localized infection of the lacrimal gland is either sclerotic or caseous. It presents with proptosis and a firm, nontender enlargement of the gland, which may result in limitation of ocular movements and ptosis (8). Both primary and secondary dacryocystitis has been attributed to tubercular infection (9,10). The patient may complain of tearing, and purulent secretions can be expressed from the lacrimal sac with gentle pressure. Secondary infection usually arises from an adjacent focus in the nose, conjunctiva, skin, or orbital bones.

CONJUNCTIVA

Tuberculosis of the conjunctiva has been the subject of numerous case reports. If the patient has no other evidence of systemic tuberculosis, the diagnosis may be obscure until a biopsy is done. Reports often describe months of unsuccessful therapeutic interventions before the correct diagnosis is made. Eyre (11) reported a large series in 1912, collecting 206 cases from the literature and his own practice in which the tubercle bacillus was demonstrated.

In primary conjunctival tuberculosis, the mucous membrane is infected through contact with organisms either by self-inoculation from sputum on a contaminated handkerchief or fingers or through contact with aerosolized droplets. Secondary tuberculous conjunctivitis develops adjacent to skin lesions, such as those from a tuberculous vesicular rash or lupus vulgaris (3,12).

The clinical presentation of conjunctival tuberculosis depends on the patient's history of infection and the virulence of the organism. Most cases have been reported in children and young adults (11,13–16). In primary conjunctival tuberculosis, patients often have a history of chronic conjunctivitis complicated by progressive lymphadenitis that can rupture and fistulize. This primary infection can result in Parinaud oculoglandular syndrome, an infectious conjunctivitis accompanied by regional adenopathy.

Eyre (11) classified conjunctival tuberculosis into four types; these classifications were modified by Duke-Elder (17):

1. *Ulcerative conjunctivitis* consists of single or multiple small ulcers that usually involve the tarsal conjunctiva and that may coalesce. These ulcers are usually painless and indolent. The preauricular node is frequently involved, and, in chronic cases, there may also be adjacent nodal involvement. Rarely, the ulcers spread and produce a corneal pannus or involve the eyelid or sclera.
2. *Nodular (miliary) conjunctivitis* consists of small, yellow or gray subconjunctival nodules that enlarge and can produce follicular conjunctivitis. These lesions commonly involve the tarsal conjunctiva; when the bulbar conjunctiva is involved, it is usually at the limbus. Regional adenopathy is less common with nodular conjunctivitis than with the ulcerative type. Cassady (14) described a 9-year-old girl with a 6-year history of a "diseased right eye." The girl underwent therapy with a variety of topical antibiotics for 6 months before referral. She had hypertrophy of the superior tarsal conjunctiva and a corneal pannus. Biopsy revealed a granulomatous lesion and the presence of acid-fast bacilli (AFBs). There was no regional adenitis; a chest radiograph demonstrated evidence of previous tuberculosis. The lesion improved with paraaminosalicylic acid and streptomycin (14).
3. *Hypertrophic papillary conjunctivitis* has large, flattened areas of granulation tissue, usually in the fornices, that may ulcerate and be accompanied by swelling of the eyelids. These lesions may enlarge, become pedunculated, and take on the appearance of a "cockscomb excrescence."
4. *Polypoid conjunctivitis* consists of a fibroma-like, pedunculated lesion that extends from the tarsal conjunctiva. Patients experience minimal symptoms.
5. *Conjunctival tuberculomas*, occurring in miliary disease, are red or yellow nonulcerative, subconjunctival nodules surrounded by normal conjunctiva.

In clinical practice, these types often overlap (11). Most reports in the current literature describe nodular or ulcerative types (13–16,18–20).

Diagnosis of conjunctival tuberculosis should be made based on culture or biopsy specimen identification of AFBs; this may be difficult in some cases. Clinical evaluation of a patient with conjunctival tuberculosis should include a search for evidence of active tuberculosis or inactive tuberculosis in the patient or active tuberculosis among close contacts of the patient. After this evaluation has been completed, systemic chemotherapy should be started. When response is delayed or systemic toxicities intervene, topical streptomycin added to the regimen may produce good results. Subconjunctival injection of streptomycin in rabbit eyes has not shown any toxic effects in the fundus (21). Topical streptomycin, in either eyedrop or ointment form, has not been shown to penetrate intact rabbit corneal epithelium (22,23). Saline solutions containing 10,000 μg/mL are well tolerated when instilled in human eyes (22).

There has been one case report of conjunctival tuberculosis secondary to *Mycobacterium bovis*. This report described bilateral, nodular ulcerative bulbar conjunctivitis in a woman with active miliary tuberculosis that involved only the lung and conjunctiva (24) (Fig. 29.1).

Phlyctenular keratoconjunctivitis is rarely found in patients with active tuberculosis (25). Helm and Holland (26) reviewed the experimental and epidemiologic evidence suggesting the association of phlyctenulosis and hypersensitivity to tuberculoprotein. The disease is most commonly found in children. Clinically, the lesions, usually located at the limbus, are elevated and pinkish white and surrounded by conjunctival hyperemia. A central ulceration may develop. Conjunctival lesions may spread to involve the cornea, but purely corneal lesions may also develop. Phlyctenular keratoconjunctivitis responds to treatment with topical corticosteroids; topical antibiotics should be used if secondary infection is present. It must be emphasized that tuberculous hypersensitivity is not the only cause of this condition.

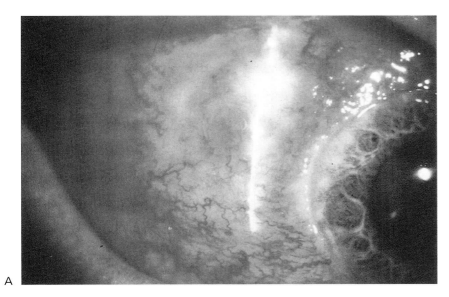

A

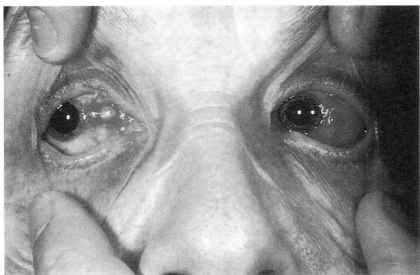

B

FIGURE 29.1. A and B: Conjunctival infection with *Mycobacterium bovis*. (From Liesegang TJ, Cameron JD. *Mycobacterium bovis* infection of the conjunctiva. *Arch Ophthalmol* 1980;98: 1764–1766, with permission.) (See Color Plate 11.)

SCLERAL DISEASE

Scleral involvement is usually secondary to endogenous spread of organisms either hematogenously or from contiguous foci within the eye. Bloomfield et al. (27) described the case of an 82-year-old patient who had active tuberculosis and a necrotic, reddish purple scleral lesion that revealed a caseating granuloma on biopsy and tuberculosis on culture. The patient was treated systemically and topical 1% streptomycin and periocular injections of streptomycin were added to the regimen (27). Nanda et al. (28) described an 81-year-old patient with a lesion initially thought to be necrotizing scleritis but grew AFBs on culture. Cases of scleral perforation secondary to intraocular tuberculosis have also been described (29,30). Involvement of the sclera in cases of episcleritis, scleritis, and sclerokeratitis has been linked to tuberculous allergy.

CORNEAL DISEASE

The cornea is rarely affected without involvement of the adjacent conjunctiva; when the cornea is involved, a pannus is typically seen (3,14). Donahue (25), in an extensive review of ocular complications seen in a tuberculosis sanitarium over 25 years, described three cases of tuberculous corneal ulcers and 14 cases of interstitial keratitis in 154 cases of ocular tuberculosis. Sheu et al. (6) described a case of chronic keratitis that grew *Mycobacterium tuberculosis* from a corneal scraping. There was no systemic evidence of tuberculosis, and the infiltrate responded to treatment.

NEUROOPHTHALMIC AND ORBITAL COMPLICATIONS

Orbital Tuberculosis

Tuberculous infection of the orbit arises from hematogenous spread or from the extension of adjacent sinus disease. Oakhill et al. (31) described an 11-year-old patient with proptosis and fever accompanying femoral swelling. A soft-tissue mass, without major bony destruction, was seen on computed tomography scan. Tuberculosis was cultured from the femoral lesion, and the orbital and femoral lesions responded to treatment (31). Khalil et al. (32) described orbital tuberculosis in two older patients: one had orbital involvement originating from pericardial tuberculosis and the other had orbital complications from extensive tuberculous sinusitis. Computed tomography scans revealed soft-tissue masses in the orbit without bony erosion. Bony erosion has also been described with sinus and orbital tuberculosis (33).

A 5-year-old boy, without previous trauma or constitutional symptoms, presented with a 4-month history of swelling of the eyelids and proptosis. There was nontender, regional lymphadenopathy and 4 mm of proptosis; motility and vision were normal. Soft-tissue window computed tomography demonstrated bony erosion of the orbital wall and roof and a large cystic mass in the orbit. Multiple AFBs were cultured from the cyst fluid. A chest radiograph was normal, and the patient responded to systemic treatment (Fig. 29.2).

Neuroophthalmic Tuberculosis

The optic nerve can be involved with tuberculosis. Miller and Frenkel (34) described a case of tuberculous retrobulbar neuritis with a central scotoma in which the diagnosis was made at surgery for tuberculous osteomyelitis. In Donahue's series (25), one case of tuberculous involvement of the optic nerve was diagnosed at autopsy. Mooney (35), in a series of 65 patients with tuberculosis meningitis, found two patients with retrobulbar neuritis. Other ocular findings in Mooney's series of tuberculosis meningitis included papilledema in 26% of cases, optic disc pallor in 20%, and

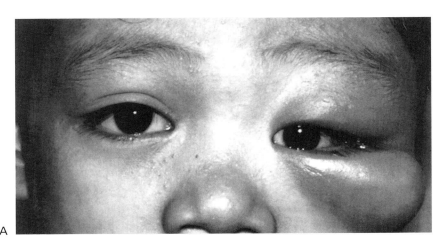

A

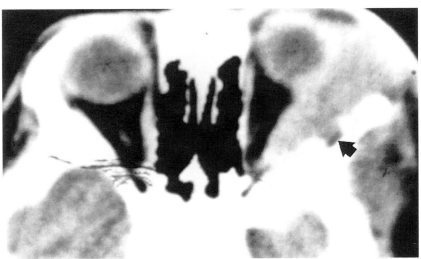

B

FIGURE 29.2. Orbital tuberculosis. **A:** Left eyelid swelling and 4 mm of proptosis. **B:** Orbital tuberculosis: axial computed tomography, soft-tissue window, shows a large mass extending into the left orbit with bony destruction of the lateral orbital wall (*arrow*). (Photographs courtesy of Heidi D. Remulla, M.D., Massachusetts Eye and Ear Infirmary, Boston, MA, U.S.A.)

transient third and sixth nerve palsies. In some cases of disc pallor, vision was severely affected, and during surgery, extensive adhesions were seen around the optic nerves (35). An optic disc tubercle has been described (36). A patient with acquired immunodeficiency syndrome (AIDS) with a pontine tuberculoma developed a gaze palsy with impaired adduction (one-and-a-half syndrome) that resolved with antituberculous treatment (37).

UVEAL TUBERCULOSIS

A diagnosis of ocular tuberculosis most often involves the uveal tract, either as chronic anterior uveitis or disseminated choroiditis (38). Fifty years ago, except for a few cases of uveitis caused by syphilis and leprosy, all other cases of uveitis were attributed to tuberculosis (39).

Tuberculous granulomatous iritis is characterized by congestion, keratic precipitates, posterior synechiae, Koeppe nodules, aqueous cells, and vitreous opacities. Posterior tuberculous uveitis can be a disseminated miliary inflammation or a solitary tuberculoma. The rich vascular supply of the anterior and posterior uveal tract predisposes these areas to tuberculous infection (25). Ciliary body tuberculosis usually affects patients younger than 30 years of age and tends to be chronic; however, patients often do not have obvious pulmonary or systemic tuberculosis (40).

The frequency of tuberculous uveitis has been a subject of controversy, in large part depending on the examiner's criteria for diagnosis. The clinical presentation is pleomorphic, and the inflammation does not have to be granulomatous in nature (41). During the early 20th century, many cases of uveitis were thought to occur in patients with a history of systemic tuberculosis or tuberculin hypersensitivity (39). In 1881, von Michael considered tuberculosis to be a common cause of uveitis and classified it into miliary, diffuse, and granulomatous types. In 1941, Woods (39) attributed 80% of granulomatous uveitis to tuberculosis, a percentage that decreased to 20% by 1960 (Table 29.1). The decline in tuberculous uveitis may be the result of recognizing other causes of uveitis, improved definitions of previously described entities, and better diagnostic laboratory techniques. In Henderly's (42) review of 600 patients with uveitis, only one case was the result of tuberculosis. Moreover, when Woods (39) reported his results in 1941, the diagnosis of idiopathic uveitis did not exist. The percentage of undetermined or idiopathic uveitis has remained high despite advances in diagnostic techniques. This, combined with stricter diagnostic criteria, has resulted in the decrease of frequency of tuberculous uveitis (26).

CHOROIDAL TUBERCULOSIS

Choroidal tubercles and tuberculomas are the most common manifestations of ocular tuberculosis. Choroidal tubercles were first recognized in 1830. Initially, they were described in terminally ill patients with acute miliary tuberculosis. However, in 1906, Cargill and Mayou (44) found choroidal tuberculomas as the first evidence of disseminated tuberculosis. In 1948, Illingworth and Wright (45) found choroidal tuberculomas early in the course of the illness. In 1983, Jabbour et al. (46) described how discovery of choroidal involvement had led to the diagnosis of pulmonary tuberculosis. In 1990, Mansour and Haymond (47) reported a case of choroidal tuberculomas without extraocular evidence of disseminated pulmonary tuberculosis. In 1989, Blodi et al. (48) reported a case of presumed choroidal tuberculosis in a patient with HIV infection.

TABLE 29.1. GRANULOMATOUS UVEITIS

Etiology	Woods, 1941 (39) 348 Patients (%)	Woods, 1960 (39) 134 Patients (%)	Weiner and BenEzra, 1991 (43) 400 Patients (%)
Tuberculosis	80	20	0.75
Syphilis	17	2	0.25
Sarcoidosis	1	3	0.5
Brucellosis	0.7	2	0.25
Histoplasmosis	0	36	3.8
Toxoplasmosis	0	13	0
Unknown	0	22	39.5
HLA-B27 positive			3.0
Behçet disease			15.3
Juvenile rheumatoid arthritis			3.3
Herpes			5.0
Trauma/surgery			8.0
Sympathetic ophthalmia			3.75
Miscellaneous	1.3	2	16.75

HLA, human leukocyte antigen.

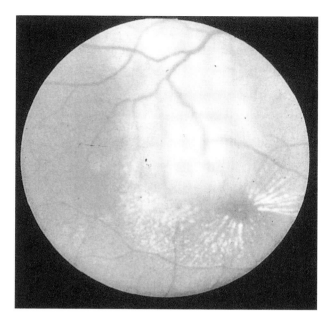

FIGURE 29.3. Miliary tuberculosis: early choroidal lesion with macular star. (From Cangemi FF, Friedman AH, Josephberg R. Tuberculoma of the choroid. *Ophthalmology* 1980;87:252–258, with permission.) (See Color Plate 12.)

Early choroidal tubercles are round or oval, white, gray-white, or yellow-white with indefinite borders (49) (Fig. 29.3). Their size ranges from 0.5 to 3.0 mm. They are usually confined to the posterior pole within two disc diameters of the optic nerve but can also be seen in the midperipheral fundus. Choroidal tubercles are usually bilateral, and there can be one to ten per eye. However, 50 to 60 tubercles have been reported in each eye (50) (Fig. 29.4). The retinal vessels overlying the lesions appear normal, but older lesions can appear elevated, causing the retinal vessels to show bowing (49,51). As the choroidal tubercles age, the pale centers become surrounded by a rim of black pigment, making the borders more distinct (50) (Fig. 29.5).

Choroidal tuberculosis is thought to occur as a result of hematogenous spread. The choroid has a greater chance of becoming infected than other portions of the eye because of its rich vascular supply and abundance of reticuloendothelial cells (50). Miliary pulmonary tuberculosis is the most common form of tuberculosis associated with choroidal involvement (52). Although the presence of choroidal tubercles is indicative of hematogenous spread, this should not be considered diagnostic for miliary tuberculosis (46,49). A prospective study of 100 patients with systemic tuberculosis documented that in patients with choroidal lesions there was a significant association with miliary disease and the presence of ocular symptoms and decreased visual acuity. HIV infection was not more common in patients with ocular involvement (53).

Choroidal tuberculomas must be differentiated from other causes of choroidal granulomas such as toxoplasmosis, syphilis, sarcoidosis, and histoplasmosis. Choroidal lesions attributed to acquired toxoplasmosis are usually solitary and larger than choroidal tuberculomas. Syphilis usually causes anterior uveitis, but chorioretinitis can accompany late secondary syphilis. In sarcoidosis, there may be an associated retinal vasculitis. Presumed ocular histoplasmosis syndrome may be suggested by history of residence in an endemic area

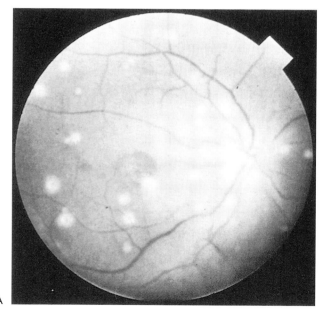

A

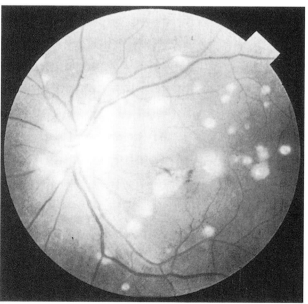

B

FIGURE 29.4. Miliary tuberculosis: multiple choroidal lesions in the right **(A)** and left **(B)** eyes. (From Chung YM, Yeh TS, Sheu SJ, et al. Macular subretinal neovascularization in choroidal tuberculosis. *Ann Ophthalmol* 1989;21:225–229, with permission.) (See Color Plate 13.)

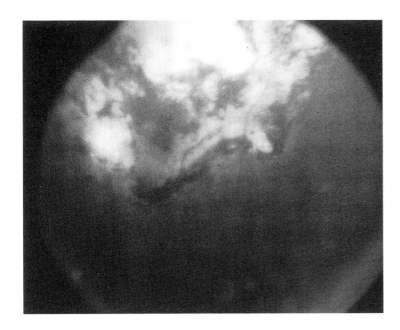

FIGURE 29.5. Late choroidal lesion with darkly pigmented borders and pale center. (Courtesy of Alan H. Friedman, M.D., Mt. Sinai School of Medicine, New York, NY, U.S.A.) (See Color Plate 14.)

or because of the presence of subretinal neovascularization. A thorough medical evaluation is vital to reach the correct diagnosis in cases of granulomas of the choroid. In most situations, biopsy of choroidal lesions in eyes with good visual acuity is too risky.

FLUORESCEIN ANGIOGRAPHY, ULTRASONOGRAPHY, AND INDOCYANINE GREEN ANGIOGRAPHY

Fluorescein angiography may be a useful diagnostic tool in choroidal tuberculosis. From the choroidal location of the lesion and the active inflammatory state, one might expect initial blocked fluorescence. However, Cangemi et al. (51) reported a choroidal tuberculoma with intense early hyperfluorescence. They postulated that the inflammatory state may wipe out the overlying retinal pigment epithelium, allowing intense fluorescence or, alternatively, that the lesion may be highly vascularized and have its own intrinsic blood supply. Jabbour et al. (46) described early hyperfluorescence of the choroidal lesion with a surrounding ring of hypofluorescence. In later phases, increased hyperfluorescence of the core lesion with late leakage was seen. Chung et al. (50), conversely, reported multiple blocked fluorescent spots in the initial phase; these became hyperfluorescent in the late phase. Some investigators believe that fluorescein angiography should be used in the follow-up of choroidal lesions for early recognition and treatment of neovascularization (52). Subretinal neovascularization has been reported in association with choroidal tuberculosis (50). Ultrasonography is helpful in diagnosing foreign bodies, choroidal melanomas, and metastatic tumors, but there

is no specific pattern for choroidal tuberculomas (46). Indocyanine green angiography can detect tuberculous lesions not visible on fundus examination. Findings on indocyanine green are not unique individually but as a pattern are strongly suggestive of granulomatous disease. The first sign consists of irregularly distributed hypofluorescent areas seen in early and intermediate frames that either become iso- or hyperfluorescent late in possibly active lesions or remain hypofluorescent in atrophic areas. These areas may appear normal on ophthalmoscopy or fluorescein angiography. The second sign, appearing on the intermediate or late angiogram, is multiple focal hyperfluorescent spots associated with long-standing disease. The third sign is fuzziness of choroidal vessels secondary to leakage that resolves after treatment. Last, there can be late diffuse zonal hyperfluorescence in areas of active lesions (54).

HISTOPATHOLOGY

Access to histopathology of choroidal or retinal lesions is mostly limited to cases from enucleations or postmortem studies. Choroidal tuberculomas are granulomatous lesions with large central areas of noncaseating necrosis surrounded by histiocytes and lymphocytes. The choroid appears thickened, and the overlying retinal pigment epithelium is absent in focal areas (55,56). Barondes et al. (55) demonstrated AFBs with a Ziehl–Neelsen stain from tissue obtained by chorioretinal endobiopsy. Although it is not always possible to demonstrate AFBs, the presence of strongly fluorescing rods, shown by use of double fluorochrome staining, provides strong evidence for tuberculosis (56). In a case of primary tuberculosis of the retina,

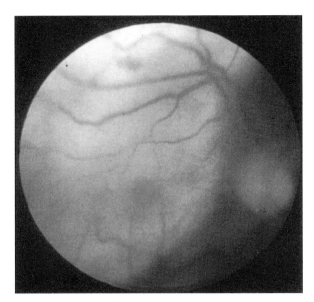

FIGURE 29.6. Choroidal tuberculoma: large subretinal mass involving the macula. (From Lyon CE, Grimson BS, Peiffer RL Jr, et al. Clinical-pathological correlation of a solitary choroidal tuberculoma. *Ophthalmology* 1985;92:845–850, with permission.) (See Color Plate 15.)

inflammatory granulomas with central areas of caseous necrosis surrounded by epithelial and giant cells and lymphocytes were seen; however, there was no evidence of AFBs (57). A case of tuberculous iridocyclitis showed granulomatous infiltration with large Langerhans cells surrounding a necrotic center (58).

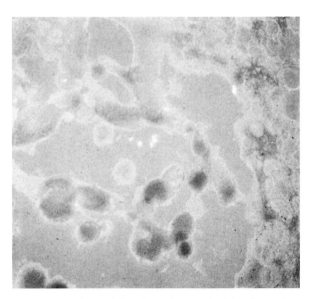

FIGURE 29.7. Choroidal tuberculoma: double fluorochrome staining with auramine and rhodamine shows strongly fluorescing rods. (From Lyon CE, Grimson BS, Peiffer RL Jr, et al. Clinical-pathological correlation of a solitary choroidal tuberculoma. *Ophthalmology* 1985;92:845–850, with permission.) (See Color Plate 16.)

A 34-year-old man with pulmonary tuberculosis treated with isoniazid (INH) and rifampin for several weeks presented with blurred vision. His vision deteriorated over the next 2 months until he had bare light perception and a large subretinal mass with a surrounding serous detachment of the retina. The blind, painful eye was enucleated. The patient had been on antituberculous medication while the lesion developed. Histopathology revealed a large granulomatous lesion of the choroid. Double fluorochrome staining revealed fluorescing rods (56) (Figs. 29.6 and 29.7).

OCULAR TUBERCULOSIS IN ACQUIRED IMMUNODEFICIENCY SYNDROME

The present resurgence of tuberculosis is largely owing to the AIDS epidemic. Extrapulmonary tuberculosis in patients with HIV became an AIDS-defining condition in 1987. The most frequent forms of extrapulmonary tuberculosis are lymphadenitis and miliary disease (59). Ocular tuberculosis remains either an underdiagnosed or underreported entity in these patients. In a review of ophthalmic findings in 28 patients with HIV infection, none was found to be the result of tuberculosis; one patient with a Roth spot had *Mycobacterium avium-intracellulare complex* pneumonia (60). There have been two reported cases of ocular tuberculosis in patients with HIV infection (48,61). Croxatto et al. (61) reported a case of a 31-year-old man with disseminated miliary tuberculosis on autopsy and two choroidal nodules. Microscopic examination of these nodules revealed caseous necrosis, monocular cells, and numerous AFBs. The second reported case was a 34-year-old man with pulmonary tuberculosis and tuberculous meningitis with visual acuity of 20/400 in the right eye and 20/40 in the left eye. Both eyes exhibited extensive granulomatous keratic precipitates. The right eye had a secluded pupil obscuring the posterior pole. Funduscopic examination of the left eye showed yellow-white choroidal infiltrates that were presumed to be tuberculous in nature (48).

The diagnosis of ocular tuberculosis in patients with HIV emphasizes the importance of considering this diagnosis when evaluating patients immunocompromised by any etiology, including organ transplantation and hyperalimentation. Mansour and Haymond (47) reported a case of histologically proven bilateral choroidal tubercles in a renal transplant recipient with fever of unknown origin.

EALES DISEASE

In 1880, Henry Eales described a syndrome of recurrent retinal and vitreous hemorrhages categorized by abnormal retinal veins and capillary dropout in the peripheral retina in young men with constipation and epistaxis. However, the entity that Eales described was considerably different from that known today as Eales disease (62).

Eales disease is an idiopathic periphlebitis of the peripheral retina, usually bilateral, seen in persons of both genders and all ages. Although typically described as a periphlebitis involving the retinal venules, evidence suggests that the inflammation affects arterioles. The disease extends posteriorly, resulting in large areas of retinal nonperfusion. In these areas, neovascularization resulting in recurrent vitreous hemorrhages can occur. Retinal and vitreous fibrous strands may develop and cause traction and result in retinal detachment (62). Treatment of Eales disease is very similar to that of other vasoproliferative disorders of the retina and includes peripheral scatter photocoagulation for neovascularization and vitrectomy for persistent vitreous hemorrhages and fibrosis.

In the past, many investigators believed there was a relationship between Eales disease and tuberculoprotein hypersensitivity (63). There has been no evidence that the ocular or retinal involvement is caused by the tubercle bacillus (62). Recently, however, polymerase chain reaction has detected *M. tuberculosis* DNA in samples of vitreous (64) and epiretinal membranes (65) in patients with Eales disease.

TUBERCULOSIS OF THE RETINA

Histopathologic studies of patients with systemic tuberculosis have shown that direct infection of the retina by *M. tuberculosis* is rare. Most cases of retinal involvement are the result of contiguous spread from adjacent choroidal lesions (66). However, in 1986, Saini et al. (57) reported a case of a 3.5-year-old child with pseudoglioma diagnosed on histopathology to have retinal tuberculosis without concomitant choroidal involvement.

DIAGNOSIS OF OCULAR TUBERCULOSIS

The diagnosis of mycobacterial infection remains a challenge in ophthalmology. A definitive diagnosis requires the identification of *M. tuberculosis* organisms in ocular fluids or tissue. In tuberculous infection of the eyelids, lacrimal system, conjunctiva, cornea, and sclera, tissue for culture and histopathology is readily available. In cases of choroidal disease, access to such samples is usually limited to tissue obtained after enucleation because of the difficulty and morbidity of intraocular biopsy.

Microscopic examination of tissue or fluid smears for the presence of AFBs provides a rapid presumptive diagnosis. Culture of aqueous or vitreous fluid specimens results in higher sensitivity but at the expense of time. Available stains include a basic AFB stain, such as Ziehl–Neelsen, or a fluorescent AFB stain. The development of the polymerase chain reaction allows amplification of mycobacterial DNA

and shortens the time required to identify mycobacteria (64,65,67,68). An enzyme-linked immunosorbent assay to detect serum antibodies against purified cord factor, a component of the wall of the tubercle bacillus, has shown promise in patients with presumed ocular tuberculosis (69).

Although definitive diagnosis can be made only with fluid or tissue, ancillary studies, such as chest radiographs and the tuberculin skin test combined with the clinical presentation, can aid in a presumptive diagnosis of ocular tuberculosis. In 1983, Abrams and Schlaegel (70) studied 18 patients with presumed tuberculous uveitis based on improvement after an INH therapeutic test and resolution of inflammation without relapse during 1 year of antituberculous treatment. Eleven of 18 patients had responses of 10 mm with 5 tuberculin units of purified protein derivative, and nine patients had responses of 5 mm or less. Abrams and Schlaegel (70) concluded that "any response of erythema or induration may be significant in the diagnosis of tuberculous uveitis." In 1982, the same investigators had stated that a negative response to an INH therapeutic test excluded a possible tuberculous cause in patients with uveitis (38). However, this view is no longer accurate because of the prevalence of multidrug-resistant tuberculosis.

OCULAR COMPLICATIONS OF ANTITUBERCULOUS THERAPY

Ethambutol

Ethambutol, introduced in 1961 as a bacteriostatic agent against tuberculosis, works as a chelating agent by depleting the eye of zinc (71). Zinc is found in high concentrations in the choroid, retina, and ganglion cells and is used by retinol dehydrogenase for the transformation of retinol (72). This last step is important for color vision.

Most cases of ocular toxicity are bilateral and result from a dose-related retrobulbar optic neuritis that can be either axial or peripheral. Axial neuritis involves the papillomacular bundle. It reduces visual acuity and causes central scotomas and color vision deficits. The peripheral form usually occurs with higher doses and results in peripheral visual field deficits but stable visual acuity and color vision (71). Because the neuritis is retrobulbar, funduscopic examination appears normal. The current regimen with 15 mg/kg of body weight daily has an incidence of ocular toxicity of 0.8% (73).

Pretreatment ophthalmologic examinations are not routinely recommended. However, patients with ocular abnormalities that make changes in vision after initiation of therapy difficult to evaluate should be examined. Patients should be advised of possible visual changes and instructed to report these in a timely fashion (73,74). Electrophysiologic tests such as flash and pattern visual-evoked potentials and flash electroretinography (72) may be helpful in the early detection of ocular abnormalities.

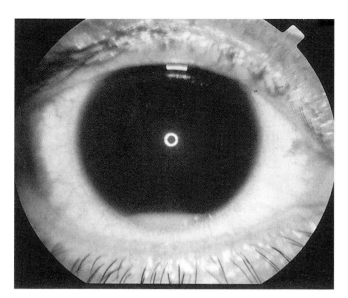

FIGURE 29.8. Rifabutin toxicity: hypopyon uveitis in an acquired immunodeficiency syndrome patient on rifabutin. (See Color Plate 17.)

Symptoms of ocular toxicity usually occur after 2 months of therapy, but Schild and Fox (71) reported a patient who developed symptoms after only 2 days of therapy at a dose of 25 mg/kg of body weight per day. Once symptoms of ocular toxicity are established, patients should be instructed to discontinue the medication. Visual recovery and resolution of visual field defects usually occur after the drug is stopped, but this may take weeks to months (75).

Isoniazid

The two most common side effects of INH are peripheral neuropathy and hepatitis (73). In 1955, Sutton and Beattie (76) reported a case of presumed INH optic neuritis and optic atrophy. In a prospective study of 1,000 patients receiving INH chemoprophylaxis, no ocular complications were found (77). This study helped to establish the rarity of ocular toxicity with INH.

Symptoms of visual loss have occurred from 10 days to 2 months after the initiation of treatment. Optic atrophy may be seen as a late finding (76). Treatment should be discontinued promptly when visual disturbance is noted.

Rifampin

Conjunctivitis is the most common ocular side effect of rifampin and varies from mild to severe. Some patients develop orange tears that can stain contact lenses and produce lens intolerance (74).

Rifabutin

Rifabutin has been implicated in the development of uveitis, in some cases severe enough to mimic infectious endophthalmitis (77,78) (Fig. 29.8).

Clofazimine

Clofazimine, which had previously been used in the treatment of dapsone-resistant leprosy, is currently used in AIDS patients with *M. avium-intracellulare complex*. Clofazimine produces brownish discoloration of the conjunctiva and brown swirls in the superficial cornea. These changes are without visual consequences (79,80). There have been two reports of a bull's eye maculopathy in patients treated with clofazimine. The patients demonstrated electrophysiologic changes consistent with generalized retinal degeneration. Patients on clofazimine should be monitored for macular pigmentary changes (81,82) (Fig. 29.9).

SUMMARY

Ocular complications of tuberculosis present a variable array of symptoms throughout the visual system. As with other extrapulmonary manifestations of the disease, diagnosis is frequently delayed, especially when there are no signs of active or past pulmonary infection. The current resurgence of tuberculosis in immunosuppressed patients with AIDS must heighten awareness of novel presentations of ocular infection. Once ocular tuberculosis is suspected and proven, treatment should be undertaken with close cooperation between the patient's internist and ophthalmologist.

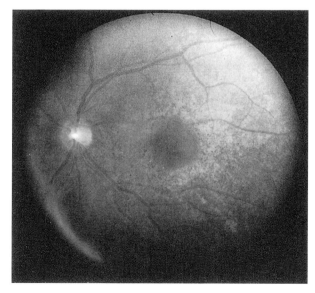

FIGURE 29.9. Clofazimine toxicity: bull's-eye maculopathy with mottled retinal pigment epithelium and central sparing. (See Color Plate 18.)

REFERENCES

1. Mifsud A. Medical history of JH Speke (1827–1864). *Practitioner* 1975;214:125–130.
2. Duke-Elder S, Perkins ES. Diseases of the uveal tract. In: Duke-Elder S, ed. *System of ophthalmology* (Vol. IX). London: Henry Kimpton, 1966:246.
3. Aclimandos WA, Kerr-Muir M. Tuberculous keratoconjunctivitis. *Br J Ophthalmol* 1992;76:175–176.
4. Duke-Elder S, MacFaul PA. The ocular adnexa: part I. Diseases of the eyelids. In: Duke-Elder S, ed. *System of ophthalmology* (Vol. XIII). London: Henry Kimpton, 1974:237.
5. Mohan K, Prasad P, Banerjee AK, et al. Tubercular tarsitis. *Ind J Opthalmol* 1985;33:115–116.
6. Sheu S-J, Shyu J-S, Chen L-M, et al. Ocular manifestations of tuberculosis. *Ophthalmology* 2001;108:1580–1585.
7. Zoric LD, Zoric DL, Zoric DM. Bilateral tuberculous abscesses on the face (eyelids) of a child. *Am J Ophthalmol* 1996;121: 717–718.
8. Mortada A. Tuberculoma of the orbit and lacrimal gland. *Br J Ophthalmol* 1971;55:565–567.
9. Sigelman SC, Muller P. Primary tuberculosis of the lacrimal sac. *Arch Ophthalmol* 1961;65:450–452.
10. Duke-Elder S, MacFaul PA. The ocular adnexa: part II. Lacrimal, orbital and para-orbital diseases. In: Duke-Elder S, ed. *System of ophthalmology* (Vol. XIII). London: Henry Kimpton, 1974: 725–728.
11. Eyre JWH. Tuberculosis of the conjunctiva: its etiology, pathology, and diagnosis. *Lancet* 1912;1:1319–1328.
12. Cook CD, Hainsworth M. Tuberculosis of the conjunctiva occurring in association with a neighbouring lupus vulgaris lesion. *Br J Ophthalmol* 1990;74:315–316.
13. Archer D, Bird A. Primary tuberculosis of the conjunctiva. *Br J Opthalmol* 1967;51:679–684.
14. Cassady JR. Tuberculosis of the conjunctiva. *Am J Ophthalmol* 1965;60:730–733.
15. Kamel S. Primary tuberculosis of the conjunctiva. *Br J Ophthalmol* 1950;34:322–327.
16. Whitford J, Hansman D. Primary tuberculosis of the conjunctiva. *Med J Aust* 1977;1:486–487.
17. Duke-Elder S. Diseases of the outer eye: part I. In: Duke-Elder S, ed. *System of ophthalmology* (Vol. VIII). London: Henry Kimpton, 1965:216–221.
18. Anhalt EF, Zavell S, Chang G, Byron HM. Conjunctival tuberculosis. *Am J Ophthalmol* 1960;50:265–269.
19. Chandler AC, Locatcher-Khorazo D. Primary tuberculosis of the conjunctiva. *Arch Ophthalmol* 1964;71:202–205.
20. Sollom AW. Primary conjunctival tuberculosis. *Br J Ophthalmol* 1967;51:685–687.
21. Gardiner PA, Michaelson IC, Rees RJW, Robson JM. Intravitreous streptomycin: its toxicity and diffusion. *Br J Ophthalmol* 1948;32:449–456.
22. Bellows JG, Farmer CJ. Streptomycin in ophthalmology. *Am J Ophthalmol* 1947;30:1215–1220.
23. Leopold IH, Nichols A. Intraocular penetration of streptomycin following systemic and local administration. *Arch Ophthalmol* 1946;35:33–38.
24. Liesegang TJ, Cameron JD. *Mycobacterium bovis* infection of the conjunctiva. *Arch Ophthalmol* 1980;98:1764–1766.
25. Donahue HC. Ophthalmic experience in a tuberculosis sanatorium. *Am J Ophthalmol* 1967;64:742–748.
26. Helm CJ, Holland GN. Ocular tuberculosis. *Surv Ophthalmol* 1993;38:229–256.
27. Bloomfield SE, Mondino B, Gray GF. Scleral tuberculosis. *Arch Ophthalmol* 1976;94:954–956.
28. Nanda M, Pflugfelder SC, Holland S. *Mycobacterium tuberculosis* scleritis. *Am J Ophthalmol* 1989;108:736–737.
29. Regillo CD, Shields CL, Shields JA, et al. Ocular tuberculosis. *JAMA* 1991;266:1490.
30. Walker C. Conglomerate tuberculosis of the iris with scleral perforation. *Br J Ophthalmol* 1967;51:256–257.
31. Oakhill A, Shah KJ, Thompson AG, et al. Orbital tuberculosis in childhood. *Br J Ophthalmol* 1982;66:396–397.
32. Khalil M, Lindley S, Matouk E. Tuberculosis of the orbit. *Ophthalmology* 1985;92:1624–1627.
33. Spoor TC, Harding SA. Orbital tuberculosis. *Am J Ophthalmol* 1981;91:644–647.
34. Miller BW, Frenkel M. Report of a case of tuberculous retrobulbar neuritis and osteomyelitis. *Am J Ophthalmol* 1971;71:751–756.
35. Mooney AJ. Some ocular sequelae of tuberculous meningitis. *Am J Ophthalmol* 1956;41:753–768.
36. Mansour AM. Optic disk tubercle. *J Neuroophthalmol* 1998;18: 201–203.
37. Minagar A, Schatz NJ, Glaser JS. Case report: one-and-a-half syndrome and tuberculosis of the pons in a patient with AIDS. *AIDS Patient Care STD* 2000;14:461–464.
38. Abrams JA, Schlaegel TF Jr. The role of the isoniazid therapeutic test in tuberculous uveitis. *Am J Ophthalmol* 1982;94:511–515.
39. Woods AC. Modern concepts of the etiology of uveitis. *Am J Ophthalmol* 1960;50:1170–1187.
40. Ni C, Papale JJ, Robinson NL, et al. Uveal tuberculosis. *Int Ophthalmol Clin* 1982;22:103–124.
41. Schlaegel TF Jr, O'Connor GR. Tuberculosis and syphilis. *Arch Ophthalmol* 1981;99:2206–2207.
42. Henderly DE, Genstler AJ, Smith RE, et al. Changing patterns of uveitis. *Am J Ophthalmol* 1987;103:131–136.
43. Weiner A, BenEzra D. Clinical patterns and associated conditions in chronic uveitis. *Am J Ophthalmol* 1991;112:151–158.
44. Cargill LV, Mayou S. A case of miliary tuberculosis in the adult. *Trans Ophthalmol Soc UK* 1906;26:101–107.
45. Illingworth RS, Wright T. Tubercles of the choroid. *BMJ* 1948;2: 365–368.
46. Jabbour NM, Faris B, Trempe CL. A case of pulmonary tuberculosis presenting with a choroidal tuberculoma. *Ophthalmology* 1985;92:834–837.
47. Mansour AM, Haymond R. Choroidal tuberculomas without evidence of extraocular tuberculosis. *Graefes Arch Clin Exp Ophthalmol* 1990;228:382–383.
48. Blodi BA, Johnson MW, McLeish WM, et al. Presumed choroidal tuberculosis in a human immunodeficiency virus infected host. *Am J Ophthalmol* 1989;108:605–607.
49. Olazábal F Jr. Choroidal tubercles. *JAMA* 1967;200:374–377.
50. Chung YM, Yeh TS, Sheu SJ, et al. Macular subretinal neovascularization in choroidal tuberculosis. *Ann Ophthalmol* 1989;21: 225–229.
51. Cangemi FF, Friedman AH, Josephberg R. Tuberculoma of the choroid. *Ophthalmology* 1980;87:252–258.
52. Gur S, Silverstone B, Zylberman R, et al. Chorioretinitis and extrapulmonary tuberculosis. *Ann Ophthalmol* 1987;19:112–115.
53. Bouza E, Merino P, Munoz P, et al. Ocular tuberculosis. *Medicine* 1997;76:53–61.
54. Wolfensberger TJ, Piguet B, Herbort CP. Indocyanine green angiographic features in tuberculous chorioretinitis. *Am J Ophthalmol* 1999;127:350–353.
55. Barondes MJ, Sponsel WE, Stevens TS, et al. Tuberculous choroiditis diagnoses by chorioretinal endobiopsy. *Am J Ophthalmol* 1991;112:460–461.
56. Lyon CE, Grimson BS, Peiffer RL Jr, et al. Clinical-pathological correlation of a solitary choroidal tuberculoma. *Ophthalmology* 1985;92:845–850.

57. Saini JS, Mukherjee AK, Nadkarni N. Primary tuberculosis of the retina. *Br J Ophthalmol* 1986;70:533–535.

58. Asensi F, Otero MC, Pérez-Tamarit D, et al. Tuberculous iridocyclitis in a three-year-old girl. *Clin Pediatr* 1991;30:605–606.

59. Barnes PF, Bloch AB, Davidson PT, et al. Tuberculosis in patients with human immunodeficiency virus infection. *N Engl J Med* 1991;324:1644–1650.

60. Humphry RC, Weber JN, Marsh RJ. Ophthalmic findings in a group of ambulatory patients infected by human immunodeficiency virus (HIV): a prospective study. *Br J Ophthalmol* 1987; 71:565–569.

61. Croxatto JO, Mestre C, Puente S, et al. Nonreactive tuberculosis in a patient with acquired immune deficiency syndrome. *Am J Ophthalmol* 1986;102:659–660.

62. Gieser SC, Murphy RP. Eales' disease. In: Albert DM, Jakobiec FA, eds. *Principles and practice of ophthalmology: clinical practice.* Philadelphia: WB Saunders, 1994:791–795.

63. Elliot AJ. 30-year observation of patients with Eales' disease. *Am J Ophthalmol* 1975;80:404–408.

64. Biswas J, Therese L, Madhavan HN. Use of polymerase chain reaction in detection of *Mycobacterium tuberculosis* DNA from vitreous sample of Eales' disease. *Br J Ophthalmol* 1999;83: 994–997.

65. Madhavan HB, Therese KL, Gunisha P, et al. Polymerase chain reaction for detection of *Mycobacterium tuberculosis* epiretinal membrane in Eales' disease. *Invest Ophthalmol Vis Sci* 2000;41: 822–825.

66. Ohmart WA. Experimental tuberculosis of the eye. *Am J Ophthalmol* 1933;16:773–778.

67. Musial CE, Tice LS, Stockman L, et al. Identification of mycobacteria from culture by using the Gen-Probe Rapid Diagnostic System for *Mycobacterium avium* complex and *Mycobacterium tuberculosis* complex. *J Clin Microbiol* 1988;26:2120–2123.

68. Bowyer JD, Gormley PD, Seth R, et al. Choroidal tuberculosis diagnosed by polymerase chain reaction. *Opththalmology* 1999; 106:290–294.

69. Sakai J-I, Matsuzawa S, Usui M, et al. New diagnostic approach for ocular tuberculosis by ELISA using the cord factor as antigen. *Br J Ophthalmol* 2001;85:130–133.

70. Abrams JA, Schlaegel F Jr. The tuberculin skin test in the diagnosis of tuberculous uveitis. *Am J Ophthalmol* 1983;96: 295–298.

71. Schild HS, Fox BC. Rapid-onset reversible ocular toxicity from ethambutol therapy. *Am J Med* 1991;90:404–406.

72. Dukes MSG. Drugs used in tuberculosis and leprosy. In: Leuenberger P, Meyer H, Baumann HR, eds. *Meyer's side effects of drugs,* 11th ed. Amsterdam: Elsevier, 1992:757–758.

73. American Medical Association. Antimycobacterial drugs. In: *Drug evaluations annual.* American Medical Association, 1994:1642–1643.

74. Fraufelder FT, Meyer SM. *Drug-induced ocular side effects and drug interaction,* 2nd ed. Philadelphia: Lea & Febiger, 1982.

75. Chatterjee VKK, Buchanan DR, Friedmann AI, et al. Ocular toxicity following ethambutol in standard dosage. *Br J Dis Chest* 1986;80:288–291.

76. Sutton PH, Beattie PH. Optic atrophy after administration of isoniazid with PAS. *Lancet* 1955;1:650–651.

77. Byrd CRB, Horn BR, Solomon DA, et al. Toxic effects of isoniazid in tuberculosis chemoprophylaxis. *JAMA* 1979;241: 1239–1241.

78. Saran BR, Maguire AM, Nicols C, et al. Hypopyon uveitis in patients with acquired immunodeficiency syndrome treated for systemic *Mycobacterium avium complex* infection with rifabutin. *Arch Ophthalmol* 1994;112:1159–1165.

79. Nêgrel AD, Chovet M, Baquillon G, et al. Clofazimine and the eye: preliminary communication. *Lepr Rev* 1984;55: 349–352.

80. Wålinder P, Gip L, Stempa M. Corneal changes in patients treated with clofazimine. *Br J Ophthalmol* 1976;60:526–528.

81. Cunningham CA, Friedberg DN, Carr RE. Clofazimine-induced generalized retinal degeneration. *Retina* 1990;10: 131–134.

82. Craythorn JM, Schwartz M, Creel D. Clofazimine induced bull's-eye retinopathy. *Retina* 1986;6:50–52.

Tuberculosis, Second Edition, edited by William N. Rom and Stuart M. Garay. Lippincott Williams & Wilkins, Philadelphia © 2004

30

TUBERCULOSIS OF THE HEAD AND NECK

**ANDREW G. SIKORA
STEPHEN G. ROTHSTEIN
KENNETH F. GARAY
RUTH SPIEGEL**

Tuberculosis (TB) of the head and neck, particularly of the larynx, was common before the marked decrease in incidence of TB in the United States beginning in the early part of the 20th century. From the years after World War I until the early 1980s, all forms of TB including TB of the larynx, ear, nose, and paranasal sinuses underwent a striking decline. This decline was reversed by the human immunodeficiency virus (HIV)/TB coepidemic beginning in the 1980s. The dramatic increase in HIV-infected patients provided a new and highly susceptible host population for *Mycobacterium tuberculosis*. Growing numbers of immigrants from areas of the world in which TB is poorly controlled, and urban poverty contributed new sources of infection and conditions favorable to the spread of TB. In parallel with the marked increase in all forms of TB, extrapulmonary TB including that of the head and neck region became more common (1,2).

The role played by HIV in producing the increase in extrapulmonary (including head and neck) TB during the 1980s and early 1990s was critical because patients with acquired immunodeficiency syndrome not only become infected with *M. tuberculosis* at a higher rate, but TB in HIV-positive patients is more likely to be extrapulmonary (2). Although head and neck TB during the pre-HIV era generally accompanied an obvious pulmonary focus of TB, HIV-infected patients with otolaryngologic manifestations of TB are likely to have atypical or even normal chest radiographs. The unreliability of classic radiographic findings,

coupled with the difficulty of accessing sites such as the larynx, middle ear, and nasal and sinus cavities for physical examination, culture, and biopsy, creates a formidable diagnostic challenge. Recent cases of head and neck TB reported in bone marrow (3) and kidney (4) transplant recipients suggest that as aggressive immunosuppressive regimens for transplant patients become more common, they may predispose to otolaryngologic TB as well.

Successful management of head and neck TB requires prompt recognition and diagnosis to facilitate the immediate institution of appropriate therapy. However, the symptoms and findings of TB in the larynx, ear, and other head and neck sites have changed, sometimes drastically, from those described in classic (preantibiotic) literature. Before widespread introduction of antituberculous chemotherapy, the patient with disease in the head and neck inevitably ran a progressively downhill course. Laryngeal, otologic, or nasal/sinus disease developed as delayed manifestations of ongoing pulmonary infection, and individual outcome generally depended on the course of the lung pathology. Tuberculous involvement of the head and neck primarily affected patients within the first three decades of life. The classic symptoms and physical findings of TB were defined during this period. Today, both classic presentations of tuberculosis and nonspecific, smoldering disorders resulting from incorrect diagnosis or unrecognized disease are seen. Because of changing demographics, the disease now occurs predominantly in the third to fifth decades (5). Dealing with an older patient population necessitates clinical differentiation of a suspected tuberculous pathology from an expanded group of other diseases such as chronic inflammatory disorders, other granulomatous diseases, and neoplasia.

From 1992 through 2000, the incidence of TB in the United States decreased by 45%, and in 2000, the rate was 5.8 cases per 100,000 population, the lowest ever recorded (6). Although extrapulmonary TB continues to account for 15% to 20% of all cases of TB, the absolute number of

A. G. Sikora: Department of Otolaryngology, New York University Medical Center, New York, New York.

S. G. Rothstein: Department of Otolaryngology, New York University Medical Center; Department of Otolaryngology, Tisch Hospital, New York, New York.

K. F. Garay: Center for Sinus and Nasal Disease, New York, New York.

R. Spiegel (Deceased): Department of Oral Pathology, Biology, and Diagnostic Science; University of Medicine and Dentistry of New Jersey; Piscataway, New Jersey.

extrapulmonary cases decreased by approximately 25% between 1994 and 2000 (from 4,265 to 3,220 cases) (7,8). If TB lymphadenitis is included, head and neck TB probably accounts for approximately one-fourth of these cases. Today, physicians rarely consider *M. tuberculosis* as a primary cause of head and neck disease. The diagnosis of head and neck TB must be based on a high index of suspicion in susceptible patients and familiarity with the new physical findings that have resulted from the widespread use of chemotherapy and changing patterns of disease spread and host resistance. Failure to understand that modern presentations of otolaryngologic TB are likely to differ from the classic presentations of the preantibiotic era can lead to missed or delayed diagnosis, with disastrous consequences for the patient. If recognized in a timely fashion, most cases can be successfully treated with anti-TB chemotherapy, sparing the patient further morbidity and allowing a return to previous function.

In this chapter, we consider otolaryngologic manifestations of TB in developed countries, focusing on the ear, nose, larynx, and other sites of the upper aerodigestive tract. We do not address neurologic, ophthalmologic, or orthopedic infections (i.e., cervical Pott disease); these are addressed elsewhere (Chapters 28, 29, and 37). Although infection with atypical mycobacteria, and mycobacterial infections of the cervical lymph nodes are briefly addressed, they are given more extensive treatment in Chapter 33.

LARYNGEAL TUBERCULOSIS

In the preantibiotic era, TB was the most common granulomatous disease involving the larynx (9). Two-thirds of all patients with tuberculous laryngeal involvement died, and

at least one-third of all patients with pulmonary TB had developed laryngeal involvement by the time of death (10). The pioneering laryngologist Chevalier Jackson estimated this number to be closer to 75% (11). Today, laryngeal TB is rare, even in HIV-infected patients. A recent case series of 146 patients with head and neck TB found that the incidence of laryngeal TB was 5.5% and was less common in HIV-infected than in immunocompetent patients (12).

Historically, laryngeal TB occurred as a secondary infection caused by an active pulmonary focus of the disease. Most, if not all, these patients had extensive cavitary pulmonary tuberculous lesions, easily documented on routine chest radiographs. The patient with laryngeal TB presented with weakness of the voice that would progress to intermittent or persistent hoarseness or to aphonia. Cough, hemoptysis, and ear pain, mediated by the superior laryngeal nerve, all became prominent symptoms with time. Although laryngeal TB could occur at any time during the course of the active pulmonary disease, most laryngeal symptoms developed within 6 to 12 months of the onset of pulmonary symptoms. The disease spread to the larynx by direct extension of organism-containing sputum from an active pulmonary focus. Virtually all patients had positive sputum smears. The bacillus invaded the laryngeal mucosa directly. Patients with cavitary lesions spent lengthy periods in bed, coughing and swallowing their infected sputum, resulting in lesions located primarily in the posterior area of the larynx (Fig. 30.1) (12a). In such a classic patient, the initial and most common laryngeal finding was a nodular swelling in the interarytenoid space that gradually spread along the aryepiglottic folds to the epiglottis.

Without antituberculous chemotherapy, there was progression of the lesion to painful ulceration, secondary bacterial or fungal infection with intense inflammation, exu-

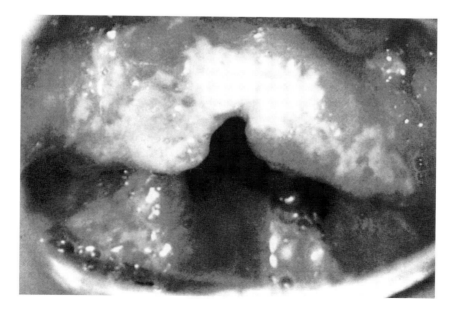

FIGURE 30.1. Tuberculous involvement of the epiglottis and aryepiglottic folds. (From Becker W, et al. *Atlas of ear, nose, and throat diseases,* 2nd ed. Stuttgart: George Thieme Verlag, 1984, with permission.)

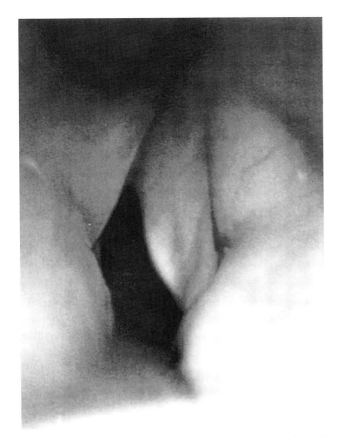

FIGURE 30.2. Diffuse laryngeal edema secondary to tuberculosis of the larynx.

berant granulomatosis and papillomatosis, and, finally, perichondritis of the underlying laryngeal framework (9). Vocal cord paralysis occurred from infiltration of the cricoarytenoid joint (9) or, more commonly, developed secondary to intrathoracic recurrent laryngeal nerve involvement by either active pulmonary lesions or fibrosis (8). Progressive, untreated laryngeal TB resulted in median fixation of the vocal cords with a characteristic, motionless glottic margin. Tubercle bacilli in sputum directly infiltrated the intrinsic laryngeal musculature. Cicatricial stenosis of the larynx inevitably occurred once the cartilaginous laryngeal framework was damaged, necessitating tracheotomy. This form of laryngeal stenosis only partially resolved with control of the disease (9). Surgical correction of laryngeal stenosis was generally unsuccessful before the development of broad-spectrum antibiotics in the 1950s. Thus, these patients were doomed to a permanent tracheotomy.

With the advent of antituberculous therapy, a markedly altered picture of laryngeal TB emerged. The infected patient is now ambulatory and does not need to be bedridden. Consequently, the intralaryngeal findings of TB are no longer restricted to lesions of the infected, sputum-drenched posterior commissure. Invasion of the local laryngeal tissues by direct extension of the bacillus is less frequent. Today, the extension of TB from its pulmonary focus may occur as miliary spread by lymphatic as well as hematogenous routes (5,13–17) and by the classic route of direct spread to the larynx in advanced pulmonary disease. The latter route occurs in most cases in nonindustrialized countries (18–20) and rarely may occur without any clinical evidence of pulmonary disease (21). Hematogenously spread TB manifests itself anywhere within the laryngeal interior (14). Although ulceration remains a finding in laryngeal locations such as the true vocal cords, in which the mucosa is adherent to the underlying structures, actual ulcers are rarely seen today (19). Edema and hyperemia are frequently the only findings in other areas of the larynx and may be the only finding in the true vocal cord in more than 50% of all cases (5, 22) (Fig. 30.2). Many patients develop multiple tuberculous lesions within anatomically distinct areas of the larynx (Fig. 30.3).

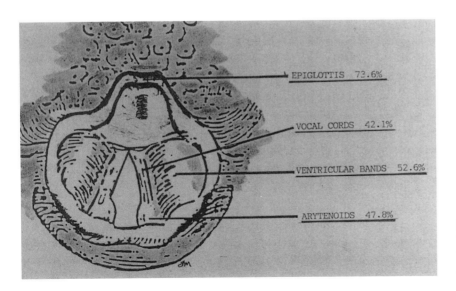

FIGURE 30.3. Locations of tuberculous infection of the larynx. (Modified from Soda A, Rubio H, Salazar M, et al. Tuberculosis of the larynx: clinical aspects in 19 patients. *Laryngoscope* 1989;99:1147–1150.)

Diffuse, edematous, nonspecific involvement has made the visual identification of laryngeal TB much more difficult than it was in the past, when the disease was characteristically a lesion of the posterior commissure (23). The diagnosis of TB of the larynx is even more difficult in the United States because of the frequent absence of a primary pulmonary focus or a suspicious or positive chest radiograph. In one contemporary study, two-thirds of patients with documented laryngeal TB seen at the Massachusetts General Hospital had either normal or minimally suspicious chest radiographs (22). In the nonindustrialized world, a positive chest radiograph continues to be a consistent finding in nearly 100% of cases. However, in industrialized society, an abnormal chest radiograph can no longer be relied on as the definitive diagnostic clue to the existence of laryngeal TB (5).

The reported significant coexistence of squamous cell carcinoma with TB in the larynx necessitates biopsy in all patients with laryngeal examinations suspicious for TB (5,22,24). In the study of Thaller et al. (22), the incidence of squamous cell carcinoma was 10%. The relationship between the two diseases remains unknown; however, both diseases share common risk factors related to substance abuse and socioeconomic status. In addition to squamous cell carcinoma, which it can resemble (25), TB of the larynx must also be differentiated pathologically from a variety of granulomatous inflammatory processes, such as sarcoidosis, polymorphic reticulosis, fungal infections, Wegener granulomatosis (26), midline granuloma, syphilis, and leprosy. Atypical mycobacteria, such as *Mycobacterium malmoense*, may rarely be the source of laryngeal infection (27); however, infection with *M. tuberculosis* is far more common. Because of its small size, the laryngeal biopsy alone may not yield sufficient histopathologic information to readily facilitate the diagnosis of TB. Although characteristic histologic evidence of granuloma formation with mononuclear lymphocyte infiltration, epithelioid and Langerhans giant cells continue to be found in two-thirds of laryngeal biopsy specimens, actual TB organisms are not always seen (5). Multiple or repeated biopsies are therefore required when suspicion has been aroused, along with both blood and sputum cultures and appropriate skin tests. Acid-fast bacillus (AFB) stains are positive in 70% to 80% of cases of laryngeal TB (15,28). Testing should continue until the diagnosis is either established or ruled out.

Early diagnosis and treatment are essential to avoid complications in the patient, to minimize exposure to patient contacts, and to protect medical personnel (22). The contagiousness of the patient with laryngeal involvement is directly related to the activity of the pulmonary process (24,29). Because laryngeal TB can be highly transmissible, scrupulous adherence to infection-control precautions is mandatory when suspicion is high. Any lesion of the larynx in a patient with a history of exposure or radiographic findings that even minimally suggest pulmonary disease should alert the examiner to the possibility of TB. In the presence of a laryngeal biopsy specimen revealing granuloma, confirmatory testing to exclude a diagnosis of TB should always be performed.

Most forms of extrapulmonary TB are sensitive to the same treatment regimens used to treat pulmonary TB in HIV-positive and -negative individuals (30). At present, the American Thoracic Society treatment recommendation for extrapulmonary TB (including laryngeal TB) is initiation of a four-drug regimen of isoniazid, rifampin, pyrazinamide, and ethambutol (31). It is important to obtain adequate cultures of sputum or biopsied tissue to guide antibiotic therapy, especially in HIV-positive individuals. Multidrug-resistant TB diagnosed by culture or disease that fails to respond to standard therapy must be treated with extended regimens. The response of the laryngeal lesions to anti-TB chemotherapy has been reported to be excellent, with most visible disease resolving within 2 months of initiation of treatment (22). Relief of symptoms such as throat pain and dysphagia usually occurs within 1 to 2 weeks of initiating antibiotics, and recovery of the voice to normal or near-normal quality is the rule (32).

In addition to antibiotics, supplementary therapies may be required for advanced disease. A short course of oral corticosteroid therapy has been suggested for rapid relief of painful dysphagia or impending airway compromise but is not necessary in most instances. A recent case report describes surgical treatment of a tubercular abscess of the larynx by incision and drainage (33). In exceptionally rare cases, tracheotomy may be required for respiratory insufficiency, either during the acute stage of the disease or after successful chemotherapy when there is glottic or cicatricial stenosis of the larynx or cervical trachea. Residual stenosis caused by loss of cartilaginous framework support by direct extension by active bacilli and subsequent intraluminal fibrosis may require reconstructive surgery to avoid a permanent tracheotomy. Laryngotracheoplasty and partial laryngectomy have been successfully performed for the correction of upper airway stenosis secondary to adequately treated TB (5). In these cases, despite excellent medical control of the active disease, extensive laryngeal fibrosis developed from mucosal invasion and cartilage exposure by the active bacillus. Prompt diagnosis and initiation of antituberculous chemotherapy are essential to minimize the potential for cartilage exposure and destruction with irreversible fibrosis.

TUBERCULOSIS OF THE EAR

Tuberculous involvement of the middle ear cleft and mastoid air cell system was responsible for 3% to 5% of all cases of both otitis media and mastoiditis at the turn of the 20th century (34). Before the advent of antituberculous chemotherapy, the bacillus was implicated as the cause of

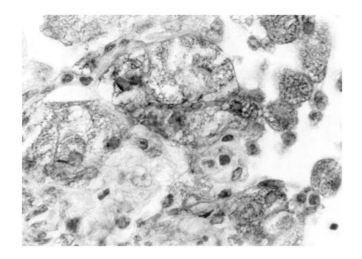

COLOR PLATE 1. Expression of inducible nitric oxide synthase (iNOS) in macrophages during infection of mice with *Mycobacterium tuberculosis*. Brown reaction product marks an immuno-histochemical reaction for iNOS in the lungs of wild-type mice. Tubercle bacilli (stained red) are contained within iNOS-positive macrophages. (From Mogues T, Goodrich ME, Ryan L, et al. The relative importance of T cell subsets in immunity and immunopathology of airborne *Mycobacterium tuberculosis* infection in mice. *J Exp Med* 2001;193:271–280, with permission.) (See Fig. 16.2 on page 221.)

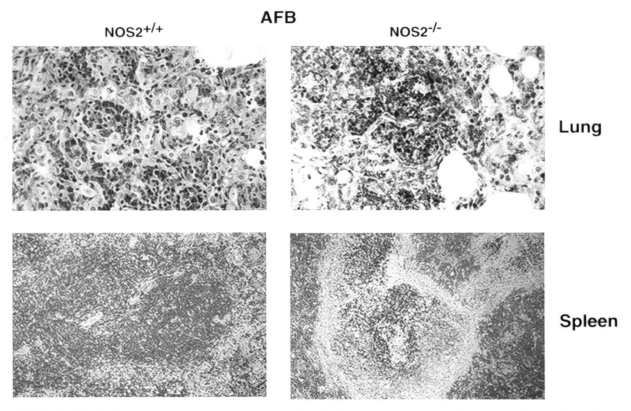

COLOR PLATE 2. Much more extensive growth of *Mycobacterium tuberculosis* in inducible nitric oxide synthase (iNOS)–deficient mice than in wild-type mice. Red-stained *M. tuberculosis* (acid-fast bacilli, *AFB*) are observed in much greater numbers in the lung and spleen 30 days after injection of 10^5 *M. tuberculosis* Erdman strain in iNOS-deficient mice ($NOS2^{-/-}$) than in wild-type mice ($NOS2^{+/+}$). (From MacMicking JD, North RJ, La Course R, et al. Identification of nitric oxide synthase as a protective locus against tuberculosis. *Proc Natl Acad Sci U S A* 1997;94:5243–5248, with permission.) (See Fig. 16.3 on page 222.)

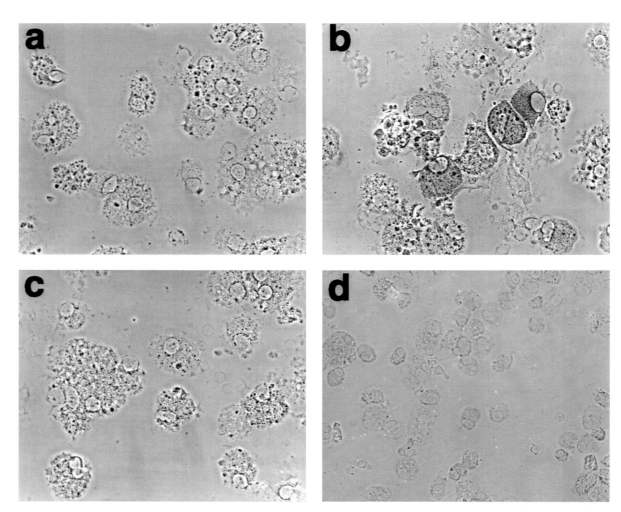

COLOR PLATE 3. Expression of inducible nitric oxide synthase (iNOS) in alveolar macrophages from human subjects with tuberculosis. **A–C:** Macrophages lavaged from the lungs of an individual with tuberculosis. **D:** Macrophages from the lungs of a normal subject. Immunocytochemistry was carried out with the following agents: **A,** preimmune serum; **B,D,** antihuman iNOS antipeptide antibody; **C,** as in **B** but with the reaction specifically blocked by the immunizing peptide. Results were similar in each of 11 patients studied. (From Nicholson S, Bonecini-Almeida MdG, Lapa e Silva JR, et al. Inducible nitric oxide synthase in pulmonary alveolar macrophages from patients with tuberculosis. *J Exp Med* 1996;183:2293–2302, with permission.) (See Fig. 16.5 on page 224.)

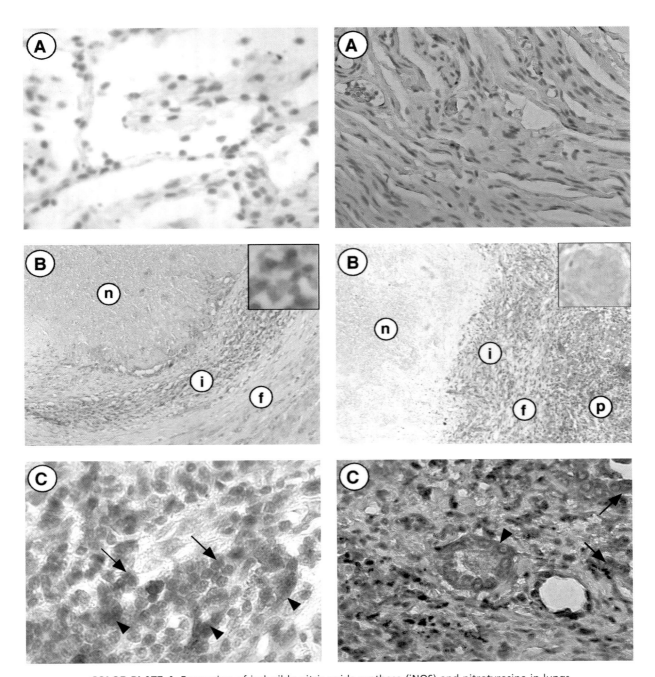

COLOR PLATE 4. Expression of inducible nitric oxide synthase (iNOS) and nitrotyrosine in lungs of patients with tuberculosis. Brown reaction product marks an immunohistochemical reaction for iNOS **(left)** or nitrotyrosine **(right)**. Each set of panels shows a field from a normal lung **(A)**, a granuloma from a surgically resected tuberculous lung **(B)**, and a field from an area of pneumonitis in a tuberculous lung **(C)** In the two panels **B**, the necrotic center (*n*), the inflammatory zone (*i*), the fibrotic capsule (*f*), and the surrounding pneumonitic area (*p*) are shown. The **insets** at higher magnification show iNOS in epithelioid macrophages **(B, left column)** and nitrotyrosine in a multinucleated giant cell **(B, right column)**. Comparison of Color Plates 1 and 3 and the present color plate indicates that tuberculosis in mice models tuberculosis in humans with respect to the expression of iNOS in *M. tuberculosis*–infected macrophages in the tissues. (From Choi HS, Rai PR, Chu HW, et al. Analysis of nitric oxide synthase and nitrotyrosine expression in human pulmonary tuberculosis. *Am J Respir Crit Care Med* 2002;166:178–186, with permission.) (See Fig. 16.6 on page 225.)

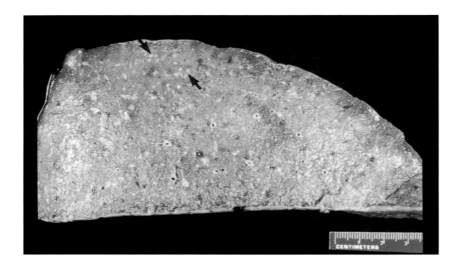

COLOR PLATE 5. Gross picture of miliary lesions in the lung parenchyma. (See Fig. 24.3 on page 325.)

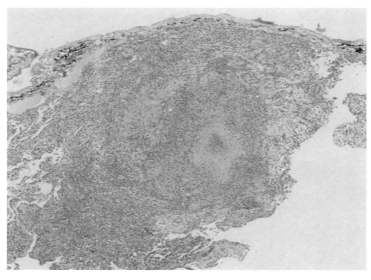

COLOR PLATE 6. Microscopic appearance of a miliary lesion on a hematoxylin–phloxine–saffranin stain. Note the central area of necrosis (original magnification ×20). (See Fig. 24.4 on page 325.)

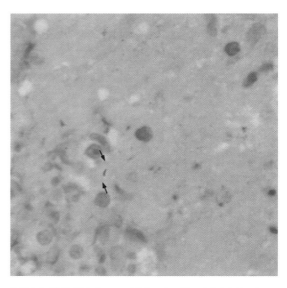

COLOR PLATE 7. Rare acid-fast bacillus (Ziehl–Neelsen, original magnification ×1,000). (See Fig. 24.14 on page 331.)

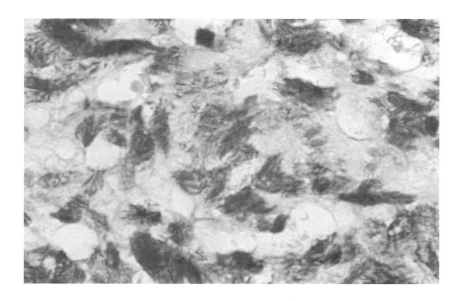

COLOR PLATE 8. Numerous acid-fast bacilli in a case of *Mycobacterium avium-intracellulare* infection (Ziehl–Neelsen, original magnification ×1,000). (See Fig. 24.15 on page 332.)

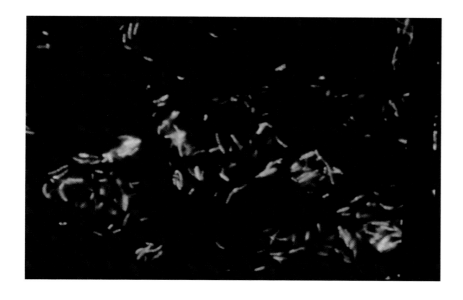

COLOR PLATE 9. Numerous mycobacteria on an auramine O stain (original magnification ×1,000). (See Fig. 24.16 on page 332.)

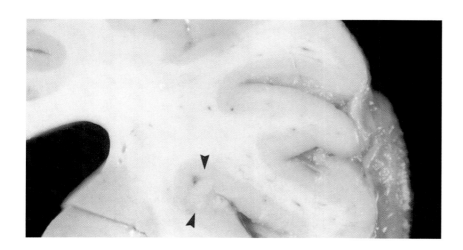

COLOR PLATE 10. Intraparenchymal necrotic lesion in the cerebral cortex of a human immunodeficiency virus–positive patient (*arrowheads*). (See Fig. 24.27 on page 341.)

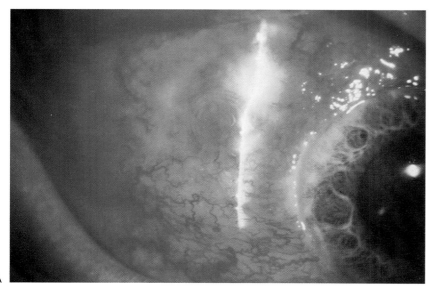

A

COLOR PLATE 11. A and B: Conjunctival infection with *Mycobacterium bovis*. (From Liesegang TJ, Cameron JD. *Mycobacterium bovis* infection of the conjunctiva. *Arch Ophthalmol* 1980;98:1764–1766, with permission.) (See Figure 29.1 on page 467.)

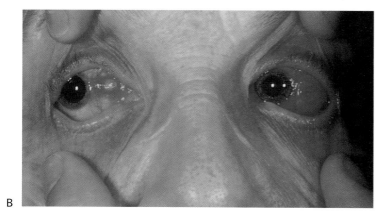

B

COLOR PLATE 11. *continued.*

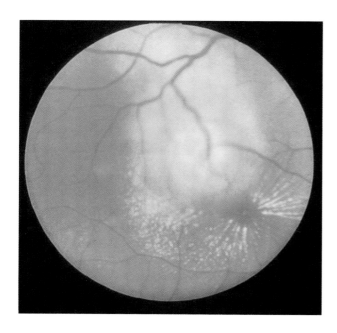

COLOR PLATE 12. Miliary tuberculosis: early choroidal lesion with macular star. (From Cangemi FF, Friedman AH, Josephberg R. Tuberculoma of the choroid. *Ophthalmology* 1980;87:252–258, with permission.) (See Figure 29.3 on page 470.)

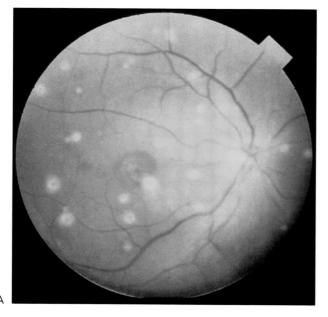

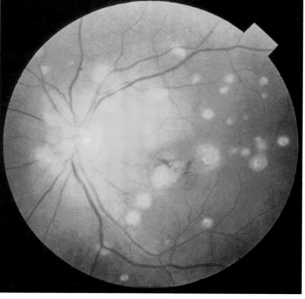

A

B

COLOR PLATE 13. Miliary tuberculosis: multiple choroidal lesions in the right **(A)** and left **(B)** eyes. (From Chung YM, Yeh TS, Sheu SJ, Liu JH. Macular subretinal neovascularization in choroidal tuberculosis. *Ann Ophthalmol* 1989;21:225–229, with permission.) (See Figure 29.4 on page 470.)

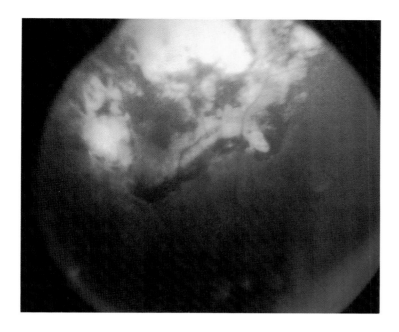

COLOR PLATE 14. Late choroidal lesion with darkly pigmented borders and pale center. (Courtesy of Alan H. Friedman, M.D., Mt. Sinai School of Medicine, New York, NY, U.S.A.) (See Figure 29.5 on page 471.)

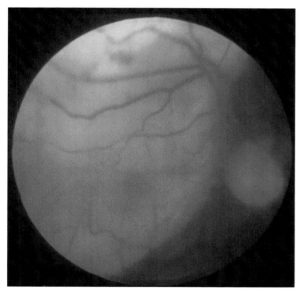

COLOR PLATE 15. Choroidal tuberculoma: large subretinal mass involving the macula. (From Lyon CE, Grimson BS, Peiffer RL Jr, Merritt JC. Clinical-pathological correlation of a solitary choroidal tuberculoma. *Ophthalmology* 1985;92:845–850, with permission.) (See Figure 29.6 on page 472.)

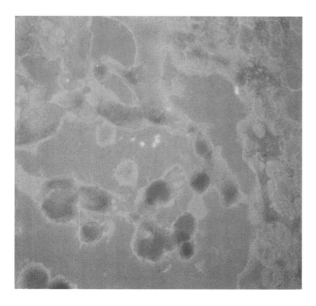

COLOR PLATE 16. Choroidal tuberculoma: double fluorochrome staining with auramine and rhodamine shows strongly fluorescing rods. (From Lyon CE, Grimson BS, Peiffer RL Jr, Merritt JC. Clinical-pathological correlation of a solitary choroidal tuberculoma. *Ophthalmology* 1985;92: 845–850, with permission.) (See Figure 29.7 on page 472.)

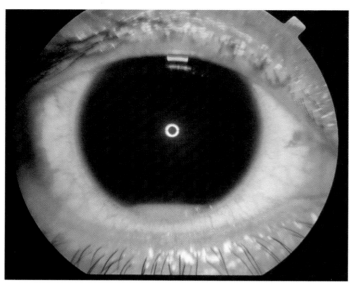

COLOR PLATE 17. Rifabutin toxicity: hypopyon uveitis in an acquired immunodeficiency syndrome patient on rifabutin. (See Figure 29.8 on page 474.)

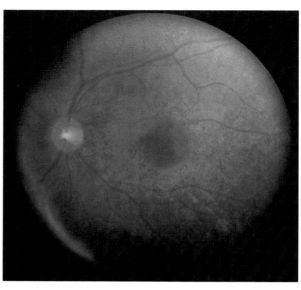

COLOR PLATE 18. Clofazimine toxicity: bull's-eye maculopathy with mottled retinal pigment epithelium and central sparing. (See Figure 29.9 on page 474.)

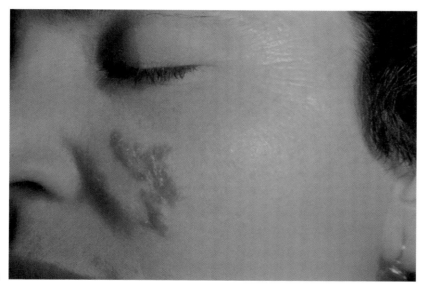

A

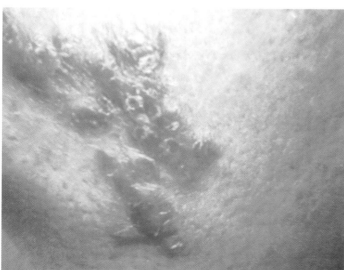

B

COLOR PLATE 19. A: Lupus vulgaris on the cheek. **B:** Close-up of lupus vulgaris. (Courtesy of Samuel Weinberg, M.D.) (See Figure 40.2 on page 597.)

15% to 50% of all cases of childhood chronic otitis media (35,36). At present, tuberculous otitis media remains a disease primarily of children and young adults (37,38). Adult-onset infections have been reported as late as 25 years after the initial development of otologic symptoms and apparently represent a failure to diagnose the tuberculous etiology initially rather than development of true adult disease (39). Today, otologic TB is extremely rare in the United States but is still prevalent in Asia and other Third World countries (40) and appears to have recently increased in frequency during the HIV/TB coepidemic. Skolnik et al. (41) found only 101 case reports of aural TB described between 1953 and 1985, whereas Mjoen et al. (42) found 93 new case reports between 1985 and 1990. Although the rarity of otologic TB precludes definitive epidemiologic study, it seems that the appearance of HIV-infected patients and increased immigration from developing countries have provided the opportunity for a recent reappearance of this disease (43).

Both direct and hematogenous routes of infection of the middle ear have been described. In the direct-spreading form, tubercle bacilli enter the eustachian tube from the nasopharynx during a cough, sneeze, or regurgitation from an active, preexisting focus in the pharynx, larynx, or lung. The shorter length and greater patency of the pediatric eustachian tube, along with its diminished angulation anatomically, predispose the middle ear of the child to infections from the nasopharynx and pharynx. This probably accounts for the much higher historic incidence of otitic TB in children compared with that in adults. The second, more common, mechanism of spread to the ear is the hematogenous route, whereby the bacillus reaches the mucosa of the middle ear through infected blood (44). Because tuberculous otitis media is primarily a mucosal disease, mastoid bone invasion and erosion develop only as a secondary process. Both middle ear cleft and mastoid air cells may become partially or completely occupied by granuloma. Extensive destruction of the ossicles, facial canal, bony labyrinth, and mastoid air cells may occur over time. Historically, facial nerve paralysis and labyrinthitis are the most common complications (45).

Myerson (45) stated "that a discharge from the middle ear appearing *without pain* in a tuberculous individual should be considered TB." Culture of this serous, *painless* otorrhea yields the bacillus if it is properly plated. Physical findings classically include multiple tympanic membrane perforations that are individually visible until there is coalescence into a large subtotal drum perforation (Fig. 30.4). However, more recent literature suggests that most patients will have progressed to a single large perforation by the time of initial presentation (46,47) The drum may be thickened with yellow areas of caseation, and pale granulation tissue may be visible in the middle ear (48). Tympanic membrane perforation, ossicular erosion, and proliferation of granulomatous tissue or ectopic bone in the middle ear (49) may

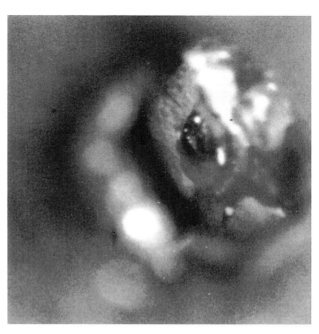

FIGURE 30.4. Tuberculous otitis media: coalesced tympanic membrane perforation with middle ear granuloma.

cause conductive hearing loss. Severe hearing loss, out of proportion with the duration of symptoms, is a common finding (45). Secondary pyogenic infection is common. Complications at this advanced stage of infection most commonly include facial nerve paralysis (50) and bony labyrinthitis (31). Petrous apicitis (51,52), direct and hematogenous extension to the middle and posterior cranial fossa, and direct extension into surrounding facial soft tissues have also been reported. All these symptoms and physical findings may be indistinguishable from otitis media or mastoiditis caused by pyogenic organisms.

Lack of consistent diagnostic features and the significant number of patients with aural TB in the absence of pulmonary infection make diagnosis challenging (53). Patients presenting with painless otorrhea, a suspicious chest radiograph, and a history of TB or exposure to TB-infected individuals are obvious candidates for diagnosis of mycobacterial disease (54). However, in the United States, only 50% of documented otitic TB patients have chest radiographic findings consistent with or suspicious of TB (41). Painless otorrhea may be the only consistent symptom of otologic TB seen today (55), and otologic symptoms have been reported as the sole manifestation of miliary TB in both immunodeficient and immunocompetent individuals (56). Although rare, atypical mycobacteria may infect the middle ear cleft as well: *Mycobacterium abscessus* has been described as a cause of otorrhea after placement of tympanostomy tubes (57).

In any unresolved case of chronic otitis, a high index of suspicion should be maintained for possible mycobacterial etiology, and both purulent discharge and abnormal mucosa should be generously sampled for AFB analysis and culture. Culture and stain of the middle ear exudate and/or a surgical biopsy of the middle ear granuloma or mucosa are usually necessary to establish the diagnosis. Culture of aural discharge has been reported to be positive in 92% of all patients with the disease (41). In culture-negative cases or in cases in which special mycobacterial cultures are not obtained, a tuberculous etiology may frequently go undetected until a surgical specimen histologically reveals the true nature of the disease (58). Antibiotic therapy is the cornerstone of treatment, with surgery generally reserved for management of complications and refractory cases. Early diagnosis is essential if successful treatment is expected with chemotherapy alone (59). Isoniazid plus rifampin is crucial for combination therapy because both enter the central nervous system. There are no large studies regarding treatment regimens for otologic TB; however, some physicians recommend 12 to 18 months of therapy.

In addition to removing tissue for diagnosis, surgical intervention may be required when otitis and mastoiditis are not confirmed as TB until after they have become well established (Fig. 30.5). At this stage, the removal of necrotic bone is usually necessary (39). A surgical approach is also indicated whenever complications, such as facial nerve paralysis, subperiosteal abscess, labyrinthitis, persistent postauricular fistula, and extension of infection into the central nervous system, occur (45,55,60). Surgery may also be required in the case of infection with strains resistant to standard chemotherapy (61,62). Elective otologic microsurgery should be delayed until a period of chemotherapy has been successfully initiated (39) or after the therapy is completed. Reconstructive procedures to improve conduc-

tive hearing disorders or restore the tympanic membrane should always be delayed until the disease is successfully controlled.

TUBERCULOSIS OF THE NOSE, NASOPHARYNX, AND PARANASAL SINUSES

Although asymptomatic infection of the adenoid pad may be common in patients with TB at other sites (63), clinical involvement of the nose, nasopharynx, and paranasal sinuses by TB is extremely rare (64,65). Nasal and sinus TB remains both silent and symptomless until it is well advanced. It almost always develops secondarily to a tuberculous focus elsewhere in the respiratory tract. Although the nasal mucosa is inherently very resistant to the tubercle bacillus, both trauma and atrophic changes facilitate the successful lodging of the bacilli within the nasal lining (66).

TB adenoiditis was once seen as a disease of children with pulmonary TB or of children whose parents had active TB. In the former, the adenoid pad and nose were bombarded by their own infected sputum, leading to a secondary focus of tuberculous infection in the nasopharynx. In the latter, the bacillus was airborne in the home environment and subsequently cultured from the nose and nasopharynx of these environmentally exposed children. This form of adenoid pad infection was uncommon even in the days of epidemic TB.

Miliary TB may produce microscopic lesions throughout the entire upper airway, but these lesions are found in the nasopharynx most frequently, if looked for postmortem (67). Today, miliary TB is primarily seen in immunosup-

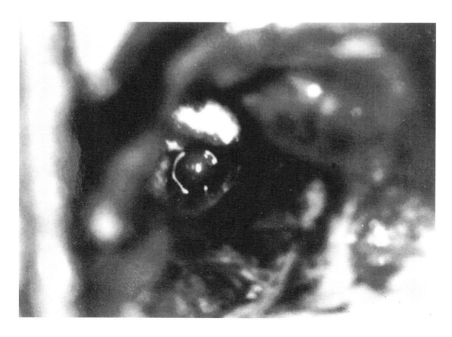

FIGURE 30.5. Tuberculous mastoiditis: large mastoid granuloma seen at surgery.

pressed or immunodeficient patients and, occasionally, in the patient on long-term steroid therapy (see Chapter 25).

The structural erosion secondary to TB in the nasopharynx, nose, and sinuses is similar to the destruction that occurs in the larynx. The direct-spreading form inevitably invades the nasopharynx, producing a characteristic ulceration and infiltration of the lymphatic tissue. Direct extension of the bacillus from the fossa of Rosenmüller to the eustachian tube and middle ear was once common (44).

Tuberculous involvement of the nasal cavity usually appears as a rapidly growing ulcer or tumor mass in the region of the quadrangular cartilage of the nasal septum. Frequently, a septal perforation develops that must be differentiated clinically from other granulomatous lesions or tumors. The anterior portions of the inferior turbinates are frequently involved in both the airborne and regurgitation varieties of the disease (66,68). TB rarely appears in the posterior nares, and the nasal floor is usually spared.

Direct extension of the tubercle bacillus from a nasal lesion into the ethmoid sinuses may occur. The organism may spread microscopically into the sphenoid, frontal, or maxillary sinuses through the sinus ducts (68). Tuberculous infection results in ulceration, formation of granulomas, and pain within the nose and infected sinus cavity. Other granulomatous disorders of the paranasal sinuses, in contrast, are frequently painless. The orbit may be invaded either by direct extension from the ethmoid or maxillary sinus or microscopically through the lacrimal duct. Direct extension of a tuberculous granuloma from a nasal focus into the cranial cavity, via the paranasal sinuses, has also been reported (67).

Bloody nasal discharge may be the earliest, possibly only, presenting symptom in nasal and paranasal sinus TB. Pain, nasal obstruction secondary to large granulomas, and dryness in the nose or throat are the classic symptoms of their involvement with the bacillus. Today, nasal endoscopy facilitates accurate evaluation of these vague symptoms. This technique allows a more thorough examination of the nasal interior and nasopharynx than previously was possible. Although culture of nasal or nasopharyngeal secretions for acid-fast organisms may yield positive results, biopsy is usually required to establish the diagnosis. Obtaining a specimen for histologic evaluation from the nose and nasopharynx is especially important because the differential diagnosis of disease may rest between TB and midline granulomas or carcinoma. Paranasal sinus endoscopy facilitates intracavity evaluation and biopsy of the mucosa or granulomatous mass. Endoscopy should always be used in the evaluation and, if indicated, biopsy of any suspicious lesion of the nasal cavity or paranasal sinuses.

As with the other forms of head and neck TB, prompt chemotherapy is the primary therapy of choice in dealing with infection of the nose, nasopharynx, and paranasal sinuses. A 9-month, three-drug protocol has been recommended (60). Before chemotherapy was introduced, cautery of nasopharyngeal or nasal ulcerations was recommended for pain relief, coupled with a regimen of strict nasal hygiene to minimize mucosal destruction (67). Although these treatments were symptomatically helpful, they have little application in modern management of the disease.

TUBERCULOSIS OF THE SALIVARY GLANDS

Tuberculous sialoadenitis may develop secondarily to infection in the oral cavity. Direct extension to salivary gland parenchyma by the bacillus may occur via the gland's ductular system. The parotid is the major salivary gland most commonly infected in this manner. Tuberculous disease is impossible to distinguish clinically from other diffuse inflammatory diseases of the salivary glands if a culture of the glandular secretions from Stensen duct or saliva is negative for acid-fast organisms. Computed tomography may reveal a diffuse enlargement of the infected gland, indistinguishable from other inflammatory pathology. Gland excision, for both biopsy and therapy, has long been accepted as the appropriate modality with which to deal with salivary gland disease (69). Superficial parotid lobectomy or total submandibular salivary gland excision provides the necessary tissue to establish an accurate pathologic diagnosis. However, subsequent prolonged chemotherapy is required to effect a cure.

Both the sublingual and minor salivary glands may become infected by direct extension from other oral cavity foci. Individual gland involvement without concurrent oral TB has not been reported (70,71). The primary treatment of choice for all forms of tuberculous sialoadenitis remains chemotherapy once the diagnosis has been made.

An unusual form of tuberculous lymphadenitis may involve the parotid salivary gland (72). Intraparotid and periparotid lymph nodes may become infected either by lymphatic drainage from the oral cavity or hematogenously from a pulmonary focus. The clinical picture varies from that of an acute infectious process to an indolent chronic one. Computed tomography may reveal discrete intraparotid adenopathy mimicking either benign or malignant tumor. Fine needle aspiration (FNA) of the intraparotid adenopathy may establish a diagnosis. If not, a parotidectomy may be warranted. When intraparotid lymphadenopathy is the result of an infection by atypical mycobacterium, total gland excision without awaiting trial of chemotherapy is recommended to eradicate the disease (73), although the lesion may infrequently resolve with antibiotics alone (74).

TUBERCULOUS CERVICAL LYMPHADENITIS

A tuberculous infection within the head and neck may result in involvement of the cervical nodes. Spread to the lymph nodes of the neck may occur secondarily to lymphatic drainage from an oral or pharyngeal tuberculous infection, hematogenously from a primary tubercular focus elsewhere in the body, or by direct extension from an adjacent infected organ. Cervical lymphadenitis is the most common head and neck manifestation of TB, and the cervical nodes are the most common site of tuberculous lymphadenitis (46,58,75). Whereas in adults, mycobacterial lymphadenitis is more likely to be caused by *M. tuberculosis* and accompanied by pulmonary findings and a positive purified protein derivative result, children are more likely to yield atypical mycobacteria and have negative purified protein derivative result and chest radiograph (76–78).

A neck node may be the first manifestation of a TB infection in the head and neck, but in an adult, cervical adenopathy must be considered a neoplastic lymphatic metastasis until proven otherwise. Consequently, some patients have had the diagnosis of tuberculous lymphadenitis made initially at radical neck dissection. The reported association of squamous cell carcinoma with laryngeal TB (5,22) and the increased incidence of all forms of TB in patients with head and neck cancer in general (79) complicates the diagnosis of TB lymphadenitis in adults and underscores the importance of bacteriologic and pathologic sampling.

Incisional biopsy (i.e., partial removal of the lymph node) has been associated with increased risk of chronic draining fistulae (80,81). Whereas the literature has classically supported excisional biopsy as the definitive diagnostic (and sometimes therapeutic) procedure, recent experience has shown the utility of FNA in the diagnosis of both tuberculous and nontuberculous mycobacterial lymphadenitis (75,82,83). FNA has excellent sensitivity and specificity for the diagnosis of mycobacterial lymphadenitis and should be used as the initial diagnostic test in suspected cases, along with a chest radiograph and purified protein derivative placement. Aspirated material is sent for AFB staining, mycobacterial culture and sensitivity testing, and cytology. Although not currently in wide use, polymerase chain reaction analysis of FNA aspirates is a promising technique that may soon allow identification and genetic typing of TB when only small amounts of sample are obtained or AFB and mycobacterial culture fail to yield the diagnosis (84). Open biopsy is reserved for patients with a negative FNA despite high clinical suspicion, when FNA is inadequate for drug sensitivity testing after failure of standard treatment, or in patients for whom treatment failure could be catastrophic (i.e., HIV infection).

In most cases, chemotherapy has proven quite successful in treating the bacillus within the lymph node, even in the absence of surgical intervention. Although treatment guidelines originally recommended extended courses of treatment, recent studies have demonstrated that short-course (6-month) treatment with multiple antibiotics is adequate treatment for most cases of tuberculous lymphadenitis (84,85). Infrequently, surgical excision may be performed as treatment for patients who fail chemotherapy or who present with advanced disease or tuberculous abscess (see Chapter 43 for additional discussion).

TUBERCULOSIS IN THE ORAL CAVITY AND OROPHARYNX

Tuberculous oral lesions are a relatively rare occurrence. Studies vary, but the incidence has usually been reported as less than 1% of the TB-infected population (86–89). Oral lesions may be either primary or secondary and may occur in both normal and immunocompromised hosts. Primary lesions are rare and usually occur in younger patients. Although the mechanism of primary inoculation is not completely established, it is believed that the organisms enter the mucosa through a small break in the surface (90–92). Oral lesions usually present as single or multiple painless ulcers and are often associated with enlargement of the regional lymph nodes. The ulcer frequently exhibits undermined edges with minimal induration and a granular or pseudomembranous base. Dimitrakopoulos et al. (93) reported two cases of primary oral TB. In both cases, patients exhibited painless ulceration of long duration and enlargement of the regional lymph nodes. The first case occurred as a painless gingival ulcer of approximately 2 months duration in a 17-year-old female patient. The second case started as a chronic gingival inflammation with bleeding around a mandibular molar and progressed, after extraction of the tooth, to an ulcer extending from the socket of the extracted tooth to the sulcus. The size of the ulcers ranged from 1×0.5 cm to 1×0.8 cm. The secondary (and more common) form of oral TB is often associated with pulmonary disease (91). Self-inoculation by the patient results from infected sputum or from hematogenous or lymphatic dissemination. Oral lesions present as single or multiple indurated, irregular, painful ulcers covered by an inflammatory exudate. A discrete bulging mass with granular or eroded and hyperemic surface may also be seen (91). Although secondary oral lesions may occur in any age group, middle-age and older individuals are usually involved (91–93).

Oral tuberculous lesions may occur at any location on the oral mucous membrane, but the tongue is most commonly affected. Other sites include the palate, lips, buccal mucosa, floor of the mouth, and gingiva. The oral lesions may present in a variety of forms, such as ulcers, nodules, tuberculomas, and periapical granulomas (93–95). The most common clinical presentation is odynophagia, with a duration ranging from 1 week to several years (91). The typical physical finding is of a single, painful ulcer with irregular borders covered by an inflammatory exudate, but atypical cases with multiple lesions or asymptomatic ulcers have been described (95). TB of the tongue has been reported in approximately 0.2% of all cases of TB (96,97). Prada et al. (98) described two cases (0.14%) in 1,471 patients. Both patients presented with a single painful ulcer diagnosed by biopsy, and in both patients, the tongue lesions were secondary to pulmonary TB. Tongue lesions are usually secondary, although primary TB of the tongue can occur (99). Saliva is believed to have a protective effect on the tongue, which may explain the paucity of tuberculous tongue lesions, despite the large numbers of bacilli contacting the tongue mucosa in a typical case of pulmonary TB (96–98,100–103).

An unusual case of secondary oral TB of the palatine tonsil was reported by Adiego et al. (87). A 50-year-old alcoholic man presented with a 1 × 0.7 cm left palatine tonsillar ulcer. Further examination revealed advanced pulmonary and multiple cerebral asymptomatic lesions. The identification of a tuberculous lesion in any location in the mouth is an unusual finding and its discovery is usually indicative of underlying pulmonary disease. Tonsillar TB is extremely rare but, if diagnosed, is usually a secondary finding. The tonsils can be involved in primary TB when there is a lack of host reaction or if the patient is immunosuppressed owing to chronic alcoholism, HIV infection, or the like (87,104).

Tuberculous gingivitis is an unusual form of TB that can present in a variety of ways, such as diffuse, hyperemic, nodular, or papillary proliferation of the gingival tissues (95). The previously discussed case reported by Dimitrakopoulos et al. (93) of an initial primary gingival lesion around a mandibular molar and subsequent ulceration is an example of one type of presentation.

It is difficult to differentiate oral TB from other conditions based on clinical signs and symptoms alone. Evaluation of the most common presentation, a chronic indurated ulcer, should prompt a clinician to consider both infectious processes, such as primary syphilis and deep fungal diseases, and noninfectious processes, such as chronic traumatic ulcer and squamous cell carcinoma (93,105). In the absence of other systemic involvement, excisional biopsy for histopathologic and bacteriologic examination with culture and sensitivity testing is often necessary for a definitive diagnosis (93,105).

The oral lesions of TB pose a potential infectious hazard to both patients and medical personnel unless barrier techniques are used. The bacilli are present at the base of most commonly encountered oral ulcers and other oral lesions. An outbreak of 14 cases of oral TB occurred after dental manipulation at two community dental clinics (99). A dentist who worked at both clinics had active TB. Mycobacteria were presumably deposited in the tooth socket at the time of extraction. The mycobacteria came from the dentist's fingers or from droplets expelled after coughing. Medical personnel are also at risk, as illustrated by the case of a physician who developed nasolabial infection after mouth-to-mouth resuscitation on a tuberculous patient (106).

Practicing infection control techniques can limit the threat posed to medical personnel (105).

OTHER HEAD AND NECK MANIFESTATIONS OF TUBERCULOSIS

Lupus vulgaris is a cutaneous tuberculous lesion in which tubercles occupy the upper layer of the dermis and extend peripherally until they coalesce with other areas in the skin (see Chapter 40). After tissue breakdown, healing occurs with significant fibrosis, scarring, and deformity. The external auditory canal, the pinna of the external ear, and the cartilaginous portion of the external nose may all be affected within the head and neck. The disease develops when contaminated exudate from tuberculous otitis media or intranasal granuloma infects the surrounding facial soft tissues. Lupus vulgaris of both the nose and ear has been successfully treated with antituberculous chemotherapy.

TB also occurs in the maxilla and mandible. Bony lesions are often the result of hematogenous spread of pulmonary TB. In a study reported by Meng (107), approximately 43% of patients with mandibular TB exhibited bony tuberculous lesions in other sites. Fukuda et al. (108) reported an unusual primary mandibular osteomyelitis in a patient with no history of pulmonary or bony tuberculous lesions. The infection spread from a periapical granuloma containing tuberculous granulation tissue when an infected tooth was extracted. Bhatt and Jayakrishnan (109) reported a case of tuberculous osteomyelitis of the mandible in a young child. The clinical presentation was similar to that of a dentoalveolar abscess.

Dilkes et al. (110) reported a case of primary TB of the cervical trachea presenting with dysphagia and a right supraclavicular lymph node. Bronchoscopy revealed a friable upper tracheal mass, and FNA revealed AFB (110).

TB rarely involves the thyroid gland, although it may present as a manifestation of miliary disease, as thyroiditis, and, uncommonly, as an abscess (111–113). As is the case in mycobacterial lymphadenopathy, FNA can be extremely useful in the workup of suspected TB of the thyroid (114,115). In a recent case report, an 11-year-old girl presented with a nontender nodular thyroid with a nuclear study consistent with a cold nodule. Surgical exploration revealed a cystic nodule with 30 mL of necrotic material that was consistent with *M. tuberculosis* (112).

SUMMARY

With the exception of cervical lymphadenopathy, TB rarely presents in the head and neck. Diagnosis may be challenging because suspicion of TB is usually low, otolaryngologic sites are frequently difficult to inspect or biopsy, and clinical presentations vary greatly and may overlap with those of nontuberculous causes of disease. The cornerstone of appropriate diagnosis is maintaining a high index of suspicion, understanding that modern presentations may differ considerably from classic descriptions of otolaryngologic TB, and ensuring that appropriate culture or biopsy material are sent for mycobacterial analysis. After the correct diagnosis is made, most head and neck TB can be successfully treated with anti-TB chemotherapy. Surgery is usually reserved for cases in which biopsy material is required for diagnosis, management of complications, and infections that fail to respond to antibiotics alone.

REFERENCES

1. Snider DE, Raviglione M, Kochi A. Global burden of tuberculosis. In: Bloom BR, ed. *Tuberculosis: pathogenesis, protection, and control*. Washington, DC: ASM Press, 1994: 3–11.
2. Hopewell PC. Overview of clinical tuberculosis. In: Bloom BR, ed. *Tuberculosis: pathogenesis, protection, and control*. Washington, DC: ASM Press, 1994:25–46.
3. George B, Mathews V, Srivastava V, et al. Tuberculosis among allogeneic bone marrow transplant recipients in India. *Bone Marrow Transplant* 2001;27:973–975.
4. Ishikawa K, Hoshinaga K, Maruyama T, et al. *Mycobacterium tuberculosis* infection of bilateral cervical lymph nodes after renal transplantation. *Int J Urol* 2001;8:640–642.
5. Soda A, Rubio H, Salazar M, et al. Tuberculosis of the larynx: clinical aspects in 19 patients. *Laryngoscope* 1989;99: 1147–1150.
6. Jereb J. Progressing toward tuberculosis elimination in low-incidence areas of the United States: recommendations of the Advisory Council for the Elimination of Tuberculosis. *MMWR Morb Mortal Wkly Rep* 2002;51:1–16.
7. Centers for Disease Control. *Reported tuberculosis in the United States, 1994*. Atlanta: CDC: Atlanta, GA, 1995.
8. Centers for Disease Control. *Reported tuberculosis in the United States, 2000*. Atlanta: CDC, 2001.
9. Jackson C, Jackson C. *Diseases of the nose, throat, and ear*. Philadelphia: WB Saunders, 1959:604–607.
10. Auerbach O. Laryngeal tuberculosis. *Arch Otolaryngol* 1946;44: 191–201.
11. Jackson C, Jackson CL. *The larynx and its diseases*. Philadelphia: WB Saunders, 1937:555.
12. Singh B, Balwally AN, Nash M, et al. Laryngeal tuberculosis in HIV-infected patients: a difficult diagnosis. *Laryngoscope* 1996; 106:1238–1240.
12a. Becker W, et al. *Atlas of ear, nose, and throat diseases*, 2nd ed. Stuttgart: George Thieme Verlag, 1984.
13. Vrabeck DP, Davidson FW. Inflammatory diseases of the larynx. In: English G, ed. *Otolaryngology*. Philadelphia: JB Lippincott, 1991.
14. Bull TR. Tuberculosis of the larynx. *BMJ* 1966;2:991–992.
15. Hunter AM, Millar JW, Wightman AJ, et al. The changing pattern of laryngeal tuberculosis. *J Laryngol Otol* 1981;95: 393–398.
16. Ramadan HH, Tarazi AW, Baroudy FM. Laryngeal tuberculosis: presentation of 16 cases and review of the literature. *J Otolaryngol* 1993;22:39–41.
17. Travis LW, Hybel SRL, Newman HM. Tuberculosis of the larynx. *Laryngoscope* 1976;86:549–558.
18. Rohwedder JJ. Upper respiratory tract tuberculosis: 16 cases in a general hospital. *Ann Intern Med* 1974;80:807–813.
19. Levenson M, Ingerman M, Grimes C. Laryngeal tuberculosis: review of 20 cases. *Laryngoscope* 1984;94:1094–1097.
20. Rupa V, Bhanu TS. Laryngeal tuberculosis in the eighties-an Indian experience. *J Laryngol Otol* 1989;103:864–868.
21. Kilgore T, Jenkins DW. Laryngeal tuberculosis. *Chest* 1983;83: 139–141.
22. Thaller SR, Gross JR, Pilch BZ, et al. Laryngeal tuberculosis as manifested in the decades 1963–1983. *Laryngoscope* 1987;97: 848–850.
23. Galli J, Nardi C, Contucci AM, et al. Atypical isolated epiglottic tuberculosis: a case report and a review of the literature. *Am J Otolaryngol* 2002;23:237–240.
24. Smallman LA, Clark DR, Raine CH, et al. The presentation of laryngeal tuberculosis. *Clin Otolaryngol* 1987;12:221–225.
25. Delap TG, Lavy JA, Alusi G, et al. Tuberculosis presenting as a laryngeal tumour. *J Infect* 1997;34:139–141.
26. Couldery AD. Tuberculosis of the upper respiratory tract misdiagnosed as Wegener's granulomatosis—an important distinction. *J Laryngol Otol* 1990;104:255–258.
27. McEwan JA, Mohsen AH, Schmid ML, et al. A hoarse voice: atypical mycobacterial infection of the larynx. *J Laryngol Otol* 2001;115:920–922.
28. Bailey CM, Windle-Taylor PC. Tuberculous laryngitis: a series of 37 patients. *Laryngoscope* 1981;91:93–100.
29. Omerod FC. Tuberculosis of the larynx. *Arch Otolaryngol* 1946; 44:191–201.
30. Horsburgh CR Jr, Feldman S, Ridzon R. Practice guidelines for the treatment of tuberculosis. *Clin Infect Dis* 2000;31: 633–639.
31. American Thoracic Society. Treatment of tuberculosis and tuberculosis infection in adults and children. *Am J Respir Crit Care Med* 1994;149:1359–1374.
32. Rohwedder JJ. Upper respiratory tract tuberculosis. In: Schlossberg D, ed. *Tuberculosis and nontuberculous mycobacterial infection*. Philadelphia: WB Saunders, 1999:154–160.
33. Muranjan SN, Kirtane MV. Tubercular laryngeal abscess. *J Laryngol Otol* 2001;115:660–662.
34. Jeanes A, Friedman I. Tuberculosis of the middle ear. *Tubercle* 1960;41:109–116.
35. Turner AL, Fraser JS. Reports for the year 1914 from the Ear and Throat Infirmary, Edinburgh Tuberculosis of the middle ear cleft in children. A clinical and pathological study. *J Laryngol Rhinol Otol* 1915;30:209–247.
36. Cox G, Swyer JG. Tuberculosis of the middle ear. *Arch Otolaryngol* 1929;9:414–421.
37. Hawkins D, Dru D, House JW, et al. Acute mastoiditis in children: a review of 54 cases. *Laryngoscope* 1983;93:568–572.
38. Plester D, Pusalkar A, Steinbach E. Middle ear tuberculosis. *J Laryngol Otol* 1980;94:1415–1421.
39. Sahn SA, Davidson PT. *Mycobacterium tuberculosis* infection of the middle ear. *Chest* 1974;66:104–106.
40. Case records of the Massachusetts General Hospital (case 27-1989). *N Engl J Med* 1989;321:34–43.
41. Skolnick PR, Nadol JB, Baker AS. Tuberculosis of the middle ear: review of the literature with an instructive case report. *Rev Infect Dis* 1986;8:403–410.
42. Mjoen S, Grontved A, Holth V, et al. Tuberculous otomastoiditis. *ORL J Otorhinolaryngol Relat Spec* 1992;54:57–59.
43. Centers for Disease Control. Diagnosis and management of mycobacterial infection and disease in persons with human immunodeficiency virus infection. *Ann Intern Med* 1986;106: 254–256.
44. Lincoln E, Sewell EM. *Tuberculosis in children*. New York: McGraw-Hill, 1963:220–222.
45. Myerson MC, Gilbert JG. Tuberculosis of the middle ear and mastoid. *Arch Otolaryngol* 1941;33:231–250.

46. Williams RG and Douglas-Jones T. *Mycobacterium* marches back. *J Laryngol Otol* 1995;109:5–13.

47. Windle-Taylor PC, Bailey CM. Tuberculous otitis media: a series of 22 patients. *Laryngoscope* 1980;90:1039–1044.

48. McHill TJI. Mycotic infection of the temporal bone. *Arch Otolaryngol* 1978;104:140–144.

49. Linthicum F. Temporal bone histopathology case of the month: tuberculous otitis media. *Otol Neurol* 2002;23:235–236.

50. Samuel J and Fernandes CMC. Tuberculous mastoiditis. *Ann Otol Rhinol Laryngol* 1986;95:264–266.

51. Kearns DB, Coker NJ, Pitcock JK, et al. Tuberculous petrous apicitis. *Arch Otolaryngol* 1985;111:406–408.

52. Kumar S, Puri V, Malik R, et al. Tuberculosis of petrous apex. *Indian Pediatr* 1991;28:407–409.

53. Robertson K, Kumar A. Atypical presentations of aural tuberculosis. *Am J Otolaryngol* 1995;16:294–302.

54. Case records of the Massachusetts General Hospital (case 25-1987). *N Engl J Med* 1987;316:1589–1597.

55. Glover S, Tranter RMD, Innes JA. Tuberculous otitis media—a reminder. *J Laryngol Otol* 1981;95:1261–1264.

56. Vomero E, Ratner SJ. Diagnosis of miliary tuberculosis by examination of middle ear discharge. *Arch Otolaryngol* 1988;114:1029–1030.

57. Franklin DJ, Starke JR, Brady MT, et al. Chronic otitis media after tympanostomy tube placement caused by *Mycobacterium abscessus*: a new clinical entity? *Am J Otol* 1994;15:313–320.

58. Lee KC, Schecter G. Tuberculous infections of the head and neck. *Ear Nose Throat J* 1995;74:395–399.

59. Wallner LJ. Tuberculosis otitis media. *Laryngoscope* 1953;63:1058–1077.

60. Lucente F, Tobias GW, Parisier SC. Tuberculous otitis media. *Laryngoscope* 1978;88:1107–1116.

61. Ma KH, Tang PS, Chan KW. Aural tuberculosis. *Am J Otol* 1990;11:174–177.

62. Weiner GM, O'Connell JE, Pahor AL. The role of surgery in tuberculous mastoiditis: appropriate chemotherapy is not always enough. *J Laryngol Otol* 1997;111:752–753.

63. Lugton I. Mucosa-associated lymphoid tissues as sites for uptake, carriage and excretion of tubercle bacilli and other pathogenic mycobacteria. *Immunol Cell Biol* 1999;77:364–372.

64. Lau S, Kwan S, Lee J, et al. Source of tubercle bacilli in cervical lymph nodes: a prospective study. *J Laryngol Otol* 1991;105:558–561.

65. Jang YJ, Jung SW, Koo TW, et al. Sinonasal tuberculosis associated with osteomyelitis of the ethmoid bone and cervical lymphadenopathy. *J Laryngol Otol* 2001;115:736–739.

66. Hyams VJ. Pathology of the nose and paranasal sinuses. In: English GM, ed. *Otolaryngology*. Philadelphia: JB Lippincott, 1991:24–25.

67. Leukins RM. Tuberculosis of the nose and nasopharynx. In: Jackson CJ, ed. *Diseases of the nose, throat, and ear*. Philadelphia: WB Saunders, 1959:36–39.

68. Page JR, Jash DK. Tuberculosis of the nose and paranasal sinuses. *J Laryngol Otol* 1974;88:579–583.

69. Rankow R, Polayas I. *Diseases of the salivary glands*. Philadelphia: WB Saunders, 1976:165–183.

70. Donohue W, Bolden TE. Tuberculosis of the salivary glands: a collective review. *Oral Surg* 1961;14:576.

71. Epker BN. Obstructive inflammatory disease of the major salivary glands. *Oral Surg Oral Med Oral Pathol* 1972;33:2–27.

72. Tunkel DE. Atypical mycobacterial adenitis presenting as a parotid abscess. *Am J Otolaryngol* 1995;16:428–432.

73. Waldman RH. Tuberculosis and the atypical mycobacteria. *Otolaryngol Clin North Am* 1982;15:581–596.

74. Jervis PN, Lee JA, Bull PD. Management of non-tuberculous mycobacterial peri-sialadenitis in children: the Sheffield otolaryngology experience. *Clin Otolaryngol* 2001;26:243–248.

75. Lee KC, Tami TA, Lalwani AK, et al. Contemporary management of cervical tuberculosis. *Laryngoscope* 1992;102:60–64.

76. Kanlikama M, Mumbuc S, Bayazit Y, et al. Management strategy of mycobacterial cervical lymphadenitis. *J Laryngol Otol* 2000;114:274–278.

77. Tunkel DE, Baroody FM, Sherman ME. Fine-needle aspiration biopsy of cervicofacial masses in children. *Arch Otolaryngol Head Neck Surg* 1995;121:533–536.

78. Rahal A, Abela A, Arcand PH, et al. Nontuberculous mycobacterial adenitis of the head and neck in children: experience from a tertiary care pediatric center. *Laryngoscope* 2001;111:1791–1796.

79. Libshitz HI, Pannu HK, Elting LS, et al. Tuberculosis in cancer patients: an update. *J Thorac Imaging* 1997;12:41–46.

80. Cantrell RW, Jensen JH, Reid D. Diagnosis and management of tuberculous cervical adenitis. *Arch Otolaryngol* 1975;101:53–57.

81. Hooper AA. Tuberculous peripheral lymphadenitis. *Br J Surg* 1972;59:353–359.

82. Lau SK, Wei WI, Hsu C, et al. Efficacy of fine needle aspiration cytology in the diagnosis of tuberculous cervical lymphadenopathy. *J Laryngol Otol* 1990;104:24–27.

83. Jha BC, Dass A, Nagarkar NM, et al. Cervical tuberculous lymphadenopathy: changing clinical pattern and concepts in management. *Postgrad Med J* 2001;77:185–187.

84. Yuen AP, Wong SH, Tam CM, et al. Prospective randomized study of thrice weekly six-month and nine-month chemotherapy for cervical tuberculous lymphadenopathy. *Otolaryngol Head Neck Surg* 1997;116:189–192.

85. van Loenhout-Rooyackers JH, Laheij RJ, Richter C, et al. Shortening the duration of treatment for cervical tuberculous lymphadenitis. *Eur Respir J* 2000;15:192–195.

86. Haddad N, Zaytoun GM, Hadi U. Tuberculosis of the soft palate: an unusual presentation of oral tuberculosis. *Otolaryngol Head Neck Surg* 1987;97:91–92.

87. Adiego M, Millan J, Royo J, et al. Unusual association of secondary tonsillar and cerebral tuberculosis. *J Otolaryngol Oncol* 1994;108:348–349.

88. Anim J, Daulatly EE. Tuberculosis of the tonsil revisited. *West Afr J Med* 1991;10:194–197.

89. Anil S, Ellepola AN, Samaranayake LP, et al. Tuberculous ulcer of the tongue as presenting feature of pulmonary tuberculosis and HIV infection. *Gen Dent* 2000;48:458–461.

90. Mignogna MD, Muzio LL, Favia G, et al. Oral tuberculosis: a clinical evaluation of 42 cases. *Oral Dis* 2000;6:25–30.

91. Eng HL, Lu SY, Yang CH, et al. Oral tuberculosis. *Oral Surg Oral Med Oral Pathol Oral Radiol Endod* 1996;81:415–420.

92. Sierra C, Fortun J, Barros C, et al. Extra-laryngeal head and neck tuberculosis. *Clin Microbiol Infect* 2000;6:644–648.

93. Dimitrakopoulos I, Zouloumis L, Lazaridis N, et al. Primary tuberculosis of the oral cavity. *Oral Surg Oral Med Oral Pathol* 1991;72:712–715.

94. Lathan SR. Tuberculosis of the palate [Letter]. *JAMA* 1971;216:521.

95. Shafer WG, Hine MK, Levy MB. *A textbook of oral pathology*. Philadelphia: WB Saunders, 1983:340–440.

96. Komer H, Shaefer RF, Mahoney PL. Bilateral tuberculous granulomas of the tongue. *Arch Otolaryngol* 1965;82:649–651.

97. Hashimoto Y, Tanioka H. Primary tuberculosis of the tongue: report of a case. *J Oral Maxillofac Surg* 1989;47:744–746.

98. Prada JI, Kindelan JM, Villanueva JL, et al. Tuberculosis of the tongue in two immunocompetent patients [Letter]. *Clin Infect Dis* 1994;19:200–202.

99. Gupta A, Shinde KJ, Bhardwaj I. Primary lingual tuberculosis: a case report. *J Laryngol Otol* 1998;112:86–87.

100. Weaver RA. Tuberculosis of the tongue. *JAMA* 1976;235:2418.
101. Molina M, Ortega G, Montoya JJ, et al. Tuberculosis de la lengua. Presentacion de 2 casos. [Letter]. *Med Clin (Barcelona)* 1987;88:212.
102. Engleman W, Putney FJ. Tuberculosis of the tongue. *Trans Am Acad Ophthalmol Otolaryngol* 1972;76:1384–1386.
103. Ladron de Guerva R. Tuberculosis ulcer of the tongue: clinical case. *Odontol Chil* 1989;37:277–279.
104. Kardon DE, Thompson LD. A clinicopathologic series of 22 cases of tonsillar granulomas. *Laryngoscope* 2000;110:476–481.
105. Regezi J, Sciubba JJ. *Oral pathology: clinical-pathological correlations*. Philadelphia: WB Saunders, 1989.
106. Heilman KM, Muschenheim C. Primary cutaneous tuberculosis resulting from mouth-to-mouth respiration. *N Engl J Med* 1965;273:1035–1036.
107. Meng CM. Tuberculosis of the mandible. *J Bone Joint Surg* 1940;22:17–27.
108. Furuda J, Shingo Y, Miyako H. Primary tuberculous osteomyelitis of the mandible: a case report. *Oral Surg Oral Med Oral Pathol* 1992;73:278–280.
109. Bhatt AP, Jayakrishnan A. Tuberculous osteomyelitis of the mandible: a case report. *Int J Paediatr Dent* 2001;11:304–308.
110. Dilkes MG, Gautama P, Knowles CH, et al. Primary tracheal tuberculosis in an otherwise healthy 65-year-old Caucasian woman. *J Laryngol Otol* 1993;107:1052–1053.
111. Barnes P, Weatherstone R. Tuberculosis of the thyroid: two case reports. *Br J Dis Chest* 1979;73:187–191.
112. Surer I, Ozturk H, Cetinkursun S. Unusual presentation of tuberculosis reactivation in childhood: an anterior neck mass. *J Pediatr Surg* 2000;35:1263–1265.
113. Khan EM, Haque I, Pandey R, et al. Tuberculosis of the thyroid gland: a clinicopathological profile of four cases and review of the literature. *Aust N Z J Surg* 1993;63:807–810.
114. Mondal A, Patra DK. Efficacy of fine needle aspiration cytology in the diagnosis of tuberculosis of the thyroid gland: a study of 18 cases. *J Laryngol Otol* 1995;109:36–38.
115. Das DK, Pant CS, Chachra KL, et al. Fine needle aspiration cytology diagnosis of tuberculous thyroiditis. A report of eight cases. *Acta Cytol* 1992;36:517–522.

MYCOBACTERIAL LYMPHADENITIS

MARK F. SLOANE

Mycobacterial lymphadenitis has plagued humanity since prerecorded times (1). The classic term *scrofula* is derived from the Latin for *glandular swelling* or from the French *full-necked sow*. Diagnosis and treatment have varied widely over the centuries. Whereas Herodotus suggested the isolation of these afflicted souls (2,3), the European kings of the Middle Ages imparted the royal touch to cure the "King's evil," to which mycobacterial lymphadenitis was referred (4). In contrast, Albucasis in his *Practica* included surgical excision of involved glands (3,5,6). In the 17th century, digitalis was used in therapy (7). Lugol, in the 18th century, believed the origin of scrofula to be similar to that of a goiter and so recommended an iodine-rich solution (Lugol solution) as a cure (2,4). The microbiologic cause of scrofula was first appreciated by Bollinger, May, and Demme in the mid- to late-19th century, when they noted that *Mycobacterium bovis* from cows was the cause of this ailment (2). In 1882, Robert Koch identified the tubercle bacillus.

EPIDEMIOLOGY

Tuberculosis of the peripheral lymph nodes is one of the most common forms of extrapulmonary tuberculosis (8–10). Cervical lymph nodes are the most common site of involvement, with or without associated disease of other lymphoid tissue (11,12). The causes of mycobacterial lymphadenitis include *Mycobacterium tuberculosis*, *M. bovis*, *Mycobacterium africanum*, and the atypical mycobacteria [often collectively referred to as nontuberculous mycobacteria (NTM)]. Three of the atypical mycobacteria are known to cause lymphadenitis: *Mycobacterium scrofulaceum*, *Mycobacterium avium-intracellulare complex*, and *Mycobacterium kansasii*. There is significant geographic variation in the prevalence of the atypical mycobacteria. For

example, in Australia (13) and British Columbia (14), these atypical organisms were detected ten times more frequently than *M. tuberculosis*. In contrast, in Kenya *M. tuberculosis* was found to be the pathogen in 72% of cases of cervical mycobacterial lymphadenitis (15). Additionally, there have been changing trends in the prevalence of pathogens over time. In southeast England, for example, there has been a decrease in *M. tuberculosis* lymphadenitis and an increase in lymphadenitis caused by the atypical organisms (16). Similarly, in Japan, where many cases of cervical lymphadenitis have been described, no cases were noted until 1867 (15). In the United States, *M. tuberculosis* accounts for approximately 95% of mycobacterial lymphadenitis in adults, whereas *M. bovis* is rarely seen in the United States today (17,18). In children, however, 92% of cases of mycobacterial lymphadenitis are caused by NTM, and the remainder are owing to *M. tuberculosis* (19). Of note, *M. scrofulaceum* is the most common cause of NTM lymphadenitis in the United States (2).

Peripheral mycobacterial lymphadenitis most frequently affects patients in their second and third decades but may afflict patients of any age. In numerous studies, there is a female predominance (approximately 2:1) (9,20–23). Additionally, the prevalence of disease varies by ethnic group, that is, a significantly higher frequency of disease is noted in populations extracted from endemic regions. Thompson et al. (12), in a review of 67 patients with mycobacterial lymphadenitis from the United Kingdom, found that 81% of patients were of Indian, Pakistani, or Bangladeshi origin, whereas less than 10% of their region's overall population was from the Indian subcontinent. Similar ethnic predispositions have been observed regarding patients from Southeast Asia and Africa, and Native Americans (24). Lee et al. (25) found a high frequency of disease in Asian and Hispanic patients in the San Francisco area. Several authors suggested that in addition to an increased frequency of tuberculosis in patients of Asian origin, there appears to be a predilection for lymphatic involvement in these populations (4,26). Similarly, blacks appear to have a predilection for tuberculous lymphadenitis as well (27,28). Finally, infection with the human immunodeficiency virus (HIV) is

M. F. Sloane: Department of Medicine, Division of Pulmonary and Critical Care Medicine, New York University School of Medicine; Medical Intensive Care Unit, Division of Pulmonary and Critical Care Medicine, New York University Medical Center; New York Pulmonary Associates, New York, New York.

associated with an increased frequency of mycobacterial infections in general and lymph node involvement in particular (25,29–32). Soriano et al. (33) compared tuberculosis in HIV-seropositive and HIV-seronegative patients in Spain; lymphadenitis was present in 25 (39%) of 65 HIV-seropositive patients, whereas none of the 65 seronegative patients had lymph node involvement.

PRESENTATION

Tuberculous lymphadenitis is generally thought to be a local manifestation of a systemic disease. *M. tuberculosis* generally enters the human body via the respiratory tract and undergoes lymphohematogenous dissemination. Given the pulmonary route of organism entry, the first lymphoid tissues encountered are presumably hilar and mediastinal lymph nodes. These nodes, however, are rarely reported as the site of *M. tuberculosis* lymphadenitis. Peripheral lymph nodes, especially in the cervical regions, are the most common sites of lymphadenopathy caused by *M. tuberculosis* (11,12,18,24). Peripheral lymphadenitis may occur at the time of initial infection (as seen in young children or the immunocompromised) or may reflect a reactivation of a prior primary infection. Host factors such as age, gender, race, and immunocompetence affect the clinical presentation. In contrast, lymphadenitis owing to NTM appears to be the result of a local infection in which the pathogens enter via oropharyngeal mucosa, salivary glands, tonsils, gingiva, or conjunctiva (18,34).

Clinical presentation differs significantly between *M. tuberculosis* and NTM lymphadenitis. NTM lymphadenitis commonly involves upper cervical lymph nodes, salivary glands, and surrounding nodes (24,35,36). Lymph node enlargement may appear rapidly and may be associated with fistula formation (19). Systemic symptoms are not a prominent feature (3,37,38). In contrast, lymphadenitis caused by *M. tuberculosis* generally presents with enlarging neck lesions over weeks to months and is generally painless. These masses commonly involve the jugular, posterior triangle, or supraclavicular lymph nodes (11,12). In combination, axillary, inguinal, and mediastinal lymph node involvement has been observed in approximately 14% to 30% (11,12,18,24). In *M. tuberculosis* lymphadenitis, systemic symptoms are commonly seen. Review of the literature reveals a significant variation of presentation. This may relate, in large part, to differences in geography or ethnic background. Classically, patients with *M. tuberculosis* lymphadenitis present with associated fever, weight loss, and fatigue and somewhat less frequently with night sweats (11,25,38). Cough is a less prominent feature, seen in approximately 10% of patients (11,25), although Kheiry and Ahmed (39) reported a rate as high as 35% in their Sudanese population. Although most authors find systemic symptoms to be a prominent feature associated with *M.*

tuberculosis lymphadenitis, Lee et al. (25) (in San Francisco) reported that 57% of patients had no systemic symptoms. There is a wide variation in authors' reports regarding chest radiograph results. Dandapat et al. (11) reported pleuroparenchymal abnormalities in four (5%) of 80 radiographs, whereas Wong and Jafek (3) reported that 68% of patients had abnormalities attributable to *M. tuberculosis*. Thompson et al. (12) (in Wales) found an ethnic difference in frequency of abnormal-appearing chest radiographs. Forty-four percent of Indian patients had tuberculosis lesions compared with only 18% of whites. In that study, the nature of the lesions was further characterized. Of the 23 abnormal-appearing chest radiographs, healed pulmonary lesions were seen in ten patients (43%), active pulmonary tuberculosis was seen in five (22%), and hilar or paratracheal lymphadenopathy was noted in seven (32%). Of note, the frequency of thoracic lymphadenopathy in association with peripheral lymphadenitis appears higher in this study than in those reported by other authors (11,12,18,24). In contrast to the high prevalence in this study of abnormal chest radiographs in specifically the Indian population in Wales (12), Jha et al. (40) recently described 60 cases of cervical tuberculous lymph node enlargement in India. Chest lesions on radiography were evident in only 16% of the patients, which is similar to the prevalence in the white population in Wales (12).

Geldmacher et al. (41) performed a retrospective analysis of 60 patients with lymph node tuberculosis who were hospitalized between 1992 and 1999 in Germany. Seventy percent were immigrants (predominantly of Afghani, Pakistani, or Indian origin) and 30% were native Germans. The cervical lymph nodes were most frequently involved (63.3%), followed by the mediastinal lymph nodes (26.7%) and the axillary lymph nodes (8.3%). According to the German Central Bureau of Statistics, the incidence of lymph node tuberculosis among immigrants is significantly higher (6.6 cases per 100,000 population) than that in the native German population (0.9 per 100,000 population) (41). Of interest is that none of the patients in this study were immigrants from the former Soviet Union, despite being from regions with the same overall incidence of tuberculosis as in Southeast Asia. One potential explanation might be a predisposition for lymph node tuberculous involvement in the populations of Southeast Asia and the Indian subcontinent or other demographic factors within these populations. An additional factor relevant to the presentation of a patient with mycobacterial lymphadenitis is the reaction to the Mantoux skin test. The presence of a reaction to purified protein derivative in patients with tuberculous lymphadenitis is generally reported as high [e.g., 92% (18), 74% (11), 98% (41)], whereas a tuberculin reaction is somewhat less frequently seen in patients with lymphadenopathy owing to NTM. Additionally, the history of known tuberculous exposure may be useful in the presentation of a patient with lymphadenitis. However, this history is often inconsistent.

Clinical presentation varies with the nature and location of *M. tuberculosis* lymphadenitis. Cervical lymphadenopathy is generally described as a painless, slowly growing neck mass or masses developing over weeks to months. Jones and Campbell (42) classified peripheral tuberculous lymph nodes into five stages ranging from enlarged, discrete, firm, and mobile nodes (stage I) to advancing nodal and perinodal involvement to frank sinus tract formation (stage V). Tuberculous mediastinal lymphadenitis rarely causes local symptoms in the adult. There have been case reports, however, of symptomatic tracheoesophageal involvement. Macchiarini et al. (43) reported a case of mediastinal tuberculosis causing a tracheoesophageal fistula that clinically and radiographically mimicked a malignant tracheoesophageal fistula. Similarly, Lee et al. (44) described a tuberculous tracheoesophageal fistula that responded to medical therapy alone. Gupta et al. (45) reported a case of esophageal compression and invasion by mediastinal tuberculosis. Adkins et al. (46) observed an esophageal perforation owing to erosion from *M. tuberculosis* in an HIV-seropositive patient. Im et al. (47) reported five patients with tuberculous esophagomediastinal fistula formation. This was detected by computed tomography with the presence of mediastinal gas noted. Two of these five patients were immunosuppressed. Other uncommon presentations of mycobacterial lymphadenitis include suppurative lymphadenitis in bacille Calmette–Guérin–vaccinated newborns in Austria (48), jaundice caused by biliary obstruction (49,50), chyluria caused by thoracic duct obstruction (51), chest pain owing to tuberculosis of the intercostal lymph nodes (52), and cardiac tamponade owing to a tension pneumopericardium associated with tuberculous mediastinal lymphadenitis (53).

DIAGNOSIS

Lymphadenopathy is an entity with an extensive differential diagnosis. In developing nations where tuberculosis remains common, tuberculous lymphadenitis continues to be one of the most frequent causes of lymphadenopathy (30% to 52%) (54). In contrast, in developed nations, tuberculosis is clearly found less frequently to be the cause of lymphadenopathy (as low as 1.6% in one series) (54–56). Mycobacterial lymphadenitis can mimic a variety of ailments, including sarcoidosis, carcinoma, lymphoma or sarcoma, viral or bacterial adenitis, fungal diseases, toxoplasmosis, catscratch fever, collagen vascular diseases, and diseases of the reticuloendothelial system. Traditionally, excisional biopsy was required to diagnose tuberculous lymphadenitis. Diagnosis is established by visualizing mycobacteria either by histopathology or by smears subjected to acid-fast stains or mycobacterial cultures. Histopathology revealing caseating granulomas is highly suggestive of mycobacterial infection, but other factors may produce

similar histology. Over the past decade, the role of fine needle aspiration (FNA) has become increasingly important in the evaluation of peripheral lymphadenopathy. Its high sensitivity and specificity for diagnosing cervical malignancies have been demonstrated (57,58). Several authors promoted FNA as the initial technique in the diagnosis of mycobacterial lymphadenitis. Specimens are routinely evaluated by cytology, acid-fast bacillus (AFB) smear, and AFB culture. The cytologic criteria for diagnosis have been well described. The diagnostic findings on cytology are epithelioid cell granulomas with or without multinucleate giant cells and caseation necrosis (32,54,59,60). Lau et al. (60) (Hong Kong) reported 108 patients whose FNA samples showed granulomatous changes. Sixty-eight of these patients underwent surgical excision. Of note, in 63 (93%), the diagnosis of tuberculosis was confirmed. In the remaining five patients, three nonspecific abscesses, one nonspecific lymphadenitis, and one metastatic mucoepidermoid carcinoma were found. Thus, the specificity of FNA was 93%. To address the sensitivity of FNA, Lau et al. (60) evaluated the FNA results of 90 patients who ultimately had histologically confirmed tuberculous lesions. The FNA material from 63 patients showed granulomatous features, with 21% of those demonstrating a positive AFB smear. An additional six patients with nondiagnostic FNA cytology revealed positive FNA AFB smears. Thus, the overall sensitivity of FNA was 77%. Of note, evaluation of AFB smear results revealed a high positive rate (47%) when necrosis was present, whereas the absence of necrosis on FNA was predictive of a low yield on AFB smear (15%), even in the patients with documented tuberculosis (60). Dandapat et al. (11) (India) performed FNA on 80 patients with biopsy-proven tuberculous lymphadenitis. Evaluation of the FNA material revealed a positive cytology finding in 83% of patients (false negative in 14%, equivocal in 3%, no false positives noted). AFB cultures were positive in 65% of patients. Radhika et al. (61) (India) performed FNA on 390 patients with tuberculous lymphadenitis. Diagnosis of tuberculosis was made by cytology and AFB staining. Overall, 24% of aspirates demonstrated positive AFB smears (33% in specimens with granuloma and necrosis). AFB cultures were positive in 35% overall (40% growth from caseating lesions, 9% from noncaseating samples). Caseating lesions with granulomas yielded positive AFB smear, culture, or both in 52% of patients. Gupta et al. (59) (Kuwait) subjected 272 FNA cytology-proved tuberculous lymphadenitis samples to mycobacterial smear and culture examination. AFB was present in 30% of direct and concentrated smears. Cultures were positive for 49%. The rate for combined AFB smear and culture positivity was 57%. The presence of necrosis yielded the highest culture results, 57% positivity (combined smear and culture was 63% positivity). Weiler et al. (62) (Israel) recently described 21 patients with cervical tuberculous lymphadenitis. Sixteen patients were of Ethiopian origin, three were from the former Soviet Union, and two were Israeli women (one of Indian and one of Moroccan origin). The authors found that FNA of the cervical lymph nodes was the most reliable method to confirm the bacteriologic agent causing the lymphadenopathy. AFB smears of the aspirate were positive in 18 of the 21 patients. Of interest, histologic examination of the lymph nodes yielded diagnostic results in only two-thirds of the cases examined. These representative studies demonstrate the role of FNA in the diagnosis of tuberculous lymphadenitis. The sensitivity and specificity are high, especially when cytology is combined with AFB stain or culture.

Given the rising frequency of HIV infection and its impact on tuberculosis, specific attention has been paid to the presentation and diagnostic evaluation of tuberculous lymphadenitis in the HIV host. Finfer et al. (32) (New York) retrospectively reviewed FNA samples of cervical or supraclavicular masses that revealed purulent, acute, or granulomatous inflammation. Thirty patients were studied: eight patients had acquired immunodeficiency syndrome (AIDS), five had AIDS-related complex or AIDS risk factors, and 17 were non-AIDS patients. Twenty-two of these 30 patients were ultimately diagnosed with *M. tuberculosis* lymphadenitis by either AFB stain of FNA or biopsy samples or AFB cultures of specimens from any body site. In this study, caseous material was a prominent finding on FNA and was associated with a high AFB smear positivity rate. AFB smears were positive in seven of eight patients with AIDS, two of five patients with AIDS-related complex or AIDS risk factors, and only one of ten of the non-AIDS patients. AFB cultures were positive in 18 of 22 patients. Of note, AFB cultures were positive for 20% of patients with negative AFB smears. These authors emphasized the role of performing AFB smears and cultures on all FNA specimens that show a purulent pattern, especially those that also contain caseous material or granulomas or are derived from patients with HIV risk factors. Similarly, Pithie and Chicksen (63) (Zimbabwe) performed FNA on extrathoracic lymph nodes (predominantly supraclavicular or cervical) in 28 HIV-positive patients with suspected tuberculosis. AFB stains were found to be positive in 20 of 23 patients in whom a diagnosis of tuberculosis was confirmed. Bem et al. (64) (Zambia) performed wide needle aspirates (no. 19 gauge) on 304 patients, 85% of whom were HIV positive. A total of 188 patients had biopsy-proven tuberculous lymphadenitis. These authors sought a rapid diagnostic procedure that did not need a trained histologist. They raised the issue that many countries in which tuberculosis is prevalent have a shortage of trained scientists and laboratory technicians. Microscopic caseation was demonstrated in 125 (73%) of 172 of tuberculous lymph nodes. AFB smears for 44 (28%) of 157 of aspirates were positive. Of the 85 lymph nodes that were found to be nontuberculous, two revealed necrotic changes that were misinterpreted as caseation in this study. These authors suggested that in

regions where trained histologists and mycobacterial cultures are difficult to obtain, the presence of caseation on microscopic examination (which was thought to be easily seen), especially in the presence of AFB smear positivity, yielded a good diagnostic sensitivity. They also noted that specificity was acceptable as well.

Other diagnostic approaches to tuberculous lymphadenitis have been suggested. In addition to FNA of peripheral lymph nodes, transbronchial needle aspiration of mediastinal lymph nodes has been reported to yield a diagnosis of tuberculous lymphadenitis (65,66). Several authors suggested the utility of nuclear medicine scans and computed tomography to aid in the evaluation and detection of extrapulmonary tuberculosis or tuberculous lymphadenitis (67–70). Although these may aid the clinician, a formal bacteriologic or histologic diagnosis is crucial.

In summary, FNA of lymph nodes has been well studied over the past decade and appears to be the diagnostic procedure of choice, when obtainable, in documenting tuberculous lymphadenitis. Incisional biopsy is associated with sinus tract and fistula formation and therefore is contraindicated (2,36,37,71,72). Surgical excisional lymph node biopsy requires a more involved procedure including the use of anesthesia. This technique is best reserved for patients for whom FNA fails to be diagnostic or in isolated patients for treatment. FNA is a safe and limited procedure; its sensitivity is quite high (higher than 80%) (11,32,54,60,63,64), whereas its specificity is excellent (59,60). Aspirates should be examined cytohistologically. Regardless of the cytologic findings, it is advisable to proceed with AFB staining and culture both for confirmation and to increase the diagnostic yield of FNA. It has been demonstrated that the yield of AFB positivity increases when a specimen has necrotic features. This observation may aid in choosing a site for aspiration. Additionally, a lymph node aspirate that appears purulent must be evaluated for *M. tuberculosis* rather than assuming a bacteriologic etiology. Although epithelioid granuloma formation, especially with caseation, is classic for *M. tuberculosis*, other entities may produce similar histopathology. AFB staining and culture will provide diagnostic certainty and will differentiate between *M. tuberculosis* and NTM disease (with treatment implications). Additionally, AFB culture offers mycobacterial drug sensitivities that may become crucial in the patient's treatment, especially with the emergence of multidrug-resistant tuberculosis.

TREATMENT

Most authors agree that lymphadenitis caused by NTM is generally treated effectively by surgical excision of the affected node or gland (42,73–78). Pang (24) reported 86 patients with NTM lymphadenitis in whom 12-month follow-up was obtainable. All were treated surgically. Of 15 patients who had incisional drainage, 12 (80%) failed compared with seven (10%) of 71 patients who had total excision of the affected tissue. Flint et al. (79) (New Zealand) recently performed a retrospective study of 57 children presenting with NTM lymphadenitis of the head and neck. Cultures revealed 56 *M. avium-intracellulare complex* and one *M. kansasii*. Based on the initial operation, the patients were placed into two groups. Group 1 (11 patients) had an excision, and group 2 (46 patients) had incision and drainage (30 patients), incision and curettage (13 patients), or aspiration (three patients). Group 1 had a significantly lower number of reoperations than group 2 and achieved a significantly greater healing rate than group 2. In group 2, those who had an excision after failure of the first operation were more likely to heal than those who did not. Surgical excision was associated with a lower rate of reoperation and a higher rate of healing than other procedures. Of note, antimycobacterial agents were used in only seven of the 56 patients. These studies, along with those of other authors, emphasize the need for adequate local excision in NTM lymphadenitis (42,75–78).

The treatment of tuberculous lymphadenitis has generated more debate over the years. The treatment of tuberculous lymphadenitis was not systematically studied until the 1970s. Before that time, treatment comprised varying combinations of surgical excision and chemotherapy (73). Kilpatrick and Douglas (80), in 1957, suggested chemotherapy with two drugs for at least 12 to 18 months. Surgical drainage was reserved for fluctuant lesions, whereas excision was recommended for large masses that failed to show a response to chemotherapy. In 1974, Iles and Emerson (81), in a London retrospective review, reported that relapse occurred in ten of 12 patients treated by surgical excision alone, whereas no relapses occurred in 24 patients who received excision along with chemotherapy. Other authors confirmed a high treatment failure or recurrence rate with surgical therapy alone. Wong and Jafek (3) reported a 31% relapse rate, and Thompson et al. (12) showed a 90% relapse rate. Several studies supported more promising results from chemotherapy alone, approaching a 90% cure rate (3,80). Recent attention has centered on the appropriate medical regimen, that is, the number of drugs and length of treatment course. Campbell (73) compared the results of two 18-month regimens: rifampin and isoniazid for 18 months with an initial 2-month course of streptomycin ands ethambutol and isoniazid for 18 months with an initial 2-month course of streptomycin. In the treatment of 108 patients with *M. tuberculosis* lymphadenitis, there were no differences between these two regimens. Although in 65% of patients, lymph nodes resolved after the 18-month course of therapy, the remaining 35% had varied lymph node responses to treatment. Some nodes increased in size, new nodes developed in some patients, and sinus tract formation developed in some. At the end of chemotherapy, 13% of patients were left with residual lymph nodes. Over the next 18 months after the discontinuation of therapy, lymph nodes further decreased in size or resolved in three-fourths of these patients. No bacteriologic relapses were documented. In a follow-up study, Campbell (73) found similar results in a comparison of two additional regimens: rifampin and isoniazid for 9 months with an initial 2-month treatment course with ethambutol and rifampin and isoniazid for 18 months with an initial 2-month treatment course with ethambutol. Eighty-four (74%) of 113 patients experienced resolution of lymph nodes during treatment. Varied lymph node responses were noted in the remaining 26% of patients, and there were no mycobacteriologic relapses. It was noted that initial surgery or aspiration did not affect the final outcome. McCarthy and Rudd (82) performed a retrospective analysis of 41 patients treated with rifampin and isoniazid for 6 months with an initial 2-month course of pyrazinamide for tuberculous lymphadenitis. While on therapy, six patients (15%) demonstrated either new or residual nodes or sinus tract formation that resolved after the initial treatment course. In one patient, a new node developed after therapy, and although AFB cultures were negative, the patient was treated again with resolution of the lymphadenopathy. More recently, Campbell et al. (83) performed a prospective comparison of three regimens for the treatment of tuberculous lymphadenitis in 157 patients. The three regimens under evaluation were isoniazid and rifampin for 9 months with an initial 2-month course of ethambutol (E2H9R9), isoniazid and rifampin for 9 months with an initial 2-month course of pyrazinamide (Z2H9R9), and isoniazid and rifampin for 6 months with an initial 2-month course of pyrazinamide (Z2H6R6). Patients received follow-up for 30 months. A small percentage of patients in each group was noted to have new nodes, enlargement of existing nodes, or sinus tract formation. At the end of therapy, residual lymph nodes were present in six (12%) patients in the E2H9R9 group, ten (17%) in the Z2H9R9 group, and ten (17%) in the Z2H6R6 group. Nine patients, four from the E2H9R9 group, two from the Z2H9R9 group, and three from the Z2H6R6 group, were ultimately retreated for presumed relapses, although mycobacteriology did not document active disease in any of the patients tested. The treatment success rate was 94% overall. There were no differences among the three regimens except for an increased need for aspiration of lesions in the ethambutol-treated group. van Loenhout-Rooyackers et al. (84) (The Netherlands) recently performed a metaanalysis of studies published between 1978 and 1997 that included patients with predominantly cervical tuberculous lymphadenitis. Patients with resistance to rifampicin and pyrazinamide and previous treatment for tuberculosis were excluded. Treatment management had to include at least isoniazid, rifampicin, and pyrazinamide and a follow-up of at least 12 months after the termination of therapy. Eight suitable articles were analyzed. There were eight treatment schedules of

6 months' duration and three schedules of 9 months' duration. Treatment for 6 months resulted in a tuberculous lymphadenitis relapse rate of 13 of 422 (3.1% with a mean follow-up of 31 months after completion of therapy. Treatment for 9 months resulted in a relapse rate of three of 112 (2.7%) with a mean follow-up of 20 months. Six months of therapy appeared to be sufficient for treatment of cervical tuberculous lymphadenitis.

In summary, although surgical lymph node excision is the treatment for NTM lymphadenitis, chemotherapy is the preferred treatment for tuberculous lymphadenitis. Whereas most patients respond with gradual resolution of their lymphadenopathy, a significant minority of patients develops either new lesions or increasing lymph node enlargement during therapy, which generally resolve over time. This phenomenon has recently been reemphasized in both immunocompetent and immunosuppressed patients (85). Although the pathogenesis is not well characterized, immune factors are implicated. Some authors successfully followed persistent lymphadenopathy for spontaneous resolution, and others advocated retreatment despite negative cultures. There is an excellent overall response to chemotherapy, yielding approximately a 90% cure rate. Recent studies supported the efficacy of the short course of chemotherapy, that is, isoniazid and rifampin for 6 months with an initial 2-month course of pyrazinamide (82,83). Surgical treatment alone yields poor results. Adjuvant surgical intervention should be reserved for lymph nodes that do not resolve with chemotherapy, for symptomatic relief (rare in the adult), for drainage of persistent fluctuant lesions, or for diagnosis if the FNA is nondiagnostic or not available.

SUMMARY

Tuberculous lymphadenopathy is one of the most common extrapulmonary manifestations of tuberculosis. Although any age, gender, or ethnic group may be affected, there appears to be a predilection for young women, especially Asian, Indian, black, or Hispanic women. Geldmacher et al. (41) observed a Southeast Asian predominance in the cases of tuberculous lymphadenitis among the immigrant population in northern Germany, where there were no cases among the immigrants from the former Soviet Union. Scrofula owing to *M. tuberculosis* is generally thought to be a local manifestation of a systemic disease. The most common lymph nodes involved are in the cervical regions. Lymphadenitis caused by *M. tuberculosis* generally presents with enlarging neck lesions over weeks to months with associated fever, weight loss, and fatigue. A reactive tuberculin skin test is common, and the history of tuberculosis exposure is not infrequent. Mycobacterial lymphadenitis owing to NTM, in contrast, is believed to be the result of local infection. NTM lymph node enlargement often appears rapidly and may be associated with fistula for-

mation. Systemic symptoms are not a prominent feature. Traditionally, excisional biopsy was required to diagnose tuberculous lymphadenitis. Over the past decade, FNA of affected lymph nodes has been shown to yield high sensitivity and specificity in the diagnosis of tuberculous lymphadenitis. Specimens should be examined cytologically as well as by AFB smear and cultures. Given the risk of sinus tract formation associated with incisional biopsy and the invasive nature of excisional lymph node biopsy, FNA of affected lymph nodes appears to be the procedure of choice to document tuberculous lymphadenitis. Lymphadenopathy caused by NTM is generally treated effectively by surgical excision of the affected tissue. In contrast, tuberculous lymphadenitis is treated with a combination of antituberculous medications. Although surgical treatment alone yields poor results, the overall response to chemotherapy yields an excellent cure rate. In isolated patients, adjuvant surgical intervention may become necessary for symptomatic relief or to aid in resolution of disease.

REFERENCES

1. Ayvazian LF. History of tuberculosis. In: Reichman LB, Hershfield ES, eds. *Tuberculosis: a comprehensive international approach.* New York: Marcel Dekker, 1993:1–20.
2. Appling D, Miller HR. Mycobacterial cervical lymphadenopathy: 1981 update. *Laryngoscope* 1981;91:1259–1266.
3. Wong ML, Jafek BW. Cervical mycobacterial disease. *Trans Am Acad Ophthalmol Otolaryngol* 1974;78:75–87.
4. Cantrell R, Jensen JH, Reid D. Diagnosis and management of tuberculous cervical adenitis. *Arch Otolaryngol* 1975;101:53–57.
5. Brothwell D, Sandinson AT. *Diseases in antiquity.* Springfield, IL: Charles C Thomas Publisher, 1967:263.
6. Castiglioni A, *A history of medicine*, 2nd ed. New York: Knopf, 1947:385–388. Krumbhaar EB, translator.
7. Talmi YP, Cohen AH, Finkelstein Y, et al. *Mycobacterium tuberculosis* cervical adenitis: diagnosis and management. *Clin Pediatr* 1989;28:408–411.
8. Weir MR, Thornton GF. Extrapulmonary tuberculosis. Experience of a community hospital and review of the literature. *Am J Med* 1985;79:467–476.
9. Hooper AA. Tuberculous peripheral lymphadenitis. *Br J Surg* 1972;59:353–359.
10. Krishnaswamy H, Koshi G, Dash SP, et al. Tuberculous lymphadenitis in South India—a histopathological and bacteriological study. *Tubercle* 1972;52:215–220.
11. Dandapat MC, Mishra BM, et al. Peripheral lymph node tuberculosis: a review of 80 cases. *Br J Surg* 1990;77:911–912.
12. Thompson MM, Underwood MJ, Sayers RD, et al. Peripheral tuberculous lymphadenopathy: a review of 67 cases. *Br J Surg* 1992;79:763–764.
13. Llewelyn DM, Dorman D. Mycobacterial lymphadenitis. *Aust Paediatr J* 1971;7:97–102.
14. Roba-Kiewicz M, Grzybowski S. Epidemiologic aspects of nontuberculous mycobacterial diseases and of tuberculosis in British Columbia. *Am Rev Respir Dis* 1974;109:613–620.
15. Yamamoto M, Sudo K, Taga M, et al. A study of diseases caused by atypical mycobacteria in Japan. *Am Rev Respir Dis* 1967;96:779–787.
16. Yates MD, Grange JM. Bacteriological survey of tuberculous

lymphadenitis in Southeast England, 1981–1989. *J Epidemiol Commun Health* 1992;46:332–335.

17. Shikhani A, Hadi UM, Mufarrij AA, et al. Mycobacterial cervical lymphadenitis. *Ear Nose Throat J* 1989;68:660–672.
18. Manolidis S, Frenkiel S, Yoskovitch A,et al. Mycobacterial infections of the head and neck. *Otolaryngol Head Neck Surg* 1993; 109:427–433.
19. Kwan LK, Stottmeier KD, Sherman IH, et al. Mycobacterial cervical lymphadenopathy, relation of etiologic agents to age. *JAMA* 1984;251:1286–1288.
20. Ord RF, Matz GJ. Tuberculous cervical lymphadenitis. *Arch Otolaryngol* 1974;99:327–329.
21. Enarson DA, Ashley MJ, Grzybowski S, et al. Nonrespiratory tuberculosis in Canada: epidemiologic and bacteriologic features. *Am J Epidemiol* 1980;112:341–351.
22. Campbell LA, Dyson IA. Lymph nodes tuberculosis: a comparison of treatments 18 months after completion of chemotherapy. *Tubercle* 1979;60:95–98.
23. Farer LS, Lowell AM, Meador MP. Extrapulmonary tuberculosis in the United States. *Am J Epidemiol* 1979;109:205–217.
24. Pang SC. Mycobacterial lymphadenitis in Western Australia. *Tubercle Lung Dis* 1992;73:362–367.
25. Lee KC, Tami TA, Lalwani AK, et al. Contemporary management of cervical tuberculosis. *Laryngoscope* 1992;102:60–64.
26. Comstock GW, Edwards LB, Livesay VT. Tuberculosis morbidity in the US Navy: its distribution and decline. *Am Rev Respir Dis* 1974;110:571–580.
27. Rich AR, ed. *The pathogenesis of tuberculosis*. Springfield, IL: Charles C Thomas Publisher, 1950.
28. Kent DC. Tuberculous lymphadenitis: not a localized disease process. *Am J Med Sci* 1967;254:866–874.
29. Stoneburner RL. Tuberculosis and acquired immunodeficiency syndrome—New York City. *JAMA* 1988;259:338–340.
30. Department of Public Health. Reported cases of certain notifiable diseases. *San Francisco Epidemiol Bull* 1989;5:4.
31. Aguado JM, Castrillo JM. Lymphadenitis as a characteristic manifestation of disseminated tuberculosis in intravenous drug abusers infected with human immunodeficiency virus. *J Infect* 1987;14:191–193.
32. Finfer M, Perchick A, Burstein DE. Fine needle aspiration biopsy diagnosis of tuberculous lymphadenitis in patients with and without the acquired immune deficiency syndrome. *Acta Cytol* 1991;35:325–332.
33. Soriano E, Mallolas J, Gatell JM, et al. Characteristics of tuberculosis in HIV-infected patients: a case-control study. *AIDS* 1988;2:429–432.
34. Olson RN. Nontuberculous mycobacterial infections of the face and neck—practical considerations. *Laryngoscope* 1981;91: 1714–1726.
35. Stanley BR, Fernandez AJ, Peppard BS. Cervicofacial mycobacterial infections presenting as major salivary gland disease. *Laryngoscope* 1983;93:1271–1275.
36. Wolinsky E. Nontuberculous mycobacteria and associated diseases. *Am Rev Respir Dis* 1979;119:107–159.
37. Levin-Epstein AA, Lucente FE. Scrofula—the dangerous masquerader. *Laryngoscope* 1982;92:938–943.
38. Deitel M, Saldanha CF, Borowy JZ, et al. Treatment of tuberculous masses in the neck. *Can J Surg* 1984;27:90–93.
39. Kheiry J, Ahmed ME. Cervical lymphadenopathy in Khartoum. *J Trop Med Hyg* 1992;95:416–419.
40. Jha BC, Dass A, Nagarkar NM, et al. Cervical tuberculous lymphadenopathy: changing clinical pattern and concepts in management. *Postgrad Med J* 2001;77:185–187.
41. Geldmacher H, Taube C, Kroeger C, et al. Assessment of lymph node tuberculosis in northern Germany: a clinical review. *Chest* 2002;121:1177–1182.

42. Jones PG, Campbell PE. Tuberculous lymphadenitis in childhood: the significance of anonymous mycobacteria. *Br J Surg* 1962;50:302–314.
43. Macchiarini P, Delamare N, Beuzeboc P, et al. Tracheoesophageal fistula caused by mycobacterial tuberculous adenopathy. *Ann Thorac Surg* 1993;55:1561–1563.
44. Lee JH, Shin DH, Kang KW, et al. The medical treatment of a tuberculous tracheo-oesophageal fistula. *Tuber Lung Dis* 1992;73:177–179.
45. Gupta SP, Arora A, Bhargava DK. An unusual presentation of oesophageal tuberculosis. *Tuber Lung Dis* 1992;73:174–176.
46. Adkins MS, Raccuia JS, Acinapura AJ. Esophageal perforation in a patient with acquired immune deficiency syndrome. *Ann Thorac Surg* 1990;50:299–300.
47. Im JG, Kim JH, Han MC. Computed tomography of esophagomediastinal fistula in tuberculous mediastinal lymphadenitis. *J Comput Assist Tomogr* 1990;14:89–92.
48. Allerberger F. An outbreak of suppurative lymphadenitis connected with BCG vaccination in Austria, 1990/1991 [Letter]. *Am Rev Respir Dis* 1991;144:469.
49. Kohn MD, Altman KA. Jaundice due to rare causes: tuberculous lymphadenitis. *Am J Gastroenterol* 1973;59:48–53.
50. Poon RT, Lo CM, Fan ST. Diagnosis and management of biliary obstruction due to periportal tuberculous adenitis. *Hepatogastroenterology* 2001;48:1585–1587.
51. Wilson RS, White RJ. Lymph node tuberculosis presenting as chyluria. *Thorax* 1976;31:617–620.
52. Subramanian S, Mazumder PR, Vijaya S, et al. Tuberculosis of the intercostal lymph nodes: an unusual presentation. *Tubercle* 1974;55:163–166.
53. Paredes C, DelCampo F, Zamarron C. Cardiac tamponade due to tuberculous mediastinal lymphadenitis. *Tubercle* 1990;71: 219–220.
54. Gupta AK, Nayar M, Chandra M. Critical appraisal of fine needle aspiration cytology in tuberculous lymphadenitis. *Acta Cytol* 1992;36:391–394.
55. Dandapat MC, Patra BK, et al. Diagnosis of tubercular lymphadenitis by fine needle aspiration cytology. *Indian J Tuberc* 1987;34:139–142.
56. Kline TS. Lymph nodes and superficial masses. In: Lotz JE, ed. *Handbook of fine needle aspiration cytology*. St Louis: Mosby, 1981:23–64.
57. Feldman PS, Kaplan MJ, Johns ME, et al. Fine needle aspiration in squamous cell carcinoma of the head and neck. *Arch Otolaryngol* 1983;109:735–742.
58. Young JEM, Archibald SD, Shier KJ. Needle aspiration cytologic biopsy in head and neck masses. *Am J Surg* 1981;142:484–489.
59. Gupta SK, Chugh TD, Sheikh ZA, et al. Cytodiagnosis of tuberculous lymphadenitis: a correlative study with microbiologic examination. *Acta Cytol* 1993;37:329–332.
60. Lau SK, Wei WI, Hsu C, et al. Efficacy of fine needle aspiration cytology in the diagnosis of tuberculous cervical lymphadenopathy. *J Laryngol Otol* 1990;104:24–27.
61. Radhika S, Gupta SK, et al. Role of culture for mycobacteria in fine-needle aspiration diagnosis of tuberculous lymphadenitis. *Diagn Cytopathol* 1989;5:260–262.
62. Weiler Z, Nelly P, Baruchin AM, et al. Diagnosis and treatment of cervical tuberculous lymphadenitis. *J Oral Maxillofac Surg* 2000;58:477–481.
63. Pithie AD, Chicksen B. Fine-needle extra-thoracic lymph-node aspiration in HIV-associated sputum-negative tuberculosis. *Lancet* 1992;340:1504–1505.
64. Bem C, Patil PS, Elliott AM, et al. The value of wide-needle aspiration in the diagnosis of tuberculous lymphadenitis in Africa. *AIDS* 1993;7:1221–1225.
65. Simecek C. Diagnosis of mycobacterial mediastinal lym-

phadenopathy by transbronchial needle aspiration (Letter). *Chest* 1992;102:1919.

66. Baron KM, Aranda CP. Diagnosis of mediastinal mycobacterial lymphadenopathy by transbronchial needle aspiration. *Chest* 1991;100:1723–1724.

67. Pombo F, Rodriguez E, Mato J, et al. Patterns of contrast enhancement of tuberculous lymph nodes demonstrated by computed tomography. *Clin Radiol* 1992;46:13–17.

68. Prat L, Bajen MT, Ricart Y, et al. Ga-67 citrate and Tc-99m HMPAO leukocyte scanning in extrapulmonary tuberculosis. *Clin Nucl Med* 1991;16:865–866.

69. Palestro C, Swyer A, Kim CK, et al. Tuberculous lymphadenitis: In-111 leukocyte and Ga-67 imaging. *Clin Nucl Med* 1991;16:857–858.

70. Yang S-O, Lee YI, Chung DH, et al. Detection of extrapulmonary tuberculosis with gallium-67 scan and computed tomography. *J Nucl Med* 1992;33:2118–2123.

71. Castro JD, Hoover L, Castro DJ, et al. Cervical mycobacterial lymphadenitis. *Arch Otolaryngol* 1985;111:816–819.

72. Siu KF, Ng A, Wong J. Tuberculous lymphadenopathy: a review of results of surgical treatment. *Aust NZ J Surg* 1983;53:253–257.

73. Campbell IA. The treatment of superficial tuberculous lymphadenitis. *Tubercle* 1990;71:1–3.

74. White MP, Bangash H, et al. Nontuberculous mycobacterial lymphadenitis. *Arch Dis Child* 1986;61:368–371.

75. Harris BH, Webb HW, Wilkinson AH Jr, et al. Mycobacterial lymphadenitis. *J Pediatr Surg* 1982;17:589–590.

76. MacKellar A, Hilton HB, Masters PL. Mycobacterial lymphadenitis in childhood. *Arch Dis Child* 1967;42:70–74.

77. MacKellar A. Diagnosis and management of atypical mycobacterial lymphadenitis in children. *J Pediatr Surg* 1976;11:85–89.

78. Joshi W, Davidson PM, Jones PG, et al. Non-tuberculous mycobacterial lymphadenitis in children. *Eur J Pediatr* 1989;148:751–754.

79. Flint D, Mahadevan M, Barber C, et al. Cervical lymphadenitis due to non-tuberculous mycobacteria: surgical treatment and review. *Int J Pediatr Otorhinolaryngol* 2000;53:187–194.

80. Kilpatrick GS, Douglas AC. Superficial glandular tuberculosis treatment with chemotherapy. *BMJ* 1957;2:612–614.

81. Iles PB, Emerson PA. Tuberculous lymphadenitis. *BMJ* 1974;1:143–145.

82. McCarthy OR, Rudd RM. Six months' chemotherapy for lymph node tuberculosis. *Respir Med* 1989;83:425–427.

83. Campbell IA, Ormerod LP, Friend JA, et al. Six month versus nine months chemotherapy for tuberculosis of lymph nodes: final results. *Respir Med* 1993;87:621–623.

84. van Loenhout-Rooyackers JH, Laheij RJ, Richter RJ, et al. Shortening the duration of treatment for cervical tuberculous lymphadenitis. *Eur Respir J* 2000;15:192–195.

85. Hill AR, Mateo F, Hudak A. Transient exacerbation of tuberculous lymphadenitis during chemotherapy in patients with AIDS. *Clin Infect Dis* 1994;19:774–776.

PLEURAL TUBERCULOSIS

STEPHAN L. KAMHOLZ

Tuberculosis (TB) (consumption, phthisis) and empyema of the pleural cavity were known to physicians since antiquity, having been well described (although not clearly separated from other diseases) by Hippocrates and Celsus (1). Involvement of the pleural surfaces in patients with TB is still one of the two most common extraparenchymal manifestations of pulmonary TB, the other being lymphatic involvement (2). Frequently, patients present for medical attention because of symptoms attributable to pleural involvement, including chest pain of a sharp pleuritic quality, dyspnea, or, less commonly, chest wall masses or draining sinus tracts (3). Although the cough, fever, sweats, and weight loss that characteristically accompany parenchymal pulmonary involvement often coexist in patients with pleural TB, symptoms referable to pleural involvement may be preeminent. Historically, recognition of the tuberculous etiology of so-called idiopathic pleural effusion was delayed by the frequent spontaneous resolution of this common form of pleural involvement (postprimary lymphocytic exudative tuberculous pleural effusion). However, the fact that 30% to 50% of these individuals later developed active parenchymal TB contributed to the current recommendations that such patients be treated for TB, even if the microbiologic diagnosis cannot be established (4). Despite the frequency with which pleural TB occurs as a postprimary manifestation, it may be seen at any phase of the disease. To further complicate the diagnosis, the cytologic characteristics of the pleural fluid may vary widely, depending on the phase of TB in which the pleural effusion develops. As with pulmonary TB, the time course and characteristics of pleural TB have also been altered by human immunodeficiency virus (HIV) coinfection.

CURRENT EPIDEMIOLOGY

The resurgence of TB in the United States from the mid-1980s through the mid-1990s was fueled, at least in part,

by the epidemic of HIV infection and acquired immunodeficiency syndrome (AIDS) and was accompanied by an increase in the number of cases of pleural TB reported annually (5). Although it was not possible to determine the relationship to HIV/AIDS for all cases of pleural TB, extrapulmonary involvement is certainly suggestive of coinfection. In one large study of disseminated (miliary) TB, pleural involvement occurred more frequently in the HIV/AIDS patient group than in those without immunodeficiency (6). It has been suggested that cell-mediated immune responses are reduced in the pleural space in HIV-associated tuberculous pleural effusion (7), and although interferon gamma (IFN-γ) levels in the HIV-positive TB pleural effusions are high, the source of the IFN-γ is suppressor CD8+ T cells, which may allow *Mycobacterium tuberculosis* to proliferate despite high levels of proinflammatory cytokines. In reviewing data for the peak year (1992) of the TB epidemic in the United States, serologic data on HIV coinfection with TB in New York City revealed only 33.6% seropositive patients, HIV status was unknown in approximately 50% of the TB cases in New York City (5), and most experts believed that, at that time, at least half of New York's TB cases were HIV related. However, the TB epidemic (in New York and the United States) waned during the closing years of the 20th century, and along with it, the number of cases of tuberculous pleural effusion decreased. In 2001, the New York City Department of Health reported 1,261 cases of TB, for the first time decreasing to below the previous nadir (1,307 cases) that had been reached in 1978 (8). TB cases in immigrants now constitute the majority of cases, in contrast to the situation during the recent epidemic.

PLEURAL DISEASE IN THE INDIVIDUAL

Classic tuberculous pleurisy occurs 3 to 7 months (4) after initial infection with *M. tuberculosis* and is well recognized as a manifestation of postprimary TB in children and young adults. In a recent series (9) from Spain, 39 (22.1%) of 175 patients with TB younger than 18 years of age had pleural effusion, and of that group, effusion was the sole

S. L. Kamholz: Department of Medicine, New York University School of Medicine, New York, New York; Department of Medicine, North Shore University Hospital, Manhasset, New York; Long Island Jewish Medical Center, New Hyde Park, New York.

radiographic finding in 41%. However, the development of pleurisy is often delayed as long as 2 years after initial infection and may occur at any time in the course of the disease. Indeed, an upward shift in the patient age spectrum (with average ages in the fifth or sixth decade not uncommon) of pleural TB and an increasingly frequent association with reactivation disease have been highlighted in several series (10–12) in non-AIDS patients. The initial infection often goes unrecognized, although in retrospect, the patient may recall a mild respiratory tract illness reminiscent of viral infection (4). It has been traditionally taught that this post-primary manifestation of TB is not frequently accompanied by clinically and radiographically apparent parenchymal pulmonary involvement. In geographic areas with a high prevalence of TB, TB pleurisy may more commonly be seen in primary/postprimary disease. A recent report (13) from Malaysia indicated that 61.4% of patients with pleural TB did not have parenchymal infiltrates and were younger (*p* = 0.041) than patients with effusions accompanying reactivation TB, both observations consistent with primary/post-primary disease. However, several reports suggest an increasing incidence of pleural effusion accompanying reactivation TB and an increase in the average age of patients with pleural TB (11,12). The coexistence with significant parenchymal lung disease is much more prevalent in HIV/AIDS (14,15). In one series involving non-AIDS patients, approximately half of the cases of pleural TB (in patients with an average age of 47 years) were accompanied by active parenchymal (often cavitary) involvement. Acid-fast bacilli are more frequently isolated from sputum cultures and identified in pleural tissue specimens from AIDS patients with tuberculous pleurisy (15). Occasionally, effusions are bilateral, and the development of contralateral TB effusion during early therapy of pleural (and parenchymal) TB has been reported (16–18).

IMMUNOPATHOGENESIS OF TUBERCULOUS PLEURAL EFFUSION

The traditional explanation for the development of a tuberculous pleural effusion is that a small subpleural focus of *M. tuberculosis* ruptures into the pleural space, setting up an interaction between the live bacilli (or its specific antigens) and sensitized CD4+ T lymphocytes. The clinical syndrome is a reflection of an *in situ* delayed-type hypersensitivity reaction in which plasma proteins exude into the pleural space and CD4+ T helper cells accumulate, proliferate, and produce and release inflammatory mediators (19). In the rabbit model of bacille Calmette–Guérin–induced experimental tuberculous pleurisy, a normal pH, normal glucose exudative effusion develops rapidly in which the predominant cells are polymorphonuclear leukocytes for the first 24 hours, followed by macrophages on days 2 through 4, and lymphocytes there-

after, with granuloma formation present by day 10 (20). Mononuclear cell migration from the peripheral blood to the pleural space occurs as peripheral blood monocytes traverse the mesothelial lining of the pleural cavity. Recent evidence (21) suggests that mesothelial cells release chemotactic factors (induced by the presence of *M. tuberculosis*), which regulate this process, and mesothelial cell–derived intercellular adhesion molecule-1 has been shown to play a critical role in this cellular recruitment process. Additionally, other cytokines play a key role in monocyte chemotaxis into the pleural space. The C-C chemokines macrophage inflammatory protein-1α and monocyte chemoattractant protein-1 are responsible for 42.4% and 29.65%, respectively, of the biologic chemotactic activity of human tuberculous pleural effusions (22). Numerous studies have demonstrated that the T lymphocytes found in the pleural fluid of patients with tuberculous effusions are specifically reactive to purified protein derivative (PPD) of *M. tuberculosis* and produce IFN when cultured with PPD (23–25). This is in contrast to peripheral blood lymphocytes from the same patients that are hyporesponsive when cultured in the presence of PPD.

Indeed, the occasional observation of cutaneous anergy to intradermal injection of PPD in patients with TB pleural effusion has been explained by the preferential sequestration of antigen-specific T cells in the pleural space (or by the presence of suppressor cells in the blood) (19,25). Enumeration of lymphocyte subsets in TB pleural effusions has revealed a range of CD4+ T cells, with ratios as high as 65%, and CD8+ T cells as high as 19% (20). IFN-γ production was attributed to the CD4+ T cells in one study (26) because treatment with anti-CD4+ monoclonal antibody and complement markedly decreases IFN-γ production, whereas treatment with anti-CD8+ monoclonal antibody did not significantly reduce IFN production (26). Subsequent studies have confirmed high levels of IFN-γ in tuberculous effusions but did not find a correlation with the distribution of lymphocyte subsets (27), nor was the higher CD4/CD8 ratio in tuberculous effusions statistically significant (28). More recently, memory T cells (CD4+CDw29+ T) from tuberculous effusions have been shown to produce IFN-γ specifically in response to PPD of *M. tuberculosis* (26) but not when stimulated by an irrelevant antigen. Additionally, IFN-γ levels were markedly elevated in the pleural fluid, suggesting local production of the lymphokine; immunofluorescent studies of pleural tissue also confirmed the predominance of memory T cells (see previously) at the site of active inflammation (29). Mean levels of IFN-γ (1,493 pg/mL) far exceed those found (80 pg/mL) in nontuberculous (malignant or inflammatory) effusions (30). The ratio of pleural fluid IFN-γ to serum IFN-γ is also significantly higher in tuberculous versus malignant effusions (31). One recent study (32) demonstrated that IFN-γ level [compared with adenosine deaminase (ADA) level, tumor necrosis factor-α and interleukin (IL)-8] was most highly correlated (0.875, by analysis of the receiver operating characteristic curve) with the tuberculous etiology of pleural effusion. Tumor necrosis factor-α in the pleural space may subsequently "drive" an increase in plasminogen activator inhibitor-1 levels and decrease tissue plasminogen activator levels, leading to fibrin deposition and pleural thickening (33).

Tuberculous pleural fluid lymphocytes produce more IFN-τ than those derived from nontuberculous effusions in individuals with positive tuberculin skin tests (34). PPD-stimulated release of the lymphokine IL-1 from pleural fluid macrophages and peripheral blood monocytes obtained from patients with pleural TB was greater than that for cells obtained from the pleural fluid and blood of patients with effusions of other etiologies (35). In addition, the pleural macrophages derived from patients with TB pleural effusion prompted the greatest IL-2 production from pleural T lymphocytes. Elevated levels of natural killer cell activity have also been described in tuberculous effusions (36,37), with increased numbers of IL-2 receptors (IL-2R) being expressed on CD16⁺ (Leu 11⁺) cells in the effusions, expression that increased on exposure (in culture) to PPD (37). Additionally, monoclonal antibody to IL-2R inhibited the cytotoxicity otherwise enhanced by culture. Thus, it was suggested that IL-2R played an important role in activation of NK cells (37). Cytotoxic T cells are thought to be important in the eradication of *M. tuberculosis*–infected macrophages and generation of PPD-specific cytotoxic T cells at the site of pathology (38), and local elaboration of the Th1 cytokines IFN-γ, IL-2 and IL-10 have been described (39). Elevated levels of soluble IL-2R have also been demonstrated (40), reflecting local proliferation of T cells in tuberculous effusions (41–43). Levels of soluble IL-2R exceeding 4,700 U/mL are highly correlated (44) with a tuberculous etiology of pleural effusion (sensitivity, 0.91; specificity, 0.94; accuracy, 0.94). Higher levels of IFN-γ and soluble IL-2R are associated with posttreatment pleural thickening (45). Matrix metalloproteinase (MMP) levels (particularly surplus levels of MMP-1, MMP-2, MMP-8, and MMP-9) in the pleural space are also associated with the ultimate development of pleural thickening and fibrosis (46). Evidence that tuberculous pleuritis represents a resistant response manifested by mild disease is provided by the demonstration of expansion of the γδ-positive T-cell population, which produces IFN-γ, granulocyte-macrophage colony-stimulating factor, IL-3, and tumor necrosis factor-α, cytokines that stimulate macrophages and may enhance mycobacterial elimination (42). Pleural fluid CD-26 levels (expressed on CD4⁺ lymphocytes) are higher in tuberculous pleural effusions and may represent a component of a Th1 cytokine response (47). Pleural fluid IL-6 levels are also elevated in tuberculous effusions and may help to differentiate TB from malignant and parapneumonic effusions (48). Elevated vitamin D, 1,25-dihydroxycholecalciferol levels have been demonstrated in tuberculous effusions (5.3-fold

higher compared with blood), probably representing local production by pleural tissue–based inflammatory cells (43). Vitamin D inhibition of proliferation by patient-derived, PPD-responsive cell lines (mononuclear and lymphocyte) that express high-affinity intracellular binding moieties for vitamin D has prompted the suggestion that modulation of the pleural inflammatory response in TB effusion is, at least in part, attributable to vitamin D (43). Transforming growth factor β plays an immunosuppressive role in inflammatory responses and may additionally be responsible for regression of granulomatous inflammation in tuberculous pleurisy (49). Determination of antimycobacterial antibody in TB pleural effusion has been shown to have potential diagnostic utility. However, passive diffusion of antibody into the pleural space and occasional false-positive results owing to malignant effusions limit the utility of such tests (50–52). Although tuberculous pleural effusion accompanying both postprimary and reactivation TB is most often of the immunologically mediated, lymphocyte-predominant type just described (12), hematogenous dissemination to the pleura is another route of formation (4).

CLINICAL MANIFESTATIONS

The presenting symptoms, signs, and radiographic findings of pleural TB now characteristically encountered in the inner city municipal hospital are illustrative of the clinical picture.

Case Report 1

A 26-year-old woman with a long history of intravenous drug abuse presented to the hospital with 2 months of fever, cough productive of greenish blood-tinged sputum, drenching night sweats, mild exertional dyspnea, and 7-kg weight loss. Physical examination revealed a 39°C temperature, 110 per minute pulse, 24 respirations per minute, and 98/60 mm Hg blood pressure. Oral thrush and diffuse cervical lymphadenopathy were present, scattered rales and coarse rhonchi were noted posteriorly over the right upper lobe, and diminished breath sounds, absent tactile fremitus, and marked percussion dullness were noted at the right lung base. Tender hepatomegaly (14-cm span by percussion) and multiple skin popping and needle track scars were present. Chest radiograph (Fig. 32.1) revealed extensive right upper lobe infiltration and partly loculated right pleural effusion. Abnormalities of routine laboratory data included hematocrit of 0.28, leukocyte count of 3.1×10^3 cells/μL, and serum sodium of 129 mEq/L. Sputum and pleural fluid stains were positive for acid-fast bacilli, subsequently proven to be *M. tuberculosis* on culture (sensitive to all antimycobacterial agents tested). Histopathologic examination of the closed needle pleural biopsy specimen revealed chronic inflammatory cells and multiple, poorly

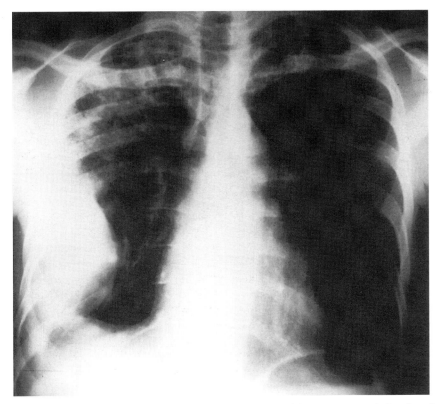

FIGURE 32.1. Posteroanterior chest radiograph of 26-year-old woman reveals loculated right pleural effusion owing to tuberculosis accompanied by extensive right upper lobe fibrocavitary infiltrate.

formed granulomata characterized by a paucity of giant cells. Respiratory isolation and four-drug therapy with isoniazid, rifampin, pyrazinamide, and ethambutol were initiated immediately on admission. Slow clinical improvement (defervescence, improved appetite, weight gain, and decreased cough) occurred over the next 7 weeks. Serologic studies revealed antibody to HIV-1. The intermediate strength tuberculin test was negative, and the patient was nonreactive to a panel of other delayed-type hypersensitivity skin test antigens.

Case Assessment

The presentation of this patient with cutaneous anergy to tests of delayed-type hypersensitivity, serologic evidence of HIV infection, pulmonary infiltrates, and exudative pleural effusion is very characteristic. In the pre-AIDS era, initial tuberculin skin tests were reported negative in as many as one-third of patients presenting with pleural effusions (53), but repeat testing within 6 to 8 weeks of the development of symptoms (or use of second-strength PPD) almost always results in a positive test in this population. In contrast, as many as 60% of HIV-positive patients with pleural TB have negative PPD skin tests (54). The pathogenesis of the negative tuberculin test in pleural

TB has been debated, with some evidence that circulating adherent monocytic cells exert a suppressor mechanism that inhibits cutaneous reactivity to PPD, and it was postulated that such suppressor cells are excluded from the pleural space (54). Other data support the sequestration of the majority of specifically sensitized T cells (reactive to PPD) within the pleural space and cast some doubt on the validity of the suppressor cell mechanism (25). Acid-fast bacteria are demonstrable on staining of pleural fluid in 10% to 15% of AIDS patients (sputum acid-fast smears positive in as many as 50%) with TB (14,15). The hemogram, serum chemistries, and other indirect indices of infection, such as the erythrocyte sedimentation rate, may all be abnormal in patients with pleural TB but are clearly nonspecific. The characteristics of the pleural fluid itself do, however, provide great assistance in the diagnosis (see previously). A contrasting clinical picture is provided by the subsequent clinical vignette.

Case Report 2

A 61-year-old recent immigrant from Eastern Europe presented because of nagging left chest pain and cough. He had a 50-pack per year smoking history and had lost 3.2 kg in the past month. Nightly temperature elevations to

38.5°C have been accompanied by drenching sweats. Physical examination was unremarkable except for diminished breath sounds and percussion dullness over the lower two-thirds of the left hemithorax. Intermediate PPD revealed 19-mm induration at 72 hours. A chest radiograph revealed a large left pleural effusion. Routine laboratory examination was within normal limits. Sputum cytologic examination and acid-fast stains were negative. Thoracentesis yielded 400 mL of yellow, slightly turbid fluid; pH 7.37; protein, 4.9 g/dL; glucose, 87 mg/dL; lactate dehydrogenase, 449 IU/L. Pleural fluid leukocyte count was 1,100 cells/μL (89% lymphocytes). Acid-fast stains and cytologic examination of the fluid were negative. Histopathologic examination of pleural tissue obtained by closed needle (Abrams) biopsy revealed chronic inflammation and multiple caseating and noncaseating granulomas. Four-drug antituberculous therapy was instituted with symptomatic improvement noted within 7 days. Acid-fast stains of pleural tissue were negative, but 8-week culture of the biopsy specimen yielded *M. tuberculosis*. Mycobacterial cultures of sputum and pleural fluid were negative. Results of drug sensitivity testing revealed pansensitive organisms, and, in view of the excellent therapeutic response, the initial four-drug regimen (isoniazid, rifampin, ethambutol, pyrazinamide) was adjusted to two drugs (isoniazid, rifampin) when these results were known.

Case Assessment

This presentation of pleural TB is characteristic of that seen in patients without HIV infection. These patients are often older (8,10–12,53), have positive tuberculin skin tests (15), relatively normal routine laboratory data (53), less commonly have positive sputum and pleural fluid acid-fast stains (14,15), and are often initially suspected to have other causes of pleural effusion (e.g., neoplastic disease). Although direct stain of pleural tissue may not frequently reveal acid-fast bacilli in HIV-negative patients, pleural tissue culture may be positive for *M. tuberculosis* in more than 80% of patients (10,15). A rapid response to treatment may also be expected.

CHARACTERISTICS OF PLEURAL FLUID

Serous pleural effusions with total protein in the range of 4 to 5 (or more) g/dL are characteristic (4,15), although lower protein content may be found in patients with AIDS. The fluid is occasionally serosanguinous and rarely frankly bloody. Pleural fluid pH is usually more than 7.30, although it may be less than 7.30 in 20% (4,15,55,56). High lactate levels (81 mg/dL; range, 45 to 200 mg/dL) have been found in tuberculous and bacterial effusions (57). Low pleural fluid glucose (<40 mg/dL) can also be seen in TB, although it is rarely less than 20 mg/dL (4,12,53), and

in one large study, it averaged 81 mg/dL (58). Mixed tuberculous and bacterial pleural effusions do occur (often with very low glucose levels), and the diagnosis of TB cannot be excluded solely based on extremely low glucose. Total pleural fluid leukocyte counts usually range from several hundred to approximately 5,000/μL (4). Patients with AIDS often have a lower pleural fluid leukocyte count with a median of 720/μL (15). Cytologic analysis usually reveals lymphocyte predominance (4,12,53,59,60), although the range is quite wide. It is unusual to find fewer 50% lymphocytes, and in many instances, 90% to 95% lymphocytes may be found (53,59,60). Some recent reports have suggested that polymorphonuclear leukocytes may occasionally predominate in as many as 38% of cases (12); in exceptional cases, the fluid is frankly purulent (61). Reactive mesothelial cells are rarely (1.2%) prevalent in tuberculous effusions (62), although one recent report casts some doubt on the rarity of this finding (63). As described previously, mesothelial cells are centrally involved in the cell–cell signaling intrinsic to the development of tuberculous pleurisy (21,22).

PLEURAL FLUID BIOCHEMISTRY

Intense interest in the biochemical components of tuberculous pleural effusions has evolved out of the desire to find specific correlates for the diagnosis of TB. Attempts to detect tuberculostearic acid in tuberculous effusions by the use of gas chromatography/mass spectrometry have had very limited success and cannot be recommended (64). ADA has received much attention. Several studies have consistently shown higher levels of ADA in the pleural fluid and serum of patients with TB effusion (41), attributed, at least in part, to a strongly positive correlation of increased CD4+ T cells and ADA levels in the effusions (41,65). Although several studies (66–68) have touted the positive predictive value of pleural fluid ADA determination (with cutoff levels greater than 47 to 53 U/L being strongly associated with TB), limitations of the assay have been emphasized by other investigators (69–71). A metaanalysis (70) suggested that pleural fluid ADA levels lower than the discriminative point ruled out pleural TB but that values higher than that point were of limited value. Other attempts to correlate ADA level with numbers of T lymphocytes were unsuccessful (71). It has not been possible to demonstrate increased ADA levels in the culture supernatants from *M. tuberculosis* isolates, indicating that the organism is not the source of the enzyme (72). Isoenzyme-2 of ADA has been associated with granulocyte-predominant tuberculous effusions that are acid-fast positive on smear or culture (73). Isoenzyme-2 of ADA has a higher positive predictive value (92%) and higher sensitivity (93%) and specificity (92%) for tuberculous effusion than does total ADA or ADA-1 (74). The pleural/serum ADA ratio was greater than 1.5 in 85.7% of tuberculous effusions in another study, which also revealed the same sensitivity as pleural fluid lysozyme determination (75). The diagnostic value of pleural fluid ADA levels is independent of HIV serologic status (76). It has been suggested (77) that the combination of polymerase chain reaction for the IS6110 sequence of *M. tuberculosis*, in combination with the measurement of ADA and IFN-γ levels, allowed a selective increase in the sensitivity and specificity of the diagnosis of tuberculous pleurisy. Lysozyme is also elevated in empyema of the pleural cavity; thus, its diagnostic utility in TB depends on the absence of empyematous fluid (78). The presence of various components of the complement cascade (79) with high levels of low molecular weight breakdown products C3d and properdin factor Ba suggests that intrapleural activation of the complement system is an important aspect of the inflammation of tuberculous pleurisy. Elevated complement activation product SC5b-9 that is 1,500 μ/L or more, accompanied by a pleural monocyte percentage greater than 90%, has an 88.5% accuracy for the identification of tuberculous effusion (80). In tuberculous pleurisy, the fibrinolytic system is also very active, with high levels of fibrinopeptide A, fibrinolytic products, and antiplasmin present in fluid; acute effusions demonstrate greater activity than chronic effusions (81). The potential diagnostic utility of measuring specific antibody to mycobacterial antigens A60 and P32 by enzyme-linked immunosorbent assay or dot-blot assay (82,83) has received much attention recently. Demonstration of mycobacterial antigens in pleural fluid by enzyme-linked immunosorbent assay (84) or radioimmunoassay (85) has also been described, and, more recently, polymerase chain reaction has been used to detect the IS6110 insertion element of mycobacterial DNA in pleural fluid (86,87) or for assay of 16S-23S rRNA gene spacer sequences (88), which improved sensitivity compared with standard mycobacterial culture of pleural fluid. These are extremely promising techniques that have not yet achieved widespread clinical use.

Radiographic Findings

In tuberculous pleural disease, plain chest radiographs most often reveal unilateral pleural effusions, more often involving the right pleural cavity; bilateral involvement may also be noted in as many as 10% of cases (20,23,89). Spontaneous resolution of tuberculous effusions has been well documented (89). Tuberculous effusions may occasionally be massive, occupying the entire hemithorax (90). As indicated above, the coexistence of pleural effusion and parenchymal disease has been increasingly observed in the AIDS era (8,11,12,14,15,17–19). Ultrasonography of the pleural cavity may be helpful in suspected tuberculous pleurisy, demonstrating winding structures of different lengths (presumably fibrin bands), mobile delicate septations, regular pleural thickening, and occasional nodularity

amidst the effusion (90–92). Computed tomography examination may be helpful in demonstrating otherwise occult areas of cavitation in the underlying lung by detecting or confirming intrathoracic lymphadenopathy (92). The latter finding is especially convincing when the use of intravenous contrast demonstrates ring enhancement of low-density (necrotic) nodes (93). Multiple pleural nodules without effusion (94,95) and discrete pleural nodules with a parasternal mass (96) have recently been reported as unusual manifestations of pleural TB. In the presence of chronic tuberculous empyema, a computed tomography scan may demonstrate a narrow (2-mm) layer of low attenuation within the parietal pleural peel, probably attributable to different episodes of pleural space infection (97).

DIAGNOSIS

The definitive diagnosis of pleural TB still rests on demonstration of the causative organism *M. tuberculosis* in culture of pleural fluid (23% to 67% yield) or of tissue obtained at pleural biopsy (90% to 97%) (10,14,53,98–101). When reviewing data regarding the yield of pleural biopsy, it is important to distinguish histopathologic demonstration of granulomas from the growth of *M. tuberculosis* from culture of biopsy material, although either is generally accepted as diagnostic. In one report (101), culture of the pleural biopsy in untreated patients with tuberculous pleurisy had a yield of 80%. Traditional open pleural biopsy has a yield similar to that of closed needle biopsy of the pleura (102). *M. tuberculosis* can be detected in formalin-fixed, paraffin-embedded tissues using commercial ribosomal RNA and DNA amplification kits, with a sensitivity ranging from 53% to 62% and a specificity of 100% (103). This technique may prove useful in the analysis of archival tissue specimens and may be more widely applied as the sensitivity of the technique improves.

Thoracoscopy (video-assisted thoracoscopic surgery) may be of value in difficult cases, demonstrating yellow-white miliary granulomas on the parietal pleura in more than 85% of cases and permitting directed biopsy of specific lesions (104,105). The other manifestation that may be noted thoracoscopically is a generalized reddening of the pleura, also associated with demonstration of granulomas on biopsy. Caution must be exercised in interpreting the presence of granulomas in pleural biopsy, however, because other diseases, e.g., plague (106), fungal infection, rheumatoid arthritis, and sarcoidosis (4) have variously been reported to cause the same histopathology. Demonstration of acid-fast bacilli on stained smears of sputum or pleural fluid, in a setting in which clinical parameters are compatible with pleural TB, is very highly suggestive. The yield of mycobacterial growth from both pleural fluid cultures and sputum in cases of pleural TB had generally been low (<30%), although higher yields have been reported in the

AIDS era (14,15). This phenomenon is attributable to low bacillary counts in the fluid and the diminished likelihood of sputum recovery of acid-fast bacilli in the absence of apparent parenchymal disease (4,107). An improved total recovery rate (57.1% compared with a historic maximum of 47%) of tubercle bacilli from pleural liquid aspirates has been demonstrated when (a) aliquots are directly injected into BACTEC (12B or 13A) (BD Diagnostic Systems, Sparks, MD, U.S.A.) broth media at the bedside, (b) aliquots of aspirates are placed in a sterile heparinized (versus plain) container, and (c) radiometric liquid culture media (rather than conventional solid media) are used in the laboratory (108). Thus, when TB is clinically likely, demonstration of granulomatous inflammation (caseating or noncaseating) on histopathologic examination of pleural biopsy tissue has traditionally been accepted as the single best test, essentially proof positive of pleural TB. The combined yield of direct acid-fast stains of pleural fluid and biopsy tissue, coupled with mycobacterial culture of pleural fluid and biopsy tissue, has exceeded 90% in some series (53,98).

THERAPY

Therapy for pleural TB must be guided by (a) the patient's general condition, (b) HIV status (either serologically determined or assumed based on risk profile), (c) presence of associated parenchymal pulmonary disease, (d) history of treatment with antituberculous chemotherapeutic agents or chemoprophylaxis, and (e) likelihood of drug-resistant organisms (based on prior isolates, prior therapy or risk group). In most instances, there is no difference in treatment of pulmonary and pleural TB. When TB pleural effusion is the first manifestation of mycobacterial disease in a locale with a low prevalence of resistant strains and occurs in an individual with low HIV risk, short-course therapy is adequate (109,110). This approach to treatment was established by the studies of Dutt et al. (107), in which a total of 201 patients with pleural TB was treated with either 9-month short-course chemotherapy regimens (143 patients) of isoniazid (INH) and rifampin (RIF) or conventional multidrug therapy (58 patients) for 18 to 24 months; results were equivalent in both groups. Similar results were reported from the United Kingdom (110). The importance of the inclusion of RIF in the three-drug (INH, RIF, and ethambutol), 9-month short-course chemotherapy of TB pleural effusion was highlighted by the results of a study from India (111). More recently, the results of 6-month treatment of tuberculous pleural effusion with two drugs (300 mg INH/600 mg RIF daily for 1 month, followed by twice-weekly therapy with 900 mg INH/600 mg RIF) were reported (107); in this study, follow-up to 133 months (median, 46 months) revealed no relapses among the 161 patients completing this therapy

for pleural TB. In locales where drug-resistant isolates are common, initial therapy for new patients with pleural TB should include four drugs (INH, RIF, ethambutol, and pyrazinamide) until results of sensitivity testing are available (112). The duration of therapy must be extended in immunosuppressed patients (including those with HIV), usually to at least 12 months (or more). Similarly, TB (pleural or other sites) occurring in patients who have received extensive prior therapy or who have known drug resistance must be treated appropriately with multidrug regimens (often five or six drugs) that include at least two (new) bactericidal agents (112a). Adjunctive treatment with corticosteroids (in addition to appropriate antituberculous chemotherapy) has been shown to accelerate both the resolution of symptomatology and reabsorption of pleural effusion (113); however, this treatment must be used judiciously and probably should be withheld in patients with HIV or HIV risk. A recent review of three small trials (*n* = 236) of adjunctive corticosteroid therapy in non-HIV–related tuberculous pleurisy indicated that there was a trend toward benefit for secondary outcomes (reduction in pleural thickening and adhesions), but it was not statistically significant (114).

TREATMENT OF COMPLICATED PLEURAL TUBERCULOSIS

Tube thoracostomy is usually reserved for complicated tuberculous effusion because of tuberculous empyema, pneumothorax, pyopneumothorax, or mixed bacterial-tuberculous empyema (56). Occasionally, however, protracted antituberculous chemotherapy and repetitive needle drainage may suffice to eradicate TB empyema (115,116). Failure to improve with appropriate antituberculous chemotherapy may occasionally be attributable to concurrent mixed infection (parenchymal, pleura, or pleuro-parenchymal) with anaerobic bacteria, e.g., *Bacteroides* species, which requires specific therapy, e.g., metronidazole (117). One of the common sequelae of pleural TB is residual pleural thickening, which may occur in as many as 50% of patients with TB pleurisy (118). Neither patient clinical characteristics nor pleural fluid biochemistry/cytology are predictive of the ultimate development of pleural thickening (118), and neither corticosteroid therapy nor repeated therapeutic thoracentesis prevents this complication (114,115).

Chronic TB empyema presents a much more difficult problem, with the approach to surgical therapy governed, at least in part, by the extent of pathology in the ipsilateral lung (119–121). Surgical decortication may be indicated when chronic empyema is accompanied by significant restriction of function (119–123) or when persistent infection in the pleural space has not been adequately eradicated by chemotherapy and other measures.

Tuberculous and posttuberculous bronchopleural fistula is often a sequelae of prior therapeutic pneumothorax (or inadequate antituberculous chemotherapy) and may present many years after the initial infections (119,124). A recent review from Italy suggests an average latent period of 44 years between the acute tuberculous illness and the presentation with empyema and/or bronchopleural or bronchocutaneous fistula (125). Chemotherapy with tube drainage, open-window thoracostomy, decortication, and pleuropneumonectomy (124,126,127) may be required to eradicate the bronchopleural fistula and empyema space. The optimal timing of surgical intervention is debated, and some patients may respond to aggressive medical therapy for primary tuberculous empyema, thus avoiding surgical intervention (128). Pleuropneumonectomy (extrapleural pneumonectomy) may be the procedure of choice when chronic empyema and ipsilateral advanced cavitary disease or bronchiectasis (with or without hemoptysis) preclude successful nonoperative management (124,126,127). Finally, tuberculous empyema may present as a chest wall mass or draining sinus tract (tuberculous empyema necessitatis), which is becoming increasingly common in this era of resurgent TB (3).

REFERENCES

1. Mettler CC. *History of medicine*. New York: Classics of Medicine Library, 1986:339.
2. Rieder HL, Snider DE Jr, Cauthen GM. Extrapulmonary tuberculosis in the United States. *Am Rev Respir Dis* 1990;141: 347–351.
3. Glicklich M, Mendelson DS, Gendal ES, et al. Tuberculous empyema necessitatis. *Clin Imaging* 1990;14:23–25.
4. Sahn SA. State of the art—the pleura. *Am Rev Respir Dis* 1988; 138:184–234.
5. Bureau of Tuberculosis Control. *Tuberculosis in New York City 1992*. New York: Bureau of Tuberculosis Control, New York City Department of Health, 1992.
6. Hill AR, Premkumar S, Brustein S, et al. Disseminated tuberculosis in the acquired immunodeficiency syndrome era. *Am Rev Respir Dis* 1991;144:1164–1170.
7. Hodsdon WS, Luzze H, Hurst TJ, et al. HIV-1-related pleural tuberculosis; elevated production of IFN-γ, but failure of immunity to *Mycobacterium tuberculosis*. AIDS 2001;15: 467–475.
8. New York City Department of Health. Office of Public Affairs. Mayor's press release (58a). Commissioner's remarks for Corona clinic opening, March 20, 2002 (T. Frieden, M.D.), 2002.
9. Merino JM, Carpintero I, Alvarez T, et al. Tuberculous pleural effusion in children. *Chest* 1999;115:26–30.
10. Chan CH, Arnold M, Chan CY, et al. Clinical and pathologic features of tuberculous pleural effusion and its long-term consequences. *Respiration* 1991;58:171–175.
11. Antoniskis D, Amin K, Barnes PF: Pleuritis as a manifestation of reactivation tuberculosis. *Am J Med* 1990;89:447–450.
12. Epstein DM, Kline LR, Albelda SM, et al. Tuberculous pleural effusions. *Chest* 1987;91:106–109.
13. Liam CK, Lim KH, Wong CM. Tuberculous pleurisy as a manifestation of primary and reactivation disease in a region with a high prevalence of tuberculosis. *J Tuberc Lung Dis* 1999;3: 816–822.
14. Ankobiah WA, Finch P, Powell S, et al. Pleural tuberculosis in patients with and without AIDS. *J Assoc Acad Minor Phys* 1990; 1:20–23.
15. Relkin F, Aranda C, Garay S, et al. Pleural tuberculosis and human immunodeficiency virus infection. *Chest* 1994;105: 1338–1341.
16. Al-Ali MA, Almasri NM. Development of contralateral pleural effusion during chemotherapy for tuberculous pleurisy. *Saudi Med J* 2000;21:574–576.
17. Vilaseca J, Lopez-Vivancos J, Arnau J, et al. Contralateral pleural effusion during drug therapy for tuberculous pleurisy. *Tubercle* 1984;65:209–210.
18. Matthay RA, Neff TA, Iseman MD. Tuberculous pleural effusions developing during chemotherapy for pulmonary tuberculosis. *Am Rev Respir Dis* 1974;109:469–472.
19. Ellner JJ, Barnes PF, Wallis RS, et al. The immunology of tuberculous pleurisy. *Semin Respir Infect* 1988;3:335–342.
20. Antony VB, Repine JE, Harada RN, et al. Inflammatory responses in experimental tuberculosis pleurisy. *Acta Cytol* 1983; 27:355–361.
21. Nasreen N, Mohammed K, Ward M, et al. *Mycobacterium*-induced transmesothelial migration of monocytes into pleural space: role of ICAM-1 in tuberculous pleurisy. *J Infect Dis* 1999; 180:1616–1623.
22. Mohammed KA, Nasreen N, Ward M, et al. *Mycobacterium*-mediated chemokine expression in pleural mesothelial cells: role of C-C chemokines in tuberculous pleurisy. *J Infect Dis* 1988; 178:1450–1456.
23. Fujiwara H, Okuda Y, Fukukawa T, et al. *In vitro* tuberculin reactivity of lymphocytes from patients with tuberculous pleurisy. *Infect Immun* 1982;35:402–409.
24. Shimokata K, Kawachi H, Kishimoto H, et al. Local cellular immunity in tuberculous pleurisy. *Am Rev Respir Dis* 1982;126: 822–824.
25. Rossi GA, Balbi B, Manca F. Tuberculous pleural effusions—evidence for selective presence of PPD-specific T-lymphocytes at site of inflammation in the early phase of the infection. *Am Rev Respir Dis* 1987;136:575–579.
26. Shimokata K, Kishimoto H, Takagi E, et al. Determination of the T-cell subset producing gamma-interferon in tuberculous pleural effusions. *Microbiol Immunol* 1986;30:353–361.
27. Ribera E, Ocana I, Martinez-Vazquez JM, et al. High level of interferon gamma in tuberculous pleural effusion. *Chest* 1988; 93:308–311.
28. Guzman J, Bross KJ, Wurtemberger G, et al. Tuberculous pleural effusions: lymphocyte phenotypes in comparison with other lymphocyte-rich effusions. *Diagn Cytopathol* 1989;5: 139–144.
29. Barnes PF, Mistry SD, Cooper CL, et al. Compartmentalization of a CD4+ T lymphocyte subpopulation in tuberculous pleuritis. *J Immunol* 1989;142:1114–1119.
30. Wongtim S, Silachamroon U, Ruxrungtham K, et al. IFN-γ for diagnosing tuberculous effusions. *Thorax* 1999;54:921–924.
31. Chen YM, Yang WK, Whang-Peng J, et al. An analysis of cytokine status in the serum and effusions of patients with tuberculous and lung cancer. *Lung Cancer* 2001;31:25–30.
32. Yamada Y, Nakamura A, Hosoda M, et al. Cytokines in pleural liquid for diagnosis of tuberculous pleurisy. *Respir Med* 2001; 95:577–581.
33. Hua C-C, Chang L-C, Chen Y-C, et al. Proinflammatory cytokines and fibrinolytic enzymes in tuberculous and malignant pleural effusions. *Chest* 1999;116:1292–1296.
34. Ribera E, Espanol T, Martinez-Vazquez JM, et al. Lymphocyte proliferation and gamma-interferon production after "*in-vitro*";

stimulation with PPD. Differences between tuberculous and nontuberculous pleurisy in patients with positive tuberculin skin test. *Chest* 1990;97:1381–1385.

35. Kurasawa T, Shimokata K. Cooperation between accessory cells and T lymphocytes in patients with tuberculous pleurisy. *Chest* 1991;100:1046–1052.

36. Okubo Y, Nakata M, Kuroiwa Y, et al. NK cells in carcinomatous and tuberculous pleurisy. Phenotypic and functional analyses of NK cells in peripheral blood and pleural effusions. *Chest* 1987;92:500–504.

37. Ota T, Okubo Y, Sekiguchi M. Analysis of immunologic mechanisms of high natural killer cell activity in tuberculous pleural effusions. *Am Rev Respir Dis* 1990;142:29–33.

38. Lorgat F, Keraan MM, Lukey PT, et al. Evidence for *in vivo* generation of cytotoxic T cells. PPD-stimulated lymphocytes from tuberculous pleural effusions demonstrate enhanced cytotoxicity with accelerated kinetics of induction. *Am Rev Respir Dis* 1992;145:418–423.

39. Barnes PF, Lu S, Abrams JS, et al. Cytokine production at the site of disease in human tuberculosis. *Infect Immun* 1993;61:3482–3489.

40. Ito M, Kojiro N, Shirasaka T, et al. Elevated levels of soluble interleukin-2 receptors in tuberculous pleural effusions. *Chest* 1990;97:1141–1143.

41. Shimokata K, Saka H, Murate T, et al. Cytokine content in pleural effusion. Comparison between tuberculous and carcinomatous pleurisy. *Chest* 1991;99:1103–1107.

42. Barnes PF, Grisso CL, Abrams JS, et al. Gamma delta T lymphocytes in human tuberculosis. *J Infect Dis* 1992;165:506–512.

43. Barnes PF, Modlin RL, Bikle DD, et al. Transpleural gradients of 1,25 dihydroxyvitamin D in tuberculous pleuritis. *J Clin Invest* 1989;83:1527–1532.

44. Porcel JM, Gazquez I, Vives M, et al. Diagnosis of tuberculous pleuritis by the measurement of soluble interleukin 2 receptor in pleural fluid. *Int J Tuberc Lung Dis* 2000;4:975–979.

45. Kim YK, Lee SY, Kwon SS, et al. Gamma-interferon and soluble interleukin 2 receptor in tuberculous pleural effusion. *Lung* 2001;179:175–184.

46. Hoheisel G, Sack U, Hui DS, et al. Occurrence of matrix metalloproteinases and tissue inhibitors of metalloproteinases in tuberculous pleuritis. *Tuberculosis (Edinb)* 2001;81:203–209.

47. Oshikawa K, Sugiyama Y. Elevated soluble CD26 levels in patients with tuberculous pleurisy. *Int J Tuberc Lung Dis* 2001;5:868–872.

48. Xirouchaki N, Tzanakis N, Bouros D, et al. Diagnostic value of interleukin-1-alpha, interleukin-6 and tumor necrosis factor in pleural effusions. *Chest* 2002;121:815–820.

49. Maeda J, Ueki N, Ohkawa T, et al. Local production and localization of transforming growth factor-beta in tuberculous pleurisy. *Clin Exp Immunol* 1993;92:32–38.

50. Levy H, Wayne LG, Anderson BE, et al. Antimycobacterial antibody levels in pleural fluid as reflection of passive diffusion from serum. *Chest* 1990;97:1144–1147.

51. Dhand R, Ganguly NK, Vaishnavi C, et al. False-positive reactions with enzyme-linked immunosorbent assay of *Mycobacterium tuberculosis* antigens in pleural fluid. *J Med Microbiol* 1988;26:241–243.

52. Baig MM, Pettengell KE, Simjee AE, et al. Diagnosis of tuberculosis by detection of mycobacterial antigen in pleural effusions and ascites. *S Afr Med J* 1986;69:101–102.

53. Berger HW, Mejia E: Tuberculous pleurisy. *Chest* 1973;63:88–93.

54. Ellner JJ. Pleural fluid and peripheral blood lymphocyte function in tuberculosis. *Ann Intern Med* 1978;89:932–933.

55. Good JT, Taryle DA, Maulitz RM, et al. The diagnostic value of pleural fluid pH. *Chest* 1980;78:55–59.

56. Chavalittamrong B, Angsusingha K, Tuchinda M, et al. Diagnostic significance of pH, lactic acid dehydrogenase, lactate and glucose in pleural fluid. *Respiration* 1979;38:112–120.

57. Brook I. Measurement of lactic acid in pleural fluid. *Respiration* 1980;40:344–348.

58. Light RW, Ball WC. Glucose and amylase in pleural effusions. *JAMA* 1973;225:257–260.

59. Spieler P. The cytologic diagnosis of tuberculosis in pleural effusions. *Acta Cytol* 1979;23:374–379.

60. Yam LT. Diagnostic significance of lymphocytes in pleural effusions. *Ann Intern Med* 1967;66:972–982.

61. Carli P. Purulent forms of tuberculous serositis. *Med Trop (Marseille)* 1989;49:193–196.

62. Hurwitz S, Leiman G, Shapiro C. Mesothelial cells in pleural fluid: TB or not TB? *S Afr Med J* 1980;57:937–939.

63. Lau K-Y. Numerous mesothelial cells in tuberculous pleural effusions. *Chest* 1989;96:438–439.

64. Yew WW, Chan C, Kwan SY, et al. Diagnosis of tuberculous pleural effusion by the detection of tuberculostearic acid in pleural aspirates. *Chest* 1991;100:1261–1263.

65. Baganha MF, Pego A, Lima MA, et al. Serum and pleural adenosine deaminase. Correlation with lymphocytic populations. *Chest* 1990;97:605–610.

66. Banales JL, Pineda PR, Fitzgerald JM, et al. Adenosine deaminase in the diagnosis of tuberculous pleural effusions. A report of 218 patients and review of the literature. *Chest* 1991;99:355–357.

67. Maritz FJ, Malan C, Le Roux I. Adenosine deaminase in the differentiation of pleural effusions. *S Afr Med J* 1982;62:556–558.

68. Strankinga WF, Nauta JJ, Straub JP, et al. Adenosine deaminase in tuberculous pleural effusions: a diagnostic test. *Tubercle* 1987;68:137–140.

69. Van Keimpema AR, Slaats EH, Wagenaar JP. Adenosine deaminase activity, not diagnostic for tuberculous pleurisy. *Eur J Respir Dis* 1987;71:15–18.

70. Ena J, Valls V, Perez de Oteyza C, et al. The usefulness and limitations of adenosine deaminase in the diagnosis of tubercular pleurisy. A meta-analytical study. *Med Clin (Barcelona)* 1990;95:333–335.

71. Ocana I, Martinez-Vazquez JM, Segura RM, et al. Adenosine deaminase in pleural fluids. Test for diagnosis of tuberculous effusion. *Chest* 1983;84:51–53.

72. Banales JL, Rivera-Martinez E, Perez-Gonzalez I, et al. Evaluation of adenosine deaminase activity in the *Mycobacterium tuberculosis* culture supernatants. *Arch Med Res* 1999;30:358–359.

73. Kurata N, Kihara M, Matsubayashi K, et al. Activities and isoenzymes of adenosine deaminase and lactate dehydrogenase in tuberculous pleural effusion with special reference to the presence of *Mycobacterium tuberculosis*. *Rinsho Byori* 1992;40:670–672.

74. Gorguner M, Cerci M, Gorguner I. Determination of adenosine deaminase activity and its isoenzymes for diagnosis of pleural effusions. *Respirology* 2000;5:321–324.

75. Valdes L, San Jose E, Alvarez D, et al. Diagnosis of tuberculous pleurisy using the biologic parameters adenosine deaminase, lysozyme and interferon gamma. *Chest* 1993;103:458–465.

76. Riantawan P, Chaowalit P, Wongsangiem M, et al. Diagnostic value of pleural fluid adenosine deaminase in tuberculous pleuritis with reference to HIV coinfection and a Bayesian analysis. *Chest* 1999;116:3–5.

77. Villegas MV, Labrada LA, Saravia NG. Evaluation of polymerase chain reaction, adenosine deaminase and interferon-γ in

pleural fluid for the differential diagnosis of pleural tuberculosis. *Chest* 2000;118:1355–1364.

78. Verea Hernando HR, Masa Jiminez JF, Dominguez Juncal L, et al. Meaning and diagnostic value of determining the lysozyme level of pleural fluid. *Chest* 1987;91:342–345.

79. Lew DP, Perrin LH, Vassalli JD, et al. High levels of complement breakdown products in tuberculous pleural effusions. *Clin Exp Immunol* 1983;52:569–574.

80. Vives M, Porcel JM, Gazquez I, et al. Usefulness of pleural complement activation products in differentiating tuberculosis and malignant effusions. *Int J Tuberc Lung Dis* 2000;4:76–82.

81. Widstrom O, Egberg N, Chmielewska J, et al. Fibrinolytic and coagulation mechanisms in stages of inflammation: a study of BCG-induced pleural exudate in guinea pig. *Thromb Res* 1983; 29:511–519.

82. Caminero JA, Rodriguez de Castro F, Carrillo T, et al. Diagnosis of pleural tuberculosis by detection of specific IgG anti-antigen 60 in serum and pleural fluid. *Respiration* 1993;60:58–62.

83. Van Vooren JP, Farber CM, De Bruyn J, et al. Antimycobacterial antibodies in pleural effusion. *Chest* 1990;97:88–90.

84. Murate T, Mizoguchi K, Amano H, et al. Antipurified-protein-derivative antibody in tuberculous pleural effusions. *Chest* 1990;97:670–673.

85. Straus E, Wu N. Radioimmunoassay of tuberculoprotein derived from *Mycobacterium tuberculosis*. *Proc Natl Acad Sci U S A* 1980;77:4301–4304.

86. De Lassence A, Lecossier D, Pierre C, et al. Detection of mycobacterial DNA in pleural fluid from patients with tuberculous pleurisy by means of the polymerase chain reaction: comparison of two protocols. *Thorax* 1992;47:265–269.

87. Pasrandaman V, Narayanan S, Narayanan PR. Utility of polymerase chain reaction using two probes for rapid diagnosis of tubercular pleuritis in comparison to conventional methods. *Indian J Med Res* 2000;112:47–51.

88. Reechaipichitkul W, Lulitanond V, Sungkeeree S, et al. Rapid diagnosis of tuberculous pleural effusion using polymerase chain reaction. *Southeast Asian J Trop Med Public Health* 2000; 31:509–514.

89. Roper WH, Waring JJ. Primary serofibrinous pleural effusion in military personnel. *Am Rev Tuberc* 1955;71:616–635.

90. Maher GG, Berger HW. Massive pleural effusion-malignant and nonmalignant causes in 46 patients. *Am Rev Respir Dis* 1972;105:458–460.

91. Carazo Martinez O, Vargas Serrano B, Rodriguez Romero R, et al. Real-time ultrasound evaluation of tuberculous pleural effusions. *J Clin Ultrasound* 1989;17:407–410.

92. Hulnick DH, Naidich DP, McCauley DI. Pleural tuberculosis evaluated by computed tomography. *Radiology* 1983;149: 759–765.

93. Pastores SM, Naidich DP, Aranda CP, et al. Intrathoracic adenopathy associated with pulmonary tuberculosis in patients with HIV infection. *Chest* 1993;103:1433–1437.

94. Tang XN, Chu KA, Lu JY, et al. Multiple pleural nodules without effusion—a rare presentation of tuberculous pleurisy. *Zhonghua Yi Xue Za Zhi* 2001;64:187–190.

95. Ariyurek OM, Cil BE. A typical presentation of pleural tuberculosis: CT findings. *Br J Radiol* 2000;73:209–210.

96. Atasoy C, Kaya A, Fitoz S, et al. Discrete pleural nodules associated with a parasternal mass: an unusual manifestation of tuberculosis. *J Thorac Imaging* 2002;7:74–77.

97. Kim HY, Song KS, Lee HJ, et al. Parietal pleura and extrapleural space in chronic tuberculous empyema: CT-pathologic correlation. *J Comput Assist Tomogr* 2001;25:9–15.

98. Poe RH, Israel RH, Utell MJ, et al. Sensitivity, specificity and predictive values of closed pleural biopsy. *Arch Intern Med* 1984; 144:325–328.

99. Levine H, Metzger W, Lacera D, et al. Diagnosis of tuberculous pleurisy by culture of pleural biopsy specimen. *Arch Intern Med* 1970;126:269–271.

100. Sharer L, McClement JH. Isolation of tubercle bacilli from needle biopsy specimens of parietal pleura. *Am Rev Respir Dis* 1968;97:466–468.

101. Scerbo J, Keltz H, Stone DJ. A prospective study of closed pleural biopsies. *JAMA* 1971;218:377–380.

102. Thompson DH, Edwards A, Mills AE. An open technique of pleural biopsy in the diagnosis of tuberculous effusions. *Ann R Coll Surg Engl* 1979;61:215–216.

103. Ruiz-Manzano J, Manterola J-M, Gamboa F, et al. Detection of *Mycobacterium tuberculosis* in paraffin-embedded pleural biopsy specimens by commercial ribosomal RNA and DNA amplification kits. *Chest* 2000;118:648–655.

104. Suzuki H, Tanaka K, Tonozuka H, et al. Clinical study of tuberculous pleuritis, diagnosed by thoracoscopy using flexible fiberoptic bronchoscope. *Nippon Kyobu Shikkan Gakkai Zasshi* 1993;31:139–145.

105. Blanc FX, Atassi K, Bignon J, et al. Diagnostic value of medical thoracoscopy in pleural disease: a 6-year retrospective study. *Chest* 2002;121:1677–1683.

106. Schmid GP, Catino D, Suffin SC, et al. Granulomatous pleuritis caused by *Francisella tularensis*: possible confusion with tuberculous pleuritis. *Am Rev Respir Dis* 1983;128:314–316.

107. Dutt AK, Moers D, Stead WW. Tuberculous pleural effusion: 6-month therapy with isoniazid and rifampin. *Am Rev Respir Dis* 1992;145:1429–1432.

108. Cheng AFB, Tai VHB, Li MSK, et al. Improved recovery of *Mycobacterium tuberculosis* from pleural aspirates: bedside inoculation, heparinized containers and liquid culture media. *Scand J Infect Dis* 1999;31:485–487.

109. Dutt AK, Moers D, Stead WW. Short-course chemotherapy for pleural tuberculosis. Nine years experience in routine treatment service. *Chest* 1986;90:112–116.

110. Ormerod LP, Horsfield N. Short-course antituberculous chemotherapy for pulmonary and pleural disease: 5 years experience in clinical practice. *Br J Dis Chest* 1987;81:268–271.

111. Malik SK, Behera D, Gilhotra R. Tuberculous pleural effusion and lymphadenitis treated with rifampin-containing regimen. *Chest* 1987;92:904–905.

112. Chawla P, Klapper P, Kamholz S, et al. Drug resistant tuberculosis in an urban population including patients at risk for HIV infection. *Am Rev Respir Dis* 1992;146:280–284.

112a. Law KF, Weiden M. Streptomycin, other aminoglycosides, and capreomycin. In: Rom WN, Garay S, eds. *Tuberculosis*. Boston: Little, Brown and Company, 1996:785–797.

113. Lee CH, Wang WJ, Lan RS, et al. Corticosteroids in the treatment of tuberculous pleurisy. A double-blind, placebo-controlled, randomized study. *Chest* 1988;94:1256–1259.

114. Matchaba PT, Volmink J. Steroids for treating tuberculous pleurisy. *Cochrane Database Syst Rev* 2000;2:CD001876.

115. Large SK, Levick RK. Aspiration in the treatment of primary tuberculous pleural effusion. *BMJ* 1958;1:1512–1514.

116. Neihart RE, Hof DG. Successful nonsurgical treatment of tuberculous empyema in an irreducible pleural space. *Chest* 1985;88:792–794.

117. Singh PP, Sridharan KB, Bhagi RP, et al. Anaerobic infection of the lung and pleural space in tuberculosis. *Indian J Chest Dis Allied Sci* 1989;31:85–89.

118. Barbas CS, Cukier A, de Varvalho CR, et al. The relationship between pleural fluid findings and the development of pleural thickening in patients with pleural tuberculosis. *Chest* 1991; 100:1264–1267.

119. Gaensler EA. The surgery for pulmonary tuberculosis. *Am Rev Respir Dis* 1982;125:73–84.

120. Toomes H, Vogt-Moykopf I, Ahrendt J. Decortication of the lung. *Thorac Cardiovasc Surg* 1983;31:338–341.
121. Nakaoka K, Nakahara K, Iioka S, et al. Postoperative preservation of pulmonary function in patients with chronic empyema thoracis: a one-stage operation. *Ann Thorac Surg* 1989;47:848–852.
122. Tatsumura T, Koyama S, Yamamoto K, et al. A new technique for one-stage radical eradication of long-standing chronic thoracic empyema. *J Thorac Cardiovasc Surg* 1990;99:410–415.
123. Al-Kattan KM. Management of tuberculous empyema. *Eur J Cardiothorac Surg* 2000;17:251–254.
124. Donath J, Khan FA. Tuberculous and posttuberculous bronchopleural fistula. *Chest* 1984;86:697–703.
125. Mancini P, Mazzei L, Zarzana A, et al. Post-tuberculous chronic empyema of the "forty years after." *Eur Rev Pharmacol Sci* 1998;2:25–29.
126. Odell JA, Henderson BJ. Pneumonectomy through an empyema. *J Thorac Cardiovasc Surg* 1985;89:423–427.
127. Naumov VN, Abramov EL, Tokaev KV, et al. New surgical tactics in the treatment of patients with complicated tuberculosis of the lungs and pleura. *Probl Tuberk* 1992;1–2:28–31.
128. Long R, Fanning A, McNamee C, et al. Medical versus surgical treatment of primary tuberculous peel. *Can Respir J* 2001;8:449–453.

33

CARDIOVASCULAR TUBERCULOSIS

JUNE E. S. ABADILLA
ALBERT E. HEURICH

Tuberculous pericarditis is a relatively rare infection that can be associated with significant morbidity and mortality (1–4). Before antibiotics were available, tuberculous pericarditis was present in 0.71% of all autopsies (5,6). Tuberculous pericarditis is an unusual manifestation of tuberculosis in much of the Western world. Pericardial involvement occurs in 1% to 4% of all patients with tuberculosis (3,5,6) and accounts for 2% to 3% of patients with extrapulmonary tuberculosis (7,8). A tuberculous etiology is established in 4% to 10% of patients with acute pericarditis (9,10), although in some parts of the world, it accounts for approximately 80% of cases (11–13). Tuberculosis is also frequently implicated as the cause of constrictive pericarditis. In the United States, tuberculosis accounts for approximately one-fifth of cases of chronic constrictive pericarditis (1–4,9,14). From reports in endemic areas, tuberculosis has accounted for 46% to 63% of etiologies of constrictive pericarditis (15–17). Histopathologic changes diagnostic of tuberculosis may be lost with chronic disease; therefore, tuberculosis may account for many cases of idiopathic constrictive pericarditis.

The acquired immunodeficiency syndrome epidemic has contributed to the worldwide resurgence in tuberculosis. Tuberculous pericarditis has been documented in patients with acquired immunodeficiency syndrome, with several cases reported as the first manifestation of human immunodeficiency virus (HIV) infection (7,18–23), including infection with multidrug-resistant strains (19). Tuberculosis accounts for as much as 93% of causes of pericardial effusions in patients coinfected with HIV disease in African countries, where both HIV and tuberculosis are epidemic (19,24,25). In the United States, it has been reported to account for anywhere from 19% to 57% (26,27). Pericardial involvement occurs in 1.5% of HIV-infected patients with extrapulmonary tuberculosis compared with 2.5% of HIV-

negative patients from the same period and area (7). In one report involving patients with HIV infection and cardiac tamponade, seven of 13 patients had tuberculosis (28).

PATHOPHYSIOLOGY

There are four stages in the evolution of tuberculous pericarditis. Initially, a fibrinous stage in which diffuse deposits of fibrin develop together with a granulomatous reaction occurs. This stage may often be clinically silent because it is not commonly observed. After this, a second stage of effusion within the pericardial sac occurs. Hypersensitivity reaction to tuberculoprotein, impaired resorptive ability, and vascular injury are believed to be mechanisms of fluid production. The pericardial surfaces become thickened and gray with a shaggy appearance owing to a fibrinous exudate (29) (Fig. 33.1). The effusion can progress through the following phases: serous, serosanguinous, turbid, or bloody. Serosanguinous pericardial fluid has been detected in 91% of HIV-seropositive patients but was described as serofibrinous in corresponding HIV-seronegative patients (19). In the turbid phase, fluid contains flakes of fibrin (9). It may revert to a clear amber to lemon color and can become a chronic cholesterol effusion (30). Cholesterol crystals induce a cellular reaction resulting in pericardial thickening (30,31). Rarely, chylopericardium occurs when there is accompanying thoracic duct disease (32). The earliest cellular reaction in the fluid consists of polymorphonuclear cells. After several days, lymphocytes predominate. Total cell count usually ranges from 500 to 10,000/mm^3 (33,34). Typical chemical changes consist of low glucose and high protein. Massive effusions, as large as 4 L, can occur (9). Tracheobronchial tuberculous lymphadenitis is associated with the largest and most rapidly accumulating effusions (9). The second stage is most likely to yield organisms.

As the effusion resolves, pericardial thickening may develop. The thickened pericardium contains fibrous tissue and granulomas; this condition characterizes the third stage. Fibrous tissue may replace the granulomas and leave no clues to the original tuberculous etiology of the pericar-

J. E. S. Abadilla: Department of Medicine, State University of New York Health Science Center at Brooklyn; Division of Pulmonary and Critical Care Medicine, Downstate Medical Center, Brooklyn, New York.
A. E. Heurich: Department of Medicine, State University of New York Health Science Center at Brooklyn; Department of Medicine, Kings County Hospital Center, Brooklyn, New York.

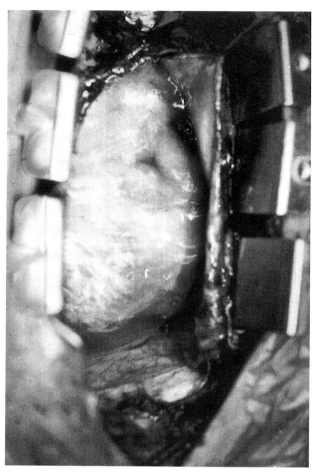

FIGURE 33.1. A view of shaggy, fibrinous pericarditis seen at the time of surgery in a patient with tuberculous pericarditis.

dial disease. With parietal pericardial thickening, myocardial constriction can occur, characteristic of stage four. Deposition of calcium in the pericardium can further complicate this stage. Progression through all four stages does not always occur clinically. The myocardium may also be affected by the pericardial disease. This may manifest initially as myocardial hypertrophy but then become myocardial atrophy (9). A postmortem study of eight patients with tuberculous constrictive pericarditis showed significant endocardial thickening in four patients and myonecrosis, lymphohistiocytic cellular infiltration, and myofibrosis in seven, suggesting that all layers of the myocardium can be involved (35).

CLINICAL PRESENTATION

The clinical presentation of patients with acute tuberculous pericarditis is quite variable. Tuberculous pericarditis occurs most often in young to middle-age adults (36,37), although there have been pediatric and geriatric cases. Some reports

document an overrepresentation of black patients (1,29). Whether enhanced susceptibility to infection with tuberculosis (38) or environmental factors account for this observation is not known. In series describing patients with mostly effusive disease, dyspnea and chest pain are present in most patients (Table 33.1). Other common symptoms are cough, weight loss, dyspnea, orthopnea, and pedal edema (1,39–42). The latter three symptoms are more specific indicators of pericardial disease. Orthopnea is present in only a minority of patients, but its presence in a patient with tuberculosis should raise concern for pericardial involvement. Cough is present in 48% to 94% of patients (1,29,43–45). Fever is usually present, occurring in 80% to 100% of patients (1,40,43–45). Signs related to a pericardial effusion occur less frequently (Table 33.1). Jugular venous distention typically occurs in 46% to 74% (1,11,29,43,45), and ankle edema is present in 24% to 64% (1,11,29,43,45). Overall, approximately 10% to 38% of patients present with evidence of pericardial tamponade (11,37).

In approximately half of the patients with chronic tuberculous pericarditis, the disease presents insidiously with no history of acute pericarditis (9). Dyspnea, jugular venous distention, hepatomegaly, ascites, and edema occur in the majority of patients, and a pericardial knock may be heard in approximately 20% (12). When hepatic circulation becomes obstructed, collateral vessels in the form of prominent superficial abdominal veins may become evident (9).

A tuberculin skin test is positive in most patients, according to series comprising mainly immunocompetent patients (1,3,11). However, this is likely not to be the case in patients coinfected with HIV, in whom tuberculin skin tests are positive in only 24% of patients with extrapulmonary tuberculosis (7). Although the skin test can help point toward the diagnosis, unless pulmonary tuberculosis is present, an evaluation of pericardial fluid, tissue, or both is necessary to establish the diagnosis.

Changes in ST and T waves on the electrocardiogram are present in 65% to 91% of patients, and low voltage in 29% to 75% (1,29,40,43). In acute pericarditis, there is characteristically initial diffuse ST segment elevation with tall, peaked or domed T waves in most leads except aVR. Subsequently, this returns to baseline and T-wave inversion may occur. Electrical alternans can develop with large effusions (46). Arrhythmias during acute pericarditis are predominantly atrial and occur primarily when there is underlying disease of the myocardium, valves, or coronary arteries (47).

In chronic tuberculous pericarditis, voltage is low with the R wave, seldom more than 6 mm. The T wave is usually inverted. The P wave becomes broad and notched in most patients. Approximately 25% of patients have axis deviation, and 33% have arrhythmias. Atrial fibrillation occurs in one-fifth of patients (9).

Radiographically, acute effusive tuberculous pericarditis typically presents teardrop- or water bottle–shaped car-

TABLE 33.1. SYMPTOMS AND SIGNS RELATING TO PERICARDITIS AS REPORTED IN SERIES OF PATIENTS WITH TUBERCULOUS PERICARDITIS

Ref.	Dyspnea (%)	Chest Pain (%)	Orthopnea (%)	Distant Heart Sound (%)	Paradoxical Pulse (%)	Pericardial Rub (%)
37	54	70	NR	NR	NR	77
43	64	42	18	NR	51	27
29	80	39	39	52	45	41
1	74	57	66	46	23	37
44	71	NR	NR	NR	47	NR
45	88	76	53	56	71	84
3	42	50	25	42	58	42
40	NR	65	47	24	53	41

NR, not reported.

diomegaly. As many as 95% of patients have cardiomegaly (11,32,39,40,45), and concomitant pleural effusion is present in 39% to 71% (11,40). The pleural effusion is most commonly left sided. A parenchymal infiltrate is present in only 29% to 32% of patients (11,45). Radiolucent fat lines in a lateral chest radiograph can be helpful in detecting an effusion. This is indicative of a radiolucent layer of epicardial fat between the myocardium and the pericardial fluid (48). Pericardial calcification is observed in 5% to 30% of patients (12,49).

Two-dimensional echocardiography provides excellent visualization of the pericardium and pericardial space in patients with tuberculous pericarditis (50,51) (Fig. 33.2). It can safely, accurately, and rapidly confirm the extent and distribution of pericardial effusions as small as 20 mL (3,40, 45,52,53) and provide evidence of tamponade. In advanced infections, "shaggy echoes" from pericardial thickening or

fibrinous exudates may be detected (45,53). The presence of exudative coating or shaggy echoes was shown in one study to have a sensitivity of 100% but a lower specificity of 22% for the diagnosis of tuberculous pericardial effusion (54). Echocardiographic findings in constrictive pericarditis may reveal the heart size to be normal or decreased with small ventricles and enlarged atria. The pericardium may be immobile and seen as a single (or double), dense, rigid shell surrounding both ventricles and the apex. Demonstration of pericardial thickening is very important because the clinical presentation of restrictive cardiomyopathy and that of tuberculous constrictive pericarditis are similar. In addition, both may reveal endocardial thickening, myofibrosis, and cellular infiltration on endomyocardial biopsy (35). Unfortunately, echocardiographic interpretation of pericardial thickening may be difficult; detectable disease shows in less than half the patients (17).

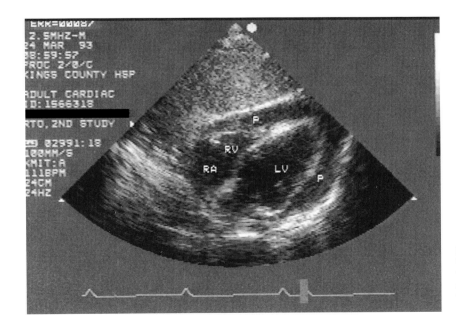

FIGURE 33.2. Echocardiographic demonstration of tuberculous pericarditis seen in subcostal view. Note the wide distance between the parietal pericardium and the epicardium of the right ventricle. *P*, pericardium; *RA*, right atrium; *RV*, right ventricle; *LV*, left ventricle.

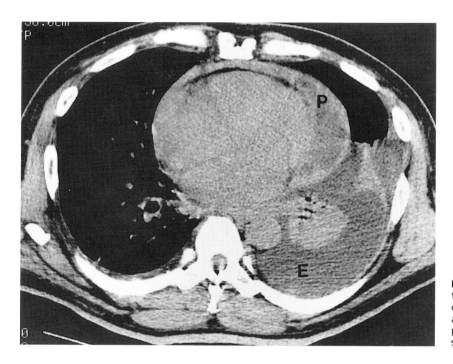

FIGURE 33.3. Computed tomography scan of the chest in a patient with tuberculous pericarditis. A thickened pericardium (*P*) is visible anteriorly. In addition, there is accompanying pleural disease bilaterally, with that on the left showing a large effusion (*E*).

Computed tomography is a reliable alternative technique useful when echocardiography is nondiagnostic for pericardial thickening (Fig. 33.3). Computed tomography may define the pericardial thickness, degree of calcification, and presence of loculated fluid. A pericardial thickness of 3 to 4 mm in adults with a clinical picture compatible with constriction, with or without angulation or sinuous config-

uration of the interventricular septum, has been successfully used to make a diagnosis of constrictive pericarditis (55). Magnetic resonance imaging can image the pericardium and yield information similar to that of computed tomography (56–58) (Fig. 33.4). Magnetic resonance imaging has limited utility in detecting calcifications (59) but may delineate the type of fluid present: transudative, exudative,

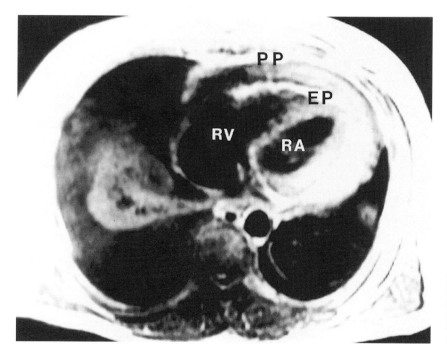

FIGURE 33.4. Magnetic resonance imaging of the chest in a patient with tuberculous pericarditis. The parietal pericardium (*PP*) is seen anteriorly. An increased distance can be seen between it and the epicardial surface (*EP*) of the right ventricle (*RV*). *RA*, right atrium.

or hemorrhagic (60). Nuclear imaging techniques using gallium 67 scintigraphy, indium 111 leukocyte imaging, and pertechnetate pyrophosphate myocardial scintigraphy have been reported to be useful in the early detection of inflammation and pericardial calcification, providing supporting evidence for tuberculous pericarditis in case reports (61,62).

DIAGNOSIS

Differential diagnosis of acute pericarditis usually includes viral, bacterial, or neoplastic pericarditis. Occasionally, radiation therapy, uremia, or collagen vascular diseases need to be considered as etiologies. Because of the variable and nonspecific features of tuberculous pericarditis, establishing the diagnosis on clinical grounds alone is impossible. A diagnosis of tuberculous pericarditis usually can be made if the *Mycobacterium tuberculosis* organism is cultured from pericardial tissue or fluid; if a pericardial biopsy shows caseating granulomas, acid-fast bacilli, or both; or if pericardial effusion or thickening occurs in a patient with bacteriologic or histologic evidence of active tuberculosis at some other tissue site (33). Rarely, other organisms with acid-fast bacilli staining properties may infect the immunodeficient patient with pericarditis. *Nocardia asteroides* may cause pericarditis, and *Mycobacterium avium-intracellulare* has been reported to cause pericarditis in patients with acquired immunodeficiency syndrome (63,64).

Sputum cultures are positive for *M. tuberculosis* in only approximately half the patients from whom they are sent (37,40). In most reports, acid-fast bacilli are rarely seen in pericardial fluid obtained from pericardiocentesis (40,43). Cultures of pericardial fluid are positive in approximately 42% to 86% of patients but are not helpful for rapid diagnosis (1,3,11,37,40). One report, in which bedside culture of pericardial effusion was used, compared double-strength liquid Kirchner culture medium, conventional Lowenstein–Jensen medium, and the radiometric medium and found positive results of 75%, 53%, and 54%, respectively (65). Pericardial biopsies in patients with acute pericarditis frequently establish the diagnosis, giving histologic evidence of tuberculosis in 70% to 83% (1,11,40) and providing tissue for culture as well. Pericardioscopy is a technique that permits direct visualization of the epicardial and pericardial surfaces, biopsies, and examination of the effusion (66). A similar diagnostic approach for visualizing the pericardium and obtaining specimens has been described involving thoracoscopic pericardial fenestration aided by a videoendoscope (67). New methods are needed for rapidly establishing the diagnosis of tuberculous involvement.

Measurement of the enzyme adenosine deaminase may be a useful aid in the early diagnosis of tuberculous infection. Adenosine deaminase has been found to be elevated in several body fluids that are commonly infected by *M. tuberculosis* (37,68–75). An elevated pericardial fluid adenosine deaminase level has been shown in several studies to be a reliable marker for the rapid diagnosis of pericardial tuberculosis. Levels higher than 40 to 70 µL had a sensitivity of 93% to 100% and specificity of 91% to 97% for tuberculous pericarditis (76–80). DNA amplification techniques including polymerase chain reaction have allowed rapid and accurate identification of tuberculosis in various clinical samples (81), including pericardial fluid (82,83) and tissue (84) and may become the procedure of choice for rapid diagnosis.

THERAPY

The risks of eventual constrictive disease and of death from acute tuberculous pericarditis underscore the need for aggressive therapy and management. Without treatment, the mortality rate of acute tuberculous pericarditis exceeds 80%. With treatment, the mortality rate ranges from 14% to 40% (1,2,9,11,29,33). Approximately 12% to 17% of patients die before diagnosis is made (1,40). Echocardiography should be routinely performed. Hemodynamic monitoring is indicated for patients with clinical or echocardiographic evidence of tamponade, patients considered at risk of tamponade, or patients with suspected constrictive pericarditis. In one protocol, a diagnostic pericardiocentesis was performed for all patients with suspected purulent pericarditis or patients with an effusion persisting for more than 7 days (10). A diagnostic pericardial biopsy was performed for illness persisting for 3 weeks (10). A search for tuberculous involvement of other systems (e.g., lungs, lymph nodes, pleura) should be undertaken. Initiation and duration of antituberculous therapy should reflect recommendations from the Centers for Disease Control and Prevention (85). Knowledge of the local community rates of resistance is especially important because cases of tuberculous pericarditis resistant to isoniazid, rifampin, streptomycin, pyrazinamide, and ethambutol have been reported (86).

The role of antituberculous therapy in tuberculous pericarditis is unquestioned. Data for the role of corticosteroids are less well defined but indicate that these agents may be beneficial in the acute phases of the disease (1,87). In a large, randomized study (11), corticosteroids significantly reduced the risk of death from pericarditis from 14% to 3% and the need for repeated pericardiocentesis from 23% to 9% but did not significantly reduce the need for open surgical drainage or eventual pericardiectomy. These findings are similar to those of smaller retrospective studies in which acute mortality was reduced (1,44), but the need for eventual pericardiectomy was unchanged (1,37,44). Corticosteroids appear to enhance resorption of the pericardial fluid and lessen (but do not eliminate) the risk of pericardium-related mortality in acute disease but do not affect long-term constrictive complications. A more recent systematic review of available data, however, questions the validity of the evidence of the reduction in mortality attributed to corticosteroids (88). Most of these investigations of adjunctive corticosteroids for tuberculous pericarditis have been done on immunocompetent patients. In one study involving HIV-positive patients with tuberculous pericarditis given corticosteroids, a reduction in mortality rate was evident but did not show a difference in the rate of resolution of the pericardial effusion or in the rate of development of constriction (89). Data from large-scale studies of the role of such treatment in HIV-positive patients, however, are scarce. An initial regimen of 60 to 80 mg prednisone per day has been used, with tapering over 8 to 11 weeks (1,11). Doses of as high as 120 mg prednisone daily resulted in a more rapid resolution of the effusion in one report, suggesting that the duration of steroid therapy could be reduced without adversely affecting outcome (90). Steroid metabolism is increased when rifampin is coadministered, and the dose may need to be increased (91).

Over time, there has been a gradual decline in mortality from the acute complications of tuberculous pericarditis (Table 33.2). This trend is probably multifactorial and related to improved detection and monitoring, liberal use of corticosteroids, and the addition of rifampin to the antituberculous regimen. However, the percentage of patients undergoing pericardiectomy has not changed appreciably.

Invasive or surgical procedures are generally recommended for three groups of patients (40): patients with cardiac tamponade, patients on medical therapy with recurrent or progressive pericardial effusion or pericardial thickening, and patients with constrictive pericarditis. Early surgical intervention has also been advocated when close follow-up of patients is difficult or impossible (92). Interventions for cardiac tamponade include pericardiocentesis, pericardiostomy, and limited or extensive pericardiectomy. Pericardiocentesis is a temporary intervention; it may be lifesaving,

but recurrence of tamponade develops in 62% to 100% of patients (11,29,37,40,43). Also, immediate diagnosis is usually not established with routine methods.

Pericardial drainage, also termed pericardiotomy or pericardial window, involves resection of a small portion of the pericardium, usually less than 4 × 4 cm, and external drainage or drainage into a nearby pleural space (93). The surgery is performed through a limited incision, most commonly a subxiphoid approach (40,93–95). Limited left anterior thoracotomy or video-assisted thoracic surgical thoracotomy have been used for pericardial drainage (96,97). These alternative incisions permit access and inspection of the pleural space and the ability to manage a pleural effusion or a pleural decortication. Mortality directly related to pericardial drainage for tuberculosis has not been observed in recent series (40,94).

Open surgical drainage by a pericardial window on admission of the patient virtually eliminates the need for pericardiocentesis and usually allows histologic confirmation of tuberculosis but does not change the acute death rate from pericarditis or alter the risk of constrictive pericarditis (11). The thickness of the pericardium obtained by biopsy may also provide useful information (40); in one series, the thickness of the pericardium in patients undergoing pericardiectomy was 10 to 13 mm compared with 2 to 6 mm in patients not requiring pericardiectomy (50).

The role of routine pericardiectomy has been controversial. Some investigators have advocated pericardiectomy during the effusive stage of the disease because it can be performed safely despite the presence of active tuberculosis (29,98) and the patient's hospital stay may be shortened (3). Also, it is impossible to reliably predict which patients will develop constrictive disease. One study showed that cardiac tamponade in the early clinical stage of tuberculous pericarditis is the factor most predictive factor of the subsequent development of constrictive pericarditis, even though

TABLE 33.2. OUTCOME OF PATIENTS TREATED FOR TUBERCULOUS PERICARDITIS

Ref.	Years	Antituberculous Therapy	Death from Pericarditis (%)	Eventual Pericardiectomy (%)
29	1952–1955	INH/STM/PAS	8/44 (18)	21/44 (48)
1	1960–1966	INH/STM/PAS	2/10 (20)	4/10 (40)
1	1960–1966	INH/STM/PAS + Pred	0/18 (0)	4/18 (22)
44	1955–1972	NR	NR	31/62 (50)
43	1973–1977	INH/STM/PAS ± Pred	16/100 (16)	19/100 (19)
3	1967–1978	INH/RIF/EMB/STM/PAS ± Pred	1/12 (8)	4/12 (33)
50	1970–1986	INH/RIF/STM ± Pred	0/16 (0)	4/16 (25)
37	1977–1987	INH/RIF/EMB	0/6 (0)	3/6 (50)
37	1977–1987	INH/RIF/EMB + Pred	0/7 (0)	4/7 (57)
11	1980–1984	INH/RIF/STM/PZA	10/74 (14)	9/74 (12)
11	1980–1984	INH/RIF/STM/PZA + Pred	2/76 (3)	6/76 (8)
40	1980–1986	INH/RIF/EMB + Pred	0/15 (0)	5/15 (33)

EMB, ethambutol; INH, isoniazid; NR, not reported; PAS, paraaminosalicylic acid; Pred, prednisone; PZA, pyrazinamide; RIF, rifampin; STM, streptomycin.

signs of tamponade resolved after pericardiocentesis (99). Myocardial atrophy develops in chronic constrictive pericarditis (100), and its perioperative mortality is related to the degree of preoperative cardiomyopathy (101,102). Detection and surgical intervention before the onset of significant cardiomyopathy has been emphasized (52,101, 102). A clinical decision analysis that assumed a 10% mortality rate from tamponade, 31% risk of constrictive disease (17% with corticosteroids), and 12% surgical mortality favored early pericardiectomy over medical therapy alone (103). Others have reserved pericardiectomy for patients with effusive disease only if there is increasing central venous pressure, despite decreasing heart size, persistent effusive disease, persistent elevation of central venous pressure despite pericardiocentesis, or pericardial thickening on biopsy (2,9,36,40,50).

The management of patients with constrictive pericarditis is mainly oriented toward surgery. For patients with a clinical diagnosis of tuberculous pericarditis with a subacute presentation, the addition of corticosteroids to antituberculous therapy may lead to a more rapid decrease in venous congestion, reduce the mortality rate from 11% to 4%, and lower the need for pericardiectomy from 30% to 21% (104). For patients with constrictive pericarditis, the surgical mortality rate is 4% to 16% (17,101,102,105). Surgery has been recommended for patients with constrictive pericarditis if there is pericardial calcification or no clinical improvement after 4 to 6 weeks of antituberculous therapy (12). The finding of pericardial calcification and atrial fibrillation or myocardial atrophy on endomyocardial biopsy has been thought to portend a poor surgical outcome (12). Although complete pericardiectomy usually resolves the problem of constrictive pericarditis, recurrent restriction has been known to occur. In such instances, the use of corticosteroids may be beneficial in reversing the constriction (106).

Most series use left anterolateral thoracotomy (17,96) or median sternotomy (105) for pericardiectomy (Table 33.3). The pericardium is generally excised from the diaphragm to the great vessels and from phrenic nerve to phrenic nerve (Fig. 33.5); decortication of the atria and great vessels is infrequently needed (Fig. 33.6). Failure to decorticate the diaphragmatic and anterolateral surfaces diminishes the surgical results. Epicardial dissection is indicated when constriction from the visceral pericardium is suspected (96).

The long-term results of a group of patients who had undergone pericardiectomy for tuberculous pericarditis were compiled from several series (3,29,37,107) (Table 33.4). Thirty-three patients closely followed for an average of 5 years (range, 1 to 13 years) had complete resolution of cardiac symptoms in 94% of cases. After successful pericardiectomy, most patients did not require medical therapy and could anticipate normal life expectancy.

Tuberculous involvement of the cardiovascular system is a relatively rare event. The distribution of reported lesions has extended from the atrium–vena cava junction to aortic arterial branches.

Tuberculous mycotic aneurysm of the aorta has been reported in 41 published cases for the period 1945 to 1999 (111). These occurred secondary to tuberculous aortitis, which was first described by Weigert (112) in 1882. The high risk of sudden rupture in the absence of appropriate treatment in the past has been uniformly fatal. Erosion of the aortic wall by a contiguous focus occurred in 75% of the cases (adenopathy in 63%), and in 25%, direct seeding of the intima, adventitia, or media was the mode of entry. Disseminated tuberculosis was present in 46% of patients. Most aneurysms were saccular and false and equally distributed between the thoracic and abdominal aortas. Disseminated tuberculosis was present in almost half of the patients. The diagnosis should be suspected in the setting of persistent pain, bleeding, a paraaortic mass, fever, shock, hoarseness and dysphasia, or hemoptysis. Recurrent gastrointestinal bleeding can also be the presenting symptom. The highest survival (87%) occurred with combined medical and prompt surgical intervention. There was no survival with a single intervention or no therapy. Results were equally good with either reconstruction with a prosthetic graft or extraanatomic bypass (111).

After nonspecific respiratory tract inflammations and neoplasms, tuberculosis is the third most common cause of hemoptysis (113). Vascular erosions in cavities (Rasmussen aneurysms) and posttuberculous bronchiectasis are the most frequent causes of tuberculous hemoptysis. Tuberculosis remains the most frequent cause of massive hemoptysis. Tuberculous aortitis is an infrequent but crucial factor

TABLE 33.3. INCISIONS FOR PERICARDIAL SURGERY

Incision	Anesthesia	Exposure	Advantage
Subxiphoid drainage	Local	Limited	Expedient
Left thoracotomy	General	Very good, except right atrium	Minimal cardiac manipulation, left decortication possible left pleural access
Median sternotomy	General	Excellent, except lateral portion left ventricle	Cardiopulmonary bypass possible

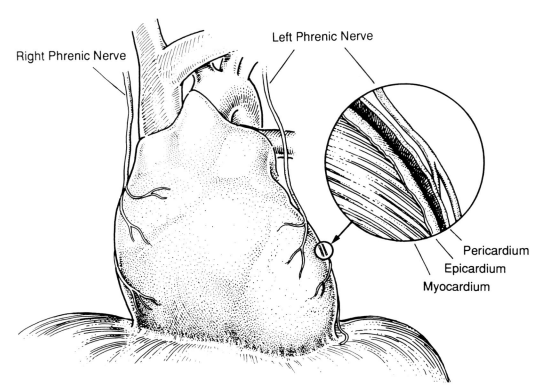

FIGURE 33.5. Normal anatomy of the anterior pericardial surface and its relationship to the diaphragm and phrenic nerves. These are important borders in pericardiectomy.

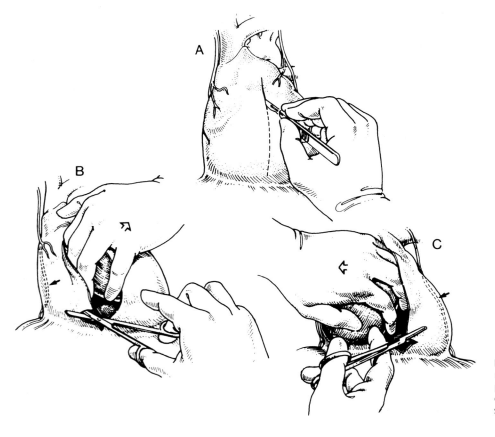

FIGURE 33.6. Incisions used to separate the myocardium from the parietal pericardium. **A:** Incision for subxiphoid drainage. **B:** Left thoracotomy incision. **C:** Median sternotomy incision.

TABLE 33.4. RESULTS OF PERICARDIECTOMY FOR TUBERCULOUS PERICARDITIS

Ref.	Center	Year	Effusion (No. of Patients)	Mortality (No. of Patients)	Constriction (No. of Patients)	Mortality (No. of Patients)
44	Chapel Hill, NC	1974	12	0	19	3
03	Galveston, TX	1980	2	0	2	0
108	Atlanta, GA	1982	6	0	2	0
102	East London, South Africa	1982	—	—	109	3
109	Los Angeles, CA	1984			6	1
21	Miami, FL	1985	2	0	6	1
40	Brooklyn, NY	1987	2	0	2	0
37	Barcelona, Spain	1988	1	0	6	0
50	Manitoba, Canada	1989	—	—	4	0
110	Baltimore, MD	1991	1	1	2	0
Total			26	1 (3.8%)	158	8 (5.1%)

in these life-threatening situations. Aortic erosions develop near lymph nodes, cold abscesses, tuberculous spondylitis, esophagitis, empyema, paravertebral abscess, and pericarditis (114). A hematogenous source for tuberculous aortitis is extremely rare. The consequences of aortitis are perforation with massive hemorrhage or formation of a perivascular hematoma (pseudoaneurysm), development of an aneurysm, or both. Tuberculous aneurysms can enlarge even with adequate chemotherapy. Rupture, bleeding, and asphyxiation can occur. Ruptures into the stomach, duodenum, jejunum, sigmoid colon, heart, pericardium, and tracheobronchial system have been described (115,116). Thoracic and abdominal aortic aneurysms predominate, but aneurysms involving the subclavian, carotid, common iliac, femoral, and innominate arteries have been reported. Almost all segments of the aorta have been involved (117) [ascending (10.2%), arch (11.4%), descending thoracic (28.4%), abdominal (42%)]. Arterial involvement includes (a) miliary tuberculosis of the intima, (b) tubercular polyps attached to the intima, (c) tuberculosis involving several layers of the arterial wall, (d) aneurysm formation, and (e) stenosing tubercular aortoarteritis. Tubercular aneurysms are mostly pseudoaneurysms (87%) and rarely true (9%) or dissecting (4%). In most patients, the aneurysm is saccular in shape. Multiple tubercular aneurysms are uncommon (117). HIV positivity can result in mycobacterial infestation of an atheromatous aorta (118).

Previously, aortography was the main diagnostic technique for demonstrating aneurysms, but this has been replaced by ultrasonography, computed tomography, and nuclear magnetic resonance imaging (119). Surgery must be urgently performed for symptomatic aneurysms. Surgical management of aneurysms has most frequently been by resection and graft placement. Other treatments have included aneurysmorrhaphy, exclusion and bypass, direct closure, and patch closure. Active infection at the surgical site requires excision of the infected material. Appropriate management includes resection of the aneurysm, repair of vessel continuity, and perioperative antituberculous chemo-

therapy. Careful clinical follow-up is needed because of the risk of recurrence in another vessel and of an anastomotic aneurysm or aortoenteric fistula (117).

With the recent increased incidence of tuberculosis related to immunosuppressed states such as HIV infection, an increase in tuberculous aortitis may be anticipated. The index of suspicion for this entity must be increased. A combination of surgical intervention and long-term chemotherapy can yield survival rates in excess of 80%. The mortality rate for surgery in tuberculous rupture is 50%. As many as one-third of these patients die during or after surgery from bleeding or rupture of another tuberculous aneurysm (120). Where feasible, *in situ* reconstruction is recommended for repair of ruptures (121).

Cardiac tuberculosis, and particularly endocardial involvement, is seen in the context of disseminated disease. The relative rarity of endocardial tuberculosis may be related to the relatively slow growth of the organism, the organism's unique fatty acid surface, and the complex interaction with immune defenses (122). Cardiac muscle has been thought to be highly resistant to tuberculosis (123–126). Tuberculoma of the myocardium is an extremely rare condition with involvement of the myocardium in fewer than 0.30% of patients dying of tuberculosis (126,127). In heart valve replacement and other forms of cardiac surgery, mycobacterial infection is very uncommon and has a poor prognosis. Most mycobacterial valvular infections appear to involve the rapid mycobacterial growers (128). Morbidity and mortality from myocardial tuberculosis have been related to conduction disturbances, ventricular aneurysms and pseudoaneurysms, ventricular rupture, aortic valve endocarditis, aortic insufficiency, superior vena cava obstruction, coronary artery occlusion, systemic embolization, obstruction to pulmonary valves, the pulmonary outflow tract, and impaired myocardial contractility (129–133). The distribution of tuberculomas in the myocardium is greatest in the right atrium and right ventricle and may be associated with atrial fibrillation. The interventricular septum is also involved and presents as conduction disturbances. The right ventricular outflow tract can be involved and manifests as outflow obstruction. Left ventricular tuberculomas occur but usually in conjunction with other cardiac sites of involvement. The differential diagnosis encompasses other diseases with granulomas such as sarcoidosis, granulomatous giant cell myocarditis, syphilitic gummas, fungal infections, rheumatic fever, rheumatoid arthritis, metastatic tumors with giant cells such as osteosarcoma and Hodgkin disease, and abscesses (133). A diagnosis of myocardial tuberculosis requires (a) histologic evidence of typical granulomas composed of a circumference of lymphocytes, epithelioid cells with Langhans giant cells, and central caseation, (b) demonstration of *M. tuberculosis*, and (c) tuberculous involvement of other organs. Demonstration of acid-fast bacilli in cardiac granulomas is very infrequent even when demonstrable in other involved organs (133).

Three types of myocardial tuberculosis have been described: miliary, isolated caseous tumor (nodular, tuberculoma), and diffuse interstitial myocarditis (infiltrative) (134). Tuberculomas can be single or multiple. Nodular and miliary lesions are the more common forms. The mediastinal and bronchial lymph nodes lie closest to the right atrium, which thus is the area of the heart most often involved (123). Besides infection via contiguous mediastinal lymph nodes or from the pericardium, hematogenous sources must also be considered. In generalized miliary tuberculosis, myocardial involvement has been found in one-third of cases (135). Solitary caseous tumors of the myocardium are very rare. Tuberculous carditis is invariably a postmortem diagnosis. The clinical features suggest myocarditis with either rapid deterioration and fatal outcome or sudden death (134).

Echocardiography and magnetic resonance imaging have been useful imaging techniques for demonstrating myocardial tuberculoma (136).

REFERENCES

1. Rooney JJ, Crocco JA, Lyons HA. Tuberculous pericarditis. *Ann Intern Med* 1970;72:73–81.
2. Ortbals DW, Avioli LV. Tuberculous pericarditis. *Arch Intern Med* 1979;139:231–234.
3. Larrieu AJ, Tyers GF, Williams EH, et al. Recent experience with tuberculous pericarditis. *Ann Thorac Surg* 1980;29:464–468.
4. Blake S, Bonor S, O'Neill H, et al. Aetiology of chronic constrictive pericarditis. *Br Heart J* 1983;50:273–276.
5. Osler W. Tuberculous pericarditis. *Am J Med Sci* 1893;105:20–37.
6. Norris GW. Tuberculous pericarditis. *Univ Penn Med Bull* 1904;17:155–170.
7. Shafer RW, Kim DS, Weiss JP, et al. Extrapulmonary tuberculosis in patients with human immunodeficiency virus infection. *Medicine* 1991;70:384–397.
8. Alvarez S, McCabe WR. Extrapulmonary tuberculosis revisited: a review of experience at Boston City and other hospitals. *Medicine* 1984;63:25–55.
9. Schepers GWH. Tuberculous pericarditis. *Am J Cardiol* 1962;9:248–276.
10. Permanyer-Miralda G, Sagrista-Sauleda J, Soler-Soler J. Primary acute pericardial disease: a prospective series of 231 consecutive patients. *Am J Cardiol* 1985;56:623–630.
11. Strang JIG, Kakaza HHS, Gibson DG, et al. Controlled clinical trial of complete open surgical drainage and of prednisolone in treatment of tuberculous effusion in Transkei. *Lancet* 1988;2:759–764.
12. Strang JIG. Tuberculous pericarditis in Transkei. *Clin Cardiol* 1984;7:667–670.
13. Dalvi BV, Kaneria VK, Thawani AJ, et al. Prospective study of 35 patients of exudative pericardial effusion with clinical and investigatory features. *Indian Heart J* 1988;40:306(abst).
14. Krumbhaar EB. The history of the pathology of the heart. In: Gould SE, ed. *The pathology of the heart.* Springfield, IL: Charles C Thomas Publisher, 1953.
15. Das PB, Gupta RP, Sukumar IP, et al. Pericardiectomy: indication and results. *J Thorac Cardiovasc Surg* 1973;66:58–70.
16. Dayem MKA, Wasfi FM, Bentall HH, et al. Investigation and treatment of constrictive pericarditis. *Thorax* 1967;22:242–52.
17. Bashi VV, John S, Ravikunar E, et al. Early and late results of pericardiectomy in 118 cases of constrictive pericarditis. *Thorax* 1988;43:637–641.
18. Supervia A, Campodarve I, Shaath M, et al. Tuberculous pericarditis as the first manifestation of AIDS. The indication for diagnostic pericardiocentesis. *Rev Clin Esp* 1993;192:150–151.
19. Taelman H, Kagame A, Batungwanayo J, et al. Pericardial effusion and HIV infection. *Lancet* 1990;335:924.
20. de Miguel J, Pedreira JD, Campos V, et al. Tuberculous pericarditis and AIDS. *Chest* 1990;97:1273.
21. Dalli E, Quesada A, Juan G, et al. Tuberculous pericarditis as the first manifestation of the acquired immunodeficiency syndrome. *Am Heart J* 1987;114:905–906.
22. Antony S, Haas DW. Tuberculous pericarditis in an HIV-infected patient. *Scand J Infect Dis* 1995;27:411–413.
23. Serrano-Heranz R, Camino A, Vilacosta I, et al. Tuberculous cardiac tamponade and AIDS. *Eur Heart J* 1995;16:430–432.
24. Cegielski JP, Lwakatare J, Dukes CS, et al. Tuberculous pericarditis in Tanzanian patients with and without HIV infection. *Tuber Lung Dis* 1994;75:429–434.
25. Pozniak AL, Weinberg J, Mahari M, et al. Tuberculous pericardial effusion associated with HIV infection: a sign of disseminated disease. *Tuber Lung Dis* 1994;75:297–300.
26. Reynolds MM, Hecht SR, Berger M, et al. Large pericardial effusions in the acquired immunodeficiency syndrome. *Chest* 1992;102:1746–1747.
27. Chen Y, Brennessel D, Walters J, et al. Human immunodeficiency virus-associated pericardial effusion: report of 40 cases and review of literature. *Am Heart J* 1999;137:516–521.
28. Kwan T, Karve MM, Emerole O. Cardiac tamponade in patients infected with HIV. *Chest* 1993;104:1059–1062.
29. Hageman JH, D'Esopo ND, Glenn WWL. Tuberculosis of the pericardium: a long-term analysis of forty-four proved cases. *N Engl J Med* 1964;270:327–332.
30. Brown AK. Chronic idiopathic pericardial effusion. *Br Heart J* 1966;28:609–614.
31. Spodick DH. Pericardial diseases. In: Spodick DH, ed. *Cardiovascular clinics.* Philadelphia: FA Davis, 1976:1–10.
32. Fowler NO. *The pericardium in health and disease.* Mount Kisco, NY: Futura, 1985.
33. Crocco JA. Cardiovascular tuberculosis. In: Schlossberg D, ed. *Tuberculosis.* New York: Springer-Verlag, 1988:133–137.
34. Delacroix I, Thomas F, Godart J, et al. Purulent tuberculous pericarditis with cardiac tamponade. *Am J Med* 1992;93:105.
35. Dave T, Narula JP, Chopra P. Myocardial and endocardial involvement in tuberculous constrictive pericarditis: difficulty

in biopsy distinction from endomyocardial fibrosis as a cause of restrictive heart disease. *Int J Cardiol* 1990;28:245–251.

36. Fowler NO. Tuberculous pericarditis. *JAMA* 1991;266:99–103.

37. Sagrista-Sauleda J, Permanyer-Miralda G, Soler-Soler J. Tuberculous pericarditis: ten-year experience with a prospective protocol for diagnosis and treatment. *J Am Coll Cardiol* 1988;11:724–728.

38. Stead WW, Senner JW, Reddick WT, et al. Racial differences in susceptibility to infection by *Mycobacterium tuberculosis*. *N Engl J Med* 1990;332:422–427.

39. Martin RP, Bowden, Filly K, et al. Intrapericardial abnormalities in patients with pericardial effusion: findings by two-dimensional echocardiography. *Circulation* 1980;61:568–572.

40. Quale JM, Lipschik GY, Heurich AE. Management of tuberculous pericarditis. *Ann Thorac Surg* 1987;43:653–655.

41. Harris LF. Tuberculous pericarditis, a unique experience. *Alabama Med* 1987;57:16–23.

42. Girling DJ, Darbyshire JH, Humphries MJ, et al. Extrapulmonary tuberculosis. *Br Med Bull* 1988;44:738–756.

43. Desai HN. Tuberculous pericarditis. A review of 100 cases. *S Afr Med J* 1979;55:877–880.

44. Carson TJ, Murray GP, Wilcox BR, et al. The role of surgery in tuberculous pericarditis. *Ann Thorac Surg* 1974;17:163–167.

45. Fowler NO, Manitsas GT. Infectious pericarditis. *Prog Cardiovasc Dis* 1973;16:323–336.

46. Pudifin D. Total electrical alternans in a patient with tuberculous pericarditis. *S Afr Med J* 1976;50:1249–1251.

47. Spodick DH. Arrhythmias during acute pericarditis. A prospective study of 100 consecutive cases. *JAMA* 1976;235:39–41.

48. Heinsimer JA, Collins GJ, Burkman MH, et al. Supine cross-table lateral chest roentgenogram for the detection of pericardial effusion. *JAMA* 1987;257:3266–3268.

49. Gimlette TMD. Constrictive pericarditis. *Br Heart J* 1959;21:9–16.

50. Long R, Younes M, Patton N, et al. Tuberculous pericarditis: long-term outcome in patients who received medical therapy alone. *Am Heart J* 1989;117:1133–1139.

51. Chandraratna PA. Echocardiography and doppler ultrasound in the evaluation of pericardial disease. *Circulation* 1991;84 (Ssuppl 3):1103–1110.

52. Berger M, Bobak L, Jelveh M, et al. Pericardial effusion diagnosed by echocardiography. *Chest* 1978;74:174–179.

53. Chia BL, Chod M, Tan H, et al. Echocardiographic abnormalities in tuberculous pericardial effusion. *Am Heart J* 1984;107:1034–1035.

54. Liu PY, Li YH, Tsai WC, et al. Usefulness of echocardiographic intrapericardial abnormalities in the diagnosis of tuberculous pericardial effusion. *Am J Cardiol* 2001;87:1133–1135.

55. Suchet IB, Horwitz TA. CT in tuberculous constrictive pericarditis. *J Comput Assist Tomogr* 1992;16:391–400.

56. Winkler M, Higgins CB. Suspected intracardiac masses: evaluation by MR imaging. *Radiology* 1987;165:117–122.

57. Stark DD, Higgins CB, Lanzer P, et al. Magnetic resonance imaging of the pericardium: normal and pathologic findings. *Radiology* 1984;150:469–474.

58. Soulen RL, Stark DD, Higgens CB. Magnetic resonance imaging of constrictive pericardial disease. *Am J Cardiol* 1985;55:480–484.

59. Hammersmith SM, Colletti PM, Norris SL, et al. Cardiac calcifications: difficult MRI diagnosis. *Magn Reson Imaging* 1991;9:195–200.

60. Naidich DP, Zerhouni EA, Siegalman SS. Heart and pericardium. In: *Computed tomography and magnetic resonance of the thorax*, 2nd ed. New York: Raven Press, 1991:557–587.

61. Ishino Y, Shiozaki H, Nakata AH. Positive Tc-99m pyrophosphate myocardial scintigraphy in a patient with tuberculous pericarditis. *Clin Nucl Med* 1992;17:515–517.

62. Schmidt U, Rebarber IF. Tuberculous pericarditis identified with gallium-67 and indium-111 leukocyte imaging. *Clin Nucl Med* 1994;19:146–147.

63. Poland GA, Jorgensen CR, Sarosi GA. Nocardia asteroides pericarditis: report of a case and review of the literature. *Mayo Clin Proc* 1990;65:819–824.

64. Woods GL, Goldsmith JC. Fatal pericarditis due to *Mycobacterium avium-intracellulare* in acquired immunodeficiency syndrome. *Chest* 1989;95:1355–1357.

65. Strang G, Latouf S, Commerford P. Bedside culture to confirm tuberculous pericarditis. *Lancet* 1991;338:1600–1601.

66. Maisch B, Drude L. Pericardioscopy—a new diagnostic tool in inflammatory diseases of the pericardium. *Eur Heart J* 1991;12(Suppl D):2–6.

67. Maisch B. Pericardial diseases, with a focus on etiology, pathogenesis, pathophysiology, new diagnostic imaging methods, and treatment. *Curr Opin Cardiol* 1994;9:379–388.

68. Telenti M, Fdez J, de Quiros B, et al. Tuberculous pericarditis: diagnostic value of adenosine deaminase. *Presse Med* 1991;20:637–640.

69. Martinez-Vazquez JM, Ribera E, Ocana I, et al. Adenosine deaminase activity in tuberculous pericarditis. *Thorax* 1986;41:888–889.

70. Isaka N, Tanaka R, Nakamura M, et al. A case of tuberculous pericarditis—use of adenosine deaminase activity (ADA) in early diagnosis. *Heart Vessels* 1990;5:247–248.

71. Ocana I, Martinez-Vazquez JM, Segura RM, et al. Adenosine deaminase in pleural fluids. Test for diagnosis of tuberculous pleural effusion. *Chest* 1983;84:51–53.

72. Piras MA, Gakis C, Budroni A, et al. Adenosine deaminase activity in pleural effusions: an aid to differential diagnosis. *BMJ* 1978;2:1751–1752.

73. Pettersson T, Ojala K, Weber TH. Adenosine deaminase in the diagnosis of pleural effusion. *Acta Med Scand* 1984;215:299–304.

74. Martinez-Vazquez JM, Ocana I, Ribera E, et al. Early diagnosis of pleuroperitoneal tuberculosis by the determination of adenosine deaminase. *Med Clin (Barcelona)* 1984;83:578–580.

75. Piras MA, Gakis C. Cerebrospinal fluid adenosine deaminase activity in tuberculous meningitis. *Enzyme* 1973;14:314–317.

76. Aggeli C, Pitsavos C, Brili S, et al. Relevance of adenosine deaminase and lysozyme measurements in the diagnosis of tuberculous pericarditis. *Cardiology* 2000;94:81–85.

77. Dogan R, Demircin M, Sarigul A, et al. Diagnostic value of adenosine deaminase activity in pericardial fluids. *J Cardiovasc Surg* 1999;40:501–504.

78. Koh KK, In HH, Lee KH, et al. New scoring system using tumor markers in diagnosing patients with moderate pericardial effusions. *Int J Cardiol* 1997;61:5–13.

79. Koh KK, Kim EJ, Cho CH, et al. Adenosine deaminase and carcinoembryonic antigen in pericardial effusion diagnosis, especially in suspected tuberculous pericarditis. *Circulation* 1994;89:2728–2735.

80. Komsuoglu B, Goldeli O, Kulan K, et al. The diagnostic and prognostic value of adenosine deaminase in tuberculous pericarditis. *Eur Heart J* 1995;16:1126–1130.

81. Brisson-Noel A, Gicquel B, Lecossier D, et al. Rapid diagnosis of tuberculosis by amplification of mycobacterial DNA in clinical samples. *Lancet* 1991;338:364–366.

82. Godfrey-Faussett P, Wilkins EG, Khoo S, et al. Tuberculous pericarditis confirmed by DNA amplification. *Lancet* 1991;337:176–177.

83. Tzoanonopoulos D, Stakos D, Hatseras D, et al. Detection of *Mycobacterium tuberculosis* complex DNA in pericardial fluid, bone marrow and peripheral blood in a patient with pericardial tuberculosis. *Neth J Med* 2001;59:177–180.

84. Cegielski JP, Devlin BH, Morris AJ, et al. Comparison of PCR, culture, and histopathology for diagnosis of tuberculous pericarditis. *J Clin Microbiol* 1997;35:3254–3257.

85. Initial therapy for tuberculosis in the era of multidrug resistance. Recommendations of the Advisory Council for the Elimination of Tuberculosis. *MMWR Morb Mortal Wkly Rep* 1993;42:1–8.

86. Horn DL, Hewlett D Jr, Alfalla C, et al. Fatal hospital acquired multidrug-resistant tuberculous pericarditis in two patients with AIDS. *N Engl J Med* 1992;327:1816–1817.

87. Bhan GL. Tuberculous pericarditis. *J Infect* 1980;2:360–364.

88. Mayosi BM, Volmink JA, Commerford PJ. Interventions for treating tuberculous pericarditis. *Cochrane Database of Syst Rev* 2000;2:CD000526.

89. Hakim JG, Ternouth I, Mushangi E, et al. Double blind randomized placebo controlled trial of adjunctive prednisolone in the treatment of effusive tuberculous pericarditis in HIV seropositive patients. *Heart* 2000;84:183–188.

90. Strang JIG. Rapid resolution of tuberculous pericardial effusion with high dose prednisone and anti-tuberculous drugs. *J Infect* 1994;28:251–254.

91. McAllister WA, Thompson PJ, Al-Habet SM, et al. Rifampicin reduces effectiveness and bioavailability of prednisolone. *BMJ* 1983;286:923–925.

92. Gabriel L, Shelburne JC. "Acute" granulomatous pericarditis, clinical and hemodynamic correlate. *Chest* 1977;71:473–478.

93. Santos GH, Frater RWM. The subxiphoid approach in the treatment of pericardial effusion. *Ann Thorac Surg* 1977;23:467–470.

94. Prager RL, Wilson CH, Bender HW. The subxiphoid approach to pericardial disease. *Ann Thorac Surg* 1982;34:6–9.

95. Palatianos GM, Thurer RJ, Pompeo MQ, et al. Clinical experience with subxiphoid drainage of pericardial effusions. *Ann Thorac Surg* 1989;48:381–385.

96. Piehler JM, Pluth JR, Schatt HV, et al. Surgical management of effusive pericardial disease: influence of extent of pericardial resection on clinical course. *J Thorac Cardiovasc Surg* 1985;90:506–515.

97. Caccavale RJ. Video assisted thoracic surgery for pericardial disease. *Chest Surg Clin North Am* 1993;3:271–281.

98. Holman E, Willett P. Treatment of active tuberculous pericarditis by pericardiectomy. *JAMA* 1951;146:1–7.

99. Suwan PK, Potjalongsilp S. Predictors of constrictive pericarditis after tuberculous pericarditis. *Br Heart J* 1995;73:187–189.

100. Dines DE, Edwards JE, Burchell HB. Myocardial atrophy in constrictive pericarditis. *Mayo Clin Proc* 1958;33:93–99.

101. McCaughan BC, Schaff HV, Piehler JM, et al. Early and late results of pericardiectomy for constrictive pericarditis *J Thorac Cardiovasc Surg* 1985;89:340–350.

102. Fennell WMP. Surgical treatment of constrictive tuberculous pericarditis. *S Afr Med J* 1982;62:353–355.

103. Sonnenberg FA, Pauker SG. Elective pericardiectomy for tuberculous pericarditis: should the snappers be snipped? *Med Decis Making* 1986;6:110–123.

104. Strang JIG, Kakaza HHS, Gibson DG, et al. Controlled trial of prednisolone as adjuvant in treatment of tuberculous constrictive pericarditis in Transkei. *Lancet* 1987;2:1418–1422.

105. Cameron J, Oesterle SN, Baldwin JC, et al. The etiologic spectrum of constrictive pericarditis. *Am Heart J* 1987;113:354–360.

106. Kashani IA, Higgins CB, Utley JR. Inflammatory constriction following complete pericardiectomy in tuberculous constrictive pericarditis. *Clin Pediatr* 1983;22:219–221.

107. Gooi HC, Smith JM. Tuberculous pericarditis in Birmingham. *Thorax* 1978;33:94–96.

108. Miller JI, Mansour KA, Hatcher CR Jr. Pericardiectomy: current indications, concepts and results in a university center. *Ann Thorac Surg* 1982;34:40–45.

109. Robertson JM, Mulder DG. Pericardiectomy: a changing scene. *Am J Surg* 1984;148:86–90

110. DeValeria PA, Baumgartner WA, Casale AS, et al. Current indications, risks and outcome after pericardiectomy. *Ann Thorac Surg* 1991;52:219–224.

111. Long R, Guzman R, Greenberg H, et al. Tuberculous mycotic aneurysm of the aorta. *Chest* 1999;115:522–531.

112. Weigert C. Uber Venetuberkel und ihre Beziehung zur Tuberkulosen Blutinfection. *Virchows Arch Pathol Anat* 1882;88:307–309.

113. Muller-Wening D, Becker HM, Blaha H, et al. Tuberculous aneurysm of the descending aorta with an aorto-bronchial fistula. *Praxis Klin Pneumol* 1982;36:22–26.

114. Golzarian J, Cheng J, Giron F, et al. Tuberculous pseudoaneurysm of the descending thoracic aorta. *Texas Heart Inst J* 1999;26:232–235.

115. Robbs JV, Bhoola KD. Aorto-oesophageal fistula complicating tuberculous aortitis. *S Afr Med J* 1976;50:702–704.

116. Takahashi K, Maruyama A, Aini S, et al. A case of tuberculous abdominal aortic aneurysm which ruptured and perforated the sigmoid. *Nippon Geka Gakkai Zasshi* 1986;87:99–104.

117. Choudhary SK, Bhan A, Talwar S, et al. Tubercular pseudoaneurysms of aorta. *Ann Thorac Surg* 2001;72:1239–1244.

118. Gouny P, Valverde A, Vincent D, et al. Human immunodeficiency virus and infected aneurysm of the abdominal aorta. *Ann Vasc Surg* 1992;6:239–243.

119. Ikezawa T, Iwatsuka Y, Naiki K, et al. Tuberculous pseudoaneurysm of the descending thoracic aorta: a case report and literature review of surgically treated cases. *J Vasc Surg* 1996;24:693–697.

120. Nachega JB, Vandercam Y, d'Udekem R, et al. Chronic dissection of the thoracic aorta in a patient with tuberculous pleuropericarditis. *Acta Clin Belg* 1998;53:53–54.

121. Allins AD, Wagner WH, Cossman DV, et al. Tuberculous infection of the descending thoracic and abdominal aorta: case report and literature review. *Ann Vasc Surg* 1999;13:439–444.

122. Cope AP, Heber M, Wilkins EG. Valvular tuberculous endocarditis: a case report and review of the literature. *J Infect* 1990;21:293–296.

123. Liau CS, Chiou HC, Wang TC. Inflammatory tumor of the myocardium. *J Formosan Med Assoc* 1980;79:1057–1069.

124. Diefenbach WCL. Tuberculosis of the myocardium: a review. *Am Rev Tuberc* 1950;62:390–402.

125. Gouley BA, Bellet S, McMillan TM. Tuberculosis of the myocardium. *Arch Intern Med* 1933;51:244–263.

126. Horn H, Saphir O. The involvement of the myocardium in tuberculosis. *Am Rev Tuberc* 1935;32:492–506.

127. Auerbach O, Guggenheim A. Tuberculosis of the myocardium: a review of the literature and a report of six new cases. *Q Bull SeaView Hosp* 1937;2:264.

128. Grange JM. Mycobacterial infections following heart-valve replacement. *J Heart Valve Dis* 1992;1:102–109.

129. Kapoor OP, Mascarenhas E, Rananaware MM, et al. Tuberculoma of the heart. Report of nine cases. *Am Heart J* 1973;86:334–340.

130. Soyer R, Brunnet A, Chevalier B, et al. Tuberculous aortic insufficiency. *J Thorac Cardiovasc Surg* 1981;82:254–256.

131. Human DG, Rose A, Fraser CB. Tuberculous aneurysm of the left ventricle. A case report. *S Afr Med J* 1983;64:26–28

132. Halim MA, Mercer EM, Guinn GE. Myocardial tuberculoma

with rupture and pseudoaneurysmal formation—successful surgical treatment. *Br Heart J* 1985;54:603–604.

133. Baretti R, Eckel L, Beyersdorf F. Isolated myocardial tuberculoma in the left ventricle. *Dtsch Med Wochenschr* 1994;119:102–106.

134. Parafiniuk W. Tuberculosis of the myocardium. *Pol Med J* 1968;8:641–646.

135. Parafiniuk W. Histomorphological and histochemical studies of the myocardial stroma in miliary tuberculosis in children. *Pol Med J* 1962;3:1078.

136. Immer FF, Pirovino M, Saner H. Isolated tuberculosis of the heart. Observation of the clinical and echocardiographic course. *Z Kardiol* 1997;86:15–19.

INTESTINAL AND PERITONEAL TUBERCULOSIS

STEVEN FIELD
STUART LEWIS

Tuberculosis of the gastrointestinal tract was once a common and feared disease. It was considered incurable. When cures did occur, physicians more often believed that their diagnoses were in error rather than accept that their conscientious care was effective or that good luck had befallen their patient. This, of course, is no longer true. In industrialized nations, successful public health campaigns and efficient diagnostic and therapeutic tools have made gut tuberculosis a relative rarity. Unfortunately, the clinician must still remain vigilant because the appearance of this disease as gastrointestinal tuberculosis is still prevalent in nonindustrialized nations, recent immigrants, and perhaps in human immunodeficiency virus (HIV)–infected individuals.

INTESTINAL TUBERCULOSIS

Historical Perspectives

Brown and Sampson (1) divided the history of intestinal tuberculosis into four distinct periods: the "dysentery period," the "period of tuberculous diarrhea," the "period of pathologic study," and the "period of roentgenologic diagnosis." The "dysentery period" was essentially the age of clinical observation and extended from the early Law of Manu (1000 B.C.), which described the phthisis as an unclean and incurable illness, through the time of Hippocrates and until Bayle (1810). Although much was written during this period, there was little speculation that the pulmonary and enteric symptoms might be the same disease in different organs. This all began to change beginning with Viorordt's 1643 description of a large pulmonary cavity and intestinal tuberculosis found at the autopsy of 33-year-old Louis XIII of France (2).

S. Field: Department of Medicine, Division of Gastroenterology, New York University School of Medicine; Department of Medicine, New York University–Tisch Hospital, New York, New York.
S. Lewis: Department of Environmental Medicine, New York University School of Medicine, New York, New York.

In 1700, Manget (3) reported a case of a man who died of phthisis who at autopsy had "hailstones" in his lungs, liver, spleen, mesenteric glands, and intestines. These hailstones' were likened to millet seed. Later in 1715, Brunner (4), a Swiss physician, described a case of enteric tuberculosis in which he found 60 intestinal ulcers, many of these in Peyer patches, in a patient who died of pulmonary tuberculosis.

The era of clinical observation gave way to the 15-year period called the "period of tuberculous diarrhea." It was during this time that the phthisis and diarrhea accompanying it were found to be of the same origin. This correlation was made by Bayle (5), in 1810, in his *Recherches sur la phthisie pulmonaire*. Bayle described the lesion of "the tubercle in cervical and mesenteric glands and . . . of the mucous membrane of the intestine which is affected with (the) same disease." He went on to state "of all the changes . . . there are perhaps none more remarkable than this ulceration, on account of the diarrhea which it frequently causes." Although the exclusion of Bayle's work from the following "period of pathologic study" seems somewhat arbitrary, Brown and Sampson date the beginning of this period with the 1825 publication of the anatomic pathologic series of Louis (6) and the later work of Rokitansky (7).

The work of Louis and of Rokitansky attempted to connect the varying symptoms of tuberculosis with the pathologic changes found at autopsy. This type of investigation represented a dramatic paradigmatic shift from the purely observational analyses that preceded it. It was the precise and painstaking anatomic observations of Louis and others that provided the foundation for modern scientific medicine and for the investigations of the pathogenesis of tuberculosis that would follow over the next 100 years. It did, as Bichat predicted, "[change] the confusion . . . in the symptoms which refusing to yield up their meaning, offer you a succession of incoherent phenomena. Open up a few corpses . . . (and) dissipate at once the darkness that observation alone could not dissipate" (8).

At the beginning of the 20th century, a great deal was known about the pathogenesis of tuberculosis, although significant gaps existed with regard to the early diagnosis of intestinal tuberculosis. It was the attitude of clinicians that "in pulmonary tuberculosis it was impossible to diagnose intestinal tuberculosis with any degree of certainty . . . and often doubt was expressed in an individual case even when the intestinal disease seemed . . . advanced" (9). Intestinal tuberculosis was considered a uniformly fatal disease and "if perchance a patient . . . recovered, the diagnosis was considered to be in error" (9). This changed with the 1919 report by Brown and Sampson (10) of a series of patients with ulcerative tuberculous colitis diagnosed by barium meal/barium enema examinations.

The publication of their study marks the beginning of the fourth period, or the "period of roentgenologic diagnosis." Although Stierlin was the first to report on the use of radiographic studies for the diagnosis of tuberculous colitis, the work of Brown and Sampson (1) was the first to be widely accepted. By 1926, 2,595 patients with pulmonary tuberculosis had been studied at the Trudeau Institute (Saranac Lake, NY, U.S.A.). Of those, 869 demonstrated evidence of intestinal tuberculosis. Although pathologic diagnoses were not obtained in all patients, 62 of the 869 who went to surgery or autopsy had evidence of tuberculous colitis.

With the advent of effective antimycobacterial medications, widespread use of skin testing, chest radiographic studies, and the pasteurization of milk, the incidence of intestinal tuberculosis decreased rapidly in industrialized nations. Mitchell and Bristol (11), analyzing more data from the Trudeau Institute, noted that only 6.3% of all cases of pulmonary tuberculosis between 1924 and 1949 were complicated by intestinal involvement and the incidence had decreased to 1% by 1949. This "period of pharmacotherapy" extended until very recently when the epidemiology of tuberculosis again changed, predominantly owing to the effects of the HIV epidemic and the increased prevalence of multidrug-resistant organisms. Thus, we have now entered the sixth period of tuberculosis: "the age of immunosuppression."

Epidemiology

Before the introduction of effective antituberculosis medications, effective public health initiatives, and the routine pasteurization of milk, intestinal tuberculosis was the most frequent complication of pulmonary tuberculosis. Autopsy series performed in the late 19th and early 20th centuries demonstrated that 3% to 90% of all cases of pulmonary tuberculosis were complicated by intestinal disease (12). The introduction of barium roentgenology afforded the opportunity to assess the frequency of disease in patients with a broad spectrum of pulmonary involvement. As mentioned, Brown and Sampson (1) found intestinal involvement in 33% of patients with pulmonary tuberculosis.

However, early studies on incidence probably included Crohn disease, which was not described until the 1930s. The severity of pulmonary disease was related to the frequency of intestinal involvement. Five percent to 8% of patients with early disease had enteric involvement; for those with moderately advanced disease, the rate rose to 14% to 18%, and 70% to 80% of patients with advanced pulmonary disease demonstrated radiographic abnormalities consistent with intestinal tuberculosis. Mitchell and Bristol (11) analyzed 346 cases of intestinal tuberculosis diagnosed by routine radiography in 5,529 patients with pulmonary tuberculosis between 1924 and 1949. During this 25-year period, 1% of patients with minimal disease, 4.5% of patients with moderately advanced disease, and 24.7% of patients with far-advanced pulmonary disease demonstrated evidence of intestinal tuberculosis. By 1949, only 1% of all patients admitted to the Trudeau Sanitorium had the complication of enteric disease.

The current incidence of intestinal tuberculosis in the industrialized world is not well characterized but is considerably less than that found in the preantibiotic era. Unfortunately, however, tuberculosis continues to be a major public health problem in many underdeveloped countries, and enteric disease is commonplace in these regions. In Delhi, India, abdominal tuberculosis comprises an estimated 0.8% of all hospital admissions, and large numbers of patients still present with obstruction or perforation requiring emergency laparotomy (13).

Few large-scale studies exist on the incidence of intestinal tuberculosis in the United States. Sherman et al. (14) studied 4,222 patients with tuberculosis who were admitted to the University of Michigan Hospital between 1956 and 1977. Only 15 were believed to have intestinal tuberculosis (0.4%). More extensive data exist regarding the incidence in Canada, the United Kingdom, and South Africa. Jakubowski et al. (15) reviewed 341 cases of abdominal tuberculosis in Canada between 1970 and 1981. The computed incidence rate decreased from two per one million per year to one per one million per year over this period, although the proportion of cases of abdominal tuberculosis remained stable at 0.8%. This study did not differentiate between peritoneal tuberculosis, mesenteric lymphadenitis, or intestinal disease. A follow-up study of residents of British Columbia, Canada, described 81 patients with abdominal tuberculosis, 33 of whom had ileocecal or anorectal disease. Among those patients, 54% had active pulmonary tuberculosis at the time of presentation (16).

Several studies published over the past 10 years detailed the incidence of abdominal tuberculosis in the United Kingdom. Klimach and Ormerod (17) reviewed 109 patients with abdominal tuberculosis (95 intestinal, 14 tuberculous peritonitis) who met strictly defined clinical and laboratory criteria and were admitted to Blackburn, Hyndburn, and Ribble Valley District hospitals between 1970 and 1984. Most of these patients were immigrants from India, Pakistan, or Bangladesh who had resided in the district for an average of 7.5 years. The computed incidence rates were 35.7 per 100,000 per year for the immigrant population and 0.43 per 100,000 per year for the native population. Palmer et al. (18), studying admissions to a West London hospital over a 10-year period (1973 to 1983), found 90 patients with abdominal tuberculosis (42 with enteric disease), 74 (82%) of whom were immigrants living in the United Kingdom for an average of 4 years. The estimated incidence rate of five per 100,000 per year was computed for the entire study population, although the rate for the immigrant subgroup was likely to be much higher.

Probert et al. (19) demonstrated a dramatic decline in incidence in immigrant populations from 22.3 per 100,000 per year in the 1970s to 9.2 per 100,000 per year in the late 1980s. During the same period, the standardized incidence in the "European population" was 0.2 per 100,000 per year. Sheldon et al. (20) found similar data for the London Borough of Tower Hamlets, where the crude incidence rate was 7.7 per 100,000 per year for the Bangladeshi population and 0.3 per 100,000 per year for the "European population." There was no difference in mortality between the immigrant and native populations. Of interest, most cases occurred among immigrants rather than their offspring, which suggests that the observed decline in incidence rates was owing to reductions in the number of new immigrants rather than inherent differences in the populations studied.

Lingenfelser et al. (21) recently reported on abdominal tuberculosis at the Groote Schuur Hospital in Cape Town, South Africa. Between 1986 and 1989, 82 patients with abdominal tuberculosis were identified, with an overall incidence rate of 20 per 100,000 per year. This incidence rate was double that found in a prior series covering the years 1962 to 1971 (22). Of patients with intestinal disease (only 14 patients in this series), 57% also had evidence of active pulmonary tuberculosis by chest radiographic study. No information was obtained on the incidence of drug-resistant organisms or HIV disease in this population.

Other data from South Africa come from the study by Pettengell et al. (23), which represents the only modern prospective analysis of the frequency of abdominal tuberculosis in patients with pulmonary tuberculosis. They studied 50 randomly chosen patients with smear-positive, cavitary tuberculosis and performed upper endoscopy, colonoscopy, double-contrast barium enemas, and small-bowel radiology on all. Proven or suspected intestinal tuberculosis was diagnosed in 23 (46%) of the patients, and the frequency of proven gastrointestinal tuberculosis increased with the severity of the pulmonary disease. This study suggests that unsuspected intestinal tuberculosis may still be a common occurrence and that the use of short treatment regimens may be inadequate in treating these patients (24).

The impact of HIV infection and the rise of multidrug-resistant organisms on the epidemiology of gastrointestinal tuberculosis is not known. Although both factors are play-ing a significant role in shaping the present epidemic of pulmonary tuberculosis, few data exist on the frequency of drug-resistant organisms isolated from patients with abdominal disease or on the effect of HIV disease on either the incidence or the course of this illness. Barnes et al. (25) noted that despite clear increases in the frequency of extra-pulmonary tuberculosis in HIV-infected patients, clinical features of gastrointestinal tuberculosis are rarely seen. At the present, only two small series have addressed this issue. At Mt. Sinai Hospital in New York City, Guth and Kim (26) found 17 patients with abdominal tuberculosis over a 5-year period, five of whom were HIV infected. Rosengart and Coppa (27) retrospectively reviewed 21 patients with abdominal mycobacterial infections admitted to Bellevue Hospital in New York City between December 1986 and June 1988. Of these patients, eight had peritoneal involvement, seven had ileocecal, three hepatic, and three had psoas abscesses. Cultures grew *Mycobacterium tuberculosis* in 17 of the cases and *Mycobacterium avium-intracellulare complex* in the other four. Twelve of the 17 patients with abdominal tuberculosis secondary to *M. tuberculosis* were either at risk of HIV infection or met Centers for Disease Control–defined criteria for acquired immunodeficiency syndrome. More recent reports have confirmed a marked increase in extrapulmonary tuberculosis in HIV-infected patients, but only a relatively modest increase in intestinal tuberculosis has been noted (28). Intestinal tuberculosis may also be associated with immunodeficiency unrelated to HIV infection; Hirasaki et al. (29) reported a case of an 85-year-old woman with idiopathic $CD4^+$ T lymphopenia with no evidence of HIV infection who presented with bloody diarrhea and high fever and had positive acid-fast cultures of stool and positive polymerase chain reaction on biopsy specimens.

Pathogenesis

Although the acrimonious debates of the 19th century on the origin and development of intestinal tuberculosis have been all but forgotten, the pathogenesis of the disease remains incompletely understood. Enteric disease can result from primary infection of the gastrointestinal tract or from secondary infection from a focus elsewhere in the body, usually the lungs. By definition, primary gastrointestinal tuberculosis occurs in the absence of clinically apparent pulmonary infection.

The likely mechanisms for infection of the bowel include direct ingestion of tubercle bacilli from either infected sputum or dairy products, hematogenous spread from foci elsewhere in the body, bile containing bacilli, or direct extension from contiguous organs (30).

The role of infected sputum in the pathogenesis of enteric disease is suggested by the frequent association of tuberculous enteritis and tuberculous laryngitis (31). The lipid-laden mycobacterial cell wall is relatively resistant to acid digestion, and this allows ingested organisms to reach and invade the bowel wall. This hypothesis also clarifies why primary intestinal tuberculosis owing to *Mycobacterium bovis*, which was caused by direct ingestion of contaminated dairy products, has been virtually eradicated by the widespread pasteurization of milk.

Hematogenous infection of the intestine is also the presumed cause of some cases of tuberculous enteritis. Calmette was a strong advocate of this mode of infection and believed that all intestinal tuberculosis was produced by hematogenous spread. This has not been supported by either experimental or clinical evidence, except in some circumstances. In miliary disease, diffuse involvement of the intestines has been described and experimental intestinal tuberculosis has been produced by direct injection of bacilli into the mesenteric arteries of animals (32,33). The importance of the seeding of the gastrointestinal tract by "silent" bacillemia in primary pulmonary tuberculosis is not clear. Recently, the frequency of bacillemia was shown to be even higher than what had been previously suspected. In a small group of patients, evidence of *M. tuberculosis* infection of peripheral blood mononuclear cells was demonstrated in eight of eight patients with only pulmonary disease (34).

The direct extension of disease from contiguous infected organs may also play a role in some patients. Primary or secondary infection of the female urogenital tract is known to occur and may cause intestinal disease. However, invasion of the bowel from tuberculous involvement of the peritoneum is not believed to occur (35). The inverse, however, is true; tuberculous peritonitis can occur after the ulceration of an abdominal lymph node or after free perforation of a tuberculous intestinal ulcer or as a consequence of transmural infection of the bowel without perforation (36).

Anatomic Distribution

Tuberculosis can affect any region of the gastrointestinal tract from the mouth to the anus. As Table 34.1 demonstrates, the ileocecal region is the most commonly affected

TABLE 34.1. ANATOMIC DISTRIBUTION OF ABDOMINAL TUBERCULOSIS

Site	Frequency (%) (Autopsy)	Clinical Reports (%)
Esophagus	0.14	0.3
Stomach	0.69	2
Duodenum	2.50	0.3
Jejunum	24.3	35[a]
Ileum	72.0	
Ileocecum	66.1	42
Appendix	25.2	1
Colon	53.8	12
Anorectum	11.9	7

[a]Includes jejunum and ileum.

site, as determined by both autopsy series and clinical reports. The striking predilection for this region is thought to be a consequence of the abundance of lymphoid tissue (Peyer patches) therein, with the increased physiologic stasis, increased rate of fluid and electrolyte absorption, and minimal digestive activity permitting greater contact time between the organism and the mucosal surface.

Another explanation for the observed frequency of ileocecal involvement may relate directly to the role of Peyer patches and their associated M cells in antigen sampling of intestinal contents. Bacille Calmette–Guérin is selectively taken up by Peyer patches without any evidence of epithelial inflammation. This is consistent with the histologic observations of isolated lymphoid involvement and little epithelial involvement in early tuberculous disease (37). As the disease progresses, the lymphoid follicles become infiltrated and inflammation extends throughout the submucosa. Eventually the epithelial layer above the Peyer patch may ulcerate, forming the characteristic histologic appearance of ulcerative tuberculous enteritis. Although it has been suggested that the bacillus is transported from epithelial mucosal glands to lymphoid follicles via phagocytes, recent data suggest that there is direct transport of bacilli from the intestinal lumen to the antigen-presenting cells of the lymphoid follicle (38).

Electron microscopy has clearly demonstrated that bacille Calmette–Guérin is taken up by M cells and transported to antigen-presenting cells in Peyer patches. Bacille Calmette–Guérin was found only to have been phagocytized by M cells, and no evidence was found for direct invasion into enterocytes (39). Other investigators demonstrated that *Mycobacterium paratuberculosis* (the etiologic agent in Johne disease of ruminants) is also selectively transported by M cells without the apparent involvement of epithelial enterocytes or intraepithelial lymphocytes (40). Although specific data for *M. tuberculosis* do not exist, the mechanism of initial infection is likely to be the same.

Although its most common site of presentation is ileocecal, tuberculosis may also involve other regions of the gastrointestinal tract. Tuberculous colitis can mimic Crohn disease of the colon and even occasionally ulcerative colitis (41), and gastric involvement takes the form of a hypertrophic antral gastritis with circumferential thickening and cicatrization, indistinguishable from sarcoidosis, idiopathic granulomatous gastritis, syphilitic gastritis, and the linitis plastica variant of gastric carcinoma. Tuberculous involvement of the esophagus (42), appendix, and perianal areas occurs as well. Anal tuberculosis, including tuberculous fistula and fissure-in-ano (43), has also been reported, although rarely, as have been (more commonly) rectal strictures (44,45) and perirectal soft-tissue masses (46). In patients infected with HIV, acute tuberculous pancreatitis and appendicitis have been noted (47,48). Pancreatic tuberculosis may present with pain, fever, weight loss, diabetes, or segmental portal hypertension; the appearance of the pancreas radiographically or at laparotomy is indistinguishable from that of pancreatic carcinoma (49–51).

Pathologic Appearance

The earliest gross changes occur most frequently in the terminal ileum or cecum where scattered nodules project into the intestinal lumen. Careful examination frequently reveals that these nodules show evidence of early ulceration and that they are generally found overlying lymphoid follicles or Peyer patches. As the inflammatory process progresses, the characteristic morphologic changes of ulcerative, ulcerohypertrophic, or hypertrophic disease occur and infection may extend to the mesenteric lymph nodes (35). The gross pathologic changes are not correlated with the presence or absence of pulmonary disease, as had been thought in the past, but more likely represent the result of a complex interaction between individual host responses and bacterial virulence (52).

In ulcerative intestinal tuberculosis, there are induration and edema of the diseased segment, with an increase in serosal fat, serosal studding with nodules, and the presence of large ulcers, characteristically transverse and circumferential, which are presumed to be formed by the coalescence of multiple smaller ones. The ulcers often have thickened, infiltrated, everted, indented, and gnawed edges, and skip areas of normal-appearing mucosa may occur. An endarteritis with subsequent deprivation of blood flow to the mucosal surface is believed to be an important factor in the pathogenesis of ulcer formation (52,53). The ulcers are believed to form relatively slowly and generally do not penetrate the muscularis propria. This, along with the fact that there is often an inflammatory wall ahead of the enlarging ulcer, makes perforation a relatively rare occurrence. When perforations do occur, they are ordinarily confined by the inflammatory tissue and fibrosis that accompany tissue perforation. As ulcers heal, the extensive fibrosis may result in strictures ("napkin ring") and cause obstructive symptoms.

The hypertrophic form (seen in 10% of patients) is characterized by extensive inflammation and fibrosis in the submucosa and subserosa (54). This often results in the adherence of bowel, mesentery, and lymph nodes into a mass. This mass may occasionally appear to be an exophytic neoplasm from the mucosal surface. As with the ulcerative form, strictures may occur and result in bowel obstruction.

Ulcerohypertrophic intestinal tuberculosis (approximately 30% of patients) displays characteristics of both forms of disease. Another much less common form of intestinal tuberculosis is diffuse colitis. Diffuse colitis is endoscopically very similar to ulcerative colitis and cannot be easily distinguished based on the mucosal appearance alone (55).

Fistulas, enteroenteric, enterovesicular, and enterocutaneous, can occur and are thought to be a consequence of secondary bacterial infection of necrotic tissue causing penetrating abscesses. Luminal narrowing can rarely be caused by extrinsic compression by lymph nodes but is more commonly caused by adjacent tuberculous adenitis, which causes colonic traction, diverticula, narrowing, fixation, and sinus tract formation.

Two recent reports have called attention to tuberculous changes in the mesenteric vasculature, including granulomas of the vessel wall, intraluminal thrombi, aneurysms, and perivascular cuffing, suggesting that a tuberculous vasculitis or vasculopathy may contribute to schemia, stricture, and hemorrhage (56,57).

Histologic Features

Caseating granulomas are the most distinctive histologic finding in tuberculous enteritis, although in a number of patients, there may only be nonspecific changes in the bowel wall, with caseating granulomas restricted to regional lymph nodes. If they are not found, it may be difficult to distinguish between Crohn disease and tuberculous enteritis. There are, however, several characteristic histologic findings that can be helpful in distinguishing between these two diseases (58). The presence of caseating granulomas is indicative of tuberculosis. Large, variably appearing, confluent granulomas strongly suggest tuberculosis as does the presence of multinucleated giant cells. The granulomas of tuberculosis are always surrounded by inflammatory cells, in contrast to those of Crohn disease, which may be seen in otherwise normal biopsy specimens. Submucosal widening and transmural follicular hyperplasia, which are common in Crohn disease, are generally absent in tuberculous colitis, whereas epithelial regeneration and glandular metaplasia are more frequent in tuberculosis.

Other findings in tuberculous enteritis include ulceration, clusters of epithelioid cells that may be oval or spindle shaped, Langhans giant cells, and chronic nonspecific inflammation. There can be a variable degree of fibrosis extending from the submucosa into the muscularis layer. The effect of HIV infection on the histopathology of *M. tuberculosis* of the gut is not well described, although granulomas tend to be more poorly formed.

Careful analysis of biopsy specimens for the presence of acid-fast bacilli is essential when tuberculous colitis is suspected. Bacilli can occasionally be found in the bowel wall, although they are more frequently observed in regional lymph nodes. A recent series of patients with colonic tuberculosis diagnosed by colonoscopy and endoscopic mucosal biopsy demonstrated ulcers in 37 of 40 specimens, Langhans giant cells in 24, focal areas of caseation in nine, and nonspecific inflammation in three (59). No bacilli were observed in any smears obtained from tissue homogenates. The use of polymerase chain reaction testing of endoscopic specimens may be of further use in diagnosing tuberculosis and in differentiating it from Crohn disease (60).

Clinical Features

Signs and Symptoms

Intestinal tuberculosis is a protean disease with no distinct pathognomonic symptom or sign. It affects both men and women without any apparent bias and tends to present in the third and fourth decades of life. Nonspecific abdominal complaints predominate and may be present for as little as 1 month to as much as a year in most patients (61).

Pulmonologists have taught that gastrointestinal symptoms may be the first and sometimes only sign of pulmonary tuberculosis (62); this is especially important in view of the resurgence of tuberculosis in the past decade.

Abdominal pain, weight loss, fever, weakness, and multiple other symptoms and signs are frequently observed (Table 34.2), although they vary dramatically from patient to patient. When present, the abdominal pain tends to be in the right lower quadrant, although a significant proportion of patients will have diffuse, central, epigastric, or left lower quadrant symptoms. It is occasionally described as cramping or colicky and may be exacerbated by eating and alleviated by vomiting or defecation. A significant number of patients will present with bowel obstruction and undergo emergency laparotomy. In Bhansali's (13) series of 300 patients with surgically proven abdominal tuberculosis (in an endemic region), 31% presented with acute obstruction and emergent laparotomy was performed on 25% of these patients. This is in agreement with the study of Palmer et al. (18) from the Central Middlesex Hospital in London where ten of 42 patients underwent emergent laparotomy for obstruction or perforation.

Diarrhea, once considered the mortal symptom of tuberculosis, is now observed relatively infrequently. When it occurs, it is symptomatically similar to that seen in Crohn disease: mucousy, liquid to semisolid stools occurring less than six to eight times per day, rarely with gross pus or blood. It is almost always associated with intestinal ulcera-

tions, although it can occur in the absence of any mucosal disease. The etiology of the diarrhea has not been clarified but most likely relates to the generalized inflammatory response in the intestine and the subsequent effect of cytokines, leukotrienes, and prostaglandins on fluid and electrolyte transport. There also may be an effect on intestinal motility, but this has never been evaluated adequately. There is a single report of secretory diarrhea in a patient with ileocecal tuberculosis (63). In that instance, intestinal perfusion studies demonstrated active chloride secretion by an endoscopically normal-appearing terminal ileum. The diarrhea resolved after 4 weeks of treatment with antituberculosis medications, and follow-up perfusion studies appeared normal after 3 months.

Weight loss is a common complaint whose etiology is likely multifactorial. Malabsorption may be related to decreased total absorptive area owing to extensive ulceration, lymphatic obstruction, or bacterial overgrowth. Bacterial overgrowth secondary to "stagnant loop" syndrome was found in 15 of 20 patients presenting with intestinal tuberculosis and obstruction. In the same series, four of ten patients with intestinal tuberculosis without obstruction had evidence of malabsorption, although only one had evidence of bacterial overgrowth. A cause could not be determined for the other three (64). Hemorrhage is uncommon, although there are case reports of melena and massive rectal bleeding owing to intestinal tuberculosis (65–68). Spontaneous intestinal perforation may occur in untreated (69) and treated (70) tuberculosis, and in one case report (71), it occurred during immune reconstitution in a patient coinfected with HIV and tuberculosis after 1 year of successful antiretroviral therapy. Portal hypertension has also been reported owing to compression of the portal vein by tuberculous lymphadenitis at the hepatic and splenic hila (72) and by splenic vein compression in tuberculous pancreatitis (49). Upper gastrointestinal obstruction has been reported caused by ulcerohypertrophic antroduodenal tuberculosis (73).

Physical Findings

Most patients appear systemically ill and malnourished, and there may be concomitant evidence of pulmonary or other extraintestinal tuberculosis. Examination of the abdomen generally reveals tenderness, most frequently in the right lower quadrant, and a palpable mass may be present in 25% to 50% of patients. The classic "doughy" abdomen (owing to extensive intraabdominal fibrous adhesion and inflammation) is uncommon and found in only 5% to 8% of all patients. Abdominal distention with increased peristaltic activity generally is associated with intestinal obstruction. Peritoneal signs may occur, and there has been free perforation of the bowel. Examination of the perineum occasionally reveals anal cryptitis, fissures, perianal abscesses, and fistula-in-ano (74).

TABLE 34.2. INTESTINAL TUBERCULOSIS: SYMPTOMS AND SIGNS

Symptom or Sign	Incidence (%)
Abdominal pain	60
Weight loss	59
Fever	47
Weakness	45
Nausea	44
Anorexia	38
Vomiting	38
Distention	24
Night sweats	23
Constipation	21
Diarrhea	18
Amenorrhea	18
Hemorrhage	4

Laboratory Findings

There is no laboratory finding characteristic of intestinal tuberculosis. The hematologic findings are most consistent with those of a chronic inflammatory disease; the leukocyte count is generally normal, although it may be elevated if obstruction or perforation has occurred. Many patients are anemic, but only a small number are truly iron deficient. Serum transaminase levels tend to be normal, although serum alkaline phosphatase and γ-glutamyl transpeptidase levels may be increased (generally implying cholestatic liver disease). The serum albumin level tends to be depressed, and coagulopathies are uncommon unless there is malabsorption or secondary infection. Stool examination for occult blood or fecal leukocytes is generally not worthwhile because negative results are frequently obtained despite extensive ulceration.

Concomitant Human Immunodeficiency Virus Infection

The epidemic of acquired immunodeficiency syndrome has been accompanied by a resurgence of tuberculosis, and the most striking feature of this resurgence is the high frequency of extrapulmonary, including gastrointestinal, involvement (25). Although the disease presentation is often similar in HIV-infected and -uninfected patients, one recent study has noted a number of important differences (75). HIV-infected patients were slightly younger; less likely to have abused alcohol (33% vs. 74%); more likely to have fevers, night sweats, and weight loss; and less likely to manifest ascites or jaundice. Tuberculin skin tests and chest radiographs were positive in equal numbers of patients in each group. Intraabdominal lymphadenopathy on computed tomography (CT) was significantly more common in the HIV-infected patients (94% vs. 36%), but central lucencies in the nodes, indicating necrosis, were equally common in both groups. Disseminated tuberculosis was present in 93% of the HIV-infected patients but only 31% of HIV-negative patients. Acid-fast smears were positive in 63% of stool specimens and 72% of abdominal lymph node aspirates in HIV-positive patients but in only 20% of stool specimens and 40% of node aspirates in the HIV-negative patients. Interesting, the overall death rates in the groups were similar.

Diagnosis

Differential Diagnosis

In nonendemic areas, the most important factor in making the diagnosis of enteric tuberculosis is to maintain a high degree of clinical suspicion for the disease. Multiple diagnostic methods are available to establish the diagnosis, and guidelines have been established to ensure that an accurate diagnosis can be made.

In a significant proportion of patients, a definitive diagnosis cannot be made and empirical treatment is the only option. Crohn disease is the most crucial diagnosis to exclude in these circumstances, although *Yersinia enterocolitica* infection, gastrointestinal histoplasmosis, actinomycosis, amebic colitis, lymphoma or other neoplasms, vascular insufficiency, periappendiceal abscesses, sarcoidosis, and rectosigmoid lymphogranuloma venereum must also be considered. The inverse of this is also true: In patients from endemic areas, great caution must be exercised when the diagnosis of Crohn disease is considered because tuberculosis will not respond to 5-aminosalicylate or its analogs and in fact may be exacerbated by glucocorticoid therapy. This caveat is even more important with the advent of infliximab (antitumor necrosis factor α monoclonal antibody) therapy in Crohn disease because such therapy cannot only reactivate pulmonary tuberculosis in these patients (76) but will exacerbate *M. tuberculosis* enteritis misdiagnosed as Crohn disease (77).

Stool Studies

Acid-fast bacilli can routinely be isolated from the stool of normal individuals. This generally represents colonization by nonpathogenic environmental strains of mycobacteria or, as in HIV-infected patients, of *M. avium-intracellulare complex*. Cultures can document the presence of active *M. tuberculosis*, but this generally implies the ingestion of infected sputum and not the presence of intestinal disease.

Radiologic Studies

Barium studies of the small intestine and colon may aid in the diagnosis. Although there are no pathognomonic radiographic features of intestinal tuberculosis, several findings are highly suggestive of disease. Increased transit time with hypersegmentation and flocculation of barium is one of the earliest signs of intestinal involvement (78). Thickening of the mucosal folds with scalloping and spiculation may also occur, and in severe disease, ulcers may be present. The exclusion of barium from an involved segment of bowel (ileum, cecum, or ascending colon) with normal-appearing segments adjacent is Stierlin sign and reflects bowel hypermotility with possible spasm of involved segments (79). The ileocecal valve is often involved with disease on both small bowel and colonic sides and may be patulous secondary to ulcerations and fibrosis (Fleischner sign). This may be a useful point of differentiation from Crohn disease, in which the valve is characteristically stenotic. Conversely, there may be valvular and ileal stenosis, which renders the differentiation more difficult.

Abdominal CT is useful in the diagnosis of intestinal tuberculosis, although again there are no pathognomonic findings. Many patients will have peripancreatic, porta hepatis, mesenteric/omental, or retroperitoneal adenopathy. Thickening of the bowel wall with associated adenopathy is

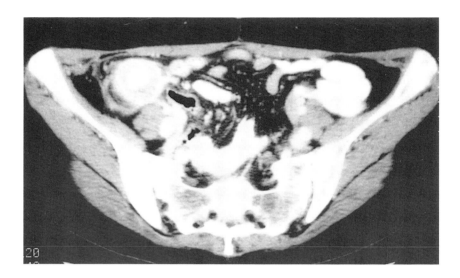

FIGURE 34.1. Ileal tuberculosis. A loop of distal ileum is thickened and hyperemic with a "target" sign.

commonly observed (Figs. 34.1 and 34.2). The presence of enlarged nodes with low-density centers (suggesting necrosis) strongly suggests *M. tuberculosis* infection. These findings have been observed in many patients with HIV infection (80–82).

Extrapulmonary disease can also be detected with gallium 67 scanning, although this is unlikely to provide sufficient specificity to become widely useful. It may be most appropriate, however, for determining the extent of disease and the presence of previously unrecognized abdominal lymph node involvement. Its advantage over abdominal CT is not clear at this time (83).

Endoscopic Diagnosis

Colonoscopy is the easiest and most direct method for establishing the diagnosis of tuberculous colitis. Unlike laparotomy, it does not require inpatient care and when combined with directed endoscopic mucosal biopsy, it has clear advantages over solely radiographic approaches. The safety of colonoscopy in patients with tuberculosis is well established. With adequate precautions and disinfection procedures, transmission to other patients or medical personnel is unlikely to occur (84,85).

As with most diagnostic procedures in intestinal tuberculosis, endoscopic findings are not pathognomonic. The ileocecal valve may be edematous or deformed. Occasionally nodules 2 to 4 mm in diameter or superficial ulcers can be found on the valve folds. Small nodules (2 to 6 mm) with a pink surface may be present in the cecum, although they can be found at any point in the colon. These nodules tend not to be friable, although areas of ulceration can be observed between them. Pseudopolypoid folds and strictures have also been observed in patients with colonic

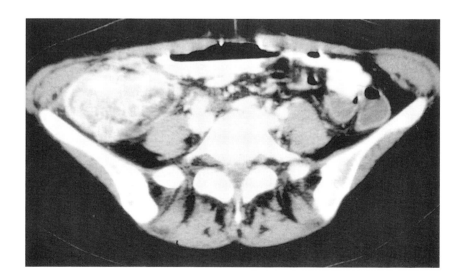

FIGURE 34.2. Ileocecal tuberculosis. A right lower quadrant inflammatory mass is present with matted bowel loops, mesentery, and nodes.

tuberculosis. Ulcerated tuberculous polypoid masses, although rare, also occur, and it is impossible, based on appearance alone to distinguish them from neoplasms of the colon (86).

Ulcerations are the most common finding and are most frequently observed in the ileocecal region. The ulcers range from 2 to 3 mm to more than 3 cm in length, tend to be linear and superficial, and have irregular margins. Segmental involvement of the colon without cecal disease was believed to be rare but is now being observed more frequently because of the widespread use of colonoscopy (87).

The yield of endoscopic biopsy ranges from 30% to 80% and relates to the number of biopsy specimens taken, whether they are from the ulcer margin, and how they are processed. Bhargava et al. (88) recommend eight to ten biopsy specimens from each patient for histology and three to four specimens for culture. The "well technique" should be used so that the submucosal layer can be sampled and the biopsy specimens should be collected in sterile saline solution and then homogenized to increase the yield from culture (88). Recently, Anand et al. (89) used polymerase chain reaction on endoscopic biopsy specimens to diagnose intestinal tuberculosis in a patient with chronic diarrhea; the usefulness of this modality has been confirmed by Moatter et al. (90).

Tuberculous enteritis also has been diagnosed by colonoscopic fine needle aspiration cytology in two patients (91). This technique may be useful for nodular lesions, but its overall utility has not been evaluated in a rigorous manner.

Direct percutaneous fine needle aspiration cytology was described recently as a method of diagnosis in the setting of a palpable abdominal mass. The report by Radhika et al. (92) (Chandigarh, India) demonstrated acid-fast bacilli in 45% of patients and epithelioid granulomas in 82%. No complications were noted, but the applicability of this technique in nonendemic regions appears limited.

Laparotomy

A surgical approach may still be necessary when there is significant uncertainty about the correct diagnosis. Fortunately, this has become much less frequent as the accuracy and efficacy of more noninvasive methods have improved. Exploratory laparotomy will, however, still be necessary in patients presenting with obstruction or free perforation.

TUBERCULOUS PERITONITIS

The first well-documented case of tuberculous peritonitis was described in 1843 at the autopsy of a 40-year-old seaman (93). It has long been considered an enigmatic, puzzling, and elusive disease that could easily be overlooked by the unsuspecting clinician. The origins of this probably lie with its insidious nature, nonspecific clinical manifesta-

tions, low prevalence, and difficulty of finding the tubercle bacillus in ascitic fluid. Some of this elusiveness has changed with the use of laparoscopy and other specific serologic tests that provide a rapid diagnosis of tuberculous peritonitis, but the varied clinical challenges of making the diagnosis still remain.

Epidemiology

Peritonitis is an uncommon manifestation of tuberculous disease, but it occurs as frequently as intestinal disease (30). As with intestinal disease, tuberculous peritonitis is more common in nonindustrialized nations, recent immigrants from endemic regions, and perhaps HIV-infected individuals. It is also a reported complication in patients undergoing peritoneal dialysis (94).

Tuberculous peritonitis is estimated to occur as a complication in 0.1% to 3.5% of all patients with pulmonary disease and represents 4% to 10% of all extrapulmonary disease. Although considered rare, it is regularly diagnosed in nonendemic regions (95). The effect of HIV infection on this complication is not known. In the small series of Rosengart and Coppa (27), the frequency of peritonitis was equally distributed between HIV- and non–HIV-infected patients.

Pathogenesis

The two most accepted mechanisms for the pathogenesis of tuberculous peritonitis are the activation of long-latent foci of tuberculous infection of the peritoneum and the hematogenous spread of bacilli from active pulmonary lesions (96). Support for these hypotheses comes from several clinical series of patients with tuberculous peritonitis (93,95,96). In these series, the frequency of concurrent active pulmonary disease ranged from 4% to 33%, and the frequency of radiographic abnormalities suggestive of old disease was much higher (37% to 63%). The occurrence of pulmonary and peritoneal disease could also, conceivably, be the result of simultaneous reactivation of disease at several sites.

Contiguous spread from lesions in the intestine or fallopian tubes, although long considered possible, only plays a role in a small number of patients. In the prospective series of Singh et al. (96) of 47 patients with tuberculous peritonitis, no patient had evidence of intestinal or female genital tract involvement as assayed by barium studies of the upper and lower gastrointestinal tract and by salpingography.

Ascites, which is present in an overwhelming majority of patients, is the result of studding of the parietal and visceral peritoneum with tuberculous nodules. It is generally exudative in nature, with features suggestive of a delayed-type hypersensitivity reaction in the abdominal cavity. The level of interferon gamma, a cytokine characteristic of the Th1 lymphocyte response and crucial in the activation of macrophage tuberculocidal activity, is elevated in patients with tuberculous peritonitis (97).

Clinical Features

As is the rule with tuberculous infections of the gastrointestinal tract, there is no pathognomonic symptom or sign of tuberculous peritonitis. Abdominal swelling and anorexia are the most frequent symptoms, whereas ascites is the most frequent sign in patients presenting with this illness.

Most patients are in their 30s or 40s, and there appears to be a slight predilection for women. The reason for this is not well understood, but it does not appear to be related to infection of the female urogenital tract. Tuberculous peritonitis is an insidious disease that progresses over the course of weeks to months, although most patients present after 6 weeks of symptoms (98). Fever, weight loss, abdominal pain, and diarrhea commonly occur but are not necessary features of the disease. Patients with underlying cirrhosis present a particularly difficult problem because their ascites is often attributed to portal hypertension and the possibility of tuberculous peritonitis is not considered. At least partly as a consequence of this, the mortality rates of cirrhotic patients tend to be higher because of delays in both diagnosis and treatment (99).

The physical examination is also not particularly useful in establishing the diagnosis. Abdominal tenderness may or may not be present, and in many patients, the presence of ascites is believed to be secondary to cirrhosis (usually alcoholic). Only a very small number (approximately 8%) presents with the characteristic doughy abdomen found in fibroadhesive or "dry" peritonitis.

Routine laboratory tests generally demonstrate evidence of a chronic inflammatory disease. Anemia, when present, is mild. The leukocyte count is often normal (more than 85% of cases) (99,100), and typically only the erythrocyte sedimentation rate is elevated. On average, most patients will have a positive reaction to PPD placed intradermally, but a negative result has little predictive value, especially in HIV-infected individuals.

Chest radiographs, ultrasonography, and abdominal CT have an adjunctive role in establishing the diagnosis. Approximately one-half of patients will have evidence of old pulmonary disease and one-sixth active disease on chest radiographs. When associated with exudative ascites, these findings may provide enough correlative clinical evidence to institute treatment in endemic regions. Characteristic ultrasound findings include fixed membranes, septa, and debris; floating debris; mobile strands; omental "cake"; thickened mesentery with adherent loops of bowel; and lymphadenopathy (101). These findings, however, are not specific for tuberculous peritonitis but, as with chest radiographs, may provide enough support for empirical treatment.

Abdominal CT has a more clearly defined role in the evaluation of abdominal tuberculosis. The presence of high-density ascites and abdominal lymphadenopathy with low-density centers (suggestive of necrosis) is highly correlated with tuberculous peritonitis. CT not only provides a more sensitive means of assessing lymph node involvement but can also better evaluate diseased mesentery, omentum, and the female urogenital tract.

Diagnostic Strategies

Paracentesis

Paracentesis is essential in the evaluation of the patient with suspected tuberculous peritonitis. The ascitic fluid is generally straw colored, although it may be blood stained in approximately 10% of patients (99). It is predominantly exudative with a protein content of more than 2.5 gm/dL. There is an important subgroup of patients who have low-protein ascites (102). These patients tend to have underlying cirrhosis (usually related to alcohol abuse), and the diagnosis of tuberculous peritonitis is often only made at autopsy. Routine use of the serum–ascites albumin gradient (exudative <1.1 g/dL) may be preferable in these patients. In the small series of Marshall and Vogele (103) of six patients, the two patients who had low ascites protein content had a narrowed albumin gradient.

The leukocyte count in tuberculous ascites ranges from 150 to 4,000 cells/mm^3, although patients with more and fewer cells have been described (101,104). Lymphocytes predominate except in patients on peritoneal dialysis who may have a neutrophilic response (94). Red blood cells are also commonly found and reflect the generalized inflammatory response of the peritoneum.

Unfortunately, direct examination and culture of ascitic fluid for acid-fast bacilli are unreliable. Acid-fast smears of ascitic fluid are diagnostic in approximately 3% of patients, and cultures are positive in 10% to 20%. Some investigators noted greater success by culturing as much as 1 L of ascitic fluid (83% positive in one report), but this has not been widely reproducible (100,102,104). The fundamental limitation of culturing ascitic fluid for acid-fast bacilli is the long time needed to obtain results.

In the past, much had been written on the use of adenosine deaminase (ADA) activity in ascitic fluid as a sensitive and specific marker for tuberculous peritonitis (105,106). ADA is an enzyme found at the cell surface of lymphocytes and macrophages. It catalyzes the conversion of adenosine to inosine and is generally elevated in regions of active lymphocyte proliferation.

Voigt et al. (105), using a cutoff value of 32 U/L, found a sensitivity and specificity of 95% and 98%, respectively, whereas others (106) noted sensitivities and specificities approaching 100% using other cutoff values. In patients with low-protein ascites (often cirrhotic in whom an accurate diagnosis may be even more crucial), the ADA activity is also lower and false-negative results are more frequent (107). Some data (108) also suggest that in HIV-infected patients with tuberculous peritonitis, ADA levels may be diminished compared with those in non–HIV-infected individuals. Most recently, work by Kaur et al. (108) demonstrated poor reliability of this assay in 140 patients with ascites, 12 of whom had proven tuberculous peritonitis. This work is in agreement with other studies of tuberculous meningitis and pleuritis that cast significant doubts on the diagnostic value of ADA determinations (108). Although ADA determinations may eventually prove to be useful, more direct methods of diagnosis are currently available (laparoscopy) and more sensitive indirect methods will likely become available in the near future (DNA amplification of mycobacteria-specific sequences by polymerase chain reaction from ascitic fluid of patients with tuberculous peritonitis). One report noted that polymerase chain reaction study of ascitic fluid was 69% sensitive for the detection of tuberculous peritonitis (109).

Laparoscopy and Blind Percutaneous Peritoneal Biopsy

Direct laparoscopic inspection and biopsy of the peritoneum are perhaps the most effective methods of diagnosing tuberculous peritonitis. Direct inspection alone will allow an accurate presumptive diagnosis in 80% to 95% of patients, whereas biopsy specimens may demonstrate acid-fast bacilli in 75% and caseating granulomas in 85% to 90% (99,110,111). One recent study (112) concluded that peritoneal biopsy was a safe and precise way to diagnose tuberculosis peritonitis and that such early diagnosis had a significant positive effect on mortality rates because a large number of patients died while waiting for peritoneal cultures to return after cell counts and chemistries were nonspecific; this study did not, however, include the use of polymerase chain reaction testing in its analysis.

Characteristic laparoscopic findings include multiple, yellow-white, "miliary" nodules over the visceral and parietal peritoneum, scattered erythematous patches, thickened and hyperemic peritoneum, turbid ascites, and adhesions. The safety of laparoscopy in both HIV- and non–HIV-infected patients thought to have tuberculous peritonitis has been well established; however, complications (perforated viscus, intraperitoneal bleeding requiring transfusion, subcutaneous hematoma) and death have occurred (101).

TREATMENT

The treatment for abdominal tuberculosis is no different than that for extrapulmonary tuberculosis at other sites. The mainstay of therapy is medical, using standard regimens for 9- or 12-month courses. Surgery has generally been reserved for patients with obstruction, free perforation, confined perforation, fistulas, or strictures. Recent evidence suggests, however, that some fistulas and strictures will respond to medical treatment alone. In fact, some tracheoesophageal and bronchoesophageal fistulas may heal solely with long courses of medical therapy (113,114).

The experience with medical treatment of strictures is more considerable. Anand et al. (115) prospectively treated 39 patients with symptoms of bowel obstruction and radiographic evidence of intestinal strictures with conventional medical therapy. At the end of 1 year of treatment, 91% demonstrated significant clinical improvement, 76% were symptom free, and only 8% did not respond and required surgery.

REFERENCES

1. Brown L, Sampson HL. *Intestinal tuberculosis: its importance, diagnosis and treatment*. New York: Lea & Febiger, 1926.
2. Harris WC. Intestinal tuberculosis with stenosis and obstruction. *Tubercle* 1952;33:50–52.
3. Manget JJ. *Theophili boneti sepulcretum sive anatomica practica (etc) Editio altera, quam novis commentariis et observationibus innumeris illustravit, actertia ad minimum*. Genevae, 1700.
4. Brunner JC. *Glandulae duodeni seu pankreas sucundarium in intesino duodeno hominis primum*, 1715.
5. Bayle GL. *Recherches sur la phthisie pulmonaire*, Paris: Gabon, 1810.
6. Louis PCA. *Recherches anatomico-pathologiques sure la phtisie*. Paris: Gabon, 1825.
7. Rokitansky C. *Manual of pathological anatomy*, vol. 2. London: Sydenham Society, 1849:46–109. Esieveking R, Translator.
8. Foucault M. *The birth of the clinic*. New York: Pantheon, 1973.
9. Walsh J. Diagnosis of intestinal tuberculosis. *Natl Assoc Study Prev Tuberc* 1909;5:217–222.
10. Brown L, Sampson HL. Early roentgen diagnosis of ulcerative tuberculous colitis. *JAMA* 1919;73:77–85.
11. Mitchell RS, Bristol LJ. Intestinal tuberculosis: an analysis of 346 cases diagnosed by routine intestinal radiography on 5529 admissions for pulmonary tuberculosis, 1929–1949. *Am J Med Sci* 1954;227:241–249.
12. Granet E. Intestinal tuberculosis: a clinical, roentgenological and pathological study of 2086 patients affected with pulmonary tuberculosis. *Am J Dig Dis* 1935;2:209–214.
13. Bhansali SK. Abdominal tuberculosis: experiences with 300 cases. *Am J Gastroenterol* 1977;67:324–337.
14. Sherman S, Rohwedder JJ, Ravikrishnan KP, et al. Tuberculous enteritis and peritonitis. *Arch Intern Med* 1980;140:506–508.
15. Jakubowski A, Elwood RK, Enarson DA. Active abdominal tuberculosis in Canada in 1970–1981. *CMAJ* 1987;137:897–900.
16. Jakubowski A, Elwood RK, Enarson DA. Clinical features of abdominal tuberculosis. *J Infect Dis* 1989;158:687–692.
17. Klimach OE, Ormerod LP. Gastrointestinal tuberculosis: a retrospective review of 109 cases in a district general hospital. *Q J Med* 1985;56:569–578.
18. Palmer KR, Patil DH, Basran GS, et al. Abdominal tuberculosis in urban Britain—a common disease. *Gut* 1985;26:1296–1305.
19. Probert CS, Jayanthi V, Wicks AC, et al. Epidemiological study of abdominal tuberculosis among Indian migrants and the indigenous population of Leicester, 1972. *Gut* 1989;33:1085–1088.
20. Sheldon CD, Probert CS, Cock H, et al. Incidence of abdominal tuberculosis in Bangladeshi migrants in east London. *Tuber Lung Dis* 1993;74:12–15.

21. Lingenfelser T, Zak J, Marks IN, et al. Abdominal tuberculosis: still a potentially lethal disease. *Am J Gastroenterol* 1993;88:744–750.
22. Novis BH, Bank S, Marks IN. Gastrointestinal and peritoneal tuberculosis: a study of cases at Groote Schuur Hospital 1962–1971. *S Afr Med J* 1973;47:365–372.
23. Pettengell KE, Larsen C, Garb M, et al. Gastrointestinal tuberculosis in patient with pulmonary tuberculosis. *Q J Med* 1990;74:303–308.
24. Cooke NJ. Treatment of tuberculosis. *BMJ* 1985;291:497–498.
25. Barnes PF, Bloch AB, Davidson PT, et al. Tuberculosis in patients with human immunodeficiency virus infection. *N Engl J Med* 1991;325:1882–1884.
26. Guth AA, Kim U. The reappearance of abdominal tuberculosis. *Surg Gynecol Obstet* 1991;172:432–436.
27. Rosengart TK, Coppa GF. Abdominal mycobacterial infections in immunocompromised patients. *Am J Surg* 1990;159:125–131.
28. Antinori S, Galimerti L, Parente F. Intestinal tuberculosis as a cause of chronic diarrhea among patient with human immunodeficiency virus infection: a report of two cases. *Dig Liver Dis* 2001;33:63–67.
29. Hirasaki S, Koide N, Ogawa H, et al. Active intestinal tuberculosis with esophageal candidiasis due to idiopathic CD4(+) T-lymphocytopenia in an elderly woman. *J Gastroenterol* 2000;35:47–51.
30. Marshall JB. Tuberculosis of the gastrointestinal tract and peritoneum. *Am J Gastroenterol* 1993;88:989–999.
31. Crawford PM, Sawyer HP. Intestinal tuberculosis in 1400 autopsies. *Am Rev Tuberc* 1934;30:568–583.
32. Stead WW, Bates JH. Evidence of a silent bacillemia in primary tuberculosis. *Ann Intern Med* 1971;74:559–561.
33. Das P, Shukla HS. Abdominal tuberculosis: demonstration of tubercle bacilli in tissue and experimental production of hyperplastic enteric lesions. *Br J Surg* 1975;62:610–617.
34. Schluger N, Condos R, Lewis S, et al. DNA amplification using the polymerase chain reaction in blood of patients with pulmonary tuberculosis. *Lancet* 1994;344:232–233.
35. Paustian FF, Bockus HL. So called primary ulcerohypertrophic ileocecal tuberculosis. *Am J Med* 1959;27:509–518.
36. Hyman S, Villa F, Alvarez S, et al. The enigma of tuberculous peritonitis. *Gastroenterology* 1962;42:1–6.
37. Abrams JS, Holden WD. Tuberculosis of the gastrointestinal tract. *Arch Surg* 1964;89:282–293.
38. Sneller MC, Strober W. M cells and host defense. *J Infect Dis* 1986;154:737–741.
39. Fujimura Y. Functional morphology of microfold cells (M cells) in Peyer's patches—phagocytosis and transport of BCG by M cells into rabbit Peyer's patches. *Gastroenterol Jpn* 1986;21:325–335.
40. Momotani E, Whipple DL, Thiermann AB, et al. Role of M cells and macrophages in the entrance of *M. paratuberculosis* into domes of ileal Peyer's patches in calves. *Vet Pathol* 1988;25:131–137.
41. Dagli AJ. Colonic tuberculosis mimicking ulcerative colitis. *J Assoc Phys India* 1999;47:939.
42. Jain SK, Jain S, Jain M, et al. Esophageal tuberculosis: is it so rare? Report of 12 cases and a review of the literature. *Am J Gastroenterol* 2002;97:287–291.
43. Myers SR. Tuberculous fistula-in-ano. *J R Soc Med* 1994;87:46.
44. Das PC, Radhakrishna K, Rao PL. Rectal stricture: a complication of tuberculosis. *J Pediatr Surg* 1996;31:983–984.
45. Sultan S, Azria F, Bauer P, et al. Anoperineal tuberculosis: diagnostic and management considerations in 7 cases. *Dis Colon Rectum* 2002;45:407–410.
46. Koniaris LG, Seibel JL. Tuberculosis presenting as a perirectal mass: report of a case. *Dis Colon Rectum* 2000;43:1604–1605.
47. Mokoena T, Bairagi N. Acute tuberculous pancreatitis associated with HIV infection. *Trop Doct* 1994;24:172–173.
48. Dezfuli M, Oo MM, Jones BE, et al. Tuberculosis mimicking acute appendicitis in patients with human immunodeficiency virus infection. *Clin Infect Dis* 1994;18:650–651.
49. Ladas SD, Vaidakis E, Lariou C, et al. Pancreatic tuberculosis in non-immunocompromised patients: reports of two cases, and a literature review. *Eur J Gastroenterol Hepatol* 1998;10:973–976.
50. Baba RD, John V. Pancreatic tuberculosis: case report and review of the literature. *Trop Gastroenterol* 2001;22:213–214.
51. Schneider A, von Birgelen C, Duhrsen U, et al. Two cases of pancreatic tuberculosis in nonimmunocompromised patients. A diagnostic challenge and a rare cause of portal hypertension. *Pancreatology* 2002;2:69–73.
52. Howell JS, Knapton PJ. Ileocecal tuberculosis. *Gut* 1964;5:524–529.
53. Malik AK, Bhasin DK, Pal L, et al. Does vasculitis occur in abdominal tuberculosis? *J Clin Gastroenterol* 1992;15:355–356.
54. Theoni RF, Margulis AR. Gastrointestinal tuberculosis. *Semin Roentgenol* 1979;14:283–294.
55. Balikian JP, Uthman SM, Kabakian HA. Tuberculous colitis. *Am J Proctol* 1977;28:75–79.
56. Kuwajerwala NK, Bapat RD, Joshi AS. Mesenteric vasculopathy in intestinal tuberculosis. *Indian J Gastroenterol* 1997;16:134–136.
57. Oran I, Parildar M, Memis A. Mesenteric artery aneurysms in intestinal tuberculosis as a cause of lower gastrointestinal bleeding. *Abdom Imaging* 2001;26:131–133.
58. Pulimood AB, Ramakrishna BS, Kurian G, et al. Endoscopic mucosal biopsies are useful in distinguishing granulomatous colitis due to Crohn's disease from tuberculosis. *Gut* 1999;45:537–541.
59. Shah S, Thomas V, Mathan M, et al. Colonoscopic study of 50 patients with colonic tuberculosis. *Gut* 1992;33:347–351.
60. Gan HT, Chen YQ, Ouyang Q, et al. Differentiation between intestinal tuberculosis and Crohn's disease in endoscopic biopsy specimens by polymerase chain reaction. *Am J Gastroenterol* 2002; 97:1446–1451.
61. Das P, Shukla HS. Clinical diagnosis of abdominal tuberculosis. *Br J Surg* 1976;63:941–946.
62. McGee GS, Williams LF, Potts J, et al. Gastrointestinal tuberculosis: resurgence of an old pathogen. *Am Surg* 1989;55:16–20.
63. Davis GR, Corbett DB, Krejs GJ. Ileal chloride secretion as a cause of secretory diarrhea in a patient with primary intestinal tuberculosis. *Gastroenterology* 1979;76:829–835.
64. Tandon RK, Basnal R, Kapur BML, et al. A study of malabsorption in intestinal tuberculosis: stagnant loop syndrome. *Am J Clin Nutr* 1980;33:244–250.
65. Verma P, Kapur BML. Massive rectal bleeding due to intestinal tuberculosis. *Am J Gastroenterol* 1979;71:217–219.
66. Posniak AL, Dalton-Clarke HJ, Ralphs DNL. Colonic tuberculosis presenting with massive rectal bleeding. *Tubercle* 1985;66:295–299.
67. Monkemuller KE, Lewis JB Jr. Massive rectal bleeding from colonic tuberculosis. *Am J Gastroenterol* 1996;91:1439–1441.
68. Watanabe T, Kudo M, Kayaba M, et al. Massive rectal bleeding due to ileal tuberculosis. *J Gastroenterol* 1999;34:525–529.
69. Sefr R, Rotterova P, Konecny J. Perforation peritonitis in primary intestinal tuberculosis. *Dig Surg* 2001;18:475–479.
70. Scriven JM, Berry D. Multiple small bowel perforations in a patient on treatment of tuberculosis. *J R Coll Surg Edinb* 1996;41:353.
71. Guex AC, Bucher HC, Demartines N, et al. Inflammatory bowel perforation during immune restoration after one year of antiretroviral and antituberculous therapy in an HIV-1-infected patient: report of a case. *Dis Colon Rectum* 2002;45:977–978.
72. Dutta U, Bhutani V, Nagi B, et al. Reversible portal hyper-

tension due to tuberculosis. *Indian J Gastroenterol* 2000;19: 136–137.

73. Gheorghe L, Bancila II, Gheorghe C, et al. Antro-duodenal tuberculosis causing gastric outlet obstruction—a rare presentation of a protean disease. *Rom J Gastroenterol* 2002;11:149–152.

74. Harland RW, Varkey B. Anal tuberculosis: report of two cases and literature review. *Am J Gastroenterol* 1992;87:1488–1491.

75. Fee MJ, Oo MM, Gabayan AE, et al. Abdominal tuberculosis in patients infected with the human immunodeficiency virus. *Clin Infect Dis* 1995;20:938–944.

76. De Rosa FG, Bonora S, Di Perri G. Tuberculosis and treatment with infliximab. *N Eng J Med* 2002;346:623–626.

77. Wagner TE, Huseby ES, Huseby JS. Exacerbation of *Mycobacterium tuberculosis* enteritis masquerading as Crohn's disease after treatment with a tumor necrosis factor-alpha inhibitor. *Am J Med* 2002;112:67–69.

78. Brombart M, Massion J. Radiologic differences between ileocecal tuberculosis and Crohn's disease. *Am J Dig Dis* 1961;6:589–622.

79. Stierlin E. Die Radiographie in der Diagnostik Ileozoekalertuberkulose und anderer Krankheiten des Dickdarms. *Munchen Med Wochenschr* 1911;58:1231–1235.

80. Radin DR. Intraabdominal *M. tuberculosis* vs. *M. avium* in patients with AIDS: distinction based on CT findings. *AJR Am J Roentgenol* 1991;156:487–491.

81. Balthazar EJ, Gordon R, Hulnick D. Ileocecal tuberculosis: CT and radiologic evaluation. *AJR Am J Roentgenol* 1990;154: 499–503.

82. Hulnick DH, Megibow AJ, Naidich DP, et al. Abdominal tuberculosis: CT evaluation. *Radiology* 1985;157:199–204.

83. Yang SO, Lee YI, Chung DH, et al. Detection of extrapulmonary tuberculosis with gallium-67 scan and computed tomography. *J Nucl Med* 1992;33:2118–2123.

84. Kalvaria I, Kottler RE, Marks IN. The role of colonoscopy in the diagnosis of tuberculosis. *J Clin Gastroenterol* 1988;10: 516–523.

85. Spach DH, Silverstein FE, Stamm WE. Transmission of infection by gastrointestinal endoscopy and bronchoscopy. *Ann Intern Med* 1993;118:117–128.

86. Bhargava DK, Tandon HD, Chawla TC, et al. Diagnosis of ileocecal and colonic tuberculosis by colonoscopy. *Gastrointest Endosc* 1985;31:68–70.

87. Medina E, Orti E, Tome A, et al. Segmental tuberculosis of the colon diagnosed by colonoscopy. *Endoscopy* 1990;22:188–190.

88. Bhargava DK, Kushwaha AK, Dasarathy S, et al. Endoscopic diagnosis of segmental colonic tuberculosis. *Gastrointest Endosc* 1992;38:571–574.

89. Anand BS, Schneider FE, El-Zaatari FA, et al. Diagnosis of intestinal tuberculosis by polymerase chain reaction on endoscopic biopsy specimens. *Am J Gastroenterol* 1994;89: 2248–2249.

90. Moatter T, Mirza S, Siddiqui MS, et al. Detection of Mycobacterium tuberculosis in paraffin embedded intestinal tissue specimens by polymerase chain reaction: characterization of IS6110 element negative strains. *J Pak Med Assoc* 1998;48:174–178.

91. Kochhar R, Rajwanshi A, Goenka MK, et al. Colonoscopic fine needle aspiration cytology in the diagnosis of ileocecal tuberculosis. *Am J Gastroenterol* 1991;86:102–104.

92. Radhika S, Rajwanshi A, Kochhar R, et al. Abdominal tuberculosis. Diagnosis by fine needle aspiration cytology. *Acta Cytol* 1993;37:673–678.

93. Dineen P, Homan W, Grafe WR. Tuberculous peritonitis: 43 years' experience in diagnosis and treatment. *Ann Surg* 1976; 184:717–722.

94. Cheng IKP, Chan PCK, Chan MK. Tuberculous peritonitis complicating long term peritoneal dialysis. *Am J Nephrol* 1988;9:155–161.

95. Sochocky S. Tuberculous peritonitis: a review of 100 cases. *Am Rev Respir Dis* 1967;95:398–401.

96. Singh MM, Bhargava AN, Jain KP. Tuberculous peritonitis: an evaluation of pathogenic mechanisms, diagnostic procedures, and therapeutic measures. *N Engl J Med* 1969;281:1091–1094.

97. Ribera E, Martinez-Vasquez JM, Ocana I, et al. Diagnostic value of ascites gamma interferon levels in tuberculous peritonitis. Comparison with adenosine deaminase activity. *Tubercle* 1991;72:193–197.

98. Manohar A, Simjee AE, Haffejee AA, et al. Symptoms and investigative finding in 145 patients with tuberculous peritonitis diagnosed by peritoneoscopy and biopsy over a five year period. *Gut* 1990;10:1130–1132.

99. Aguado JM, Pons F, Casafont F, et al. Tuberculous peritonitis: a study comparing cirrhotic and noncirrhotic patients. *J Clin Gastroenterol* 1990;12:550–554.

100. Bastani B, Shariatzadeh MR, Dehdashti F. Tuberculous peritonitis—report of 30 cases and review of the literature. *Q J Med* 1985;56:549–557.

101. Lee DH, Lim JH, Ko YT, et al. Sonographic finding in tuberculous peritonitis of wet-ascitic type. *Clin Radiol* 1991;44: 306–310.

102. Burack WR, Hollister RM. Tuberculous peritonitis: a study of 47 proved cases encountered by a general medical unit in twenty-five years. *Am J Med* 1960;29:510–523.

103. Marshall JB, Vogele KA. Serum-ascites albumin difference in tuberculous peritonitis. *Am J Gastroenterol* 1988;83:1259–1261.

104. Martin RE, Bradsher RW. Elusive diagnosis of tuberculous peritonitis. *South Med J* 1986;79:1076–1079.

105. Voigt MD, Kalvaria I, Trey C, et al. Diagnostic value of ascites adenosine deaminase in tuberculous peritonitis. *Lancet* 1989; 1:751–754.

106. Bhargava DK, Nijhawan S, Gupta M. Adenosine deaminase and tuberculous peritonitis. *Lancet* 1989;1:1260–1261.

107. Fernandez-Rodriguez CM, Perez-Arguelles BS, Ledo L, et al. Ascites adenosine deaminase activity is decreased in tuberculous ascites with low protein content. *Am J Gastroenterol* 1991; 86:1500–1503.

108. Kaur A, Basha A, Ranjan M, et al. Poor diagnostic value of adenosine deaminase in pleural, peritoneal and cerebrospinal fluids in tuberculosis. *Indian J Med Res* 1992;95:270–277.

109. Gau H, Ouyang Q, Ba H. Laboratory diagnosis of tuberculous peritonitis (abstract in English). *Zhangha Jin He He Hu Xi Za Zhi* 1997;20:149–152.

110. Wolfe JHN, Behn AR, Jackson BT. Tuberculous peritonitis and role of diagnostic laparoscopy. *Lancet* 1979;1:852–853.

111. Bhargava BK, Shriniwas MD, Chopra P, et al. Peritoneal tuberculosis: laparoscopic patterns and its diagnostic accuracy. *Am J Gastroenterol* 1992;87:109–112.

112. Chow KM, Chow VC, Hung LC, et al. Tuberculous peritonitis-associated mortality is high among patients waiting for the results of mycobacterial cultures of ascitic fluid samples. *Clin Infect Dis* 2002;35:409–413.

113. Lee JH, Shin DH. The medical treatment of a tuberculous tracheoesophageal fistula. *Tubercle Lung Dis* 1992;73: 177–179.

114. Conjalka MS, Usselman J. Successful medical treatment of a tuberculosis B-E fistula. *Mt Sinai J Med* 1980;47:283–284.

115. Anand BS, Nanda R, Sachdev GK. Response of tuberculous stricture to antituberculous treatment. *Gut* 1988;29:62–69.

HEPATOBILIARY TUBERCULOSIS

HILLEL TOBIAS
ALEX SHERMAN

The resurgence of tuberculosis (TB) in industrialized nations, in part as a result of its prominence in patients with acquired immunodeficiency syndrome (AIDS), has led to an increased awareness of the potential involvement of the liver and biliary tract by TB. Until relatively recently, extrapulmonary TB in the United States was considered to be rare and was found predominantly in immigrants from Third World nations. Two reports from the early 1990s, however, document the increasing incidence of abdominal and hepatobiliary TB, especially in urban inner city populations (1,2). The migration of populations from areas of high TB prevalence to the West has also been emphasized (3).

Liver involvement is common, whether the infection is apparently confined to the lung or is systemic. Klatskin (4) demonstrated that as many as two-thirds of patients with primary pulmonary TB have some evidence of liver involvement. Hepatic granulomas have been found in as many as 80% of patients with chronic pulmonary TB. This was confirmed in autopsy studies of patients dying of chronic pulmonary TB (5). Hepatic lesions have similarly been described in more than 90% of miliary or widespread infection (6).

Although involvement of the liver by TB is common, clinical manifestations of this involvement are not. Primary hepatic TB, however, is a well-described syndrome in which hepatic involvement overwhelmingly dominates the clinical picture (7). Jaundice and death from hepatic failure have been reported (8–10).

Another manifestation of the interrelationship of TB and the liver results from the potential of current antitubercular chemotherapeutic agents to produce hepatic toxicity. Both isoniazid and rifampin, the mainstays of TB treatment, can cause hepatotoxicity (11). Second-tier antituberculous drugs, increasingly used in complex multidrug regimens, also have hepatotoxic potential (12). Thus, the liver can play a prominent role in the patient with TB.

CLINICAL SYMPTOMS

Most patients with hepatic TB manifest no symptoms specifically referable to the hepatobiliary tract but present with nonspecific symptoms, such as fever, malaise, fatigue, night sweats, anorexia, and weight loss. Patients with prominent hepatic complaints represent a minority of patients with hepatic TB. In these patients, abdominal pain, jaundice, or ascites may occur.

In a series of 200 predominantly black South African patients, 86% of whom had miliary TB and 14% of whom had "local hepatic tuberculosis," nonspecific symptoms were common in both groups (13). Abdominal pain was present in approximately half of both groups. Jaundice was not uncommon in those with localized hepatic TB but was unusual in the group with miliary disease (13). Alvarez and Carpio (14) reported on 130 patients with hepatic TB in the Philippines. Jaundice was common, involving 35% of patients. Abdominal pain was present in 39% of the non-jaundiced group.

Abdominal pain appears to be the most important specific symptom of hepatic TB in several series, including 96 cases of so-called *tuberculous hepatitis* (15). Right upper quadrant or diffuse abdominal pain, changed bowel habits, and even acute abdomen may be present. Abdominal symptoms frequently occur in combination with respiratory symptoms or weight loss. In another series of 41 patients with hepatic TB diagnosed by liver biopsy, 15% presented with jaundice (16). Recently, Bernhard et al. (17) reported their experience with 18 cases of gastrointestinal TB in San Jose, CA. The most common clinical presentation was a triad of abdominal pain, fever, and weight loss. The mean time to diagnosis was 50 days. The authors emphasize the importance of a high index of clinical suspicion to avoid diagnostic delay.

H. Tobias: Department of Medicine, New York University School of Medicine; Transplant Service, New York University Medical Center, New York, New York.
A. Sherman: Department of Medicine, New York University School of Medicine; Department of Medicine, New York University Medical Center, New York, New York.

SIGNS

Although jaundice occurs in a minority of patients with TB involving the liver, organomegaly is common. Hersch (13) reported hepatomegaly in 71% of patients with miliary TB and 95% of patients with local hepatic TB. Half of the patients with hepatomegaly exhibited hepatic tenderness. Splenomegaly was apparent in 32% of patients with miliary and 57% of those with localized hepatic TB. In Filipino patients with hepatic involvement, essentially all patients exhibited hepatomegaly (14). Hepatic tenderness was noted in one-third of them, and splenomegaly in one-fourth. The liver was enlarged and firm in more than 80% of the patients of Essop et al. (15). Hepatic tenderness was evident in 60% and splenomegaly in 40%. Maharaj et al. (16) found hepatomegaly in 95% and splenomegaly in 32% of their patients with hepatic TB. Ascites was noted in one-fourth of the patients (16). Others have not reported this finding (13–15).

LABORATORY

The most common specific hepatic biochemical abnormalities are elevations of serum alkaline phosphatase and γ-glutamyl transpeptidase levels. The alkaline phosphatase level was abnormal in more than 75% and 90% of patients from the Filipino and South African series, respectively (13,14). This abnormality is likely to be secondary to the presence of multiple intrahepatic granulomas. The involvement of the extrahepatic biliary tree by TB or extrahepatic common bile duct obstruction by tuberculous lymph nodes at the porta hepatis is a rare cause of cholestasis (14).

Serum transaminase levels may also be elevated. Tuberculous hepatitis has been reported (15). In the series of 96 patients by Essop et al. (15), alanine aminotransferase and aspartate aminotransferase levels were elevated in 70%, with an alanine aminotransferase/aspartate aminotransferase ratio of 1.5:1. Alvarez and Carpio (14) reported almost universal transaminase elevations in the jaundiced patients but variable elevations in the nonicteric. Parenchymal inflammation reported in histologic descriptions of tuberculous granulomatous hepatitis may be responsible (18).

Hyperbilirubinemia can be seen in some patients with hepatic TB; several large series reported an incidence of less than 20% (14,19,20). With primary hepatic TB, the incidence is 35% to 50% (13,14). Hyperbilirubinemia is usually owing to intrahepatic cholestasis and only occasionally reflects extrahepatic biliary obstruction. Jaundice in these patients is only rarely an indicator of hepatic failure associated with overwhelming hepatic TB involvement.

Alterations in albumin/globulin ratios are common. Hypoalbuminemia and hyperglobulinemia are present in approximately 80% of patients with hepatobiliary TB,

reflecting the systemic chronic disease rather than hepatic synthetic dysfunction (13,15,16).

IMAGING

Radiographic investigations in patients with hepatobiliary TB may suggest the diagnosis, but the findings are usually nonspecific. In older series, most patients with hepatobiliary TB had chest radiographic studies indicating TB (14–16). In modern series of abdominal TB, however, concomitant pulmonary disease is much less common, occurring in as few as 10% of patients (1). Thus, the absence of pulmonary disease no longer reliably excludes the diagnosis of hepatobiliary TB. The increased frequency of extrapulmonary presentations of TB in AIDS patients has made this increasingly true (21).

Calcifications of the liver on abdominal radiographs are highly suggestive of hepatobiliary TB. Both Alvarez and Carpio (14) and Maglinte et al. (22) reported hepatic calcifications in approximately 50% of patients with hepatobiliary TB. Multiple chalky or powdery calcifications in the liver and nodal calcifications along the course of the common bile duct are highly suggestive of hepatobiliary TB and allow it to be reliably differentiated from other causes of liver calcification (22,23).

Specific imaging modalities of the liver reveal hepatobiliary involvement by TB in one of two forms. The more common form of hepatic involvement is miliary. The liver is diffusely involved by small nodules ranging from 0.5 to 2.0 mm in size. The much rarer so-called macronodular or pseudotumoral form consists of tuberculous nodules larger than 2.0 mm in diameter. These larger nodules are space-occupying lesions that can mimic neoplasms. These abnormalities are being increasingly described owing to the more frequent use of newer imaging techniques (24).

Technetium–sulfa colloid liver scans were used more frequently in older series but have generally been supplanted by ultrasonography and computed tomography.

Abdominal ultrasonography is now almost universally used as the initial imaging modality for suspected hepatic disease. The sonographic appearance of the miliary form of hepatic involvement is nonspecific and consists of either a homogeneously enlarged liver or a "bright echo" pattern of increased hepatic echogenicity (25). The macronodular or pseudotumoral form appears on ultrasonography as either single or multiple hypoechoic lesions (25). Tan et al. (26), however, described an unusual case of macronodular TB presenting as a hyperechoic lesion mimicking an infiltrative hepatic tumor. Sonography may also demonstrate extrahepatic biliary obstruction secondary to lymphadenopathy at the porta hepatis.

Computed tomography provides a detailed evaluation of the hepatic parenchyma. The more common diffuse miliary involvement appears as small, low-density foci widely scattered throughout the hepatic substance. The rarer macronodular variety appears as single or multiple low-density intrahepatic masses (27,28).

Endoscopic retrograde cholangiography and percutaneous transhepatic cholangiography provide direct visualization of the biliary tree and are commonly used in jaundiced patients with hepatobiliary TB. Maglinte et al. (22) performed direct cholangiography on 22 patients with obstructive jaundice. The obstruction was found at the porta hepatis in 86% and in the distal common bile duct in 14% of patients. Biliary involvement ranged from mild narrowing to severe irregular tortuous strictures with marked proximal dilation. Biliary involvement in this series was owing to extrinsic compression of the common bile duct by tuberculous lymph nodes. Fan et al. (29) described involvement of the biliary epithelium by TB, as confirmed by choledochoscopic biopsy of a common hepatic duct stricture. Bearer et al. (30) detailed the case of a woman with obstructive jaundice caused by a bile duct stricture. The diagnosis of TB was made by the observation of acid-fast bacillus (AFB) in bile aspirated during endoscopic retrograde cholangiopancreatography. Successful relief of jaundice was accomplished by the placement of an expandable metal stent across the narrowing. This report illustrates the therapeutic and diagnostic role of endoscopic retrograde cholangiopancreatography in the rare cases of TB involving the biliary tree.

CLINICAL SYNDROMES

Miliary involvement of the liver generally produces mild or nonspecific symptoms and laboratory abnormalities and requires no special attention other than that directed against the systemic infection itself. Liver involvement can, however, play an important role in the diagnosis and prognosis of this systemic syndrome. This is demonstrated by the series of Maartens et al. (31), who reviewed 109 cases of miliary TB observed over a 10-year period at their community-based teaching unit. Liver biopsy was diagnostic in all ten patients in whom it was performed. Overall, 24% of the patients died. An elevated serum transaminase level was one of several independent predictors of mortality (31).

Hepatobiliary involvement by TB can, at times, dominate the clinical picture and lead to unusual clinical presentations.

Congenital Tuberculosis

The liver is often involved in congenital TB. This is defined as TB acquired by the fetus in intrauterine life. It is rare; fewer than 200 cases have been reported. The liver is involved in approximately 80% of patients (32). Specific hepatic signs include hepatomegaly and jaundice. Foo et al. (33) described an infant with congenital TB presenting with poor feeding, jaundice, and hepatosplenomegaly. The infant died in hepatic failure on day 36 of life. The reported

mortality rate for congenital TB is high, despite modern chemotherapy (34). The diagnosis is frequently made only at postmortem examination. Hepatic involvement recently was incorporated into the revised diagnostic criteria for congenital TB (35).

Focal Liver Lesions

Rarely, hepatic TB lesions appear as masses larger than 2 mm in diameter. Involvement of the liver by space-occupying TB lesions may mimic primary or metastatic hepatic tumor or pyogenic abscess. These lesions have been referred to by a variety of names, including tuberculoma, macronodular TB, or pseudotumoral TB. In an individual patient, lesions may be single or multiple. Lesions as large as 12 cm in size have been reported (36). The rarity of this presentation is emphasized by Herman et al. (37), who reviewed the global literature. Since 1950, only 23 cases of isolated nodular TB have been reported; nearly all were suspected of having a hepatic neoplasm.

Visualization of the liver by modern imaging techniques raises the suspicion of neoplasia in patients with tuberculoma. Although percutaneous aspiration of the lesion under imaging guidance is theoretically the diagnostic procedure of choice, this has only occasionally resulted in definitive diagnosis. An open biopsy is frequently required (36). Macronodular TB may also resemble pyogenic abscess (38–41). Balsarkar and Joshi (39) report the case of a 38-year-old woman with epigastric pain, fever, and jaundice. Imaging studies demonstrated a multiseptate abscess. AFBs were identified in the purulent fluid obtained at laparotomy. A large liver abscess with a thick, fibrous capsule may be particularly difficult to treat with systemic anti-TB medications; these medications may not penetrate to the core of the cavity. The infusion of antibiotics directly into the abscess cavity by means of a percutaneously placed catheter may offer a therapeutic advantage (42).

Local Hepatic Tuberculosis (Primary Hepatic Tuberculosis)

Involvement of the hepatobiliary tract by TB, either without apparent involvement elsewhere or only with local lymph node and splenic involvement, has been termed primary or local hepatic TB (43). This was first reported by Bristowe (44) in 1858 and remains a rare presentation. Essop et al. (43) estimated an incidence of approximately 1% in patients with hepatic TB.

The liver is usually extensively involved in local hepatic TB. Symptoms, signs, laboratory abnormalities, and imaging studies are similar to those for miliary TB (45).

The pathogenesis of local hepatic TB is unclear. In contrast to patients with miliary spread, in which the tubercle bacillus is thought to reach the liver via the hepatic artery, in local hepatic TB, the bacillus may gain direct access to the liver from the portal vein via the gastrointestinal tract.

This difference in pathogenesis may explain the observation that in miliary TB, lesions are concentrated near the hepatic veins, although in the local form, they are usually found periportally (46). The rarity of the local variety may be because the liver is an inhospitable place for the tubercle bacillus owing to its low tissue oxygen level (46). Alternatively, the tubercle bacillus may reach the liver by hematogenous or lymphatic spread, with failure of the organism to lodge elsewhere, or regression of involvement at other sites, leaving only the hepatic lesions as clinically evident. Because of the uncertainty regarding pathogenesis, the term primary hepatic TB, implying that the infection arose in the liver, may be inappropriate. The term local hepatic TB is preferred (43).

Hepatic Failure

Despite the common involvement of the liver in miliary TB and the often extensive distribution of TB lesions within the liver, a significant decline in hepatic function is unusual in hepatic TB. Rare cases of hepatic failure owing to massive TB infiltration of the liver, however, have been sporadically described. Sharma et al. (8), in 1981, reported the presentation of a 36-year-old woman with massive hepatosplenomegaly and liver failure. Liver failure was evidenced by jaundice, ascites, and hepatic encephalopathy. The woman died of upper gastrointestinal hemorrhage and progressive hepatic coma. Autopsy revealed massive involvement of the liver and spleen with tuberculous granulomas. Asada et al. (9) described a 58-year-old Japanese man with jaundice and fulminant hepatic failure that progressed to hepatic coma and death. Pathologic examination revealed dense studding of the liver with granulomas. More recently, Hussain et al. (10) described fulminant hepatic failure in an Asian woman. She died despite the prompt institution of anti-TB medications and intensive supportive therapy. Postmortem evaluation showed widespread miliary TB.

The rarity of liver failure in hepatic TB may be owing to the fact that the presence of the tuberculous granulomas, even if massive, does not directly result in the extensive destruction of hepatocytes. The liver may be massively enlarged by the presence of granulomas, yet liver metabolic function remains normal.

Ruttenberg et al. (47) reported portal hypertension in two patients with abdominal TB. Neither resulted from hepatic failure. In the first case, a 26-year-old man developed portal hypertension from a segmental splenic vein occlusion by a tuberculous lymph node. In the second, a 42-year-old woman developed portal and splenic vein thrombosis secondary to pancreatic TB.

Biliary Tuberculosis

Obstructive jaundice in hepatobiliary TB only rarely results from intrinsic involvement of the bile ducts. Fan et al. (29), however, described the occurrence of a biliary stricture in a 46-year-old Filipino woman caused by granulomatous involvement of the biliary epithelium.

Tuberculous cholangitis is extremely rare (48). It is thought to occur as a result of rupture of a caseating granuloma from the portal tract into the bile duct. Clinical features resemble bacterial cholangitis, with right upper quadrant pain, fever, and jaundice. Tuberculous involvement of the gallbladder is also rare but was chronicled in a large Chinese series (49). A rare case of hepatobiliary TB presenting as a gallbladder tumor has also been described (50).

HISTOPATHOLOGY

The pathologic hallmark of hepatic TB is the granuloma (Fig. 35.1). A granuloma is a characteristic collection of inflammatory cells, arising in response to a variety of inciting agents. TB is one of the major causes of hepatic granulomas and enters into the differential diagnosis of so-called granulomatous hepatitis (see later).

Granulomas in the liver are structurally similar to granulomas in other organs and tissues. They are discrete, usually sharply defined aggregates of inflammatory cells, generally 1 to 2 mm in diameter. Epithelioid cells or macrophages make up the bulk of the granuloma, surrounded by a ring of mononuclear cells, predominantly lymphocytes. Multinucleated giant cells may be seen as well as fibroblasts, eosinophils, mast cells, and basophils. Central caseation necrosis may be present (51). Hepatic granulomas are most frequently found periportally. The lobular architecture and function of the liver are only rarely affected. Healing of granulomas occurs by fibrosis and hyalinization and may result in eventual calcification.

The epithelioid cell (so-called because of its structural similarity to epithelial cells) is an invariable component of granulomas. Granuloma formation is thought to be initiated when an initial stimulus (i.e., infection by the tubercle bacillus) results in the focal recruitment of mononuclear cells. The key step in granuloma formation appears to be the differentiation of the monocyte or macrophage into an epithelioid cell. The pathogenesis of granulomas remains the subject of continuing study (51).

The liver is rich in reticuloendothelial tissue (i.e., Kupffer cells). The abundance of immunologic tissue makes the liver important in the clearance of pathogens. The facilitation of the immunologic response to pathogens within the liver explains why the liver is a prime site for the development of granulomas.

"Granulomatous Hepatitis"

Hepatic granulomas are common; they have been found in as many as 30% of liver biopsy specimens (51). Strictly speaking, the term granulomatous hepatitis is a misnomer; the granulomatous inflammation does not usually result in

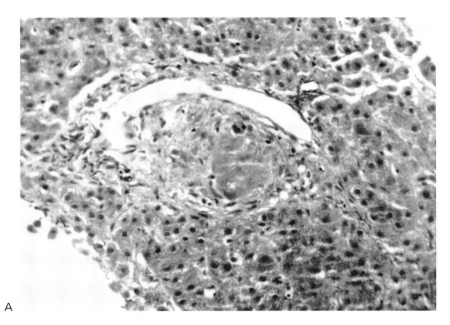

A

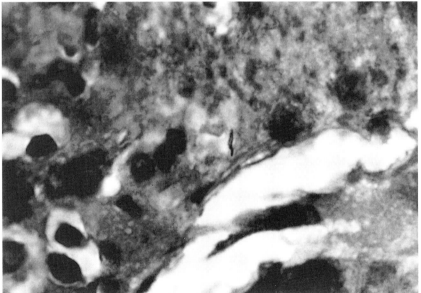

B

FIGURE 35.1. *Mycobacterium tuberculosis.* **A:** Medium-power photomicrograph of needle biopsy specimen of liver shows a well-formed epithelioid granuloma with multinucleated Langhans-type giant cells within a portal triad (trichrome stain, original magnification ×160). **B:** Oil immersion photomicrograph of the same biopsy specimen as in **A** shows a single acid-fast bacillus (acid-fast stain, original magnification ×1,000). (Courtesy of Dr. John V. Scholes, Department of Pathology, New York University Medical Center, New York, NY.)

the destruction of hepatocytes and therefore should not be thought of as hepatitis. Hepatic granulomatous disease is a more logical term.

The list of causes of hepatic granulomas is long and includes infectious and noninfectious factors. Harrington et al. (51) listed 88 specific disease entities associated with hepatic granulomas.

Although TB is a major cause of hepatic granulomas in most series, its frequency is highly variable and depends on the population studied. Sartin and Walker (52) reported only a 3% incidence of TB in a series of 88 patients with granulomas at the Mayo Clinic. Other series reported higher frequencies ranging from 10% to 53% of patients (51). In a review of granulomatous hepatitis by Harrington

et al. (51) in 1982, TB was responsible for approximately 20% of hepatic granulomas in eight series totaling 1,129 patients. Indian investigators established a tubercular cause of granulomatous hepatitis in 55% of 51 patients (53). TB is by far the most common infectious cause of hepatic granulomas. Conversely, hepatic granulomas are present in more that 90% of cases of miliary TB, 70% of cases of extrapulmonary TB, and 25% of apparently isolated pulmonary TB (6).

Sherlock (54) suggested several features of hepatic granulomas owing to TB that allow them to be differentiated from granulomas of other causes. These features include (a) AFBs within the granuloma, (b) central caseation necrosis, (c) irregularity of the granuloma contour, with a particularly dense rim of lymphocytes surrounding the granuloma, and (d) relatively few granulomas, with a tendency to coalesce. These criteria are by no means universal, and strict reliance on them may be misleading. AFBs may be seen in tuberculous granulomas in 0% to 35% of patients (51). Their frequency is highest in patients with miliary disease. The presence of AFBs, although highly suggestive of TB, cannot be relied on with certainty because atypical mycobacterioses are an increasing cause of hepatic granulomas, especially with the advent of AIDS (see later). Although definitive diagnosis by culture is desired, cultures of liver biopsy specimens are positive for only a small percentage of patients (51). The presence of caseation necrosis in tuberculous granulomas has been highly variable, with rates ranging from 0% to 100% in various series (51). This classic finding is highly suggestive of TB; however, it is nonspecific. Johnson et al. (55) reported the occurrence of caseating hepatic granulomas in a patient with Hodgkin disease. Other causes include coccidiomycosis and brucellosis. The pathologic features of tuberculous granulomas are not specific and require confirmation by culture of *Mycobacterium tuberculosis*.

As previously mentioned, macroscopic lesions larger than 2 mm may also be found in hepatic TB. These represent the coalescence of two or more granulomas into a larger lesion and may be referred to as tuberculomas.

Nonspecific Pathologic Changes

In addition to specific histologic evidence of hepatic TB (i.e., caseating granulomas with AFBs), several nonspecific hepatic pathologic changes have been described. Korn et al. (5), in 1959, described liver biopsies in 30 patients with extrapulmonary (not necessarily hepatic) TB. Granulomas were seen in 80% of the specimens. All patients exhibited nonspecific inflammatory infiltration of the hepatic parenchyma. Ninety percent of patients exhibited foci of Kupffer cell hyperplasia, generally in distended sinusoids, often accompanied by adjacent inflammatory infiltration and hepatocyte necrosis. Fibrosis was observed in two-thirds of biopsy specimens. This was generally portal or periportal and mild in degree. Architectural distortion characteristic of cirrhosis was not observed. Mild fatty change was seen in 30% of biopsies; fatty change was marked in only one patient. Similar nonspecific lesions have been described more recently in a series of 71 cases of pulmonary and extrapulmonary TB (56).

Popper and Schaffner (18) described nonspecific hepatic changes of miliary TB. These include areas of focal necrosis and portal inflammation, Kupffer cell proliferation, and fatty liver. Hersch (13) found fatty liver in 14% of liver biopsies and 28% of autopsied subjects with hepatic TB. The origin of these nonspecific alterations in hepatic structure is not clear. Concomitant alcoholism and malnutrition may be contributory. Cirrhosis found in

patients with hepatic TB is likely to be coincidental. Hepatic amyloidosis may occur in 5% to 10% of patients with fatal TB (57,58). The liver is diffusely enlarged by the deposition of amyloid between the hepatocytes and the sinusoidal epithelium. Hepatic amyloidosis causes remarkably little hepatocellular dysfunction, despite often massive hepatomegaly.

Passive congestion of the liver secondary to right-sided congestive heart failure in association with advanced pulmonary TB has been described (58).

ACQUIRED IMMUNODEFICIENCY SYNDROME AND HEPATOBILIARY TUBERCULOSIS

AIDS patients have a relatively high incidence of TB, which may run an unusually aggressive course (21). Extrapulmonary involvement in AIDS patients is common, occurring in approximately half of the patients. Louie et al. (59), in 1986, reported that approximately 50% of AIDS patients diagnosed with TB at Bellevue Hospital in New York City from 1979 to 1985 had extrapulmonary involvement compared with a 20% incidence in nonimmunocompromised populations. In comparison, the incidence of extrapulmonary TB in a 1964 series was 7.7% (60). In the setting of AIDS and extrapulmonary TB, hepatic involvement is common. Abdel-Dayem et al. (61), in 1997, documented liver involvement at autopsy in 45% of 29 patients dying of AIDS with confirmed TB. Symptoms and signs of hepatic involvement and laboratory abnormalities tend to be similar to those in patients without AIDS (61).

Reports from the early 1990s document the rise of abdominal TB, especially in poor inner city populations (1,2). The liver in AIDS patients with TB is only one of several sites of abdominal involvement; other sites of intraabdominal involvement include the peritoneum, lymph nodes, and psoas muscle.

Atypical mycobacterioses, in particular *Mycobacterium avium-intracellulare complex* infection, are also commonly found in patients with AIDS. These disseminated infections commonly involve the liver. The differentiation of these mycobacterial infections, both producing AFB-positive hepatic granulomatous disease, may occasionally be challenging. Usually, however, clinical and pathologic findings allow the distinction with a reasonable degree of confidence, even before confirmatory culture results become available.

The comparative incidence of *M. tuberculosis* versus *M. avium-intracellulare complex* in various series differs greatly (see later). This may be owing to the fact that these infections occur in different stages of immunocompromise. Infection with *M. tuberculosis* occurs relatively early in the course of AIDS, whereas disseminated *M. avium-*

intracellulare complex usually indicates profound immunosuppression. Geographic, racial, and socioeconomic factors may also influence these differences in comparative incidence.

MYCOBACTERIUM TUBERCULOSIS AND ATYPICAL MYCOBACTERIOSES IN ACQUIRED IMMUNODEFICIENCY SYNDROME

Prego et al. (62), in 1990, reported the yield of various diagnostic modalities in the evaluation of fever of undetermined origin in patients with AIDS. Liver biopsy was the most efficient diagnostic modality, revealing AFBs in a higher percentage of patients (75%) than bone marrow biopsy (25%). Mycobacterial infections were ultimately diagnosed in 75% of patients: *M. avium-intracellulare complex* in 42% and *M. tuberculosis* in 25%.

Orenstein et al. (63), in 1985, reviewed liver biopsies in ten patients with AIDS or suspected AIDS at the Downstate Medical Center in Brooklyn, NY. Nine of the ten patients had a history of intravenous drug use. All ten patients had hepatic granulomas. Only one patient was ultimately diagnosed as having *M. tuberculosis* infection; five had confirmed *M. avium-intracellulare complex* infections. Conversely, Comer et al. (64) found *M. tuberculosis* to be a more common pathogen than *M. avium-intracellulare complex*. In a retrospective series of 48 liver biopsies performed at Harlem Hospital in New York City, serving an inner city, predominantly indigent population, granulomas owing to mycobacteria were seen in one-third of specimens. Eleven patients were ultimately diagnosed with *M. tuberculosis* infection, and five patients were found to have *M. avium-intracellulare complex* infection (64).

The differentiation of *M. avium-intracellulare complex* from *M. tuberculosis* has important clinical and prognostic consequences. *M. tuberculosis* infection, reflecting less immunosuppression, has a relatively good response to antituberculous chemotherapy. Disseminated *M. avium-intracellulare complex* infection, conversely, responds poorly to prolonged multidrug regimens.

Hepatic granulomas owing to *M. tuberculosis* in patients with AIDS may be surprisingly well developed because immunocompromise is relatively mild. Few AFBs are seen within these lesions (65). By contrast, noncaseating granulomas owing to *M. avium-intracellulare complex* are generally poorly formed and exhibit large numbers of AFBs. Large, foamy macrophages and a paucity of lymphocytes have also been described as characteristic of these lesions (66) (Fig. 35.2).

Unusual forms of hepatic TB may be seen more commonly in patients with AIDS. Pottipati et al. (67) described two patients with tuberculous liver abscesses. Patients with

AIDS may have a predilection for visceral mycobacterial abscesses (68). This may be owing to the rapid, unchecked proliferation of mycobacteria in a setting of immunocompromise.

TUBERCULOSIS AND LIVER TRANSPLANTATION

Orthotopic liver transplantation has become the procedure of choice for many patients with end-stage liver disease of diverse etiologies. High-level immunosuppression is required after transplantation to prevent graft rejection. In this setting, the risk of activation of latent TB is substantial. Higgins et al. (69) reported TB in five of 2,380 liver transplant recipients at the University of Pittsburgh. Of these five patients, only one had had a positive tuberculin test response. Salizzoni et al. (70) reported the death of a liver transplant recipient with multiple infections, among them disseminated TB. Liver biopsy revealed hepatic granulomas that were AFB negative.

The issue of prophylactic treatment of patients with a positive tuberculin test preoperatively is problematic. Prophylactic therapy involves isoniazid, a known hepatotoxin. In fact, severe isoniazid-associated hepatitis requiring liver transplantation has been reported (71). Conversely, reactivated TB, especially in the setting of immunosuppression, may be fatal. In addition, the incidence of previous TB exposure may be underestimated, as most patients with TB in the series of Higgins et al. (69) were either not tested or tuberculin negative (i.e., anergic).

Salizzoni et al. (70) recommend routine preoperative screening for TB via tuberculin skin testing, with prophylactic treatment of patients with positive results. In addition, patients with negative tuberculin test results may be prophylactically treated if there is (a) a history of contact with a patient with active TB, (b) radiographic evidence of disease, or (c) a history of residence or extensive travel in endemic areas.

Experience at the New York University Liver Transplant Service illustrates the potential pitfalls in the management of these patients A 55-year-old Dominican man was found preoperatively to be purified protein derivative positive. The purified protein derivative response was attributed to previous bacille Calmette–Guérin vaccination and not treated. A preoperative chest radiograph was normal. Six months after liver transplantation, a cavitary lesion developed in the left upper pulmonary lobe; the specimen obtained by percutaneous needle aspiration of the lesion was positive for AFB. The patient was treated with isoniazid, ethambutol, and rifampin. Increasingly abnormal liver enzyme levels and jaundice developed; isoniazid and rifampin were discontinued. A pleural effusion and hypotension rapidly ensued; second-line triple therapy with ethambutol, amikacin, and ciprofloxacin was initiated.

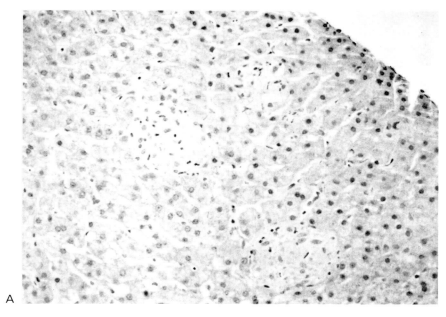

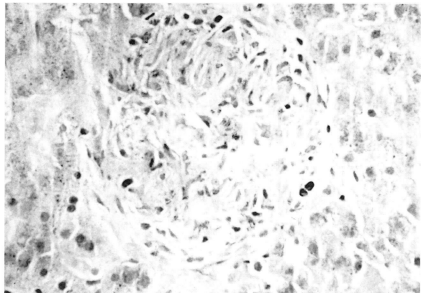

FIGURE 35.2. *Mycobacterium avium-intracellulare complex.* **A:** Medium-power photomicrograph of needle biopsy specimen of liver shows two small aggregates of epithelioid histiocytes (poorly formed epithelioid granulomas) within hepatic lobular parenchyma (hematoxylin–eosin, original magnification ×200). **B:** High-power photomicrograph of a histiocytic aggregate (poorly formed granuloma) from same biopsy specimen as in **A** shows numerous acid-fast bacilli, including clumps and clusters, within histiocytes and macrophages of granuloma (acid-fast stain, original magnification ×400). (Courtesy of Dr. John V. Scholes, Department of Pathology, New York University Medical Center, New York, NY.)

Simultaneously, the immunosuppressive medications were drastically cut back to minimal levels. Reduction of immunosuppression appears to be critical in this setting. Nonetheless, active TB in an immunosuppressed hepatic transplant recipient is associated with a high mortality (L. Teperman, *personal communication*, 1994).

DIAGNOSIS

Hepatobiliary TB should be considered in the patients with compatible symptoms and signs and biochemical evidence of liver disease. Imaging studies may suggest miliary or pseudotumoral hepatic involvement. The lack of pulmonary disease should not deter a consideration of hepatobiliary TB. This is especially true in patients with AIDS.

Liver biopsy is essential to the diagnosis. The demonstration of *M. tuberculosis* by culture of liver tissue makes the diagnosis most certain. The yield of culture is variable, ranging from 0% to 43% in various series (51). The yield of culture is highest in miliary disease and when granulomas show central caseation. Positive cultures may be obtained even in the absence of granulomas or AFBs on histologic examinations (62). Alternatively, caseating granulomas with AFBs may fail to yield positive cultural confirmation of *M. tuberculosis*.

The presence of hepatic caseating granulomas containing AFBs is highly suggestive of *M. tuberculosis* infection. These classic findings are highly variable, however, and found in 0% to 100% of patients in various series (51). Caseating granulomas, however, may rarely be seen in other conditions (55). AFBs are reported to be present in 0% to 35% of liver biopsy specimens from patients with hepatic TB (51). Although some features of AFB-containing granulomas may suggest *M. tuberculosis*, cultural confirmation is helpful to exclude *M. avium-intracellulare complex*.

The polymerase chain reaction for the detection of *M. tuberculosis* has the potential to increase diagnostic sensitivity and accuracy in hepatic TB, without the long interval required for *M. tuberculosis* culture. Diaz et al. (72), in Mexico City, evaluated the utility of this technology in the diagnosis of hepatic granulomas. Forty-three liver specimens were characterized as having definitive or probable tuberculosis based on clinical and microbiologic data. Sensitivity of the polymerase chain reaction assay was 58% in the diagnosis of hepatic granulomas; specificity was 96% (72). The ultimate role for this developing technology in the diagnosis of hepatic TB has yet to be fully delineated.

TREATMENT

The therapy of TB with hepatobiliary involvement does not differ from that used in patients without such involvement (73). Five first-line antituberculous agents are the mainstay of current regimens. Second-line agents should be used only in patients with organisms demonstrated to be resistant to first-line drugs or in those who cannot tolerate these medications. Isoniazid is almost always used in combination with other drugs. Isoniazid and rifampin for 9 months is curative in the absence of resistance. The addition of pyrazinamide for the initial 2 months of therapy allows a 6-month duration of therapy. No currently acceptable regimen for TB is shorter than 6 months in duration. Compliance with the antituberculous regimen is critical to its success. Patients with extrapulmonary TB appear to respond to standard antituberculous regimens as well as those with disease apparently localized to the lungs. Therapy of patients with drug-resistant TB should be guided by the results of culture and sensitivity testing. The therapy of those with AIDS and TB may be complicated by the well-known interactions of rifampin and antiretroviral therapy; rifabutin may be substituted in this setting (74). A detailed description of current antituberculous regimens is beyond the scope of this chapter.

Hepatic toxicity is common with currently used antituberculous agents. Patients with hepatic TB in whom liver biochemical abnormalities are often present at the start of therapy may present a diagnostic dilemma as therapy progresses. Clinical symptoms and signs may be slow to regress, and biochemical parameters may often worsen with adequate therapy. A liver biopsy may clarify the issue of whether worsening hepatic parameters represent progression of hepatic TB or are owing to drug toxicity.

Jaundice in the patient with hepatobiliary TB may be a result of biliary obstruction. Ultrasonography of the liver, showing dilation of the intrahepatic or extrahepatic biliary ductal system (or both), can delineate the presence of biliary obstruction and its anatomic location. Biliary drainage, by either percutaneous or endoscopic access, is indicated in these patients. Surgical decompression is rarely necessary.

PROGNOSIS

Hepatobiliary TB is a treatable infection. Successful therapy, however, requires an accurate microbiologic diagnosis and compliance with a regimen of demonstrated efficacy. The latter in particular is often not possible in indigent patients of low socioeconomic status in whom the incidence of hepatobiliary TB is rapidly increasing. Drug-resistant strains, requiring complex multidrug regimens, are especially difficult to eradicate.

Patients with hepatobiliary involvement by TB may have a worse prognosis than patients without such involvement (31). This may be owing to the fact that hepatobiliary involvement generally is a result of more widespread, advanced disease. Clinical series have shown variable mortality rates. Hersch (13), in 1964, found a mortality rate of 75% in jaundiced patients with hepatic TB. Alvarez and Carpio (14), in 1983, found an overall mortality rate of 12% despite antituberculous therapy. One-third of their deaths were reported to be owing to esophageal variceal bleeding resulting from portal hypertension not directly attributable to the TB. Most of these patients had associated cirrhosis. Essop et al. (15) reported a cumulative mortality rate of 42%. Poor prognostic factors included age younger than 20 years, acute hepatic TB, coagulopathy, and high mean caseation score. Jaundice per se was not associated with high mortality.

The outlook of patients with hepatic TB and AIDS is problematic. TB is generally treatable, and its presence speaks to a relatively low level of immunosuppression. Conversely, successful therapy of TB does not affect the progressive immunosuppression owing to human immunodeficiency virus infection. The latter factor would appear to be the most important variable influencing long-term survival. The outlook of patients with *M. avium-intracellulare complex* infection remains poor.

REFERENCES

1. Guth AA, Kim U. The reappearance of abdominal tuberculosis. *Surg Gynecol Obstet* 1991;172:432–436.
2. Rosengart TK, Coppa G. Abdominal mycobacterial infections in immunocompromised patients. *Am J Surg* 1990;159:125–131.

3. Jayanthi V, Probert CS, Sher KS, et al. The renaissance of abdominal tuberculosis. *Dig Dis* 1993;11:36–44.
4. Klatskin G. Hepatitis associated with systemic infection. In: Schiff L, ed. *Diseases of the liver*, 2nd ed. Philadelphia: JB Lippincott Co, 1963:539–572.
5. Korn RJ, Kellow WF, Heller P, et al. Hepatic involvement in extrapulmonary tuberculosis; histologic and functional characteristics. *Am J Med* 1959;27:60–71.
6. Klatskin G. Hepatic granulomata: problems in interpretation. *Mt Sinai J Med* 1977;44:798–812.
7. Terry RB, Gunnar RM. Primary miliary tuberculosis of the liver. *JAMA* 1957;164:150–157.
8. Sharma SK, Shamim SQ, Bannerjee CK, et al. Disseminated tuberculosis presenting as massive hepatosplenomegaly and hepatic failure. *Am J Gastroenterol* 1981;76:153–156.
9. Asada Y, Hayashi T, Sumiyoshi A, et al. Miliary tuberculosis presenting as fever and jaundice with hepatic failure. *Hum Pathol* 1991;22:92–94.
10. Hussain W, Mutimer D, Harrison R, et.al. Fulminant hepatic failure caused by tuberculosis. *Gut* 1995;36:792–794.
11. Steele MA, Burk RF, DesPrez RM. Toxic hepatitis with isoniazid and rifampin. A meta-analysis. *Chest* 1991;99:465–471.
12. Zimmerman HT, Maddrey WC. Toxic and drug induced hepatitis. In: Schiff L, Schiff ER, eds. *Diseases of the liver*, 7th ed. Philadelphia: JB Lippincott Co, 1993:707–783.
13. Hersch C. Tuberculosis of the liver: a study of 200 cases. *S Afr Med J* 1964;38:857–863.
14. Alvarez SZ, Carpio R. Hepatobiliary tuberculosis. *Dig Dis Sci* 1983;28:193–200.
15. Essop AR, Posen JA, Hodkinson JH, et al. Tuberculosis hepatitis: a clinical review of 96 cases. *Q J Med* 1984;53:465–477.
16. Maharaj B, Leary WP, Pudifen DJ. A prospective study of hepatic tuberculosis in 41 black patients. *Q J Med* 1987;242:517–522.
17. Bernhard JS, Bhatia G, Knauer CM. Gastrointestinal tuberculosis: an eighteen-patient experience and review. *J Clin Gastroenterol* 2000;31:339–340.
18. Popper H, Schaffner F. *Liver: structure and function*. New York: McGraw-Hill, 1957.
19. Bowry S, Chan CH, Weiss H, et al. Hepatic involvement in pulmonary tuberculosis: histologic and functional characteristics. *Am Rev Respir Dis* 1970;101:941–948.
20. Munt PW. Miliary tuberculosis in the chemotherapy era: with a clinical review in 69 American adults. *Medicine* 1971;51:139–155.
21. Daniel TM, Fauci AS. Multidrug-resistant tuberculosis. In: Wilson JD, et al., eds. *Harrison's principles of internal medicine, supplement 5*. New York: McGraw-Hill, 1993.
22. Maglinte DT, Alvarez SZ, Ng AC, et al. Patterns of calcifications and cholangiographic findings in hepatobiliary tuberculosis. *Gastrointest Radiol* 1988;13:331–335.
23. Alvarez SZ. Hepatobiliary tuberculosis. *J Gastroenterol Hepatol* 1998;13:833–839.
24. Zipser RD, Rau JE, Ricketts RR, et al. Tuberculous pseudotumors of the liver. *Am J Med* 1976;61:946–951.
25. Blangy S, Cornud F, Sibert A, et al. Hepatic tuberculosis presenting as tumoral disease on ultrasonography. *Gastrointest Radiol* 1988;13:52–54.
26. Tan TC, Cheung AY, Wan WY, et al. Tuberculoma of the liver presenting as a hyperechoic mass on ultrasound. *Br J Radiol* 1997;70:1293–1295.
27. Levine C. Primary macronodular hepatic tuberculosis: US and CT appearances. *Radiology* 1990;15:307–309.
28. Hulnick DH, Megibow AJ, Naidich DP, et al. Abdominal tuberculosis: CT evaluation. *Radiology* 1985;157:199–204.
29. Fan ST, Ng IOL, Choi TK, et al. Tuberculosis of the bile duct: a

rare cause of biliary stricture. *Am J Gastroenterol* 1989;84:413–414.
30. Bearer EA, Savides TJ, McCutchan JA. Endoscopic diagnosis and management of hepatobiliary tuberculosis. *Am J Gastroenterol* 1996;91:2602–2604.
31. Maartens G, Wilcox PA, Benatar SR. Miliary tuberculosis: rapid diagnosis, hematologic abnormalities, and outcome in 109 treated adults. *Am J Med* 1990;89:291–296.
32. Siegel M. Pathological findings and pathogenesis of congenital tuberculosis. *Am Rev Tuberc* 1934;29:297–308.
33. Foo AL, Tan KK, Chay OM, et al. Congenital tuberculosis. *Tuber Lung Dis* 1993;74:59–61.
34. Hageman J, Shulman S, Schreiber M, et al. Congenital tuberculosis: critical reappraisal of clinical findings and diagnostic procedure. *Pediatrics* 1980;66:980–984.
35. Cantwell MF, Shehab ZM, Costello AM, et al. Brief report: congenital tuberculosis. *N Engl J Med* 1994;330:1051–1054.
36. Achem SR, Kolts BE, Grisnik J, et al. Pseudotumoral hepatic tuberculosis. Atypical presentation and comprehensive review of the literature. *J Clin Gastroenterol* 1992;14:72–77.
37. Herman P, Pugliese V, Laurino NR, et al. Nodular form of local hepatic tuberculosis: case report. *J Trop Med Hyg* 1995;98:141–142.
38. Mahajan SK, Kishore K, Chugh SN, et al. Subcapsular tubercular liver abscess. *J Assoc Phys India* 1998;46:657–658.
39. Balsarkar D, Joshi MA. Isolated tuberculous hepatic abscess in a non-immunocompromised patient. *J Postgrad Med* 2000;46:108–109.
40. Rahmatulla RH, al-Mofleh IA, al-Rashed RS, et al. Tuberculous liver abscess: a case report and review of the literature. *Eur J Gastroenterol Hepatol* 2001;13:437–440.
41. Amarapurkar DN, Chopra KB, Phadke AY, et al. Tubercular abscess of the liver associated with HIV infection. *Indian J Gastroenterol* 1995;14:21–22.
42. Kubota H, Ageta M, Kubo H, et al. tuberculosis liver abscess treated by percutaneous infusion of antituberculous agents. *Intern Med* 1994;33:351–356.
43. Essop AR, Moosa MR, Segal I, et al. Primary tuberculosis of the liver—a case report. *Tubercle* 1983;64:291–293.
44. Bristowe JS. On the connection between abscess of the liver, and gastrointestinal ulceration. *Trans Pathol Soc* 1858;9:241.
45. Chien RN, Lin PY, Liaw YF. Hepatic tuberculosis: comparison of military and local form. *Infection* 1995;23:5–8.
46. Gallinger S, Strasberg SM, Marcus HI, et al. Local hepatic tuberculosis, the cause of a painful hepatic mass: case report and review of the literature. *Can J Surg* 1986;29:451–452.
47. Ruttenberg D, Graham S, Burns D, et al. Abdominal tuberculosis—a cause of portal vein thrombosis and portal hypertension. *Dig Dis Sci* 1991;36:112–115.
48. Sherlock S. The liver in infections. In: Sherlock S, ed. *Diseases of the liver and biliary system*, 7th ed. Oxford: Blackwell Science, 1985:460–461.
49. Wang CT. Hepatobiliary tuberculosis. *Chin J Tuberc Respir Dis* 1991;14:40–41.
50. Ben RJ, Young T, Lee HS. Hepatobiliary tuberculosis presenting as a gall bladder tumor. *Scand J Infect Dis* 1995;27:415–417.
51. Harrington PT, Gutierrez JJ, Ramirez-Ronda CH, et al. Granulomatous hepatitis. *Rev Infect Dis* 1982;4:638–655.
52. Sartin JS, Walker RC. Granulomatous hepatitis: a retrospective review of 88 cases at the Mayo Clinic. *Mayo Clin Proc* 1991;66:914–918.
53. Sabharwal BD, Malhotra N, Garg R, et al. Granulomatous hepatitis: a retrospective study. *Indian J Pathol Microbiol* 1995;38:413–416.
54. Sherlock S. Hepatic granulomas. In: Sherlock W, ed. *Diseases of

the liver and biliary system, 5th ed. Oxford: Blackwell Science, 1975:598–606.

55. Johnson LN, Iser O, Knodell RG. Caseating hepatic granulomas in Hodgkin's lymphoma. *Gastroenterology* 1990;99:1837–1840.

56. Gupta S, Meena HS, Chopra R. Hepatic involvement in tuberculosis. *J Assoc Phys India* 1993;41:20–22.

57. Jones JM, Peck WM. Incidence of fatty liver in tuberculosis with special reference to tuberculous enteritis. *Arch Intern Med* 1994; 74:371–374.

58. Ullom JT. The liver in tuberculosis. *Am J Med Sci* 1909;137: 694–699.

58. Louie E, Rice LB, Holzman RS. Tuberculosis in non-Haitian patients with acquired immunodeficiency syndrome. *Chest* 1986; 90:542–545.

60. Das P, Shukla HS. Clinical diagnosis of abdominal tuberculosis. *Br J Surg* 1976;63:941–946.

61. Abdel-Dayem HM, Naddaf S, Aziz M, et al. Sites of tuberculous involvement in patients with AIDS. Autopsy findings and evaluation of gallium imaging. *Clin Nucl Med* 1997;22: 310–314.

62. Prego V, Glatt AE, Roy V, et al. Comparative yield of blood culture for fungi and mycobacteria, liver biopsy, and bone marrow biopsy in the diagnosis of fever of undetermined origin in human immunodeficiency virus-infected patients. *Arch Intern Med* 1990;150:333–336.

63. Orenstein MS, Tavitian A, Yonk B, et al. Granulomatous involvement of the liver in patients with AIDS. *Gut* 1985;26:1220–1225.

64. Comer GM, Mukherjee S, Scholes JV, et al. Liver biopsies in the acquired immune deficiency syndrome: Influence of endemic disease and drug abuse. *Am J Gastroenterol* 1989;84: 1525–1531.

65. Gordon SC, Reddy KR, Gould EE, et al. The spectrum of liver disease in the acquired immunodeficiency syndrome. *J Hepatol* 1986;2:475–484.

66. Farhi DC, Mason UG, Horsburgh CR. Pathologic findings in disseminated *Mycobacterium avium-intracellulare* infection. A report of 11 cases. *Am J Clin Pathol* 1986;85:67–72.

67. Pottipati AR, Dave PB, Gumaste V, et al. Tuberculous abscess in acquired immunodeficiency syndrome. *J Clin Gastroenterol* 1992;14:72–77.

68. Capell MS. Hepatobiliary manifestations of the acquired immune deficiency syndrome. *Am J Gastroenterol* 1991;86:1–15.

69. Higgins R, Kusne S, Reyes J, et al. Mycobacterium infection after liver transplantation. Presented at the XIII International Congress of the Transplant Society, San Francisco, CA, August 19–24, 1990(abst).

70. Salizzoni P, Tiruviuamala P, Reichman LB. Liver transplantation: an unheralded probable risk for tuberculosis. *Tuber Lung Dis* 1992;73:232–238.

71. Severe isoniazid-associated hepatitis. *MMWR* 1993;42:545–547.

72. Diaz ML, Herrera T, Lopez-Vidal Y, et al. Polymerase chain reaction for the detection of Mycobacterium tuberculosis DNA in tissue and assessment of its utility in the diagnosis of hepatic granulomas. *J Lab Clin Med* 1996;127:359–363.

73. Small PM, Fujiwara PI. Management of tuberculosis in the United States. *N Engl J Med* 2001; 345:189–200.

74. Havlir DV, Barnes PF. Tuberculosis in patients with human immunodeficiency virus infection. *N Engl J Med* 340;5:367–373.

TUBERCULOSIS OF THE GENITOURINARY TRACT

DAVID S. GOLDFARB
LISA SAIMAN

TUBERCULOSIS OF THE KIDNEY, URETERS, AND BLADDER

Epidemiology

Tuberculosis (TB) of the kidney is usually a disease of young to middle-age people, involving men more than women at nearly a 2:1 ratio (1–3). It rarely occurs in children. The true incidence and prevalence of genitourinary TB are difficult to estimate because many patients remain asymptomatic with respect to the genitourinary tract because the disease is often not looked for in these asymptomatic patients and because urine can become sterilized relatively rapidly after institution of chemotherapy.

As the incidence of TB in the developed world decreased during the 1950s, 1960s, and 1970s, there was a parallel decrease in the incidence of genitourinary TB. In the United States, there was a steady decline in the number of cases reported (776 in 1977, 476 in 1986, 227 in 2000) (4,5). A large European urology department reported that 4.0% of all patients seen in the department between 1935 and 1958 had genitourinary TB, with the percentage steadily declining to 0.6% between 1981 and 1986 (6).

Most data suggest that not only is the absolute number of cases of genitourinary TB decreasing but that the incidence of genitourinary disease, in relation to the number of TB cases and compared with other causes of extrapulmonary disease, has been decreasing. According to the Centers for Disease Control and Prevention data, the proportion of all patients with extrapulmonary TB who had genitourinary disease decreased from 17.9% in 1977 to 11.9% in 1986 and to 7% in 2000 (4,5). When expressed as a percentage of all TB cases, the proportion with genitourinary disease decreased slightly from 2.5% to 2.0%. Conversely, in one German autopsy study, the proportion with renal TB, including miliary disease, among all TB cases was constant: 23.2% between 1928 and 1949 and 24.0% between 1976 and 1989 (7). Although autopsy data may not accurately reflect the clinical situation, the German study reported that the proportion of patients with genital disease (male or female) decreased from 11% in the earlier period to 3.9% in the later one. Data from Great Britain also clearly show the decline in genitourinary disease: 472 cases reported in 1980 and 204 reported in 1987, 7.1% and 5.1%, respectively, of the number of pulmonary cases reported in those years (3).

Although the incidence of pulmonary TB rebounded in the 1990s owing to the acquired immunodeficiency syndrome (AIDS) epidemic, adverse socioeconomic conditions, and the spread of drug-resistant organisms, there is some scanty evidence that the incidence of genitourinary disease is also increasing. This is especially true among patients coinfected with human immunodeficiency virus (HIV). At King's County Hospital in New York City, the proportion of patients with TB at any site who had concomitant genitourinary disease was 37% among AIDS patients and 25% among non–HIV-infected patients ($p < 0.02$) (8). These patients had more involvement of the kidney, bladder, and male genitalia specifically. Similarly, in Atlanta, GA, 24 of 1,282 patients diagnosed with TB from 1991 to 1997 had positive urine cultures for *Mycobacterium tuberculosis* (9). Of these 24 patients, 16 were coinfected with HIV. However, there were no differences in clinical presentations or mortality rates when HIV-infected patients were compared with HIV-negative patients.

In Canada, there was a 25% reduction in the incidence of genitourinary TB in the period 1991 to 1995 compared with 1986 to 1990. An interesting speculation attributed this decline to the antimycobacterial activity of quinolones, which were used progressively over these

D. S. Goldfarb: Department of Medicine, New York University School of Medicine; Nephrology Section, New York Harbor Department of Veterans Affairs Medical Center, New York, New York.
L. Saiman: Department of Pediatrics, Columbia University College of Physicians and Surgeons; Department of Pediatrics, New York Presbyterian Medical Center, New York, New York.

periods for the treatment of bacterial urinary tract infections (10).

The overall proportion of U.S.-born AIDS patients with presumptive extrapulmonary TB rose from 2.8% in 1988 to 4.0% in 1991 in New York City (11). These data are not site specific and therefore do not include estimates of the proportion with genitourinary disease. In Tennessee, where the number of AIDS patients is relatively small, the proportion of all TB cases with extrapulmonary disease remained the same, although the incidence of genitourinary disease decreased significantly from 1977 to 1986 (12). In Great Britain, for another example, rates of extrapulmonary disease remained constant during the 1980s, whereas that of genitourinary disease decreased continually (3). Therefore, one cannot extrapolate from statistics on extrapulmonary disease to estimate trends in the incidence of genitourinary disease. In addition, differences in susceptibility of different extrapulmonary sites to TB by age, race or ethnicity, gender, and country of origin are seen in the Centers for Disease Control and Prevention data (13). Genitourinary disease was less common in blacks than in non-Hispanic whites and more common in foreign-born and female patients.

Pathogenesis and Pathology

The usual pathogen of urinary tract TB is *M. tuberculosis*, but other nontuberculous mycobacteria can infect the genitourinary tract as well. *Mycobacterium bovis* was once an important organism, but since the advent of pasteurization of milk, this is now unusual, even in England and Scotland where this organism has always been more prevalent (14). As late as 1987, *M. bovis* accounted for 1% of all TB cases in Southeast England, with genitourinary involvement second to pulmonary involvement (15). There are occasional case reports of renal infection with *Mycobacterium kansasii* (16) and *Mycobacterium avium-intracellulare complex* (17), particularly in patients with immunologic deficiencies. The latter complex might be expected to be isolated with greater frequency from the urine because *M. avium-intracellulare complex* is commonly isolated from the blood of patients with advanced HIV infection (18).

We are not aware of any reports in the literature documenting the clinical significance or pathology of *M. avium-intracellulare complex* in the genitourinary tract of HIV-infected patients. Yet, as expected, it is often cultured from the urine of patients with disseminated infection. One report found that in patients with disseminated *M. avium-intracellulare complex* infection, the yield of positive urine cultures for the organism was 43% (12 of 28 patients) (18). Of 40 patients with renal tissue obtained at autopsy, 22 (55%) had positive culture results. However, the clinical effects of infection of the urinary tract were not documented. The paucity of reports on infection with *M. avium-intracellulare complex* at this site might suggest that

the poorly formed granulomas typical of the immune response of HIV-infected patients to this organism (19) are associated with a lesser degree of renal destruction or that short life expectancies limit the manifestations of the disease.

Renal TB is always the result of hematogenous spread of the organism from the lungs. This may occur at the time of the primary pulmonary infection or at the time of secondary infection (reactivation) in the lungs. With 20% of the cardiac output and the resultant high cortical oxygen tension, the kidney is a favored site for deposition and reproduction of the bacillus. Initial infection occurs in the capillaries of the renal cortex. At this stage, there may be multiple tubercles throughout the kidneys. If in the course of primary infection, cell-mediated immunity develops and the proliferation of the organism is halted by competent macrophages, as demonstrated by granuloma formation, fibrous scars can form and harbor dormant bacilli for as long as 40 years. With reactivation caused by diabetes mellitus, corticosteroid administration, old age, and other forms of immunosuppression, these foci may begin once more to proliferate. From cases in which the primary infection was clinically apparent, it is known that the clinical appearance of renal disease can occur as much as 10 to 25 years later (1,3).

As the process of granuloma formation and necrosis progresses, the organisms are shed into the lumens of the tubules and thereby spread into the deeper regions of the medulla. Here, hypertonicity may impair macrophage function and allow the continued destructive proliferation of the organism (20). Multiple microscopic foci coalesce to form larger areas of caseating necrosis or cavitary disease. Progression to macroscopic lesions soon involves the renal papillae, causing them to slough as well and produce debris capable of causing caliceal and occasionally ureteral obstruction. Bacilli appear in the urine, and "sterile" pyuria is evident. The calices become ulcerated and deformed by both mass lesions and fibrotic scarring. Even with treatment, continued fibrous scarring leads to further distortion of the collecting system architecture. Stenosis and stretching of the calices owing to this deformation lead to many of the radiographic manifestations (discussed later). An important feature of the disease in the kidney is calcification, seen with both progressive necrosis and healing of lesions. These calcifications are plainly seen on radiographs and can be quite extensive (see discussion of radiographic manifestations) (21–23). When ureteral obstruction and hydronephrosis occur, the renal parenchyma can be reduced to a thin shell surrounding a large, heavily calcified caseous mass filling the dilated pelvis and calices ("pyonephrosis" or "putty kidney") (24). A total loss of function, called *autonephrectomy*, is often the result.

The advent of bacilluria leads to distribution of the organism to the ureters and bladder. The ureteral mucosa may become ulcerated, thickened, and noncontractile owing to fibrosis of the wall (24), with resultant pelvic–ureteral junction obstruction, vesicoureteral reflux, and hydronephrosis. A similar process affects the urinary bladder, leading to contraction and fibrosis of the wall, sometimes with calcification. Cystoscopy may demonstrate patchy cystitis, bullous granulations near the ureteral orifices, and, rarely, tuberculous ulcerations. Portions of the genital tract may become involved by exposure to the urine or, more frequently, by local hematogenous or lymphatic spread of the organism (see later).

The treatment of bladder neoplasia with bacille Calmette–Guérin instillation is sometimes complicated by a more severe cystitis than desired, and systemic dissemination is possible. Cases of ureteral obstruction have also been described (25).

Case Report

The patient was first seen in 1972 with dysuria at the age of 68. Intravenous pyelography (IVP) disclosed decreased function of the left kidney and a possible bladder mass. Urinalysis was notable for 30 to 40 leukocytes per high-power field with occasional red blood cells. A chest radiograph appeared normal. Cystoscopy was performed, and a biopsy specimen demonstrated granulomatous, highly vascular tissue diffusely infiltrated with lymphocytes, neutrophils, and plasma cells. There was no evidence of malignancy, and the diagnosis was chronic cystitis. Multiple acid-fast bacillus (AFB) smears of the urine were negative, as were two urine cultures for AFBs. There was no record of a purified protein derivative (PPD) test being performed. The patient had no history of TB.

The patient eventually developed low-volume urinary frequency and nocturia, voiding every 30 minutes. At age 74, he developed anorexia and was found to have severe azotemia: blood urea nitrogen, 160 mg/dL; creatinine, 4.4 mg/dL, potassium, 6.0 mEq/L. He was normotensive. Urinalysis demonstrated 2+ protein and five to ten leukocytes per high-power field. IVP showed no demonstrable flow to the left kidney with no visualization, consistent with autonephrectomy. There was good flow to the right kidney. Reflux from the bladder into the left ureter was noted. There was mild hydronephrosis with ureterovesical obstruction of the right kidney. The chest radiograph results were again negative. Another bladder biopsy was performed, and the specimen demonstrated marked polymorphonuclear infiltrate and lymphoplasmacytic infiltrate and hemorrhage in the mucosa, lamina propria, and muscularis. AFB stains were positive in the focally necrotic areas, and nonnecrotizing granulomas were seen in the lamina propria. Urine AFB smears and cultures were positive at that time. The patient began treatment with isoniazid, rifampin, and ethambutol and underwent sigmoid cystoplasty with implantation of the right ureter into the sigmoid loop. One month later, he had significantly improved renal function: blood urea nitro-

gen, 34 mg/dL; creatinine, 1.5 mg/dL. Urine AFB cultures became negative within several months. He had gradual improvement in urinary frequency, but in the next year, urinary incontinence developed. Cystoscopy showed further bladder shrinkage. Retrograde pyelography was performed and demonstrated no obstruction of the right kidney (Fig. 36.1). Serum bicarbonate concentration was 14 to 21 mEq/L and chloride was 110 to 118 mEq/L, with a urine pH of 6 to 7, consistent with renal tubular acidosis associated with ureterosigmoidostomy. Chemotherapy was continued for 2 years. The patient had some decline in renal function over the ensuing years and died at age 86 of com-

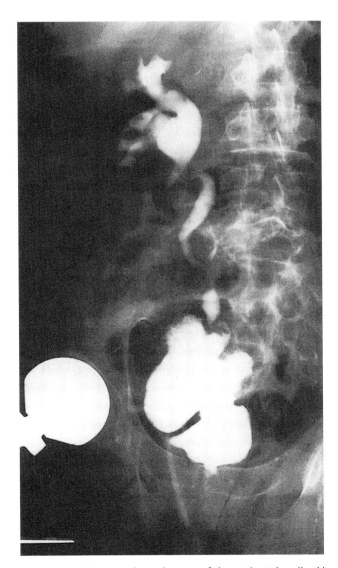

FIGURE 36.1. Retrograde pyelogram of the patient described in the text. The right collecting system is visualized owing to reflux up a dilated, somewhat tortuous ureter and dilated pelvis. The collecting system empties into a loop of colon augmenting a contracted native bladder after sigmoid cystoplasty. The calices have normal architecture. The patient had a prosthetic hip, unrelated to tuberculosis.

plications from congestive heart failure. His creatinine concentration at that time was 3.2 mg/dL.

This case report illustrates a number of important points. Despite a very suggestive biopsy specimen, albeit with negative urine cultures, and a history of bladder involvement highly suspicious for TB, the diagnosis was not made for 6 years. Severe renal involvement was present for some time before the diagnosis was finally made.

Clinical Presentations

Many patients with renal TB remain asymptomatic, and early in the course often have no radiographic signs. As described already, when renal TB is suspected owing to an incidental finding of sterile pyuria, extensive spread and necrosis may already have occurred before the disease is discovered. This is particularly true of miliary TB, which occurs with massive hematogenous spread from pulmonary TB. The clinical presentation is then dominated by the patient's grave systemic illness. Despite numerous granulomas in the kidney, there may be no specific manifestations of renal infection (1).

Series reporting symptoms of genitourinary TB yielded varied results depending on the method of case finding. Summaries of urologic experience stress the high incidence (as high as 70%) (1) of urologic complaints including dysuria, flank pain, and hematuria. Back or flank pain is not common and can reflect caliceal or ureteral obstruction. Other symptoms include nocturia, urinary frequency, and urgency. Such symptoms may be partly attributable to defects of urinary concentration. Often, as in the patient described here, they reflect bladder involvement, with resultant diminished bladder capacity and inability to empty completely. These symptoms may also represent, and must be distinguished from, bacterial cystitis or upper urinary tract infection, which frequently complicates genitourinary TB (26). Failure of antibacterial antibiotics to resolve pyuria and lower tract symptoms should lead to consideration of tuberculous urinary tract infection.

In contrast, surveys for urinary TB in patients with pulmonary disease have found patients in earlier stages of infection and therefore asymptomatic with respect to the genitourinary tract. In one series of 328 inpatients with pulmonary TB, 10% had positive urine cultures for *M. tuberculosis*, and two-thirds of those occurred in patients with no clinical features of urinary tract disease (27). One study of HIV-infected patients with extrapulmonary TB was typical in that the patients' presenting symptoms rarely reflected genitourinary involvement (8). Instead, they presented frequently with lymphadenopathy, respiratory symptoms, or constitutional symptoms such as fever, night sweats, and weight loss. Such constitutional symptoms are less common with genitourinary TB (14%) than with pulmonary TB and less common than presentation with no symptoms at all (20%) (1). Findings on physical examination are almost always lacking.

Hypertension has long been thought to be a manifestation of renal TB, with some reports claiming cure of hypertension after unilateral nephrectomy (28,29). However, these studies estimated the incidence of hypertension from renal TB to be 5% to 10% but did not control adequately for the relatively high incidence of hypertension in the general population. The etiologic association is therefore in doubt (30) but may be somewhat stronger for those with unilateral nonfunctioning kidneys (29).

Often reactivation of the renal lesions occurs when little evidence of active pulmonary disease is still present, reflecting the long dormancy of the organism. Most studies find that the minority (≤40%) of patients has active pulmonary TB, although a majority (≥60%) does have abnormal-appearing chest radiographs usually suggestive of inactive pulmonary disease (1,2). Similarly, only a minority (<30%) has any history of diagnosed TB (1,6).

Despite widespread dissemination of the organism, severe renal involvement is often asymmetric and therefore renal failure is uncommon. The incidence of azotemia (blood urea nitrogen >25 mg/dL) with urinary tract TB is 5% to 12% (1,2,31). TB accounted for 0.65% of end-stage renal disease diagnoses in Europe and only 0.004% of renal failure diagnoses in the United States (32). As in the patient described here, the potential for more severe renal insufficiency arises especially when bilateral vesicoureteral reflux occurs or when ureteral involvement leads to hydronephrosis. In patients with severe disease, progressive renal insufficiency can also result from destruction of glomeruli, segmental obstruction of calices, and necrosis of the medullary interstitium and tubules. A more chronic form of tuberculous tubulointerstitial nephritis associated with progressive renal insufficiency has also been described (33).

Abnormalities of the urinary sediment are seen in more than 90% of patients. In descending order of frequency, these include pyuria, pyuria with hematuria, and hematuria alone (1). Investigators stress that the diagnosis of TB may be delayed because a significant number of patients has positive bacterial cultures that presumably represent superinfection of an anatomically distorted urinary tract. Persistence of pyuria after appropriate antibiotic therapy should lead to an evaluation for genitourinary TB (2). Rarely, long-standing disease may cause amyloidosis and present with proteinuria or the nephrotic syndrome. Mild proteinuria (<1 g per 24 hours) may be seen in as many as 50% of patients, whereas approximately 15% excrete more than 1 g of protein per 24 hours (31). Anemia is seen in less than 20% of patients with nonmiliary disease.

Besides the variable loss of glomerular filtration, abnormalities in renal tubular functions are commonly observed. These include urinary concentrating defects (in as many as 84% of patients) (31) owing to destruction of the terminal collecting ducts and distortion of the medullary architecture. Few patients have polyuria and nephrogenic diabetes insipidus. Renal tubular acidosis occurs as well, although its frequency has not been ascertained. Although there are no reports of hyperkalemia associated with TB, it should be expected because hyporeninemic hypoaldosteronism is a common manifestation of various tubulointerstitial diseases, including obstructive uropathy (34). Hyperkalemia and hyperchloremic metabolic acidosis may also suggest glucocorticoid or mineralocorticoid deficiency, which can be manifestations of adrenal destruction by TB.

Radiographic Findings

Several radiology textbooks offer excellent compilations of the varied radiographic manifestations of urinary tract TB (21–23). Most literature contains descriptions of the abnormalities present on IVP, with the relative scarcity of reports and reviews of more modern techniques [sonography, computed tomography (CT), and magnetic resonance imaging], reflecting the declining incidence of genitourinary disease in the years in which those techniques were popularized. Most authorities have considered IVP to be the radiographic procedure of choice, giving unrivaled views of the collecting system, particularly with early and minor papillary and urothelial changes. Improvements in the resolution of sonographic equipment may allow detection of smaller focal lesions that previously were missed (35). CT is particularly useful for visualization of these focal lesions, nonfunctioning segments of the urinary tract, and perirenal or abdominal masses (tuberculomas) (36). Helical or spiral CT scanning continues to improve and has probably replaced IVP as the procedure of choice, although administration of nephrotoxic radiocontrast is still required (37). CT particularly excels at demonstrating caliceal involvement, cortical thinning, parenchymal abscesses, and the involvement of other organs and the retroperitoneum (23). Magnetic resonance imaging does not appear to offer specific benefits in the imaging of urinary tract TB. Angiography is rarely used, although it is occasionally helpful in distinguishing a tuberculoma or focal obstruction from a more vascularized neoplasm (3,23,38). The utility of gallium scanning to detect genitourinary TB is unproved. In one study, the test demonstrated 83% sensitivity in detecting TB at other extrapulmonary sites but missed the one case of proved renal TB (by urine culture) (39).

In the early stages of the disease, or with miliary disease, most radiographic evaluations are unrevealing. With more advanced disease, IVP may demonstrate a variety of distortions of the collecting system from the calices to the bladder (23,40). These include cortical fibrosis leading to distortion, stretching, dilation (caliectasis), and occlusion of the calices and renal pelvis; obstruction at any level of the urinary tract; cavitation in the renal parenchyma, with parenchymal and papillary necrosis leading to filling defects; and masses (tuberculoma) at any level that must sometimes be distinguished from neoplasia. In as many as 50% of patients, plain films demonstrate calcifications that

may be focal or diffuse, lobar, or reniform involving the entire kidney in the case of autonephrectomy (40) (Figs. 36.2 through 36.4). In some patients, these will be indistinguishable from renal stones without further evaluation. Nonfunction is manifested by the absence of a nephrogram in the renal phase of IVP. Autonephrectomy is particularly well visualized by CT (Fig. 36.5), demonstrating the kidney to be a sac of caseous material usually surrounded by a calcified rim. Occasionally, a small, fibrotic kidney is seen instead (22).

Ureteral involvement may include strictures, with or without obstruction; "corkscrewing" or "beading" owing to alternating constrictions and dilations; pipestem formation (rigid, fibrotic, straight); ulcerations; hydroureter; and, rarely, calcification (41,42). Bladder involvement is detected by luminal irregularities caused by ulceration and filling defects caused by granulomas. More frequently, bladder disease is manifested by thickened, fibrotic walls

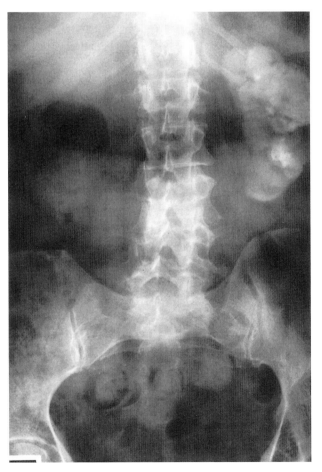

FIGURE 36.2. Plain film of the abdomen (without intravenous administration of contrast material) demonstrates a left "putty kidney": a large mass of caseous material, demonstrating diffuse and focal areas of calcification. Administration of contrast material demonstrated its complete lack of function. Also seen is fusion of the left hip owing to old tuberculous arthritis.

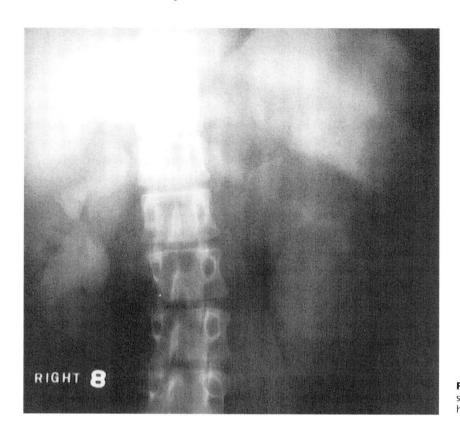

FIGURE 36.3. A nephrotomogram demonstrates a rim of calcification around a left hydronephrotic, nonfunctioning kidney.

leading to a markedly diminished capacity. In the developing world, bladder calcification may simulate schistosomiasis. Retrograde pyelography, as performed in the patient described here (Fig. 36.1), may be helpful in delineating ureteral involvement in the patient with a poorly functioning kidney.

Diagnosis

Unexplained urinary symptoms or persistent pyuria in patients with any history of TB or radiographs suggesting active or inactive disease should lead to an evaluation for genitourinary TB. All patient series have demonstrated the high rate (80% to 90%) of positive urinary cultures in patients with TB of the urinary tract. This test remains the mainstay of diagnosis, although cultures may require several weeks to become positive. Three to five first morning urine specimens should be cultured to give the highest yields (43). Acid-fast stains of the urine should be performed but are less reliable. In one study, only 50% of urine specimens demonstrating positivity on cultures for any mycobacteria showed positivity on AFB smears (44). This is in part owing to false-negative findings arising from the scant amount of bacilli in the urine in some patients. False-positive AFB smears may result from colonization of the external genitalia by nonpathogenic mycobacteria. This problem can be minimized by prompt culturing of specimens, as opposed to the older practice of concentrating 24-hour specimens,

which may have allowed proliferation of skin contaminants (43,44). The superiority of this technique is demonstrated by the study cited above in which all but one of 23 patients with positive smears or cultures were judged to have clinically established urinary tract disease (44).

However, cultures from the urine require weeks to grow and may be negative. Polymerase chain reaction (PCR) has been used in efforts to obtain an earlier diagnosis of TB of the genitourinary tract. In an Indian study, 42 patients with suspected genitourinary TB underwent several diagnostic evaluations including urinary PCR for *M. tuberculosis* (45). Urinary PCR was positive in 81% of cases, urine cultures were positive in 31%, bladder biopsy was positive in 46%, and 88% of IVP was suggestive but not diagnostic. Similarly, authors in Egypt demonstrated the potential utility of PCR in rapidly diagnosing TB of the genitourinary tract (46). As many as 10% of patients may have inhibitory substances in the urine interfering with detection, and spot samples are less reliable than 24-hour collections (47).

Urine cultures will be positive in only 25% of patients with miliary disease, some of whom will have a normal urinary sediment (1). In those with active pulmonary disease, the high rates of culture-positive or smear-positive sputum will, of course, be helpful in making the diagnosis if the urine study results are negative. In addition, more than 90% of patients with urinary tract TB will have a positive PPD test response, assuming that anergy is not present (1,6). Among all AIDS patients with TB at any site who

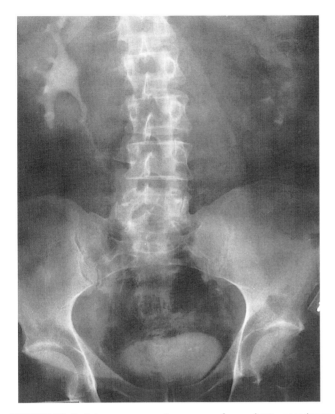

FIGURE 36.4. Intravenous pyelogram performed 10 years later in the same patient examined in Fig. 36.3. The hydronephrosis has resolved, and the left nonfunctioning kidney now contains diffuse calcification. Curvilinear calcifications outline several tuberculomas. The right side shows a normal collecting system except for the most inferior calix, which shows slight distortion associated with a loss of the normal rounded contour of the inferior pole. This suggests focal scarring by tuberculosis. The right kidney is slightly large because of compensatory hypertrophy.

had a urine culture for AFB performed, there was a positive result in 77% (8); only 24% of these HIV-infected patients had a positive PPD test response.

Except for the few examples just cited of urinary tract infection with nontuberculous mycobacteria, positive cultures for organisms other than *M. tuberculosis* and rarely *M. bovis* represent nonpathogens, either skin contaminants or colonizers of the urethra. Examples include *Mycobacterium xenopi*, *Mycobacterium fortuitum*, and *Mycobacterium smegmatis*. In one report of 572 positive urine cultures for nontuberculous mycobacteria, only six appeared to be clinically important (48). Criteria suggested to select clinically important disease caused by nontuberculous mycobacteria are (a) symptoms of chronic or recurrent genitourinary infection, (b) endoscopic or radiographic evidence of genitourinary disease, (c) abnormal urinary sediment, (d) absence of other urinary pathogens, (e) repeated isolation of the same organism, and (f) histologic evidence of granulomatous disease, particularly in the presence of AFBs (49). The first four criteria raise the possibility, the fifth raises the probability, and the sixth may be considered diagnostic. These potentially useful criteria have not been tested prospectively.

Because urine cultures may take several weeks to give positive results and may remain negative for as many as 10% of patients and because urine AFB smears are unreliable as well, other more invasive techniques have been advocated. In eight patients with suspected renal TB who had at least five negative AFB smears and negative cultures, with radiographic abnormalities demonstrated by CT or sonography, cytodiagnosis was accomplished by fine needle aspiration under ultrasound guidance (50). In seven patients, the material demonstrated Langhans giant histiocytes,

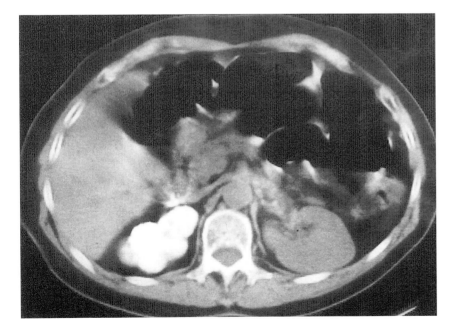

FIGURE 36.5. Computed tomography of the abdomen without intravenous contrast material demonstrates a small, densely calcified right kidney, typical of autonephrectomy. The left kidney is normal. The left kidney of the patient described in the text would have had a similar appearance on computed tomography.

caseous debris, and epithelioid histiocyte aggregates. In all eight patients, positive cultures were obtained. In another series using a similar technique, 19 patients with sonographic abnormalities were studied. Fifteen of these, including six with negative urinary AFB cultures, had a positive result by aspiration cytology (51).

Treatment

Medical Therapy

Two trends in the treatment of urinary tract TB have been evident in the past 30 years: shorter courses using multiple-drug therapy and fewer indications for surgery, particularly for nephrectomy. The general recommendations of the American Thoracic Society, the World Health Organization, and the Centers for Disease Control and Prevention regarding the treatment of genitourinary TB have been that extrapulmonary disease does not require a different or more prolonged course of therapy than does pulmonary disease (52–54). The details of the principles and recommendations regarding therapy are described in Chapter 47. Care should be taken with drugs, such as aminoglycosides and ethambutol, which are eliminated by the kidneys in patients with renal insufficiency or taking cyclosporine.

Recommendations regarding initial therapy and duration of treatment may change as the incidence of drug-resistant infections increases. There have been no significant changes in the recommended treatment of genitourinary TB specifically in recent years. It is important to note that none of the summaries of treatment recommendations for TB (53) or nontuberculous mycobacteria (55) makes explicit reference to the treatment of the kidney and genitals, instead combining them with other causes of extrapulmonary disease. This appears to be a reasonable practice because most evaluations of treatment with chemotherapy support the use of relatively short courses of therapy (≤1 year) compared with the longer courses routinely recommended years ago (1,3,53,54). Other authors suggest that the possibility of covert prostatic infection, which is more difficult to eradicate, might be appropriately dealt with by treating all patients with renal TB for as long as 2 years (20). No data exist to support this point of view, and most estimates of the incidence of prostatic infection are low enough to suggest that this is an unnecessary precaution (56) (see later). Furthermore, longer courses might be associated with patient noncompliance and prolonged risk of the side effects of the drugs. However, adequately controlled, randomized studies specific to genitourinary disease comparing different treatment regimens have not been performed. Such studies would be difficult to complete given the overall satisfactory nature of current chemotherapy and the relatively low current incidence of isolated genitourinary disease. Furthermore, the follow-up periods after trials of short-course therapy may not be adequate to ensure the

eradication of extrapulmonary disease. Vigilance is required to detect failures of therapy in the genitourinary tract. In 174 cases of genitourinary TB diagnosed in Turkey, the relapse rate after 12 months of chemotherapy was 19% (57). The authors suggested that poor nutritional status and challenging social situations may have contributed to the high relapse rate.

Surgical Therapy

Another unresolved but related issue is the role of nephrectomy in the treatment of the nonfunctioning kidney. One prevalent belief is that nephrectomy accomplishes removal of the bulk of caseous material, allowing a much shorter course of therapy (3,58). In part, this belief is based on the finding of viable AFB in kidneys resected after at least 3 months of chemotherapy (58). If one favors longer treatment courses over surgery, 3 months would seem to be an arbitrarily short period of follow-up for judging the adequacy of renal sterilization. In another series, flank sinuses or abscesses developed in three of four patients who did not undergo nephrectomy (29). There are also claims that exploration will occasionally disclose kidneys with obstructive lesions that, when repaired, lead to restoration of some renal function (59). Improved CT visualization of the nonfunctioning kidney may find these rare cases and eliminate the need for exploration.

More recently, the modern technique of laparoscopic nephrectomy makes removal of an affected kidney less onerous with shorter recovery time. The procedure has been done with the same very low rates of complications seen when the procedure is performed for noninfectious indications (60,61). Initial concerns regarding the use of the laparoscopic technique in this setting were that fibrous adhesions and spillage of caseous material would lead to worse outcomes, and conversion to open nephrectomy may be required for some difficult cases (62,63).

Conversely, authors have repeatedly stated that nephrectomy is rarely needed and that a longer course of therapy, as long as 2 years, is sufficient to eradicate the organism from even these massively infected organs, reserving nephrectomy for those with persistent hematuria, pain, or bacterial urinary tract infection, suspected cancer, or rare cases of new hypertension (64–66). Observation for as long as 22 years of 25 patients with nonfunctioning kidneys disclosed no failures of chemotherapy. This approach must take into account the problems of compliance and drug toxicity. To summarize, the need for nephrectomy should be infrequent and then only if there are strong indications for using a shorter course of therapy.

Because postinflammatory scarring with obstruction of the collecting system at any level can occur as treatment proceeds, periodic radiographic imaging has been advocated, perhaps as frequently as every 3 to 4 months until the course is completed (26). The efficacy of such an approach has not been demonstrated in other than an anecdotal fashion, and the incidence of such an effect may be low in the era of multiple-drug chemotherapy, allowing longer intervals between studies (67). (Note that the patient described previously had progressive bladder symptoms continuing through the course of therapy.) IVP has been the traditional examination for this purpose, but ultrasonography might suffice and spare the patient the exposure to contrast agents and radiation. After completion of therapy, imaging can be done at yearly intervals.

The role of surgery in preserving renal function when disease of the collecting system leads to obstructive uropathy is unquestioned. Should evidence of hydrocalix, hydronephrosis, or hydroureter appear, obstruction should be relieved. Usually this would entail procedures such as pyeloplasty, ureteral dilation, and, if the latter fails, ureteral reimplantation. No convincing evidence of the utility of steroids to prevent stricture formation during the course of therapy has been reported (20,68).

Also useful when bladder capacity fails to increase in response to therapy is bladder augmentation with loops of ileum or colon to diminish the symptoms of chronic bladder involvement, as in the patient described previously (69–71). Occasionally, when ureteral stricture is present, ureteral reimplantation into a loop of bowel is necessary. Urinary diversion with ureteral reimplantation into an ileal conduit is rarely required.

TUBERCULOSIS OF THE FEMALE GENITOURINARY TRACT

TB of the female genitourinary tract has been an increasingly rare presentation of TB among women in developed nations (72–74) but has remained an important cause of infertility in the developing world (75–79). Despite an increase in active TB infections and coinfection with HIV, pelvic TB has become rare in the United States as evidenced by the lack of a reported clinical series since the 1970s (1,74). However in an era of frequent immigration and international travel, American health care providers still do encounter women with pelvic TB. Therefore, it is important that clinicians, particularly obstetricians and gynecologists, be familiar with the potential presentations, diagnostic evaluation, treatment, and outcome of TB within the female genital tract.

Epidemiology

Genital TB is most commonly diagnosed in women of childbearing age from developing countries who have never been pregnant (72–74,76,77,79). Pelvic TB can also be diagnosed in older women, as demonstrated by a large Swedish retrospective study performed from 1968 to 1977 in which most patients with pelvic TB were post-

menopausal, suggesting a long latent period before the onset of symptoms (80,81). Throughout the world, most women with pelvic TB have not had a previous diagnosis of pulmonary TB. When there is a history of pulmonary TB, the diagnosis has been made years earlier (72,74). The lung disease may be active or quiescent or have healed without radiographic residua (72,74,76,80).

The incidence of pelvic TB as reported from infertility clinics around the world varies. In developed countries such as Australia and the United States, fewer than 1% of women presenting to infertility clinics are diagnosed with pelvic TB. In the United States, these women are usually foreign born (72,74). In the developing world, approximately 5% to 10% of infertile women are found to have pelvic TB, and in some regions of India, 19% of infertile women have been found to have pelvic TB (77–79). However, it is difficult to establish the true incidence and prevalence of pelvic TB because asymptomatic, latent cases predominate over symptomatic disease. In a 1960s autopsy study of women who died with pulmonary TB in the United States, 8% were found to have unsuspected pelvic disease as determined by careful histologic examination of the fallopian tubes (72). In a study performed in the late 1980s in India, 37 (60%) of 62 women aged 15 to 45 years with active pulmonary TB had evidence of unsuspected pelvic TB on laparoscopy. Of these, 15 (41%) of 37 had fallopian tubercles, including four with coexisting endometrial disease and two with ovarian tubercles (82). The duration of pulmonary symptoms did not correlate with the presence of pelvic TB.

Overall, the incidence of pelvic TB is decreasing throughout the world. Although this decline is not well understood, it is likely that improved diagnosis and treatment of pulmonary TB are responsible. Earlier diagnosis of pulmonary TB and more successful treatment with shorter courses of multidrug regimens may be having a favorable impact on the incidence of pelvic TB.

Pathogenesis

The pathogenesis of TB of the female genitourinary tract is similar to that of other forms of extrapulmonary TB. Most commonly, pelvic TB occurs after hematogenous spread of *M. tuberculosis* from a primary pulmonary site (1,72). Approximately 5% of pelvic TB cases are thought to occur secondary to direct spread from the bladder, rectum, or intestine along the peritoneal surface to the pelvis. Rarely, cervical, vulvar, and vaginal TB may result from direct sexual contact with a partner with TB of the genitourinary tract.

Almost all patients (90% to 100% of patients with pelvic TB) have disease of the fallopian tube, and both tubes are usually involved (72,80,83). The cause of the predilection of *M. tuberculosis* for the fallopian tubes is unknown. The infectious process within the tubes may remain dormant for years and then reactivate years later. From the tubes, secondary spread can cause peritonitis (45% of patients with pelvic TB) or ovarian disease (10% to 30%) or can involve the endometrium (50% to 80%) or less commonly the cervix (<5%) or vagina (<1%).

Pathology

Generally, pelvic TB mimics chronic nontuberculous salpingitis (72,84,85). The tubes become thickened, the fimbriated end of the tubes remains everted, and the orifice remains patent. With time, the tubes become adherent to the surrounding pelvic structures. Macroscopically, the appearance of the fallopian tubes becomes distinctive for TB during later stages when the tubal peritoneum is studded with tubercles. Microscopically, caseating granulomas form within the fallopian tubes. Serial sections of the tubes may be required to detect granulomas (72,83). Hyperplastic and adenomatous mucosa are also very suggestive of TB (73).

Uterine involvement is usually limited to the endometrium rather than the myometrium (83,84). The endometrium may not exhibit tubercles because the monthly sloughing of the endometrium during menstruation does not allow adequate time for tubercles and caseating granulomas to form. Biopsy of the endometrium reveals epithelioid and giant cells, but AFBs are rarely seen.

Ovarian pathology demonstrates periovarian adhesions rather than parenchymal granulomas (73,83). Cervical involvement is generally limited to the endocervical canal. Vulvovaginal lesions typically present as small, shallow ulcers with sinus tracts and scar formation (73,86,87).

Clinical Presentations

Case Report

A 31-year-old Korean-born patient was seen in 1990 in an infertility clinic in the United States with a chief complaint of infertility during a 10-year marriage. She reported dysmenorrhea and scant menstrual bleeding. She had no pelvic pain but had been treated in Korea with five shots of penicillin for a pelvic infection 5 years previously. She did not have a history of pulmonary TB; her mother had TB during this patient's childhood. During her evaluation for infertility, laparoscopy demonstrated bilateral tubal obstruction and hysterosalpingography showed a normal uterine cavity with classic changes of salpingitis isthmica nodosa (SIN). The tubes are only visualized for approximately half their extent. The impression was bilateral SIN (Fig. 36.6). TB remained unsuspected until tuboplasty, when tubercles of the tubes and ovaries were found, multiple adhesions of the bowel to the pelvis were noted, and caseous material was seen throughout the pelvis. Histopathology revealed noncaseating granulomas, but AFB staining was negative. The skin response to PPD

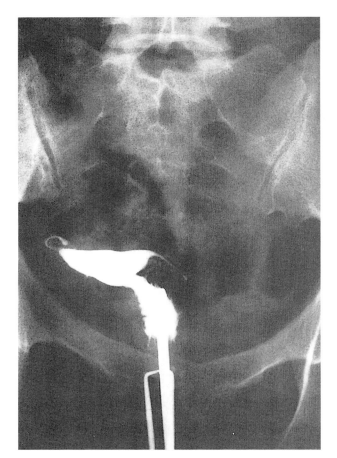

FIGURE 36.6. Hysterosalpingography of the patient described in the text. The uterine cavity is normal. The tubes show the classic changes of salpingitis isthmica nodosa. The tubes are only visualized for approximately half their extent. No spillage is documented.

placed at this time was 20 mm of induration, and the chest radiograph showed left apical pleural thickening without an infiltrate, adenopathy, or a cavity. Urinalysis revealed no leukocytes and IVP appeared normal. She was treated empirically with isoniazid, rifampin, and pyrazinamide and intraoperative cultures of her fallopian tubes grew *M. tuberculosis*. She received treatment for 18 months and remained infertile.

As illustrated by this case report, pelvic TB is most commonly diagnosed during a workup for infertility or during evaluation of abnormal uterine bleeding, pelvic pain, or adnexal masses. Menstrual irregularities occur in as many as 40% of patients and may be minimal in early disease because the endometrium retains its secretory ability. Amenorrhea is present in approximately one-half of patients, usually secondary to endometrial fibrosis or owing to primary ovarian failure caused by active tuberculous involvement. Menorrhagia, metrorrhagia, and postmenopausal bleeding also have been described. Dysmenorrhea or diffuse abdominal discomfort occurs as inflammatory exudate from the tubes enters the pelvis. Patients may appear to have pelvic inflammatory disease unresponsive to antimicrobial therapy. Some patients have had pelvic TB diagnosed during evaluation for weight loss, fatigue, and low-grade fever. However, genital TB may be asymptomatic (74).

Unsuspected pelvic TB has been diagnosed intraoperatively during evaluation for a pelvic mass or during laparotomy for fallopian tube reconstructive surgery, as in the patient described here (80). An ectopic pregnancy may also be the initial clinical presentation. Renal involvement may occur simultaneously with pelvic TB in 10% of women.

Physical Examination

Approximately one-half of patients with pelvic TB have normal findings on physical examinations. The most common finding is uterine or adnexal enlargement, but there are no specific physical findings diagnostic of pelvic TB.

Diagnosis

The diagnosis of pelvic TB usually requires a combination of microbiologic, histologic, and radiographic techniques. Supportive studies such as the PPD test and chest radiographs are also useful. Most patients with pelvic TB have a reactive skin test. Chest radiographs are often normal, although some patients have undiagnosed active pulmonary disease and others have evidence of previous healed TB.

Microbiologic Studies

Cultures of *M. tuberculosis* can be obtained from several sources, including endometrial biopsy specimens, menstrual blood, or, less commonly, peritoneal fluid (74–76). To ensure maximal yield, several specimens of menstrual blood at the time of maximal flow should be collected either via vaginal washings or in a cervical cap. However, if disease is limited to the fallopian tubes, these cultures will be negative.

Histologic Studies

A definitive diagnosis of pelvic TB is most often made histologically. Typically, granulomas are seen on biopsy or curettage of the endometrium immediately before the onset of menses. However, endometrial biopsies may not be suggestive of TB. Infection may be limited to the fallopian tubes in 50% of patients. The endometrium is sloughed monthly with menstruation, and granulomas may not have enough time to form. The specimen obtained by biopsy may be small or blood flow may be scant. Thus, histopathologic examination and culture of serial sections of both fallopian tubes are the most effective means of diagnosing pelvic TB (83).

Radiographic Studies

Radiographic evaluation usually includes hysterosalpingography with water-soluble contrast material and chest radiographs (73,88). Hysterosalpingography typically appears abnormal in patients with pelvic TB and may exhibit the following features: multiple constrictions of the fallopian tubes, obstruction of the fallopian tube in the zone of transition between the isthmus and the ampulla, endometrial adhesions, distortion or even frank obliteration of the uterine cavity, and, less commonly, irregular calcifications in the adnexal area or calcified lymph nodes. Occasionally, there may be vascular or lymphatic intravasation of contrast material (88).

Hysterosalpingography may also show nonspecific changes such as SIN, as demonstrated in the patient described earlier (89). SIN is a radiographic term that refers to nodular outpouchings, diverticula, and inflammation. SIN does not identify an etiology for the inflammation but can occur with bacterial infection and tuberculous involvement of the fallopian tubes. A very high incidence of infertility and ectopic pregnancy occurs in patients with SIN.

There has been some concern voiced in the literature that hysterosalpingography should not be performed for evaluation of pelvic TB because of the risk of disseminating *M. tuberculosis* into the abdominal cavity. However, most series do not demonstrate adverse events after this radiographic procedure (73,74).

There has also been some recent interest in the use of ultrasonography for evaluation of pelvic TB (35), but there have been no comparative studies of hysterosalpingography and ultrasonography. Thus, although most women diagnosed with pelvic TB have had abnormal-appearing hysterosalpingography, confirmatory histopathologic or microbiologic studies should still be performed. Any woman with pelvic TB should also be studied for renal involvement.

Treatment

Medical

In general, treatment of pelvic TB is derived from treatment regimens for pulmonary disease, and there seems to be an excellent response to antimicrobial agents (74,76,90). Although most of the reports in the literature predate the use of pyrazinamide, a few published series used short-course regimens. A successful 6-month, four-drug regimen including rifampin, isoniazid, pyrazinamide, and ethambutol was used in 34 women in South Africa (76). In India, 14 women with endometrial TB were successfully treated with isoniazid and rifampin for 9 months; repeat endometrial cultures were negative after 3 months of treatment (79). However, the patients in both studies were followed for only 3 to 6 months after therapy was complete. A short duration of follow-up may be inadequate to document relapse. No published reports have described management of infection caused by multidrug-resistant organisms.

Surgery

Surgery, particularly radical excision of the uterus, tubes, and ovaries, may be required if microbiologic cure cannot be obtained. This may occur if large adnexal masses or tuboovarian abscesses are present. Surgical interventions may be indicated for chronic pelvic pain, recurrent disease after medical management, pelvic TB in a postmenopausal woman, and persistent fistulous tracts. These recommendations predate multidrug therapeutic regimens but still appear valid. Most experts advise initiating chemotherapy for 2 to 4 weeks before surgery and continuing treatment for at least 6 to 12 months after surgery.

Long-Term Sequelae

Patients treated for pelvic TB achieve microbiologic and clinical cure, but neither medical nor surgical treatment has been shown to improve fertility. Intrauterine pregnancy after pelvic TB is rare, and posttreatment fertility rates with successful pregnancy range from 0% to 10% (72,80,90). Ectopic pregnancies and early miscarriages are common (73,78). If a patient has had prolonged amenorrhea, it is unlikely that normal menses will occur.

Tubal reconstruction is usually ineffective (91). Despite restoring tubal patency, the tubal and endometrial damage resulting from TB usually prevents normal conception and implantation. Thus, it is critical to counsel women with pelvic TB that tuboplasty is most likely fruitless and, when attempted, should be delayed until medical management is complete. *In vitro* fertilization techniques may improve fertility. Frydman et al. (92) reported that six (27%) of 22 women had successful pregnancies after *in vitro* fertilization. Similarly, in South Africa, 13 (38%) of 34 women from 1986 to 1987 achieved intrauterine pregnancies (90).

TUBERCULOSIS OF THE MALE GENITALIA
Epididymis and Testes

TB of the epididymis and testes probably occurs via hematogenous spread of the organism from the lungs. Because most patients with epididymal disease have positive urine cultures, it was thought possible that the genital disease might arise from the urine, necessitating its retrograde passage through the vas deferens. This notion was supported by the autopsy finding that miliary renal disease was associated with an incidence of epididymal disease of 13%, whereas 52% of those with caseous renal disease and 100% of those with cavitary renal disease had epididymal infection (93). However, 11% of those with genital lesions had no renal lesions, suggesting hematogenous spread (3,94).

These findings might be as supportive of hematogenous spread as of urinary tract dissemination. Infection of the testes probably arises often directly from the epididymis. Apparent venereal transmission from or to a woman with pelvic infection has been reported (95,96). The disease is most common between the ages of 20 and 40 years (97). More than 70% of patients have a history of TB, with most having pulmonary infection. The disease has been reported in HIV-positive patients (98,99). Rare cases have been caused by *M. xenopi*, *M. kansasii*, and other nontuberculous organisms (16,17,100,101). As many as 50% of patients also have positive urine cultures, often with no clinical evidence of renal disease. In one study, only 26% of patients with epididymal disease had normal-appearing IVP (102).

Most patients present with scrotal swelling, sometimes with pain, and, less frequently, the appearance of acute epididymitis (6,97). Occasionally, abscess or scrotal sinus formation is also present (97,102). The differential diagnosis includes testicular tumors and bacterial infection. In the past, 34% of patients had bilateral involvement, although this now may be infrequent (3) and both the right and left organs are equally affected. On examination, the epididymis is often rubbery or nodular. Between 50% and 75% of patients have palpable thickening of the vas deferens; rarely, this has a "beaded" consistency and may be associated with secondary hydrocele. Calcification of the vas deferens is occasionally seen on radiographs, and because it often involves the lumen, it has a solid, beaded appearance (21). This may distinguish it from the calcification of the vas deferens seen with diabetes, which involves only the wall and resembles a railroad track. Scrotal sonography may show heterogeneous and hypoechoic swelling of the epididymis and an associated sinus tract or extratesticular calcifications (103).

The diagnosis is often based on the clinical context. Ultimately, however, epididymal biopsy is often necessary. Fine needle aspiration has been successfully used in this setting as well (95). A few patients have positive semen cultures, often with nontuberculous mycobacteria. This may be an important cause of male infertility in affected populations. The disease causes changes in the seminal fluid composition and thereby adversely influences sperm motility and agglutination (104).

Treatment consists of chemotherapy, with epididymectomy or orchiectomy performed less frequently. Surgery is indicated only if there is a lack of clinical response (3,105). Treatment may restore the patency of the epididymis but often leaves behind a thickened, scarred cord. There is no evidence of a significant effect of treatment on semen quality or infertility. Testicular sperm extraction may restore fertility (106).

Prostate

TB of the prostate is now quite unusual: five of 2,599 patients with prostatitis were diagnosed at the Mayo Clinic in a 10-year period (56). Three of the patients had no evidence of renal disease. The disease was common in the prechemotherapy era (94). Most authors believe that the disease occurs from hematogenous dissemination rather than from exposure to the urine (3,94). Patients may present with symptoms of prostatic enlargement such as nocturia, frequency, and dysuria (56,107). Physical examination may demonstrate a minimally abnormal gland with slight enlargement or nodularity (26,56). The diagnosis can be made by transrectal needle biopsy or transurethral resection and has been an incidental finding after prostatic resection for other indications. Radiographic visualization of the prostate demonstrates enlargement of the gland and bilateral low-density lesions (107). Ultrasonography has demonstrated periprostatic fluid collection and urethral fistulas (108). CT allows better visualization of the seminal vesicles (23,42). Sonography can demonstrate dilation of the seminal vesicles as well, but such changes are not clearly pathognomonic for TB (35). Treatment with courses of therapy for as long as 2 years may be necessary (20).

Penis

TB of the penis is extremely unusual, with 139 cases reported as of 1971 (109) and only isolated case reports since then. It was once seen after ritual circumcision (110). It may occur in association with disease elsewhere in the urinary tract (111). Venereal transmission has been reported, including a case in which molecular typing was used to document infection passing from husband to wife, resulting in endometrial TB (112). The lesion appears as a superficial ulcer of the glans and responds well to chemotherapy. Penile infection with *Mycobacterium celatum* has been reported in a patient with HIV infection (113). Infection of the penis with bacille Calmette–Guérin has occurred after intravesical instillation of the organism in the treatment of bladder neoplasia (114).

Urethra

Urethral TB is also quite rare and is usually associated with involvement of other parts of the genitourinary tract. It may present as a chronic discharge or a mass caused by abscess formation or cause strictures and sinus tracts, leading to symptoms of lower tract obstruction (115).

REFERENCES

1. Simon HB, Weinstein AJ, Pasternak MS, et al. Genitourinary tuberculosis. Clinical features in a general hospital population. *Am J Med* 1977;63:410–420.
2. Christensen W. Genitourinary tuberculosis: review of 102 cases. *Medicine* 1974;53:377–390.
3. Gow JG. Genitourinary tuberculosis. In: Walsh PC, Retik AB, Vaughan ED, eds. *Campbell's urology*. Philadelphia: WB Saunders, 1998:807–836.
4. Snider DE. *Tuberculosis statistics: states and cities—1982–1987.* Atlanta: US Department of Human Services/Public Health Service, Centers for Disease Control, 1988;8429:1–82.
5. Centers for Disease Control and Prevention. *Reported tuberculosis in the United States* (http://www.cdc.gov/nchstp/tb/surv/surv2001/default.htm), Atlanta, 2001.
6. Poulios C, Malovrouvas D. Progress in the approach of tuberculosis of the genitourinary tract. *Acta Urol Belg* 1990;58:101–123.
7. Schubert GE, Haltaufderheide T, Golz R. Frequency of urogenital tuberculosis in an unselected autopsy series from 1928 to 1949 and 1976 to 1989. *Eur Urol* 1992;21:216–223.
8. Shafer RW, Kim DS, Weiss JP, et al. Extrapulmonary tuberculosis in patients with human immunodeficiency virus infection. *Medicine* 1991;70:384–397.
9. Nzerue C, Drayton J, Oster R, et al. Genitourinary tuberculosis in patients with HIV infection: clinical features in an inner-city hospital population. *Am J Med Sci* 2000;320:299–303.
10. Fanning A. Tuberculosis: 6. Extrapulmonary disease. *CMAJ* 1999;160:1597–1603.
11. Slutsker L, Castro KG, Ward JW, et al. Epidemiology of extrapulmonary tuberculosis among persons with AIDS in the United States. *Clin Infect Dis* 1993;16:513–518.
12. Mehta JB, Dutt A, Harvill L, et al. Epidemiology of extrapulmonary tuberculosis. *Chest* 1991;99:1134–1138.
13. Rieder HL, Snider DE, Cauthen GM. Extrapulmonary tuberculosis in the United States. *Am Rev Respir Dis* 1990;141:347–351.
14. Bruce LG. The incidence of genitourinary tuberculosis in the western region of Scotland. *Br J Urol* 1970;42:637–641.
15. Yates MD, Grange JM. Incidence and nature of human tuberculosis due to bovine tubercle bacilli in South-East England: 1977–1987. *Epidemiol Infect* 1988;101:225–229.
16. Woods LE, Butler VB, Pollak A. Human infection with the yellow acid fast bacillus. A report of fifteen additional cases. *Am Rev Tuberc* 1956;73:917.
17. Pergament M, Gonzales R, Fraley EE. Atypical mycobacteriosis of the urinary tract—a case report of extensive disease caused by the Battey bacillus. *JAMA* 1974;229:816–817.
18. Hawkins CC, Gold JW, Whimbey E, et al. *Mycobacterium avium* complex infections in patients with the acquired immunodeficiency syndrome. *Ann Intern Med* 1986;105:184–188.
19. Pitchenik AE, Fertel D. Tuberculosis and nontuberculous mycobacterial disease. *Med Clin North Am* 1992;76:121–171.
20. Pasternack MS, Rubin RH. Urinary tract tuberculosis. In: Schrier RW, ed. *Diseases of the kidney and urinary tract*, 7th ed. Philadelphia: Lippincott Williams & Wilkins, 2001:1017–1037.
21. Friedland GW, Filly R, Goris ML, et al. Infection and Infestations. In: Friedland GW, Filly R, Goris ML, et al., eds. *Uroradiology*. New York: Churchill Livingstone, 1983:381–393.
22. Ney C, Friedenberg RM. Tuberculosis of the kidney. In: Ney C, Friedenberg RM, eds. *Radiographic atlas of the genitourinary system*. Philadelphia: JB Lippincott Co, 1981:373–409.
23. Kim SH. Urogenital tuberculosis. In: Pollack HM, McClennan BL, Dyer RK, et al., eds. *Clinical urography*. Philadelphia: WB Saunders, 2000:1193–1228.
24. Cavallo T. Tubulointerstitial nephritis. In: Jennette JC, Olson JL, Schwartz MM, eds. *Heptinstall's pathology of the kidney*, New York: Lippincott–Raven, 1998:667–679.
25. Lamm DL. Complications of bacillus Calmette–Guerin immunotherapy. *Urol Clin North Am* 1992;19:565–572.
26. Cos LR, Cockett ATK. Genitourinary tuberculosis revisited. *Urology* 1982;20:111–117.
27. Bentz RR, Dimcheff DG, Nemiroff MJ, et al. The incidence of urine cultures positive for *Mycobacterium tuberculosis* in a gen-

eral tuberculosis patient population. *Am Rev Respir Dis* 1975;
111:647–650.

28. Nesbitt RM, Ratliff RK. Hypertension associated with unilateral nephropathy. *J Urol* 1940;437:427.

29. Flechner SM, Gow JG. Role of nephrectomy in the treatment of non-functioning or very poorly functioning unilateral tuberculosis kidney. *J Urol* 1980;123:822–825.

30. Schwartz DT, Lattimer JK. Incidence of arterial hypertension in 540 patients with renal tuberculosis. *J Urol* 1968;98:651–653.

31. Wisnia LG, Jukolj S, Lopez de Santa Maria J, et al. Renal function damage in 131 cases of urogenital tuberculosis. *Urology* 1978;11:457–461.

32. Eastwood JB, Maidi M, Maxwell JD, et al. Tuberculosis as primary renal diagnosis in end-stage uraemia. *J Nephrol* 1994;7: 290–293.

33. Eastwood JB, Corbishley CM, Grange JM. Tuberculosis and the kidney. *J Am Soc Nephrol* 2001;12:1307–1314.

34. Defronzo RA. Hyperkalemia and hyporeninemic hypoaldosteronism *Kidney Int* 1980;17:118–134.

35. Das KM, Indudhara R, Vaidyanathan S. Sonographic features of genitourinary tuberculosis. *AJR Am J Roentgenol* 1992;158: 327–329.

36. Merenich WM, Popky GL. Radiology of renal infection. *Med Clin North Am* 1991;75:425–469.

37. Kaplan DM, Rosenfield AT, Smith RC. Advances in the imaging of renal infection. Helical CT and modern coordinated imaging. *Infect Dis Clin North Am* 1997;11:681–705.

38. Giustra PE, Watson RC, Shulman H. Arteriographic finding in the various stages of renal tuberculosis. *Radiology* 1971;100: 597–602.

39. Yang S, Lee YI, Chung DG, et al. Detection of extrapulmonary tuberculosis with gallium-67 scan and computed tomography. *J Nucl Med* 1992;33:2118–2123.

40. Kollins SA, Hartman GW, Carr DT, et al. Roentgenologic findings in urinary tract tuberculosis: a 10 year investigation. *AJR AM J Roentgenol* 1974;121:487–500.

41. Friedenberg RM, Ney C, Stachenfeld RA. Roentgenologic manifestations of tuberculosis of the ureter. *J Urol* 1968;99: 25–29.

42. Birnbaum BA, Friedman JP, Lubat E, et al. Extrarenal genitourinary tuberculosis: CT appearance of calcified pipe-stem ureter and seminal vesicle abscess. *J Comput Assist Tomogr* 1990; 14:653–655.

43. Kenney M, Loechel AB, Lovelock FJ. Urine cultures in tuberculosis. *Am Rev Respir Dis* 1960;82:564.

44. Klotz SA, Penn RL. Acid-fast staining of urine and gastric contents is an excellent indicator of mycobacterial disease. *Am Rev Respir Dis* 1987;136:1197–1198.

45. Hemal AK, Gupta NP, Rajeev TP, et al. Polymerase chain reaction in clinically suspected genitourinary tuberculosis: comparison with intravenous urography, bladder biopsy, and urine acid fast bacilli culture. *Urology* 2000;56:570–574.

46. Moussa OM, Eraky I, El Far MA, et al. Rapid diagnosis of genitourinary tuberculosis by polymerase chain reaction and nonradioactive DNA hybridization. *J Urol* 2000;164:584–588.

47. van Vollenhoven P, Heyns CF, de Beer PM, et al. Polymerase chain reaction in the diagnosis of urinary tract tuberculosis. *Urol Res* 1996;24:107–111.

48. Grange JM, Yates MD. Survey of mycobacteria isolated from urine and the genitourinary tract in South-East England from 1980 to 1989. *Br J Urol* 1992;69:640–646.

49. Brooker WJ, Aufderheide AC. Genitourinary tract infections due to atypical mycobacteria. *J Urol* 1980;124:242–244.

50. Baniel J, Manning A, Leiman G. Fine needle cytodiagnosis of renal tuberculosis. *J Urol* 1991;146:689–691.

51. Das KM, Vaidyanathan S, Rajwanshi A, et al. Renal tuberculosis: diagnosis with sonographically guided aspiration cytology. *AJR Am J Roentgenol* 1992;158:571–573.

52. O'Brien RJ. The treatment of tuberculosis. In: Reichman LB, Hershfield ES, eds. *Tuberculosis: a comprehensive international approach*. New York: Marcel Dekker, 1993:207–240.

53. American Thoracic Society. Treatment of tuberculosis and tuberculosis infection in adults and children. *Am J Respir Crit Care Med* 1994;149:1359–1374.

54. Centers for Disease Control and Prevention. *Core curriculum on tuberculosis* (http://www.cdc.gov/nchstp/tb/pubs/corecurr/default. htm), Atlanta, 2001.

55. American Thoracic Society. Diagnosis and treatment of disease caused by nontuberculous mycobacteria. *Am J Respir Crit Care Med* 1997;156:S1–S25.

56. O'Dea MJ, Moore SB, Greene LF. Tuberculosis prostatitis. *Urology* 1978;11:483–485.

57. Gokce G, Kilicarslan H, Ayan S, et al. Genitourinary tuberculosis: a review of 174 cases. *Scand J Infect Dis* 2002;34:338–340.

58. Gow JG. The surgery of genitourinary tuberculosis. *Br J Surg* 1966;53:210–216.

59. Wong SH, Lau WY. The surgical management of non-functioning tuberculous kidneys. *J Urol* 1980;124:187–191.

60. Lee K, Kim H, Byun S, et al. Laparoscopic nephrectomy for tuberculous nonfunctioning kidney: comparison with laparoscopic simple nephrectomy for other diseases. *Urology* 2002;60:411–414.

61. Kim HH, Lee KS, Park K, et al. Laparoscopic nephrectomy for nonfunctioning tuberculous kidney. *J Endourol* 2000;14:433–437.

62. Rassweiler J, Fornara P, Weber M, et al. Laparoscopic nephrectomy: the experience of the laparoscopy working group of the German Urologic Association. *J Urol* 1998;160:18–21.

63. Gupta NP, Agrawal AK, Sood S. Tubercular pyelonephritic nonfunctioning kidney—another relative contraindication for laparoscopic nephrectomy: a case report. *J Laparoendosc Adv Surg Tech A* 1997;7:131–134.

64. Bloom S, Wechsler H, Lattimer JK. Results of long-term study of nonfunctioning tuberculous kidneys. *J Urol* 1970;104: 654–657.

65. Wechsler H, Lattimer JK. An evaluation of the current therapeutic regimen for renal tuberculosis. *J Urol* 1975;113:760–761.

66. Horne NW, Tulloch WS. Conservative management of renal tuberculosis. *Br J Urol* 1975;47:481–487.

67. Iseman MD. Extrapulmonary tuberculosis. In: Barondess JA, ed. *The clinical management and control of tuberculosis*. New York: New York Academy of Medicine, 1992:143–157.

68. Gow JG. Results of treatment in a large series of cases of genitourinary tuberculosis and the changing pattern of the disease. *Br J Urol* 1970;42:647–655.

69. Kerr WK, Gale GL, Struthers NW, et al. Prognosis in reconstructive surgery for urinary tuberculosis. *Br J Urol* 1970;42: 672–678.

70. Wesolowski S. Later results of cystoplasty in chronic tuberculosis cystitis. *Br J Urol* 1970;42:697–703.

71. Dounis A, Gow JG. Bladder augmentation—a long-term review. *Br J Urol* 1979;51:264–268.

72. Schaefer G. *Davis' gynecology and obstetrics*. Hagerstown, MD: Harper & Row, 1976.

73. Schaefer G. Female genital tuberculosis. *Clin Obstet Gynecol* 1976;19:223–239.

74. Klein TA, Richmond JA, Mishell DR. Pelvic tuberculosis. *Obstet Gynecol* 1976;48:99–104.

75. Emembolu JO. Endometrial flora of infertile women in Zaria, northern Nigeria. *Int J Gynaecol Obstet* 1989;30:155–159.

76. De Vynck WE, Kruger TF, Joubert JJ, et al. Genital tuberculosis associated with female infertility in the western Cape. *S Afr Med* 1990;77:630–631.

77. Oosthuizen AP, Wessels PH, Hefer JN. Tuberculosis of the female genital tract in patients attending an infertility clinic. *S Afr Med* 1990;77:562–564.
78. Varma TR. Genital tuberculosis and subsequent fertility. *Int Gynaecol Obstet* 1991;35:1–11.
79. Jindal UN, Jindal SK, Dhall GI. Short course chemotherapy for endometrial tuberculosis in infertile women. *Int J Gynaecol Obstet* 1990;32:75–76.
80. Falk V, Ludviksson K, Agren G. Genital tuberculosis in women: analysis of 187 newly diagnosed cases from 47 Swedish hospitals during the ten-year period from 1968–1977. *Am J Obstet Gynecol* 1980;138:974–977.
81. Dhillon SS, Gosewehr JA, Julian TM, et al. Genital tuberculosis: case report and literature review. *Wisc Med J* 1990;89:14–17.
82. Tripathy SN. Laparoscopic observations of pelvic organs in pulmonary tuberculosis. *Int J Gynaecol Obstet* 1990;32:129–131.
83. Nogales-Ortiz F, Taracon I, Nogales F. The pathology of female genital tuberculosis: a 32 year study of 1436 cases. *Obstet Gynecol* 1979;53:422–428.
84. Novak ER, Woodruff JD. Granulomatous salpingitis. In: Novak ER, ed. *Novak's gynecologic and obstetric pathology*. Philadelphia: WB Saunders, 1979:328–333.
85. Gompel C, Silverberg SG. The fallopian tube. In: Gompel C, Silverberg SG, eds. *Pathology in gynecology and obstetrics*. Philadelphia: JB Lippincott Co, 1994:284–312.
86. Vani R, Kuntal R, Pralhad K. A rare location of extrapulmonary tuberculosis: the vulva. *Tuber Lung Dis* 1993;74:64.
87. Husemeyer RP. Postmenopausal tuberculosis of the cervix: case report and review. *Br J Obstet Gynaecol* 1977;84:153–154.
88. Siegler AM, Kontopoulos V. Female genital tuberculosis and the role of hysterosalpingography. *Semin Roentgenol* 1979;14:295–304.
89. Anderson JR. Genital tuberculosis. In: Jones HW, Wentz AC, Burnett LS, eds. *Novak's textbook of gynecology*. Baltimore: Williams & Wilkins, 1988:557–569.
90. Sunderland AM. The treatment of tuberculosis of female genital tract with streptomycin, PAS, isoniazid. *Tubercle* 1963;57:137–140.
91. Sunderland AM. Surgical treatment of tuberculosis of the female genital tract. *Br J Obstet Gynaecol* 1980;87:610–615.
92. Frydman R, Eibschitz I, Belaishc-Allart JC, et al. *In vitro* fertilization in tuberculous infertility. *J In Vitro Fertil Embryo Transfer* 1985;2:184–188.
93. Medlar EM, Spain DM, Holliday RW. Post-mortem compared with clinical diagnosis of genitourinary tuberculosis in adult males. *J Urol* 1949;61:1078.
94. Sporer A, Auerbach O. Tuberculosis of prostate. *Urology* 1978;11:362–365.
95. Wolf JS, McAninch JW. Tuberculosis epididymo-orchitis: diagnosis by fine needle aspiration. *J Urol* 1991;145:836–838.
96. Lattimer JK. Renal tuberculosis. *N Engl J Med* 1965;273:208–211.
97. Ross JC, Gow JG, St Hill CA. Tuberculous epididymitis. A review of 170 patients. *Br J Surg* 1961;48:663–666.
98. Desmond N, Lynch M, Murphy D, et al. Tuberculous epididymitis: a case report in an HIV seropositive male. *Int J STD AIDS* 1993;4:178–179.
99. Goodman P, Maklad NF, Verani RR, et al. Tuberculous abscess of the testicle in AIDS: sonographic demonstration. *Urol Radiol* 1990;12:53–55.
100. Hepper NGG, Karlson AG, Leary FJ, et al. Genitourinary infection due to *Mycobacterium kansasii*. *Mayo Clin Proc* 1971;46:387–390.
101. Clark R, Cardona L, Valainis G, et al. Genitourinary infections caused by mycobacteria other than *Mycobacterium tuberculosis*. *Tubercle* 1989;70:297–300.
102. Ferrie BG, Rundle JSH. Tuberculous epididymo-orchitis. A review of 20 cases. *Br J Urol* 1983;55:437–439.
103. Chung JJ, Kim MJ, Lee T, et al Sonographic findings in tuberculous epididymitis and epididymo-orchitis. *J Clin Ultrasound* 1997;25:390–394.
104. Razic MMA, El-Morsy FE. Genitourinary mycobacteria in infertile Egyptian men. *Fertil Steril* 1990;54:713–717.
105. O'Flynn D. Surgical treatment of genito-urinary tuberculosis. A report on 762 cases. *Br J Urol* 1970;42:667–671.
106. Lenk S, Schroeder J Genitourinary tuberculosis. *Curr Opin Urol* 2001;11:93–98.
107. Wang J, Chang T. Tuberculosis of the prostate: CT appearance. *J Comput Assist Tomogr* 1991;15:269–270.
108. Tikkakoski T, Karstrup S, Lohela P, et al. Tuberculosis of the lower genitourinary tract: Ultrasonography as an aid to diagnosis and treatment. *J Clin Ultrasound* 1993;21:269–271.
109. Lal MM, Sekhan GS, Dhall JC. Tuberculosis of the penis. *J Indian Med Assoc* 1971;56:316–317.
110. Lewis EL. Tuberculosis of the penis. A report of 5 new cases and a complete review of the literature. *J Urol* 1946;56:737.
111. Jitpraphai P, Glasberg S, Wise GJ. Penile tuberculosis. *Urology* 1973;1:145–147.
112. Angus BJ, Yates M, Conlon C, et al. Cutaneous tuberculosis of the penis and sexual transmission of tuberculosis confirmed by molecular typing. *Clin Infect Dis* 2001;33:E132–E134.
113. Dahl DM, Klein D, Morgentaler A. Penile mass caused by the newly described organism *Mycobacterium celatum*. *Urology* 1996;47:266–268.
114. Ribera M, Bielsa J, Manterola JM, et al. *Mycobacterium bovis*-BCG infection of the glans penis: a complication of intravesical administration of bacillus Calmette–Guerin. *Br J Dermatol* 1995;132:309–310.
115. Indudhara R, Vaidyanathan S, Radotra BD. Urethral tuberculosis. *Urol Int* 1992;48:436–438.

SPINAL TUBERCULOSIS

ERIC LEIBERT
GEORGE HARALAMBOU

HISTORY

Spinal tuberculosis (TB) has affected humans for millennia. Skeletal lesions suggestive of Pott disease have been found in Egyptian mummies (1). Recent testing using DNA amplification on a specimen dating to 5200 B.C. has confirmed what was long suspected, that the lesions were caused by *Mycobacterium tuberculosis* (2). Skeletal lesions suspected to represent Pott disease have been found in pre-Columbian new world sites as well (3–5). These, too, have been confirmed by polymerase chain reaction (6,7). That TB was documented to have existed in the New World before it was reintroduced by the Europeans is part of the puzzle of the history of humans in the New World.

Sir Percivall Pott (8) first associated the spinal deformity with the neurologic deficit and proposed treatment by drainage in 1779. He cites a description by Hippocrates of recovery of neurologic function after spontaneous drainage of an abscess as his inspiration:

> . . . and the late Dr. Cameron, of Worcester, who told me, that remarked in Hippocrates, an account of a paralysis of the lower limbs, cured by an abscess in the back he had in a case of useless limbs attended, with a curvature of the spine, endeavored to imitate this act of nature by exciting a purulent discharge, and that it had proved very beneficial . . .

The skeletal form was not linked to the disease known as consumption or pthisis until after the description of the tubercle bacillus in 1882.

EPIDEMIOLOGY

The epidemiology of Pott disease follows the epidemiology of TB as a whole. As rates of TB decreased in the United

States through most of the past century, both before and after the introduction of antituberculous chemotherapy, rates of spinal TB decreased as well. Spinal TB has been noted to account for approximately half of cases of bone and joint TB in many series (9–11) and between 1% and 5.4% of cases of TB (12–14). Articular infection is the next most frequent and involves the knees, hips, sacroiliac joint, shoulder, elbow, and ankle (15,16).

As rates of TB in developed countries decrease, the average age of TB patients increases, reflecting reactivation of infection acquired in the past when the disease was more prevalent (17). Immigrants from a developing country to a Western country are more likely to have epidemiologic characteristics of their countries of origin and so immigrants with TB are younger, reflecting more recent transmission. The same phenomenon is observed in spinal TB (18). A Swiss report from 1988 of 26 cases noted that although the mean age of the 12 Swiss nationals was 69 years, the mean age of the 14 immigrants, many from developing countries, was 30 years (19).

When increased numbers of TB cases were described in the United States in the 1980s and 1990s, the number of cases of spinal TB increased as well (20). The increase in incidence of TB in the United States in the 1980s and 1990s is attributed in large part to the human immunodeficiency virus (HIV) epidemic (21). In New York City in 1992, 34% of TB cases were in known HIV-positive individuals (22). It is estimated that a more accurate percentage is closer to 40% (23). HIV-positive individuals are at a dramatically higher risk of developing TB. It is not known whether they are more or less likely to have spinal TB. Jellis (24), in Zambia, reported on 159 patients with skeletal TB and a known HIV test result. He noted that 60% of adults with spinal TB were HIV positive. In contrast, he estimates that one-third of the adult population of Lusaka, Zambia, is HIV positive. Early reports suggested that extrapulmonary TB was more common in HIV-infected individuals (25). The data from Bellevue Hospital in New York City (14) suggest that HIV-positive patients were not overrepresented (27%) among cases of

E. Leibert: Department of Medicine, Division of Pulmonary and Critical Care Medicine, New York University School of Medicine; Chest Service, Bellevue Hospital, New York, New York.

G. Haralambou: Department of Medicine, Division of Pulmonary and Critical Care Medicine, New York University Medical Center, New York, New York.

spinal TB compared with their representation among total cases of TB (34%).

PATHOPHYSIOLOGY

Tuberculous spondylitis is a slowly progressive, destructive infection of one or more vertebrae. In the classic presentation, the infection involves two adjacent vertebral bodies with intervening disc space destruction (15). An abscess may form adjacent to the primary site that can track along tissue planes, compress vital organs, invade remote sites, or rupture to the skin surface (15).

Mycobacteria are believed to reach the vertebral column via the hematogenous route, either via the intercostal arteries or the venous plexus of Batson (26–28). However, it is likely that the lymphatic system can also be a route of entry (16,26,29). The infection usually begins in the cancellous bone in the subchondral region of the vertebral body (15). Progression of infection leads to vertebral body weakening, collapse, and disc space narrowing. Herniation of the intervertebral disc into the weakened bone causes loss of vertebral height. The anterior portion of the vertebral body is typically involved, either superiorly or inferiorly, causing anterior wedging, kyphosis, and sharp angulation of the spine (15,29,30). This pattern of vertebral body destruction is responsible for the characteristic gibbus deformity (31). Involvement of the intervertebral disc is variable. Because it is relatively avascular, it may be spared even when adjacent vertebrae are involved (29). However, it is often invaded and destroyed secondarily by direct spread of the advancing infection in the contiguous vertebral body (15,29).

Tuberculous spondylitis most commonly affects the thoracic and lumbar regions. In a study of 103 patients with spinal TB by Pertuiset et al. (29), the thoracic or lumbar regions were nearly equally affected and were the site of involvement in at least 80% of cases. Cervical and sacral vertebral lesions are also well described (27). Involvement of adjacent vertebrae is the familiar presentation, but a multifocal pattern in which multiple, isolated, nonadjacent vertebrae are affected is also common. Involvement of the posterior vertebral elements (i.e., the laminae, transverse processes, pedicles and spinous processes) is infrequent, occurring in 0.2% to 10% of cases according to several reports (32, 33). Isolated infection of the posterior elements is extremely rare. However, the incidence of neurologic deficits is much higher when these structures are involved (34). Involvement of the pedicle in the thoracic spine may present with destruction of the adjoining rib (34).

Examination of bone samples from patients with tuberculous spondylitis demonstrates relatively small numbers of mycobacterial organisms. Bone cultures from tuberculous spinal lesions show growth of 30 to 100 colonies per culture of tissue. In comparison, expectorated sputum from patients with pulmonary TB shows growth of several hundred thousand colonies per culture. The destructive process in tuberculous spondylitis progresses at a slower rate than pyogenic infections, and this characteristic has been suggested as a distinguishing feature between these types of infection (16,34). The affected area of bone tissue has an opaque, "cheesy" appearance composed of coalescent abscess and granulation tissue (35). Microscopically, the exudate contains Langerhans-type giant cells, epithelioid cells, and lymphocytes surrounding a zone of central necrosis and fibrosis (26). Because the infection does not produce proteolytic enzymes, there is localized bone resorption and osteoporosis with little periosteal inflammation or sclerosis. Progression of the infection to the cortical surface raises the periosteum, causing devascularization and necrosis (35). New bone formation, which occurs during healing, may lead to fusion of adjacent vertebra (16,27,30). Bone fusion was a marker of healing dating back to the 1930s (36,37).

The formation of a paravertebral abscess is a common complication of tuberculous spondylitis. This develops as the infectious process ruptures through the vertebral body and advances beneath the anterior and posterior longitudinal ligaments. The incidence of paravertebral abscess in one study of patients with spinal TB was 57% (19). The abscess contains tubercle bacilli, infected material, and fragments of destroyed bone. It usually also contains calcified material, a characteristic that, when visible radiographically, is considered strongly suggestive of a tuberculous rather than a pyogenic process (15,38). Abscesses may track extensively along tissue planes, carrying bone fragments along. Abscesses in the thoracic region may form adjacent to the pleura, extend into the pleural space to form an empyema, and may invade the lung. In the lumbar region, the abscess may track along the psoas sheath to enter the femoral trigone. Sacral lesions may extend into the perineum or gluteal region (35). Abscesses of the cervical vertebrae may track into the retropharyngeal space or posterior triangle (27,39). Other sites secondarily involved are the esophagus, liver, kidney, bladder, rectum, vagina, and aorta (34). The rim of hypervascularity and inflammation around the abscess leads to scalloping of the lateral and anterior aspects of the vertebral bodies (34). In essentially any region, the abscess may form a sinus tract with drainage of purulent material out to the skin.

Neurologic deficits are common in tuberculous spondylitis, occurring in 23% to 76% of cases according to various studies (19,29,40,41). Extrinsic compression of the spinal cord may result from extradural abscess, subluxation, granulation tissue formation, vertebral body collapse, and stretching of the cord over bony ridges in the spinal canal (27). Posterior rupture of the vertebral body may injure the spinal cord by the release of infected debris and bone fragments. Vascular compression or thrombosis may also occur. Direct infection of neural structures from a contiguous focus is also well described (42,43). Localized arachnoiditis, focal demyelination, inflammation of the spinal cord and nerve roots, and vasculitis are usually present around areas of tuberculous spondylitis, even in the absence of direct compression. These lesions often extend beyond the vertebral segment involved. These inflammatory effects may be more important than direct-pressure effects in causing neurologic deficits (19).

CLINICAL PRESENTATION

Low-grade fever, weight loss, malaise, night sweats, and vague back pain characterize the early stages of spinal TB. This indolent course may persist for months to years before complications arise.

More advanced infection presents as localized pain over the affected vertebrae, kyphoscoliosis, and neurologic complications such as neuralgia, sensory loss, paraplegia, and cauda equina syndrome. Formation and tracking of a paravertebral abscess may cause pain, a palpable mass at a distant site, or a cutaneous draining sinus (35).

Laboratory tests generally are nonspecific and unhelpful in diagnosis. The erythrocyte sedimentation ratio is usually elevated with an average of 44 mm per hour in the series of Lifeso et al. (44) of 107 patients. However, an erythrocyte sedimentation rate of less than 10 mm per hour was seen in six patients and a rate between 10 and 20 mm per hour was seen in five patients. The leukocyte count is usually normal but can be elevated. Skin testing with purified protein derivative is usually positive but can be negative, especially in debilitated, immunosuppressed, or elderly patients. In the series of Lifeso et al., 14% of patients had negative tests in the setting of proven spinal TB. In endemic areas, the high prevalence of purified protein derivative reactivity negates the diagnostic value of a positive test. In fact, as many as 50% of elderly patients with spinal TB may have negative skin tests (15,45).

The chest radiograph is abnormal, with evidence of either active or prior pulmonary disease in 35% to 70% of cases (20,46–50).

RADIOGRAPHY

A plain radiograph is the most common initial test but is often negative in the earlier disease stages before the destructive process has advanced. As the disease progresses, radiographs of the vertebral body show collapse, loss of vertebral body height, disc space narrowing, bone erosion, demineralization, and loss of definition of the end plates. Destruction and collapse of the anterior aspect of the vertebral body is the predominant pattern, resulting in the anterior angulation (i.e., gibbus deformity). Paravertebral abscess formation appears on plain radiograph as soft-tissue swelling along the vertebral column. In the thoracic spine,

a fusiform density appears. In the lumbar spine, psoas abscess appears as a lateral bowing of the psoas shadow. A distinguishing characteristic of psoas abscess owing to tuberculous infection is the finding of calcification within the abscess (15,28,44,51).

Computed tomography (CT) is more sensitive than plain radiograph in demonstrating evidence of early infection. Early foci of infection within the bone, end plate destruction, fragmentation of the vertebrae, and elevation of the periosteum are demonstrated more easily (34). Involvement of the posterior elements, which is usually not visible on plain radiograph, can be demonstrated using CT (29). Extension into the spinal canal with impending spinal cord compression may be detected and treated earlier, before severe neurologic deficits ensue (16). In addition, CT with use of intravenous contrast can detect and trace the extent of an associated paravertebral abscess (16,29). CT examination of the abscess reveals low attenuation, multiloculated fluid collections with a surrounding thick rim of enhancement (34). CT is also useful for guiding percutaneous biopsy (15).

Magnetic resonance imaging (MRI), which affords better definition of soft tissues, has been considered the optimal imaging choice for spinal TB owing to its increased sensitivity and multiplanar capability (16,52). MRI evaluation of tuberculous spondylitis demonstrates focal decreased signal on T1-weighted images and increased signal on T2-weighted images (29,34). Contrast enhancement further improves definition. Cortical bone involvement and calcification within a paravertebral abscess are not demonstrated as well as with CT (34). However, MRI allows excellent tissue detail that enables accurate detection of abscess formation and extension. Involvement of the posterior vertebral elements, spinal canal narrowing, thecal sac displacement, meningeal involvement, and spinal cord compression are also easily demonstrated (26).

Bone scan using technetium-99m pyrophosphate has shown variable sensitivity and utility. In the series of Lifeso et al. (44), 35% of patients showed no evidence of increased uptake despite known disease demonstrable by other means. Gallium 67 scanning also had poor sensitivity (44). In the study of Pertuiset et al. (29), technetium-99m scan detected infection in 58 of 63 patients with known disease.

DIAGNOSIS

Tuberculous spondylitis often eludes diagnosis owing to the slowly progressing, indolent nature and nonspecific manifestations of the early stages of infection. The diagnostic process is often initiated once recognition of characteristic clinical symptoms prompts radiographic evaluation and subsequent diagnostic procedure to obtain histologic material. Growth of *M. tuberculosis* or demonstration of typical caseating granulomata in histologic specimens in the appropriate clinical setting establishes the diagnosis.

Clinical presentation, laboratory examination, and radiographic imaging can be highly suggestive of spinal TB. In endemic areas, this may be sufficient for empirical treatment (13). Definitive diagnosis of tuberculous spinal infection requires growth of *M. tuberculosis* on culture of material from a suspected site or demonstration of typical findings on histologic specimens. Diagnostic techniques include open surgical biopsy, percutaneous needle biopsy, and percutaneous needle aspiration. CT or ultrasound guidance is used for percutaneous procedures. Masood (53) reported on specimens obtained by fine needle aspiration. In this series, specimens revealed positive acid-fast bacillus (AFB) stain in 64%, growth of *M. tuberculosis* in 83%, and caseating granulomas on histologic examination in 73%. In the series of Pertuiset et al. (29), percutaneous needle biopsy and surgical biopsy yielded positive AFB smears in 20% and 25% of specimens, respectively. Percutaneous aspirate of a paravertebral abscess yielded a positive smear in 59%. AFB culture in percutaneous biopsy, surgical biopsy, and needle aspirate of an abscess was positive in 76%, 81%, and 93%, respectively. Surgical and percutaneous biopsy was diagnostic on histologic examination in 62% and 68%, respectively (29). Histologic examination is frequently advantageous in that it may establish the diagnosis of tuberculous infection before growth on culture.

THE EVOLUTION OF TREATMENT

Treatment of spinal TB in the preantibiotic era included bedrest, prolonged immobilization, or surgery (11). Many surgical treatments were attempted for spinal TB in the preantibiotic era. Early promising results of both costotransversectomy and spinal fusion were not borne out by subsequent series that demonstrated secondary infection, dissemination of TB, and excess mortality (54,55). The conclusion of one series from 1937 was that surgery for stabilization should only be done after the infection was quiescent (37).

In 1951, Dobson (11) reported 914 patients treated between 1932 and 1948. None received antituberculous chemotherapy. All were treated with prolonged immobilization (average of 39 months) in a brace or plaster cast. Fifty-four underwent subsequent spinal fusion after the infection was thought to have become quiescent. The mortality rate on the initial hospitalization was 19%. Sixty-two percent had no active disease at discharge, although 22% (137 patients) of these were subsequently readmitted for active disease. The results at 3 years had 366 patients able to work, 306 dead, and the remainder lost, disabled, or with active disease.

The discovery of antituberculous chemotherapy in the late 1940s revolutionized the treatment of TB (56). The question of the relative roles of medication and spinal surgery in spinal TB arose quickly.

In 1956, Hodgson and Stock (57) described the use of an anterior approach to the spine with decompression of neural elements and autologous bone grafting to promote fusion. All patients were treated antituberculous chemotherapy for 18 to 24 months. In subsequent reports in 1960 and 1964, they reported that 94% of treated patients made complete recoveries (58,59). They acknowledged that this was a major operation and not to be undertaken lightly and without appropriate resources.

In 1962, Konstam and Blesovsky (60) reported on the management results of 207 patients with spinal TB who were treated with isoniazid (INH) and paraaminosalicylic acid (PAS) without streptomycin. Medications were given for a minimum of 12 months and continued until there was radiographic evidence of healing. Twenty-seven patients underwent surgical abscess drainage. Patients were allowed to ambulate without bracing. One hundred seventy-eight (86%) of patients recovered completely; 109 patients were healed by 12 months, 172 by 18 months, and the rest by 24 months. This study represented an important advance in the management of Pott disease because it was the first to show that chemotherapy without surgery or long-term immobilization could be highly successful. This aroused widespread interest in the use of ambulatory outpatient chemotherapy. It is interesting to note that a 1-year regimen of INH and PAS had an unacceptably high relapse rate of 22% in a 1962 study of patients with cavitary pulmonary TB (61).

EARLY BRITISH MEDICAL RESEARCH COUNCIL WORKING PARTY ON TUBERCULOSIS OF THE SPINE STUDIES

These discrepant approaches to the treatment of spinal TB led the British Medical Research Council Working Party on Tuberculosis of the Spine (MRC) to conduct a series of randomized clinical trials with long follow-up to assess the various available treatments (46–49,62–66). These studies were carried out in Korea, Rhodesia (now Zimbabwe), South Africa, and Hong Kong. All patients received antituberculous chemotherapy. In reports one through nine, treatment was with INH and PAS, with some patients randomized to the addition of streptomycin for the first 3 months. The methods of treatment were determined by locally available resources and included outpatient chemotherapy, chemotherapy with immobilization by bed rest or body casts, chemotherapy, and conservative debridement of obviously infected bone without fusion, and, in Hong Kong and South Africa, chemotherapy with radical surgery consisting of anterior resection, debridement of granulation tissue and nonviable bone, and autologous bone strut grafting (Table 37.1).

Favorable outcome was defined as "full physical activity with clinically and radiographically quiescent disease, with no sinuses, abscesses, or myelopathy with functional impairment, all without modification of the allocated regimen" (46).

TABLE 37.1. EARLY BRITISH MEDICAL RESEARCH COUNCIL WORKING PARTY ON TUBERCULOSIS OF THE SPINE STUDIES

Location	MRC Report No.	Groups	% Favorable at 18 Mo	% Favorable at 3 Yr	% Favorable at 5 Yr	% Favorable at 10 Yr	% Favorable at 15 Yr
Korea, Masan	1,5,9	Inpatient bed rest	66	84	91	92	
		Outpatient ambulatory	58	88	89	88	
		SPH[a]	56	82	86[b]	85[b]	
		PH[c]	67	90	92	91	
Korea, Pusan (children)	2,5,9	Plaster jacket	68	86	90	89	
		No jacket	60	82	84	83	
		SPH[a]	65	80			
		PH[c]	63	87			
Rhodesia	3,6	Debridement	81	85	84		
		Ambulatory	79	86	83		
		SPH[a]	84	84			
		PH[c]	76	86			
Hong Kong	4,6,8,13	Debridement	79	86	88	89	87
		Radical surgery	89	87	89	86	85
South Africa	7	Debridement	69	88			
		Radical surgery	64	81			

[a]18 months of isoniazid (H) and paraaminosalicylic acid (P) with and without streptomycin (S) for 3 months.
[b]Data pooled from Masan and Pusan, Korea.
[c]18 months of isoniazid and paraaminosalicylic acid.
MRC, British Medical Research Council Working Party on Tuberculosis of the Spine.

There was no advantage to immobilization by either hospitalization or plaster jacket. There was no long-term advantage to debridement, although patients had earlier resolution of abscesses (49). There was no advantage to radical anterior surgery in terms of favorable outcome (48,64,65).

Radical operation in South Africa was no better than debridement, but radical operation done in Hong Kong had distinct advantages. Patients in groups treated without radical surgery experienced an average increase in kyphosis of 10 degrees in those with thoracic lesions and 8 degrees in those with lumbar lesions; some patients had significantly more. Patients treated with radical surgery in Hong Kong had more rapid abscess resolution and bony fusions. Kyphosis improved on average by 1.4 degrees in the thoracic region and 0.5 degree in the lumbar region (65).

Based on these results, the MRC (65) recommended the following:

> When appropriate facilities and enough hospital beds are available, together with experienced spinal surgeons and good postoperative nursing, the modified Hong Kong operation as performed by its originators, has definite advantages . . . it has produced substantially earlier bony fusion, vertebral reconstitution and no increase in kyphosis . . . .When adequate facilities are lacking, reliance should be placed on ambulant chemotherapy alone.

This conclusion shaped both how spinal TB was treated in developed countries and how subsequent research was conducted.

BRITISH MEDICAL RESEARCH COUNCIL WORKING PARTY ON TUBERCULOSIS OF THE SPINE TRIALS BASED ON RIFAMPIN-CONTAINING REGIMENS

Starting with the tenth report in 1986, the MRC reported on patients treated with short-course regimens containing rifampin (67–71). Centers in Hong Kong, India (Madras),

and Korea were included. In Hong Kong, all patients underwent radical surgery. The comparison was of 6 and 9 months of INH and rifampin along with 6 months of streptomycin. In India, INH plus rifampin for 6 or 9 months was compared with surgery plus INH and rifampin for 6 months. In Korea, surgery was not done. Various combinations of chemotherapy regimens were compared. Results at 5 years were appeared in the 14th report (Table 37.2).

Patients in all groups except those who received short-course therapy without rifampin had excellent results in terms of favorable status. Surgery in India was no better than ambulatory chemotherapy, both in terms of favorable status and progression of kyphosis. The fact that surgical outcomes were better in Hong Kong than in India was attributed to less extensive initial disease and to difficulty in introducing a major surgical procedure even in an orthopedic center.

The conclusion of the MRC (69) regarding the role of surgery in the era of effective short-course chemotherapy is as follows:

> Short term chemotherapy based upon rifampicin in patients ambulatory from the start would appear to be the best available method of treatment for this disease. Indeed, the main indication for any form of surgery would appear to be difficulty in diagnosis. . . .The advantages of radical surgery do not seem to justify its widespread adoption; it should be confined to centres adequately equipped in all respects.

CHEMOTHERAPY

Appropriate chemotherapy is central to the treatment of spinal TB. MRC report 14 showed that short-course ambulant chemotherapy with a rifampin-containing regimen leads to favorable outcomes in more than 91% (227 of 247) of patients and that there was no advantage to surgery in the studied groups. The current standard regimen in the devel-

TABLE 37.2. BRITISH MEDICAL RESEARCH COUNCIL WORKING PARTY ON TUBERCULOSIS OF THE SPINE STUDIES OF RIFAMPIN-CONTAINING REGIMENS

Location	MRC Report No.	Groups	% Favorable at 18 Mo	% Favorable at 3 Yr	% Favorable at 5 Yr	% Favorable at 10 Yr
Korea	12,14	6 HR	49	82	90	
		9 HR	56	75	85	
		9 P/E, H	40	73	73	
		18 P/E, H	48	79	90	
Madras, India	Indian Council, 14, Parthasarathy	Radical surgery, 6 HR	58	80	88	90
		6 HR	58	87	91	94
		9 HR	60	96	98	99
Hong Kong	10,14	Radical surgery 6 HRS	76	96	96	
		Radical surgery 9 HRS[a]	85	92	96	

[a]Streptomycin given for 6 months.
MRC, British Medical Research Council Working Party on Tuberculosis of the Spine; H, isoniazid; R, rifampin; S, streptomycin.

oped world is INH, rifampin, pyrazinamide, and ethambutol as initial empirical therapy with ethambutol discontinued as soon as cultures confirm susceptibility and pyrazinamide discontinued at 2 months. INH and rifampin are continued for the duration of treatment. (Doses in both adults and children are the same as for pulmonary TB and are discussed elsewhere in this text.) It is very likely that the current regimens that include pyrazinamide would have outcomes at least as good as those in both recent MRC studies, which used INH and rifampin alone, and the original MRC 18-month regimens. It is interesting that in the new series of MRC spinal TB studies, INH and rifampin alone for 6 months, which is associated with an unacceptably high failure rate in pulmonary TB, had as good an outcome at 5-year follow-up as the 9-month regimen.

There has been a tendency to treat spinal TB for far longer than pulmonary TB. Many of the recently published case series describe treatment for 12 months or longer (29,72,73). The 1994 Centers for Disease Control and Prevention guidelines recommend 12 months of therapy for bone TB (74). There is little in the modern literature to support this (75). The MRC studies showed that a 6-month regimen of INH and rifampin was associated with outcomes as good as a 9-month regimen.

The International Union Against Tuberculosis and Lung Disease has recommended a regimen of INH and thiacetazone in the continuation phase of therapy in patients with pulmonary TB in the developing world. This allows an inexpensive empirical regimen that is likely to be successful in most cases but that will not risk the development of resistance to rifampin (76). Use of thiacetazone in spinal TB has not been extensively investigated. In one report from 1975, the authors mention that they had switched from a regimen of INH and PAS to one of INH and thiacetazone because of cost concerns (77). They do not analyze thiacetazone-treated patients as a separate group. There is nothing in the literature regarding use of this sort of regimen and its outcomes in spinal TB. It is likely that patients are being treated with the International Union Against Tuberculosis and Lung Disease regimen for spinal TB in places where the regimen has been adopted. A report of outcomes of these patients would be of interest. Thiacetazone has been associated with a significant rate of toxic skin reactions in HIV-positive individuals. If HIV infection is likely, ethambutol is often substituted (78,79).

There have been only a few case reports of patients with spinal TB and multidrug-resistant organisms (80,81). Most authorities would advise treatment with a regimen such as one used for pulmonary multidrug-resistant TB. It is likely that drugs penetrate well. Using radiolabeled drug, INH, PAS, and streptomycin have all been shown to penetrate infected bone well (77). PAS and streptomycin have been highly successful when they were components of standard therapy. Some have argued that drug resistance is a surgical indication (20). In the preantibiotic era, there was no advantage to surgery (36). In the era before the routine use of rifampin, there was an advantage with surgery in Hong Kong but not South Africa (63,64).

Directly observed therapy (DOT) is the standard of care in treatment of pulmonary TB because it is associated with better outcomes (82,83). A major benefit of these improved outcomes is the reduction of transmission of infection and secondary cases. For this reason, it is possible to mandate DOT for pulmonary TB (84). Resources required are quite modest and in most settings are cost-effective (85). DOT likely leads to similar improvement in outcomes in spinal TB. Because spinal TB is not contagious, adherence cannot be coerced, and the benefit to the community of the expense of DOT is less compelling.

Intermittent therapy is highly effective in pulmonary TB (86). It has the advantage of being cheaper and easier to supervise by DOT. The MRC (69) explicitly states that development of intermittent regimens is a widely accepted need. There have been no large studies of intermittent therapy in spinal TB. In absence of studies, some treatment guidelines recommend treatment with the same regimen that is used for pulmonary TB (87).

SURGICAL INDICATIONS

Paresis occurs in 11% to 35% of cases of spinal TB (88). Although the MRC results seem to suggest that chemotherapy rather than surgery should be the standard of care, their results may not be applicable to all situations. The MRC studies excluded patients too neurologically impaired to walk across a room. In the newer studies, only two of 60 patients in Hong Kong had myelopathy, none with functional impairment. In India, 19 of 304 had myelopathy, 13 with functional impairment. In Korea, 33 of 359 had myelopathy, 22 with functional impairment (69).

Patients with advanced neurologic deficits who would have been excluded from MRC studies are described in a number of series (89–91). In general, these describe surgical approaches without a control group and have good results. There are no controlled studies of outcome in severe paresis. Seddon (36) noted in the 1930s that most patients with Pott paralysis recovered with prolonged bed rest in an open-air hospital. Authors of some series advocate aggressive surgery for everyone with paresis, citing the risk of progression or irreversible neurologic deficit or kyphosis (20,92). Others advocate a less aggressive approach. Jain (89) recently published an algorithm that includes a trial of medications for 3 weeks to be followed by surgery for those who fail to improve.

Patients with three or more vertebral bodies involved were excluded from the early MRC studies in Hong Kong. Several studies suggest that risk of deformity, instability, and progression to neurologic deficit correlates with the size of the vertebral lesion (31,93,94). These lesions, larger than those considered by the MRC, are potentially an indication for surgery to ensure stability and prevent progression of kyphosis and subsequent paresis.

MRC studies were done in patients with active spinal TB. Patients who develop paresis long after treatment because of progression of kyphosis will not improve with chemotherapy. The management is surgery to relieve compression (89).

The MRC concluded that a nondiagnostic biopsy was an indication for surgical biopsy. Resistance to chemotherapy, failed chemotherapy, severe kyphosis, cord compression, progressive pulmonary impairment, and progressive kyphosis have all been considered surgical indications (95).

SURGICAL MANAGEMENT AND TECHNIQUE

All patients who undergo surgical procedures should receive full courses of antituberculous chemotherapy. No series or study of surgical techniques has had satisfactory outcomes without antituberculous chemotherapy.

The factors that influence the selection of a surgical approach include the location of the disease focus, the extent of vertebral destruction, neurologic deficit, and spinal deformity. It is common to underestimate the extent of disease based on plain films (15). Modern imaging with MRI can allow more accurate preoperative planning (96).

Laminectomy is commonly used for lesions located posteriorly. It allows rapid and easy access for tissue diagnosis, débridement, and neural decompression. Laminectomy is of limited utility for anteriorly located lesions because access to the anterior spinal column is limited and because, in patients with extensive involvement of the anterior spinal elements, laminectomy increases the risk of further instability (89).

The posterolateral approach (costotransversectomy) provides access to the posterior spinal column and the lateral aspect of the vertebral body. This can be particularly useful for upper thoracic lesions. The approach is usually extrapleural and, if extended, the anterior part of the vertebral body can be accessed.

The anterior and anterolateral approaches allow good access to the vertebral body, the most common site of disease. This facilitates radical surgery with vertebrectomy and bone grafting. The details of the approach vary based on the level of the spinal involvement.

After the diseased area is reached, resection can be performed. All affected bone is resected. Resection is extended until normal bone is exposed both superiorly and inferiorly. If the entire vertebral body is affected, the adjacent disc space is resected, even if the disc is normal, along with the end plates of the adjacent normal vertebral body to create a surface suitable for autologous bone grafting. Enough bone should be resected to relieve all compression of the posterior longitudinal ligament. To allow decompression of neural

tissue, the dura may be inspected and explored. After débridement, vertebrectomy, and decompression, an autologous bone graft is placed to allow fusion. Iliac crest, rib, and fibular grafts have all been used. An iliac crest graft is preferred if the space to be filled is small. Rib and fibular grafts can fill longer gaps but are limited by the increased risk of stress fracture (94).

Spinal instrumentation may provide additional stabilization, especially if the anterior disease and subsequent surgery are extensive. This is more commonly an issue in the lumbar region because the thoracic spine above T11 is inherently more stable because of fixation by the rib cage. Because of concerns about introducing a foreign body into an infected area, posterior instrumentation, which keeps the hardware far away from the site of infection, has been preferred. Anterior instrumentation would have a biomechanical advantage of stabilizing the spine anteriorly, where forces are greater and where the weakness is located. The advantage in stability, especially when compared with rib or fibular bone grafts, has led to many reports on the use of anterior instrumentation (97–99). They describe improved stability and no excess infectious complications. One study suggests that *M. tuberculosis* is less adherent to stainless steel discs *in vitro* than is *Staphylococcus epidermidis* (100).

EXTERNAL BRACING

In MRC patients who did not undergo surgery, bracing had no role. The surgical arm was managed postoperatively on plaster beds in early reports, but in later reports, this was allowed but not encouraged (67). In most series reporting on radical surgery, all patients who underwent a radical procedure were managed with external bracing or some form of immobilization (101).

The exact length of time for bracing depends on the surgical procedure, the use of instrumentation, clinical judgment, and the radiographic appearance of bony fusion. Longer periods of bracing are used for patients who do not have instrumentation or who had two or more vertebral bodies resected. Immobilization is generally continued until there is either bony fusion or at least stability, a period often in the range of 6 to 12 months (101).

CERVICAL TUBERCULOSIS

TB of the cervical spine represents 3% to 5% of cases of spinal TB (11,43,102,103). Pain and limited range of motion are common. Hoarseness and dysphagia may occur. Disease in the cervical spine does not produce as severe a progression of the deformity as in the thoracic spine (89). Diagnosis is often delayed until the patient has neurologic complications. Hsu and Leong (43) reported a 42.5% spinal cord compression rate in 40 patients.

Cervical TB was not included in the MRC studies. Treatment practice is based on case series (43,104). Although bed rest and plaster jackets added nothing to ambulant chemotherapy in other areas of the spine in the MRC studies, immobilization is widely used in cervical spine TB being treated medically and is universal in postoperative patients. Hsu and Leong (43) found differences between children younger than 10 years and older patients. Younger patients had more diffuse involvement and larger abscesses. Drainage and chemotherapy were adequate for the younger patients. For older patients, they recommended radical anterior débridement and strut grafting followed by chemotherapy. Results with cervical laminectomy and/or posterior cervical fusion were poor. Jain (89) reported that approximately 60% to 65% of the patients have neural recovery with nonoperative treatment. The remaining patients require surgical decompression. He advocates the same "middle path" approach for patients with cervical spinal TB and paresis as he does for spinal TB elsewhere.

Atlantoaxial TB (C1-2) represented six of 46 cases of cervical TB in the series of Hsu and Leong (43). TB of the upper cervical spine may be complicated by the formation of a paravertebral abscess in the retropharyngeal space or posterior triangle of the neck, occasionally with a draining sinus. The patient may present with severe neck pain, limitation of movement, local tenderness, instability of the neck, difficulty in swallowing, hoarseness, or stridor (105). Particularly if TB causes ligamentous injury and instability, there is risk of atlantoaxial subluxation and upward movement of the dens (106). Neurologic deficit is common, although not universal (104,107,108).

External bracing is universal for atlantoaxial TB. If with time, bracing, and antituberculous chemotherapy, the spine is considered unstable, posterior spinal fusion should be contemplated. Surgical decompression is indicated when a retropharyngeal abscess produces dysphagia or hoarseness or if the patient does not have an adequate clinical response and neural recovery with nonoperative treatment.

The anterior approach to C1-2 is via a transoral route. Fine needle aspiration can be done for diagnosis by this route (89). Although transoral débridement is a simple procedure for decompression and obtaining a biopsy specimen, transoral surgery for reduction of subluxation or dislocation is a major procedure and has a 50% failure rate (104). Therefore, anterior operations are not commonly performed.

HUMAN IMMUNODEFICIENCY VIRUS

Defects in cell-mediated immunity in HIV-positive patients make reactivation of latent infection or progressive primary TB extremely common. There have, however, been a few reported series of patients with HIV infection and spinal TB (14,98,109).

A series from Bellevue Hospital in New York City identified seven HIV-positive patients with spinal TB (14). The patients had signs and symptoms on presentation typical of Pott disease, with back pain in all patients. Interestingly, the development of spinal TB did not seem to be related to the degree of immunosuppression present. The range of $CD4^+$ cell counts was wide, with several patients having counts in the normal or near-normal range. Preservation of cell-mediated immunity (as reflected by delayed-type hypersensitivity reactions to tuberculin) was also noted in six of the seven patients, and only one patient in the series had a history of an opportunistic infection. The two patients who underwent surgery were also similar to HIV in clinical behavior.

Govender et al. (98) described 39 patients with spinal TB and HIV who were all managed surgically. Again, patients had relatively high CD4 cell counts, a lack of other AIDS-defining illnesses, and clinical behavior similar to HIV negative.

Jellis (110) reported on a large group of HIV-positive patients with spinal TB. He noted that there was more lumbar disease in HIV-positive patients. Risk of surgery for bone TB is doubled in asymptomatic HIV-positive patients and tripled in those manifesting clinical signs and symptoms. He notes that early HIV infection should not preclude surgery for those who would benefit from it.

The clinical characteristics of spinal TB in HIV-positive patients on highly active antiretroviral therapy have yet to be reported.

Although the MRC studies showed that therapy for spinal TB is effective when given as a 6-month course and guidelines for treatment of TB in HIV-positive patients allow short-course therapy, recent failures of regimens for pulmonary TB in HIV-positive patients during the continuation phase (111) highlight the fact that TB in HIV-infected patients is different. A prolonged course may be reasonable from a bacteriologic standpoint.

PREGNANCY

In the developing world, spinal TB is a disease of younger people. Because it frequently strikes during childbearing years, spinal TB in pregnancy should not be uncommon. There have been few reports (112–114). Issues in the management of paraplegia during pregnancy include the development of pressure ulcers, the effect of sensory or motor deficits during labor, and autonomic dysreflexia. In spinal TB, additional concerns include that the mother might be contagious (because many patients with spinal TB have concomitant pulmonary TB), the potential for a paraspinal abscess to complicate epidural or spinal anesthesia, and the need to avoid drugs that might harm the fetus.

Govender et al. (112) described four patients with paraplegia who were treated conservatively until delivery and underwent anterior surgery with good outcomes postpartum. Vaidya et al. (113) reported on two patients with cervical TB who underwent termination of pregnancy followed by anterior fusion because of rapidly progressive neurologic condition.

REFERENCES

1. Derry D. Pott's disease in ancient Egypt. *Med Pres Circ* 1938; 197:196–199.
2. Crubezy E, Ludes B, Poveda JD, et al. Identification of *Mycobacterium* DNA in an Egyptian Pott's disease of 5,400 years old. *Comptes Rendus Acad Sci* 1998;321:941–951.
3. Morse D. Prehistoric tuberculosis in America. *Am Rev Respir Dis* 1961;83:489–504.
4. Allison MJ, Mendoza D, Pezzia A. Documentation of a case of tuberculosis in pre-Columbian America. *Am Rev Respir Dis* 1973;107:985–991.
5. Klepinger L. Tuberculosis in the New World: more possibilities, probabilities and predictions. *Am J Phys Anthropol* 1982;57:203.
6. Salo WL, Aufderheide AC, Buikstra J, et al. Identification of *Mycobacterium tuberculosis* DNA in a pre-Columbian Peruvian mummy. *Proc Natl Acad Sci U S A* 1994;91:2091–2094.
7. Christensen D. Pre-Columbian mummy lays TB debate to rest. *Sci News* 1994;145:181.
8. Pott P. Remarks on that kind of palsy of the lower limb, which is frequently found to accompany a curvature of the spine, and is supposed to be caused by it. Together with its method of cure. In: *Medical classics* (Vol. 1, no. 4). Baltimore: Williams & Wilkins, 1936, 1779:269–337.
9. Davidson P, Horowitz, I. Skeletal tuberculosis. *Am J Med* 1970; 48:77–84.
10. Davies P, Humphries MJ, Byfied SP, et al. Bone and joint tuberculosis. A survey of notifications in England and Wales. *J Bone Joint Surg [Br]* 1984;66:326–330.
11. Dobson J. Tuberculosis of the spine. *J Bone Joint Surg [Br]* 1951;33:517–531.
12. O'Malley B, Zeft HJ. Disseminated bone tuberculosis without pulmonary manifestations. *Am J Med* 1965;38:932–936.
13. Alothman A, Memish ZA, Awada A, et al. Tuberculous spondylitis: analysis of 69 cases from Saudi Arabia. *Spine* 2001; 26:E565–E570.
14. Leibert E, Schluger NW, Bonk S, et al. Spinal tuberculosis in patients with human immunodeficiency virus infection: clinical presentation, therapy and outcome. *Tuber Lung Dis* 1996;77:329–334.
15. Moore SL, Rafii M. Imaging of musculoskeletal and spinal tuberculosis. *Radiol Clin North Am* 2001;39:329–342.
16. Yao DC, Sartoris DJ. Musculoskeletal tuberculosis. *Radiol Clin North Am* 1995;33:679–689.
17. Härö AS. Tuberculosis in Finland. Dark past—promising future. In: *Tuberculosis and respiratory diseases yearbook, volume 24*. Helsinki: The Finnish Lung Health Association, 1998:1–151.
18. Paus B. The changed pattern of bone and joint tuberculosis in Norway. *Acta Orthop Scand* 1977;48:277–279.
19. Janssens JP, de Haller R. Spinal tuberculosis in a developed country. A review of 26 cases with special emphasis on abscesses and neurologic complications. *Clin Orthop* 1990:67–75.
20. Rezai AR, Lee M, Cooper PR, et al. Modern management of spinal tuberculosis. *Neurosurgery* 1995;36:87–98.
21. Brudney K, Dobkin J. Resurgent tuberculosis in New York City. Human immunodeficiency virus, homelessness, and the decline of tuberculosis control programs. *Am Rev Respir Dis* 1991;144:745–749.
22. Bureau of Tuberculosis Control. *Information summary, 2000*. New York: New York City Department of Health, 2001.
23. Fujiwara PI. Tide pools: what will be left after the tide has turned? *Int J Tuberc Lung Dis* 2000;4:S111–S1116.
24. Jellis JE. Orthopaedic surgery and HIV disease in Africa. *Int Orthop* 1996;20:253–256.
25. Chaisson RE, Schecter GF, Theuer CP, et al. Tuberculosis in patients with the acquired immunodeficiency syndrome. Clinical features, response to therapy, and survival. *Am Rev Respir Dis* 1987;136:570–574.
26. Narlawar RS, Shah JR, Pimple MK, et al. Isolated tuberculosis of posterior elements of spine: magnetic resonance imaging findings in 33 patients. *Spine* 2002;27:275–281.
27. Gorse GJ, Pais MJ, Kusske JA, et al. Tuberculous spondylitis. A report of six cases and a review of the literature. *Medicine* 1983; 62:178–193.
28. Antunes JL. Infections of the spine. *Acta Neurochir* 1992;116:179–186.
29. Pertuiset E, Beaudreuil J, Liote F, et al. Spinal tuberculosis in adults. A study of 103 cases in a developed country, 1980–1994. *Medicine* 1999;78:309–320.
30. Boxer DI, Pratt C, Hine AL, et al. Radiological features during and following treatment of spinal tuberculosis. *Br J Radiol* 1992;65:476–479.
31. Rajasekaran S. The problem of deformity in spinal tuberculosis. *Clin Orthop* 2002:85–92.
32. Babhulkar SS, Tayade WB, Babhulkar SK. Atypical spinal tuberculosis. *J Bone Joint Surg [Br]* 1984;66:239–242.
33. Travlos J, du Toit G. Spinal tuberculosis: beware the posterior elements. *J Bone Joint Surg [Br]* 1990;72:722–723.
34. Sharif HS, Morgan JL, al Shahed MS, et al. Role of CT and MR imaging in the management of tuberculous spondylitis. *Radiol Clin North Am* 1995;33:787–804.
35. Boachie-Adjei O, Squillante RG. Tuberculosis of the spine. *Orthop Clin North Am* 1996;27:95–103.
36. Seddon H. Pott's paraplegia: prognosis and treatment. *Br J Surg* 1935;22:769–799.
37. McKee G. A comparison of the results of spinal fixation operations and non-operative treatment in Pott's disease in adults. *Br J Surg* 1937;24:456.
38. Cordova F, Criner GJ. A 25-year-old man with back pain and an abnormal chest radiograph. *Chest* 1996;109:559–561.
39. Naim Ur R, El-Bakry A, Jamjoom A, et al. Atypical forms of spinal tuberculosis: case report and review of the literature. *Surg Neurol* 1999;51:602–607.
40. Hayes AJ, Choksey M, Barnes N, et al. Spinal tuberculosis in developed countries: difficulties in diagnosis. *J R Coll Surg Edinb* 1996;41:192–196.
41. Azzam NI, Tammawy M. Tuberculous spondylitis in adults: diagnosis and treatment. *Br J Neurosurg* 1988;2:85–91.
42. Tuli SM, Srivastava TP, Varma BP, et al. Tuberculosis of spine. *Acta Orthop Scand* 1967;38:445–458.
43. Hsu LC, Leong JC. Tuberculosis of the lower cervical spine (C2 to C7). A report on 40 cases. *J Bone Joint Surg [Br]* 1984;66:1–5.
44. Lifeso RM, Weaver P, Harder EH. Tuberculous spondylitis in adults. *J Bone Joint Surg [Br]* 1985;67:1405–1413.
45. Evanchick CC, Davis DE, Harrington TM. Tuberculosis of peripheral joints: an often missed diagnosis. *J Rheumatol* 1986; 13:187–189.
46. Anonymous. A controlled trial of ambulant out-patient treatment and in-patient rest in bed in the management of tubercu-

losis of the spine in young Korean patients on standard chemotherapy a study in Masan, Korea. First report of the Medical Research Council Working Party on Tuberculosis of the Spine. *J Bone Joint Surg [Br]* 1973;55:678–697.

47. Anonymous. A controlled trial of plaster-of-paris jackets in the management of ambulant outpatient treatment of tuberculosis of the spine in children on standard chemotherapy. A study in Pusan, Korea. Second report of the Medical Research Council Working Party on Tuberculosis of the Spine. *Tubercle* 1973; 54:261–282.

48. Anonymous. A controlled trial of anterior spinal fusion and debridement in the surgical management of tuberculosis of the spine in patients on standard chemotherapy: a study in Hong Kong. *Br J Surg* 1974;61:853–866.

49. Anonymous. A controlled trial of debridement and ambulatory treatment in the management of tuberculosis of the spine in patients on standard chemotherapy. *J Trop Med Hyg* 1974;77: 72–92.

50. Omari B, Robertson JM, Nelson RJ, et al. Pott's disease. A resurgent challenge to the thoracic surgeon. *Chest* 1989;95: 145–150.

51. Slater RR Jr, Beale RW, Bullitt E. Pott's disease of the cervical spine. *South Med J* 1991;84:521–523.

52. Desai SS. Early diagnosis of spinal tuberculosis by MRI. *J Bone Joint Surg [Br]* 1994;76:863–869.

53. Masood S. Diagnosis of tuberculosis of bone and soft tissue by fine-needle aspiration biopsy. *Diagn Cytopathol* 1992;8: 451–455.

54. Kohli S. Radical surgical approach to spinal tuberculosis. *J Bone Joint Surg [Br]* 1967;49:668–673.

55. Ito H, Tsuchiya J, Asami G. A new radical operation for Pott's disease. *J Bone Joint Surg* 1934;16:499.

56. Ryan F. *The forgotten plague: how the battle against tuberculosis was won and lost.* Boston: Little, Brown, 1992.

57. Hodgson A, Stock FE. Anterior spinal fusion. Preliminary communication on the radical treatment of Pott's paraplegia. *Br J Surg* 1956;44:266–275.

58. Hodgson A, Stock FE. Anterior spine fusion for the treatment of tuberculosis of the spine. *J Bone Joint Surg [Am]* 1960;42: 295–310.

59. Hodgson A, Yan A, Kwon JS. A clinical study of 100 consecutive cases of Pott's paraplegia. *Clin Orthop* 1964;36:128–150.

60. Konstam P, Blesovsky, A. The ambulant treatment of spinal tuberculosis. *Br J Surg* 1962;50:26–38.

61. Anonymous. Long-tern chemotherapy in the treatment of chronic pulmonary tuberculosis with cavitation. A report to the Medical Research Council by their Tuberculosis Chemotherapy Trials Committee. *Tuber Lung Dis* 1962;43:201–267.

62. Anonymous. A five-year assessment of controlled trials of in-patient and out-patient treatment and of plaster-of-Paris jackets for tuberculosis of the spine in children on standard chemotherapy. Studies in Masan and Pusan, Korea. Fifth report of the Medical Research Council Working Party on tuberculosis of the spine. *J Bone Joint Surg [Br]* 1976;58:399–411.

63. Anonymous. A controlled trial of anterior spinal fusion and debridement in the surgical management of tuberculosis of the spine in patients on standard chemotherapy: a study in two centres in South Africa. Seventh Report of the Medical Research Council Working Party on tuberculosis of the spine. *Tubercle* 1978;59:79–105.

64. Anonymous. Five-year assessments of controlled trials of ambulatory treatment, debridement and anterior spinal fusion in the management of tuberculosis of the spine. Studies in Bulawayo (Rhodesia) and in Hong Kong. Sixth report of the Medical Research Council Working Party on Tuberculosis of the Spine. *J Bone Joint Surg [Br]* 1978;60:163–177.

65. Anonymous. A 10-year assessment of a controlled trial comparing debridement and anterior spinal fusion in the management of tuberculosis of the spine in patients on standard chemotherapy in Hong Kong. Eighth Report of the Medical Research Council Working Party on Tuberculosis of the Spine. *J Bone Joint Surg [Br]* 1982;64:393–398.

66. Anonymous. A 10-year assessment of controlled trials of inpatient and outpatient treatment and of plaster-of-Paris jackets for tuberculosis of the spine in children on standard chemotherapy. Studies in Masan and Pusan, Korea. Ninth report of the Medical Research Council Working Party on Tuberculosis of the Spine. *J Bone Joint Surg [Br]* 1985;67:103–110.

67. Anonymous. A controlled trial of six-month and nine-month regimens of chemotherapy in patients undergoing radical surgery for tuberculosis of the spine in Hong Kong. Tenth report of the Medical Research Council Working Party on Tuberculosis of the Spine. *Tubercle* 1986;67:243–259.

68. Anonymous. Controlled trial of short-course regimens of chemotherapy in the ambulatory treatment of spinal tuberculosis. Results at three years of a study in Korea. Twelfth report of the Medical Research Council Working Party on Tuberculosis of the Spine. *J Bone Joint Surg [Br]* 1993;75:240–248.

69. Anonymous. Five-year assessment of controlled trials of short-course chemotherapy regimens of 6, 9 or 18 months' duration for spinal tuberculosis in patients ambulatory from the start or undergoing radical surgery. Fourteenth report of the Medical Research Council Working Party on Tuberculosis of the Spine. *Int Orthop* 1999;23:73–81.

70. Parthasarathy R, Sriram K, Santha T, et al. Short-course chemotherapy for tuberculosis of the spine. A comparison between ambulant treatment and radical surgery—ten-year report. *J Bone Joint Surg [Br]* 1999;81:464–471.

71. Indian Council of Medical Research/British Medical Research Council Working Party. A controlled trial of short-course regimens of chemotherapy in patients receiving ambulatory treatment or undergoing radical surgery for tuberculosis of the spine. *Indian J Tuberc* 1989;36[Suppl]:1–21.

72. Moon MS. Tuberculosis of the spine. Controversies and a new challenge. *Spine* 1997; 22:1791–1797.

73. Roy TM, Giles C, Mendieta J, et al. Pott's disease in Kentucky: diagnosis and treatment. *J Kentucky Med Assoc* 1988;86: 499–502.

74. Bass JB Jr, Farer LS, Hopewell PC, et al. Treatment of tuberculosis and tuberculosis infection in adults and children. American Thoracic Society and The Centers for Disease Control and Prevention. *Am J Respir Crit Care Med* 1994;149: 1359–1374.

75. van LR, Verbeek AL, Jutte PC. Chemotherapeutic treatment for spinal tuberculosis. *Int J Tuberc Lung Dis* 2002;6:259–265.

76. Rieder HL, Arnadottir T, Trebucq A, et al. Tuberculosis treatment: dangerous regimens? *Int J Tuberc Lung Dis* 2001;5:1–3.

77. Tuli SM. Results of treatment of spinal tuberculosis by "middle-path" regime. *J Bone Joint Surg [Br]* 1975;57:13–23.

78. Okwera A, Whalen C, Byekwaso F, et al. Randomised trial of thiacetazone and rifampicin-containing regimens for pulmonary tuberculosis in HIV-infected Ugandans. The Makerere University-Case Western University Research Collaboration. *Lancet* 1994;344:1323–1328.

79. van Gorkom J, Kibuga DK. Cost-effectiveness and total costs of three alternative strategies for the prevention and management of severe skin reactions attributable to thiacetazone in the treatment of human immunodeficiency virus positive patients with tuberculosis in Kenya. *Tuber Lung Dis* 1996;77:30–36.

80. Lindquist SW, Steinmetz BA, Starke JR. Multidrug-resistant tuberculosis of the first cervical vertebra in an immunocompetent adolescent. *Pediatr Infect Dis J* 1997;16:333–336.

81. Cherifi S, Guillaume MP, Peretz A. Multidrug-resistant tuberculosis spondylitis. *Acta Clin Belg* 2000;55:34–36.
82. Sbarbaro JA. Of pride and program planning—a lesson in reality. *Chest* 1998;114:1229–1230.
83. Schluger N, Ciotoli C, Cohen D, et al. Comprehensive tuberculosis control for patients at high risk for noncompliance. *Am J Respir Crit Care Med* 1995;151:1486–1490.
84. Feldman G, Srivastava P, Eden E, et al. Detention until cure as a last resort: New York City's experience with involuntary in-hospital civil detention of persistently nonadherent tuberculosis patients. *Semin Respir Crit Care Med* 1997;18:493–501.
85. Moore RD, Chaulk CP, Griffiths R, et al. Cost-effectiveness of directly observed versus self-administered therapy for tuberculosis. *Am J Respir Crit Care Med* 1996;154:1013–1019.
86. Cohn DL, Catlin BJ, Peterson KL, et al. A 62-dose, 6-month therapy for pulmonary and extrapulmonary tuberculosis. A twice-weekly, directly observed, and cost-effective regimen. *Ann Intern Med* 1990;112:407–415.
87. Bureau of Tuberculosis Control. *Clinical policies and protocols.* New York: New York City Department of Health, 1999.
88. Chakirgil GS. Evaluation of anterior spinal fusion for treatment of vertebral tuberculosis. *Orthopedics* 1991;14:601–607.
89. Jain AK. Treatment of tuberculosis of the spine with neurologic complications. *Clin Orthop* 2002;398:75–84.
90. Louw JA. Spinal tuberculosis with neurological deficit. Treatment with anterior vascularised rib grafts, posterior osteotomies and fusion. *J Bone Joint Surg [Br]* 1990;72:686–693.
91. Martin NS. Pott's paraplegia. A report on 120 cases. *J Bone Joint Surg [Br]* 1971;53:596–608.
92. Altman GT, Altman DT, Frankovitch KF. Anterior and posterior fusion for children with tuberculosis of the spine. *Clin Orthop* 1996;325:225–31.
93. Korkusuz F, Islam C, Korkusuz Z. Prevention of postoperative late kyphosis in Pott's disease by anterior decompression and intervertebral grafting. *World J Surg* 1997;21:524–528.
94. Rajasekaran S, Shanmugasundaram TK. Prediction of the angle of gibbus deformity in tuberculosis of the spine. *J Bone Joint Surg [Br]* 1987;69:503–509.
95. Yau AC, Hodgson AR. Penetration of the lung by the paravertebral abscess in tuberculosis of the spine. *J Bone Joint Surg [Br]* 1968;50:243–254.
96. Mehta JS, Bhojraj SY. Tuberculosis of the thoracic spine. A classification based on the selection of surgical strategies. *J Bone Joint Surg [Br]* 2001;83:859–863.
97. Yilmaz C, Selek HY, Gurkan I, et al. Anterior instrumentation for the treatment of spinal tuberculosis. *J Bone Joint Surg [Br]* 1999;81:1261–1267.
98. Govender S, Parbhoo AH, Kumar KP, et al. Anterior spinal decompression in HIV-positive patients with tuberculosis. A prospective study. *J Bone Joint Surg [Br]* 2001;83:864–867.
99. Chen WJ, Wu CC, Jung CH, et al. Combined anterior and posterior surgeries in the treatment of spinal tuberculous spondylitis. *Clin Orthop* 2002;398:50–59.
100. Oga M, Arizono T, Takasita M, et al. Evaluation of the risk of instrumentation as a foreign body in spinal tuberculosis. Clinical and biologic study. *Spine* 1993;18:1890–1894.
101. Wood GWI. Infections of spine. In: Canale ST, ed. *Campbell's operative orthopaedics.* St. Louis: Mosby, 1998:3113–3121.
102. Martin NS. Tuberculosis of the spine. A study of the results of treatment during the last twenty-five years. *J Bone Joint Surg [Br]* 1970;52:613–628.
103. Guirguis AR. Pott's paraplegia. *J Bone Joint Surg [Br]* 1967;49:658–667.
104. Jain AK, Kumar S, Tuli SM. Tuberculosis of spine (C1 to D4). *Spinal Cord* 1999;37:362–369.
105. Fang D, Leong JC, Fang HS. Tuberculosis of the upper cervical spine. *J Bone Joint Surg [Br]* 1983;65:47–50.
106. Lifeso R. Atlanto-axial tuberculosis in adults. *J Bone Joint Surg [Br]* 1987;69:183–187.
107. Tuli S. Management and results. In: Tuli S, ed. *Tuberculosis of the skeletal system.* New Delhi: Jaypee Brothers Medical Publishers Ltd, 1997:240–261.
108. al Arabi KM, al Sebai MW. Bifacetal dislocation following tuberculosis of the cervical spine. *Tubercle* 1991;72:294–298.
109. Jones BE, Young SM, Antoniskis D, et al. Relationship of the manifestations of tuberculosis to CD4 cell counts in patients with human immunodeficiency virus infection. *Am Rev Respir Dis* 1993;148:1292–1297.
110. Jellis JE. Human immunodeficiency virus and osteoarticular tuberculosis. *Clin Orthop* 2002;398:27–31.
111. Anonymous. Acquired rifamycin resistance in persons with advanced HIV disease being treated for active tuberculosis with intermittent rifamycin-based regimens. *MMWR Morb Mortal Wkly Rep* 2002;51:214–215.
112. Govender SM, Moodley SC, Grootboom, MJ. Tuberculous paraplegia during pregnancy. A report of 4 cases. *S Afr Med J* 1989;75:190–192.
113. Vaidya MS, Shah GV, Bharucha, KE. Pregnancy and its outcome in quadriplegia due to Pott's spine. *Int J Gynaecol Obstet* 1995;49:319–321.
114. Casper GH, Heath P, Garland SM. A pain in the neck in pregnancy: cervical spinal tuberculosis. *Aust N Z J Obstet Gynaecol* 1995;35:398–400.

38

NONVERTEBRAL INFECTIONS OF THE MUSCULOSKELETAL SYSTEM BY *MYCOBACTERIUM TUBERCULOSIS*

SARA B. KRAMER
SICY H. S. LEE
STEVEN B. ABRAMSON

Involvement of the musculoskeletal system is a rare extrapulmonary complication of *Mycobacterium tuberculosis*. The clinical presentation is often insidious and nonspecific and may occur without overt pulmonary tuberculosis (TB) or other organ involvement. Therefore, the diagnosis is often difficult and the treatment is frequently delayed such that at the time of diagnosis osseous destruction is often present. Knowledge of the disease and an index of suspicion are essential to making a prompt diagnosis. Vertebral infection (Pott disease) is the most common form of musculoskeletal TB, accounting for nearly 50% of all cases. This entity is discussed in Chapter 37. Peripheral joint, tendon, muscular, osteomyelitis, and bursal involvement are addressed in this chapter.

EPIDEMIOLOGY

The incidence of TB in the United States significantly declined in the 1950s until the early 1980s, from 84,000 reported cases in 1953 to a nadir of approximately 22,000 cases in 1984. From 1985 to 1991, however, the number of reported TB cases increased: 39,000 more cases were reported than would have been expected had the previous downward trend continued (1). This resurgence is attributed to the occurrence of TB among human immunodeficiency virus–infected individuals and the increase of drug-resistant

S. B. Kramer: Department of Medicine, New York University School of Medicine; Department of Medicine, New York University Medical Center, New York, New York.

S. H. S. Lee: Department of Medicine, Division of Rheumatology, New York University School of Medicine; New York University–Hospital for Joint Diseases, New York, New York.

S. B. Abramson: Department of Medicine, New York University School of Medicine; Division of Rheumatology and Medicine, New York University–Hospital for Joint Diseases, New York, New York.

TB. Along with the increased frequency of pulmonary TB, there is also a disproportionate increased rate of extrapulmonary TB, and among the cases of extrapulmonary TB, the incidence of osteoarticular TB has also increased. In the United States, extrapulmonary TB accounted for 7.8% of all TB cases and the number increased to 13.0% in 1973 and 18.5% in 1989 (2,3). Correspondingly, the percentage for osteoarticular TB was 1.1% in 1973 and increased to 1.8% by 1989, accounting for 10% of all extrapulmonary TB. Half of these had no evidence of pulmonary involvement (2,3). These increases appear to be more pronounced among immigrants and minority groups including blacks, Hispanics, Asians, and Native Americans (4). From 1993 to 1996, new cases of TB were reported to have fallen again, except in foreign-born individuals (2). Several studies reported the epidemiologic differences between immigrant and native populations in industrialized countries. In a 1978 to 1987 study conducted at Saroka Medical Center, Beer Sheva, Israel, among 279 patients with TB, 33% also had extrapulmonary involvement. Of these, 51% were Jews of Ethiopian origin. Of the individuals with extrapulmonary TB, osteoarticular TB occurred in 8% (5). Another study reported the results of a national survey in Wales and England in a 6-month period in 1978 to 1979. Of the 4,172 patients reported to have TB during that period, 58% were white and 34% were immigrants primarily from India. There was a relative increased incidence of extrapulmonary TB among immigrants (40% among whites versus 55% among Indians) (6). Another study conducted at Blackburn, United Kingdom, surveyed 1,120 reported patients with TB from 1978 to 1987. Among these patients, 6.3% had osteoarticular TB, and this occurred two times more often among patients of Indian subcontinent ethnic origin compared with native-born whites. Two percent to 3% of immigrants accounted for one-third of the total TB cases and more than 50% had manifestations of extrapulmonary involvement (7).

In recent years, there has been a decrease in the incidence of TB in the United States. In 2000, a total of 16,377 cases representing a 39% decrease from 1992 when the number of cases peaked in the United States. (8). There are no data on the rate of musculoskeletal TB during this period.

Several underlying diseases have also been implicated to increase the risk of mycobacteria infections and include diabetes mellitus, long-term corticosteroid use, chronic renal failure, blood dyscrasias, chronic obstructive pulmonary disease, peptic ulcer disease, gastrectomy, alcoholism, cirrhosis, Paget disease, drug abuse, the use of antibody against tumor necrosis factor for the treatment of rheumatoid arthritis and Crohn disease, and HIV infection (9–11). The risk of developing active TB in patients with acquired immunodeficiency syndrome not receiving isoniazid chemoprophylaxis was higher in those with a positive tuberculin purified protein derivative (PPD) skin test result (10.4 cases per 100 person-years) and in anergic patients (12.4 cases per 100 person-years) than in nonanergic patients with a negative PPD test result (5.4 cases per 100 person-years) (12). Among patients with acquired immunodeficiency syndrome infected with TB, extrapulmonary involvement is extremely common, occurring in 30% to 70% of patients, although osteoarticular involvement is less common (4).

Articular TB affects both genders equally, although there may be a slight increase in incidence among males (3). In the past, it has been considered a disease affecting primarily the very young, although in industrialized and developed countries, the incidence has been increasing with age and is found to be most frequent in the 25- to 44-year age group (4,6,13,14). Among less developed countries, an analysis of 194 patients with osteoarticular TB in Meerut, India, reported that the highest incidence was in the second decade (30%), followed by the first (22%), the third (18%), and then the fourth decade (14%) (15). In another study conducted in Tunisia, 4% of patients were children or adolescents, 75% were 20 to 60 years old, and 10% were 60 to 80 years old. In the United States, the incidence in the 25- to 44-year age group is increased among blacks (2,898 cases in 1985 to 4,628 cases in 1991, an increase of 59.7%) and Hispanics (1,153 cases in 1985 to 2,257 cases in 1991, an increase of 95.8 %) (16).

CLINICAL PRESENTATION

Osteoarticular TB occurs primarily by lymphohematogenous spread from a primary focus. It also can occur, infrequently, by contiguous spread from adjacent tissues or direct inoculation (17). The onset of osteoarticular TB is usually insidious, with the infection remaining latent for years before it becomes active (average of 6 to 24 months) (9). Systemic symptoms of fever, night sweats, and weight loss may or may not be present during active osteoarticular

TB. Fewer than 50% of individuals with osteoarticular TB have detectable active pulmonary TB at the time of diagnosis. The symptoms often mimic more common forms of inflammatory arthritis including juvenile rheumatoid arthritis (18) or coexist with another process such as gout (19). Local pain is the most common symptom followed by impairment of movement of the affected area. Local swelling of superficial joints and bone is a frequent manifestation and regional muscle wasting and deformity may occur. In other cases, painless cold abscess was the only presenting clinical feature (15). Involvement of multiple sites is seen in 5% to 30% of cases of articular TB (8,9). Reactivation after treatment occurs in 17% to 34% of individuals, most commonly in the hip (20).

Tuberculosis of Peripheral Joints

Tuberculous arthritis occurs primarily in weight-bearing joints, the most commonly involved being the hips and knees, ankles, and feet, in descending order. Among non-weight-bearing joints, the most commonly involved in descending order are the elbows, wrists, joints in the hands (dactylitis), and shoulders (15,21,22). In a recent series of 18 patients from Spain with extraspinal tuberculous musculoskeletal involvement, 22% had infection in the lower limbs, followed by 16.6% in the upper limbs and the same number in the pelvis. More than half (55.5%) had isolated soft-tissue involvement including muscle, synovial tendon sheath, synovial bursa, and fascial tissue. Half of the patients in this series had involvement in more than one location (22). The period from the onset of initial symptoms to clinical confirmation ranges from 12 to 36 months, with a mean duration of 19.5 months (23). In one series, the diagnosis was made after a mean duration of 6.5 ± 7 years (range, 2 weeks to 20 years) from the onset of disease to the time of diagnosis with chronic progressive joint pain seen in all (24). Limitation of motion is seen in 80% and joint swelling in 40%. Chronic sinus formation is reported in 25% to 50%, and periarticular abscesses in 50%. More than 80% of patients have monoarticular involvement. Evidence for extraarticular postprimary TB is present in more than 50% of the patients, with pulmonary involvement being the most prevalent; extrapulmonary nonarticular TB such as lymphadenopathy, kidney, and skin involvement has also been reported (20,24,25). Systemic features of mild fever, weight loss, and fatigue are present in approximately 50% of the patients. Results of skin tests with five tuberculin units of PPD are positive in more than 90% of the patients (20).

Osteomyelitis

Bone involvement is usually by hematogenous spread but can occur by lymphatic or local extension secondary to contiguous tuberculous synovitis, or, conversely, osteomyelitis may lead to a septic joint (26). Osteomyelitis comprises 2%

to 3% of all cases of musculoskeletal TB. It usually presents with pain and swelling with abscess and sinus formation (27). Appendicular tuberculous osteomyelitis can occur without joint involvement. In adults, it usually occurs as a single lesion, with a predilection for metaphysis of long bones including the femur, tibia, and ulna, with the ribs, pubis, and skull being less common sites. In children, multiple lesions in the long bones predominate, but the short tubular bones of the hands and feet may be infected (tuberculous dactylitis), although the latter is rarely seen in adults (4%). Contiguous sinus tracts and cold soft-tissue abscesses often occur. TB infection can be masked by staphylococcal infection and therefore should be suspected and excluded in individuals who have staphylococcal osteomyelitis and respond poorly to antistaphylococcal agents (28). Diagnosis is frequently delayed in patients with widespread lytic lesions of TB because it occurs rarely and multiple osteolytic lesions are usually regarded as highly suggestive of malignancy. Radiographs typically reveal lytic lesions with variable degrees of sclerosis and periosteal reaction. If the lesion is complicated by secondary infection, there may be more sclerosis, making it even more difficult to differentiate the lesion from pyogenic osteomyelitis (27). Tubercular osteomyelitis can at times present as closed cystic TB or closed tubercular diaphysitis, both of which lack abscess or sinus formation. Closed cystic TB is a well-defined cystic lesion in the bone without sclerosis, generalized osteopenia, or sinus formation. There is pain and swelling away from the joint. This type of radiographic finding is more common in male patients younger than 40 years of age. After treatment with antituberculous drugs, the lesion heals with sclerosis (27)

TB of the rib is an uncommon form of osteoarticular TB, although TB is the most common inflammatory lesion of the ribs (second only to metastatic neoplasm as a cause for a destructive rib lesion). TB of the rib can be pure tuberculous osteomyelitis of the ribs or juxtacostal TB with or without rib destruction. The pathogenesis is by either direct contiguous or hematogenous spread of the tubercle bacilli. The presenting symptoms are painful or nontender chest wall mass or chest pain. By computed tomography, lesions appear as well-defined juxtacostal soft-tissue masses with central low attenuation and peripheral rim enhancement, the so-called cold abscess with frequent evidence of rib destruction. The most frequent site of involvement is the rib shaft (61%), followed by the costovertebral joint (35%) and the costochondral junction (13%), although in other series, the costochondral junction was thought to be most commonly involved. Thirty percent to 60% of cases of rib TB are associated with active or healed TB. Direct extension into the lung parenchyma and pleura is uncommon but has been reported (29).

Less frequent tuberculous osteomyelitis in the head and neck region includes chronic mastoiditis after otitis media and presenting as complete facial paralysis (30). Tuberculous osteomyelitis of the mandible also has been reported

and occurs through a carious tooth or an area of gingivitis or, more commonly, is the result of the hematogenous spread of pulmonary TB. Meng (31) reported that approximately 43% of the patients with TB of the mandible had tuberculous lesions in the bones elsewhere in the body.

Reid first reported TB of the skull in 1842 (32) as an uncommon entity and accounts for 0.2% to 1.3% of all tubercular osteitis. Strauss (33), in 1933, reviewed all 220 cases in the literature at that time and added three of his own. Since then, Meng (31) described 40 cases in 1940 from China, and Mohanty et al. (33a) reported 22 cases in 1981 from India. Apart from these, sporadic reports, predominantly from the developing world, have been published (34–37). To date, TB of the skull remains uncommon, often with a delay in diagnosis. Skull lesions usually present as painless swelling or discharging sinuses. Headache is uncommon but if present is usually localized to the site of infection. Neurologic symptoms and seizures are uncommon. Trauma has been proposed but has not been substantiated to be a predisposing risk factor for TB of the skull. TB of the skull is commonly associated with TB elsewhere in the body, with the lung as the most common site of primary involvement. Calvarial involvement occurs on average more than 1 year after primary active TB infection. TB of the skull develops after breakdown of a focus elsewhere in the body, and seeding of the bacillus occurs hematogenously rather than by lymphatic spread as more commonly seen in other bones. Further development depends on host resistance and virulence of the bacillus. As the lesion develops, it perforates the inner and outer tables. The dura is extremely resistant to cranial TB. In Strauss' (33) review of 223 patients, only ten had associated tuberculous meningitis and five had cerebral TB. Contiguous spread of infection from sinuses also can occur. TB of the skull is often a disease of childhood and early adolescence but is rare in those younger than 1 year. It is prevalent equally in both sexes.

Tuberculous Tenosynovitis

Tuberculous tenosynovitis is usually secondary to involvement of adjacent bone. At least two distinctive processes may result from involvement of the hand: carpal tunnel syndrome and compound palmar ganglion, a distinctive bilobed swelling on either side of the volar carpal ligament (38,39). The clinical picture is usually swelling above the flexor retinaculum, with marked limitation in flexion and extension of the fingers, and intense local osteoporosis. The incidence of tuberculous flexor tenosynovitis is very low, and the differential diagnosis includes other causes of carpal tunnel syndrome: trauma (e.g., Colle fracture, carpal bone dislocation), tumors, myxedema, acromegaly, diabetes, pregnancy, amyloidosis, sarcoidosis, and pyogenic infection. Diagnosis is by identification of the tubercle bacilli by culture and typical granulomas histologically (40).

Childhood Osteoarticular Tuberculosis

Skeletal TB continues to be a major health hazard among children in the developing countries. The therapy of osteoarticular TB is difficult in children because the diagnosis is often delayed, resulting in more severe disease with marked deformities.

Lymphohematogenous dissemination at the time of primary infection is the most common source of extrapulmonary TB in children. Spread from established pulmonary or extrapulmonary TB is less common (41). The thoracolumbar region is the most common site and is involved in approximately 50% of reported patients, followed by the hip (15%), and the knee joint (10%) of patients. Among hospitalized patients, however, involvement of the hip joint leads to more incapacitating and crippling disease (42). Osteomyelitis without involvement of a joint occurs in 20% of the patients. In general, patients with appendicular osteoarticular TB present with deformity, limp, stiffness, pain, and discharging sinuses. Patients with spinal TB present with kyphosis, pain, spasm of paraspinal muscles, and paraparesis. The main features of tubercular osteomyelitis are pain, discharging sinuses, and thickening of the diaphyseal region on radiographic examination. Involvement of the growth plate and premature fusion is seen radiographically in more than 60% of patients. There is a male preponderance, with a male/female ratio of 2 to 3:1. The duration of symptoms at the time of presentation varies from 3 weeks to 20 months, with 70% of patients presenting 3 months after the onset of symptoms. Active or inactive pulmonary disease is found in fewer than 30% of patients, with 75% having a positive PPD skin test response and mild to moderate elevation of the erythrocyte sedimentation rate (43). Tubercular sinuses start healing within 3 to 4 months of initiation of therapy. Clinically and radiographically, the disease appears to heal at approximately 12 to 14 months in 78%. However, deformities and stiffness of the joints can persist, and kyphosis may worsen and cause permanent deformity. Patients with growth plate involvement showed shortening of the limbs. Early diagnosis is important to avoid permanent disability but is possible only with a good history, complete physical examination, and a high index of suspicion. These may be supported by a positive PPD test response, elevated erythrocyte sedimentation rate, and chest radiographs. Radiographs of the involved joints are not useful in the early stage and may even be misleading. Diagnosis is by culture of joint fluid, which usually only yields 20% to 40% positivity. Culture of synovial biopsy specimen has a higher yield with classic histologic changes (42,43).

Although the usual presentation of TB arthritis is usually insidious with synovial fluid showing predominantly mononuclear cells, Zahraa et al. (44) reported three pediatric patients in Chicago, two with an acute presentation. These two, both Hispanic boys, one 11 months and the other 4 years old, also had TB otitis media, an extrapulmonary infection occurring in less than 1% of cases. These patients had a presentation typical of an acute bacterial infection with an acutely warm swollen joint, fever, peripheral leukocytosis, and elevated erythrocyte sedimentation rate. Synovial fluid analysis showed an elevated leukocyte count with a predominance of neutrophils. PPDs, planted after the children did not respond to antibiotics, were positive and key to the diagnosis and institution of anti-TB therapy. Synovial biopsy confirmed the diagnosis in one patient. Both responded to antituberculous chemotherapy with restoration of hearing (44).

An unusual presentation of tubercular osteomyelitis was observed in nine children who presented with a long period of ill health including low-grade fever, cough, and malnutrition. Clinical examination showed bilateral thickening of the tibia and ulna with no warmth or tenderness. Radiographs showed generalized thickening and sclerosis in the diaphysis of the involved bones. All had positive PPD, and only five of the nine had chest radiograph findings for TB. Diagnosis was made by open biopsy, and all responded to appropriate therapy (27).

Poncet Disease

Although Poncet disease was originally described by Charcot in 1864 and Lancereaux in 1871, Anton Poncet first gave a detailed description of this syndrome (45). It denotes a reactive polyarthritis associated with visceral or disseminated TB in the absence of any evidence of bacteriologic infection of the joints themselves. There have been other case reports primarily involving individuals from Asian countries. Pathogenesis is unclear. Chemotherapy with antituberculous drugs has been effective and resulted in long remissions in all patients (46,47).

DIAGNOSIS

Tuberculous Arthritis

Synovial fluid aspiration with or without synovial biopsy is important in the diagnosis of TB of the joints. The synovial fluid is usually turbid or cloudy, with an elevated leukocyte count of 2,500 to 100,000 cells/mm^3, with an average of 20,000 cells/mm^3 consisting of approximately 60% neutrophils. The protein concentration is usually elevated and blood glucose–synovial fluid glucose differences were less than 50 mg/dL in 60% of reported patients (48). Results of staining of the synovial fluid are positive in approximately 20% of the patients, whereas culture yields positivity in 80% of the patients (48). Synovial biopsy specimens can reveal the histologic finding of TB in approximately 80% to 90% of the patients, although proper selection of tissue is paramount because the histologic picture can vary depending on the site of biopsy. Similarly, a synovial biopsy culture is positive in approximately 90% of the patients. The use of all three diagnostic modalities will allow the highest diagnostic yield. Sant and Bajaj (49) reported in their series of 70 patients with tuberculous synovitis that gross appearance of synovium included thickened synovial membrane in 21.4%, increased vascularity in 7.14%, grayish white appearance in 100%, caseation and destruction of cartilage in 21.4% each, and villous growth in 10.71% of patients. Microscopic appearance included the presence of fibrosis, lymphocytic infiltration, and epithelioid cells forming typical granuloma of tuberculous lesions. Caseation in 78.57%, proliferation of synovial membrane in 92.85%, and an increased number of mast cells in 82.95% of patients were observed (49). These observations corroborated with observations made by others (50,51).

Masood (52) reported the use of fine needle aspiration biopsy under radiographic guidance in the diagnosis of TB of bone and soft tissue in 11 patients. Granulomatous reaction with or without caseation necrosis was seen in 73%. The aspirated material was acellular or predominantly composed of necrotic material and inflammatory infiltrates in 27% (one-third) of the patients. Acid-fast bacilli were demonstrated by Ziehl–Neelsen staining in 64% (seven patients). Culture for *M. tuberculosis* was positive in 83%. Complemented by special stains and microbiologic culture, fine needle biopsy can be a simple alternative to open biopsy for the diagnosis of TB of bone and soft-tissue lesions. Direct amplification tests using the polymerase chain reaction have been helpful in diagnosing pulmonary TB from sputum specimens. Limited data are evaluable using this technique for extrapulmonary TB, and even less work has been done in musculoskeletal TB. A small study of tissue from patients with Pott disease showed a sensitivity of 95% and specificity of 83%. Only small series or individual case reports are available for tuberculous arthritis. These, unfortunately, have a small but disturbing number of false positives from control patients with different types of arthritis. Larger studies are needed to establish the usefulness of this technique (53).

Radiographic findings can be classified as advocated by Martini and Ouahes (54) in 1988:

- Stage I: no bony lesions, localized osteoporosis
- Stage II: one or more erosions (or cavities) in the bone, discrete diminution of the joint space
- Stage III: involvement and destruction of the whole joint without gross anatomic disorganization
- Stage IV: gross anatomic disorganization

For most patients, conventional radiographs are sufficiently reliable for the detection and follow-up of tuberculous involvement of the bone and joint. Initially, the infection may be primarily synovial, with radiographic evidence of joint swelling resulting from a combination of synovial hypertrophy and effusion. The chronic synovitis leads to hyperemia and periarticular osteoporosis. With continued growth of synovial pannus and extravascular formation of fibrin, amorphous fragments or "rice bodies" are formed. These are nonspecific for TB and have been reported in patients with rheumatoid arthritis, other fungal infections, or chronic arthritides. The normally sharp, subarticular cortical outline becomes blurred, smudged, or even invisible. Secondary marginal erosions mimic those of rheumatoid arthritis. In due course, destruction of the articular cartilage leads to narrowing of the joint space. These changes are slow compared pyogenic infection because proteolytic enzymes are absent from the tuberous exudate. Reduction in the depth of joint space is thus a late occurrence. In summary, the triad of radiographic findings (Phemister triad) consists of peripheral erosions of the synovial attachment around a joint, slow destruction of the affected joint cartilage, and considerable juxtaarticular osteoporosis (55,56).

A radionuclide bone scan is useful in the initial stages when radiographs do not yet demonstrate characteristic abnormalities. Computed tomography may be indicated if conventional radiographic techniques do not give sufficient information about bone destruction or soft-tissue involvement. Magnetic resonance imaging is a reliable modality in demonstrating early inflammation and abnormalities in the paraarticular soft tissue. Both computed tomography and magnetic resonance imaging are particularly sensitive in detecting periarticular abscesses (55). The differential diagnosis includes rheumatoid arthritis, gouty arthritis, osteoarthritis, tumors, and pyogenic arthritis. In rheumatoid arthritis, the disease is usually polyarticular and involves mainly the small bones of the hands and feet. Radiographic problems arise only when the rheumatoid arthritis is monoarticular at its onset or affects only a few medium-size joints. Osteoporosis and marginal erosions are accompanied by an early and significant narrowing of the articular space in rheumatoid arthritis, although they also produce marginal erosions resembling those in TB. In gouty arthritis, the marginal erosions usually have overhanging edges, and lobulated eccentric calcified tophi are more frequently seen. In infection, the marginal erosions are poorly defined. In osteoarthritis, subchondral bony sclerosis and osteophyte formation are usually obvious, and osteoporotic change and marginal erosions are rarely observed. In rare forms of tuberculous arthritis with extension to the neighboring bursa and tendon sheaths, swelling in the involved soft-tissue space can mimic a tumor mass. Magnetic resonance imaging can define the extent and characteristics of a tumor mass. In patients with pyogenic infection, the articular destruction can be very rapid, with complete loss of the joint space and large destructive osseous foci appearing within a period of 1 to 3 weeks; in TB, slow progression of the disease, significant osteoporosis, and mild sclerosis are more prominent. However, differentiating between tuberculous and pyogenic arthritis radiographically is still difficult, and tuberculous arthritis with secondary pyogenic infection of the sinuses is possible. In those instances, synovial fluid aspiration with or without tissue biopsy and culture would be necessary for definitive diagnosis.

Magnetic resonance imaging is a useful tool in evaluating soft-tissue involvement by TB. Pyomyositis accounted for 60% of the cases in one study of 18 patients with extraspinal osseous TB. The iliopsoas, gluteus, pectoralis, and sternocleidomastoid muscles were involved. Most muscles showed intermediate signal intensity on T1-weighted images and high or very high signal intensity on T2-weighted images (22).

In patients with TB of the skull, an area of rarefaction is evident radiographically in early disease. Commonly, this develops into a punched-out, well-circumscribed lesion with a sequestrum in its center. The less common radiographic finding is an irregular defect with widespread involvement of cancellous bone, especially of the inner table, and is seen as a large area of bone destruction with ill-defined margins, involving both the inner and outer tables at several places. The frontal and parietal bones are preferentially affected by TB because of their greater area of cancellous bone and diploic structures. Lesions may be single or multiple. Extensive sclerosis and bone reaction around the lesion, representing osteoblastic repair, are typically absent. Computed tomography shows soft-tissue swelling, cone-shaped bony defect, and bony sequestrum, and, after administration of a contrast agent, an enhanced extradural mass adjacent to the bony defect. Diagnosis is best made by biopsy and the demonstration of the tubercle bacilli by smear or culture. In the absence of this, it is essential to interpret radiographic and histologic features along with clinical findings.

TREATMENT

Although the medical literature contains multiple studies that address therapy of pulmonary TB, it contains limited studies specifically for osteoarticular TB. However, in studies (57–63) that considered the efficacy of various medical treatments, combination chemotherapy resulted in excellent cure rates. Various regimens have been proposed, from the conventional duration of 18 to 24 months to short-

term but more intensive multidrug therapy for 6 months (Table 38.1) (57–66). All regimens include isoniazid and rifampin with or without ethambutol, streptomycin, and pyrazinamide in various dosing regimens. Chemotherapy constitutes the first step in the treatment of TB (Table 38.2). For appendicular TB, immobilization and rest are reserved for relief of pain during the acute phase and should be followed by early, active mobilization without weight bearing for 4 to 6 weeks. Surgery is only indicated as a diagnostic tool and when necessary to drain an abscess unresponsive to medical treatment (67). It is not unusual for a tuberculous knee to be severely damaged. Controversy exists over the proper treatment of a knee with extensive joint damage. Arthrodesis has been considered a reasonable choice; however, patients are usually disappointed in the degree of dysfunction. Su et al. (68) reported 16 cases of TB of the knee treated with total knee replacement. Eight patients had been diagnosed before surgery and were treated with anti-TB chemotherapy for 2 to 20 months before surgery and for 1 year after arthroplasty. Eight patients were diagnosed with TB at the time of surgery and therefore were treated only postoperatively with antituberculous chemotherapy. All patients were treated with rifampicin, ethambutol, and isoniazid for 12 months after surgery. The average length of follow-up was 75 months (range, 41 to 132). Five patients cases had a recurrence of TB in the involved joint. Four of the five patients did not receive preoperative anti-TB therapy. The one patient with recurrence who had been treated preoperatively was treated with long-term corticosteroids for persistent rheumatoid synovitis after the completion of postoperative antituberculous therapy. That patient eventually required surgical removal of the prosthesis. The four remaining patients received prolonged anti-TB therapy. One developed miliary TB with lung, ankle, and knee involvement and sinus tract development. He eventually responded to antimicrobial therapy and some surgical débridement. Thus, total knee replacement is an option for patients treated pre- and postoperatively with antituberculous medications (68). For tuberculous tenosynovitis, chemotherapy often needs to be supplemented by débride-

TABLE 38.1. ANTITUBERCULOUS THERAPY

Regimen	Initial Phase		Continuation Phase	
	Drugs	Duration	Drugs	Duration
18–24 mo	INH, RMP, ± EMB or STM qd	2 mo	INH, RMP qd or b.i.w.	16–22 mo
9 mo	INH, RMP qd	1 mo	INH, RMP qd or b.i.w.	8 mo
6 mo	INH, RMP, PZA ± ETB or STM qd	2 mo	INH, RMP qd or b.i.w.	4 mo
6 mo	INH, RMP, PZA, STM qd	2 wk	INH, RMP, PZA, STM b.i.w.	6 wk
			INH, RMP b.i.w.	18 wk

b.i.w., twice weekly; ETB, ethambutol; INH, isoniazid; PZA, pyrazinamide; qd, daily; RMP, rifampin; STM, streptomycin.
Data from refs. 57–66.

TABLE 38.2. ANTITUBERCULOUS DRUGS

Drug	Daily Dose		Twice-Weekly Dose	
	Children	Adults	Children	Adults
Isoniazid	10–15 mg/kg p.o. or i.m., max. 300 mg	5 mg/kg p.o. or i.m., max. 300 mg	20–30 mg/kg p.o., max. 900 mg	15 mg/kg p.o., max. 900 mg
Rifampin	10–20 mg/kg p.o., max. 600 mg	10 mg/kg p.o., max. 600 mg	10–20 mg/kg p.o., max. 600 mg	10–20 mg/kg p.o., max. 600 mg
Pyrazinamide	15–30 mg/kg p.o., max. 2 g	—[a]	50 mg/kg p.o., max. 4 g	—[a]
Ethambutol	15–20 mg/kg p.o., max. 2.5 g	15–25 mg/kg p.o., max. 2.5 g	50 mg/kg p.o., max. 2.5 g	50 mg/kg p.o., max. 2.5 g
Streptomycin	20–40 mg/kg i.m., max. 1 g	15 mg/kg i.m., max. 1 g for age <50 yr and 10 mg/kg i.m., max. 750 mg for age >50 yr	25–30 mg/kg i.m., max. 1 g	Only after 2–4 mo, same as daily dose

[a]Daily dose ranges from 800 mg (14.5–20.0 mg/kg), 1,200 mg (16.0–21.4 mg/kg), and 1,600 mg (17.8–21.1 mg/kg) for the respective weight ranges of 40–55 kg, 56–75 kg, and 76–90 kg.
i.m., intramuscularly; max., maximum; p.o.; orally.
From American Thoracic Society/Centers for Disease Control and Prevention/Infectious Diseases Society of America. Treatment of tuberculosis. *Am J Respir Crit Care Med* 2003;167:603–662, with permission.

ment (38). Surgery is indicated for patients with vertebral TB complicated by neurologic abnormality, spinal instability, or large paravertebral or psoas abscess. Selection and subsequent adjustment of the therapeutic regimen should be based on drug resistance, side effects, compliance, and clinical response.

Treatment of skull TB includes surgery and anti-TB therapy alone or in combination. Surgery is best indicated for diagnostic purposes or removal of thick extradural granulation tissue and necrotic bone or in patients who have a sinus discharge. With the current surgical expertise and therapeutic regimens, the prognosis is good (35–37).

Individuals requiring total hip and knee arthroplasty for quiescent TB should receive perioperative antituberculous therapy (isoniazid and rifampin) 3 weeks before and 6 to 9 months after surgery to minimize risk of reactivation.

ATYPICAL MYCOBACTERIA

Atypical mycobacteria are ubiquitous in nature and are often isolated from soil, water, and animals. Some atypical mycobacteria are nonpathogenic in humans, whereas others rarely to relatively frequently cause human diseases. Some species are considered contaminants when isolated, whereas others are indicative of a disease-causing pathogen. To date, no person-to-person transmission of disease has been reported. Immunosuppressed individuals are more predisposed to such infections. Atypical mycobacterial infection of bone and joint may result from percutaneous inoculation of the organism or from hematogenous spread, and most frequently affects the tendon sheaths of the hand and wrist. Articular disease most often involves the digits, wrists, and knees. Infection of prepatellar and olecranon bursae have been reported (69,70). Atypical *Mycobacterium* species that

cause bone, joint, tendon sheath, and bursa infections can be categorized according to the Runyon classification (Table 38.3) (71–73). Among the most common atypical mycobacteria that usually cause tenosynovitis of the hands are *Mycobacterium kansasii, Mycobacterium avium-intracellulare complex, Mycobacterium fortuitum*, and *Mycobacterium chelonae*. These organisms cause infections most commonly through penetrating injuries or injections (74,75).

The diagnosis of osteoarticular atypical mycobacteria is usually established by isolation of the organism from biopsy tissue or synovial fluid and is corroborated by compatible histopathologic, clinical, and radiographic findings. Pathologic and radiographic findings for *M. tuberculosis* are usually indistinguishable from those for the atypical organisms.

M. fortuitum and *M. chelonae* are commonly found in the environment and have been reported to cause osteomyelitis and articular infections in immunocompromised individuals by hematogenous spread or direct penetration of a wound. Treatment of *M. fortuitum* infection is often difficult because the organism is usually resistant to all conventional anti-TB therapy, and treatment depends on the results of *in vitro* sensitivity studies. Current standard therapy includes surgical excision when possible plus intravenous amikacin or kanamycin and cefoxitin (with probenecid) for 2 to 6 weeks, followed by one or two oral agents with demonstrated *in vitro* efficacy for 2 to 6 months. Sulfonamides, doxycycline, and minocycline have been the most frequent oral agents (76). More recently, the fluorinated quinolone ciprofloxacin has been used effectively in combination with minocycline in the treatment of disseminated *M. fortuitum* infection (77).

M. avium-intracellulare complex infection is distributed throughout the United States, particularly the southeast. Infection of the tendon sheaths of the hand and wrist is

TABLE 38.3. ATYPICAL MYCOBACTERIA THAT ARE SKELETAL PATHOGENS

Mycobacterium Organism	Growth Rate (d)	Human Pathogen	Environmental Contaminant	Reservoir	Skeletal Infection
Photochromogens (Runyon group I)					
M. kansasii	10–21	Yes	Rarely	Water, cattle, swine (rarely)	Common
M. marinum	7–14	Yes	Rarely	Fish, water	Infrequent
Scotochromogens (Runyon group II)					
M. scrofulaceum	10–28	Yes	Yes	Soil, water, moist watery foodstuffs	Infrequent
M. flavescens	7–10	Very rarely	Yes	Soil, water	Infrequent
M. szulgai	12–28	Yes	No	Unknown	Infrequent
M. gordonae	10–28	Very rarely	Yes	Water	Infrequent
Nonchromogens (Runyon group III)					
M. avium-intracellulare	10–21	Yes	Yes	Soil, water, swine, cattle, birds, fowl	Common
M. triviale	10–21	No	Yes	Soil, water	Infrequent
M. terrae	10–21	Very rarely	Yes	Soil, water	Infrequent
M. xenopi	14–28	Yes	Yes	Water	Infrequent
M. haemophilum	56	Very rarely	Unknown	Unknown	Infrequent
Rapid growers (Runyon group IV)					
M. fortuitum	3–7	Yes	Yes	Soil, water, animals, marine life	Common
M. chelonae	3–7	Yes	Yes	Soil, water, animals, marine life	Common
M. smegmatis	3–7	Very rarely	Possibly	Moist surfaces, urogenital Flora	Infrequent

Data from Ref. 71–73.

most common, although bursitis, osteomyelitis, and septic arthritis have been reported. Surgical excision and prolonged multidrug therapy (four to five drugs for 24 to 36 months) are usually indicated because of the relative resistance of this organism to chemotherapy. Combination therapy used in the treatment includes rifampin, ethambutol, streptomycin or amikacin, clofazimine, and, more recently, ciprofloxacin and the new macrolides clarithromycin and azithromycin (78,79).

M. kansasii infection is most often found in the southwestern United States. Infection of periarticular tissue, osteomyelitis, and septic arthritis have all been reported with or without disseminated disease, particularly in immunocompromised individuals. *M. kansasii* infection responds well to combination therapy consisting of isoniazid, rifampin, and ethambutol for a period of 18 to 24 months (74,80,81).

Mycobacterium marinum is found in aquatic environments. Infection is considered occupational or hobby associated, resulting from frequent contact with fish and crustaceans. Infections occur primarily through cutaneous extension to the underlying tendon sheaths of the hand and wrist. Treatment with the combination of rifampin and ethambutol for 18 to 24 months is fairly effective. Surgery should be reserved for patients in whom chemotherapy fails or for those with adverse prognostic indicators, such as a draining sinus or persistent pain and swelling (82–85).

Mycobacterium szulgai has been reported to cause tenosynovitis and carpal tunnel syndrome. Cure can be achieved by débridement and chemotherapy with ethambutol and rifampin because this organism is resistant to isoniazid (86).

Mycobacterium haemophilum is a fastidious atypical mycobacterium that is considered an emerging pathogen in immunocompromised patients. From 1978 to 1994, there were 26 confirmed cases of infection with this organism, 11 of which were reported in the United States. In 1994, Straus et al. (87) detailed 13 more cases found in seven metropolitan hospitals in New York City between 1989 and 1991. Eight of 13 patients developed joint and bone symptoms, including tenderness and swelling. All eight individuals were human immunodeficiency virus positive and considered immunosuppressed. There are no standardized susceptibility tests for *M. haemophilum* nor is there a uniform response on susceptibility tests performed. Various regimens have been described and include isoniazid, rifampin, and ethambutol; trimethoprim-sulfamethoxazole; minocycline; erythromycin; rifampin and minocycline; rifampin and paraaminosalicylic acid; and rifampin and erythromycin. Effectiveness of the therapy frequently depends on the immunocompromised status and tolerance to therapy of the patient (87,88).

In general, medical therapy for the treatment of atypical mycobacteria infection is selected based on the species, *in vitro* susceptibilities, host immune status, and location and extent of disease. Surgical removal of affected tissue contributes significantly to clinical resolution when the organism is relatively resistant to chemotherapy.

CONCLUSION

Although tuberculous disease of bones and joints is relatively uncommon, it still occurs and can cause devastating sequelae because it is frequently not diagnosed until permanent damage has occurred. It should be considered in the differential diagnosis of monarthritis or back pain and among individuals with underlying illness or other manifestations of TB. An aggressive approach including synovial or bone biopsy is needed.

REFERENCES

1. National action plan to combat multidrug-resistant tuberculosis. *MMWR Morb Mortal Wkly Rep* 1992;41:1–48.
2. Harrington JT. Mycobacterial and fungal infections. In: Ruddy S, Harris E, Sledge C, et al. *Kelley's textbook of rheumatology.* Philadelphia: WB Saunders, 2001:1493–1505.
3. Farer LS, Lowell AM, Meador MP. Extrapulmonary tuberculosis in the United States. *Am J Epidemiol* 1979;109:205–217.
4. Rossman MD. The resurgence of tuberculous and nontuberculous mycobacteria. In: Fishman AP, ed. *Update: pulmonary disease and disorder*, vol. 2. New York: McGraw-Hill, 1992:287–297.
5. Dolberg OT, Schlaeffer F, Greene VW, et al. Extrapulmonary tuberculosis in an immigrant society: clinical and demographic aspects of 92 cases. *Rev Infect Dis* 1991;13:177–179.
6. Davies PDO, Humphries MJ, Byfield SP, et al. Bone and joint tuberculosis: a survey of notifications in England and Wales. *J Bone Joint Surg [Br]* 1984;66:326–330.
7. Hodgson SP, Ormerod LP. Ten-year experience of bone and joint tuberculosis in Blackburn 1978–1987. *J R Coll Surg Edinb* 1990;35:259–262.
8. Centers for Disease Control and Prevention. Tuberculosis morbidity among U.S.-born and foreign-born populations—United States, 2000. *MMWR Morb Mortal Wkly Rep* 2002;51:101–104.
9. Hanza M. Joint and spine tuberculosis. *Rev Rheum* 1994;60:83–86.
10. Alvarez S, McCabe WR. Extrapulmonary tuberculosis revisited: a review of experience at Boston City and other hospitals. *Medicine* 1984;63:25–55.
11. Keane J, Gershon S, Wise RP, et al. Tuberculosis associated with infliximab, a tumor necrosis factor alpha-neutralizing agent. *N Engl J Med* 2001;345:1098–1104.
12. Moreno S, Baraia-Etxburn J, Bouza E, et al. Risk for developing tuberculosis among anergic patients infected with HIV. *Ann Intern Med* 1993;119:194–198.
13. Gillespie WJ. Epidemiology in bone and joint infection. *Infect Dis Clin North Am* 1990;4:361–376.
14. Weir MR. The enigma of extrapulmonary tuberculosis. *N Y State J Med* 1989;89:251–252.
15. Agarwal RP, Mohan N, Garg RK, et al. Clinicosocial aspect of osteo-articular tuberculosis. *J Indian Med Assoc* 1990;88:307–309.
16. Barnes PF, Barrows SA. Tuberculosis in the 1990's. *Ann Intern Med* 1993;119:400–410.
17. de Jong JW, van Altena R. Non-respiratory tuberculosis with Mycobacterium tuberculosis after penetrating lesions of the skin: five case histories. *Int J Tuberc Lung Dis* 2000;4:1184–1847.
18. Al-Matar MJ, Cabral DA, Petty RE. Isolated tuberculous monoarthritis mimicking oligoarthricular juvenile rheumatoid arthritis. *J Rheumatol* 2001;28:204–206.
19. Lorenzo JP, Csuka ME, Derfus BA, et al. Concurrent gout and *Mycobacterium tuberculosis* arthritis. *J Rheumatol* 1997;24:184–186.
20. Enarson DA, Fujii M, Nakiela EM, et al. Bone and joint tuberculosis: a continuing problem. *CMAJ* 1979;120:139–145.
21. Fishman AP. Clinical forms of mycobacterial disease. In: Jeffers JD, Navrozov M, eds. *Pulmonary disease and disorders.* New York: McGraw-Hill, 1988:1851–1862.
22. Soler R, Rodriguez E, Remuinan C, et al. MRI of musculoskeletal extraspinal tuberculosis. *J Comput Assist Tomogr* 2001;25:177–183.
23. Hsu SH, Sun JS, Chen IH, et al. Reappraisal of skeletal tuberculosis: role of radiological imaging. *J Formosan Med Assoc* 1993;92:34–41.
24. Ellis ME, El-Ramahi KM, Al-Dalaan AN. Tuberculosis of peripheral joints: a dilemma in diagnosis. *Tuber Lung Dis* 1993;74:399–404.
25. Evanchick CC, Davis DE, Harrington TM. Tuberculosis of peripheral joints: an often missed diagnosis. *J Rheumatol* 1986;13:187–189.
26. Waldrogel FA, Medoff G, Swartz MN. *Osteomyelitis. Clinical features, therapeutic considerations and unusual aspects.* Springfield, IL: Charles C Thomas Publisher, 1991:78–91.
27. Babhulkar S, Pande S. Unusual manifestations of osteoarticular tuberculosis. *Clin Orthop* 2002;1:114–120.
28. Sinnott JT, Cancio MR, Frankel MA, et al. Tuberculous osteomyelitis masked by concomitant staphylococcal infection. *Arch Intern Med* 1990;150:1865–1867.
29. Lee G, Im JG, Kim JS, et al. Tuberculosis of the ribs: CT appearance. *J Comput Assist Tomogr* 1993;17:363–366.
30. Chernoff WG, Parnes LS. Tuberculous mastoiditis. *J Otolaryngol* 1992;21:290–292.
31. Meng CM. Tuberculosis of the mandible. *J Bone Joint Surg [Am]* 1940;22:17–27.
32. Ried E. Medizinisches Correspondenzblatt Bayerischer Ärzte. Erlangen, No. 33, 1842.
33. Strauss DC. Tuberculosis of the flat bones of the vault of the skull. *Surg Gynaecol Obstet* 1933;57:384–398.
33a. Mohanty S, Rao CJ, Mukherji KC. Tuberculosis of the skull. *Int Surg* 1981;66:81–83.
34. Ip M, Tsui E, Wong KL, et al. Disseminated skeletal tuberculosis with skull involvement. *Tuber Lung Dis* 1993;74:211–214.
35. Gupta PK, Kolluri VR, Chandramouli BA, et al. Calvarial tuberculosis: a report of two cases. *Neurosurgery* 1989;25:830–833.
36. Pelteret RM. Tuberculosis osteitis of the skull. *Ann Trop Paediatr* 1989;9:40–42.
37. LeRoux PD, Griffin GE, Marsh HT, et al. Tuberculosis of the skull—rare condition: case report and review of the literature. *Neurosurgery* 1990;26:851–855.
38. Wolinsky E. Disease due to mycobacteria. In: Wyngaarden JB, Smith LH, Bennett JC, eds. *Textbook of internal medicine.* Philadelphia: WB Saunders, 1992:1733–1742.
39. Klofkorn RW, Steigerwald JC. Carpal tunnel syndrome as the initial manifestation of tuberculosis. *Am J Med* 1976;60:583–586.
40. Cramer K, Seiler JG, Milek MA. Tuberculous tenosynovitis of the wrist. Two case reports. *Clin Orthop* 1991;262:137–140.
41. Jacobs JC, Li SC, Ruzal-Shapiro C, et al. Tuberculous arthritis in children. *Clin Pediatr* 1994;33:344–348.
42. Negusse W. Bone and joint tuberculosis in childhood in a children's hospital, Addis Ababa. *Ethiop Med J* 1993;31:51–61.
43. Singh SB, Saraf SK, Singh LI, et al. Osteoarticular tuberculosis in children. *Indian Pediatr* 1992;29:1133–1137.
44. Zahraa J, Johnson D, Lim-Dunham J, et al. Unusual features of osteoarticular tuberculosis in children. *J Pediatr* 1996;129:597–602.
45. Isaacs AJ, Sturrock RD. Poncet's disease: fact or fiction, a reappraisal of tuberculous rheumatism. *Tubercle* 1974;55:135–142.
46. Khoury MI. Does reactive arthritis to tuberculosis (Poncet's disease) exist? *J Rheumatol* 1989;16:1162–1164.

47. Pande D, Dubey AP, Choudhary P. Poncet's disease. *Indian Pediatr* 1988;26:828–830.

48. Wallace R, Cohen AS. Tuberculous arthritis. A report of two cases with a review of biopsy and synovial fluid findings. *Am J Med* 1976;61:277–280.

49. Sant M, Bajaj H. Role of histopathology in the diagnosis of tuberculous synovitis. *J Indian Med Assoc* 1992;90:263–264.

50. Lal KB, Gupta MN, Gupta AK. Synovial biopsy in diagnosis of tuberculosis of knee joints. *Indian J Surg* 1972;34:275–279.

51. Misgar MS, Chrungoo RK, Ashrof M. The problem in the diagnosis of chronic synovitis of knee. *J Indian Med Assoc* 1978;70:132–136.

52. Masood S. Diagnosis of tuberculosis of bone and soft tissue by fine-needle aspiration biopsy. *Diagn Cytopathol* 1992;8:451–455.

53. Harrington JT. The evolving role of direct amplification tests in diagnosing osteoarticular infections caused by mycobacteria and fungi. *Curr Opin Rheumatol* 1999;11:289–292.

54. Martini M, Ouahes M. Bone and joint tuberculosis: a review of 652 cases. *Orthopedics* 1988;11:861–866.

55. Chapman M, Murray RO, Stoher DJ. Tuberculosis of the bone and joints. *Semin Roentgenol* 1978;14:266–282.

56. Harisinghani M, McLoud T, Shepard J, et al. Tuberculosis from head to toe. *Radiographics* 2000;20:449–470.

57. American Thoracic Society. Treatment of tuberculosis and tuberculosis infection in adults and children. *Am Rev Respir Dis* 1986;134:355–366.

58. Dutt AK, Moers D, Stead WW. Short-course chemotherapy for extrapulmonary tuberculosis: nine years' experience. *Ann Intern Med* 1986;104:7–12.

59. Hannachi M, Martini M, Boulahbal F, et al. Comparison of 3 chemotherapeutic regimens of short duration (6 months) in osteoarticular tuberculosis: results after 5 years. *Bull Int Union Tuberc Lung Dis* 1988;57:46–47.

60. Tenth Report of the Medical Research Council Working Party on Tuberculosis of the Spine. A controlled trial of six-month and nine-month regimens of chemotherapy in patients undergoing radical surgery for tuberculosis of the spine in Hong Kong. *Tubercle* 1986;67:243–259.

61. Dutt AK, Stead WW. Treatment of extrapulmonary tuberculosis. *Semin Respir Infect* 1989;4:225–231.

62. Cohn DL, Catlin BJ, Peterson KL, et al. A 62-dose, 6-month therapy for pulmonary and extrapulmonary tuberculosis: a twice weekly, directly observed, and cost-effective regimen. *Ann Intern Med* 1990;112:407–415.

63. Combs DL, O'Brien RJ, Geiter LJ. USPHS Tuberculosis Short-Course Chemotherapy Trial 21: effectiveness, toxicity, and acceptability: the report of final results. *Ann Intern Med* 1990;112:397–406.

64. Moon MS, Kim I, Woo YK, et al. Conservative treatment of tuberculosis of the thoracic and lumbar spine in adults and children. *Int Orthop* 1987;11:315–322.

65. Biddulph J. Short-course chemotherapy for childhood tuberculosis. *Pediatr Infect Dis J* 1990;9:794–801.

66. Tuberculosis of the spine: a 10 year assessment of a controlled trial comparing debridement and anterior spinal fusion in the management of tuberculosis of the spine in patients on standard chemotherapy in Hong Kong. *J Bone Joint Surg [Br]* 1982;64:383–398.

67. Aguirre M, Bago J, Martin N. Tuberculosis of the knee. *Acta Orthop Belg* 1989;55:22–25.

68. Su J, Huang T, Lui S. Total knee arthroplasty in tuberculous arthritis. *Clin Orthop* 1996;323:181–187.

69. Schickendantz MS, Watson JT. Mycobacterial prepatellar bursitis. *Clin Orthop* 1990;258:209–212.

70. Marcheusky AM, Damster B, Green S. The clinicopathological spectrum of non-tuberculous/mycobacterial osteoarticular infections. *J Bone Joint Surg [Am]* 1985;67:925–929.

71. Wolinsky E. Nontuberculous mycobacteria and associated diseases. *Am Rev Respir Dis* 1979;119:107–159.

72. Saunders WE Jr, Horowitz EA. Other *Mycobacterium* species. In: Mandell GL, Douglas RG Jr, Bennett JE, eds. *Principles and practice of infectious diseases*, Vol. 3. New York: Churchill Livingstone, 1990:1914–1926.

73. Woods GL, Washington JA II. Mycobacteria other than *Mycobacterium tuberculosis*: review of microbiologic and clinical aspects. *Rev Infect Dis* 1987;9:275–294.

74. Dixon JM. Non-tuberculous mycobacterial infection of the tendon sheaths in the hand. *J Bone Joint Surg [Br]* 1980;63:542–544.

75. Wallace RJ, Swenson JR, Silcox VA, et al. Spectrum of disease due to rapidly growing mycobacteria. *Rev Infect Dis* 1983;5:657–679.

76. Ip RK, Chow SP. *Mycobacterium fortuitum* infections of the hand. Report of five cases. *J Hand Surg* 1992;17:675–677.

77. Burns DN, Rohatgi PK, Rosenthal R, et al. Disseminated *Mycobacterium fortuitum* successfully treated with combination therapy including ciprofloxacin [Erratum appears in *Am Rev Respir Dis* 1990;142:1235]. *Am Rev Respir Dis* 1990;142:468–470.

78. Ellyer JJ, Goldberger MJ, Parenti DM. *Mycobacterium avium* infection and AIDS: a therapeutic dilemma in rapid evaluation. *J Infect Dis* 1991;163:1326–1335.

79. Wolinsky E. Mycobacterial diseases other than tuberculosis. *Clin Infect Dis* 1992;15:1–12.

80. Dillon J, Millson C, Morris L. *Mycobacterium kansasii* infection in the wrist and hand. *Br J Rheumatol* 1990;29:150–153.

81. Carroll SR, Newson SW, Tenner JR. Treatment of septic arthritis due to *Mycobacterium kansasii*. *BMJ* 1984;289:591–592.

82. Chow SP, Stoebal AB, Lou JHK. *Mycobacterium marinum* infection of the hand involving deep structures. *J Hand Surg* 1983;8:568–573.

83. Jones MW, Wahid IA, Matthews JP. Septic arthritis of the hand due to *Mycobacterium marinum* in fisherman. *J Clin Microbiol* 1988;28:333–334.

84. Clark RB, Spector H, Friedman DM, et al. Osteomyelitis and synovitis produced by *Mycobacterium marinum* in fisherman. *J Clin Microbiol* 1990;28:2570–2572.

85. Donta ST, Smith PW, Levitz RE. Therapy of *Mycobacterium marinum* infections. *Ann Intern Med* 1986;146:902–904.

86. Stratton CW, Phelps DB, Relhr LB. Tuberculoid tenosynovitis and carpal tunnel syndrome caused by *Mycobacterium szulgai*. *Am J Med* 1978;65:349–350.

87. Straus WL, Ostroff SM, Jernigan DB, et al. Clinical and epidemiologic characteristics of *Mycobacterium haemophilum*, an emerging pathogen in immunocompromised patients. *Ann Intern Med* 1994;120:118–125.

88. Gupta I, Kocher J, Miller AJ, et al. *Mycobacterium haemophilum* osteomyelitis in an AIDS patient. *N J Med* 1992;89:201–202.

89. American Thoracic Society/Centers for Disease Control and Prevention/Infectious Diseases Society of America. Treatment of tuberculosis. *Am J Respir Crit Care Med* 2003;167:603–662.

ENDOCRINE AND METABOLIC MANIFESTATIONS OF TUBERCULOSIS

JOSEPH LOWY

Tuberculosis has long been known to affect the endocrine organs; historically, this infection was among the first conditions to be described with such varied endocrine metabolic disorders as adrenal insufficiency, the syndrome of inappropriate antidiuretic hormone secretion (SIADH), and hypercalcemia. Conversely, there are primary hormonal disorders and therapies that may predispose to the activation or spread of tuberculosis, such as diabetes mellitus and corticosteroid administration. Furthermore, the administration of antituberculous drugs has been associated with endocrine effects.

TUBERCULOSIS AND THE ADRENAL GLANDS

In 1855, Thomas Addison (1) wrote *On the Constitutional Effects of Diseases of the Suprarenal Capsules.* According to Addison:

> The patient . . . in most of the cases I have seen, has been observed gradually to fall off in general health; he becomes languid and weak, indisposed to either bodily or mental exertion; the appetite is impaired or entirely lost; the pulse small and feeble . . . the body wastes . . . slight pain is from time to time referred to the stomach, and there is occasionally actual vomiting . . . . We discover a most remarkable, and, so far as I know, characteristic discoloration taking place in the skin, sufficiently marked indeed . . . to have attracted the attention of the patient himself . . . . It may be said to present a dingy or smoky appearance . . . . The body wastes . . . . The pulse becomes smaller and weaker, and . . . the patient at length gradually sinks and expires.

A review of the case histories of Addison's 11 patients with adrenal insufficiency suggests that at least seven had tuberculosis. Although tuberculosis was the most common cause of adrenal insufficiency in Addison's day, in the United States, tuberculosis now causes approximately 20%

of cases. Autoimmune destruction is responsible for approximately 75% of the cases, and the balance is caused by other infections, adrenal hemorrhage, and malignancy.

Postmortem studies and more recent evaluation with computed tomography scan and magnetic resonance imaging have shed light on the course of tubercular infection of the adrenal glands. Active adrenal tuberculosis is associated with unilateral or bilateral enlargement of the adrenal glands. With healing, the adrenal glands either normalize or subsequently atrophy and develop calcification (3,4).

The incidence of true adrenal insufficiency in adrenal tuberculosis has been debated. Slavin et al. (5) detected adrenal involvement in 53% of patients with late generalized tuberculosis; only one patient was reported to show symptoms referable to adrenal disease. Clinically active, extraadrenal tuberculosis may be present before, during, or after the diagnosis of adrenal insufficiency (6). Most patients present with chronic adrenal failure, although acute adrenal failure has been reported (7).

The signs and symptoms of chronic adrenal insufficiency were well described by Addison and include fatigue, anorexia, nausea, abdominal pain, diarrhea, orthostatic hypotension, and hyperpigmentation. The acute syndrome is characterized by muscle, joint, and abdominal pains. Clinical signs include fever, hypotension, and central nervous system depression. Laboratory tests may reveal anemia, neutropenia, and eosinophilia with reactive lymphocytosis. Electrolyte abnormalities occur in most patients and include hyponatremia, primarily from glucocorticoid deficiency, and hyperkalemia, caused by aldosterone deficiency. Mild hyperchloremia acidosis and prerenal azotemia result from dehydration and decreased cardiac output (2).

Subclinical adrenal infection may be common with active tuberculosis. Ellis and Tayoub (8) found that 55% of patients with acute pulmonary tuberculosis had a suboptimal response to a short synthetic adrenocorticotropic hormone (ACTH) test, although none had clinical disease. Similar results were noted in one follow-up study (9), but a much lower incidence was found in another (10), at least in part

J. Lowy: Department of Medicine, New York University Medical Center, New York, New York.

because of different techniques and criteria for an abnormal response to ACTH. Chan et al. (11) also demonstrated a suboptimal cortisol response to ACTH. However, their data suggested that most of the patients had a hyperstimulated basal state secondary to stress, and none of their patients had subnormal basal cortisol concentrations at presentation (11). York et al. (12) used diurnal samples of cortisol as a gauge of adrenocortical function and found no difference between patients with and without active tuberculosis.

The diagnosis of adrenal insufficiency is obvious when the classic signs and symptoms of the disease are present. Conversely, patients with active tuberculosis may have many of the same constitutional symptoms but no signs of adrenal insufficiency. Thus, a high level of suspicion for this potentially life-threatening complication of tuberculosis must be maintained. Laboratory testing should include basal cortisol levels and evaluation of response to ACTH stimulation. Noninvasive imaging studies may reveal enlarged to atrophic glands, depending on the duration of the illness. The presence of calcification is said to favor a diagnosis of tuberculosis (13), although calcification may be found in other infections and hemorrhagic conditions.

Once adrenal insufficiency is established, the diagnosis of tubercular adrenalitis may be presumptive in the setting of old or current extraadrenal tuberculosis. If the cause of the adrenal insufficiency is in doubt, fine needle aspiration under fluoroscopic or computed tomography guidance may be confirmatory (14).

Suspicion of acute adrenal crisis demands immediate therapy that should not be delayed for results of diagnostic studies. After blood is drawn for electrolytes, glucose, cortisol, and ACTH levels, fluids should be administered rapidly in the form of saline or 5% dextrose in saline. Intravenous dexamethasone sodium phosphate (4 mg) or hydrocortisone (100 mg) should be injected immediately. Dexamethasone has the advantage of greater duration (12 to 24 hours), and it does not interfere with the measurement of cortisol levels during the short ACTH stimulation test. If hydrocortisone is used, 100 mg should be administered every 6 hours. Mineralocorticoid replacement with fludrocortisone (0.1 mg by mouth daily) may be initiated; however, several days are required before the sodium-retaining effects are realized. Maintenance therapy in chronic primary adrenal insufficiency involves the administration of glucocorticoid and mineralocorticoid replacement.

HYPONATREMIA AND THE SYNDROME OF INAPPROPRIATE ANTIDIURETIC HORMONE SECRETION

Case

A 51-year-old homeless chronic alcoholic was brought into Bellevue Hospital in New York by ambulance after passersby had witnessed him having a seizure on the street.

He had many past admissions for alcohol withdrawal seizures, delirium tremens, acute pancreatitis, alcoholic cirrhosis, and insulin-dependent diabetes mellitus. He was febrile and was treated for presumed aspiration pneumonia with parental antibiotics. Because he continued to have fever, erythromycin was added for a 14-day course, but fever persisted. A purified protein derivative test was placed and was nonreactive. The patient was also anergic. A gallium 67 scan revealed increased uptake in both apices. Sputum smears for acid-fast bacilli were negative five times. The patient was empirically started on isoniazid, rifampin, pyrazinamide, and ethambutol. His sputum grew *Mycobacterium tuberculosis*.

His hospital course was complicated by hyponatremia. His serum sodium was 128 mEq/L on admission, with a reduced serum osmolality of 256 mOsm (normal, 280 to 285 mOsm). His renal function was normal and serum albumin was slightly reduced. His urine osmolality was high (513 mOsm) with increased urinary sodium of 119 mEq/L. A repeat serum osmolality was 229 mOsm with a serum sodium of 118 mEq/L. A diagnosis of SIADH secondary to tuberculosis was made, and the patient was placed on fluid restriction. He was observed to be noncompliant and developed nausea with several vomiting episodes. He was started on 150 mg demeclocycline four times daily. However, his nausea and vomiting persisted, and a subsequent sodium serum level was 114 mEq/L. The patient ultimately responded to treatment with the loop diuretic furosemide and small amounts of hypertonic saline.

In 1950, after several reports of hyponatremia in pulmonary tuberculosis, Sims et al. (15) reported ten such patients in whom the absence of primary renal or adrenal disease was documented. As this syndrome occurred without the signs and symptoms characteristic of a true sodium-depleted state, it was referred to as asymptomatic hyponatremia. The pathogenesis of this syndrome was elucidated in 1957 by Schwartz et al. (16) in patients who had bronchogenic carcinoma and whose studies included the careful measurement of serum and urine osmolality and electrolytes. Schwartz et al. determined that the hyponatremia was caused by an inappropriate secretion of antidiuretic hormone. Subsequently, patients with pulmonary tuberculosis were demonstrated to fulfill the clinical criteria of SIADH (17). In 1970, Vorherr et al. (18) demonstrated the presence of a substance with antidiuretic hormone–like properties similar or identical to arginine vasopressin from tuberculous lung tissue of a patient with hyponatremia, which suggested that this tissue either produces or, less likely, absorbs inappropriately released hormone from the posterior pituitary.

Many central nervous system diseases have been associated with SIADH, presumably because of an abnormal release of arginine vasopressin from the pituitary gland. Tuberculous meningitis was reported to be associated with SIADH in a patient who also had active pulmonary disease (19).

The essential diagnostic criteria for SIADH are (a) decreased effective osmolality of the extracellular fluid (plasma osmolality less than 275 mOsm/kg H_2O), (b) inappropriate urinary concentration (urinary osmolality greater than 100 mOsm/kg H_2O with normal renal function), (c) euvolemia, (d) elevated urinary sodium excretion with normal salt and water intake, and (e) absence of other potential causes of euvolemic hypoosmolality such as hypothyroidism, adrenal insufficiency, and recent diuretic use (20).

The euvolemic hyponatremia associated with SIADH must be differentiated from the hypovolemic hyponatremia that has also been reported to occur with tuberculous meningitis (21).

Symptoms usually do not appear until the serum sodium level falls below 125 mEq/L. Their severity relates to the degree of hypoosmolality and the period over which it develops. These factors determine the degree of brain swelling owing to osmotic water shifts into the brain. Patients present with nausea, vomiting, seizures, and altered sensorium ranging from confusion to stupor and coma.

Slow correction with fluid restriction is appropriate for mild SIADH. If any central nervous system symptoms are present, rapid correction is indicated with hypertonic saline, often in combination with furosemide. Chronic SIADH has been treated successfully with demeclocycline, which induces a nephrogenic form of diabetes insipidus by the peripheral inhibition of arginine vasopressin.

TUBERCULOSIS AND HYPERCALCEMIA

Hypercalcemia has been frequently associated with tuberculosis, but it is generally asymptomatic and mild. In a 1979 study by Abassi et al. (22) of 79 patients with active pulmonary tuberculosis, 22 who were normocalcemic on admission developed hypercalcemia during their hospital course. Calcium levels were not corrected for hypoalbuminemia. There was a close correlation between the degree of hypercalcemia and amount of vitamin D supplementation. All cases were mild and responded to withdrawal of supplementation, hydration, continued antituberculous therapy, or combinations of these regimens.

A subsequent study that corrected for albumin levels found 51% of patients with tuberculosis and 26% of controls with calcium levels above the normal range on admission. In addition, patients with more severe disease, as measured by radiographic criteria, had higher levels of serum calcium (23). In a more recent study of 88 Greek patients with tuberculosis, albumin-adjusted hypercalcemia was detected in 25% of cases (24).

Most cases of hypercalcemia in tuberculosis, like those associated with sarcoidosis and other granulomatous diseases, appear to be linked to abnormal vitamin D metabolism. Levels of dihydroxyvitamin D have correlated significantly with serum calcium levels in advanced pulmonary tuberculosis (25). Hypercalcemia with elevated dihydroxyvitamin D levels has also been reported in a patient with end-stage renal disease and active tuberculosis (26). Patients who receive supplemental vitamin D are more likely to develop hypercalcemia (22).

A rare cause of hypercalcemia in patients with tuberculosis is hyperparathyroidism with parathyroid adenoma. This has occurred as a coexisting disease (27) and with evidence of tuberculous granulomatous inflammation of the adenoma (28). Disseminated skeletal tuberculosis may also be associated with hypercalcemia and may respond to therapy with corticosteroids (29).

TUBERCULOSIS AND THE PITUITARY GLAND

Pituitary gland involvement was seen in 4% of patients with late, generalized tuberculosis (5). Tuberculosis may spread hematogenously or by direct extension from the sphenoid sinus, brain, or meninges. Headache, fever, and ophthalmopathy are the most common associated symptoms (30). However, its incidence may have been grossly underestimated. Lam et al. (31) carefully studied the pituitary function of 49 patients who had tuberculous meningitis in childhood and found ten to have abnormal function. Seven had growth hormone deficiency, and a significant correlation was found between height and the age at diagnosis of meningitis. Seven patients had gonadotrophin deficiency (four of whom also had growth hormone deficiency), one had corticotropin deficiency, and one had mild hyperprolactinemia. None had diabetes insipidus.

Hypopituitarism has been reported to be associated with intrasellar calcification after tuberculous meningitis (30). Radiographic findings suggestive of an intrasellar tumor may be seen with pituitary tuberculosis and other nonmalignant diseases of the pituitary such as sarcoidosis and histiocytosis X. Tuberculoma of the pituitary is rare and, for the most part, has been diagnosed at autopsy, but it has also been described antemortem in a patient with hypopituitarism (32).

Diabetes insipidus may occur with hypopituitarism if an intrasellar process interrupts the hypothalamohypophysial tracts by suprasellar extension or by isolated hypothalamic or suprasellar disease. Tuberculosis meningitis has been reported to be associated with diabetes insipidus (33,34), presumably because of the proximity of the hypothalamohypophysial pathways to the basal cisterns, the site of maximal involvement in this form of meningitis (30).

TUBERCULOSIS AND THE THYROID GLAND

The first case of tuberculous involvement of the thyroid gland was reported in the late 1800s. In the autopsy series of Slavin et al. (5), 14 of 100 patients had evidence of tuberculosis involving the thyroid gland. Mycobacteria may spread to the thyroid gland hematogenously or from an adjacent focus such as cervical or mediastinal adenitis (35,36). The presentation may be that of a nodule, mass, thyroiditis (painful swelling), or acute or cold abscess (37). Symptoms from pressure effects include dysphagia, dyspnea, and dysphonia. Disorders of thyroid function are rare. Rankin and Graham (38) reported a relatively large series of patients with symptoms of hyperthyroidism; however, this 1932 study used basal metabolic rate. There are only isolated case reports of thyrotoxicosis (39) and hypothyroidism (40) in association with thyroid tuberculosis.

The diagnosis of tuberculosis of the thyroid gland has rarely been made clinically. Most reported cases are found based on surgical or autopsy specimens. Fine needle aspiration is currently used for the diagnosis of thyroid lesions and has been diagnostic in the setting of thyroid tuberculosis (37).

TUBERCULOSIS AND DIABETES MELLITUS

In his 1934 review of the association of diabetes and tuberculosis, Root (2) stated:

> During the latter half of the nineteenth century the diabetic patient appeared doomed to die of pulmonary tuberculosis if he succeeded in escaping coma . . . . So striking was the association in the minds of the physicians of the time that several writers believed there to be an hereditary tendency of the two.

Autopsy studies in the 1800s found evidence of tuberculosis in 38% to 50% of patients with diabetes. Root himself noted that pulmonary tuberculosis developed more than ten times as frequently in patients with diabetes and that in 85% of patients, the development of tuberculosis appeared to follow the onset of diabetes (41).

Animal studies subsequently supported the observation that patients with diabetes were susceptible to tuberculosis. These studies demonstrated that different species of animals with natural resistance to tuberculosis could be rendered sensitive to this infection with pancreatectomy or induced hyperglycemia.

Insulin deficiency results in impairment of both leukocyte- and lymphocyte-mediated responses to infection. These immunodeficiencies improve with antidiabetic treatment. The advent of effective antituberculous and antidiabetic treatment led to a decrease in the death rate from tuberculosis in patients with diabetes from 5.5% to 3% in the years 1922 through 1929 to 1956 through 1965, respectively (42).

It has been reported that the presentation of tuberculosis in patients with diabetes is different from that in patients without diabetes. In one study of 36 patients with diabetes and tuberculosis, there was a significant increase in cavitary and sputum positive disease (43). In another study, an increase in lower lobe disease was suggested (44).

There is no evidence that treatment of active tuberculosis in patients with diabetes is less effective than it is in patients without diabetes. The recommendation that tuberculin-positive adult with diabetes with negative chest radiographs receive isoniazid prophylaxis has been questioned (45).

ANTITUBERCULOUS DRUGS AND ENDOCRINE METABOLIC EFFECTS

Acute adrenal failure has been reported in patients receiving antituberculous therapy, with rifampin being most commonly implicated. This drug has marked effects on steroid metabolism and is known to be a potent inducer of the microsomal enzymes involved in drug metabolism. In the five reported cases of addisonian crisis associated with rifampin therapy, four developed signs of adrenal failure 2 weeks after the drug was started. As noted earlier, subclinical infection of the adrenal glands may be common. A limited hormonal reserve may develop into overt adrenal failure with therapy from such factors as increased steroid metabolism and paradoxical swelling (46).

Hypocalcemia was reported in a small percentage of patients treated for several months with isoniazid, rifampin, or both (47). The administration of isoniazid to normal subjects may result in transient hypocalcemia, apparently in response to a change in vitamin D levels (48). Rifampin may also affect vitamin D metabolism, although this was not demonstrated to be clinically significant (49). Concern has been raised regarding the risk of hypocalcemia and osteomalacia in patients treated with these drugs, especially in the setting of malnutrition (50).

The administration of paraaminosalicylic acid has been associated with hypoglycemia (51) and goiter (52).

REFERENCES

1. Addison T. On the constitutional and local effects of diseases of the suprarenal capsules. (London: Samuel Highley, 1855). In: Kelly EC, ed. *Medical classics* (Vol. 2). Baltimore: Williams & Wilkins, 1937:233–280.
2. Root HF. The association of diabetes and tuberculosis. *N Engl J Med* 1934;210:1–13.
3. Tarvinder BSB, Vohra RB, Sujatha, et al. CT in adrenal enlargement due to tuberculosis: a review of the literature with five new cases. *Clin Imaging* 1992;16:102–108.
4. Vita JA, Silverberg SJ, Goland RS, et al. Clinical clues to the cause of Addison's disease. *Am J Med* 1985;78:461–466.
5. Slavin RE, Walsh TJ, Pollack AD. Late generalized tuberculosis: a clinical pathologic analysis and comparison of 100 cases in the preantibiotic and antibiotic eras. *Medicine* 1980;59:352–356.
6. Sadler MR, Beresford OD. Miliary tuberculosis associated with Addison's disease. *Tubercle* 1971;52:208–300.
7. Kelestimur F, Ozbakir O, Saglam A, et al. Acute adrenocortical failure due to tuberculosis. *J Endocrinol Invest* 1993;16:281–284.

8. Ellis ME, Tayoub F. Adrenal function in tuberculosis. *Br J Dis Chest* 1986;80:7–12.

9. Sarma GR, Immanuel C, Ramachandran G, et al. Adrenocortical function in patients with pulmonary tuberculosis. *Tubercle* 1990;71:277–282.

10. Barnes DJ, Naraqi S, Temu P, et al. Adrenal function in patients with active tuberculosis. *Thorax* 1989;44:422–424.

11. Chan CHS, Arnold M, Mak TWL, et al. Adrenocortical function and involvement in high risk cases of pulmonary tuberculosis. *Tuber Lung Dis* 1993;74:395–398.

12. York EL, Enarson DA, Nobert EJ. Adrenocortical function in patients investigated for active tuberculosis. *Chest* 1992;101: 1338–1341.

13. Wilms GE, Baert AL, Kint EJ, et al. Computed tomographic findings in bilateral adrenal tuberculosis. *Radiology* 1983;146: 729–730.

14. Yee ACN, Gopinath N, Ho CS, et al. Fine needle aspiration biopsy of adrenal tuberculosis. *J Can Assoc Radiol* 1986;37: 287–289.

15. Sims EAH, Welt LG, Orloff J, et al. Asymptomatic hyponatremia in pulmonary tuberculosis. *J Clin Invest* 1950;29:1545–1557.

16. Schwartz WB, Bennett W, Curelop S, et al. A syndrome of sodium loss and hyponatremia probably resulting from inappropriate secretion of antidiuretic hormone. *Am J Med* 1957;23: 529–542.

17. Weiss H, Katz S. Hyponatremia resulting from apparently inappropriate secretion of antidiuretic hormone in patients with pulmonary tuberculosis. *Am Rev Respir Dis* 1965;92: 609–616.

18. Vorherr H, Massry SG, Fallet R, et al. Antidiuretic principle in tuberculous lung tissue. *Ann Intern Med* 1970;72:383–387.

19. Stein DH, Seriff NS, Khan I. Transient errthrocytosis and inappropriate antidiuretic hormone secretion in a patient with tuberculous meningitis. *Mt Sinai J Med* 1972;39:265–270.

20. Verbalis JG. Inappropriate antidiuresis and other hypo-osmolar states. In: Becker KL, ed. *Principles and practice of endocrinology and metabolism.* Philadelphia: JB Lippincott Co, 1990.

21. Ti LK, Kang SC, Cheong KF. Acute hyponatremia secondary to cerebral salt wasting syndrome in a patient with tuberculous meningitis. *Anaesth Intensive Care* 1998;26:420–423.

22. Abassi A, Chemplavil JK, Farah S, et al. Hypercalcemia in active tuberculosis. *Ann Intern Med* 1979;90:324–328.

23. Need AG, Phillips AJ, Chin FTS, et al. Hypercalcemia associated with tuberculosis. *BMJ* 1980;280:831.

24. Rousses A, Lagogianni I, Gonis A, et al. Hypercalcemia in Greek patients with tuberculosis before the initiation of anti-tuberculosis treatment. *Respir Med* 2001;95:187–190.

25. Bell NH, Shary J, Shaw S, et al. Hypercalcemia associated with increased circulating 1,25 dihydroxyvitamin in a patient with pulmonary tuberculosis. *Calcif Tissue Int* 1985;3:588–591.

26. Gkonos PJ, London R, Hendler ED. Hypercalcemia and elevated 1,25-dihydroxyvitamin levels in a patient with end-stage renal disease and active tuberculosis. *N Engl J Med* 1984;311:1683–1685.

27. Kipnis S, Rajn L. Hypercalcemia in tuberculosis: a case with proved hyperparathyroidism. *N Y State J Med* 1981;81:1517–1518.

28. Kar DK, Agarwal G, Mehta B et al. Tuberculosis granulomatous inflammation associated with adenoma of parathyroid gland manifesting as primary hyperparathyroidism. *Endocr Pathol* 2001;12:355–359.

29. Braman SS, Goldman AL, Schwarz MI. Steroid-responsive hypercalcemia in disseminated bone tuberculosis. *Arch Intern Med* 1973;132:269–271.

30. Berger SA, Edberg SC, David G. Infectious disease in the sella turcica. *Rev Infect Dis* 1986;8:747–755.

31. Lam KSL, Sham MMK, Tam SCF, et al. Hypopituitarism after tuberculous meningitis in childhood. *Ann Intern Med* 1993; 118:701–706.

32. Brooks MH, Dumlao JS, Bronsky D, et al. Hypophysial tuberculoma with hypopituitarism. *Am J Med* 1973;54:777–781.

33. Levin AR. Diabetes insipidus associated with tuberculous meningitis. *BMJ* 1959;2:1061–1063.

34. Hay DR. Diabetes insipidus after tuberculous meningitis. *BMJ* 1960;1:707.

35. Sachs MK, Dickinson G, Amazon K. Tuberculous adenitis of the thyroid mimicking subacute thyroiditis. *Am J Med* 1988;85: 573–575.

36. Liote HA, Spaulding C, Bazelly B, et al. Thyroid tuberculosis associated with mediastinal lymphadenitis. *Tubercle* 1987;68:229–231.

37. Magboo MLC, Clark OH. Primary tuberculous thyroid abscess mimicking carcinoma diagnosed by fine needle aspiration biopsy. *West J Med* 1990;153:657–659.

38. Rankin FW, Graham AS. Tuberculosis of the thyroid gland. *Ann Surg* 1932;96:625–646.

39. Kapoor VK, Subramani K, Das AK, et al. Tuberculosis of the thyroid gland associated with thyrotoxicosis. *Postgrad Med J* 1985;61:339–340.

40. Barnes P, Weatherstone R. Tuberculosis of the thyroid: two case reports. *Br J Dis Chest* 1979;73:187–191.

41. Zack MB, Fulkerson LL, Stein E. Glucose intolerance in primary tuberculosis. *Am Rev Respir Dis* 1973;108:1164–1169.

42. Bagdade JD. Infection in diabetes: predisposing factors. *Postgrad Med J* 1976;59:160–161.

43. Hendy M, Stableforth D. The effect of established diabetes mellitus on the presentation of infiltrative pulmonary tuberculosis in the Asian community of an inner city area of the United Kingdom. *Br J Dis Chest* 1983;77:87–90.

44. Weaver AR. Unusual radiographic presentation of pulmonary tuberculosis in diabetic patients. *Am Rev Respir Dis* 1974;109: 162–163.

45. Rose DN, Silver AL, Schecter CB. Tuberculosis chemoprophylaxis for diabetics: Are the benefits worth the risk? *Mt Sinai J Med* 1985;52:253–258.

46. Wilkins EGL, Hnizdo E, Cope A. Addisonian crisis induced by treatment with rifampicin. *Tubercle* 1989;70:69–73.

47. British Thoracic Association. A controlled trial of six months chemotherapy in pulmonary tuberculosis. *Br J Dis Chest* 1981;75:141–153.

48. Brodie MJ, Boobis AR, Hillyard CJ, et al. Effect of isoniazid on vitamin D metabolism and hepatic mono-oxygenase activity. *Clin Pharmacol Ther* 1981;30:363–370.

49. Brodie MJ, Boobis AR, Dollery CT, et al. Rifampicin and vitamin D metabolism. *Clin Pharmacol Ther* 1980;27:810–814.

50. Arnsten AR. Endocrine and metabolic aspects of tuberculosis. In: Schlossberg D, ed. *Tuberculosis*, 3rd ed. New York: Springer-Verlag, 1994:247–256.

51. Dandona P, Greenbury E, Beckett AG. Para-aminosalicylic acid-induced hypoglycaemia in a patient with diabetic nephropathy. *Postgrad Med J* 1980;56:135–136.

52. Munkner T. Studies on goitre due to para-aminosalicylic acid. *Scand J Respir Dis* 1969;50:212–226.

40

MYCOBACTERIA AND THE SKIN

SUSAN BURGIN
MIRIAM KELTZ POMERANZ
PHILIP ORBUCH
JEROME L. SHUPACK
RENA S. BRAND

Mycobacterium tuberculosis was first identified by Koch in 1882. However, clinicians had described lesions in the skin before the organism was isolated. René Théophile Hyacinthe Laënnec (1781–1826) described a lesion in his own finger, which he attributed to "direct inoculation" of "tuberculous matter" (1).

Tuberculosis (TB) affecting the skin can be divided into two broad categories: cutaneous TB and tuberculids (2–6) (Table 40.1). Cutaneous TB can be thought of as *M. tuberculosis* infecting the skin; tuberculids may be considered cutaneous reactions to extracutaneous TB. Cutaneous TB can be further subdivided by the source of the organism, that is, exogenous or endogenous. Tuberculous chancres and warty TB are caused by infections of the skin from outside sources. Endogenous infections can be secondary to hematogenous or lymphatic spread. Autoinoculation from underlying infected tissues, such as lymph nodes, or from bodily excretions, such as sputum, can also cause skin infections. These infections are named lupus vulgaris, acute miliary TB of the skin, tuberculous gumma, orificial TB, and scrofuloderma. There are multiple other names in the literature for these categories of cutaneous TB (1,2,7–11) (Table 40.2).

In any patient, both the source of the infection (i.e., exogenous or endogenous) and the patient's immunologic state are determinants in evaluating the clinical skin infection (12) (Table 40.3). Two aspects of a person's immune function are important in TB: sensitivity to TB (i.e., previ- ous exposure to TB) and immunocompetence. The first can be evaluated with a purified protein derivative (PPD) test. In primary infections, the PPD test result is negative, but in secondary infections in normal hosts the test is positive. The second factor, immunocompetence, is less specific and therefore harder to quantify.

This chapter presents a discussion of TB and the skin on the basis of categories. In clinical medicine, these categories may overlap and patients may not fit into any of them. However, this classification is widely used in the literature and can serve as a framework for conceptualizing TB as it affects the skin. The chapter also discusses atypical mycobacteria that often have a greater predilection for the skin than *M. tuberculosis*.

CUTANEOUS TUBERCULOSIS

Tuberculous Chancre

Clinical Characteristics

Tuberculous chancres occur as primary infections when exogenous sources inoculate damaged skin of nonsensitized individuals, most commonly children (10). Lesions are most commonly found on the face or limbs at sites of trauma but have been reported on the conjunctiva, oral mucosa, anus, genitalia, and as paronychia. Sexual transmission from a primary penile tuberculous chancre has recently been reported (13). A chancre begins as a firm nodule that ulcerates, with borders that have been variably described as sharp, ragged, and undermined (3,7,10). The ulcers are not tender. An older lesion has a firmer, less ragged edge and an adherent crust (14). Regional painless lymphadenopathy subsequently develops and may be accompanied by lymphangitis (10). The primary chancre and associated lymphadenopathy may be analogized to the Ghon complex of primary pulmonary TB. Associated sys-

S. Burgin and M. K. Pomeranz: Department of Dermatology, New York University School of Medicine; Department of Dermatology, Bellevue Hospital, New York, New York.
P. Orbuch and R.S. Brand: Department of Dermatology, New York University Medical Center, New York, New York.
J. L. Shupack: Department of Dermatology, New York University School of Medicine; Department of Dermatology, Tisch Hospital, New York, New York.

TABLE 40.1. CLASSIFICATION OF CUTANEOUS TUBERCULOSIS

Cutaneous tuberculosis
  Exogenous source
    Tuberculous chancre
    Warty tuberculosis
    (Lupus vulgaris)
    (Orificial tuberculosis)
  Endogenous source
    Hematogenous/lymphatic spread
      Lupus vulgaris
      Acute miliary tuberculosis of the skin
      Tuberculous gumma
      (Orificial tuberculosis)
    Autoinoculation/contiguous spread
      Orificial tuberculosis
      Scrofuloderma
      (Lupus vulgaris)
      (Warty tuberculosis)
Tuberculids
  True tuberculids
    Papulonecrotic tuberculid
    Lichen scrofulosorum
  Facultative tuberculids
    Erythema induratum
  Newer tuberculids
    Nodular granulomatous phlebitis
    Nodular tuberculid
  Possible tuberculids
    Erythema nodosum
  Former tuberculids
    Lupus miliaris disseminatus faciei
    Rosacea-like tuberculid
    Lichenoid tuberculid

Data from references 2–6.

TABLE 40.2. MULTIPLE NAMES FOR CUTANEOUS TUBERCULOSIS

Tuberculous chancre
  Primary inoculation (2)
  Tuberculosis primary complex (2)
  Primary inoculation tuberculosis (7)
  Primary cutaneous complex (8)
  Primary cutaneous tuberculosis (9)
Warty tuberculosis
  Tuberculosis verrucosa cutis (2)
  Tuberculosis cutis verrucosa (2)
  Lupus verrucosus (1)
  Verruca necrogenica (2)
  Prosector's wart (2)
  Anatomic tubercle (1)
Lupus vulgaris
  Tuberculosis luposa cutis (2)
Acute miliary tuberculosis of the skin
  Acute disseminated miliary tuberculosis (10)
  Tuberculosis cutis miliaris disseminata (2)
  Tuberculosis cutis acuta generalisata (2)
  Tuberculosis miliaris generalisata (9)
Tuberculous gumma
  Metastatic tuberculous abscess (2)
  Gummatous tuberculosis (7)
  Tuberculosis colliquativa (7)
  Tuberculosis locus minoris resistentia (11)
Orificial tuberculosis
  Tuberculosis cutis orificialis (2)
  Tuberculosis ulcerosa cutis et mucosae (2)
  Tuberculosis orificialis (9)
Scrofuloderma
  Tuberculosis colliquativa cutis (2)
  Tuberculosis cutis colliquativa (9)

Data from references 1, 2, 7–11.

temic symptoms, if any, are mild (3). The lesion heals over months, leaving a scar (10). Rarely, a tuberculous chancre by local or hematogenous spread can lead to lupus vulgaris, scrofuloderma, or miliary TB (3,14). Usually patients with a tuberculous chancre have an overall intact immune system; the PPD test result is negative at first but eventually turns positive because the patient has been exposed to *M. tuberculosis* (5).

Pathology

The histology of a tuberculous chancre varies with the timing of a biopsy. Early lesions demonstrate an acute neutrophilic infiltrate in the dermis with necrosis (15). Bacilli are easily seen with the Ziehl–Neelsen stain. These bacilli are thin, curved rods, approximately 4 μm long and 1 μm wide (16). After about 2 weeks of lesional development, monocytes and macrophages are present, along with areas of necrosis. When the lesion has matured at 3 to 6 weeks, more epithelioid and giant cells are present, with less necrosis and fewer bacilli (12). The epidermis frequently is hyperplastic but ulceration may also be present (16).

Warty Tuberculosis

Clinical Characteristics

Warty TB, like a tuberculous chancre, occurs from an exogenous source that inoculates the skin; however, unlike a tuberculous chancre, warty TB occurs in people who have had previous exposure to TB and is caused by repeated infection (3,10). Warty TB is the most prevalent form of cutaneous TB in Hong Kong, where it was reported predominantly in children (17). Elsewhere, it occurs most commonly in adult men (9). Three modes of transmission are seen (14). Inoculation via trauma possibly from expectorated sputum in the environment and autoinoculation from one's own sputum are most commonly encountered. Physicians and butchers may develop warty TB through occupational exposure (thus, the terms "prosector's wart," "anatomic tubercle," and "verruca necrogenica") (1,2). Lesions have been found on hands, wrists, dorsa of the feet, knees, ankles, and buttocks (3,9). In adults, it is more common on hands; in children, on legs (18). Warty TB begins as a reddish brown or purple papule or papulopustule that grows by peripheral extension to a warty plaque (3,10) (Fig.

TABLE 40.3. CLINICAL CHARACTERISTICS OF CUTANEOUS TUBERCULOSIS

	Type of Infection	PPD Test	Immune Function	Bacilli in Biopsy	Common Age Group	Gender Predilection
Tuberculous chancre	Primary	–(later ++)	Good	Common	Children	—
Warty tuberculosis	Secondary	++	Moderate to good	Occasional	Adults	Male
Lupus vulgaris	Secondary	++	Moderate to good	Rare	Children and adults	Female
Acute miliary tuberculosis	Primary or secondary	–	Poor	Common	Children	—
Tuberculous gumma	Secondary	+	Poor to moderate	Occasional	Children and adults	—
Orificial tuberculosis	Secondary	– or ++	Poor	Common	Adults	Male
Scrofuloderma	Secondary	++	Poor to good	Occasional	Children and adults	—
Papulonecrotic tuberculid		++	Good	None	Children and young adults	Female
Lichen scrofulosorum		++	Good	None	Children and young adults	—
Erythema induratum		++	Good	None	Young adults and adults	Female
Erythema nodosum		++	Good	None	Young adults and adults	Female

Modified from Moschella SL, Cropley TG. Diseases of the mononuclear phagocytic system. In SL Moschella, HJ Hurley, eds. *Dermatology*, 3rd ed. Philadelphia: WB Saunders, 1992:1031–1141.
PPD, purified protein derivative.

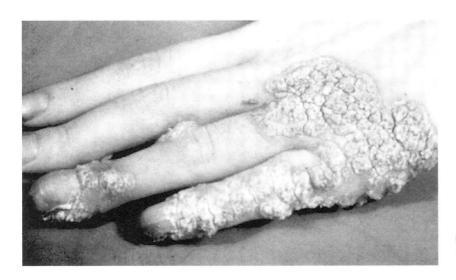

FIGURE 40.1. Warty tuberculosis on the hand. (Courtesy of Samuel Weinberg, M.D., New York University School of Medicine, New York, NY.)

40.1). The lesion may be active at the periphery as it resolves in its center (9), or it may form a uniformly papillomatous plaque (14). The surface may have clefts and fissures that may discharge pus (3,10). Usually only one or two lesions are present (7). Lymphadenopathy is generally not seen unless secondary pyogenic infection is present (7); however, true tuberculous lymphadenitis has rarely been reported (19). The lesions may heal spontaneously over years or they may progress slowly (10,18). Atrophic scars remain after healing (3). Warty TB occurs in patients with moderate-to-good overall immune systems and positive PPD skin test result (7,9,20).

Pathology

Warty TB causes both epidermal and dermal changes. The epidermis develops hyperkeratosis, acanthosis, and papillomatosis. An inflammatory infiltrate, occasionally with abscess formation, appears in the upper dermis. The tuberculoid granuloma (i.e., irregular accumulation of epithelioid and inflammatory cells, with or without giant cells and caseation necrosis) is present in the middermis (15). Ackerman placed warty TB in the category "suppurative granulomatous dermatitis" because there may be both granulomatous (histiocytic) inflammation and a suppurative (neutrophilic) infiltrate (16). Bacilli may be seen with special stains. Although mycobacteria are more commonly found than in cases of lupus vulgaris, bacilli often cannot be identified (7,15,18).

Lupus Vulgaris

Clinical Characteristics

Lupus vulgaris results from spread of TB from an endogenous reservoir to the skin via hematogenous or lymphatic

routes or by contiguous extension. However, the primary infection is not always documented. A noncutaneous tuberculous focus is found in less than 50% of patients (3,7,21), which is usually tuberculous lymphadenitis (18). Rarely, lupus vulgaris is acquired from an exogenous source, such as bacille Calmette–Guérin (BCG) vaccination (22). This type of cutaneous TB occurs in both children and adults and is perhaps slightly more prevalent in females (3,7). It is the most common type of cutaneous TB in the West (3). In Europe, more than 80% of cases occur on the face and neck, frequently around the nose (3,7). In India, many cases occur on the trunk (3). In a study from South Africa, 13 of 18 cases involved the face, three the ears, and two the chest, abdomen, or scrotum (7). The lesions begin as reddish brown, soft, gelatinous papules that coalesce to form a plaque with serpiginous borders (3,7,10,14) (Fig. 40.2). The plaque grows by peripheral extension with a scar in the center. Apple-jelly–colored nodules are classically seen at the periphery by diascopy, which entails pressing a glass slide against the skin (10). Other clinical variants include hypertrophic, ulcerative, vegetative, papular, and nodular as well as mucosal (nasal, oral, conjunctival) lesions (2,3,10).

Single lesions usually occur, but there can also be multiple lesions (5,21). The lesions heal with scarring and can be mutilating. Cartilage of the nose, ear, or both was destroyed in seven of 18 cases reported by Visser and Heyl (7). Squamous cell carcinoma may occur in the scars of lupus vulgaris (2,7,23).

According to Sehgal et al. (20), a patient with lupus vulgaris has better cell-mediated immunity than that in patients with warty TB or scrofuloderma. The PPD test result should be positive; however, in two of the cases presented by Marcoual et al. (21), the result was negative. Culturing for mycobacteria is more sensitive than histologic staining, but culturing is not diagnostic in 100% of cases (2,21). Inoculation of biopsy material into guinea pigs has

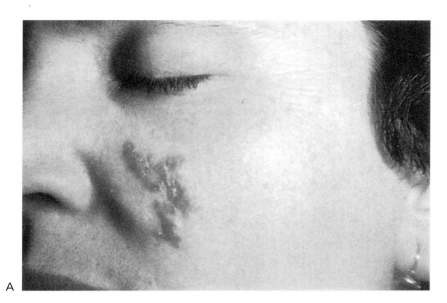

A

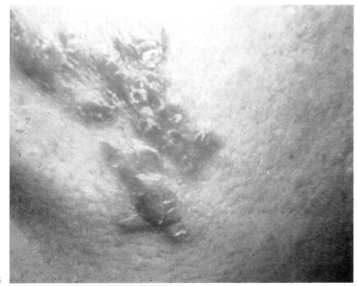

B

FIGURE 40.2. **A:** Lupus vulgaris on the cheek. **B:** Close-up of lupus vulgaris. (Courtesy of Samuel Weinberg, M.D.) (See Color Plate 19.)

been used to demonstrate the presence of *M. tuberculosis*; more recently, polymerase chain reaction (PCR) on fixed tissue has been employed (9,24,25).

Pathology

The histologic changes of lupus vulgaris occur in both the epidermis and the dermis. The changes in the epidermis depend on the morphology of the lesion—either atrophy or hyperplasia is prominent. Pseudoepitheliomatous hyperplasia is seen at the borders of ulcerated lesions (15). In the upper dermis, there may be a typical tubercle (or true tuberculous infiltrate) characterized by epithelioid cells surrounded by mononuclear cells with giant cells and some caseation necrosis. However, in other cases, lupus vulgaris is better described as a "tuberculoid" infiltrate with irregular

granulomatous inflammation with or without giant cells and necrosis (15). Acid-fast bacillus (AFB) cannot usually be found in the histologic sections (2,3,7,15,16). In long-standing lesions, telangiectasia and fibrosis may be present (16).

Acute Miliary Tuberculosis of the Skin

Clinical Characteristics

Acute miliary TB of the skin is a disseminated eruption caused by the hematogenous spread of mycobacteria, usually in a primary (first) infection. This eruption is seen mostly in children and infants (2,10) and may have been what McCray and Esterly described in two cases of congenital TB (26). Miliary TB has been reported to occur after infections such as measles and scarlet fever. A rise in the number of adult cases has been seen in the last decade in association with human immunodeficiency virus (HIV) infection, specifically in acquired immunodeficiency syndrome (AIDS). Furthermore, acute miliary TB is the form of cutaneous TB that has been most commonly reported in association with HIV infection. Stack et al. (8) reported miliary TB of the skin in a patient with AIDS in 1990. Since then at least 15 additional cases in AIDS patients have been reported (27). Surprisingly, in one review of patients older than 15 years, the presence of other underlying systemic illnesses was rare (26). Nevertheless, miliary TB is generally believed to occur in patients with poor immune function and is often fatal (2,3).

The primary site of infection is frequently the lung, with dissemination to multiple organs, including the skin. Discrete, pinhead-sized, blue–red papules form, often with vesicles in the center. The lesions may appear umbilicated (10). Although generalized, there are no more than 20 to 30 papules (28). Other morphologic lesions, such as ulcers, nodules, or macules, may result (3,9,28). The lesions heal with a white scar surrounded by a brown halo (10). Healing usually occurs in 4 to 6 weeks but can range from 2 weeks to 10 months (27). The PPD test result in these patients is almost always negative (3). Lesional cultures are regularly positive; however, in the absence of cultures, PCR may be employed to detect the presence of mycobacterial DNA (29).

Pathology

Histologic sections of acute miliary TB of the skin often reveal a nonspecific neutrophilic infiltrate in the dermis with cellular debris and bacilli found in the necrotic center of the lesion. There may be some hint of a tubercle formation around the microabscesses (15,16).

Tuberculous Gumma

Clinical Characteristics

Hematogenous spread of TB during a period of lowered immunity may result in a local abscess or tuberculous gumma. Undernourished children or immunodeficient adults are usually affected. There may be concomitant underlying progressive noncutaneous TB, acute miliary TB, or no obvious underlying tuberculous focus (4). The lesions may occur anywhere on the limbs and trunk, often at sites of previous trauma (2,3,11); however, lesions with no antecedent trauma have been described (30). A nontender, fluctuant, subcutaneous nodule breaks down, developing undermined ulcers, sinuses, or both. At this stage the lesion may resemble scrofuloderma (14). Occasionally, the surface is verrucous (3). Patients usually have a positive PPD test result (3).

Pathology

Tuberculous gummas represent abscesses with central massive necrosis and a rim of epithelioid and giant cells. The histologic characteristics may be nonspecific. Tuberculoid inflammation may be found in the subcutaneous tissue and the deep dermis with only a chronic infiltration in the upper dermis. Bacilli are often difficult to find (3).

Orificial Tuberculosis

Clinical Characteristics

Orificial TB arises from autoinoculation around body orifices as patients expectorate or excrete *M. tuberculosis* (2). This type of eruption is rare, even in countries in which TB is relatively common (3). Patients are usually middle-aged to older men with advanced visceral disease (2,9). The ulcers develop at the mucocutaneous border of the mouth, nose, anus, vagina, or urinary meatus (9). Lesions on the hard palate have also been described (7). Painful, ulcerative lesions develop from yellowish brown nodules (2,3,10). The ulcers, with an undermined, bluish edge, are shallow and usually smaller than 2 cm in diameter (3,9). These lesions do not heal spontaneously (3). The overall immune status of these patients is usually poor, although PPD skin test results are usually positive (2,3).

Pathology

The histologic specimen from a case of orificial TB may reveal tuberculoid inflammation in the deep dermis beneath an ulcerated epidermis or may have a nonspecific inflammatory infiltrate. However, with Ziehl–Neelsen staining, bacilli can be found (3,15).

Scrofuloderma

Clinical Characteristics

Scrofuloderma results from contiguous spread of infection from an underlying focus, usually lymph node but also bone, joint, or epididymis (10,14). Visser and Heyl (7) described scrofuloderma in a broad age range: 18 months to 66 years; however, it is most prevalent in children, adolescents, and the elderly (4). It was the most common type of cutaneous TB seen in children from northern India (31). Scrofuloderma is most commonly seen overlying lymph nodes in the neck, but the chest and axillae are also common sites (3,7) (Fig. 40.3). Soft or indurated nodules or plaques develop from harder subcutaneous nodules (7,10). Eventually, ulcers (which may be linear or serpiginous, and with prominent granulation tissue) or sinus tracts form. Scrofuloderma can heal, leaving hypertrophic and cordlike scars (9). Patients developing scrofuloderma usually have weakened cell-mediated immunity overall but often maintain a positive PPD (20).

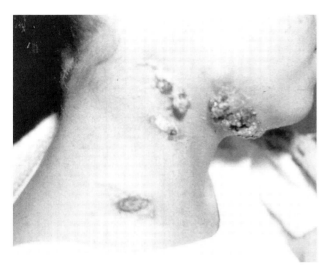

FIGURE 40.3. Scrofuloderma on the neck. (Courtesy of Samuel Weinberg, M.D.)

Pathology

The center of a lesion of scrofuloderma demonstrates nonspecific abscess formation, often with overlying ulceration of the epidermis. In the periphery and deep to the abscess, a tuberculoid infiltrate with necrosis can sometimes be seen (15). Visser and Heyl considered tuberculous gumma and scrofuloderma unworthy of distinction from each other. Although articles frequently state that bacilli are demonstrable, Visser and Heyl (7) found bacilli in only 25% (two of eight) of the patients they observed.

Other Primary Forms: Tuberculous Cellulitis

A single case report describes cutaneous TB manifesting as cellulitis. Tender erythematous plaques developed on the abdomen of an immunosuppressed woman with diabetes mellitus taking corticosteroids. She had a remote history of adequately treated pulmonary TB. The PPD test result was negative. The caseating granulomas on skin biopsy stained positively with Ziehl–Neelsen, and results of both culture and PCR with mycobacterial DNA were positive (32).

TUBERCULIDS

The definition of a tuberculid and its precise relationship to TB is constantly evolving. A tuberculid is best considered as a cutaneous immunologic response to an extracutaneous tuberculous infection. While the primary focus of infection may not be evident at the time of presentation, collateral evidence of a tuberculous etiology, such as strong PPD reactivity and response to antituberculous medication, is a nec-

essary concomitant (4). Historically, it was believed that a tuberculid develops after hematogenous dissemination of "toxins" of tuberculous bacilli (33). In general, bacilli are not identifiable by AFB stains or culture; therefore, diagnosis was based on the above criteria. With the advent of PCR, however, mycobacterial DNA has been identified in skin lesions of the tuberculids (29, 34–37; this finding obviously provides stronger proof of cause but argues against the tuberculids being conceptualized as a group distinct from true cutaneous infection. Classically, papulonecrotic tuberculid and lichen scrofulosorum are considered true tuberculids because there is strong evidence of a tuberculous cause in most cases, whereas erythema induratum is deemed a facultative tuberculid because *M. tuberculosis* is one of many etiologic agents.

Papulonecrotic Tuberculid

Clinical Characteristics

Although papulonecrotic tuberculid most commonly affects young adults, children are frequently affected, and only one third of patients are older than 30 years (38,39). Females outnumber males by about 3:1 (7,40).

The classic description is an asymptomatic, symmetric papular eruption that develops over the extensor surfaces of the body, including arms, legs and buttocks, as well as ears, face, and penis (7,23). The hands, feet, or both were involved in 10 of 12 cases reviewed by Wilson-Jones and Winkelman (40). Individual papules, 2 to 8 mm in diameter, develop in crops and eventuate in pustules, ulcers, or crusts (3,7) (Fig. 40.4). Spontaneous healing occurs, typically leaving atrophic, varioliform scars (7,40). Rarely, larger nodules that ulcerate have been described (40). The course of the eruption may extend from months to years

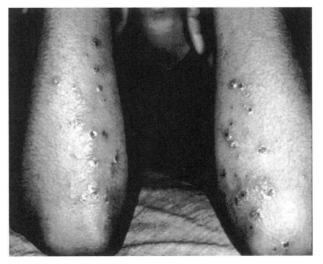

FIGURE 40.4. Papulonecrotic tuberculid on the arms. (Courtesy of Samuel Weinberg, M.D.)

(3). Lupus vulgaris lesions have arisen from papulonecrotic tuberculid lesions. With antituberculosis drug therapy, lesions heal in 1 to 2 months (38). Theoretically, the diagnosis rests on a strongly positive PPD test result, evidence of TB elsewhere in the patient, and good response to antituberculosis medication. However, active TB has been demonstrated in only 30% to 40% of patients (7,40).

The proposed cause of the skin lesions is hematogenous spread of bacilli that causes an Arthus reaction and delayed hypersensitivity (40). These patients' active immune systems destroy all evidence of the bacilli in the skin, making stains and cultures negative (39). However, lesions examined by PCR may reveal evidence of *M. tuberculosis* (35,36), and in the majority of cases in some series (34). This latter phenomenon has lead contemporary authors to reclassify papulonecrotic tuberculid as true cutaneous TB (29).

Pathology

Early lesions of papulonecrotic tuberculid demonstrate a leukocytoclastic vasculitis (38) with fibrin deposition and thrombotic occlusion of vessels. Wilson-Jones and Winkelman (40) described a lymphocytic vasculitis. A subsequent area of wedge-shaped necrosis forms in the dermis. Later lesions demonstrate epithelioid and giant cells accumulating around the wedge, which is eventually shed (15). Biopsy does not reveal bacilli (40).

Lichen Scrofulosorum

Clinical Characteristics

Lichen scrofulosorum occurs most commonly in association with TB of lymph node or bone or both (14,41). This tuberculid occurs predominantly in children and young adults where it manifests mainly on the trunk. In adults, women are more commonly affected, and trunk, limbs, and face may be involved (7,42).

Lichen scrofulosorum is an asymptomatic eruption of minute lichenoid papules that may be flesh-colored, red–brown, or gray–brown (Fig. 40.5). The papules are usually follicular or perifollicular in distribution, and may appear in groups or have an annular configuration (42,43). Other forms of cutaneous TB may be present concurrently, such as lupus vulgaris (44), tuberculous gumma and tuberculosis cutis verrucosa (45), and erythema induratum (46). Like papulonecrotic tuberculid, patients with lichen scrofulosorum exhibit a strongly positive PPD test result (3,7). A patient with lichen scrofulosorum and AIDS reportedly manifested a negative PPD test result (47). Where PCR has been employed, mycobacterial DNA is detectable in lesions of lichen scrofulosorum (35). Without antituberculous therapy the lesions will undergo involution over months, whereas appropriate treatment leads to prompt resolution within weeks (4,14).

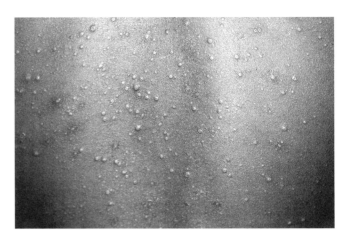

FIGURE 40.5. Lichen scrofulosorum on the back. (Courtesy of Deepak Modi, M.D., Medical School of University of the Witwatersrand, Johannesburg, South Africa.)

Pathology

Superficial dermal granulomas are present in the pathologic sections of lichen scrofulosorum. Caseation necrosis may or may not be present, and histologic distinction of this lesion from cutaneous sarcoidosis may be impossible (3,7,15). Some report the granulomas as contiguous with hair follicles or sweat ducts (3,15). Others describe them as "unrelated to appendageal structures" (7). Bacilli are not found.

Facultative Tuberculids: Erythema Induratum

Clinical Characteristics

Erythema induratum of Bazin was described by its namesake in 1861 as associated with TB. Many clinicians no longer believe there is a true association between TB and what is also called nodular vasculitis (48). However, because cases have been described in patients who have strongly positive PPD reactions and who recover after antituberculous treatment, nodular vasculitis or erythema induratum may occasionally be a true tuberculid. There is also evidence from lesions examined by PCR that *M. tuberculosis* may be causative (35,37). The lesions of erythema induratum occur in crops of painful, 1- to 2-cm nodules, usually on the posterolateral calves (4,49). Lesions have also been described on the arms, thighs, feet, and buttocks (48). Young women are most commonly affected (7,9,48). The lesions are firm, blue–red nodules that ulcerate (4). They may heal spontaneously in 3 to 4 months but may also persist for years (7,48). PPD skin test results are strongly positive in all cases associated with TB (48).

Pathology

Nodular vasculitis is the more common term used in pathology literature to describe the histologic findings of these lesions. Arteritis, lobular panniculitis, and fat necrosis are the diagnostic features (16). Bacilli are not found in sections of erythema induratum (i.e., in cases of nodular vasculitis purportedly associated with TB) (7).

Newly Described Tuberculids: Nodular Granulomatous Phlebitis and Nodular Tuberculid

Two distinct new entities have been recently described. Nodular granulomatous phlebitis, or phlebitic tuberculid, was first described by Hara et al. in 1997 (5). It presents as nonulcerating subcutaneous nodules on the anteromedial aspects of the legs (29). Histologically, epithelioid cell granulomas are found in walls of the cutaneous veins. Mycobacterial DNA was detected in four of five cases (5).

Nodular tuberculid was delineated from papulonecrotic tuberculid and erythema induratum by Jordaan et al. (6) in 2000. It presents as leg nodules, most commonly in children. The diagnosis is based on histopathologic grounds: there is granulomatous inflammation with or without vasculitis at the junction of the dermis and the subcutaneous fat. Kumar et al. (49) questioned this disease as a new entity and suggested that nodular tuberculid should be conceptualized as a superficial variant of erythema induratum or erythema nodosum.

Possible Tuberculids: Erythema Nodosum

Clinical Characteristics

Erythema nodosum clinically resembles erythema induratum in that it causes formation of tender, red nodules, usually on the legs of women. However, erythema nodosum is more common on anterior legs and rarely ulcerates. Erythema nodosum, although not a rare entity, is rarely associated with TB (7). In the United States, it is more commonly associated with other infectious diseases, sarcoidosis, and medications (16).

Pathology

Erythema nodosum is a septal panniculitis. Early lesions may have neutrophils in the fat septa; older lesions have lymphohistiocytic infiltrates. Histologically, erythema nodosum is clearly distinguished from erythema induratum by the absence of significant lobular infiltrates, necrosis, and vasculitis (16).

Former Tuberculids

Clinical Characteristics

Multiple skin lesions have historically been associated with TB, but the relationship is no longer believed. Lupus miliaris disseminatus faciei is now considered a form of granu-

lomatous rosacea, an acneiform condition. Rosacea-like tuberculid also represents a form of rosacea. Lichenoid tuberculid has been described as a symmetric eruption usually affecting the extremities but sometimes generalizing over the body (4).

Pathology

These lesions all have granulomatous histology, which explains the confusion with tuberculids. In cases now believed to be forms of rosacea, the granulomas tend to be associated with hair follicles (16).

BACILLE CALMETTE–GUÉRIN VACCINATION

Bacille Calmette–Guérin (BCG) vaccination is an attenuated bovine *Mycobacterium* injection used to immunize people against *M. tuberculosis*. Most people develop a positive PPD test result 5 to 6 weeks after injection (3). At the site of injection, an enlarging papule usually develops within 10 to 14 days and ulcerates at 6 weeks (Fig. 40.6). It

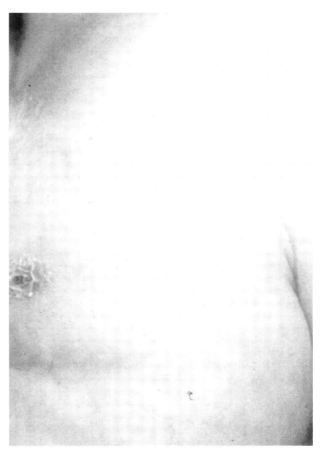

FIGURE 40.6. Bacille Calmette–Guérin vaccination reaction with lymphadenopathy. (Courtesy of Samuel Weinberg, M.D.)

then heals with scarring. Regional lymph nodes may be transiently inflamed (50).

Complications from the vaccine are rare. Kakakhel and Fritsch (3) divided skin complications into local and generalized forms. At the site of injection one can develop a keloid, an abnormally large ulcer, a subcutaneous abscess, an epithelial cyst, an eczematous reaction, a granulomatous reaction, lupus vulgaris, or warty TB (3,50). The rate of development of localized abscess or ulcer formation, or regional lymphadenitis, in a cohort of infants was reported as 0.4 per 1,000 vaccines (51). Izumi and Matsunaga (52) believe that lupus vulgaris is more likely to occur if vaccination is repeated. More generalized skin disease, secondary to BCG vaccination, includes erythema nodosum, tuberculids, scrofuloderma, or nonspecific hemorrhagic or papular eruptions (3,50,53). Possible systemic complications include lymphadenitis, osteitis, hepatic dysfunction, anaphylaxis, flulike symptoms, metastatic tuberculous foci, and widespread dissemination (which is usually fatal in immunosuppressed individuals) (3,53). Disseminated disease has been reported at a rate of 4.3 per million infants vaccinated. These patients may or may not have cutaneous disease as a concomitant factor, variably described as "subcutaneous nodules" or "multiple papular skin nodules" (53).

DIAGNOSIS AND TREATMENT

As with any other medical problem, history and physical examination have an important role in the diagnosis of cutaneous TB. One must ascertain the patient's history of TB as well as exposure to infectious contacts. Symptoms associated with the skin lesions and the time course help narrow the differential. One must look closely at the morphology and distribution of the lesion(s) and examine for associated adenopathy. When cutaneous TB is expected, a PPD test should be done and a chest radiograph obtained. A skin biopsy (often with subcutaneous tissue) is almost always necessary. The biopsy should be processed for both routine histology (formalin fixed) and culture (fresh tissue). Although Ziehl–Neelsen staining or auramine/rhodamine fluorescence may reveal AFBs, culture is needed to properly identify the organism. There are numerous reports of identification of the organism in the skin by the use of the PCR methodology, including that in lupus vulgaris, scrofuloderma, orificial TB, primary inoculation TB, and miliary TB, as well as in the tuberculids as seen above (24,29,34–37,54, 55). PCR offers a more rapid diagnosis than conventional culture [5 days as opposed to 2 weeks with the Bactec (Becton, Dickinson and Company, Franklin Lakes, NJ, U.S.A.) system] and is useful in the differentiation of cutaneous TB from atypical mycobacterial infections. However, widespread routine use of the technique is precluded by the variability of sensitivity and specificity even in specialized laboratories and its variable

cost effectiveness (54,55). Sometimes response to antituberculous therapy helps to clarify the diagnosis (3,24,35, 36,40).

The management of cutaneous TB is modeled after treatment regimens tested for pulmonary TB. The American Thoracic Society recommends that extrapulmonary TB be managed "according to the principles and with the drug regimens outlined for pulmonary TB" (56). Isoniazid and rifampin are the pillars around which treatment is built. In 6-month regimens, pyrazinamide and either ethambutol or streptomycin is added for the first 2 months. In 9-month regimens, only three drugs are used in the first 2 months, and isoniazid and rifampin are continued for another 7 months. After the first 2 months of therapy, twice-weekly dosing regimens have been established in the hopes of increasing compliance by directly observed therapy (56,57). Children with miliary tuberculosis should receive 12 months of treatment (56). Cutaneous TB and tuberculids have both been reported to recur when inadequate antituberculous chemotherapy regimens were used (21,40,48).

Cases of multidrug-resistant TB have been recognized in the skin, both in the presence of the HIV virus and in its absence, underscoring the importance of culturing the affected tissue. Isolates from three of four patients with acute miliary TB and AIDS were resistant to isoniazid, rifampin, and ethambutol (two of the three were also resistant to ethionamide) (28); and a plaque of warty TB in a 13-year-old HIV-negative boy grew a multidrug-resistant strain that was resistant to isoniazid and rifampin (58).

Adjuvant surgical therapy may be helpful in the management of cutaneous TB. Drainage, débridement, or both may accelerate healing in scrofuloderma, tuberculous gumma, and orificial TB (3). Surgical excision may be indicated in early lesions of lupus vulgaris. Plastic surgery can correct the mutilating effects of advanced lupus vulgaris (57).

ATYPICAL MYCOBACTERIA

Atypical mycobacteria can be defined most simply as mycobacteria other than *M. tuberculosis* organisms (59). Atypical mycobacteria usually do not include *M. bovis*, *M. africanum*, or *M. leprae*. In the 1950s, Runyon (60) classified them on the basis of pigmentation and growth rates as photochromogens, scotochromogens, nonchromogens, and rapid growers. In more recent literature, atypical mycobacteria are broadly grouped into pathogens and nonpathogens (with the understanding that nonpathogens rarely become pathogens) (59,61–70) (Tables 40.4 and 40.5).

Atypical mycobacteria are different from *M. tuberculosis* in several ways. Perhaps the most important difference is the fact that person-to-person transmission is rare. The organisms are found in the environment and can colonize humans without causing true infection. Underlying circumstances, such as chronic pulmonary disease, trauma, or

TABLE 40.4. INFECTION FROM ATYPICAL MYCOBACTERIA

Mycobacterium Pathogen	Frequent Skin Infection	Rare Skin Infection	Lymphadenitis
M. avium-intracellulare		+	+
M. fortuitum-chelonae complex	+		+
M. haemophilum	+		+
M. kansasii		+	+
M. malmoense			+
M. marinum	+		
M. scrofulaceum		+	+
M. shimoidei[a]			
M. simiae[a]			
M. szulgai		+	+
M. ulcerans	+		
M. xenopi[a]			

[a]Pathogens not causing skin or lymph node infections.
Data from references 59, 61–63.

TABLE 40.5. NONPATHOGENIC ATYPICAL MYCOBACTERIA[a]

Name	Skin Lesions Reported
M. asiaticum	
M. flavescens	+
M. gastri	
M. gordonae	+
M. neoaurum	
M. para-fortuitum complex	
M. phlei	
M. smegmatis	+
M. terrae complex	
M. thermoresistible	+
M. vaccae	+

[a]These mycobacteria are usually (but not exclusively) nonpathogenic.
Data from references 59, 64–70.

immunosuppression, are frequently necessary precursors to pathogenic infection (59).

The skin is one of the common sites of infection for several atypical mycobacteria: *M. marinum, M. ulcerans,* the rapid growers (*M. fortuitum, M. chelonae,* and *M. abscessus*), and *M. haemophilum*. Many of the other mycobacteria have been reported in skin lesions, and the skin can be involved in disseminated infections.

Mycobacterium marinum

M. marinum infection in humans was originally described in the skin (71). Other names for this organism are *M. balnei* and *M. platypoecilus* (59). The source of the infection is freshwater or saltwater from pools or aquariums; hence the name "swimming pool granuloma" (72). *M. marinum* commonly causes formation of a nodule on the arm or hand (72,73) (Fig. 40.7). Sporotrichoid spread with nodules fol-

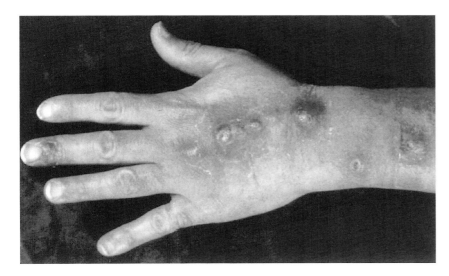

FIGURE 40.7. *Mycobacterium marinum* infection on the arm. (Courtesy of Department of Dermatology, New York University.)

lowing the course of the lymphatics is not unusual (73). Disseminated skin lesions have been reported in nonimmunosuppressed individuals, but most patients with disseminated disease have underlying disease (74).

On histologic sections, it is difficult to find bacilli in the lesions, but in immunocompromised patients numerous bacilli may be present (72). When found, the mycobacteria are often in histiocytes. These mycobacteria are longer and broader than those of *M. tuberculosis* and have crossbanding. The organisms grow best at 31°C to 33°C (59). Clarithromycin, minocycline, doxycyline, and trimethoprim–sulfamethoxazole all are effective as monotherapy, as are rifampin and ethambutol in combination. Therapy should be continued for at least 3 months (75). Because lesions can heal spontaneously, critical evaluation of therapy is difficult.

Mycobacterium ulcerans

M. ulcerans causes skin ulcers in humans. These ulcers have been described in people from Australia ("Bairnsdale ulcer"), Uganda ("Buruli ulcer") and other parts of Africa, as well as in Malaysia, New Guinea, Guyana, and Mexico (76). The natural habitat for *M. ulcerans* appears to be swampy areas (72). Lesions usually occur on the extremities of children after minor trauma, although in Australia the mean age for these lesions is 28.6 years. An enlarging nodule may be noticed at 3 weeks, but incubation usually occurs 6 to 12 weeks after inoculation (59,76). Ulceration ensues.

The borders of the ulcer are ragged and undermined. Often the ulcer is painless and not associated with lymphadenopathy. The lesion may resolve spontaneously, but can be scarring and deforming. AFBs are often seen in ulcer drainage and usually in histologic section (76). Infarction of the tissue infected with *M. ulcerans* occurs. Cultures of the tissue should be incubated at 30°C to 33°C. Preferred treatment, when possible, is excision and grafting. Chemotherapeutic regimens with combinations of trimethoprim–sulfamethoxazole, rifampin, streptomycin, dapsone, and ethambutol have been used. Because *M. ulcerans* is sensitive to heat, local measures to increase the temperature of the lesion have also been tried (71).

Mycobacterium fortuitum, Mycobacterium chelonae, and Mycobacterium abscessus

M. fortuitum, *M. chelonae*, and *M. abscessus* may be grouped as the *M. fortuitum* complex, but today these rapid growers are recognized as separate species (4). The organisms are found in soil, dust, and water (78,79). These mycobacteria can cause localized skin lesions in surgical wounds or after trauma (80). Patients infected in a community outbreak of *M. fortuitum* secondary to contamination of footbaths at a nail salon presented with furunculosis (81). A case mimicking lupus vulgaris has been described (82), as has one with

a sporotrichoid pattern of nodules (83). When disseminated skin lesions are found, the patient is almost always immunosuppressed (77).

Biopsies of these lesions reveal mycobacteria with special stains in less than one third of patients, but a higher rate is found in immunocompromised patients (59). When found, the organisms are clumped extracellularly with surrounding neutrophils (79,83,84). Cultures of rapid growers grow at 25°C to 40°C and usually appear within a week, although they can take many weeks to grow (78). Cultures are needed to identify the organism and allow for antibacterial sensitivities to be determined. A combination of amikacin and cefoxitin with probenecid, followed by oral antibiotics for several weeks, has been used to manage these infections. Recently, the new macrolide antibiotic clarithromycin has been successfully used to manage *M. chelonae* and *M abscessus* infections. Other antibiotics used for these infections are erythromycin, doxycycline, tetracycline, minocycline, tobramycin, trimethoprim–sulfamethoxazole, ciprofloxacin, clofazimine, and azithromycin (59,77–79). Linezolid may also prove useful (85). Antimicrobial sensitivity testing is essential because of resistance; for example, *M. chelonae* is often resistant to cefoxitin, and *M. abscessus* is frequently resistant to ciprofloxacin and may prove resistant to clarithromycin (75,82).

Mycobacterium scrofulaceum

M. scrofulaceum is so named because it causes lesions that mimic true tuberculous scrofuloderma. The organism may be found in dairy products, oysters, soil, and water (59). Enlarged cervical lymph nodes infected with this organism tend to open and drain. Children are most commonly affected with lymphadenitis. Lymphadenitis may also be caused by *M. kansasii*, *M. szulgai*, *M. avium-intracellulare*, *M. malmoense*, *M. fortuitum* complex, and *M. haemophilum* (59,61). An adult with sporotrichoid lesions has been described (62). Rarely, skin lesions secondary to hematogenous spread have been reported (86). The organism may be cultured at 25°C, 31°C, or 37°C (59). Either surgical intervention or antituberculous chemotherapy may be used as treatment (86).

Mycobacterium szulgai

M. szulgai is rarely pathogenic in humans. Its natural environment is unknown. When humans are infected, the lungs are most commonly involved. However, there have been cases in which the skin was involved without evidence of pulmonary disease. Biopsy does not always reveal mycobacteria. Cultures grow at both 25°C and 37°C in approximately 14 days (60). The organism is usually sensitive to ethionamide, ethambutol, isoniazid, and rifampin (64,86,88), but streptomycin, capreomycin, and viomycin have also been tried (59).

Mycobacterium kansasii

M. kansasii most commonly causes pulmonary infections in men but rarely can cause skin infections (72). The morphology of the skin infection can be quite variable, with localized lesions, scattered lesions, and multiple sporotrichoid lesions (72,88,89). Verrucous, cellulitic, papulopustular, nodular, and ulcerative lesions have also been described (90). In immunosuppressed patients, extracutaneous foci are often present. The organism grows best at 37°C in 10 to 14 days (72). The treatment involves the use of antituberculous chemotherapy such as isoniazid, rifampin, and ethambutol, or clarithromycin as an alternative (75).

Mycobacterium avium Complex

M. avium complex is found in numerous environmental sources: fresh water and saltwater, soil, house dust, dried plants, dairy products, and animal tissue (71,91). There have been rare cases of primary infection of the skin, with both plaques and ulcers. More commonly, the lungs are infected and the skin is infected because of hematogenous dissemination. Nodular, pustular, and ulcerative lesions have been described (91,92). A single case mimicked lupus vulgaris (94). Disseminated disease may be more common now because of the AIDS epidemic (Fig. 40.8). Skin lesions may be seen in the immune reconstitution syndrome associated with the induction of highly active antiretroviral therapy. These have been described as tender and erythematous with a pustular center (94). On histologic examination, the bacilli may be found intracellularly (59). These bacilli grow best at 37°C (72). While tuberculids are rarely seen in atypical mycobacterial infections, both papulonecrotic tuberculid and lichen scrofulosorum have been reported in association with *M. avium* complex (95,96). The new macrolides, either clarithromycin or azithromycin, form the basis of therapy for these infections. Rifabutin, or rifampin, and ethambutol are given in combination. Treatment may be necessary for up to 2 years, but with localized disease shorter courses are acceptable (85).

Mycobacterium haemophilum

M. haemophilum is a rare cause of skin lesions in humans; most often the infection is found in immunosuppressed patients (97), where it may be the sole manifestation of disease (98). In patients with AIDS, *M. haemophilum* may cause disseminated disease (61). Nodules occur most often on the extremities, but the face or chest can also be involved. On histologic examination, AFBs are often found (59). The most common histologic pattern is a mixed suppurative and granulomatous reaction, but a nongranulomatous pattern has been recognized (99). Diagnosis depends on culturing the organism, which requires a hemin or ferric ammonium citrate–enriched media and a temperature of 28°C to 32°C. Therapy with macrolides, ciprofloxacin, trimethoprim–sulfamethoxazole, doxycycline, antituberculous agents, and surgical excision has been used (100,101).

Mycobacteria malmoense

M. malmoense is a rare pathogen that usually infects the lungs. There is no known inanimate source; it is found in wild armadillos. The most common extrapulmonary infection is cervical adenitis in children. Cases of tenosynovitis

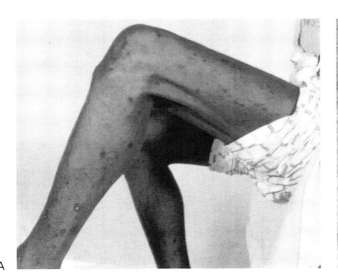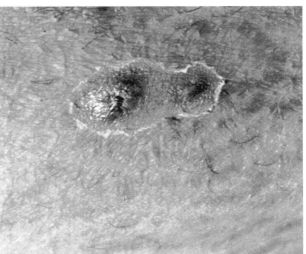

FIGURE 40.8. A: Disseminated *Mycobacterium avium* complex in a patient with acquired immunodeficiency syndrome. **B:** Close-up of cutaneous *Mycobacterium avium* complex. (Courtesy of Mary Ruth Buchness, M.D., New York Medical College, Valhalla, NY.)

in adults with overlying soft-tissue swelling, draining sinuses, or both have been reported. Disseminated disease has been found in immunosuppressed patients and can result in dermatologic findings (61). The organism grows at 22°C to 37°C (60). Special media at a lower pH may be necessary (67). Almost all *M. malmoense* isolates are resistant to isoniazid but are usually sensitive to rifampin and ethambutol (61,85).

Nonpathogens

The nonpathogens usually do not cause clinical disease. *M. thermoresistible*, *M. flavescens*, *M. gordonae*, *M. vaccae*, and *M. smegmatis* have been reported in skin lesions (64–70).

Summary of Atypical Mycobacteria

Atypical mycobacteria must be considered as causative organisms in unusual skin infections. Although histologic sections may suggest the diagnosis, culture of tissue is necessary even when AFBs are seen. Tissue cultures should be incubated at two temperatures (e.g., 30°C and 35°C) at least, and, if *M. haemophilum* or *M. malmoense* is suspected, in special medium. Cultures need to be incubated for as long as 12 weeks (67). Culture allows identification of the organism and drug sensitivity testing. Appropriate treatment regimens, whether watchful waiting, surgery, chemotherapy, or all of these, can then be determined.

REFERENCES

1. Marmelzat WL. Laennec and the "prosector's wart." *Arch Dermatol* 1962;86:74–76.
2. Beyt BE, Ortbals DW, Santa Cruz DJ, et al. Cutaneous mycobacteriosis: analysis of 34 cases with a new classification of the disease. *Medicine* 1981;60:95–109.
3. Kakakhel KV, Fritsch P. Cutaneous tuberculosis. *Int J Dermatol* 1989;28:355–362.
4. Tappeiner G, Wolff K. Tuberculosis and other mycobacterial infections. In: Freedberg IM, Eisen AZ, Wolff K, et al., eds. *Dermatology in general medicine*, 5th ed. New York: McGraw-Hill, 1999:2274–2290.
5. Hara K, Tsuzuki T, Takagi N, et al. Nodular granulomatous phlebitis of the skin: a fourth type of tuberculide. *Histopathology* 1997;30:129–134.
6. Jordaan HF, Schneider JW, Abdulla EAK. Nodular tuberculide: a report of four patients. *Pediatr Dermatol* 2000;17:183–188.
7. Visser VJ, Heyl T. Skin tuberculosis as seen at Ga-Rankuwa hospital. *Clin Exp Dermatol* 1993;18:507–515.
8. Stack R, Bickley LK, Coppel IG. Miliary tuberculosis presenting as skin lesions in a patient with acquired immunodeficiency syndrome. *J Am Acad Dermatol* 1990;23:1031–1035.
9. Harahap M. Tuberculosis of the skin. *Int J Dermatol* 1983;22:542–545.
10. Sehgal VN, Bhattacharya SN, Jain S, et al. Cutaneous tuberculosis: the evolving scenario. *Int J Dermatol* 1994;33:97–104.
11. Vidal D, Barnadas M, Perez M, et al. Tuberculous gumma following venepuncture. *Br J Dermatol* 2001;144:601–603.
12. Moschella SL, Cropley TG. Diseases of the mononuclear phagocytic system. In: Moschella SL, Hurley HJ, eds. *Dermatology*, 3rd ed. Philadelphia: WB Saunders, 1992:1031–1141.
13. Angus BJ, Yates M, Conlon C, et al. Cutaneous tuberculosis of the penis and sexual transmission of tuberculosis confirmed by molecular typing. *Clin Infect Dis* 2001;33:132–134
14. Gawkrodger DJ. Mycobacterial infections. In: Champion RH, Burton JL, Burns DA, et al., eds. *Textbook of dermatology*, 6th ed. Oxford: Blackwell Science, 1998:1181–1214.
15. Lever WF, Schaumberg-Lever G. In: Elder *Histopathology of the skin*. 8th ed. Philadelphia: JB Lippincott, 1997:468–477.
16. Ackerman B. *Histologic diagnosis of inflammatory skin diseases*. Philadelphia: Lea & Febiger, 1978:397–402, 454–456.
17. Wong KO, Lee KP, Chin SF. Tuberculosis of the skin in Hong Kong (a review of 160 cases) *Br J Dermatol* 1968;180:424–429.
18. Wortman PD. Pulmonary and cutaneous tuberculosis. *J Am Acad Dermatol* 1992;27:459–460.
19. Pereira MB, Gomes MK, Pereira F. Tuberculosis verrucosa cutis associated with tuberculous lymphadenitis. *Int J Dermatol* 2000;39:856–858.
20. Sehgal VN, Gupta R, Bose M, et al. Immunohistopathological spectrum in cutaneous tuberculosis. *Clin Exp Dermatol* 1993;18:309–313.
21. Marcoual J, Seruitje O, Moreno A, et al. Lupus vulgaris: clinical, histopathologic, and bacteriologic study of 10 cases. *J Am Acad Dermatol* 1992;26:404–407.
22. Handjani F, Delir M, Sodaifi P, et al. Lupus vulgaris following bacilli Calmette–Guérin vaccination. *Br J Dermatol* 2001;144:444–445.
23. Gooptu C, Marks N, Thomas J, et al. Squamous cell carcinoma associated with lupus vulgaris. *Clin Exp Dermatol* 1999;23:99–102.
24. Steidl M, Neubert U, Volkenardt M, et al. Lupus vulgaris confirmed by polymerase chain reaction. *Br J Dermatol* 1993;129:314–318.
25. Margall N, Baselga E, Coll P, et al. Detection of *Mycobacterium tuberculosis* complex DNA by polymerase chain reaction for rapid diagnosis of cutaneous tuberculosis. *Br J Dermatol* 1996;135:231–236.
26. McCray MK, Esterly NB. Cutaneous eruptions in congenital tuberculosis. *Arch Dermatol* 1981;117:460–464.
27. Daikos GL, Uttamchandani RB, Tuda C, et al. Disseminated miliary tuberculosis of the skin in patients with AIDS: report of four cases. *Clin Infect Dis* 1998;27:205–208.
28. Rietbrock RC, Dahlmans RPM, Smedts F, et al. Tuberculosis cutis miliaris disseminata as a manifestation of miliary tuberculosis: literature review and report of a case of recurrent skin lesions. *Rev Infect Dis* 1991;13:265–269.
29. Barbagallo J, Tager P, Ingleton R, et al. Cutaneous tuberculosis: diagnosis and treatment. *Am J Clin Dermatol* 2002;3:319–328.
30. Miller FSW, Cashman M. Metastatic tuberculous abscesses. *Arch Dis Child* 1955;30:169–173.
31. Kumar B, Rai R, Kaur I, et al. Childhood cutaneous tuberculosis: a study over 25 years from northern India. *Int J Dermatol* 2001;40:26–32.
32. Lee NH, Choi EH, Lee WS, et al. Tuberculous cellulitis. *Clin Exp Dermatol* 2000;25:222–223.
33. Kumar B, Kaur S. Papulonecrotic tuberculid. *Indian J Dermatol Venereol Leprol* 1977;43:212-213.
34. Victor T, Jodaan HF, van Niekerk DJT, et al. Papulonecrotic tuberculide: identification of mycobacterial tuberculous DNA by polymerase chain reaction. *Am J Dermatopathol* 1992;14:492–495.
35. Degitz K, Steidl M, Thomas P, et al. Aetiology of tuberculids (letter). *Lancet* 1993;341:239–240.
36. Schneider JW, Geiger DH, Rossouw DJ, et al. *Mycobacterium*

tuberculosis DNA in erythema induratum of Bazin (letter). *Lancet* 1993;342:747–748.

37. Baselga E, Margall N, Barnadas MA, et al. Detection of *Mycobacterium tuberculosis* DNA in lobular granulomatous panniculitis (erythema induratum-nodular vasculitis). *Arch Dermatol* 1997;133:457–462.

38. Morrison JGL, Fourie ED. The papulonecrotic tuberculid. *Br J Dermatol* 1974;91:263–270.

39. Sloan JB, Medenica M. Papulonecrotic tuberculid in a 9-year-old American girl: case report and review of the literature. *Pediatr Dermatol* 1990;7:191–195.

40. Wilson-Jones E, Winkelman RK. Papulonecrotic tuberculid: a neglected disease in Western countries. *J Am Acad Dermatol* 1986;14:815–826.

41. Ramdial PK, Mosam A, Pillay T, et al. Childhood lichen scrofulosorum revisited. *Pediatr Dev Pathol* 2000;3:211–215.

42. Torrelo A, Valverde E, Mediero IG, et al. Lichen scrofulosorum. *Pediatr Dermatol* 2000;17:373–376.

43. Beena KR, Ramesh V, Mukherjee A. Lichen scrofulosorum: a series of eight cases. *Dermatology* 2000;201:272–274.

44. Sehgal VN, Srivastava G, Sharma VK. Lupus vulgaris, caries of the spine and lichen scrofulosorum: an intriguing association. *Clin Exp Dermatol* 1987;12:280–282.

45. Kakakhel K. Simultaneous occurrence of tuberculous gumma, tuberculosis verrucosa cutis and lichen scrofulosorum. *Int J Dermatol* 1998;37:860–869.

46. Park YM, Hong JK, Cho SH, et al. Concommitant lichen scrofulosorum and erythema induratum. *J Am Acad Dermatol* 1998;38:841–843.

47. Arianayagam AV, Ash S, Russel Jones R. Lichen scrofulosorum in a patient with AIDS. *Clin Exp Dermatol* 1994;19:74–76.

48. Rademaker M, Lowe DG, Munro DD. Erythema induratum (Bazin's disease). *J Am Acad Dermatol* 1989;21:740–745.

49. Kumar B, Parsad D. Is "nodular tuberculide" a distinct entity? (letter) *Pediatr Dermatol* 2001;18:164–165.

50. Dostrovsky A, Sagher F. Dermatological complications of BCG vaccination. *Br J Dermatol* 1963;75:180–192.

51. Lotte A, Wasz-Hockeert O, Poisson N, et al. Second IUATLD study on complications induced by intradermal BCG-vaccination. *Bull Int Union Tuberc* 1988;63:47–59.

52. Izumi AK, Matsunaga J. BCG vaccine–induced lupus vulgaris. *Arch Dermatol* 1982;118:171–172.

53. Antanya RJ, Gardner ES, Bettencourt MS, et al. Cutaneous complications of BCG vaccination in infants with immune disorders: two cases and a review of the literature. *Pediatr Dermatol* 2001;18:205–209.

54. Tan SH, Tan BH, Goh CL, et al. Detection of *Mycobacterium tuberculosis* DNA using polymerase chain reaction in cutaneous tuberculosis and tuberculids. *Int J Dermatol* 1999;38:122–127.

55. Nachbar E, Classen V, Nachbar T, et al. Orificial tuberculosis: detection by polymerase chain reaction. *Br J Dermatol* 1996;135:106–109.

56. Bass JB Jr, Farer LS, Hopewell PC, et al. Treatment of tuberculosis and tuberculous infection in adults and children. American Thoracic Society and the Centers for Disease Control and Prevention. *Am J Respir Crit Care Med* 1994;149:1359–1374.

57. Corsello BF. New approach to treatment of pulmonary and extrapulmonary tuberculosis. *Int J Dermatol* 1987;26:185–189.

58. Ramesh V, Murlidhar S, Kumar J, et al. Isolation of drug-resistant tubercule bacilli in cutaneous tuberculosis. *Pediatr Dermatol* 2001;18:393–395.

59. Woods GL, Washington JA III. Mycobacteria other than *Mycobacterium tuberculosis*: review of microbiologic and clinical aspects. *Rev Infect Dis* 1987;9:275–299.

60. Runyon EH. Anonymous mycobacteria in pulmonary disease. *Med Clin North Am* 1959;43:273–290.

61. Zaugg M, Salfinger M, Opravil M, et al. Extrapulmonary and disseminated infections due to *Mycobacterium malmoense*: case report and review. *Clin Infect Dis* 1993;16:540–549.

62. Sowers WF. Swimming pool granuloma due to *Mycobacteria scrofulaceum*. *Arch Dermatol* 1972;105:760–761.

63. Cross GM, Guill MA, Aton JK. Cutaneous *Mycobacteria szulgai* infection. *Arch Dermatol* 1985;121:247–249.

64. Starke JR. Nontuberculous mycobacterial infections in children. *Adv Pediatr Infect Dis* 1992;7:123–159.

65. Wallace RJ, Nash DR, Tsukamura M, et al. Human disease due to *Mycobacterium smegmatis*. *Infect Dis* 1988;158:52–59.

66. Neeley SP, Denning DW. Cutaneous *Mycobacterium thermoresistible* infection in a heart transplant recipient. *Rev Infect Dis* 1989;11:608–611.

67. Wayne LG, Sramek HA. Agents of newly recognized or infrequently encountered mycobacterial diseases. *Clin Microbiol* 1992;5:1–25.

68. Shelley WB, Folkens AT. *Mycobacterium gordonae* infection of the hand. *Arch Dermatol* 1984;120:1064–1065.

69. Hachem R, Raad I, Rolston KVI, et al. Cutaneous and pulmonary infections caused by *Mycobacterium vaccae*. Clin Infect Dis 1996;23:173–175.

70. del Giudice P, Bernard E, Pinier Y, et al. Cutaneous infection due to *Mycobacterium gordonae* in a human immunodeficiency virus–infected patient. *Clin Infect Dis* 1998;26:1486–1487.

71. Linell F, Norden A. *Mycobacterium balnei*. A new acid-fast bacillus occurring in swimming pools and capable of producing skin lesions in humans. *Acta Tuberc Scand* 1954;33:1–84.

72. Street ML, Umbert-Millet IJ, Roberts GD, et al. Nontuberculous mycobacterial infections of the skin: report of fourteen cases and review of the literature. *J Am Acad Dermatol* 1991;24:208–215.

73. Edelstein H. *Mycobacterium marinum* skin infections. Report of 31 cases and review of the literature. *Arch Intern Med* 1994;154:1359–1364.

74. King AJ, Fairley JA, Rasmussen JE. Disseminated cutaneous *Mycobacterium marinum* infections. *Arch Dermatol* 1983;119:268–270.

75. Medical Section of the American Lung Association. Diagnosis and treatment of disease caused by nontuberculous mycobacteria. This official statement of the American Thoracic Society was approved by the board of directors, March 1997. *Am J Respir Crit Care Med* 1997;156:S1–S5.

76. Clancy JK, et al. Mycobacterial skin ulcers in Uganda. *Lancet* 1961;2:951–954.

77. Wallace RJ, Tanner D, Brennan PJ, et al. Clinical trial of clarithromycin for cutaneous (disseminated) infection due to *Mycobacterium chelonae*. *Ann Intern Med* 1993;119:482–486.

78. Rotman DA, Blauvelt A, Kerdel FA. Widespread primary cutaneous infection with *Mycobacterium fortuitum*. *Int J Dermatol* 1993;32:512–514.

79. Swetter SM, Kindel SE, Smollen BR. Cutaneous nodules of *Mycobacterium chelonae* in an immunosuppressed patient with pre-existing pulmonary colonization. *J Am Acad Dermatol* 1993;28:352–355.

80. Wallace RJ Jr, Swenson HM, Silcox VA, et al. Spectrum of disease due to rapidly growing *Mycobacterium*. *Rev Infect Dis* 1983;5:657–679.

81. Winthrop K, Abrams M, Yakrus M, et al. An outbreak of mycobacterial furunculosis associated with footbaths at a nail salon. *N Engl J Med* 2002;346:1366–1371.

82. Lin YC, Chiu HC, Hsiao CH, et al. Cutaneous *Mycobacterium fortuitum* infection mimicking lupus vulgaris. *Br J Dermatol* 2002;147:170–173.

83. Franck N, Cabie A, Villette B, et al. Treatment of *Mycobacterium chelonae*–induced skin infection with clarithromycin. *J Am Acad Dermatol* 1993;28:1019–1021.
84. Drabick JJ, Duffy PE, Samlosker CP, et al. Disseminated *M. chelonae* subspecies *chelonae* infections with cutaneous and osseous manifestation. *Arch Dermatol* 1990;126:1064–1067.
85. Brown-Elliot BA, Wallace RJ, Blinkholm R, et al. Successful treatment of disseminated *Mycobacterium chelonae* infection with linezolid. *Clin Infect Dis* 2001;33:1433–1434.
86. Murray-Leisure KA, Egan N, Weite Kamp MR. Skin lesions caused by *Mycobacterium scrofulaceum*. *Arch Dermatol* 1987;123:369–370.
87. Sybert A, Tsoue E, Garagusi UF. Cutaneous infection due to *Mycobacterium szulgai*. *Am Rev Respir Dis* 1977;115:695–698.
88. Owens DW, McBride ME. Sporotrichoid cutaneous infection with *Mycobacterium kansasii*. *Arch Dermatol* 1969;100:54–58.
89. Hirsh FS, Saffold OE. *Mycobacterium kansasii* infection with dermatologic manifestations. *Arch Dermatol* 1976;112:706–708.
90. Hanke CW, Temofeew RK, and Slama SL. *Mycobacterium kansasii* infection with multiple cutaneous lesions. *J Am Acad Dermatol* 1987;16:1122–1128.
91. Cox SK, Strausbough LJ. Chronic cutaneous infection caused by *Mycobacterium intracellulare*. *Arch Dermatol* 1981;117:794–796.
92. Ichiki Y, Hirose M, Akiyama T, et al. Skin infection caused by *Mycobacterium avium*. *Br J Dermatol* 1997;136:260–263.
93. Kullavanijaya P, Sirimachan S, Surarak S. Primary cutaneous infection with *Mycobacterium avium intracellulare* complex resembling lupus vulgaris. *Br J Dermatol* 1997;136:264–266.
94. Brown M, Williams IG, Miller RF. Deterioration of disseminated cutaneous *Mycobacterium avium* complex infection with a leukemoid reaction following institution of highly active antiretroviral therapy. *Sex Transm Infect* 2001;77:149–150.
95. Williams JT, Pulitzer DR, Devillez RL. Papulonecrotic tuberculide secondary to disseminated *Mycobacterium avium* complex. *Int J Dermatol* 1994;33:109–112.
96. Komatsu H, Terinuma A, Tabata N, et al. *Mycobacterium avium* infection of the skin associated with lichen scrofulosorum: report of three cases. *Br J Dermatol* 1999;141:554–557.
97. Dautzenberg B, Truffot C, Legris S, et al. Activity of clarithromycin against *Mycobacterium avium* infection in patients with the acquired immune deficiency syndrome. *Am Rev Respir Dis* 1991;144:564–569.
98. Shah MK, Sebti A, Kiehn TE, et al. *Mycobacterium hemophilum* in immunocompromised patients. *Clin Infect Dis* 2001;33:330–337.
99. Busam KJ, Kiehn TE, Salob SP, et al. Histologic reactions to cutaneous infections by *Mycobacterium hemophilum*. *Am J Surg Pathol* 1999;23:1379-1385.
100. McGovern J, Bix BC, Webster G. *Mycobacterium haemophilum* skin disease successfully treated with excision. *J Am Acad Dermatol* 1994;30:269–270.
101. Saubolle MA, Kiehn TE, White MH, et al. *Mycobacterium hemophilum*: microbiology and expanding clinical and geographic spectra of disease in humans. *Clin Microbiol Rev* 1996;9:435–437.

TUBERCULOSIS IN CHILDREN

MONA RIGAUD
WILLIAM BORKOWSKY

The World Health Organization (WHO) has estimated that in 1990 alone there were more than 8 million new cases of tuberculosis (TB) worldwide and 2.9 million deaths caused by TB. Approximately 1.3 million of these new cases and 450,000 deaths occurred in children younger than 15 years (1). TB remains a health threat globally. WHO estimated the prevalence of TB in 1997 at 16.2 million, including 8 million new cases (2). Based on a steady 3% annual increase of TB in the world, 10.2 million new TB infections are projected for the year 2005. The state of TB in children reflects the same trend found in adults. Some experts attribute 10% of the global TB burden to children, and 1 million children were projected to have TB in 2000 (3). As in the adult population, the burden of caring for children with TB is found primarily in countries with the fewest resources to face such public health challenges.

The basic process of infection and disease caused by *Mycobacterium tuberculosis* and the concepts of diagnosis and management of TB are the same for children and adults. Accurate diagnosis and effective treatment of TB disease and the identification of TB infection without disease, along with successful completion of preventive therapy, are as important for children as for adults. Furthermore, adequate preventive therapy can block the development of TB disease in most individuals and interrupt potential transmission of TB. However, there are several differences in the epidemiology, clinical manifestations, and management of TB in children (Table 41.1). These differences are highlighted throughout the chapter.

EPIDEMIOLOGY

In the United States, the dramatic increase in the incidence of TB (54.5%) in young adults 25 to 44 years of age (prime childbearing/rearing years) from 1985 to 1992 was paral-

leled by marked increases in the incidence of TB in children. Cases of TB in persons 14 years of age and under increased by 34.1% during the same period (4). The public health measures taken to halt the resurgence of TB in the United States resulted in a steady decline of new cases. Approximately 17,000 new cases of TB were reported in the year 2000, indicating a drop of 39% since 1992 (5). An overall decline of TB was also seen in children as the number of reported cases in children younger than 14 years decreased from 1,696 in 1992 to 1,252 in 1997 (6). However, TB remains prevalent in foreign-born individuals living in the United States (7) and continues to be a problem in specific U.S.-born populations (8).

Children at High Risk of Tuberculosis Infection

Although children are no more likely than adults to develop TB infection when exposed to a person with infectious TB, they are at substantially greater risk of developing TB disease, especially miliary disease and meningitis. Factors that determine the risk of TB infection are the same for children and adults: the possibility of exposure to a person with active, infectious TB; the infectivity and treatment status of the person with TB; and the degree of exposure to the infectious individual. Children exposed to adults with increased risk of TB infection are also at increased risk of infection. This includes children exposed to persons from countries with a high prevalence of TB, incarcerated adults, residents of nursing homes, homeless persons, illicit-drug–using adults, and poor or medically indigent persons. The more prolonged and close the exposure to the infectious case, the greater the risk of infection. For children, this specifically includes exposure to caregivers with TB, such as relatives, neighbors, babysitters, day care providers, or teachers (9).

A disproportionate number of cases of TB occur in urban areas in both children and adults. Poverty, with resultant poor nutrition, overcrowded living conditions, and inadequate medical care, has a major role in the occurrence of TB. Immigrants to the United States represent another population in which the number of cases of TB is increasing. This includes adopted and foreign-born children (10,11).

M. Rigaud: Department of Pediatrics, New York University Medical Center; Department of Pediatrics, Bellevue Hospital–Tisch Hospital, New York, New York.
W. Borkowsky: Department of Pediatrics, New York University School of Medicine, New York, New York.

TABLE 41.1. CHARACTERISTICS OF TUBERCULOSIS IN CHILDREN AS OPPOSED TO THAT IN ADULTS

1. There are variations in the risk of developing active tuberculosis and in the likelihood of transmission of infection based on a child's age.
2. Children rarely develop cavitary lesions.
3. Extrapulmonary disease is more common in children.

Increased incidence rates of TB in adults may be the result of primary infection or reactivation disease, but increased incidence rates in children are generally caused by recent transmission of TB, thus representing a primary infection in the child. The occurrence of a recent TB infection (tuberculin skin test (TST) conversion, with or without evidence of disease in the past 2 years) should be considered a sentinel event indicating recent transmission of *M. tuberculosis* from an infectious adult or adolescent to the identified child.

Tuberculosis Infection Versus Disease

The diagnostic standards and classification of TB set forth by the American Thoracic Society (12) are applicable to children and adults. The distinction between infection and disease is an important one for many reasons, including the fact that children are more likely than adults to develop disease after primary infection with TB.

TB infection without disease is the stage in which an individual has a positive TST result but no signs or symptoms of disease and the chest roentgenogram is normal. TB represents clinical disease when the primary infection is not contained by the host response or when the latent infection reactivates and clinical signs and symptoms are apparent. While estimates suggest that 5% to 10% of adults with *M. tuberculosis* infection progress to active disease at some time during their life, a child's risk may exceed the 10% upper limit (13).

The risk of active disease is greatest in the first few years after infection and greater in persons who are malnourished (body weight 10% less than ideal), are immunosuppressed because of illness such as human immunodeficiency virus (HIV) infection or medications, or have other medical conditions (e.g., silicosis, sarcoidosis, or diabetes mellitus). The risk of developing TB is greater for children, especially infants, and varies with age. Children younger than 6 years have the highest rates of tuberculous disease and also have the most severe disease (advanced pulmonary disease, miliary or tuberculous meningitis) (13). The younger the child, the greater the risk of developing active disease; as many as 43% of children younger than 1 year, 24% of children 1 to 5 years, and 15% of adolescents develop active TB at some time after the primary infection (14).

Transmission

Children usually acquire TB from adults or adolescents. Children younger than 10 years are usually not considered to be contagious (15). There are several reasons for this: children rarely have cavitary lesions; their pulmonary lesions generally contain fewer *M. tuberculosis* organisms (therefore, they are more often culture negative); many children with TB have no or little cough; and younger children are less capable of forcefully coughing and aerosolizing organisms in droplet nuclei. There is, however, one case report of two children younger than 2 years who had extensive endobronchial TB with positive cultures and positive smears. Transmission of TB apparently occurred in a few of the health care workers providing care for these hospitalized children (16). More recently, transmission of TB by a non-hospitalized child was reported in the United States. A 9-year-old boy from Marshall Island with extensive cavitary disease and positive cultures and smears transmitted TB to contacts at home, in the same classroom, and on the same bus route (17). Therefore, children with evidence of clinical TB (either signs or symptoms) or abnormal chest roentgenograms, especially those with cavitary lesions, should be appropriately isolated until they have three consecutive negative acid-fast bacillus (AFB) smears, receive appropriate antituberculosis treatment, and have decreased cough.

The decision to isolate a specific patient should be individualized depending on the estimated degree of infectiousness. The duration of isolation should be based on the clinical response to therapy (diminished sputum production, cough, fever, etc.), laboratory assessment (AFB smears of sputum or cutaneous lesions), and the risk to those exposed. Adolescents are more like adults in their ability to transmit TB and should be treated as adults with regard to transmission and isolation. Since children get infection from adults, household contacts may have a greater propensity to transmit infection than the hospitalized infected child and must be screened for active disease prior to coming into the hospital setting.

Human Immunodeficiency Virus Infection and Tuberculosis in Children

Despite the fact that coinfection with HIV and *M. tuberculosis* is common in adults (18), very few children have been identified with both infections (19–21). Retrospective data from New York City during the late 1980s, a period of resurgence of TB, revealed that 3% of HIV-infected children had TB and that these were more likely to have extrapulmonary TB and specimens positive for cultures and smears (22). The risk of coinfected adults developing active TB is estimated at 10% per year (23). Children who have close contact with these coinfected adults are at high risk of becoming infected with TB regardless of their own HIV status. In investigations of contacts or associates, inquiry about any factors that may place children at greater risk of TB infection, including HIV infection in family members or close contacts, is appropriate. Furthermore, children with TB should be evaluated for HIV infection.

CLINICAL ASPECTS OF TUBERCULOSIS IN CHILDREN

The presentation of TB is extremely variable. It depends on the age of the host, the organ systems involved, the stage of infection (primary vs. reactivation), the host immune response, and the reproduction and spread of the organism. The lungs are the most commonly involved sites because the most common form of transmission is through organisms inhaled as droplet nuclei. Lymphohematogenous spread occurs more commonly in children and causes extrapulmonary disease in approximately 30% of children with TB (24). The propensity for lymphohematogenous spread places children at greater risk not only for extrapulmonary disease in general, but also for the more serious forms of TB, such as miliary TB and tuberculous meningitis.

Tuberculosis Infection Without Disease

Primary TB infection is usually a preclinical state marked by an absence of clinical symptoms, a normal chest roentgenogram, and a positive TST reaction. After infection with *M. tuberculosis*, a person may take 3 to 12 weeks to develop delayed-type hypersensitivity to the tuberculin proteins. During that time, identification of the infected individual, if he or she remains asymptomatic, is almost impossible. Most children remain asymptomatic during the primary infection, although a few may manifest nonspecific symptoms such as fever, malaise, and fatigue; these symptoms are rarely recognized as being caused by TB. Most children diagnosed with TB infection without disease are identified during contact investigations or skin test screening. Preventive therapy should begin in a timely fashion at this stage to block progression to active disease.

Active Tuberculosis Disease

Children with active TB tend to have clinical symptoms depending on their age and the degree of dissemination of the infection. However, more than half of the children may have few symptoms or be completely asymptomatic (25). One case series of children younger than 1 year with culture-proven TB reported presenting symptoms (primarily consisting of cough, fever, and poor feeding, and secondarily rales and localized pulmonary findings) in

79% of their cohort (26). In addition, a more recent review reported that symptoms of fever, weight loss, night sweats, cough, and hemoptysis were also encountered in older children (21).

Pulmonary Tuberculosis

Depending on its progression, active pulmonary TB in children manifests in a variety of forms, including endobronchial disease with focal lymph adenopathy, progressive pulmonary disease, pleural involvement, and reactivated pulmonary disease. The most common form is endobronchial disease with focal lymphadenopathy resulting from spread of the tubercle bacillus from the alveoli to both the bronchioles and the lymphatics. Subsequent drainage to the lymph nodes, along with the host response of activated macrophages and delayed hypersensitivity, leads to a significant inflammatory response and lymph node enlargement (Fig. 41.1). Lymph node enlargement can impinge on proximal anatomic sites and cause various clinical manifestations, such as bronchial obstruction (26), odynophagia with esophageal compression, and vocal cord or hemidiaphragmatic paralysis caused by local nerve compression. Bronchial obstruction can lead to a "collapse–consolidation" picture on chest roentgenogram, usually with minimal symptoms or signs suggestive of foreign body aspiration or simply a persistent cough (Fig. 41.2).

Progressive primary pulmonary TB occurs when the focal lesion progresses to a large caseous mass, which often drains into proximal bronchi and cavitates. This form of pulmonary disease is rare in children but more common in young infants or persons with abnormal cell-mediated immunity. These young children often appear very ill, with marked weight loss, fever, and cough. Classic signs of pneumonia are often evident consistent with the progressive lesions: dullness to percussion, egophony, decreased breath sounds, and rales.

Pleural involvement in primary pulmonary TB is generally uncommon, occurring more often in older children and adolescents (27,28). Their clinical presentation is usually one of pneumonia with a pleural effusion and persistent fever. However, pleural effusion without radiologic manifestation can occur (28). Mediastinal shifting along with marked shortness of breath and tachypnea can occur with large effusions.

Reactivation of TB occurs primarily in older children and adolescents. It is the result of activation of an old, latent focus of *M. tuberculosis* infection spread to that site via a lymphohematogenous route. Generally, this is a focal process, limited by previous host response and sensitivity to *M. tuberculosis* such that the reactivated infection undergoes caseation and liquefaction. The clinical presentation is usually subacute with weight loss, fatigue, fever, cough, and (rarely) hemoptysis.

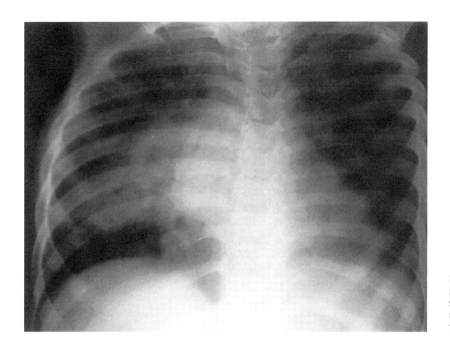

FIGURE 41.1. Roentgenogram of a child with primary tuberculosis. Posteroanterior view shows a hazy area of consolidation in the right midlung field in association with right hilar fullness (adenopathy).

Extrapulmonary Tuberculosis

Extrapulmonary TB includes peripheral lymph adenopathy in approximately 65% of patients, tuberculous meningitis in 10% to 15%, infection of bones or joints in 4%, and miliary TB (infection at several distant sites) in 5% (29).

Adenitis

Peripheral tuberculous lymphadenitis generally is the result of local spread from the primary site of infection, especially to supraclavicular or paratracheal nodes.

Lymphohematogenous dissemination can spread infection to distant lymph nodes from the primary infection. Rarely, peripheral adenitis is the result of a primary extrapulmonary site of infection. Tuberculous lymphadenitis usually presents as enlarged, firm, nontender lymph nodes with little erythema or fluctuance (30). Weight loss, fatigue, malaise, and fever are either absent or minimal. The adenitis can progress to caseation and necrosis and cause erythema, fluctuance, and, occasionally, spontaneous drainage. The lymph nodes most commonly involved are the anterior or posterior cervical and supraclavicular lymph nodes; less commonly, the submandibular, submental, axillary, and inguinal nodes are involved. *Scrofula* is a term applied to mycobacterial adenitis in the neck with marked lymph node enlargement. Often a biopsy and culture are necessary to distinguish other common causes of lymphadenitis and tuberculous or nontuberculous mycobacterial lymphadenitis. (31)

Meningitis

Tuberculous meningitis is the most common cause of death from TB because of the delay that usually occurs in making the diagnosis. It occurs most commonly in children younger than 6 years and more often in children younger than 2 years (32). Lymphohematogenous spread seeds foci in the brain, meninges, or both, and caseation can lead to extension into the subarachnoid space. Hydrocephalus occurs if there is obstruction of cerebrospinal fluid flow. Extension to the basilar meninges can cause compression of the third, sixth, and seventh nerves, resulting in paresis, paralysis, or both.

The clinical signs and symptoms of tuberculous meningitis are insidious, necessitating a high index of suspicion to make a timely diagnosis. Initially, nonspecific signs and symptoms (fever, vomiting, decreased appetite, behavioral changes) predominate (32,33). After 1 to 2 weeks, focal signs are evident, including vomiting, stiff neck, altered alertness, or seizures. Altered deep tendon reflexes, cranial nerve palsies, or unintelligible speech may appear. The illness can progress to severe cerebral damage despite early diagnosis and intervention, causing decerebrate or decorticate positioning, opisthotonos, deteriorating mental status, coma, and death.

Miliary

Miliary TB occurs in approximately 5% to 6% of patients manifesting extrapulmonary disease. It is caused by the rupture of caseous material into a blood vessel, resulting in hematogenous spread to numerous sites throughout the body. Like tuberculous meningitis, miliary TB is a complication of primary TB in young children. Approximately one third of children with miliary TB present with meningitis as one of the many involved sites.

The presentation of miliary TB depends on the specific sites involved (34). It occurs either subacutely with weight

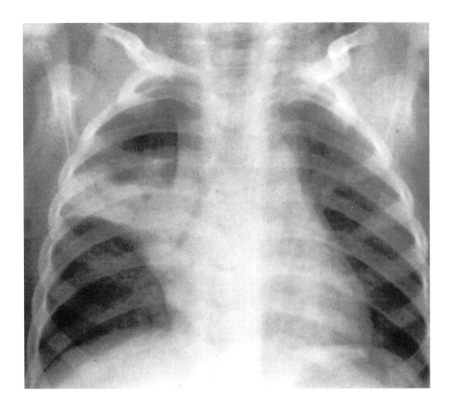

FIGURE 41.2. Roentgenogram showing collapse–consolidation in a child with pulmonary tuberculosis. Posteroanterior view shows an area of dense consolidation in association with volume loss and mediastinal adenopathy. Note elevation of the minor fissure.

loss, fatigue, malaise, and low-grade fever, or acutely with high fever and rapid onset of associated symptoms. The child usually has lymphadenopathy, hepatosplenomegaly, and a paucity of respiratory signs. Respiratory manifestations often evolve and include cough, tachypnea, cyanosis, and respiratory distress. Subtle findings, such as papular, necrotic, or purpuric lesions on the skin or choroidal tubercles on the retina, should be carefully sought during the physical examination.

Bone and Joints

Skeletal TB is a late complication of lymphohematogenous spread of bacilli, usually presenting years after the primary infection. Infants and young children are at greater risk of developing TB of the bone or joints because of the increased likelihood of lymphohematogenous dissemination and the increased vascularity of their bones during growth. The focal infection often begins in the metaphysis due to bacilli seeding the endarteries. Endarteritis leads to local bony destruction and subsequent drainage into the adjacent joint capsule or through a sinus tract to the skin. The most common sites involved are the large weight-bearing bones or joints such as the vertebrae (40% to 50% of patients), hip, knee, and elbow (35). TB of the bone or joint presents acutely or subacutely, as do the other common pyogenic bacterial skeletal infections, and is diagnosed in the context of seeking evidence for pyogenic bacterial bone and joint infection. Vertebral TB may be very insidi-

ous, presenting with signs of referred pain, abnormal posturing, or even a paravertebral abscess. Bony destruction with bone deformity is a late sign of skeletal TB.

Rarer sites of extrapulmonary TB include the genitourinary system (36), middle ear or mastoid, pericardium, eyes, and skin.

Tuberculosis in the Newborn Infant

TB in the newborn infant can be either congenital or the result of postnatal acquired infection.

Congenital Tuberculosis

Congenital TB is rare. Several hundred cases have been reported in the literature. Infection of the fetus can occur by transplacental spread of bacilli through the umbilical vein; bacilli reaching the amniotic fluid from tuberculous endometritis, placentitis, or both; or ingestion of infected amniotic fluid at the time of delivery. The clinical presentation of congenital TB commonly begins in the second or third week of life and is similar to that of bacterial sepsis and other congenital infections. Signs and symptoms often include poor feeding and poor weight gain, jaundice, hepatosplenomegaly, abdominal distention, cough, tachypnea, irritability, lethargy, and lymphadenopathy (37). The diagnosis of TB disease in the mother is often overlooked, yet it is essential to the diagnosis of congenital TB in the infant.

The TST is usually negative in the infant, especially in the first 6 to 8 weeks of life, but should be performed at the first suspicion of the illness and repeated if possible. Most infants have an abnormal chest roentgenogram, and almost half demonstrate a miliary pattern. Culturing for AFB from any site suspected to be involved is essential, including gastric aspirates, urine, cerebrospinal fluid, liver biopsy, and bone marrow aspirates. Examination and culture of the placenta is appropriate when the diagnosis is suspected or when the mother has had active TB during pregnancy. In nearly half the cases the diagnosis is made at autopsy.

Diagnostic criteria for congenital TB require the illness to have begun in the first weeks of the infant's life, the mother to have documented TB, and the infant to have a positive culture for *M. tuberculosis* or, preferably, histologic evidence of caseating granuloma or a primary hepatic complex (38). Ideally, postnatal transmission can be excluded.

Perinatal Tuberculosis

Perinatal TB is more common than congenital TB. Although it has a lower mortality rate, the morbidity of perinatal TB can be significant, especially when it leads to miliary or tuberculous meningitis. The route of infection is most commonly inhalation of tuberculous bacilli from any caregiver with active pulmonary TB. Infection rarely occurs by ingestion of infected breast or cow's milk or by direct inoculation through traumatized skin or mucous membranes (e.g., at ritual circumcision).

Clinical presentation is usually delayed until the patient is 1 to 3 months old and varies according to the infecting dose of bacillus and the sites involved. The clinical presence of meningitis, miliary, or primary pulmonary TB does not help to differentiate perinatal from congenital TB.

Diagnosis of active TB in the mother or other close contacts of the infant is essential, particularly in documenting postnatal transmission. The timing of acquisition of TB in the newborn does not affect treatment decisions.

DIAGNOSIS OF TUBERCULOSIS IN CHILDREN

Tuberculin Skin Test

Tuberculin skin testing was the first diagnostic tool for identifying tuberculous infection or disease in children and remains today the cornerstone of TB control programs. The Mantoux test, the most reliable of the TSTs, involves the intradermal injection of 5 units of purified protein derivative (PPD) prepared from supernatant extracts of cultures of *M. tuberculosis*. The American Academy of Pediatrics defines 5 mm or greater, 10 mm or greater, and 15 mm or greater induration thresholds to be used to determine a positive tuberculin reaction in different groups

at risk to develop TB (39,40). For children at high risk (e.g., those who are contacts of adults with infectious TB, who are immunosuppressed, who have clinical evidence of TB, or have abnormalities consistent with TB on chest roentgenogram), a TST reaction of 5 mm or greater of induration should be interpreted as a positive test result. For infants or for children who are living with adults in high-risk groups, induration of 10 mm or greater is considered positive; for all other persons who are considered to be at low risk for TB, induration of 15 mm or greater is classified as positive. The sensitivity and specificity of the Mantoux test can be problematic in establishing the diagnosis of TB. False-positive results of the Mantoux tests can be seen after recent vaccination with bacille Calmette–Guérin (BCG) or when previous infection with a nontuberculous mycobacteria causes cross-reactivity between similar antigens. Possible causes for false-negative tuberculin tests include transient anergy from TB infection itself, anything that decreases the host response to the skin test (i.e., other infections, vaccines, illnesses, malnutrition, stress, medications, young age); or, more commonly, factors that cause improper preparation, administration, measurement, or interpretation of the test (41). To ensure accurate reading of the Mantoux test, careful placement, standardized measurement of the induration, and practiced interpretation of the reacting size of the Mantoux test relative to the age of the patient, risks factors for testing, pertinent epidemiologic factors, and the specific medical history of the patient must be taken into consideration (4). Moreover, multiple puncture skin tests, which have been widely used in children for the ease of placement, should rarely if ever be used. The lack of standardization of the exact dose of antigen delivered and the variability of interpreting results (e.g., parents have been allowed to interpret the results themselves and report them to the physician) leads to a substantial incidence of false-positive and false-negative readings.

The Committee on Infectious Diseases of the American Academy of Pediatrics has stated that BCG vaccination is not a contraindication to tuberculin testing and that the Mantoux test be interpreted in a similar fashion regardless of the patient's history of BCG vaccination (40). However, the role of BCG vaccination as a possible confounder of a positive TST reaction has been debated over the years as BCG vaccination can lead to a reactive TST because of cross-reactivity of antigens. To differentiate skin reaction to BCG or infection with *M. tuberculosis*, a TST reaction of less than 10 mm in diameter is usually attributed to BCG reactivity. However, several reports have shown that the 10-mm induration is not a firm benchmark in differentiating TB infection from BCG reactivity (42). The age of the child at the time of the BCG vaccination and the number of doses of vaccines received may determine the size of the TST response, which can exceed 10 mm in diameter (43). It is, however, useful to know that the induration response to tuberculin testing after BCG declines over time, and the decline is more acute in children who have received the vaccine perinatally. Overall, only 5% of persons have a reactive tuberculin test 5 years after BCG vaccination (44). A child who received a BCG vaccination more than 5 years before presentation and who responds to skin testing with an induration of 10 mm or greater should be considered infected with *M. tuberculosis*. Further evaluation by chest roentgenography and administration of preventive isoniazid therapy are generally indicated. A child who received BCG vaccination less than 5 years before presentation and who demonstrates a TST reaction of 10 to 15 mm of induration should undergo a careful review of exposure risk, of results of previous tuberculin tests, of clinical signs or symptoms, and of a chest roentgenogram to assess the likelihood of tuberculous infection (45,46). Documented PPD conversion, clinical symptomatology, or radiologic evidence of TB should be considered confirmation of infection, which necessitates appropriate chemotherapy. Children who previously received BCG and who have a TST reaction of 5 to 10 mm, in the absence of confirmatory evidence of infection or exposure to infectious TB, should have tuberculin testing repeated over time because those children are at continued high risk of TB infection.

Case Finding Versus Screening/Targeted Tuberculin Skin Test

The usefulness of any test, such as the tuberculin test, depends on its sensitivity, its specificity, and the prevalence of the illness to be detected. The higher the prevalence of the illness, the greater the positive predictive value of the test. Using the tuberculin test for case finding, as part of the evaluation of children with clinical manifestations suggestive of TB or in children who have been exposed to adults with active disease, increases its positive predictive value. Contact investigation and associate investigation (discussed later) are occasions in which the Mantoux test has a higher positive predictive value because there is an increased likelihood of TB infection in these situations.

Routine screening in situations in which the prevalence of TB is low results in more false-positive reactions and diminishes the positive predictive value of the Mantoux test. Targeted screening, using the tuberculin test, to check children at high risk in a community with a proven high prevalence of TB enhances the utility of the test and is a useful way of identifying individuals with asymptomatic TB infection. The goal for using Mantoux testing in contact or associate investigations or in selective screening is to identify individuals who have asymptomatic TB infection and to provide preventive therapy to limit the occurrence of active TB.

In general, routine tuberculin skin testing in children living in areas with a low prevalence of TB, in the absence of specific risk factors, is not indicated. Children who are exposed to TB, who are at high risk for TB infection, or who live in communities with a high prevalence of TB should be tested yearly with the Mantoux test. In other communities in which the prevalence of TB is high, but the children have no risk factors or their risk cannot be assessed, periodic screening at specific times (e.g., before starting school or day care, or when changing schools) may be indicated.

Radiologic Diagnosis

Radiologic imaging is an essential step in the workup and in diagnosis of TB. Imaging of the chest helps to evaluate lung involvement in an asymptomatic patient and, as most children have TB infection without disease, the chest roentgenogram may be normal. Yet, in investigating for possible active tuberculous pulmonary disease, the chest roentgenogram may be the most useful tool because children with disease have a positive culture only 40% of the time (25). Moreover, often the chest roentgenogram shows evidence of more disease than is clinically evident. Radiologic images reflect the relationship between the dividing mycobacteria, the cellular host response, and the destruction of the lung parenchyma that may result from such interaction (47).

The most common radiologic finding in children with pulmonary TB is the primary complex consisting of a density of any lobe of the lung parenchyma and regional lymph node enlargement (hilar and paratracheal) (48) (Fig. 41.1). Primarily in children younger than 3 years, lymphadenopathy as the sole lung finding may be the hallmark of primary disease (49). Resolution of the parenchymal lesion and lymphadenopathy is later seen as focal scarring on imaging studies or as calcification in lymph nodes. All other radiologic abnormalities are the result of complications from the primary complex reflecting inadequate containment of *Mycobacterium* by the host. Progression of parenchymal lesion can lead to cavity formation, which is rarely seen in children. Local spreading of the primary complex is evident on chest roentgenogram as infiltrates in contiguous lobules or lobes. Lymph node enlargement, which is common in young children, often obstructs adjacent bronchi and leads to the "collapse–consolidation" picture shown in Figure 41.2. Pleural or pericardial effusion results from the rupture of the primary complex into these spaces.

Lymphohematogenous spread of disease can manifest radiographically in the thorax in various ways. This includes miliary (seedlike) lesions throughout the lungs (Fig. 41.3), pericardial or pleural involvement, and even endogenous reinfection in adolescents with evidence of disease long after the primary infection, often seen as involvement of the upper lobes. Diagnosis of extrapulmonary TB in the bones, kidney, liver, and spleen requires the use of other radiologic modalities, such as sonography, nuclear imaging, computed tomography (CT), and magnetic resonance imaging.

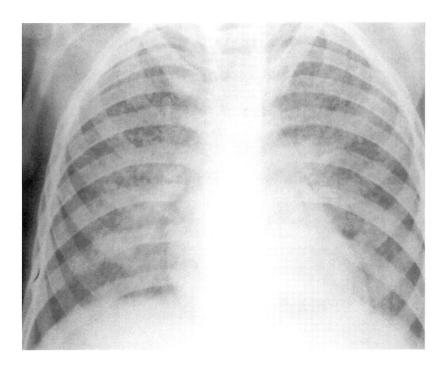

FIGURE 41.3. Miliary tuberculosis in an infant. Chest roentgenogram shows a diffuse, bilateral, reticular-nodular pattern with interstitial thickening. There is no focal consolidation.

Recent advances in the use of chest CT to diagnose pulmonary TB have allowed improvements in the resolution of suspected parenchymal lesions and lymphadenopathy; have permitted clinicians to follow the complications of disease; and, perhaps most importantly, have made it possible to evaluate children whose chest roentgenograms are normal but who nonetheless are suspected of having pulmonary TB (50,51). In one report, CT detection of lung lesions not visualized by chest roentgenogram affected the treatment of 37% of evaluable children (52).

The newest high-resolution, low-dose, computed tomography (HRLDCT) scanners are useful not only because of their dramatic sensitivity but also because of their decreased motion artifact and low radiation exposure. Using HRLDCT scanning (120 kV, 80 milliamperes, single-slice imaging) with the General Electric HiSpeed Advantage Scanner (Milwaukee, WI, U.S.A.) for a noncontrast scan of the thorax exposes the child to radiation equivalent to that of four chest roentgenograms. HRLDCT scanning has been most useful in confirming the diagnosis of TB while smears and cultures are pending (Bellevue Hospital experience to date). Identification of the primary complex (demonstrating lymph node enlargement not evident on chest roentgenogram) and documenting multiple small areas of consolidation as evidence of endobronchial spread are two clear advantages of HRLDCT scanning over chest roentgenography (Fig. 41.4).

Laboratory Tests

Bacteriologic evaluation of clinical specimens is the gold standard for diagnosis of TB in children and is crucial in studies of mycobacterial resistance to antimycobacterial drugs. A Ziehl–Neelsen stain for AFB should be performed on all specimens. These should be processed as well for culture. As in adults, the traditional culture methods and media (Lowenstein–Jensen and Middlebrook solid media) require 4 to 10 weeks for results and have been replaced by liquid culture broth methods. These newer techniques utilize radiometric analysis and liquid media, with the release of $^{14}CO_2$ from fatty acids labeled with carbon 14 metabolized by the growing mycobacteria, and yield culture and sensitivity results in 7 to 21 days.

Obtaining adequate specimen for analysis in children is a daunting task. Despite the fact that there is approximately 60% concordance between the mycobacterial culture and sensitivity results for the identified source case and the child (53), every child suspected of having TB should undergo mycobacterial culturing and sensitivity testing. It is important to culture all appropriate body sites and fluids because 30% of children with TB have extrapulmonary disease. Children younger than 10 years have difficulty producing sputum on command for analysis; therefore, aspiration of the gastric content for bacteriologic studies for AFB is the procedure of choice in this age group. Aspiration of the gastric content should be performed in the early morning before the patient gets out of bed, immediately following a period of 8 to 10 hours in which he or she had nothing by mouth. The gastric contents should be washed out with a large volume of sterile water with a neutral pH and delivered promptly to the laboratory. Even in the best of hands, gastric aspirate culture is positive in children with pulmonary TB approxi-

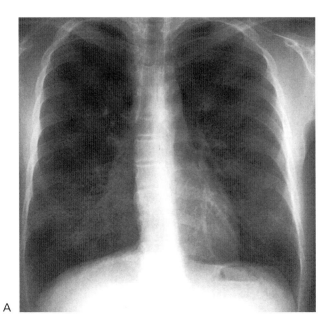

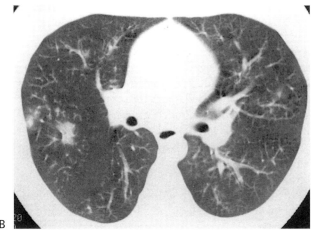

FIGURE 41.4. A: Normal chest roentgenogram in a child with a positive tuberculin skin test reaction and documented exposure to active pulmonary tuberculosis. There are no infiltrates or adenopathy evident. **B:** Computed tomography scan of the chest of the same child. There are multiple focal areas of consolidation seen in a distribution consistent with endobronchial spread of tuberculosis. Additional lobular consolidations and adenopathy were evident on other cuts.

mately 20% to 52% of the time, and 10% of such children have a positive AFB smear (54).

A recent pediatric case series reported a 49% overall sensitivity of all clinical and laboratory studies (sputum, gastric aspirate, pleural fluid, biopsy specimen). The successful recovery of bacteriologic specimen was most often found in children older than 10 years (55). Bronchoscopy has been used to enhance recovery of mycobacteria in lung tissue. However, bronchoscopy is invasive and with current culture techniques its yield is at best equivalent to a correctly performed gastric aspiration (56,57). Bronchoscopy is indicated as a therapeutic or diagnostic procedure to determine the extent of endobronchial disease or bronchial obstruc-

tion and to evaluate the potential for bronchiectasis or bronchial stenosis.

Newer methods of mycobacterial detection, such as (a) polymerase chain reaction (PCR) amplification or detection of structural components of *M. tuberculosis* in patient samples and (b) DNA probes for direct detection of nucleic acid sequences of *M. tuberculosis* in clinical specimens and detection of drug resistance, are presently being used. The Food and Drug Administration has approved two commercial nucleic acid amplification (NAA) tests—MTD (amplified *Mycobacterium tuberculosis* Direct Test; Gen-Probe Inc., San Diego, CA, U.S.A.) and Amplicor (Roche, Diagnostic Systems, Inc., Indianapolis, IN, U.S.A.)—for smear-negative and positive specimens in suspected tuberculous patients. Guidelines have been issued by the Centers for Disease Control and Prevention for their use (58): presumption of TB is established if the first sputum specimen is smear and NAA positive. If the specimens are negative for both tests or they exhibit discordant results, the repetition of NAA tests up to three times is suggested before any conclusions can be reached. Problems with the tests in patients previously or presently treated with antimycobacterial chemotherapy are underscored. A positive *M. tuberculosis* culture and the patient's response to antimycobacterial chemotherapy substantiate a diagnosis of TB infection. Obvious reasons to use the NAA assays are their quick turn-around time (48 hours), and, perhaps, their reported increased sensitivity to detect *M. tuberculosis* as compared with standard bacteriologic tests (59). In general, the commercial assays can diagnose 50% of smear-negative, culture-positive cases of pulmonary TB (60). Gomez-Pastrana et al. (61) reported that PCR had a sensitivity of 56.8% in children with clinically active disease as compared with 37.8% culture-positive and 13.5% smear-positive children. The specificity of the NAA approached 100%. Most of the benefit of using NAA as a diagnostic test was seen in a patient who had a positive TST, a negative chest roentgenogram, and a negative culture and smear. Of these patients, 29.8% had a positive NAA and were found to have pulmonary lymphadenopathy when screened by CT (52). The management of these cases is problematic, and whether to treat the patients with more than one drug is not known. Furthermore, the use of NAA in the diagnosis of extrapulmonary TB is not well delineated. For example, a negative NAA test of cerebrospinal fluid does not exclude a diagnosis of tuberculous meningitis. On the other hand, a positive test cannot be ignored.

The diagnosis of latent TB depends primarily on an imprecise test, the TST. The role of more specific assays is being evaluated. Measurement of interferon gamma production by peripheral blood mononuclear cells (i.e., Quantiferon; Cellestis, Melbourne, Australia) indicates that BCG recipient are seven times more likely to have a positive TST reaction and no production of interferon than patients who are not BCG recipients and have a positive TST reaction (62). The performance of this test in children is unknown.

Other tests, such as white blood cell count, differential, and sedimentation rate, are nonspecific and serve only in a supportive role. Examination and testing of specific sites, e.g., liver (liver function tests), kidneys (urinalysis), or AFB culture of specific sites as appropriate, is indicated to determine whether there is evidence of extrapulmonary disease.

Once TB infection has been identified in a child, the question is not whether the child should be treated but whether TB disease is present and how many drugs should be used. The goal of the other tests is to diagnose the existence and extent of disease and to facilitate an appropriate therapeutic decision.

MANAGEMENT OF TUBERCULOSIS IN CHILDREN

The therapeutic principles for the management of TB are the same for adults and children. Differences in the practice of TB treatment in children are related to numerous factors: (a) the pharmacokinetics of various antituberculous medications is different in children; (b) children generally have fewer mycobacterial organisms (caseous lesions instead of cavities) and, therefore, are less likely to develop secondary resistance; (c) extrapulmonary disease is more common in children, and so medications used for children must penetrate specific body sites and tissues; (d) children tolerate higher doses of antituberculous medications per kilogram of body weight with fewer side effects; and (e) because the commercial preparations of antituberculous medications were formulated for adults (pills, capsules, dosage sizes) (Table 41.2), often the formulations must be specially modified for children, which can cause problems with stability, bioavailability, tolerance, and compliance.

Recommended Treatment Regimens

Treatment regimens have evolved over the last decade as a result of numerous studies on the efficacy of short-course multidrug regimens. The Committee on Infectious Diseases of the American Academy of Pediatrics published recommendations for the management of TB in children (Table 41.3) (54). The regimen consists of an intense early (1 to 2 months) therapy of three or four drugs. It is continued as daily or twice-weekly therapy (of at least two drugs) under the direct observation of a health care worker for a period of treatment of 6 to 12 months. Crucial to these recommendations are the concepts that (a) the mycobacterial organisms must be sensitive to at least two or more of the prescribed drugs and (b) compliance is ensured through a combination of sensitive and culturally appropriate education, close medical follow-up, and directly observed therapy (DOT).

Various studies have documented the efficacy of shorter, more intense courses of chemotherapy and the benefits of DOT to ensure compliance (47). Recently, an observational study showed that 93% of 142 children improved after a shortened intense daily therapy of 2 weeks followed by twice-weekly therapy with three drugs for 6 weeks and finished with two drugs to complete 24 weeks of therapy (64). Longer courses of treatment are indicated for skeletal TB (9 to 12 months), tuberculous meningitis (12 months), or drug-resistant TB (12 to 18 months).

Although there have been no prospective studies on the management of TB in children with HIV infection, prudence suggests treating for 9 to 12 months, or at least 6 months, after negative cultures, with particular attention to the sensitivity pattern of the identified source's isolate and the risk of multidrug-resistant tuberculosis.

Drug-resistant TB occurs either because a strain of *M. tuberculosis* is already resistant to one or more drugs or because an emergent drug-resistant organism has evolved during therapy (secondary resistance). Inadequate or incorrect management by the physician and poor adherence to the treatment regimen by the patient can lead to secondary drug resistance. Children, infected by generally smaller populations of organisms, rarely develop secondary drug resistance. Children are at higher risk of drug-resistant TB when they are exposed to adults at high risk for drug resistance, such as immigrants from regions of high prevalence of drug-resistant TB, adults who have a history of treatment for TB (especially adults with incomplete or inadequate therapy, those with HIV infection or a history of drug use, and homeless or imprisoned adults). Steiner et al. (53) demonstrated that the pattern of primary drug resistance in children was similar to that found in the presumed source case of TB.

When drug resistance is suspected, therapy should be individualized on the basis of information about the presumed source case and the resistance pattern of that *M. tuberculosis* isolate. Initial therapy should include four or five drugs and vigorous efforts to isolate and test the susceptibility of the organism from the child. Subsequent adjustment of the regimen should include any new information on the resistance pattern and the assistance of an expert in the management of TB. Treatment should last for 12 to 18 months and should include DOT to protect against noncompliance, possible failure, or the emergence of additional resistance. The role of newer drugs, such as linezolid, should be determined after consultation with a physician expert in the management of TB. The propensity of this drug to act as a bone marrow suppressor undoubtedly may limit its usefulness in long-term therapy.

Corticosteroids (dexamethasone or prednisone) are used mainly in the treatment of TB of the central nervous system (65). The purpose of the corticosteroids is to diminish the host inflammatory response that may be producing additional tissue damage. Corticosteroids have documented benefits in reducing inflammation and increased intracranial pressure (66) and, when used as adjunctive therapy in the treatment of tuberculous meningitis, lead to lower mor-

TABLE 41.2. DRUGS FOR THE MANAGEMENT OF TUBERCULOSIS IN CHILDREN

Drugs	Dose Forms	Daily Dose (mg/kg)	Twice-a-Week Dose (mg/kg)	Maximal Dose
		First-Line Drugs		
Isoniazid[a]	Scored tablets 100 mg; 300 mg Syrup 10 mg/mL[c]	10–15[b]	20–30	Daily: 300 mg Twice a week: 900 mg
Rifampin	Capsules 150 mg; 300 mg syrup formulated from capsules[d]	10–20	10–20	600 mg
Pyrazinamide	Scored tablets 500 mg[e]	20–40 given o.d.	50	2 g
Ethambutol[f]	Tablets 100 mg 400 mg	15–25**	50	2.5 g
Streptomycin[g]	Vials: 1 g, 4 g	20–40	20–40 intramuscular	1 g
		Second-Line Drugs		
Capreomycin	Vials: 1 g	15–30 given o.d.	15–30 intramuscular	1 g
Ciprofloxacin[h]	Tablets 250 mg 500 mg 750 mg	Adults 500–1,500 mg/d Pediatrics 20–30 given b.i.d.		1.5 g
Ofloxacin[h]	Tablets 200 mg 300 mg 400 mg	Adults 400–800 mg total/d (given twice daily)		0.8 g
Levofloxacin[h]	Tablets 250 mg 500 mg Vials: 25 mg/mL	Adults 500–1,000 given once daily		1 g
Cycloserine	Capsules 250 mg	10–20		1 g
Ethionamide	Tablets 250 mg	15–20 given in 2 or 3 divided doses		1 g
Kanamycin	Vials 75 mg/mL 500 mg/2 mL 1 g/3 mL	15–30 intramuscular		1 g
Paraaminosalicylic acid	Tablets 500 mg, 1 g Bulk powder Delayed-release granules	200–300 3 or 4 times daily		10 g

[a]Rifamate is a capsule containing 150 mg isoniazid and 300 mg rifampin. Rifater is a capsule containing 50 mg isoniazid, 120 mg rifampin and 300 mg pyrazinamide.
[b]Dosage for isoniazid in combination with rifampin should be limited to 10 mg/kg per day to prevent hepatotoxicity.
[c]Liquid preparations may be unstable if not freshly prepared each month; they may also cause diarrhea.
[d]Instability may be a problem with formulated liquid preparations.
[e]For small children, preparations of crushed tablets may be necessary.
[f]Ethambutol should be used with caution in children, with frequent monitoring of color discrimination, visual acuity, and fundoscopic exam.
[g]If streptomycin is not available, kanamycin, capreomycin, and amikacin are alternatives.
[h]Fluoroquinolones are not approved for use in persons younger than 18 years; their use in children necessitates assessment of the potential risks and benefits.
*Bacteriostatic; **Bacteriocidal.
b.i.d., twice daily; o.d., once daily.
Adapted from *2000 Red Book: Report of the Committee on Infectious Diseases.* Elk Grove Village, IL: American Academy of Pediatrics, 2000.

TABLE 41.3. RECOMMENDED TREATMENT REGIMENS FOR CHILDREN WITH DRUG-SUSCEPTIBLE TUBERCULOSIS

Infection or Disease Category	Regimen	Remarks
Latent Tuberculosis		
Isoniazid susceptible	9 mo once a day	Twice a week treatment DOT for 9 mo; 9–12 mo treatment for HIV-infected children
Isoniazid resistant	6 mo of R daily	
Isoniazid–rifampin resistant	Consult specialist	
Pulmonary	6 mo regimens: 2 mo of I, R, P once a day followed by 4 mo I and R daily	If possibility of drug resistance add another drug (E or S) to initial 3 drugs until drug susceptibilities are known
	OR	
	2 mo of I, R, P daily followed by 4 mo of I, R daily	If nonadherence is likely in the initial phase, drugs can be given 2 or 3 times/wk under DOT
	OR	
	9 mo regimens: for hilar adenopathy only, 9 mo of I, R daily	6 mo of I, R once daily, 1 mo of I, R daily, followed by 5 mo of I, R DOT twice a week has been used in areas of rare drug resistance
	OR	
	1 mo of I, R daily, followed by 8 mo of I, R twice a week	
Extrapulmonary:	2 mo of I, R, P, and S once a day followed by 7–10 mo of I, R once a day for 9–12 mo total	Streptomycin is given until drug susceptibilities are known
Meningitis		
Miliary		
Bone/joint	OR	
	2 mo of I, R, P, and S once a day followed by 7–10 mo of I, R twice a week for 9–12 mo total	For patients from areas where streptomycin resistance is common capreomycin or kanamycin may be used instead of streptomycin
Other (e.g., cervical lymph adenopathy)	Same as for pulmonary disease	

DOT, directly observed therapy; HIV, human immunodeficiency virus; I, isoniazid; P, pyrazinamide; R, rifampin; S, streptomycin.
Adapted from *2000 Red Book: Report of the Committee on Infectious Diseases.* Elk Grove Village, IL: American Academy of Pediatrics, 2000.

tality, neurologic morbidity, and improved clinical outcome (67). Prednisone, 1 to 2 mg per kilogram of body weight daily for 4 to 6 weeks with a 2-week taper, can be started after antituberculous treatment has begun.

Follow-up Care

Compliance remains the largest problem in effective management of TB. Language-specific, culturally sensitive material, appropriate for the educational level of the patient and family, must be provided. An early educational effort facilitates contact or associate investigations that must accompany effective therapy. Written instructions for medication administration, duration of therapy, renewal of prescriptions, and the name, telephone number, and location of a health care worker to serve as a resource for addressing emergent problems or questions should be distributed to each patient. Medical follow-up every 4 to 8 weeks should be scheduled to monitor the side effects of medications, compliance, and response to therapy. An organized system of recalls for missed appointments should also be arranged.

Notification and involvement of local public health authorities should occur for all cases of TB disease. Depending on available resources, notification of authorities may enhance the contact investigation and prevention. DOT should be used for the management of all tuberculous disease in children and is mandatory in the management of any case involving congenital TB, tuberculous meningitis, multidrug-resistant TB, or coexistent HIV infection.

Routine testing of liver function before or during therapy is not indicated except in situations of multidrug therapy, severe TB disease (miliary, meningitis), malnutrition, or coexistence of other liver disease or hepatotoxic treatments. Transient transaminase elevation occurs in less than 5% of children and in 5% to 10% of adolescents receiving isoniazid alone. The transaminase value returns to normal without any change in treatment (68,69). Clinical hepatitis in children receiving isoniazid alone or in conjunction with rifampin or pyrazinamide occurs rarely, although data on the frequency of hepatitis in large populations of children are not available. If clinical symptoms of hepatitis (nausea, vomiting, decreased appetite, abdominal pain, fatigue, or jaundice) occur in association with the use of isoniazid, rifampin, or pyrazinamide, the medications should be stopped, liver function assessed, and the cause of symptoms investigated. If liver function test results are normal or return to normal when therapy is stopped, treatment can be reinitiated, one drug at a time. When liver function remains abnormal, an alternative regimen should be chosen. Occasionally, transaminase elevations of greater than four to five times normal are discovered without clinical symptomatology. In these instances, the medications should be stopped until the laboratory values return to normal; then therapy can be restarted.

Follow-up chest roentgenograms should be obtained as needed to follow documented abnormalities. Intrathoracic lymphadenopathy requires a resolution period of 2 to 3 years. Follow-up chest roentgenography at the end of therapy is appropriate to confirm either resolution or no change as well as to produce a baseline if future evaluation is clinically indicated. Although a small number of persons become TST negative during therapy, there is no correlation between follow-up skin tests and the adequacy of therapy or the state of TB infection. Routine repeat Mantoux skin testing is not indicated.

Preventive Therapy

There are numerous ways to prevent the spread of TB, such as effective management of active, infectious, pulmonary TB; environmental controls (masks, adequate ventilation, ultraviolet lighting, isolation); contact or associate investigation; and vaccination with BCG. Approaches to prevention that are particularly important in pediatrics include administration of prophylactic isoniazid to high-risk contacts of a patient with contagious TB, treatment with isoniazid in a person with tuberculin conversion (to prevent the development of TB disease), and BCG vaccination in areas with a high prevalence of TB.

Prophylactic Therapy

An infant or child (especially one younger than 5 years) who is exposed to active pulmonary TB and whose initial TST result is negative should receive isoniazid for 3 to 6 months until repeat skin testing is done, in an attempt to prevent infection. Because TB infection is a sentinel case for infection in an adult, efforts to effectively manage active TB in the adult must be undertaken at the same time to reduce the risk of transmission. If the adult is adequately treated and is culture negative, and if the child remains healthy and has a negative reaction to Mantoux tests at 3 and 6 months after the initial test, isoniazid can be stopped.

There is a long history of therapy with isoniazid to block the progression from the preclinical stage of TB infection without disease (latent TB) to the clinical stage of active TB. Twelve months of isoniazid therapy alone in children with good compliance has been demonstrated to be more than 95% effective in preventing reactivation over a period of 20 to 30 years (70). Current recommendations for the management of TB by the American Academy of Pediatrics are isoniazid 10 mg/kg of body weight (300 mg maximum) per day for 9 months or rifampin 10 mg/kg of body weight per day for 6 to 9 months if resistance to isoniazid exists in a close contact (63) (Table 41.3). There are no comparative studies in children for shorter courses of isoniazid, for intermittent dosing two or three times weekly, or for alternative regimens when the presumed source of the TB infection has multidrug-resistant TB.

Bacille Calmette–Guérin Vaccination

BCG vaccination is routinely used throughout the world, but not in the United States. There is good evidence that BCG vaccination in children younger than 2 months protects them from miliary TB or tuberculous meningitis (71). The data concerning the efficacy of the various strains of BCG vaccination in preventing TB vary tremendously, with estimated protection reported as low as 0% and as high as 80% in published studies (72). To elucidate the efficacy of BCG, Brewer et al. conducted a meta-analysis of 1,412 case-control studies and 14 prospective trials and concluded that BCG reduces the risk of pulmonary and extrapulmonary TB by approximately 50% (73).

Adverse reactions to BCG vaccination include local reactions, lymphadenitis, and dissemination of *Mycobacterium bovis* infection. Local reactions include subcutaneous abscesses, delayed healing, excessive scarring, or keloid formation. In general, appropriate intradermal vaccination causes initial ulceration, then crusting and healing for 2 to 3 months. Usually a permanent scar that is round, depressed, and approximately 4 to 8 mm in diameter results. Lymphadenitis, either axillary or cervical, occurs infrequently. Its occurrence depends on the strain of BCG used, the dose, and the person's age at vaccination. Lymphadenitis can heal spontaneously, and systemic antituberculous therapy is usually ineffective. If the lymph nodes become adherent or drain, surgical drainage is appropriate. Disseminated infection from BCG occurs rarely; its occurrence is generally related to severe immunodeficiency. Although BCG vaccination in children with HIV infection is a theoretical concern, prospective studies from Africa have not reported an increase in disseminated BCG disease (74). Most children born to HIV-infected mothers are not infected with HIV, yet TB infection remains a high risk in these families and BCG vaccination could provide protection. In areas with a high prevalence of TB, BCG vaccination continues to provide some degree of protection, especially in young children prone to miliary or tuberculous meningitis.

Contact Investigation

Contact investigation and associate investigation are essential components of any program of TB prevention (4). A contact investigation is the systematic evaluation of the TB status of the contacts of an identified case of active TB. The investigation is prioritized to assess, first, persons with the greatest relative risk of infection depending on the degree of exposure (close contacts, e.g., in the household or at work) and, second, casual contacts if the risk of infection is proven to be high among close contacts.

An associate investigation examines the TB status of all close contacts of a child with a positive TST to identify the source case and other infected contacts. Nemir and Krasinski reported that a source case could be identified for two thirds of the patients when the child was younger than 10 years, but for only one third of the patients when an adolescent was the sentinel case (75). The urgency and the extent of the investigation should be individualized for each patient on the basis of the apparent infectiousness of the person with active TB.

Treatment of an Infant Born to a Mother with Tuberculosis

Each case of an infant born to a mother who is suspected of having TB must be managed in an individualized fashion. To prevent the spread of the disease, the TB status of the mother and close contacts must be fully evaluated. Although separation of the infant from the mother (or family) should be minimized, evidence of communicable TB (cavitary lesions, endobronchial disease, positive AFB smear, etc.) warrants such separation (63).

If the mother has evidence of hematogenous spread of TB (bone, renal, meningeal involvement, or miliary disease), the infant and placenta (if possible) should be evaluated for evidence of congenital TB (see "Tuberculosis in the Newborn Infant"). The mother and infant should be separated until the mother is documented to be noninfectious by negative AFB smears and is receiving an effective antituberculous regimen. If there is any evidence of placental involvement or of TB in the infant, treatment of the infant with four antituberculous medications should begin immediately. If the evaluation of the infant is negative, the infant should receive isoniazid until 6 months of age, along with close medical follow-up, repeat Mantoux testing, and chest roentgenography at 3 and 6 months. Complete evaluation of all household contacts of the infant must be completed before the infant is discharged from the hospital.

If the mother or a close contact of the infant has newly diagnosed TB disease, the infant and mother (or contact) must be separated until the case is determined to be noninfectious. All household contacts should be evaluated in a timely fashion. Separation of the mother and infant is not necessary if the mother is not infectious and has been receiving adequate therapy for 2 weeks and continued compliance is ensured. Breast-feeding can occur. The infant should begin isoniazid before discharge, should undergo Mantoux testing and chest roentgenography at 6 weeks of age, and be followed closely for the first 3 to 6 months of life. If the Mantoux test and chest roentgenographic results are negative at 6 weeks and 3 months of life, if the child remains clinically well, and if the identified source continues adequate therapy, isoniazid can be stopped. If the identified source continues to have positive AFB smears or cultures, or noncompliance is evident, BCG vaccination of the infant is another option to prevent TB disease.

In the case of a mother or household contact with a positive tuberculin test, prompt and complete evaluation of the case and all contacts is mandatory to ensure that the infant is not exposed to active TB. If there is no evidence of active TB in the mother or close contacts, then there is no reason for separation of the infant. If the contacts cannot be completely evaluated in a timely fashion, prophylactic isoniazid for the infant should be considered until exclusion of the possibility of exposing the infant to active disease can be accomplished. The infant should be evaluated with the Mantoux test at 6 weeks and 3 months of age.

Ideally, the TB status of the mother should be determined before pregnancy or during pregnancy, along with complete evaluation of all contacts, long before delivery of the infant. Treatment of a pregnant woman with active disease can be accomplished with isoniazid, rifampin, ethambutol, or paraaminosalicylic acid without adverse effects to the fetus or infant. A pregnant woman with evidence of recent PPD conversion (more recent than 2 years) and no disease should receive preventive isoniazid therapy for 6 months beginning as early as the second trimester.

REFERENCES

1. Kochi A. The global tuberculosis situation and the new control strategy of the World Health Organization. *Tubercle* 1991; 71:1–6.
2. Cegielski JP. The global tuberculosis situation. *Infect Dis Clin North Am* 2002;16: 1-58.
3. Donald PR. Childhood tuberculosis: out of control? *Curr Opin Pulmon Med* 2002;8:178–182.
4. American Thoracic Society, Medical Section of the American Lung Association. Control of tuberculosis in the United States. *Am Rev Respir Dis* 1992;146:1623–1633.
5. Bloom BR. Tuberculosis: the global view. *N Engl J Med* 2002; 346:1434–1435.
6. Tuberculosis morbidity–United States, 1997. *MMWR Morb Mortal Wkly Rep* 1998;47:253–257.
7. Recommendations for prevention and control of tuberculosis among foreign-born persons. *MMWR Morb Mortal Wkly Rep* 1998;47:1–29.
8. Tuberculosis outbreak on an American Indian reservation—Montana, 2000–2001. *MMWR Morb Mortal Wkly Rep* 2002;51: 232–234.
9. Leggiardo RJ, Callory B, Dowdy S, et al. An outbreak of tuberculosis in a family day care home. *Pediatr Infect Dis J* 1989; 8:52–54.

10. Lange WR, Warnock-Eckhart E, Bean ME. *Mycobacterium tuberculosis* infection in foreign-born adoptees. *Pediatr Infect Dis J* 1989;8:625–629.

11. Saiman L. Risk factors for latent tuberculosis infection among children in New York City. *Pediatrics* 2001;107:999–1003.

12. American Thoracic Society. Diagnostic standards and classification of tuberculosis in adults and children. *Am J Respir Crit Care Med* 2000;149:1359–1374.

13. Comstock GW, Livesay VT, Woolpert SF. The prognosis of a positive tuberculin reaction in childhood and adolescence. *Am J Epidemiol* 1974;99(2):131–138.

14. Miller FJW, Seale RME, Taylor MD. *Tuberculosis in children.* Boston: Little, Brown and Company, 1963.

15. Wallgren A. On the contagiousness of childhood tuberculosis. *Acta Pediatrica* 1937;22:229–234.

16. Rabalais G, Adams G, Stover B. PPD skin test conversion in health-care workers after exposure to *Mycobacterium tuberculosis* infection in infants. *Lancet* 1991;338:826.

17. Curtis AB. Extensive transmission of *Mycobacterium tuberculosis* from a child. *N Engl J Med* 1999;341:1491–1495.

18. Friedman W, et al. Tuberculosis, AIDS, and deaths among substance abusers on welfare in New York City. *N Engl J Med* 1996;334:828–833.

19. Moss WJ, Dedyo T, Suarez M, et al. Tuberculosis in children infected with human immunodeficiency virus: a report of five cases. *Pediatr Infect Dis J* 1992;11:114–120.

20. Bakshi SS, Alvarez D, Hilfer DL, et al. Tuberculosis in human immunodeficiency virus–infected children. A family infection. *Am J Dis Child* 1993;147:320–324.

21. Burroughs M. Clinical presentation of tuberculosis in culture-positive children. *Pediatr Infect Dis J* 1999;18:440–446.

22. Thomas P. Tuberculosis in human immunodeficiency virus–infected and human immunodeficiency virus–exposed children in New York City. *Pediatr Infect Dis J* 2000;19:700–706.

23. Selwyn PA, et al. A prospective study of tuberculosis among intravenous drug abusers with human immunodeficiency virus infection. *N Engl J Med* 1990;320:545–550.

24. Wier MR, Thornton GF. Extrapulmonary tuberculosis: experience of a community hospital and review of the literature. *Am J Med* 1985;79:467–478.

25. Starke JR, Taylor-Watts KT. Tuberculosis in the pediatric population of Houston, Texas. *Pediatrics* 1989;84:28–35.

26. Vallejo, JG. Clinical features, diagnosis, and treatment of tuberculosis in infants. *Pediatrics* 1994:84:1–7.

27. Schaaf HS, Beyers N Respiratory tuberculosis in childhood: the diagnostic value of clinical features and special investigations. *Pediatr Infect Dis J* 1995:14:189–194.

28. Merino JM, Carpintero I. Tuberculosis pleural effusion in children. *Chest* 1999;115:26–30.

29. Smith KC. Tuberculosis in children. *Curr Probl Pediatr* 2001;31:1–34.

30. Dandapat MC. Peripheral lymph node tuberculosis: a review of 80 cases. *Br J Surg* 1990;77:911–912.

31. Nataraj G, Kurup S. Correlation of fine needle aspiration cytology, smear and culture in tuberculous lymphadenitis: a prospective study. *J Postgrad Med* 2002;48:113–116.

32. Waecker JN, Connor JD. Central nervous system tuberculosis in children: a review of 30 cases. *Pediatr Infect Dis J* 1990;9:539–543.

33. Farinha NJ, Razali KA. Tuberculosis of the central nervous system in children a 20-year survey. *J Infect* 2000;41:61–68.

34. Janner K, Kirk S. Cerebral tuberculosis without neurologic signs and with normal cerebrospinal fluid. *Pediatr Infect Dis J* 2000;19:763–764.

35. Tuli SM. General principles of osteoarticular tuberculosis. *Clin Orthop* 2002:1(398):11–19.

36. Chattopadhyay A, Bhatnagar S. Genitourinary tuberculosis in pediatric surgical practice. *J Pediatr Surg* 1997;32:1283–1286.

37 Smith KC. Congenital tuberculosis: a rare manifestation of a common infection. *Curr Opin Infect Dis* 2002;15:269–274.

38. Nemir RL, O'Hare D. Congenital tuberculosis: review and diagnostic guidelines. *Am J Dis Child* 1985;139:284–287.

39. Committee on Infectious Diseases of the American Academy of Pediatrics. Screening for tuberculosis in infants and children. *Pediatrics* 1994;93:131–134.

40. Committee on Infectious Diseases of the American Academy of Pediatrics. Update on tuberculosis skin testing of children. *Pediatrics* 1996;97:282.

41. Starke JR, Jacobs RF, Jereb J. Resurgence of tuberculosis in children. *J Pediatr* 1992;120(6):839–855.

42. Besser ER. Risk factors for positive Mantoux tuberculin skin tests in children in San Diego, California: evidence for boosting and possible foodborne transmission. *Pediatrics* 2001;108:305–310.

43. Menzies D. What does tuberculin reactivity after Bacille Calmette–Guérin vaccination tell us. *CID* 2000;31:S71–S74.

44. Karalliede S, Katugha LP, Uragoda CG. The tuberculin response of Sri Lankan children after BCG vaccination at birth. *Tubercle* 1987;68:33–38.

45. Nemir RL, Teichner A. Management of tuberculin reactions in children and adolescents previously vaccinated with BCG. *Pediatr Infect Dis J* 1983;2:446–451.

46. Fox AS, Lepow ML. Tuberculin skin testing in Vietnamese refugees with a history of BCG vaccination. *Am J Dis Child* 1983;137:1093–1094.

47. Mc Adams HP. Radiologic manifestations of pulmonary tuberculosis. *Radiol Clin North Am* 1995;33:655–675.

48. Stanberry SD. Tuberculosis in infants and children. *J Thor Imaging* 1990;5:17-27.

49. Leung AN. Primary tuberculosis in childhood: radiographic manifestations. *Radiology* 1992;182:87–91.

50. Neu N. Diagnosis of pediatric tuberculosis in the modern era. *Pediatr Infect Dis J* 1999;18:122–126.

51. Delacourt C. Computed tomography with normal chest radiograph in tuberculosis infection. *Arch Dis Child* 1993;69:430–432.

52. Kim AJR. Pulmonary tuberculosis in children: evaluation with CT. *AJR Am J Roentgenol* 1997;168:1005–1009.

53. Steiner P, Rao M, Mitchell M. Primary drug-resistant tuberculosis in children: correlation of drug susceptibility patterns of matched patient and source-case strains of *Mycobacterium tuberculosis. Am J Dis Child* 1985;139:780–782.

54. Pompitus WF. Standardization of gastric aspirate technique improves yield in the diagnosis of tuberculosis in children. *Pediatr Infect Dis J* 1997;16:222–226.

55. Merino JM. Microbiology of pediatric primary pulmonary tuberculosis. *Chest* 2001;119:1434–1438.

56. Abadco DL, Steiner P. Gastric lavage is better than bronchoalveolar lavage for isolation of *Mycobacterium tuberculosis* in childhood pulmonary tuberculosis. *Pediatr Infect Dis J* 1992;11:735–738.

57. de Blic J, Azevedo I, Burren CP, et al. The value of flexible bronchoscopy in childhood pulmonary tuberculosis. *Chest* 1991;100:688–692.

58. Uptdate: Nucleic acid amplification tests for tuberculosis. *MMWR Morb Mortal Wkly Rep* 2000;49:593–594.

59. Gomez-Pastrana D, Torronteras R, Caro, P, et al. Comparison of Amplicor, in-house polymerase chain reaction, and conventional culture for the diagnosis of tuberculosis in children. *Clin Infect Dis* 2001;32:17–22.

60. Schluger NW. Changing approaches to the diagnosis of tuberculosis. *Am J Respir Crit Care Med* 2001;164:2020–2024.

61. Gomez-Pastrana D, Torronteras R, Caro, P, et al. Diagnosis of tuberculosis in children using a polymerase chain reaction. *Pediatr Pulmonol* 1999;28:344–351.
62. Mazurek GH. Comparison of a whole-blood interferon assay with tuberculin skin testing for detecting latent *Mycobacterium tuberculosis* infection. *JAMA* 2001;286:1740–1747.
63. Red Book Committee on Infectious Diseases of the American Academy of Pediatrics. *Tuberculosis. Report of the Committee on Infectious Diseases of the American Academy of Pediatrics.* 2000: 593–613.
64. Al-Dossary FS, Ong LT, Correa AG, et al. Treatment of childhood tuberculosis with a six month directly observed regimen of only two weeks of daily therapy. *Pediatr Infect Dis J* 2002;21: 91–97.
65. Waecker NJ. Tuberculous meningitis in children. *Curr Treat Opt Neurol* 2002;4:249–257.
66. Girgis NI, et al. Dexamethasone as an adjunct to treatment of tuberculous meningitis. *Pediatr Infect Dis J* 1991;10:179–183.
67. Schoeman J, Van Zyl LE. Effect of corticosteroids on intracranial pressure, computed tomographic findings, and clinical outcome in young children with tuberculous meningitis. *Pediatrics* 1997; 99:226–231.
68. Nakajo MM, Rao M, Steiner P. Incidence of hepatotoxicity in children receiving isoniazid chemoprophylaxis. *Pediatr Infect Dis J* 1989;8:649–650.
69. Litt IF, Cohen MI, McNamara H. Isoniazid hepatitis in adolescents. *J Pediatr* 1976;89:133–135.
70. Hsu KHK. Thirty years after isoniazid: its impact on tuberculosis in children and adolescents. *JAMA* 1984;251:1283–1285.
71. Ten Dam HG, Hitze KL. Does BCG vaccination protect the newborn and young infants? *Bull WHO* 1980;58:37–41.
72. Fine PEM. The BCG story: lessons from the past and implications for the future. *Rev Infect Dis* 1989;11(Suppl 2):S353–S359.
73. Brewer TF. Preventing tuberculosis with bacillus Calmette–Guérin vaccine: a meta-analysis of the literature. *Clin Infect Dis* 2000;31(Suppl 3):S64–S67.
74. Ten Dam HG. BCG vaccination and HIV infection. *Bull Int Union Tuberc Lung Dis* 1990;65:38–39.
75. Nemir RL, Krasinski K. Tuberculosis in children and adolescents in the 1980s. *Pediatr Infect Dis J* 1988;7:375–379.

42

TUBERCULOSIS, PREGNANCY, AND TUBERCULOUS MASTITIS

STUART M. GARAY

Much of the early literature regarding tuberculosis (TB) and pregnancy is difficult to interpret because of changes in diagnostic and therapeutic practices. This chapter presents current concepts with respect to the diagnosis and management of TB in pregnancy. The presentation and outcome for pregnant women with TB may vary according to the country of origin. Women from developed countries, such as the United States and England, may have a better prognosis than those from the less developed countries of Africa, Asia, and Latin America. The differences may be secondary to the ability to access care, the trimester of pregnancy in which the diagnosis of TB was made, as well as the complicating variable of human immunodeficiency virus (HIV) coinfection. In the United States, important factors regarding presentation and outcome appear to be recent immigration status and country of origin, race and ethnicity, socioeconomic level, as well as HIV status (1). The resurgence of TB in the United States peaked in 1992 (1). Between 1985 and 1992 the incidence of TB in persons aged 25 to 45 years (the peak age group for reproductive-aged women) increased by 44% (2). A study of two urban hospitals in New York City revealed that the incidence of TB in pregnant women increased between 1985 and 1992 (3). There were 12.4 cases per 100,000 births from 1985 to 1990 and 94.8 cases per 100,000 births from 1991 to 1992. This increase was largely attributed to the rise in the number of HIV-infected pregnant women. Since 1992 there has been a significant decline in the number of new cases of TB in the United States (decreasing 39% by the year 2000), primarily reflecting a 55% decrease in the number of cases among U.S-born persons (1). By 2000 there had been a proportionate decrease in the number of cases in persons aged 25 to 44 years, but this age group still comprised 34% of the new TB cases. The proportion of individuals with TB and HIV coinfection in persons aged 25 to 44 also declined from 29% in 1993/94 to 19% in 1999 (1,4). These data

suggest a concomitant decline may have occurred in the incidence of TB in pregnancy. However, during this period there has been a significant increase in TB in foreign-born individuals (4% increase since 1992), with a proportionate increase in the number of foreign-born women aged 25 to 44 with newly diagnosed TB (1). These women may have contributed to an increase in the number of pregnant patients with TB. The net result of these findings is unclear because there are no national statistics regarding the incidence of TB in pregnant women.

EFFECT OF PREGNANCY ON THE PROGNOSIS OF TUBERCULOSIS

The role of pregnancy in the reactivation or progression of TB has been intensely debated for centuries. From early antiquity Hippocrates and Galen believed that pregnancy improved the prognosis of TB. As late as the 19th century, a German physician named Ramody recommended that young women with TB marry and become pregnant to slow disease progression (5). Increased abdominal and thoracic pressure in pregnancy was believed to help close tuberculous cavities. However, in 1850 a review of 24 patients by Grisolle demonstrated that TB worsened during pregnancy (6). This view became the dominant teaching by the beginning of the 20th century and held until about 1950. As a result, many experts recommended therapeutic abortion for women with TB.

In 1953, Hedvall reviewed the literature regarding pregnancy and TB (7). He found 1,000 women who had progression of TB during pregnancy, but he found an equal number of women in whom pregnancy seemed to affect the disease beneficially. In an independent study, Hedvall followed 250 women with TB through pregnancy (7). He found that radiographic abnormalities remained stable in 84% of patients. Seven percent of patients had radiographic progression of disease, whereas 9% of the women improved. Schaefer et al. reviewed 506 patients treated at New York Lying-In Hospital before 1955 (8). Four hundred

S. M. Garay: Division of Pulmonary and Critical Care Medicine, New York University School of Medicine, New York, New York.

eighty-six patients had inactive disease, that is, they had a positive tuberculin skin test result with radiographic abnormalities but were asymptomatic and had negative sputum cultures. Only 3.7% of these women progressed to active disease during pregnancy. The rate of disease progression was not significantly different in the nonpregnant controls.

Although the opinion regarding the effect of pregnancy on TB was changing by the middle of the 20th century, there was new concern regarding the postpartum period. Investigators proposed that TB could progress as a result of the postpartum descent of the diaphragm (which could affect intrathoracic pressures and, in turn, cavitary closure), hormonal fluctuations, nutritional deprivation, and altered immunity. Hedvall (7) found that during the first postpartum year 76% of patients were stable, 15% worsened, and 9% improved. Subsequently, Crombie (9) noted a higher risk of relapse during the first postpartum year. He found that 31 of 101 pregnant women with inactive disease developed active disease after delivery; 20 of these 31 cases occurred during the first postpartum year. In contrast, Edge (10) found no increased risk of TB in postpartum English women compared with aged-matched women in the general population. Several other studies in the United States by Cohen et al. (11,12) and Rosenbach et al. (13) also failed to demonstrate increased risk of progression of TB during the postpartum period. More recently, as a result of a study in Kenya, Gilks et al. (14) suggested that recent pregnancy in HIV-infected women predisposed them to active TB.

With the arrival of antituberculosis agents, the controversy regarding the effects of pregnancy and the postpartum period has declined. DeMarch (15) followed two groups of women who had completed therapy for TB. He found that the 100 women who became pregnant were no more likely to have reactivation of their disease than were nulliparous women. Pridie and Stradling (16) also found that pregnancy did not change the course of TB in appropriately treated patients. From 1955 to 1972, Schaefer et al. (8) described a 0.8% reactivation rate among pregnant patients who had previously received two antituberculous medications for a year. This was comparable to the rate of reactivation in nonpregnant patients. Mehta (17) compared 53 patients with active TB to controls matched for age and extent of disease. He found no significant differences between pregnant and nonpregnant patients in rapidity of sputum conversion, radiographic improvement, cavitary closure, or relapse rate. Thus, at the present time it appears that pregnancy does not adversely affect the natural course of TB or its management.

In the prechemotherapy era, advanced TB in a pregnant woman carried a high risk of mortality—as high as 30% to 40% (8). Today the prognosis is significantly better in developed countries utilizing multidrug therapy. However, recent reports from developing countries suggest a considerable mortality in pregnant TB patients. In Zambia, TB accounts for 25% of the nonobstetric deaths in pregnant women (18). Pillay et al. (19) reviewed their experience at a university hospital in Durban, South Africa where of 146 pregnant women with TB, 15 (10%) died; almost all of those who died were coinfected with HIV.

One final concern regarding the effect of TB on pregnancy is the impact of TB on the type of delivery, on pregnancy-related complications, and on the fetus and/or newborn. Schaefer et al. found that normal, spontaneous delivery occurred with equal frequency among patients with or without TB (8). There was no significant difference in the use of general anesthesia or cesarean section. The infants of women with inactive or mild disease did not have a significantly increased incidence of prematurity or low birth weight. Bjerkedal et al. (20) published a review of their experience in Norway. Between 1967 and 1968 there were 134,368 pregnancies with pulmonary TB diagnosed in 542 pregnancies (16). Some complications were greater in women with TB, such as toxemia of pregnancy (7.4% vs. 4.7%) and vaginal bleeding (4.4% vs. 2.2%). The rate of miscarriage was greater in pregnant women with TB (20.1 per 1,000 total births vs. 2.3 per 1,000 in controls). However, there were no differences in prematurity, low birth weight, or perinatal mortality in the two groups. In 1994 Jana et al. (21) reviewed the perinatal outcome of 79 pregnant women with TB compared with 316 nontuberculous pregnant women in India. TB did not affect the mode of delivery (C-section vs. vaginal delivery). The frequency of acute fetal distress was significantly higher (15.2% vs. 6.3%, $p < 0.01$). Preterm labor was found twice as frequently (22.8% vs. 11.5%, $p < 0.01$) in pregnant women with TB, whereas perinatal death (10.1% vs. 1.6%, $p < 0.01$) was observed six times as frequently. In addition, the average weight of newborns was 215 g lower in TB-infected women (21).

Recently, maternal and fetal outcome have been shown to be related to whether TB is diagnosed late in pregnancy, whether the mother has advanced pulmonary disease, as well as whether the presentation of TB is pulmonary or extrapulmonary (21). In a matched control study from Mexico, Figueroa-Damian (22,23) found that obstetric morbidity was significantly higher in pregnant women who initiated therapy late in pregnancy. Obstetric complications included preterm labor, preeclampsia, premature rupture of membranes, and fetal growth retardation. The risk of neonatal mortality was also high, though congenital TB was not. Newborns of women with TB had a higher risk of prematurity, perinatal death, and birth weight less than 2,500 g (23). Jana et al. (24) found that the effects of extrapulmonary TB on pregnancy depend on the sites involved, as well as the severity and duration of the disease. TB lymphadenitis had no significant effect on maternal and fetal outcome. In contrast, other sites of TB involvement, such as intestinal, spinal, and meningeal, were associated with increased maternal disability, fetal growth retardation, and neonates with low Apgar scores.

Finally, pregnant patients with multidrug-resistant TB (MDR-TB) have an increased risk of neonatal complications. Good et al. (25) suggested that maternal infection with drug-resistant TB poses a greater risk to the fetus. Mothers with MDR-TB had more advanced disease with more extensive radiographic changes and longer sputum conversion times. Nonetheless, in a recent small series (four patients) of pregnant women with MDR-TB, all newborns were born healthy and free of TB (26).

CLINICAL MANIFESTATIONS

Case Study

A 20-year-old Hispanic, HIV-negative woman presented in the 28th week of pregnancy complaining of 2 months' duration of fevers, night sweats, and a cough productive of thick, green sputum. Her brother had recently been diagnosed with active TB. Physical examination revealed respirations of 21/minute; inspiratory crackles were auscultated at the base of the left lung. Abdominal girth was consistent with 28 weeks of pregnancy. Laboratory examination revealed white blood cell count of 30,000 cells/mm³. A sputum smear revealed numerous acid-fast bacilli. Chest radiograph revealed a cavitary infiltrate in the apical and posterior segment of the right upper lobe. The lingula and superior segment of the left lower lobe were also involved (Fig. 42.1). Treatment consisted of isoniazid (INH), rifampin, and ethambutol for 2 months, at which time sensitivity studies revealed that the organisms were pansensitive. INH and rifampin were continued for an additional 7 months. The patient had an uncomplicated delivery at the 40th week of gestation. The infant was of normal weight and without congenital malformations. The infant had a negative tuberculin test, normal chest radiograph, and negative gastric smears 1 week after birth. A repeat purified protein derivative (PPD) test performed on the newborn was negative at 3 months.

Clinical Presentation

Although pregnancy should not obscure the clinical presentation of TB, early disease and symptoms may mimic the physiologic changes that occur in pregnancy, including fatigue, malaise, and tachypnea. Wilson et al. (27) found that at least 50% of pregnant women with new onset of TB were unaware of their disease and had few, if any, symptoms. Sixty-five percent of pregnant TB patients in the study by Schaefer et al. (8) were asymptomatic. The clinical presentation of TB in pregnant women may be similar to that in nonpregnant patients. Good et al. (25) reviewed the frequency of symptoms in 27 patients who developed TB during pregnancy or the first 12 months postpartum. Eleven had drug-sensitive TB, whereas 16 had drug-resistant TB (rifampin was not part of standard chemotherapy at the time

of the study, i.e., 1965–1974). They found cough in 74% of patients, weight loss in 41%, fever in 30%, malaise and fatigue in 30%, and hemoptysis in 19%. Approximately 19% of patients were asymptomatic at the time of diagnosis, but chest radiographs were abnormal. Good found that tuberculin skin tests were positive in all except one pregnant patient. These results are in contrast to the previously cited studies by Wilson (27) and Schaefer (8) in which most patients diagnosed during pregnancy were asymptomatic or diagnosed on routine prenatal screening. More recently, two smaller studies by Carter (28) and Doveren (29) found that pregnant TB patients more often are smear negative (culture positive) with minimal radiographic findings, usually unilateral noncavitary disease. An unusual presentation is that of persistent postpartum fever, which may be found in both pulmonary and extrapulmonary TB (30,31).

The diagnosis of TB may be delayed because pregnant women and their physicians are more likely to defer a chest radiograph. Proper shielding reduces the amount of radiation exposure to the fetus (32). While pulmonary TB is most common in pregnant women, extrapulmonary TB may also occur. Wilson et al. reported extrapulmonary disease in 10% of pregnant women with TB in their series, a proportion comparable to nonpregnant women of the same age (27). This is similar to the general population, except for individuals who are coinfected with HIV, who have a greater incidence of extrapulmonary TB. More recently, several studies have noted a higher incidence of extrapulmonary TB (23,33). Llewelyn et al. (33) reported that nine of 13 pregnant patients with TB diagnosed during a 30-month period had extrapulmonary TB. All patients were recent immigrants from Africa or the sub-Saharan continent. Pillay et al. (19) found no difference in the incidence of extrapulmonary TB between HIV- and non–HIV-infected pregnant women, occurring in 20% to 25% of cases. Jana et al. (24) presented a detailed review of 33 extrapulmonary TB cases from a major referral center in Chandigarh, India. TB lymphadenitis was the most common form of extrapulmonary (12 of 33 cases). It was diagnosed early, was easily treated, and had no significant effect on maternal and fetal outcome. Disease in other sites was more difficult to diagnose, including intestinal (nine cases), skeletal/vertebral (seven cases), renal (two cases), meningeal (2 cases), and endometrial (one case). Extrapulmonary TB in these sites resulted in more adverse consequences for both mother and newborn.

EVALUATION OF THE HIGH-RISK PATIENT DURING PREGNANCY

Screening

Many women come to medical attention for the first time to seek prenatal care. As noted earlier, between 19% and 65% of pregnant patients presenting with pulmonary TB

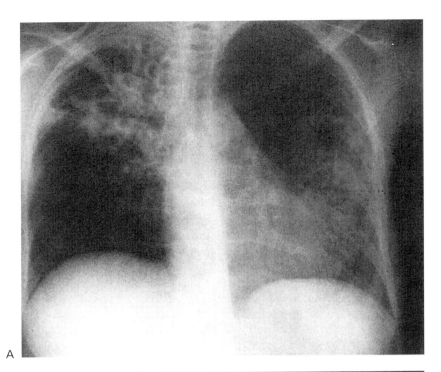

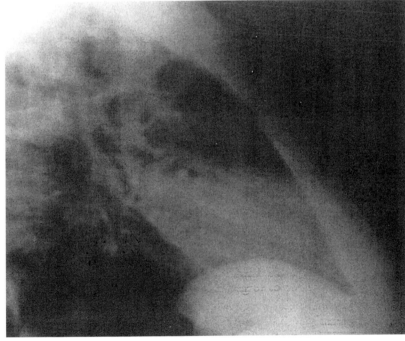

FIGURE 42.1. A: Posteroanterior radiographs of 20-year-old, Hispanic, human immunodeficiency virus–negative, pregnant woman discussed in the case study in text. **B:** Lateral radiographs of the same patient.

are unaware of their disease and have no significant symptoms (8,25,27–29,33). For this reason, all women who are at high risk for tuberculous infection, active disease, or both should be questioned carefully about symptoms and routinely receive a tuberculin skin test during prenatal evaluation. If the tuberculin skin test reaction is greater than 10 mm induration, a chest radiograph should be obtained to exclude the possibility of active disease. If the patient does not have symptoms, the radiograph may be delayed until

after the 12th week of gestation and should be performed with proper abdominal shielding. A doubtfully positive reading with an induration of 5 to 10 mm without a history of recent exposure requires retesting after 3 months (34). In pregnant women with known HIV infection or those with recent close contact with a person with active disease, ≥5 mm induration is considered positive (2). However, routine screening by chest radiograph is not indicated—not only because of its potential radiation risk but also because of its low yield as a screening device. Hadlock et al. (35) obtained screening chest radiographs in 5,422 pregnant women. Only 19 women had radiographic changes consistent with TB; three were unsuspected on the basis of history and physical examination; and only two had active disease. Bonebrake et al. (36) obtained screening chest radiographs in 11,725 pregnant women and found only one patient with evidence of TB: it was inactive. During posteroanterior chest radiograpy 50 mrad is delivered, that is, less than the dose thought to be hazardous to the fetus, especially if abdominal shielding is used. Appropriate shielding limits the fetal radiation exposure to less than 0.3 mrad and should not harm the fetus (37). However, controversy exists regarding the potential hazard of even small amounts of radiation to the fetus, particularly during the first trimester of gestation (38,39). Caution should be used whenever chest radiographs are obtained.

There has been some debate in the literature about the sensitivity of the tuberculin test during pregnancy. Finn et al. (40) reported that there was a lower prevalence of positive tuberculin skin tests in pregnant women than in a control population, suggesting that tuberculin sensitivity may be diminished during pregnancy. This study was flawed since patients did not serve as their own controls. Other studies in which women served as their own controls have noted no difference in tuberculin reactivity during pregnancy (41,42). Present and Comstock (41) compared 226 pregnant women who had taken two tuberculin skin tests (with an interval of 1 year between tests) with an equal number of matched controls who were not pregnant during either test. Minimal and similar increases were seen in both groups in the median diameter of induration during the 1-year interval. Pregnancy did not affect the tuberculin skin test response. Covelli and Wilson (43) found that 172 of 1,420 (12.2%) pregnant women were tuberculin positive, an incidence approximating that of nonpregnant young women. The utility of tuberculin skin testing has been demonstrated recently in both HIV- and non–HIV-infected pregnant women (44–47). There is no evidence that the tuberculin skin test has an adverse effect on the mother (by reactivating quiescent foci) or on the fetus (48).

Preventive Therapy

Preventive therapy with INH should usually be delayed until after delivery for women who have a positive tuberculin test reaction and a normal chest radiograph. However, pregnant women with positive tuberculin skin test reactions and normal radiographs, or radiographs with only a calcified lymph node or Ghon complex, should receive preventive therapy with INH during pregnancy if they are recent convertors who have documentation of a nonreactive tuberculin skin test within 2 years of the positive test; or if they are close contacts of a person with active disease; or if they are immunocompromised (49,50). Any patient who is HIV

seropositive and has a history of positive tuberculin test result (even if the patient is subsequently found to be anergic) should be treated with preventive therapy during pregnancy (49).

Moulding et al. (51) described 20 deaths from INH-associated hepatitis that occurred during a 14-year period in California. Four of the deaths occurred in women who began INH during pregnancy and continued INH therapy postpartum. The basis for their apparent increased risk could not be explained. Subsequently, Franks et al. (52) found that pregnant Hispanic women had a 2.5-fold increased risk of developing INH hepatitis and a 4-fold risk of dying from hepatitis. However, these findings were not statistically significant.

Snider and Caras (53) analyzed the subject of INH-associated deaths from hepatitis. They reviewed the published literature as well as the databanks of the Food and Drug Administration, the Lexis file (litigation), and the National Center for Health Statistics for INH-related deaths. In addition, they conducted a mail survey of state and territorial epidemiologists. They found 177 deaths. Postpartum status and indication for preventive therapy was available in only 21 of 32 female patients aged 15 to 44 years. Of these, only eight (38%) were reported to be within a year postpartum when they died. Despite the scanty data, Snider and Caras concurred with the previously cited studies suggesting that the postpartum period may represent a time when women are especially vulnerable to INH hepatotoxicity. Thus, postpartum women should be monitored carefully when they are treated with prophylactic INH.

The standard dosage of INH for preventive therapy is a single 5-mg dose per kilogram of body weight per day (usually 300 mg/day). Patients should be treated for 9 months. HIV-infected pregnant women with positive PPD reaction should receive INH and pyridoxine for 12 months. Pregnant women receiving INH should have baseline and follow-up liver function studies, preferably on a monthly basis. Pyridoxine should be given to pregnant patients receiving INH to decrease the incidence of INH-induced neuropathy (54).

MANAGEMENT OF TUBERCULOSIS DURING PREGNANCY

Adherence to treatment is especially difficult in pregnancy because of general concerns about the effect of medication on the fetus. In addition, pregnancy-related nausea may lead to poor compliance, and antituberculosis therapy may contribute to the nausea. Supervised treatment is especially helpful in encouraging adherence. The indications for management of active TB in a pregnant woman are the same as for a nonpregnant woman. Because many of the antituberculous drugs have not been used in large numbers of pregnant patients, the recommended therapeutic regimen differs slightly. According to the most recent recommendations of the Centers for Disease Control and Prevention (CDC) and the American Thoracic Society, the treatment regimen for the pregnant patient consists of at least INH and rifampin (49,55). In addition, ethambutol is recommended initially until sensitivity testing results show that INH and rifampin are effective. After 3 months of treatment with three drugs, another 6 months of INH and rifampin is recommended (provided the organisms are sensitive). HIV-infected patients with active TB should receive treatment with INH, rifampin, and ethambutol, and a fourth drug, such as pyrazinamide, for 9 to 12 months, or until sputum cultures have been negative for 6 months. The need for additional second-line drugs should be considered in light of the potential of MDR-TB. Patients must be informed about their therapeutic options and the potential teratogenicity of the second-line drugs (26,55).

Numerous data on the use of INH during pregnancy have been reported. Although it crosses the placenta, INH does not appear to be teratogenic, even when administered during the first trimester. Demyelination, depending on which day of gestation the drug was given, has been reported in chick embryos. However, this can be blocked by the *in vivo* administration of pyridoxine (vitamin B_6) (56,57). In two U.S. Public Health Service trials in the 1970s, 14 pregnant women were inadvertently treated with INH and rifampin for 20 to 24 weeks and with INH and ethambutol for 8 to 18 months (58). Of the 11 live births (three women elected to have therapeutic abortion), there were no complications of pregnancy or abnormalities in the children.

Hammond et al. (59) reported on 502 women who received INH for various periods during pregnancy. A total of 667 fetuses were exposed to INH: two were aborted; six infants were stillborn; four died less than 1 month after birth; 665 lived. Records were available 1 to 13 years after birth in 660 children: no malignancies were found. Snider et al. (58) in reviewing TB management during pregnancy reported on 1,302 published accounts of pregnant women who received INH during 1,480 pregnancies. More than 400 women had received INH during the first trimester. Almost 96% of pregnancies resulted in normal births, while 1% were abnormal. Of the remaining pregnancies, 0.7% were electively aborted, 0.3% were aborted spontaneously, 0.6% were stillborn, and approximately 1.4% were premature. Many of the published reports were drawn from different countries and spanned three decades; therefore, finding a comparable control group was difficult. Nevertheless, the reported 1% incidence of abnormalities in infants of mothers who were treated with INH falls well below the 1.2% to 6% incidence of fetal malformations that has been cited in the population at large (58). Multiple studies have examined the use of INH during pregnancy, with the general consensus that any potential side effects (such as central nervous system malfunctions and increased seizure activity) can be significantly reduced by supplementation with 50 mg/day of pyridoxine (60).

Because rifampin inhibits DNA-dependent RNA polymerase, there is some fear that it may interfere with fetal development. Snider et al. (58) reviewed published reports of 442 women who received rifampin in 446 pregnancies. They found a rate of congenital malformation of 3.35% in infants of mothers who received rifampin, which is within the range described for the entire population (58). A variety of malformations were described, including limb reductions, central nervous system lesions, and hemorrhagic complications. An association between rifampin and hemorrhagic disease of the newborn has been suggested, and prophylactic vitamin K is recommended in the infants of mothers treated for TB (60).

The third drug used most frequently during pregnancy is ethambutol. Lewitt et al. studied embryos up to 12 weeks after conception obtained from women who had therapeutic and elective abortions (61). None of the embryos appeared to have gross malformations. Bobrowitz (62) reported 42 pregnancies in 38 women who received ethambutol in doses from 15 to 25 mg per kilogram of body weight. Eight infants were born with a variety of abnormalities. Although it was feared that ethambutol might interfere with ophthalmologic development, this was not observed. Snider et al. (58) also found 650 reports of ethambutol use during pregnancy (320 in the first trimester), and reported the incidence of malformation was 2%.

Pyrazinamide is used as a bactericidal drug in most first-line regimens in nonpregnant women. Essentially, no studies have been done to prove its safety during pregnancy. Jana et al. (24) followed six women in an advanced stage of pregnancy with extrapulmonary TB who received pyrazinamide because of its bactericidal effects and its penetration of cerebrospinal fluid (63). They found no adverse fetal effects. As discussed above, the routine use of pyrazinamide in pregnancy is recommended by various international organizations, but its use in the United States has not been recommended because the available data on teratogenicity are inadequate (55). The lack of sufficient published data regarding the teratogenicity of pyrazinamide has led the CDC and the American Thoracic Society to refrain from recommending it as the fourth drug in standard therapy for pregnant women (55). However, Davidson (65) noted that it has been used during pregnancy around the world without significant adverse effects reported. He has endorsed the use of pyrazinamide in pregnancy despite the absence of animal studies to support its lack of teratogenicity. The British Thoracic Society recommends use of pyrazinamide during pregnancy (64).

Streptomycin is the only first-line antituberculous drug that has been shown to cause significant fetal malformation (66–69). In 40 pregnancies, 82% of women delivered normal babies. However, 17% of the babies had eighth nerve palsies with deficits ranging from mild hearing loss to bilateral deafness (66). Thirty-five fetuses were found to have abnormalities after streptomycin was given to 203 women with 206 pregnancies, 72 whom received the drug during the first trimester (60,69). Congenital deafness has been reported in infants with *in utero* exposure to streptomycin, although there is no consistent relationship between ototoxicity and the gestational age of exposure (67,68). Streptomycin is potentially teratogenic throughout pregnancy. Other aminoglycosides, including kanamycin, amikacin, and capreomycin, are also contraindicated during pregnancy.

Because of the emergence of MDR-TB, pregnant women must sometimes be treated with second-line antituberculous agents. Unfortunately, not much is known about the safety during pregnancy of most second-line drugs. Overall management of MDR-TB has a poor prognosis, with a mortality of 37% and a projected cure rate of 56% (70). Paraaminosalicylic acid (PAS) was commonly used in conjunction with INH during the 1950s and 1960s. Of the 1,302 pregnant women who were reported as receiving INH, 495 also received PAS (58). There did not appear to be an increase in the incidence of malformations among the infants of mothers treated with this drug. PAS often causes gastrointestinal side effects and is difficult to tolerate during pregnancy.

There is not enough information to determine the risk of cycloserine or ethionamide during pregnancy, although nonspecific teratogenic effects have been attributed to ethionamide (71). A review of ethionamide exposure in 1,082 pregnancies found a very high malformation rate of 30%; four of five individuals exposed to ethionamide during the first trimester had central nervous system defects (72). Sporadic case reports indicated no associated birth defects (72).

Little is known about the use of the fluoroquinolones (ofloxacin and ciprofloxacin) during pregnancy. However, they may cause arthropathies in immature animals as well as children. A review of 200 women treated with fluoroquinolones (ciprofloxacin, 105; norfloxacin, 93; and ofloxacin, 2) during the first trimester did not find any musculoskeletal abnormalities (73). Those treated with fluoroquinolones had a higher rate of therapeutic abortion. Their use during pregnancy must be weighed against the risk to the fetus and should be considered only in patients with MDR-TB (49). No guidelines exist for the treatment of pregnant women with drug-resistant TB. Because the safety and efficacy of many second-line drugs has not been determined, some clinicians have suggested that elective abortion be considered when treating a pregnant woman with MDR-TB (25).

Recent experience with MDR-TB in pregnant women is limited (73a,73b). Shin et al. reported seven pregnant patients with extensive parenchymal disease due to MDR-TB who were successfully treated utilizing individualized regimens consisting of multiple second-line drugs. There were no obstetrical complications. Perinatal transmission of MDR-TB did not occur. Excellent outcomes were achieved for the women and their children.

BREAST-FEEDING

Another issue that must be addressed in the postpartum patient with TB is the safety of breast-feeding. Several studies have measured the concentration of antituberculous drugs in breast milk (74–77). This entire topic has been recently reviewed in great detail (77–79). INH concentration in breast milk peaks 3 hours after ingestion and reaches a concentration of 16.6 μg/mL with a 300-mg dose (74). The potential dose that the infant would be exposed to from beast milk is 2.49 mg/kg per day (80), which is approximately 12% to 25% of the usual therapeutic infant dose of 10 to 20 mg/kg per day (79). Potential dose exposure to the infant is calculated by multiplying the highest recorded milk concentration by the average daily milk intake of 150 ml/kg per day (80). Drug toxicity may occur in the breast-fed infant when both mother and infant are receiving INH (see below).

Rifampin has peak milk concentrations of 1 to 3 μg/mL with a 600-mg dose (75). The percentage of rifampin transferred to breast milk is 0.05% (75). The potential dose to the infant from breast milk is 0.45 to 0.735 mg/kg per day, which is 2.2% to 7.3% of the infant therapeutic dose of 10 to 20 mg/kg per day (80).

Milk concentration of ethambutol after an oral dose of 15 mg/kg during a 2-hour period was 1.4 μg/mL, which is similar to that found in maternal plasma (1.5 μg/mL) (79). The potential dose to the infant from breast milk is 0.69 mg/kg per day (80). This is approximately 2.8% to 6.9% of the pediatric therapeutic dose.

Streptomycin breast milk concentrations measured 30 minutes after an intramuscular injection of 1 g of streptomycin were 0.3 to 0.6 μg/mL. At 6 hours milk concentrations were 1.1 to 1.3 μg/mL, which is 12% to 47% of maternal plasma levels (76,77). The potential dose exposure to the breast-feeding infant is 1.5 to 4.5 mg/kg per day, which is approximately 3.8% to 22.5% of the infant therapeutic dose (79,80). Aminoglycoside antibiotics such as streptomycin (and kanamycin) are poorly absorbed via the gastrointestinal tract. Therefore, potential for systemic absorption into breast milk is low. While streptomycin use is not recommended routinely for pregnancy, it is compatible with breast-feeding (81).

Pyrazinamide excretion into breast milk is minimal with a maximum estimate of 0.3% of the weight-adjusted dose ingested by the infant (82). Maximal pyrazinamide breast milk concentration was 1.5 μg/mL measured 3 hours after maternal ingestion of a single 1-g dose as compared with maternal plasma concentration of 42 μg/mL at 2 hours after dosing. The potential infant exposure dose is 0.225 mg/kg per day, which is approximately 0.75% to 1.5% of the usual pediatric therapeutic dose.

Although it has been suggested that mothers receiving antituberculous medications substitute commercially available formula for breast milk, most authorities believe this to be unnecessary in light of the absence of reports of adverse effects among infants of nursing mothers and the relatively small doses that infants receive (49,77). If both mother and infant are taking INH, the drug may reach supratherapeutic doses in the nursing infant. In this circumstance, bottle-feeding is recommended. Supplemental pyridoxine should be given to an infant who is taking INH or whose mother (who is breast-feeding) is taking INH. Pyridoxine deficiency may cause seizures in the newborn (83). In summary, at the present time, INH, rifampin, ethambutol, streptomycin, and kanamycin are considered by the American Academy of Pediatrics to be compatible with breast-feeding (79,81). Although pyrazinamide is not "approved," outside of the United States it is accepted. The other agents are of questionable compatibility because of a lack of adequate studies.

CONGENITAL TUBERCULOSIS

Congenital TB is rare; fewer than 300 cases have been reported in the literature. Because the diagnosis is often missed, a new sign of congenital TB in the differential diagnosis of fever and respiratory failure in a newborn is important. During pregnancy, TB may infect the placenta or the female genital tract. Two scenarios have been proposed to describe the pathogenesis of intrauterine infection. In the first scenario, the fetus is infected hematogenously through the umbilical vein. Under these circumstances *Mycobacterium tuberculosis* has been identified in the amnion, decidua, and the chorionic villi (84,85). When this occurs, a primary focus develops in the liver with involvement of the periportal lymph nodes, and tubercle bacilli infect the lungs secondarily. In the second scenario, the fetus is infected as a result of aspiration or ingestion of amniotic fluid that was contaminated by hematogenous dissemination of TB to the placenta. When the fetus has multiple primary foci in the gut or the lungs, the mode of transmission often cannot be determined. Furthermore, differentiating between congenital TB and disease acquired early in the postpartum period is difficult. The criteria for making the diagnosis of congenital TB were originally defined by Beitzki in 1935 (86). However, these criteria were generated from review of autopsy material. They include (a) bacteriologic proof of *M. tuberculosis* infection, (b) a primary complex in the liver, (c) exclusion of extrauterine infection, and (d) occurrence of the disease during the first few days of life.

Cantwell et al. (85) believe that these criteria have lost their clinical usefulness. Only three of 29 cases reported in the literature since 1980 fulfill Beitzke's criteria. On the basis of findings in reported cases since 1980, Cantwell et al. proposed revised diagnostic criteria for congenital TB (85). The infant must have proven TB lesions and at least one of the following: (a) lesions in the first week of life; (b) a primary hepatic complex or caseating hepatic granulomas;

(c) tuberculous infection of the placenta or the maternal genital tract; or (d) exclusion of the possibility of postnatal transmission.

Until Cantwell's group described two cases of congenital TB in 1994, the most recent case in the United States had been reported in 1982. Review of the 29 reported cases published since 1980 revealed that the median age at presentation was 24 days (range, 1 to 84 days) (85). The presenting signs and symptoms were often nonspecific, although hepatosplenomegaly (76% of patients) and respiratory distress (72% of patients) occurred most often. Fever (48% of patients) and lymphadenopathy (38% of patients) occurred less frequently. Abdominal distention, lethargy, irritability, ear discharge, and skin lesions occurred in less than 25% of patients.

Symptoms of congenital TB usually begin within the second and third weeks of life. The chest radiograph may be normal immediately after birth, but progresses rapidly with occasional cavitation being described (88). If possible, the placenta should be examined and cultured for tubercle bacilli. In a review published in 1980 by Hageman et al. (84), a miliary pattern was observed in 50% of patients. Radiographic abnormalities consistent with primary TB were also seen. In the recent review by Cantwell et al. (85), chest radiographic findings were abnormal in 80% of infants and nonspecific in 18 of 23 patients (78%).

The reaction to the tuberculin skin test is usually negative initially, but may become positive within 4 to 8 weeks. Because it is often difficult to obtain sputum from infants, *M. tuberculosis* is more easily cultured from gastric aspirates (89). Hageman (84) found that gastric aspirates provided the diagnosis of TB in 10 of 12 patients. Similarly high yields were found by Cantwell et al. (85). Direct smears from the middle ear and bone marrow, as well as tracheal aspirates, may also show acid-fast bacilli. Culture of cerebrospinal fluid is also recommended but has a lower yield (84,90). Open lung biopsy has also been used to establish the diagnosis (91). Obtaining a maternal history of exposure to TB is an important diagnostic tool, although mothers are often diagnosed with TB after the diagnosis has been made in the infant.

The mortality of congenital TB is very high, approaching 50% in most reviews (87,90). Delay in diagnosis is a significant cause of mortality. In Hageman's study, nine of the 12 patients who died were diagnosed at autopsy. Early diagnosis resulted in a better prognosis, with 14 of 17 patients surviving (84). Treatment is discussed in Chapter 41.

TREATMENT OF THE NEWBORN INFANT WHOSE MOTHER HAS TUBERCULOSIS

When an infant is born to a PPD-positive mother, separation of mother and infant is rarely indicated. Possible exceptions would include a mother infected with multidrug-resistant organisms or a contagious family member known to be noncompliant with treatment. A mother whose tuberculin test is positive but who has a normal chest radiograph requires INH as preventive therapy postpartum if she did not begin therapy during pregnancy. However, an infant does not require special evaluation for TB if the mother is asymptomatic. A mother who has been diagnosed with active TB during pregnancy and has been culture negative for 3 months before delivery poses little risk of infection to the newborn. The child should have a PPD placed at birth and at 3-month intervals but does not require treatment or further evaluation unless the tuberculin test result is positive. If, however, the mother has not been culture negative for 3 months before delivery, or if she has had less than 2 weeks of treatment and is AFB smear positive, the child should be evaluated for active disease with a chest radiograph, have serial cultures of sputum and gastric washings, and undergo tuberculin testing at 6 weeks (92). If there is no evidence of disease, the child should receive INH (5 mg/kg) until the mother has been culture negative for 3 months. Separation of the infant from the mother is likely to be required if the mother has MDR-TB because of the prolonged infectivity and the lack of an effective chemoprophylaxis regimen (64). Separation should be considered if the mother does not comply with treatment.

A South African study found that infants who were given INH while their mothers had active TB did not develop disease (93). After 3 months, if the mother is culture negative and the child remains PPD negative, INH can be stopped. If the child becomes tuberculin positive, INH should be continued for an additional 6 to 9 months after evaluation for active disease. If the mother has INH-resistant TB, the infant should receive rifampin provided the mother is infected with rifampin-sensitive TB (49,94). In the neonate with TB, it is essential to begin appropriate therapy as soon the diagnosis is suspected and cultures have been obtained. The drug regimen for the infant is similar to that for the adults (see Chapter 41).

Bacille Calmette–Guérin (BCG) vaccination of the newborn infant may be considered under special circumstances. An early study by Kendig (95) of infants born to mothers with TB revealed no TB in 30 infants who were vaccinated with BCG. Thirty-eight of 75 infants who were not vaccinated and did not receive INH prophylaxis developed TB; three of those infants died. Similarly, studies from Canada and England demonstrated a protective effect for BCG against the development of TB in infants living in households with a risk of TB exposure (96,97). Colditz et al. (98) performed an extensive metaanalysis on the efficacy of BCG vaccination in newborns and infants. They found that BCG reduces the risk of TB by greater than 50%. As a result of these and other studies, in 1996 the Advisory Council for the Elimination of Tuberculosis and the Advisory Committee on Immunization Practices issued a joint statement regarding the role of BCG for infants and children (99).

They recommended that BCG be considered in an infant with a negative tuberculin skin test under the following circumstances: a) the child is exposed continually to an untreated patient/mother, and the child can neither be separated from this patient nor given long-term INH preventive therapy; or b) the infant is exposed continually to a mother who has INH- and rifampin-resistant TB, and the child cannot be separated from the mother. Infants who test HIV-positive should not be given BCG, because it is a live vaccine that can potentially cause disseminated BCG infection. See Chapter 41 for further details.

TUBERCULOUS MASTITIS

Tuberculous mastitis was first described by Sir Astley Cooper in a treatise on breast disease published in 1829 (100). Cooper wrote, "In young women who have enlargement of the cervical absorbent glands, I have sometimes, though rarely, seen tumours of a scrofulous nature form in their bosoms" (100).

In the past, tuberculous mastitis was a rare disease occurring in only 0.1% of all breast lesions (101,102). Recently, it has been suggested that tuberculous mastitis constitutes approximately 3.0% of surgically managed breast diseases in developing countries (103). It is extremely rare in developed countries. In the prechemotherapy era, Raw found only seven cases of TB involving the breast among 10,000 autopsies performed on TB sanatorium patients (104). Shaefer's review of surgical lesions of the breast at New York Hospital from 1949 to 1954 revealed only two cases in 2,141 breast specimens (105). Subsequently, Haagensen (106) reviewed 8,000 breast specimens from 1938 to 1967 at Columbia–Presbyterian Medical Center in New York and found only five cases of tuberculous mastitis. At the Institut Curie in Paris, only six cases were reported between 1970 and 1981 (107). In 1985, Hale et al. (108) reviewed a 10-year study at Baylor University Medical Center in Dallas comprising 6,000 patients admitted for breast disease: only one case of mammary TB was found. The low incidence of tuberculous mastitis may be due to the high resistance offered by breast tissue to the survival and multiplication of tubercle bacillus (102). Similar resistance to *M. tuberculosis* infection is exhibited by skeletal muscle and spleen (102,109).

Tuberculous mastitis is almost exclusively found in females in the reproductive age group, especially during the lactation period (109–111) Nonetheless, tuberculous mastitis has been reported in female patients aged 6 months to 84 years (102,112). Khanna et al. (103) reported that 30% of their 52 patients with tuberculous mastitis encountered over a 15-year period were lactating. In contrast, only 7% of patients (100-patient series) treated by Shinde et al. (113) presented with lactation. Tuberculous mastitis in a male patient is a rarity. In a series from India, Khana et al. (103)

found that 4% of their patients were male. Tuberculous mastitis has been described as a presenting manifestation of acquired immunodeficiency syndrome (AIDS) (114).

Tuberculous mastitis presents in one of three ways: a painless breast mass, edema of the breast, or a localized abscess (102,103). The lump is usually solitary, ill defined, and occasionally hard and may be difficult to differentiate from carcinoma. Pain in the tuberculous lump is present more frequently than in carcinoma, often being a dull, constant, and nondescript ache. Regional lymph node involvement is very common. Breast abscess with or without sinus tract drainage is the least common presentation. Patients with a lump and associated discharge sinuses are easily diagnosed but need to be differentiated from actinomycosis by the absence of sulfur granules in the discharge and by fungal culture (103). Bilateral disease is extremely rare. Both breasts are affected equally, and the upper outer quadrant appears to be the most frequently involved area.

Tuberculous mastitis may be classified as either primary or secondary disease. Primary involvement is confined only to the breast. It is extremely uncommon and is seen in those rare cases of direct inoculation of the breast by tuberculous bacilli through abrasions of the skin or duct openings in the nipple (102,111,115). Secondary involvement of the breast occurs with evidence of other organ involvement, even when it is clinically unapparent. Major routes of dissemination include lymphatic, hematogenous, and contiguous spread. The most common route is lymphatic spread by retrograde extension from axillary nodes (102,106). Between 50% and 75% of patients have axillary node involvement at the time of presentation (102,105). Domingo et al. (116) utilized contrast material to radiographically demonstrate communication between tuberculous inflammation of the breast and axillary nodes. Occasionally spread is from cervical or mediastinal nodes. Hematogenous spread is the mechanism for disseminated TB. However, Nagashima (117) performed autopsies on 34 patients who died of miliary TB and none had breast involvement, suggesting that hematogenous spread is an unusual mechanism for tuberculous mastitis. Contiguous spread from the ribs, pleural space, or through the rectus sheath from an intraabdominal source has also been reported (106,117).

McKeown and Wilkinson (118) classified tuberculous mastitis into several pathologic categories: (a) Nodular tuberculous mastitis is the most common type, presenting as a localized mass with extensive caseation and little fibrosis with or without sinuses. This variant is often mistaken for fibroadenoma or carcinoma. (b) Disseminated tuberculous mastitis is the second most common type, involving the entire breast with multiple sinuses. (c) Sclerosing tuberculous mastitis contains minimal caseation with extensive hyalinization of the stroma and rare sinus formation; it afflicts older women, is slow growing, and is also often mistaken for carcinoma on initial pathologic examination (103).

The clinical presentation apart from the breast findings is usually unremarkable; constitutional findings and pulmonary TB are often lacking. In the series by Khanna at al. (103) these findings were found to be associated in only 21% and 10% of patients, respectively. While tuberculin skin tests results are often positive, chest radiographs and sputum results are frequently negative. Banerjee et al. (102) found abnormal chest radiographs in only three of 18 patients, while in no patient could tubercle bacilli be cultured from sputum (102). In contrast, Dent and Webber (119) found evidence of TB elsewhere in the body in eight of 21 patients, including lungs (five patients), spine (one patient), and genitalia (one patient) (119). Four of the six patients with pulmonary disease had acid-fast bacilli in their sputa; in two patients the chest radiograph suggested previous TB. Tuberculous mastitis may occur years after its presentation elsewhere in the body, though evidence of this is scanty (120).

Diagnosis is made by demonstration of acid-fast bacilli in breast tissue obtained by biopsy, wedge resection, or needle aspiration (102,103,108,113,121–124). Fine-needle aspiration biopsy can be used to differentiate between cancer and infection, and eliminates the need for open biopsy and mastectomy in these patients (121). Granulomata and caseous necrosis with or without acid-fast bacilli are usually seen. Lack of caseation excludes the possibility of a tuberculous lesion. Other causes for granulomatous diseases must then be considered: histoplasmosis, sarcoidosis, and erythema nodosum. These are excluded by use of appropriate stains. Culture confirms the diagnosis. Unfortunately, bacteriologic confirmation is obtained in only a minority of suspected cases. Tubercle bacilli were isolated in only 25% to 50% of tuberculous mastitis cases (111,123,125). Therefore, the cytologic presence of caseation and epithelioid cell granulomata are usually sufficient for diagnosis. However, careful review of the pathologic findings is necessary because coexistent breast carcinoma has been reported (126). Radiologic imaging modalities, such as mammography and ultrasonography, are unreliable in distinguishing tuberculous mastitis from carcinoma. This is because of the nonspecific and variable pattern of the tuberculous inflammatory lesion (127). Similarly, computed tomography scanning and magnetic resonance imaging are not diagnostic without histologic confirmation. However, these modalities may be used to demonstrate continuity with the chest wall or pleura and may indicate the presence of asymptomatic pulmonary lesions (128–131).

In the older literature, mastectomy (108,111) or wedge resection plus chemotherapy (110) was recommended for the management of tuberculous mastitis. Surgery is now limited to removal of extensive necrotic tissue or if chemotherapy fails (102,112). In the patient who presents with a breast lump requiring excision for diagnosis, standard chemotherapy should follow.

Data on chemotherapy for tuberculous mastitis have shown variable results (102,132,133). Most patients have had wedge resection surgery followed by chemotherapy. Dent and Webber (119) reported success in 20 patients treated with INH, streptomycin, and PAS in whom surgery was limited to a diagnostic biopsy. Banerjee et al. (102) reported on 18 patients who underwent wedge or excisional biopsy with subsequent chemotherapy consisting of INH, streptomycin, and thiacetazone (or PAS in three cases) for 18 months. There was complete resolution in 16 patients. Optimal duration of therapy is similar to that in other forms of extrapulmonary TB, which is usually 9 months unless drug resistance is present (120). Occasionally, chemotherapy fails despite organism susceptibility. McMeeking et al. (134) reported chemotherapy failure in a middle-aged woman despite 4-month treatment with INH, rifampin, and ethambutol. Subsequent partial mastectomy was necessary. Possible mechanisms for failure include poor drug absorption into the infected area as well as defective cellular immunity. Finally, relapse may occur despite adequate therapy. This has been documented following short-course (6-month) treatment protocols (116).

REFERENCES

1. Centers for Disease Control and Prevention. Reported tuberculosis in the United States, 2000. Atlanta, Georgia: US Department of Health and Human Services, August 2001.
2. Centers for Disease Control and Prevention. Tuberculosis among pregnant women—New York City, 1985–1992. *MMWR Morb Mortal Wkly Rep* 1993;42:605–611.
3. Margono F, Mroyeh J, Garely A, et al. Resurgence of active tuberculosis among pregnant women. *Obstet Gynecol* 1994;83: 911–914.
4. Moore M, McCray E, Onorato IM. Cross-matching TB and AIDS registries: TB patients with HIV co-infection, United States, 1993–1994. *Public Health Rep* 1999;114:269–277.
5. Snider DE Jr. Pregnancy and tuberculosis. *Chest* 1984;3S: 10S–13S.
6. Grisolle A. De l'influence que la grossesse et la phthisie pulmonaire exerçant réciproquement l'une sur l'autre. *Arch Gen Med* 1850;22:41.
7. Hedvall E. Pregnancy and tuberculosis. *Acta Med Scand* 1953;147(Suppl 286):1–101.
8. Schaefer G, Zervoudakis I, Fuchs F, et al. Pregnancy and pulmonary tuberculosis. *Obstet Gynecol* 1975;46:706–715.
9. Crombie JB. Pregnancy and pulmonary tuberculosis. *Br J Tuberc* 1954;48:97–101.
10. Edge JR. Pulmonary tuberculosis and pregnancy. *BMJ* 1952;1:845–847.
11. Cohen RC. Effect of pregnancy and parturition on pulmonary tuberculosis. *BMJ* 1943;2:775–783.
12. Cohen JD, Patton EA, Badger TL. The tuberculous mother. *Am Rev Respir Dis* 1952;65:1–23.
13. Rosenbach LM, Gangemi CR. Tuberculosis and pregnancy. *JAMA* 1956;161:1035–1038.
14. Gilks CF, Brindle RJ, Otieno LS, et al. Extrapulmonary and disseminated tuberculosis in HIV-1 seropositive patients presenting to the acute medical service in Nairubi. *AIDS* 1990;4: 981–985.
15. DeMarch P. Tuberculosis and pregnancy. *Chest* 1975;68: 800–804.
16. Pridie R, Stadling P. Management of pulmonary tuberculosis during pregnancy. *BMJ* 1961;3;78–79.
17. Mehta B. Pregnancies and tuberculosis. *Dis Chest* 1961;39: 505–511.
18. Ahmed Y, Mwamba P, Chintu C, et al. A study of maternal mortality at the University Teaching Hospital, Lusaka, Zambia: the emergence of tuberculosis as a major non-obstetric cause of maternal death. *Int J Tuberc Lung Dis* 1999;3:675–680.
19. Pillay T, Khan M, Moodley J, et al. The increasing burden of tuberculosis in pregnant women, newborns and infants under 6 months of age in Durban, Kwazulu-Natal. *S Afr Med J* 2001; 91:983–987.
20. Bjerkedal T, Bahna S, Lehman EH. Course and outcome of pregnancy in women with pulmonary tuberculosis. *Scand J Respir Dis* 1975;56:245–250.
21. Jana N, Vasishta K, Jindal SK, et al. Perinatal outcome in pregnancies complicated by pulmonary tuberculosis. *Int J Gynecol Obstet* 1994;44:119–124.
22. Figueroa-Damian R, Arredondo-Garcia JL. Pregnancy and tuberculosis: influence of treatment on perinatal outcome. *Am J Perinatal* 1998;15:303–306.
23. Figueroa-Damian R, Arredondo-Garcia JL . Neonatal outcome of children born to women with tuberculosis. *Arch Med Res* 2001;32:66–69.
24. Jana N, Vasishta K, Saha S, et al. Obstetrical outcomes among women with extrapulmonary tuberculosis. *N Engl J Med* 1999; 341:645–649.
25. Good J, Iseman M, Davidson P, et al. Tuberculosis in association with pregnancy. *Am J Obstet Gynecol* 1981;140:492–498.
26. Nitta AT, Milligan D. Management of four pregnant women with multidrug-resistant tuberculosis. *Clin Infect Dis* 1999;28: 1298–1304.
27. Wilson E. Thelin T, Dilts P. Tuberculosis complicated by pregnancy. *Am J Obstet Gynecol* 1972;115:526–531.
28. Carter EJ, Mates S. Tuberculosis during pregnancy: the Rhode Island experience, 1987 to 1991. *Chest* 1994;106:1466–1470.
29. Doveren RFC, Block R. Tuberculosis and pregnancy: a provincial study (1990–1996). *Neth J Med* 1998;52:100–106.
30. Brar HS, Golde SH, Egan JE. Tuberculosis presenting as puerperal fever. *Obstet Gynecol* 1987;70:488–490.
31. Kuppuswmi N, Powell L, Freese V. Extrapulmonary tuberculosis as a cause of unexplained postpartum fever. *J Reprod Med* 1995;40:232–234.
32. Toppenberg KS, Hill DA, Miller DP. Safety of radiographic imaging during pregnancy. *Am Fam Physician* 1999;59: 1813–1838.
33. Llewelyn M, Cropley I, Wilkinson R, et al. Tuberculosis diagnosed during pregnancy: a prospective study from London. *Thorax* 2000;55:129–132.
34. Centers for Disease Control and Prevention. Anergy skin testing and tuberculosis preventive therapy for HIV infected persons: revised recommendations. *MMWR Morb Mortal Wkly Rep* 1997;46:1–10.
35. Hadlock FP, Park SK, Wallace R. Routine radiographic screening of the chest in pregnant women: is it indicated? *Obstet Gynecol* 1979;54:433–436.
36. Bonebrake CR, Noller KL, Lochman CP, et al. Routine chest roentgenography in pregnancy. *JAMA* 1978;240:2747–2748.
37. American College of Obstetricians and Gynecologists. Committee on Obstetric Practice. *Guidelines for diagnostic imaging during pregnancy.* ACOG Committee Opinion 158. Washington, DC, 1995.
38. Swartz HM, Reichling BA. Hazards of radiation exposure for pregnant women. *JAMA* 1978; 239:1907–1908.
39. Brent RL. The effect of embryonic and fetal exposure to x-ray, microwaves, and ultrasound: counseling the pregnant and non-

pregnant patient about these risks. *Semin Oncol* 1989;16: 347–368.

40. Finn R, St. Hill CA, Govan AJ, et al. Immunological responses in pregnancy and survival of fetal homograft. *BMJ* 1972;3: 150–152.

41. Present P, Comstock GW. Tuberculin sensitivity in pregnancy. *Am Rev Respir Dis* 1975;112:413–416.

42. Montgomery W, Young R, Allen M, et al. The tuberculin test in pregnancy. *Am J Obstet Gynecol* 1968;10:829–831.

43. Covelli HD, Wilson RT. Immunologic and medical considerations in tuberculin-sensitized pregnant patients. *Am J Obstet Gynecol* 1978;132:256–259.

44. Mofenson LM, Rodriguez EM, Hershaw, et al. *Mycobacterium tuberculosis* infection in pregnant and non-pregnant women infected with HIV in the Women and Infants Transmission Study. *Arch Intern Med* 1995;156:1066–1071.

45. Eriksen NL, Helfgott AW. Cutaneous anergy in pregnant and nonpregnant with human immunodeficiency virus. *Infect Dis Obstet Gynecol* 1998;6:13–17.

46. Nolan TE, Espinosa TL, Pastorek JG. Tuberculin skin testing in pregnancy: trends in a population. *J Perinatol* 1997;17:199–201.

47. Schulte JM, Bryan P, Dodds S et al. Tuberculosis skin testing among HIV-infected pregnant women in Miami, 1995 to 1996. *J Perinatol* 2002;22:159–162.

48. Snider DE, Farer LS. Package inserts of antituberculosis drugs and tuberculin. *Am Rev Respir Dis* 1985;131:809–810.

49. American Thoracic Society. Targeted tuberculin testing and treatment of latent tuberculosis infection. *Am J Respir Crit Care Med* 2000;161:5221–5247.

50. Raucher H, Gribetz I. Care of the pregnant woman with tuberculosis and her newborn infant: a pediatrician's perspective. *Mt Sinai J Med* 1986;53:70–76.

51. Moulding TS, Redeker AG, Kanel GC. Twenty isoniazid-associated deaths in one state. *Am Rev Respir Dis* 1989;140:700–705.

52. Franks A, Binkin N, Snider DE, et al. Isoniazid hepatitis among pregnant and postpartum Hispanic patients. *Public Health Rep* 1989;104:151–155.

53. Snider DE Jr, Caras GJ. Isoniazid-associated hepatitis deaths: a review of available information. *Am Rev Respir Dis* 1992;145: 494–497.

54. Snider DE Jr. Pyridoxine supplementation during isoniazid therapy. *Tubercle* 1980;61:191–196.

55. American Thoracic Society/Centers for Disease Control and Prevention/Infectious Diseases Society of America. Treatment of tuberculosis. *Am J Respir Crit Care Med* 2003;167:603–662.

56. Levene CI, Carrington MJ. The inhibition of protein-lysine 6-oxidase by various lathyrogens: evidence for two different mechanisms. *Biochem J* 1985; 232:293–296.

57. Pandet SK, Sensharma S. Neuroembryopathic effect of INH on the cerebellum of chick embryo. *Indian J Med Sci* 1988;42: 291–293.

58. Snider DE Jr, Layde P, Johnson M, et al. Treatment of tuberculosis during pregnancy. *Am Rev Respir Dis* 1980;122:65–79.

59. Hammond EC, Selikoff IJ, Robitzek E. Isoniazid therapy in relation to later occurrence of cancer in adults and children. *BMJ* 1967;2:792–795.

60. Bothamley G. Drug treatment for tuberculosis during pregnancy. *Drug Safety* 2001;24:553–565.

61. Lewit T, Nebel L, Terracina S, et al. Ethambutol in pregnancy; observations on embryogenesis. *Chest* 1974;66:25–26.

62. Bobrowitz I. Ethambutol in pregnancy. *Chest* 1974;66:20–24.

63. Kingdom JCP, Kennedy DH. Tuberculous meningitis in pregnancy. *Br J Obstet Gynaecol* 1989;96:233–235.

64. Joint Tuberculosis Committee of the British Thoracic Society. Chemotherapy and management of tuberculosis in the United Kingdom: recommendations 1998. *Thorax* 1998;53:536–548.

65. Davidson PT. Treating tuberculosis: what drugs, for how long? *Ann Intern Med* 1990;112:393–394.

66. Varpela E, Hietalalahti J, Aro M. Streptomycin and dihydrostreptomycin during pregnancy and their effect on the child's inner ear. *Scand J Respir Dis* 1969;50:101–109.

67. Donald PR, Sellers SL. Streptomycin ototoxicity in the unborn child. *S Afr Med J* 1981;60:316–318.

68. Robinson G, Cambon KG. Hearing loss in infants of tuberculous mothers treated with streptomycin during pregnancy. *N Eng J Med* 1964;271:949–951.

69. Conway N, Birt BD. Streptomycin in pregnancy: effect on the fetal ear. *BMJ* 1965;2:260–263.

70. Goble M, Iseman MD, Madsen LA, et al. Treatment of 171 patients with pulmonary tuberculosis resistant to isoniazid and rifampin. *New Engl J Med* 1993;328:527–532.

71. Potworowska M, Sianozecko E, Szuflodowica R. Ethionamide treatment and pregnancy. *Polish Med J* 1966;5:1153–1158.

72. Schardein JL. Chemically induced birth defects. New York: Marcel Dekker, 1993:378.

73. Loebstein R, Addis A, Ho E, et al. Pregnancy outcome following gestational exposure to fluoroquinolones: a multicenter, prospective, controlled study. *Antimicrob Agents Chemother* 1998;42:1336–1339.

73a. Nitta A, Milligan D. Management of four pregnant women with multidrug-resistant tuberculosis. *Clin Infect Dis* 1999;28: 1298–1304.

73b. Shin S, Guerra D, Rich M, et al. Treatment of multidrug-resistant tuberculosis during pregnancy: a report of 7 cases. *Clin Infect Dis* 2003;326:996–1003.

74. Berlin C, Lee C. Isoniazid and acetylisoniazid disposition in human milk, saliva, and plasma. *Fed Proc* 1979;38:426.

75. Vorherr H. Drug excretion in breast milk. *Postgrad Med J* 1974;56:97–104.

76. Fujimori H, Imai S. Studies on dihydrostreptomycin administered to the pregnant and transferred to their fetuses. *Jpn Obstet Gynecol Soc* 1957;4:133–149.

77. Snider DE Jr, Powell K. Should women taking antituberculosis drugs breast-feed? *Arch Intern Med* 1984;144:589–590.

78. Brost BC, Newman RB. The maternal and fetal effects of tuberculosis therapy. *Obstet Gynecol Clin N Am* 1997;24: 659–673.

79. Tran JH, Montakantikul P. The safety of antituberculosis medications during breast-feeding. *J Hum Lact* 1998;14:337–340.

80. Fulton B, Moore LL. Antiinfectives in breast milk. III. Antituberculars, quinolones and urinary germicides. *J Hum Lact* 1993;9:43–46.

81. American Academy of Pediatrics. The transfer of drugs and other chemicals into human milk. *Pediatrics* 1994;93:137–150.

82. WHO Working Group, Bennet PN, ed. *Drugs and human lactation.* New York: Elsevier, 1988:281–282.

83. McKenzie SA, Macnab NJ, Katz G. Neonatal pyridoxine responsive convulsions due to isoniazid therapy. *Arch Dis Child* 1976;51:567–568.

84. Hageman J, Shulman S, Schreiber M, et al. Congenital tuberculosis: critical reappraisal of clinical findings and diagnostic procedures. *Pediatrics* 1980;66:980–984.

85. Cantwell MR, Shehab ZM, Costello AM, et al. Brief report: congenital tuberculosis. *N Engl J Med* 1994;330:1051–1054.

86. Beitzke H. Uber die angeborene Tuberkulose Infektion. *Ergeb Tuberk Forsch* 1935;7:1–30.

87. Gogus S, Uner H, Akcoren Z, et al. Neonatal tuberculosis. *Pediatr Pathol* 1993;13:299–304.

88. Cunningham DG, μgraw TT, Griffin AJ, et al. Neonatal tuberculosis: with pulmonary cavitation. *Tubercle* 1987;63:217–219.

89. Foo A, Tan K, Chay O. Congenital tuberculosis. *Tuber Lung Dis* 1993;74:59–61.

90. Nemir RL, O'Hare D. Congenital tuberculosis. *Am J Dis Child* 1985;139:284–287.

91. Stallworth JR, Brasfield DM, Tiller RE. Congenital miliary tuberculosis proven by open lung biopsy specimen and successfully treated. *Am J Dis Child* 1980;134:320–321.

92. Joint Tuberculosis Committee of the British Thoracic Society. Control and Prevention of tuberculosis in the United Kingdom: code of practice 2000. *Thorax* 2000;55:887–901.

93. Dormer B, Swart J, Harrison I, et al. Prophylactic isoniazid protection of infants in a tuberculosis hospital. *Lancet* 1959;2: 902–903.

94. Villarino MER, Rizdon R, Weismuller M, et al. Rifampin preventive therapy for tuberculosis infection: experience with 157 adolescents. *Am J Respir Crit Care Med* 1997;155: 1735–1738,

95. Kendig E. The place of BCG vaccine in the management of infants born of tuberculous mothers. *N Engl J Med* 1969;281: 520–523.

96. Curtis H, Leck I, Bamford F. Incidence of childhood tuberculosis after neonatal BCG vaccination. *Lancet* 1984;1:145–148.

97. Young T, Hershfield E. A case-control study to evaluate the effectiveness of mass neonatal BCG vaccination among Canadian Indians. *Am J Public Health* 1986;76:783–786.

98. Colditz G, Berkey C, Mosteller F, et al. The efficacy of BCG vaccination in preventing tuberculosis in newborns and infants. *Pediatrics* 1995;96:29–35.

99. Centers for Disease Control and Prevention. The role of BCG vaccine in the prevention and control of tuberculosis in the United States: a joint statement by the Advisory Council for the Elimination of Tuberculosis and the Advisory Committee on Immunization Practices. *MMWR Morb Mortal Wkly Rep* 1996; 45:1–18.

100. Cooper A. *Illustrations of the diseases of the breast.* Part 1. London: Longman, Rees Orme, Brown and Green, 1829:73.

101. Hamit HF, Ragsdale TH. Mammary tuberculosis. *J R Soc Med* 1982;75:764.

102. Banerjee SN, Ananthakrichnan N, Mehta RB, et al. Tuberculous mastitis: a continuing problem. *World J Surg* 1987;11: 105–109.

103. Khanna R, Prasanna G, Gupta P, et al. Mammary tuberculosis: report on 52 cases. *Postgrad Med J* 2002;78:422–424.

104. Raw N. Tuberculosis of the breast. *BMJ* 1924;1:657–658.

105. Schaefer G. Tuberculosis of the breast. *Am Rev Tuberc Pulm Dis* 1955;72:810–824.

106. Haagensen CD. Infections in the breast. In: Haagensen CD, ed. *Diseases of the breast*, 3rd ed. Philadelphia: WB Saunders, 1986:384–393.

107. Guillet JL, Salmon RJ, Durand JC, et al. Mammary tuberculosis. *Lancet* 1982;2:166.

108. Hale JA, Peters GN, Cheek JH. Tuberculosis of the breast: rare but still extent. *Am J Surg* 1985;150:620–624.

109. Mukerjee P, George M, Maheswasi HB, et al. Tuberculosis of the breast. *J Indian Med Assoc* 1974;62:410.

110. Wilson TS, MacGregor JW. The diagnosis and treatment of tuberculosis of the breast. *Can Med Assoc J* 1963;89:1118–1124.

111. Morgen M. Tuberculosis of the breast. *Surg Gynecol Obstet* 1931;53:593–605.

112. Goldman KP. Tuberculosis of the breast. *Tubercle* 1978;59: 41–45.

113. Shinde SR, Chandawarkar RY, Deshmukh SP. Tuberculosis of the breast masquerading as carcinoma: a study of 100 patients. *World J Surg* 1995;19:379–381.

114. Hartstein M, Leaf HL. Tuberculosis of the breast as a presenting manifestation of AIDS. *Clin Infect Dis* 1992;15:692–693.

115. Wilson JP, Chapman SW. Tuberculous mastitis. *Chest* 1990;98: 1505–1509.

116. Domingo CH, Ruiz J, Roig J, et al. Tuberculosis of the breast: a rare modern disease. *Tubercle* 1990;71:221–223.

117. Nagashima Y. The role of the female breast in the presence of tuberculosis of the internal organs and especially in miliary tuberculosis. *Virchows Arch Pathol Anat* 1925;254:184.

118. McKeown KC, Wilkinson KW. Tuberculosis of the breast. *Br J Surg* 1952;39:420–429.

119. Dent DM, Webber BL. Tuberculosis of the breast. *S Afr Med J* 1977;51:611–614.

120. Wapnir IL, Pallan TM, Gaudino J, et al. Latent mammary tuberculosis: a case report. *Surgery* 1985;98:976–978.

121. Thompson K, Donzelli J, Jensen J, et al. Breast and cutaneous mycobacteriosis: diagnosis by fine-needle aspiration biopsy. *Diagn Cythopathol* 1997;17:45–49.

122. Jayaram G. Cytomorphology of tuberculous mastitis. *Acta Cytol* 1985;29:974–978.

123. Ikard RW, Perkins D. Mammary tuberculosis: a rare disease. *S Med J* 1977;70:208–221.

124. Gupta D, Rajwanashi A, Gupta SK, et al. Fine needle aspiration cytology in the diagnosis of tuberculous mastitis. *Acta Cytol* 1999;43:191–194.

125. Goksoy E, Duren M, Durgun V, et al. Tuberculosis of the breast. *Eur J Surg* 1995;161:471–473.

126. Miller RE, Salomon PF, West JP. The coexistence of carcinoma and tuberculosis of the breast and axillary lymph nodes. *Am J Surg* 1971;121:338–340.

127. Zandrino F, Monetti F, Candolfo N. Primary tuberculosis of the breast. A case report. *Acta Radiol* 2000;41:61–63.

128. Arslan A, Ciftci E, Yildiz F, et al. Multifocal bone tuberculosis presenting as a breast mass: CT and MRI findings. *Eur Radiol* 1999;9:1117–1119.

129. Goyal M, Sharma R, Shaaarma A, et al. Chest wall tuberculosis simulating breast carcinoma. *Australas Radiol* 1998;42:86–87.

130. Schnarkowski P, Schmidt D, Kessler M, et al. Tuberculosis of the breast: US, mammographic and CT findings. *J Comput Assist Tomogr* 1994;185:970–975.

131. Oh KK, Kim JH, Kook SH. Imaging of tuberculous disease involving breast. *Eur Radiol* 1998;8:1475–1480.

132. Alagaratnam TT, Ong GB. Tuberculosis of the breast. *Br J Surg* 1980;67:611–614.

133. Apps MCP, Harrison NK, Blauth CIA. Tuberculosis of the breast. *Br Med J* 1984;288:1874–1875.

134. McMeeking AA, Gonzalez R, Hanna B. Mammary tuberculosis. *NY State J Med* 1989;89:288–289.

43

SURGICAL THERAPY OF TUBERCULOSIS

ARTHUR D. BOYD
BERNARD K. CRAWFORD, JR.
LAWRENCE GLASSMAN

Evidence of tuberculous infection found in ancient Egyptian (1) and South American mummies (2) demonstrates that tuberculosis (TB) has been a scourge of mankind for thousands of years. In 400 B.C., Hippocrates (3) wrote extensively about TB ("phthisis," as TB was named in Greek), making references to injection of air into the chest cavity for therapeutic purposes. Throughout the centuries, the pathophysiology of TB ("consumption," based on the Latin synonym for TB) was little understood, and until the 1800s effective treatment was nonexistent. The early treatment of TB in the 19th century and the first half of the 20th century provided the stimulus for the development of general thoracic surgery. Today, with the recrudescence of TB in debilitated and immunocompromised hosts, the lessons learned during the developing years once again assume significance.

Before the development of antituberculous drugs in the middle of the 20th century, bed rest and collapse therapy were the only available treatments for pulmonary TB. These "magic mountain" methods were developed on the basis of autopsy observations showing necrosis with cavitation in the upper third of the lung of consumptive patients. The elastic recoil characteristic of pulmonary tissue and the augmentation of traction on these cavities with the act of breathing and the decrease in blood supply to the apical portions of the lung were all factors understood to contribute to the persistence of tuberculous disease in the upper parts of the lung (4). Consequently, mechanical interventions that would cause the tuberculous cavities to collapse and thus allow healing were developed.

BED REST THERAPY

Bed rest was the first successful therapy widely used in the management of TB. Bed rest reduces the functional residual capacity of the lung, thereby decreasing static tension on the walls of the tuberculous cavities. It also reduces dynamic traction on the cavity walls by decreased ventilation and increased blood flow to the apices of the lung, allowing the cavities to collapse and healing to take place.

Around 1880, Dettweiler in Germany and Turban in Switzerland introduced bed rest for the management of tuberculosis. At Davos Platz, Turban followed 396 patients treated with bed rest and documented that TB was not always fatal. After 3 years, 44% (175 patients) of these patients were well and at normal activity, 35% (140 patients) had died, and 21% (81 patients) remained symptomatic (4,5). Trudeau at the Cottage Sanatorium in the Adirondacks in upstate New York introduced bed rest therapy into the United States in 1900. Because bed rest failed to arrest TB in a high percentage of patients and because relapse was common, collapse therapy was used with increasing frequency.

COLLAPSE THERAPY

Artificial Pneumothorax

In 1821, James Carson of Liverpool, England was the first to advocate artificial pneumothorax as a treatment for TB:

> The sides of the abscess are prevented from falling into a salutary contact, not by the matter which lodges between them, but by the powerful elasticity and retraction of the surrounding substance. As soon, expect healing in a divided tendo Achilles without mechanical aid. By collapse of the lung, on the other hand, the diseased part would be placed in a quiescent state, receiving little or no disturbance from the movement of respiration which would be performed solely by the other lung, and the divided surfaces would be brought into close contact by the same resilient power which before had kept them asunder. An abscess in this lung would be placed in

---

A. D. Boyd: Department of Surgery, New York University School of Medicine; Department of Surgery, New York University Medical Center, New York, New York.

B. K. Crawford, Jr.: Department of Cardiothoracic Surgery, New York University School of Medicine; Department of Thoracic Surgery, New York University Tisch Hospital, New York, New York.

L. Glassman: Department of Cardiothoracic Surgery, North Shore University Hospital, Manhasset, New York.

circumstances at least as favorable to the healing process as the same affections on any other part of the body. In those cases of consumption in which the disease is placed in one of the lungs only, the remedy would appear to be simple, safe and complete. Furthermore, a hemorrhage from one of the lungs, the frequent prelude of consumption, if not immediately fatal, would be as certainly stopped by the collapse of that lung, as the flooding consequent upon parturition by the contraction or rather the resilience of the womb. The state of collapse must be by degrees only. It has long been my opinion that if ever phthisis is to be cured, and it is an event of which I am by no means disposed to despair, it must be accomplished by mechanical means, or in other words by a surgical operation (6).

Subsequently, clinical improvement of TB was occasionally observed when a pleural effusion or a spontaneous pneumothorax occurred in a patient with TB. In 1892, Forlanini was the first to introduce nitrogen into the pleural space as therapy for pulmonary TB (7). However, his experience, as innovative and significant as it was, was not widely recognized. In 1898, Murphy, of Chicago, reviewed observations of 11,540 Civil War patients with chest injuries and noticed that only minimal symptoms occurred in many of these pneumothorax patients. He became a strong advocate of artificial pneumothorax in the management of tuberculosis (8). Not only did Murphy use this treatment extensively, but he also recognized the usefulness of the recently discovered chest radiograph in evaluating and following patients with TB.

In the first half of the 20th century, pneumothorax was widely used, usually as an adjunct to bed rest. By the end of World War II it was recognized that a satisfactory pneumothorax could be maintained in only 25% of patients and that tuberculous empyema developed in 20% (Fig. 43.1).

At least 20% of patients treated with artificial pneumothorax were dead after 10 to 20 years (9). The era of pneumothorax ended with the development of plombage and more effective forms of collapse therapy.

Pneumonolysis

Artificial pneumothorax frequently was ineffective because of the presence of adhesions that prevented the diseased lung from collapsing. In 1912, Jacobaeus (10), a Scandinavian pulmonologist, used a modified cystoscope as a thoracoscope and divided pulmonary adhesions with a cautery, thereby permitting collapse of the diseased lung. However, Jacobaeus's procedure never attained wide usage in the treatment of patients with TB. It is interesting to note, however, that the thoracoscope he improvised provided the prototype for today's instrument. Augmented by fiberoptic lighting, video imaging, and specially designed complementary instrumentation, the thoracoscope is now widely used in general thoracic surgery.

Pneumoperitoneum and Phrenic Nerve Paralysis

Pneumoperitoneum and phrenic nerve paralysis, either temporary or permanent, were also used in the management of TB. These techniques caused the diaphragm to elevate and compress the lower lung, and there was some effect on apical cavities. Pneumoperitoneum was shown to reduce the functional residual capacity that seemed to be additive to the reduction obtained by bed rest. This suggested that pneumoperitoneum augmented and reinforced the effects of bed rest (11).

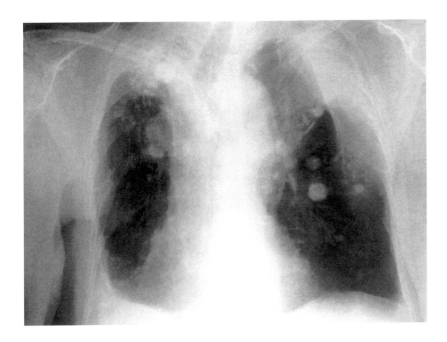

FIGURE 43.1. Chest radiograph showing a loculated pleural effusion with calcified wall secondary to chronic pneumothorax therapy.

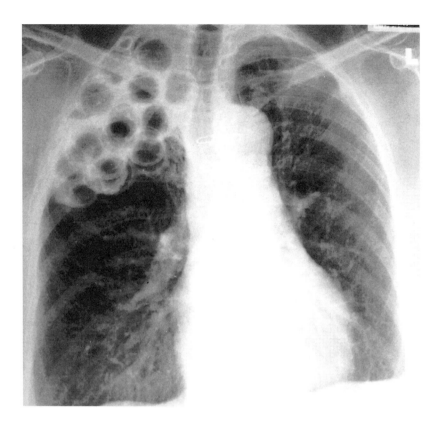

FIGURE 43.2. Lucite balls at right apex.

Although used extensively, phrenic nerve paralysis had no physiologic basis to support its use. Eventually, bronchospirometric studies showed that diaphragmatic paralysis caused mediastinal flutter that interfered with ventilation of both lungs. This observation caused phrenic nerve paralysis to fall into disuse (12).

Extrapleural Pneumothorax or Plombage

In the early 1900s, Tuffier (13) created an extrapleural space that he filled with air; later, he inserted a free-fat graft. He hoped that the creation of an extrapleural space would provide a convenient and permanent method for compressing the underlying diseased lung. However, prolonged maintenance of the extrapleural space required either repeat injections of air or insertion of a foreign material (or plomb) into the extrapleural space. No truly satisfactory material for plombage was available, as is indicated by the number of substances that were tried, such as paraffin, bone fragments, Lucite balls (Figs. 43.2 and 43.3), gauze, and oil (14). All of these materials tended to migrate or become infected. In addition, the external walls of large peripheral tuberculous cavities received their blood supply from the pleura, and opening the extrapleural space divided these vessels, which often resulted in necrosis of the cavity walls and subsequent fistula formation with the development of empyema. Therefore, use of the extrapleural space was abandoned (15).

Around 1937, interest in extrapleural pneumothorax was rekindled (16). Results were encouraging in patients who had been properly selected. When patients with large peripheral cavities were excluded, and when air was used as the plomb, results were satisfactory. Because extrapleural pneumothorax was less radical, many preferred it to thoracoplasty (see below) (17). However, shortly thereafter, with the introduction of antituberculous drugs, resectional therapy was introduced; thus, extrapleural pneumothorax was never widely used.

Subcostal and Extraperiosteal Plombage

Concurrent with the renewed interest in extrapleural pneumothorax, several groups (18–20) concluded that the plane outside the periosteum and intercostal muscle would be more secure than the extrapleural space. They dissected the periosteum from the ribs, creating a pocket inside the ribs and outside the periosteum and intercostal muscles into which they placed a polyethylene bag containing plastic balls (Figs. 43.2 and 43.3). This procedure actively compressed the underlying lung but spared pulmonary function by avoiding paradoxical motion of the chest wall. However, as happened with extrapleural pneumothorax, pulmonary resection soon became popular, and subcostal extraperiosteal plombage was not widely used except for patients in whom resection was impossible.

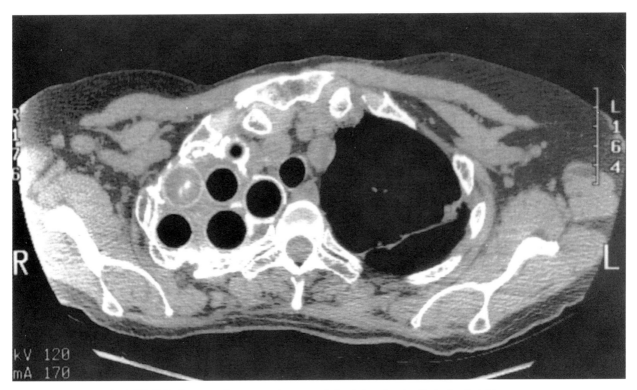

FIGURE 43.3. Computed tomography scan of chest showing Lucite balls at right apex.

Thoracoplasty

Thoracoplasty was initially used in the 1880s for the management of empyema (21). In 1885 in Lausanne, de Cerenville (22) removed anterior portions of the second and third ribs in an attempt to collapse underlying tuberculous cavities. Other variations of thoracoplasty were also tried, but none was sufficiently extensive to achieve collapse of the underlying tuberculous cavities.

Brauer (23), an internist, was the first to advocate extensive rib resections sufficient to collapse the diseased lung. In 1907, Friederich, at Brauer's urging, began resection of the second through the ninth ribs, along with their periosteum and intercostal muscles using a U-shaped incision. Brauer recognized the physiologic problems resulting from this extensive procedure. He described that a flutter of the chest wall and mediastinum—"pendulum respiration"—resulted in imperfect aeration. It is indeed surprising that a large percentage of these patients survived. The mortality rate of this extensive resection was 30%. As a result of his observations on these patients, Brauer made many suggestions that influenced the development of thoracoplasty during the next 30 years. He recommended staging the procedure (two to three stages), and hypothesized that preserving the periosteum and intercostal muscles would stabilize the chest wall. He also advised limiting thoracoplasties to the upper ribs, including the first rib. In addition, he advised using "positive-pressure breathing" during the postoperative period to control flutter of the chest wall and mediastinum. This suggestion preceded by 45 years the description by Avery, Morch, and Benson of internal pneumatic stabilization in the management of flailed chest (24).

In 1873, Wilms (25) reported on paravertebral thoracoplasty, resecting ribs posteriorly from the angle back to the transverse process. This less radical procedure was associated with a much lower mortality than Brauer and Friederich's procedure, and was more effective than de Cerenville's technique. Sauerbruck described numerous variations of thoracoplasty, reported in great detail in 1925 by John Alexander (26).

Alexander, from the University of Michigan, is recognized as the father of thoracoplasty in the United States and was one of the early leaders in the development of thoracic surgery. During his early career, Alexander himself contracted active TB, for which he was hospitalized and prescribed bed rest. During this hospitalization, although physically inactive, he was mentally very productive and wrote the first English text on the surgical management of TB. This accomplishment is reminiscent of that of Chevalier Jackson, the father of American endoscopy, who produced several texts on endoscopy during long periods of treatment for pulmonary TB (27).

By 1935, Alexander (28) had perfected the posterior lateral method of thoracoplasty, and it was widely used from then on. The procedure was done in three or four stages. The first rib, in addition to the next five to seven ribs, was resected. The transverse processes and underlying ribs were resected to prevent the formation of a residual space in the posterior gutter. The anterior ribs were resected only in the region of the underlying disease. The operative mortality with this staged thoracoplasty was 2% or less and resulted in cavity closure and disappearance of tuberculous bacilli from the sputum in 80% of patients. With the introduction of streptomycin (SM) in 1945 (29), resectional surgery became safe, and thoracoplasty was used less frequently; in fact, its use in the management of TB became almost obsolete.

RESECTIONAL THERAPY

Successful pulmonary resection for the management of bronchiectasis and carcinoma in the latter part of the 19th century and the first half of the 20th century led surgeons to try these techniques on patients with TB. However, the results of resection for TB were disappointing, as there were frequent complications and a high mortality rate (30).

In 1897, Tuffier (31) first successfully performed local excision of tuberculous nodules in several patients. However, successes were few and for many years no reports of resection for TB appeared in medical literature. Then, in the mid-1930s, a successful lobectomy (32) and pneumonectomy (33) were reported for TB in patients who were thought to have had bronchiectasis. In 1940, a survey study reported on 50 patients who had pulmonary resection for TB. Of 19 patients who had pneumonectomies, eight died (40%) and only three patients were well. Of 31 patients who had lobectomies, six died (20%) and 16 were classified as well (30).

Before 1940, most pulmonary resections were performed by the tourniquet technique of mass ligation. Around 1940, Reinhoff (34), Blade and Kemp (35), and Churchill and Klopstock (36) reported on the technique of individual ligation for pulmonary resection, which led to a renewed interest in resectional therapy for TB. However, it soon became apparent that bronchi involved with TB did not hold sutures well and that frequently the disease spreads to the opposite lung during the operation. Thus, the results of resection were not greatly improved by the technique of individual ligation (15).

After the introduction of SM in 1945, pulmonary resection of localized TB was performed with excellent results and an acceptable morbidity and mortality, but resistance of tuberculous organisms to SM developed rapidly when this drug was used alone. Fortunately, other antituberculous drugs were developed. When they were used simultaneously with SM, significant delay in the development of resistant organisms occurred (29).

Frequently, TB has a regional distribution in the lung, not a lobar distribution. Consequently, development of techniques of wedge resection and segmental resection, in addition to lobectomy and pneumonectomy, permitted the

complete resection of TB and the preservation of as much normal lung tissue as possible. As more effective drugs became available, tuberculous infections were managed satisfactorily with drug therapy and resection was not necessary for most patients, including those left with open, negative cavities. By the mid-1960s, resectional surgery for TB was so uncommon that it seemed that all treatment for TB would become nonsurgical.

In recent years, however, the increase in the number of patients who are immunosuppressed or infected with atypical TB and drug-resistant organisms has resulted in a dramatic increase in the number of operations being performed for TB. More than 60 patients with TB have been operated on at the New York University Medical Center since 1990. This is more than four times as many as were operated on during the previous similar period. Representative of the current population with TB is a 43-year-old, noncompliant man with bilateral disease and a large cavity at the left apex (Figs. 43.4 and 43.5). At presentation, his organism was resistant to isoniazid (INH), rifampin (RIF), kanamycin, and SM. He was started on a regimen of paraaminosalicylic acid (PAS), ethambutol (EMB), and ethionamide. Six months later, the infecting organism was resistant not only to INH, RIF, and kanamycin but also to EMB. However, it was sensitive to ciprofloxacin and PAS. He was prescribed pyrazinamide, PAS, capreomycin, and ciprofloxacin. After 3 months of this regimen, his sputum remained positive and a left upper lobe resection was carried out. At operation, his latissimus dorsi muscle and serratus anterior muscle were placed in the apex of the left pleural space for coverage of his bronchial stump and for control of air leaks. Postoperatively, his course was uneventful. He was maintained on a strict antituberculous regimen and after 1 year was sputum negative and in good health. Noncompliance and drug resistance demonstrate two current indications for pulmonary resection in tuberculous patients (Table 43.1).

Indications for Resectional Surgery
Drug-Resistant Mycobacterium tuberculosis

Patients infected with TB organisms with high levels of resistance to RIF, INH, and to all or most other first-line drugs (SM, pyrazinamide, EMB) are considered to have drug-resistant tuberculosis. Because these patients have a high likelihood of failure with medical therapy (37), they should undergo surgical resection if their disease is sufficiently localized and they have adequate cardiopulmonary reserve.

A regimen of drugs to which the organism is fully or partially susceptible should be given for 3 months, followed by operation. A report from the National Jewish Medical and Research Center in Denver (38) showed that patients at that center, on average, received 5.8 drugs preoperatively. In

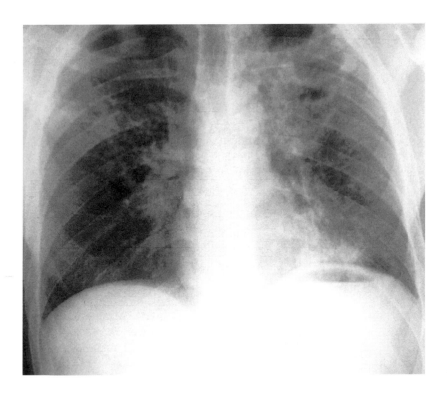

FIGURE 43.4. Chest radiograph showing bilateral infiltrates and a large cavity at left apex.

spite of this aggressive therapy, nearly half of the patients undergoing surgery had positive sputum at the time of operation. An integral part of the management is aggressive antituberculous regimen continued after resection. In the most recent series from the University of Colorado (39), 172 patients underwent 180 pulmonary resections for multidrug-resistant TB. Operative mortality was 3.3% (six of 180) and the morbidity rate was 12% (20 of 166). Nearly 95% of the patients were rendered sputum negative; only four of 91 patients with preoperative positive sputum cultures tested positive after resection. Overall mortality for this difficult group has been excellent, comparing favorably with that of a comparable group treated with medication alone.

Mycobacterial Infections Other Than Tuberculosis

Patients with mycobacterial infections other than TB are usually treated with three- or four-drug regimens for 18 to 24 months. A success rate of 40% to 60% can be expected in these patients. Patients in whom this treatment fails are left with stable but chronically active disease (40). Resectional therapy should be considered for these patients if

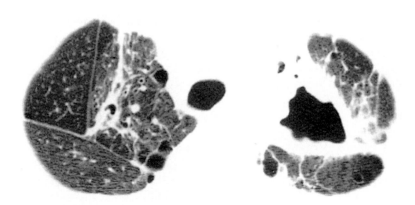

FIGURE 43.5. Computed tomography scan showing large left apical cavity.

TABLE 43.1. INDICATIONS FOR PULMONARY RESECTION IN TUBERCULOUS PATIENTS

Absolute Indications	Relative Indications
Massive hemoptysis (600 cm³/24 h)	Hemoptysis
Destroyed lung, positive sputum	Drug-resistant TB
Bronchopleural fistula	Bronchial stenosis
Suspicion of carcinoma	Persistent positive sputum
	Open, negative cavity
	TB empyema
	Atypical tuberculous infections

TB, tuberculosis.

their disease is localized and their overall condition is satisfactory (38,40). The most common causative agent in these patients is *Mycobacterium avium-intracellulare* complex. Some patients have *M. kansasii, M. chelonae,* or *M. xenopi.* Intensive, drug-specific therapy should be administered to these patients for 3 months before surgery.

Pomerantz et al. (38) reported on 38 patients resected for mycobacteria other than *M. tuberculosis,* 26 of whom had positive sputum at the time of operation. Although mortality rates for operative procedures have been reported from 0 to 7% (41,42), which is quite acceptable, the complication rate in patients with mycobacterial infections other than TB was high (29 of 41 patients). Bronchopleural fistula, prolonged air leaks, and space problems may occur. Current thinking is that chemotherapy combined with resection may be preferable to chemotherapy alone in patients with atypical TB if the patient has localized pulmonary disease and adequate cardiopulmonary status.

Hemoptysis

Moderate hemoptysis is common in patients with tuberculous infections. In most instances, sedation, bed rest, and antituberculous medications control the bleeding. Since tuberculous involvement is frequently diffuse and often bilateral, bronchoscopy should be performed early to localize the site of bleeding. If bleeding becomes massive (600 cm³/24 hours) or severe (200 cm³/24 hours) and recurrent, resection of the site of bleeding is indicated (43–45). Since bleeding is usually from bronchial arteries in cavitary lesions, bronchial artery embolization is sometimes helpful in slowing or stopping hemorrhage preoperatively. Bronchial embolization as definitive therapy should be considered in patients with such poor pulmonary reserve that pulmonary resection is not possible (46). Bronchial artery angiography in this setting reveals bronchial artery hypertrophy in 88% of cases. Embolization is generally only a temporizing measure as most patients will ultimately require surgery or die of complications of the underlying disease (47).

Aspergillomas (fungus balls) frequently grow in old tuberculous cavities and can cause massive hemorrhage. Because systemic antifungal therapy is not effective in controlling bleeding in this situation, pulmonary resection is usually required. Preoperative embolization of the bronchial artery and subclavian artery branches supplying the cavity should be considered in these patients. Intracavitary amphotericin B has been utilized in inoperable situations (48).

At the time of pulmonary resection for hemoptysis, insertion of a double-lumen endotracheal tube or placement of a bronchial occluding balloon catheter helps to prevent contamination of the opposite lung by blood or infectious materials. Preventing blood from spilling into the contralateral lung allows ventilation to continue normally during and after pulmonary resection. Bronchoscopy must be performed immediately after every resection to remove all blood and clots from the remaining tracheobronchial tree.

Persistent Positive Sputum

Persistently positive sputum cultures after 6 months of documented chemotherapy is a relative indication for surgical resection. This regimen requires that two or more first-line drugs, including INH and RIF, be given and that the infective organisms be susceptible to these drugs. Destroyed lung with severe cavitation, bronchial stenosis, or bronchiectasis is usually present in these persistently sputum-positive patients (49). Occasionally, bronchial stenosis without positive sputum may develop as a late sequela of endobronchial TB. In this setting, sleeve resection (if anatomically feasible) or parenchymal resection is indicated.

Mass Lesions

A mass lesion that cannot be diagnosed by percutaneous needle biopsy or transbronchial biopsy, especially if it shows radiographic evidence of enlargement, should be resected because of the possibility of carcinoma. Often these indeterminant nodules prove to be tuberculomas, not carcinomas. Positron emission tomography, which often gives a positive result in active tuberculous lesions, may fail to differentiate these entities.

A radiographic change, especially enlargement of an old tuberculous scar, is worrisome because such a change often is due to development of a carcinoma. Biopsy or resection of these lesions is indicated.

Bronchopleural Fistula

A mixed tuberculous and pyogenic empyema may result from a bronchopleural fistula in tuberculous patients. If the underlying lung is incapable of reexpansion, lobectomy or extrapleural pneumonectomy may be required to cure this condition. Among the late sequelae of extrapleural plombage may be a bronchopleural fistula caused by erosion of the Lucite balls (50). Operation with removal of the foreign bodies and muscle flap is indicated.

Operative Management

Before thoracotomy, all patients must be evaluated to ensure that their cardiovascular, pulmonary, and nutritional status is adequate to withstand a major operative procedure. It is imperative to determine that the patient will be left with adequate pulmonary reserve to allow a reasonable lifestyle after pulmonary resection. Pulmonary function studies should be performed; if these are not obviously adequate, differential quantitative ventilation perfusion scanning should also be carried out. In general, the patient should be left with a postoperative forced expiratory volume in 1 second of at least 800 to 1,000 cm^3. If the patient will not be left with this minimal reserve, resectional surgery should be considered only if no alternative exists. At or before operation, the surgical team should perform bronchoscopy to determine that there is no endobronchial disease. Presence of endobronchial disease greatly increases the risk of bronchopleural fistula after resection. A double-lumen endobronchial tube should be used to prevent contamination of the contralateral lung and make the operative procedure easier by collapsing the operated lung.

The goal of surgery is to excise all gross disease. In some instances this can be achieved by means of a wedge resection with surgical staples, but in most instances a lobectomy or pneumonectomy is required. Sometimes the superior segment of the lower lobe is removed along with an upper lobe by means of a wedge or segmental resection. Bilateral staged procedures may be required. A pneumonectomy should be done only if the entire lung is involved or if the remaining portion of the lung will not adequately fill the pleural space. Lungs involved with TB are typically densely adherent to the pleura. Freeing the apex of the lung in the extrapleural plane is often much easier than trying to excise the lung intrapleurally. However, particular care must be exercised in freeing the lung above the first rib because the subclavian vessels and brachial plexus can easily be injured.

In recent years, the use of muscle-sparing thoracotomy has been considered for all patients undergoing resection. This permits use of muscle flaps to reinforce the bronchial closure and control leaks from lung parenchyma and to prevent space problems (51) (Fig. 43.6). At New York Univer-

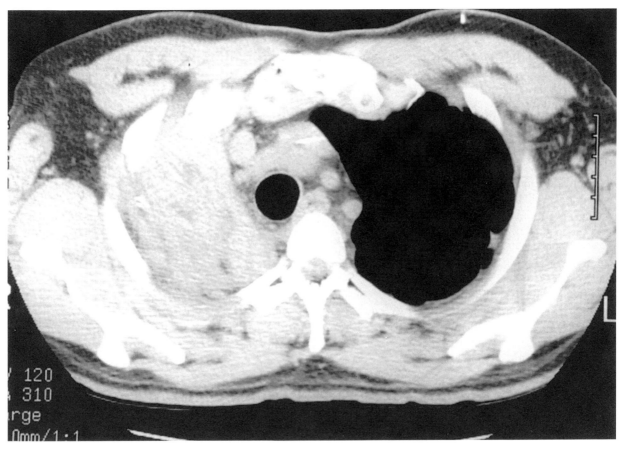

FIGURE 43.6. Latissimus dorsi and serratus anterior muscle flaps in the right upper pleural space.

sity Medical Center in the last 4 years, muscle flaps have been used with excellent results in 16 patients having resections for TB. Transposition of the latissimus and/or serratus muscles via a small chest wall defect with resection of a 3- to 4-cm portion of the second rib allows easy insertion toward the apex and obliteration of the potential apical space.

Patients with TB with chronic empyema and destroyed lungs frequently require extrapleural pneumonectomy to control the infection (52) (Fig. 43.7). The extrapleural pneumonectomy is carried out most easily through the bed of the resected fifth rib. The empyema pocket is separated from the chest wall in the extrapleural plane; every effort to stay out of the empyema pocket must be taken. The dissection at the apex of the chest above the first rib is often extremely difficult. In some instances, the pleura has to be left adherent to the subclavian vessels in this area. Dissection of the pleura from the diaphragm is also frequently difficult. Usually, on the mediastinal aspect of the lung, the adhesions are less dense and the dissection easier, but care

must be taken not to injure the underlying esophagus, as well as the phrenic and vagus nerves. A tube in the esophagus is helpful for identification and avoidance of that organ. The hilar structures can usually be handled in a standard fashion, although intrapericardial resection may occasionally be required.

Pleural Disease

A pure tuberculous effusion usually responds to antituberculous therapy. Because of the risk of secondary infection, chest tube drainage is contraindicated. A simple pneumothorax resulting from TB usually responds to insertion of a chest tube and antituberculous chemotherapy. Persistent air leak is uncommon but often can be reconciled with a VATS approach. A mixed tuberculous and pyogenic empyema is generally secondary to a bronchopleural fistula. Simple tube insertion and antituberculous therapy usually does not resolve a mixed empyema because of failure of the lung to expand. Decortication is required if the underlying

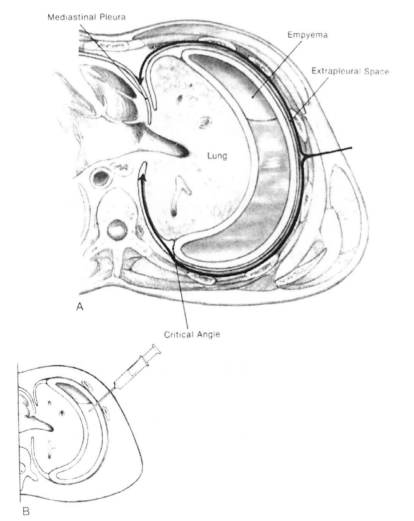

FIGURE 43.7. Principle of extrapleural pneumonectomy. **A:** Through a standard thoracotomy incision, the dissection is begun in the extrapleural plane and carried to the mediastinal level. Usually, although lightly fused, the pleura in this area is not involved in the empyema. Pulmonary vascular and bronchial dissection can be accomplished in a relatively normal fashion. **B:** Technique of aspirating the contents of the empyema to reduce its bulk and facilitate dissection. (From Hood RM. Pleural infections. In: Hood RM, et al., eds. *Surgical diseases of the pleura and chest wall.* Philadelphia: WB Saunders, 1986:126, with permission.)

lung can expand normally. Extrapleural pneumonectomy is required if the underlying lung is destroyed and cannot expand adequately. If the patient's general condition does not permit this extensive surgical procedure, open drainage of the pleural space by means of an Eloesser flap (53) may have to be accepted as definitive therapy (Fig. 43.8).

Results of Resectional Therapy

The availability of effective antituberculous drugs has made curative resectional therapy for TB possible and relatively safe. The risk of bronchopleural fistula after resection for TB is approximately 3%. Positive sputum at the time of operation and endobronchial disease increase the risk of a bronchopleural fistula. Historically, a residual apical space after pulmonary resection occurred in as much as 20% of patients and half of these developed an empyema or bronchopleural fistula (49). In recent years, particularly in drug-resistant patients, the use of muscle flaps to reinforce the bronchial stump, to control air leaks, and to fill the apical space appears to have reduced the risk of these complications (38).

The mortality rate of patients undergoing resectional surgery varies greatly. In patients having elective surgery and whose organisms are drug sensitive, the mortality rate approaches 0% (42). In patients with drug resistance, the mortality rate is approximately 3.3% (39). Those patients undergoing emergency resections for hemoptysis have a mortality rate of 15% or higher (43–45). Pneumonectomy for TB, especially extrapleural pneumonectomy, has a higher mortality rate than that for carcinoma. Morbidity rates are higher as well, with postpneumonectomy empyema, bleeding, and bronchopulmonary fistula being the most often reported (54). Despite this, the long-term outlook for patients who survive resectional surgery is excellent, approaching 95%, 5 years after surgery (49).

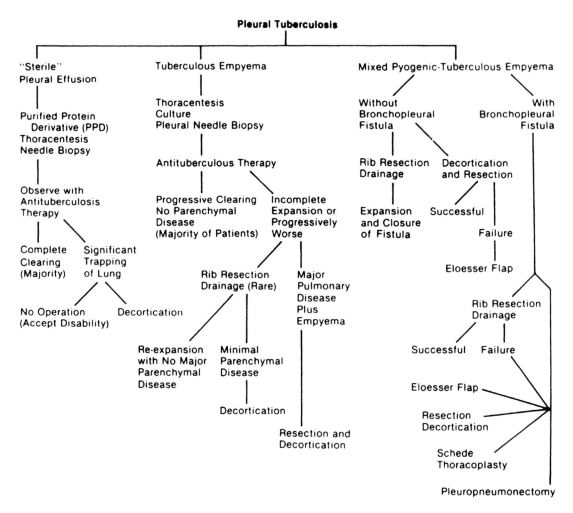

FIGURE 43.8. Algorithm for the management of pleural tuberculosis. (From Hood RM. Pleural infections. In: Hood RM, et al., eds. Surgical diseases of the pleura and chest wall. Philadelphia: WB Saunders, 1986:117, with permission.)

REFERENCES

1. Morse D, Brothwell DR, Ucko PJ, Tuberculosis in Ancient Egypt. *Am Rev Respir Dis* 1964; 90:524–541.
2. Morse D. Prehistoric tuberculosis in America. *Am Rev Tuberc* 1961;83:489–504.
3. Kraus AK. A Note on the practice of artificial pneumothorax by the Hippocratic school. *Am Rev Tuberc* 1922;6:327–330.
4. Dock W. Apical localization of phthisis: its significance in treatment by prolonged rest in bed. *Am Rev Tuberc* 1946;53:297–305.
5. Pratt JH. The Evolution of the rest treatment of pulmonary tuberculosis. *Am Rev Tuberc* 1944;50:185–201.
6. Carson J. *Essays, physiological and practical.* Liverpool: BF Wright, 1822.
7. Forlanini C. Zur Behandlung der Lungenschwind Sucht durch Kunstlich Erzeugten Pneumothorax. *Dtsch Med Wochenschr* 1906;32:1401–1406.
8. Murphy JB. Surgery of the lung. *JAMA* 1898;31:151, 165, 208–216, 281–297, 341–356.
9. Mitchell RS. Artificial pneumothorax: a statistical analysis of 557 cases initiated in 1930–1939 and followed in 1949. *Am Rev Tuberc* 1951;64:1–158.
10. Jacobaeus HC. Endopleurale Operationen unter der Leitung des Thorakoskops. *Beitr Kin Tuberk,* 1915;35:1–36.
11. Wright GW, Place R, Princi F. The physiological effects of pneumoperitoneum upon the respiratory apparatus. *Am Rev Tuberc* 1949;60:706–714.
12. Gaensler EA, Cugell DW. Bronchospirometry. V. Differential residual volume determination. *J Lab Clin Med* 1952;49:558–578.
13. Tuffier T. *Etat Actuel de la Chirurgie Intrathoracique.* Paris: Masson, 1914:90–105, 163–172.
14. Baer G. Uber Extrapleurale Pneumolyse mit Sofortiger Plombierung bei Lungentuberkulose. *Munch Med Wochenschr* 1913;60:1587–1590.
15. Gaensler EA. The surgery for pulmonary tuberculosis. *Am Rev Respir Dis* 1982;125:73–84.
16. Graf W. Ausblick auf neue Wege in der Chirurgischen Kollapstherapie der Lungentuberkulose. *Dtsch Med Wochenschr* 1937;63:4–7.
17. Advantages of surgical treatment of tuberculous cavities (editorial). *JAMA* 1950;142:905–906.
18. Lucas BGB, Cleland WP. Thoracoplasty with plombage: a review of the early results in 125 cases. *Thorax* 1950;5:248–256.
19. Woods FJ, Walker JH, Schmidt L. Extraperiosteal temporary plombage in thoracoplasty: a preliminary report. *Dis Chest* 1950;18:401–402.
20. Watson TR Jr, Gaensler EA. Immediate and late respiratory impairment due to selective staged thoracoplasty, extraperiosteal plombage and extrapleural conversion thoracoplasty. *Trans Natl Tuberc Assoc* 1952;48:288–304.
21. Schede M. Die Behandlung der Empyema. Verhandl *Cong Innere Med* 1890;9:41–141.
22. de Cerenville. De intervention operatoire dans les mal-adies du poumon. *Rev Med Suisse Rom,* 1885;5:441–467.
23. Brauer L. Erfahrungen und Uberlegungen zur Lungen Kollapstherapie. *Beitr Klin Tuberk* 1909;12:49–154.
24. Avery EE, Morch ET, Benson DW. Critically crushed chests: a new method of treatment by internal "pneumatic" stabilization with continuous mechanical hyperventilation. *J Thorac Surg* 1956;32:291–311.
25. Wilms M. Die Pfeilerresektion der Rippen zur Verengerung des Thorax bei Lungentuberkulose. *Therap Gegenw* 1913;54:17–24.
26. Alexander J. *The surgery of pulmonary tuberculosis.* Philadelphia: Lea & Febiger, 1925.
27. Boyd AD. Chevalier Jackson: the father of American bronchoesophagoscopy. *Ann Thorac Surg* 1994;57:502–505.
28. Alexander J. *The collapse therapy of pulmonary tuberculosis.* Springfield, IL: Charles C Thomas, 1937.
29. Weinstein L. Antimicrobial agents. Drugs used in the chemotherapy of tuberculosis and leprosy. In: Goodman LS, Gillman A, eds. *Pharmacological basis of therapeutics*, 5th ed. New York: Macmillan, 1975.
30. Jones JC. Early experience with resection in pulmonary tuberculosis in the surgical management of pulmonary tuberculosis. In: Steele JD, ed. *The surgical management of pulmonary tuberculosis.* Springfield, IL: Charles C Thomas, 1957.
31. Tuffier M. *Chirurgie de Poumon, en Particulier dans les Cavernes Tuberculeuses et la Gangrene Pulmonaire.* Paris: Masson, 1897.
32. Beye HL. Discussion of SO Freedlander, lobectomy in tuberculosis: report of a case. *J Thorac Surg* 1935;5:18–26.
33. Lindskog GE. Total pneumonectomy in pulmonary tuberculosis: report of a case. *J Thorac Surg* 1937;7:102–106.
34. Reinhoff WF Jr. Pneumonectomy: a preliminary report of the operative technique in two successful cases. *Bull Johns Hopkins Hosp* 1933;53:390–393.
35. Blades B, Kent EM. Individual ligation technique for lower lobe lobectomy. *J Thorac Surg* 1940;10:84–101.
36. Churchill ED, Klopstock R. Lobectomy for pulmonary tuberculosis. *Ann Surg* 1943;117:641–669.
37. Goble M, Hersburg CR, Waite D, et al. Treatment of isoniazid and rifampin resistant tuberculosis. *Am Rev Respir Dis* 1988;4(Suppl):24.
38. Pomerantz M, Madsen L, Goble M, et al. Surgical management of resistant mycobacterial tuberculosis and other mycobacterial pulmonary infections. *Ann Thorac Surg* 1991;52:1108–1112.
39. Pomerantz BJ, Cleveland JC Jr, Olson HK, et al. Pulmonary resection for multi-drug resistant tuberculosis. *J Thorac Cardiovasc Surg* 2001;121:448–453.
40. Iseman MD, Corpe RF, O'Brien RF, et al. Disease due to *Mycobacterium avium-intracellulare.* *Chest* 1985;87(Suppl):1395–1495.
41. Corpe RF. Surgical management of pulmonary disease due to *Mycobacterium avium-intercellulare.* *Rev Infect Dis* 1981;3:1064.
42. Moran JF, Alexander LG, Staub EW, et al. Long-term results of pulmonary resection for atypical mycobacterial disease. *Ann Thorac Surg* 1983;35:597–604.
43. Conlan AA, Hurwitz SS, Krige L, et al. Massive hemoptysis. *J Thorac Cardiovasc Surg* 1983;85:120–124.
44. Corey R, Hla KM. Major and massive hemoptysis: reassessment of conservative management. *Am J Med Sci* 1987;249:301–309.
45. Garzon AA, Cerruti MM, Goldring ME. Exsanguinat-ing hemoptysis. *J Thorac Cardiovas Surg* 1982;84:829–833.
46. Eckstein MR, Waltman AC, Athanasoulis CA. The management of massive hemoptysis: control by angiographic methods. In: Kittle CF, ed. *Current controversies in thoracic surgery.* Philadelphia: WB Saunders, 1986:255–260.
47. Yu-Tang Goh P, Lin M, Teo N, et al. Embolization for hemoptysis: a six year review. *Cardiovasc Intervent Radiol* 2002;25:17–25.
48. Battaglini JW, Murray GF, Keagy BA, et al. Surgical management of symptomatic pulmonary aspergilloma. *Ann Thorac Surg* 1985;39:512–516.
49. Moran JF. Surgical treatment of pulmonary tuberculosis. In:

Spencer FC, Sabiston D, eds. *Surgery of the chest*, 5th ed. Philadelphia: WB Saunders, 1990.

50. Weissberg D. Weissberg D. Late Complications of collapse therapy for pulmonary tuberculosis. *Chest* 2001;120:847–851.

51. Pairolero PC, Arnold PG, Piehler JM. Intrathoracic transposition of extrathoracic skeletal muscle. *J Thorac Cardiovasc Surg* 1983; 86:809–817.

52. Hood RM. Pleural infections. In: Hood RM, et al, *Surgical diseases of the pleura and chest wall.* Philadelphia: WB Saunders, 1986.

53. Eloesser L. Of an operation for tuberculous empyema. *Ann Thorac Surg* 1969;8:355–357.

54. Blyth DF. Pneumonectomy for inflammatory lung disease. *Eur J Cardiothorac Surg* 2000;18:429–434.

44

NONTUBERCULOUS MYCOBACTERIAL INFECTIONS IN THE HUMAN IMMUNODEFICIENCY VIRUS–NEGATIVE HOST

RICHARD J. WALLACE, JR.

Although not as important worldwide as tuberculosis, diseases due to mycobacteria other than *Mycobacterium tuberculosis* are almost certainly more common than tuberculosis in the United States. However, such has not always been the case. The recognition of the organisms as pathogens is relatively recent, with series of patients with chronic pulmonary disease not being reported in the literature until the mid-1950s (1–3). Recognition that these organisms, known initially as the *yellow bacillus* (*Mycobacterium kansasii*), the *Battey bacillus* (*Mycobacterium avium* complex, after the Battey Sanatorium in Georgia where it was first recognized), or collectively as *anonymous* mycobacteria (4), were true pathogens took significant time. Early scientists and clinicians such as Ernest Runyon (the Runyon classification system) (3), William Shaffer (serotyping of *Mycobacterium avium-intracellulare-scrofulaceum*), John Chapman, Emanuel Wolinsky (the major treatise on these organisms as pathogens) (4), and Chai Ahn (diagnostic criteria and drug trials) (5) were major participants in the effort to bring deserved recognition to these organisms.

Currently categorized as the nontuberculous mycobacteria (NTM), this group of organisms shares a number of features. Unlike *M. tuberculosis*, these organisms are normal inhabitants of the environment. Also unlike tuberculosis, pulmonary disease and other infections due to the NTM are not contagious so patients with diseases are not generally isolated. Because these organisms frequent the environment, infections of the skin and soft tissue following local trauma occur much more frequently. Many clinicians consider these organisms as opportunists rather than virulent pathogens, as some local or systemic immune impairment is

required for them to cause disease. As with *M. tuberculosis*, little is known of virulence genes or specific cellular products that result in tissue invasion and subsequent disease. No known toxins are produced by these species with the exception of *M. ulcerans*. This lack of knowledge reflects the limited research and general lack of knowledge about the pathogenesis of mycobacterial infections, including leprosy and tuberculosis.

The earliest classification of the NTM focused on laboratory features of these organisms, especially their growth rate and pigment production (Runyon classification system) (3). With greater knowledge of these organisms and the disease they produce, most current evaluation of the NTM focuses on the clinical rather than the laboratory aspect of the organisms (Table 44.1). This presentation is no different. After a brief discussion of disease epidemiology and the laboratory, the remaining discussion focuses on the major diseases produced by these organisms: chronic pulmonary disease, cutaneous infections, lymphadenitis, and disseminated infections (Table 44.2).

EPIDEMIOLOGY

The general environmental reservoirs of the common NTM pathogens, especially *M. avium* complex, have been studied in detail. *M. avium* complex is readily recovered from natural water supplies, especially those along the coastline that have a partial mixture of saltwater (estuaries) (6,7). This organism also has been recovered from tap water, including hospital water supplies (8), and from soil (9). *M. avium* is a recognized pathogen of animals and birds, although these strains appear genetically distinct form strains causing human disease. Skin testing with an antigen preparation derived from *Mycobacterium intracellulare* (the Battey antigen) was performed on more than 250,000 naval recruits

R. J. Wallace, Jr.: Department of Microbiology, The University of Texas Health Center at Tyler, Tyler, Texas.

TABLE 44.1. SPECIES OF NONTUBERCULOUS MYCOBACTERIA ENCOUNTERED IN CLINICAL DISEASE SETTINGS

Common Pathogens	Rare Pathogens
M. avium-intracellulare	M. immunogenum
M. kansasii	M. asiaticum
M. marinum	M. mageritense
M. fortuitum	M. simiae
M. chelonae	M. nonchromogenicum
M. abscessus	M. smegmatis group
M. ulcerans[a]	M. peregrinum
M. malmoense[a]	M. mucogenicum
M. xenopi[a]	M. fortuitum third biovariant complex
	M. szulgai
	M. haemophilum
	M. lentiflavum
	M. triplex
	M. genavense

Probable Nonpathogens[b]
Pigmented rapidly growing mycobacteria
M. terrae complex
M. gordonae
M. scrofulaceum

[a]These species are rare in the United States but are common pathogens in other areas of the world.
[b]Under unique circumstances these species can probably cause disease as well.

who had spent their entire lives in a single county, and the results were reported as a map of skin test reactivity over the entire United States (Fig. 44.1) (10). This map showed skin test reactivity to be greatest in the southeastern region of the United States, the area that has generally reported the largest number of cases of chronic pulmonary disease (4).

M. kansasii has been much more difficult to recover from natural water supplies. Piped water systems are considered the major reservoir for this species, with disease focused in major urban areas in the United States, Europe, and Japan. Five genotypes of *M. kansasii* are recognized, with type I organisms responsible for more than 90% of disease worldwide (11). In the United States, *M. kansasii* is concentrated in the midwest; thus, its name is a fair reflection of the major areas of disease (4).

TABLE 44.2. COMMON CLINICAL DISORDERS DUE TO NONTUBERCULOUS MYCOBACTERIA IN THE HUMAN IMMUNODEFICIENCY VIRUS–NEGATIVE HOST

Chronic pulmonary disease
Cutaneous disease
Lymphadenitis (cervical)
Disseminated disease (cutaneous, systemic)

Rapidly growing species are also readily recovered from soil and natural water (4,9), and these presumably serve as the major source of community-acquired human infections. These species, especially *Mycobacterium fortuitum*, *Mycobacterium mucogenicum*, and *Mycobacterium abscessus*, have been recovered from injection solutions (12), distilled water, hospital tap water (13,14), or ice prepared from hospital tap water (13,15), where it served as a source of health care–associated (nosocomial) disease or contamination (12–18). Contaminated automated bronchoscope washing machines seem especially prone to pseudo-outbreaks with the *M. abscessus*-like species *M. immunogenum* (17). Rapidly growing mycobacteria are relatively resistant to chlorine and glutaraldehyde and survive well in distilled water; these features probably contribute to their presence in these health care–associated settings. DNA fingerprinting studies have shown identity between the environmental isolates and those causing disease (13–15,18–21). Disease rates due to rapidly growing mycobacteria are highest in the southeastern region of the United States, although disease has been reported from almost all areas (4).

Some epidemiologic information is available on NTM other than *M. avium* complex, *M. kansasii*, and the rapidly growing mycobacteria, but these organisms have been studied in much less detail. *Mycobacterium xenopi* grows optimally at higher temperatures than do most mycobacteria (42°C), and piped hot water systems are considered its major reservoir. Occasionally, pseudo-outbreaks have been reported as a result of contamination of hospital hot water systems with *M. xenopi* (22,23).

Disease due to *Mycobacterium simiae* in the United States has been concentrated in a few geographic areas, primarily central Texas (San Antonio) (24) and areas of Arizona and New Mexico (25). As with the prior two species, similar or identical organisms were identified by molecular techniques in the municipal or hospital water supply, suggesting that water is the major reservoir (4,26,27).

Mycobacterium marinum is usually associated with freshwater and saltwater, and has been recovered on a number of occasions from unchlorinated swimming pools or hot springs, tropical fish, or fish tank water that was the apparent source of human disease (4). Other NTM species recently identified within natural water supplies include *M. malmoense* and *M. ulcerans*, whereas *Mycobacterium genavense* has been found in psittacine birds. Some fastidious pathogens, such as *Mycobacterium haemophilum* and *M. genavense*, have never been recovered from the environment. The development of DNA amplification systems such as the polymerase chain reaction (PCR) may allow for much better detection of these organisms in the future, when they exist in complex biologic systems and are difficult if not impossible to grow in isolation. Such investigations have been performed with the fastidious species *Mycobacterium ulcerans* (28).

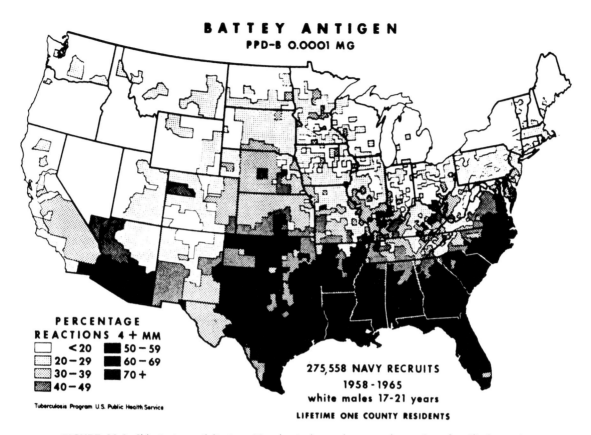

BATTEY ANTIGEN
PPD-B 0.0001 MG

PERCENTAGE
REACTIONS 4 + MM
<20   50 − 59
20 − 29   60 − 69
30 − 39   70 +
40 − 49

Tuberculosis Program U.S. Public Health Service

275,558 NAVY RECRUITS
1958 - 1965
white males 17-21 years
LIFETIME ONE COUNTY RESIDENTS

FIGURE 44.1. Skin test reactivity to a *Mycobacterium avium* complex antigen [purified protein derivative type B (*PPD-B*)] of naval recruits who were lifetime residents of a single county. (From Edwards LB, et al. An atlas of sensitivity to tuberculin, PPD-B, and histoplasmin in the United States. *Am Rev Respir Dis* 1969;99:1–132, with permission.)

LABORATORY FEATURES

Details about the laboratory features of the NTM are given elsewhere. However, some features of the NTM deserve mention. In general, the acid-fast staining and culture techniques adopted for *M. tuberculosis* work satisfactorily for the NTM (4). These organisms are more likely to be missed with fluorochrome staining than is *M. tuberculosis*. For *M. avium* complex, this usually relates to the small coccobacillary form of the organism that is readily missed. On acid-fast bacillus (AFB) smears, some species, especially *M. kansasii*, appear as large, long-beaded organisms that make the presence of NTM highly likely. The NTM are more susceptible to the sodium hydroxide decontamination procedures, especially the rapidly growing species. In general, the common pathogenic species of NTM grow well on egg-based (Löwenstein-Jensen) and agar-based (Middlebrook 7H10) solid media, and in broth culture systems. As with *M. tuberculosis*, culturing should include both broth and solid media.

Several organisms require special attention to be grown. *M. marinum* grows only at 28°C to 30°C on primary isolation, and *M. chelonae*, *M. abscessus*, and *M. haemophilum* all

generally grow better at this temperature. For this reason, all skin cultures (or when these species are the expected pathogens) should be incubated at these low temperatures. *M. haemophilum* requires the addition of a hemin disk (or its equivalent) to the surface of the agar isolation plate, and *Mycobacterium genavense* must be incubated in broth culture bottles for a minimum of 6 weeks.

Growth rates and the presence or absence of pigmentation continue to provide useful early information, but the classic Runyon classification method is no longer used. With approximately 90 species of NTM and the desire for more rapid identification than the Runyon method allows, commonly encountered NTM are now generally identified directly to species or complex (Table 44.1) by the use of more rapid techniques, such as DNA probe or high-performance liquid chromatography. Susceptibility testing is performed on selected drugs for NTM utilizing standards published by the NCCLS (National Committee for Clinical Laboratory Standards) in 2000 (29). Currently, *M. kansasii* is routinely tested only against rifampin, and *M. avium* complex only against a newer macrolide (usually clarithromycin), whereas rapidly growing mycobacteria are generally tested against multiple drugs.

Fingerprinting of the NTM in outbreak or pseudo-outbreak situations can be performed by a number of techniques. Pulsed-field gel electrophoresis is most commonly utilized, followed by arbitrarily primed PCR and hybridization with a repetitive insertional element (19–21,30,31).

LYMPHADENITIS

The most common form of NTM lymphadenitis is childhood cervical lymphadenitis. This disease typically occurs in previously healthy children between 1 and 5 years of age (32). The disease is localized to one side of the face and neck, and most often involves the submandibular and preauricular lymph nodes. Mediastinal or hilar nodes may be involved. Parotid gland enlargement occasionally occurs due to involvement of intraparotid lymph nodes (33). A unilateral mass with or without associated overlying erythematous skin changes is the usual presentation. With time, the lymph nodes undergo suppuration and drain. Systemic symptoms are usually absent, and the chest radiograph appears normal. The most commonly recovered organism from the involved lymph nodes is currently *M. avium* complex (85%) (32–35). Some lymph nodes are AFB smear positive but culture negative (as many as 50% in older series). In some recent studies, poorly growing organisms such as *M. haemophilum* and *M. genavense* have been recovered, while other studies have shown *M. avium* DNA by PCR despite the negative cultures. Another one third of affected patients have a typical presentation, consisting of caseating granulomas on histology, but negative AFB smears and cultures (32). The disease pathogenesis is unknown, but the location and clinical setting suggest regional lymphadenitis from an occult intraoral inoculation (33).

The diagnosis of the disease is based on a high index of suspicion, sometimes a weakly reactive (<10 mm) or strongly reactive (≥15 mm) response to purified protein derivative (PPD), and culture and histopathologic examination of the lymph node. The major (preoperative) differential diagnosis includes tuberculosis, cat scratch disease, cutaneous nocardiosis, tularemia, and, rarely, malignant disease of the nodes. The excised lymph nodes usually show caseating granulomas indistinguishable from tuberculosis, with about 20% of patients also showing some combination of acute inflammation ("dimorphic inflammatory response") (36).

The treatment for the disease is excision of the major involved nodes, which is curative in more than 90% of patients (32,37). Involved areas of the skin and fistulous tract are also excised. Incision and drainage is a poor treatment, usually being followed by chronic fistulas and sinus tract formation (32,37). Treatment with standard tuberculosis drugs has not been useful. Clarithromycin, in combination with ethambutol or rifabutin, should be considered for patients with minor disease or when recurrence of disease follows surgery. This recommendation is based on the success of clarithromycin drug combinations in the management of pulmonary or disseminated *M. avium-intracellulare* complex disease (38,39) and uncontrolled reports of success when treating lymph node disease, as use of these drugs in cervical lymphadenitis has been limited (40). However, the large, sometimes fluctuant character of the lymph nodes makes surgical excision important, even with highly active drugs such as the newer macrolides.

Infrequently, other forms of NTM lymphadenitis involve either peripheral or central lymph nodes. Such disease can involve the rapidly growing mycobacteria (*M. chelonae* and *M. abscessus*) (41), *M. avium* complex, *M. haemophilum*, *M. marinum* (42), or, rarely, other species (4).

CUTANEOUS DISEASE

The best-known disease other than chronic lung disease caused by the NTM is skin or soft-tissue disease. The major players are *M. marinum*; the rapidly growing species *M. fortuitum* and *M. abscessus,* and *M. ulcerans*.

Infection due to *M. marinum* usually follows accidental trauma of the hand or fingers, followed by placement of the hand in a fish tank or aquarium that is contaminated with *M. marinum* ("fish tank granuloma"). More than 90% of cases involve the hands, and approximately 80% relate to fish tanks (43). Disease may also follow trauma in freshwater or saltwater settings, especially in southeastern United States (4,23,42). Hence, the key to diagnosis of this pathogen is a good history. The disease usually presents as a chronic localized superficial papule, nodule, cellulitis, or pyoderma following accidental trauma in or around saltwater or a fish tank. Occasionally proximal nodular lesions that mimic sporotrichosis develop. Tenosynovitis is also a common presentation. Osteomyelitis and septic arthritis also occur but much less frequently. The disease remains localized and the patient is usually asymptomatic. Diagnosis is based on a history of water exposure and a biopsy specimen that grows the organism. The key to recovery of the organism is to remember that primary isolation of *M. marinum* requires incubation at 28°C to 30°C. There is no drug treatment of choice for *M. marinum* infection. Commonly used regimens include minocycline or doxycycline, trimethoprim–sulfamethoxazole, rifampin plus ethambutol, or, more recently, clarithromycin given for a minimum of 3 months (Table 44.3) (43,44). Routine susceptibility testing of this species is not required because all isolates have comparable drug susceptibilities (29). Surgical débridement may be required in about 10% of patients (4, 23,43).

Skin and soft-tissue disease is also the most common disease presentation of the rapidly growing mycobacteria. The development of local pain, swelling, and drainage 4 to 8 weeks following accidental trauma with potential wound

TABLE 44.3. DRUGS USED FOR THE MANAGEMENT OF NONTUBERCULOUS MYCOBACTERIA

Slowly growing species	**M. marinum**
Clarithromycin or azithromycin	Doxycycline (minocycline)
Rifampin or rifabutin	Trimethoprim–sulfamethoxazole
Ethambutol	Clarithromycin
Streptomycin	Rifampin
Amikacin	Ethambutol
Rapidly growing species	
Clarithromycin or azithromycin	
Amikacin	
Cefoxitin	
Imipenem	
Doxycycline (minocycline)	
Sulfamethoxazole or trimethoprim–sulfamethoxazole	
Ciprofloxacin, levofloxacin, newer quinolones	
Tobramycin (*M. chelonae* only)	
Linezolid	

contamination with little or no systemic symptoms is the classic presentation. Typical community-acquired injuries include stepping on a nail, other metal puncture wounds, or motor vehicle accidents (41,45). Cellulitis with serous drainage is the usual presentation, although abscess formation, synovitis or arthritis, and osteomyelitis can also occur. Most patients are otherwise healthy. Both adults and children are affected, with the extremities (hands or feet or legs) being the usual site of infection (41,45). Patients are usually afebrile, with a normal white blood cell count, and are otherwise not ill. Diagnosis is usually readily made by culture of drainage or a biopsy specimen. *M. fortuitum* and *M. abscessus* are the usual pathogens (41), followed by *M. fortuitum* third-biovariant complex (45), *M. chelonae* (46), and the *Mycobacterium smegmatis* group (47).

Health care–associated surgical or catheter-related infections due to the rapidly growing mycobacteria are also recognized. Mycobacterial surgical infections first came to medical attention in 1976 with the report of an outbreak of *M. abscessus* sternal wound infections following cardiac surgery in North Carolina. Subsequently, outbreaks of sternal wound infections were reported in three other states as well as Hungary (13,48). Most outbreaks involved *M. fortuitum* or *M. abscessus*, and in one outbreak in Texas the same organisms were recovered from the incoming municipal water supply as well as from tap water and ice used in the hospital operating room (13,19,20,48), suggesting tap water and hospital ice machines as the likely reservoir for the mycobacteria. Sporadic sternal wound disease also occurs in similar geographic areas as the epidemic disease.

Surgical wound infections following augmentation mammaplasty are also recognized, with patients concentrated in North Carolina, Florida, and Texas (49,50). These patients usually present with serous, watery drainage and breakdown of the surgical incision site 4 to 8 weeks following surgery. Almost 90% of cases are due to *M. fortuitum* and, interestingly, are usually unilateral (49,50).

Currently, the major health care–associated disease of the rapidly growing mycobacteria is catheter-related sepsis (41,51). This disease initially came to medical attention in patients receiving hemodialysis or automated peritoneal dialysis where processed tap water contaminated with mycobacteria was being used. *M. fortuitum*, *M. chelonae*, *M. abscessus* (41,46,51), and *M. mucogenicum* are the usual pathogens. Other health care–associated cutaneous infections can occur in sporadic or outbreak form, and these include surgical wound infections following other surgical or cosmetic procedures (41), postinjection abscesses (12,16), and middle ear infections following the use of chronic drainage tubes (53). Recent sporadic and outbreak disease has been associated with injections of alternative medicines (12,16), liposuction (14), and the use of footbaths (18). Where studied and identified, contaminated tap water or fluids for medical use have been the identified source of infection. No chronic human carrier or contaminated dust samples have been identified. The use of DNA fingerprinting using pulsed-field gel electrophoresis (20,21) or random amplified polymorphic DNA (RAPID) PCR (19) have provided evidence or proof of definite clonal relationships between environmental and disease-producing strains in many of these outbreaks (13,14,18–21).

Drug susceptibility patterns of the three common pathogenic species of rapidly growing mycobacteria are unique among the slowly growing NTM in their resistance to primary antituberculous agents juxtaposed to their susceptibility to a variety of traditional antibacterial agents (Table 44.3) (45–47,51,54–58). This *in vitro* susceptibility applies to such agents as amikacin (54), cefoxitin (54,57), imipenem (57), doxycycline (minocycline) (54), sulfamethoxazole (54), the newer quinolones (56), and clarithromycin (55). The species vary remarkably in their susceptibility to these agents, with *M. fortuitum* being the most drug susceptible of the common pathogenic species. Oral agents useful for *M. fortuitum* include doxycycline (40% of isolates), clarithromycin (80%), sulfamethoxazole (95%), and the newer quinolones (100%). In contrast, the only oral agent to which untreated isolates of *M. chelonae* and *M. abscessus* are uniformly susceptible is clarithromycin (and presumably azithromycin) (46,55). Recent studies have suggested that linezolid and the 8-methoxyquinolones (gatifloxacin and moxifloxacin) are active against most isolates of *M. chelonae* and some isolates of *M. abscessus* (58). Therapy based on *in vitro* susceptibilities, though not done in a randomized, controlled trial format, has demonstrated the usefulness of those drugs not only for *M. fortuitum*, *M. abscessus*, and *M. chelonae* (56,59,60) but also for other rapidly growing species, such as the *M. smegmatis* group (47), *M. fortuitum* third-biovariant complex (45), and *M. mucogenicum* (52). Determination of drug susceptibilities is essential, as susceptibilities to most of the mentioned agents are variable both between taxonomic groups and (in the case of the tetracyclines) within the same species or subgroup.

M. ulcerans is endemic in tropical areas such as the rural western coast of Africa (61), where the ulcerated skin lesion is referred to as Buruli ulcer, and Australia, where it is called Bairnsdale ulcer (62). It is nonendemic in the United States but very common in these tropical areas. The organism produces nodular skin lesions, which, if not treated, lead to slowly enlarging skin ulcers. These lesions can result in severe functional loss of an extremity (62). Early lesions may respond to antimicrobials (63), but large ulcerated lesions require surgical excision and skin grafting (61–63).

Rarely, species of NTM other than *M. marinum*, *M. ulcerans*, or rapidly growing species are associated with skin or soft-tissue disease. Localized disease due to *M. kansasii*, *M. avium-intracellulare*, or *Mycobacterium nonchromogenicum* (*Mycobacterium terrae* complex) is well described (4,64). This disease can involve the skin or the skeletal system, including tendon sheaths (tenosynovitis is the typical disease for *M. nonchromogenicum*), joints, bones, and bursae (4,33,64). Most patients are normal hosts, and localized disease develops following penetrating trauma to an extremity. Surgical biopsy is almost always required to make a diagnosis. Given the known presence of most of these organisms in the environment, the existence of such disease is not surprising.

DISSEMINATED DISEASE

In the HIV-negative patient, disseminated disease due to NTM is relatively rare (4,64). Most patients are immunosuppressed. Two types of disease are seen. Disseminated cutaneous disease involves the skin and adjacent soft tissues almost exclusively; it rarely involves bone. Involvement of the lung, bone marrow, blood, liver, spleen, and visceral lymph nodes is rare. The major pathogens in this syndrome are the rapidly growing species *M. chelonae* (46) and, more rarely *M. abscessus* (65), *M. marinum* (4,66), and *M. haemophilum* (23,33,64).

Disseminated cutaneous disease due to *M. chelonae* presents as multiple peripheral subcutaneous nodules that eventually drain. The number of lesions ranges from four or five to innumerable, almost confluent masses. The lesions are concentrated on the extensor surfaces of the legs but can occur on the extensor surfaces of the forearm and rarely elsewhere. The patients are almost always taking low-dose corticosteroids (90%), with the most common underlying conditions being rheumatoid arthritis, organ transplantation, and miscellaneous autoimmune disorders (46). Symptoms of disseminated cutaneous disease with *M. chelonae* are usually minimal. The disease is easily diagnosed by evaluation of drainage or biopsy material by AFB stain and culture. The treatment of choice is clarithromycin 500 mg twice a day for 6 months (60), with a course of imipenem, linezolid, or tobramycin given initially (2 to 6 weeks) to reduce the risk of clarithromycin resistance. Approximately 25% of strains are also susceptible to doxycycline and up to 90% to the 8-methoxyquinolone gatifloxacin, which may replace the injectable imipenem or aminoglycoside in initial combination treatment (46,54).

Disseminated cutaneous disease due to *M. marinum* or *M. haemophilum* is most commonly encountered in HIV-positive patients, usually those who are severely immune suppressed. It less commonly occurs in HIV-negative hosts with other types of immune suppression. In both, the disease presents as chronic skin lesions with few systemic symptoms and is readily diagnosed if the appropriate culture conditions are used.

The other type of disseminated NTM disease is disseminated systemic disease, which usually involves the lungs, liver, spleen, and bone marrow, and only infrequently involves the skin and then usually as no more than one or two lesions. Typical pathogens in this group are *M. kansasii* and, rarely, *M. avium* complex (64). One organism that produces a combination of both syndromes is the rapidly growing *M. abscessus*. This organism typically causes disease in patients with leukemia or lymphoma, and patients have multiple skin lesions as well as positive cultures of blood, bone marrow, and occasionally other deep tissues (65).

PULMONARY DISEASE

The best-recognized clinical disease attributable to NTM is chronic pulmonary disease. The major pathogens causing this disease, which are discussed in some detail, are *M. avium-intracellulare*, *M. kansasii*, and *M. abscessus* (4,33,64).

Mycobacterium avium-intracellulare

The most frequently encountered NTM lung disease is due to *M. avium-intracellulare* complex. Current studies suggest that approximately 80% of cases can be attributed to *M. intracellulare*. From an epidemiologic standpoint, three major syndromes or clinical presentations are seen. The best known, which represents about 40% to 50% of clinical cases, is upper lobe cavitary lung disease that radiographically and clinically mimics reactivation tuberculosis. These patients are predominantly male alcoholics and/or smokers with coexistent chronic obstructive pulmonary disease. The patients are generally older than 50 years, white, and present with cough, weight loss, and hemoptysis. Upper lobe cavitary lung disease was the first type of lung disease due to *M. avium-intracellulare* to be described and represents the predominant type reported in case summaries through the early 1980s (67,68).

The second group of patients with *M. avium-intracellulare* infection, which also represents about 40% to 50% of clinical cases, comprise those with no underlying disease other than bronchiectasis. Prince et al. (69) first drew attention to recent increases in *M. avium-intracellulare* disease and the importance of this patient group. These patients are predominantly white (95%), women (80%), are nonsmokers, and have interstitial rather than cavitary radiographic changes. The disease is often focused in the lingula and right middle lobes, a feature referred to as *Lady Windermere's syndrome* (70). Prince et al. (69) noted the potentially serious nature of this disease, as four (19%) of 21 patients died of respiratory failure during the study follow-up. This is a significant finding, as this type of disease was often referred to as airway *colonization* in the past, with the real disease considered to be bronchiectasis (71). Utilizing high-resolution computed tomography, Williams et al. (72,73) defined the radiographic features of this form of *M. avium-intracellulare* lung disease. The lungs typically show nodular disease and cylindrical bronchiectasis, often in the same lung segment. Hence, this form of disease is usually referred to as nodular bronchiectatic disease. Clinical disease can also be seen in association with other types of bronchiectasis in patients with previous viral, bacterial, or tuberculosis-related damage, and patients with cystic fibrosis (CF) (Table 44.4). The latter group is one of the most recently

recognized groups with *M. avium-intracellulare* disease. Studies of young adults with CF showed that 10% to 20% of individuals in many areas of the country will have positive mycobacterial sputum cultures, primarily *M. avium-intracellulare* (74). The disease may be hard to separate from exacerbators of the underlying CF. Fever refractory to antibiotic therapy is a major sign of progressive disease.

A third form of disease, only recognized in the past few years, is a diffuse manifestation with a ground-glass appearance that mimics hypersensitivity pneumonitis (75–77). Patients present with fever, cough, shortness of breath, and hypoxia, and have no underlying disease, including bronchiectasis. All have used a hot tub, and the disease is referred to as hot-tub lung (77). Presumably this is a diffuse disease related to inhalation of heavily contaminated water from the hot tub. It appears to represent both infection (since the organism can be seen and grown from lung tissue) and a hypersensitivity reaction.

Therapy for *M. avium-intracellulare* lung disease, until the introduction of the macrolides, was only partially effective (67,68,78). The newer macrolides, with initial studies focusing on clarithromycin, are highly active in the management of *M. avium-intracellulare* (38,39) and appear more active as monotherapy than multidrug regimens without a macrolide. A study by Wallace et al. (39) showed that initial clarithromycin monotherapy at 500 mg twice a day for 4 months resulted in sputum conversion in approximately 60% of HIV-negative patients with chronic lung disease. A similar study with azithromycin showed a lower sputum conversion rate after 4 months of initial monotherapy but comparable conversion rates at 6 months after the addition of other drugs (74% with clarithromycin, 58% with azithromycin) (79).

Although administered as part of these initial trials, clarithromycin or azithromycin for *M. avium-intracellulare* lung disease should *never* be given as monotherapy because of the risk of mutational resistance. They should be given in combination with ethambutol and a rifamycin (rifampin or rifabutin). The current preferred treatment regimen for patients with the first two types of lung disease who weigh at least 50 kg and have normal renal function (recommended by the American Thoracic Society) (64) is clarithromycin 500 mg in the morning and evening or 1,000 mg single dose, rifampin 600 mg, and ethambutol 25 mg/kg given three times weekly (Monday–Wednesday–Friday). Azithromycin 500 mg three times weekly with the same doses of ethambutol and rifampin is a reasonable alternative, although it appears less active than clarithromycin. Streptomycin should be considered for patients with extensive disease, especially cavitary disease, or for those who fail initial three-drug therapy. Streptomycin should be given for the first 2–4 months. The dose and dosing interval depends on the patient's age, weight, and renal function (Table 44.5). An effective drug regimen for clarithromycin-resistant isolates has not been established. Toxicity screens should be done to watch for liver

TABLE 44.4. ASSOCIATED UNDERLYING DISEASES OR RISK FACTORS IN HUMAN IMMUNODEFICIENCY VIRUS–NEGATIVE PATIENTS WITH CHRONIC LUNG DISEASE DUE TO NONTUBERCULOUS MYCOBACTERIA

Preexisting bronchiectasis due to
  Idiopathic factor(s) (most cases)
  Prior *M. tuberculosis* infection
  Previous bacterial or viral infections
  Cystic fibrosis
Pneumoconiosis (especially silicosis and coal miner's disease)
Cigarette abuse, usually with chronic lung disease
Alcohol abuse
Achalasia (rapidly growing species)
Lipoid pneumonia (rapidly growing species)
Hot-tub use (*M. avium-intracellulare*)

TABLE 44.5. CURRENT TREATMENT RECOMMENDATION FOR NONTUBERCULOUS MYCOBACTERIAL LUNG DISEASE IN HUMAN IMMUNODEFICIENCY VIRUS–NEGATIVE PATIENTS

Organism	Drug Doses	Frequency	Duration	Surgery
M. avium complex	Clarithromycin 500 mg b.i.d. *or* azithromycin 500 mg	t.i.w.	Until culture negative for 1 yr based on monthly sputum cultures	Consider resection for localized disease if isolate becomes macrolide resistant
	Ethambutol 25 mg/kg	t.i.w.		
	Rifampin 600 mg	t.i.w.		
	All three drugs given t.i.w. (Monday–Wednesday–Friday)			
	± Streptomycin (dosing based on age, body weight, renal function) considered for severe/advanced disease	t.i.w.	First 2–4 mo	
M. kansasii	Isoniazid 300 mg	Daily	18–24 mo (culture negative at least 1 yr)	Not routinely indicated
	Rifampin 600 mg	Daily		
	Ethambutol 15 mg	Daily		
M. abscessus	Clarithromycin 500 mg b.i.d.	Daily	2–6 wk for symptomatic or progressive disease (suppressive therapy)	Consider resection for localized disease
	Amikacin (once daily, peaks of approximately 20 µg/mL) *plus*	Daily		
	Cefoxitin 4 g t.i.d. *or*	Daily		
	Imipenem 750 mg t.i.d. *or*	Daily		
	Linezolid 600 mg (if susceptible)	Daily	Consider 6–12 mo of clarithromycin plus linezolid if tolerated	

b.i.d., twice daily; t.i.d., three times daily; t.i.w., three times per week.

function abnormalities (first 6 months), leukopenia (rifabutin), visual changes (ethambutol), and hearing alterations (streptomycin, azithromycin). These should be done monthly and whenever potentially related symptoms occur. Monthly sputum cultures should be obtained on therapy, and patients are treated until they are culture negative for 1 year. It is this author's opinion that additional drugs, such as the newer quinolones, minocycline, cycloserine, and clofazimine, add little to these regimens based on human and *in vitro* studies. Rifampin is preferred over rifabutin in that it has fewer side effects, especially in women with nodular bronchiectasis where adverse events are (unfortunately) very frequent.

Treatment for hot-tub lung is not yet established, but likely requires both prednisone and the three-drug antimicrobial regimen, at least initially.

The role of surgical resection for *M. avium-intracellulare* lung disease remains controversial since it was first proposed and discussed in detail by Corpe (80), who worked at the Battey Sanatorium in Georgia. The current initial success with drug therapy alone using the macrolides suggests that this should be first-line therapy. Patients whose isolates become macrolide resistant or fail therapy with these agents could then be considered for surgery if they have localized disease, especially upper lobe cavitary disease. There should be aggressive attempts to make the patient's sputum culture negative preoperatively (to prevent intraoperative spread), and drug therapy should be continued until the patient is culture negative for 1 year.

Routine susceptibility testing of *M. avium-intracellulare* is probably not necessary as all untreated isolates of *M. avium-intracellulare* are macrolide susceptible. For patients who do not respond or who relapse on clarithromycin or azithromycin, susceptibility testing to these agents becomes critical as point mutations that affect the adenine at positions 2058 or 2059 of the 23S ribosomal binding site for the macrolides can occur on therapy (81) and result in high minimal inhibitory concentrations (MICs) (>64 µg/mL) for clarithromycin that are never seen with untreated strains (usual MICs 1–4 µg/mL) (81,82). Macrolide resistance invariably results in treatment failure with the standard three-drug regimen. For patients who fail to show a microbiologic response with 6 months of standard multidrug therapy, other drugs, such as streptomycin and rifabutin in place of rifampin, should be considered along with referral to an expert in the clinical management of this disease. All patients with a macrolide-resistant strain of *M. avium-intracellulare* should be referred to such an expert.

Mycobacterium kansasii

The second most common NTM lung disease is caused by *M. kansasii* (4). The typical patient is older than 50 years with a history of cigarette abuse. Other potential risk factors include pneumoconiosis, elderly white female with nodular bronchiectasis, and HIV infection, although the risk for the latter is small in comparison with the risk for disseminated *M. avium-intracellulare*. Many patients, perhaps as many as 50%, have no identifiable risk other than living in a geographic area with known disease. The presentation of *M. kansasii* lung disease is similar to that of tuberculosis, with cough, weight loss, and hemoptysis. Fever may be present but is much less common than with tuberculosis. Fibronodular or fibrocavitary upper lobe disease is the usual radiographic finding (5). Thin-walled cavities mimicking bullae are seen with a much higher frequency than with tuberculosis.

The current treatment for *M. kansasii* lung disease recommended by the American Thoracic Society (64) is a three-drug regimen consisting of isoniazid 300 mg, ethambutol 15 mg/kg, and rifampin 600 mg given for 18 to 24 months (Table 44.5). Patients should be culture negative for a minimum of 12 months. For patients unable to tolerate these three drugs, clarithromycin 500 mg twice a day offers exciting potential based on low MICs and its successful use with other mycobacteria (64). A recent short-course treatment trial using the same regimen of drugs given three times weekly for *M. avium-intracellulare* and the same end point showed a sputum conversion rate of 100% and a success rate of 95% (83). However, more experience with this regimen is needed before it can be routinely recommended. Other alternative drugs include streptomycin, sulfamethoxazole or trimethoprim–sulfamethoxazole, the newer quinolones, and linezolid. Rifampin resistance develops in some patients on therapy, especially those taking only one or two effective drugs (isoniazid is much less active against *M. kansasii* than against *M. tuberculosis*). HIV infection was responsible for one third of recent cases of rifampin-resistant *M. kansasii* in one series from Texas, probably related to noncompliance (84). Management of rifampin-resistant disease (in compliant patients) has an approximate 90% success rate without surgery using high-dose isoniazid (900 mg), sulfamethoxazole, ethambutol, and streptomycin (84). Clarithromycin, although not studied, probably will contribute to even better success in management of this disease.

Mycobacterium abscessus

The third most common cause of NTM lung disease in the United States is *M. abscessus* (formerly *M. chelonae* subspecies *abscessus*). A review of 145 cases of lung disease by Griffith et al. (85) provided a good clinical picture but a relatively bleak therapeutic picture for *M. abscessus* lung disease. Preexisting lung disease, especially bronchiectasis, is the major risk factor for the disease (Table 44.4). Most patients have no other recognizable risk factors. These patients are white (90%), female, nonsmokers who present only with cough. Cavitary disease is not usually seen with *M. abscessus* infection. Rather the chest radiograph usually shows patchy interstitial disease, often bilateral, often interpreted as scarring or fibrosis. High resolution computed tomography almost always shows right middle lobe and/or lingular nodular disease with associated bronchiectasis (86). These patients are remarkably similar to the patients with nodular bronchiectasis and *M. avium-intracellulare*, and as many as 20% of patients with *M. abscessus* will have *M. avium-intracellulare* at some time as well. The disease is generally a slowly progressive one, although some patients will ultimately die of the disease. Because of drug resistance to all antituberculous drugs and most antibacterial agents, cure of *M. abscessus* disease is possible only with surgical resection. Short courses (2 to 6 weeks) of clarithromycin, amikacin, and cefoxitin (Table 44.5) provide symptomatic and bacteriologic and radiographic improvement but are not curative. The newer 8-methoxyquinolones and linezolid offer some promise for some patients (58), but use of these drugs to date has been limited.

A number of other NTM species have been reported as a cause of chronic lung disease. These include rapidly growing species, such as *M. fortuitum*, and slowly growing mycobacterial species, including *M. xenopi*, *M. szulgai*, *M. simiae*, and *M. malmoense* (Table 44.1) (4,23,33,64). In general, these species have been identified as causing disease in fewer than 50 patients in the United States, although *M. xenopi* and *M. malmoense* are relatively common in other areas of the world (4,23,64). There are no unique features of their disease to distinguish them in presentation or radiographic features from other NTM lung pathogens. Therapy for these diseases is uncertain because of the infrequent character of the infections. These less well-known lung pathogens were well reviewed in a study by Wayne and Sramek (23).

REFERENCES

1. Christianson LC, Dewlett HJ. Pulmonary disease in adults associated with unclassified mycobacteria. *Am J Med* 1960;29: 980–991.
2. Crow HE, King CT, Smith E, et al. A limited clinical, pathologic, and epidemiologic study of patients with pulmonary lesions associated with atypical acid-fast bacilli in the sputum. *Am Rev Tuberc* 1957;75:199–222.
3. Timpe A, Runyon EH. The relationship of "atypical" acid-fast bacteria to human disease: a preliminary report. *J Lab Clin Med* 1954;44:202.
4. Wolinsky E. Nontuberculous mycobacteria and associated disease. *Am Rev Respir Dis* 1979;119:107–159.
5. Ahn CH, McLarty JW, Ahn SS, et al. Diagnostic criteria for pul-

monary disease caused by *Mycobacterium kansasii* and *Mycobacterium intracellulare. Am Rev Respir Dis* 1982;125:388–391.

6. Gruft H, Falkinham JO, Parker BC. Recent experience in the epidemiology of disease caused by atypical mycobacteria. *Rev Infect Dis* 1981;3:990–996.

7. Meissner G, Anz W. Sources of *Mycobacterium avium* complex infection resulting in human disease. *Am Rev Respir Dis* 1977; 116:1057–1064.

8. du Moulin GC, Stottmeier KD, Pelletier PA, et al. Concentration of *Mycobacterium avium* by hospital hot water systems. *JAMA* 1988;260:1599–1601.

9. Wolinsky E, Rynearson TK. Mycobacteria in soil and their relation to disease-associated strains. *Am Rev Respir Dis* 1968;97: 1032–1037.

10. Edwards LB, Aquaviva F, Livesay V, et al. An atlas of sensitivity to tuberculin, PPD-B, and histoplasmin in the United States. *Am Rev Respir Dis* 1969;99:1–132.

11. Picardeau M, Prod'Hom G, Raskine L, et al. Genotypic characterization of five subspecies of *Mycobacterium kansasii. J Clin Microbiol* 1997;35:25–32.

12. Galil K, Miller LA, Yakrus MA, et al. Abscesses due to *Mycobacterium abscessus* linked to injection of unapproved alternative medication. *Emerg Infect J* 1999;5:681–687.

13. Kuritsky JN, Bullen MG, Broome CV, et al. Sternal wound infections and endocarditis due to organisms of the *Mycobacterium fortuitum* complex: a potential environmental source. *Ann Intern Med* 1983;98:938–939.

14. Meyers H, Brown-Elliott BA, Moore D, et al. An outbreak of *Mycobacterium chelonae* infection following liposuction. *Clin Infect Dis* 2002;34:1500–1507.

15. Gebo KA, Srinivasan A, Perl TM, et al. Pseudo-outbreak of *Mycobacterium fortuitum* on a human immunodeficiency virus ward: transient respiratory tract colonization from a contaminated ice machine. *Clin Infect Dis* 2002;35:32–38.

16. Villaneuva A, Calderon RV, Vargas BA, et al. Report on an outbreak of post-injection abscesses due to *Mycobacterium abscessus*, including management with surgery and clarithromycin therapy and comparison of strains by random amplified polymorphic DNA polymerase chain reaction. *Clin Infect Dis* 1997;24: 1147–1153.

17. Wilson RW, Steingrube VA, Böttger EC, et al. *Mycobacterium immunogenum* sp. nov., a novel species related to *Mycobacterium abscessus* and associated with clinical disease, pseudo-outbreaks, and contaminated metalworking fluids: an international cooperative study on mycobacterial taxonomy. *Int J Syst Evol Microbiol* 2001;51:1751-1764.

18. Winthrop KL, Abrams M, Yakrus M, et al. An outbreak of mycobacterial furunculosis associated with footbaths at a nail salon. *N Engl J Med* 2002;346:1366–1371.

19. Zhang Y, Rajagopalan M, Brown BA, et al. Randomly amplified polymorphic DNA PCR for comparison of *Mycobacterium abscessus* strains from nosocomial outbreaks. *J Clin Microbiol* 1997;35:3132–3139.

20. Hector JSR, Pang Y, Mazurek GH, et al. Large restriction fragment patterns of genomic *Mycobacterium fortuitum* DNA as strain-specific markers and their use in epidemiologic investigation of four nosocomial outbreaks. *J Clin Microbiol* 1992;30: 1250–1255.

21. Wallace RJ Jr, Zhang Y, Brown BA, et al. DNA large restriction fragment patterns of sporadic and epidemic nosocomial strains of *Mycobacterium chelonae* and *Mycobacterium abscessus. J Clin Microbiol* 1993;31:2697–2701.

22. Sniadack DH, Ostroff SM, Karlix MA, et al. A nosocomial pseudo-outbreak of *Mycobacterium xenopi* due to a contaminated potable water supply: lessons in prevention. *Infect Control Hosp Epidemiol* 1993;14:636–641.

23. Wayne LG, Sramek HA. Agents of newly recognized or infrequently encountered mycobacterial disease. *Clin Microbiol Rev* 1992;5:1–25.

24. Valero G, Peters J, Jorgensen JH, et al. Clinical isolates of *Mycobacterium simiae* in San Antonio, Texas. *Am J Respir Crit Care Med* 1995;152:1555–1557.

25. Rynkiewica DL, Cage GD, Butler WR, et al. Clinical and microbiological assessment of *Mycobacterium simiae* isolates from a single laboratory in southern Arizona. *Clin Infect Dis* 1998;26: 625–630.

26. Conger NG, Laurel V, Oliver K, et al. *Mycobacterium simiae* pseudo-outbreak among hospitalized patients. The 40th Annual Meeting of the Infectious Disease Society of America, October 24–27, 2002, Chicago, Abstract 422, p 118.

27. Crossey MJ, Yakrus MA, Cook MB, et al. Isolation of *Mycobacterium simiae* in a southwestern hospital and typing by multilocus enzyme electrophoresis. American Society of Microbiology conference, Las Vegas, NV, 1994, Abstract U38.

28. Roberts B, Hirst R. Immunomagnetic separation and PCR for detection of *Mycobacterium ulcerans. J Clin Microbiol* 1997;35: 2709–2711.

29 National Committee for Clinical Laboratory Standards. *Susceptibility testing of mycobacteria, nocardia and other aerobic actinomycetes: tentative standard*, 2nd ed. 2000:M24–T2.

30. Coffin JW, et al. Use of restriction fragment length polymorphisms resolved by pulsed-field gel electrophoresis for subspecies identification of mycobacteria in the *Mycobacterium avium* complex and for isolation of DNA probes. *J Clin Microbiol* 1992;30: 1829–1836.

31. Mazurek GH, Hartman S, Zhang Y-S, et al. Large DNA restriction fragment polymorphism in the *Mycobacterium avium–M. intracellulare* complex: a potential epidemiologic tool. *J Clin Microbiol* 1993;31:390–394.

32. Schaad UB, Votteler TP, McCracken GH, et al. Management of atypical mycobacterial lymphadenitis in childhood. *J Pediatr* 1979;95:356–360.

33. Wolinsky E. Mycobacterial disease other than tuberculosis. *Clin Infect Dis* 1992;15:1–12.

34. Pang SC. Mycobacterial lymphadenitis in western Australia. *Tuber Lung Dis* 1992;73:362–367.

35. Lai KK, Stottmeier KD, Sherman IH, et al. Mycobacterial cervical lymphadenopathy. *JAMA* 1984;251:1296.

36. Reid JD, Wolinsky M. Histopathology of lymphadenitis caused by atypical mycobacteria. *Am Rev Respir Dis* 1969;99:8–12.

37. Taha AM, Davidson PT, Bailey WC. Surgical treatment of atypical mycobacterial lymphadenitis in children. *Pediatr Infect Dis* 1985;4:664–667.

38. Dautzenberg B, Truffot C, Legris S, et al. Activity of clarithromycin against *Mycobacterium avium* infection in patients with the acquired immune deficiency syndrome. *Am Rev Respir Dis* 1991;144:564–569.

39. Wallace RJ Jr, Brown BA, Griffith DE, et al. Initial clarithromycin monotherapy for *Mycobacterium avium-intracellulare* complex lung disease. *Am Rev Respir Dis* 1994;149:1335–1341.

40. Green PA, Fordham von Reyn C, Smith RP Jr. *Mycobacterium avium* complex parotid lymphadenitis: successful therapy with clarithromycin and ethambutol. *Pediatr Infect Dis* 1993;12: 615–617.

41. Wallace RJ Jr, Swenson JM, Silcox VA, et al. Spectrum of disease due to rapidly growing mycobacteria. *Rev Infect Dis* 1983;5: 657–679.

42. Collins CH, Grange JM, Noble WC, et al. *Mycobacterium marinum* infections in man. *J Hyg* 1985;94:135–149.

43. Casal M, del Mar Casal M. Multicenter study of incidence of *Mycobacterium marinum* in humans in Spain. *Int J Tuberc Lung Dis* 2001;5:197–199.

44. Edelstein H. *Mycobacterium marinum* skin infections. *Arch Intern Med* 1994;154:1359–1364.
45. Wallace RJ Jr, Brown BA, Silcox VA, et al. Clinical disease, drug susceptibility and biochemical patterns of the unnamed third biovariant complex of *Mycobacterium fortuitum. J Infect Dis* 1991;163:598–603.
46. Wallace RJ Jr, Brown BA, Onyi G. Skin, soft tissue, and bone infections due to *Mycobacterium chelonae* subspecies *chelonae*—importance of prior corticosteroid therapy, frequency of disseminated infections, and resistance to oral antimicrobials other than clarithromycin. *J Infect Dis* 1992;166:405–412.
47. Wallace RJ Jr, Nash DR, Tsukamura M, et al. Human disease due to *Mycobacterium smegmatis. J Infect Dis* 1988;158:52–59.
48. Szabo I. *Mycobacterium chelonei* endemy after heart surgery with fatal consequences. *Am Rev Respir Dis* 1980;121:607.
49. Clegg HW, Foster MT, Sanders WE Jr, et al. Infection due to organisms of the *Mycobacterium fortuitum* complex after augmentation mammaplasty: clinical and epidemiologic features. *J Infect Dis* 1983;147:427–433.
50. Wallace RJ Jr, Steele LC, Labidi A, et al. Heterogeneity among isolates of rapidly growing mycobacteria responsible for infections following augmentation mammaplasty despite case clustering in Texas and other southern coastal states. *J Infect Dis* 1989;160:281–288.
51. Raad II, Vartivarian S, Khan A, et al. Catheter-related infections caused by the *Mycobacterium fortuitum* complex: 15 cases and review. *Rev Infect Dis* 1991;13:1120–1125.
52. Wallace RJ Jr, Silcox VA, Tsukamura M, et al. Clinical significance, biochemical features, and susceptibility patterns of sporadic isolates of the *Mycobacterium chelonae*-like organisms. *J Clin Microbiol* 1993;31:3231–3239.
53. Franklin DJ, Starke JR, Brady MT, et al. Chronic otitis media after tympanostomy tube placement caused by *Mycobacterium abscessus*: a new clinical entity? *Am J Otol* 1994;15:313–320.
54. Swenson JM, Wallace RJ Jr., Silcox VA, et al. Antimicrobial susceptibility of 5 subgroups of *Mycobacterium fortuitum* and *Mycobacterium chelonae. Antimicrob Agents Chemother* 1985;28:807–811.
55. Brown BA, Wallace RJ Jr, Onyi GO, et al. Activities of four macrolides, including clarithromycin, against *Mycobacterium fortuitum, Mycobacterium chelonae*, and *M. chelonae*–like organisms. *Antimicrob Agents Chemother* 1992;36:180–184.
56. Wallace RJ Jr, Bedsole G, Sumter G, et al. Activities of ciprofloxacin and ofloxacin against rapidly growing mycobacteria with demonstration of acquired mutational resistance following single-drug therapy. *Antimicrob Agents Chemother* 1990;34:65–70.
57. Wallace RJ Jr, Brown BA, Onyi G. Susceptibilities of *Mycobacterium fortuitum* biovar *fortuitum* and the two subgroups of *Mycobacterium chelonae* to imipenem, cefmetazole, cefoxitin, and amoxicillin–clavulanic acid. *Antimicrob Agents Chemother* 1991;35:773–775.
58. Wallace RJ Jr, Brown-Elliott BA, Ward SC, et al. Activities of linezolid against rapidly growing mycobacteria. *Antimicrob Agents Chemother* 2001;45:764–767.
59. Wallace RJ Jr, Swenson Jm, Silcox VA, et al. Treatment of nonpulmonary infections due to *Mycobacterium fortuitum* and *Mycobacterium chelonei*: on the basis of *in vitro* susceptibilities. *J Infect Dis* 1985;152:500–514.
60. Wallace RJ Jr, Tanner D, Brennan PJ, et al. Clinical trial of clarithromycin for cutaneous (disseminated) infection due to *Mycobacterium chelonae. Ann Intern Med* 1993;119:482–486.
61. Marston BJ, Diallo MO, Horsburgh CR Jr, et al. Emergence of Buruli ulcer in the Daloa region of Cote d'Ivoire. *Am J Trop Med Hyg* 1995;52:219–224.
62. Goutzamanis JJ, Gilbert GL. *Mycobacterium ulcerans* infection in

Australian children: report of eight cases and review. *Clin Infect Dis* 1995;21:1186–1192.
63. Portaels F, Traore H, De Ridder K, et al. *In vitro* susceptibility of *Mycobacterium ulcerans* to clarithromycin. *Antimicrob Agents Chemother* 1998;42:2070–2073.
64. Wallace RJ Jr, Cook JL , Glassroth J, et al. American Thoracic Society Statement: diagnosis and treatment of disease caused by nontuberculous mycobacteria. *Am Respir Crit Care Med* 1997;156:S1–S25.
65. Ingram CW, Tanner DC, Durack DT, et al. Disseminated infection with rapidly growing mycobacteria. *Clin Infect Dis* 1993;16:463–471.
66. Parent LJ, Salam MM, Appelbaum PC, et al. Disseminated *Mycobacterium marinum* infection and bacteremia in a child with severe combined immunodeficiency. *Clin Infect Dis* 1995;21:1325–1327.
67. Yeager H Jr, Raleigh JW. Pulmonary disease due to *Mycobacterium intracellulare. Am Rev Respir Dis* 1973;108:547–552.
68. Davidson PT, Khanijo V, Goble M, et al. Treatment of disease due to *Mycobacterium intracellulare. Rev Infect Dis* 1981;3:1052–1059.
69. Prince DS, Peterson, DD, Steiner RM, et al. Infection with *Mycobacterium avium* complex in patients without predisposing conditions. *N Engl J Med* 1989;321:863–868.
70. Reich JM, Johnson RE. *Mycobacterium avium* complex pulmonary disease presenting as an isolated lingular or middle lobe pattern. *Chest* 1992;101:1605–1609.
71. Wallace RJ Jr. *Mycobacterium avium* complex lung disease and women—now an equal opportunity disease. *Chest* 1994;105:6–7.
72. Hartman TE, Swensen SJ, Williams DE. *Mycobacterium avium-intracellulare* complex: evaluation with CT. *Radiology* 1993;187:1–4.
73. Swensen SJ, Hartman TE, Williams DE. Computed tomographic diagnosis of *Mycobacterium avium-intracellulare* complex in patients with bronchiectasis. *Chest* 1994;105:49–52.
74. Kilby JM, Gilligan PH, Yankaskas JR, et al. Nontuberculous mycobacteria in adult patients with cystic fibrosis. *Chest* 1992;102:70–75.
75. Embil J, Warren P, Yakrus M, et al: Pulmonary illness associated with exposure to *Mycobacterium avium* complex in hot tub water: hypersensitivity pneumonitis or infection? Chest 1997;111:813–816.
76. Kahana LM, Kay JM, Yakrus MA, et al. *Mycobacterium avium* complex infection in an immunocompetent young adult related to hot tub exposure. Chest 1997;111:242–245.
77. Khoor A, Leslie KO, Tazelaar HD, et al. Diffuse pulmonary disease caused by nontuberculous mycobacteria in immunocompetent people (hot tub lung). *Am J Clin Pathol* 2001;115:755–762.
78. Ahn CH, Ahn SS, Anderson RA, et al. A four-drug regimen for initial treatment of cavitary disease caused by *Mycobacterium avium* complex. *Am Rev Respir Dis* 1986;134:438–441.
79. Griffith DE, Wallace RJ Jr, Brown BA, et al: Azithromycin (Azith) monotherapy (mono-Rx) for HIV (–) patients with *Mycobacterium avium intracellulare* complex (MAI) lung disease. *Am J Respir Crit Care Med* 1995;151:A477, Abstract.
80. Corpe RF. Surgical management of pulmonary disease due to *Mycobacterium avium-intracellulare. Rev Infect Dis* 1981;3:1064–1067.
81. Meier A, Kirschner P, Burkhardt S, et al. Identification of mutations in 23S rRNA gene of clarithromycin-resistant *Mycobacterium intracellulare. Antimicrob Agents Chemother* 1994;38:121–122.
82. Heifets L, Mor N, Vanderkolk J. *Mycobacterium avium* strains resistant to clarithromycin and azithromycin. *Antimicrob Agents Chemother* 1994;37:2364–2370.

83. Griffith DE, Brown-Elliott BA, Wallace RJ Jr. An intermittent clarithromycin-containing regimen for *Mycobacterium kansasii* lung disease. *Am J Respir Crit Care Med* 2001;163:A762.

84. Wallace RJ Jr, Dunbar D, Brown BA, et al. Rifampin-resistant *Mycobacterium kansasii*. *Clin Infect Dis* 1994;18:736–743.

85. Griffith DE, Girard WM, Wallace RJ Jr. Clinical features of pulmonary disease caused by rapidly growing mycobacteria: "Analysis of 154 patients." *Am Rev Respir Dis* 1993;147: 1271–1278.

86. Hazelton TR, Newell JD, Cook JL, et al. CT findings in 14 patients with *Mycobacterium chelonae* pulmonary infection. *AJR Am J Roentgenol* 2000;175:413–416.

45

TUBERCULOSIS AND THE HUMAN IMMUNODEFICIENCY VIRUS INFECTION

JOSEPH N. BURZYNSKI
NEIL W. SCHLUGER
STUART M. GARAY

Infection with the human immunodeficiency virus (HIV) has transformed tuberculosis (TB) from an endemic disease into a worldwide epidemic. HIV is the most important known risk factor that promotes progression to active TB in people with *Mycobacterium tuberculosis* infections. Instead of a 5% to 10% lifetime risk for persons with latent TB infection that their disease will progress to active TB, persons coinfected with HIV have a 5% to 15% annual risk of developing active TB disease (1,2). The World Health Organization (WHO) estimates that one third to one half of persons with HIV will develop TB disease. In 2002, more than 630,000 new cases of TB/HIV were reported worldwide and 450,000 deaths were attributed to TB/HIV (3). In many areas of Asia and Africa, TB control efforts have been challenged by the high number of patients coinfected with HIV and TB. For example, despite the successful efforts of the Revised National Tuberculosis Control Program in India, including improved access to care for TB patients and vastly improved directly observed therapy (DOT) services, it is predicted that the HIV epidemic will lead to an additional 200,000 cases of TB per year in India, even at the current relatively low rate of HIV infection (4).

Early in the course of the acquired immunodeficiency syndrome (AIDS) epidemic, the link between HIV and TB was not clearly recognized. Indeed, in 1983 at the first National Heart, Lung, and Blood Institute workshop on the pulmonary complications of AIDS, this possibility was not mentioned (5). Later that same year, in three separate reports—Vieira et al. (6), Pitchenik et al. (7), and Pape et al. (8)—noted an increased incidence of TB in HIV-infected Haitians living in Haiti or the United States. During the past decade, TB has become the major opportunistic infection complicating the HIV epidemic worldwide, although other infections remain more common in some geographic areas.

By the year 2000, the prevalence of HIV and TB continued to climb worldwide, with HIV largely fueling the increased incidence of TB. In 2000, the Global Programme on AIDS of the World Health Organization estimated that the prevalence of HIV infection among adults and children worldwide was 36.1 million (9). At the same time, about 2 billion people (one third of the human population) had latent infection with *M. tuberculosis* and approximately 11.8 million people were coinfected. Currently 12% of TB patients are HIV positive and 22.5% of deaths from TB are due to TB/HIV worldwide. In some regions, such as Africa, the rates are dramatically higher. Of 2 million cases of TB in Africa in 1999, some researchers estimate that two thirds were HIV positive. The number of TB cases is predicted to increase 10% per year in Africa because of HIV and will reach 3.3 million by 2005 and surpass 4 million shortly thereafter.

The converging epidemics of AIDS and TB have been complicated by the emergence of a third epidemic, that of multidrug-resistant TB (MDR-TB) (10,11). The difficulty in diagnosing TB in HIV-infected persons has been compounded by the potential for TB to progress rapidly in these patients.

This review summarizes the knowledge obtained during the past decade regarding the interaction between HIV and TB. Although the emphasis is on the United States, reference is made to differences in the remaining industrialized as well as the nonindustrialized world.

J. N. Burzynski: Department of Pulmonary Medicine, Columbia University College of Physicians and Surgeons; Tuberculosis Control Program, Washington Heights Chest Center, New York City Department of Health and Mental Hygiene, New York, New York.

N. W. Schluger: Department of Medicine, Columbia University College of Physicians and Surgeons; Department of Medicine, Division of Pulmonary, Allergy, and Critical Care Medicine, Columbia Presbyterian Medical Center, New York, New York.

S. M. Garay: Division of Pulmonary and Critical Care Medicine, New York University Medical Center, New York, New York.

EPIDEMIOLOGY

United States

In the United States between 10 and 19 million people harbor the tubercle bacillus, whereas approximately 1 million (only some of whom have been infected with *M. tuberculosis*) are HIV seropositive (10,12,13). The year 1985 marks a historical milestone. In that year the number of new TB cases began to deviate from the previously consistent yearly decline. Between 1953 (when national reporting began) and 1984, there had been a constant decrease in the TB case rate of approximately 5% per year (13,14). Between 1984 and 1985 the decline became negligible (0.2%, or 54 cases), and in 1986 there was an increase in the number of new TB cases (up 2.6%, or 567 cases) from the previous year. This marked the first increase in TB cases in more than 30 years. After 1986 the number of newly reported TB cases continued to increase until 1992. By 1992, the number of new cases of TB peaked at 26,673 (10.5 cases per 100,000 population) and represented a 20% increase from 1985. The largest increases occurred in New York City (approximately 80%), California (approximately 50%), and Texas (approximately 30%). Had the previously noted decline been observed through 1992, approximately 52,000 fewer cases than what was reported would have been expected between 1985 and 1992 (15). From 1992 to 1994, the number of TB cases reported annually decreased by 8.7% (16,17) (and this trend continued throughout the decade). In 1994, a total of 24,361 cases of TB (9.4 cases per 100,000 population) were reported (17). By 2001, the number of reported cases had declined to 15,989, representing a rate of 5.6 per 100,000. While the increase in TB cases resulted from a combination of factors, including immigration from countries with a high incidence of TB, intravenous drug use, homelessness, poverty, and a significant decline in local TB control programs, HIV infection was one of the leading causes of this unexpected change (10,18–21). The decrease in TB cases reported since 1993 reflects the impact of federal, state, and local TB control efforts, including DOT and support for programs to prevent TB disease among HIV-infected persons (17).

As early as 1983 it was suggested that TB was common among AIDS patients who came from areas with a recognized high prevalence of TB (6–8). Pitchenik et al. (7) described 10 of 20 severely immunosuppressed AIDS patients who had TB; TB was discovered concomitant with or prior to the AIDS diagnosis. A subsequent more detailed report by Pitchenik et al. (22) in 1984 revealed that 27 (60%) of 45 Haitian patients with AIDS also had TB. TB preceded the diagnosis of AIDS by a mean of 6 months in 22 patients. Similarly, reports from other parts of the country but from areas with populations at risk for TB (such as minority populations, foreign immigrants, and intravenous drug users) supported the association between AIDS and TB (23–26).

Matching of TB and AIDS registries in 43 states by the Centers for Disease Control and Prevention (CDC) revealed that 3.8% of AIDS cases appeared on TB registries. The percentage varied widely: 5% in New York to 10% in Florida. In 1988, the CDC initiated a sampling of 3,077 patients in 20 urban TB clinics in 14 cities to determine the prevalence of HIV infection among patients with TB (27). The median rate of seropositivity was 3.4%, with the highest rates reported in New York City (46%), Newark (34%), Boston (27%), Miami (24%), and Baltimore (13%).

In the United States, the most striking effects of HIV infection on the incidence of TB come from New York City. Between 1978 and 1991, New York City's proportion of total U.S. TB cases rose from 4.6% to 14.0%. Between 1984 and 1991 the TB case rate increased from 19.9 to 50.2 per 100,000 population, an 81% increase (28). Most strikingly, case rates in Central Harlem in 1989 reached 169 per 100,000 persons, rivaling case rates in Africa (20). Concomitant with this rise in the number of TB cases was the progressive increase in the number of HIV-infected individuals throughout the city, especially in areas with increased TB case rates. After peaking in 1992 this trend has reversed. Some of the credit for the turning the tide against the TB epidemic must go to the intensive effort by local health departments by increasing the emphasis of DOT, the standardization of treatment regimens, and improved infection control measures. The New York City Department of Health (NYCDOH) estimated that the cost of caring for patients in the New York City outbreak was roughly $1 billion. However, the cost of controlling the outbreak was a small fraction of this, and the cost of preventing it would have been even smaller (29). In New York City the proportion and number of persons with TB who are coinfected with HIV declined from 33.6% and 1,281 cases in 1992 to 14.6% and 184 cases in 2001 (30). This same trend occurred nationally, with a lower proportion of HIV-positive individuals every year from 1993 to 2000 even though HIV testing has been more widespread. In 1993, 30% of all TB patients were tested for HIV and 15% tested positive. By 2000, 49% of TB patients were tested for HIV and only 9% tested positive (CDC:http://www.cdc.gov/nchstp/tb/surv/surv2001/content/T1.htm).

The decline in the number of HIV cases was illustrated by a study of TB transmission patterns in New York City over the decade of the 1990s. In the early 1990s, cases of TB were clustered, that is, groups of TB isolates with identical restriction fragment length polymorphism (RFLP) patterns were identified, indicating recent TB transmission. The clusters, identifying recent TB transmission, had a high incidence of HIV-positive persons (40%). By the end of the decade, TB cases were much more likely to be single events without clustering, demonstrating a shift to more cases in the foreign-born with reactivation TB, whereas cases involving HIV infection and recent transmission became less frequent (31).

Braun et al. (32) demonstrated a change in TB mortality in the United States during the AIDS epidemic between 1980 and 1990. A bimodal age distribution spanning ages 20 to 49 years accompanied the preexisting peak in the elderly. In 1990, 54% (729 of 1,344) of deaths with TB in persons 20 to 49 years old occurred in persons who also had AIDS. These statistics were not surprising in light of a CDC survey of TB clinics demonstrating an HIV prevalence of 47% in individuals with TB aged 25 to 44 years (15). As a result of the data cited here, the CDC instituted a new surveillance definition for AIDS that included pulmonary TB. This was revised from the 1987 definition, which recognized extrapulmonary TB as an AIDS-related diagnosis.

Africa

Even before the AIDS epidemic, the annual incidence of TB in Africa was exceedingly high, with the sub-Saharan African case rate approximating 200 per 100,000 per year (33–35). By 2002 the incidence rate in sub-Saharan Africa had climbed to 259 per 100,000 cases. In a report on the global burden of TB from WHO, Africa had the highest rate (1.2%) of HIV/TB coinfection (HIV-positive patients with latent TB infection) in the general population, and Africa also had the highest percentage of persons with TB who were HIV positive (32%). Of the ten countries with the highest incidence rates per capita, nine were in Africa. They included Botswana, Namibia, South Africa, Zambia, and Zimbabwe with incidence rates of 400 per 100,000 persons or more (36). Early reports from Africa had suggested a possible association between HIV infection and TB (37,38). Many subsequent studies found high levels of HIV seroprevalence in TB patients, averaging 40% with a range of 20% to 73% (39–49). For example, in Uganda and Zambia more than 60% of TB patients were HIV seropositive, whereas 30% of newly diagnosed TB patients in Kenya were HIV seropositive (39–41,48). A notable exception to the high seroprevalence rates had been Lagos, Nigeria, where a 5% rate was reported in the early 1990s (50).

By 1999 the WHO estimated that 11.8 million people were living with HIV/TB coinfection, and the majority were in Africa. These individuals are at extraordinarily high risk for developing clinical TB in comparison with HIV-seronegative patients who are purified protein derivative (PPD) positive. Cohort studies from Zaire and Rwanda confirmed this risk (51,52). In a retrospective cohort study in Zaire, Braun et al. (51) followed HIV-seropositive and HIV-seronegative women of childbearing age for a median period of 32 months. TB developed in 7.6% of 249 HIV-seropositive women (3.1 cases per 100 person-years) compared to 0.3% of 310 HIV-seronegative women (0.12 cases per 100 person-years); the relative risk was 26. Assuming that 50% of the population was infected with TB (i.e., PPD positive), the annual risk in the two groups can be calculated to be 6.2% and 0.2%, respectively (53). Similar statistics come from

Rwanda, where Allen et al. (52) studied the incidence of TB in a cohort of 1,470 women (473 HIV seropositive and 997 HIV seronegative). During a 2-year follow-up period, TB developed in 20 HIV-seropositive and two HIV-seronegative women. The annual incidence was 2.5% and 0.1%, respectively, with a relative risk of 23. The annual incidence among HIV-seropositive patients with a positive tuberculin skin test result was 5.5%, assuming a prevalence of tuberculous infection of 50% (53). These studies demonstrated that the risk of progression to TB among HIV-seropositive patients is similar to that found in the United States. Selwyn et al. (1) prospectively studied HIV-seropositive intravenous drug users in New York City. Over a 2-year period, TB developed in seven of 49 HIV-seropositive persons with a positive tuberculin skin test result, compared with none of 62 HIV-seronegative drug users, yielding a rate of 7.9% per year and a risk ratio of 24.0.

The number of cases of TB in Africa is skyrocketing upward, which is evident from data available on the reported numbers of TB cases in Africa. Burundi, Malawi, Tanzania, Zambia, and Uganda have experienced dramatic increases in the number of reported cases. Whereas Tanzania had an 86% increase in reported cases, even greater increases of 140%, 154%, and 180% were observed in Burundi, Zambia, and Malawi, respectively (53).

Because 70% of coinfected individuals live in sub-Saharan Africa, this region has felt the overwhelming brunt of the epidemic of HIV-related TB. A small glimmer of hope came from a study of highly active antiretroviral therapy (HAART) on the incidence of TB in South Africa. This study examined 264 HIV-infected patients receiving HAART and found a lower incidence of TB than in non-HAART HIV-infected patients. HAART reduced the incidence of HIV-associated TB by more than 80% in an area endemic for TB and HIV. Widespread effective HAART treatment might help to combat the increasing incidence of HIV-related TB in sub-Saharan Africa (54).

Asia

Southeast Asia and the western Pacific regions contributed more than 60% of the global TB incidence in 1990 (33). However, the spread of HIV infection through this area occurred later than in the United States, Europe, and Africa (55,56). As of early 1995, the HIV epidemic has had only a mild impact on TB in this region. Of the 4.9 million cases of TB in 1990, only 85,000 were attributable to HIV infection (33). However, as of 1994, the WHO estimated that more than 850,000 people were coinfected with TB and HIV in South and Southeast Asia, creating a huge potential for HIV-related TB cases in the near future (57). The rates of increase for HIV-related TB have been high. In 1989, 5% of TB patients in Chiang Rai, northern Thailand, were HIV seropositive; this incidence increased to 25% in 1993 and to 70% by 1998. From 1990 to 1998, the number of new TB cases at the Chiang Rai Hospital increased more than three-fold (58). In Bombay, 2.3% of TB patients were HIV seropositive in 1989, compared with 9% in 1993. TB is the most common life-threatening opportunistic infection associated with HIV in Asian patients: 82% of patients with AIDS in Myanmar, 56% in India, and 52% in Thailand have TB (57). The incidence of TB will continue to increase among Asian HIV patients (33,57,59,60). In 2002, India was estimated to have the highest incidence of TB with 1.8 million new cases. At that time, the number of HIV-positive cases was a relatively low 45,000. However, the relatively small percentage of HIV-related TB cases may change soon because although TB/HIV coinfection rates were higher in Africa, the number of people coinfected in India was greater than in any other country (1.8 million in 2002). China was estimated to have 1.4 million new cases of TB in 2002 but only 5,000 cases were HIV related. For the western Pacific region that includes China, the Philippines, Vietnam, Cambodia, Korea, Japan, and Malaysia, less than 1% of TB cases were HIV related. The only exception was Cambodia where 3% of cases were HIV related. The epidemiology is likely changing, as pointed out in a recent study from Vietnam. In Ho Chi Minh City, HIV prevalence among TB patients has increased steadily from 0.5% in 1995 to 4% in 2000 (61).

Central and South America

As of 1990, Central America, South America, and the Caribbean islands accounted for 569,000 cases of TB, 20,000 of which were related to HIV infection (33). By 1992 it was estimated that more than 300,000 individuals were coinfected with HIV and TB in this region, suggesting that HIV-related TB will become a greater problem in the future (53). As noted earlier, some of the initial reports regarding the association between HIV and TB come from studies on Haitian patients residing in the United States as well as in Haiti (6–8). TB has developed in 25% to 60% of Haitians with AIDS. In rural Haiti, 24% of patients with TB were HIV seropositive (62). Throughout Latin America the seroprevalence rate of HIV among TB patients ranges from 2% to 31% (63–65). Studies from Mexico, Brazil, and Argentina reported that 7% to 25% of patients with AIDS develop TB at some time during their illness (66). The possibility of underdiagnosis is demonstrated by a recent study from Brazil reported that, among TB patients, poor women and those who sought TB treatment in their own residential neighborhood rather than in a district health center were less likely to receive testing for HIV (67).

Europe

The impact of the AIDS epidemic on TB in western Europe has varied from country to country (68). In France, AIDS has had an important impact on TB in the Paris area, where HIV-infected TB patients alone accounted for the increase

in the number of cases over that expected. The HIV-seropositive rate among TB patients in Paris was much higher than that of all other areas of the country (12% vs. 1%). Approximately 40% of all HIV-infected patients with TB were foreign-born (almost half were from sub-Saharan Africa). In contrast, a multicenter retrospective study conducted at nine university hospitals in southern France revealed that only 121 (2.1%) of 5,730 HIV-seropositive inpatients and outpatients had TB (69). Similarly, a study of the TB registry in the Rhône district of France failed to demonstrate a significant overlap between patients with HIV and those with TB (70). Antonucci et al. (71) reported on a retrospective multicenter study involving 40% of the total number of HIV-infected patients in Italy cared for by the national health service between 1985 and 1989. The proportion of HIV-infected subjects diagnosed with TB increased during the study period from three (0.2%) of 1,380 in 1985 to 152 (2.3%) of 6,504 in 1989 ($p < 0.0001$). Of all the European countries, Spain appears to have the highest incidence of TB in AIDS patients; three studies documented that TB developed in 21% to 36% of AIDS patients (72–74). As in the Italian study, most of these patients were intravenous drug users. In Frankfurt, Germany, TB developed in more than 10% of AIDS patients between 1984 and 1988 (68). In the Netherlands, the incidence of TB among Dutch men aged 25 to 49 years residing in Amsterdam increased from 16.1 to 34.7 per 100,000; this has been attributed to HIV infection (75,76). Other studies indicate that rates of coinfection in some parts of Europe have continued to increase. In an anonymous seroprevalence study in an inner-city hospital in London, blood samples from 157 consecutive TB patients were tested, yielding an HIV infection prevalence of 24.8% (77). In a prison in Spain, it has been reported that 20.1% of new inmates were coinfected with TB and HIV (78).

In western Europe, where HAART is widely available for HIV-infected patients, Kirk et al. (79) have reported on the impact of HAART in a large multicenter cohort of more than 7,000 patients followed from 1994 to 1999. The overall incidence of *M. tuberculosis* decreased from 1.8 cases per 100 years of person follow-up to 0.3 cases per 100 person-years of follow-up during the period of observation. The reduction in TB was associated with the introduction of HAART and changes in the CD4 count.

Eastern Europe and the countries of the former Soviet Union in particular have gained increasing attention as reports of increasing rates of HIV, TB, and especially MDR-TB warn of a public health disaster threatening to spin out of control. In Russia, there was a doubling of the number of newly detected TB cases from 1991 to 2000 (80). The situation has been particularly bleak in the prison system. The International Committee of the Red Cross noted in a 1998 report that the case rate per year in prisons in Georgia was 5,995 per 100,000, which was 60 times that of the civilian population and a major cause of death there.

The rate of multidrug resistance in prisons in Georgia was 13%, at least 20% in Russia, and 23% in Azerbaijan. HIV rates in Russian prisons are known to be increasing, with 3,500 HIV-positive prisoners identified in 2000 compared with 2,661 the year previously. Together with chronic over-crowding and poor ventilation, the increasing incidence of HIV infection and extraordinarily high incidence of TB disease are certain to leave a huge public health dilemma for the foreseeable future (81). The explanation for the increasing incidence of TB in Russia is familiar to anyone who worked in TB control in New York City in the 1990s: deterioration of living conditions and social factors, inadequate management of TB services, lack of strict monitoring of TB patients, underfunding of the TB control service, and the spread of HIV infection (80).

IMMUNOPATHOGENESIS

Cellular Immune Response

The impact of HIV and TB coinfection is bidirectional. That is, TB affects the natural history of HIV infection, and HIV infection affects the presentation and natural history of TB. Substantial evidence exists that the consequences of HIV and TB coinfection are greater than would be the case for either condition singly. A study from several hospitals in the United States examined survival in a cohort of HIV-infected patients who had been successfully treated for TB and compared that survival to a cohort HIV-infected persons who had never had TB but were matched for CD4 count. At every level of CD4 count, survival in a Kaplan–Meier life table analysis was worse for patients who had had TB than those who had not (82). From this study it appeared that TB accelerates the natural history of HIV infection and leads to earlier death. Another study examined the impact of concomitant TB on the course of HIV infection by comparing 70 HIV-positive patients with TB and 120 HIV-positive patients without TB who were matched by CD4 count. In this study, TB was not an independent predictor of increased mortality but was associated with an *increased* risk of the development of other opportunistic infections (83).

More direct evidence of accelerated HIV progression from TB is provided by several *in vitro* studies examining the interaction between *M. tuberculosis* and HIV at the molecular level. Zhang et al. (84) demonstrated that both cell-wall components and whole *M. tuberculosis* organisms increased transcription of the long terminal repeat (LTR) of HIV *in vitro*. This seems to be mediated through activation of the transcription factors nuclear factor κB (NF-κB) and interleukin-6 (IL-6). The same investigators demonstrated this *in vivo* by comparing HIV viral copies taken from bronchial alveolar lavage (BAL) samples from radiographically abnormal areas of lungs of TB patients with those from radiographically normal segments and with samples

taken from patients without TB. Branched DNA levels of HIV were highest in samples taken from radiographically abnormal segments of lungs of HIV-positive TB patients compared with controls. In addition, branched DNA levels of HIV declined over time with TB treatment (85).

CD4+ T lymphocytes and macrophages have a central role in the immune response to mycobacterial infection. HIV infection results in progressive depletion and dysfunction of CD4+ cells with defects in macrophage and monocyte function (86). As a result, HIV-infected patients have an increased risk of reactivation of latent TB as well as an increased risk of disease from new infection (1,87,88). In a prospective longitudinal study, Guelar et al. (87) found a mean CD4+ count of 77 ± 103 cells/mm^3 (range, 1 to 400 cells/mm^3) in 23 (3.1%) of 733 HIV-infected, PPD-negative patients who ultimately developed TB. The mean CD4+ cell count of the entire group was 377 ± 260 cells/mm^3.

Macrophage-based resistance against TB is due to its ability to control intracellular mycobacterial growth. CD4+ lymphocytes prime macrophages to control intracellular growth by releasing cytokines such as interferon-γ (IFN-γ), IL-1 and IL-2, and tumor necrosis factor-α (TNF-α), which activate blood-borne macrophages (89). An additional protective mechanism may be the generation of cytolytic T cells in response to mycobacteria (90). CD4+ T cells and γ/δ T cells kill autologous infected macrophages (91–93). Forte et al. (94) demonstrated decreased cytolytic T-cell activity in HIV-infected patients. The continued loss of CD4+ cells in HIV-seropositive patients and their reduced production of IL-2 may be the cause of decreased cytolytic T-lymphocyte activity (95). While the CD4+ cell count declines during progressive HIV infection, the numbers of CD8+ cells and γ/δ T cells often increase (96). Their role in the development of TB in HIV-infected patients remains to be defined.

TB can accelerate the course of HIV infection (82,97,98). Toossi et al. (99) demonstrated enhanced susceptibility of blood monocytes from patients with TB to produce infection with HIV-1. As noted previously, infection with *M. tuberculosis* stimulates release of mononuclear cytokines such as IL-1, IL-2, IL-6, and TNF-α. *M. tuberculosis* up-regulates the genes for these cytokines (100). These cytokines enhance replication of HIV-1 *in vitro* using several lines (101). The mechanism of this stimulation has been localized to the 5′ LTR of HIV-1; more specifically to the NF-κB transcription enhancer site (102). Recently, Zhang et al. (84) demonstrated that *M. tuberculosis* and its major antigenic cell wall component lipoarabinomannan were potent inducers of HIV-1 replication and LTR transcription via nuclear factors NF-κB and IL-6 sites. This was through direct and indirect stimulation by the cytokines IL-1 and TNF-α. These data suggest that the cytokines involved in defense against TB may be deleterious in seropositive patients. The interaction between TB and HIV may increase viral burden, accelerating progression to advanced stages of HIV disease (103).

There is also a major impact of HIV infection on the natural history of TB. The major defect in immune function in patients with HIV infection is related mainly, though not entirely, to the decline in numbers and impairment of function of CD4$^+$ T lymphocytes. There is now substantial evidence from studies in humans that CD4$^+$ T cells are of crucial importance in initiating and maintaining an effective host immune response against TB. CD4$^+$ T cells (sometimes called T-helper cells or T$_H$ lymphocytes) are now classified into at least two types, namely, T$_H$1 and T$_H$2 cells. T$_H$1 and T$_H$2 cells have different phenotypes based on the patterns of cytokines which they secrete (104). T$_H$1 cells primarily secrete IFN-γ, whereas T$_H$2 cells secrete IL-4, IL-5, and IL-10. It had previously been shown that a T$_H$1-type response represented a favorable immune response in patients with leprosy, as compared to a T$_H$2 response in patients with the same disease. Yamamura et al. (105) took biopsy specimens from tuberculoid leprosy lesions (characterized by paucibacilliary lesions without a great deal of tissue necrosis) and compared the cytokine gene expression patterns with those seen in specimens from lepromatous leprosy lesions (multibacillary lesions characterized by extensive tissue necrosis). In the tuberculoid lesions, the inflammatory infiltrate consists of T lymphocytes with a high level of mRNA transcripts for IFN-γ and IL-1. By contrast, in the lepromatous lesions, the infiltrate is characterized by T cells with high levels of mRNA transcripts for IL-4, IL-5, and IL-10. These findings suggested that a T$_H$1-type response is beneficial in response to infectious disease. Direct evidence of the beneficial nature of a T$_H$1-type response in TB comes from studies by Condos et al. (106), who examined local immune responses in the lungs of patients with active pulmonary TB. In patients with radiographically and clinically minimal disease [i.e., noncavitary infiltrates and sputum samples that were negative for acid-fast bacillus (AFB) on smear] there was a lymphocytic alveolitis characterized by cells that produced locally high amounts of IFN-γ. In contrast, patients with advanced, cavitary, smear-positive TB did not produce high levels of IFN-γ. The significance of IFN-γ was further demonstrated by the same group of investigators who showed that exogenously administered IFN-γ had beneficial effects in patients with MDR-TB (107). These clinical studies support a large number of *in vitro* and animal studies that also demonstrate an important role for IFN-γ in host defense against TB. These studies have established that this proinflammatory cytokine has several effects at the cellular level that are important in host defense against intracellular pathogens, including the activation of alveolar macrophages (leading to the production of reactive oxygen and reactive nitrogen species considered important in growth inhibition and/or killing of *M. tuberculosis*), increased expression of major histocompatibility complex class II molecules, and increased migration of lymphocytes.

As CD4$^+$ cells are the major source of IFN-γ in the body, and CD4$^+$ cell counts and function are depressed in patients with HIV infection, it stands to reason from the foregoing discussion that HIV-infected persons would be especially susceptible to TB infection and disease.

Tuberculin Skin Reactivity

Tuberculin skin reactivity is dependent on lymphokine release. The tuberculin skin test is a delayed-type hypersensitivity reaction that generally parallels cellular immunity. Anergy, which develops as a consequence of progressive HIV infection, undermines efforts to detect occult TB infection in those who are at greatest risk for active disease. Johnson et al. (108) demonstrated that among patients with active TB, approximately 30% of those who were HIV seropositive and more than 60% of those with AIDS had tuberculin skin reactions to 5-tuberculin units comprising less than 10 mm of induration. Retesting 1 week later did not increase the rate of positive response.

Similarly, Huebner et al. (109) found that anergy was four times and 15 times as likely for persons with CD4$^+$ counts of 200 to 400 cells/mm^3 and less than 200 cells/mm^3, respectively, as for persons with more than 499 CD4$^+$ cells/mm^3. However, 40% of patients with counts less than 200 cells/mm^3 were not anergic, suggesting that a CD4$^+$ cutoff for assuming anergy could be misleading.

Because of increased anergy, reactions of 5 mm of induration or larger are considered positive. However, in a community-based study in Baltimore, Graham et al. (110) showed that skin test positivity varied markedly between HIV-seropositive patients (14%) and HIV-seronegative patients (25%), suggesting a cutoff definition of 2 mm of induration or more in HIV-positive patients. In contrast, Huebner et al. (111) found that small (1 to 4 mm) tuberculin skin test reactions in HIV-infected patients did not represent diminished reactivity due to HIV. Of 329 nonanergic patients, 58 (18%) demonstrated at least 5 mm of induration in response to tuberculin. Sixteen patients had 1 to 4 mm of induration. Of these 16 patients, 13 (81%) showed at least 5 mm of induration in response to either *Candida* antigen, tetanus toxoid, or mumps antigen, and nine (56%) had an induration of at least 10 mm. They concluded that individuals who react to other delayed-type hypersensitivity antigens should also mount a significant reaction ($\geq$5 mm) to tuberculin if they are truly infected with *M. tuberculosis*. Any test in an HIV-positive person with a reaction of 5 mm or greater should be considered positive.

As discussed earlier, Selwyn et al. (1) prospectively demonstrated that there is an increased risk for active TB in HIV-positive patients who are PPD positive. Several studies have demonstrated that anergic HIV-infected persons are not at a high risk of developing active TB (112,113), reversing trends seen in earlier studies (114,115). Also, several trials have demonstrated that treatment of anergic HIV-infected individuals did not result in decreased mortality (112,116). In general, anergy testing does not provide useful information at the time of tuberculin skin testing.

CLINICAL PRESENTATION

Most opportunistic infections in patients with AIDS occur late in the course of HIV infection. Thus, significant CD4⁺ cell depletion is necessary for clinical disease from *Pneumocystis* species or *Mycobacterium avium-intracellulare* complex (MAC) to occur (117). Although TB disease can occur concomitantly with or after other AIDS-related opportunistic infections, it often precedes these by 1 month to 2 years. In an early CDC analysis of 159 AIDS patients with TB diagnosed between 1981 and 1986 in the state of Florida, Rieder et al. (118) found that TB preceded AIDS diagnosis by more than 1 month in 80 patients (50%), presented within 1 month of the diagnosis of AIDS in 47 patients (30%), and was diagnosed more than 1 month after diagnosis of AIDS in only 32 patients (20%). In some areas of the world, TB is often the index diagnosis for HIV infection and presents over a wide spectrum of immunodeficiency (119,120).

The literature is replete with case reports regarding the "atypical presentation" of HIV-related TB (121–126). Early descriptions suggested a propensity for negative tuberculin skin test results; radiographic features suggesting primary TB (such as mediastinal adenopathy and lack of apical infiltrates); and a high rate of extrapulmonary TB resulting in brain abscesses, tuberculomas, meningitis, pericarditis, and gastric, peritoneal, and bone TB. In contrast, several studies reported "classic" or "usual" features. The patients in these studies were presumably more immunocompetent. Some of these series were prospective; most assessed HIV seropositivity and tuberculin status while following patients for the development of TB (127–131). Four of these studies attempted some correlation with CD4⁺ cell counts. The following discussion focuses on consensus findings based on these latter studies as well as selected other reports.

Case Study

A 45-year-old black man presented to Bellevue Hospital complaining of fever, night sweats, and a 10-lb (4.5-kg) weight loss over the preceding 2 months. A mildly productive cough developed 3 weeks previously and the expectorated material became blood tinged 2 days prior to admission. He smoked cigarettes (1 pack a day for 20 years) and was formerly an intravenous drug user. HIV seropositivity was documented 1 year previously. The following were noted on physical examination: temperature, 39.4°C; respirations, 19 breaths per minute; pulse, 85 beats per minute; and blood pressure, 115/80 mm Hg. Oral thrush was present. Chest examination was unre-

markable. Abdominal examination revealed no organomegaly. Examination of the extremities revealed no cyanosis or clubbing. Laboratory data revealed a white blood cell count of 11,200/mm³ with 73% polymorphonuclear cells, 18% lymphocytes, and 9% monocytes; sedimentation rate of 83 mm/hour; sodium level of 131 mEq/L; potassium concentration of 4.1 mEq/L; and CD4⁺ cell count of 125 cells/mm³. A chest radiograph revealed bilateral hilar adenopathy with right upper lobe parenchymal nodularity (Fig. 45.1A). Subsequently, chest computed tomography (CT) demonstrated hilar and mediastinal adenopathy with central necrosis (Fig. 45.1B). The right upper lobe nodularity was seen more clearly and conformed to a "tree-in-bud" appearance (Fig. 45.1C). A tuberculin skin test result was positive with 18 mm of induration. Three sputum samples obtained for AFB staining were negative. Because of the negative sputum smears and a differential diagnosis that included lung carcinoma, the patient underwent fiberoptic bronchoscopy. The BAL fluid revealed 380 × 10³ cells/mL with 89% macrophages, 7% lymphocytes, 3% neutrophils, and 1% eosinophils. The transbronchial needle aspirate of the mediastinal nodes recovered numerous tubercle bacilli as shown on AFB staining; AFB staining of the lavage fluid was negative. A transbronchial biopsy of the right upper lobe parenchymal abnormality revealed caseating granulomas without AFB organisms. Cultures of the sputum, BAL fluid, transbronchial needle aspirate, and transbronchial biopsy all yielded tubercle bacilli.

This case report represents a typical patient with HIV-related TB. Symptoms are significant but nonspecific. Except for fever and oral thrush, the physical findings are unremarkable. TB presented in this patient early in the course of his HIV infection, with a relatively high CD4⁺ cell count and positive tuberculin skin test result suggesting less immunosuppression. Indeed, this patient had no significant opportunistic infections prior to the onset of TB. The radiographic pattern is suggestive of TB in light of the right upper lobe nodular infiltrate as well as the adenopathy. The chest CT scan is quite characteristic of TB (see below). Bronchoscopy proved useful by providing an early diagnosis: Cultures were confirmatory but unfortunately not timely.

Pulmonary involvement occurs in at least 75% of all HIV-infected patients with TB. Symptoms and physical findings are usually not predictive of TB in HIV-seropositive patients. Unfortunately, fever, sweats, fatigue, weight loss, anorexia, and cough are very common symptoms in all HIV-seropositive patients and are suggestive of diseases such as *P. carinii* pneumonia, histoplasmosis, lymphoma, wasting syndrome, and MAC disease. *M. tuberculosis* infection is now regarded as the most common cause of fever of unknown origin in HIV-infected patients (132,133). Modilevsky et al. (134) found fever (91%) and cough (84%) to be the most common presenting symptoms in a retrospective study of 39 patients in Los Angeles. Other symptoms included a mean weight loss of 11.4 ± 7.2 kg, dyspnea (64%), chest pain (25%), as well as extrapulmonary symp-

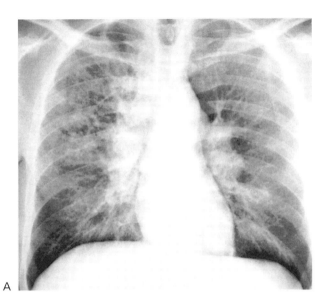

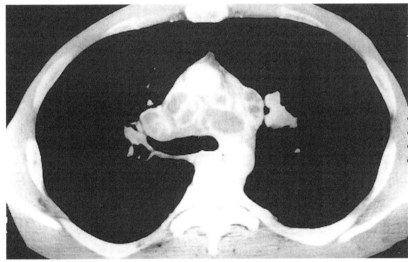

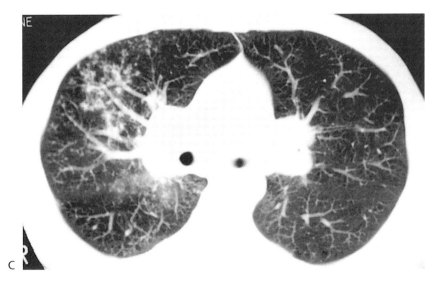

FIGURE 45.1. A: Chest radiograph reveals bilateral mediastinal and hilar adenopathy with diffuse interstitial infiltrates. **B:** Chest computed tomography scan reveals rim enhancement of the nodes with central necrosis. **C:** Characteristic "tree-in-bud" appearance in the right upper lobe is typical of tuberculosis.

toms of diarrhea (54%) and abdominal pain (26%). On physical examination the mean temperature was 39.2 ± 0.8°C. Tachypnea was observed in only 36% of patients.

Because signs and symptoms are so nonspecific, tuberculin skin testing could be a useful part of the clinical evaluation. However, more than 50% of patients with active TB and another AIDS-defining diagnosis are anergic (22,24, 108). Jones et al. (131) retrospectively categorized 97 HIV-infected patients with TB from Los Angeles. Utilizing a cutoff of induration diameter of at least 5 mm, they found positive tuberculin test results in zero of 13 patients with fewer than 100 CD4+ cells/mm³, eight (61%) of 13 patients with a CD4+ count of 101 to 200 cells/mm³, five (42%) of 12 with a CD4+ count of 201 to 300 cells/mm³, and 10 (91%) of 11 patients with a CD4+ count of more than 300 cells/mm³. Mukadi et al. (130) studied consecutive HIV-seropositive patients in Zaire who had recently received the diagnosis of pulmonary TB. Negative PPD test results and anergy were more common with increasing immunodeficiency as measured by CD4+ cell counts. Sixty (28%) of 211 patients had negative tuberculin test results despite the diagnosis of TB. When these patients were stratified according to CD4+ counts, negative PPD test results were observed in more than 50% of patients with fewer than 200 CD4+ cells/mm³, in 25% of patients with 200 to 499 CD4+ cells/mm³, and in less than 10% of patients with more than 500 CD4+ cells/mm³.

Markers of severity, such as mycobacteremia and positive AFB smears, were more common in patients with markedly depressed CD4+ cell counts, according to Jones et al. (131). In contrast, tuberculous pleuritis and positive tuberculin skin test results, which are dependent on the integrity of cellular immunity, were more common in patients with higher CD4+ cell counts. In most industrialized countries, the clinical features of TB vary according to the degree of immunosuppression, and atypical presentations are more commonly found among the most immunosuppressed patients. This may not be true for extrapulmonary TB (see below). In sub-Saharan Africa, patients with HIV-related TB are more likely to present with extrapulmonary disease, miliary infiltrates, and nonreactive tuberculin test responses than are those without HIV infection (39–42,44,48,135). Few African studies have provided clinical correlation with CD4+ cell counts. Whether patients who have been reported in African series were more immunosuppressed is unknown.

The spectrum of radiologic findings for TB in HIV-infected patients is similar to that observed in seronegative patients. A compilation of reported radiographic findings from 15 studies involving 457 HIV-positive patients in the United States revealed that more than 30% of patients presented with hilar or mediastinal adenopathy (1, 22–25,127–131,136–139). Cavitation was present in only 18% of patients, while apical or upper lobe infiltrates were seen in slightly more than 25%. Lower lobe infiltrates

(10%), diffuse (7%) or miliary patterns (7%), and pleural effusions (17%) were also observed. Normal-appearing chest radiographs were found in 6% of patients with proved TB. However, these statistics are misleading. As with clinical findings, radiographic manifestations appear to correlate with the degree of immunosuppression. Greenberg et al. (136) correlated radiographic findings with CD4+ cell counts in 68 patients. Fifty-five percent of patients with CD4+ cell counts greater than 200/mm³ showed a typical postprimary pattern compared with only 23% of those with CD4+ cell counts less than 200/mm³. Jones et al. (131) found mediastinal adenopathy in 21 of 58 patients (30% with fewer than 200 CD4+ cells/mm³ compared with only four (13%) of 30 patients with more than 200 CD4+ cells/mm³). In contrast, pleural effusions were present in six of 58 (10%) patients with ≤200 CD4+ cells/mm³ versus eight (27%) of 30 patients with more than 200 CD4+ cells/mm³.

Thus, HIV-seropositive patients with less immunosuppression (i.e., higher CD4+ cell counts) often have radiographic findings typical for reactivation. These include infiltrates in the posterior segment of the upper lobes or superior segment of the lower lobe. Cavitation may be present. As immunosuppression increases with falling CD4+ counts, "atypical" findings occur more frequently. Infiltrates can be focal, occurring in the middle and lower lobes more frequently, or can be diffuse, reticular, nodular, or even miliary. Upper lobe infiltrates and cavitation are unusual. Chest radiographs may also appear normal in 7% to 14% of patients (136,140). The clinician must maintain a high index of suspicion for TB in a patient who presents with cough and sputum production but a normal-appearing chest radiograph (141).

Unilateral and bilateral pleural effusions occur with varying frequency, ranging from 10% to 38% (22–25,128,130, 131,136,140,142–144). In a series from the United States, 44% to 50% had associated infiltrates, and 5% to 20% presented with hilar/mediastinal adenopathy. Effusions were bilateral in 10% to 28% of patients (145,146). Similarly, Batungwanayo et al. (147), in a study of HIV-related tuberculous effusions in Kigali, Rwanda, found associated localized infiltrates (28%), miliary patterns (14%), and adenopathy (11%) in 57 patients with AIDS. Richter et al. (148) in a prospective study of HIV-seropositive patients with tuberculous effusions in Dar es Salaam, Tanzania reported that one third of the patients had evidence of disseminated tuberculosis disease.

Radionucleotide studies are not routinely performed in patients with TB; however, in the workup of AIDS patients presenting with pulmonary complications, gallium scans have proved useful in distinguishing different manifestations (149). TB and lymphomas commonly show focal uptake in the hila, mediastinum, and lung parenchyma. Thallium shows high avidity for certain tumors, such as Kaposi sarcoma and lymphoma. Lee et al. (150) have demonstrated that sequential thallium–gallium scans display a focal mismatch that is specific for mycobacterial infections though fungal disease due to cryptococcosis, histoplasmosis, and coccidioidomycosis cannot be excluded.

The role of CT of the chest is limited because findings are usually nonspecific (see Chapter 26). However, subtle abnormalities, such as a miliary pattern or unsuspected cavitation, may be found. A highly characteristic finding is the presence of "low-density" hilar and mediastinal nodes (Fig. 45.1B). Peripheral enhancement of enlarged nodes is observed following the intravenous administration of contrast material. The low-density areas located centrally within the nodes are presumably due to caseation or liquefaction necrosis. Pastores et al. (151) in a retrospective study found that 20 (80%) of 25 patients with documented *M. tuberculosis* infection had low-density nodes. Although intrathoracic adenopathy has been observed in AIDS patients with lymphoma, MAC infection, fungal infection, Kaposi sarcoma, and, rarely, *P. carinii* pneumonia, low-density nodes are much less frequently present in these diseases.

DIAGNOSIS

It is estimated that sputum AFB smears are positive in 65% to 75% of HIV-seronegative patients who have had multiple specimens and in 30% to 40% of those with a single specimen (152–154). In a non-HIV setting, Kim et al. (152) found positive smears in 20% to 40% of patients with minimal disease, in 60% to 70% of patients with moderate disease, and 90% to 95% of patients with advanced cavitary disease. Similarly, Greenbaum et al. (154) reported positive smears in 52% of patients with cavitary disease but in only 32% with local infiltrates. Barnes et al. (155) found positive smears in 90% of patients with radiographic findings typical of adult reactivation; for 98% of patients with cavitary TB, AFB was found on sputum smear.

Sputum culture for *M. tuberculosis* remains the gold standard for diagnosis of pulmonary TB. In resource-poor countries the diagnosis is heavily dependent on the sputum AFB smear. HIV-positive patients have been reported to have a lower yield on AFB smears. Brindle et al. (156) measured the concentration of viable tubercle bacilli in sputum; HIV-positive patients excreted slightly fewer organisms per milliliter of sputum than did HIV-negative patients with culture-confirmed TB. Positive AFB smears were observed in 31% to 89% of patients; cultures were positive in 85% to 100% of patients. Klein et al. (157) found that only 11 (29%) of 38 patients with AIDS or AIDS-related complex had an initial positive smear compared with 35 (61%) of 57 control patients. Repeated sputum samples (up to five) brought the yield to 45%. In a study by Kramer et al. (13) analyzing the reasons for delayed diagnosis of TB, the most frequent problem was that too few (fewer than three) sputum samples were obtained for mycobacterial studies in patients with respiratory symptoms and radiographic findings suggestive of TB.

The sensitivity of sputum smears may be greater in those patients with less immunosuppression because they present with chest radiographs typical of reactivation (i.e., there is often evidence of cavitation). In contrast, patients who are more immunocompromised have chest radiographs typical of primary or miliary TB without evidence of cavitation. Close to 90% of patients with pulmonary TB have an abnormal chest radiograph whereas up to 10% have a normal chest radiograph. Findings of classic TB, such as apical infiltrates and cavitation, are less common in HIV-infected patients; mid- and lower-lung disease is more common as are lymphadenopathy, pleural effusions, and interstitial infiltrates (158).

Fiberoptic bronchoscopy is a useful means of making a rapid diagnosis of TB in selective patients. Miro et al. (159) studied 27 high-risk patients for HIV infection (only 18 of 27 patients had clinical evidence of HIV infection). Positive AFB smears were found in the sputum, BAL fluid, and/or bronchial washings in 30% of patients, compared with a 37% positive yield from bronchial brushings and/or transbronchial biopsy specimens (*p* value not significant). The addition of the transbronchial biopsy specimen increased the culture yield from 96% to 100% (*p* value not significant). They concluded that transbronchial biopsy did not contribute significantly to the diagnosis of TB. In contrast, in a retrospective study, Kennedy et al. (160) found an immediate diagnosis (positive acid-fast smear of the BAL fluid or granulomas in biopsy specimens) in 23 (34%) of 67 HIV-infected patients and 20 (44%) of 45 HIV-negative patients who had negative sputum smears prior to bronchoscopy. Transbronchial biopsy provided the exclusive means for rapid diagnosis in six (10%) of 59 patients by demonstrating granulomas. BAL provided a diagnosis exclusively in seven (12%) of 60 patients. Both techniques together provided the sole means of diagnosis in 13 (22%) of 60 patients. Salzman et al. (161) retrospectively studied 31 HIV-positive patients with smear-negative TB who underwent bronchoscopy and obtained similar results (161). An immediate diagnosis was made by evaluation of bronchoscopic specimens in 15 (48%) of 31 patients. Transbronchial biopsy was the sole positive specimen in seven patients (23%). Transbronchial needle biopsy of mediastinal adenopathy has also proved useful for diagnosing TB in otherwise sputum-negative and bronchoscopy-negative (negative findings on BAL and transbronchial biopsy) patients (162).

Interestingly, in the study by Kennedy et al. (160), 91% of prebronchoscopy sputum samples (all smear negative) yielded positive culture results, but only 63% of lavage specimens from this same group were positive. There are several factors that may explain this finding. The topical lidocaine used for local anesthesia during bronchoscopy may inhibit the growth of AFBs in culture (163). Salzman et al. (161) also analyzed bronchoscopic specimens from 40 patients in whom MAC grew in culture. An immediate identification of AFB was made in only four patients (10%). When bronchoscopy is performed, appropriate infection control practices for both HIV and TB must be followed. Proper ventilation, ultraviolet lights, filtration of air, and use of particulate respirators have been recommended to reduce nosocomial transmission of TB due to bronchoscopy (164–166).

The diagnostic approach that has elicited the most excitement recently is the polymerase chain reaction (PCR) (see Chapter 12). Diagnostic PCR is a DNA amplification technique that utilizes specific DNA sequences to serve as markers for the presence of organisms. Theoretically, PCR may detect fewer than 10 organisms in a specimen in contrast to the 10,000 organisms per milliliter necessary for smear positivity. Early experience utilizing the mycobacterial insertion element IS*6110*, a DNA sequence that is present in *M. tuberculosis*, yielded high sensitivity and specificity (167,168). However, one large clinical trial failed to demonstrate superiority over sputum AFB smears (168). Furthermore, Walker et al. (169) found that the IS*6110* sequence was found in sputum from patients with active TB as well as from a majority (75%) of patients with a history of TB. Similarly, in a study of 65 patients undergoing PCR, Schluger et al. (170) found 37 positive test results though only 23 patients had evidence of active disease. Whereas the overall sensitivity was 100%, specificity was only 70%. In this same study, Schluger et al. analyzed the use of PCR in HIV-infected patients. A subgroup of 12 patients in whom AFB smears were negative but cultures were positive had PCR evidence of *M. tuberculosis.* Eight of these patients were HIV positive; seven of eight patients had either hilar or mediastinal adenopathy as the predominant chest radiographic abnormality. All HIV-positive patients had undergone transbronchial lung or lymph node biopsy. Thus, in a small subset of HIV-infected patients PCR may prove diagnostic. Because of the limited clinical experience as well as its cost and required technical expertise, routine use of PCR cannot be recommended at this time in all patients, although it is unquestionably true that this techniques represents a substantial improvement over AFB smears alone for the diagnosis of active TB in previously untreated patients (171). This may change in some industrialized countries in light of the recent reported success by a "routine" mycobacteriology laboratory provided standardization of samples and techniques can be achieved (172–174).

Relkin et al. (145) analyzed the yield from pleural specimens in HIV-infected patients. AFB smears of pleural fluid were positive in six (15%) of 40 specimens, whereas AFB culture of the fluid was positive in 36 (91%) patients. Granulomatous changes were found in 14 (88%) of 16 patients who underwent pleural biopsy; 11 (69%) had positive AFB smears on pleural tissue, and in seven (47%) of 15 the pleural tissue cultures were positive for *M. tuberculosis.* Only the percentages for AFB on pleural tissue and the positive AFB cultures were statistically greater in HIV-positive than HIV-negative patients (145).

Although not common practice prior to the AIDS epidemic, blood culturing for mycobacteria growth is routine in HIV-infected patients. Blood cultures employing Bactec radiometric broth (Becton, Dickinson, and Company, Franklin Lakes, NJ, U.S.A.) in conjunction with an isolation lysis centrifugation system (see Chapter 11) are positive for *M. tuberculosis* in 26% to 42% of HIV-infected patients with TB (134,175–177). The frequency of positive blood cultures is inversely related to the CD4$^+$ cell count. Jones et al. (131) found that blood cultures were the only extrapulmonary source of *M. tuberculosis* in 13 of 43 patients with no more than 100 CD4$^+$ cells/mm^3. Blood cultures were positive in 18 (49%) of 37 patients with CD4$^+$ counts of 100 cells/mm^3 or less; in three (20%) of 15 patients with CD4$^+$ counts of 101 to 200 cells/mm^3, one (7%) of 15 patients with 201 to 300 CD4$^+$ cells/mm^3, and zero of eight patients with more than 300 CD4$^+$ cells/mm^3. Schluger et al. (178) performed PCR on the peripheral blood of eight patients with active TB, six of whom had HIV infection (178). There was no evidence of disseminated or extrapulmonary TB. All eight had circulating *M. tuberculosis* detected by PCR. A larger study by the same group confirmed this finding (179).

Extrapulmonary Tuberculosis

Since 1987, extrapulmonary TB has been accepted as an AIDS-defining diagnosis. The frequency of diagnosing extrapulmonary TB in HIV-infected patients may be related to the degree of immunosuppression as well as to the extent of diagnostic assessment (131,180). The frequency of extrapulmonary TB has ranged from 25% to 66% (7, 22–25,69,128,131,134,137,180–186).

Shafer et al. (180) retrospectively found extrapulmonary TB in 199 (43%) of 464 consecutive patients diagnosed at one medical center in Brooklyn, New York between 1983 and 1988. Disseminated TB (defined as being present in blood, bone marrow, or liver) was found in 76 patients (38%). Other significant extrapulmonary sites included genitourinary tract (37%), peripheral lymph nodes (22%), pleura (16%), central nervous system (14%), abdomen including nodes or peritoneum (14%), and mediastinum (12%). Only a small subset of patients (15) had CD4$^+$ cell counts; these were significantly reduced (median of 92 cells/mm^3 with a range of 11 to 677). Jones et al. (131) retrospectively found extrapulmonary TB in 30 of 97 patients with HIV-related TB diagnosed at a municipal hospital in Los Angeles, California, between 1990 and 1991. Extrapulmonary TB correlated with the degree of immunosuppression, increasing as CD4$^+$ cell counts fell. Most patients (47 of 79, or 59%) had CD4$^+$ cell counts lower than 300/mm^3.

Only five (28%) of 18 had more than 300 CD4$^+$ cells/mm^3. Positive blood cultures were the only extrapulmonary source in 14 patients (15%). Hill et al. (181) retrospectively reviewed 79 patients presenting with disseminated TB between 1984 and 1987 at two municipal hospitals in Brooklyn. Dissemination was categorized either as miliary TB (miliary pattern on chest radiograph, or miliary lesions on liver, bone marrow biopsy, or autopsy) or "focal disseminated" (concurrent involvement of at least two noncontiguous organ sites). HIV-disseminated disease caused major constitutional symptoms, occurring in 8% of all patients with newly diagnosed TB with a high short-term mortality rate (25%). Of note, a miliary chest radiographic pattern was observed in 20 patients (20%); pleural effusions in 12 (15%); and a normal chest radiograph in 7 (9%).

Not all studies found a progressive increase in the frequency of extrapulmonary TB with decreasing CD4$^+$ cell counts (69,182,183,186). Llibre et al. (182) reviewed their experience with 73 HIV-infected patients admitted to a hospital in Barcelona, Spain between 1984 and 1990. TB was extrapulmonary in 47% of patients in whom it was the first opportunistic HIV infection and in 47% with previously diagnosed AIDS. The location of TB and its dissemination were not significantly linked to a more profound reduction in CD4$^+$ cell counts. CD4$^+$ counts were 294 ± 101, 229 ± 96, and 205 ± 110 cells/mm^3 for pulmonary, extrapulmonary, and disseminated TB, respectively. Of patients without a previous diagnosis of AIDS (58/73), pulmonary TB appeared in only 31 (53%). Extrapulmonary involvement included peripheral lymph nodes in nine (15.5%), miliary TB in nine (15.5%), meninges in five (8.6%), and skeleton in one (1.7%). All of these extrapulmonary localized or disseminated forms of TB occurred when the patients were less immunocompromised. Perrone et al. (183) reported similar findings from Paris in a study of 56 HIV-related TB patients followed between 1983 and 1989. Forty-two of 56 had extrapulmonary involvement, including 37 patients (66%) in whom TB occurred before the diagnosis of AIDS. Seventy-six percent of this latter group had extrapulmonary involvement. The mean CD4$^+$ count in this group was 281 cells/mm^3. There was no significant difference in the mean CD4$^+$ count in patients with pulmonary (232 cells/mm^3) versus those with extrapulmonary (243 cells/mm^3) TB. In this series, tuberculous hepatitis was the most common extrapulmonary diagnosis (32%), owing to the frequent use of needle biopsy of the liver. In southern France TB presented as pulmonary in 53 patients, extrapulmonary in 36 patients (29.3%), and combined in 34 patients (27.6%) (69). There was no statistically significant difference among these locations as to the mean CD4$^+$ cell count (155 ± 27, 157 ± 26, and 181 ± 33 cells/mm^3, respectively). Cervical lymph nodes were the most common extrapulmonary site in this study.

Sub-Saharan African patients with HIV-related TB are more likely to present with extrapulmonary disease

(39,42,46,48,135). Significant extrapulmonary disease has been seen in Malawi (57%), Nairobi, Kenya (57%), Zambia (60%), as well as Kinshasa, Zaire (48%) (42,46,48,184, 187). Lymphadenopathy, both intrathoracic and extrathoracic, is the most common extrapulmonary manifestation.

In patients with extrapulmonary TB, normal-appearing chest radiographs are found for 10% to 15% of patients, which is similar in frequency to that for non-HIV TB (180,181). Although respiratory secretions from 71% of patients grew *M. tuberculosis,* only 25% had a positive AFB smear. Acid-fast smears of stool are positive in 40% of patients with HIV infection and TB (134). This probably represents organisms in swallowed sputum, since these patients have positive sputum smears and rarely exhibit gastrointestinal TB.

An unusual extrapulmonary manifestation is the formation of TB abscesses. Lupatkin et al. (185) described tuberculous abscess formation in atypical locations in AIDS patients. These patients represented 12% of the AIDS-associated TB cases diagnosed over a 2-year period. Abscesses were found in the neck, mediastinum, liver, abdominal wall, pancreas, and psoas muscle (without vertebral involvement). In some patients abscess was the initial presentation of tuberculous disease as well as the first AIDS-defining illness.

Multidrug-Resistant Tuberculosis Outbreaks

HIV-infected patients are more likely to acquire TB when exposed to other patients with TB (188). Indeed, the infection can progress rapidly to cause clinical disease (189). Two recent studies—one from San Francisco (190) and one from New York City (191)—suggested that in most HIV-infected persons, TB might be due to a recent transmission rather than reactivation.

The emergence of MDR-TB has drawn considerable media as well as scientific attention, as New York City had the misfortune of becoming the epicenter of the MDR-TB epidemic. A nationwide survey found that more than 60% of all cases in the United States were located in New York City (192). In 1993, Frieden et al. (193) reported that 33% of new isolates in New York City (during a 1-month observation period in 1991) were resistant to at least one drug; 26% were resistant to isoniazid (INH) and 19% to both INH and rifampin. Some individual hospitals have also observed a striking increase in MDR-TB. At Bellevue Hospital Center, 16% of patients were resistant to both INH and rifampin (11). This represented a dramatic increase from 1971, when 2.5% of isolates had combined resistance to INH and rifampin. Similarly, at Kings County Hospital Center, another large municipal hospital in Brooklyn, New York, the overall resistance rate was 31% (194). By 1996, Frieden et al. (195) reported that a multiinstitutional outbreak of highly drug-resistant TB in New York City accounted for nearly one fourth of cases of MDR-TB in the

United States during a 43-month period. Of 267 patients with an identical or nearly identical strain of drug resistant TB, 96% had nosocomially acquired disease at 11 hospitals in New York City. Of the 267 patients, 86% were infected with the human immunodeficiency virus.

Because of the increased susceptibility of HIV-infected individuals, nosocomial transmission has been reported with drug-sensitive TB and MDR-TB (189). The latter is characterized by rapid progression from exposure to active disease as well as a high rate of mortality. Small et al. (88) reported exogenous reinfection with MDR-TB organisms in patients with advanced TB, utilizing analysis of restriction fragment length polymorphisms on serial isolates obtained in hospitalized patients. Exogenous reinfection occurred either during therapy for the original infection or after therapy had been completed.

Since 1990, several outbreaks of MDR-TB have been reported to the CDC: 8 hospital clusters, 1 prison outbreak, and 1 community-acquired outbreak (196). They spread rapidly, involved large numbers of patients, and occurred in either hospitals or prisons (196–202). The reported outbreaks have occurred mostly in New York, New Jersey, and Florida. The total number of all cases is approximately 300. Transmission has occurred from patient to patient as well as from patient to health care worker.

Factors that have led to these MDR-TB outbreaks are multiple. The increased incidence of TB in areas with a high prevalence of HIV infection resulted in the placement of highly contagious persons (TB) with highly susceptible immunocompromised patients. This resulted in close confinement of these two populations in hospitals, homeless shelters, and prisons. It has become evident that most of these institutions had inadequate infection control practices. Failure to observe isolation practices as well as lack of adequate negative-pressure ventilation in isolation rooms was the norm. Even in hospitals that have had prior outbreaks of MDR-TB, the infection control processes were not adequate. In one study of two hospitals, 19% of MDR-TB patients were not isolated on the first day of admission to the hospital (203). Finally, delayed diagnosis of TB as well as failure to recognize the potential for drug resistance has resulted in ineffective therapy. Failure to recognize drug resistance was often due to the delay in obtaining drug susceptibility tests. Failure to diagnose TB was due to failure to suspect TB and obtain appropriate smears and cultures as well as the result of coexisting infection in the lungs (such as with *Pneumocystis* organisms). In one outbreak, transmission was associated with the administration of aerosolized pentamidine to patients with active TB (197). The rooms used for pentamidine aerosolization had positive air pressure relative to the adjacent clinic areas.

Recently, Jacobs et al. (204) reported on a new culture assay utilizing a light-producing reaction catalyzed by the firefly enzyme luciferase. Drug susceptibility was assessed by a method based on the efficient production of photons by viable mycobacteria infected with a specific reporter phage expressing the firefly luciferase gene. Culture of conventional drug-susceptible strains with antituberculosis drugs such as INH and rifampin resulted in light extinction. In contrast, light signals persisted after luciferase reporter phage infection of drug-resistant strains. This technique may reduce the time required for drug sensitivity studies from weeks to days, a necessary improvement in the management and prevention of MDR-TB (205). Other technologies, such as those employing molecular beacons for rapid identification of drug resistance, are also under investigation (206).

Increased attention and improved infection control techniques have greatly reduced the incidence of MDR-TB outbreaks in the United States. Outbreaks in other areas of the world demonstrate that without vigilance this issue will continue to complicate TB control efforts. In Argentina, the high prevalence of primary multidrug resistance in Argentina may be related to outbreaks among HIV-infected patients in metropolitan hospitals (207). In Russia, outbreaks have been demonstrated in the prison system (80). In other countries, MDR-TB is becoming more prevalent in the general population while HIV rates are increasing too. High rates of MDR-TB were shown by Pablos-Mendez in New Dehli in the WHO's global surveillance for drug resistance project in 1994 to 1997 (207).

TREATMENT

The treatment of persons coinfected with HIV and TB can be a clinically rewarding experience but one that has become increasingly complex in the era of HAART. Although the initiation of therapy for HIV-related TB follows the general principles for the management of TB in the HIV-uninfected person, special considerations include the following: (a) the potential for drug–drug interactions when antituberculosis therapy and HIV-related antiretrovirals are coadministered; (b) timing for the initiation of HIV-related therapy for persons diagnosed with both infections simultaneously; and (c) the potential for prolongation of therapy in persons with advanced immunosuppression due to HIV infection.

Therapy for TB should be instituted rapidly when the disease is suspected in an HIV-infected person. A brisk clinical response to standard antituberculosis therapy has been observed in many series of HIV-infected patients (208–213). Therapy for TB leads to an improvement in TB-related symptoms but also in markers of HIV disease as CD4 counts rise and viral loads fall independent of specific therapy for HIV (103).

Most published series regarding therapy demonstrated a good response utilizing regimens containing both INH and rifampin (7,22,24,72,127,128,183,186,214–216). Current recommendations from the CDC are to use an initial regimen of INH, rifampin, and pyrazinamide. A fourth drug, most often ethambutol, is used in areas with drug resistance rates ≥4%. No adjustment in dosage of antituberculosis medications is necessary for HIV-infected persons. Although the poor absorption of antituberculosis drugs in HIV-infected patients has been a theoretical concern, poor absorption leading to treatment failure has been rarely reported and for most patients is thought not to be clinically significant. Even patients documented to have low drug levels have had excellent clinical outcomes (217). Therapeutic drug monitoring is recommended only for patients with failure or relapse where malabsorption is suspected.

Time to defervescence, sputum conversion, and resolution of radiographic abnormalities occurs as rapidly with HIV-infected patients as in noninfected patients (156,186,214). One recent study demonstrated high culture conversion rates; an incredible 97.3% of HIV-infected patients had converted sputum cultures to negative at 2 months with the standard four-drug regimen (218). Other studies have also demonstrated high rates of culture conversion (208,209).

One of the first series with detailed information on the response of HIV-infected patients to antituberculosis therapy came from a retrospective cohort study by Small et al. (186) of 132 patients. Most patients were treated with INH, rifampin, and pyrazinamide or ethambutol. Therapy resulted in sterilization of sputum in a median of 10 weeks, and treatment failures or relapses occurred in only 6% of patients, comparing favorably with results in non–HIV-infected patients. Seven deaths occurred in untreated patients (five related to TB). Of 125 treated patients, an additional 96 patients had died by the time of analysis; TB was the cause of death in only four patients and a contributory factor in an additional four patients.

Several prospective studies have now confirmed the efficacy of antituberculosis therapy in HIV-seropositive patients with drug-susceptible TB (210–212, 219,220). Jones et al. (208) prospectively evaluated 89 patients of whom 82 received daily INH, rifampin, and pyrazinamide with or without ethambutol for 2 months followed by daily INH plus rifampin for 7 months. Therapy was self-administered in two thirds and directly observed in one third of cases. All patients demonstrated rapid clinical improvement within the first month of therapy; sputum cultures reverted to negative after 3 months of therapy in 52 of 54 patients from whom specimens were obtained. Treatment failure occurred in only five (6%) patients, four of whom were noncompliant. Of the 66 patients who completed therapy, none relapsed.

Perriëns et al. (219) prospectively studied the efficacy of a short-course regimen consisting of 2 months of daily INH, rifampin, pyrazinamide, and ethambutol with subsequent twice-weekly INH and rifampin for 4 months. Following completion of this phase of therapy, the HIV-seropositive patients who had no evidence of TB were randomized to receive INH plus rifampin or placebo for an additional 6 months. A total of 260 HIV-seropositive and 186 HIV-seronegative patients were evaluated. Sputum smear conversion occurred in 88% of patients after 2 months of therapy and 99% after 4 months of therapy. Cultures were negative in 93% of patients after 2 months. There was no difference between HIV-seropositive and seronegative patients.

At the end of the 6-month treatment more HIV-seropositive than HIV-seronegative patients continued to cough (17% vs. 8%) and continued to produce sputum (21% vs. 11%). The rate of treatment failure was similar in both groups: 3.8% among HIV-seropositive patients and 2.7% among HIV-seronegative patients. At the end of 24 months, HIV-seropositive patients who received extended therapy with INH and rifampin had a significantly lower relapse rate (1.9%) than patients who received placebo (9%) ($p < 0.01$). However, there was no difference in overall survival between those assigned to INH plus rifampin and those assigned to placebo (83% and 84%, respectively).

Most experts now believe that the initial treatment regimen for TB for all patients (including HIV-negative patients) in large urban areas (where primary resistance may be greater than 4%) should include INH, rifampin, pyrazinamide, and ethambutol. After 2 months of therapy, drug susceptibility information should determine the subsequent therapy. In HIV-positive patients with drug-susceptible organisms, the CDC and American Thoracic Society (ATS) recommend that INH and rifampin be continued to complete a total of 6 months of therapy for most patients (221). DOT has been recommended for all patients with HIV-related TB. Response to therapy should be assessed by clinical, bacteriologic, and radiographic examinations.

Intermittent therapy for pansusceptible TB, at least in the continuation phase of therapy, has become the standard of care for most patients with TB treated in local health departments. Intermittent therapy improves adherence, is less costly, and has had high success rates (222). However, two recent trials have dampened the enthusiasm for intermittent therapy in patients treated for HIV-related TB. In U.S. Public Heath Service Study 22, a trial that compared rifapentine and INH given once a week with rifampin and INH given twice a week in the continuation phase of therapy, persons with HIV infection were removed from further participation in the study when four of 30 patients in the rifapentine arm relapsed with rifampin-resistant TB (223). In another study, U.S. Public Health Service Study 23, patients with HIV-related pansusceptible TB were treated with an intermittent rifabutin–based regimen in the continuation phase of treatment (after the first 2 months). The trial's data safety monitoring board advised suspending enrollment in the trial because of the occurrence of five cases of failure/relapse with acquired rifamycin resistance (224). Although the rate of treatment failure or relapse in the study was low, all five patients with failure/relapse had acquired rifamycin resistance. Common features in patients with acquired rifamycin resistance were low CD4 counts and twice-weekly therapy in the continuation phase of therapy (after the first 2 months). Whether or not a similar phenomenon will occur with rifampin, which has a shorter half-life, is not clear.

In a study that used INH and rifampin twice a week in the continuation phase of therapy, two patients relapsed with rifampin-resistant TB (210). One patient had received a total of 6 months of therapy and the other 9 months. For one patient thought to have a relapse, the "relapse" organism had a different restriction fragment length polymorphism analysis of chromosomal DNA indicating that it was a new infection rather than a relapse. The other relapse case did not have an organism available for DNA fingerprinting. Until more data are available, CDC has recommended that persons with HIV–TB coinfection and CD4 cell counts less than 100/mm^3 not be treated with highly intermittent (once or twice weekly) regimens. These patients should receive daily therapy during the intensive phase, and daily or three-times-a-week therapy during the continuation phase (224).

HAART, which usually includes protease inhibitors or nonnucleoside reverse transcriptase inhibitors, has radically changed the care of persons with HIV disease. In populations with access to these medications it has improved the clinical prognosis, leading to a decreased rate of hospitalizations and a decline in morbidity and mortality (225,226). However, the potential for complicated drug–drug interactions when treating a patient with TB and HIV, particularly the interactions of the rifamycins with protease inhibitors and nonnucleoside reverse transcriptase inhibitors, could be an obstacle for patients requiring treatment for both. Many patients are first diagnosed with AIDS at the time of TB diagnosis. For these patients starting therapy for TB is urgent because TB is a public health threat and can lead to death if not managed promptly. For patients who receive a diagnosis of TB and HIV simultaneously, treatment for TB must be initiated but the decision about when to start antiretroviral therapy is more difficult.

The major obstacle in the concurrent management of HIV and TB stems from the significant drug interactions of the rifamycins and two classes of antiretroviral medications: the nonnucleoside reverse transcriptase inhibitors and HIV protease inhibitors. Rifampin is a key component of the antituberculosis regimen, but rifampin is a significant inducer of the cytochrome P450 system, CYP3A, and therefore greatly increases the metabolism of many drugs, including protease inhibitors and nonnucleoside reverse transcriptase inhibitors. Increased metabolism of these drugs can lead to decreased blood levels, and low levels of antiretrovirals may lead to HIV treatment failure and development of HIV drug resistance (227).

The CDC has published guidelines for the use rifamycins for the management of TB among HIV-infected patients taking protease inhibitors or nonnucleoside reverse

transcriptase inhibitors (228). Because these drug interactions are complex and data on their use are limited, therapy should be guided by expert consultation. As new antiretroviral drugs are developed and data are obtained, recommendations for use of these drugs in combination with antituberculosis medications will change. An initial report from New York City demonstrated that most health care providers were recommending combination regimens inappropriately using rifampin in combination with antiretroviral regimen containing protease inhibitors, contrary to established recommendations (229). Some data indicate that rifampin can be used in specific instances for the management of active TB, as was specified in a CDC recommendation. If a patient must receive antiretrovirals and a rifamycin simultaneously, use of rifampin may be considered in the following situations: (a) in patients taking the nonnucleoside reverse transcriptase inhibitor efavirenz and two nucleoside reverse transcriptase inhibitors; (b) in patients whose antiretroviral regimen includes the protease inhibitor ritonavir and one or more nucleoside reverse transcriptase inhibitors; or (c) in patients whose antiretroviral regimen includes the combination of two protease inhibitors, such as ritonavir and saquinavir (230). Of the three available rifamycins, rifampin is the most potent inducer of the CYP3A, rifapentine intermediate, and rifabutin the least. Rifampin leads to markedly decreased levels (75% to 90%) of the protease inhibitors other than ritonavir and would almost certainly lead to decreased antiviral effects (231). Because rifabutin has been used with success in the management of active TB in patients without HIV (232,233) and has less of an effect on blood levels of the antiretroviral agent(s), its use has also been recommended when treatment is coadministered. Rifabutin can be used with all of the currently approved protease inhibitors (indinavir, nelfinavir, saquinavir, ritonavir, amprenavir, and the fixed combination lopinavir/ritonavir) and with certain nonnucleoside reverse transcriptase inhibitors (efavirenz and nevirapine) (228).

Protease inhibitors are potent inhibitors of the P450 system and therefore increase the serum concentrations of drugs metabolized by that enzyme system. Rifabutin is a substrate of CYPA3, and inhibitors of that system, like the protease inhibitors, can increase concentrations of rifabutin and one of its metabolites to toxic levels. To avoid toxic concentrations the daily dose of rifabutin should be adjusted to 150 mg except with saquinavir hard-gel capsules where the dose remains at 300 mg. For nelfinavir, indinavir, and amprenavir. The dose of rifabutin can be 300 mg two or three times a week for patients receiving an intermittent regimen (not recommended for patients with CD4 cell counts less than 100/mm^3). Because ritonavir substantially increases the levels of rifabutin, the dose of rifabutin should be adjusted to 150 mg two or three times a week when given with ritonavir.

For the nonnucleoside reverse transcriptase inhibitors, nevirapine can be given with a daily rifabutin dose of 300 mg. Concentrations of nevirapine are slightly decreased as are concentrations of rifabutin when they are coadministered. When used with nevirapine, rifabutin might also be prescribed as 300 mg two or three times a week. Because efavirenz is a CYP3A inducer, the daily dose of rifabutin should be adjusted to 450 or 600 mg when they are used together. Rifabutin may be given at 600 mg two or three times a week when prescribed with efavirenz. Delaviridine should not be used with the rifamycins (228).

To date little clinical information for patients treated simultaneously for both infections has been published. One series from the A. G. Holley State Tuberculosis Hospital in Florida examined the effects of rifabutin in patients receiving HAART. All 25 patients receiving therapy for TB were culture negative within 2 months of the initiation of therapy, and 20 of 25 patients had undetectable viral loads (<500 copies/mL) during therapy (232). The paucity of data and lack of long-term follow-up has led some experts to urge caution regarding coadministration of these therapies. One expert in TB control has advised avoiding the use of rifabutin in patients receiving protease inhibitors or nonnucleoside reverse transcriptase inhibitors, at least until more data are available (234). Additional clinical trials using these drugs in combination, including pharmacokinetic studies, are in progress.

Beyond the complexities of the drug–drug interactions, in many instances starting therapy for both conditions is impractical. The pill burden is large at the beginning of treatment for TB and the additional pill burden for HIV infection can be overwhelming. In addition, overlapping toxicities make the sorting out of any side effects extremely difficult. In a study from London of patients with dual infection, 99 (54%) of 183 patients had adverse events during therapy requiring change or interruption of HIV treatment, TB treatment, or both. Patients on concomitant antiretroviral and antituberculosis therapy were significantly more likely to suffer an adverse event (223). For most patients who have highly effective therapy available for both conditions, it is better to delay antiretroviral therapy. After the second month of TB therapy the treatment is simplified for most patients at least by having a decreased pill burden, which may allow the initiation of antiretroviral treatment at that time.

The optimal time to start antiretroviral therapy in coinfected patients has not been determined. HIV-infected persons may present with relatively high CD4 counts where HIV therapy may not even be indicated according to current guidelines. Some studies have shown advanced immunosuppression in most HIV-infected patients presenting with TB, and for these patients starting an effective antiviral therapy is more critical. In a study in London by Dean et al. (233), 39% of patients with a CD4 count of fewer than 100×10^6 cells/L that were not receiving antiretrovirals had an additional AIDS-defining illness during treatment for TB. This led to their recommendation of

early initiation of HAART in TB patients with CD4 counts less than 100×10^6 cells/L.

An additional concern in starting antiretroviral therapy in the coinfected patient is the possibility of a paradoxical reaction. Paradoxical reactions are transient worsening of signs or symptoms related to TB that do not represent failure of treatment or a second process. Paradoxical reactions were described prior to the era of HIV disease; a small percentage of patients may have developed symptomatic tuberculomas or increased lymphadenopathy, worsening fever, cough, or infiltrates on chest radiograph with the start of antituberculosis therapy (235–247). This syndrome is common in coinfected patients, most often after the start of HAART (238,239). The incidence of paradoxical reactions is probably related to the reconstitution of T-cell proliferation and function leading to increased interferon-γ secretion after initiation of HAART (240). These symptoms can be significant and distressing to the patient and must be a consideration in the decision of when to start antiretroviral treatment.

As noted above, relapse rates after standard therapy have been acceptably low, and in most studies rates have been similar to those in uninfected populations. A review of studies showing low relapse rates led to the current CDC/ATS recommendation of 6 months of standard therapy in patients with pansusceptible TB (222). However, isolated reports with small numbers of patients have documented relapses after completion of therapy (241–243), and some lingering concern exists regarding the optimal duration of therapy in these patients. A large study in Zaire demonstrated a high relapse rate of 9% in HIV-infected patients with TB treated with a standard 6-month regimen (219). However, in this study only one half of the doses in the continuation phase were observed and the authors did not determine if relapses were from recurrence of disease with the same strain of *M. tuberculosis* or if there was reinfection with a new strain. There was no significant difference in the mortality rates between the patients who were treated for 6 months and those treated for 12 months.

A recent retrospective review from New York City showed a significantly higher relapse rate in HIV-infected patients compared to uninfected patients and a relapse rate of 7.9% for HIV-infected patients treated for less than 36 weeks (221). Some authorities have remained skeptical about 6-month therapy for TB in HIV-infected patients, and the CDC/ATS guidelines do recommend prolonging treatment for patients who have had a delayed clinical and bacteriologic response to antituberculosis therapy (222). Relapse rates among patients with HIV-associated TB should be interpreted with caution, however, as several studies using restriction fragment length polymorphism analysis have demonstrated that many cases initially classified as relapses are in fact caused by exogenous reinfection (244,245).

The mortality rate from HIV-related TB has ranged from 14% to 44%. Studies from Africa suggested that HIV-seropositive patients have a 5-fold to 14-fold greater risk of dying during treatment than HIV-seronegative patients (246,247). However, recent reports have been more encouraging. A study from Grady Memorial Hospital in Atlanta showed improved survival rates in the decade from 1991 to 2000 (248). The 1-year survival rates in patients with both HIV and TB was 58% in 1991 and increased to 83% in 1997. This improvement was attributed to improvements in TB and HIV therapy. Death occurring early in the course of treatment for TB is more likely attributable to TB (or failure to diagnose TB) than that occurring later in the course of treatment. Bacterial superinfections as well as other HIV-related opportunistic diseases are more likely to occur late in the course of treatment. Even in Africa the increased mortality appears to be mostly due to bacterial infections with *Salmonella typhimurium*, other gram-negative rods, and *Streptococcus pneumoniae;* hypersensitivity reactions; and cerebral space-occupying lesions (41,247).

Prior to initiation of therapy, it is crucial to consider whether a patient is likely to be infected with a drug-resistant organism. The prevalence of drug-resistant TB is falling in most of the large urban areas of the United States. In New York City, the 25 cases of MDR-TB reported in 2000 represented a 94.3% decrease from the 441 cases reported in 1992. However, a therapeutic regimen should be designed to cover this possibility if (a) there has been close contact with a patient known to have MDR-TB within the previous 6 months; (b) previous treatment was consistent with an inadequate regimen (based on knowledge of prior culture and sensitivity results); (c) relapse occurs after an apparent initial clinical response; and (d) rapid progressive clinical and radiologic deterioration occurs within the first 4 weeks of therapy (138).

By definition, multidrug-resistant organisms are resistant to at least two drugs, usually INH and rifampin. In patients suspected of having MDR-TB, various five- and six-drug regimens have been advocated. Fischl et al. (200,249) from Jackson Memorial Hospital in Florida reported response to therapy in 62 HIV-positive patients with MDR-TB who were diagnosed between 1988 and 1990. Of the 62 patients, only four (7%) converted to smear negative whereas 11 (18%) who were smear negative remained so. Seven (11%) had persistently positive smears and 39 (63%) had intermittent smears throughout the course of therapy. Only 30 patients were treated for longer than 2 months; 25 received two or more effective drugs. Of these patients, only two had three consecutive negative cultures. It took a mean of 273 days to become culture negative. The median survival time was 2.1 months. Similar poor prognosis has been experienced elsewhere. At Bellevue Hospital, 88 HIV-positive patients with MDR-TB were treated from 1983 through 1992 (250). The mortality rate at 12 months was 61%.

Effective therapy for MDR-TB requires utilization of "second-line drugs" such as ethionamide, capreomycin,

cycloserine, paraaminosalicylic acid, as well as ethambutol, pyrazinamide, and streptomycin (see Chapter 48) (251). Alternative aminoglycosides, such as kanamycin and amikacin, have been utilized. A minimum of three new drugs that the patient has not received (and for which *in vitro* susceptibilities are known) should be initiated. Most often a fourth drug, usually a fluoroquinolone such as ciprofloxacin, ofloxacin, or levofloxacin, is used. Because levofloxacin can be given once a day, is generally well tolerated and has superior bactericidal activity in animal models (252). It is the quinolone most frequently used by the New York City Department of Health and Mental Hygiene. It is frequently helpful to include one parenteral drug in the prescribed regimen to be used for the first several months. The New York City Department of Health and Mental Hygiene has recommended that an aminoglycoside or capreomycin be continued until 6 months after culture conversion and that the total length of therapy should be extended to 24 months (253). These recommendations are similar to those published by WHO (254). In most situations, patients with MDR-TB will begin therapy under hospital observation so as to monitor potential toxicity as well as to isolate the patient until there is a response to therapy.

A relatively high rate of adverse reactions in HIV-positive patients due to TB chemotherapy has been reported. In Africa there has been an extraordinarily high rate of mucocutaneous reactions due to thiacetazone, requiring discontinuation (255,256). Occasionally, toxic epidermal necrolysis and death have been reported. In the recent study from Zaire by Perriëns et al. (209), 11% of patients developed a papular pruritic rash but did not require cessation of therapy. In the United States, Small et al. (186) reported that 18% of patients required alteration of their antituberculosis chemotherapy due to adverse reactions such as rash, gastrointestinal intolerance, and hepatitis. This compares to a 4% incidence in a non–HIV-infected population (257). Adverse effects were attributed to rifampin in 12%, pyrazinamide in 6%, INH in 4%, and ethambutol in 2% of patients. Most adverse effects occurred within the first 2 months of therapy. In the study by Jones et al. (208), only 5% of patients developed adverse reactions requiring alteration of therapy. Almost all reactions occurred within the first month of therapy and included jaundice, hepatitis, and rash.

In areas of the world where HAART is not widely available, another therapy option has been immunotherapy with heat-killed *Mycobacterium vaccae* (SRL172) organisms. However, a recent trial showed no improvements in bacteriologic outcomes or in survival in treated patients (258).

LATENT TUBERCULOSIS INFECTION

INH has proven effective for the management of latent TB in individuals with HIV infection (1,259). However, prior to therapy, TB must be excluded by means of history, chest radiography, and sputum culture. Inadvertent use of INH alone in a patient with TB disease may lead to drug resistance. All HIV-positive patients with a positive tuberculin skin test result, defined as 5 mm or greater, should receive treatment regardless of age.

Due to insensitivity and unreliability, anergy testing is no longer used routinely in the evaluation of tuberculin skin test reactions (260). In addition, patients may have selective anergy for the tuberculin skin test at the time of active TB disease. A negative tuberculin skin test reaction does not exclude either latent TB or active TB, even in the presence of a reaction to other antigens (261). Several recent studies have shown that anergic HIV-infected persons are not at high risk of developing active TB, which reverses earlier assumptions (112,113).

Selwyn et al. (1) found that none of 27 HIV-infected patients with a positive tuberculin test result developed TB after completing 12 months of INH therapy, at a median follow-up time of 25 months. Guelar et al. (87) prospectively studied 839 HIV-infected patients, 106 of whom had a positive tuberculin test result, Active TB developed in seven of 26 patients not receiving INH chemoprophylaxis, in four of 61 patients 3 to 27 months after completing 9 months of prophylaxis with INH (8.9 per 100 patient-years), and in none still receiving INH. Unfortunately, there was a high rate of discontinuation of INH due to intolerance (eight of 43 patients) mostly due to hepatitis. The authors suggested that the benefit of INH prophylaxis might be of short duration in HIV-infected patients. Finally, Pape et al. (259) conducted a randomized trial of INH and pyridoxine versus pyridoxine alone for 12 months. When the subset of PPD-positive patients was analyzed, TB developed in six (24%) of 25 patients who received pyridoxine alone versus two (5%) of 38 who received INH and pyridoxine. Thus, there were 5.7 versus 3.2 cases per 100 person-years. INH reduced the risk of TB by 83%.

The efficacy of INH alone has had limited success in part due to poor tolerance and poor patient acceptance and adherence of a lengthy regimen (262–265). Two trials have compared regimens of 2 months of rifampin and pyrazinamide to INH therapy (266,267). In a multicentered trial conducted in the United States, Brazil, Haiti, and Uganda, rifampin at a dosage of 10 to 20 mg/kg daily with a maximal dose of 600 mg and pyrazinamide at 15 to 25 mg/kg daily was compared with 12 months of INH 300 mg daily. The 2-month regimen was well tolerated, and both treatments had similar rates of adverse side effects. In the 3-year follow-up, both arms had similar rates of active TB (267). Enthusiasm for this regimen has been dampened by reports of 21 cases of liver injury including five deaths in HIV-negative patients taking the 2-month regimen of rifampin and pyrazinamide for the management of latent TB infection (268). Other investigators have also found an increased risk

of serious hepatotoxicity with the 2-month regimen of rifampin and pyrazinamide (269). This regimen may also be contraindicated for some patients receiving certain antiretrovirals due to drug–drug interactions, as discussed in the section on treatment. Other short multidrug regimens that include rifampin have been tested (116,270). In Uganda, Johnson et al. (270) found that both INH and short multidrug regimens of INH and rifampin or INH, rifampin, and pyrazinamide were effective in preventing active TB in the short term. However, the effect of INH was lost after the first year of treatment, whereas the effect in the short multidrug regimens containing rifampin was sustained for up to 3 years. These studies have not yet affected the ATS and CDC recommendations for the management of latent TB infection.

Currently, the ATS and the CDC recommend 9 months of INH. The 2-month regimen of rifampin and pyrazinamide may be considered in HIV-positive persons, but careful monitoring guidelines should be followed (268). The British Thoracic Society recommends a 6-month regimen of INH or a 3-month regimen of INH and rifampin (271). A current trial by the Tuberculosis Trials Consortium at the CDC is evaluating tolerance and efficacy of 3 months of INH and rifapentine given once a week versus 9 months of daily INH.

A more difficult problem arises in the HIV-positive patient exposed to persons with drug-resistant pulmonary TB. The CDC published extensive guidelines to assess the nature of the contact, the likelihood that the strain is that of MDR-TB, and the patient's risk for developing active TB. All high-risk contacts (shared household, close social contact) should be presumed infected with drug-resistant organisms, even if tuberculin negative. The regimen for the management of latent TB infection will vary depending on the susceptibilities of the isolate from the source case. With INH resistance only, rifampin may be used. For contacts to MDR-TB, the treatment regimen is speculative. The combined use of pyrazinamide and either ethambutol or a fluoroquinolone may be used.

INFECTION CONTROL

Transmission of TB is influenced by the infectiousness of the source patient as well as the susceptibility of the contact. Two conflicting theories pertain to this issue. First, HIV-infected TB patients may be less contagious since cavity formation is less frequent. Alternatively, these patients may be more infectious because the diminished cell-mediated immunity caused by HIV may allow extensive replication of tubercle bacilli in the lungs that could be expectorated in droplet form.

Many studies have attempted to answer this question (40,43,127). Pitchenik et al. (127) in Florida observed no significant difference in the unadjusted tuberculin rate among 102 home contacts of HIV-positive and HIV-negative patients. However, the HIV status of the contacts was not known, which may have led to a significant false-negative rate. The frequency of positive acid-fast smears is a marker of infectivity. As discussed earlier, HIV-positive and HIV-negative patients have a similar percentage of positive smears. Elliott et al. (272) conducted a cross-sectional tuberculin study among household contacts of HIV-positive and HIV-negative patients with bacteriologically confirmed TB in Zambia. A total of 207 contacts of 43 HIV-positive patients and 141 contacts of 28 HIV-negative patients were compared. Fifty-two percent of contacts of HIV-positive patients developed a positive tuberculin test result compared with 71% of contacts of HIV-negative patients ($p < 0.001$). A positive tuberculin response was related to the number of bacilli seen in the sputum smear of the index case patient. This group speculated that HIV-positive patients carry a lower bacillary load in their sputum and therefore may be less infectious. Nunn et al. (43) conducted a similar study in Kenya. They diagnosed TB in 13 (5.1%) of 255 contacts of HIV-negative index patients in contrast to eight (7.8%) of 102 contacts of HIV-positive patients. The difference was not statistically different. However, HIV-positive contacts were more likely to develop TB. These authors concluded that HIV-1 did not enhance the infectiousness of TB.

A recent meta-analysis that included data from 11 studies found that the prevalence of skin test positivity and active disease were similar regardless of the HIV status in the index case. The authors also concluded that TB patients with HIV infection were not intrinsically more infectious to their contacts than were HIV-negative TB patients (273).

Bacille Calmette–Guérin Vaccination

Bacille Calmette–Guérin (BCG) is a live attenuated strain of *Mycobacterium bovis* used throughout the world for vaccinating newborns against *M. tuberculosis*. The protection obtained has varied from zero to 80%, and a meta-analysis of 26 BCG trials concluded that the most consistent benefit is a reduction in the incidence of disseminated TB in infants and children (274). There is no evidence that BCG vaccine is protective in HIV-infected persons. Concerns regarding its safety in HIV-positive patients have been raised (275,276). Weltman and Rose (277) reviewed the reported BCG complications in HIV-infected patients. Complications included regional suppurative adenitis months after vaccination, local ulceration at the injection site, and disseminated disease (277–281). Serious BCG complications have not occurred in prospective studies of HIV-infected infants (282,283). The WHO recommends vaccination for asymptomatic HIV-infected children who are at risk for TB (284). The WHO does not recommend BCG vaccination for children or adults with asymptomatic HIV infection or for persons suspected of being HIV

infected with minimal risk for *M. tuberculosis*. In the United States, there is minimal indication for BCG vaccination. Furthermore, both the CDC and the ATS find HIV infection to be a contraindication for BCG vaccination (285,286).

REFERENCES

1. Selwyn PA, Hartel D, Lewis VA, et al. A prospective study of the risk of tuberculosis among intravenous drug users with human immunodeficiency virus infection. *N Engl J Med* 1989; 320:545–550.
2. World Health Organization TB Program: www.who.int/gtb/policyrd. TBHIV.htm, 2002.
3. World Health Organization. *Global tuberculosis control: surveillance, planning, financing.* Geneva: WHO Report, 2002:15–39.
4. Khatri GR, Frieden TR. Controlling tuberculosis in India. *N Engl J Med* 2002;347:1420–1425.
5. Murray JF, Felton CP, Garay SM, et al. Pulmonary complications of the acquired immunodeficiency syndrome. Report of a National Heart, Lung, and Blood Institute workshop. *N Engl J Med* 1984;310:1682–1688.
6. Vieira J, Frank E, Spira TJ, et al. Acquired immune deficiency in Haitians: opportunistic infections in previously healthy Haitian immigrants. *N Engl J Med* 1983; 308:125–129.
7. Pitchenik AE, Fischl MA, Dickinson GM, et al. Opportunistic infections and Kaposi's sarcoma among Haitians: evidence of a new acquired immunodeficiency state. *Ann Intern Med* 1983; 98:277–284.
8. Pape JW, Liautaud B, Thomas F, et al. Characteristics of the acquired immunodeficiency syndrome (AIDS) in Haiti. *N Engl J Med* 1983;309:945–950.
9. World Health Organization. *Global tuberculosis report 2000.* Geneva, WHO Report, 2000:20–45.
10. Bloom BR, Murray CJ. Tuberculosis: commentary on a reemergent killer. *Science* 1992;257:1055–1064.
11. Neville K, Bromberg A, Bromberg R, et al. The third epidemic—multidrug-resistant tuberculosis. *Chest* 1994;105: 45–48.
12. HIV prevalence estimates and AIDS case projections for the United States: report based upon a workshop. *MMWR Recomm Rep* 1990;39:1–31.
13. Rieder HL, Cauthen GM, Comstock GW, et al. Epidemiology of tuberculosis in the United States. *Epidemiol Rev* 1989;11: 79–98.
14. Rieder HL, Cauthen GM, Kelly GD, et al. Tuberculosis in the United States. *JAMA* 1989;262:385–389.
15. Tuberculosis morbidity—United States, 1992. *MMWR Morb Mortal Wkly Rep* 1993;42:363–364.
16. Expanded tuberculosis surveillance and tuberculosis morbidity—United States, 1993. *MMWR Morb Mortal Wkly Rep* 1994; 43:361–366.
17. Tuberculosis morbidity—United States, 1994. *MMWR Morb Mortal Wkly Rep* 1995;44:387–389, 395.
18. Snider DE Jr, Roper WL. The new tuberculosis. *N Engl J Med* 1992;326:703–705.
19. Cantwell MF, Snider DE Jr, Cauthen GM, et al. Epidemiology of tuberculosis in the United States, 1985 through 1992. *JAMA* 1994;272:535–539.
20. Brudney K, Dobkin J. Resurgent tuberculosis in New York City. Human immunodeficiency virus, homelessness, and the decline of tuberculosis control programs. *Am Rev Respir Dis* 1991;144: 745–749.

21. Landesman SH. Commentary: tuberculosis in New York City—the consequences and lessons of failure. *Am J Public Health* 1993;83:766–768.

22. Pitchenik AE, Cole C, Russell BW, et al. Tuberculosis, atypical mycobacteriosis, and the acquired immunodeficiency syndrome among Haitian and non-Haitian patients in south Florida. *Ann Intern Med* 1984;101:641–645.

23. Sunderam G, McDonald RJ, Maniatis T, et al. Tuberculosis as a manifestation of the acquired immunodeficiency syndrome (AIDS). *JAMA* 1986;256:362–366.

24. Louie E, Rice LB, Holzman RS. Tuberculosis in non-Haitian patients with acquired immunodeficiency syndrome. *Chest* 1986;90:542–545.

25. Chaisson RE, Schecter GF, Theuer CP, et al. Tuberculosis in patients with the acquired immunodeficiency syndrome. Clinical features, response to therapy, and survival. *Am Rev Respir Dis* 1987;136:570–574.

26. Handwerger S, Mildvan D, Senie R, et al. Tuberculosis and the acquired immunodeficiency syndrome at a New York City hospital: 1978–1985. *Chest* 1987;91:176–180.

27. Onorato IM, McCray E. Prevalence of human immunodeficiency virus infection among patients attending tuberculosis clinics in the United States. *J Infect Dis* 1992;165:87–92.

28. New York City Department of Health. *Tuberculosis in New York City, 1991*. New York: New York City Department of Health, 1991:1–40.

29. Frieden TR, Fujiwara PI, Washko RM, et al. Tuberculosis in New York City—turning the tide. *N Engl J Med* 1995;333:229–233.

30. New York City Department of Health. *Tuberculosis information summary, 2001*. New York: New York Department of Health, 2002:1–43.

31. Geng E, Kreiswirth B, Driver C, et al. Changes in the transmission of tuberculosis in New York City from 1990 to 1999. *N Engl J Med* 2002;346:1453–1458.

32. Braun MM, Cote TR, Rabkin CS. Trends in death with tuberculosis during the AIDS era. *JAMA* 1993;269:2865–2868.

33. Dolin PJ, Raviglione MC, Kochi A. Global tuberculosis incidence and mortality during 1990–2000. *Bull WHO* 1994;72:213–220.

34. Grzybowski S. Tuberculosis in the Third World. *Thorax* 1991;46:689–691.

35. Murray CJ, Styblo K, Rouillon A. Tuberculosis in developing countries: burden, intervention and cost. *Bull Int Union Tuberc Lung Dis* 1990;65:6–24.

36. Dye C, Scheele S, Dolin P, et al. Consensus statement. Global burden of tuberculosis: estimated incidence, prevalence, and mortality by country. WHO Global Surveillance and Monitoring Project. *JAMA* 1999;282:677–686.

37. Piot P, Quinn TC, Taelman H, et al. Acquired immunodeficiency syndrome in a heterosexual population in Zaire. *Lancet* 1984;2:65–69.

38. Mann J, Snider DE Jr, Francis H, et al. Association between HTLV-III/LAV infection and tuberculosis in Zaire. *JAMA* 1986;256:346.

39. Eriki PP, Okwera A, Aisu T, et al. The influence of human immunodeficiency virus infection on tuberculosis in Kampala, Uganda. *Am Rev Respir Dis* 1991;143:185–187.

40. Elliott AM, Luo N, Tembo G, et al. Impact of HIV on tuberculosis in Zambia: a cross sectional study. *BMJ* 1990;301:412–415.

41. Nunn P, Gicheha C, Hayes R, et al. Cross-sectional survey of HIV infection among patients with tuberculosis in Nairobi, Kenya. *Tuber Lung Dis* 1992;73:45–51.

42. Colebunders RL, Ryder RW, Nzilambi N, et al. HIV infection in patients with tuberculosis in Kinshasa, Zaire. *Am Rev Respir Dis* 1989;139:1082–1085.

43. Nunn P, Kibuga D, Elliott A, et al. Impact of human immunodeficiency virus on transmission and severity of tuberculosis. *Trans R Soc Trop Med Hyg* 1990;84 Suppl 1:9–13.

44. Richards SB, St Louis ME, Nieburg P, et al. Impact of the HIV epidemic on trends in tuberculosis in Abidjan, Cote d'Ivoire. *Tuber Lung Dis* 1995;76:11–16.

45. Standaert B, Niragira F, Kadende P, et al. The association of tuberculosis and HIV infection in Burundi. *AIDS Res Hum Retroviruses* 1989;5:247–251.

46. Kelly P, Burnham G, Radford C. HIV seropositivity and tuberculosis in a rural Malawi hospital. *Trans R Soc Trop Med Hyg* 1990;84:725–727.

47. Migliori GB, Borghesi A, Adriko C, et al. Tuberculosis and HIV infection association in a rural district of northern Uganda: epidemiological and clinical considerations. *Tuber Lung Dis* 1992;73:285–290.

48. Elliott AM, Halwiindi B, Hayes RJ, et al. The impact of human immunodeficiency virus on presentation and diagnosis of tuberculosis in a cohort study in Zambia. *J Trop Med Hyg* 1993;96:1–11.

49. Kamanfu G, Mlika-Cabanne N, Girard PM, et al. Pulmonary complications of human immunodeficiency virus infection in Bujumbura, Burundi. *Am Rev Respir Dis* 1993;147:658–663.

50. Idigbe EO, Nasidi A, Anyiwo CE, et al. Prevalence of human immunodeficiency virus (HIV) antibodies in tuberculosis patients in Lagos, Nigeria. *J Trop Med Hyg* 1994;97:91–97.

51. Braun MM, Badi N, Ryder RW, et al. A retrospective cohort study of the risk of tuberculosis among women of childbearing age with HIV infection in Zaire. *Am Rev Respir Dis* 1991;143:501–504.

52. Allen S, Batungwanayo J, Kerlikowske K, et al. Two-year incidence of tuberculosis in cohorts of HIV-infected and uninfected urban Rwandan women. *Am Rev Respir Dis* 1992;146:1439–1444.

53. Narain JP, Raviglione MC, Kochi A. HIV-associated tuberculosis in developing countries: epidemiology and strategies for prevention. *Tuber Lung Dis* 1992;73:311–321.

54. Badri M, Wilson D, Wood R. Effect of highly active antiretroviral therapy on incidence of tuberculosis in South Africa: a cohort study. *Lancet* 2002;359:2059–2064.

55. John TJ, Babu PG, Jayakumari H, et al. Prevalence of HIV infection in risk groups in Tamilnadu, India. *Lancet* 1987;1:160–161.

56. Solomon S, Anuradha S, Rajasekaran S. Trend of HIV infection in patients with pulmonary tuberculosis in south India. *Tuber Lung Dis* 1995;76:17–19.

57. Narain JP, Pattanayak S. AIDS and tuberculosis in Asia: a public health priority. In: *Proceedings of Tenth International Conference on AIDS*, Yokohama, Japan, August 7–11, 1994, Vol. 10.

58. Siriarayapon P, Yanai H, Glynn JR, et al. The evolving epidemiology of HIV infection and tuberculosis in northern Thailand. *J Acquir Immune Defic Syndr* 2002;31:80–89.

59. Lalit K. Upsurge in tuberculosis: HIV effect. *Indian J Tuberc* 1993;40:43–46.

60. Transuphaswadikul S, Limpakarnjanarat K, Lohsomboon P, et al. The clinical presentation of AIDS in Thailand. In: *Proceedings of the Eighth International Conference on AIDS, Amsterdam, July 19–24, 1992*. PoC4078:C258.

61. Quy HT, Nhien DT, Lan NT, et al. Steep increase in HIV prevalence among tuberculosis patients in Ho Chi Minh City. *AIDS* 2002;16:931–932.

62. Long R, Scalcini M, Manfreda J, et al. Impact of human immunodeficiency virus type 1 on tuberculosis in rural Haiti. *Am Rev Respir Dis* 1991;143:69–73.

63. Casiro A. Extrapulmonary tuberculosis: impact of an old disease in a new epidemic. In: *Proceedings of the Eighth International*

Conference on AIDS, Amsterdam, July 19–24. 1992:8:B99 (abstract no. PoB 3075).

64. Kritski AL, Werneck-Barroso E, Vieira MA, et al. HIV infection in 567 active pulmonary tuberculosis patients in Brazil. *J Acquir Immune Defic Syndr* 1993;6:1008–1012.

65. Perez-Gomez HR, Ortiz-Covarrubias A, Leon-Garcia A. Tuberculosis and human immunodeficiency virus in Mexican patients. In: *Proceedings of the 32nd Interscience Conference on Antimicrobial Agents and Chemotherapy, Anaheim, CA, October 11–14.* 1992;1641:384.

66. Jessurun J, Angeles-Angeles A, Gasman N. Comparative demographic and autopsy findings in acquired immune deficiency syndrome in two Mexican populations. *J Acquir Immune Defic Syndr* 1990;3:579–583.

67. DeRiemer K, Soares EC, Dias SM, et al. HIV testing among tuberculosis patients in the era of antiretroviral therapy: a population-based study in Brazil. *Int J Tuberc Lung Dis* 2000; 4:519–527.

68. Raviglione MC, Sudre P, Rieder HL, et al. Secular trends of tuberculosis in western Europe. *Bull WHO* 1993;71:297–306.

69. Dupon M, Ragnaud JM. Tuberculosis in patients infected with human immunodeficiency virus 1. A retrospective multicentre study of 123 cases in France. The Groupe des Infectiologues du Sud de la France. *Q J Med* 1992;85:719–730.

70. Liard R, Harf R, Korobaeff M, et al. HIV infection and tuberculosis: an epidemiological study from a French register. *Tuber Lung Dis* 1994;75:291–296.

71. Antonucci G, Girardi E, Armignacco O, et al. Tuberculosis in HIV-infected subjects in Italy: a multicentre study. The Gruppo Italiano di Studio Tubercolosi e AIDS. *AIDS* 1992;6: 1007–1013.

72. Laguna F, Adrados M, Diaz F, et al. AIDS and tuberculosis in Spain. A report of 140 cases. *J Infect* 1991;23:139–144.

73. Bouza E, Martin-Scapa C, Bernaldo de Quiros JC, et al. High prevalence of tuberculosis in AIDS patients in Spain. *Eur J Clin Microbiol Infect Dis* 1988;7:785–788.

74. Berenguer J, Moreno S, Laguna F, et al. Tuberculous meningitis in patients infected with the human immunodeficiency virus. *N Engl J Med* 1992;326:668–672.

75. van Deutekom H, Warris-Versteegen AA, Krijnen P, et al. The HIV epidemic and its effect on the tuberculosis situation in The Netherlands. *Tuber Lung Dis* 1993;74:159–162.

76. van Deutekom H, Manos GE, Danner SA, et al. AIDS and tuberculosis. Results of a retrospective study in 225 AIDS patients. *Bull Int Union Tuberc Lung Dis* 1990;65:33–34.

77. Bowen EF, Rice PS, Cooke NT, et al. HIV seroprevalence by anonymous testing in patients with *Mycobacterium tuberculosis* and in tuberculosis contacts. *Lancet* 2000;356:1488–1489.

78. Martin V, Guerra JM, Cayla JA, et al. Incidence of tuberculosis and the importance of treatment of latent tuberculosis infection in a Spanish prison population. *Int J Tuberc Lung Dis* 2001;5: 926–932.

79. Kirk O, Gatell JM, Mocroft A, et al. Infections with *Mycobacterium tuberculosis* and *Mycobacterium avium* among HIV-infected patients after the introduction of highly active antiretroviral therapy. EuroSIDA Study Group JD. *Am J Respir Crit Care Med* 2000;162:865–872.

80. Yerokhin VV, Punga VV, Rybka LN. Tuberculosis in Russia and the problem of multiple drug resistance. *Ann N Y Acad Sci* 2001;953:133–137.

81. Stern V. Problems in prisons worldwide, with a particular focus on Russia. *Ann N Y Acad Sci* 2001;953:113–119.

82. Whalen C, Horsburgh CR, Hom D, et al. Accelerated course of human immunodeficiency virus infection after tuberculosis. *Am J Respir Crit Care Med* 1995;151:129–135.

83. Munsiff SS, Alpert PL, Gourevitch MN, et al. A prospective study of tuberculosis and HIV disease progression. *J Acquir Immune Defic Syndr Hum Retrovir* 1998;19:361–366.

84. Zhang Y, Nakata K, Weiden M, et al. *Mycobacterium tuberculosis* enhances human immunodeficiency virus-1 replication by transcriptional activation at the long terminal repeat. *J Clin Invest* 1995;95:2324–2331.

85. Nakata K, Rom WN, Honda Y, et al. *Mycobacterium tuberculosis* enhances human immunodeficiency virus-1 replication in the lung. *Am J Respir Crit Care Med* 1997;155:996–1003.

86. Bender BS, Davidson BL, Kline R, et al. Role of the mononuclear phagocyte system in the immunopathogenesis of human immunodeficiency virus infection and the acquired immunodeficiency syndrome. *Rev Infect Dis* 1988;10:1142–1154.

87. Guelar A, Gatell JM, Verdejo J, et al. A prospective study of the risk of tuberculosis among HIV-infected patients. *AIDS* 1993; 7:1345–1349.

88. Small PM, Shafer RW, Hopewell PC, et al. Exogenous reinfection with multidrug-resistant *Mycobacterium tuberculosis* in patients with advanced HIV infection. *N Engl J Med* 1993;328: 1137–1144.

89. Orme IM, Andersen P, Boom WH. T cell response to *Mycobacterium tuberculosis*. *J Infect Dis* 1993;167:1481–1497.

90. Orme IM, Miller ES, Roberts AD, et al. T lymphocytes mediating protection and cellular cytolysis during the course of *Mycobacterium tuberculosis* infection. Evidence for different kinetics and recognition of a wide spectrum of protein antigens. *J Immunol* 1992;148:189–196.

91. Kumararatne DS, Pithie AS, Drysdale P, et al. Specific lysis of mycobacterial antigen-bearing macrophages by class II MHC-restricted polyclonal T cell lines in healthy donors or patients with tuberculosis. *Clin Exp Immunol* 1990;80:314–323.

92. Kaufmann SH. CD8$^+$ T lymphocytes in intracellular microbial infections. *Immunol Today* 1988;9:168–174.

93. Munk ME, Gatrill AJ, Kaufmann SH. Target cell lysis and IL-2 secretion by gamma/delta T lymphocytes after activation with bacteria. *J Immunol* 1990;145:2434–2439.

94. Forte M, Maartens G, Rahelu M, et al. Cytolytic T-cell activity against mycobacterial antigens in HIV. *AIDS* 1992;6:407–411.

95. Spickett GP, Dalgleish AG. Cellular immunology of HIV-infection. *Clin Exp Immunol* 1988;71:1–7.

96. De Maria A, Ferrazin A, Ferrini S, et al. Selective increase of a subset of T cell receptor gamma delta T lymphocytes in the peripheral blood of patients with human immunodeficiency virus type 1 infection. *J Infect Dis* 1992;165:917–919.

97. Lederman MM, Georges DL, Kusner DJ, et al. *Mycobacterium tuberculosis* and its purified protein derivative activate expression of the human immunodeficiency virus. *J Acquir Immune Defic Syndr* 1994;7:727–733.

98. Wallis RS, Vjecha M, Amir-Tahmasseb M, et al. Influence of tuberculosis on human immunodeficiency virus (HIV-1): enhanced cytokine expression and elevated beta 2-microglobulin in HIV-1-associated tuberculosis. *J Infect Dis* 1993;167: 43–48.

99. Toossi Z, Sierra-Madero JG, Blinkhorn RA, et al. Enhanced susceptibility of blood monocytes from patients with pulmonary tuberculosis to productive infection with human immunodeficiency virus type 1. *J Exp Med* 1993;177: 1511–1516.

100. Schauf V, Rom WN, Smith KA, et al. Cytokine gene activation and modified responsiveness to interleukin-2 in the blood of tuberculosis patients. *J Infect Dis* 1993;168:1056–1059.

101. Koyanagi Y, O'Brien WA, Zhao JQ, et al. Cytokines alter production of HIV-1 from primary mononuclear phagocytes. *Science* 1988;241:1673–1675.

102. Osborn L, Kunkel S, Nabel GJ. Tumor necrosis factor alpha and interleukin 1 stimulate the human immunodeficiency virus

enhancer by activation of the nuclear factor kappa B. *Proc Natl Acad Sci U S A* 1989;86:2336–2340.

103. Goletti D, Weissman D, Jackson RW, et al. Effect of *Mycobacterium tuberculosis* on HIV replication. Role of immune activation. *J Immunol* 1996;157:1271–1278.

104. Modlin RL. Th1-Th2 paradigm: insights from leprosy. *J Invest Dermatol* 1994;102:828–832.

105. Yamamura M, Uyemura K, Deans RJ, et al. Defining protective responses to pathogens: cytokine profiles in leprosy lesions. *Science* 1991;254:277–279.

106. Condos R, Rom WN, Liu YM, et al. Local immune responses correlate with presentation and outcome in tuberculosis. *Am J Respir Crit Care Med* 1998;157:729–735.

107. Condos R, Rom WN, Schluger NW. Treatment of multidrug-resistant pulmonary tuberculosis with interferon-gamma via aerosol. *Lancet* 1997;349:1513–1515.

108. Johnson MP, Coberly JS, Clermont HC, et al. Tuberculin skin test reactivity among adults infected with human immunodeficiency virus. *J Infect Dis* 1992;166:194–198.

109. Huebner RE, Schein MF, Bass JB Jr. The tuberculin skin test. Clinical Infectious Diseases 1993;17:968-75.

110. Graham NM, Nelson KE, Solomon L, et al. Prevalence of tuberculin positivity and skin test anergy in HIV-1-seropositive and -seronegative intravenous drug users. *JAMA* 1992;267:369–373.

111. Huebner RE, Schein MF, Hall CA, Barnes SA. Delayed-type hypersensitivity anergy in human immunodeficiency virus–infected persons screened for infection with *Mycobacterium tuberculosis*. *Clin Infect Dis* 1994;19:26–32.

112. Gordin FM, Matts JP, Miller C, et al. A controlled trial of isoniazid in persons with anergy and human immunodeficiency virus infection who are at high risk for tuberculosis. Terry Beirn Community Programs for Clinical Research on AIDS. *N Engl J Med* 1997;337:315–320.

113. Daley CL, Hahn JA, Moss AR, et al. Incidence of tuberculosis in injection drug users in San Francisco: impact of anergy. *Am J Respir Crit Care Med* 1998;157:19–22.

114. Moreno S, Baraia-Etxaburu J, Bouza E, et al. Risk for developing tuberculosis among anergic patients infected with HIV. *Ann Intern Med* 1993;119:194–198.

115. Selwyn PA, Sckell BM, Alcabes P, et al. High risk of active tuberculosis in HIV-infected drug users with cutaneous anergy. *JAMA* 1992;268:504–509.

116. Whalen CC, Johnson JL, Okwera A, et al. A trial of three regimens to prevent tuberculosis in Ugandan adults infected with the human immunodeficiency virus. Uganda-Case Western Reserve University Research Collaboration. *N Engl J Med* 1997;337:801–808.

117. Masur H, Ognibene FP, Yarchoan R, et al. CD4 counts as predictors of opportunistic pneumonias in human immunodeficiency virus (HIV) infection. *Ann Intern Med* 1989;111:223–231.

118. Rieder HL, Cauthen GM, Bloch AB, et al. Tuberculosis and acquired immunodeficiency syndrome—Florida. *Arch Intern Med* 1989;149:1268–1273.

119. Mocroft A, Youle M, Phillips AN, et al. The incidence of AIDS-defining illnesses in 4883 patients with human immunodeficiency virus infection. Royal Free/Chelsea and Westminster Hospitals Collaborative Group. *Arch Intern Med* 1998;158:491–497.

120. Daley CL, Mugusi F, Chen LL, et al. Pulmonary complications of HIV infection in Dar es Salaam, Tanzania. Role of bronchoscopy and bronchoalveolar lavage. *Am J Respir Crit Care Med* 1996;154:105–110.

121. Fischl MA, Pitchenik AE, Spira TJ. Tuberculous brain abscess and Toxoplasma encephalitis in a patient with the acquired immunodeficiency syndrome. *JAMA* 1985;253:3428–3430.

122. Bishburg E, Sunderam G, Reichman LB, et al. Central nervous system tuberculosis with the acquired immunodeficiency syndrome and its related complex. *Ann Intern Med* 1986;105:210–213.

123. D'Cruz IA, Sengupta EE, Abrahams C, et al. Cardiac involvement, including tuberculous pericardial effusion, complicating acquired immune deficiency syndrome. *Am Heart J* 1986;112:1100–1102.

124. Brody JM, Miller DK, Zeman RK, et al. Gastric tuberculosis: a manifestation of acquired immunodeficiency syndrome. *Radiology* 1986;159:347–348.

125. Barnes P, Leedom JM, Radin DR, et al. An unusual case of tuberculous peritonitis in a man with AIDS. *West J Med* 1986;144:467–469.

126. Mallolas J, Gatell JM, Rovira M, et al. Vertebral arch tuberculosis in two human immunodeficiency virus-seropositive heroin addicts. *Arch Intern Med* 1988;148:1125–1127.

127. Pitchenik AE, Burr J, Suarez M, et al. Human T-cell lymphotropic virus-III (HTLV-III) seropositivity and related disease among 71 consecutive patients in whom tuberculosis was diagnosed. A prospective study. *Am Rev Respir Dis* 1987;135:875–879.

128. Theuer CP, Hopewell PC, Elias D, et al. Human immunodeficiency virus infection in tuberculosis patients. *J Infect Dis* 1990;162:8–12.

129. Shafer RW, Chirgwin KD, Glatt AE, et al. HIV prevalence, immunosuppression, and drug resistance in patients with tuberculosis in an area endemic for AIDS. *AIDS* 1991;5:399–405.

130. Mukadi Y, Perriens JH, St Louis ME, et al. Spectrum of immunodeficiency in HIV-1-infected patients with pulmonary tuberculosis in Zaire. *Lancet* 1993;342:143–146.

131. Jones BE, Young SM, Antoniskis D, et al. Relationship of the manifestations of tuberculosis to CD4 cell counts in patients with human immunodeficiency virus infection. *Am Rev Respir Dis* 1993;148:1292–1297.

132. Bissuel F, Leport C, Perronne C, et al. Fever of unknown origin in HIV-infected patients: a critical analysis of a retrospective series of 57 cases. *J Intern Med* 1994;236:529–535.

133. Miralles P, Moreno S, Perez-Tascon M, et al. Fever of uncertain origin in patients infected with the human immunodeficiency virus. *Clin Infect Dis* 1995;20:872–875.

134. Modilevsky T, Sattler FR, Barnes PF. Mycobacterial disease in patients with human immunodeficiency virus infection. *Arch Intern Med* 1989;149:2201–2205.

135. Batungwanayo J, Taelman H, Dhote R, et al. Pulmonary tuberculosis in Kigali, Rwanda. Impact of human immunodeficiency virus infection on clinical and radiographic presentation. *Am Rev Respir Dis* 1992;146:53–56.

136. Greenberg SD, Frager D, Suster B, et al. Active pulmonary tuberculosis in patients with AIDS: spectrum of radiographic findings (including a normal appearance). *Radiology* 1994;193:115–119.

137. Given MJ, Khan MA, Reichman LB. Tuberculosis among patients with AIDS and a control group in an inner-city community. *Arch Intern Med* 1994;154:640–645.

138. Lessnau KD, Gorla M, Talavera W. Radiographic findings in HIV-positive patients with sensitive and resistant tuberculosis. *Chest* 1994;106:687–689.

139. Kramer F, Modilevsky T, Waliany AR, et al. Delayed diagnosis of tuberculosis in patients with human immunodeficiency virus infection (see comments). *Am J Med* 1990;89:451–456.

140. Long R, Maycher B, Scalcini M, et al. The chest roentgenogram in pulmonary tuberculosis patients seropositive for human immunodeficiency virus type 1. *Chest* 1991;99:123–127.

141. Pedro-Botet J, Gutierrez J, Miralles R, et al. Pulmonary tuberculosis in HIV-infected patients with normal chest radiographs. *AIDS* 1992;6:91–93.

142. Saks AM, Posner R. Tuberculosis in HIV positive patients in South Africa: a comparative radiological study with HIV negative patients. *Clin Radiol* 1992;46:387–390.

143. Pitchenik AE, Rubinson HA. The radiographic appearance of tuberculosis in patients with the acquired immune deficiency syndrome (AIDS) and pre-AIDS. *Am Rev Respir Dis* 1985;131: 393–396.

144. Shafer RW, Edlin BR. Tuberculosis in patients infected with human immunodeficiency virus: perspective on the past decade. *Clin Infect Dis* 1996;22:683–704.

145. Relkin F, Aranda CP, Garay SM, et al. Pleural tuberculosis and HIV infection. *Chest* 1994;105:1338–1341.

146. Ankobiah WA, Finch P, Powell S, et al. Pleural tuberculosis in patients with and without AIDS. *J Assoc Acad Minor Phys* 1990; 1:20–23.

147. Batungwanayo J, Taelman H, Allen S, et al. Pleural effusion, tuberculosis and HIV-1 infection in Kigali, Rwanda. *AIDS* 1993;7:73–79.

148. Richter C, Perenboom R, Mtoni I, et al. Clinical features of HIV-seropositive and HIV-seronegative patients with tuberculous pleural effusion in Dar es Salaam, Tanzania. *Chest* 1994; 106:1471–1475.

149. Kramer EL, Sanger JJ, Garay SM, et al. Gallium-67 scans of the chest in patients with acquired immunodeficiency syndrome. *J Nucl Med* 1987;28:1107–1114.

150. Lee VW, Cooley TP, Fuller JD, et al. Pulmonary mycobacterial infections in AIDS: characteristic pattern of thallium and gallium scan mismatch. *Radiology* 1994;193:389–392.

151. Pastores SM, Naidich DP, Aranda CP, et al. Intrathoracic adenopathy associated with pulmonary tuberculosis in patients with human immunodeficiency virus infection. *Chest* 1993;103:1433–1437.

152. Kim TC, Blackman RS, Heatwole KM, et al. Acid-fast bacilli in sputum smears of patients with pulmonary tuberculosis. Prevalence and significance of negative smears pretreatment and positive smears post-treatment. *Am Rev Respir Dis* 1984;129:264–268.

153. Levy H, Feldman C, Sacho H, et al. A reevaluation of sputum microscopy and culture in the diagnosis of pulmonary tuberculosis. *Chest* 1989;95:1193–1197.

154. Greenbaum M, Beyt BE Jr, Murray PR. The accuracy of diagnosing pulmonary tuberculosis at a teaching hospital. *Am Rev Respir Dis* 1980;121:477–481.

155. Barnes PF, Verdegem TD, Vachon LA, et al. Chest roentgenogram in pulmonary tuberculosis. New data on an old test. *Chest* 1988;94:316–320.

156. Brindle RJ, Nunn PP, Githui W, et al. Quantitative bacillary response to treatment in HIV-associated pulmonary tuberculosis. *Am Rev Respir Dis* 1993;147:958–961.

157. Klein NC, Duncanson FP, Lenox TH III, et al. Use of mycobacterial smears in the diagnosis of pulmonary tuberculosis in AIDS/ARC patients. *Chest* 1989;95:1190–1192.

158. Perlman DC, el-Sadr WM, Nelson ET, et al. Variation of chest radiographic patterns in pulmonary tuberculosis by degree of human immunodeficiency virus-related immunosuppression. The Terry Beirn Community Programs for Clinical Research on AIDS (CPCRA). The AIDS Clinical Trials Group (ACTG). *Clin Infect Dis* 1997;25:242–246.

159. Miro AM, Gibilara E, Powell S, et al. The role of fiberoptic bronchoscopy for diagnosis of pulmonary tuberculosis in patients at risk for AIDS. *Chest* 1992;101:1211–1214.

160. Kennedy DJ, Lewis WP, Barnes PF. Yield of bronchoscopy for the diagnosis of tuberculosis in patients with human immunodeficiency virus infection. *Chest* 1992;102:1040–1044.

161. Salzman SH, Schindel ML, Aranda CP, et al. The role of bronchoscopy in the diagnosis of pulmonary tuberculosis in patients at risk for HIV infection. *Chest* 1992;102:143–146.

162. Harkin TJ, Ciotoli C, Addrizzo-Harris DJ, et al. Transbronchial needle aspiration (TBNA) in patients infected with HIV. *Am J Respir Crit Care Med* 1998;157:1913–1918.

163. Schmidt RM, Rosenkranz HS. Antimicrobial activity of local anesthetics: lidocaine and procaine. *J Infect Dis* 1970;121: 597–607.

164. Dooley SW Jr, Castro KG, Hutton MD, et al. Guidelines for preventing the transmission of tuberculosis in health-care settings, with special focus on HIV-related issues. *MMWR Recomm Rep* 1990;39:1–29.

165. Agerton T, Valway S, Gore B, et al. Transmission of a highly drug-resistant strain (strain W1) of *Mycobacterium tuberculosis*. Community outbreak and nosocomial transmission via a contaminated bronchoscope. *JAMA* 1997;278:1073–1077.

166. Michele TM, Cronin WA, Graham NM, et al. Transmission of *Mycobacterium tuberculosis* by a fiberoptic bronchoscope. Identification by DNA fingerprinting. *JAMA* 1997;278: 1093–1095.

167. Brisson-Noel A, Gicquel B, Lecossier D, et al. Rapid diagnosis of tuberculosis by amplification of mycobacterial DNA in clinical samples. *Lancet* 1989;2:1069–1071.

168. Eisenach KD, Sifford MD, Cave MD, et al. Detection of *Mycobacterium tuberculosis* in sputum samples using a polymerase chain reaction. *Am Rev Respir Dis* 1991;144: 1160–1163.

169. Walker DA, Taylor IK, Mitchell DM, et al. Comparison of polymerase chain reaction amplification of two mycobacterial DNA sequences, IS6110 and the 65kDa antigen gene, in the diagnosis of tuberculosis. *Thorax* 1992;47:690–694.

170. Schluger NW, Kinney D, Harkin TJ, Rom WN. Clinical utility of the polymerase chain reaction in the diagnosis of infections due to *Mycobacterium tuberculosis*. *Chest* 1994;105:1116–1121.

171. Schluger NW. Changing approaches to the diagnosis of tuberculosis. *Am J Respir Crit Care Med* 2001;164:2020–2024.

172. Clarridge JE III, Shawar RM, Shinnick TM, et al. Large-scale use of polymerase chain reaction for detection of *Mycobacterium tuberculosis* in a routine mycobacteriology laboratory. *J Clin Microbiol* 1993;31:2049–2056.

173. Forbes BA, Hicks KE. Direct detection of *Mycobacterium tuberculosis* in respiratory specimens in a clinical laboratory by polymerase chain reaction. *J Clin Microbiol* 1993;31:1688–1694.

174. Noordhoek GT, Kolk AH, Bjune G, et al. Sensitivity and specificity of PCR for detection of *Mycobacterium tuberculosis*: a blind comparison study among seven laboratories. *J Clin Microbiol* 1994;32:277–284.

175. Shafer RW, Goldberg R, Sierra M, Glatt AE. Frequency of *Mycobacterium tuberculosis* bacteremia in patients with tuberculosis in an area endemic for AIDS. *Am Rev Respir Dis* 1989;140: 1611–1613.

176. Barber TW, Craven DE, McCabe WR. Bacteremia due to *Mycobacterium tuberculosis* in patients with human immunodeficiency virus infection. A report of 9 cases and a review of the literature. *Medicine (Baltimore)* 1990;69:375–383.

177. Bouza E, Diaz-Lopez MD, Moreno S, et al. *Mycobacterium tuberculosis* bacteremia in patients with and without human immunodeficiency virus infection. *Arch Intern Med* 1993;153:496–500.

178. Schluger NW, Condos R, Lewis S, et al. Amplification of DNA of *Mycobacterium tuberculosis* from peripheral blood of patients with pulmonary tuberculosis (see comments). *Lancet* 1994; 344:232–233.

179. Condos R, McClune A, Rom WN, et al. Peripheral-blood-based PCR assay to identify patients with active pulmonary tuberculosis. *Lancet* 1996;347:1082–1085.

180. Shafer RW, Kim DS, Weiss JP, et al. Extrapulmonary tuberculosis in patients with human immunodeficiency virus infection. *Medicine (Baltimore)* 1991;70:384–397.

181. Hill AR, Premkumar S, Brustein S, et al. Disseminated tuberculosis in the acquired immunodeficiency syndrome era. *Am Rev Respir Dis* 1991;144:1164–1170.

182. Llibre JM, Tor J, Manterola JM, Carbonell C, Roset J. Risk stratification for dissemination of tuberculosis in HIV-infected patients. Q J Med 1992;82:149–157.

183. Perronne C, Ghoubontni A, Leport C, et al. Should pulmonary tuberculosis be an AIDS-defining diagnosis in patients infected with HIV? *Tuber Lung Dis* 1992;73:39–44.

184. Gilks CF, Brindle RJ, Otieno LS, et al. Extrapulmonary and disseminated tuberculosis in HIV-1-seropositive patients presenting to the acute medical services in Nairobi. *AIDS* 1990;4:981–985.

185. Lupatkin H, Brau N, Flomenberg P, et al. Tuberculous abscesses in patients with AIDS. *Clin Infect Dis* 1992;14:1040–1044.

186. Small PM, Schecter GF, Goodman PC, et al. Treatment of tuberculosis in patients with advanced human immunodeficiency virus infection. *N Engl J Med* 1991;324:289–294.

187. Elliott AM, Halwiindi B, Hayes RJ, et al. The impact of human immunodeficiency virus on response to treatment and recurrence rate in patients treated for tuberculosis: two-year follow-up of a cohort in Lusaka, Zambia. *J Trop Med Hyg* 1995;98:9–21.

188. Daley CL, Small PM, Schecter GF, et al. An outbreak of tuberculosis with accelerated progression among persons infected with the human immunodeficiency virus. An analysis using restriction-fragment-length polymorphisms. *N Engl J Med* 1992;326:231–235.

189. Di Perri G, Cruciani M, Danzi MC, et al. Nosocomial epidemic of active tuberculosis among HIV-infected patients. *Lancet* 1989;2:1502–1504.

190. Small PM, Hopewell PC, Singh SP, et al. The epidemiology of tuberculosis in San Francisco. A population-based study using conventional and molecular methods. *N Engl J Med* 1994;330:1703–1709.

191. Alland D, Kalkut GE, Moss AR, et al. Transmission of tuberculosis in New York City. An analysis by DNA fingerprinting and conventional epidemiologic methods. *N Engl J Med* 1994;330:1710–1716.

192. Bloch AB, Cauthen GM, Onorato IM, et al. Nationwide survey of drug-resistant tuberculosis in the United States (see comments). *JAMA* 1994;271:665–671.

193. Frieden TR, Sterling T, Pablos-Mendez A, et al. The emergence of drug-resistant tuberculosis in New York City (published erratum appears in N Engl J Med 1993 Jul 8;329(2):148) (see comments). *N Engl J Med* 1993;328:521–526.

194. Chawla PK, Klapper PJ, Kamholz SL, et al. Drug-resistant tuberculosis in an urban population including patients at risk for human immunodeficiency virus infection. *Am Rev Respir Dis* 1992;146:280–284.

195. Frieden TR, Woodley CL, Crawford JT, Lew D, Dooley SM. The molecular epidemiology of tuberculosis in New York City: the importance of nosocomial transmission and laboratory error. *Tuber Lung Dis* 1996;77:407–113.

196. Villarino ME, Geiter LJ, Simone PM. The multidrug-resistant tuberculosis challenge to public health efforts to control tuberculosis. *Public Health Rep* 1992;107:616–625.

197. Beck-Sague C, Dooley SW, Hutton MD, et al. Hospital outbreak of multidrug-resistant *Mycobacterium tuberculosis* infections. Factors in transmission to staff and HIV-infected patients. *JAMA* 1992;268:1280–1286.

198. Edlin BR, Tokars JI, Grieco MH, et al. An outbreak of multidrug-resistant tuberculosis among hospitalized patients with the acquired immunodeficiency syndrome. *N Engl J Med* 1992;326:1514-21.

199. Pearson ML, Jereb JA, Frieden TR, et al. Nosocomial transmission of multidrug-resistant *Mycobacterium tuberculosis*. A risk to patients and health care workers. *Ann Intern Med* 1992;117:191–196.

200. Fischl MA, Daikos GL, Uttamchandani RB, et al. Clinical presentation and outcome of patients with HIV infection and tuberculosis caused by multiple-drug-resistant bacilli. *Ann Intern Med* 1992;117:184–190.

201. Centers for Disease Control and Prevention. Multidrug-resistant tuberculosis outbreak on an HIV ward—Madrid, Spain, 1991–1995. *MMWR Morb Mortal Wkly Rep* 1996;45:330–333.

202. Centers for Disease Control and Prevention. Meeting the challenge of multidrug-resistant tuberculosis: summary of a conference. *MMWR Morb Mortal Wkly Rep* 1992;41:51–57.

203. Tokars JI, McKinley GF, Otten J, et al. Use and efficacy of tuberculosis infection control practices at hospitals with previous outbreaks of multidrug-resistant tuberculosis. *Infect Control Hosp Epidemiol* 2001;22:449–455.

204. Jacobs WR Jr, Barletta RG, Udani R, et al. Rapid assessment of drug susceptibilities of *Mycobacterium tuberculosis* by means of luciferase reporter phages (see comments). *Science* 1993;260:819–822.

205. Riska PF, Su Y, Bardarov S, et al. Rapid film-based determination of antibiotic susceptibilities of *Mycobacterium tuberculosis* strains by using a luciferase reporter phage and the Bronx Box. *J Clin Microbiol* 1999;37:1144–1149.

206. Piatek AS, Tyagi S, Pol AC, et al. Molecular beacon sequence analysis for detecting drug resistance in *Mycobacterium tuberculosis*. *Nat Biotechnol* 1998;16:359–363.

207. Pablos-Mendez A, Raviglione MC, Laszlo A, et al. Global surveillance for antituberculosis-drug resistance, 1994–1997. World Health Organization–International Union against Tuberculosis and Lung Disease Working Group on Anti-Tuberculosis Drug Resistance Surveillance (see comments) (published erratum appears in *N Engl J Med* 1998;339:139). *N Engl J Med* 1998;338:1641–1649.

208. Jones BE, Otaya M, Antoniskis D, et al. A prospective evaluation of antituberculosis therapy in patients with human immunodeficiency virus infection. *Am J Respir Crit Care Med* 1994;150:1499–1502.

209. Perriens JH, St Louis ME, Mukadi YB, et al. Pulmonary tuberculosis in HIV-infected patients in Zaire. A controlled trial of treatment for either 6 or 12 months. *N Engl J Med* 1995;332:779–784.

210. el-Sadr WM, Perlman DC, Matts JP, et al. Evaluation of an intensive intermittent-induction regimen and duration of short-course treatment for human immunodeficiency virus–related pulmonary tuberculosis. Terry Beirn Community Programs for Clinical Research on AIDS (CPCRA) and the AIDS Clinical Trials Group (ACTG). *Clin Infect Dis* 1998;26:1148–1158.

211. Chaisson RE, Clermont HC, Holt EA, et al. Six-month supervised intermittent tuberculosis therapy in Haitian patients with and without HIV infection. *Am J Respir Crit Care* Med 1996;154:1034–1038.

212. Kennedy N, Berger L, Curram J, et al. Randomized controlled trial of a drug regimen that includes ciprofloxacin for the treatment of pulmonary tuberculosis. *Clin Infect Dis* 1996;22:827–833.

213. Kassim S, Sassan-Morokro M, Ackah A, et al. Two-year follow-up of persons with HIV-1- and HIV-2-associated pulmonary tuberculosis treated with short-course chemotherapy in West Africa. *AIDS* 1995;9:1185–1191.

214. Githui W, Nunn P, Juma E, et al. Cohort study of HIV-positive and HIV-negative tuberculosis, Nairobi, Kenya: comparison of bacteriological results. *Tuber Lung Dis* 1992;73:203–209.

215. Schurmann D, Bergmann F, Jautzke G, et al. Acute and long-term efficacy of antituberculous treatment in HIV-seropositive

patients with tuberculosis: a study of 36 cases. *J Infect* 1993; 26:45–54.

216. Grosset JH. Treatment of tuberculosis in HIV infection. *Tuber Lung Dis* 1992;73:378–383.

217. Peloquin CA, Nitta AT, Burman WJ, et al. Low antituberculosis drug concentrations in patients with AIDS. *Ann Pharmacother* 1996;30:919–925.

218. El-Sadr WM, Perlman DC, Matts JP, et al. Evaluation of an intensive intermittent-induction regimen and duration of short-course treatment for human immunodeficiency virus–related pulmonary tuberculosis. Terry Beirn Community Programs for Clinical Research on AIDS (CPCRA) and the AIDS Clinical Trials Group (ACTG) (In Process Citation). *Clin Infect Dis* 1998;26:1148–1158.

219. Perriens JH, St. Louis ME, Mukadi YB, et al. Pulmonary tuberculosis in HIV-infected patients in Zaire. A controlled trial of treatment for either 6 or 12 months (see comments). *N Engl J Med* 1995;332:779–784.

220. Sterling TR, Alwood K, Gachuhi R, et al. Relapse rates after short-course (6-month) treatment of tuberculosis in HIV-infected and uninfected persons. *AIDS* 1999;13:1899–1904.

221. Driver CR, Munsiff SS, Li J, Kundamal N, Osahan SS. Relapse in persons treated for drug-susceptible tuberculosis in a population with high coinfection with human immunodeficiency virus in New York City. *Clin Infect Dis* 2001;33:1762–1769.

222. Prevention and treatment of tuberculosis among patients infected with human immunodeficiency virus: principles of therapy and revised recommendations. Centers for Disease Control and Prevention. *MMWR Recomm Rep* 1998;47:1–58.

223. Vernon A, Burman W, Benator D, et al. Acquired rifamycin monoresistance in patients with HIV-related tuberculosis treated with once-weekly rifapentine and isoniazid. Tuberculosis Trials Consortium. *Lancet* 1999;353:1843–1847.

224. Acquired rifamycin resistance in persons with advanced HIV disease being treated for active tuberculosis with intermittent rifamycin-based regimens. *MMWR Morb Mortal Wkly Rep* 2002;51:214–215.

225. Palella FJ Jr, Delaney KM, Moorman AC, et al. Declining morbidity and mortality among patients with advanced human immunodeficiency virus infection. HIV Outpatient Study Investigators. *N Engl J Med* 1998;338:853–860.

226. Detels R, Munoz A, McFarlane G, et al. Effectiveness of potent antiretroviral therapy on time to AIDS and death in men with known HIV infection duration. Multicenter AIDS Cohort Study Investigators. *JAMA* 1998;280:1497–1503.

227. Burman WJ, Gallicano K, Peloquin C. Therapeutic implications of drug interactions in the treatment of human immunodeficiency virus-related tuberculosis. *Clin Infect Dis* 1999; 28:419–429;quiz 430.

228. Centers for Disease Control and Prevention. Updated guidelines for the use of rifabutin or rifampin for the treatment and prevention of tuberculosis among HIV-infected patients taking protease inhibitors or nonnucleoside reverse transcriptase inhibitors. *MMWR Morb Mortal Wkly Rep* 2000;49:185–189.

229. Sundaram V, Driver CR, Munsiff SS. Tuberculosis treatment practices in the era of protease inhibitors: a provider survey. *AIDS* 1999;13:149–150.

230. Lopez-Cortes LF, Ruiz-Valderas R, Viciana P, et al. Pharmacokinetic interactions between efavirenz and rifampicin in HIV-infected patients with tuberculosis. *Clin Pharmacokinet* 2002; 41:681–690.

231. Burman WJ, Jones BE. Treatment of HIV-related tuberculosis in the era of effective antiretroviral therapy. *Am J Respir Crit Care Med* 2001;164:7–12.

232. Narita M, Stambaugh JJ, Hollender ES, et al. Use of rifabutin with protease inhibitors for human immunodeficiency

virus–infected patients with tuberculosis. *Clin Infect Dis* 2000; 30:779–783.

233. Dean GL, Edwards SG, Ives NJ, et al. Treatment of tuberculosis in HIV-infected persons in the era of highly active antiretroviral therapy. *AIDS* 2002;16:75–83.

234. Iseman M. Tuberculosis in relation to human immunodeficiency virus and acquired immunodeficiency syndrome. In: *A clinician's guide to tuberculosis.* Philadelphia: Lippincott Williams & Wilkins, 2000:199–252.

235. Smith H. Paradoxical responses during the chemotherapy of tuberculosis. *J Infect* 1987;15:1–3.

236. Teoh R, Humphries MJ, O'Mahony G. Symptomatic intracranial tuberculoma developing during treatment of tuberculosis: a report of 10 patients and review of the literature. *Q J Med* 1987;63:449–460.

237. Race EM, Adelson-Mitty J, Kriegel GR, et al. Focal mycobacterial lymphadenitis following initiation of protease-inhibitor therapy in patients with advanced HIV-1 disease. *Lancet* 1998;351:252–225.

238. Narita M, Ashkin D, Hollender ES, et al. Paradoxical worsening of tuberculosis following antiretroviral therapy in patients with AIDS. *Am J Respir Crit Care Med* 1998;158:157–161.

239. Crump JA, Tyrer MJ, Lloyd-Owen SJ, et al. Military tuberculosis with paradoxical expansion of intracranial tuberculomas complicating human immunodeficiency virus infection in a patient receiving highly active antiretroviral therapy. *Clin Infect Dis* 1998;26:1008–1009.

240. Schluger NW, Perez D, Liu YM. Reconstitution of immune responses to tuberculosis in patients with HIV infection who receive antiretroviral therapy. *Chest* 2002;122:597–602.

241. Sunderam G, Mangura BT, Lombardo JM, et al. Failure of "optimal" four-drug short-course tuberculosis chemotherapy in a compliant patient with human immunodeficiency virus. *Am Rev Respir Dis* 1987;136:1475–1478.

242. Shafer RW, Jones WD. Relapse of tuberculosis in a patient with the acquired immunodeficiency syndrome despite 12 months of antituberculous therapy and continuation of isoniazid. *Tubercle* 1991;72:149–151.

243. Dylewski J, Thibert L. Failure of tuberculosis chemotherapy in a human immunodeficiency virus–infected patient. *J Infect Dis* 1990;162:778–779.

244. van Rie A, Warren R, Richardson M, et al. Exogenous reinfection as a cause of recurrent tuberculosis after curative treatment. *N Engl J Med* 1999;341:1174–1179.

245. Sonnenberg P, Murray J, Glynn JR, et al. HIV-1 and recurrence, relapse, and reinfection of tuberculosis after cure: a cohort study in South African mineworkers. *Lancet* 2001;358:1687–1693.

246. Nunn P, Brindle R, Carpenter L, et al. Cohort study of human immunodeficiency virus infection in patients with tuberculosis in Nairobi, Kenya. Analysis of early (6-month) mortality. *Am Rev Respir Dis* 1992;146:849–854.

247. Perriens JH, Colebunders RL, Karahunga C, et al. Increased mortality and tuberculosis treatment failure rate among human immunodeficiency virus (HIV) seropositive compared with HIV seronegative patients with pulmonary tuberculosis treated with "standard" chemotherapy in Kinshasa, Zaire. *Am Rev Respir Dis* 1991;144:750–755.

248. Leonard MK, Larsen N, Drechsler H, et al. Increased survival of persons with tuberculosis and human immunodeficiency virus infection, 1991–2000. *Clin Infect Dis* 2002;34:1002–1007.

249. Fischl MA, Uttamchandani RB, Daikos GL, et al. An outbreak of tuberculosis caused by multiple-drug-resistant tubercle bacilli among patients with HIV infection (see comments). *Ann Intern Med* 1992;117:177–183.

250. Park MM, Davis AL, Schluger NW, Cohen H, Rom WN. Outcome of MDR-TB patients, 1983–1993. Prolonged survival

with appropriate therapy. *Am J Respir Crit Care Med* 1996;153:317–324.

251. National action plan to combat multidrug-resistant tuberculosis. *MMWR Recomm Rep* 1992;41:5–48.

252. Ji B, Lounis N, Truffot-Pernot C, Grosset J. *In vitro* and *in vivo* activities of levofloxacin against *Mycobacterium tuberculosis. Antimicrob Agents Chemother* 1995;39:1341–1344.

253. New York city Department of Health Tuberculosis Control Program. *Tuberculosis: clincal procedures and protocols.* New York, 1999.

254. Crofton J, Chaulet P, Maher D. *Guidelines for the management of drug resistant tuberculosis.* Geneva: World Health Organization, 1997:1–49.

255. Nunn P, Kibuga D, Gathua S, et al. Cutaneous hypersensitivity reactions due to thiacetazone in HIV-1 seropositive patients treated for tuberculosis. *Lancet* 1991;337:627–630.

256. Kelly P, Buve A, Foster SD, McKenna M, Donnelly M, Sipatunyana G. Cutaneous reactions to thiacetazone in Zambia—implications for tuberculosis treatment strategies. *Trans R Soc Trop Med Hyg* 1994;88:113–115.

257. Slutkin G, Schecter GF, Hopewell PC. The results of 9-month isoniazid-rifampin therapy for pulmonary tuberculosis under program conditions in San Francisco. *Am Rev Respir Dis* 1988;138:1622–1624.

258. Mwinga A, Nunn A, Ngwira B, et al. *Mycobacterium vaccae* (SRL172) immunotherapy as an adjunct to standard antituberculosis treatment in HIV-infected adults with pulmonary tuberculosis: a randomised placebo-controlled trial. *Lancet* 2002;360:1050.

259. Pape JW, Jean SS, Ho JL, et al. Effect of isoniazid prophylaxis on incidence of active tuberculosis and progression of HIV infection. *Lancet* 1993;342:268–272.

260. Centers for Disease Control and Prevention. Anergy skin testing and tuberculosis (corrected) preventive therapy for HIV-infected persons: revised recommendations. *MMWR Recomm Rep* 1997;46:1–10.

261. Slovis BS, Plitman JD, Haas DW. The case against anergy testing as a routine adjunct to tuberculin skin testing. *JAMA* 2000;283:2003–2007.

262. Codecasa LR, Besozzi G. Acceptance of isoniazid preventive treatment by close contacts of tuberculosis cases: a 692-subject Italian study. *Int J Tuberc Lung Dis* 1998;2:208–212.

263. Bock NN, Metzger BS, Tapia JR, et al. A tuberculin screening and isoniazid preventive therapy program in an inner-city population. *Am J Respir Crit Care Med* 1999;159:295–300.

264. Camins BC, Bock N, Watkins DL, et al. Acceptance of isoniazid preventive therapy by health care workers after tuberculin skin test conversion. *JAMA* 1996;275:1013–1015.

265. Ngamvithayapong J, Uthaivoravit W, Yanai H, et al. Adherence to tuberculosis preventive therapy among HIV-infected persons in Chiang Rai, Thailand. *AIDS* 1997;11:107–112.

266. Halsey NA, Coberly JS, Desormeaux J, et al. Randomised trial of isoniazid versus rifampicin and pyrazinamide for prevention of tuberculosis in HIV-1 infection. *Lancet* 1998;351:786–792.

267. Gordin F, Chaisson RE, Matts JP, et al. Rifampin and pyrazinamide vs isoniazid for prevention of tuberculosis in HIV-infected persons: an international randomized trial. Terry Beirn Community Programs for Clinical Research on AIDS, the Adult AIDS Clinical Trials Group, the Pan American Health Organization, and the Centers for Disease Control and Prevention Study Group. *JAMA* 2000;283:1445–1450.

268. Update: Fatal and severe liver injuries associated with rifampin and pyrazinamide for latent tuberculosis infection, and revisions in American Thoracic Society/CDC Recommendations—

United States, 2001. This official American Thoracic Society/Centers for Disease Control and Prevention (ATS/CDC) update was approved by the ATS executive committee, August 2001. *Am J Respir Crit Care Med* 2001;164:1319–1320.

269. Jasmer RM, Saukkonen JJ, Blumberg HM, et al. Short-course rifampin and pyrazinamide compared with isoniazid for latent tuberculosis infection: a multicenter clinical trial. *Ann Intern Med* 2002;137:640–647.

270. Johnson JL, Okwera A, Hom DL, et al. Duration of efficacy of treatment of latent tuberculosis infection in HIV-infected adults. *AIDS* 2001;15:2137–2147.

271. Control and prevention of tuberculosis in the United Kingdom: code of practice 2000. Joint Tuberculosis Committee of the British Thoracic Society. *Thorax* 2000;55:887–901.

272. Elliott AM, Hayes RJ, Halwiindi B, et al. The impact of HIV on infectiousness of pulmonary tuberculosis: a community study in Zambia. *AIDS* 1993;7:981–987.

273. Cruciani M, Malena M, Bosco O, et al. The impact of human immunodeficiency virus type 1 on infectiousness of tuberculosis: a meta-analysis. *Clin Infect Dis* 2001;33:1922–1930.

274. Colditz GA, Brewer TF, Berkey CS, et al. Efficacy of BCG vaccine in the prevention of tuberculosis. Meta- analysis of the published literature (see comments). *JAMA* 1994;271:698–702.

275. Boudes P, Sobel A, Deforges L, et al. Disseminated *Mycobacterium bovis* infection from BCG vaccination and HIV infection. *JAMA* 1989;262:2386.

276. Reichman LB. Why hasn't BCG proved dangerous in HIV-infected patients? *JAMA* 1989;261:3246.

277. Weltman AC, Rose DN. The safety of Bacille Calmette-Guerin vaccination in HIV infection and AIDS. *AIDS* 1993;7:149–157.

278. Lumb R, Shaw D. *Mycobacterium bovis* (BCG) vaccination. Progressive disease in a patient asymptomatically infected with the human immunodeficiency virus. *Med J Aust* 1992;156:286–287.

279. Smith E, Thybo S, Bennedsen J. Infection with *Mycobacterium bovis* in a patient with AIDS: a late complication of BCG vaccination. *Scand J Infect Dis* 1992;24:109–110.

280. Reynes J, Perez C, Lamaury I, et al. Bacille Calmette–Guérin adenitis 30 years after immunization in a patient with AIDS. *J Infect Dis* 1989;160:727.

281. Armbruster C, Junker W, Vetter N, Jaksch G. Disseminated bacille Calmette–Guérin infection in an AIDS patient 30 years after BCG vaccination. *J Infect Dis* 1990;162:1216.

282. BCG vaccination and pediatric HIV infection—Rwanda, 1988–1990. *MMWR Morb Mortal Wkly Rep* 1991;40:833–836.

283. Lallemant-Le Coeur S, Lallemant M, Cheynier D, et al. Bacillus Calmette–Guérin immunization in infants born to HIV-1-seropositive mothers. *AIDS* 1991;5:195–199.

284. Tuberculosis and AIDS. Statement on AIDS and tuberculosis. Geneva, March 1989. Global Programme on AIDS and Tuberculosis Programme, World Health Organization, in collaboration with the International Union Against Tuberculosis and Lung Disease. *Bull Int Union Tuberc Lung Dis* 1989;64:8–11.

285. Bass JB Jr, Farer LS, Hopewell PC, et al. Treatment of tuberculosis and tuberculosis infection in adults and children. American Thoracic Society and the Centers for Disease Control and Prevention (see comments). *Am J Respir Crit Care Med* 1994;149:1359–1374.

286. Tuberculosis and human immunodeficiency virus infection: recommendations of the Advisory Committee for the Elimination of Tuberculosis (ACET). *MMWR Morb Mortal Wkly Rep* 1989;38:236–238, 243–250.

MYCOBACTERIUM AVIUM-INTRACELLULARE COMPLEX AND OTHER NONTUBERCULOUS MYCOBACTERIAL INFECTIONS IN HUMAN IMMUNODEFICIENCY VIRUS–INFECTED PATIENTS

MARK PARTA
STUART M. GARAY

During the past 20 years, acquired immunodeficiency syndrome (AIDS) has become one of the principal infectious causes of death in the world (1). The protean manifestations of human immunodeficiency virus (HIV) infection are rivaled in complexity by the spectrum of opportunistic infections that accompany HIV-associated immunologic dysfunction. Mycobacterial infections are inextricably woven into the fabric of HIV infection throughout the world. HIV-related *Mycobacterium tuberculosis* is dealt with in Chapter 45. This chapter will deal with *Mycobacterium avium-intracellulare* complex (MAC) and other mycobacteria that have been identified as clinical problems in HIV infection.

The manifestations of some mycobacterial species (MAC predominantly) in advanced HIV infection suggests that there is a synergistic effect of these organisms in driving the progression of AIDS and that HIV impairs immunity to mycobacterial infections (2). The inherent pathogenicity of mycobacteria and the stage of immunosuppression caused by HIV interact in a complex and poorly understood manner to cause disease in AIDS.

The individual characteristics of mycobacteria as per the classic Runyon scheme are of some usefulness in the clinical microbiology laboratory and provide a basic context for epidemiology. New tools for characterizing species and strains have emerged. These also contribute to the basic science of pathogenesis (3,4). For the purposes of understanding the role of mycobacteria in HIV infection, clinical considerations should predominate. Organisms that are pathogenic in the nonimmunosuppressed host will cause disease in HIV-infected persons. Although microbiologic advances have broadened the spectrum of organisms reported in HIV-infected persons, many mycobacterial species occur rarely. Limited reporting provides insufficient evidence that such organisms are pathogens with specific characteristics in the HIV-infected patient.

The sections of this chapter dedicated to individual organisms will stress two characteristics of mycobacteria in the HIV-infected host. First, organisms that have classically been pulmonary pathogens have retained that status in HIV infection, although the rate of progression of disease, burden of organisms, and the propensity to disseminate may be greater in the HIV-infected host. The second characteristic of mycobacterial infections in the HIV-infected host is the common occurrence of manifestations that were rare before the advent of HIV-related disease in the early 1980s (5). The first reports of disseminated MAC (DMAC) from New York heralded this important and almost new pathogenic potential (6). MAC infection has become the most reported and studied bacterial complication of advanced AIDS (7). Once considered a pulmonary commensal in patients with some predisposing (usually structural) lung disease, two parallel developments have redefined the importance of MAC as a pathogen. More intense analysis of the "colonized" patient without HIV infection has often revealed tissue pathology. New antimicrobial agents that are practical to use and effective against MAC have established that clinical symptoms and pathologic findings regress with treatment (8). This scenario recurs *in extremis* in the context of HIV infection. Once the most common cause of bacteremia in AIDS patients, MAC infection nevertheless was

M. Parta: AIDS Program, Bellevue Hospital Center, New York, New York.
S.M. Garay: Department of Medicine, New York University School of Medicine, New York, New York.

often not treated. Early studies often found that patients died in the interval between presentation and diagnosis, but the severity of immunosuppression and the innumerable other infectious and malignant complications of end-stage HIV disease made it difficult to establish the role of MAC in morbidity and mortality (9–11).

Other species that are commonly isolated but uncommonly associated with disease in the non–HIV-infected patient have been reassessed. El-Solh et al. (12) reviewed nontuberculous mycobacteria (NTM) pulmonary isolates (exclusive of MAC and *Mycobacterium kansasii*) from AIDS patients (12). They found that no specific radiographic findings characterized NTM infections in AIDS. *Mycobacterium xenopii* accounted for 66% of these cases, and a survival advantage was associated with treatment.

MYCOBACTERIUM AVIUM-INTRACELLULARE

Taxonomy and Epidemiology

MAC consists of *M. intracellulare*, *M. lepraemurium* (only a pathogen in animals), and three subspecies of *M. avium*: *M. sylvaticum*, *M. paratuberculosis*, and *M. avium*. Guthertz et al. (13) found that *M. avium* subsp. *avium* accounted for 98% of strains from AIDS patients. This relationship has held for almost a decade, with a 1997 report from Brazil identifying *M. avium* as the pathogen in 88% of patients with MAC (14). The medical literature variably refers to *M. avium* or *M. avium-intracellulare* (MAI) or MAC as the pathogen. Unless noted, the term MAC will be used throughout this chapter.

As environmental and clinical isolates of mycobacteria are studied throughout the world, increasing variability in the utility of classic speciation and strain typing has been noted (15). Greater specificity associated with new typing methods may contribute to our understanding of new disease-associated phenotypes. Mycobacteria are common environmental saprophytes and are found throughout the world. There is a close relationship between many of the organisms that cause human disease and those most commonly found in animals, suggesting that some infections qualify as a zoonosis (16). The evolution in mycobacterial epidemiology is well illustrated in the case of MAC. Serologic reactivities with surface glycopeptidolipids (GPLs) define 28 MAC serovars (17). However, this test is not routinely available, and classical biochemical typing is not always accurate. Current techniques used to analyze MAC include nucleic acid probing (AccuProbe, Gen-Probe Inc., San Diego, CA, U.S.A.) or sequencing of 16S ribosomal DNA (rDNA), or hsp65 amplification with sequencing or restriction fragment length polymorphism analysis (3,17). 16S–23S rRNA internal transcribed spacer (ITS) analysis demonstrates identity among isolates from AIDS patients but variety in isolates from elderly persons with pulmonary disease (18). Genetic heterogeneity is present within MAC

serovars by these techniques, providing a more sensitive epidemiologic tool (19,20). Newer techniques allow for the discrimination of isolates not typed by commercially available molecular probes, such as some Indian subcontinent *M. intracellulare* (19). Pulse-field gel electrophoresis patterns tend to be unique in MAC infections, but polyclonal infection (up to 20%) has been reported in a series that analyzed isolates from 12 AIDS patients (21). Various techniques provide different answers as to the clonality of isolates in patients with AIDS. A study of patients failing therapy found that drug-susceptible and resistant isolates were genetically related by rRNA analysis in six of eight patients (22).

The epidemiology of mycobacterial infections in AIDS is critically influenced by rates of endemic tuberculosis. Geographic trends in MAC infections seem to be influenced by major histocompatibility complex class II alleles such as DR2, which may have the same influence in DMAC as reported for tuberculosis and leprosy (23). A protective role of previous tuberculous infection against MAC disease has been proposed but remains unproven (24). Areas of high tuberculosis prevalence continue to report high rates of tuberculous complications in HIV-infected persons. Regions where tuberculosis is rare have increased rates of disease caused by NTM (25). A common condition such as mycobacterial lymphadenitis may be caused by *MAC* in as few as 2% of cases in a country with high tuberculosis prevalence, such as India (26). Early reports from Africa reported no disease due to MAC, but in 1992 a study of 48 patients in Kenya found MAC in three of 14 patients with mycobacteremia (27,28). A recent study from South Africa that assessed the utility of blood cultures for the diagnosis of mycobacterial disease found that DMAC was isolated half as often as tuberculosis (29). No cases of tuberculosis are reported in an autopsy series of AIDS patients from Japan, consistent with the low prevalence of tuberculosis in the general population (30).

MAC has been identified as an environmental isolate from the United States to Finland and eastern and southern Africa (31). By 1997, analysis of environmental isolates of MAC in Zaire revealed that these were similar to organisms causing disseminated disease in AIDS patients in that country (32). MAC is most commonly isolated from water, and hospital water systems have been suggested as a potential threat. However, the organism can be found in soil, and the ingestion of certain foods has been identified as a risk for infection (33,34). The differential prevalence of species colonization of biofilms in drinking water distribution systems has been reported (35). With such a ubiquitous organism, the principal epidemiologic factor in the presence of disease associated with MAC and HIV remains the degree of immunosuppression associated with HIV infection. Trends throughout the world support the contention that both site of disease and stage of HIV infection contribute to defining the risk of tuberculous versus NTM infection. Lung disease and acid-fast bacillus (AFB)–positive sputum smears favor the diagnosis of tuberculosis, whereas a CD4$^+$ T-lymphocyte (CD4$^+$ T cell) count of less than 50/mL favors DMAC (36). These T-cell concentrations are the most consistently documented indicator of risk for DMAC; levels of viremia contribute but are less firmly categorized (37). Prophylaxis for *Pneumocystis jiroveci* pneumonia (formerly *Pneumocystis carinii* pneumonia, PCP) and improved medical care of HIV persons in general allows more patients to progress to degrees of immunosuppression associated with a risk of MAC (38). Surveys of the incidence of DMAC may be confounded by study design. MAC will appear more frequently in surveys of disease in known HIV-infected persons than in those that identify first illnesses leading to the diagnosis of HIV infection (39).

Microbiology and Pathogenesis

Mycobacterial infections in HIV-infected persons occur in every conceivable form and in every type of tissue. Species-specific trends sometimes mimic the pathogenic potential of the organisms in non–HIV-infected persons. MAC may cause pulmonary disease in HIV patients that is similar to the chronic pulmonary infections described before the HIV epidemic, but its most salient characteristic is its propensity to disseminate with advanced immunosuppression.

The obligate intracellular nature of many mycobacterial pathogens is important in identifying host defects in containment and pathogen-specific pathways for exploiting them. Once internalized, mycobacteria compartmentalize in phagosomes that provide sanctuary sites for persistence and replication (40,41). Pathogenic strains of MAC may not induce macrophage apoptosis. Impairment of phagosome–lysosome fusion is a much discussed pathogenic mechanism (42). The signal defect in HIV infection, namely, the loss of CD4$^+$ T cells, reduces the ability of macrophages to become activated to kill or control mycobacteria. Some defects may be different with regard to *M. tuberculosis* versus other organisms. These differences are best defined with MAC. For instance, animal models demonstrate antagonism of host defenses against MAC by the up-regulation of inducible nitric oxide synthase. The opposite effect is seen with *M. tuberculosis* (43).

Cytokines, which are autocrine and intercellular signaling molecules, have been intensively studied in mycobacterial infections in HIV-infected and uninfected hosts. The reader is referred to an excellent review of cytokines as they relate to HIV infection (44). Cytokine production is dysregulated in HIV infection, both in the total host and at the level of the host cell, parasitized or not by mycobacteria. Inflammatory cytokines have various roles in MAC and HIV infection. Tumor necrosis factor-α (TNF-α) production is necessary for defense against intracellular MAC infection, and inhibitors of TNF-α impair macrophage killing and increase interleukin-6 (IL-6) production, which

correlates with increased growth of MAC (45,46). *In vitro* infection of macrophages induces the production of IL-10, IL-6, and TNF-α. Studies in patients with DMAC confirm that elevated levels of these cytokines are present in serum and decrease with successful treatment (47).

The role of mycobacterial infections in accelerating the progression of HIV disease is documented at every level. HIV levels have been reported to increase by a median of 0.4 log10 at the onset of MAC bacteremia (48). Important histologic studies show that macrophages infected with MAC have increased levels of HIV replication (49). *In vitro*, increased levels of HIV production from HIV-infected macrophages occur in the presence of MAC antigen and may increase CCR5 expression, thereby increasing targets for HIV infection (50). Matrix metalloproteinases have been implicated in the stimulation of HIV production from MAC-infected macrophages (51). The synergy of HIV and MAC infection at the cellular level is well documented. Coinfected cultures had threefold increased HIV replication and contained more HIV-infected cells (2). HIV-infected cells showed significant enhancement of MAC growth compared with controls.

Tissue pathology in mycobacterial infections generally represents the state of host defenses (52). Even *M. tuberculosis* may be found in poorly formed granulomas in advanced HIV infection. Immune reconstitution may allow MAC to be the stimulus for discreet and well-formed granulomatous inflammation (53). The most common organ pathology in disseminated mycobacterial infections, for which MAC will be the surrogate, is the poorly formed granuloma with a heavy infestation of organisms inside macrophages and throughout the parenchyma (54).

The predominance of *M. avium* in HIV infection, both among NTM and in comparison with other members of the MAC, suggests that some characteristics associated with speciation such as cell wall GPLs have a pathologic role in disease (55). These components may contribute to immunosuppression, as suggested by their inhibition of cytokine production by T$_H$1 CD4$^+$ T cells from normal volunteers (56). Serovar or species-specific GPL content is represented microbiologically by changes in colony morphology. These changes can be accentuated by passage through animals, and a rough/transparent (RgT) isolate obtained in this fashion multiplied faster with increased mortality (60% to 80%) compared with smooth/transparent (SmT) colonies (10%) in a murine model. These cell wall changes may represent the presence of specific molecules that modulate macrophage function and defense. The colonial morphotypes differ in their drug susceptibilities, perhaps on the basis of changes in cell wall permeability (57). Adherence to epithelial cells and persistence in biofilms may be other important functions of these changes in cell wall content. This may be apparent on gross inspection of colony morphology, or it can be accentuated by the use of selective agars incorporating dyes such as Congo red (58,59).

Clinical Manifestations and Diagnosis

Autopsy series have confirmed that mycobacteria cause disease in every organ and body site. The most common sites of identification in DMAC are lymph nodes (74%), spleen (74%), liver (52%), lungs (22%), colon (13%), small bowel (11%), and bone marrow (9%) (60). These manifestations are best considered as inoculation phenomena (cutaneous disease when the skin is the site of entry) with concomitant hematogenous or lymphatic spread, as noted for the gastrointestinal (GI) tract. Autopsy studies in MAC patients have demonstrated that the GI tract is often the site of entry and dissemination. These studies suggest that the presence of organisms in blood is subsequent to replication in viscera and lymphatic tissue (61).

Pulmonary disease caused by MAC is more common in AIDS than was previously thought. Fever, cough, and nodular infiltrates predominate and may be indistinguishable from tuberculosis. Pulmonary MAC may be an AIDS-defining illness early after infection, presenting with consolidation, nodular infiltrates, and cavitation (62,63). A retrospective survey of cases at Bellevue Hospital with sputum cultures that grew MAC found that HIV-infected patients were more likely to meet American Thoracic Society (ATS) criteria for MAC-related pulmonary disease than non–HIV-infected patients. However, even among HIV-infected patients, the majority of those with MAC in the sputum would not be considered to have disease by ATS criteria. The majority of these exclusions were for the presence of another diagnosed pulmonary infection (64). At Bellevue, the isolation of MAC from the sputum of patients with pulmonary tuberculosis was not clearly linked to outcome except in patients with DMAC, multidrug-resistant tuberculosis, or advanced AIDS (65). These observations underline the difficulty in defining the context in which MAC is a pulmonary pathogen. It is likely that ATS criteria in the setting of advanced HIV infection are too rigorous a standard. Patients with profound immunosuppression often harbor multiple pathogens that contribute to pulmonary disease at the same time.

Focal adenopathy may not present with systemic symptoms; fungal infections and lymphoid malignancies are important considerations in a differential diagnosis. The GI tract portal of entry for MAC explains the frequent fever, abdominal pain, diarrhea, and organomegaly. Reticuloendothelial system concentrations of organisms may reach 6.9 log10 colony-forming units (CFU) per gram (61). GI hemorrhage has been reported as an initial sign (66). Endoscopic inspection may reveal characteristic findings, and tissue pathology resembles that of Whipple disease (67). Hepatosplenomegaly and elevations in alkaline phosphatase and γ-glutamyltransferase suggest focal involvement of the biliary tract (68).

Although no retinal finding was noted as an ocular manifestation of DMAC in a series that mainly assessed *Toxo-plasma* infection, antiretroviral therapy (ART) unmasked latent choroidal infection (53,69). Septic arthritis and osteomyelitis, central nervous system disease (ranging from meningoencephalitis to spinal cord compression), pericarditis, liver abscess, appendicitis, pancreatitis, and involvement of every other segment of the GI tract, from the esophagus to the colon, suggest that any site may be involved (70–79).

Dermatologic manifestations are protean. Varioliform pustular eruptions, papulonecrotic tuberculid, "red nodules," and spindle cell tumors that might otherwise suggest Kaposi sarcoma are described (80–83).

One characteristic presentation of disseminated disease in advanced HIV infection is a febrile wasting syndrome without immediately apparent focal clinical pathology (84). Blood cultures may contain 10^4 CFU/mL, although quantitative yields from bone marrow are more likely to be prognostic than those from blood (82). Anemia, as an additional predictive feature that suggests DMAC, may be profound and disproportionate to the other cytopenias that accompany advanced HIV infection. A hemolysin has been isolated from *M. avium* that might represent the microbial cause of this particularly common manifestation (85).

Before proceeding to the specifics of diagnosis, several general points about DMAC in HIV infection should be made. Recent advances in the reversal of HIV-associated immunosuppression and effective prophylaxis and management of MAC itself have changed clinical decision making. The time needed for a diagnosis may cause difficulties due to cost constraints. The most efficient diagnostic modalities are expensive and require considerable expertise. Furthermore, although the sensitivity of diagnostics is enhanced with more extensive disease, successful treatment should be improved by earlier interventions (86). Horsburgh et al. (87) reviewed cases of DMAC that presented to Grady Memorial Hospital from 1985 to 2000. They suggested that detection was occurring earlier in the course of infection, attributable to heightened clinical suspicion of DMAC. Survival trends improved in inverse relation to the detection of systemic symptoms most consistent with advanced dissemination, such as anemia, night sweats, weight loss, and an elevated alkaline phosphatase level.

MAC isolated from a normally sterile site is diagnostic of dissemination. The presence of MAC in stool and sputum, while not inevitably diagnostic of dissemination, is sufficiently predictive of the risk of dissemination to change prophylactic measures in many clinical settings. Relative hazards over a year for dissemination in patients with respiratory tract and GI tract colonization were 2.3 and 6.0, respectively (88). Blood cultures are the most common site of identification of dissemination, both because of the frequency of mycobacteremia and because of the less invasive sampling and advances in the laboratory in culturing blood. Clinical prediction models can be used to decrease the number of blood cultures that are obtained from low-risk patients. Factors that contributed to positive and negative predictive values of 30% and 98% were the low CD4+ T-cell levels present at dissemination (≤50/mL), the duration of fever (>30 days in 3 months), and laboratory values (hematocrit <30% and albumin <3 g/dL) as sensitive predictors (89%) of DMAC (89).

The most common current diagnostic modalities are based on radiometric or nonradiometric detection of growth, either directly from blood or from other processed body fluids inoculated onto indicator media, with subsequent speciation by the use of molecular probes. Current methods of blood culture vary by species and technique, and generally yield a result in 9 to 26 days. The average time to detection in one recent report was 13 days for MAC and 26 days for *M. tuberculosis* (90–92).

As in many other settings, diagnostic microbiology is compromised by antecedent antibiotic administration (93). Furthermore, there may be fluctuating levels of bacteremia that make the comparison of unpaired techniques unreliable (94). In a setting in which 17% of blood cultures obtained with the ISOLATOR blood culture system (E. I. DuPont de Nemours, Wilmington, DE, U.S.A.) had less than 1 CFU/mL, the sensitivity of two sequential blood cultures to detect DMAC was 98% (95). Polymerase chain reaction (PCR) may decrease the detection time to as little as 1 day, but is still not generally available and not as sensitive as culture. The sensitivity of PCR may be as high as 96%, depending on methodology and the number of samples analyzed (96).

Radiologic studies provide important guidelines for the identification of sites of pathology in the patient with disseminated but clinically nonfocal infection. Certain radiographic findings may differ among mycobacterial species. In a report on pulmonary radiographic findings, patients with *M. kansasii* and *M. xenopi* had more cavitation, "tree-in-bud" appearance, and preexisting emphysema, whereas severe bronchiectasis and nodular infiltrates characterized the computed tomography (CT) appearance of pulmonary MAC (97). However, this study did not distinguish between HIV- and non–HIV-infected patients. Improvements in the radiofrequency of ultrasound from 3.5 MHz to 5 MHz may increase its sensitivity in the detection of visceral abscesses (98). CT can be used to identify body cavity adenopathy that otherwise eludes detection. These nodes may have homogeneous soft-tissue attenuation. Hepatomegaly and splenomegaly are common (50% and 42%). A recent report found a decreased frequency of mesenteric and retroperitoneal lymphadenopathy with MAC bacteremia, but this finding may represent earlier detection of bacteremia (99). Nuclear medicine imaging modalities may provide some added sensitivity and even specificity in certain settings. Focal gallium uptake in the mediastinal and hilar nodes without thallium uptake (thallium–gallium mismatch) may be specific for mycobacterial infection in immunodeficient patients (100).

Cultures of stool and sputum are relatively insensitive (20% and 22%, respectively) but have strong positive predictive values (60%) for DMAC over a 1-year interval (88). When GI or biliary tract signs and symptoms predominate, endoscopy and biopsy may have appreciable yields (101). Elevations in alkaline phosphatase and γ-glutamyltransferase suggest liver disease. Liver biopsy may provide an early histologic diagnosis in that setting (102). When diarrheal symptoms predominate in disseminated disease, endoscopy may provide important visual clues to the diagnosis. Massive infiltration and expansion of intestinal villi cause the mucosa to appear coarsely granular, although mucosal exudation is lacking (103).

MAC in other tissue sites is variably associated with dissemination, and the clinical syndrome and stage of CD4+ T-cell depletion must be taken into consideration. The examination of bone marrow is not inherently more sensitive than blood culture. However, it permits detection of some infections that blood cultures miss and provides additional as well as early histologic information that is useful in narrowing the differential diagnosis of disseminated disease (104). Quantitative cultures of bone marrow may be 3 log10 higher than concomitant blood cultures. Hafner et al. (86) suggested that length of survival correlated with the intensity of bone marrow infection rather than blood.

Some lymph nodes, such as submandibular or cervical glands, may be sites of localized disease even in advanced HIV infection. However, infection of other sites in the reticuloendothelial system, especially intrathoracic and intraabdominal lymph nodes, spleen, and liver, suggests dissemination. Finally, the profound immunosuppression that makes the host susceptible to DMAC confounds any attempt at making a simple, unifying diagnosis. MAC may exist concomitantly with other opportunistic infections, such as *Cryptococcus neoformans*, *Histoplasma capsulatum*, cytomegalovirus, and lymphoid malignancies. Thoroughness and care in the histologic examination and processing of specimens is of the utmost importance in establishing the full panoply of diagnoses associated with any form of tissue disease (105–107).

Management

Management of mycobacterial infections in the HIV-infected host has changed drastically secondary to certain developments. The availability of new drugs, specifically clarithromycin and azithromycin, has allowed establishment of generally well-tolerated and effective antimicrobial regimens. The true role of MAC in the progression, morbidity, and mortality of HIV infection was only clarified once these agents allowed management of DMAC infection (108). The presence of effective therapy for HIV infection itself has clearly established that the restoration of host immunity, associated with the suppression of viral replication, can lead to a cure for these infections (109). Choices of therapy are critically influenced by drug interactions specific to the classes of antiretroviral agents that have led to reduced morbidity and mortality even in advanced HIV infection (110).

Three drugs dominated early clinical trials that found that patients with DMAC and AIDS could be successfully treated and established that treatment was associated with better survival. Rifabutin, a rifamycin S derivative, demonstrated increased efficacy against MAC, and the use of rifabutin in anti-MAC regimens, when treatment led to negative cultures, was associated with significant decreases in morbidity and survival increases of 195 days (111,112). Clarithromycin and azithromycin (strictly an azalide) were initially developed to increase the class's spectrum against respiratory tract gram-negative pathogens such as *Haemophilus influenzae*. Their activity against MAC and tolerability quickly made them the cornerstone of therapy. Other members of the extended-spectrum macrolide class are still not approved for use in the United States, although some *in vitro* and animal model data suggest that telithromycin (technically a ketolide) and roxithromycin may have activity against *M. avium* (113,114).

The progress of the AIDS epidemic and the evolution of MAC as a significant pathogen created a critical niche for these drugs. Their unusual pharmacokinetic properties of intracellular accumulation make them ideal agents. The specifics of drug pharmacokinetics and pharmacodynamics have been reviewed elsewhere (115,116). While these observations related to drug absorption, *in vitro* activity and intracellular disposition, and pH-related activity are especially important for the development of new drugs, large clinical trials have defined the use of the available agents (117).

Early clinical trials in DMAC demonstrated both the clinical and microbiologic benefit of managing DMAC, with a relative hazard of death of 0.45 in treated patients (118). However, when used in patients with high organism burdens, the emergence of drug resistance and the failure to clear infections was evident (119,120). Subsequent trials applied information generated from animal models and *in vitro* to formulate effective combination therapies (121,122). Ethambutol, an effective agent *in vitro*, has been the most studied and is the most accepted agent for use in combination with a macrolide (123). Clofazimine is no longer recommended because of increased mortality in the clofazimine-containing arm of a combination drug trial (124). The spectrum of aminoglycosides that pertain to the management of DMAC has narrowed. The only agent presently used is amikacin. A small study suggests it might be useful in an "induction" phase to improve clearance of organisms from the blood because the aminoglycosides are generally ineffective in clearing other tissues (125). The number of available quinolones has increased, but there is little information on the use of any but ciprofloxacin, ofloxacin, or levofloxacin. There are no compelling data to

suggest that the addition of a quinolone in the majority of cases improves outcome. A retrospective survey suggested a significant improvement in time to death with the addition of ciprofloxacin to clarithromycin/ethambutol (126,127).

There are new additions to the armamentarium against mycobacterial infections. Oxazalidinones have been studied *in vitro* , and there are reports of clinical success with the currently available agent, linezolid. Mefloquine has *in vitro* activity and has been used in combination with linezolid in the management of refractory MAC infection in a non–HIV-infected patient (128–130).

Immunotherapies have not been reported with sufficient frequency in HIV-infected persons to justify their use. A case report showed no benefit from the use of interferon-γ (131). Granulocyte-macrophage colony-stimulating factor (CSF) enhanced the mycobactericidal activity of cells but had no effect on bacteremia, and granulocyte-CSF was retrospectively associated with improved survival (132,133).

Management of MAC infections, localized or systemic, should include clarithromycin (500 mg b.i.d.) or azithromycin (600 mg q.d) usually in combination with ethambutol. Guidelines from the ATS in 1997 and the British Thoracic Society in 2000 recommend the use of a rifamycin in combination therapy. Rifampin is included in the British Thoracic Society guidelines (134,135). These recommendations must be interpreted with caution due to interactions of rifamycins with HIV protease inhibitors and nonnucleoside reverse transcriptase inhibitors. Antiretroviral drug interactions with rifamycins have been extensively discussed in the context of the management of tuberculosis (136). Macrolides are not active against *M. tuberculosis*, but their effectiveness against MAC makes rifamycins unnecessary in most cases (137). The necessity for adjustments to macrolide/ethambutol therapy may be indicated by level of CD4+ T-cell cytopenia. The addition of a quinolone or addition of early aminoglycoside therapy has been advocated (125,127). Single-drug trials have demonstrated improvement with increasing doses of clarithromycin. However, multidrug regimens utilizing clarithromycin at dosages exceeding 1,000 mg/day were associated with increased mortality (138).

Direct comparative trials of clarithromycin and azithromycin have been inadequate in size or have been compromised by epidemiologic problems (decreased frequency of disease in the era of prophylaxis, for instance) (139,140). A general consensus has arisen that clarithromycin is the more potent agent based on *in vitro* activity, animal models, and noncomparative trials (141). However, azithromycin does have advantages, such as activity against *Toxoplasma gondii* and fewer reported interactions with other drugs that are metabolized by the cytochrome P450 system. Caution should be exercised in interpreting a lack of systematic reporting as indicating a lack of interaction. Documented interactions make clarithromycin an awkward agent when rifabutin must be used (usually in the period when the differential diagnosis of AFB-positive pulmonary disease still includes *M. tuberculosis*). Simplification of therapies at some reasonably early time remains important when ART is still pending. Even without drug interactions, pill burdens in advanced HIV infection can make the strongest person lose heart.

Management of DMAC as a disease that occurs before the institution of effective antiretroviral therapy poses some problems not addressed by current clinical trials. Control of HIV infection is without doubt the major contributor to long-term outcome. It would still seem prudent to seek a "cooling off" period for any opportunistic infection. The goal would be to abrogate the increased HIV replication induced by MAC and increase the likelihood that ART will succeed (142). Defervescence and some resolution of any localized syndrome associated with MAC would be worth a period of several weeks before ART is added. The judicious use of prophylaxis and management of other conditions should accompany this preparation for the use of ART, which is the key to the successful prevention or eradication of DMAC. Effective ART induces reductions in the systemic levels of TNF-α, TNF-α receptors, and IL-10 associated with DMAC. It also tends to normalize the distorted cellular profiles of TNF-α production that characterize peripheral blood mononuclear cells from HIV-infected persons (143,144).

Few characteristics of DMAC in HIV infection have dominated the literature as have localized and systemic complications related to immune reconstitution. This can be measured both by *in vitro* responses to mycobacterial antigen and by clinical findings. A previously ineffectual or absent immune response can return with a vengeance and create local syndromes at the site of infestation. These can be devastating, disfiguring, and can make continued therapy difficult. MAC infections may be inapparent until ART unveils an immune response that is more sensitive than the best diagnostics. The manifestations of these infections include suppuration (usually most marked in patients with the most vigorous cellular responses to HIV treatment), obstruction of viscera, and constitutional syndromes that have no specific features to distinguish them from new and aggressive pathologic entities (145–149). Diagnosis of these infections should be sought with biopsies guided by signs and symptoms of local involvement.

Until microbiologic confirmation is obtained, the presumptive diagnosis of tissue pathology with AFBs will continue to be tuberculosis. When necessary, it is possible to construct a regimen that minimizes drug interactions and is effective against both MAC and tuberculosis. When microbiologic information is complete, a clinical decision can be made that allows for tailoring of therapy. Rifabutin in adjusted doses serves this purpose but with the caveats stressed above (Table 46.1). Recent recommendations from the U.S. Public Health Service have warned of failure of antituberculous chemotherapy in AIDS patients with fewer than 60 CD4+ T cells/mL when intermittent dosing of the rifamycin (once or twice weekly) is used (150). As noted above, azithromycin is not reported to interfere with rifabutin metabolism in the same fashion as clarithromycin, but its addition to these complex regimens has not been assessed in any clinical trial. Caution should be exercised regarding the addition of clarithromycin, particularly in this setting. Clarithromycin inhibits the metabolism of rifabutin and leads to increased rifabutin levels. This will increase rifabutin's interactions with many effective antiretroviral agents, potentially compromising their effectiveness. Recent recommendations include available information on the adjustment of rifabutin doses for administration with antiretroviral agents (151,152). These recommendations do not take into account the concomitant administration of clarithromycin, so that they may not apply with this combination. Furthermore, all protease inhibitors in current use, with the exception of nelfinavir, are commonly administered with variable doses (from 100 to 400 mg

TABLE 46.1. RIFABUTIN INTERACTIONS WITH SELECTED ANTIRETROVIRAL AGENTS

	Nev	Efav	Nelf	Lop/rit	Ind.
Δ with Rif 300 (mg/qd)	Decr. 16%		Decr. 32%		Decr. 32%
Rif level Δ		Decr. 35%	Incr. 2×	Incr. 3×[a]	Incr. 2×
Rec. Δ Rif (mg/q.o.d)		450–600	150	150 q.o.d.	150
Rec. Δ Rif (mg/int)[b]		600 2–3×/wk			300 mg 2–3×/wk

Efav, efavirenz; Ind, indinavir; Lop/rit, lopinavir/ritonavir; Nelf, nelfinavir; Nev, nevirapine; Rif, rifabutin.
[a]Rifabutin 25-O-desacetyl metabolite increased 47.5-fold.
[b]Note caution on the intermittent dosing of rifamycin in patients with CD4+ T-cell/mL less than 60 (148).
Adapted from Centers for Disease Control and Prevention. Acquired Rifamycin resistance in persons with advanced HIV disease being treated for active tuberculosis with intermittent rifamycin–based regimes. *MMWR Surveill Summ* 2002;51:214–215.

b.i.d.) of ritonavir for pharmacologic boosting. This creates another daunting and generally unassessed interaction with rifabutin. The clarithromycin–rifabutin interaction may also increase the incidence of rifabutin-associated uveitis, a problem also seen with concomitant fluconazole and rifabutin (153,154). Therapeutic drug monitoring might help avoid some of these problems, but its lack of general availability and expense precludes its common use.

Management of DMAC in the patient with failing ART is largely unassessed. Clinical benefit is still present when HIV treatment does not suppress viremia (155). However, the success of therapy for opportunistic infections will be inversely proportional to the degree of immunosuppression and the burden of organisms. These factors combine to make the emergence of isolates resistant to available therapies inevitable. Temporary benefit may be obtained from modification or intensification of drug combinations. Neither susceptibility testing nor clinical trials of salvage therapies are sufficiently related to long-term clinical outcome to be useful (156).

The relationship of drug resistance to clinical failure in MAC infections is complex and incompletely understood. Noncompliance is a prominent feature in many reports of treatment failure (157,158). Clarithromycin remains the only agent for which susceptibility testing has sufficient clinical correlation to be useful (117). Whether clinical failure is due to the emergence of latent, clonally related, drug-resistant populations, polyclonal initial infection, or reinfection with drug-resistant organisms is unclear. However, principles derived from animal models and *in vitro* testing are consistent with clinical results (159). Macrolide resistance occurs when the population of MAC exceeds 10^8 organisms. This high mycobacterial burden is most likely in patients with extreme immunosuppression. This is confirmed by the increased incidence of resistance in prophylaxed or treated patients with fewer then 25 CD4+ T cells. Although reports of initial infection with clarithromycin-resistant MAC have appeared, this problem remains insufficiently common to justify baseline susceptibility testing even to this agent (160).

The microbiologic basis for resistance to macrolides has been elucidated, and specific nucleotide changes in ribosomal RNA have been identified that lead to resistance (161). Changes that affect the utility of other classes of drugs, such as rifamycins, are less well understood. The defined mechanism of resistance to rifamycins in *M. tuberculosis* does not seem to be operative in MAC (162). Studies in which microbiologic resistance and outcome of treatment in animal models are inconsistent continue to appear (163). Clinicians should bear in mind that this contradiction may represent the evolution of microbiologic standards for reporting resistance.

Prophylaxis

Multiple strategies have been considered to control the impact of MAC in advanced HIV infection, from preven-

tion of contamination to bacteriologic or clinical monitoring. Chemoprophylaxis, now the recommended approach, not only decreases the incidence of disseminated infection but has an impact on mortality as well (164). The benefits of prophylaxis extend to the incidence of other important clinical events in advanced HIV infection, such as PCP, community-acquired pneumonia, and neoplastic disease, again confirming the synergy of DMAC in accelerating immunologic deterioration (158). In the absence of effective ART, the effectiveness of prophylaxis wanes with time and degree of immunosuppression. In one study, the median time to DMAC with clarithromycin prophylaxis versus no prophylaxis was 217 days versus 199 days with clarithromycin-susceptible MAC and 385 days with clarithromycin-resistant MAC. Clarithromycin resistance occurred disproportionately in patients with fewer than 20 CD4+ T cells/mL (165). The incidence of resistance to rifabutin in groups receiving prophylaxis has varied. Initial assessments suggested that the development of resistance should not affect the continuation of therapy (166). Since resistance testing for rifabutin is still not standardized, the lack of *in vitro* resistance in the face of clinical failure remains an unsolved problem.

Rifabutin was the first agent reported to be effective in the prevention of DMAC. Early trials of rifabutin alone demonstrated a decrease in the incidence of DMAC, with relative risks decreased up to 3.1 versus placebo recipients (167). Concerns arose very early thereafter about the utility of the drug, which was the first to benefit from the obscurity surrounding the emergence of drug-resistant isolates. Additionally, the chronic administration of a rifamycin alone in areas of prevalence of *M. tuberculosis* caused considerable alarm. Rifamycin-resistant tuberculosis has been reported in a patient receiving MAC prophylaxis with rifabutin (168).

The macrolides utilized for the treatment of MAC are also effective prophylactic agents. The combination of azithromycin and rifabutin had greater efficacy than either drug alone (DMAC in 3% at one year for the combination, 15% for rifabutin alone, 8% with azithromycin alone) (169). A companion trial of azithromycin alone showed a statistically significant improvement with a hazard ration of 0.34 versus placebo (11% developed MAC with azithromycin, 25% with placebo at 18 months) (170). The combination of clarithromycin and rifabutin was more effective (not statistically significant) than either drug alone and was associated with more adverse events (171). The trial of clarithromycin alone was stopped at the first interim analysis due to an adjusted hazard ratio of 0.31 (6% with drug versus 16% for placebo) in favor of clarithromycin (158). The final and most salient reason to avoid rifamycins in the treatment of HIV-infected persons came with the advent of protease-inhibitor based therapy. Rifamycin-induced metabolism of these agents, as noted above, leads to decreases in protease-inhibitor serum levels that would predict loss of activity (172). This has led to the general recommendation that rifabutin be avoided if possible and replaced as a prophylactic and therapeutic agent by azithromycin or clarithromycin. The ease of administration, efficacy, and tolerability of once-weekly 1200 mg of azithromycin have made this the prophylactic regimen of choice in most settings (173).

Prophylaxis is most effective when given early, but successive reports of risk have established the current threshold of 75 CD4+ T-cells/ml as the common time to initiate MAC prophylaxis. Clinical considerations may suggest that more intense prophylaxis would be appropriate with more advanced immunosuppression or other factors (sputum or stool-culture positive patients) that increase the risk of dissemination. Since the disease in this circumstance will proceed along a continuum, it is reasonable to intensify prophylaxis after risk assessment. Daily clarithromycin with or without ethambutol may be used in patients at highest risk or with suspected subclinical disease.

Discontinuation of Treatment and Prophylaxis

The need to include a section on successful treatment and discontinuation of prophylaxis is the greatest evidence for the remarkable strides made in understanding and controlling both HIV infection and DMAC. Fivefold reductions in the incidence of MAC in patients on ART have been reported (174). Susceptibility to MAC disease may still be present within 2 months of initiation of ART and in patients with suboptimal CD4+ T-cell responses.

Cessation of primary prophylaxis is easiest to assess. With effective ART, the recrudescence to CD4+ T cells to levels that exceed 100/mL on a repeated basis (>6 months) is considered sufficient grounds to lessen the risk of DMAC and discontinue primary prophylaxis (175–177). Standards for the completion of therapy (or cessation of secondary prophylaxis) are more difficult to establish. Clearance of mycobacteremia would seem to be a desirable goal, but no reports have so far established that this is a sufficiently sensitive marker of clinical success. Local complications such as lymphadenitis may persist for prolonged periods of time and actually represent more troublesome sites of clinical involvement in patients who have better immune reconstitution. There have been reports of recrudescent disease with both continuation and cessation of mycobacterial therapy, further underscoring our lack of understanding of all the specific elements that lead to control and eradication of MAC. Rates of relapse have varied from 0.9 to 4 per 100 person-years. Manifestations have included systemic deterioration as well as worsening localized disease (178–184). The interpretive pitfalls of this data are well illustrated in a case reported by Murray et al. (185). Isolated cerebral *M. avium* resistant to clarithromycin occurred in a patient with good cellular and virologic responses to HIV therapy. The

lesion was characterized by granulomatous inflammation. Prolonged prior therapy (>6 years) with clarithromycin and ethambutol and continued secondary prophylaxis with azithromycin had been used in this patient with prior mycobacteremia. This clinical failure may represent the selection of resistant isolates because of the high burden of organisms initially and successful immune reconstitution directed at the residual drug-resistant population.

The general standard for cessation of primary prophylaxis may apply to cessation of therapy. Successful therapy should lead to the resolution of symptoms referable to MAC, such as fever, inanition, and diarrhea. The utilization of viral load in the decision process regarding cessation of DMAC therapy has not been reported. Shafran et al. (186) reviewed 52 cases of cessation of therapy for DMAC. The median follow-up after stopping antimycobacterial therapy was 20 months. Only one patient had MAC disease in the follow-up period. This failure occurred 37 months after cessation of antimycobacterial therapy and 2 months after cessation of ART that was not suppressing viremia. The prolonged period without recrudescent disease in the one failure reported may have represented reacquisition rather than recrudescent infection, as noted by the authors. It is notable that fewer patients with a history of DMAC that recrudesced after cessation of secondary prophylaxis had undetectable viral loads (31%) than those with successful cessation of secondary prophylaxis for *Toxoplasma* encephalitis (68%) (179).

MYCOBACTERIUM KANSASII

Horsburgh and Selik (187), in a 1989 review, reported that *M. kansasii* was the second most common cause of NTM disease in AIDS patients in the United States (3% of disseminated cases of NTM). The appearance, course, and response to therapy have been clarified in the last decade. *M. kansasii* in regions where it is common behaves predominantly as a pulmonary pathogen with a propensity to disseminate at the extremes of immunosuppression (188). Identification has been improved by the standard use of molecular probes in microbiologic processing. An Italian study of clinical isolates noted failures to hybridize with commercial probes (AccuProbe *M. kansasii* Culture Identification Test). These isolates clustered as a biotype by phenotypic traits. There was a significant association with isolation from AIDS patients and this novel biotype (189).

A slow-growing photochromogen, *M. kansasii* is endemic in the central United States, down the Mississippi Valley and from east to west coasts, but disease has been reported in HIV-infected persons from nonendemic areas such as New York City (190). It is present in Europe as represented by series from London, Amsterdam, Spain, and Paris (191–195). Series from England found that it was less common than *M. xenopi* in both HIV-infected and non–HIV-infected patients (196,197). It is a common pathogen in South Africa, and although present in Japan, no cases in HIV infection (consistent with a low endemic prevalence of HIV in Japan) are reported. It is rare in Australia. As with other mycobacteria, unusual manifestations in HIV infection are more likely with greater degrees of immunosuppression. Bloch et al. (198) reviewed all positive sputum cultures for *M. kansasii* in three California counties from 1992 to 1996. Rates per 100,000 persons were 115 with HIV infection (median CD4$^+$ T cells 290/mL) and 647 for those with AIDS (median CD4$^+$ T cells 20/mL). African Americans with AIDS, women with AIDS, and African-American women with AIDS had rates of 1,533, 1,450, and 2,137 cases per 100,000 population. Mycobacteremia was present in 20% of those from whom blood cultures were taken. The authors made note of a possible association with poverty.

M. kansasii tends to be a pathogen in urban areas, and isolation from water supplies suggests that the aerosol route accounts for acquisition of the organism (199). Pulmonary disease predominates in that setting, with radiographic appearances characterized as upper lobe infiltrates, diffuse interstitial infiltrates, and thin-walled cavitary lesions, which may predispose to pneumothoraces. Endobronchial lesions occur and may resolve with treatment and without residual bronchial abnormalities (200). Pulmonary disease is often complicated by the presence of other pathogens. A series from New Orleans reported concomitant MAC in respiratory specimens of 13 of 49 patients with 13 other pulmonary microbiologic isolates (201). Corbett et al. (202) followed a cohort of South African miners for 1 year for the development of disease secondary to NTM. *M. kansasii* was common, and 34% of patients were HIV infected. HIV-associated disease occurred at a median CD4$^+$ T-cell count of 381/mL, and 83% of patients were cured after 12 months of treatment. A second report from South Africa emphasizes the prevalence of silicosis and/or old tuberculous scarring in this same population (203). These miners underwent active radiographic surveillance, and patients with HIV and *M. kansasii* infections were more likely to have a normal premorbid chest radiograph, with less cavitation (55% vs. 78%) and more hilar adenopathy. This suggests that occupationally acquired lung damage created a setting in which mycobacterial disease occurred at earlier stages of immunosuppression.

Disseminated disease is represented by bloodstream infection, central nervous system disease, and bone and joint infections. Pericarditis, osteomyelitis, arthritis, and tenosynovitis have been reported from Spain (204–207). A retrospective review of *M. kansasii* septic arthritis from France emphasized the prevalence (four of seven patients) of HIV infection with this complication (208). Poor outcomes with dissemination were reported in the first 10 years of the HIV epidemic, usually in patients with advanced HIV disease (209). English reports of disseminated disease

also note frequent isolation from the GI tract, suggesting that this is sometimes the site from which the organism disseminates (192).

Treatment proceeds along lines established by the ATS (134). MICs for isoniazid are higher for *M. kansasii* than for *M. tuberculosis*, but effective levels can be achieved. Rifamycins are a mainstay of treatment. Rifampin-resistant isolates have occurred, and HIV infection was common in these patients (210). Responses to four-drug therapy based on *in vitro* susceptibilities remained acceptable, with sputum cultures converting to negative in 90% of patients. Bacteriologic relapse occurred in 80% of patients who withdrew from therapy after less than 6 months of culture negativity. Macrolides are highly active *in vitro* (211), and either these or rifabutin (see cautions above) are suggested as substitutes for rifampin in the HIV-infected patient due to interactions with antiretroviral drugs (134). Management of pulmonary disease in the nonimmunosuppressed patient is generally for 18 months, with a minimum of 12 months of culture negativity. No clear experience justifies modification of that recommendation in either the context of HIV infection or dissemination.

MYCOBACTERIUM XENOPI

An organism of uncertain pathologic potential in the nonimmunosuppressed patient, *M. xenopi* is the second most common NTM isolate in various regions of the world, from Canada to England. Uncertainty as to its clinical importance has been exacerbated by improvements in detection and its presence in hospital water supplies, especially hot water (it is an obligate thermophile). For these reasons, it has dominated many reports of contaminating microbiology or mycobacterial isolates with a dubious pathogenic role (212,213).

In the rare circumstance when the organism causes disease, it is predominantly a pulmonary pathogen. Its presentation is similar to that of MAC in the nonimmunosuppressed patient with preexisting lung conditions. In AIDS patients there is a high prevalence of coinfection. One series reported *P. carinii* (nine cases), cytomegalovirus (five), MAC (two), and bacterial (four) and fungal (two) pathogens from 17 patients (214). Three fourths of these patients were thought to be colonized with *M. xenopi*, with disease prominent in those with more advanced HIV (four of seven with CD4$^+$ T cells ≤50/mL). Disseminated disease is reported in HIV infection, but rarely so. More recently, disease in HIV-infected persons has occurred in the context of antiretroviral treatment, suggesting that the organism may be a target of immune reconstitution (215).

Therapy should consist of a macrolide with ethambutol and a rifamycin. Clarithromycin is the most studied macrolide in non–HIV-infected persons. Caution about the use of rifamycins in HIV-infected patients on ART has been noted above.

MYCOBACTERIUM HAEMOPHILUM

First identified in 1978 in Israel as a cause of cutaneous ulcers in a patient with Hodgkin disease, *M. haemophilum* has been disproportionately studied and reported due to its microbiologic characteristics rather than its propensity to cause disease (216,217). Reports remain rare enough to make geographic considerations difficult; the organism is reported from every continent except Africa. Two cases reported from Brazil (a nasal ulcer and elbow osteomyelitis) represent the first cases from South America (218). The authors emphasize the laboratory variability in culture attributes. They suggest that blood from cultured tissue may have accounted for growth on primary isolation. The possibility of *M. haemophilum* as a cause of a syndrome characteristic of disseminated NTM infection in an AIDS patient is reinforced by smear positivity with a lack of growth on solid media. Both temperature-dependent growth (optimal at 28°C to 33°C) and the requirement for supplemented media (either with commercial paper containing hemin or the addition of ferric ammonium citrate to the medium) are critical in achieving growth.

Cutaneous disease has been the principal manifestation in AIDS patients. Subcutaneous abscesses or erythematous, tender nodules, especially over joints, may occur. Lymphadenitis, and occasionally osteomyelitis or arthritis, may also be explained by temperature-dependent growth (219). Pulmonary disease may have a disproportionately poor outcome (220), with five deaths among six patients in a series of 23 cases from a cancer center in New York. The organism may account for localized syndromes following immune reconstitution (221).

Recommendations for therapy are based on case reports. Generally, rifabutin [the rifamycin with lowest minimal inhibitory concentrations (MICs)] as well as a quinolone and a macrolide are used in combination. An aminoglycoside and tetracycline might be added in disseminated or pulmonary disease (220,222). Of note, there are reports of resolution without specific antimicrobial therapy in AIDS patients who succeed with ART (223). No clear recommendation on duration of therapy is possible. In the severely compromised patient 12 to 18 months of treatment is often the goal. This may be modified in the HIV-infected patient in whom reversal of immunosuppression (return of CD4+ T cells to >100/mL for >6 months) is achieved.

MYCOBACTERIUM GENAVENSE

First reported clinically and subsequently characterized microbiologically in the early 1990s by a group in Geneva, *M. genavense* causes a syndrome generally indistinguishable from that of DMAC (224).

The first series of patients presented with widely disseminated GI and lymphoid tissue involvement, accompanied by fever, diarrhea, and weight loss (225). Subsequent reports have broadened the geography of infection, to areas throughout Europe, North America, Australia, and Taiwan. A bias to detecting MAC and the more advanced technologies necessary for identification may have limited reporting (226–232). Furthermore, as noted below, susceptibility to macrolides and the use of that class for prophylaxis against DMAC may limit further cases. Isolation from birds has been noted, and the question of *M. genavense* being an avian zoonosis has been raised but not confirmed (233). The organism has been identified in hospital tap water (234).

Standard cultures are negative in up to 50% of autopsy-proven cases. Recent clinical reports have emphasized the appearance of disease in advanced HIV infection (CD4+ T-cell counts <100/mL). Abdominal pain, organomegaly, diffuse lymphadenopathy, as well as focal findings in the liver and spleen have been reported (235,236). Some patients have diffuse nodular pulmonary infiltrates (237). One case of an isolated brain mass has been reported (238). Stool smears showed AFB significantly more often than in DMAC in one series, but cultures were positive in only 15% of cases, as opposed to 71% with MAC (239).

A syndrome consistent with disseminated mycobacterial disease in patients with advanced AIDS should alert the clinician to search for *M. genavense*. This is especially true when smears from tissue are positive (small coccobacillary AFB) and there is no growth. Liquid medium growth is enhanced by acidity (pH 6.0), and inhibitors commonly used in the mycobacteriology laboratory (PANTA and polyoxyethylene stearate) reduce yields (240). Microaerophilic conditions (2.5% to 5% O_2) may enhance growth (241). The organisms are inhibited by NAP. Nucleic amplification techniques provide greatest sensitivity (242).

In vitro susceptibility is not standardized, but a murine model suggested that clarithromycin, rifabutin, ethambutol, and ciprofloxacin are effective. The first two drugs gave earlier reductions in spleen CFUs than the latter two (243). Clinical success has been reported with the use of clarithromycin (244). Clarithromycin MICs have been reported to be ≤0.06 to 0.25 μg/mL (245). Treatment may proceed based on principles enumerated for MAC, as fluoroquinolones, macrolides, and rifamycins are effective *in vitro*. The utility of ethambutol and aminoglycosides is not clear.

SAV

The *SAV* group, including *Mycobacterium simiae-avium* and *Mycobacterium triplex*, is a newly formed consortium of organisms that have biochemical similarities but can be genetically distinguished by nucleic acid amplification and high-performance liquid chromatography. They are slow growing but do not fall into one Runyon classification (246).

M. simiae was first identified in an HIV-infected patient early in the epidemic. A native of the Congo, the patient received medical care in France and had concomitant disseminated *M. simiae* and MAC infection (247). Cases have been reported over a broad geographic distribution, including Malawi, Israel, and Thailand (248,249). Clinical reports have continued to emphasize the similarity to and the frequent occurrence of coinfection with MAC (250,251).

Growth characteristics in the laboratory are similar to those of MAC, but the organisms are broadly resistant to antimicrobials except for clarithromycin and ethionamide. No report has defined clinical responses because therapy with these agents did not prevent recrudescence of disease with an isolate that had an unchanged susceptibility profile (252).

OTHER NONTUBERCULOUS MYCOBACTERIA

Mycobacterium gordonae, a saprophytic scotochromogen, is a rare cause of disease. Early reports suggested that it is pathogenic in advanced HIV infection, with some pulmonary disease and rare cases of dissemination. However, pulmonary isolates often occur in the presence of other pathogens. Management of disseminated disease has been successful with antituberculous agents (253,254). A patient with isolated cutaneous disease responded well to therapy (255).

Mycobacterium celatum has been reported in a handful of cases. Pneumonia and bacteremic dissemination have occurred. It is important to note that clinical improvement has occurred with the administration of isoniazid, rifampin, and ethambutol, although this was not suggested by *in vitro* testing (256,257). Disease has been reported with rifabutin-resistant (MIC 8 mg/L) isolates in AIDS patients, both with CD4+ T cell counts less than 10/mL, receiving rifabutin prophylaxis (258). Some mention should be made about laboratory identification and *in vitro* studies. Conventional assays may misidentify the organism as *M. xenopi* or *MAC* (259). *M. celatum* type 1 has been reported to cross-react with the AccuProbe *M. tuberculosis* complex assay, and this may be temperature dependent (260,261). Microbiologic, cell-based, and animal studies have demonstrated colony morphology–associated virulence and drug susceptibilities similar to those noted for MAC. In the murine model, the more virulent forms were most reduced by macrolides (262).

Classically a cause of cervical lymphadenitis in children, *M. scrofulaceum* has caused pulmonary, cutaneous (chronic ulcerative and nodular skin lesions), and disseminated disease in AIDS patients (263–265). Once considered a member of the MAC, it is now classified as a separate species. Its similarity to *M. avium* in many respects and the rarity of reports of disease associated with *M. scrofulaceum* serve to reinforce the specific pathogenic role or broad geographic range of *M. avium* in HIV infection. Susceptibility to clarithromycin, ethambutol, and clofazimine have been

demonstrated *in vitro*, and the general similarity to *M. avium* susceptibilities suggests that treatment regimens similar to those used for MAC would be appropriate.

Common isolates but uncommon pathogens, members of the *Mycobacterium terrae complex* are reported in a single case of disseminated infection with pulmonary (diffuse interstitial involvement) and skin manifestations (painless, nonpruritic papulonodular lesions) in an AIDS patient. The organism was broadly susceptible to antimicrobials, but the patient died before therapy could be instituted (266). We have seen one case of symptomatic urethritis with urine cultures positive for *M. terrae* in a patient with advanced AIDS at Bellevue Hospital. However, the patient was lost to follow-up before specific chemotherapy could be started or its effectiveness assessed.

Mycobacterium szulgai has been reported to cause pulmonary infection, disseminated disease, and osteomyelitis in AIDS patients (267–270). Pulmonary infection is clinically indistinguishable from tuberculosis. The organism has a worldwide distribution but is a rarely reported pathogen even in nonimmunocompromised patients. Pulmonary disease is the predominant manifestation. Both increased and decreased susceptibility to antituberculous agents has been reported. Macrolides have been used with success in the management of isolated cutaneous disease in a non–HIV-infected patient (271). At Bellevue, we have treated a Vietnamese immigrant with disseminated disease (suppurative lymphadenopathy, cutaneous and bone disease without pulmonary involvement). The patient's first isolate, from a lymph node biopsy, was susceptible to first-line antituberculous agents. Treatment with clarithromycin, ethambutol, and ART led to initial resolution of local symptoms. ART was also successful, but recrudescence of the *M. szulgai* infection occurred at 4 months with a clarithromycin-resistant isolate. A year-long course of multidrug therapy led to resolution of the mycobacterial infection.

Although highly endemic in Africa and present in Australia, *M. ulcerans* as a specific pathogen in HIV infection is represented by a single case report, although HIV infection has been present in series of cases of Buruli ulcer. Both standard excisional therapy and antimycobacterial agents (rifampin, ethambutol, and clarithromycin) did not arrest the progression of disseminated cutaneous and bone lesions (272).

Mycobacterium malmoense, a slow-growing nonchromogenic organism, is more common in Europe than in the United States. Presenting as a tumorlike mass in the lung or as a disseminated pathogen (pulmonary and GI disease) at late stages of HIV infection, therapy was successful in one case with rifabutin, clofazimine, and isoniazid. Sputum smears have been positive for AFB without concomitant radiographic abnormalities (273–275). Earlier reports have not been followed by additional information that would suggest that this organism has a special role in HIV infection even in endemic areas (276).

Mycobacterium marinum is an organism that grows in brackish waters. It has limited pathogenicity because its growth is contingent on low temperature. Reports of clinical disease in HIV infection (sporotrichoid spread) do not identify any special prevalence or characteristics in AIDS patients (277–279).

Mycobacterium shimoidei has been reported in only a few cases of lung disease worldwide. Two cases of AIDS patients with disseminated disease (positive blood cultures) are described, one from Australia and one from Switzerland. The organism is often misidentified by biochemicals as *M. terrae*, but restriction fragment length polymorphism and PCR of ribosomal DNA allow for proper speciation (280,281). The organism is too rarely encountered for therapeutic recommendations to be available.

Rapidly growing mycobacteria are rarely reported in HIV infection. Most cases involve *Mycobacterium fortuitum*. The clinical characteristics of these reports do not suggest that these infections are markedly different in the HIV-infected host. Cases similar to those in nonimmunosuppressed persons include a catheter-related infection, an intragluteal injection site abscess (*Mycobacterium chelonae*) accompanied by lymph node involvement, and cutaneous disease (282, 283). *M. fortuitum* caused one case of osteomyelitis from India (in this case reported as *M. fortuitum-chelonae*), one of pulmonary disease from Benin, and one urinary tract infection from Turkey (284–286). Isolated cervical adenitis responded to incision, drainage, and therapy with ciprofloxacin and clarithromycin in a report of two cases from Louisiana (287). A pseudo-outbreak of *M. fortuitum* on an HIV hospital ward was traced to a contaminated ice machine and the contaminated sputum specimens were not associated with progressive pulmonary disease (288). A review of rapidly growing mycobacteria isolated over 11 years in Sweden identified only one case of disseminated *M. fortuitum* and one sputum isolate of *M. chelonae* in HIV-infected persons (289). No change from standard therapy for these organisms has been suggested.

Among the rapidly growing mycobacteria, *M. fortuitum* dominates reports of dissemination. Cases have occurred in North and South America (290–292). A pathologic series from Texas reported 11 cases, nine with cervical lymphadenitis and two with dissemination (293). Advanced HIV infection was present in the patients, and a relative (seven of 11) or absolute (four of 11) monocytosis was the only laboratory abnormality noted. Inflammation tended to be suppurative with or without a granulomatous reaction. The authors noted a tendency to early misidentification of the organism as *Nocardia*. Clinical responses to therapy were curative in ten of 11 cases. *M. chelonae* was isolated from a bone marrow culture in one AIDS patient from a series of 1,225 specimens in North Carolina (294). Central nervous system infection occurs with *M. fortuitum* and has been associated with poor outcomes (295,296).

Wallace et al. (297) reported on *M. chelonae*-like organisms in a series that reviewed 87 microbiologic isolates. The respiratory tract was the source in 54 cases, but disease was present only in two AIDS patients. These organisms were subsequently reclassified as *Mycobacterium mucogenicum* (298). Posttraumatic wound infections and catheter-related sepsis were the other manifestations of clinical disease in nonimmunosuppressed patients.

REFERENCES

1. Report on the global HIV/AIDS epidemic. The Barcelona report. UNAIDS at Barcelona. XIV International Conference on AIDS, Barcelona, 7–12 July 2002.
2. Ghassemi M, Andersen BR, Reddy VM. Human immunodeficiency virus and *Mycobacterium avium* complex coinfection of monocytoid cells results in reciprocal enhancement of multiplication. *J Infect Dis* 1995;171:68–73.
3. Springer, B, Stockman L, Teschner K, et al. Two-laboratory collaborative study on identification of mycobacteria: molecular versus phenotypic methods. *J Clin Microbiol* 1996;34: 296–303.
4. Lévy-Frébault V, Portaels F. Proposed minimal standards for the genus *Mycobacterium* and for description of newly slowly growing *Mycobacterium* species. *Int J Syst Bacteriol* 1992;42: 315–323.
5. Horsburgh CR Jr, Mason UG III, Farhi DC, et al. Disseminated infection with *Mycobacterium avium-intracellulare*. A report of 13 cases and a review of the literature. *Medicine* 1985; 64:36–48.
6. Greene JB, Sidhu GS, Lewin S, et al. *Mycobacterium avium-intracellulare*: a cause of disseminated life-threatening infection in homosexuals and drug abusers. *Ann Intern Med* 1982;97: 539–546.
7. Nightingale DS, Byrd LT, Southern PM, et al. Incidence of *Mycobacterium avium-intracellulare* complex bacteremia in human immunodeficiency virus–positive patients. *J Infect Dis* 1992;165:1082–1085.
8. Asnis DS, Bresciani AR, Cohn M. *Mycobacterium avium-intracellulare* complex pneumonia in a non–HIV-infected individual: an increasingly recognized disease. *South Med J* 1996;89 (5):522-5.
9. Ives DV, Davis RB, Currier JS. Impact of clarithromycin and azithromycin on patterns of treatment and survival among AIDS patients with disseminated *Mycobacterium avium* complex. *AIDS* 1995;9:261–266.
10. Horsburgh CR. *Mycobacterium avium* complex infection in the acquired immunodeficiency syndrome. *N Engl J Med* 1991; 324:1332–1338.
11. Chin DP, Reingold AL, Stone EN, et al. The impact of *Mycobacterium avium* complex bacteremia and its treatment on survival of AIDS patients—a prospective study. *J Infect Dis* 1994;170:578–584.
12. El-Solh AA, Nopper J, Abul-Khoudoud MR, et al. Clinical and radiographic manifestations of uncommon pulmonary nontuberculous mycobacterial disease in AIDS patients. *Chest* 1998; 114:138–145.
13. Guthertz LS. Damsker B, Bottone EJ, et al. *Mycobacterium avium* and *Mycobacterium intracellulare* infections in patients with and without AIDS. *J Infect Dis* 1989;160:1037–1041.
14. Saad MH, Vincent V, Dawson DJ, et al. Analysis of *Mycobacterium avium* complex serovars isolated from AIDS patients

from southeast Brazil. *Mem Inst Oswaldo Cruz* 1997;92: 471–475.

15. Wong DA, Yip PC, Cheung DT, et al. Simple and rational approach to the identification of *Mycobacterium tuberculosis*, *Mycobacterium avium* complex species, and other commonly isolated mycobacteria. *J Clin Microbiol* 2001;39:3768–3771.

16. Thorel MF, Huchzermeyer HF, Michel AL. *Mycobacterium avium* and *Mycobacterium intracellulare* infection in mammals. *Rev Sci Tech* 2001;20:204–218.

17. Denner JC, Tsang AY, Chatterjee D, et al. Comprehensive approach to identification of serovars of *Mycobacterium avium* complex. *J Clin Microbiol* 1992;30:473–478.

18. De Smet KA, Brown IN, Yates M, et al. Ribosomal internal transcribed spacer sequences are identical among *Mycobacterium avium-intracellulare* complex isolates from AIDS patients, but vary among isolates from elderly pulmonary disease patients. *Microbiology* 1995;141:2739–2747.

19. Devallois A, Picardeau M, Paramasivan CN, et al. Molecular characterization of *Mycobacterium avium* complex isolates giving discordant results in AccuProbe tests by PCR-restriction enzyme analysis, 16S rRNA gene sequencing, and DT1-DT6 PCR. *J Clin Microbiol* 1997;35:2767–2772.

20. Beggs ML, Stevanova R, Eisenach KD. Species identification of *Mycobacterium avium* complex isolates by a variety of molecular techniques. *J Clin Microbiol* 2000;38:508–512.

21. Slutsky AM, Arbeit RD, Barber TW, et al. Polyclonal infections due to *Mycobacterium avium* complex in patients with AIDS detected by pulsed-field gel electrophoresis of sequential clinical isolates. *J Clin Microbiol* 1994;32:1773–1778.

22. Matsiota-Bernard P, Zinzendorf N, Onody C, et al. Comparison of clarithromycin-sensitive and clarithromycin-resistant *Mycobacterium avium* strains isolated from AIDS patients during therapy regimens including clarithromycin. *J Infect* 2000; 40:49–54.

23. LeBlanc SB, Naik EG, Jacobson L, et al. Association of DRB1*1501 with disseminated *Mycobacterium avium* complex infection in North American AIDS patients. *Tissue Antigens* 2000;55:17–23.

24. Sterling TR, Moore RD, Graham NM, et al. *Mycobacterium tuberculosis* infection and disease are not associated with protection against subsequent disseminated *M. avium* complex disease. *AIDS* 1998;12:1451–1457.

25. Stankova M, Rozsypal H, Kubin M, et al. Mycobacterial infections in patients with AIDS in a low HIV prevalence area. *Cent Eur J Public Health* 1994;2:100–102.

26. Shenoy R, Kapadi SN, Pai KP, et al. Fine needle aspiration diagnosis in HIV-related lymphadenopathy in Mangalore, India. *Acta Cytol* 2002;46:35–39.

27. Colebunders R, Nembunzu M, Portaels F, et al. Isolation of mycobacteria from stools and intestinal biopsies from HIV seropositive and HIV seronegative patients with and without diarrhea in Kinshasa, Zaire. Preliminary results. *Annales de la Societé Belge de Médecine Tropicale* 1990;70:303–309.

28. Gilks CF, Brindle RJ, Mwachari C, et al. Disseminated *Mycobacterium avium* infection among HIV-infected patients in Kenya. *J Acquir Immune Defic Syndr Hum Retrovirol* 1995;8:195–198.

29. von Gottberg A, Sacks L, Machala S, et al. Utility of blood cultures and incidence of mycobacteremia in patients with suspected tuberculosis in a South African infectious disease referral hospital. *Int J Tuberc Lung Dis* 2001;5:80–86.

30. Ohtomo K, Wang S, Masunaga A, et al. Secondary infections of AIDS autopsy cases in Japan with special emphasis on *Mycobacterium avium-intracellulare* complex infection. *Tohoku J Exp Med* 2000;192:99–109.

31. von Reyn CF, Waddell RD, Eaton T, et al. Isolation of *Mycobac-*

terium avium complex from water in the United States, Finland, Zaire, and Kenya. *J Clin Microbiol.* 1993;31:3227–3230.

32. Fonteyne PA, Kunze ZM, De Beenhouwer H, et al. Characterization of *Mycobacterium avium* complex related mycobacteria isolated from an African environment and patients with AIDS. *Trop Med Int Health* 1997;2:200–207.

33. von Reyn CF, Maslow JN, Barber TW, et al. Persistent colonisation of potable water as a source of *Mycobacterium avium* infection in AIDS. *Lancet* 1994;343:1137–1141.

34. Yajko DM, Chin DP, Gonzalez PC, et al. *Mycobacterium avium* complex in water, food, and soil samples collected from the environment of HIV-infected individuals. *J Acquir Immune Defic Syndr Hum Retrovirol* 1995;9:176–182.

35. Falkinham JO III, Norton CD, LeChevallier MW. Factors influencing numbers of *Mycobacterium avium*, *Mycobacterium intracellulare*, and other mycobacteria in drinking water distribution systems. *Appl Environ Microbiol* 2001;67:1225–1231.

36. Yajko DM, Nassos PS, Sanders CA, et al. High predictive value of the acid-fast smear for *Mycobacterium tuberculosis* despite the high prevalence of *Mycobacterium avium* complex in respiratory specimens. *Clin Infect Dis* 1994;19:334–336.

37. Williams PL, Currier JS, Swindells S. Joint effects of HIV-1 RNA levels and CD4 lymphocyte cells on the risk of specific opportunistic infections. *AIDS* 1999;13:1035–1044.

38. Hoover DR, Saah AJ, Bacellar H, et al. Clinical manifestations of AIDS in the era of pneumocystis prophylaxis. Multicenter AIDS Cohort Study. *N Engl J Med* 1993;329:1922–1926.

39. Jones JL, Hanson DL, Chu SY, et al. Surveillance of AIDS-defining conditions in the United States. Adult/Adolescent Spectrum of HIV Disease Project Group. *AIDS* 1994;8: 1489–1493.

40. Armstrong JA, Hart PDA. Response of cultured macrophages to *Mycobacterium tuberculosis*, with observations on fusion of lysosomes with phagosomes. *J Exp Med* 1971;134:713–740.

41. Horsburgh CR Jr. The pathophysiology of disseminated *Mycobacterium avium* complex disease in AIDS. *J Infect Dis* 1999;179(Suppl 3):S461–S465.

42. Balcewicz-Sablinska MK, Gan H, Remold HG. Interleukin 10 produced by macrophages inoculated with *Mycobacterium avium* attenuates mycobacteria-induced apoptosis by reduction of TNF-alpha activity. *J Infect Dis* 1999;180:1230–1237.

43. Gomes MS. Florido M, Pais TF, et al. Improved clearance of *Mycobacterium avium* upon disruption of the inducible nitric oxide synthase gene. *J Immunol* 1999;162:6734–6739.

44. Cohen OJ, Kinter A, Fauci AS. Host factors in the pathogenesis of HIV disease. *Immunol Rev* 1997;159:31–48.

45. Sathe SS, Sarai A, Tsigler D, et al. Pentoxifylline aggravates impairment in tumor necrosis factor-alpha secretion and increases mycobacterial load in macrophages from AIDS patients with disseminated *Mycobacterium avium-intracellulare* complex infection. *J Infect Dis* 1994;170:484–487.

46. Denis M, Ghadirian E. *Mycobacterium avium* infection in HIV-1-infected subjects increases monokine secretion and is associated with enhanced viral load and diminished immune response to viral antigens. *Clin Exp Immunol* 1994;97:76–82.

47. Havlir DV, Torriani FJ, Schrier RD, et al. Serum interleukin-6 (IL-6), IL-10, tumor necrosis factor (TNF) alpha, soluble type II TNF receptor, and transforming growth factor beta levels in human immunodeficiency virus type 1–infected individuals with *Mycobacterium avium* complex disease. *J Clin Microbiol* 2001;39:298–303.

48. Havlir DV, Haubrich R, Hwang J, et al. Human immunodeficiency virus replication in AIDS patients with *Mycobacterium avium* complex bacteremia: a case control study. California Collaborative Treatment Group. *J Infect Dis* 1998;177:595–599.

49. Orenstein JM, Fox C, Wahl SM. Macrophages as a source of HIV during opportunistic infections. *Science* 1997;276:1857–1861.

50. Wahl SM, Greenwell-Wild T, Peng G, et al. *Mycobacterium avium* complex augments macrophage HIV-1 production and increases CCR5 expression. *Proc Natl Acad Sci U S A* 1998;95:12574–12579.

51. Dezzutti CS, Swords WE, Guenthner PC, et al. Involvement of matrix metalloproteinases in human immunodeficiency virus type 1–induced replication by clinical *Mycobacterium avium* isolates. *J Infect Dis* 1999;180:1142–1152.

52. Lawn SD, Butera ST, Shinnick TM. Tuberculosis unleashed: the impact of human immunodeficiency virus infection on the host granulomatous response to *Mycobacterium tuberculosis*. *Microbes Infect* 2002;4:635–646.

53. Zamir E, Hudson H, Ober RR, et al. Massive mycobacterial choroiditis during highly active antiretroviral therapy: another immune-recovery uveitis? *Ophthalmology* 2002;109:2144–2148.

54. Farhi DC, Mason UG III, Horsburgh CR Jr. Pathologic findings in disseminated *Mycobacterium avium-intracellulare* infection. A report of 11 cases. *Am J Clin Pathol* 1986;85:67–72.

55. Fattorini L, Xiao Y, Li B, et al. Induction of IL-1 beta, IL-6, TNF-alpha, GM-CSF and G-CSF in human macrophages by smooth transparent and smooth opaque colonial variants of *Mycobacterium avium*. *J Med Microbiol* 1994;40:129–33.

56. Horgen L, Barrow ELW, Barrow WW, et al. Exposures of human peripheral blood mononuclear cells to total lipids and serovar-specific glycopeptidolipids from *Mycobacterium avium* serovars 4 and 8 results in inhibition of TH1-type responses. *Microb Pathog* 2000;29:9–16.

57. Kansal RG, Gomez-Flores R, Mehta RT. Change in colony morphology influences the virulence as well as the biochemical properties of the *Mycobacterium avium* complex. *Microb Pathog* 1998;25:203–214.

58. Cangelosi GA, Palermo CO, Laurent JP, et al. Colony morhotypes on Congo red agar segregate along species and drug susceptibility lines in the *Mycobacterium avium-intracellulare* complex. *Microbiology* 1999;145:1317–1324.

59. Reddy VM, Luna-Herrera J, Gangadharam PR. Pathobiological significance of colony morphology in *Mycobacterium avium* complex. *Microb Pathog* 1996;21:97–109.

60. Abdel-Dayem HM, Omar WS, Aziz M, et al. Disseminated *Mycobacterium avium* complex. Review of Ga-67 and Tl-201 scans and autopsy findings. *Clin Nucl Med* 1996;21:547–556.

61. Torriani FJ, Behling CA, McCutchan JA, et al. Disseminated *Mycobacterium avium* complex: correlation between blood and tissue burden. *J Infect Dis* 1996;173:942–949.

62. Kalayjian RC, Toossi Z, Tomashefski JF Jr, et al. Pulmonary disease due to infection by *Mycobacterium avium* complex in patients with AIDS. *Clin Infect Dis* 1995;20:1186–1194.

63. Primack SL, Logan PM, Hartman TE, et al. Pulmonary tuberculosis and *Mycobacterium avium-intracellulare*: a comparison of CT findings. *Radiology* 1995;194:413–417.

64. Raju B, Schluger NW. Significance of respiratory isolates of *Mycobacterium avium* complex in HIV-positive and HIV-negative patients. *Int J Infect Dis* 2000;4:134–139.

65. Epstein MD, Aranda CP, Bonk S, et al. The significance of *Mycobacterium avium* complex cultivation in the sputum of patients with pulmonary tuberculosis. *Chest* 1997;111:142–147.

66. Collazos J, Blanco MS, Mayo J, et al. Gastrointestinal hemorrhage due to gastroduodenal involvement by *Mycobacterium avium* complex in a patient with acquired immune deficiency syndrome. *J Clin Gastroenterol* 1998;26:84–85.

67. Poorman JC, Katon RM. Small bowel involvement by *Mycobacterium avium* complex in a patient with AIDS: endoscopic, his-

68. Cavicchi M, Pialoux G, Carnot F, et al. Value of liver biopsy for the rapid diagnosis of infection in human immunodeficiency virus–infected patients who have unexplained fever and elevated serum levels of alkaline phosphatase or gamma-glutamyl transferase. *Clin Infect Dis* 1995;20:606–610.

69. Arevalo JF, Quiceno JI, Garcia RF, et al. Retinal findings and characteristics in AIDS patients with systemic *Mycobacterium avium-intracellulare* complex and toxoplasmic encephalitis. *Ophthalmic Surg Lasers* 1997;28:50–54.

70. Sheppard DC, Sullam PM. Primary septic arthritis and osteomyelitis due to *Mycobacterium avium* complex in a patient with AIDS. *Clin Infect Dis* 1997;25:925–926.

71. Hadad DJ, Petry TC, Maresca AF, et al. *Mycobacterium avium* complex (MAC): an unusual potential pathogen in cerebrospinal fluid of AIDS patients. *Rev Inst Med Trop Sao Paulo* 1995;37:93–98.

72. Rotstein AH, Stuckey SL. *Mycobacterium avium* complex spinal epidural abscess in an HIV patient. *Australas Radiol* 1999;43:554–557.

73. Woods GL, Goldsmith JC. Fatal pericarditis due to *Mycobacterium avium-intracellulare* in acquired immunodeficiency syndrome. *Chest*. 1989;95:1355–1357.

74. Casado JL, Pintado V, Gomez-Mampaso E, et al. Mycobacterial liver abscess in a patient with AIDS. *Postgrad Med J* 1998;74:181–183.

75. Domingo P, Ris J, Lopez-Contreras J, et al. Appendicitis due to *Mycobacterium avium* complex in a patient with AIDS. *Arch Intern Med* 1996;156:1114.

76. Albu E, Yousuf AM, Swaminathan K, et al. Tuberculous and nontuberculous mycobacterial infection of the pancreas in a patient with AIDS. *Pancreas* 1996;12:412–413.

77. El-Serag HB, Johnston DE. *Mycobacterium avium* complex esophagitis. *Am J Gastroenterol* 1997;92:1561–1563.

78. Wu ML, Poles MA, Thompson AD, et al. Enterocolonic *Mycobacterium avium-intracellulare*. *Arch Pathol Lab Med* 2002;126:381.

79. Huh JJ, Panther LA. *Mycobacterium avium* complex peritonitis in an AIDS patient. *Scand J Infect Dis* 2001;33:936–938.

80. Bachelez H, Ducloy G, Pinquier L, et al. Disseminated varioliform pustular eruption due to *Mycobacterium avium intracellulare* in an HIV-infected patient. *Br J Dermatol* 1996;134:801–803.

81. Taylor CR, Bailey EM. Red nodule on the forearm of an HIV-positive man. Isolated cutaneous *Mycobacterium avium-intracellulare* infection. *Arch Dermatol* 1998;134:1279–1284.

82. Williams JT, Pulitzer DR, DeVillez RL. Papulonecrotic tuberculid secondary to disseminated *Mycobacterium avium* complex. *Int J Dermatol* 1994;33:109–112.

83. Corkill M, Stephens J, Bitter M. Fine needle aspiration cytology of mycobacterial spindle cell pseudotumor. A case report. *Acta Cytol* 1995;39:125–128.

84. Gordin FM, Cohn DL, Sullam PM, et al. Early manifestations of disseminated *Mycobacterium avium* complex disease: a prospective evaluation. *J Infect Dis* 1997;176:126–132.

85. Deshpande RG, Khan MB, Bhat DA, et al. Haemolysin from *Mycobacterium avium* complex isolates from AIDS patients. *J Med Microbiol* 1998;47:365–367.

86. Hafner R, Inderlied CB, Peterson DM, et al. Correlation of quantitative bone marrow and blood cultures in AIDS patients with disseminated *Mycobacterium avium* complex infection. *J Infect Dis* 1999;180:438-447.

87. Horburgh CR Jr, Gettings J, Alexander LN, et al. Disseminated *Mycobacterium avium* complex disease among patients infected

with human ommunodeficiency virus, 1985–2000. *Clin Infect Dis* 2001;33:1938–1943.

88. Chin DP, Hopewell PC, Yajko DM, et al. *Mycobacterium avium* complex in the respiratory or gastrointestinal tract and the risk of *M. avium* complex bacteremia in patients with human immunodeficiency virus infection. *J Infect Dis* 1994;169: 289–295.

89. Chin DP, Reingold AL, Horsburgh CR Jr, et al. Predicting *Mycobacterium avium* complex bacteremia in patients infected with human immunodeficiency virus: a prospectively validated model. *Clin Infect Dis* 1994;19:668–674.

90. Hanna BA, Walters SB, Bonk SJ, et al. Recovery of mycobacteria from blood in mycobacteria growth indicator tube and Lowenstein-Jensen slant after lysis-centrifugation. *J Clin Microbiol* 1995;33:3315–3316.

91. Kanchana MV, Cheke D, Natyshak I, et al. Evaluation of the BACTEC MGIT 960 system for the recovery of mycobacteria. *Diagn Microbiol Infect Dis* 2000;37:31–36.

92. Esteban J, Fernandez-Roblas R, Cabria F, et al. Usefulness of the BACTEC MYCO/F lytic system for detection of mycobacteremia in a clinical microbiology laboratory. *J Microbiol Meth* 2000;40:63–66.

93. Lebrun L, Livartowski J, May T, et al. Failure of the radiometric Bactec method to detect *Mycobacterium avium* complex in the blood of patients infected with human immunodeficiency virus who were treated with antibiotics. *Clin Infect Dis* 1995;21: 1343–1344.

94. Kemper CA, Havlir D, Bartok AE, et al. Transient bacteremia due to *Mycobacterium avium* complex in patients with AIDS. *J Infect Dis* 1994;170:488–493.

95. Yagupsky P, Menegus MA. Cumulative positivity rates of multiple blood cultures for *Mycobacterium avium-intracellulare* and *Cryptococcus neoformans* in patients with the acquired immunodeficiency syndrome. *Arch Pathol Lab Med* 1990;114: 923–925.

96. Rodrigues Vde F, Queiroz Mello FC, Ribeiro MO, et al. Detection of *Mycobacterium avium* in blood samples of patients with AIDS by using PCR. *J Clin Microbiol* 2002;40:2297–2299.

97. Hollings NP, Wells AU, Wilson R, et al. Comparative appearances of non-tuberculous mycobacteria species: a CT study. *Eur Radiol* 2002;12:2211–2217.

98. Murray JG, Patel MD, Lee S, et al. Microabscesses of the liver and spleen in AIDS: detection with 5-MHz sonography. *Radiology* 1995;197:723–727.

99. Pantongrag-Brown L, Krebs TL, Daly BD, et al. Frequency of abdominal CT findings in AIDS patients with *M. avium* complex bacteraemia. *Clin Radiol* 1998;53:816–819.

100. Lee VW, Cooley TP, Fuller JD, et al. Pulmonary mycobacterial infections in AIDS: characteristic pattern of thallium and gallium scan mismatch. *Radiology* 1994;193:389–392.

101. Bosch O, Porres JC, Martinez Quesada G, et al. Endoscopic appearance of a duodenal infection by *Mycobacterium avium-intracellulare* in AIDS. *Endoscopy* 1994;26:506.

102. Cavicchi M, Pialoux G, Carnot F, et al. Value of liver biopsy for the rapid diagnosis of infection in human immunodeficiency virus–infected patients who have unexplained fever and elevated serum levels of alkaline phosphatase or gamma-glutamyl transferase. *Clin Infect Dis* 1995; 20:606–610.

103. Cappell MS, Philogene C. The endoscopic appearance of severe intestinal *Mycobacterium avium* complex infection as a coarsely granular mucosa due to massive infiltration and expansion of intestinal villi without mucosal exudation. *J Clin Gastroenterol* 1995;21:323–326.

104. Hussong J, Peterson LR, Warren JR, et al. Detecting disseminated *Mycobacterium avium complex* infections in HIV-positive patients. The usefulness of bone marrow trephine biopsy specimens, aspirate cultures, and blood cultures. *Am J Clin Pathol* 1998;110:806–809.

105. Duong M, Piroth L, Chavanet P, et al. A case of rhombencephalitis with isolation of *cytomegalovirus* and *Mycobacterium avium* complex in a woman with AIDS. *AIDS* 1994;8: 1356–1357.

106. Arasteh K, Cordes C, Futh U, et al. Co-infection by *Cryptococcus neoformans* and *Mycobacterium avium intracellulare* in AIDS. Clinical and epidemiological aspects. *Mycopathologia* 1997–98; 140:115–120.

107. Moulignier A, Eliaszewicz M, Mikol J, et al. Spinal cord compression due to concomitant primary lymphoma and *Mycobacterium avium-intracellulare* infection of the paravertebral muscles in an AIDS patient. *Eur J Clin Microbiol Infect Dis* 1996; 15:891–893.

108. Ives DV, Davis RB, Currier JS. Impact of clarithromycin and azithromycin on patterns of treatment and survival among AIDS patients with disseminated *Mycobacterium avium* complex. *AIDS* 1995;9:261–266.

109. Rossi M, Flepp M, Telenti A, et al. Swiss HIV Cohort Study. Disseminated *M. avium* complex infection in the Swiss HIV Cohort Study: declining incidence, improved prognosis and discontinuation of maintenance therapy. *Swiss Med Wkly* 2001; 131:471–477.

110. Palella FJ Jr, Delaney KM, Moorman AC, et al. Declining morbidity and mortality among patients with advanced human immunodeficiency virus infection. *N Engl J Med* 1998;338: 853–860.

111. O'Brien RJ, Lyle MA, Snider DE Jr. Rifabutin (ansamycin LM 427): A new rifamycin-S derivative for the treatment of mycobacterial diseases. *Rev Infect Dis* 1987;9:519–530.

112. Olliaro P, Dautzenberg B. Control of the body burden of *M. avium* complex is associated with improved quality of life and prolonged survival of patients with AIDS: a prospective trial with rifabutin combined with isoniazid, clofazimine, ethambutol. *J Chemother* 1994;6:189–196.

113. Young LS, Bermudez LE, Wu M, et al. Potential role of roxithromycin against the *Mycobacterium avium* complex. *Infection* 1995;23 (Suppl 1):S28–S32.

114. Bermudez LE, Inderlied CB, Kolonoski P, et al. Telithromycin is active against *Mycobacterium avium* in mice despite lacking significant activity in standard *in vitro* and macrophage assays and is associated with low frequency of resistance during treatment. *Antimicrob Agents Chemother* 2001;45:2210–2214.

115. Peters DH, Clissold SP. Clarithromycin. A review of its antimicrobial activity, pharmacokinetic properties and therapeutic potential. *Drugs* 1992;44:117–164.

116. Peters DH, Friedel HA, McTavish D. Azithromycin. A review of its antimicrobial activity, pharmacokinetic properties and clinical efficacy. *Drugs* 1992;44:750–799.

117. Peloquin, CA *Mycobacterium avium* complex infection. Pharmacokinetic and pharmacodynamic considerations that may improve clinical outcomes. *Clin Pharmackokinet* 1997;32:132–144.

118. Chin DP, Reingold AL, Stone EN, et al. The impact of *Mycobacterium avium* complex bacteremia and its treatment on survival of AIDS patients—a prospective study. *J Infect Dis* 1994;170:578–584.

119. Husson RN, Ross LA, Sandelli S, et al. Orally administered clarithromycin for the treatment of systemic *Mycobacterium avium* complex infection in children with acquired immunodeficiency syndrome. *J Pediatr* 1994;124:807–814.

120. Chaisson RE, Benson CA, Dube MP, et al. Clarithromycin therapy for bacteremic *Mycobacterium avium* complex disease. A randomized, double-blind, dose-ranging study in patients with AIDS. AIDS Clinical Trials Group Protocol 157 Study Team. *Ann Intern Med* 1994;121:905–911.

121. Doucet-Populaire F, Truffot-Pernot C, Grosset J, et al. Acquired resistance in *Mycobacterium avium complex* strains isolated from AIDS patients and beige mice during treatment with clarithromycin. *J Antimicrob Chemother* 1995;36:129–136.

122. Yajko DM, Sanders CA, Madej JJ, et al. *In vitro* activities of rifabutin, azithromycin, ciprofloxacin, clarithromycin, clofazimine, ethambutol, and amikacin in combinations of two, three, and four drugs against *Mycobacterium avium*. *Antimicrob Agents Chemother* 1996;40:743–749.

123. Dube MP, Sattler FR, Torriani FJ, et al. A randomized evaluation of ethambutol for prevention of relapse and drug resistance during treatment of *Mycobacterium avium* complex bacteremia with clarithromycin-based combination therapy. California Collaborative Treatment Group. *J Infect Dis* 1997;176:1225–1232.

124. Chaisson RE, Keiser P, Pierce M, et al. Clarithromycin and ethambutol with or without clofazimine for the treatment of bacteremic *Mycobacterium avium* complex disease in patients with HIV infection. *AIDS* 1997;11:311–317.

125. Roger PM, Carles M, Agussol-Foin I, et al. Efficacy and safety of an intravenous induction therapy for treatment of disseminated *Mycobacterium avium* complex infection in AIDS patients: a pilot study. *J Antimicrob Chemother* 1999;44: 129–131.

126. Tomioka H, Sato K, Kajitani H, et al. Comparative antimicrobial activities of the newly synthesized quinolone WQ-3034, levofloxacin, sparfloxacin, and ciprofloxacin against *Mycobacterium tuberculosis* and *Mycobacterium avium* complex. *Antimicrob Agents Chemother* 2000;44:283–286.

127. Keiser P, Nassar N, Skiest D, et al. A retrospective study of the addition of ciprofloxacin to clarithromycin and ethambutol in the treatment of disseminated *Mycobacterium avium* complex infection. *Int J STD AIDS* 1999;10:791–794.

128. Peters J, Kondo KL, Lee RK, et al. *In-vitro* activity of oxazolidinones against *Mycobacterium avium* complex. *J Antimicrob Chemother* 1995;35:675–679.

129. Nannini EC, Keating M, Binstock P, et al. Successful treatment of refractory disseminated *Mycobacterium avium* complex infection with the addition of linezolid and mefloquine. *J Infect* 2002;44:201–203.

130. Bermudez LE, Kolonoski P, Wu M, et al. Mefloquine is active *in vitro* and *in vivo* against *Mycobacterium avium* complex. *Antimicrob Agents Chemother* 1999;43:1870–1874.

131. Lauw FN, van Der Meer JT, de Metz J, et al. No beneficial effect of interferon-gamma treatment in 2 human immunodeficiency virus–infected patients with *Mycobacterium avium* complex infection. *Clin Infect Dis* 2001;32:81–82.

132. Kemper CA, Bermudez LE, Deresinski SC. Immunomodulatory treatment of *Mycobacterium avium* complex bacteremia in patients with AIDS by use of recombinant granulocyte-macrophage colony-stimulating factor. *J Infect Dis* 1998; 177:914–920.

133. Keiser P, Rademacher S, Smith J, et al. G-CSF association with prolonged survival in HIV-infected patients with disseminated *Mycobacterium avium* complex infection. *Int J STD AIDS* 1998;9:394–399.

134. American Thoracic Society. Diagnosis and treatment of disease caused by nontuberculous mycobacteria. *Am J Respir Crit Care Med* 1997;156:S1–S25.

135. British Thoracic Society. Subcommittee of the Joint Tuberculosis Committee of the British Thoracic Society. Management of opportunist mycobacterial infections: Joint Tuberculosis Committee Guidelines 1999. *Thorax* 2000;55:210–218.

136. Centers for Disease Control and Prevention. Prevention and treatment of tuberculosis among patients infected with human immunodeficiency virus: principles of therapy and revised recommendations *MMWR Morb Mortal Wkly Rep* 1998;47:1–51.

137. Gordin FM, Sullam PM, Shafran SD, et al. A randomized, placebo-controlled study of rifabutin added to a regimen of clarithromycin and ethambutol for treatment of disseminated infection with *Mycobacterium avium complex*. *Clin Infect Dis* 1999;28:1080–1085.

138. Cohn DL, Fisher EJ, Peng GT, et al. A prospective randomized trial of four three-drug regimens in the treatment of disseminated *Mycobacterium avium* complex disease in AIDS patients: excess mortality associated with high-dose clarithromycin. Terry Beirn Community Programs for Clinical Research on AIDS. *Clin Infect Dis* 1999;29:125–133.

139. Dunne M, Fessel J, Kumar P, et al. A randomized, double-blind trial comparing azithromycin and clarithromycin in the treatment of disseminated *Mycobacterium avium* infection in patients with human immunodeficiency virus. *Clin Infect Dis* 2000;31:1245–1252.

140. Ward TT, Rimland D, Kauffman C, et al. Randomized, open-label trial of azithromycin plus ethambutol vs. clarithromycin plus ethambutol as therapy for *Mycobacterium avium* complex bacteremia in patients with human immunodeficiency virus infection. Veterans Affairs HIV Research Consortium. *Clin Infect Dis* 1998;27:1278–1285.

141. Steele-Moore L, Stark K, Holloway WJ. *In vitro* activities of clarithromycin and azithromycin against clinical isolates of *Mycobacterium avium–M. intracellulare* [letter]. *Antimicrob Agents Chemother* 1999;43:1530.

142. Aukrust P, Muller F, Lien E, et al. Tumor necrosis factor (TNF) system levels in human immunodeficiency virus–infected patients during highly active antiretroviral therapy: persistent TNF activation is associated with virologic and immunologic treatment failure. *J Infect Dis* 1999;179:74–82.

143. Franco JM, Rubio A, Rey C, et al. Reduction of immune system activation in HIV-1-infected patients undergoing highly active antiretroviral therapy. *Eur J Clin Microbiol Infect Dis* 1999;18: 733–736.

144. MacArthur RD, Lederman MM, Benson CA, et al. Effects of *Mycobacterium avium* complex infection treatment on cytokine expression in human immunodeficiency virus–infected persons: results of AIDS clinical trials group protocol 853. *J Infect Dis* 2000;181:1486–1490.

145. Aberg JA, Chin-Hong PV, McCutchan A, et al. Localized osteomyelitis due to *Mycobacterium avium* complex in patients with human immunodeficiency virus receiving highly active antiretroviral therapy. *Clin Infect Dis* 2002;35:E8–E13.

146. Race EM, Adelson-Mitty J, Kriegel GR, et al. Focal mycobacterial lymphadenitis following initiation of protease-inhibitor therapy in patients with advanced HIV-1 disease. *Lancet* 1998;351:252–255.

147. Foudraine NA, Hovenkamp E, Notermans DW, et al. Immunopathology as a result of highly active antiretroviral therapy in HIV-1-infected patients. *AIDS* 1999;13:177–184.

148. Phillips P, Kwiatkowski MB, Copland M, et al. Mycobacterial lymphadenitis associated with the initiation of combination antiretroviral therapy. *J Acquir Immune Defic Syndr Hum Retrovirol* 1999;20:122–128.

149. Brown M, Williams IG, Miller RF. Deterioration of disseminated cutaneous *Mycobacterium avium* complex infection with a leukaemoid reaction following institution of highly active antiretroviral therapy. *Sex Transm Infect* 2001;77:149–150.

150. Centers for Disease Control and Prevention. Acquired rifamycin resistance in persons with advanced HIV disease being treated for active tuberculosis with intermittent rifamycin–based regimens. *MMWR Morb Mortal Wkly Rep* 2002;51:214–215.

151. Hafner R, Bethel J, Power M, et al. Tolerance and pharmacokinetic interactions of rifabutin and clarithromycin in human immunodeficiency virus–infected volunteers. *Antimicrob Agents Chemother* 1998;42:631–639.

152. Centers for Disease Control and Prevention. Guidelines for using antiretroviral agents among HIV-infected adults and adolescents. Recommendations of the Panel on Clinical Practices for Treatment of HIV. *MMWR Morb Mortal Wkly Rep* 2002; 51:1–64.

153. Shafran SD, Singer J, Zarowny DP, et al. Determinants of rifabutin-associated uveitis in patients treated with rifabutin, clarithromycin, and ethambutol for *Mycobacterium avium complex* bacteremia: a multivariate analysis. Canadian HIV Trials Network Protocol 010 Study Group. *J Infect Dis* 1998;177: 252–255.

154. Piscitelli SC, Gallicano KD. Interactions among drugs for HIV and opportunistic infections. *N Engl J Med* 2001; 344:984–996.

155. Deeks, SG, Wrin T, Liegler T, et al. Virologic and immunologic consequences of discontinuing combination antiretroviral-drug therapy in HIV-infected patients with detectable viremia. *N Engl J Med* 2001;344:472–480.

156. Dube MP, Torriani FJ, See D, et al. Successful short-term suppression of clarithromycin-resistant *Mycobacterium avium* complex bacteremia in AIDS. California Collaborative Treatment Group. *Clin Infect Dis* 1999;28:136–138.

157. Burman WJ, Stone BL, Rietmeijer CA, et al. Long-term outcomes of treatment of *Mycobacterium avium* complex bacteremia using a clarithromycin-containing regimen. *AIDS* 1998;12:1309–1315.

158. Pierce M. Crampton S. Henry D, et al. A randomized trial of clarithromycin as prophylaxis against disseminated *Mycobacterium avium complex* infection in patients with advanced acquired immunodeficiency syndrome. *N Engl J Med* 1996; 335:384–391.

159. Grosset J, Ji B. Prevention of the selection of clarithromycin-resistant *Mycobacterium avium-intracellulare* complex. *Drugs* 1997;54(Suppl 2):23–27.

160. Goujard C, Lebrun L, Doucet-Populaire F, et al. Clarithromycin-resistant *Mycobacterium avium* strain in a clarithromycin-naive AIDS patient. *Clin Infect Dis* 1998;26:186.

161. Meier A, Heifets L, Wallace RJ Jr, et al. Molecular mechanisms of clarithromycin resistance in *Mycobacterium avium*: observation of multiple 23S rDNA mutations in a clonal population. *J Infect Dis* 1996;174:354–360.

162. Guerrero C, Stockman L, Marchesi F, et al. Evaluation of the rpoB gene in rifampicin-susceptible and -resistant *Mycobacterium avium* and *Mycobacterium intracellulare*. *J Antimicrob Chemother* 1994;33:661–663.

163. Bermudez LE, Nash K, Petrofsky M, et al. Clarithromycin-resistant *Mycobacterium avium* is still susceptible to treatment with clarithromycin and is virulent in mice. *Antimicrob Agents Chemother* 2000;44:2619–2622.

164. McNaghten AD, Hanson DL, Jones JL, et al. Effects of antiretroviral therapy and opportunistic illness primary chemoprophylaxis on survival after AIDS diagnosis. Adult/Adolescent Spectrum of Disease Group. *AIDS* 1999;13:1687–1695.

165. Craft JC, Notario GF, Grosset JH, et al. Clarithromycin resistance and susceptibility patterns of *Mycobacterium avium* strains isolated during prophylaxis for disseminated infection in patients with AIDS. *Clin Infect Dis* 1998;27:807–812.

166. Böttger EC, Wallace RJ Jr. Lack of rifabutin resistance with prophylaxis for disseminated *Mycobacterium avium* complex. *Lancet* 1994;344:1506–1507.

167. Nightingale SD, Cameron DW, Gordin FM, et al. Two controlled trials of rifabutin prophylaxis against *Mycobacterium avium* complex infection in AIDS. *N Engl J Med* 1993;329: 828–833.

168. Bishai WR, Graham NMH, Harrington G, et al. Rifampicin-resistant tuberculosis in a patient receiving rifabutin prophylaxis. *N Engl J Med* 1996;334:1573–1576.

169. Havlir DV, Dube MP, Sattler FR, et al. California Collaborative Treatment Group. Prophylaxis against disseminated *Mycobacterium avium* complex with weekly azithromycin, daily rifabutin, or both. *N Engl J Med* 1996;335:392–398.

170. Oldfield EC III, Fessel WJ, Dunne MW, et al. Once weekly azithromycin therapy for prevention of *Mycobacterium avium* complex infection in patients with AIDS: a randomized, double-blind, placebo-controlled multicenter trial *Clin Infect Dis* 1998;26:611–619.

171. Benson CA, Williams PL, Cohn DL. The AIDS Clinical Trials Group 196/Terry Beirn Community Programs for Clinical Research on AIDS 009 Protocol Team. Clarithromycin or rifabutin alone or in combination for primary prophylaxis of *Mycobacterium avium* complex disease in patients with AIDS: a randomized, double-blind, placebo-controlled trial. *J Infect Dis* 2000;181:1289–1297.

172. Centers for Disease Control and Prevention. Updated guidelines for the use of rifabutin or rifampin for the treatment and prevention of tuberculosis among HIV-infected patients taking protease inhibitors or nonnucleoside reverse transcriptase inhibitors. *MMWR Morb Mortal Wkly Rep* 2000;49:185–189.

173. Kaplan JE, Masur H, Holmes KK; USPHS; Infectious Disease Society of America. Recommendations of the U.S. Public Health Service and the Infectious Disease Society of America. Guidelines for preventing opportunistic infections among HIV-infected persons—2002. *MMWR Morb Mortal Wkly Rep* 2002;51:1–52.

174. Baril L, Jouan M, Agher R, et al. Impact of highly active antiretroviral therapy on onset of *Mycobacterium avium* complex infection and cytomegalovirus disease in patients with AIDS. *AIDS* 2000;14:2593–2596.

175. Cinti SK, Kaul DR, Sax PE, et al. Recurrence of *Mycobacterium avium* infection in patients receiving highly active antiretroviral therapy and antimycobacterial agents. *Clin Infect Dis* 2000;30: 511–514.

176. El-Sadr WM, Burman WJ, Grant LB, et al. Discontinuation of prophylaxis for *Mycobacterium avium* complex disease in HIV-infected patients who have a response to antiretroviral therapy. Terry Beirn Community Programs for Clinical Research on AIDS. *N Engl J Med* 2000;342:1085–1092.

177. Currier JS, Williams PL, Koletar SL, et al. AIDS Clinical Trials Group 362 Study Team. Discontinuation of *Mycobacterium avium* complex prophylaxis in patients with antiretroviral therapy-induced increases in CD4$^+$ cell count. A randomized, double-blind, placebo-controlled trial. *Ann Intern Med* 2000;133: 493–503.

178. Kirk O, Reiss P, Uberti-Foppa C, et al. European HIV Cohorts. Safe interruption of maintenance therapy against previous infection with four common HIV-associated opportunistic pathogens during potent antiretroviral therapy. *Ann Intern Med* 2002;137:239–250.

179. Zeller V, Truffot C, Agher R, et al. Discontinuation of secondary prophylaxis against disseminated *Mycobacterium avium* complex infection and toxoplasmic encephalitis. *Clin Infect Dis* 2002;34:662–667.

180. Aberg JA, Yajko DM, Jacobson MA. Eradication of AIDS-related disseminated *mycobacterium avium* complex infection after 12 months of antimycobacterial therapy combined with highly active antiretroviral therapy. *J Infect Dis* 1998;178: 1446–1449.

181. Hadad DJ, Lewi DS, Pignatari AC, et al. Resolution of *Mycobacterium avium* complexbacteremia following highly active antiretroviral therapy. *Clin Infect Dis* 1998;26:758–789.

182. Cabie A, Abel S, Brebion A, et al. Mycobacterial lymphadenitis after initiation of highly active antiretroviral therapy. *Eur J Clin Microbiol Infect Dis* 1998;17:812–813.

183. Boyd AE, Brettle RP. Localized *Mycobacterium avium intracellulare* psoas abscess in patients with AIDS after antiretroviral therapy. *AIDS* 1999;13:2185–2186.

184. Bartley PB, Allworth AM, Eisen DP. *Mycobacterium avium* complex causing endobronchial disease in AIDS patients after partial immune restoration. *Int J Tuberc Lung Dis* 1999;3:1132–1136.

185. Murray R, Mallal S, Heath C, et al. Cerebral *Mycobacterium avium* infection in an HIV-infected patient following immune reconstitution and cessation of therapy for disseminated *Mycobacterium avium* complex infection. *Eur J Clin Microbiol Infect Dis* 2001;20:199–201.

186. Shafran SD, Mashinter LD, Phillips P, et al. Successful discontinuation of therapy for disseminated *Mycobacterium avium* complex infection after effective antiretroviral therapy. *Ann Intern Med* 2002;137:734–737.

187. Horsburgh CR, Selik RM. The epidemiology of disseminated nontuberculous mycobacterial infection in the acquired immunodeficiency syndrome (AIDS). *Am Rev Respir Dis* 1989;139:4–7.

188. Levine B, Chaisson RE. *Mycobacterium kansasii*: a cause of treatable pulmonary disease associated with advanced human immunodeficiency virus (HIV) infection. *Ann Intern Med* 1991;114:861–868.

189. Tortoli E, Simonetti MT, Lacchini C, et al. Tentative evidence of AIDS-associated biotype of *Mycobacterium kansasii*. *J Clin Microbiol* 1994;32:1779–1782.

190. Ciotoli C, Schluger N, Harkin T, et al. Isolation of *Mycobacterium kansasii* from patients with human immunodeficiency virus (HIV). *Am Rev Respir Dis* 1994;149:A686.

191. Lortholary O, Deniel F, Boudon P, et al. Groupe d'Etude Des Mycobacteries de la Seine-Saint-Denis. *Mycobacterium kansasii* infection in a Paris suburb: comparison of disease presentation and outcome according to human immunodeficiency virus status. *Int J Tuberc Lung Dis* 1999;3:68–73.

192. Klein JL, Corbett EL, Slade PM, et al. *Mycobacterium kansasii* and human immunodeficiency virus co-infection in London. *J Infect* 1998;37:252–259.

193. van der Meer JT, Kerssemakers SP, van Steenwijk RP, et al. [Infections with *Mycobacterium kansasii* in the Academic Medical Center in Amsterdam: the changing clinical spectrum since the start of the HIV epidemic]. *Ned Tijdschr Geneeskd* 1998;142:965–969. [In Dutch.]

194. Rooney G, Nelson MR, Gazzard B. *Mycobacterium kansasii*: its presentation, treatment and outcome in HIV infected patients. *J Clin Pathol* 1996;49:821–823.

195. Urkijo JC, Montejo M, Aguirrebengoa K, et al. [Disease caused by *Mycobacterium kansasii* in patients with HIV infection]. *Enferm Infecc Microbiol Clin* 1993;11:120–125. [In Spanish.]

196. Yates MD, Grange JM, Collins CH. The nature of mycobacterial disease in south east England, 1977–84. *J Epidemiol Community Health* 1986;40:295–300.

197. Yates MD, Pozniak A, Grange JM. 1993. Isolation of mycobacteria from patients seropositive for the human immunodeficiency virus (HIV) in southeast England: 1984–1992. *Thorax* 1993;48:990–995.

198. Bloch KC, Zwerling L, Pletcher MJ, et al. Incidence and clinical implications of isolation of *Mycobacterium kansasii*: results of a 5-year, population-based study. *Ann Intern Med* 1998;129:698–704.

199. Joseph O. Falkinham III. Epidemiology of infection by nontuberculous mycobacteria. *Clin Microbiol Rev* 1996;9:177–215.

200. Connolly MG Jr, Baughman RP, Dohn MN. *Mycobacterium kansasii* presenting as an endobronchial lesion. *Am Rev Respir Dis* 1993;148:1405–1407.

201. Witzig RS, Fazal BA, Mera RM, et al. Clinical manifestations

202. Corbett EL, Blumberg L, Churchyard GJ, et al. Nontuberculous mycobacteria. defining disease in a prospective cohort of South African miners *Am J Respir Crit Care Med* 1999;160:15–21.

203. Corbett EL, Churchyard GJ, Hay M, et al. The impact of HIV infection on *Mycobacterium kansasii* disease in South African gold miners. *Am J Respir Crit Care Med* 1999;160:10–14.

204. Pintado V, Fortun J, Casado JL, et al. *Mycobacterium kansasii* pericarditis as a presentation of AIDS. *Infection* 2001;29:48–50.

205. Casado Burgos E, Muga Bustamante R, Olive Marques A, et al. [Infectious arthritis by *Mycobacterium kansasii* in a patient with human immunodeficiency virus]. *Med Clin (Barc)* 2001;116:237–238. [In Spanish.]

206. Pintado V, Antela A, Corres J, et al. [Arthritis and tenosynovitis caused by *Mycobacterium kansasii* associated with human immunodeficiency virus infection] *Rev Clin Esp* 1999;199:863. [In Spanish.]

207. Martinez T, Creagh R, Saavedra JM, et al. [*Mycobacterium kansasii* osteomyelitis in a patient infected by the human immunodeficiency virus]. *Enferm Infecc Microbiol Clin* 2000;18:148-9. [In Spanish.]

208. Bernard L, Vincent V, Lortholary O, et al.*Mycobacterium kansasii* septic arthritis: French retrospective study of 5 years and review. *Clin Infect Dis* 1999;29:1455–1460.

209. Bamberger DM, Driks MR, Gupta MR, et al. *Mycobacterium kansasii* among patients infected with human immunodeficiency virus in Kansas City. *Clin Infect Dis* 1994;18:395–400.

210. Wallace RJ Jr, Dunbar D, Brown BA, et al. Rifampin-resistant *Mycobacterium kansasii*. *Clin Infect Dis* 1994;18:736–743.

211. Biehle J, Cavalieri SJ. *In vitro* susceptibility of *Mycobacterium kansasii* to clarithromycin. *Antimicrob Agents Chemother* 1992;36:2039–2041.

212. Donnabella V, Salazar-Schicchi J, Bonk S, et al. Increasing incidence of *Mycobacterium xenopi* at Bellevue Hospital: an emerging pathogen or a product of improved laboratory methods? *Chest* 2000;118:1365–1370.

213. Jiva TM, Jacoby HM, Weymouth LA, et al. *Mycobacterium xenopi*: innocent bystander or emerging pathogen? *Clin Infect Dis* 1997;24:226–232.

214. el-Helou P, Rachlis A, Fong I, et al. *Mycobacterium xenopi* infection in patients with human immunodeficiency virus infection. *Clin Infect Dis* 1997;25:206–210.

215. Bachmeyer C, Blum L, Stelianides S, et al. *Mycobacterium xenopi* pulmonary infection in an HIV infected patient under highly active antiretroviral treatment. *Thorax* 2001;56:978–979.

216. Sompolinsky D, Lagziel A, Naveh D, et al. *Mycobacterium haemophilum* sp. nov., a new pathogen of humans. *Int J Syst Bacteriol* 1978;28:67–75.

217. Rogers PL, Walker RE, Lane HC, et al. Disseminated *Mycobacterium haemophilum* infection in two patients with the acquired immunodeficiency syndrome. *Am J Med* 1988;84:640–642.

218. Sampaio JLM, Alves VAF, LeãoSC, et al. *Mycobacterium haemophilum*: emerging or underdiagnosed in Brazil? *Emerg Infect Dis* 2002;8: 1359–1360.

219. Dever LL, Martin JW, Seaworth B, et al. Varied presentations and responses to treatment of infections caused by *Mycobacterium haemophilum* in patients with AIDS. *Clin Infect Dis* 1992;14:1195–1200.

220. Shah MK, Sebti A, Kiehn TE, et al. *Mycobacterium haemophilum* in immunocompromised patients. *Clin Infect Dis* 2001;33:330–337.

221. Kuijper EJ, Wit FW, Veenstra J, et al. Recovery of *Mycobac-*

terium haemophilum skin infection in an HIV-1-infected patient after the start of antiretroviral triple therapy. *Clin Microbiol Infect.* 1997;3:584–585.

222. Atkinson BA, Bocanegra R, Graybill JR. Treatment of *Mycobacterium haemophilum* infection in a murine model with clarithromycin, rifabutin, and ciprofloxacin. *Antimicrob Agents Chemother* 1995;39:2316–2319.

223. Paech V, Lorenzen T, von Krosigk A, et al. Remission of cutaneous *Mycobacterium haemophilum* infection as a result of antiretroviral therapy in a human immunodeficiency virus—infected patient. *Clin Infect Dis* 2002;34:1017–1019.

224. Hirschel B, Chang HR, Mach N, et al. Fatal infection with a novel unidentified mycobacterium in a man with the acquired immunodeficiency syndrome. *N Engl J Med* 1990;323:109–113.

225. Böttger EC, Teske A, Kirschner P, et al. Disseminated "*Mycobacterium genavense*" infection in patients with AIDS. *Lancet* 1992;340:76–80.

226. Rodriguez P, March F, Garrigo M, et al. [Disseminated *Mycobacterium genavense* infection in patients with HIV infection. Description of 5 cases and review of the literature] *Enferm Infecc Microbiol Clin* 1996;14:220–226. [In Spanish.]

227. Coyle MB, Carlson LC, Wallis CK, et al. Laboratory aspects of "*Mycobacterium genavense*," a proposed species isolated from AIDS patients. *J Clin Microbiol* 1992;30:3206–3212.

228. Gaynor CD, Clark RA, Koontz FP, et al. Disseminated *Mycobacterium genavense* infection in two patients with AIDS. *Clin Infect Dis* 1994;18:455–457.

229. Yan JJ, Ko WC, Tsai HM, et al. Disseminated *Mycobacterium genavense* infection in a patient with acquired immunodeficiency syndrome: first case report in Taiwan. *J Formos Med Assoc* 1999;98:62–65.

230. Shafran SD, Taylor GD, Talbot JA. Disseminated *Mycobacterium genavense* infection in Canadian AIDS patients. *Tuber Lung Dis* 1995;76:168–170.

231. Pechere M, Opravil M, Wald A, et al. Clinical and epidemiologic features of infection with *Mycobacterium genavense*. Swiss HIV Cohort Study. *Arch Intern Med* 1995;155:400–404.

232. Kirschner P, Vogel U, Hein R, et al. Bias of culture techniques for diagnosing mixed *Mycobacterium genavense* and *Mycobacterium avium* infection in AIDS. *J Clin Microbiol* 1994;32:828–831.

233. Boian M, Avaniss-Aghajani E, Walker R, et al. Identification of *Mycobacterium genavense* in intestinal tissue from a parakeet using two polymerase chain reaction methods: are pets a reservoir of infection in AIDS patients? *AIDS* 1997;11:255–256.

234. Hillebrand-Haverkort ME, Kolk AH, Kox LF, et al. Generalized *Mycobacterium genavense* infection in HIV-infected patients: detection of the mycobacterium in hospital tap water. *Scand J Infect Dis* 1999;31:63–68.

235. Böttger EC. *Mycobacterium genavense*: an emerging pathogen. *Eur J Clin Microbiol Infect Dis* 1994;13:932–936.

236. Monill JM, Moreno A, Clotet M, et al. *Mycobacterium genavense* enteritis in a patient with AIDS: radiologic features. *AJR Am J Roentgenol* 1999;172:1143–1144.

237. Monill JM, Franquet T, Sambeat MA, et al. *Mycobacterium genavense* infection in AIDS: imaging findings in eight patients. *Eur Radiol* 2001;11:193–196.

238. Berman SM, Kim RC, Haghighat D, et al. *Mycobacterium genavense* infection presenting as a solitary brain mass in a patient with AIDS: case report and review. *Clin Infect Dis* 1994;19:1152–1154.

239. Thomsen VO, Dragsted UB, Bauer J, et al. Disseminated infection with *Mycobacterium genavense*: a challenge to physicians and mycobacteriologists. *J Clin Microbiol* 1999;37:3901–3905.

240. Realini L, Van Der Stuyft P, De Ridder K, et al. Inhibitory effects of polyoxyethylene stearate, PANTA, and neutral pH on

growth of *Mycobacterium genavense* in BACTEC primary cultures. *J Clin Microbiol* 1997;35:2791–2794.

241. Realini L, De Ridder K, Palomino J, et al. Microaerophilic conditions promote growth of *Mycobacterium genavense*. *J Clin Microbiol* 1998;36:2565–2570.

242. Klein JL, Brown TJ, Dean GL, et al. *Mycobacterium genavense* infection in a UK based patient with AIDS: diagnosis using molecular techniques. *Sex Transm Infect* 1998;74:306.

243. Vrioni G, Nauciel C, Kerharo G, et al. Treatment of disseminated *Mycobacterium genavense* infection in a murine model with ciprofloxacin, amikacin, ethambutol, clarithromycin and rifabutin. *J Antimicrob Chemother* 1998;42:483–487.

244. Matsiota-Bernard P, Thierry D, De Truchis P, et al. *Mycobacterium genavense* infection in a patient with AIDS who was successfully treated with clarithromycin. *Clin Infect Dis* 1995;20:1565–1566.

245. Carlson LD, Wallis CK, Coyle MB. Standardized BACTEC method to measure clarithromycin susceptibility of *Mycobacterium genavense*. *J Clin Microbiol* 1998;36:748–751.

246. Tortoli E, Piersimoni C, Kirschner P, et al. Characterization of mycobacterial isolates related to, but different from, *Mycobacterium simiae*. *J Clin Microbiol* 1997;35:697–702.

247. Lévy-Frébault V, Pangon B, Bure A, et al. *Mycobacterium simiae* and *Mycobacterium avium–M. intracellulare* mixed infection in acquired immune deficiency syndrome. *J Clin Microbiol* 1987;25:154–157.

248. Centers for Disease Control and Prevention. Disseminated infection with *Simiae-Avium* group mycobacteria in persons with AIDS—Thailand and Malawi, 1997. *MMWR Morb Mortal Wkly Rep* 2002;51:501–502.

249. Munier D, Dux S, Samra Z, et al. *Mycobacterium simiae* infection in Israeli patients infected with AIDS. *Clin Infect Dis* 1993;17:508–509.

250. Torres RA, Nord J, Feldman R, et al. Disseminated mixed *Mycobacterium simiae–Mycobacterium avium* complex infection in acquired immune deficiency syndrome. *J Infect Dis* 1991;164:432–433.

251. Koeck JL, Debord T, Fabre M, et al. Disseminated *Mycobacterium simiae* infection in a patient with AIDS: clinical features and treatment. *Clin Infect Dis* 1996;23:832–833.

252. Cingolani A, Sanguinetti M, Antinori A, et al. Disseminated mycobacteriosis caused by drug-resistant *Mycobacterium triplex* in a human immunodeficiency virus–infected patient during highly active antiretroviral therapy. *Clin Infect Dis* 2000;31:177–179.

253. Chan J, McKitrick JC, Klein RS. *Mycobacterium gordonae* in the acquired immunodeficiency syndrome. *Ann Intern Med* 1984;101:400.

254. Lessnau KD, Minanese S, Talavera W. *Mycobacterium gordonae*: a treatable disease in HIV-positive patients. *Chest* 1993;104:1779–1785.

255. del Giudice P, Bernard E, Pinier Y, et al. Cutaneous infection due to *Mycobacterium gordonae* in a human immunodeficiency virus–infected patient. *Clin Infect Dis* 1998;26:1486–1487.

256. Piersimoni C, Tortoli E, De Sio G. Disseminated infection due to *Mycobacterium celatum* in patient with AIDS [letter]. *Lancet* 1994;344:332.

257. Tortoli E, Piersimoni C, Bacosi D, et al. Isolation of the newly described species *Mycobacterium celatum* from AIDS patients. *J Clin Microbiol* 1995;33:137–140.

258. Gholizadeh Y, Varnerot A, Maslo C, et al. *Mycobacterium celatum* infection in two HIV-infected patients treated prophylactically with rifabutin. *Eur J Clin Microbiol Infect Dis* 1998;17:278-281.

259. Zurawski CA, Cage GD, Rimland D, et al. Pneumonia and bacteremia due to *Mycobacterium celatum* masquerading as *Mycobacterium xenopi* in patients with AIDS: an underdiagnosed problem? *Clin Infect Dis* 1997;24:140–143.

260. Butler WR, O'Connor SP, Yakrus MA, et al. Cross-reactivity of genetic probe for detection of *Mycobacterium tuberculosis* with newly described species *Mycobacterium celatum. J Clin Microbiol* 1994;32:536–538.

261. Somoskovi A, Hotaling JE, Fitzgerald M, et al. False-positive results for *Mycobacterium celatum* with the AccuProbe *Mycobacterium tuberculosis complex* assay. *J Clin Microbiol* 2000;38:2743–2745.

262. Fattorini L, Baldassarri L, Li YJ, et al. Virulence and drug susceptibility of *Mycobacterium celatum. Microbiology* 2000;146:2733–2742.

263. Sanders JW, Walsh AD, Snider RL, et al. Disseminated *Mycobacterium scrofulaceum* infection: a potentially treatable complication of AIDS. *Clin Infect Dis* 1995;20:549.

264. Nunez Fernandez MJ, Ojea de Castro R, Anibarro Garcia L, et al. [Disseminated infection by *Mycobacterium scrofulaceum* in an infected HIV patient]. *An Med Interna* 2002;19:381–382. [In Spanish.]

265. Shay WE, LaBombardi VJ. Diagnosis of disseminated *Mycobacterium scrofulaceum* infection in an AIDS patient using a continuously monitored culture system. *Int J STD AIDS* 1999;10:413–416.

266. Carbonara S, Tortoli E, Costa D, et al. Disseminated *Mycobacterium terrae* infection in a patient with advanced human immunodeficiency virus disease. *Clin Infect Dis* 2000;30:831–835.

267. Zamboni M, Igreja RP, Bonecker C, et al. [*Mycobacterium szulgai* infection in a patient with hemophilia and AIDS]. *Rev Assoc Med Bras* 1992;38:150–152. [In Portuguese.]

268. Luque AE, Kaminski D, Reichman R, et al. *Mycobacterium szulgai* osteomyelitis in an AIDS patient. *Scand J Infect Dis* 1998;30:88–91.

269. Newshan G, Torres RA. Pulmonary infection due to multidrug-resistant *Mycobacterium szulgai* in a patient with AIDS. *Clin Infect Dis* 1994;18:1022–1023.

270. Roig P, Nieto A, Navarro V, et al. [Mycobacteriosis from *Mycobacterium szulgai* in a patient with human immunodeficiency virus infection]. *An Med Interna* 1993;10:182–184. [In Spanish.]

271. Shimizu T, Kodama K, Kobayashi H, et al. Successful treatment using clarithromycin for a cutaneous lesion caused by *Mycobacterium szulgai. Br J Dermatol.* 2000;142:838–840.

272. Johnson RC, Ifebe D, Hans-Moevi A, et al. Disseminated *Mycobacterium ulcerans* disease in an HIV-positive patient: a case study. *AIDS* 2002;16:1704–1705.

273. Jenkins PA. *Mycobacterium malmoense. Tubercle* 1985;66:193–195.

274. Jenkins PA, Tsukamura M. Infections with *Mycobacterium malmoense* in England and Wales. *Tubercle* 1979;60:71–76.

275. Yoganathan K, Elliott MV, Moxham J, et al. Pseudotumor of the lung caused by *Mycobacterium malmoense* infection in an HIV positive patient. *Thorax* 1994;49:179–180.

276. Claydon EJ, Coker RJ, Harris JRW. *Mycobacterium malmoense* infection in HIV positive patients. *J Infect* 1991;23:191–194.

277. Lambertus MW, Mathisen GE. *Mycobacterium marinum* infection in a patient with cryptosporidiosis and the acquired immunodeficiency syndrome. *Cutis* 1988;41:38–40.

278. Ries KM, White GL Jr, Murdock RT. Atypical mycobacterial infection caused by *Mycobacterium marinum* [letter]. *N Engl J Med* 1990;322:633.

279. Zukervar P, Canillot S, Gayrard L, et al. [Sporotrichoid *Mycobacterium marinum* infection in a patient infected with human immunodeficiency virus] *Ann Dermatol Venereol* 1991;118:111–113. [In French.]

280. Furrer H, Bodmer T, von Overbeck J. [Disseminated nontuberculous mycobacterial infections in AIDS patients] *Schweiz Med Wochenschr* 1994;124:89–96. [In German.]

281. Mayall B, Gurtler V, Irving L, et al. Identification of *Mycobacterium shimoidei* by molecular techniques: case report and summary of the literature. *Int J Tuberc Lung Dis* 1999;3:169–173.

282. Brady MT, Marcon MJ, Maddux H. Broviac catheter–related infection due to *Mycobacterium fortuitum* in a patient with acquired immunodeficiency syndrome. *Pediatr Infect Dis J* 1987;6:492–494.

283. Eichmann A, Huszar A, Bon A. *Mycobacterium chelonae* infection of lymph nodes in an HIV-infected patient. *Dermatology* 1993;187:299–300.

284. Anagonou SY, Gninafon M, Kinde-Gazard D, et al. [*Mycobacterium fortuitum* in a patient with human immunodeficiency syndrome (AIDS) in Benin)] *Med Trop (Mars)* 1992;52:303–305. [In French.]

285. Gadre DV. HIV associated chronic atypical osteomyelitis by *Mycobacterium fortuitum—chelonae group*—a case report. *Indian J Med Sci* 1997;51:161–163.

286. Ersoz G, Kaya A, Cayan S, et al. Urinary *Mycobacterium fortuitum* infection in an HIV-infected patient. *AIDS* 2000;14:2802–2803.

287. Butt AA. Cervical adenitis due to *Mycobacterium fortuitum* in patients with acquired immunodeficiency syndrome. *Am J Med Sci* 1998;315:50–55.

288. Gebo KA, Srinivasan A, Perl TM, et al. Pseudo-outbreak of *Mycobacterium fortuitum* on a human immunodeficiency virus ward: transient respiratory tract colonization from a contaminated ice machine. *Clin Infect Dis* 2002;35:32–38.

289. Svahn A, Hoffner SE, Petrini B, et al. *Mycobacterium fortuitum* complex in Sweden during an 11-year period. *Scand J Infect Dis* 1997;29:573–577.

290. Corti M, Soto I, Villafane F, Esquivel P, Di Lonardo M. [Disseminated infection due to *Mycobacterium fortuitum* in an AIDS patient]. *Medicina (B Aires)* 1999;59:274–276. [In Spanish.]

291. Sack JB. Disseminated infection due to *Mycobacterium fortuitum* in a patient with AIDS. *Rev Infect Dis* 1990;12:961–963.

292. Shafer RW, Sierra MF. *Mycobacterium xenopi, Mycobacterium fortuitum, Mycobacterium kansasii,* and other nontuberculous mycobacteria in an area of endemicity for AIDS. *Clin Infect Dis* 1992;15:161–162.

293. Smith MB, Schnadig VJ, Boyars MC, et al. Clinical and pathologic features of *Mycobacterium fortuitum* infections. An emerging pathogen in patients with AIDS. *Am J Clin Pathol* 2001;116:225–232.

294. Talbot EA, Reller LB, Frothingham R. Bone marrow cultures for the diagnosis of mycobacterial and fungal infections in patients infected with the human immunodeficiency virus. *Int J Tuberc Lung Dis* 1999;3:908–912.

295. Smith MB, Boyars MC, Woods GL. Fatal *Mycobacterium fortuitum* meningitis in a patient with AIDS. *Clin Infect Dis* 1996;23:1327–1328.

296. Jacob CN, Henein SS, Heurich AE, et al. Nontuberculous mycobacterial infection of the central nervous system in patients with AIDS. *South Med J* 1993;86:638–640.

297. Wallace RJ Jr, Silcox VA, Tsukamura M, et al. Clinical significance, biochemical features, and susceptibility patterns of sporadic isolates of the *Mycobacterium chelonae*-like organism. *J Clin Microbiol* 1993;31:3231–3239.

298. Springer B, Böttger ED, Kirschner P, et al. Phylogeny of the *Mycobacterium chelonae-like* organism based on partial sequencing of the 16S rRNA gene and proposal of *Mycobacterium mucogenicum* sp. nov. *Int J Syst Baceriol* 1995;45:262–267.

THERAPY

PRINCIPLES OF TUBERCULOSIS MANAGEMENT

ERIC LEIBERT
WILLIAM N. ROM

OVERVIEW OF PRINCIPLES OF TREATMENT

The principles of tuberculosis (TB) management are straightforward. Violation of these principles continues to contribute to the morbidity of TB. Diagnosis must be made quickly so that infectious individuals do not continue to spread disease. Treatment with appropriate drugs must be initiated. The regimen should rapidly render the patient noninfectious. The regimen should be the shortest course that is safe and effective. The regimen must not promote drug resistance. There must be a reliable supply of medication. Medication must be reliably taken, even if this requires extra resources for directly observed therapy (DOT). All of these goals are more readily ensured by programmatic guidelines. The principles of management also apply to drug-resistant TB. Violation of these rules in drug-resistant TB may lead to disaster.

DIAGNOSIS

A prompt and accurate diagnosis is important both to the treatment of the individual and to TB control in the community. The incidence of active, smear-positive pulmonary disease varies from less 4 cases per 100,000 in some Western countries to more than 250 cases per 100,000 in parts of sub-Saharan Africa (1). In the West, TB is sufficiently uncommon that it is often not suspected, particularly when it presents with an uncommon manifestation. When TB is not suspected or when appropriate precautions are omitted, there is a risk of nosocomial and community transmission (2–4).

E. Leibert: Department of Medicine, Division of Pulmonary and Critical Care Medicine, New York University School of Medicine, New York, New York.

W. N. Rom: Department of Medicine, Division of Pulmonary and Critical Care Medicine, New York University School of Medicine; Bellevue Chest Service, New York, New York.

In the developing world where TB is extremely common but resources scarce, the challenge is to devise a program to diagnose and manage the most infectious cases as cheaply as possible. In this setting, the World Health Organization (WHO) recommends a diagnostic program centered on microscopy, which requires less expensive equipment and can be performed by persons with only modest training (5). By targeting the most infectious people, secondary cases can be avoided, leading to the biggest gains given available resources (6). Chest x-ray technology is relatively expensive and is nonspecific as a diagnostic tool (7).

Other issues hamper diagnosis in the developing world. There is often limited access to health care because of travel distance and cost (8). Unfortunately, war is a common cause of lack of access to health care in parts of the developing world. War is associated with increases in TB mortality in patients on therapy (9), though possibly not with increased rates (10). Alternate providers are often sought out before presentation to government clinics (11). There are poorly understood gender differences that result in longer delays in diagnoses for women (12). There is a perception in certain places that TB is incurable (13) and that as a result there is no benefit to diagnosis. There are cultural differences in the understanding of TB (14,15) that can delay presentation for care. This is true of many other conditions (16).

THE BEGINNINGS OF TUBERCULOSIS MANAGEMENT

Important lessons about TB management have been learned at every step in its development. These principles remain relevant and inform many aspects of modern tuberculosis management.

Until the 1940s, there was no medication effective against TB in humans (17). Standard treatment included rest and fresh air (18). Lung rest was encouraged by having the patient lie down on the affected side so as to limit chest wall and air movement on that side. If cavitation was present, closure of the cavity was considered essential to any chance of cure. Collapse therapy using phrenic nerve ligation, pneumothorax, or thoracoplasty was done to bring about closure of the cavity (19).

Effective antituberculous medication was introduced in 1944 with streptomycin. Hinshaw described rapid and dramatic improvement in the first patients treated (20). This led to a change in expectations regarding the management of TB. Medication rapidly became the accepted form of therapy and the possibility of cure was raised. This is our first principle, that *TB is a treatable disease.* While this seems obvious now, many decades after the discovery of effective antituberculous therapy, it was not always so. There is still the perception in the third world that TB is incurable (13). This will needlessly hamper efforts at developing effective TB control programs.

From the beginning, it was clear that streptomycin was an imperfect treatment. Although many of the first 16 patients to receive streptomycin improved, some with more chronic or extensive disease remained bacteriologically positive. Their organisms were later shown to have become resistant to streptomycin even when exposed to high concentrations *in vitro* (21). Large-scale studies of streptomycin confirmed unacceptably high failure rates and rates of streptomycin resistance (22,23). It became clear that the prospect of controlling TB with streptomycin would be limited by these factors.

Paraaminosalicylic acid (PAS) was introduced in 1945. Early results suggested that its efficacy was similar to that of streptomycin. This drug, too, fostered the emergence of resistance and, ultimately, treatment failure (24,25).

With two competing drugs available, and uncertainty about optimal treatment, the British Medical Research Council (BMRC) organized a study of the roles of streptomycin and PAS. [This was the first of dozens of landmark studies of antituberculous therapy conducted by the BMRC over the years. It would be impossible to overstate their contribution to the field (26,27).] Patients were randomized to streptomycin alone, PAS alone, or streptomycin plus PAS. Streptomycin alone was superior to PAS alone. The dual regimen was comparable to streptomycin alone, but the emergence of streptomycin-resistant organisms was reduced from 70% with streptomycin alone to 9% when PAS was combined with streptomycin (28). This was the first demonstration of the benefits of multidrug therapy in TB. This concept is central to TB management: *Always treat with multiple drugs to which the organism is susceptible.*

Isoniazid (INH) was introduced in 1951. It had early spectacular results (31), but monotherapy rapidly led to resistance and failures (32). Large, well-done studies confirmed that the preceding principle (stated differently) applies to INH as well (33,34): *Multidrug therapy prevents the emergence of resistance.*

Early experience suggested that the time frame for biologic cure was measured in months to years. A BMRC study addressed this question directly. They followed 387 patients with cavitary disease treated with combination therapy for 1, 2, or 3 years. Patients treated for 1 year had a relapse rate of 22%; those treated for 2 years had a relapse rate of 4%. There was no benefit from the addition of a third year (36). This leads to the important principle that *TB therapy must be of sufficient duration.* This important idea was firmly established early. Defining the shortest effective regimen motivated many subsequent trials.

With the realization that a multidrug regimen would be required for management of TB, and with the availability of multiple medications, TB could be managed effectively. By 1963, Hinshaw and Garland in their textbook *Diseases of the Chest* advocated a TB regimen of combination therapy with INH and PAS for at least 24 months, with streptomycin given for the first 3 to 6 months (37). These drugs were to remain the standard treatment regimen well into the 1970s. The regimen was highly effective at leading to initial biologic cure; it had an acceptably low relapse rate and was associated with low emergence of resistant organisms (38).

With the availability of multiple drugs, questions about the details of the best regimen arose. There is theoretical justification for using more than two drugs. Larger numbers of organisms contain greater numbers of bacilli that may be resistant to initial agents, so that by using several agents at once in the initial phase, more efficient killing can be achieved (39,40).

In the 1960s, several controlled trials of the best available agents provided strong evidence for the concept of an initial intensive phase (36,41). These studies showed that outcomes both in terms of time to culture conversion and in terms of relapse were better when 6 weeks of streptomycin was added to a 12-month regimen of INH and PAS. Additional studies also confirmed the value of multiple drugs in the initial phase of treatment (42,43). In the continuation phase fewer drugs could be given. By the mid- to late 1960s, this principle of therapy when applied to patients with advanced disease had been firmly established. *There is benefit to additional medication in the initial phase of treatment, particularly when the organism burden is high.*

TOWARD SHORT-COURSE THERAPY

As additional drugs were developed, many additional trials were organized to determine their place in the antituberculosis armamentarium (44). Rifampin was introduced for clinical use in 1966. It showed excellent bactericidal activity *in vitro* (45) and in early animal studies (46,47). Early experience in humans suggested that it might be a candidate for a short-course trial (48,49).

47: Principles of Tuberculosis Management   **715**

The recognition that multiple drugs given together would allow the most efficient bacterial killing led to the testing of a variety of short-course regimens that today form the cornerstone of our approach to management of active disease (50,51). A significant motive behind developing short-course regimens was the realization that long-term therapy (18 to 24 months), though extremely effective, was expensive and difficult to administer with any degree of confidence in terms of patient adherence to the regimen (52). Several major large-scale field trials of short-course chemotherapy provide the data that inform current treatment regimens.

The first East African/BMRC trials (53–55) examined several 6-month regimens and compared them to a reference regimen of 18 months of treatment with INH and thiacetazone, with streptomycin given for the first 2 months of therapy. The regimen of INH, rifampin, and streptomycin daily injections for 6 months had an acceptably low relapse rate of 2%. This rate is dramatically better than the same study with pyrazinamide (PZA) (11% relapse) or thiacetazone (22% relapse) instead of rifampin, and better than the 4% relapse rate in the 18-month regimen. Relapses that occurred using short-course regimens tended to occur within the first year after completion of therapy. Relapses were with organisms that retained their initial susceptibility, reemphasizing that multiagent therapy is extremely effective in preventing the emergence of drug-resistant strains of mycobacteria. Regimens were well tolerated. In only 14 (2.5%) of 540 patients was it necessary to discontinue any drug during therapy (Table 47.1).

The fact that a rifampin-containing regimen could allow effective short-course therapy of active, smear-positive, cavitary disease provided the framework for future investigations in the field. *Rifampin is the cornerstone of short-course therapy.*

Both the rifampin- and the PZA-containing regimens were more effective in rapidly rendering patients culture negative than either the two-drug regimen or the regimen containing thiacetazone. This foreshadowed the special place that PZA would eventually have in the initial phase of therapy.

The major impediment to the wide use of short-course therapy was the need for daily injections of streptomycin. Daily injections require availability of skilled health care workers. The injections are painful and are resisted by patients. Streptomycin is expensive and has high toxicity. The next step was to develop regimens that could be given intermittently or did not contain streptomycin at all.

The second East African/BMRC trial (56) involved more than 700 patients with smear-positive disease and tested four 6-month regimens. All regimens achieved excellent bacteriologic response by the end of the 6-month treatment period. The relapse rate was 7% or below for all regimens tested, and relapses involved organisms that were susceptible to all drugs contained in the treatment regimen.

Patients who relapse after treatment with an appropriate multidrug regimen relapse with susceptible organisms. The group receiving twice-weekly INH, streptomycin, and PZA in the continuation phase had excellent response rates and an acceptable relapse rate of 4%. The group receiving INH and rifampin for 6 months had a 7% relapse rate. Acceptable relapse rates have been defined as less than 5% (57).

This trial demonstrated that a rifampin-containing regimen could be effective in just 6 months without streptomycin and that *a regimen based on intermittent therapy can be highly effective.* Finally, although the addition of streptomycin seemed to confer some advantage in lowering the 1-year relapse rate from 5% to 2% in 6-month daily regimens, the benefit of adding this inconvenient and uncomfortable drug was small.

By the end of the 1970s short-course therapy was well established. Standard therapy consisted either of INH (300 mg) and rifampin (600 mg) daily for 9 months, or daily for 1 month followed by twice-weekly rifampin (600 mg) and INH (900 mg) for 8 additional months. The intermittent regimen comprises a total of 99 doses given over 9 months (58). This regimen had a success rate of more than 98%, sputum conversion within 2 months in more than 80% of patients, and a relapse rate after treatment of less than 1%. Patients who relapsed retained susceptibility to INH and rifampin. In many areas this approach to therapy remained standard for several years. When an organism is known to be susceptible, this approach remains completely reasonable.

CURRENT SHORT-COURSE REGIMENS

The British Thoracic Association studied 6-month regimens of daily INH and rifampin with 2 months of PZA plus streptomycin or PZA plus ethambutol (59,60). Bacteriologic cure was essentially 100%. Relapses were noted in only one of 125 patients treated with the former regimen and three of 132 patients treated with the latter regimen. This study confirmed that PZA and ethambutol could substitute for PZA and streptomycin with no appreciable loss of efficacy or increase in relapse rates, allowing a toxic and difficult-to-administer drug to be replaced without harm.

TABLE 47.1. THE FIRST EAST AFRICAN BRITISH MEDICAL RESEARCH COUNCIL SHORT-COURSE CHEMOTHERAPY TRIALS

Regimen	Months	No. Relapses (%)	No. Resistant
SMN/INH/RIF	6	2 (2)	2
SMN/INH/PZA	6	12 (11)	3
SMN/INH/T	6	23 (22)	1
SMN/INH	6	33 (29)	1
SMNx2/INH/T	18	4 (4)	0

INH, isoniazid; PZA, pyrazinamide; RIF, rifampin; SMN, streptomycin; T, thioacetazone.

The Hong Kong Chest Service/BMRC studied more than 900 patients with a variety of 6-month regimens (61,62). Several regimens included INH, rifampin, and streptomycin, and varied the duration of treatment with PZA for 2, 4, or 6 months. Virtually all patients had bacteriologic response. In the 5-year follow-up period, relapses were rare; for regimens containing PZA, the relapse rates were between 1% and 4%, even if streptomycin was excluded. By contrast, a regimen of INH, rifampin, streptomycin, and ethambutol for 6 months was associated with a 10.3% relapse rate. (It should be noted that INH, rifampin, and daily streptomycin in the first East African study had a relapse rate of 2%.) This study provided further evidence that *there is an important benefit from the inclusion of PZA in the initial phase of 6-month regimens.* In this trial, all medications were given three times per week for the duration of treatment, further supporting the role of intermittent therapy.

The U.S. Public Health Service Trial 21 (USPHS 21) used daily, self-administered INH and rifampin for 6 months, supplemented by daily PZA for the first 2 months of treatment (63). (Ethambutol was added to the regimen if patients had a history of prior treatment with INH or had immigrated to the United States within the past 30 years from a country where a high proportion of patients had drug-resistant disease.) The rate of adverse drug reactions for the 6-month regimen was 7.7%, with a relapse rate of 3.5% after 24 months of follow-up. These are excellent results in a trial compromised by the fact that 16.8% of patients on the 6-month regimen were judged to be non-compliant with therapy.

A study from the Denver Department of Health and the University of Colorado examined the efficacy of an entirely intermittent, directly observed, 6-month regimen consisting of INH, rifampin, and PZA for 2 months (drugs were given daily for 2 weeks and twice weekly thereafter) followed by twice-weekly INH and rifampin for an additional 4 months (64). In 101 patients enrolled, only two relapses were noted. The study consisted of just 62 total doses of medication.

Based on these studies (and many others conducted throughout the world), 6-month intermittent regimens are now considered standard and effective therapy in most of the world, and they form the foundation of the current recommendations of the American Thoracic Society (ATS) and the U.S. Centers for Disease Control and Prevention (CDC) (29).

The CDC recommended addition of ethambutol to the standard treatment in the United States in 1993 because of an increasing incidence of drug-resistant TB (35). They noted that this regimen would be highly effective even in cases of INH resistance. They also cite evidence from USPHS 21 (63) that the four-drug regimen converted the sputum more rapidly than a three-drug regimen.

Current ATS/CDC guidelines recommend initial treatment with INH, rifampin, PZA, and ethambutol. Ethamb-

utol may be discontinued once resistance is excluded. PZA may be discontinued after 8 weeks. INH and rifampin are continued for an additional 4 months. These guidelines apply to the vast majority of patients and, if followed, lead to excellent outcomes (29) (Table 47.2).

Several trials in the 1980s tried to shorten therapy beyond 6 months using more intensive treatment. Many different 2-, 3-, 4-, and 5-month regimens were tested (65–67). Initial response to therapy was excellent. Rifampin-containing regimens were associated with more rapid culture conversion than regimens without rifampin. Initial therapy with PZA was effective in rapidly achieving bacteriologic conversion. All regimens were associated with unacceptably high relapse rates. *No trial has demonstrated*

TABLE 47.2. SUMMARY RECOMMENDATIONS OF THE AMERICAN THORACIC SOCIETY AND THE CENTERS FOR DISEASE CONTROL AND PREVENTION FOR INITIAL THERAPY OF ACTIVE PULMONARY TUBERCULOSIS IN ADULTS

1. A 6-month regimen consisting of isoniazid (INH), rifampin, pyrazinamide, and ethambutol (or streptomycin in children too young to be monitored for visual acuity) given for 2 months, followed by INH and rifampin for 4 months is the preferred treatment for patients with fully susceptible organisms who adhere to treatment. Ethambutol may be discontinued when susceptibility testing reveals that the organism is susceptible to INH and rifampin. Treatment may be daily, 5x/ week on directly observed therapy (DOT), 3x/ week on DOT or twice/week on DOT, with daily therapy for the first 2 weeks. This four-drug regimen is effective even when the infecting organism is resistant to INH.
2. Alternatively, a 9-month regimen of INH, rifampin, and ethambutol (or streptomycin in children too young to be monitored for visual acuity) is acceptable for persons who cannot or should not take pyrazinamide. The initiation phase of this regimen is given daily. The continuation phase may be daily, 5x/ week on DOT, or twice/ week on DOT. If INH resistance is demonstrated, rifampin and ethambutol should be given for a minimum of 12 months.
3. Multiple drug–resistant tuberculosis (i.e., resistance to at least isoniazid and rifampin) presents difficult treatment problems. Treatment must be individualized and based on susceptibility studies. In such cases, consultation with an expert is recommended.
4. A continuation phase of INH and rifampin for only 2 months is acceptable therapy for adults who have active tuberculosis and are sputum smear and culture negative.
5. The major determinant of the outcome of treatment is adherence to the drug regimen. Careful attention should be paid to measures designed to foster adherence. DOT is the preferred initial strategy to insure adherence. The use of fixed drug combinations may enhance patient adherence, may reduce the risk of inappropriate monotherapy, and may prevent the development of secondary drug resistance. For this reason, the use of such fixed drug combinations is strongly encouraged in adults.

that therapy for periods shorter than 6 months is effective for smear-positive patients. Studies in smear- and culture-negative active-TB patients have shown excellent results with regimens of INH, rifampin, and PZA for 3 (68) or 4 (69) months—a fact that is recognized in CDC/ATS guidelines (29).

Not all regimens will be effective. A "failing regimen" is defined as failure to convert sputum to smear negative after 5 months of treatment (29). A major possibility in a patient with a failing regimen is that the organism has become resistant to one or more drugs in the regimen. (Nonadherence and problems with absorption should also be considered.) When this is suspected, the regimen is compromised. We cannot know initially to which drugs, if any, the organism remains sensitive. The principle for the approach to a failing regimen is simple: *Never add a single drug to a failing regimen.* When adding drugs to a failing regimen, always add a minimum of two drugs to which the organism is sensitive (or highly likely to be sensitive) and which have not been compromised. If these data are not available or if the drugs to be added are insufficiently potent, it is conventional to add drugs (29,30).

The emergence of resistance follows a predictable pattern. The spontaneous rate of mutation to INH resistance in a wild-type pansusceptible population of TB is roughly 1 in 10^6. The rate for rifampin is roughly 1 in 10^8. While a person might have 10^6 or even 10^8 organisms, 10^{14} organisms (the number of organisms one would need to harbor a single organism that is resistant to both drugs) is beyond the number of organisms in even advanced disease (35). The rate of selection for an organism resistant to both drugs in a patient treated with both drugs should be very small indeed.

MONOTHERAPY

Monotherapy during the intensive phase leads to the development of resistance and treatment failure. Monotherapy in the continuation phase is a more complex issue. Few organisms remain during the continuation phase, fewer than would be expected to produce a substantial number of resistant mutants in an organism that was initially pansusceptible and was managed with a multidrug-intensive phase (70). Furthermore, it is unclear how much each drug contributes to bactericidal activity in the continuation phase. Mitchison (70) believes that INH adds little to rifampin but that it is the major sterilizing component of a non–rifamycin-containing regimen. In a BMRC trial in Tanzania in 1985, INH monotherapy was compared to INH plus thiacetazone in the continuation phase after 2 months of therapy with INH, rifampin, PZA, and streptomycin (71). There was no development of resistance or treatment failure, though the relapse rate was substantially higher in the INH monotherapy group (11 of 100) than in the INH and thiacetazone group (three of 105).

Mitchison (70) reviewed BMRC studies of regimens of INH/thiacetazone in the continuation phase. He noted that 7.7% of organisms that are fully susceptible relapse with such a regimen, compared with 31% of those initially INH resistant. Sixteen percent (ten of 67) of relapsed organisms among initially INH-resistant organisms became resistant to thiacetazone.

A study in Hong Kong compared rifapentine and INH weekly or less with rifampin and INH three times weekly in the continuation phase of treatment. Patients who were drug resistant from the start of treatment were not excluded. There was no emergence of resistance even among patients who received rifamycin alone in the continuation phase. Treatment failure or relapse rate was 4.2% (seven of 165) for patients with fully susceptible organisms treated with INH and rifampin. There were no treatment failures or relapses among seven patients whose organism was initially INH resistant treated with INH and rifampin. The rate of adverse outcome was similar for patients on rifapentine and INH with a fully susceptible organism at the start of treatment (11%, 38 of 346) to the rate among those on this regimen whose organism was initially INH resistant (72). This supports the concept that monotherapy is well tolerated in the continuation phase.

Both the International Union Against Tuberculosis and Lung Disease (IUATLD) and WHO recommend a continuation phase of only two drugs in the empiric management of TB in the third world, even when resistance to one of the drugs is possible (73,74). The IUATLD regimen does not include rifampin in the continuation phase. As long as rifampin is not subjected to potential monotherapy in the continuation phase, it would not be compromised, and a retreatment regimen containing the most important drug would remain an option for that small subset of patients who might become resistant to the drugs used in the continuation phase. WHO includes INH, plus either rifampin for those countries with adequate resources or ethambutol for those without.

Monotherapy in the continuation phase is a complex issue. *Program guidelines might call for an empiric therapy regimen that may lead to monotherapy in the continuation phase after consideration of local resources and with a plan for a retreatment regimen.*

Mitchison (70) pointed out that virtually all of INH's bactericidal activity occurs very early in the intensive phase. Thereafter, rifamycin becomes the active drug. He noted that outcomes are similar in patients who received monotherapy in the continuation phase to those of patients who did not. He recommended a trial of higher doses of rifamycin alone in the continuation phase.

However, these arguments must be applied with great caution. USPHS 22 treated patients in the continuation phase with weekly rifapentine and INH. Because the half-life of rifapentine is dramatically longer than that of INH, this is essentially monotherapy for a large part of each week.

In human immunodeficiency virus (HIV)–infected individuals this led to significant acquired rifamycin resistance (75,76).

HUMAN IMMUNODEFICIENCY VIRUS

It was recognized early in the HIV epidemic that there was a strong and important association between acquired immunodeficiency syndrome (AIDS) and reactivation of latent TB (77). In 1983, Vieira et al. (78) described ten Haitian immigrants with AIDS, six of whom had active TB. In 1984, Pitchenik et al. (79) described 45 Haitian immigrants with AIDS, 27 of whom (60%) had active TB.

Selwyn et al. (80) prospectively followed 49 tuberculin skin test–positive patients with AIDS who attended a methadone maintenance program. He found that seven of 36 who did not receive INH developed active TB over 22 months. None of the 13 who received INH developed active TB.

Well-documented nosocomial outbreaks highlighted the frequency with which progressive primary TB can occur in AIDS patients. Di Perri et al. (81) described a patient with AIDS, on an HIV ward, who had cough and fever, but a normal chest radiograph and negative sputum smears for acid-fast organisms. Sputum cultures were positive. Seven of 18 AIDS patients on the ward developed active pulmonary TB within 60 days.

Daley et al. (82) described an outbreak investigation at a housing facility for HIV-positive patients. Twelve patients developed active pulmonary TB over 5 months. All 11 who had positive cultures had the same restriction fragment length polymorphism pattern, different from that of two other patients from the same facility who had active TB 6 months earlier. This confirmed recent transmission and very rapid progression to active disease.

The rise in the incidence of TB in the United States in the 1980s and 1990s is attributed in large part to the HIV epidemic. In New York City in 1992, 34% of TB cases involved known HIV-positive individuals. It is estimated that a more accurate figure would be close to 40%.

The association between AIDS and TB is attributed to defects in cell-mediated immunity in HIV-positive patients. HIV causes depletion of lymphocytes, particularly CD4 lymphocytes, in the lungs of persons with TB. This failure of CD4 alveolitis limits effective immune response to TB infection (83). It is now clear that TB within the lung creates conditions favorable to local HIV replication (84).

While HIV-positive individuals are at dramatically higher risk for development of TB, the degree of immunosuppression at which this "opportunistic infection" occurs can be significantly earlier in the course of HIV disease than other AIDS-defining illnesses (85). Clinical presentations are different in those with advanced HIV from those with early HIV disease and relatively preserved immunity. Those

with early disease have clinical presentations more like conventional TB. Upper lobe disease is predominant and cavitation is common (86). In contrast, in late HIV, upper lobe disease is less common. The patient with active reactivation pulmonary TB may have infiltrates in the lower lung zones, or may even have clear lungs (87). Lymphadenopathy (which is typically low density on computed tomography scan, consistent with necrosis) is common (88). *In a patient with HIV and unexplained pulmonary symptoms, TB must be suspected, even with a normal chest radiograph.*

Early in the TB epidemic of the 1980s and 1990s, the prognosis for HIV-infected TB patients was particularly poor. Median survival for a patient with TB after the diagnosis of AIDS was 8 months (77). The cause of death was usually an AIDS-related complication, not TB.

In persons with AIDS coinfected with multidrug-resistant TB, the outlook was universally dismal (89–91). A study from Bellevue Hospital showed that early diagnosis and institution of appropriate therapy could lead to significantly improved survival (92).

Early guidelines for the treatment of people with TB coinfected with HIV recommended prolongation of treatment (85,93). By the mid-1990s, with universal sensitivity testing, careful attention to the details of the treatment, and DOT, and following significant infusion of resources, reports began to emerge suggesting that such patients did well when treated with an appropriate regimen (91). In all cases, an appropriate regimen should include DOT (94). Guidelines for treatment of HIV/TB-coinfected individuals shifted, and recommended regimens and courses became the same as those for HIV-negative patients (29).

The introduction of protease inhibitors (PIs) in 1996 and multidrug highly active antiretroviral therapy (HAART) revolutionized the prognosis for HIV-infected people (95,96). HAART brings some challenges to the management of TB. Interactions among rifamycins, protease inhibitors, and nonnucleoside reverse transcriptase inhibitors (NNRTIs) are complex and clinically very relevant. Many combinations are possible.

Rifamycins are potent inducers of the cytochrome P450-3A (CYP3A) system. Of these, rifampin is most potent and rifabutin least. Rifabutin, but seemingly not rifampin or rifapentine, is metabolized by CYP3A (97). Protease inhibitors inhibit CYP3A and are metabolized by CYP3A. NNRTIs induce CYP3A and are metabolized by CYP3A (98).

Because rifampin is a potent inducer of CYP3A, use of rifampin with both PIs and NNRTIs was formerly felt to be contraindicated (99). Rifabutin has a similar activity profile to that of rifampin. The fact that rifabutin is a less potent inducer of CYP3A means that it causes less instability of levels of NNRTIs and PIs. This makes it a preferred choice for use in most patients on HAART. Even with rifabutin, important interactions occur. Dosage of rifabutin must be reduced when it is used with (most) PIs and increased when it is used with (most) NNRTIs. Use of rifabutin can be recommended only with those drugs for which the interaction has been characterized and for which dosage can be adjusted. CDC guidelines were published in 1998 (99) and updated in 2000 (100).

The updated guidelines list specific instances in which rifampin can safely be used concurrently with HAART. Rifampin may be used along with ritonavir because the action of ritonavir to inhibit CYP3A may offset rifampin's effect (101). Saquinavir may be used along with rifampin as long as ritonavir is also used. Rifampin may be used along with efavirenz as long as the efavirenz dose is increased (100).

Both rifampin and rifabutin decrease delavirdine concentration unacceptably. Delavirdine cannot be used safely with any rifamycin. Rifabutin remains the preferred drug in most instances. The updated guidelines include the use of rifabutin with ritonavir as long as the rifabutin dose is decreased considerably. Rifabutin can now be used with all PIs and all NNRTIs except delavirdine. The dosage of rifabutin should be decreased by half to 150 mg/day when rifabutin is used with PIs other than ritonavir or saquinavir to avoid rifabutin toxicity. When rifabutin is used with NNRTIs, the dose of rifabutin should be adjusted upward (100) (Table 47.3).

The option of discontinuing HAART during TB treatment is appealing as this would avoid potential drug interactions and allow conventional treatment with rifampin. For patients with advanced HIV disease and those already on HAART, this is problematic. For these patients a common solution is to choose a regimen of HAART compatible with rifabutin (or rifampin) and to adjust the dosage of the medications according to guidelines. In a patient not previously on HAART, withholding HAART for the first 2 months of TB therapy minimizes the risk of immune restoration syndrome, polypharmacy, and misattribution of an effect of TB medication to HAART or the combination (98). *Treatment of patients receiving HAART and antituberculous chemotherapy is complex. Guidelines exist for managing drug interactions. Patients should be treated in consultation with physicians experienced in managing both conditions. Communication between physicians managing the TB and the HIV is essential.*

Another option for treating a patient with TB coinfected with HIV is to use a non–rifamycin-containing regimen. Although the regimen of streptomycin, PZA, and INH was effective, with relapse rates between 5% and 6% when given for 9 months in an HIV-negative population in Hong Kong (102), this regimen has not been extensively used in HIV-positive individuals. Because it is generally felt to be an inferior regimen, most experts avoid this approach (100).

It is generally believed that the immune restoration syndrome represents an immune reaction to antigens released by treated TB. The syndrome manifests as a worsening of clinical or radiographic findings upon initiation of appropriate anti-tuberculosis treatment. The immune restoration syndrome has recently been associated with the initiation of HAART in HIV-positive patients taking TB medications (103–106).

Narita et al. (104) described worsening findings in 12 of 33 HIV-infected patients started on HAART. The syndrome was associated with conversion of tuberculin skin test to positive. Outcomes were not affected though three reactions were severe enough to warrant systemic steroids.

Wendel et al. (103) found paradoxical worsening in six of the 62 cases. It was present in three of 28 patients receiving HAART and in three of 44 patients not receiving HAART. She also noted that TB relapse occurred in two of

TABLE 47.3. GUIDELINES FOR COADMINISTRATION OF RIFAMYCINS WITH HIGHLY ACTIVE ANTIRETROVIRAL THERAPY[a]

Drug	Drug Dose	RBT	RBT Dose	Drug Dose	RIF	RIF Dose
PIs						
Saquinavir Hard-gel	No change	Y[b]	300	No change	Y[b]	600
Saquinavir Soft-gel	Increase	Y	150 intermittent	No change	Y[b]	600
Ritonavir	No change	Y	150 intermittent	No change	Y	600
Lopinavir/Ritonavir	No change	Y	150 intermittent	N/A	N	N/A
Indinavir	Increase	Y	150 daily 300 intermittent	N/A	N	N/A
Nelfinavir	Increase	Y	150 daily 300 intermittent	N/A	N	N/A
Amprenavir	No change	Y	150 daily 300 intermittent	N/A	N	N/A
NNRTIs						
Nevirapine	No change	Y	No change	No change	Y	?
Delaviadine	N/A	N	N/A	N/A	N	N/A
Efavirenz	Increase	Y	No change	No change	Y	600

N, no; NNRTI, nonnucleoside reverse transcriptase inhibitor; PI, protease inhibitor; RBT, rifabutin; RIF, rifampin; Y, yes.
[a]These recommendations change rapidly. Always consult updated guidelines.
[b]If used with ritonavir.

the six patients who had paradoxical worsening compared to 476 patients who did not have paradoxical worsening. She concludes that paradoxical worsening of TB occurs less frequently and that it is less strongly associated with HAART, but that it appears to be associated with an increased risk of TB relapse.

Fishman (106) described worsening chest x-ray in 14 of 31 (45%) HIV-positive TB patients on HAART, in contrast to 20% of TB patients who were either HIV positive and not on HAART or who were HIV negative. Kunimoto et al. (105) described a patient who developed respiratory failure when HAART was started 2 months into TB therapy. The reaction has been described in HIV-negative patients and in HIV-positive patients not on HAART (103,104,107).

Although guidelines for the management of TB in an HIV-coinfected individual are largely the same as for TB alone, there is evidence that the disease is different biologically. Malabsorption of medication is common in HIV-positive patients with TB. This may be a risk factor for the emergence of drug resistance (108). USPHS 22 investigated the use of weekly rifapentine in the continuation phase. Patients were treated either with rifapentine 600 mg and INH 900 mg once per week or with INH 900 mg and rifampin 600 mg twice weekly after a 2-month induction phase of INH, rifampin, PZA, and ethambutol given either daily or three times per week (75).

The HIV-positive arm of USPHS 22 was closed early after five of 30 HIV-positive patients treated with rifapentine relapsed, 4 with rifamycin-resistant organisms. Three of 31 HIV-positive patients receiving rifampin relapsed, all with susceptible organisms (75). The emergence of resistance was not described in HIV-negative patients taking rifapentine (109).

Because of differences in drug half-life, patients were essentially receiving rifapentine monotherapy for a large part of the week. The fact that HIV-positive patients do, in fact, develop resistance to a monotherapy drug even during the continuation phase, whereas HIV-negative patients under similar circumstances do not, tells us that HIV-positive patients are different. The fact that there was sufficient organism load for selection of resistant organisms implies that in these patients the intensive phase was less effective at sterilizing TB. There was an association with lower CD4 count.

In the developing world, the IUATLD has recommended treatment in the continuation phase with INH and thiacetazone (73). This strategy is inexpensive and highly effective (56). However, this regimen, because it is designed for use without susceptibility testing, has a certain risk for the patient receiving monotherapy in the continuation phase. In HIV-positive patients on such a regimen, by analogy to USPHS 22, there should be concern about possible treatment failure with a resistant organism. Use of the most important class of drugs, the rifamycins, would not be potentially compromised (76). Thiacetazone has been associated with a significant rate of toxic skin reactions in HIV-positive individuals (110,111). If HIV infection is likely, ethambutol is often substituted.

USPHS 23 is a study of twice-weekly rifabutin use in HIV-positive patients with TB. In March 2002, enrollment in USPHS 23 was halted because five patients developed rifamycin resistance. All five had low CD4 counts. Four of the five received twice-weekly therapy in the intensive phase. Because both the HIV-positive arm of USPHS 22 and a prior trial using twice-weekly rifampin and INH in HIV (112) had similar emergence of rifamycin resistance in HIV-positive patients with low CD4 counts on intermittent therapy, CDC recommends more frequent therapy in that group (113). *HIV-positive patients are different from HIV-negative ones in their responses to therapy. Treatment guidelines must be assessed separately.*

NEW DRUGS

Rifapentine is a long-acting rifamycin. It, together with its active metabolite, 25-desacetylrifapentine, has a half-life of elimination of 26 to 42 hours (114). In 1998 the Food and Drug Administration (FDA) approved rifamycin for twice-weekly use in the intensive phase and for weekly use in the continuation phase of therapy. A weekly dosing regimen would be a tremendous advantage in terms of providing medication by DOT. Data provided to the FDA in support of approval of rifapentine indicated that at the approved dose of 600 mg rifapentine was slightly less effective than rifampin (115). The expected improved adherence to the regimen and to DOT is a potential advantage of rifapentine (116).

A study of 672 newly diagnosed TB patients in Hong Kong compared a continuation phase of INH and rifampin dosed three times weekly with a continuation phase of INH and rifapentine dosed either weekly or 2 of every 3 weeks (72,117). No comment is made about HIV status, but drug users and people in poor medical condition or with serious non-TB disease were excluded. At 30 months follow-up, the rates of adverse treatment events (relapse plus failure) were 4.2% for the rifampin regimen, 10.2% for the weekly rifapentine arm, and 11.2 % for the 2-of-3-weeks arms (72).

This study was somewhat compromised by concerns about incomplete absorption and the quality of the rifapentine preparation used (118,119). The dosage was increased during the study to compensate (120). Interestingly, the outcome was independent of initial INH resistance and rate of INH acetylation, though the numbers are small (72).

Mitchison (119) has pointed out that no rigorous study of early bactericidal activity has been done. The dose of 600 mg was chosen based on animal and pharmacokinetic data. One area of concern is that high levels of protein binding might lead to poor concentrations of free drug. A recent dose finding study was conducted because of these concerns and because of disappointing efficacy of rifapentine in both studies (72,109). This study suggests that doses of 900 mg and possibly 1,200 mg are safe. There were no reports of flulike illness with rifapentine in the dose finding study or the clinical trials with the 600-mg dose. Whether there are clinical advantages to the higher doses remains to be seen (121).

To date, no long-acting companion drug exists. Since the half-life of INH is only 1 hour in rapid acetylators and 3 hours in slow acetylators (122), a patient on a continuation phase of INH and rifapentine weekly would essentially be receiving rifapentine monotherapy for a large part of the week. Based on USPHS 22, such a regimen cannot be used in HIV-positive patients (75). Whereas USPHS 22 showed the rifapentine regimen to have similar efficacy to a rifampin one in HIV-negative patients, the study in Hong Kong did not (72).

Absorption of rifapentine is significantly enhanced when it is taken with food. Mitchison (120) argues that since the study in Hong Kong shows that a less bioavailable rifapentine is inferior at current doses, caution is needed before it can be introduced in places where a fatty meal cannot be assured before each dose (119).

The need for new classes of medication for the management of TB has been recognized for years (123). The last new class of antibiotics useful in TB was the quinolones, introduced in the 1980s. While these are not FDA approved for TB, they have been widely used in multidrug-resistant TB patients (29). Ofloxacin and levofloxacin are quinolones that have better activity than ciprofloxacin (124). Sparfloxacin is even more highly active against *Mycobacterium tuberculosis*, but its use is significantly limited by toxicity, photosensitivity, and prolongation of the QT interval with torsades des pointes (125). Moxifloxacin is a newer quinolone with a better safety profile. *In vitro* data suggest that it may be as active as INH, and early clinical reports are promising (126,127).

The oxazolidinones are a new and novel class of ribosome-binding protein synthesis–inhibiting antibiotics (128). Linezolid is the first of these and is approved for use in drug-resistant gram-positive infections. It has significant activity against gram-positive bacteria (129) and excellent activity against *M. tuberculosis in vitro* (130). It has been used in a limited number of TB patients, sometimes with great success (131). Linezolid may become an important component of salvage therapy for multidrug-resistant TB, although at current pricing its usefulness will be limited. Other oxazolidinones have even better activity against *M. tuberculosis in vitro* (130).

Drugs in the isonicotinoylhydrazone family show promise (132) The macrolides have activity against *Mycobacterium avium* complex but not against *M. tuberculosis* (123). Reports that combination with other agents may improve macrolide activity against TB bear investigation (133).

PREDICTORS OF OUTCOME

A highly effective TB regimen may still have a failure rate of several percentage points (57). Longer courses of treatment have been associated with reduced relapse rates (102,134). Defining risk factors would allow identification of those people at increased risk of relapse whose course should be lengthened. Patients with silicotuberculosis (135) benefit from longer treatment, with relapse rates falling from 20% to less than 5% with an increase in treatment from 6 to 8 months. Several studies (136,137) have defined cavitation and prolonged culture positivity as risk factors for poor outcome. ATS guidelines (29) recommend prolonging therapy for patients with cavitary disease who are still smear positive after 2 months of therapy. They recommend carefully monitoring those with only one of those factors and prolonging therapy if response to therapy is unsatisfactory. HIV-positive patients, those with extensive disease and those with low body weight, should also be carefully monitored.

The HIV-negative arm of USPHS 22 was large enough to allow for investigation into risks of relapse or failure. Five risk factors for relapse were identified in the study overall: white, non-Hispanic; underweight; bilateral disease; radiographic evidence of cavitation; and sputum culture still positive at 2 months. Of these, bilateral disease and race were no longer risk factors when analyzed in the rifampin-only arm. Smear-positive status at 2 months was not a good predictor of treatment failure or relapse (109) (Table 47.4).

DIRECTLY OBSERVED THERAPY

Many studies have shown patient adherence rates below 70% for a variety of conditions (138–140). This percentage has been remarkably consistent across age, racial, ethnic, gender, and socioeconomic groups (94). In fact, the only group with significantly higher reported adherence rates is patients who are symptomatic (141).

TABLE 47.4. RISK FACTORS FOR TREATMENT FAILURE IN U.S. PUBLIC HEALTH SERVICE TRIAL 22

Risk Factor	Hazard Ratio
Non-Hispanic white	1.8
Underweight	2.8
Cavitation	3.0
Bilateral abnormalities	1.8
Positive sputum culture	2.8

Adapted from the Tuberculosis Trials Consortium CDC. Rifapentine and isoniazid once a week versus rifampicin and isoniazid twice a week for treatment of drug-susceptible pulmonary tuberculosis in HIV-negative patients: a randomized clinical trial. *Lancet* 2002;360:528–534.

Given these consistently low adherence rates, cure rates for TB in the range of 70% for an organism susceptible to the prescribed treatment would be no surprise. Such rates would, however, be a public health disaster. Cure rates for TB when the therapy is observed using a properly functioning DOT system are in excess of 90%. With state, city, and private funding, 113 patients were referred for DOT at the Bellevue Chest Service with only 11 nonadherent and lost to follow-up. Ninety-nine percent of the remainder achieved bacteriologic cure (142). Cure rates are important for both the patient and the community. *DOT is the standard of care for the provision of TB treatment*. Providing treatment to a TB patient without DOT is a deviation from the standard of care (94,143). There are those who point out that the benefits realized by a well-functioning DOT program may come not only from the act of observing the swallowing of the pill, but also from the many other components of the program of treatment (144). This point bears further discussion. Refinement of programmatic activities will continue. For now, completion rates and cure rates improve with the application of resources implied by the term DOT.

While DOT is standard of care, it is frequently neglected and frequently resisted. Patients are often offended by discussion of DOT. They sense a lack of trust. They feel inconvenienced. The initial discussion of the diagnosis and management of TB is the best time for the first discussion of DOT. This is the time to address concerns about DOT. A policy of universal DOT helps to prevent a patient from feeling singled out. Studies have shown that providers are no better than chance at predicting which patients will adhere to their regimen. Providers who "trust" a patient and decide that the patient doesn't need DOT are more likely to have identified a patient similar to themselves in some demographic category than one who will be adherent (143,145). Arranging for the provision of DOT is an important programmatic function and has priority in even the most resource-poor environment.

The logistics of providing DOT are complex. Patients have jobs. They work long hours. They work irregular hours. They work far away. They may not want family or co-workers or associates to know their diagnosis. The provision of DOT requires working with the patient to overcome these many obstacles and arrange a DOT system that can work for him or her. To this end, there is no substitute for working closely with the patient.

Patients often have very reasonable concerns and barriers that significantly interfere with DOT adherence. Programs should create enablers to help overcome barriers, as well as incentives or other rewards for adherence. A simple enabler is to remove or reduce the cost of transportation. In New York City, the majority of patients on DOT receive subway fare with each DOT visit (146). Provision of incentives has been shown to improve patient adherence to treatment (147,148).

Perhaps the most important aspect of a DOT program, and the most difficult to institute in a bureaucracy, is flexibility. Patients must get their medication. The dosages must be observed. The doses need not be given only in a particular location or at a particular time. The DOT program must accommodate any reasonable request, as well as some requests that aren't reasonable. This may require extended hours. This may require partnerships with other health care institutions or community agencies (149). New York City has had great success with field DOT programs that accommodate people at work and at home. It has had great success with weekend and evening DOT hours (150,151).

ROLE OF PUBLIC HEALTH PROGRAMS

Incidence rates of TB in the United States declined steadily through the 20th century. The rate of decline changed little with the introduction of antituberculous chemotherapy (152). By the late 1980s an excellent drug regimen was available that is effective and easy to administer. In spite of this, the decline in TB rates reversed itself in the late 1980s and early 1990s. The epidemic was concentrated in inner cities. In New York City, the number of cases almost tripled (150). The HIV epidemic has been blamed for much of this rise, as HIV-infected individuals are particularly susceptible to progression from infection to active disease. At least 34% of cases during that time were in HIV-positive individuals. But it was not the HIV epidemic alone that caused the increase. There were serious problems with TB control programs in New York and other big cities. Funding was down, staffing was down, and systems were not in place for case management or DOT (153).

It was entirely predictable that such a system would have an unacceptably high failure rate and that many of the individuals who had experienced treatment failure would emerge drug resistant and secondarily infect others. *Multidrug-resistant TB is a marker of a failing public health program*. The errors were magnified by the fact that the drug resistant cases occurred in HIV infected and disadvantaged individuals who were most vulnerable and who were frequently housed in congregate settings (153)

What was lacking was the sort of intervention that could have been provided by a well-functioning Department of Health. A mechanism was needed to report and track cases. A system of case management was needed that could assign one public health staffer to be responsible for the success of the patient's treatment even when the patient signed out against medical advice. A mechanism was needed to use legal means to detain patients who had repeatedly failed to complete a course of therapy and ensure that they would complete their treatment.

While this epidemic is clearly associated with the HIV epidemic, control of the TB epidemic preceded breakthroughs in HAART. Epidemic control was associated with revitalization of the TB control program. The situation began to improve rapidly in 1992 with a massive infusion of funding, primarily from the CDC (150). This provided the resources to hire a cadre of public health advisors. A case management system was put into place along with a system of accountability. A commitment was made to provide DOT both in city clinics and in the field, whether at work, at home, or at any other location acceptable to the patient. This system succeeded in persuading 73% of all TB patients in New York City and 85% of all patients treated at New York Department of Health clinics to enroll in DOT (154). All cases were discussed at a patient review conference providing an opportunity for the director of the TB control program to review every case in the city. This provided both education and accountability (151). Outreach to non–Department of Health providers allowed opportunities for partnerships, education, and training. A system of regulatory affairs was set up to allow for warnings, court-ordered DOT, and even detention in the case of nonadherence to therapy despite court order (155,156). With these interventions, TB rates in New York City dropped rapidly, now down to the lowest rates ever (157), demonstrating that *there is a crucial role for a well-functioning public health program.*

Frieden et al. (158) have noted that the challenges in the developing world at the end of the 20th century parallel those in New York City at the end of the 19th century. They noted that the epidemiology, in terms of both case rates and demographics, were similar. They stated that in both cases a programmatic response to diagnostic modalities, case management, and public education were important in efforts to control TB.

WHO has listed government commitment, case detection, standardized short-course chemotherapy, regular drug supply, and a monitoring system as five elements of a TB control policy package. In addition, they have outlined key operations for a national TB program (74). CDC has published a similar list of program guidelines (159)

Local government and departments of health have an important role in the prevention of monotherapy. Too often in the developing world, needed drugs are unavailable. Inattentiveness, cost, and logistic constraints all play a role. Under these circumstances, well-meaning health care providers often treat patients with inappropriate regimens of whatever medications are available. Assuring drug availability is a key role for government (74).

The promulgation of a standardized regimen appropriate to the circumstances of the population is a critical function of government. Such a regimen might allow for use of resources where they are clearly needed and facilitate inexpensive, yet appropriate, program-wide treatment. The desirable regimen is one that allows rapid bacteriologic conversion, is cheap and easily administered, and may be given for a short duration with an acceptable failure and relapse rate. A perfect example of such an approach is the adoption of IUATLD guidelines for low-income countries (73). The alternative to a standardized government-promulgated reg-

imen is therapeutic anarchy. When a wide variety of regimens are used, there is a high risk of treatment errors that allow the emergence of resistant organisms, a potentially disastrous result (160–163) *Having a standard regimen prevents therapeutic anarchy.*

Local guidelines should be developed based on local susceptibility data. Ideally susceptibility is tested on every patient's isolate. If this is not practical, some form of susceptibility surveillance should be in place to allow selection of empiric therapy (74). In all patients, initial therapy will be empiric until culture results are available. Multiple drugs must be provided to which the organism is likely to be susceptible.

A case management system has worked very well in a number of programs (143,164,165). Public health workers can be assigned to follow particular patients. Case managers would be expected to know the details of their patients' illness, treatment, living arrangements, and how they get their medication. Such a worker provide a patient with an ally in the often bewildering health care system and should be an individual on whom the patient can call for information or assistance. The case manager function works best when the worker is from the patient's own community. This arrangement often helps to overcome language and cultural barriers (151). Case management can allow better coordination of DOT and more thorough contact investigation.

When case management, DOT, education, efforts to address the patient's concerns and obstacles, warnings, and sometimes outright bribery have failed to get the patient to take his or her medicine, and when the patient remains infectious, the public health must be protected. Many jurisdictions have regulations that allow the TB control program to use the legal system to intervene when a patient fails to take required medications (166). Such systems should never be used as a substitute for maximal effort to understand and accommodate the needs of patients, but is a way to protect the public health when all other efforts have failed. New York City recently published their experiences with such a regulatory system (167). Regulatory affairs is a programmatic function. In all cases due process is required. In all cases it must be clear that detention must be the last and only resort. Details of such a program will have to be adjusted to the needs of the community, but all communities must ensure adherence to and completion of the treatment regimen.

Because TB is a public health threat, and because DOT improves cure rates, it is possible to discuss mandating DOT. Denver has a system in which every patient is served with an order of quarantine (166). This order mandates quarantine unless the Department of Health states otherwise. The price of suspension of this order of quarantine is adherence to DOT. Noncompliance with a commissioner's order for DOT is grounds for detention in New York City (167). It should be emphasized that the need for detention should be viewed as a failure of other interactions with the patient.

One of the important functions of a TB control program is to recognize infectious individuals so as to prevent them from transmitting infection to others (2). In the developing world sputum microscopy has been used to identify patients who are most infectious and therefore most in need of medication to prevent infection of others (74).

Although patients who are sputum smear positive are certainly more infectious than those who are smear negative, patients who are smear negative can still transmit disease. In a study by Gryzbowski et al. (168), smear-negative, culture-positive patients accounted for about 40% of cases of active TB. Seven percent of purified protein derivative–positive close contacts of smear-positive patients had active TB, compared with 4% of contacts among smear-negative culture-positive patients. A recent study by Behr et al. (169) used DNA fingerprinting to establish clusters of probable recent transmission. Behr et al. could then investigate the transmission rate among smear-negative and positive patients. They found that smear-negative culture-positive cases appear to be responsible for at least 17% of TB transmission, a number not substantially changed by modeling and sensitivity analysis to account for potential bias. They conclude with what should be an important principle:

> We propose that the limitations of the sputum acid-fast smear be respected . . . if diagnosis of TB remains a clinical possibility despite a negative smear, isolation should be continued until there is a response to treatment or the diagnosis is ruled out.

The dissemination of information is another useful role for government. A well-functioning program can quickly alert the local physicians to any change in drug availability, susceptibility patterns, or treatment recommendations. Such a program can ensure that accurate information and treatment recommendations are made available to health care providers in the community. It can educate patients about their condition and its treatment. It can facilitate educational and outreach activities in the community. The New York City Department of Health Tuberculosis Control Program maintains a computerized registry of all cases of suspected or confirmed TB since 1985. It allows physicians to quickly find out about the patient's previous treatment regimen, duration of treatment, adherence, and mycobacteriology results. This system also serves to prevent overtreatment of persons who have been previously evaluated. It allows for more prompt discovery and treatment of those who have not yet completed an adequate course. It can be invaluable in cases of nonadherence or interrupted treatment, or in cases in which treatment is complicated by other factors, such as drug resistance.

REFERENCES

1. World Health Organization. *Global tuberculosis control: surveillance, planning, financing*. WHO Report 2002. Geneva, 2002.
2. Centers for Disease Control and Prevention. Guidelines for preventing the transmission of *Mycobacterium tuberculosis* in health-care facilities. *MMWR Morb Mortal Wkly Rep* 1994; 43.
3. Frieden TR, Sherman LF, Maw KL, et al. A multi-institutional outbreak of highly drug-resistant tuberculosis: epidemiology and clinical outcomes. *JAMA* 1996;276:1229–1235.
4. Griffith DE, Hardeman JL, Zhang Y, et al. Tuberculosis outbreak among healthcare workers in a community hospital. *Am J Respir Crit Care Med* 1995;152:808–811.
5. Toman K. *Tuberculosis case-finding and chemotherapy*. Geneva: World Health Organization, 1979.
6. WHO Tuberculosis Programme. *Framework for effective tuberculosis control*. Geneva, 1994.
7. Styblo K. *Epidemiology of tuberculosis*. Jena: VEB Gustav Fisher, 1984.
8. Van der Werf TS , Dade, GK, van der Mark TW. Patient compliance with tuberculosis treatment in Ghana: factors influencing adherence to therapy in a rural service programme. *Tuber Lung Dis* 1990;71:247–252.
9. Gustafson P, Gomes VF, Vieira CS, et al. Tuberculosis mortality during a civil war in Guinea-Bissau. *JAMA* 2001;286:599–603.
10. Drobniewski FA, Verlander NQ. Tuberculosis and the role of war in the modern era. *Int J Tuberc Lung Dis* 2000;4: 1120–1125.
11. Yamada N, Osuga K, Shimouchi A, et al. Gender difference in delays to diagnosis and health care seeking behaviour in a rural area of Nepal. *Int J Tuberc Lung Dis* 2001;5:24–31.
12. Uplekar MW, Rangan S, Weiss MG, et al. Attention to gender issues in tuberculosis control. *Int J Tuberc Lung Dis* 2001;5: 220–224.
13. Khan A, Walley J, Newell J, et al. Tuberculosis in Pakistan: socio-cultural constraints and opportunities in treatment. *Social Sci Med* 2000;50:247–254.
14. Caprara A, Abdulkadir N, Idawani C, et al. Cultural meanings of tuberculosis in Aceh Province, Sumatra. *Med Anthropol.* 2000;19:65–89.
15. Banerjee A, Harries AD, Nyirenda T, et al. Local perceptions of tuberculosis in a rural district in Malawi. *Int J Tuberc Lung Dis* 2000;4:1047–1051.
16. Fadiman A. *The spirit catches you and you fall down: a Hmong child, her American doctors, and the collision of two cultures*. New York: Farrar, Straus and Giroux, 1997.
17. Ryan F. *The forgotten plague: how the battle against tuberculosis was won and lost*. Boston: Little, Brown and Company, 1992.
18. Francine AP. *Pulmonary tuberculosis. Its modern and specialized treatment*. Philadelphia: Lippincott, 1906.
19. Morgan R. Artificial pneumothorax in a group of cases of pulmonary tuberculosis formerly looked upon as hopeless. *Am J Roentgenol Radium Ther* 1933;30:309–314.
20. Hinshaw HC, Feldman WH. Streptomycin in the treatment of clinical tuberculosis a preliminary report. *Proc Staff Meet Mayo Clin* 1945;20:313–331.
21. Feldman WH. Streptomycin: some historical aspects of its development as a chemotherapeutic agent in tuberculosis. *Am Rev Tuberc* 1954;69:859–868.
22. Streptomycin Committee central office, Veterans Administration. The effect of streptomycin upon pulmonary tuberculosis. Preliminary report of a cooperative study of 223 patients by the Army, Navy and Veterans Administration. *Am Rev Tuberc* 1947; 56:485–507.
23. British Medical Research Council. Streptomycin treatment of pulmonary tuberculosis. A Medical Research Council investigation. *BMJ* 1948;2:769–782.
24. Lehmann J. Para-aminosalicylic acid in the treatment of tuberculosis. *Lancet* 1946;1:15–16.
25. Lehmann J. Twenty years afterward: historical notes on the discovery of the antituberculous effect of para-amino-salicylic acid (PAS) and the first clinical trials. *Am Rev Respir Dis* 1964;90: 953–956.

26. Iseman MD, Sbarbaro JA. Short-course chemotherapy of tuberculosis. Hail Britannia (and friends)! [letter comment]. *Am Rev Respir Dis* 1991;143:697–698.

27. Fox W, Ellard GA, Mitchison DA. Studies on the treatment of tuberculosis undertaken by the British Medical Research Council tuberculosis units, 1946–1986, with relevant subsequent publications. *Int J Tuberc Lung Dis* 1999;3:S231–S279.

28. British Medical Research Council. Treatment of pulmonary tuberculosis with streptomycin and para-amino-salicylic acid: a Medical Research Council investigation. *BMJ* 1950;2:1073–1085.

29. American Thoracic Society/Centers for Disease Control and Prevention/Infectious Diseases Society of America: Treatment of tuberculosis. *Am J Respir Crit Care Med* 2003;167:603–662.

30. Bureau of Tuberculosis Control. *Clinical policies and protocols*. New York: New York City Department of Health, 1999.

31. Robitzek EH, Selikoff IJ. Hydrazine derivatives of isonicotinic acid (Rimifon, Marsilid) in the treatment of active progressive caseous-pneumonic tuberculosis. A preliminary report. *Am Rev Tuberc* 1952;65:402–428.

32. Hobby GL, Lenert TF. Resistance to isonicotinic acid hydrazide. *Am Rev Tuberc* 1952;65:771–774.

33. British Medical Research Council. Various combinations of isoniazid with streptomycin or with PAS in the treatment of pulmonary tuberculosis: seventh report to the Medical Research Council by their Tuberculosis Chemotherapy Trials Committee. *BMJ* 1955;1: 435–445.

34. U.S. Public Health Service Cooperative Investigation of Antimicrobial Therapy of Tuberculosis. Report on thirty-two week observations on combinations of isoniazid, streptomycin and para-amino salicylic acid. *Am Rev Tuberc* 1954;70: 521–526.

35. Initial therapy for tuberculosis in the era of multidrug resistance. Recommendations of the Advisory Council for the Elimination of Tuberculosis. *MMWR Morb Mortal Wkly Rep* 1993; 42:1–8.

36. British Medical Research Council. Long-term chemotherapy in the treatment of chronic pulmonary tuberculosis with cavitation: a report to the Medical Research Council by their Tuberculosis Chemotherapy Trials Committee. *Tuber Lung Dis* 1962; 43:201–219.

37. Hinshaw H, Garland, LH. *Diseases of the chest*. Philadelphia: WB Saunders, 1963:542.

38. Results at 5 years of a controlled comparison of a 6-month and a standard 18-month regimen of chemotherapy for pulmonary tuberculosis. *Am Rev Respir Dis* 1977;116:3–8.

39. Canetti G. The eradication of tuberculosis: theoretical problems and practical solutions. *Tuber Lung Dis* 1962;43:301–321.

40. Mitchison DA. Chemotherapy of tuberculosis: a bacteriologist's viewpoint. *BMJ* 1965;1:1333–1340.

41. MacDonald FW. Study of triple versus double drug therapy of cavitary tuberculosis. Study 29. Second preliminary report. 27th Pulmonary Disease Research Conference, 1968. Veterans Administration–Armed Forces.

42. Livings GD. Results of original course of chemotherapy for tuberculosis: data from cooperative study, general regimens. *Transactions of the 18th conference on chemotherapy of tuberculosis. VA conferences in pulmonary diseases*. 1959;18:18.

43. Isoniazid with thiacetazone (thioacetazone) in the treatment of pulmonary tuberculosis in East Africa—third investigation: the effect of an initial streptomycin supplement. *Tubercle* 1966;47: 1–32.

44. D'Esopo ND. Clinical trials in pulmonary tuberculosis. *Am Rev Respir Dis* 1982;125:85–93.

45. Verbist L, Gyselen A. Antituberculous activity of rifampin *in vitro* and *in vivo* and the concentrations attained in human blood. *Am Rev Respir Dis* 1968;98:923–932.

46. Batten J. Rifampicin in the treatment of experimental tuberculosis in mice: sterilization of tubercle bacilli in the tissues. *Tubercle* 1970;51:95–99.

47. Grumbach F. Experimental *"in vivo"* studies of new antituberculosis drugs: capreomycin, ethambutol, rifampicin. *Tubercle* 1969;50(Suppl):12–21.

48. Gyselen A, Verbist L, Cosemans J, et al. Rifampin and ethambutol in the retreatment of advanced pulmonary tuberculosis. *Am Rev Respir Dis* 1968;98:933–941.

49. Nitti V, Catena E, Delli Veneri F, et al. Rifampin in association with isoniazid, streptomycin, and ethambutol, respectively, in the initial treatment of pulmonary tuberculosis. *Am Rev Respir Dis* 1971;103:329–337.

50. Dickinson JM, Mitchison DA. Suitability of rifampicin for intermittent administration in the treatment of tuberculosis. *Tubercle* 1970;51:82–94.

51. Grosset J. The sterilizing value of rifampicin and pyrazinamide in experimental short-course chemotherapy. *Bull IUAT* 1978; 53:5–12.

52. Fox W. Realistic chemotherapeutic policies for tuberculosis in the developing countries. *BMJ* 1964:135.

53. Controlled clinical trial of short-course (6-month) regimens of chemotherapy for treatment of pulmonary tuberculosis. *Lancet* 1972;1:1079–1085.

54. Controlled clinical trial of four short-course (6-month) regimens of chemotherapy for treatment of pulmonary tuberculosis. Second report. *Lancet* 1973;1:1331–1338.

55. Controlled clinical trial of four short-course (6-month) regimens of chemotherapy for treatment of pulmonary tuberculosis. Third report. East African/British Medical Research Councils. *Lancet* 1974;2:237–240.

56. Controlled clinical trial of four 6-month regimens of chemotherapy for pulmonary tuberculosis. Second report. Second East African/British Medical Research Council Study. *Am Rev Respir Dis* 1976;114:471–475.

57. American Thoracic Society. Medical Section of the American Lung Association: treatment of tuberculosis and tuberculosis infection in adults and children. *Am Rev Respir Dis* 1986;134: 355–363.

58. Dutt AK, Stead WW. Chemotherapy of tuberculosis for the 1980's. *Clin Chest Med* 1980;1:243–252.

59. A controlled trial of six months chemotherapy in pulmonary tuberculosis. First report: results during chemotherapy. British Thoracic Association. *Br J Dis Chest* 1981;75:141–153.

60. A controlled trial of six months chemotherapy in pulmonary tuberculosis. Second report: results during the 24 months after the end of chemotherapy. British Thoracic Association. *Am Rev Respir Dis* 1982;126:460–462.

61. Five-year follow-up of a controlled trial of five 6-month regimens of chemotherapy for pulmonary tuberculosis. Hong Kong Chest Service/British Medical Research Council. *Am Rev Respir Dis* 1987;136:1339–1342.

62. Hong Kong Chest Service/British Medical Research Council. Controlled trial of 2, 4, and 6 months of pyrazinamide in 6-month, three-times-weekly regimens for smear-positive pulmonary tuberculosis, including an assessment of a combined preparation of isoniazid, rifampin, and pyrazinamide. Results at 30 months. *Am Rev Respir Dis* 1991;143:700–706.

63. Combs DL, O'Brien RJ, Geiter LJ. USPHS Tuberculosis Short-Course Chemotherapy Trial 21: effectiveness, toxicity, and acceptability. The report of final results. *Ann Intern Med* 1990; 112:397–406.

64. Cohn DL, Catlin BJ, Peterson KL, et al. A 62-dose, 6-month therapy for pulmonary and extrapulmonary tuberculosis. A twice-weekly, directly observed, and cost-effective regimen. *Ann Intern Med* 1990;112:407–415.

65. Long-term follow-up of a clinical trial of six-month and four-month regimens of chemotherapy in the treatment of pulmonary tuberculosis. Singapore Tuberculosis Service/British Medical Research Council. *Am Rev Respir Dis* 1986;133: 779–783.

66. A controlled clinical trial of 3- and 5-month regimens in the treatment of sputum-positive pulmonary tuberculosis in South India. Tuberculosis Research Centre, Madras, and National Tuberculosis Institute, Bangalore. *Am Rev Respir Dis* 1986;134: 27–33.

67. Controlled clinical trial of five short-course (4-month) chemotherapy regimens in pulmonary tuberculosis. Second report of the fourth study. East African/British Medical Research Councils Study. *Am Rev Respir Dis* 1981;123:165–170.

68. A controlled trial of 2-month, 3-month, and 12-month regimens of chemotherapy for sputum-smear-negative pulmonary tuberculosis. Results at 60 months. *Am Rev Respir Dis* 1984; 130:23–28.

69. Dutt AK, Moers D, Stead WW. Smear- and culture-negative pulmonary tuberculosis: four-month short-course chemotherapy. *Am Rev Respir Dis* 1989;139:867–870.

70. Mitchison DA. Role of individual drugs in the chemotherapy of tuberculosis. *Int J Tuberc Lung Dis* 2000;4:796–806.

71. Controlled clinical trial of two 6-month regimens of chemotherapy in the treatment of pulmonary tuberculosis. Tanzania/British Medical Research Council Study. *Am Rev Respir Dis* 1985;131:727–731.

72. Tam CM, Chan SL, Kam KM, et al. Rifapentine and isoniazid in the continuation phase of a 6-month regimen. Interim report: No activity of isoniazid in the continuation phase. *Int J Tuberc Lung Dis* 2000;4:262–267.

73. Enarson DA, Rieder HL, Arnadottir T, et al. *Management of tuberculosis: a guide for low income countries.* International Union Against Tuberculosis and Lung Disease, 2000.

74. World Health Organization. *Treatment of tuberculosis: guidelines for national TB programmes.* Geneva, 1997.

75. Vernon A, Burman W, Benator D, et al. Acquired rifamycin monoresistance in patients with HIV-related tuberculosis treated with once-weekly rifapentine and isoniazid. Tuberculosis Trials Consortium. *Lancet* 1999;353:1843–1847.

76. Rieder HL, Arnadottir T, Trebucq A, et al. Tuberculosis treatment: dangerous regimens? *Int J Tuberc Lung Dis* 2001;5:1–3.

77. Chaisson RE, Schecter GF, Theuer CP, et al. Tuberculosis in patients with the acquired immunodeficiency syndrome. Clinical features, response to therapy, and survival. *Am Rev Respir Dis* 1987;136:570–574.

78. Vieira J, Frank E, Spira TJ, et al. Acquired immune deficiency in Haitians: opportunistic infections in previously healthy Haitian immigrants. *N Engl J Med* 1983;308:125–129.

79. Pitchenik AE, Cole C, Russell BW, et al. Tuberculosis, atypical mycobacteriosis, and the acquired immunodeficiency syndrome among Haitian and non-Haitian patients in South Florida. *Ann Intern Med* 1984;101:641–645.

80. Selwyn PA, Hartel D, Lewis VA, et al. A prospective study of the risk of tuberculosis among intravenous drug users with human immunodeficiency virus infection. *N Engl J Med* 1989; 320:545–550.

81. Di Perri G, Cruciani M, Danzi MC, et al. Nosocomial epidemic of active tuberculosis among HIV-infected patients. *Lancet* 1989;2:1502–1504.

82. Daley CL, Small PM, Schecter GF, et al. An outbreak of tuberculosis with accelerated progression among persons infected with the human immunodeficiency virus. An analysis using restriction-fragment-length polymorphisms. *N Engl J Med* 1992;326:231–235.

83. Law KF, Jagirdar J, Weiden MD, et al. Tuberculosis in HIV-positive patients: cellular response and immune activation in the lung. *Am J Respir Crit Care Med* 1996;153:1377–1384.

84. Nakata K, Rom WN, Honda Y, et al. *Mycobacterium tuberculosis* enhances human immunodeficiency virus-1 replication in the lung. *Am J Respir Crit Care Med* 1997 155:996–1003.

85. Barnes PF, Bloch AB, Davidson PT, et al. Tuberculosis in patients with human immunodeficiency virus infection. *N Engl J Med* 1991;324:1644–1650.

86. Theuer CP, Hopewell PC, Elias D, et al. Human immunodeficiency virus infection in tuberculosis patients. *J Infect Dis* 1990 162:8–12.

87. Pitchenik AE, Rubinson HA. The radiographic appearance of tuberculosis in patients with the acquired immune deficiency syndrome (AIDS) and pre-AIDS. *Am Rev Respir Dis* 1985 131: 393–396.

88. Harkin TJ, Ciotoli C, Addrizzo-Harris DJ, et al. Transbronchial needle aspiration (TBNA) in patients infected with HIV. *Am J Respir Crit Care Med* 1998;157:1913–1918.

89. Frieden TR, Sterling T, Pablos-Mendez A, et al. The emergence of drug-resistant tuberculosis in New York City. *N Engl J Med* 1993;328:521–526.

90. Fischl MA, Daikos GL, Uttamchandani RB, et al. Clinical presentation and outcome of patients with HIV infection and tuberculosis caused by multiple-drug-resistant bacilli. *Ann Intern Med* 1992;117:184–190.

91. Small PM, Schecter GF, Goodman PC, et al. Treatment of tuberculosis in patients with advanced human immunodeficiency virus infection. *N Engl J Med* 1991;324:289–294.

92. Park MM, Davis AL, Schluger NW, et al. Outcome of MDR-TB patients, 1983–1993. Prolonged survival with appropriate therapy. *Am J Respir Crit Care Med* 1996;153:317–324.

93. Tuberculosis and human immunodeficiency virus infection: recommendations of the Advisory Committee for the Elimination of Tuberculosis (ACET). *MMWR Morb Mortal Wkly Rep* 1989;38:236–238, 243–250.

94. Sbarbaro JA. Of pride and program planning—a lesson in reality. *Chest* 1998;114:1229–1230.

95. Mocroft A, Vella S, Benfield TL, et al. Changing patterns of mortality across Europe in patients infected with HIV-1. EuroSIDA Study Group. *Lancet* 1998;352:1725–1730.

96. Palella FJ Jr, Delaney KM, Moorman AC, et al. Declining morbidity and mortality among patients with advanced human immunodeficiency virus infection. HIV Outpatient Study Investigators. *N Engl J Med* 1998;338:853–860.

97. Burman WJ, Gallicano K, Peloquin C. Comparative pharmacokinetics and pharmacodynamics of the rifamycin antibacterials. *Clin Pharmacokinet* 2001;40:327–341.

98. Burman WJ, Jones BE. Treatment of HIV-related tuberculosis in the era of effective antiretroviral therapy. *Am J Respir Crit Care Med* 2001;164:7–12.

99. Prevention and treatment of tuberculosis among patients infected with human immunodeficiency virus: principles of therapy and revised recommendations. Centers for Disease Control and Prevention. *MMWR Morb Mortal Wkly Rep* 1998; 47:1–58.

100. Centers for Disease Control and Prevention. Updated guidelines for the use of rifabutin or rifampin for the treatment and prevention of tuberculosis among HIV-infected patients taking protease inhibitors or nonnucleoside reverse transcriptase inhibitors. Centers for Disease Control and Prevention. *MMWR Morb Mortal Wkly Rep* 2000;49:185–189.

101. Moreno S, Podzamczer D, Blazquez R, et al. Treatment of tuberculosis in HIV-infected patients: safety and antiretroviral efficacy of the concomitant use of ritonavir and rifampin. *AIDS* 2001 15:1185–1187.

102. Controlled trial of 6-month and 9-month regimens of daily and

intermittent streptomycin plus isoniazid plus pyrazinamide for pulmonary tuberculosis in Hong Kong. The results up to 30 months. *Am Rev Respir Dis* 1977;115:727–735.

103. Wendel KA, Alwood KS, Gachuhi R, et al. Paradoxical worsening of tuberculosis in HIV-infected persons. *Chest* 2001;120: 193–197.
104. Narita M, Ashkin D, Hollender ES, et al. Paradoxical worsening of tuberculosis following antiretroviral therapy in patients with AIDS. *Am J Respir Crit Care Med* 1998;158:157–161.
105. Kunimoto DY, Chui L, Nobert E, et al. Immune mediated "HAART" attack during treatment for tuberculosis. Highly active antiretroviral therapy. *Int J Tuberc Lung Dis* 1999;3: 944–947.
106. Fishman JE, Saraf-Lavi E, Narita M, et al. Pulmonary tuberculosis in AIDS patients: transient chest radiographic worsening after initiation of antiretroviral therapy. *AJR Am J Roentgenol* 2000;174:43–49.
107. Choremis CB, Padiatellis C, Zoumboulakis D, et al. Transitory exacerbation of fever and roentgenographic findings during treatment of tuberculosis in children. *Am Rev Tuberc* 1955;72:527–536.
108. Sandman L, Schluger NW, Davidow AL, et al. Risk factors for rifampin-monoresistant tuberculosis: a case-control study. *Am J Respir Crit Care Med* 1999;159:468–472.
109. The Tuberculosis Trials Consortium CDC. Rifapentine and isoniazid once a week versus rifampicin and isoniazid twice a week for treatment of drug-susceptible pulmonary tuberculosis in HIV-negative patients: a randomised clinical trial. *Lancet* 2002; 360:528–534.
110. Okwera A, Whalen C, Byekwaso F, et al. Randomised trial of thiacetazone and rifampicin-containing regimens for pulmonary tuberculosis in HIV-infected Ugandans. The Makerere University–Case Western University Research Collaboration. *Lancet* 1994;344:1323–1328.
111. van Gorkom J, Kibuga DK. Cost-effectiveness and total costs of three alternative strategies for the prevention and management of severe skin reactions attributable to thiacetazone in the treatment of human immunodeficiency virus positive patients with tuberculosis in Kenya. *Tuber Lung Dis* 1996;77:30–76.
112. el-Sadr WM, Perlman DC, Matts JP, et al. Evaluation of an intensive intermittent-induction regimen and duration of short-course treatment for human immunodeficiency virus–related pulmonary tuberculosis. Terry Beirn Community Programs for Clinical Research on AIDS (CPCRA) and the AIDS Clinical Trials Group (ACTG). *Clin Infect Dis* 1998;26:1148–1158.
113. Acquired rifamycin resistance in persons with advanced HIV disease being treated for active tuberculosis with intermittent rifamycin-based regimens. *MMWR Morb Mortal Wkly Rep* 2002;51:214–215.
114. Keung A, Eller MG, McKenzie KA, et al. Single and multiple dose pharmacokinetics of rifapentine in man: part II. *Int J Tuberc Lung Dis* 1999;3:437–444.
115. Package insert rifapentine (Priftin). Kansas City: Hoechst Marion Roussel, 1998.
116. Temple ME, Nahata MC. Rifapentine: its role in the treatment of tuberculosis. *Ann Pharmacother* 1999;33:1203–1210.
117. Tam CM, Chan SL, Lam CW, et al. Rifapentine and isoniazid in the continuation phase of treating pulmonary tuberculosis. Initial report. *Am J Respir Crit Care Med* 1998;157:1726–1733.
118. Kanyok T. A lesson to be learned. *Int J Tuberc Lung Dis* 1997; 1:490–492.
119. Mitchison DA. Development of rifapentine: the way ahead. *Int J Tuberc Lung Dis* 1998 2:612–615.
120. Tam CM, Chan SL, Lam CW, et al. Bioavailability of Chinese rifapentine during a clinical trial in Hong Kong. *Int J Tuberc Lung Dis* 1997;1:411–416.

121. Bock NN, Sterling TR, Hamilton CD, et al. A prospective, randomized, double-blind study of the tolerability of rifapentine 600, 900, and 1,200 mg plus isoniazid in the continuation phase of tuberculosis treatment. *Am J Respir Crit Care Med* 2002;165:1526–1530.
122. Weber WW, Hein DW. Clinical pharmacokinetics of isoniazid. *Clin Pharmacokinet* 1979;4:401–422.
123. O'Brien RJ, Vernon AA. New tuberculosis drug development. How can we do better? *Am J Respir Crit Care Med* 1998; 157:1705–1707.
124. Ji B, Lounis N, Maslo C, et al. In vitro and in vivo activities of moxifloxacin and clinafloxacin against *Mycobacterium tuberculosis*. *Antimicrob Agents Chemother* 1998;42:2066–2069.
125. Stahlmann R. Clinical toxicological aspects of fluoroquinolones. *Toxicol Lett* 2002;127:269–277.
126. Alvirez-Freites EJ, Carter JL, Cynamon MH. In vitro and in vivo activities of gatifloxacin against *Mycobacterium tuberculosis*. *Antimicrob Agents Chemother* 2002;46:1022–1025.
127. Tomioka H. Prospects for development of new antimycobacterial drugs. *J Infect Chemother* 2000;6:8–20.
128. Swaney SM, Aoki H, Ganoza MC, et al. The oxazolidinone linezolid inhibits initiation of protein synthesis in bacteria. *Antimicrob Agents Chemother* 1998;42:3251–3255.
129. Noskin GA, Siddiqui F, Stosor V, et al. In vitro activities of linezolid against important gram-positive bacterial pathogens including vancomycin-resistant enterococci. *Antimicrob Agents Chemother* 1999;43:2059–2062.
130. Cynamon MH, Klemens SP, Sharpe CA, Chase S. Activities of several novel oxazolidinones against *Mycobacterium tuberculosis* in a murine model. *Antimicrob Agents Chemother* 1999;43: 1189–1191.
131. Hadjiangelis NP, Leibert E, Harkin TJ, et al. Linezolid: a promising new agent for multi-drug resistant tuberculosis treatment (abstract A868). ATS 99th International Conference, May 16–21, Seattle, WA.
132. De Logu A, Onnis V, Saddi B, et al. Activity of a new class of isonicotinoylhydrazones used alone and in combination with isoniazid, rifampicin, ethambutol, para-aminosalicylic acid and clofazimine against *Mycobacterium tuberculosis*. *J Antimicrob Chemother* 2002;49:275–282.
133. Bosne-David S, Barros V, Verde SC, et al. Intrinsic resistance of *Mycobacterium tuberculosis* to clarithromycin is effectively reversed by subinhibitory concentrations of cell wall inhibitors. *J Antimicrob Chemother* 2000;46:391–395.
134. Long-tern chemotherapy in the treatment of chronic pulmonary tuberculosis with cavitation. A report to the Medical Research Council by their Tuberculosis Chemotherapy Trials Committee. *Tuber Lung Dis* 1962;43:201–267.
135. A controlled clinical comparison of 6 and 8 months of antituberculosis chemotherapy in the treatment of patients with silicotuberculosis in Hong Kong. Hong Kong Chest Service/ Tuberculosis Research Centre, Madras/British Medical Research Council. *Am Rev Respir Dis* 1991;143:262–267.
136. Aber VR, Nunn AJ. [Short term chemotherapy of tuberculosis. Factors affecting relapse following short term chemotherapy]. *Bull Int Union Against Tuberc* 1978 53:276–280.
137. Zierski M, Bek E, Long MW, et al. Short-course (6 month) cooperative tuberculosis study in Poland: results 18 months after completion of treatment. *Am Rev Respir Dis* 1980;122:879–889.
138. Davis MS. Predicting non-compliant behavior. *J Health Social Behav* 1967;8:265–271.
139. Sumartojo E. When tuberculosis treatment fails. A social behavioral account of patient adherence. *Am Rev Respir Dis* 1993; 147:1311–1320.
140. Sbarbaro JA. The patient–physician relationship: compliance revisited. *Ann Allergy* 1990;64:325–331.

141. Bergman AB, Werner RJ. Failure of children to receive penicillin by mouth. *N Engl J Med* 1963;268:1334–1338.

142. Schluger N, Ciotoli C, Cohen D, et al. Comprehensive tuberculosis control for patients at high risk for noncompliance. *Am J Respir Crit Care Med* 1995;151:1486–1490.

143. Chaulk CP, Kazandjian VA. Directly observed therapy for treatment completion of pulmonary tuberculosis: Consensus Statement of the Public Health Tuberculosis Guidelines Panel. *JAMA* 1998;279:943–948.

144. Volmink J, Matchaba P, Garner P. Directly observed therapy and treatment adherence. *Lancet* 2000;355:1345–1350.

145. Wardman AG, Knox AJ, Muers MF, et al. Profiles of non-compliance with antituberculous therapy. *Br J Dis Chest* 1988;82: 285–289.

146. Davidson H, Smirnoff M, Klein SJ, et al. Patient satisfaction with care at directly observed therapy programs for tuberculosis in New York City. *Am J Public Health* 1999;89:1567–1570.

147. Davidson H, Schluger NW, Feldman PH, et al. The effects of increasing incentives on adherence to tuberculosis directly observed therapy. *Int J Tuberc Lung Dis* 2000;4:860–865.

148. Bock NN, Sales RM, Rogers T, DeVoe B. A spoonful of sugar …: improving adherence to tuberculosis treatment using financial incentives. *Int J Tuberc Lung Dis* 2001;5:96–98.

149. CDC Division of Tuberculosis Elimination. *Treatment of TB disease. Core curriculum on tuberculosis.* Atlanta: CDC Division of Tuberculosis Elimination, 2000, Chapter 7.

150. Frieden TR, Fujiwara PI, Washko RM, Hamburg MA. Tuberculosis in New York City—turning the tide. *N Engl J Med* 1995;333:229–233.

151. Dorsinville MS. Case management of tuberculosis in New York City. *Int J Tuberc Lung Dis* 1998;2:S46–S52.

152. Summary of notifiable diseases, United States, 1990. *MMWR Morb Mortal Wkly Rep* 1991;39:1–61.

153. Brudney K, Dobkin J. Resurgent tuberculosis in New York City. Human immunodeficiency virus, homelessness, and the decline of tuberculosis control programs. *Am Rev Respir Dis* 1991; 144:745–749.

154. New York City Department of Health. Bureau of Tuberculosis Control. *Information summary, 1999.* New York, 2000.

155. Feldman G, Srivastava P, Eden E, et al. Detention until cure as a last resort: New York City's experience with involuntary in-hospital civil detention of persistently nonadherent tuberculosis patients. *Semin Respir Crit Care Med* 1997;18:493–501.

156. New York City Department of Health Tuberculosis Control Program. *Commissioner's orders for adherence to anti-TB treatment.* TB Fact Sheet 5a. New York, 2000.

157. New York City Department of Health. Bureau of Tuberculosis Control. *Information summary, 2000.* New York, 2001.

158. Frieden TR, Lerner BH, Rutherford BR. Lessons from the 1800s: tuberculosis control in the new millennium. *Lancet* 2000;355:1088–1092.

159. Essential components of a tuberculosis prevention and control program. Recommendations of the Advisory Council for the Elimination of Tuberculosis. *MMWR Recommend Rep* 1995;44:1–16.

160. Satcher D. From the surgeon general. Tuberculosis—battling an ancient scourge. *JAMA* 1999;282:1996.

161. Walton D, Farmer P. MSJAMA: the new white plague. *JAMA* 2000;284:2789.

162. Kimerling ME. The Russian equation: an evolving paradigm in tuberculosis control. *Int J Tuberc Lung Dis* 2000;4:S160–S167.

163. Portaels F, Rigouts L, Bastian I. Addressing multidrug-resistant tuberculosis in penitentiary hospitals and in the general population of the former Soviet Union. *Int J Tuberc Lung Dis* 1999; 3:582–588.

164. Klopf LC. Tuberculosis control in the New York State Department of Correctional Services: a case management approach. *Am J Infect Control* 1998 26:534–537.

165. Mathema B, Pande SB, Jochem K, et al. Tuberculosis treatment in Nepal: a rapid assessment of government centers using different types of patient supervision. *Int J Tuberc Lung Dis* 2001;5:912–919.

166. Burman WJ, Cohn DL, Rietmeijer CA, et al. Short-term incarceration for the management of noncompliance with tuberculosis treatment. *Chest* 1997;112:57–62.

167. Gasner MR, Maw KL, Feldman GE, et al. The use of legal action in New York City to ensure treatment of tuberculosis. *N Engl J Med* 1999;340:359–366.

168. Grzybowski S, Barnett GD, Styblo K. Contacts of cases of active pulmonary tuberculosis. *Bull IUAT* 1975;50:90–106.

169. Behr MA, Warren SA, Salamon H, et al. Transmission of *Mycobacterium tuberculosis* from patients smear-negative for acid-fast bacilli. *Lancet* 1999;353:444–449.

MANAGEMENT OF MULTIDRUG-RESISTANT TUBERCULOSIS

TIMOTHY J. HARKIN
RANY CONDOS

In the United States a recent epidemic of tuberculosis that peaked in 1992 is now waning. The epidemic was accompanied by a striking upswing in the prevalence of multidrug-resistant strains of *Mycobacterium tuberculosis* (1). New York City had the misfortune to be the epicenter of an epidemic of multidrug-resistant tuberculosis (MDR-TB), defined as a strain resistant to at least isoniazid and rifampin *in vitro* (2,3). A nationwide survey in 1991 found that more than 60% of all cases in the United States were located in New York City (1). At Bellevue Hospital Center, which treats approximately 10% of all of the tuberculosis patients in New York City, combined resistance to isoniazid and rifampin increased from 2.5% of *M. tuberculosis* isolates in 1971 to 16% in 1991 (2). The response by the city of increased funding for tuberculosis control programs, particularly the emphasis on providing directly observed therapy (DOT) to as many tuberculosis patients as possible, successfully combined with increased physician awareness and education to stem the epidemic. In 1992, of the 3,811 cases of tuberculosis in New York, 441 were MDR-TB (11.6%); in 2001, only 24 of 1,261 cases (1.9%) were multidrug-resistant—a remarkable decrease of 95% in only 9 years (4).

EVOLUTION OF MULTIDRUG-RESISTANT STRAINS

Acquired drug resistance is the means by which the overwhelming majority of multidrug-resistant strains of *M. tuberculosis* emerge, as spontaneous mutation causing resistance to more than one drug is a relatively uncommon occurrence. Human error on the part of the tuberculosis control program, the physician directing treatment, or the

patient with tuberculosis (frequently all play a role) is the major factor in the appearance of multidrug-resistant strains. Understanding how an organism may acquire resistance to multiple drugs is essential in the prevention of the emergence of a multidrug-resistant organism in an individual receiving antituberculous chemotherapy. Acquired drug resistance was first noted during the early trials of streptomycin in the management of tuberculosis (5). Isolates from tuberculosis patients were susceptible to streptomycin prior to treatment; after a period of clinical improvement, many patients relapsed with organisms that were resistant to streptomycin. Thus arose the concept that single-drug therapy for tuberculosis selects out drug-resistant organisms. This phenomenon is explained by the rates of spontaneous mutation of drug resistance in *M. tuberculosis*. For example, spontaneous resistance to isoniazid occurs in approximately 1 in 10^6 organisms and to rifampin in 1 in 10^8. The incidence of spontaneous mutation of resistance to both drugs is the product of the incidences of resistance to the individual drugs, that is, 1 in $10^6 \times 1$ in 10^8, or 1 in 10^{14} (6). A tuberculous cavity in a patient's lung may contain as many as 10^9 organisms. If the infecting organism was originally susceptible to both drugs, one may therefore predict that the cavity harbors several hundred organisms resistant to isoniazid, as well as a few resistant to rifampin, but none resistant to both drugs. Administration of both isoniazid and rifampin should lead to a cure, as isoniazid-resistant organisms will be killed by rifampin, and rifampin-resistant organisms will be killed by isoniazid. However, if the infecting organism was resistant to isoniazid, all organisms in the cavity will be isoniazid resistant, and a small number will spontaneously mutate and develop rifampin resistance as well. Administration of isoniazid and rifampin in this setting is equivalent to monotherapy with rifampin alone, for isoniazid will not be effective against any of the organisms. Nonetheless, as rifampin will kill almost all of the organisms, initial clinical improvement may occur. Killing of the rifampin-sensitive organisms will provide a selection bias

T. J. Harkin: Department of Medicine, New York University School of Medicine; Chest Service, Bellevue Hospital Center, New York, New York.

R. Condos: Division of Pulmonary and Critical Care Medicine, New York University School of Medicine, New York, New York.

for the few organisms resistant to both drugs, allowing them to flourish in the cavity, and eventually the disease will reoccur as MDR-TB (7).

The patient's contribution to the selection of drug-resistant strains comes in the form of erratic compliance with drug therapy. Different types of noncompliance are possible, with different impacts on the course of disease. A patient receiving an adequate regimen of chemotherapy who stops taking all medications before an appropriate duration of treatment has been completed is at increased risk of recurrent disease, but this behavior should not change the susceptibility patterns of the infecting organism (8). Usually such a patient can be successfully treated with the same drug regimen previously prescribed. More worrisome is the patient who omits one or more drugs from an adequate regimen; if this individual takes only a single drug, or changes the regimen so that it contains only one drug to which the organism is susceptible (effectively equivalent to monotherapy), the risk of selecting out an organism resistant to the single drug is high. The patient may not acknowledge this type of erratic drug administration, and even if a history of irregular dosing is obtained, the specific details are often difficult or impossible to reconstruct. Because early clinical, radiologic, or bacteriologic improvement may temporarily occur despite monotherapy or irregular therapy, noncompliance may be unsuspected; the first evidence of noncompliance to appear during the course of therapy may be the emergence of drug resistance, manifested by failure of bacteriologic conversion of sputum or by recurrence of positive sputum cultures after initial sputum conversion.

The above scenarios may also be interpreted as failures of the tuberculosis control program. The responsibilities of the program (in addition to administering appropriate therapy) include educating the patient regarding the importance of taking all doses of all the medications for the appropriate duration of time, as well as providing as much opportunity as possible for the patient to do so (9). DOT programs may be the best means of providing maintenance therapy; therefore, their use is strongly encouraged (10). They provide assurance that the patient is taking multidrug therapy as well as timely information if the patient stops taking medication before the prescribed duration. This allows early contact of the patient to reinforce the need to continue therapy.

Management of active tuberculosis provides many challenges to the physician in terms of choosing an appropriate drug regimen because there are significant pitfalls that can result in the emergence of drug-resistant organisms. Widely recognized risk factors for drug resistance include previous treatment for tuberculosis, residence in an area endemic for drug resistance, and close contact with a known case of active MDR-TB (2,11). However, a recent nationwide study found that only 40% of isolates resistant to isoniazid and/or rifampin had one of these risk factors (1). Therefore,

M. tuberculosis isolates from initial episodes as well as from relapses should always be tested for susceptibility to all first-line drugs.

While awaiting results of susceptibility testing, the patient must receive a multiple-drug regimen based on knowledge of the prevailing drug susceptibilities in the community. Current recommendations call for regimens containing a minimum of four drugs in communities where at least 4% of isolates are drug resistant (10). If the initial susceptibility tests show resistance or if resistance is suspected due to a lack of bacteriologic response to treatment, and a decision is made that the regimen should be expanded, a minimum of two new drugs must be added. The new drugs must be chosen from those to which the organism is known to be sensitive or those that the patient has never received (10). It cannot be overemphasized that *a single drug must never be added to a failing regimen*. This cardinal rule may not be as simple to follow as it first appears. Among New York City's large homeless or transient population, it is not uncommon to find patients with MDR-TB who have been treated in several different hospitals with several different regimens and who are unable to provide a detailed treatment history; it may be clear that a regimen is failing, while unclear just what that regimen is! In such situations considerable investigation may be required prior to designing a new regimen to ensure the minimum of two new drugs. Recognizing this problem, in 1993 the New York City Department of Health established a centralized database wherein the results of each patient's smears, cultures, and drug susceptibilities are recorded, in addition to treatment histories and outcomes (12). This approach enhances the possibility of choosing an effective retreatment regimen when confronted with such a situation.

The contribution of physicians to the development of MDR-TB should not be minimized. A telling study of MDR-TB patients referred to the National Jewish Center for Immunology and Respiratory Medicine found a disturbingly high average of 3.9 physician treatment errors per case. The most common errors were addition of a single drug to a failing regimen; failure to identify preexisting or acquired drug resistance; and administration of an initial regimen inadequate in number of drugs or duration of therapy, or both (13). The results of this study emphasize the need for physicians caring for patients with active tuberculosis to be well versed in the basic principles of treatment.

When a patient relapses with tuberculosis after previous treatment, the likelihood that he or she is harboring an organism with newly acquired drug resistance depends on several factors. One is the duration of previously inadequate therapy, as the risk of acquired resistance increases with length of treatment. The hazards of even brief courses of monotherapy in the setting of active tuberculosis were strikingly illustrated in a study by the Centers for Disease Control and Prevention, which found resistance to isoniazid in 25% of isolates from patients who had previously received up to 2 weeks of treatment with isoniazid alone (14). Isoniazid resistance increased to more than 60% among patients receiving 6 months of monotherapy and to more than 80% after 2 years.

Patient compliance patterns are clearly important but are difficult to ascertain precisely. In addition, the number of drugs in the initial regimen, the initial resistance pattern, and the characteristics of the individual drugs themselves interact in a complex manner to prevent or promote the development of additional drug resistance. For instance, Mitchison and Nunn (15) studied the effect of initial drug resistance on the efficacy of short-course chemotherapy in 12 trials conducted by the British Medical Research Council. Of patients with initial resistance to isoniazid alone or streptomycin alone, treatment with a regimen of isoniazid, streptomycin, and pyrazinamide failed in 12 (21%) of 57, in contrast to only two failures among 235 patients who received any multidrug regimen containing rifampin.

PRINCIPLES OF MEDICAL TREATMENT

A review of the literature on the management of drug-resistant tuberculosis provides some guidelines for potentially effective treatment for MDR-TB in addition to warnings of pitfalls to avoid. Three pieces of information are essential to design a salvage regimen of chemotherapy for an individual with MDR-TB:

1. *Results of prior susceptibility tests.* If available, these results provide information necessary for the design of a new regimen. While this may seem to be an obvious statement, all too often an inadequate effort is made to obtain results from tests performed at another treatment site. A problem may arise if different susceptibility patterns are found at different times in the treatment course, particularly resistances that appear to come and go. This phenomenon may be due to sampling of different populations of organisms in a patient with a large bacillary load or to different techniques of testing in different labs. The best course in such a situation is not clear; the most conservative approach, which we advocate, is to assume that the worst combination of resistances that has been found is correct and design a new regimen accordingly. In addition, the experience and quality of the microbiology laboratory must be taken into account. When an experienced laboratory reports consistent susceptibility results, and a less experienced laboratory reports results at variance, it is usually prudent to accept the results of the more experienced laboratory. An important point to appreciate is that susceptibility testing should be used to guide choices of chemotherapy but should not be used in isolation to dictate therapy; one must take into account the clinical response to treatment. A patient who has persistently positive smears and cultures despite a regimen to which *in vitro* susceptibility has been demonstrated merits a complete reevaluation of the treatment strategy, and such a situation in particular requires confirmation that the individual has adhered to the prescribed regimen.

2. *Treatment history.* When one assembles the components of a salvage regimen, the efficacy of any drug that was used in a previous inadequate treatment regimen must be regarded with suspicion, even if no resistance was demonstrated at that time. (For the purpose of this discussion, an adequate regimen is one that would be expected to cure when administered for an appropriate duration. An inadequate regimen is one that would be not be expected to have a high response rate regardless of treatment duration, due to the presence of resistance to some drug or drugs in the regimen and the relative weaknesses of the remaining drugs in the regimen.) Even when *in vitro* sensitivities to previously used agents are demonstrated, these agents may not prove as effective in a salvage regimen as the *in vitro* susceptibility pattern predicts (16). At times it is appropriate to assume resistance to a particular drug even when sensitivity testing cannot be done or will not be available for some time. For example, consider a patient for whom the sputum smear or culture fails to convert to negative during a regimen consisting of isoniazid, rifampin, pyrazinamide, and ethambutol. When susceptibility testing results become available 2 months into treatment, initial resistance to isoniazid, rifampin, and ethambutol is found. Susceptibility testing for pyrazinamide, which is not widely available, was not performed. In this setting of 2 months of monotherapy with pyrazinamide, it is safest to assume that, if not initially present, resistance to pyrazinamide has developed.

3. *Susceptibility patterns in the community.* This issue becomes a factor in choosing a salvage regimen only if a treatment failure occurs during chemotherapy and no prior susceptibility tests are available. If available, results of an individual's susceptibility tests should take precedence over local susceptibility patterns.

SELECTING A DRUG REGIMEN

It hardly needs to be stated that the cardinal rule dictating that effective drug treatment of tuberculosis requires the use of multiple agents is particularly imperative in the case of MDR-TB. Implementation of this rule is complicated because the optimal number of drugs is unclear and the choice of drugs is limited by the resistance pattern of the individual strain. Because the drugs used in retreatment regimens are generally less effective, most authorities recommend a minimum of three or four agents, and possibly as many as six or seven (10,17,18). The duration of medical therapy required is uncertain. In treating a patient with MDR-TB, a minimum of 18 months is usually necessary, but 24 months may be preferable; longer courses may be required for severe disease.

Decisions regarding optimal drug selection for the management of MDR-TB are best made with the aid of drug susceptibility testing, which reliably predicts an organism's response to particular agents. Unfortunately, it is rare that such results would be available before therapy is implemented. Only if no intervening treatment was given after prior drug susceptibilities were obtained, or if intervening treatment consisted only of multiple drugs to which all prior testing had shown susceptibility, could the earlier test results be expected to continue to apply to the susceptibilities of the organism at the time of the current episode. However, the usual circumstance requires therapy that must include a minimum of three drugs that ideally meet two criteria: the organism is known to be susceptible to the drugs and the patient has never received the drugs. If both criteria cannot be met, then therapy must be empiric, with the latter criterion taking precedence. Patients with active tuberculosis who are close contacts of patients known to have MDR-TB should be treated according to the susceptibility patterns of the index patient, pending the results of susceptibility tests on their organism.

Second-line agents receive this designation because they are less effective and more toxic than first-line agents; difficulty can arise in designing the least toxic regimen expected to have maximal efficacy. At the present time, if the patient has not received a quinolone before, this class of drug best serves as a crucial member of a salvage regimen (10,17), particularly when used in combination with a parenteral agent. Specific regimens recommended for patients with various drug resistance patterns will be outlined subsequently. The incidence of toxicity that necessitates discontinuation of one or more agents is increased when such regimens are employed and may necessitate choosing substitutions from an even smaller pool of remaining drugs. For complete discussions of the relative merits and disadvantages of individual agents, the reader is referred to chapters on specific drug types (Chapters 50–52).

In essence, choosing a salvage regimen can seem relatively simple: eliminate from the list of potential agents all drugs to which resistance is known, regard with suspicion any other drug that the patient has received in a failing or inadequate regimen (at least until results from new susceptibility tests are available), and then construct a regimen centered around the drugs that remain.

RECENT EXPERIENCE WITH NEWER AGENTS

Rifabutin

Rifabutin is a spiropiperidyl derivative of rifamycin S that is more active than rifampin against slow-growing mycobacteria including *M. tuberculosis* and *M. avium-intracellulare.* In liquid culture, the minimal inhibitory concentration (MIC) for rifamycin-susceptible strains of *M. tuberculosis* range from 0.003 to 0.006 µg/mL (19) Rifabutin acts by inhibiting mycobacterial DNA–dependent RNA polymerase in a way similar to that of other rifamycins and is

bactericidal for bacilli. The bioavailability of rifabutin is 10% to 20%, and absorption is relatively rapid with peak serum concentrations 2 to 3 hours after dosing (20). Food delays absorption but does not affect the peak serum concentration or area under the curve (21). Rifabutin is bound to serum proteins and penetrates well into all tissues. Rifabutin is extensively metabolized in the liver, and its major metabolites have activity against *M. tuberculosis* (22). Like rifampin, rifabutin induces its own metabolism and has a half-life of 36 hours. Rifabutin serum concentrations are increased when the drug in administered with inhibitors of cytochrome P450, and can result in increased activity of rifabutin or increases in rates of rifabutin toxicity (23).

Rifabutin has been used extensively in patients with human immunodeficiency virus (HIV) infection; the greatest clinical experience has been to prevent *M. avium* complex (MAC) disease in patients with advanced acquired immunodeficiency syndrome (AIDS) (24). Doses of rifabutin used in the human trials ranged from 150 to 300 mg given daily or twice weekly. In one study of HIV-infected tuberculosis patients, sputum culture conversion was similar to rifampin (25).

Rifamycin resistance in *M. tuberculosis* correlates closely with genetic alterations in the RNA polymerase β subunit gene (26). There has been significant though not complete cross-resistance between rifampin and rifabutin in *M. tuberculosis* strains (27). *In vitro* studies have identified MDR-TB isolates that are resistant to rifampin but sensitive to rifabutin. It is in these cases that rifabutin has been suggested to play a role in the management of MDR-TB. In Taiwan, rifabutin has been included in the management of susceptible MDR-TB strains in combination with ofloxacin. Suo et al. (28) reported a 73% sputum culture conversion rate in these difficult cases. Achievable cerebrospinal fluid and serum concentrations have been documented with rifabutin in another case report suggesting rifabutin's usefulness (29). Although no case controlled studies have been performed, rifabutin is recommended in cases of MDR-TB where drug sensitivity has been documented. Due to the high level of cross-resistance with rifampin, empiric treatment in cases of rifampin resistance is not recommended.

Fluoroquinolones

Another group of recently developed drugs with promising antituberculous activity are the fluoroquinolones, including ciprofloxacin, ofloxacin, levofloxacin, and moxifloxacin (10,30–33). Fluoroquinolones act by the inhibition of DNA gyrase. Two randomized controlled studies suggest that fluoroquinolones may be effective when used as first-line agents against tuberculosis. Ofloxacin was as effective as ethambutol in a 6-month, three-drug regimen (31), and ciprofloxacin was nearly as effective as rifampin in a 6-month, four-drug regimen (32). Both studies were small and excluded patients with drug-resistant tuberculosis. Until larger, controlled studies can be performed to clearly delineate how these important agents best fit into the overall strategy in managing both susceptible and drug-resistant tuberculosis, judicious use of fluoroquinolones is advisable. Currently, the most prudent course is probably to reserve fluoroquinolones for use in multidrug salvage regimens for patients with known or suspected MDR-TB (10).

Over the past decade, most of the published experience in the management of MDR-TB has involved ciprofloxacin and ofloxacin. In a number of recent uncontrolled studies comprising several hundred patients with severe MDR-TB, one of these two agents was used in a multidrug regimen, usually in conjunction with a parenteral agent and one to three others (34–36). Cure rates in the some of the most recent studies have been in the 75% to 80% range, in comparison with a study published only few years earlier reporting a 56% cure rate among patients whose treatment had occurred prior to the introduction of fluoroquinolones (15). Although the evidence may not be conclusive, there is widespread consensus that fluoroquinolones are important components of treatment regimens for MDR-TB. A newer agent, levofloxacin, the L isomer of ofloxacin, is twice as active *in vitro* against *M. tuberculosis* (37), and its use is currently recommended. Unfortunately, resistance of *M. tuberculosis* to fluoroquinolones is increasing. A recent study from the Philippines reports resistance to ciprofloxacin in 27%, to ofloxacin in 35%, and to both in 17% of *M. tuberculosis* isolates (38). This may be due to widespread use of fluoroquinolones in diseases other than tuberculosis, at times inappropriately.

Interferon-γ

The ability of macrophages to inhibit the growth of *M. tuberculosis* seems to depend on the state of activation of the effector cell. Great attention has recently been focused on the role of the cytokine interferon-γ (IFN-γ) and its ability to inhibit mycobacterial growth. A major role for IFN-γ in mycobacterial host defense has been suggested by a variety of *in vitro* and animal experiments. Genetically altered mice that lack IFN-γ or its receptor are extraordinarily susceptible to infection with *M. bovis*, though the mechanism of this susceptibility is not precisely known (39). Jaffe (40) demonstrated that IFN-γ administered by aerosol to normal human subjects is capable of activating alveolar macrophages.

Holland et al. (41) have used systemically administered IFN-γ to successfully treat a group of patients with systemic infections caused by *M. avium* complex and other nontuberculous mycobacteria. In addition, a cohort of patients have recently been described in whom a genetic defect in IFN-γ receptor function is present, leading to infections with mycobacteria that are usually nonpathogenic (42). Taken together, these experiments suggest an important

role for IFN-γ in host defense, and it is certainly possible that this cytokine acts primarily as a macrophage activator.

Early clinical experience with IFN-γ in the management of mycobacterial disease has come from studies in leprosy where low doses of IFN-γ were given by subcutaneous injection to patients with lepromatous leprosy. These patients received IFN-γ in combination with regular antimycobacterial treatment and were found to have increased granuloma formation suggesting a more effective immune response (43).

Our group studied the effects of IFN-γ delivered directly to the lung by aerosol in patients with active MDR-TB despite long-term drug therapy with regimens tailored to the pattern of drug resistance of *M. tuberculosis* isolates (44). Patients received aerosolized IFN-γ at a dose of 500 μg three times per week for 1 month. All patients tolerated the treatment well. Sputum smears became negative in all patients and the time to a positive sputum culture increased, suggesting a decrease in mycobacterial burden. The size of cavitary lesions was reduced in all patients and sputum smears remained negative for up to 3 months after discontinuation of IFN-γ treatment. These exciting preliminary studies suggest that IFN-γ may indeed augment immune defenses in pulmonary tuberculosis and may act in conjunction with conventional therapy as an immunomodulator.

Linezolid

Linezolid is a member of a new class of antimicrobial agents, the oxazolidinones, that inhibit bacterial protein synthesis. *In vitro* studies have demonstrated significant activity against *M. tuberculosis* with MIC in the range of 0.5 to 2.0 μg/mL, including multidrug-resistant strains (45–47).

We recently presented our early experience with the use of linezolid in the management of MDR-TB at the 2003 annual meeting of the American Thoracic Society in Seattle (47a). Five patients had MDR-TB resistant to all first-line agents and the aminoglycosides; one patient also resistant to capreomycin; one patient also to ciprofloxacin; and three patients also to ciprofloxacin and capreomycin. Two patients had relapsed after pneumonectomy, and one had a pneumonectomy immediately prior to starting on a salvage regimen. All five received linezolid 600 mg orally twice daily, in addition to the previous failing regimen, and four also received aerosolized IFN-γ three times weekly. Four patients had sputum culture conversion to negative in 7 to 97 days, and the fifth had radiographic improvement despite intermittently positive cultures. We conclude that linezolid was safe and well tolerated, and contributed to culture conversion in this small group of patients with severe MDR-TB. Further studies will determine if linezolid truly has a role in the management of MDR-TB.

Cross-Resistance, Drug Interactions, and Bioavailability

Fortunately, little cross-resistance is found among most antituberculous drugs. This is true even of the aminoglycosides; it should also be remembered that, although capreomycin is often grouped with the aminoglycosides, it is structurally unrelated and therefore exhibits no cross-resistance. Cross-resistance is also uncommon between isoniazid and ethionamide, another nicotinic acid–related compound. On the other hand, as much as 80% of organisms resistant to rifampin will be resistant to rifabutin as well.

Ethionamide or paraaminosalicylic acid (PAS) individually can cause hypothyroidism, and this side effect is more common when the two drugs are given simultaneously. These two drugs frequently cause severe gastrointestinal upset, and many patients cannot tolerate their combination for this reason. Giving these drugs at bedtime 1 hour after an antiemetic and with a hypnotic may improve tolerance. In extreme circumstances, one may be forced to use capreomycin and an aminoglycoside together; despite the lack of cross-resistance, side effects of eighth nerve and renal toxicities are shared, which generally precludes their combination. Cycloserine, which commonly causes psychiatric disturbances, must be used with extreme caution to prevent the exacerbation of preexisting disorders of this nature, particularly depression; suicides have occurred in patients receiving this medication.

Malabsorption of antituberculous agents has been raised as a potential mechanism for both acquisition of resistance and failure of retreatment regimens (48,49). Monitoring of drug serum levels to assure adequate dosing and absorption recently was advocated (17,48,50). This issue may be of particular concern in patients with AIDS, who are at risk for a wide range of gastrointestinal disorders that can interfere with drug absorption. The practicality and clinical relevance of these tests, which are not widely available, requires further study. The interaction of medications in a treatment regimen is another area that merits more investigation, as studies have suggested that some drugs may affect the bioavailability of other drugs administered simultaneously (49,51). If effects of drug combinations on bioavailability are found to be clinically significant or unpredictable, monitoring of drug levels may indeed be crucial in guaranteeing dosing that achieves target serum levels.

In addition, it should be remembered that the parenteral drugs may be administered intravenously as well as intramuscularly (although this is difficult with streptomycin); this option may be useful in the initial therapy of a cachectic patient with little muscle mass who cannot tolerate the painful injections. Similarly, if there is concern about oral absorption due to nausea and vomiting from other medications, a fluoroquinolone may be administered intravenously in conjunction with an aminoglycoside or capreomycin to ensure delivery of what may be the two most important drugs in the regimen.

SURGICAL MANAGEMENT

In the early part of this century, surgical treatment of patients with tuberculosis constituted the only active intervention the clinician could offer that had a reasonable chance of altering the course of the disease. Unfortunately, the rise in MDR-TB has again provided the need for surgery as an adjunct to retreatment with medical regimens (52–54).

The most extensive experience with surgical intervention in MDR-TB recently reported comes from the National Jewish Center in Denver (52,53). Patients were selected for surgery based on extensive drug resistance, poor response to medical therapy, and disease sufficiently localized to permit resection of the bulk of involved lung with enough remaining functioning lung to predict recovery without respiratory insufficiency. Importantly, most patients had some degree of bilateral disease. Of 57 patients, there was one postoperative death, and six patients were left with some degree of respiratory insufficiency. However, 49 of 50 long-term survivors remained smear and culture negative.

In a report by Chiang et al. (54) from Taiwan, 24 of 27 patients with MDR-TB who underwent pulmonary resection converted to or maintained negative sputum cultures with one perioperative death and one relapse after completion of treatment.

Clearly, in appropriate cases, surgical resection can have an important role in the management of MDR-TB. Selection of surgical candidates and timing of adjunctive surgery must be performed on a case-by-case basis. Only those patients whose organisms demonstrate drug resistance patterns that predict a high probability of treatment failure should be considered for resection. Nonetheless, unless the organism is still sensitive to at least two drugs that are likely to be effective, surgery will probably be futile. The goal of surgery must be to remove as much diseased lung as possible, particularly cavities, while not creating crippling respiratory impairment. This does not preclude such procedures as bilateral upper lobectomy. The anticipated site of the surgical stump must be evaluated by bronchoscopy immediately prior to surgery to ensure the absence of endobronchial tuberculosis, which would guarantee poor healing and a persistent bronchopleural fistula. The most difficult decision is the optimal timing of surgery. Ideally some degree of clinical response to the drug regimen is desirable; this must be balanced against the potential for emergence of further resistance and spread of disease to involve a proportion of lung that would preclude surgery.

SUGGESTED TREATMENT REGIMENS FOR SPECIFIC DRUG RESISTANCE PATTERNS

Recommended regimens for the management of MDR-TB have been published elsewhere. The following discussion describes the approach taken on the Bellevue Chest Service in various clinical settings, employing the reasoning detailed previously in this chapter. The aim is to provide the reader with examples of the application of general guidelines, not rigid protocols. Indeed, the key to successful management of MDR-TB is individualization of therapy and the ability to adapt treatment strategy in response to changing clinical situations. One blanket statement that may be safely made is that no treatment regimen will be successful unless the patient actually receives the medications. For this reason, essentially all patients with MDR-TB are best treated by means of some type of DOT program to ensure compliance with what are frequently unpleasant drug regimens. (Note also that in the following discussions, though we consider levofloxacin to be the fluoroquinolone of choice for reasons outlined above, other fluoroquinolones may be used as well.)

Suspected Resistance to a Standard Four-Drug Oral Regimen Due to Persistently Positive Cultures After 2 to 3 Months of Treatment or Clinical and Radiographic Deterioration Before Initial Susceptibility Results Are Available

We add three drugs in this setting, usually streptomycin, levofloxacin, and ethionamide. If the susceptibility tests reveal resistance to all first-line agents, including streptomycin, we stop the streptomycin, and add capreomycin (at least until subsequent tests demonstrate microbial susceptibility to kanamycin and amikacin, one of which may then be substituted) and PAS, and, if the illness is severe, cycloserine as well.

Resistance to Isoniazid Alone, or in Combination with Resistance to Streptomycin

Effective treatment regimens for isolated isoniazid resistance are well established. The combination of rifampin, pyrazinamide, and ethambutol is effective when all three drugs are given for 6 to 9 months (55). Rifampin and ethambutol may also be effective when administered for 12 months (56). The presence of streptomycin resistance does not affect the efficacy of these regimens.

In practice, some clinicians advocate continuing isoniazid in the regimen despite documented resistance in the hope that an undetected subpopulation of isoniazid-susceptible organisms is present. As there is no evidence that continuing isoniazid in this setting improves the outcome of therapy, we discontinue the drug if an experienced and reliable laboratory has reported resistance.

Resistance to Rifampin Alone

Isolated resistance to rifampin is unusual. Because rifampin is a potent antituberculous drug that made effective short-course therapy possible, resistance to this agent prolongs the duration of treatment. Isoniazid and ethambutol are effective when administered for 18 months; it is advisable to include streptomycin until bacteriologic conversion has occurred, and often 2 to 3 months after (57,58). The benefit of adding pyrazinamide in this setting is unknown, but we believe it is desirable to include it for the entire treatment period, or at least for the first 2 months to expedite conversion to a noninfectious state.

Resistance to Isoniazid and Ethambutol, With or Without Resistance to Streptomycin

Rifampin and pyrazinamide should be combined with levofloxacin and streptomycin. If a good clinical response is achieved, the streptomycin may be stopped at a total dose of 120 g to decrease toxicity. In this setting, as in the remainder of the resistance patterns to be discussed, resistance to streptomycin necessitates the substitution of one of the second-line aminoglycosides (kanamycin or amikacin) or capreomycin. The remaining drugs should be continued either for 9 months or for at least 6 months after cultures convert to negative—whichever is longer.

Resistance to Isoniazid and Rifampin, With or Without Resistance to Streptomycin

When the two most important antituberculous drugs are not effective, we prefer a regimen of four drugs. The remaining first-line drugs—pyrazinamide, ethambutol, and streptomycin—are used in conjunction with a levofloxacin to make a potent combination. In the setting of MDR-TB, ethambutol should be used at a dose of 25 mg/kg (rather than 15 mg/kg), which may be bactericidal. The higher dose increases the risk of retrobulbar neuritis from 1% to about 5%, requiring close monitoring for this side effect (58–60). The regimen should be continued for at least 18 months after cultures convert to negative.

Resistance to Isoniazid, Rifampin, and Ethambutol, With or Without Resistance to Streptomycin

If a reliable laboratory reports susceptibility to pyrazinamide, this drug may be combined with a quinolone, streptomycin or one of the second-line parenteral drugs, and ethionamide. In general, however, reliable information on susceptibility to pyrazinamide is not widely available, in which case PAS or cycloserine should be included. Treatment should be continued for a minimum of 18 months after cultures are negative. Adjunctive surgical management should be strongly considered in this setting.

Resistance to All First-Line Drugs and Any Second-Line Drugs

In this setting, we consider a fluoroquinolone and a parenteral agent to be the primary drugs around which to design a retreatment regimen, with the remaining two or three drugs serving to protect against the emergence of resistance to the first two. In practice, the choices are so limited that such regimens are usually made up of all drugs to which resistance has not yet been demonstrated. Strong consideration must be given to surgery. We would also advocate consideration of IFN-γ and linezolid if resistance to the fluoroquinolones or capreomycin or both is demonstrated. Treatment should be administered for a minimum of 18 to 24 months after cultures are negative.

OUTCOMES OF TREATMENT

Not surprisingly, patients who are immunosuppressed by HIV appear to fare particularly poorly when coinfected with MDR-TB (61–64). In an article describing 62 such patients, Fischl et al. (61) report a median survival of 2.1 months from time of diagnosis with tuberculosis. MDR-TB was not suspected early in the course for these patients, and many patients died before drug susceptibility tests were available. We reviewed 173 patients with MDR-TB treated at Bellevue Hospital from 1983 to 1993, of whom 52% were coinfected with HIV (66). Mortality was significantly greater for HIV-infected patients than for HIV-negative patients (72% vs. 20%). In HIV-infected patients, only appropriate therapy was associated with improved survival, with a median survival of 14.1 months. This emphasizes the need for high suspicion of MDR-TB in the HIV-infected patient to enable early institution of appropriate therapy.

A report from the National Jewish Center regarding the outcome of treatment in 171 MDR-TB patients who were HIV negative is only moderately more encouraging (17). Of 134 patients with adequate follow-up, 87 (65%) responded with negative sputum cultures. Twelve of these patients subsequently relapsed, yielding an overall response rate of only 56%. Tuberculosis was the cause of death in 22% of patients.

More recent studies have demonstrated improved results as experience with the management of MDR-TB increased. In a study from Korea, Park et al. (34) reported an 82% response to treatment with 17 months follow-up. Yew et al. (35) reported an 81% cure rate in patients who received either ofloxacin or levofloxacin as part of a four- or five-drug regimen. A study from Turkey by Tahaoglu (36) described an overall success rate of 77%, although one third of these "successes" were "probable" cures.

In summary, the outlook for clinicians struggling with the management of MDR-TB today remains extremely challenging but with evidence of hope for the future. The number of available effective drugs is limited, most of these are poorly tolerated, and duration of treatment is quite long. Even with aggressive therapy that may include surgery, it appears that we can only hope to cure about 50% to 75% of patients. There is evidence that more effective and more tolerable drugs are being developed. This and improved case detection, increased awareness of the potential for acquiring drug resistance, and enhanced infection control are our primary weapons in controlling this deadly disease.

ACKNOWLEDGMENT

The authors wish to acknowledge the contribution of H. William Harris, M.D.

REFERENCES

1. Bloch AB, Cauthen GM, Onorato IM, et al. Nationwide survey of drug-resistant tuberculosis in the United States. *JAMA* 1994; 271:665–671.
2. Neville K, Bromberg A, Bromberg R, et al. The third epidemic—multidrug-resistant tuberculosis. *Chest* 1994;105:45–48.
3. Frieden TR, Sterling T, Pablos-Mendez A, et al. The emergence of drug-resistant tuberculosis in New York City. *N Engl J Med* 1993;328:521–526.
4. New York City Department of Health, Tuberculosis Bureau. *Information summary.* New York: New York Department of Health, 2001.
5. McDermott W, Muschenheim C, Hadley SJ, et al. Streptomycin in the treatment of tuberculosis in humans. *Ann Intern Med* 1947;27:769–822.
6. David HL. Probability distribution of drug-resistant mutants in unselected populations of *Mycobacterium tuberculosis. Appl Microbiol* 1970;20:810–814.
7. Iseman MD, Madsen LA. Drug-resistant tuberculosis. *Clin Chest Med* 1989;10:341–353.
8. Snider DE Jr, Long MW, Cross FS, et al. Six-months isoniazid-rifampin therapy for pulmonary tuberculosis. *Am Rev Respir Dis* 1984; 129:573
9. Iseman M. Tailoring a time bomb. *Am Rev Respir Dis* 1985; 132:735.
10. American Thoracic Society. Treatment of tuberculosis and tuberculosis infection in adults and children. *Am J Respir Crit Care Med* 1994; 149:1359–1374.
11. Barnes PF. The influence of epidemiologic factors on drug resistance rates in tuberculosis. *Am Rev Respir Dis* 1987;136:325–328.
12. New York City Department of Health, Tuberculosis Bureau. *Information summary.* New York, NY: New York Department of Health, 1993.
13. Mahmoudi A, Iseman MD. Pitfalls in the care of patients with tuberculosis. *JAMA* 1993;270:65–68.
14. Costello HD, Caras GJ, Snider DE Jr. Drug resistance among previously treated tuberculosis patients: a brief report. *Tubercle* 1980;121:313–316.
15. Mitchison DA, Nunn AJ. Influence of initial drug resistance on the response to short-course chemotherapy of pulmonary tuberculosis. *Am Rev Respir Dis* 1986;133:423–430.
16. Goble M, Iseman MD, Madsen LA, et al. Treatment of 171 patients with pulmonary tuberculosis resistant to isoniazid and rifampin. *N Engl J Med* 1993;328:527–532.

17. Iseman MD. Treatment of multidrug-resistant tuberculosis. *N Engl J Med* 1993;329:784–791.

18. World Health Organization. *Guidelines for the management of drug-resistant tuberculosis.* Geneva: World Health Organization, 1997.

19. Della Bruna C, Schioppacassi G, Ungheri D, et al. LM 427, a new spiropiperadylrifamycin: *in vitro* and *in vivo* studies. *J Antibiot* 1983;36:1502–1506

20. Blashke TF, Skinner MH. The clinical pharmacokinetics of rifabutin. *Clin Infect Dis* 1996;22: S15–S22.

21. Narang PK, Lewis RC, Bianchine JR. Rifabutin absorption in humans: relative bioavailability and food effect. *Clin Pharmacol Ther* 1992;52:335–341.

22. Battaglia R, Pianezzola E, Salgarollo G, et al. Absorption, disposition and preliminary pathway of ^{14}C-rifabutin in animals and man. *J Antimicrob Chemother* 1990;26:813–822.

23. Brindle RJ, Nunn PP, Githiu G, et al. Quantitative bacillary response to treatment in HIV-associated pulmonary tuberculosis. *Am Rev Respir Dis* 1993;147:958–961.

24. Nightingale SD, Cameron DW, Gordin FM, et al. Two randomized trials of rifabutin prophylaxis against *Mycobacterium avium* complex infection in AIDS. *N Engl J Med* 1993;329: 828–833.

25. Schwander S, Rusch-Gerdes S, Mateega A, et al. A pilot study of antituberculosis combinations comparing rifabutin with rifampicin in the treatment of HIV-1 associated tuberculosis: a single-blind randomized evaluation in Ugandan patients with HIV-1 infection and pulmonary tuberculosis. *Tuber Lung Dis* 1995;76:210–218.

26. Kapur V, Li LL, Iordanescu S, et al. Characterization by automated DNA sequencing of mutations in the gene (rpoB) encoding the RNA polymerase beta-subunit in rifampin-resistant *Mycobacterium tuberculosis* strains from New York City and Texas. *J Clin Microbiol* 1994;32:1095–1098.

27. Uzun M, Erturan Z, Ang O. Investigation of cross-resistance between rifampin and rifabutin in *Mycobacterium tuberculosis* complex strains. *Int J Tuberc Lung Dis* 2002;6: 164–165.

28. Suo J, Yu MC, Lee CN, et al. Treatment of multidrug-resistant tuberculosis in Taiwan. *Chemotherpy* 1996;42(Suppl3):20–23.

29. DeVincenzo JP, Berning SE, Peloquin CA, et al. Multidrug-resistant tuberculosis meningitis: clinical problems and concentrations of second-line antituberculous medications. *Ann Pharmacother* 1999;33:1184–1188.

30. Hong Kong Chest Service/British Medical Research Council. A controlled study of rifabutin and an uncontrolled study of ofloxacin in the retreatment of patients with pulmonary tuberculosis resistant to isoniazid, streptomycin and rifampicin. *Tuber Lung Dis* 1992; 73:59–67.

31. Kohno S, Koga H, Kaku M, et al. Prospective comparative study of ofloxacin or ethambutol for the treatment of pulmonary tuberculosis. *Chest* 1992;102:1815–1818.

32. Mohanty KC, Dhamgaye TM. Controlled trial of ciprofloxacin in short-term chemotherapy for pulmonary tuberculosis. *Chest* 1993;104:1194–1198.

33. Peloquin CA, Berning SE, Huitt GA, et al. Levofloxacin for drug-resistant *Mycobacterium tuberculosis. Ann Pharmacother* 1998;32:268–269.

34. Park SK, Kim CT, Song SD. Outcome of chemotherapy in 107 patients with pulmonary tuberculosis resistant to isoniazid and rifampin. *Int J Tuberc Lung Dis* 1998;2:877–884.

35. Yew WW, Chan CK, Chau CH, et al. Outcomes of patients with multidrug-resistant pulmonary tuberculosis treated with ofloxacin/levofloxacin-containing regimens. *Chest* 2000;117: 744–751.

36. Tahaoglu K, Torun T, Sevim T, et al. The treatment of multi-drug resistant tuberculosis in Turkey. *N Engl J Med* 2001;345:170–174.

37. Mor N, Vanderkolk J, Heifets L. Inhibitory and bacterial acitivities of levofloxacin against *Mycobacterium tuberculosis in vitro* and in human macrophages. *Antimicrob Agents Chemother* 1994; 38:1161–1164.

38. Grimaldo ER, Tupasi TE, Rivera AB, et al. Increased resistance to ciprofloxacin and ofloxacin in multidrug-resistant *Mycobacterium tuberculosis* isolates from patients seen at a tertiary hospital in the Philippines. *Int J Tuberc Lung Dis* 2001;5:546–550.

39. Cooper AM, Dalton DK, Stewart TA, et al. Disseminated tuberculosis in interferon gamma gene disrupted mice. *J Exp Med* 1993;178:2243–2247

40. Jaffe HA, Buhl R, Mastrangeli A, et al. Organ specific cytokine therapy. Local activation of mononuclear phagocytes by delivery of an aerosol of recombinant interferon gamma to the human lung. *J Clin Invest* 1991;88:297–302.

41. Holland SM, Eisenstein EM, Kuhns DB, et al. Treatment of refractory disseminated nontuberculous mycobacterial infection with interferon gamma. A preliminary report. *N Engl J Med* 1994;330:1348–1355.

42. Newport MJ, Huxley CM, Huston S et al. A mutation in the interferon-gamma-receptor gene and susceptibility to mycobacterial infection. *N Engl J Med* 1996;335:1941–1949.

43. Nathan CF, Kaplan G, Levis WR, et al. Local and systemic effects of intradermal recombinant interferon gamma in patients with lepromatous leprosy. *N Engl J Med* 1986;315:6–15.

44. Condos R, Rom WN, Schluger NW. Treatment of multi-drug resistant pulmonary tuberculosis with interferon-γ via aerosol. *Lancet* 1997;349:1513–1515.

45. Brickner SJ, Hutchinson DK, Barbachyn MR, et al. Synthesis and antibacterial activity of U-100592 and U-100766, two oxazolidinone antibacterial agents for the potential treatment of multidrug-resistant gram-positive bacterial infections. *J Med Chem* 1996;39:673–679.

46. Zurenko GE, Yagi BH, Schaadt, et al. *In vitro* activities of U-100592 and U-100766 novel oxazolidinone antibacterial agents. *Antimicrob Agents Chemother* 1996;40:839–845.

47. Cynamon MH, Klemens SP, Sharpe CA, et al. Activities of several novel oxazolidinone against *Mycobacterium tuberculosis* in a murine model. *Antimicrob Agents Chemother* 1999;43:1189–1195.

47a. Hadjiangelis NP, Leibert E, Harkin TJ, et al. Linezolid: a promising new agent for multidrug-resistant tuberculosis treatment. *Am J Respir Crit Care Med* 2003;167:A868.

48. Berning SE, Huitt GA, Iseman MD, et al. Malabsorption of antituberculous medications by a patient with AIDS. *N Engl J Med* 1992;327:1817–1818.

49. Turner M, McGowan C, Nardell E, et al. Serum drug levels in tuberculosis patients. *Am J Respir Crit Care Med* 1994;149:A527.

50. Peloquin CA. Using therapeutic drug monitoring to dose the antimycobacterial drugs. *Clin Chest Med* 1997;18:79–87.

51. Jain V, Mehta VL, Kulshrestha S. Effect of pyrazinamide on rifampicin kinetics in patients with tuberculosis. *Tuber Lung Dis* 1993;74:87–90.

52. Iseman MD, Madsen L, Goble M, et al. Surgical intervention in the treatment of pulmonary disease caused by drug-resistant *Mycobacterium tuberculosis. Am Rev Respir Dis* 1990;141:623–625.

53. Mahmoudi A, Iseman MD. Surgical intervention in the treatment of drug-resistant tuberculosis: update and extended follow-up. *Am Rev Respir Dis* 1992;145:A816.

54. Chiang CY, Yu MC, Bai KJ, et al. Pulmonary resection in the treatment of patients with pulmonary multidrug-resistant tuberculosis in Taiwan. *Int J Tuberc Lung Dis* 2001;5:272–277.

55. Hong Kong Chest Service/British Medical Research Council. Five-year followup of a controlled trial of five 6-month regimens of chemotherapy for pulmonary tuberculosis. *Am Rev Respir Dis* 1987;136:1339–1342.

56. Zierski M. Prospects of retreatment of chronic resistant pulmonary tuberculosis: a critical review. *Lung* 1977;154:91.

57. McDonald FW. *Study of triple versus double drug therapy of cavitary tuberculosis. Study 29. Preliminary report.* 27th Pulmonary Disease Research Conference, VA–Armed Forces, Washington, DC, 1968.

58. Bobrowitz ID. Ethambutol-isoniazid vs. streptomycin-ethambutol-isoniazid in original treatment of cavitary tuberculosis. *Am Rev Respir Dis* 1974;109:548–553.

59. Liebold JE. The ocular toxicity of ethambutol and its relation to dose. *Ann N Y Acad Sci* 1966;135:904–914.

60. Donomae I, Yamamoto K. Clinical evaluation of ethambutol in pulmonary tuberculosis. *Ann N Y Acad Sci* 1966;135:849–881.

61. Fischl M, Daikos GL, Uttamchandani RB, et al. Clinical presentation and outcome of patients with HIV infection and tuberculosis by multidrug-resistant bacilli. *Ann Intern Med* 1992;117:184–190.

62. Nosocomial transmission of multidrug-resistant tuberculosis among HIV-infected persons—Florida and New York, 1988–1991. *MMWR Morb Mortal Wkly Rep* 1991;40:585–591.

63. Chawla PK, Klapper PJ, Kamholz SL, et al. Drug-resistant tuberculosis in an urban population including patients at risk for human immunodeficiency virus infection. *Am Rev Respir Dis* 1992;146:280–284.

64. Busillo CP, Lessnau K-D, Sanjana V, et al. Multidrug resistant *Mycobacterium tuberculosis* in patients with human immunodeficiency virus infection. *Chest* 1992;102:797–801.

65. Soeiro R. A tale of two mutants. *N Engl J Med* 1993;328:1192–1193.

66. Park MM, Davis AL, Schluger NW, et al. Outcome of MDR-TB patients, 1983–1993: prolonged survival with appropriate therapy. *Am J Respir Crit Care Med* 1994;153:317–324.

ISONIAZID

YING ZHANG

Isoniazid [isonicotinic acid hydrazide (INH)] is the most widely used of all antituberculosis (anti-TB) drugs. INH (Fig. 49.1) was first chemically synthesized from ethyl isonicotinate and hydrazine hydrate in 1912 by Meyer and Mally (1) at Charles University in Prague for their doctoral theses in chemistry. However, the antituberculosis activity of INH was not recognized until 40 years later. In 1952, three drug companies, Hoffmann-La Roche, E. R. Squibb & Sons, and Bayer AG, simultaneously discovered INH as a highly active antituberculosis drug (2–4). Fox et al. (2) discovered INH based on the observation by Chorine (5) that nicotinamide (Fig. 49.1) had particular anti-TB activity. Offe (4) and Domagk (6) discovered INH based on their earlier work on the anti-TB activity of thiosemicarbazone (Fig. 49.1). The first clinical study of INH was reported in 1952, conducted at Sea View Hospital in New York by Robitzek and Selikoff (7). The trial was so successful that the patients were overjoyed and "dancing in the wards" (8). Because INH is very inexpensive to manufacture, the use of INH greatly reduced the cost of the streptomycin and paraaminosalicylic acid–based chemotherapy. The discovery of INH represented a major milestone in the conquest of tuberculosis (TB), which led to the 1955 Lasker Award being given to Hoffmann-La Roche Research Laboratories, Squibb Institute for Medical Research, and Edward Robitzek, Irving Selikoff, Walsh McDermott, and Carl Muschenheim for establishing the remarkable efficacy of INH in the treatment of TB (9). INH has since been a mainstay TB drug and is the cornerstone of all effective regimens for the prevention and treatment of TB.

The recent emergence and outbreak of multidrug-resistant TB (MDR-TB) (resistant to at least INH and rifampin) (10–14) have stimulated renewed interest in understanding the mechanisms of drug action and resistance in *Mycobacterium tuberculosis* (15). The outbreak of MDR-TB in human immunodeficiency virus (HIV)–positive individuals in New York City in the late 1980s and early 1990s attracted particular public attention (11–14). The cloning of the *katG* gene, encoding catalase-peroxidase involved in INH activation, and the demonstration of the *katG* mutation as a cause for INH resistance represented the first molecular study elucidating the mechanism of INH resistance (16). The identification of InhA, an enzyme involved in mycolic acid synthesis, provided the first molecular target for INH (17). Significant progress has been made in our understanding of the mechanisms of INH action and resistance in the past decade. Because of the importance of INH in the treatment of TB, there is a vast body of literature on INH (in fact, more than any TB drug) since its introduction for the treatment of TB in the 1950s. INH has been reviewed many times in the past (18–23) and several times in more recent years when the molecular basis of INH action and resistance became available (24–32). The purpose of this chapter is to (a) provide an update on the mechanisms of INH action and resistance, (b) highlight the gaps in our knowledge and areas that need further research, and (c) provide a brief account of the clinical aspects of INH.

CHEMISTRY AND STRUCTURE ACTIVITY RELATIONSHIP

INH has a simple structure consisting of a pyridine ring and a hydrazide group (Fig. 49.1). INH is colorless or white crystalline powder with a chemical formula of $C_6H_7N_3O$ and a molecular weight of 137.14. It is readily soluble in water to as much as 140 mg/mL at 25°C but is much less soluble in organic solvents (33). The basic method of manufacture is condensation of hydrazine with γ-substituted pyridine (33).

Both the pyridine and hydrazide moieties are essential for the high level of activity of INH against *M. tuberculosis*. Various derivatives of INH were either less active or have less favorable pharmacologic properties than INH (3). Among the INH derivatives, it is worth noting the different sensitivity between *M. tuberculosis* and *Mycobacterium bovis* to several hydrazides such as thiophen-2-carboxylic acid

Y. Zhang: Department of Molecular Microbiology and Immunology, Johns Hopkins Bloomberg School of Public Health, Baltimore, Maryland.

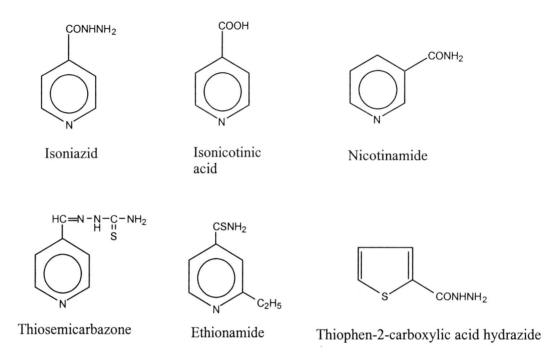

FIGURE 49.1. Structure of isoniazid and related compounds.

hydrazide (TCH) (Fig. 49.1), 2-furoic acid hydrazide, and benzylhydrazide (34). *M. tuberculosis* is typically resistant to TCH with a minimal inhibitory concentration (MIC) of more than 25 μg/mL, whereas *M. bovis* is sensitive (MIC <1 μg/mL) (34,35). This feature is commonly used to distinguish *M. bovis* from *M. tuberculosis* (36). However, some variants of *M. tuberculosis*, such as those from Asia, are often sensitive to TCH (37,38). There is some cross-resistance between INH and TCH resistance in *M. bovis* strains (35,38). The basis for the differential sensitivity between *M. bovis* and *M. tuberculosis* and the cross-resistance between INH and TCH in bovine strains is unknown.

SPECTRUM OF ACTIVITY AND FACTORS AFFECTING THE ACTIVITY

M. tuberculosis is highly susceptible to INH with MIC values in the range of 0.01 to 0.25 μg/mL being reported in the literature, depending on the type of media, inocula, and incubation times (39). Approximately 50% strains are susceptible to 0.06 μg/mL and 80% are susceptible to 0.1 μg/mL INH (39). *M. bovis* strains are slightly less susceptible to INH than to *M. tuberculosis* (40). Other mycobacteria, such as *Mycobacterium smegmatis*, *Mycobacterium phlei*, and *Mycobacterium avium* are less susceptible, with an MIC in the range of 10 to 100 μg/mL INH (19). However, *Mycobacterium aurum* (MIC = 0.3 to 1 μg/mL) (41), *Mycobacterium kansasii*, *Mycobacterium gastri*, and *Mycobacterium xenopi* (MIC = 1 to 5 μg/mL) (42) are more suscep-

tible to INH than other nontuberculous mycobacteria. Other bacterial species outside the mycobacterial genera are highly resistant to INH with an MIC of at least 600 μg/mL (43).

INH is active against growing tubercle bacilli but not resting bacilli (44). Oxygen plays an important role in INH action (44), probably because of the oxygen requirement for KatG-mediated INH activation (45). INH has no activity against *M. tuberculosis* under anaerobic conditions (44), presumably because KatG-mediated INH activation is affected without oxygen. The activity of INH is most obvious at 37°C but is greatly reduced at 4°C (46,47), presumably a reflection of optimal temperature requirement for the KatG-mediated INH activation. Structurally related organic acid hydrazides such as benzoic acid hydrazide and nicotinic acid hydrazide reduce INH activity (48). This antagonism is likely owing to competition for KatG-mediated drug activation and inactivation of KatG enzyme by related hydrazide (49). Pyruvic acid, α-ketoglutaric acid, acetone, and pyridoxal (but not pyridoxine) interfere with INH activity through the formation of hydrazone with INH (50,51), which inactivates INH and interferes with KatG-mediated activation. In addition, pyruvic acid, α-ketoglutaric acid may also destroy peroxide needed for the INH activation. Despite the structural similarity and the nicotinamide origin (Fig. 49.1), unlike pyrazinamide (PZA), which requires acid pH for activity (52), the activity of INH is not influenced by pH between 5.0 and 8.0 (53). It is noteworthy that despite the production of weak acid isonicotinic acid (INA) during INH activation, the

INH activity is not enhanced by acid pH. This is presumably because INA (pK$_a$ ~ 5) is a much weaker acid than pyrazinoic acid (pK$_a$ = 2.9), the active derivative of PZA. Metal ions such as Cu^{2+} and Fe^{2+} enhance the activity of INH (19) (see Mechanism of Action section). Culture supernatant and cell extracts of *M. tuberculosis* were found to contain factors that antagonize the activity of INH *in vitro* (54) and in mice (55). The identity of the antagonist is yet to be elucidated.

ACTIVITY IN MACROPHAGES AND IN ANIMALS

Because INH penetrates host cells readily, it has essentially the same high activity against intracellular *M. tuberculosis* as against extracellular bacilli *in vitro* (56,57). INH at 10 mg/kg is highly active against *M. tuberculosis* in various animal models, such as guinea pigs, mice, and monkeys (39). At doses as high as 100 mg/kg, INH is no more effective than 10 mg/kg, which is the equivalent of 5 mg/kg in humans (39). In the mouse model of TB infection, bacterial colony counts in infected organs decrease quickly in the first few days of INH treatment. However, the early bactericidal activity of INH becomes slower after the first 2 to 3 weeks in mice. The number of colony-forming units stabilizes at a low level after 2 to 3 months of treatment with INH. Longer treatment with INH monotherapy may lead to the emergence of INH-resistant organisms and the number of colony-forming unit in the infected organs may increase again. The addition of a second antituberculous drug, such as paraaminosalicylic acid or streptomycin, prevents the emergence of INH-resistant organisms. INH + PZA showed the best sterilizing activity in mice when compared with other drug combinations (58,59), which is the basis for the modern short-course chemotherapy. [For more information on the INH activity in animal models, refer to Bartmann (39).]

MECHANISM OF ACTION

Despite the seemingly simple structure of INH, its mode of action is one of the most complex of all antibiotics. This is shown by the large amount of literature that deals with different aspects of the INH action (19–23). INH interferes with nearly every metabolic pathway in *M. tuberculosis*. The current model of how INH works is shown in Figure 49.2. The following deals with different steps of INH action.

Isoniazid Uptake

INH gets into *M. tuberculosis* through diffusion (60–62). Earlier studies have shown that INH uptake appeared to be inhibited by cyanide and azide (48). The lower intracellular

radioactivity in the cells in the presence of cyanide or azide does not necessarily indicate that uptake of INH requires energy but may be explained by the inhibitory effect of these agents on the KatG enzyme involved in INH activation. Using INH labeled with radioactive carbon (^{14}C), it was shown that INH sensitive *M. tuberculosis* strains accumulate significant amounts of radioactivity in the cells, whereas INH-resistant strains usually have much less radioactivity associated with the cells (46,47,60,63). The degree of INH accumulation in *M. tuberculosis* correlates with the catalase-peroxidase activity (61). It is unlikely that KatG is involved directly in the transport of INH into the cell. The most likely explanation is that INH-derived radicals or anions produced during INH activation by KatG are trapped inside the cell in susceptible organisms. In contrast, in the resistant organisms with deficient KatG activity, there is very little or no reactive form of INH being produced intracellularly. The free unconverted INH without KatG activation diffuses out of the cell readily, giving the impression of no INH uptake in the resistant bacilli. Nonsusceptible bacteria such as *Escherichia coli*, *Staphylococcus aureus*, *Corynebacterium xerosis*, and *M. phlei* took up little radioactive INH (47,61), and their lack of accumulation of INH is likely to be owing to more active efflux mechanisms (see later).

Isoniazid Activation

INH is a prodrug that has to be activated by *M. tuberculosis* catalase-peroxidase enzyme (KatG) encoded by the *katG* gene (16) to generate a range of highly reactive species for bactericidal activity. The *M. tuberculosis* KatG is a bifunctional enzyme that has both catalase and peroxidase activity with a molecular weight of 80 kd (16,64). The native KatG enzyme is a dimer that contains one heme per subunit (65). In addition to catalase and peroxidase activity (16), *M. tuberculosis* KatG has been shown to have Mn^{2+}-dependent peroxidase (66), peroxynitritase (67), and cytochrome P-450–like oxygenase activities (68). The process of INH activation is not well understood. The availability of cloned KatG has stimulated a great deal of recent interest in understanding the mechanism of INH activation by KatG (45,49,66,67,68–75). Several modes of INH activation by KatG have been proposed (45,68,71,75). The first uses molecular oxygen and produces superoxide that is thought to generate a cytochrome P-450–like oxyferrous intermediate at the KatG active site. The second uses peroxide to oxidize INH through the peroxidase compound I/II pathway. INH activation could also be initiated by superoxide anion in the presence of KatG (71). In addition, manganese was shown to enhance the KatG-mediated INH activation and production of the InhA inhibitor isonicotinic acyl–nicotinamide adenine dinucleotide (reduced form) (NADH), but manganese was not essential to the process (74). The KatG-mediated INH activation can also be produced by man-

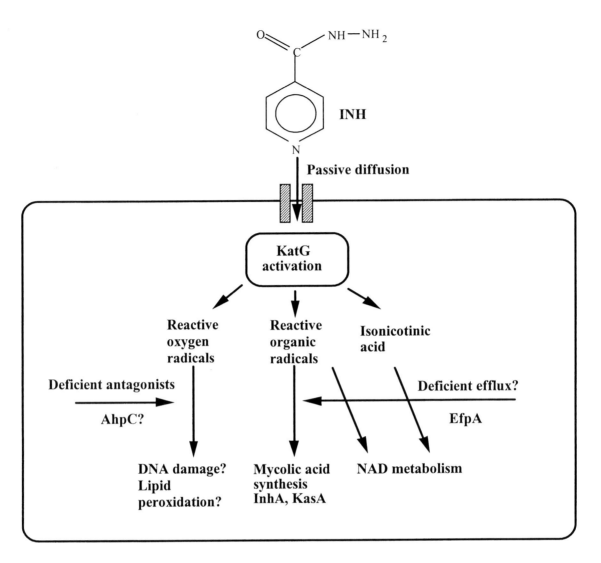

FIGURE 49.2. Isoniazid (*INH*) enters tubercle bacilli by passive diffusion and is activated by KatG to a range of reactive species or radicals and isonicotinic acid. These reactive species and radicals include both reactive oxygen species (hydrogen peroxide, superoxide, peroxynitrite, hydroxyl radical) and organic radicals (e.g., isonicotinic acyl radical). These species and radicals then attack multiple targets, e.g., mycolic acid synthesis, DNA damage, lipid peroxidation, and nicotinamide adenine dinucleotide metabolism in the cell. Deficient efflux and insufficient antagonism of INH-derived radicals such as defective antioxidative defense may underlie the unique susceptibility of *Mycobacterium tuberculosis* to INH.

ganese alone *in vitro* but at a much slower rate than the KatG-mediated activation (74). It is of interest to note that manganese can indeed potentiate INH sensitivity in INH-resistant (presumably KatG-deficient) strains (76), most likely through KatG-independent activation of INH by manganese (66,74).

The radicals produced by KatG-mediated INH activation include both reactive oxygen species such as superoxide, peroxide, and hydroxyl radical (77,78) and reactive organic species such as isonicotinic acyl radical or anion (79), some electrophilic species (49), and acylperoxo and pyridyl radical adducts (73). These KatG-derived reactive

species and radicals affect multiple cellular targets and are associated with the bactericidal activity of INH (Fig. 49.2). The stable end products of INH activation include INA (Fig. 49.1), isonicotinamide, 4-hydroxymethylpyridine, and hydrazone of α-ketoglutaric acid (20,49). These end products had no significant antituberculosis activity (20). Yellow pigments are produced during INH activation in an *in vitro* system containing INH, nicotinamide adenine dinucleotide (NAD), oxygen, and some trace metal (80–82). The production of the yellow pigments correlates well with catalase-peroxidase activity, and INH-resistant bacille Calmette–Guérin (BCG) failed to produce the pigments (82).

Purified catalase-peroxidase had the ability to produce the yellow pigments (83), indicating that the pigment production is a property of the KatG enzyme. The chemical identity of the yellow pigments and their role in INH action are unknown.

Target Inhibition

INH induces multiple biochemical changes (19–23), presumably through the aforementioned reactive species and radicals and product(s) derived from INH activation. INH has been shown to cause accumulation of soluble carbohydrates (84,85) and phosphate esters (85), inhibition of mycolic acid synthesis (86–89), phospholipid synthesis (90), DNA synthesis (91,92), and protein synthesis (23). The various reactive oxygen radicals produced during INH activation can also potentially damage DNA (93) and cause lipid peroxidation. The sequence of these events and their role in the bactericidal activity of INH need further evaluation. However, because the effect of INH on DNA and protein syntheses occurs much later when the bactericidal activity of INH is obvious, they are thought to be secondary and less important in INH action (20,23).

The primary target of INH inhibition is thought to be the mycolic acid synthesis pathway (86–89), which relates to the loss of acid-fastness in mycobacteria by INH treatment (94). Indeed, the InhA enzyme [enoyl acyl carrier protein (ACP) reductase], involved in elongation of fatty acids in mycolic acid synthesis, has been identified as a molecular target for INH inhibition (17). Much progress has been made in the past few years concerning how INH inhibits the InhA enzyme through a series of biochemical (69,70,74,95,96) and crystallographic studies (79,97). The overexpressed InhA was shown to be an NADH-dependent enoyl ACP reductase with a chain-length specificity of 16 carbons (95). INH did not bind or inhibit InhA enzyme in the absence of KatG (95) but did so after the addition of KatG (68,96), indicating that inhibition of InhA by INH is KatG dependent. The S94A mutant InhA identified in INH-resistant *M. bovis* (17) was found to have a five- to eightfold increase in K_m value for NADH binding over the wild-type InhA enzyme (95). Comparison of crystal structures of the wild-type and the S94A mutant InhA also confirms the reduced NADH binding of the S94A mutant InhA (97). Other mutations in InhA, such as I16T, I21V, I47T, and I95P, were also found to cause reduced NADH binding (70). One would expect that reduced NADH binding of mutant InhA proteins would impair their function as enoyl ACP reductase. Paradoxically, the reduced NADH binding of the mutant InhA enzymes did not appear to affect the maximal velocity for fatty acyl substrate (70,95). KatG-mediated InhA inhibition occurred with the wild-type InhA but less so with the S94A mutant InhA owing to reduced NADH binding of the mutant enzyme (96). The active species (isonicotinic acyl radical or anion) derived from KatG-mediated INH activation that inhibits InhA is proposed to react with the nicotinamide component of the NADH molecule bound on the InhA enzyme through covalent attachment to NADH (79), leading to inhibition of InhA function. Alternatively, isonicotinic acyl radical reacts with NAD(H) first and then attacks InhA (74). In a recent study using temperature-sensitive INH and ethionamide-resistant InhA mutants of *M. smegmatis*, Vilcheze et al. (98) showed that thermal inactivation of InhA at 42°C caused the same effects, such as accumulation of fatty acid synthase I products and cell lysis as INH treatment. The outcome of InhA inhibition or inactivation is the accumulation of C24 fatty acids in *M. smegmatis* (98), which is consistent with an earlier observation that treatment of *M. tuberculosis* with INH caused accumulation of saturated C26 or unsaturated C24 fatty acids (99). However, for technical reasons, the same experiment could not be performed with *M. tuberculosis* (98). It will be of interest to see whether replacing the wild-type *inhA* with mutant *inhA* or vice versa alters susceptibility to INH and whether there is any difference in susceptibility to KatG-mediated inactivation of InhA between the highly susceptible *M. tuberculosis* and the less susceptible *M. smegmatis*. Another enzyme KasA (β-ketoacyl ACP synthase) (100) involved in meromycolate extension of mycolic acid synthesis has been identified based on its ability to bind radioactive INH and is proposed to be a target for INH inhibition (100). The molecular basis of KasA inhibition by INH is not yet available.

In addition, INH has been proposed to interfere with NAD metabolism by incorporating into NAD through exchange of INH or its metabolic product INA or isonicotinamide with the nicotinamide component of NAD to form pseudo-NAD (18,101,102), which cannot function as an electron acceptor in the respiratory chain. This can, in turn, affect various functions of NAD such as energy metabolism and DNA repair, in which NAD is a cofactor for DNA ligase needed for the repair of nicked DNA (103). Using INH labeled with tritium, Seydel et al. (102) showed that INH was incorporated into NAD to form an NAD analog, although it is not clear whether the unaltered INH or an activated form of INH is incorporated into NAD. INH was also shown to cause NAD depletion by inhibition of NAD synthesis (104) or by indirectly activating the NAD glycohydrolase (NADase) enzyme through removal of the enzyme repressor (105–107). NADase activity is not detected under normal conditions in the cell extract owing to binding of its repressor. Heat or INH treatment can activate the NADase activity by removing its heat-labile repressor (105–107). Unfortunately, there is no recent study available on this fascinating biochemical mechanism of NADase control and its role in INH action. The importance of NAD depletion in INH action was questioned by Jackett et al. (108), who showed that NAD depletion did not correlate with loss of bacterial viability at low INH concentrations or with antibacterial activity of INH in young or old cultures. The importance of INH interference of NAD metabolism is supported by the observations that increased NADH content, owing to either exogenous addition (104) or mutations in NADH dehydrogenase (109), both cause reduced sensitivity to INH. Further molecular and biochemical studies are needed to address the effect of INH on NAD metabolism.

INH forms complexes with divalent metal ions (19,33). Fe^{2+} and Cu^{2+} have been shown to enhance the activity of INH (23). It is quite doubtful that this enhancement effect is through chelation of metal ions. The most likely explanation is that metal ions facilitate INH oxidation and generation of reactive species such as hydroxyl radical during KatG-mediated INH activation by serving as electron donors. It is important to note that INH has multiple effects on the tubercle bacillus, and it is not always easy to pinpoint which event comes first and which is the essential target whose inhibition leads to cell death. Many of the studies on INH action were done in the 1950s to 1970s before the advent of modern molecular biology and biochemical tools. It will be necessary to evaluate the relative importance of the aforementioned factors in INH action using a combination of molecular, biochemical, and structural approaches.

Using the microarray technology, Wilson et al. (110) examined the genes that are induced by INH treatment in *M. tuberculosis*. Genes encoding Fas II enzymes AcpM (ACP), KasA, KasB, FabD (malonyl coenzyme A–malonyl ACP transacylase), AccD (acetyl coenzyme A carboxylase β chain) were induced. The trehalose dimycolyltransferase C (antigen 85 C), involved in mycolate transfer (111), was also induced as reported previously (112). Two genes *fadE24* and *fadE23* encoding fatty acyl coenzyme A dehydrogenase involved in fatty acid β-oxidation were induced. Interestingly, *efpA* encoding an efflux protein (113) was also induced by INH, which presumably helps to remove toxic radicals produced during INH activation. The *ahpC* gene encoding the antioxidant enzyme hydroperoxide reductase, which is overexpressed in KatG-negative, INH-resistant strains in compensation for loss of KatG (114–116), was also up-regulated. Four genes of unknown function, *Rv1592c*, *Rv1772*, *Rv0341*, and *Rv0342*, were induced, two of which, *Rv0341* and *Rv0342*, were shown to be induced by INH in a previous study (117). However, the *inhA* gene, which encodes a target for INH, was not induced by INH. It is likely that the above INH-inducible genes play a protective role in response to the toxic effect of INH. The role of these unknown genes in an alternative mechanism of INH resistance needs further evaluation.

Unique Susceptibility of *Mycobacterium tuberculosis* to Isoniazid

Any discussion of the mechanism of INH action is incomplete without addressing the unique susceptibility of *M.*

tuberculosis to INH. Although other mycobacteria and bacteria have the KatG enzyme needed for INH activation as well as the InhA homolog, they are not susceptible to INH. The basis for this difference is complex and not well understood. The following factors may be involved.

1. Higher peroxidase activity of the KatG enzyme in *M. tuberculosis* than in other bacteria such as *E. coli* (118, 119) and *M. smegmatis* or *Mycobacterium vaccae* (Y. Zhang, unpublished observation, 1993). This can lead to increased activation of INH in *M. tuberculosis*.
2. Presence of sensitive targets. Enzymes involved in fatty acid synthesis (such as InhA) of the mycolic acid pathway may be more sensitive to INH-derived reactive species in *M. tuberculosis* than their counterparts in other mycobacteria or bacteria. This hypothesis can now be tested with the availability of cloned InhA or its homologs from different bacterial species. In addition, INH inhibited acetate oxidation in susceptible *M. tuberculosis* or BCG but not in nonsusceptible *E. coli* or *S. aureus* (120).
3. Deficient efflux of INH-derived toxic radicals or INA generated during INH activation. It is striking that only the highly susceptible *M. tuberculosis* accumulates radioactive INH, whereas naturally resistant mycobacteria or bacteria do not. This suggests that *M. tuberculosis* may have some deficiency in removing the INH-derived radicals from the cell compared with nontuberculous bacteria. A recent study showed that the less susceptible *M. smegmatis* has a demonstrable efflux mechanism for INH (121). Although *M. tuberculosis* efflux protein EfpA is induced on INH treatment (110), it remains to be demonstrated whether the *M. tuberculosis* efflux mechanism is less active compared with *M. smegmatis*, as shown for pyrazinoic acid in the case of PZA susceptibility (122).
4. Lack of antagonists. The KatE-type, heat-stable catalase (also called HP-II–type catalase) is absent in *M. tuberculosis* but present in other mycobacteria or bacteria (123,124). The KatE-type catalase may remove the toxic peroxide produced during or needed for INH activation and may provide protection against INH in nontuberculous mycobacteria or bacteria. However, overexpression of *M. avium katE* in *M. tuberculosis* did not appear to confer any resistance to INH (125). Another potential antagonist, arylamine *N*-acetyltransferase (NAT), involved in inactivation of INH (126–128) could be less active or poorly expressed in *M. tuberculosis* but more active or highly expressed in other less susceptible mycobacteria or bacteria.
5. Defective antioxidative defense. The observation that overexpression of *M. tuberculosis* KatG conferred some degree of INH sensitivity to *E. coli katG/katE* double mutant (16), prompted Rosner (129) to examine the role of OxyR, a transcriptional activator for up-regulat-

ing several antioxidant genes (e.g., *katG, ahpC*) in *E. coli* in susceptibility to INH in *E. coli* (129). Inactivation of OxyR (129) and KatG/AhpC (130) in *E. coli* caused increased susceptibility to INH. These findings led to the discovery of a defective OxyR (131,132) and the assessment of the role of AhpC in INH action in *M. tuberculosis* (114–116). *M. tuberculosis* seems to be particularly susceptible to endogenously generated reactive oxygen or organic radicals, presumably a reflection of its deficient antioxidative defense and defective efflux mechanisms. Inappropriate antioxidative defense of *M. tuberculosis* in the face of an increased oxygen radical burden produced during INH activation by KatG may be related to its usually high susceptibility to INH.

6. Inefficient NAD synthesis. *M. tuberculosis* has a defective PncB enzyme, nicotinic acid phosphoribosyltransferase, in the Preiss–Handler pathway involved in nicotinic acid recycling to make NAD (133). This deficiency in nicotinic acid recycling may render *M. tuberculosis* particularly vulnerable to NAD depletion on INH treatment (104–107) and may underlie its high susceptibility to INH.

MECHANISM OF RESISTANCE

Resistance to INH develops readily in cultures or *in vivo* during INH monotherapy. *In vitro*, mutation to INH resistance occurs at a rate of 10^{-6} per bacterium per generation in *M. tuberculosis* (19). Single-step mutation causing high levels of INH resistance usually leads to loss of catalase and peroxidase activity. However, some low-level resistant strains with catalase activity can develop a higher level of resistance through multiple mutations and may still retain catalase activity. The degree of INH resistance varies from low (0.2 μg/mL) to as high as 100 μg/mL (134). Because INH is the most commonly used antituberculosis drug, resistance to INH is also the most frequent among drug-resistant clinical isolates. INH resistance can be as high as 20% to 30% in some cities and the percentage of INH-resistant strains varies in different geographic regions (135,136).

Loss of catalase-peroxidase renders the INH-resistant organisms highly susceptible to peroxide, which can be produced during normal metabolism or inside host macrophages. INH-resistant organisms, especially with deficient catalase activity, grow and survive less well compared with INH susceptible strains *in vitro* (19,137). INH-resistant strains often have a longer lag time in culture and may have different growth requirements than susceptible strains (19,137). For example, pyruvate medium was found to be useful for isolation of INH-resistant strains (138). Some INH-resistant strains grow poorly in culture media and require additional factors such as hemin to grow

(139,140). Because catalase-deficient, INH-resistant organisms grow poorly in culture (owing to production of hydrogen peroxide), bovine catalase is added to culture media in the albumin–dextrose–catalase (ADC) supplement to improve the isolation and growth of peroxide-sensitive, catalase-deficient, INH-resistant strains. INH-resistant strains may also lose NADH dehydrogenase activity (137). INH-resistant strains are also more sensitive to nitrofuran (141), which may produce reactive radicals in bacterial cell.

A great deal of progress has been made in recent years on the molecular basis of INH resistance. Mutations in the following genes (*katG, inhA, kasA, ndh, ahpC*) are associated with INH resistance.

katG

INH-resistant clinical isolates of *M. tuberculosis* frequently lose catalase and peroxidase enzyme activities (142). There is generally a good correlation between INH resistance and loss of catalase activity, especially in high-level resistant strains with an MIC greater than 5 μg/mL (19,137). However, low-level resistant strains with an MIC of 1 μg/mL or less often still possess catalase activity (19,137). To address the role of catalase and peroxidase in INH resistance, Zhang et al. (16,118) cloned the catalase-peroxidase gene (*katG*) from *M. tuberculosis* and showed that *katG* mutations were the cause of INH resistance in INH-resistant clinical isolates. From analysis of eight INH-resistant strains in the original study (16), *katG* deletions were found in two highly resistant strains. Subsequent studies (143–157) have shown that *katG* point mutations are more frequent than deletions in INH-resistant strains (Table 49.1). That *katG* mutation is the cause of INH resistance was demonstrated by restoration of INH susceptibility to KatG-deficient (with either *katG* deletion or point mutations), INH-resistant strains by transformation with a functional *katG* gene (118). Loss of KatG causing INH resistance represents a novel mechanism of drug resistance. Mutations in KatG reduce its ability to activate the prodrug INH, thus leading to resistance. The *katG* gene forms an operon with the upstream gene *furA* in various mycobacteria including *M. tuberculosis* (158,159). FurA is a negative regulator of *katG*, and removal of *furA* caused overexpression of KatG and hypersensitivity to INH, whereas overexpression of FurA reduced the KatG expression (158,159). Mutations in *furA* may cause INH resistance through repression of KatG expression, but this has not been confirmed in INH-resistant strains (159). It is of interest to note that the *katG* gene is situated in a highly variable and unstable region of the *M. tuberculosis* genome (160). This region contains different types of repeat DNA sequences, which vary in copy number in different *M. tuberculosis* strains (160). These repeat DNA sequences may be the cause of the instability of this region and in turn may contribute to the high frequency of *katG* mutations and deletions in INH-resistant strains. For

TABLE 49.1. GENETIC POLYMORPHISMS ASSOCIATED WITH ISONIAZID RESISTANCE

Region	Amino Acid or Nucleotide	Comment	Region	Amino Acid or Nucleotide	Comment
katG	Complete or partial deletion	Complete or partial deletion of *katG* is a relatively rare event that results in high-level INH resistance.		A574V	
	M1A			L587M,P	
	T11A			G593D	
	T12P			L617del	
	N35E			L619P	
	A61T			G629S	
	D63E			L634F	
	A65ins			S700P	
	I71N			A710V	
	N88R			A714P	
	D94A		Promoter *mabAinhA*	−8 t → g,a	Numeration based on nucleotide position relative to *mabA* start codon
	G99E			−15 c → t	
	H108E,Q			−16 a → g	
	A110V			−17 g → t	
	G120del			−24 g → t	
	A122del			−55 a → g	
	G123del		InhA	I16T	Two- to 12-fold increase in K_m for NADH
	G125ins			I21V,T	
	M126I			I47T	
	N138S,H			V78A	
	A139P			I95P	
	S140N,A			S94A	
	D142A		Intergenic region *oxyR-ahpC*	−55 a → g	Numbering based on nucleotide position relative to the putative transcription start site. *ahpC* promoter mutations have been shown to increase AhpC expression, generally in the presence of a damaged KatG. An actual role of *ahpC* promoter mutation in resistance has not been proven.
	L148A			−46 g → a	
	L150A			−46 ins at	
	Y155S			−45 c → t	
	S160L			−44 t → a	
	A172T			−42 t → c	
	T180C			−39 c → t	
	W198stop			−34 t → a,c	
	V200stop			−32 g → a	
	E217del			−30 c → t	
	F252L			−15 c → t	
	T262R			−12 c → t	
	P275T			−10 c → a,t	
	E289del			−9 g → a	
	W300G,stop			−6 g → a	
	S302R			−4 a → g	
	S315T,N,I,R,G	Mutation of S315 is the most prevalent mechanism of resistance to INH. S315T mutants have a moderately competent catalase peroxidase with a reduced ability to metabolize INH		+4 c → t	
	W328L,C			+33 g → a	
	I334T		Pseudogene OxyR	18 g → a	Polymorphisms without known relation to INH resistance. 18 g → a is found in susceptible strains.
	I335T			27 g → t	
	L336R			28 c → a	
	A350S				
	I393N		AhpC	P2S	Unclear role in INH resistance or AhpC function
			KasA	D66N	The role of *kasA* mutations in INH resistance is unclear. Some polymorphisms, G269S, and G312S are present in susceptible strains.
				R121K	
	L463R	L463R most likely represents a natural polymorphism with no association with INH resistance.		G269S	
	W477stop			G312S	
	G485V			G387D	
	D511del			F413L	
	D513del		Ndh	T110A	Mutation in *ndh* causes increased NADH/NAD ratio, which leads to INH resistance in some clinical isolates.
	R515C			R268H	
	L521del				
	Q525P				
	F567S				

INH, isoniazid; NAD, nicotinamide adenine dinucleotide; NADH, nicotinamide adenine dinucleotide (reduced form).
Compiled from references 16, 17, 27, 69, 100, 109, 114–116, 143–157, 167, 171, 174–176.

example, two highly INH-resistant strains, B1453 and strain 24, were found to have 20-kilobase (kb) and 6-kb deletions including the *katG* in this region, respectively (160). In addition, an INH-sensitive Indian *M. tuberculosis* isolate with an intact *katG* had a 10-kb deletion in this region (160).

Approximately 50% to 80% of INH-resistant *M. tuberculosis* strains contain a mutation in the *katG* gene (143–157). Various mutations in *katG* have been identified in INH-resistant strains of *M. tuberculosis* (Table 49.1). The KatG S315T mutation is the most common mutation and occurs in approximately 50% to 92% of INH-resistant clinical isolates (148,152,153,155,156). The KatG S315T mutation reduces the catalase and peroxidase activity by 50% (161,162) and is associated with relatively high levels of resistance (MIC = 5 to 10 µg/mL). The S315T mutation was proposed to affect the binding of INH to KatG and cause a reduced rate of superoxide-dependent INH oxidation (71,72). KatG R463L is a polymorphism found in *M. bovis*, *Mycobacterium africanum*, and *Mycobacterium microti* (163) that is equally capable of activating INH as the wild-type KatG (64,161) and is generally considered not associated with INH resistance (161–63). However, KatG R463L may cause a very subtle change in KatG activity, which is responsible for the slightly less INH-susceptible phenotype in *M. bovis* strains.

Because of the important role KatG plays in INH activation and INH resistance, there has been intense competition in solving the crystal structure of *M. tuberculosis* KatG. However, repeated attempts to solve this structure have been unsuccessful. In fact, none of the bacterial KatG proteins has been crystallized. Determining the structure of *M. tuberculosis* KatG will help to understand the mechanism of INH activation and how KatG mutations can cause INH resistance.

An acquired higher level of resistance to INH in other mycobacteria is associated with reduced peroxidase activity, but the catalase activity appears intact owing to the presence of a second catalase (KatE) (164). For example, when *M. avium* develops a higher level of INH resistance, the peroxidase activity was reduced owing to mutations in the *katG*, but the catalase activity was apparently normal because of intact KatE activity (165).

inhA

Genetic studies in *M. smegmatis* and *M. bovis* identified InhA, a homolog of enoyl reductase (EnvM) from *E. coli* (166), as a target for INH (17). The *inhA* gene encodes the NADH-dependent enoyl ACP reductase involved in the elongation of long-chain fatty acids in mycolic acid synthesis (17). Resistance to INH can occur by mutation at the InhA active site that lowers the enzyme's affinity to NADH without affecting the enzymatic activity (70,96) or by mutations in the promoter region of the *mabAinhA* operon

causing increased expression of InhA (Table 49.1). The reduced binding of NADH to InhA is proposed to cause less vulnerability of InhA to attack by activated INH radicals (70). Mutations in the promoter region of *mabA* encoding 3-ketoacyl ACP reductase, which forms an operon with *inhA*, appear to be more frequent than mutations in the *inhA* structural gene in INH-resistant *M. tuberculosis* strains (146–148) (Table 49.1).

Mutations in *inhA* or the promoter region of the *mabAinhA* operon occur in 15% to 34% of INH-resistant strains and are usually associated with a low level of INH resistance (MIC = 0.2 to 1 µg/mL) (145–148,167). INH-resistant *M. tuberculosis* harboring *inhA* mutations could have additional mutations in *katG*, conferring a higher level of INH resistance (147). In contrast, mutations in *katG* can cause either low- or high-level of resistance, depending on the effect of mutations on the catalase-peroxidase enzyme activity required for INH activation. Mutations in *katG* leading to complete loss of enzyme activity lead to a high level of INH resistance. Mutations in *inhA* or its promoter not only cause INH resistance but also confer resistance to the structurally related second-line drug ethionamide (Fig. 49.1) (17) and the common antibacterial agent triclosan, which inhibits InhA in *M. smegmatis* (168) and *M. tuberculosis* (169,170).

kasA

Mdluli et al. (100) found that INH at 1 µg/mL induced two proteins, ACP protein AcpM and β-ketoacyl ACP synthase KasA, which are type II enzymes involved in fatty acid and mycolic acid synthesis. Mutations in the *kasA* gene have been found in INH-resistant and INH susceptible isolates (169,170) (Table 49.1). In some INH-resistant isolates containing *kasA* mutations, additional mutations in *katG* or *inhA* genes have been identified (100,171,172). The significance of *kasA* mutations in INH resistance needs careful interpretation. KasA and KasB (a similar protein with the same activity as KasA) have been shown to be targets for thiolactomycin in *M. bovis* BCG (173). According to Kremer et al. (173), overexpression of KasA, KasB, or KasA-KasB in BCG conferred resistance to thiolactomycin but not to INH (173). However, in a recent study by Slayden et al. (170), KasA overexpression was found to cause resistance to not only thiolactomycin but also INH and triclosan, which also inhibits InhA (168–170). The reason for the inconsistent results of KasA overexpression in INH susceptibility is unclear but could reflect differences in the level of KasA expression, bacterial host strains (BCG versus *M. tuberculosis* H37Rv) and different methodologies for susceptibility testing. In any event, the level of INH resistance conferred by KasA overexpression is not high, i.e., from 0.025 in the control strain to 0.125 µg/mL INH in the KasA-overexpressing strain (170). Co-overexpression of both InhA and KasA resulted in a somewhat higher level of

INH resistance (0.25 μg/mL) than the control strain (0.025 μg/mL INH), in addition to cross-resistance to both thio-lactomycin and triclosan (170). These authors suggest that InhA and KasA expression is not independently regulated and that alterations in the expression level of InhA could affect that of KasA (170). It remains to be demonstrated how the activated form of INH reacts with KasA or AcpM and if KasA promoter up-mutations can be identified in INH-resistant clinical isolates of *M. tuberculosis*. Further biochemical and structural studies are needed to elucidate the role of KasA in INH action and resistance.

ndh

NADH dehydrogenase gene (*ndh*) was determined to be involved in INH resistance by complementation of an INH-resistant, temperature-sensitive *M. smegmatis* mutant with a genomic library of *M. tuberculosis* (109). *ndh* mutations confer INH resistance in *M. smegmatis* by lowering the rate of NADH oxidation and increasing the intracellular NADH/NAD+ ratio. An increased amount of NADH may compete for the binding of the INH-NAD adduct to the active site of the InhA enzyme or may promote displacement of the isonicotinic acyl NADH from InhA. It is worth noting that early studies indicated that some INH-resistant *M. tuberculosis* strains could lose NADH dehydrogenase activity (137). Indeed, a recent study showed that *ndh* mutations were detected in eight of 84 (9.5%) INH-resistant *M. tuberculosis* clinical isolates, seven of which had the same mutation of R268H and the eighth isolate had T110A mutation (174) (Table 49.1). The eight strains with *ndh* mutations were resistant to at least 0.1 μg/mL INH, but the exact level of resistance was not reported. It is of interest to note that the two mutations in *ndh* do not occur at the NADH binding site of the enzyme (174) and are different from those identified in *M. smegmatis* (109). Another gene that also complemented the temperature-sensitive and INH-resistant phenotype was malate dehydrogenase (*mdh*) (109), which catalyzes the NADH-dependent interconversion of oxaloacetate and malate in the tricarboxylic acid cycle. Mutations in *mdh* have not yet been found in INH-resistant *M. tuberculosis* isolates.

ahpC

Overexpression of the antioxidant enzyme AhpC (alkyl hydroperoxide reductase) owing to mutations in the promoter region of *ahpC* is often found in KatG-negative, INH-resistant clinical isolates as a compensatory mechanism for the loss of KatG (114–116,165,175,176). In some INH-resistant strains, AhpC mutation was found in strains with apparently intact KatG (167), raising the possibility that AhpC may be involved in removing intracellular peroxide needed for INH activation (114,115). However, AhpC itself is not directly involved in INH resistance

(177). Mutation in the *ahpC* promoter region is a useful surrogate marker for detection of INH resistance, which occurs in approximately 16% INH-resistant strains (167).

Other Genes

Although most INH-resistant strains may be accounted for by mutations in the previously discussed genes, some catalase-positive, low-level, INH-resistant clinical isolates do not have mutations in *katG*, *inhA*, *ndh*, or *kasA* (174), indicating that additional unknown genes are involved in INH resistance. The *mdh* gene (109) and the INH-induced unknown genes identified in the microarray analysis (110) could be candidate genes for mutation search among INH-resistant strains. In addition, the uridine 5′-diphospho-galactopyranose mutase gene *glf*, conferring a low level of INH resistance to the *E. coli oxyR* mutant (178), could be another candidate gene. Arylamine NAT enzyme, which can acetylate arylamines and hydrazines and inactivate INH, could also be a candidate. Humans have two NATs, NAT1, and NAT2, and the latter enzyme is involved in inactivation of INH *in vivo* (179). NAT homologs have recently been identified from *M. smegmatis* and *M. tuberculosis*, and the purified NAT enzymes have been shown to convert INH to *N*-acetyl-INH *in vitro* (126–128). Overexpression of *nat* from *M. tuberculosis* in *M. smegmatis* caused a threefold increase in resistance to INH (126). The *M. smegmatis nat* knockout mutant had slightly increased susceptibility to INH (127). Eighteen percent of clinical isolates of *M. tuberculosis* contained a single point mutation of G207R in the NAT enzyme. The NAT G207R mutation appeared to correlate with a very slight decrease in INH susceptibility at 0.02 μg/mL in two strains that harbor the mutation compared with 0.005 μg/mL in the sensitive control strain H37Rv (128). It will be of interest to determine the level of *nat* gene expression, the intrinsic enzymatic activity of the NAT protein in *M. tuberculosis* compared with other less susceptible mycobacterial species as well as the possibility of NAT overexpression owing to promoter up-mutations being involved in INH resistance in *M. tuberculosis*.

MOLECULAR DETECTION OF ISONIAZID RESISTANCE

Molecular detection of drug resistance involves amplification by polymerase chain reaction of the genomic region conferring resistance followed by detection of mutations. Although molecular tests offer a number of advantages over conventional drug susceptibility testing, such as fast turn-around time, possibilities for automation, and reduction of biohazard (180), there are several limitations, such as mutations in multiple genes and at multiple locations within a gene, unknown genes involved in resistance, and the costs.

Polymerase chain reaction sequencing is by far the most accurate method of mutation detection. However, it is time-consuming and expensive. Polymerase chain reaction–single-strand conformation polymorphism is not sensitive enough to detect all the mutations (181). The solid-phase sequence scanning (182), the microarray technology developed by Affymetrix (183), and the peptide nucleic acid probe assay (184) offer some promise but are still in development.

Although the molecular detection of rifampin resistance is straightforward because 96% of resistant strains have mutations in an 81-base pair (bp) region of the *rpoB* gene (185), molecular detection of INH resistance is hampered by the multiple genes involved (*katG, inhA*, promoter *mabA/inhA, kasA, ndh, ahpC*) and incomplete knowledge of additional genes involved in resistance. Limited analysis at the KatG S315 region and the promoter regions of *mabA/inhA* and *ahpC* may allow detection of as many as 80% to 90% of resistant strains (167), but the percentage may be subject to geographic variations (171).

VIRULENCE OF ISONIAZID-RESISTANT STRAINS

INH resistance is the only case in which acquisition of drug resistance may affect the fitness and virulence of the organism. It is well known since the 1950s that INH-resistant strains often lose not only catalase activity but also virulence for guinea pigs (142,186). Attenuation of virulence of INH-resistant, catalase-deficient strains is somewhat less easily shown in mice than in guinea pigs (186), presumably because of the different susceptibility of the two animal species to TB infection. There is generally a good correlation between loss of catalase activity and level of INH resistance and the degree of attenuation of virulence (137). Strains resistant to 10 μg/mL or more usually lose virulence in guinea pigs (137,186). However, among strains with a level of resistance between 1 and 0.1 μg/mL INH, approximately 50% show reduced virulence and the other 50% are fully virulent (137). With the identification of the *katG* gene encoding catalase-peroxidase (16), molecular genetic studies have shown that transformation of INH-resistant, catalase-deficient strains with the *M. tuberculosis katG* restore not only INH susceptibility (118) but also virulence in guinea pigs (187,188). This clearly indicates that KatG is not only involved in INH resistance but also is a virulence factor in *M. tuberculosis*. It is most likely that the degree of the catalase activity is an important factor in determining whether an INH-resistant strain is still virulent. Low-level, INH-resistant strains with positive catalase activity are expected to be still virulent. Even when INH-resistant strains have mutations in *katG* but the mutations do not cause complete loss of catalase activity, such strains may still be somewhat virulent. It is apparent that INH-resistant strains can show a spectrum of virulence from lack of virulence to fully virulent. Thus, the answer to the frequently asked question "Do INH-resistant strains lose virulence?" is "It all depends."

The mechanisms by which tubercle bacilli develop INH resistance may influence the virulence of the organisms. It appears that *in vitro* selection for INH resistance preferentially isolates mutants with mutations in *katG* but not in other genes (165,189). This bias for KatG mutation *in vitro* is probably a reflection of the difference of *in vivo* and *in vitro* conditions and the higher INH concentrations than the *in vivo* achievable INH concentrations (2 to 5 μg/mL) used in most *in vitro* selections. INH-resistant strains owing to mutations in genes other than *katG*, such as *inhA* and *ndh*, are expected to be still virulent. In a study with a well-characterized isogenic strain of *M. bovis*, loss of virulence in guinea pigs was associated with a loss of catalase activity but not with mutations in the *inhA* (187). It is of interest to note that INH-resistant, KatG-negative strains often acquire compensatory mutation in the promoter region of *ahpC*, leading to increased expression of the AhpC enzyme to compensate for the loss of the KatG and presumably better survival *in vivo*. Although the *ahpC* compensatory mutation may be important for restoring peroxide homeostasis in the KatG-deficient organism, it did not appear to contribute to increased virulence in mice (177). However, blocking the expression of AhpC using antisense RNA caused attenuation of virulence of *M. bovis* in the guinea pig model (190), indicating that AhpC is important for virulence. The discrepant results are likely to be owing to the difference in susceptibility to TB infection between guinea pigs and mice.

The question of whether INH-resistant strains are still virulent or pathogenic for humans is very complex and more difficult to answer owing to variable host genetic susceptibility, immune status (immunocompromised versus healthy) or BCG vaccination, and mixed bacterial populations. It is quite likely that catalase-negative, high-level, INH-resistant strains are not only attenuated for virulence in animals but also in humans. Indirect evidence suggests that catalase-negative INH-resistant strains are less transmissible than sensitive strains (137) and have somewhat impaired ability to produce progressive disease in humans (191). In addition, patients excreting INH-resistant, catalase-negative guinea pig avirulent strains were found to have favorable clinical course, whereas patients excreting INH-resistant, catalase-positive guinea pig virulent strains showed progression of the disease or death (192). Unlike the *in vitro*–derived, INH-resistant mutants, the clinical specimens often contain mixed bacterial populations of both INH-sensitive and -resistant bacilli and even bacilli of varying degree of INH resistance, which will complicate the analysis. INH-resistant strains also appear to be attenuated for virulence in monkeys (137). However, monkeys infected with a guinea pig–passaged, INH-resistant strain developed TB disease (137), presumably because of the selection of INH-sensitive virulent bacilli from a mixed bacterial population in the guinea pigs. INH-resistant organisms that lose catalase activity would be at a disadvantage to survive *in vivo* so that sensitive bacterial population will take over and outgrow the resistant population. The isolation of INH-resistant and catalase-negative strains from patients does not necessarily mean that such strains are still virulent because such strains could well have developed in patients during the treatment. However, low-level, INH-resistant strains with catalase activity may not lose virulence. The particularly successful strain W, which caused the outbreak of MDR-TB in New York City, spread across the United States and abroad, and is resistant to seven antimycobacterial drugs, is clearly capable of causing active transmission of the disease, especially in HIV-positive individuals (193). It is worth noting that strain W, which is resistant to INH, harbors the common *katG* mutation S315T and still retains significant catalase activity (71,72,161,162). In a recent study from The Netherlands, INH-resistant strains with the S315T KatG mutation was found to cause secondary TB cases as often as INH-susceptible organisms (155). There is a need for molecular epidemiology studies that combine precise genetic characterization of INH resistance mechanism and IS6110 typing to understand the issue of virulence and infectivity or transmissibility of INH-resistant organisms. Loss of virulence is usually not seen for *M. tuberculosis* strains resistant to other drugs. For example, we have found an active transmission of TB owing to PZA-monoresistant strains exhibiting the same characteristic *pncA* mutation profile (an 8-bp deletion and R140S), and almost identical IS6110 fingerprints in Quebec, Canada (194).

PHARMACOKINETICS AND METABOLISM

INH is readily absorbed after oral or parenteral administration and is distributed to all body fluids and intracellular compartments (195). After oral administration of the usual dose of 5 mg/kg INH or 300 mg per day, a peak serum concentration of 5 μg/mL is achieved in 1 to 2 hours (195). INH concentrations in the lungs and cerebrospinal fluid are similar to that achieved in the serum (195). INH is minimally bound to serum proteins, crosses the placenta, and is excreted in human milk (195). INH is metabolized in the liver primarily by acetylation and dehydrazination. INH is converted by the NAT2 enzyme to acetyl-INH, which is then split into monoacetylhydrazine and INA. Monoacetylhydrazine is acetylated into diacetylhydrazine, and INA is conjugated to glycine to form isonicotinoylglycine. INH is also directly conjugated to form hydrazones. The major metabolites include acetyl-INH and INA. Other metabolites found in the urine are acid-labile hydrazones, isonicotinylglycine, monoacetylhydrazine, and diacetylhydrazine (195). None of

the metabolic products has any significant antituberculosis activity. The half-life of INH ranges from 1 to 3 hours, depending on its acetylation rate, which is controlled by genetic differences in the host *N*-acetyltransferase (NAT2) activity encoded by the *nat2* gene located on chromosome 8p22 (179). Polymorphisms at the *nat2* locus determine whether the individual is a rapid or a slow acetylator (179). Approximately 50% of blacks and whites are slow acetylators, and the rest are rapid acetylators, whereas most Eskimos and Asians (85%) are rapid acetylators (179). Most INH (70%) is excreted in metabolized form in the urine. Slow acetylators excrete 37% of the drug as free INH or its hydrazone conjugates and 63% as acetyl-INH and its metabolites (INA and monoacetylhydrazine). In contrast, rapid acetylators excrete 94% of INH as acetyl-INH and its metabolites and only 2.8% as free INH and 3.6% as hydrazone conjugates (195). Liver disease can reduce acetylation rates. The rate of acetylation does not significantly alter the efficacy of the drug with current INH dosing.

TREATMENT

INH is usually given orally but can be given intramuscularly or intravenously when appropriate or when oral administration is not feasible. The recommended daily dose of INH is 10 to 20 mg/kg for children and 5 mg/kg for adults, with a maximal dose of 300 mg (195). For most children, the daily 10 mg/kg is sufficient, but a 20-mg/kg daily dose should be used for tuberculous meningitis (195). INH can be safely used in pregnant women. INH has high, early bactericidal activity and kills actively growing bacterial populations, which causes a rapid decrease in the number of bacilli in a patient's sputum during the first 2 weeks of treatment (196). Its activity slows down for the nongrowing bacterial populations. Although INH is a powerful TB drug, it is not used alone for the treatment of TB except for chemoprophylaxis. INH is used in combination with rifampin, PZA, and ethambutol in the directly observed therapy, short course (DOTS) strategy for the treatment of TB to improve efficacy and avoid emergence of drug resistance. The recommended 6-month short-course therapy (for adults weighing more than 51 kg) consists of the initial phase of treatment daily with INH (300 mg, 5 mg/kg), rifampin (600 mg, 10 mg/kg), PZA (2,000 mg, 25 mg/kg), ethambutol (1,200 mg, 15 mg/kg) for 2 months, followed by the continuation phase of treatment three times weekly with INH (600 mg, 10 mg/kg) and rifampin (600 mg, 10 mg/kg) for 4 months (197). DOTS is recommended by the World Health Organization for the treatment of all patients with TB who are HIV negative. DOTS should be initiated as soon as the diagnosis is made, and culture/sensitivity tests should be performed on all initial specimens.

For HIV-related TB, standard 6-month DOTS is still used for patients who have not started antiretroviral therapy or whose antiretroviral regimen does not include a protease inhibitor or nonnucleotide reverse transcriptase inhibitors (such as nevirapine, delavirdine, and efavirenz) (198). In other more common situations, DOTS is used with some modifications (198). Because of drug interactions, rifampin is not recommended for patients who (a) will start treatment with an antiretroviral regimen that includes a protease inhibitor or a nonnucleotide reverse transcriptase inhibitors or (b) have established HIV infection and are on antiretroviral therapy when TB is newly diagnosed and needs to be treated. Two options are currently recommended for such patients: (a) a 6-month rifabutin-based regimen and (b) a 9-month streptomycin-based regimen when rifamycin is contraindicated (such as intolerance to rifamycins or patient/physician not to combine antiretroviral and TB therapy). For patients who have delayed response (lack of bacterial conversion from positive to negative or lack of resolution or progression of signs and symptoms of TB), the 6-month DOTS should be prolonged to 9 months, whereas the 9-month, streptomycin-containing regimen should be prolonged to 12 months. For TB disease that is resistant to INH only, a 6- to 9-month therapy with rifampin, PZA, and ethambutol should be given. Patients with MDR-TB should be managed by or in consultation with physicians experienced with management of MDR-TB. The recommended duration of treatment of MDR-TB in HIV-seropositive patients is 24 months with drug regimens containing an aminoglycoside (streptomycin, kanamycin, amikacin) or capreomycin and a fluoroquinolone (198). At least two drugs to which the organism is susceptible should be added. Pyridoxine (vitamin B_6) at 25 to 50 mg daily or 50 to 100 mg twice weekly should be given to all HIV-infected TB patients undergoing TB therapy containing INH to reduce the occurrence of INH-induced side effects in the central or peripheral nervous system.

There is some controversy as to whether patients harboring INH-resistant organisms should still be treated with INH (199). In low-level, primary INH resistance, INH treatment seemed to be beneficial (200). Because the peak serum INH concentration is 5 μg/mL (195), it is likely that low-level, INH-resistant bacilli with positive catalase activity may still respond to INH treatment, but bacilli that are highly resistant (MIC >5 μg/mL) may not. Indeed, some experts suggest that INH can still be used for low-level INH resistance (>1% of bacilli resistant to 0.2 μg/mL but susceptible to 1 μg/mL INH), whereas INH is not recommended for higher levels of resistance (>1% bacilli resistant to 1 μg/mL INH) (198). However, retreatment of secondary INH resistance with INH is more controversial (199). In one controlled retreatment trial with various combinations of ethionamide, cycloserine, and PZA, addition of INH (300 mg per day) showed no benefit (201). However, in another trial with a smaller number of patients using ethionamide and PZA, the addition of higher doses of INH (1 to 1.5 g per day) showed marked benefit (202). The reasons for the discrepant results could be owing

to different drug regimens and the INH dose being used. Whether INH treatment of resistant bacilli has any demonstrable benefit is quite complex and may depend on the level of resistance, percentage of sensitive and resistant bacilli, INH dose, drug regimens, and study design. Despite the suggestion that INH may still be used in cases of low-level, INH-resistant strains to make them highly resistant, lose catalase, and become less infectious, further studies are clearly needed.

INH is also used in combination with other antimycobacterial drugs for the treatment of infections caused by *M. kansasii* and *M. xenopi* (195) because of the INH sensitivity of the two organisms. For both *M. kansasii* and *M. xenopi* infections, treatment with INH, rifampin, and ethambutol for 12 to 24 months may be needed (195). However, *M. avium* infection cannot be treated with INH because of its high level of resistance.

Isoniazid Chemoprophylaxis

INH is used alone in the chemoprophylaxis of early-stage TB infection [also called latent TB infection (LTBI)] to prevent the development of active disease in contacts and recent tuberculin converters. LTBI can also be treated with rifampin for 4 months or rifampin and PZA for 2 months (203), but this is beyond the scope of this review and is not covered here. LTBI is diagnosed by tuberculin skin test positivity. The tuberculin test is only useful in low-incidence countries (e.g., United States, The Netherlands, United Kingdom) where BCG vaccination is not used. In the United States, targeted tuberculin testing is recommended in high- but not low-risk populations. The targeted tuberculin testing is considered an important component of the TB elimination strategy by U.S. Public Health Service Advisory Council on the Elimination of Tuberculosis (203). However, INH prophylaxis is not commonly used in developing countries. For people who are at highest risk of developing active TB (e.g., those who are HIV positive, receiving immunosuppressant therapy, in close contact with TB patients, or have abnormal chest x-rays consistent with prior TB), more than 5 mm of induration is considered positive. For other people with an increased probability of recent infection or with other clinical conditions that increase the risk of progression to active TB, more than 10 mm of induration is considered positive. These include recent immigrants from high-prevalence countries; injection drug users; health care workers with exposure to TB; TB laboratory personnel; persons with clinical conditions such as silicosis, diabetes, and chronic renal failure; and children and adolescents exposed to adults in high-risk categories. For people at low risk of TB, more than 15 mm is considered positive. INH chemoprophylaxis should be offered to persons with LTBI at increased risk of TB (active disease should be ruled out) unless there is a strong contraindication (203).

Chemoprophylaxis with INH 5 mg/kg of body weight for adults and 10 mg/kg of body weight for children (maximal 300 mg per day) is given daily for 6 to 9 months (203) for high-risk populations. The newly updated Centers for Disease Control and Prevention guidelines recommend that INH be given daily for 9 months regardless of HIV status (203). This 9-month regimen is longer than the previous 6-month regimen for HIV-negative individuals but shorter than the previous 12-month regimen for the HIV-positive individuals. The 9-month INH regimen is the preferred regimen with a recommendation level A. The 6-month INH daily regimen is an acceptable alternative with a recommendation level B (alternative, acceptable to offer) for HIV-negative individuals but level C (offer when preferred or alternative regimens cannot be given) for HIV-positive individuals (203). Persons infected with INH-resistant organisms are unlikely to benefit from INH prophylaxis. In this case, use of other TB drugs (such as rifampin and PZA) should be considered. For persons who are likely infected with MDR-TB and at a high risk of developing TB, treatment with PZA and ethambutol or PZA and a fluoroquinolone for 6 to 12 months is recommended (203).

Patients being treated for LTBI should receive clinical evaluation at least monthly. Clinical monitoring during treatment is indicated for all patients, which includes education of patients about signs and symptoms of side effects of INH including unexplained anoxia, nausea, vomiting, dark urine, rash, and persistent fatigue (203). Laboratory testing (e.g., serum glutamic-oxaloacetic transaminase, serum glutamic-pyruvic transaminase, bilirubin) is not usually recommended at the start of the prophylaxis except in HIV-infected persons, pregnant women, persons with history of liver disease, or persons who regularly use alcohol (203). The risk of liver damage by INH, especially in patients older than 35 years of age, resulted in conflicting views in the United States on the benefits of INH prophylaxis in low-risk tuberculin reactors (204). Because of this potential problem, many physicians use decision analysis of the benefits and drawbacks of treating or not treating with INH (205). It is important to involve the patient in the decision analysis whenever possible.

DRUG INTERACTIONS

INH inhibits the metabolism of the anticonvulsant drug phenytoin, which can cause phenytoin toxicity, especially in slow inactivators. INH may interfere with the metabolism of the anticonvulsant drug carbamazepine, causing carbamazepine toxicity. INH inhibits histaminase and can cause histamine toxicity when patients eat food (such as cheese and fish) that is rich in histamine (195). In addition, INH, because of its structural similarity to iproniazid, a known inhibitor of monoamine oxidase used in the treatment of some mental illnesses, may inhibit monoamine oxidase and cause hypertensive crisis in patients who take substances (cheese and red wine) rich in monoamines (195). INH may increase the anticoagulant activity of warfarin (195). The half-life of INH can be increased by drugs such as paraaminosalicylic acid, procainamide, and chlorpromazine and reduced by ethanol and other drugs that increase microsomal enzyme activity in the liver (206). No known interactions exist between INH and antiretroviral drugs for the treatment of HIV infection.

ADVERSE EFFECTS

INH is a drug that is well tolerated in most instances. The most frequent reactions are those affecting the nervous system and the liver.

Hepatic Reactions

The most serious adverse effect is damage to the liver and potentially fatal hepatitis. INH-associated hepatotoxicity was reported to result from the toxic effect of an intermediate product produced by N-hydroxylation of monoacetyl hydrazine, one of the metabolites of INH, by the liver cytochrome P-450 oxidase system (207). The frequency of liver damage increases with age and is in general less than 2% (195). In the United States, during 1-year INH treatment, INH-associated hepatitis occurred in no persons younger than age 20, in 2.4 persons aged 20 to 34, and in 19.2 persons aged 50 to 64 years of age, per 1,000 subjects (204). Slow INH acetylators owing to mutant NAT2 are at a higher risk of hepatotoxicity in recent studies (208,209), although some earlier studies did not appear to find the correlation between acetylator status and hepatotoxicity (210). Other factors that predispose to INH-associated liver damage include excessive alcohol consumption, intravenous drug abuse, and a history of liver disease. The combination of INH and rifampin causes a higher risk of hepatitis than INH or rifampin given alone. Asymptomatic elevations of serum transaminase levels may occur in some cases during the first few months of INH therapy. In most instances, abnormal enzyme levels return to normal with no need to discontinue medication (195). Routine monitoring of serum transaminase is not necessary, except in high-risk individuals, such as those who are older than 35 years of age, those who take alcohol daily or hepatotoxic medications, or those who have a history of liver disease (195). In occasional instances, progressive liver damage occurs, with accompanying symptoms. In these cases, INH, and perhaps other potentially liver damaging drugs such as rifampin and PZA, should be stopped. Drugs that cause no liver toxicities, such as streptomycin, ethambutol, and ofloxacin, can be used instead (195).

Nervous System Toxicities

Peripheral neuropathy and central nervous system symptoms can occur during INH therapy because of its interference with pyridoxine (vitamin B_6) metabolism. Vitamin B_6 is a cofactor for the synthesis of neurotransmitters in various brain areas. INH can cause vitamin B_6 deficiency by formation of INH-pyridoxine hydrazones, which lowers the effective concentration of pyridoxine in serum and tissues. Slow acetylators are at a higher risk of developing neurotoxicity. INH, at a daily dose of 5 mg/kg, rarely causes neurologic symptoms, and pyridoxine is not given routinely to patients taking the normal dose of INH. Higher doses of INH increase the risk of neurotoxicity. Symptoms can be prevented by low-dose pyridoxine at 10 to 25 mg per day when prescribing INH therapy for malnourished patients, diabetic and uremic patients, patients with chronic alcoholism, pregnant patients, and patients with a seizure disorder (195,207). Other less frequent neurologic adverse effects include toxic encephalopathy, convulsions, optic neuritis and atrophy, memory impairment, restlessness and insomnia, and psychiatric disturbances (psychosis) (195). INH overdose should be treated promptly with pyridoxine in a dose that is similar to the estimated overdose of INH (195).

Other Reactions

Gastrointestinal reactions, such as nausea, vomiting, and epigastric distress, are uncommon (195). Hypersensitivity to INH is occasionally encountered, manifesting fever, pruritus, skin eruptions (morbilliform, maculopapular, eruptive rash), lymphadenopathy, and vasculitis (195). Hematologic reactions include agranulocytosis, hemolytic, sideroblastic or aplastic anemia, thrombocytopenia, and eosinophilia. Metabolic and endocrine reactions such as pellagra, hyperglycemia, metabolic acidosis, and gynecomastia could occur (195). Rheumatic syndrome and systemic lupus erythematosus–like syndrome occur infrequently. Local irritation has been observed at the site of intramuscular injection. INH has been reported to have carcinogenic properties in mice (211), but in humans, INH has not been found to increase the risk of cancer (212).

Contraindications to Isoniazid Therapy

INH is contraindicated in patients who have had previous severe INH-associated hepatitis, acute liver disease of any etiology, and INH hypersensitivity reactions such as drug fever, chills, and arthritis (195).

CONCLUSION

INH is an important front-line anti-TB drug that forms the basis of modern TB chemotherapy. INH is almost an ideal drug for the treatment of TB because it is inexpensive, highly specific and bactericidal, easily administered, and relatively nontoxic. The introduction of INH in the clinical treatment of TB in 1952 represented a major historic advance in the fight against this disease. Despite the simple

structure of INH, its mechanism of action is highly complex because it interferes with multiple cellular processes in tubercle bacilli. The study of INH has provided an excellent opportunity to learn about the basic biology of this fascinating organism. The application of modern molecular biology, biochemistry, and structural biology in recent years has greatly improved our understanding of the molecular mechanisms of INH action and resistance. However, many aspects of INH action and resistance still remain obscure and need molecular definition and confirmation. The increasing emergence of drug-resistant strains including those resistant to INH poses a serious threat to the control of TB. It is expected that improved understanding of the mechanisms of INH action and resistance will provide new tools for more effective control such as rapid detection of INH resistance and design of new drugs active against resistant organisms.

REFERENCES

1. Meyer H, Malley J. Uber hydrazinderivate de pyridincarbonsauren. *Montashefte Chem* 1912;33:393–414.
2. Fox HH. The chemical approach to the control of tuberculosis. *Science* 1952;116:129–134.
3. Bernstein J, Lott WA, Steinberg BA, et al. Chemotherapy of experimental tuberculosis. V. Isonicotinic acid hydrazide (Nydrazid) and related compounds. *Am Rev Tuberc* 1952;65:357–364.
4. Offe HA, Siefken W, Domagk G. The tuberculostatic activity of hydrazine derivatives from pyridine carboxylic acids and carbonyl compounds. *Z Naturforsch* 1952;7b:462–468.
5. Chorine V. Action de l'amide nicotinique sur les bacilles du genre *Mycobacterium*. *CR Acad Sci (Paris)* 1945;220:150–151.
6. Domagk G. Die experimentellen Grundlagen einer Chemotherapie der Tuberkulose. *Beitr Klin Tuberk* 1948;101:367–394.
7. Robitzek EH, Selikoff IJ. Hydrazine derivatives of isonicotinic acid (Rimifon, Marsilid) in the treatment of active progressive caseous-pneumonic tuberculosis. A preliminary report. *Am Rev Tuberc* 1952;65:402–428.
8. TB—and hope. *Time Magazine* 1952; Mar 3:42–44.
9. Thomas L. *The Lasker awards: four decades of scientific medical progress*. New York: Raven Press, 1986.
10. Pablos-Mendez A, Raviglione MC, Laszlo A, et al. Global surveillance for antituberculosis-drug resistance 1994-1997. World Health Organization-International Union against Tuberculosis and Lung Disease Working Group on Anti-Tuberculosis Drug Resistance Surveillance (published erratum appears in *N Engl J Med* 1998;339:139). *N Engl J Med* 1998;338:1641–1649.
11. Nosocomial transmission of multidrug-resistant tuberculosis among HIV-infected persons—Florida and New York, 1988–1991. *MMWR Morb Mortal Wkly Rep* 1991;40:585–591.
12. Edlin BR, Tokars JI, Grieco MH, et al. An outbreak of multidrug-resistant tuberculosis among hospitalized patients with the acquired immunodeficiency syndrome. *N Engl J Med* 1992;326:1514–1521.
13. Transmission of multidrug-resistant tuberculosis among immunocompromised persons in a correctional system—New York, 1991. *MMWR Morb Mortal Wkly Rep* 1992;41:507–509.
14. Frieden TR, Sterling T, Pablos-Mendez A, et al. The emergence of drug-resistant tuberculosis in New York City (erratum

appears in *N Engl J Med* 1993;329:148). *N Engl J Med* 1993; 328:521–526.

15. Bloom BR, Murray CJ. Tuberculosis: commentary on a reemergent killer. *Science* 1992;257:1055–1064.

16. Zhang Y, Heym B, Allen B, et al. The catalase-peroxidase gene and isoniazid resistance of *Mycobacterium tuberculosis*. *Nature* 1992;358:591–593.

17. Banerjee A, Dubnau E, Quemard A, et al. *inhA*, a gene encoding a target for isoniazid and ethionamide in *Mycobacterium tuberculosis*. *Science* 1994;263:227–230.

18. Kruger-Thiemer E. Isonicotinic acid hypothesis of the antituberculosis action of isoniazid. *Am Rev Tuberc* 1958;77:364–367.

19. Winder FG. The antibacterial action of streptomycin, isoniazid and PAS. In: Barry VC, ed. *Chemotherapy of tuberculosis*. London: Butterworth, 1964:111–149.

20. Youatt J. A review of the action of isoniazid. *Am Rev Respir Dis* 1969;99:729–749.

21. Krishna Murti CR. Isonicotinic acid hydrazide. In: Corcoran VW, FE Hahn, eds. *Antibiotics III*. Berlin: Springer-Verlag, 1975:621–652.

22. Takayama K, Davidson LA. Isonicotinic acid hydrazide. In: Hahn FE, ed. *Antibiotics: mechanism of action of antibacterial agents*. Berlin: Springer-Verlag, 1979:98–119.

23. Winder FG. Mode of action of the antimycobacterial agents and associated aspects of the molecular biology of mycobacteria. In: Ratledge C, Stanford J eds. *The biology of mycobacteria*, vol. I. New York: Academic Press, 1982:354–438.

24. Zhang Y. Genetic basis of isoniazid resistance of *Mycobacterium tuberculosis*. *Res Microbiol* 1993;144:143–149.

25. Zhang Y, Young DB. Molecular mechanisms of isoniazid: a drug at the front line of tuberculosis control. *Trends Microbiol* 1993;1:109–113.

26. Sacchettini JC, Blanchard JS. The structure and function of the isoniazid target in *M. tuberculosis*. *Res Microbiol* 1996;147:36–43.

27. Ramaswamy S, Musser JM. Molecular genetic basis of antimicrobial agent resistance in *Mycobacterium tuberculosis*; 1998 update. *Int J Tuberc Lung Dis* 1998;79:3–29.

28. Miesel L, Rozwarski DA, Sacchettini JC, et al. Mechanisms for isoniazid action and resistance. *Novartis Found Symp* 1998;217:209–220.

29. Heym B, Saint-Joanis B, Cole ST. The molecular basis of isoniazid resistance in *Mycobacterium tuberculosis*. *Tuber Lung Dis* 1999;79:267–271.

30. Zhang Y, Telenti A. Genetics of drug resistance in *Mycobacterium tuberculosis*. In: Hatfull G, Jacobs WR, eds. *Molecular genetics of mycobacteria*. Washington, DC: ASM Press, 2000:235–254.

31. Slayden RA, Barry CE 3rd. The genetics and biochemistry of isoniazid resistance in *Mycobacterium tuberculosis*. *Microbes Infect* 2000;2:659–669.

32. Somoskovi A, Parsons LM, Salfinger M. The molecular basis of resistance to isoniazid, rifampin, and pyrazinamide in *Mycobacterium tuberculosis*. *Respir Res* 2001;2:164–168.

33. Brewer GA. Isoniazid. In: Florey K, ed. *Analytical profiles of drug substances*. New York: Academic Press, 1977:6:183–258.

34. Fox HH. Newer synthetic structures of interest as tuberculostatic drugs. *Science* 1953;114:497–505.

35. Bonicke R. Uber die tuberculostatische Wirksamkeit pentaheterocyclicher Carbonsaurehydrazide. *Z Hygiene* 1958;145:263.

36. Collins CH, Grange JM, Yates MD. *Tuberculosis bacteriology*. London: Butterworth, 1985:59–66.

37. Yates MD, Collins CH, Grange JM. "Classical" and "Asian" variants of *Mycobacterium tuberculosis* isolated in South East England 1977–1980. *Tubercle* 1982;63:55–61.

38. Yates MD, Grange JM, Collins CH. A study of the relationship between the resistance of *Mycobacterium tuberculosis* to isonicotinic acid hydrazide (isoniazid) and to thiophen-2-carboxylic acid hydrazide. *Tubercle* 1984;65:295–299.

39. Bartmann K. Isoniazid. In: Bartmann K, ed. *Antituberculosis drugs: handbook of experimental pharmacology*. Berlin: Springer–Verlag, 1998:113–134.

40. Knox R, King MB, Woodroffe RC. *In vitro* action of isoniazid on *Mycobacterium tuberculosis*. *Lancet* 1952;2:854–858.

41. Wheeler PR, Anderson PM. Determination of the primary target for isoniazid in mycobacterial mycolic acid biosynthesis with *Mycobacterium aurum* A+. *Biochem J* 1996;318:451–457.

42. Inderlied CB, Nash KA. Antimycobacterial agents: In vitro susceptibility testing, spectra of activity, mechanisms of action and resistance, and assays for activity in biological fluids. In: Lorian V, ed. *Antibiotics in laboratory medicine*. Baltimore: Williams & Wilkins, 1996:127–175.

43. Pansy F, Stander H, Donovick R. *In vitro* studies on isonicotinic acid hydrazide. *Am Rev Tuberc* 1952;65:761–764.

44. Mitchison DA, Selkon JB. The bactericidal activities of antituberculosis drugs. *Am Rev Tuberc* 1956;74(Suppl):109–116.

45. Zabinski RF, Blanchard JS. The Requirement for manganese and oxygen in the isoniazid-dependent inactivation of *Mycobacterium tuberculosis* enoyl reductase. *J Am Chem Soc* 1997;119:2331–2332.

46. Barclay WR, Ebert RH, Koch-Weser D. Mode of action of isoniazid. *Am Rev Tuberc* 1953;67:490–496.

47. Youatt J. The uptake of isoniazid by washed cell suspension of mycobacteria and other bacteria. *Aust J Exp Biol Med Sci* 1958;36:223–233.

48. Youatt J. The uptake of isoniazid and related compounds by mycobacteria. *Aust J Exp Biol Med Sci* 1960;38:331–338.

49. Johnsson K, Schultz PG. Mechanistic studies of the oxidation of isoniazid by the catalase-peroxidase from *Mycobacterium tuberculosis*. *J Am Chem Soc* 1994;116:7425–7426.

50. Pope H. The neutralization of isoniazid activity in *Mycobacterium tuberculosis* by certain metabolites. *Am Rev Tuberc* 1956;73:735–747.

51. Schaefer WB. The effect of ketone compounds on the inhibition of growth of tubercle bacilli by isoniazid *in vitro*. *Am Rev Tuberc* 1953;68:273–276.

52. McDermott W, Tompsett R. Activation of pyrazinamide and nicotinamide in acidic environment in vitro. *Am Rev Tuberc* 1954;70:748–754.

53. Mitchison DA. Titration of strains of tubercle bacilli against isoniazid. *Lancet* 1952;2:858–860.

54. Youmans AS, Youmans GP. The inactivation of isoniazid by filtrates and extracts of mycobacteria. *Am Rev Tuberc* 1955;72:196–203.

55. Youmans AS, Youmans GP. The effect of anti-isoniazid substance produced by mycobacteria on the chemotherapeutic activity of isoniazid in vivo. *Am Rev Tuberc* 1956;73:764–767.

56. Suter E. Multiplication of tubercle bacilli within phagocytes cultivated in vitro and effect of streptomycin and isonicotinic acid hydrazide. *Am Rev Tuberc* 1952;65:775–776.

57. Mackaness GB, Smith N. The action of isoniazid (isonicotinic acid hydrazide) on intracellular tubercle bacilli. *Am Rev Tuberc* 1952;66:125–133.

58. McCune RM, Tompsett R. The fate of *Mycobacterium tuberculosis* in mouse tissues as determined by the microbial enumeration technique. I. The persistence of drug susceptible tubercle bacilli in the tissues despite prolonged antimicrobial therapy. *J Exp Med* 1956;104:737–762.

59. McCune RM, Tompsett R, McDermott W. The fate of *Mycobacterium tuberculosis* in mouse tissues as determined by the microbial enumeration technique. II. The conversion of

tuberculous infection to the latent state by administration of pyrazinamide and a companion drug. *J Exp Med* 1956;104:763–802.

60. Tsukamura M., Tsukamura S, Nakano E. The uptake of isoniazid by mycobacteria and its relation to isoniazid susceptibility. *Am Rev Respir Dis* 1963;87:269–275.

61. Wimpenny JWT. The uptake and fate of isoniazid in *Mycobacterium tuberculosis* var *bovis* BCG. *J Gen Microbiol* 1967;47:379–388.

62. Bardou F, Raynaud C, Ramos C, et al. Mechanism of isoniazid uptake in *Mycobacterium tuberculosis*. *Microbiology* 1998;144:2539–2544.

63. Sriprakash KS, Ramakrishnan T. Isoniazid-resistant mutants of *Mycobacterium tuberculosis* H37Rv: uptake of isoniazid and the properties of NADase inhibitor. *J Gen Microbiol* 1970;60:125–132.

64. Heym B, Zhang Y, Poulet S, et al. Characterization of the *katG* gene encoding a catalase-peroxidase required for the isoniazid susceptibility of *Mycobacterium tuberculosis*. *J Bacteriol* 1993;175:4255–4259.

65. Johnsson K, Froland WA, Schultz PG. Overexpression, purification, and characterization of the catalase-peroxidase KatG from *Mycobacterium tuberculosis*. *J Biol Chem* 1997;272:2834–2840.

66. Magliozzo RS, Marcinkeviciene JA. The role of Mn(II)-peroxidase activity of mycobacterial catalase-peroxidase in activation of the antibiotic isoniazid. *J Biol Chem* 1997;272:8867–8870.

67. Wengenack NL, Jensen MP, Rusnak F, et al. *Mycobacterium tuberculosis* KatG is a peroxynitritase. *Biochem Biophys Res Commun* 1999;256:485–487.

68. Magliozzo RS, Marcinkeviciene JA. Evidence for isoniazid oxidation by oxyferrous mycobacterial catalase-peroxidase. *J Am Chem Soc* 1996;118:11303–11304.

69. Johnsson K, King DS, Schultz PG. Studies on the mechanism of action of isoniazid and ethionamide in the chemotherapy of tuberculosis. *J Am Chem Soc* 1995;117:5009–5010.

70. Basso LA, Zheng R, Musser JM, et al. Mechanisms of isoniazid resistance in *Mycobacterium tuberculosis*: enzymatic characterization of enoyl reductase mutants identified in isoniazid-resistant clinical isolates. *J Infect Dis* 1998;178:769–775.

71. Wengenack NL, Hoard HM, Rusnak F. Isoniazid oxidation by *Mycobacterium tuberculosis* KatG: a role for superoxide which correlates with isoniazid susceptibility. *J Am Chem Soc* 1999;121:9748–9749.

72. Wengenack NL, Todorovic S, Yu L, et al. Evidence for differential binding of isoniazid by *Mycobacterium tuberculosis* KatG and the isoniazid-resistant mutant KatG(S315T). *Biochemistry* 1998;37:15825–15834.

73. Wengenack NL, Rusnak F. Evidence for isoniazid-dependent free radical generation catalyzed by *Mycobacterium tuberculosis* KatG and the isoniazid-resistant mutant KatG(S315T). *Biochemistry* 2001;40:8990–8996.

74. Lei B, Wei CJ, Tu SC. Action mechanism of antitubercular isoniazid. Activation by *Mycobacterium tuberculosis* KatG, isolation, and characterization of InhA inhibitor. *J Biol Chem* 2000;275:2520–2526.

75. Chouchane S, Lippai I, Magliozzo RS. Catalase-peroxidase (*Mycobacterium tuberculosis* KatG) catalysis and isoniazid activation. *Biochemistry* 2000;39:9975–9983.

76. Cohn ML, Kovitz C, Oda U, et al. Studies on isoniazid and tubercle bacilli. *Am Rev Tuberc* 1954;70:641–664.

77. Shoeb HA, Bowman Jr BU, Ottolenghi AC, et al. Evidence for the generation of active oxygen by isoniazid treatment of extracts of *Mycobacterium tuberculosis* H37Ra. *Antimicrob Agents Chemother* 1985;27:404–407.

78. Shoeb HA, Bowman BU Jr, Ottolenghi AC, et al. Evidence for the generation of active oxygen by isoniazid treatment of extracts of *Mycobacterium tuberculosis* H37Ra. *Antimicrob Agents Chemother* 1985;27:408–412.

79. Rozwarski DA, Grant GA, Barton DHR, et al. Modification of the NADH of the isoniazid target (InhA) from *Mycobacterium tuberculosis*. *Science* 1998;279:98–102.

80. Youatt J. Pigments produced by mycobacteria exposed to isoniazid. *Aust J Exp Biol Med Sci* 1961;39:93–100.

81. Youatt J. Pigments produced by mycobacteria exposed to isoniazid. II. *Aust J Exp Biol Med Sci* 1962;40:197–200.

82. Youatt J, Tham SH. An enzyme system of *Mycobacterium tuberculosis* that reacts specifically with isoniazid. *Am Rev Respir Dis* 1969;100:25–30.

83. Gayatri Devi B, Shaila MS, Ramakrishnan T, et al. The purification and properties of peroxidase in *Mycobacterium tuberculosis* H37Rv and its possible role in the mechanism of action of isonicotinic acid hydrazide. *Biochem J* 1975;149:187–197.

84. Winder F. Early changes induced by isoniazid in the composition of *Mycobacterium tuberculosis*. *Biochim Biophys Acta* 1964;82:210–212.

85. Winder FG, Brennan PJ, McDonnell I. Effect of isoniazid on the composition of mycobacteria with particular reference to soluble carbohydrates and related substances. *Biochem J* 1967;104:385–393.

86. Winder FG, Collins PB. Inhibition by isoniazid of synthesis of mycolic acids in *Mycobacterium tuberculosis*. *J Gen Microbiol* 1970;63:41–48.

87. Takayama K, Wang L, David HL. Effect of isoniazid on the in vivo mycolic acid biosynthesis, cell growth and viability of *Mycobacterium tuberculosis*. *Antimicrob Agents Chemother* 1972;2:29–35.

88. Takayama K, Schnoes HK, Armstrong EL, et al. Site of inhibitory action of isoniazid in the synthesis of mycolic acids of *Mycobacterium tuberculosis*. *J Lipid Res* 1975;16:308–317.

89. Wang L, Takayama K. Relationship between the uptake of isoniazid and its action on in vivo mycolic acid synthesis in *Mycobacterium tuberculosis*. *Antimicrob Agents Chemother* 1972;2:438–441.

90. Brennan PJ, Rooney SA, Winder FG. The lipids of *M. tuberculosis* BCG: fractionation, composition, turnover, and effects of isoniazid. *Irish J Med Sci* 1970;3:371–390.

91. Gangadharam PR, Harold FM, Schaefer WB. Selective inhibition of nucleic acid synthesis in *Mycobacterium tuberculosis* by isoniazid. *Nature* 1963;198:712–714.

92. Wimpenny JWT. Effect of isoniazid on biosynthesis in *Mycobacterium tuberculosis* var *bovis* BCG. *J Gen Microbiol* 1967;47:379–388.

93. Ito KK, Yamamoto K, Kawanishi S. Manganese-mediated oxidative damage of cellular and isolated DNA by isoniazid and related hydrazines: non-Fenton-type hydroxyl radical formation. *Biochemistry* 1992;31:11606–11613.

94. Middlebrook G. Sterilization of tubercle bacilli by INH and incidence of variants resistant to drug *in vitro*. *Am Rev Tuberc* 1952;65:765–767.

95. Quémard A, Sacchettini JC, Dessen A, et al. Enzymatic characterization of the target for isoniazid in *Mycobacterium tuberculosis*. *Biochemistry* 1995;34:8235–8241.

96. Quémard A, Dessen A, Sugantino M, et al. Binding of catalase-peroxidase-activated isoniazid to wild-type and mutant *Mycobacterium tuberculosis* enoyl-ACP reductases. *J Am Chem Soc* 1996;118:1561–1562.

97. Dessen A, Quemard A, Blanchard JS, et al. Crystal structure and function of the isoniazid target of *Mycobacterium tuberculosis*. *Science* 1995;267:1638–1641.

98. Vilcheze C, Morbidoni HR, Weisbrod TR, et al. Inactivation of the *inhA*-encoded fatty acid synthase II (FASII) enoyl-acyl car-

rier protein reductase induces accumulation of the FASI end products and cell lysis of *Mycobacterium smegmatis. J Bacteriol* 2000;182:4059–4067.

99. Davidson LA, Takayama K. Isoniazid inhibition of the synthesis of monounsaturated long-chain fatty acids in *Mycobacterium tuberculosis* H37Ra. *Antimicrob Agents Chemother* 1979;16: 104–105.

100. Mdluli K, Slayden RA, Zhu Y, et al. Inhibition of a *Mycobacterium tuberculosis* beta-ketoacyl ACP synthase by isoniazid. *Science* 1998;280:1607–1610.

101. Zatman LJ, Kaplan NO, Colowick SP, et al. Effect of isonicotinic acid hydrazide on diphosphopyridine nucleotidases. *J Biol Chem* 1954;209:453–484.

102. Seydel JK, Tono-Oka S, Schaper K-J, et al. Mode of action of isoniazid (INH). *Arzneimittelforschung* 1976;26:477–478.

103. Moat AG, Foster JW. *Microbial physiology.* New York: Wiley-Liss, 1995.

104. Sriprakash KS, Ramakrishnan T. Isoniazid and nicotinamide adenine dinucleotide synthesis in *M. tuberculosis. Indian J Biochem* 1969;6:49–50.

105. Bekierkunst A. Nicotinamide-adenine dinucleotide in tubercle bacilli exposed to isoniazid. *Science* 1966;152:525–526.

106. Gopinathan KP, Ramakrishnan T, Vaidyanathan CS. Purification and properties of an inhibitor for nicotinamide-adenine-dinucleotidase from *M. tuberculosis* H37Rv. *Arch Biochem Biophys* 1966;113:376–382.

107. Winder F, Collins P. The effect of isoniazid on nicotinamide nucleotide levels in *Mycobacterium bovis* strain BCG. *Am Rev Respir Dis* 1968;97:719–720.

108. Jackett PS, Aber VR, Mitchison DA. The relationship between nicotinamide adenine dinucleotide concentration and antibacterial activity of isoniazid in *Mycobacterium tuberculosis. Am Rev Respir Dis* 1977;115:601–607.

109. Miesel L, Weisbrod T, Marcinkeviciene JA, et al. NADH dehydrogenase defects confer resistance to isoniazid and conditional lethality in *Mycobacterium smegmatis. J Bacteriol* 1998;180: 2459–2467.

110. Wilson M, DeRisi J, Kristensen HH, et al. Exploring drug-induced alterations in gene expression in *Mycobacterium tuberculosis* by microarray hybridization. *Proc Natl Acad Sci U S A* 1999;96:12833–12838.

111. Belisle JT, Vissa VD, Sievert T, et al. Role of the major antigen of *Mycobacterium tuberculosis* in cell wall biogenesis. *Science* 1997;276:1420–1422.

112. Garbe TR, Hibler NS, Deretic V. Isoniazid induces expression of the antigen 85 complex in *Mycobacterium tuberculosis. Antimicrob Agents Chemother* 1996;40:1754–1756.

113. Doran JL, Pang Y, Mdluli KE, et al. *Mycobacterium tuberculosis efpA* encodes an efflux protein of the QacA transporter family. *Clin Diagn Lab Immunol* 1997;4:23–32.

114. Dhandayuthapani S, Zhang Y, Mudd MH, et al. Oxidative stress response and its role in sensitivity to isoniazid in mycobacteria: characterization and inducibility of *ahpC* by peroxides in *Mycobacterium smegmatis* and lack of expression in *M. aurum* and *M. tuberculosis. J Bacteriol* 1996;178:3641–3649.

115. Wilson TM, Collins DM. *ahpC*, a gene involved in isoniazid resistance of the *Mycobacterium tuberculosis* complex. *Mol Microbiol* 1996;19:1025–1034.

116. Sherman DR, Mdluli K, Hickey MJ, et al. Compensatory *ahpC* gene expression in isoniazid-resistant *Mycobacterium tuberculosis. Science* 1996;272:1641–1643.

117. Alland D, Kramnik I, Weisbrod TR, et al. Identification of differentially expressed mRNA in prokaryotic organisms by customized amplification libraries (DECAL): the effect of isoniazid on gene expression in *Mycobacterium tuberculosis. Proc Natl Acad Sci U S A* 1998;95:13227–13232.

118. Zhang Y, Garbe T, Young D. Transformation with *katG* restores

119. Hillar A, Loewen PC. Comparison of isoniazid oxidation catalyzed by bacterial catalase-peroxidases and horseradish peroxidase. *Arch Biochem Biophys* 1995;323:438–446.

120. Meadow P, Knox R. The effect of isonicotinic acid hydrazide on the oxidative metabolism of *Mycobacterium tuberculosis* var. *bovis* BCG. *J Gen Microbiol* 1956;14:414–424.

121. Choudhuri BS, Sen S, Chakrabarti P. Isoniazid accumulation in *Mycobacterium smegmatis* is modulated by proton motive force-driven and ATP-dependent extrusion systems. *Biochem Biophys Res Commun* 1999;256:682–684.

122. Zhang Y, Scorpio A, Nikaido H, et al. Role of acid pH and deficient efflux of pyrazinoic acid in unique susceptibility of *Mycobacterium tuberculosis* to pyrazinamide. *J Bacteriol* 1999;181: 2044–2049.

123. Bartholomew WR. Multiple catalase enzymes in two species of mycobacteria. *Am Rev Respir Dis* 1968;97:710–712.

124. Loewen PC, Switala J, Triggs-Raine BL. Catalases HPI and HPII in *Escherichia coli* are induced independently. *Arch Biochem Biophys* 1985;243:144–149.

125. Milano A, De Rossi E, Gusberti L, et al. The *katE* gene, which encodes the catalase HPII of *Mycobacterium avium. Mol Microbiol* 1996;19:113–123.

126. Payton M, Auty R, Delgoda R, et al. Cloning and characterization of arylamine N-acetyltransferase genes from *Mycobacterium smegmatis* and *Mycobacterium tuberculosis*: increased expression results in isoniazid resistance. *J Bacteriol* 1999;181: 1343–1347.

127. Payton M, Gifford C, Schartau P, et al. Evidence towards the role of arylamine N-acetyltransferase in *Mycobacterium smegmatis* and development of a specific antiserum against the homologous enzyme of *Mycobacterium tuberculosis. Microbiology* 2001; 147:3295–3302.

128. Upton AM, Mushtaq A, Victor TC, et al. Arylamine *N*-acetyltransferase of *Mycobacterium tuberculosis* is a polymorphic enzyme and a site of isoniazid metabolism. *Mol Microbiol* 2001; 42:309–317.

129. Rosner JL. Susceptibility of *oxyR* regulon mutants of *Escherichia coli* and *Salmonella typhimurium* to isoniazid. *Antimicrob Agents Chemother* 1993;37:2251–2253.

130. Rosner J L, Storz G. Effects of peroxides on susceptibilities of *Escherichia coli* and *Mycobacterium smegmatis* to isoniazid. *Antimicrob Agents Chemother* 1994;38:1829–1833.

131. Deretic V, Philipp W, Dhandayuthapani S, et al. *Mycobacterium tuberculosis* is a natural mutant with an inactivated oxidative stress regulatory gene: implications for sensitivity to isoniazid. *Mol Microbiol* 1995;17:889–900.

132. Sherman DR, Sabo PJ, Hickey MJ, et al. Disparate responses to oxidative stress in saprophytic and pathogenic mycobacteria. *Proc Natl Acad Sci U S A* 1995;92:6625–6629.

133. Kasarov LB, Moat AG. Metabolism of nicotinamide adenine dinucleotide in human and bovine strains of *Mycobacterium tuberculosis. J Bacteriol* 1972;110:600–603.

134. Hobby GL, Lenert TF. Resistance to isonicotinic acid hydrazide. *Am Rev Tuberc* 1952;65:771–774.

135. Snider DE Jr, Cauthen GM, Farer LS, et al., Drug-resistant tuberculosis. *Am Rev Respir Dis* 1991;144:732.

136. Cohn DL, Bustreo F, Raviglione MC. Drug-resistant tuberculosis: review of the worldwide situation and the WHO/IUATLD Global Surveillance Project. *Clin Infect Dis* 1997;24 (Suppl 1):S121–S130.

137. Meissner G. The bacteriology of the tubercle bacillus. In: Barry VC, ed. *Chemotherapy of tuberculosis.* London: Butterworth, 1964:65–109.

138. Stonebrink B. The use of pyruvate containing egg medium in

isoniazid sensitivity in *Mycobacterium tuberculosis* isolates resistance to a range of drug concentrations. *Mol Microbiol* 1993;8: 521–524.

the culture of isoniazid resistant strains of *Mycobacterium tuberculosis* var *hominis. Acta Tuberc Scand* 1958;35:67–80.

139. Fisher MV. The altered growth characteristics of isoniazid-resistant tubercle bacilli. *Am Rev Tuberc* 1952;66:626–628.

140. Fisher MV. Hemin as a growth factor for certain isoniazid resistant strains of *M. tuberculosis. Am Rev Tuberc* 1954;69:797–805.

141. Beutner E, Doyle WM, Evander LC. Collateral susceptibility of isoniazid-resistant tubercle bacilli to nitrofuran. *Am Rev Respir Dis* 1963;88:712–715.

142. Middlebrook G. Isoniazid resistance and catalase activity of tubercle bacilli. *Am Rev Tuberc* 1954;69:471–472.

143. Heym B, Honore N, Truffot-Pernot C, et al. Implications of multidrug resistance for the future of short course chemotherapy of tuberculosis: a molecular study. *Lancet* 1994;344: 293–298.

144. Rouse DA, Morris SL. Molecular mechanisms of isoniazid resistance in *Mycobacterium tuberculosis* and *Mycobacterium bovis. Infect Immun* 1995;63:1427–1433.

145. Rouse DA, Li Z, Bai GH, et al. Characterization of the *katG* and *inhA* genes of isoniazid-resistant clinical isolates of *Mycobacterium tuberculosis. Antimicrob Agents Chemother* 1995; 39:2472–2477.

146. Morris S, Bai GH, Suffys P, et al. Molecular mechanisms of multiple drug resistance in clinical isolates of *Mycobacterium tuberculosis. J Infect Dis* 1995;171:954–960.

147. Heym B, Alzari PM, Honore N, et al. Missense mutations in the catalase-peroxidase gene, *katG*, are associated with isoniazid resistance in *Mycobacterium tuberculosis. Mol Microbiol* 1995; 15:235–245.

148. Musser JM, Kapur V, Williams DL, et al. Characterization of the catalase-peroxidase gene (*katG*) and *inhA* locus in isoniazid-resistant and -susceptible strains of *Mycobacterium tuberculosis* by automated DNA sequencing: restricted array of mutations associated with drug resistance. *J Infect Dis* 1996;173:196–202.

149. Dobner P, Rusch-Gerdes S, Bretzel G, et al. Usefulness of *Mycobacterium tuberculosis* genomic mutations in the genes *katG* and *inhA* for the prediction of isoniazid resistance. *Int J Tuberc Lung Dis* 1997;1:365–369.

150. Haas WH, Schilke K, Brand J, et al. Molecular analysis of *katG* gene mutations in strains of *Mycobacterium tuberculosis* complex from Africa. *Antimicrob Agents Chemother* 1997;41:1601–1603.

151. Nachamkin I, Kang C, Weinstein MP. Detection of resistance to isoniazid, rifampin, and streptomycin in clinical isolates of *Mycobacterium tuberculosis* by molecular methods. *Clin Infect Dis* 1997;24:894–900.

152. Marttila HJ, Soini H, Eerola E, et al. A Ser315Thr substitution in KatG is predominant in genetically heterogeneous multidrug-resistant *Mycobacterium tuberculosis* isolates originating from the St. Petersburg area in Russia. *Antimicrob Agents Chemother* 1998;42:2443–2445.

153. Escalante P, Ramaswamy S, Sanabria H, et al. Genotypic characterization of drug-resistant *Mycobacterium tuberculosis* isolates from Peru. *Tuber Lung Dis* 1998;79:111–118.

154. Gonzalez N, Torres MJ, Aznar J, et al. Molecular analysis of rifampin and isoniazid resistance of *Mycobacterium tuberculosis* clinical isolates in Seville, Spain. *Tuber Lung Dis* 1999;79: 187–190.

155. van Soolingen D, de Haas PE, van Doorn HR, et al. Mutations at amino acid position 315 of the *katG* gene are associated with high-level resistance to isoniazid, other drug resistance, and successful transmission of *Mycobacterium tuberculosis* in the Netherlands. *J Infect Dis* 2000;182:1788–1790.

156. Abate G, Hoffner SE, Thomsen VO, et al. Characterization of isoniazid-resistant strains of *Mycobacterium tuberculosis* on the basis of phenotypic properties and mutations in *katG. Eur J Clin Microbiol Infect Dis* 2001;20:329–333.

157. Siddiqi N, Shamim M, Hussain S, et al. Molecular characteri-

zation of multidrug-resistant isolates of *Mycobacterium tuberculosis* from patients in North India. *Antimicrob Agents Chemother* 2002;46:443–450.

158. Zahrt TC, Song J, Siple J, et al. Mycobacterial FurA is a negative regulator of catalase-peroxidase gene *katG. Mol Microbiol* 2001;39:1174–1185.

159. Pym AS, Domenech P, Honore N, et al. Regulation of catalase-peroxidase (KatG) expression, isoniazid sensitivity and virulence by *furA* of *Mycobacterium tuberculosis. Mol Microbiol* 2001;40:879–889.

160. Zhang Y, Young D. Strain variation in the *katG* region of *Mycobacterium tuberculosis. Mol Microbiol* 1994;14:301–308.

161. Rouse DA, DeVito JA, Li Z, et al. Site-directed mutagenesis of the *katG* gene of *Mycobacterium tuberculosis*: effects on catalase-peroxidase activities and isoniazid resistance. *Mol Microbiol* 1996;22:583–592.

162. Saint-Joanis B, Souchon H, Wilming M, et al. Use of site-directed mutagenesis to probe the structure, function and isoniazid activation of the catalase/peroxidase, KatG, from *Mycobacterium tuberculosis. Biochem J* 1999;338:753–760.

163. Sreevatsan S, Pan X, Stockbauer KE, et al. Restricted structural gene polymorphism in the *Mycobacterium tuberculosis* complex indicates evolutionarily recent global dissemination. *Proc Natl Acad Sci U S A* 1997;94:9869–9874.

164. Davis WB, Phillips DM. Differentiation of catalases in *Mycobacterium phlei* on the basis of susceptibility to isoniazid: association with peroxidase and acquired resistance to isoniazid. *Antimicrob Agents Chemother* 1977;12:529–533.

165. Mdluli K, Swanson J, Fischer E, et al. Mechanisms involved in the intrinsic isoniazid resistance of *Mycobacterium avium. Mol Microbiol* 1998;27:1223–1233.

166. Bergler H, Hogenauer G, Turnowsky F. Sequences of the *envM* gene and of two mutated alleles in *Escherichia coli. J Gen Microbiol* 1992;138:2093–2100.

167. Telenti A, Honore N, Bernasconi C, et al. Genotypic assessment of isoniazid and rifampin resistance in *Mycobacterium tuberculosis*: a blind study at reference laboratory level. *J Clin Microbiol* 1997;35:719–723.

168. McMurry LM, McDermott PF, Levy SB. Genetic evidence that InhA of *Mycobacterium smegmatis* is a target for triclosan. *Antimicrob Agents Chemother* 1999;43:711–713.

169. Parikh SL, Xiao G, Tonge PJ. Inhibition of InhA, the enoyl reductase from *Mycobacterium tuberculosis*, by triclosan and isoniazid. *Biochemistry* 2000;39:7645–7650.

170. Slayden RA, Lee RE, Barry CE 3rd. Isoniazid affects multiple components of the type II fatty acid synthase system of *Mycobacterium tuberculosis. Mol Microbiol* 2000;38:514–525.

171. Lee AS, Lim IH, Tang LL, et al. Contribution of *kasA* analysis to detection of isoniazid-resistant *Mycobacterium tuberculosis* in Singapore. *Antimicrob Agents Chemother* 1999;43:2087–2089.

172. Piatek AS, Telenti A, Murray MR, et al. Genotypic analysis of *Mycobacterium tuberculosis* in two distinct populations using molecular beacons: implications for rapid susceptibility testing. *Antimicrob Agents Chemother* 2000;44:103–110.

173. Kremer L, Douglas JD, Baulard AR, et al. Thiolactomycin and related analogues as novel anti-mycobacterial agents targeting KasA and KasB condensing enzymes in *Mycobacterium tuberculosis. J Biol Chem* 2000;275:16857–16864.

174. Lee AS, Teo AS, Wong SY. Novel mutations in *ndh* in isoniazid-resistant *Mycobacterium tuberculosis* isolates. *Antimicrob Agents Chemother* 2001;45:2157–2159.

175. Kelley CL, Rouse DA, Morris SL. Analysis of *ahpC* gene mutations in isoniazid-resistant clinical isolates of *Mycobacterium tuberculosis. Antimicrob Agents Chemother* 1997;41:2057–2058.

176. Sreevatsan S, Pan X, Zhang Y, et al. Analysis of the *oxyR-ahpC* region in isoniazid-resistant and -susceptible *Mycobacterium tuberculosis* complex organisms recovered from diseased humans

and animals in diverse localities. *Antimicrob Agents Chemother* 1997;41:600–606.

177. Heym B, Stavropoulos E, Honore N, et al. Effects of overexpression of the alkyl hydroperoxide reductase AhpC on the virulence and isoniazid resistance of *Mycobacterium tuberculosis*. *Infect Immun* 1997;65:1395–1401.

178. Chen P, Bishai WR. Novel selection for isoniazid (INH) resistance genes supports a role for NAD+-binding proteins in mycobacterial INH resistance. *Infect Immun* 1998;66: 5099–5106.

179. Sim E, Payton M, Noble M, et al. An update on genetic, structural and functional studies of arylamine *N*-acetyltransferases in eucaryotes and procaryotes. *Hum Mol Genet* 2000;9: 2435–2441.

180. Telenti A, Persing DH. Novel strategies for the detection of drug resistance in *Mycobacterium tuberculosis*. *Res Microbiol* 1996;147:73–79.

181. Victor TC, Pretorius GS, Felix JV, et al. *katG* mutations in isoniazid-resistant strains of *Mycobacterium tuberculosis* are not infrequent. *Antimicrob Agents Chemother* 1996;40:1572.

182. Head SR, Parikh K, Rogers YH, et al. Solid-phase sequence scanning for drug resistance detection in tuberculosis. *Mol Cell Probes* 1999;13:81–87.

183. Troesch A, Nguyen H, Miyada CG, et al. Mycobacterium species identification and rifampin resistance testing with high-density DNA probe arrays. *J Clin Microbiol* 1999;37:49–55.

184. Bockstahler LE, Li Z, Nguyen NY, et al. Peptide nucleic acid probe detection of mutations in *Mycobacterium tuberculosis* genes associated with drug resistance. *Biotechniques* 2002;32: 508–510, 512, 514.

185. Telenti A, Imboden P, Marchesi F, et al. Detection of rifampicin-resistance mutations in *Mycobacterium tuberculosis*. *Lancet* 1993;341:647–650.

186. Morse WC, Weiser OL, Kuhns DM, et al. Study of virulence of isoniazid-resistant tubercle bacilli in guinea pigs and mice. *Am Rev Tuberc* 1954;69:464–468.

187. Wilson TM, de Lisle GW, Collins DM. Effect of *inhA* and *katG* on isoniazid resistance and virulence of *Mycobacterium bovis*. *Mol Microbiol* 1995;15:1009–1015.

188. Li Z, Kelley C, Collins F, et al. Expression of *katG* in *Mycobacterium tuberculosis* is associated with its growth and persistence in mice and guinea pigs. *J Infect Dis* 1998;177:1030–1035.

189. Sassetti CM, Boyd DH, Rubin EJ. Comprehensive identification of conditionally essential genes in mycobacteria. *Proc Natl Acad Sci U S A* 2001;98:12712–12717.

190. Wilson T, de Lisle GW, Marcinkeviciene JA, et al. Antisense RNA to *ahpC*, an oxidative stress defense gene involved in isoniazid resistance, indicates that AhpC of *Mycobacterium bovis* has virulence properties. *Microbiology* 1998;144:2687–2695.

191. Oestreicher R, Observations on the pathogenicity of isoniazid-resistant mutants of tubercle bacilli from tuberculous patients. *Am Rev Tuberc* 1955;71:390–405.

192. Schweiger O, Vandra E. Bacteriologic and clinical significance of the catalase activity of *Mycobacterium tuberculosis*. *Am Rev Tuberc* 1958;78:735–748.

193. Agerton T, Valway S, Gore B, et al. Transmission of a highly drug-resistant strain (strain W1) of *Mycobacterium tuberculosis*. Community outbreak and nosocomial transmission via a contaminated bronchoscope. *JAMA* 1997;278:1073–1077.

194. Cheng SJ, Thibert L, Sanchez T, et al. *pncA* mutations as a major mechanism of pyrazinamide resistance in *Mycobacterium tuberculosis*: spread of a monoresistant strain in Quebec Canada. *Antimicrob Agents Chemother* 2000;44:528–532.

195. Isoniazid. In: Kucers A, Crowe SM, Grayson ML, et al. *The use of antibiotics*, 5th ed. Boston: Butterworth-Heineman, 1997: 1179–1210.

196. Mitchison D. The action of antituberculosis drugs in short course chemotherapy. *Tubercle* 1985;66:219–225.

197. World Health Organization. Treatment of tuberculosis, guidelines for national programs (http://www.who.int/gtb/publications/ttgnp/index.htm), 1997.

198. Prevention and treatment of tuberculosis among patients infected with human immunodeficiency virus: principles of therapy and revised recommendations. *MMWR Morb Mortal Wkly Rep* 1998;47:1–58.

199. Moulding TS. Should isoniazid be used in retreatment of tuberculosis despite acquired isoniazid resistance? *Am Rev Respir Dis* 1981;123:262–264.

200. Devadatta S, Bhatia AL, Andrews RH, et al. Response of patients infected with isoniazid-resistant tubercle bacilli to treatment with isoniazid plus PAS or isoniazid alone. *Bull WHO* 1961;25:807–829.

201. International Union Against Tuberculosis. A comparison of regimens of ethionamide, pyrazinamide and cycloserine in retreatment of patients with pulmonary tuberculosis. *Bull Int Union Tuberc* 1969;42:7–57.

202. Petty TL, Mitchell RS. Successful treatment of advanced isoniazid and streptomycin-resistant pulmonary tuberculosis with ethionamide, pyrazinamide, and isoniazid. *Am Rev Respir Dis* 1962;86:503–512.

203. Targeted tuberculin testing and treatment of latent tuberculosis infection. *MMWR Morb Mortal Wkly Rep* 2000;49:1–51.

204. Comstock GW, Edwards PQ. The competing risks of tuberculosis and hepatitis for adult tuberculin reactors. *Am Rev Respir Dis* 1975;111:573–577.

205. Colice GL. Decision analysis, public health policy, and isoniazid chemoprophylaxis for young adult tuberculin skin reactors. *Arch Intern Med* 1990;150:2517–2522.

206. Weber WW, Hein DW, Litwin A, et al. Relationship of acetylator status to isoniazid toxicity, lupus erythematosus, and bladder cancer. *Fed Proc* 1983;42:3080–3097.

207. Holdiness MR. Clinical pharmacokinetics of the antituberculosis drugs. *Clin Pharmacokinet* 1984;9:511–544.

208. Ohno M, Yamaguchi I, Yamamoto I, et al. Slow *N*-acetyltransferase 2 genotype affects the incidence of isoniazid and rifampicin-induced hepatotoxicity. *Int J Tuberc Lung Dis* 2000; 4:256–261.

209. Huang YS, Chern HD, Su WJ, et al. Polymorphism of the *N*-acetyltransferase 2 gene as a susceptibility risk factor for antituberculosis drug-induced hepatitis. *Hepatology* 2002;35: 883–889.

210. Gurumurthy P, Krishnamurthy MS, Nazareth O, et al. Lack of relationship between hepatic toxicity and acetylator phenotype in three thousand South Indian patients during treatment with isoniazid with tuberculosis. *Am Rev Respir Dis* 1984;129:58–61.

211. Biancifiori C, Severi L. The relation of isoniazid and allied compounds to carcinogenesis in the species of small laboratory animals. *Br J Cancer* 1966;20:528–538.

212. Campbell AH, Guilfoyle P. Pulmonary tuberculosis, INH and cancer. *Br J Dis Chest* 1970;64:141–149.

RIFAMYCIN ANTIBIOTICS, WITH A FOCUS ON NEWER AGENTS

ANDREW A. VERNON

If rifampin resistance became widespread, it would threaten the success of modern short-course treatment of tuberculosis (1).

Rifamycin antibiotics are among the most potent antituberculous agents known. Their discovery and widespread application revolutionized tuberculosis (TB) treatment, making available worldwide the use of highly effective regimens requiring only 6 months. Despite the critical importance of these drugs in the control of TB, many aspects of their function and use remain incompletely understood. More recently, interest has focused on the potential of long-acting rifamycins to reduce the number of doses required in therapy of active TB. This chapter reviews the current knowledge of available rifamycins, including recent experience with selected long-acting compounds.

HISTORY OF RIFAMYCIN DEVELOPMENT

Rifamycins were first isolated and developed by the Lepetit Research Laboratories (Milan, Italy) (2). In 1957, a Lepetit antibiotic screening program encouraged vacationing staff to collect microbiologic samples from any location. One worker returned with samples from a pine forest in St. Raphael near Nice, France. These samples yielded an organism now classified as *Amycolatopsis* (formerly *Streptomyces*) *mediterranei*, from fermentation broths of which several substances active against gram-positive bacteria and mycobacteria were obtained. The class of substances was nicknamed Riffifi, taken from the title of a then-popular French motion picture [colorful nicknames were used for many such products, but few progressed to wider use; for example, a compound nicknamed Mata Hari eventually gave rise to a short-lived antibiotic called matamycin (P. Sensi, personal communication, 2002)]. The most stable component of the complex, rifamycin B, initially appeared

relatively nontoxic and moderately therapeutic in animal models. Further work demonstrated that rifamycin B was itself inactive against bacteria but underwent transformation to a more active product, rifamcyin SV, which was highly active against gram-positive bacteria and against *Mycobacterium tuberculosis*. Lepetit collaborated with Ciba-Geigy (in Basel, Switzerland) in a fruitful effort to develop a rifamycin that was well absorbed orally, achieved sustained blood levels, and possessed greater activity against mycobacteria and gram-negative bacteria. Rifampin was selected for further clinical investigation around 1965, based on its antimycobacterial activity and (especially) its oral bioavailability. Information on its activity was presented extensively in 1966 (3). Rifampin was approved by the U.S. Food and Drug Administration in 1971. Large-scale clinical trials of rifampin-based treatment regimens for pulmonary TB began in the early 1970s, and results began to appear in the late 1970s. Within 15 years, published data from clinical trials had firmly established the efficacy of 6-month TB treatment regimens containing rifampin, isoniazid (INH), and pyrazinamide.

The activity of other rifamycins continued to be investigated in the several decades since the initial development of rifampin. Interest centered on compounds with possible activity against rifampin-resistant strains of TB, and it also centered on those with longer half-lives and thus suitable for highly intermittent dosing regimens. Three have advanced to phase 2 and 3 trials in humans, and two (rifabutin and rifapentine) have been licensed for use in the United States (rifabutin for the prevention of disseminated *Mycobacterium avium* in 1996 and rifapentine for the treatment of pulmonary TB in 1998).

STRUCTURE AND MECHANISM OF ACTION OF RIFAMYCIN ANTIBIOTICS

The rifamycins possess a unique *ansa* structure consisting of an aromatic nucleus linked on both sides by an aliphatic bridge (Fig. 50.1). Significant structural change at C-21, C-

A. A. Vernon: Office of the Director, National Center for HIV, STD, and TB Prevention, Centers for Disease Control and Prevention, Atlanta, Georgia.

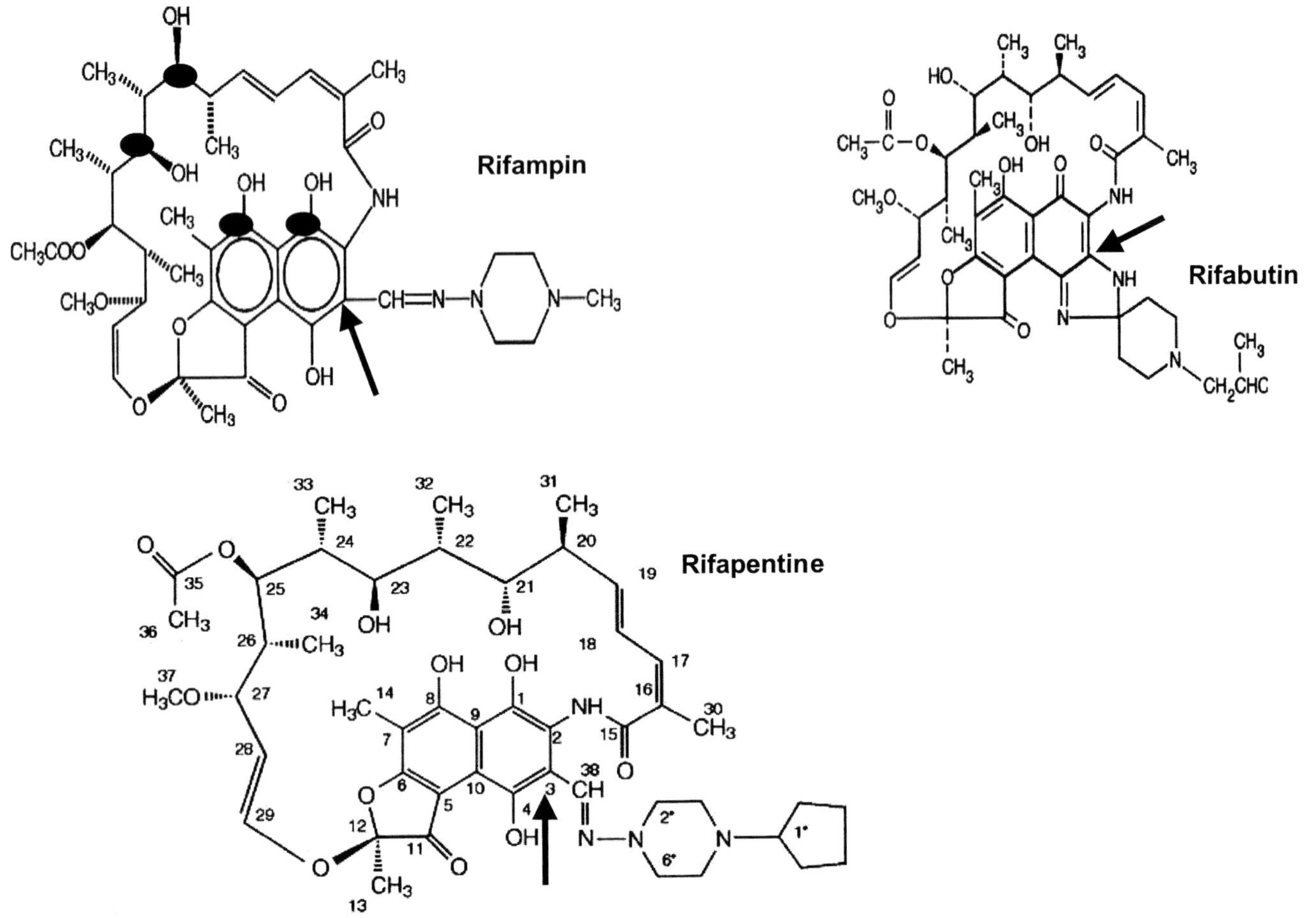

FIGURE 50.1. Structure of three rifamycins.

23, C-8, or C-1 result in markedly decreased microbiologic activity. The spatial relationships of these four sites must be maintained for antimycobacterial activity. Modifications to the side chains at C-3 are feasible without loss of activity and give rise to the three rifamycins currently in clinical use. Rifampin (or rifampicin) is a 3-formyl derivative of rifamycin S. Rifabutin is a spiropiperidyl derivative of rifamycin S. Rifapentine is cyclopentyl-substituted rifampin.

Rifamycins are bactericidal both against tubercle bacilli growing in log phase and against those in stationary phase. Studies of early bactericidal activity have demonstrated significant activity in the earlier phases of human therapy, when bacilli are multiplying most rapidly (although the activity of rifampin in this model is significantly lower than that of INH during the first 2 days of therapy) (4,5). Rifamycins are the most potent sterilizing agents used in the chemotherapy of TB. In contrast to INH, they continue to play an important role throughout the course of chemotherapy, killing tubercle bacilli for months after the start of therapy. These differences are believed to stem from the different populations of organisms thought to be pre-

sent at various times and sites during therapy (Fig. 50.2) (6). Again, in contrast to INH, the rifamycins begin to act quite rapidly after bacilli are exposed (7). After a 6- or 24-hour pulsed exposure to rifampin, surviving mycobacteria begin to grow again in 2 to 3 days (compared with a lag period of 6 to 9 days after INH pulses) (8). There is some indication that rifampin has an increased bactericidal effect if dosing is widely spaced, allowing time for bacilli to recover between doses (9,10). This observation formed the experimental basis for investigation of intermittent dosing with rifampin-based regimens.

Rifamycins share a common primary mechanism of action: they bind to and inhibit the action of the DNA-dependent RNA polymerase of mycobacteria (but not to the mammalian enzyme). This enzyme's function is to read a DNA sequence and catalyze the polymerization of the complementary RNA chain. The enzyme is composed of four subunits, to one of which [the 1,400-amino acid (β subunit)] rifamycins bind. This binding blocks elongation of the growing RNA chain (11). Resistance to rifamycins is most commonly conferred by the occurrence of single

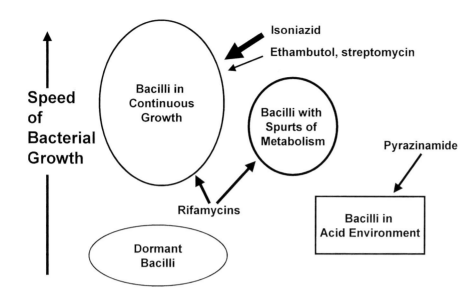

FIGURE 50.2. Hypothesized populations of tuberculosis bacilli relative to drug effects. (Adapted from Mitchison DA. How drug resistance emerges as a result of poor compliance during short course chemotherapy for tuberculosis. *Int J Tuberc Lung Dis* 1998;2:10–15.)

mutations in three limited segments of the RNA polymerase β subunit gene (rpoβ) (12,13). Most authorities consider that such rpoB mutations confer cross-resistance to all rifamycins (14,15), but there is some evidence that rifabutin may have at least partial activity against strains possessing selected rpoβ mutations that confer resistance primarily to rifampin and rifapentine (16,17). These observations have been explained recently with the description of the crystal structure of the rifampin-RNA polymerase interaction. Rifampin binds (through 6 to 12 points of hydrogen bonding) to the β subunit at a point approximately 12 Å from the DNA/RNA channel and physically obstructs elongation of the RNA chain beyond the second or third nucleotide. Resistance mutations typically replace a smaller amino acid with a bulkier one at a point of hydrogen bonding, resulting in distortion of the rifamycin binding pocket and failure of rifamycins to bind to the polymerase (11). Why inhibition of protein synthesis may result in efficient killing of mycobacteria rather than simply inhibition of growth is suggested by recent observations on the mechanism of programmed cell death, or apoptosis, in *Escherichia coli* (18). Rifampin has been shown to trigger bacterial apoptosis through an interaction with the *mazEF* addiction module, specifically by inhibiting the continued synthesis of the labile antitoxic protein *mazE*, allowing the unrestrained lethal action of the long-lived toxic protein *mazF*. Whether such mechanisms occur in *M. tuberculosis* is currently uncertain.

Other mechanisms of resistance are apparent, although not well characterized, both in *M. tuberculosis* and in nontuberculous mycobacteria. Tubercle bacilli in stationary phase (presumably similar to latent bacilli *in vivo*) are partially tolerant to rifampin, and a subpopulation of persistent but transcriptionally active bacilli are not killed by any known antituberculous agents; such bacilli do not possess

rpoβ mutations (19). Possible alternative mechanisms of resistance to rifamycins in these persistent bacilli include an alteration in drug permeability and the use of alternative sigma factors, conferring differential sensitivity of RNA polymerase to rifamycins.

PHARMACOKINETICS OF RIFAMYCINS

Absorption, Distribution, Metabolism, and Elimination of Rifamycins

Pharmacokinetic and pharmacodynamic features of the three rifamycins currently licensed in the United States are shown in Table 50.1 (20), which is adapted from a recent extensive review.

Rifampin is administered in a dose of 10 to 20 mg/kg to a maximum of 600 mg daily. The recommended dose in the United States is the same when used two or three times weekly for TB treatment (21). As noted previously, rifampin is well absorbed when taken orally. Concurrent antacids do not affect exposure; taking the drug with a high-fat meal reduces C_{max} (maximal concentration) but increases T_{max} (time to maximal concentration), with a small (6%) resultant reduction in the area under the time-concentration curve (AUC) (22).

The metabolism of rifampin is complex and remains incompletely understood. Rifampin and other rifamycins are primarily metabolized in the liver, and urinary excretion accounts for a small portion of parent drug. Acocella (23) proposed a two-compartment model to explain rifampin pharmacokinetics. Rifampin undergoes a first-pass effect in the liver where it is partly metabolized and excreted primarily into bile, competing with bilirubin. At doses of 300 to 450 mg, hepatic excretion is saturated and rifampin appears in serum (24). All three available rifamycins are

TABLE 50.1. PHARMACOLOGIC AND PHARMACODYNAMIC CHARACTERISTICS OF THE THREE CURRENTLY AVAILABLE RIFAMYCIN ANTIBIOTICS

Feature	Rifampin 600 mg (Twice Weekly)	Rifabutin 300 mg (Twice Weekly)	Rifapentine 600 mg (Once Weekly)
Bioavailability (%)	68	20	Unknown
Range of T_{max} (time to C_{max}, hr)	1.5–2.0	2.5–4.0	5–6
Range of C_{max} (mg/L)	8–20	0.2–0.6	8–30
Effect of food	Decrease AUC 6%; decrease C_{max} 36%	AUC and C_{max} unchanged; T_{max} increased	Increase AUC 40%–50%
Effect of antacids	None	None (didanosine)	Unknown
Major metabolic pathway	Deacetylation, hydrolysis to formyl derivatives	CYP 3A-mediated hydroxylation, deacetylation	Deacetylation, hydrolysis to formyl derivatives
Range of serum half-life (hr)	2–5	32–67	14–18
Effect on CYP 3A	Pronounced	Weak	Moderate
Autoinduction	Yes	Yes	No (or slight)
Effect on indinavir AUC (example of CYP 3A induction)	92% decrease	34% decrease	70% decrease
Change in AUC when given with a CYP 3A inhibitor	No effect	293% increase	No effect
Typical C_{max} (mg/L)	10.0	0.45	15.0
MIC in broth culture (mg/L)	0.15	0.06	0.04
Binding to plasma proteins (%)	85%	71%–85%	97%

AUC, area under the time-concentration curve; C_{max}, maximal drug concentration; MIC, minimal inhibitory concentration.
Adapted from Burman WJ, Gallicano K, Peloquin C. Comparative pharmacokinetics and pharmacodynamics of the rifamycin antibacterials. *Clin Pharmacokinet* 2001;40:327–341.

metabolized to a microbiologically active 25-*O*-desacetyl metabolite by an esterase enzyme. Rifampin is reabsorbed well from the gastrointestinal tract, but its major metabolite (25-*O*-desacetyl rifampin) is not, with eventual elimination both in urine and from the intestinal tract. Rifampin notably induces its own metabolism (autoinduction), with the result that AUC and plasma half-life (t) are both reduced by 20% to 40% after 7 to 10 days of daily dosing (25). Because the metabolism of rifampin is primarily hepatic, persons with severely reduced hepatic function (owing to cirrhosis, diminished blood flow, or other reasons) will obtain higher serum levels and rarely may require dose reduction. No dose modification is generally needed in the presence of renal insufficiency.

Some aspects of the metabolism of rifabutin are still more complex (26). Oral bioavailability is approximately 20% after a standard 300-mg dose. The effect of food is less compared with that on rifampin. The plasma C_{max} is quite low compared with that of rifampin (Table 50.1), whereas the plasma half-life is approximately tenfold greater. Rifabutin is considerably more lipid soluble than rifampin (with a greater than sixfold increase in the oil/water partition coefficient). Consequently, it is extensively distributed in tissues. Its time-concentration curve is biphasic, with a very long terminal half-life, possibly favoring intermittent administration. Major metabolites are 25-*O*-desacetyl rifabutin and 31-*OH*-rifabutin, which are microbiologically active and achieve plasma concentrations that are approximately 5% and 10% of the parent drug, respectively. Sev-

eral other metabolites have been identified, and only a small proportion of a radiolabeled dose is accounted for by the parent drug and the two major metabolites. Protein binding is similar to or slightly less than that of rifampin. Like rifampin, rifabutin induces its own metabolism, with a 37% decrease in the AUC and a 13% decrease in C_{max} after ten daily doses.

Rifapentine was licensed for administration at a dose of 600 mg once weekly. It is metabolized similarly to rifampin but does not significantly induce its own metabolism (27). Approximately 87% of radiolabeled rifapentine appears in urine (17%) and feces (70%), with 99% of plasma radioactivity accounted for by the parent compound and its 25-*O*-desacetyl metabolite. Dosing with food increases the AUC and C_{max} by approximately 45%. The serum half-life for rifapentine is severalfold that of rifampin, allowing less frequent dosing, and is responsible for the initial investigation of rifapentine as part of a once-weekly regimen (28).

All three rifamycins are substantially bound to plasma proteins. In theory, this may limit penetration into cerebrospinal fluid and other compartments (although rifampin is clinically effective in tuberculous meningitis). Protein binding is particularly high for rifapentine, and this may play a role in diminishing its efficacy at the 600-mg doses in persons with more advanced TB disease (29). Although intracellular penetration is high for rifabutin and uncertain for rifapentine, the importance of this observation remains unclear because debate continues whether mycobacteria are killed within macrophages or extracellularly.

Interactions with Other Drugs

Rifamycins are among the most potent known inducers of the hepatic cytochrome P-450 enzyme system, with the most marked effect on isoforms 3A4 and 2C8/9. This effect occurs within a few days of the first dose and persists for 7 to 14 days after dosing is stopped. As a consequence, the metabolism of many other drugs is affected (generally resulting in lower plasma levels of the second drug). Many drugs or drug classes are affected. This effect on other drugs has been well demonstrated for rifampin and appears to be similar in direction for rifabutin and rifapentine. However, the potency of the three rifamycins as inducers of hepatic cytochrome enzymes differs substantially, with rifampin > rifapentine > rifabutin. Judging from the effect on indinavir (Table 50.1), the magnitude of the difference is approximately 3:2:1, respectively. Several clinical situations commonly require attention. An increase in methadone dose to avoid precipitation of narcotic withdrawal symptoms is needed for persons receiving rifampin while on methadone maintenance therapy. Drug doses for persons with human immunodeficiency virus (HIV) coinfection who are being treated with highly active antiretroviral therapy may need to be adjusted when rifamycins are used concurrently. Many interaction effects are drug specific, and an effort should be made to obtain expert consultation and the latest available information to guide dosing (30). Bidirectional interactions have also been well described, and multidrug regimens for concurrent treatment of HIV and TB result in complex interaction effects whose details have not been well studied. In general, rifampin should not be coadministered with most currently available HIV protease inhibitors (Table 50.1). In its place, rifabutin may be used, with appropriate adjustment of dose and attention to dosing frequency. Rifampin may be coadministered with some nonnucleoside reverse transcriptase inhibitors (e.g., efavirenz), but the dose of the nonnucleoside reverse transcriptase inhibitor may require adjustment (e.g., efavirenz dose increases from 600 to 800 mg daily when coadministered with rifampin). Concurrent rifabutin causes a reduction in C_{max} and the AUC of zidovudine, a drug that is metabolized by glucuronidation in the liver; this effect does not appear to be clinically significant. Rifabutin exposure is not affected by concurrent zidovudine. Interactions with other currently available anti-HIV nucleoside reverse transcriptase inhibitors do not appear to be significant.

ADVERSE EFFECTS OF RIFAMYCIN ANTIBIOTICS

Adverse effects of rifamycins have been best characterized for rifampin. The major problems have been serious hypersensitivity reactions (including thrombocytopenia, acute renal failure, interstitial nephritis, shock, and hemolytic anemia as well as flu syndrome), hepatitis, and problems with concurrent medications consequent to induction of the cytochrome P-450 enzyme system (see Interactions with Other Drugs section). Most major reactions (except mild to moderate flu syndrome) should lead to permanent discontinuation of all rifamycins.

Hypersensitivity reactions to rifampin has been reported since use of the drug began in the 1960s (31,32). One study of more than 20,000 patients with leprosy receiving 600 mg rifampin daily for 3 months noted the following rates of individual hypersensitivity reaction types: flu syndrome (0.26%), acute renal failure (0.01%), thrombocytopenia (0.01%), and hypotension (0.01%) (33). Hematologic reactions begin within a few hours of administration and resolve spontaneously if subjects are not rechallenged. Flu-like syndrome includes various combinations of fever, shivering, faintness, headache, myalgia, arthralgia, and, in some patients, hypotension. It appears within hours of drug administration. It is more frequent at higher doses and with more widely spaced dosing (Table 50.2) (34). It appears to be rare with currently recommended doses and can often be eliminated by changing from intermittent to daily administration. The hypersensitivity reactions are thought to be owing to immune-mediated reactions to the drug, although detectable antibody against rifampin is not always present; investigations of possible relationships with cytokines associated with similar symptom complexes have not been reported (20).

The risk of serious liver damage owing to rifampin appears to be small. Hepatocellular reactions rather than cholestasis occur. Some data suggest that serious liver reactions are more common in persons with underlying liver injury owing to alcoholism or chronic viral hepatitis. Anecdotes abound, but few well-controlled studies allow dissection of rates owing to each of the common antituberculous drugs when used in combination. An excellent study of patients with TB in Montreal reported a rate of serious hepatitis caused by rifampin of 0.05 per 100 person-months; the rates owing to pyrazinamide and to INH were ten and three times greater, respectively (36). Experience with rifabutin and rifapentine is more limited, but neither appears to be a frequent cause of hepatitis.

Minor problems include occasional cutaneous reactions, gastrointestinal reactions, and orange-red discoloration of

TABLE 50.2. PERCENTAGE OF PATIENTS DEVELOPING FLU SYNDROME

Rifampin Dose (mg)	Twice-Weekly Dosing	Once-Weekly Dosing
600	4	10
900	8	22–31
1,200–1,800	16–22	35–57

From Grosset J, Leventis S. Adverse effects of rifampin. *Clin Infect Dis* 1983;5:S440–S446, with permission.

body fluids (notably tears and urine, providing a reliable although transient indicator of absorption). Minor reactions such as flushing, redness and watering of the eyes, and rash usually occur early in therapy and typically are mild and self-limiting. Gastrointestinal reactions most often include anorexia, nausea, and mild abdominal discomfort.

Both rifapentine and rifabutin appear to be capable of causing adverse effects similar to those caused by rifampin. Adverse effects specific to rifabutin have been described. Most of these were described during trials using rifabutin for prophylaxis against or treatment of infection with *Mycobacterium avium-intracellulare* complex in persons with advanced HIV disease. They have been associated generally with higher rifabutin doses (450 to 600 mg daily) (37) or with concomitant administration of drugs known to be potent inhibitors of the P-450 isoform CYP 3A, such as clarithromycin (38), or the HIV protease inhibitors, which partly inhibit the metabolism of rifabutin (39). These effects include uveitis, leukopenia, arthralgia, and skin discoloration. Adverse effects owing to rifapentine appear to be slightly less frequent than with rifampin (40,41). Mild hyperbilirubinemia has been described in some patients but appears to have no clinical consequence. Recognizable flu syndrome was reported in only one of 1,226 patients randomized to continuation phase therapy with 600 mg rifapentine once weekly in the three published treatment trials (42).

ANIMAL DATA

Murine models of TB treatment using rifampin were reported beginning in the late 1960s and were uniformly favorable (43). These models accurately predicted both the efficacy and necessary duration of rifampin-based regimens. Models of rifampin-based regimens for prevention of TB have been similarly useful, although potential differences between human and murine metabolism may pose occasional challenges (44). In the 1980s and 1990s, a series of murine studies examined the efficacy of regimens using rifabutin and rifapentine for the treatment and prevention of TB. These models generally demonstrated the efficacy of intermittent rifabutin- or rifapentine-based regimens in the treatment of murine TB (45–48). Studies of TB preventive therapy using a murine chronic infection model similarly suggested that intermittent regimens using rifabutin or rifapentine would be as effective as daily regimens using rifampin (49–51). After reports of suboptimal efficacy of once-weekly rifapentine-based treatment regimens (see the next section), murine studies of the combination of moxifloxacin and rifapentine suggested that this quinolone derivative might be a better companion drug in future clinical trials (52).

TUBERCULOSIS CLINICAL TRIALS INVOLVING PERSONS WITH ACTIVE DISEASE

Trials with Rifampin

Rifampin Trials in Persons with Nonhuman Immunodeficiency Virus Tuberculosis

The earliest clinical trials with rifampin rapidly established its remarkable efficacy in TB chemotherapy. Many of the trials that established its place were conducted by the British Medical Research Council (53). Table 50.3 lists British Medical Research Council studies in East and Central Africa that demonstrated early on the potent sterilizing capacity of rifampin.

A key U.S. Public Health Service trial demonstrated that a daily dose of 450 mg was significantly inferior (with regard to sputum culture conversion and occurrence of treatment failures) to a dose of 600 mg and indicated that doses of less than 9 mg/kg may be suboptimal (54). This finding was supported by pharmacokinetic data showing that serum concentrations are considerably lower with the smaller dose. Numerous subsequent trials using the 600 mg

TABLE 50.3. SHORT-COURSE CHEMOTHERAPY TRIALS OF THE BRITISH MEDICAL RESEARCH COUNCIL IN EAST AND CENTRAL AFRICA

Study No.	Year Started	Drugs in Regimen	Duration (Mo)	No. of Patients	2-Year Relapse Rate (%)
1	1970	SHR	6	152	3
		SHZ		153	8
		SH		112	29
2	1972	SHR	6	171	2
		HR		164	7
4	1978	2SHRZ/4HR	6	104	3
		2SHRZ/4H		105	10

H, isoniazid; R, rifampin; S, streptomycin; Z, pyrazinamide. Prefix numbers indicate number of months for each subregimen.
Data from Fox W, Ellard GA, Mitchison DA. Studies on the treatment of tuberculosis undertaken by the British Medical Research Council Tuberculosis Units, 1946–1986, with relevant subsequent publications. *Int J Tuberc Lung Dis* 1999; 3[suppl]:S231–S279.

dose (or approximately 10 mg/kg) established the efficacy of rifampin-based 9-month (55,56) and then 6-month regimens (53,57), established the appropriate selection and timing of companion drugs (58), and demonstrated the efficacy of intermittent (thrice- and twice-weekly) treatment regimens. (53,59,60). Together these trials have established standards by which all TB chemotherapy regimens are now measured: (a) short-course rifampin-based regimens of 6 to 9 months should result in combined rates of failure during therapy plus relapse after therapy that do not exceed 5% and (b) acquired drug resistance should be an extremely rare event (<1%) in patients on supervised therapy.

Rifampin Trials in Persons with Human Immunodeficiency Virus Tuberculosis

Several trials have reported data relevant to performance of rifampin-based regimens in patients with TB and concurrent HIV/acquired immunodeficiency syndrome. These trials are listed and described in recent reviews (61). In general, rifampin-based regimens used daily or twice or thrice weekly have performed adequately in persons with HIV-TB. Acquired rifamycin-monoresistant failure or relapse has been reported to occur in patients with HIV-TB who receive intermittent rifampin-based therapy (62). Such events appear more frequent in persons with more advanced HIV disease, but reliable data on incidence are not available.

Trials with Rifabutin

Experience with Mycobacterium avium

In the early 1990s, rifabutin was shown to be effective in the prophylaxis (63) and treatment (64) of infection owing to *M. avium-intracellulare* complex in persons with advanced HIV disease. Subsequent trials have established a preeminent role for newer macrolide drugs, but rifabutin remains an important alternative or companion drug for the management of HIV-related *M. avium-intracellulare* complex infections (65,66). As noted above, trials involving HIV-associated *M. avium-intracellulare* complex infections have provided important data concerning adverse effects of rifabutin.

Experience with Mycobacterium tuberculosis

A small number of clinical trials using rifabutin in the treatment of disease caused by *M. tuberculosis* has been published:

A multicenter trial in Argentina, Brazil, and Thailand randomized patients to daily treatment with INH, pyrazinamide, ethambutol, and either rifabutin (150 or 300 mg) or rifampin for 8 weeks, followed by INH and the same rifamycin for 16 weeks (67). Rates of bacteriologic success

(sputum negativity at last observation) were 94%, 92%, and 89%, respectively. Relapses occurred in five patients, two receiving 300 mg rifabutin, two receiving 150 mg rifabutin, and one receiving 600 mg rifampin. Two additional trials in Spain and South Africa achieved similar preliminary results but were never published in full (68).

A pilot study in Uganda compared rifabutin and rifampin in the treatment of HIV-associated TB (69). Fifty HIV-1–infected patients with culture-positive pulmonary TB were randomized to daily INH, ethambutol, pyrazinamide, and either rifabutin (150 or 300 mg) or rifampin (450 or 600 mg); the lower doses were given to persons weighing less than 50 kg. After 2 months, ethambutol and pyrazinamide were stopped, and the other drugs continued for 4 months. Treatment was observed twice weekly during the first 2 months and once weekly thereafter. Sputum smear conversion occurred in 21 patients in each arm. Rifabutin- and rifampin-containing regimens had comparable efficiency. However, rifabutin-treated patients had significantly more rapid clearance of acid-fast bacilli from sputum at 2 months ($p < 0.05$, Fisher exact test) and over the entire study period ($p < 0.05$, log-rank test) than rifampin-treated patients.

A trial conducted at eight centers in South Africa randomized 298 patients to daily supervised INH, ethambutol, pyrazinamide, and either 300 mg rifabutin or 600 mg rifampin for 8 weeks. INH and the same rifamycin were continued twice weekly for 16 weeks more. HIV testing was not done because HIV prevalence was believed to be low at the time that the study was done (late 1980s). Sputum culture conversion at 8 weeks occurred in 92.0% of the rifabutin arm and 87.7% of the rifampin arm. Six percent of patients in both arms remained culture positive at 24 weeks. Overall, 225 patients completed therapy and 95 completed 24 months of follow-up. The cumulative relapse rate at 24 months was 7.2% in the rifabutin arm and 5.0% in the rifampin arm, a difference that was not statistically significant. Adverse events were uncommon in both arms (4.2% and 2.6% in the rifabutin and rifampin arms, respectively) (89).

Preliminary results of a trial in HIV-infected TB patients were reported in 2002 (15). TB Trials Consortium study 23 was a single-arm trial that treated HIV-infected TB patients in the United States and Canada with supervised INH, pyrazinamide, ethambutol, and rifabutin. Patients were enrolled during intensive phase, and switched at enrollment to a regimen (either daily or intermittent) containing rifabutin. In the continuation phase, all patients received INH and rifabutin twice weekly. Enrollment was suspended after 180 patients had been entered. Although failure during therapy and relapse after treatment were uncommon (two failures and three relapses among 156 evaluable patients; the Kaplan–Meier rate of failure/relapse was 4.1%), all five unfavorable outcomes were associated with acquired rifamycin resistance. Failure/relapse and acquired resistance were associated with very low (<100) CD4 cell counts at the start of TB therapy.

Trials with Rifapentine

Two initial trials in China used a rifapentine formulation manufactured in Shanghai (70,71). The first trial used rifapentine only twice weekly and the second used rifapentine both once and twice weekly, each compared with a standard rifampin-based regimen. All regimens were administered for 9 months. Both trials gave all companion medications on a daily basis. Both trials found no difference in efficacy or safety between the rifapentine-based and rifampin-based regimens. Thus, these trials suggested the safety of rifapentine, but neither demonstrated a regimen offering any practical advantage to the use of rifapentine, and microbiologic monitoring in these two trials was not optimal.

Three large clinical trials have assessed the efficacy of a once-weekly rifapentine-based regimen using a dose of 600 mg (Table 50.4):

The first once-weekly rifapentine trial began in 1990 in Hong Kong, enrolling patients with pulmonary TB (72). Participants all received a standard thrice-weekly induction (intensive phase) with INH, rifampin, pyrazinamide, and streptomycin and were then randomized to 4 months of once-weekly INH and rifampin, 4 months of the same regimen with every third dose omitted (to simulate nonadherence), or standard thrice-weekly INH and rifampin. This trial used the noncommercial formulation of rifapentine manufactured in Shanghai. Pretrial data indicated that bioavailability was equivalent to the then-available commercial product (73). However, studies while the trial was ongoing demonstrated that the bioavailability of the trial medication was only approximately 65% to 70% of the commercial product, despite its being given with a high-fat breakfast to maximize absorption (74). Consequently, the dose of rifapentine was increased from 600 mg to 750 to

900 mg. HIV testing was not done, but HIV infection was believed to be rare because injection drug users were excluded and HIV prevalence in Hong Kong was very low. Life table rates of failure/relapse after 2 years of follow-up were 4.2%, 10.2%, and 11.1% in the three arms, respectively, with a small number of late relapses in the once-weekly arms (Table 50.4). Serious side effects were uncommon in all three arms. The response in patients with baseline resistance to INH was similar to that of patients with fully susceptible isolates. *N*-acetyltransferase-2 genotyping of a small number of patients found no evidence of increased relapse among rapid acetylators of INH (75). These two findings suggested that INH was playing no role in the continuation phase of this regimen. An analysis of risk factors for relapse implicated age, radiographic extent of disease, and treatment arm as independently associated with failure/relapse in the Hong Kong trial (76). These authors concluded that a once-weekly continuation regimen based on rifapentine at a dose of 600 mg was not sufficiently efficacious.

A second trial was conducted by the commercial manufacturer in South Africa (90%) and North America (10%). This trial enrolled 722 HIV-negative patients with pulmonary TB and randomized them to one of two regimens: either $2(HZE)_7P_2/4HP_1$ or $2(HRZE)_7/4HR_2$. Treatment was supervised only twice weekly during induction; all dosing was supervised during continuation. After 6 months of follow-up, the crude rates of failure were 1% (four of 286) and 3% (eight of 284), and the crude relapse rates were 10% (25 of 249) and 5% (11 of 229), respectively (40). An analysis of risk factors for failure/relapse implicated male gender, inadequate dosing with nonrifamycin drugs during induction, and sputum culture positivity at 2 months as independently associated with unfavorable outcome. This trial was the primary basis for rifapentine licensure in the United States in 1998.

A third trial (using a commercially formulated drug) was conducted by the TB Trials Consortium in the United

TABLE 50.4. COMPARISON OF THREE RIFAPENTINE TRIALS IN HUMAN IMMUNODEFICIENCY VIRUS–NEGATIVE PATIENTS WITH TUBERCULOSIS

Feature	Hong Kong	HMR 008	TB Trials Consortium Study 22
Induction	2 (HRZS)$_3$	2 HRZE, or 2 (HZE)$_7$P$_2$	2 (HRZE/S)$_7$, or ½ (HRZE/S)$_7$ 1½ HRZE/S)$_2$
No. of doses	72, 40, 35	88, 72	58–88, 42–72
Continuation	4 (HR)$_3$	4 (HR)$_2$	4 (HR)$_2$
	4 (HP)$_1$	4 (HP)$_1$	4 (HP)$_1$
	4 (HP)$_{1:2/3}$		
Risk factors for F/R	Age, radiographic extent, treatment arm	Gender, 2-mo sputum culture, adherence in intensive phase	2-mo sputum culture, cavitation, underweight, bilateral disease, white race ethnicity
Life table rate of F/R in 4 (HR)$_{2\ or\ 3}$	4.2%	Approx. 8%	5.9%
Life table rate of F/R in 4 (HP)$_1$	10.2%	Approx. 14%	10.3%

E, ethambutol; F/R, failure or relapse; H, isoniazid; HMR, Hoechst Marion Roussel; P, rifapentine; R, rifampin; S, streptomycin; Z, pyrazinamide. Prefix numbers indicate number of months for each subregimen. Subscripts indicate number of administrations per week (see text).

States and Canada. This trial enrolled both 71 HIV-positive and 1,004 HIV-negative patients with pulmonary TB at the end of standard intensive phase therapy and randomized them to one of two continuation phase regimens: either 2HRZE/4HP$_1$ or 2HRZE/4HR$_2$ (41). The HIV-positive (n = 71) arm was terminated early because of acquired rifamycin-resistant relapse among four of five relapsed patients receiving once-weekly INH/rifapentine in continuation; relapse with rifamycin monoresistance was associated with very low CD4 cell counts. No resistance was seen among three relapsed HIV-positive patients receiving twice-weekly INH/rifampin (90).

In the HIV-negative arm, the life table rates of failure/relapse after 2 years of follow-up were 10.3% in the INH/rifapentine arm and 5.9% in the INH/rifampin arm. In the HIV-negative arm of the trial, acquired rifamycin resistance occurred in only one relapsed patient who received twice-weekly INH/rifampin. In a multivariate analysis, five factors were identified as independently associated with failure/relapse: sputum culture positivity at 2 months, cavitation on chest radiograph, being underweight at diagnosis, bilateral pulmonary involvement, and non-Hispanic white race. Among participants without pulmonary cavitation, the crude rates of failure/relapse were six of 210 (2.9%) in the once-weekly arm and six of 241 (2.5%) in the twice-weekly arm. These authors recommended use of the once-weekly, rifapentine-based continuation regimen in HIV-negative patients who have no cavitation on chest radiograph. In this study, failure/relapse occurred in both treatment arms in more than 20% of patients with both radiographic cavitation and 2-month culture positivity, indicating that a subgroup of patients are at especially high risk of adverse treatment outcome (Table 50.5) (41).

A pharmacokinetic substudy associated with the TB Trials Consortium study found that failure/relapse in the once-weekly INH/rifapentine was significantly associated with lower exposure to INH (i.e., lower INH AUC) and with rapid INH acetylator genotype (77). In contrast to findings of the Hong Kong trial, these TB Trials Consortium data suggest a substantive role for INH in the continuation phase of once-weekly, rifapentine-based therapy. A similar association was not seen in the twice-weekly, rifampin-

based arm, and neither arm displayed a significant association of outcome with any rifamycin pharmacokinetic parameter, suggesting that rifamycin pharmacokinetics were adequate in the majority of study patients.

CLINICAL TRIALS OF TREATMENT OF LATENT TUBERCULOSIS INFECTION USING RIFAMYCINS

Several formal clinical trials have investigated use of rifamycins in the treatment of latent TB infection (or preventive therapy). These have been summarized in recent guidelines (78). Rifampin has been used alone for the treatment of latent TB infection (79), in combination with INH (79,80), or in combination with pyrazinamide (rifampin/pyrazinamide) (81–84). Although the available data are far fewer than those supporting use of INH, they suggest that rifampin, alone (for 4 months) or in combination with INH (for 3 months), is an effective therapy for latent TB infection. Several studies in the 1990s demonstrated the efficacy of rifampin/pyrazinamide given for 2 months to TB-infected persons with HIV. Recently, however, in HIV-negative persons with TB infection, rifampin/pyrazinamide given for 2 months has been associated with five deaths caused by severe hepatotoxicity, leading to revision of guidelines and recommendation of intensive biweekly monitoring in persons receiving the rifampin/pyrazinamide for 2 months regimen (85). It is thought likely that the pyrazinamide component is primarily responsible for the hepatotoxicity. Interest in rifamycin-based treatment of latent TB infection remains high. Studies are underway in several areas to assess the efficacy of a 3-month, 12-dose treatment of latent TB infection regimen of INH and rifapentine, and results will be available in 5 to 7 years.

CURRENT APPROACHES AND REMAINING CHALLENGES TO OPTIMAL USE OF RIFAMYCINS

Current recommendations for use of rifamycins in TB treatment and prevention are available from the Centers for Disease Control and Prevention [available at http://www.cdc.gov/nchstp/tb (accessed on 22 April 2002)], the American Thoracic Society [available at http://www.thoracic.org/statements/ (accessed on 22 April 2002)], the Infectious Disease Society of America [available at http://www.idsociety.org/ (accessed on 22 April 2002)], and the American Pediatric Association [available at http://www.aap.org/ (accessed on 22 April 2002)]. These guidelines are frequently updated. Current expert opinion supports the use of rifampin or rifabutin in daily or thrice-weekly regimens and use of any of the available rifamycins in twice-weekly regimens; it calls for adjusted-dose regimens containing rifabutin when drug interactions with anti-HIV drugs are likely to be of significant concern and

TABLE 50.5. RATE OF UNFAVORABLE EVENTS BY CAVITATION, 2-MONTH CULTURE, AND TREATMENT

Cavitation	Two-Month Culture	HP1 (%)	HR2 (%)	% of Total (n)
Negative	Negative	2.4	2.1	42 (360)
Negative	Positive	11.1	5.0	4 (38)
Positive	Negative	9.1	6.2	38 (327)
Positive	Positive	26.8	21.8	16 (137)

HP1, once-weekly isoniazid plus rifapentine; HR2, twice-weekly isoniazid plus rifampin.

TABLE 50.6. SUMMARY OF CLINICAL EXPERIENCE IN ACTIVE TUBERCULOSIS (TB) WITH THREE RIFAMYCINS

	Rifampin	Rifabutin	Rifapentine
Efficacy	<5% failure/relapse	<5% failure/relapse	Modest increase in failure/relapse when used once weekly, but only 3% failure/relapse in noncavitary HIV-negative patients
Rhythm of administration	Daily, thrice weekly, twice weekly	Daily, thrice weekly, twice weekly	Once weekly
Risk factors for failure/relapse	Positive sputum culture at 2 months, cavitation on chest X-ray, underweight, advanced HIV	Advanced HIV; other factors not assessed	Positive sputum culture at 2 months, cavitation on chest X-ray, underweight, advanced HIV
Adverse effects	Hypersensitivity, flu syndrome	Uveitis, leucopenia, arthralgia, bronzing, plus same effects as rifampin	Same effects as rifampin, perhaps at slightly reduced rate
Drug interactions	Substantial	Less	Intermediate
Risk of rifamycin monoresistant relapse	Yes: Reported in HIV-positive TB with CD4 count <100, and rarely in HIV-negative TB	Yes: In HIV-positive TB with CD4 count <100	Yes: Once-weekly regimen had 14% failure/relapse, with four of five resistant in one small study. Precludes use in HIV-positive TB
Circumstances favoring use	Acceptable in most patients if unacceptable drug interactions are not present	If unacceptable drug interactions preclude use of rifampin, especially those involving anti-HIV protease inhibitors	Once-weekly is cost-effective DOT option in noncavitary HIV-negative patients

DOT, directly observed therapy; HIV, human immunodeficiency virus.

the use of daily intensive phase and at least thrice-weekly continuation phase in persons with advanced HIV disease (e.g., CD4 cell count less than 100/mm^3) and allows use of a once-weekly continuation phase with rifapentine-based regimens only in low-risk HIV-negative patients who have noncavitary pulmonary TB. Table 50.6 provides a summary of clinical trial experience with these three licensed rifamycins in treatment of active TB and indicates circumstances in which each drug may be used.

The remaining challenges to the optimal and desirable use of the rifamycins are several. Despite 30 years experience, rifamycin-based treatment regimens still require at least 6 months, most still require dosing at least twice or thrice weekly, and many still fail to cure a substantial proportion of high-risk patients with more extensive disease at baseline. Higher rates of cure might be achieved with higher rifamycin doses (86), if these can be tolerated without unacceptable increases in the rate of adverse reactions (87). Data from a phase 2 study of rifapentine given at doses of 600, 900, and 1,200 mg indicate that moderate dose increases of this drug may be feasible (88). Drug–drug interactions involving rifamycins are proving to be particularly problematic in the setting of HIV infection in which there is the need to use highly active antiretroviral therapy. Agents with diminished potential for interaction, such as rifabutin, are useful in this setting but may necessitate more frequent dosing to avoid acquisition of rifamycin resistance. Acquired

resistance and diminished efficacy remain obstacles to the use of once-weekly dosing. It is possible that a different companion drug, with pharmacokinetic characteristics more closely matched to those of the rifamycins, may help to avoid these problems. Current work is assessing the potential for a long-acting quinolone antibiotic such as moxifloxacin to play this role. More information is needed to understand the metabolism and pharmacodynamics of the rifamycins, including their key site of action, the impact of protein binding, and the basis for persistence. Fortunately, the cost of these agents is decreasing; rifampin is off patent, and the patent on rifabutin will soon expire. Thus, it is likely that these agents will be increasingly used in the global effort to control TB.

REFERENCES

1. Mitchison DA, Nunn AJ. Influence of initial drug resistance on the response to short-course chemotherapy of pulmonary tuberculosis. *Am Rev Respir Dis* 1986;133:423–430.
2. Sensi P. History of the development of rifampin. *Rev Infect Dis* 1983;5[Suppl 3]:S402–S406.
3. Sensi P, Maggi N, Furesz S, et al. Chemical modifications and biological properties of rifamycins. *Antimicrob Agents Chemother* 1967;1966:699–714.
4. Donald PR, Sirgel FA, Botha FJ, et al. The early bactericidal activity of isoniazid related to its dose size in pulmonary tuberculosis. *Am J Respir Crit Care Med* 1997;156:895–900.

5. Sirgel FA, Donald PR, Odhiambo J, et al. A multicentre study of the early bactericidal activity of anti-tuberculosis drugs. *J Antimicrob Chemother* 2000;45:859–870

6. Mitchison DA. How drug resistance emerges as a result of poor compliance during short course chemotherapy for tuberculosis. *Int J Tuberc Lung Dis* 1998;2:10–15.

7. Mitchison DA. Role of individual drugs in the chemotherapy of tuberculosis. *Int J Tuberc Lung Dis* 2000;4:796–806.

8. Mitchison DA. Basic concepts in the chemotherapy of tuberculosis. In: Gangadharam PRJ, Jenkins PA, eds. *Mycobacteria, volume 2. Chemotherapy*. New York: Chapman & Hall, 1998.

9. Dickinson JM, Mitchison DA. Suitability of rifampicin for intermittent administration in the treatment of tuberculosis. *Tubercle* 1970;51:82–94.

10. Mitchison DA, Dickinson JM. Laboratory aspects of intermittent drug therapy. *Postgrad Med J* 1971;47:737–741.

11. Campbell EA, Korzheva N, Mustaev A, et al. Structural mechanism for rifampicin inhibition of bacterial RNA polymerase. *Cell* 2001;104:901–912.

12. Telenti A, Imboden P, Marchesi F, et al. Detection of rifampicin-resistant mutations in *Mycobacterium tuberculosis. Lancet* 1993; 341:647–650.

13. Donnabella V, Martiniuk F, Kinney D, et al. Isolation of the gene for the beta subunit of RNA polymerase from rifampicin-resistant *Mycobacterium tuberculosis* and identification of new mutations. *Am J Respir Cell Mol Biol* 1994;11:639–643.

14. Truffot-Pernot C, Giroir AM, Maury L, et al. Study of the minimal inhibitory concentration of rifabutine (Ansamycin LM 427) for *Mycobacterium tuberculosis, Mycobacterium xenopi* and *Mycobacterium avium-intracellulare. Rev Mal Respir* 1988;5:401–406

15. Centers for Disease Control. Notice to readers: acquired rifamycin resistance in persons with advanced HIV disease being treated for active tuberculosis with intermittent rifamycin-based regimens. *MMWR Morb Mortal Wkly Rep* 2002;51:214–215.

16. Williams DL, Spring L, Collins L, et al. Contribution of rpoB mutations to development of rifamycin cross-resistance in *Mycobacterium tuberculosis. Antimicrob Agents Chemother* 1998;42:1853–1857.

17. Yang B, Koga H, Ohno H, et al. Relationship between antimycobacterial activities of rifampicin, rifabutin, and KRM-1648 and rpoB mutations of *Mycobacterium tuberculosis. J Antimicrob Chemother* 1998:42:621–628.

18. Sat B, Hazan R, Fisher T, et al. Programmed cell death in *Escherichia coli*: some antibiotics can trigger *mazEF* lethality. *J Bacteriol* 2001;183:2041–2045.

19. Hu Y, Mangan JA, Dhillon J, et al. Detection of mRNA transcripts and active transcription in persistent *Mycobacterium tuberculosis* induced by exposure to rifampin or pyrazinamide. *J Bacteriol* 2000;182:6358–6365.

20. Burman WJ, Gallicano K, Peloquin C. Comparative pharmacokinetics and pharmacodynamics of the rifamycin antibacterials. *Clin Pharmacokinet* 2001;40:327–341.

21. American Thoracic Society/Centers for Disease Control and Prevention/Infectious Diseases Society of America. Treatment of tuberculosis. *Am J Respir Crit Care Med* 2003;167:603–662.

22. Peloquin CA, Namdar R, Singleton MD, et al. Pharmacokinetics of rifampin under fasting conditions, with food, and with antacids. *Chest* 1999;115:12–18.

23. Acocella G. Pharmacokinetics and metabolism of rifampin in humans. *Rev Infect Dis* 1983;5[Suppl 3]:S428–S432.

24. Acocella G. Clinical pharmacokinetics of rifampicin. *Clin Pharmacokinet* 1978;3:108–127.

25. Acocella G, Nonis A, Perna G, et al. Comparative bioavailability of isoniazid, rifampin, and pyrazinamide administered in free combination and in a fixed triple formulation designed for daily use in antituberculosis chemotherapy. II. Two-month, daily administration study. *Am Rev Respir Dis* 1988;138:886–890.

26. Blaschke TF, Skinner MH. The clinical pharmacokinetics of rifabutin. *Clin Infect Dis* 1996;22[Suppl 1]:S15–S22.

27. Keung A, Reith K, Eller MG, et al. Enzyme induction observed in healthy volunteers after repeated administration of rifapentine and its lack of effect on steady-state rifapentine pharmacokinetics: part I. *Int J Tuberc Lung Dis* 1999;3:426–436.

28. Keung A, Eller MG, McKenzie KA, et al. Single and multiple dose pharmacokinetics of rifapentine in man: part II. *Int J Tuberc Lung Dis* 1999;3:437–444.

29. Mitchison DA. Development of rifapentine: the way ahead. *Int J Tuberc Lung Dis* 1998;2:612–615.

30. Centers for Disease Control. Notice to readers: updated guidelines for the use of rifabutin or rifampin for the treatment and prevention of tuberculosis among HIV-infected patients taking protease inhibitors or nonnucleoside reverse transcriptase inhibitors. *MMWR* 2000;49:185–189.

31. Girling DJ. Adverse reactions to rifampicin in antituberculosis regimens. *J Antimicrobial Chemother* 1977;3:115–132.

32. Martinez E, Collazos J, Mayo J. Hypersensitivity reactions to rifampin. *Medicine* 1999;78:361–369.

33. Blajchman MA, Lowry RC, Pettit JE, et al. Rifampicin-induced immune thrombocytopenia. *BMJ* 1970;3:24–26.

34. Singapore Tuberculosis Service/British Medical Research Council. Controlled trial of intermittent regimens of rifampin plus isoniazid for pulmonary tuberculosis in Singapore. The results up to 30 months. *Am Rev Respir Dis* 1977;116:807–820.

35. Grosset J, Leventis S. Adverse effects of rifampin. *Clin Infect Dis* 1983;5:S440–S446.

36. Yee D, Valiquette C, Pelletier M, et al. Incidence of side effects of anti-tuberculosis drugs among patients with active tuberculosis. *Am J Respir Crit Care Med* 2002;165[Suppl]:A17(abst).

37. Shafran SD, Singer J, Zarowny DP, et al., for the Canadian HIV Trials Network Protocol 010 Study Group. Determinants of rifabutin-associated uveitis in patients treated with clarithromycin and ethambutol for *Mycobacterium avium* complex bacteremia: a multivariate analysis. *J Infect Dis* 1998;177: 252–255.

38. Benson CA, Williams PL, Cohn DL, et al., and the ACTG196/CPCRA 009 Protocol Team. Clarithromycin or rifabutin alone or in combination for primary prophylaxis of *Mycobacterium avium* complex disease in patients with AIDS: a randomized, double-blind, placebo-controlled trial. *J Infect Dis* 2000;181:1289–1297.

39. Burman WJ, Gallicano K, Peloquin C. Therapeutic implications of drug interactions in the treatment of human immunodeficiency virus-related tuberculosis. *Clin Infect Dis* 1999;28: 419–430.

40. Rifapentine labeling information (United States). Accessed online on March 25, 2002 at http://www.fda.gov/cder/foi/label (1998/21024lbl.pdf).

41. Tuberculosis Trials Consortium. Once-weekly rifapentine and isoniazid versus twice-weekly rifampin and isoniazid in the continuation phase of therapy for drug-susceptible pulmonary tuberculosis: a prospective, randomized clinical trial among HIV-negative persons. *Lancet* 2002;360:528–534.

42. Tam CM, Chan SL, Lam CW, et al. Rifapentine and isoniazid in the continuation phase of treating pulmonary tuberculosis. Initial report. *Am J Respir Crit Care Med* 1998;157:1726–1733.

43. Grosset J. The sterilizing value of rifampicin and pyrazinamide in experimental short course chemotherapy. *Tubercle* 1978;59: 287–297.

44. Lecoeur HF, Truffot-Pernot C, Grosset J. Experimental short-course preventive therapy of tuberculosis with rifampin and pyrazinamide. *Am Rev Respir Dis* 1989;140:1189–1193. See also Mitchison DA. Pyrazinamide in the chemoprophylaxis of tuberculosis [Letter]. *Am Rev Respir Dis* 1990;142:1467.

45. Della Bruna C, Schioppacassi G, Ungheri D, et al. LM-427, a new spiropiperidyl rifamycin: *in vitro* and *in vivo* studies. *J Antibiot* 1983;36:1502–1506.

46. Dhillon J, Dickinson JM, Guy JA, et al. Activity of two long-acting rifamycins, rifapentine and FCE22807, in experimental murine tuberculosis. *Tubercle Lung Dis* 1992;73:116–123.

47. Grosset J, Lounis N, Truffot-Pernot C, et al. Once-weekly rifapentine containing regimens for treatment of tuberculosis in mice. *Am J Respir Crit Care Med* 1998;157:1436–1440.

48. Daniel N, Lounis N, Ji B, et al. Antituberculosis activity of once-weekly rifapentine-containing regimens in mice. Long-term effectiveness with 6- and 8-month treatment regimens. *Am J Respir Crit Care Med* 2000;161:1572–1577.

49. Ji B, Truffot-Pernot C, Lacroix C, et al. Effectiveness of rifampin, rifabutin and rifapentine for preventive therapy of tuberculosis in mice. *Am Rev Respir Dis* 1993;148:1541–1546.

50. Chapuis L, Ji B, Truffot-Pernot C, et al. Preventive therapy of tuberculosis with rifapentine in immunocompetent and nude mice. *Am J Respir Crit Care Med* 1994;150:1355–1362.

51. Jabes D, Della Bruna C, Rossi R, et al. Effectiveness of rifabutin alone or in combination with isoniazid in preventive therapy of mouse tuberculosis. *Antimicrob Agents Chemother* 1994;38:2346–2350.

52. Lounis N, Bentoucha A, Truffot-Pernot C, et al. Effectiveness of once-weekly rifapentine and moxifloxacin regimens against *Mycobacterium tuberculosis* in mice. *Antimicrob Agents Chemother* 2001;45:3482–3486.

53. Fox W, Ellard GA, Mitchison DA. Studies on the treatment of tuberculosis undertaken by the British Medical Research Council Tuberculosis Units, 1946–1986, with relevant subsequent publications. *Int J Tuberc Lung Dis* 1999;3[Suppl]:S231–S279.

54. Long MW, Sinder DE, Farer LS. U.S. Public Health Service Cooperative Trial of three rifampin-isoniazid regimens in treatment of pulmonary tuberculosis. *Am Rev Respir Dis* 1979;119:879–894.

55. British Thoracic Association. Short course chemotherapy in pulmonary tuberculosis. *Lancet* 1980;1:1182.

56. Dutt AK, Jones L, Stead WW. Short-course chemotherapy for tuberculosis with largely twice-weekly isoniazid-rifampin. *Chest* 1979;75:441–447.

57. Combs DL, O'Brien RJ, Geiter LJ. USPHS Tuberculosis short-course chemotherapy trial 21: effectiveness, toxicity, and acceptability. The report of final results. *Ann Intern Med* 1990;112:397–406.

58. Hong Kong Chest Service/British Medical Research Council. Controlled trial of 2, 4, and 6 months of pyrazinamide in 6-month, 3 x weekly regimens for smear-positive pulmonary tuberculosis, including an assessment of a combined preparation of isoniazid, rifampin, and pyrazinamide. *Am Rev Respir Dis* 1991;143:700–706.

59. Snider DE, Graczyk J, Bek E, et al. Supervised six-months treatment of newly diagnosed pulmonary tuberculosis using isoniazid, rifampin, and pyrazinamide with and without streptomycin. *Am Rev Respir Dis* 1984;130:1091–1094.

60. Cohn DL, Catlin BJ, Peterson KL, et al. A 62-dose, 6-month therapy for pulmonary and extrapulmonary tuberculosis. A twice-weekly, directly observed, and cost effective regimen. *Ann Intern Med* 1990;112:407–415.

61. Centers for Disease Control and Prevention. Prevention and treatment of tuberculosis among patients infected with human immunodeficiency virus: principles of therapy and revised recommendations. *MMWR Recomm Rep* 1998;47:1–58.

62. ElSadr WM, Perlman DC, Matts JP, et al., for the Terry Beirn Community Programs for Clinical Research on CAIDS, and the AIDS Clinical Trials Group. Evaluation of an intensive intermittent induction regimen and duration of short course treatment for human immunodeficiency virus related pulmonary tuberculosis. *Clin Infect Dis* 1998;26:1148–1158.

63. Nightingale SD, Cameron DW, Gordis FM, et al. Two controlled trials of rifabutin prophylaxis against *Mycobacterium avium* complex infections in AIDS. *N Engl J Med* 1993;329:828–833.

64. Sullam PM, Gordin FM, Wynne BA, and the Rifabutin Study Group. Efficacy of rifabutin in the treatment of disseminated infection due to *Mycobacterium avium* complex. *Clin Infect Dis* 1994;19:84–86.

65. Shafran SD, Singer J, Zarowny DP, et al., for the Canadian HIV Trials Network Protocol 010 Study Group. A comparison of two regimens for the treatment of *Mycobacterium avium* complex bacteremia in AIDS: rifabutin, ethambutol, and clarithromycin versus rifampin, ethambutol, clofazimine, and ciprofloxacin. *N Engl J Med* 1996;335:377–383.

66. Havlir DV, Dube MP, Sattler FR, et al., for the California Collaborative Treatment Group. Prophylaxis against disseminated *Mycobacterium avium* complex with weekly azithromycin, daily rifabutin, or both. *N Engl J Med* 1996;335:392–398.

67. Gonzalez-Montaner LJ, Natal S, Yonchaiyud P, et al. Rifabutin for the treatment of newly-diagnosed tuberculosis: a multinational, randomized, comparative study versus rifampicin. *Tuberc Lung Dis* 1994;75:341–347.

68. Grassi C, Peona V. Use of rifabutin in the treatment of pulmonary tuberculosis. *Clin Inf Dis* 1996;22[Suppl 1]:S50–S54.

69. Schwander S, Rusch-Gerdes S, Mateega A, et al. A pilot study of antituberculosis combinations comparing rifabutin with rifampicin in the treatment of HIV-1 associated tuberculosis. A single-blind randomized evaluation in Ugandan patients with HIV-1 infection and pulmonary tuberculosis. *Tuberc Lung Dis* 1995;76:210–218.

70. He GJ. A comparative study of rifapentine treatment and three years follow-up on initial pulmonary tuberculosis. *Chung Hua Chieh Ho Ho Hu Hsi Tsa Chih* 1993;16:73–76

71. Biya Y, Lizhen Z, Fengying Z, et al. A clinical comparative study of Chinese-made rifapentine on chemotherapy of tuberculosis (follow-up results after three years) National Cooperative Group on the Clinical Study of Rifapentine. *Chin Antibiot* 1992;17:313–322.

72. Tam CM, Chan SL, Lam CW, et al. Rifapentine and isoniazid in the continuation phase of treating pulmonary tuberculosis. Initial report. *Am J Respir Crit Care Med* 1998;157:1726–1733.

73. Chan SL, Yew WW, Porter JHD, et al. Comparison of Chinese and Western rifapentines and improvement of bioavailability by prior taking of various meals. *Int J Antimicrob Agents* 1994;3:267–274.

74. Tam CM, Chan SL, Lam CW, et al. Bioavailability of Chinese rifapentine during a clinical trial in Hong Kong. *Int J Tuberc Lung Dis* 1997;1:411–416.

75. Tam CM, Chan SL, Kam KM, et al. Rifapentine and isoniazid in the continuation phase of a 6-month regimen. Interim report: no activity of isoniazid in the continuation phase. *Int J Tuberc Lung Dis* 2000;4:262–267.

76. Tam CM, Chan SL, Kam KM, et al. Rifapentine and isoniazid in the continuation phase of a 6-month regimen. Final report at 5 years: prognostic value of various measures. *Int J Tuberc Lung Dis* 2002;6:3–10.

77. Weiner M, Burman W, Vernon A, et al., the Tuberculosis Trials Consortium. Low isoniazid concentrations and outcome of tuberculosis treatment with once-weekly isoniazid and rifapentine. *Am J Respir Crit Care Med* 2003;167:1341–1347.

78. American Thoracic Society, Centers for Disease Control and Prevention. Targeted tuberculin testing and treatment of latent tuberculosis infection. *Am J Respir Crit Care Med* 2000;161:S221–S247.

79. Hong Kong Chest Service, Tuberculosis Research Centre, Madras, and British Medical Research Council. A double-blind placebo controlled clinical trial of three antituberculosis chemoprophylaxis regimens in patients with silicosis in Hong Kong. *Am Rev Respir Dis* 1992;145:36–41.

80. Johnson JL, Okwera A, Hom DL, et al. Duration of efficacy of treatment of latent tuberculosis infection in HIV-infected adults. *AIDS* 2001;15:2137–2147

81. Quigley MA, Mwinga A, Hosp M, et al. Long-term effect of preventive therapy for tuberculosis in a cohort of HIV-infected Zambian adults. *AIDS* 2001;15:215–222

82. Gordin FM, Chaisson RE, Matts JP, et al. An international, randomized trial of rifampin and pyrazinamide versus isoniazid for prevention of tuberculosis in HIV-infected persons. *JAMA* 2000; 283:1445–1450.

83. Halsey NA, Coberly JS, Desormeaux J, et al. Rifampin and pyrazinamide vs. isoniazid for prevention of tuberculosis in HIV-1 infected persons: an international randomized trial. *Lancet* 1998;351:786–792.

84. Mwinga A, Hosp M, Godfrey-Faussett D, et al. Twice weekly tuberculosis preventive therapy in HIV infection in Zambia. *AIDS* 1998;12:2447–2457.

85. Centers for Disease Control. Update: fatal and severe liver injuries associated with rifampin and pyrazinamide for the treatment of latent tuberculosis infection, and revisions in American Thoracic Society/CDC Recommendations—United States, 2001. *MMWR Morb Mortal Wkly Rep* 2001;50:733–735.

86. Mitchison DA. Role of individual drugs in the chemotherapy of tuberculosis. *Int J Tuberc Lung Dis* 2000;4:796–806.

87. Kreis B, Pretet S. Two three-month regimens for pulmonary tuberculosis. *Bull Int Union Tuberc* 1976;51:71–75.

88. Bock N, Pachucki C, Vernon A, et al. A prospective, randomized, double-blind study of the tolerability of rifapentine 600 mg, 900 mg and 1200 mg plus isoniazid in the continuation phase of tuberculosis treatment. *Am J Respir Crit Care Med* 2002;165: 1526–1530.

89. McGregor MM, Olliaro P, Walmarans L, et al. Efficacy and safety of rifabutin in the treatment of patients with newly diagnosed pulmonary tuberculosis. *Am J Respir Crit Care Med* 1996;154: 1462–1467.

90. Vernon A, Burman W, Benator D, et al. and the Tuberculosis Trials Consortium. Acquired rifamycin monoresistance in patients with HIV-related tuberculosis treated with once-weekly refapentine and isoniazid. *Lancet* 1999;353:1843–1847.

PYRAZINAMIDE, ETHAMBUTOL, ETHIONAMIDE, AND AMINOGLYCOSIDES

EDWARD D. CHAN
DELPHI CHATTERJEE
MICHAEL D. ISEMAN
LEONID B. HEIFETS

According to the principles set forth by Dr. D. A. Mitchison, the *Mycobacterium tuberculosis* population *in vivo* consists of several groups based on their location and metabolic activity (Fig. 51.1) (1): (i) actively metabolizing and rapidly growing, (ii) semidormant in an acidic environment (e.g., in the early inflammation sites), (iii) semidormant in nonacidic environment with occasional spurts of metabolism, and (iv) bacilli in a dormant state. Isoniazid is most active against the rapidly growing subpopulation (i) and thus display the highest among antituberculosis (anti-TB) drugs, an effect known as early bactericidal activity (EBA). Drugs that have the highest long-term sterilizing activity (other than EBA) include pyrazinamide (against ii) and rifampin (against iii). Drugs with a sterilizing effect are believed, based on both experimental models and in extensive human clinical trials, to significantly reduce relapse rates, especially in the short-course anti-TB regimens (1). No drugs are thought to be active against truly dormant bacilli. In this chapter, we discuss the role of pyrazinamide (PZA), ethambutol (EMB), ethionamide, aminoglycosides, and capreomycin in the treatment of TB.

PYRAZINAMIDE

Structure and Pharmacologic Properties

Pyrazinamide (PZA) is an amide derivative of pyrazine-2-carboxylic acid and an analog of nicotinamide (Fig. 51.2). It is considered the third most important drug in the modern regimens for anti-TB chemotherapy, after isoniazid and rifampin (2). Its anti-TB activity was first reported in 1952 (3). It is well absorbed and well distributed when taken orally. Peak plasma concentrations are approximately 50 μg/mL and with a half-life of 10 hours; once-daily dosing is feasible (2). The concentration of PZA in the epithelial lining fluid obtained from either normal volunteers or patients with acquired immunodeficiency syndrome was more than 16-fold greater than the plasma concentrations and approximately four to 40 times the reported minimal inhibitory concentration (MIC) for PZA-susceptible strains of *M. tuberculosis* (4). PZA crosses inflamed meninges well and has been recommended for treatment of patients with TB meningitis (5). PZA is hydrolyzed by liver enzymes (as well as by *M. tuberculosis*) to pyrazinoic acid (POA) (Fig. 51.2) and excreted primarily by glomerular filtration. Thus, dose modification must accompany its use in patients with hepatic or renal dysfunction. PZA is significantly cleared by hemodialysis (6). In a study of seven patients on long-term hemodialysis, 45% of the PZA dose administered 2 hours before hemodialysis was recovered in the dialysate; the median hemodialysis clearance, calculated by dividing the amount recovered in the dialysate by the serum area under the curve during hemodialysis, was 270 mL/min for PZA (6). In general, all TB drugs in patients in end-stage renal failure should be dosed after hemodialysis. In the context of pharmacologic research studies, a chromatographic technique to rapidly and accurately measure PZA levels in

E. D. Chan: Department of Medicine, University of Colorado Health School of Medicine; Department of Medicine, National Jewish Medical and Research Center, Denver, Colorado.

D. Chatterjee: Departments of Microbiology, Immunology, and Pathology, Colorado State University, Fort Collins, Colorado.

M. D. Iseman: Department of Medicine, University of Colorado School of Medicine; Department of Medicine, National Jewish Medical and Research Center, Denver, Colorado.

L. B. Heifets: Department of Microbiology, University of Colorado Health Sciences Center; Mycobacteriology Clinical Reference Laboratory, National Jewish Medical and Research Center, Denver, Colorado.

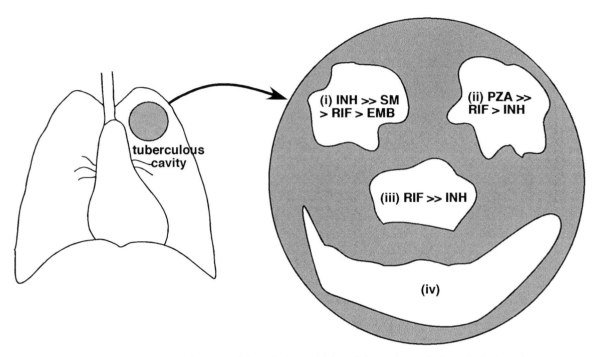

FIGURE 51.1. Schematic diagram of the relative activities of the major antituberculosis drugs in the context of the various *in vivo* populations of *Mycobacterium tuberculosis* in a tuberculous lung cavity. Isoniazid *(INH)* has the greatest early bactericidal activity against *(i)* actively metabolizing and rapidly growing mycobacteria. Pyrazinamide *(PZA)* and rifampin *(RIF)* have the greatest sterilizing activity against *(ii)* semidormant mycobacteria in an acidic environment, and *(iii)* semidormant bacteria in a nonacidic environment, respectively. *EMB*, ethambutol; *SM*, streptomycin.

human plasma, bronchoalveolar lavage fluid, and even alveolar cells was recently described (7).

Mechanisms of Action and Antimicrobial Activity

PZA is active only against *M. tuberculosis* and *Mycobacterium africanum*; it is inactive against *Mycobacterium bovis* and the nontuberculous mycobacteria. In a cell-free, acidic environment (pH 5.5), the MIC of PZA was approximately 16 μg/mL in liquid medium containing Tween-80, 8 to 16 μg/mL in high citrate medium without Tween-80, and 6.2 to 60 μg/mL in 7H12 broth (8,9). PZA displays a dramatic sterilizing activity against semidormant bacteria, induced by maintaining broth culture at pH 4.8 to 5.0. In this instance, the presence of 50 μg/mL PZA led to a sharp

decline in the number of viable bacteria by more than 1,000-fold (10). However, such an acidic environment is quite unfavorable for *M. tuberculosis*. To obviate this issue, one technique used a 7H12 broth medium with the BACTEC radiometric assay in which *M. tuberculosis* isolates were initially cultivated at pH 6.8 and, after reaching the logarithmic growth phase, the solution was made acidic to pH 5.5 and PZA added (11). This method was able to distinguish between PZA-sensitive and PZA-resistant strains. Currently, laboratory testing for PZA susceptibility uses a 7H12 broth at pH 6.0 using PZA concentrations (e.g., 100, 300, and 900 μg/mL) that far exceeds that attainable *in vivo* as measured in serum (12). The rationale for this protocol is that the major goal of susceptibility testing is to distinguish between PZA-susceptible and PZA-resistant strains. The minimal bactericidal concentration (MBC) of PZA has not been determined because even with PZA concentrations as high as 1,000 μg/mL, the proportion of the bacterial population killed was not greater than 74% (10,13). Other problematic issues with PZA susceptibility testing is that false resistance to PZA may be reported when there is excessive inoculum of *M. tuberculosis* or the medium contains excessive bovine serum albumin (BSA), either of which can lead to alkalinization of the medium and to falsely elevated MICs (9,14,15). Based on these subtle but important laboratory nuances, we believe that the

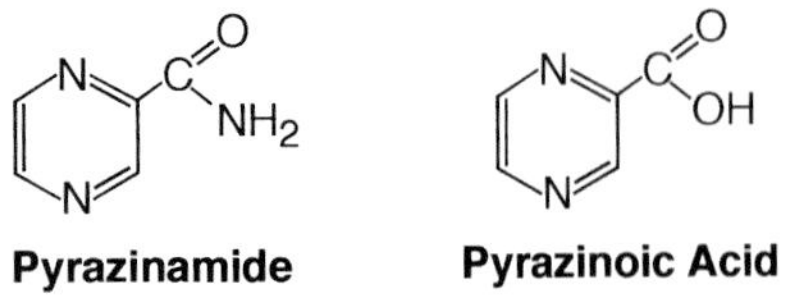

FIGURE 51.2. Structure of pyrazinamide and its metabolite, pyrazinoic acid.

Pyrazinamide   **Pyrazinoic Acid**

method for PZA drug susceptibility testing to differentiate susceptible and resistant clinical isolates should use either a 7H12 broth at a pH of 6.0 to 6.2 with three PZA concentrations of 100, 300, and 900 µg/mL or a test in this medium with 300 µg/mL or a new agar medium at pH 6.2 containing 10% fetal bovine serum with PZA concentrations of 900 and 1,200 µg/mL (14,16).

With peak concentrations attainable *in vivo* (30 to 40 µg/mL), PZA is active only in acidic environments (it has no activity measurable at pH 7.0 to 7.4), and it was suggested early that perhaps the effect of PZA *in vivo* took place in the acidic environment of phagolysosomes of macrophages. However, recent evidence indicates that the phagosomes where the bacilli reside are nearly pH neutral (17,18). This has led to the hypothesis that the *in vivo* effect of PZA is not against intracellular bacteria but rather occurs primarily in the acidic environment of the early inflammation sites. As acute inflammation and acidity decreases, the activity of PZA decreases. This hypothesis was recently corroborated by an *in vitro* experiment in which PZA had neither bacteriostatic nor bactericidal activity against *M. tuberculosis* persisting or multiplying in cultured human monocyte–derived macrophages (19). In addition, this model would explain why the main contribution of PZA is seen only in the first 2 months of therapy (1,20).

The PZA mechanism of anti-TB action is not precisely known, although it is believed to be active against a semi-dormant mycobacterial subpopulation (ii) in an acidic environment (1). Crowle et al. (21) showed that addition of a supraphysiologic concentration (4 µg/mL) of vitamin D₃ enhanced PZA killing of *M. tuberculosis*. It has been hypothesized that PZA is a prodrug and that susceptible strains of *M. tuberculosis* produce pyrazinamidase, which converts PZA to POA, the purported antimicrobial moiety of PZA (22). Although POA does display a dose-dependent antimicrobial activity against *M. tuberculosis*, the MICs of POA against *M. tuberculosis* were eight- to 16-fold greater than the

MICs of PZA and were in the range of 240 to 480 µg/mL in liquid 7H12 medium (23). In contrast, Speirs et al. (24) found comparable POA and PZA MICs in liquid Dubos medium. As revealed insightfully by Zhang et al. (15), the principal reason for this discrepancy is that in the former study (23), the stock POA concentration may have been underestimated because POA has poor solubility in water, leading to overestimation of POA MICs. Subsequently, it was shown that *M. tuberculosis* was equally susceptible to both PZA and POA on 7H11 agar medium when POA was dissolved in dimethyl sulfoxide (15). Another potential cause of the apparent discrepancy in MICs between PZA and POA is the fact that conversion of POA occurs at the surface of the bacterial cell or within it. A third reason is the presence of bovine serum albumin (BSA) in the fetal bovine serum–containing culture medium (15); at relatively high BSA concentrations greater than 0.5% (e.g., 1% or 2%), BSA binds preferentially to the weak acid POA but not neutral amide PZA, resulting in falsely elevated POA MICs. Therefore, it has become clearer in recent years that indeed POA plays an important role, directly or indirectly, in the anti-TB activity of PZA. Furthermore, acid pH enhances the uptake and accumulation of POA in *M. tuberculosis* (15). It was also shown that *M. tuberculosis* has a defective efflux mechanism for intracellular POA, as opposed to other mycobacteria, accounting for the unique susceptibility of *M. tuberculosis* to PZA (Fig. 51.3) (25). Recently, Zhang et al. (15) also showed that reserpine, a multidrug resistance efflux pump inhibitor, can enhance the susceptibility of H37Ra *M. tuberculosis* to PZA, lowering PZA MICs from more than 1,000 mg/L to 400 mg/L, even at a near-neutral pH of 6.8 (Fig. 51.3A). In contrast, reserpine had no effect on POA MICs. The reasoning is that at a near-neutral pH of 6.8, POA is charged and therefore cannot penetrate the bacterial cells easily, whereas PZA penetrates and is converted to POA intracellularly, which is then subjected to the POA efflux inhibitory effects of reserpine.

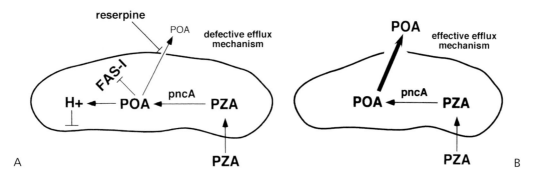

FIGURE 51.3. Proposed mechanistic action of pyrazinamide (*PZA*). PZA is converted to pyrazinoic acid (*POA*) by pyrazinamidase (*pncA*). POA is considered to play an important role, directly or indirectly, in the antimycobacterial activity of PZA. The ability of PZA to kill *M. tuberculosis* **(A)** and not the other *Mycobacteria* species **(B)** is considered to be owing to a selective defect in the POA efflux mechanism in *M. tuberculosis*. Proposed targets for PZA/POA include the mycobacterial enzyme fatty acid synthetase I (*FAS-I*), and the disruption of mycobacterial membranes by the acidic (*H+*) action of POA.

Zimhony et al. (26) showed that the target for PZA in *M. tuberculosis* was fatty acid synthetase I (Fig. 51.3A). The mechanism is likely to be more complicated because recently it was shown that although fatty acid synthetase I could be inhibited by 5-chloro-PZA, purified fatty acid synthetase I was not inhibited by POA (27). Another hypothesis of the target of PZA is that POA lowers the intracellular pH, destabilizing the mycobacterial membrane (Fig. 51.3A) (8,28).

Clinical Efficacy and Use in Tuberculosis Patients

In earlier works from East Africa, the addition of either PZA or rifampin to the basic streptomycin/isoniazid regimen substantially reduced the relapse rate, although rifampin was slightly more effective than PZA (29). Moreover, addition of *both* rifampin and PZA to the streptomycin/isoniazid regimen further lowered the relapse rate (30,31). Other studies from Hong Kong, Poland, and the United States also showed the favorable impact that PZA had on relapse rate (summarized in reference 32). Currently, the combination of PZA with isoniazid and rifampin forms the basis of the standard regimen recommended by the American Thoracic Society/Centers for Disease Control and Prevention and World Health Organization 6-month regimens (33). The addition of PZA to isoniazid and rifampin was the key step to reducing the duration of treatment from 9 to 6 months while achieving a greater than 95% cure rate. This therapeutic effect of PZA is believed to be owing to its role in augmenting the sterilizing effect on population (ii) of Mitchison's model. Multiple studies document the lack of additional benefit when PZA was given beyond the first 2 months to patients with drug-susceptible TB, a finding that would corroborate the sterilizing activity of PZA in the initially acidic inflammatory debris (32,34–36).

PZA is available in 500-mg tablets or as 300-mg fixed-dose combination tablets with isoniazid (50 mg) and rifampin (120 mg) known as Rifater. The recommended PZA dose is 15 to 30 mg/kg daily only for the first 2 months of therapy. Although PZA had no sterilizing activity in the continuation phase of therapy, it has been suggested that in patients with initial isoniazid resistance, it may be of some value beyond the initial 2 months of treatment (37). However, in the context of drugs available, these studies were suboptimal because they compared isoniazid alone with isoniazid plus PZA in the continuation phase in mycobacteria with initial resistance to streptomycin or isoniazid. PZA can also be given twice or thrice weekly after 2 weeks of a daily regimen. The twice- or thrice-weekly regimen dose is 50 mg/kg daily, not to exceed 3 g per day.

Two months of PZA combined with rifampin daily has also been recommended as an alternative to isoniazid for treatment of latent TB (38). This regimen was regarded favorably because of its potency in the mouse model (39,40). However, 20 known cases of serious hepatitis and five deaths associated with early use of the regimen led to new stringent precautions (41).

Although PZA has been shown to penetrate well into cerebrospinal fluid, its efficacy in TB meningitis has not been rigorously demonstrated. It is possible that the milieu in TB meningitis is not sufficiently acidic to promote PZA activity. A recent case report is consistent with that hypothesis (42). Meningitis evolved several months into treatment of miliary multidrug-resistant TB with isoniazid, rifampin, PZA, and EMB; the strain was resistant to isoniazid, rifampin, and EMB but susceptible to PZA (42). Although this case raises questions about the utility of PZA in central nervous system TB, it does not, in our estimation, preclude its use.

Mechanism of Resistance

A few mechanisms of resistance have been reported for PZA in mycobacteria. Scorpio and Zhang (43) showed that mutations in the gene-encoding pyrazinamidase (*pncA*) is primarily responsible for the resistance to PZA. Various types of mutations have been described, including upstream mutations, missense changes, nucleotide insertions and deletions, and termination mutations (44). Thus, in *pncA*-mutated mycobacteria, there is a lack of conversion of PZA to POA, resulting in PZA resistance. In subsequent confirmatory studies, approximately 72% to 98% of clinical isolates resistant to PZA had mutations throughout the 558-base pair (bp) *pcnA* coding region and the −11 promoter region (44–46). In one of these studies, 32 of 33 (97%) isolates with negative pyrazinamidase activity had a *pncA* gene mutation. Additionally, none of the 135 clinical isolates with positive pyrazinamidase activity had mutations in the *pncA* gene (45). Inexplicably, however, three mutants with *in vitro*–selected PZA resistance were pyrazinamidase positive and showed no mutation in the *pncA* gene, suggesting that additional mechanisms may be involved in PZA resistance (45). Alternatively, the important possibility of false resistance discussed earlier must be taken into consideration with these PZA-resistant but negative *pncA* gene mutation cases (14). Interestingly, testing of various *M. bovis* strains, which are phenotypically resistant to PZA, revealed a very high frequency of C to G substitution at position 169 of the *pncA* gene, rendering it nonfunctional (47). Boshoff and Mizrahi (48) showed that integration of the *M. tuberculosis pncA* gene or of the *Mycobacterium smegmatis pzaA* gene, which also encodes for a pyrazinamidase, into a *pncA* mutant strain of PZA-resistant *M. tuberculosis* reconstituted the susceptibility to PZA.

Adverse Reactions

Hepatotoxicity is the major concern in PZA therapy. The effect is dose related, affecting as many as 15% of patients receiving the *previously* recommended dose of 40 to 50 mg/kg daily (~3 gm/d) (20). The current recommended dose of 15 to 30 mg/kg daily has significantly less risk of hepatotoxicity. Moreover, PZA is considered to be significantly less hepatotoxic than isoniazid and rifampin because the frequency of hepatotoxicity in patients who received PZA in doses of 25 to 35 mg/kg along with isoniazid and rifampin was the same as among those who received the latter two drugs alone (2,49,50). However, a hypersensitivity-like reaction resulting in severe hepatitis may rarely occur with PZA (51).

Recently, over a 6-month period in 2001, a total of 21 cases of serious liver injury, including five deaths, was reported to the Centers for Disease Control and Prevention in patients taking the combination of rifampin and PZA for the treatment of latent TB (52). Unfortunately, the denominator (i.e., the number of patients on this regimen) is not known but is estimated to be fewer than 10,000 individuals. Nevertheless, these serious cases of hepatotoxicity have resulted in updated recommendations published jointly by American Thoracic Society/Centers for Disease Control and Prevention on the use of the short-course rifampin-PZA treatment for latent TB (41). The new recommendations are that for all individuals, regardless of human immunodeficiency virus status, 9 months of daily isoniazid is preferred over the 2-month rifampin/PZA regimen for the treatment of latent TB as long as treatment completion can be ensured. The 2-month regimen may be considered when completion of longer treatment courses is unlikely and the patient can be monitored closely (41). Manifestations of hepatotoxicity include asymptomatic elevations in serum aminotransferases, jaundice, and liver tenderness. One recommendation for monitoring for rifampin + PZA–induced hepatotoxicity is to determine the levels of serum aminotransferases at baseline and at 2, 4, and 6 weeks of treatment and to discontinue rifampin/PZA when there is (a) serum aminotransferase level that exceeds five times the upper limit of normal in an asymptomatic individual, (b) any elevation of serum aminotransferases that is accompanied by symptoms of hepatitis, or (c) any elevation in serum bilirubin (41). In considering the explanation for this unanticipated risk of severe hepatitis, it may be relevant to reexamine the serious hepatitis reported when PZA and ofloxacin were given to contacts of patients with multidrug-resistant TB in New York City (53) and Orange County, CA (54). In both of these settings, serious hepatitis led to discontinuation of treatment in approximately half of the subjects. Based on these reports, it is not unreasonable to speculate that the increased risk of hepatotoxicity from PZA may be somehow, unintuitively, be related to the *absence* of isoniazid.

Other relatively common adverse effects of PZA include nausea, vomiting, anorexia, and elevation in serum uric acid, which may be either asymptomatic or associated with polyarthralgia, especially of the shoulders (55). Less common adverse reactions to PZA include rhabdomyolysis with myoglobinuric renal failure, gouty arthritis, photosensitivity, maculopapular rash, thrombocytopenia, sideroblastic anemia, increased serum iron, urticaria, and other hypersensitivity reactions. The gastrointestinal distress is common initially but generally abate with continued therapy with or without symptomatic treatment (32). PZA-induced elevation in serum uric acid concentration is owing to the ability of POA to block renal tubular excretion of uric acid (56). The frequency of polyarthralgia is significantly decreased with intermittent PZA therapy (e.g., thrice weekly), a finding substantiated by experimental evidence that less uric acid is retained with intermittent PZA therapy (56,57).

Concomitant administration of PZA to patients on rifampicin may increase the latter's renal clearance, although no empirical dose changes in rifampicin are recommended (58).

ETHAMBUTOL

Structure and Pharmacologic Properties

EMB (dextro-2,2′-(ethylenediimino)-di-1-butanol), a synthetic compound with structural similarity to D-arabinose (Fig. 51.4), was first introduced in 1961 (59–61). EMB given orally is 75% to 80% absorbed. Food does not interfere with EMB uptake, although absorption is decreased

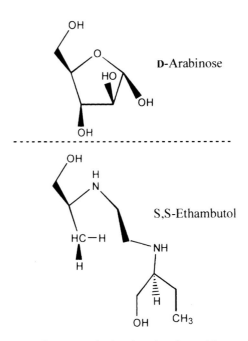

FIGURE 51.4. Structure of ethambutol and D-arabinose, the latter is present in a polymeric form in the mycobacterial cell wall components arabinogalactan and lipoarabinomannan. Ethambutol, an open chain structure, is drawn to schematically mimic D-arabinose.

with concomitant use of antacids. Peak levels correlate with dose, e.g., a 15-mg/kg dose results in a peak level of 2 to 4 μg/mL, whereas a 25-mg/kg dose results in a peak level of 4 to 6 μg/mL (62). It has rapid, good distribution throughout the body, including pulmonary macrophages (63), with the exception of the central nervous system. Thus, even with meningeal inflammation, only 10% to 50% of the plasma level is obtained in the cerebrospinal fluid. EMB is excreted mainly unchanged (~80%) by the kidneys, and therefore the dose must be reduced for patients with renal insufficiency (64). EMB is not significantly removed by hemodialysis (6). Median recovery of EMB in dialysate was only 2% of the dose administered, and the median hemodialysis clearance was 46 mL/min.

Mechanisms of Action and Antimicrobial Activity

The spectrum of activity of EMB includes *M. tuberculosis* and many of the slow-growing, nontuberculous mycobacte-

ria. The precise mode of action of EMB and the molecular basis of resistance are not fully understood. Early studies conducted with EMB demonstrated that the *S,S*, absolute stereochemistry was essential for activity and its bacteriostatic property. The effects of EMB are pleiotropic, and several hypotheses have been proposed for its mode of action. Although many of the original works were carried out on mycobacterial species other than *M. tuberculosis*, based on structure–activity studies, the effects attributed to EMB included inhibition of (a) RNA metabolism (65,66), (b) phospholipid synthesis (67), (c) transfer of mycolic acids to cell wall linked arabinogalactan (68), (d) spermidine synthesis (69), and (e) an early step of glucose conversion into monosaccharides constituting cell wall polysaccharides such as arabinogalactan and arabinomannan. As shown in Figures 51.4 and 51.5, EMB could conceivably behave as an arabinose mimetic, competitively inhibiting specific steps in the biosynthesis of cell wall components. Indeed, Takayama and Kilburn (70) showed that the primary effect of EMB is on the inhibition of synthesis of the arabinan component of the

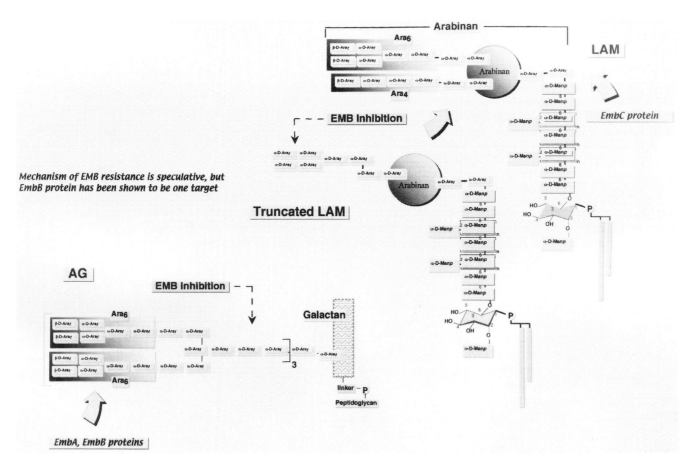

FIGURE 51.5. Schematic representation depicts the action of ethambutol (*EMB*). EMB inhibits the arabinan of lipoarabinomannan (*LAM*) and produces a discrete population of truncated LAM (75). We believe that a similar phenomenon occurs in arabinogalactan (*AG*), although a truncated AG has not been analyzed thus far. The EmbA and EmbB proteins have now been shown to participate only in AG (82) synthesis and speculated to be α-(1→3) arabinosyltransferases. EmbC, conversely, acts on LAM in an unknown manner. Zhang N, et al. *Mol Microbiol* 2003 (in press).

cell wall macromolecule arabinogalactan. Extending this observation, it was shown subsequently that this effect applied to both the arabinan of arabinogalactan and of lipoarabinomannan, but in succession such that the inhibition of radioactive carbon (^{14}C) on the arabinan of arabinogalactan was immediate, whereas that on lipoarabinomannan occurred only after 1 hour (71). This differential effect suggested that the site of action was not in the early stages of arabinan synthesis but rather in the final polymerization steps (72). In support of this, the transfer of arabinofuranose (Ara*f*) from β-D-arabinofuranosyl-P-decaprenol to the arabinan polymer was inhibited by EMB. Hence, the arabinosyltransferases were implicated as targets of EMB (73).

The inhibitory effects of EMB on the biosynthesis of arabinan have been demonstrated at several levels (70,71,74). Subsequently, the interesting phenomenon of truncated lipoarabinomannan was reported for the fast-growing, EMB-resistant *M. smegmatis* that were grown in the presence of EMB (Fig. 51.5) (75). Further studies in EMB-resistant clinical isolates of *M. tuberculosis* showed a reduction in mannose capping that decorates the terminal end of lipoarabinomannan (76), the cell wall associated macromolecule implicated in many of the pathogenic attributes of *M. tuberculosis*. It has been argued that reduction in mannose capping, resulting in a truncated lipoarabinomannan, is owing to the consequence of the disruption of the machinery that assembles a complete arabinan in lipoarabinomannan (Fig. 51.5).

During the course and description of these biochemical works, genes encoding the cellular target of EMB were simultaneously identified in *M. avium* by using drug resistance and overexpression as a selection tool. It was further established that these two genes (*embA* and *embB*) were required to confer low levels of resistance to EMB when overexpressed in an otherwise susceptible *M. smegmatis* host. These genes encode novel membrane proteins and share amino acid similarities in the range of 61% to 68%. The *embA* and *embB* genes are translationally coupled, typical for proteins with coordinated expression, and are predicted to form a multienzyme complex. Three contiguous genes encoding putative target(s) for EMB and termed *embC*, *embA*, and *embB* have since been identified in *M. tuberculosis* (77). The *embCAB* gene cluster was initially identified in an EMB-resistant strain of *M. smegmatis* and was subsequently characterized in both *M. tuberculosis* (77) and *Mycobacterium leprae* (78). Two of these genes were similar to the *embA* and *embB* genes described in *M. avium*, and the third one was termed as *embC*. These genes are likely to be organized as an operon in the order *embC*, *embA*, and *embB*. The EmbCAB proteins are predicted to be typical membrane proteins with 12-transmembrane domains and a C-terminal globular region of approximately 400 amino acids of predicted periplasmic location. These enzymes are well conserved among different mycobacteria (68,70,79,80).

It has also been shown that EmbB is the primary target of EMB. Telenti et al. (77) postulated that amino acid 306 of EmbB, the mutation of which may lead to resistance (see later), is located in a cytoplasmic loop that forms an EMB resistance–determining region. Furthermore, it has been shown that amino acids in this region are well conserved among EmbB proteins across mycobacterial species (81). This implies that natural resistance to EMB results from an accumulation of genetic events determining overexpression of the Emb proteins (EmbA, EmbB, and EmbC) and/or structural mutations in EmbB (72).

In a recent study, it was shown that inactivation of *embA* and *embB* genes in *M. smegmatis* led to severe alteration in the morphology, drug permeability, and arabinose content of cell wall arabinogalactan (82). Moreover, detailed biochemical characterization revealed that these mutants had defective terminal hexaarabinofuranosyl (Ara$_6$) arrangements. Specifically, a primary lesion in these mutants was demonstrated to be in the three-arm branch off the α-5 arabinan chain. Thus, a substantial amount of the otherwise predominant Ara$_6$ branched structure was found to be converted to the linear Ara$_4$ arrangement. The Ara$_6$ being the template for mycolylation, the mutants also contained lesser mycolates leading to altered physiologic behavior mentioned previously. Both of the *embA*−/− and *embB*−/− mutants exhibited similar defects in arabinogalactan, thereby supporting the hypothesis that EmbA and EmbB proteins share similar functions. Although these cumulative studies bring us a step closer to stating that Emb proteins are indeed arabinosyltransferases, numerous questions still remain to be addressed. For instance, the transmembrane domains present in these proteins suggest that they could also be involved in transporting arabinogalactan/lipoarabinomannan precursors across the plasma membrane, making these proteins bifunctional. Future work on delineation of the catalytic and active sites of these proteins coupled with identification of more Emb proteins in EMB-resistant clinical isolates may provide an in-depth a view of a precise role of Emb proteins and mechanism of EMB drug action and resistance.

EMB is active only against actively multiplying bacteria, although its EBA is not as potent as isoniazid (83,84). The MICs of ethambutol in various liquid and solid media were found to be 0.5 to 2 μg/mL; in 7H12 BACTEC broth and in 7H10 agar, the MICs were 0.95 to 3.8 μg/mL and 1.9 to 7.5 μg/mL, respectively (8,85,86). The MBCs ranged from 3.8 to 60 μg/mL (85). The MBC/MIC ratio is relatively high (~8), and thus it is not clear whether its early antimycobacterial activity is owing to its bactericidal or inhibitory effect (8,85).

Clinical Efficacy and Use in Tuberculosis Patients

EMB was first recommended for use in the treatment of TB in 1966 (87). In the 1970s and early 1980s, the standard treatment regimen for TB in the United States was 18 months of daily isoniazid and EMB with an initial 2-month course of streptomycin (32,88–91). In a study of patients with pulmonary TB treated initially for an average of 3.5 months with isoniazid, rifampicin, and EMB, continuation treatment for an additional year with EMB + isoniazid was as effective as rifampin + isoniazid (92). Subsequently, it was found that the addition of EMB to the superior isoniazid/rifampin/streptomycin regimen did not increase the rate of 2-month negative cultures, a marker for relapse rate (93). In fact, the replacement of PZA by EMB increased the relapse rate (94). Thus, EMB contributes only modestly to the standard regimen of isoniazid, rifampin, and PZA (32). Today, the principal value of EMB is that it is used empirically, along with isoniazid, rifampin, and PZA, in the empirical treatment of TB in individuals deemed at risk of preexisting drug resistance, especially to isoniazid and/or streptomycin (37). In *M. tuberculosis* resistant to both isoniazid and rifampin, EMB forms an important component in the armamentarium. Early studies indicated predictable additive effects of EMB with other anti-TB medications including isoniazid and rifampin (95).

EMB is available in 100- and 400-mg tablets. The dose of EMB is 25 mg/kg daily for the first 2 months, followed by 15 mg/kg daily, with efficacy comparable with that of higher dose therapy used in early studies (91).

Mechanism of Resistance

Resistance to EMB occurs mostly among the isolates that are also resistant to isoniazid and rifampin (96). Owing to the identification of the *embCAB* genes, analysis of the molecular basis of resistance of mycobacteria to EMB was made possible. Sequence analysis of a high-level, EMB-resistant mutant of *M. smegmatis* DNA and comparison with the wild-type strain revealed mutation that results in an isoleucine to phenylalanine substitution in the EmbB protein (97). This alteration (Ile289Phe) is located in the loop that is predicted to be of cytoplasmic location. Two other distinct EMB-resistant *M. smegmatis* strains carried a isoleucine to methionine (Ile289Met) or methionine to threonine (Met292Thr) substitution in EmbB (97). In *M. tuberculosis*, mutations associated with resistance involved substitution of methionine with valine, leucine, or isoleucine at position 306 of EmbB (98). This mutation was also observed in 47% of clinical isolates. It has been postulated that EMB may bind to a pocket in EmbB in the region containing Met306 and a mutation in this region would cause a lower affinity of binding of EMB to EmbB, leading to resistance (99). Although mutation in the *embB* gene has been directly correlated with EMB resistance (98), mutations in *embA* and *embC* have not been identified thus far.

Despite substantial progress made in establishing some targets of EMB, there is substantial work that is still required to establish the molecular basis of EMB resistance in *M. tuberculosis*. Future studies should include identification of mutations in discrete domains in the Emb proteins, likely arabinosyltransferases, resulting in defective EMB–Emb protein interactions.

Adverse Reactions and Drug Interactions

The major toxicities associated with EMB are optic neuritis and peripheral neuropathy owing to demyelinization. With the eye toxicity, which appears to be dose related, there are defects in both visual acuity and red-green color vision (100,101). In patients prescribed EMB, it is recommended that, after obtaining baseline visual acuity and color perception tests, these tests be repeated every 4 to 6 weeks, especially with new visual symptoms. Other less common adverse effects of EMB include gastrointestinal intolerance, hyperuricemia, and hypersensitivity reactions including rash, and, rarely, thrombocytopenia (102). In general, EMB is considered safe during pregnancy with no known teratologic effects (103,104).

There are no significant drug interactions with EMB except for decreased EMB absorption with concomitant administration of aluminum hydroxide antacids (105).

ETHIONAMIDE

Structure and Pharmacologic Properties

Ethionamide is structurally related to isoniazid (Fig. 51.6). Ethionamide was synthesized in 1956 and its anti-TB activity documented in 1959 (106). Ethionamide is absorbed well when taken orally, giving peak plasma concentrations of 1 to 5 μg/mL (32). It penetrates well into the cerebrospinal fluid, even in normal meninges. It is metabolized by the liver, and a small amount is excreted renally.

Mechanisms of Action and Antimicrobial Activity

Similar to isoniazid, ethionamide is also an inhibitor of mycolic acid synthesis, although it is less potent than isoni-

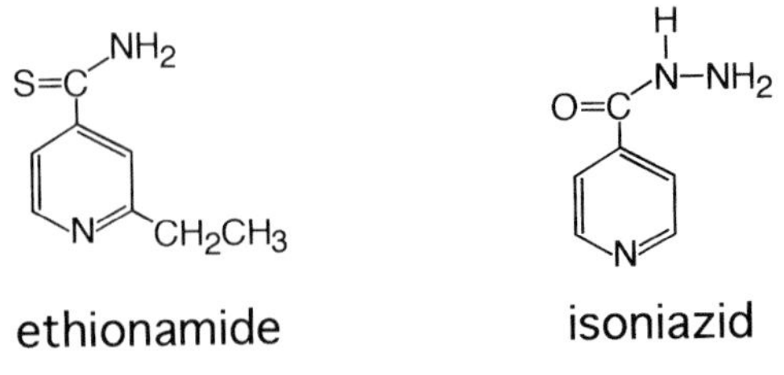

FIGURE 51.6. Structure of ethionamide and similarity to isoniazid.

azid (107). Thus, it is only active against *Mycobacteria* species. Heifets et al. (108) determined the MICs of ethionamide for 14 drug-susceptible strains of *M. tuberculosis* and found the MIC to range from 0.3 to 1.25 μg/mL in 7H12 broth. The MICs in 7H11 agar were higher at approximately 2.5 to 10 μg/mL. When three of the strains were tested simultaneously for MICs and MBCs by sampling and plating from 7H12 broth and counting the number of colony-forming units per milliliter, the MBCs were 2.5 to 5 μg/mL, giving an MBC/MIC ratio of 2 or 4. Thus, susceptible strains are defined as an MIC of 1.25 μg/mL or less, moderately susceptible as 2.5 μg/mL, moderately resistant as 5 μg/mL, and resistant as more than 10 μg/mL (109).

Clinical Efficacy and Use in Tuberculosis Patients

Ethionamide is considered a second-line agent typically used in the treatment of multidrug-resistant TB. Because ethionamide and isoniazid have structural similarity, it is a theoretical concern that concomitant use may result in interference with isoniazid acetylation. Ethionamide is available in 250-mg tablets. The recommended initial dose is 250 mg twice daily and increased as tolerated until a maximum of 1,000 mg daily is reached, although this dose is rarely tolerable.

Mechanism of Resistance

There is now a clearer understanding of the mechanism of resistance to ethionamide. Mutations within the promoter and coding regions of enoyl-acyl carrier protein reductase gene (*inhA*), which is involved in mycolic acid synthesis, confer resistance to both isoniazid and ethionamide (110). However, despite this evidence of a potential common target, there is a lack of cross-resistance between the two drugs in clinical isolates (111). More recently, Baulard et al. (112) showed that ethionamide is also a prodrug that is activated by a monooxygenase activator called EthA. A neighboring open-reading frame, termed EthR, was found to negatively regulate the production of EthA. Thus, overexpression of EthR led to decreased production of EthA, which then resulted in less activation of ethionamide, leading to ethionamide resistance. Conversely, overexpression of *ethA* led to hypersensitivity to ethionamide in mycobacteria.

Adverse Reactions and Drug Interactions

Ethionamide is associated with a very high incidence of gastrointestinal distress manifested principally by dysgeusia, anorexia, nausea, vomiting, diarrhea, and a metallic taste in the mouth. Most of the gastrointestinal intolerance can be reduced by slowly increasing the dose, e.g., 250 mg daily for a few days, then twice daily, thrice daily, and, if tolerated,

four times daily (113). Other adverse effects include hepatotoxicity, hypersensitivity reactions, worsened glucose intolerance in diabetics, hypothyroidism, gynecomastia, frozen shoulder syndrome, peripheral neuropathy, and psychiatric and other central nervous system disturbances such as headache, vision changes, and drowsiness. The hepatotoxicity may be associated with prolonged (3 to 6 weeks) elevation of hepatocellular enzymes and may increase for a time even after the drug has been discontinued (113). The risk of hypothyroidism is further increased with concomitant use of paraaminosalicylic acid. Interestingly, the neurologic sequelae may be decreased by pyridoxine or nicotinamide.

Ethionamide is relatively free of drug interactions. Central nervous system side effects may be increased when ethionamide is used in combination with cycloserine or isoniazid (114). In addition, there are theoretical concerns of decreased gastrointestinal absorption with concomitant use of antacids (114).

AMINOGLYCOSIDES AND CAPREOMYCIN

Structure and Pharmacologic Properties

The aminoglycoside antibiotics are effective against an array of bacteria including enterococci, gram-negative bacilli, and mycobacteria. Waksman's discovery of streptomycin in the early 1940s heralded the rationale for TB chemotherapy (115). Since then, several aminoglycosides have been developed with a wide spectrum of activity. Aminoglycosides are structurally defined by the presence of amino sugars bound by glycosidic linkage to a central hexose nucleus (116). The structures of streptomycin, kanamycin, and amikacin, the three aminoglycosides with more substantial activity against *M. tuberculosis*, are shown in Figure 51.7. Capreomycin is a macrocyclic polypeptide antibiotic, isolated from *Streptomyces capreolus*, and not an aminoglycoside, although it has similar activities and toxicities to the aminoglycosides. Owing to poor oral absorption, parenteral administration is required for all the aminoglycosides and for capreomycin. For an adult with normal renal function, a 1,000-mg dose of streptomycin gives a peak serum concentration between 35 and 45 μg/mL (117). This is relevant in light of the fact that aminoglycosides display concentration-dependent killing. The volume of distribution approximates the extracellular space. However, aminoglycosides cross the blood–brain barrier poorly, even with frank meningitis. Concerning pulmonary infections, the drug levels in bronchial secretions is consistently poor. After administration, the serum half-life of aminoglycosides is 2 to 4 hours in individuals with normal renal function. Aminoglycosides are eliminated predominantly by glomerular filtration. Thus, in patients with renal insufficiency, the serum half-life may be considerably prolonged. Aminoglycosides are removed efficiently by hemodialysis (118).

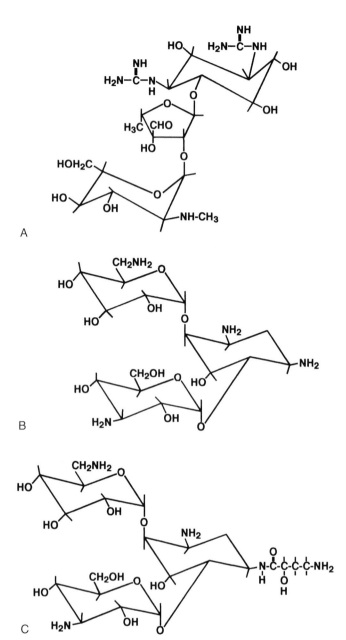

FIGURE 51.7. Structure of streptomycin **(A)**, kanamycin **(B)**, and amikacin **(C)**. Note the structural similarity of kanamycin and amikacin.

Mechanisms of Action and Antimicrobial Activity

The mode of action of the aminoglycosides is irreversible binding to a highly conserved A site of the 16S ribosomal RNA, a subcomponent of the bacterial 30S ribosomal subunit. This binding results in the misreading of messenger RNA translation and thus inhibition of bacterial protein synthesis (119). In gram-negative bacteria, the cationic aminoglycosides are also able to bind to the negatively charged lipopolysaccharide on the bacterial cell membrane, disrupting cell wall function (120). Whether such a mechanism also occurs with the mycobacterial cell wall complex

remains to be determined. The mechanism of action of capreomycin is not known but is also thought to be involved in the inhibition of protein synthesis via interaction with the 70S ribosome (72).

In general, the MICs of streptomycin, kanamycin, and amikacin are similar in various types of liquid and solid media, ranging from 0.4 to 3.0 μg/mL (86,121,122). The MBCs for four strains of mycobacteria, between 0.5 and 2.0 μg/mL, was very close to the MICs for streptomycin, kanamycin, and amikacin (121). Thus, the MICs for the aminoglycosides and for capreomycin are well below their peak plasma concentrations and the MBC/MIC ratios are relatively low (123). The MICs and MBCs for capreomycin are also similar to the aminoglycosides (Table 51.1) (121). In low pH environments or anaerobic conditions, the transport and efficacy of aminoglycosides are severely impaired. In a murine model of TB, the antimycobacterial activity of streptomycin, kanamycin, and amikacin (all at 200 mg/kg) were compared with isoniazid (25 mg/kg) in Swiss mice intravenously inoculated with H37Rv strain of *M. tuberculosis* (124). All surviving mice were killed on day 30. Based on survival rate, spleen weights, gross lung lesions, and numbers of colony-forming units in the spleens, isoniazid was more bactericidal than any of the aminoglycosides, although amikacin was the most active of the aminoglycosides. Donald et al. (125) tested amikacin for its EBA in South Africans with smear-positive pulmonary TB. Compared with isoniazid, which displayed the expected significant EBA, amikacin in doses of 5, 10, or 15 mg/kg showed essentially no EBA. This lack of EBA occurred despite serum levels that were far in excess of the MIC of 2 to 4 μg/mL. One possible explanation for this seeming paradox between the poor *in vivo* EBA compared with the excellent *in vitro* activity of the aminoglycosides is that activity in the *in vivo* acidic environment is likely decreased because aminoglycoside activity is critically dependent on pH.

Clinical Efficacy and Use in Tuberculosis Patients

The two aminoglycosides with the greatest *in vitro* activity against *M. tuberculosis* are streptomycin and amikacin (Table 51.2). Streptomycin was the subject of the first controlled treatment trial for TB, in which patients were randomized to either bed rest alone or bed rest plus streptomycin (126). Although streptomycin-treated patients initially improved, their course was characterized by the now expected development of streptomycin-resistant TB (127). Subsequently, streptomycin-containing regimens, with rare exceptions, formed the basis of the many randomized short-course trials carried out in East and Central Africa, Hong Kong, Singapore, and India (1). Overall, the addition of streptomycin to isoniazid, rifampin, and PZA during the initial phase modestly enhanced the outcome (32). In fact, although EMB is commonly used as the

TABLE 51.1. SUSCEPTIBILITY AND PEAK PLASMA CONCENTRATIONS

Drug	Peak Plasma Concentration (μg/mL)	Susceptible (MIC μg/mL)	Moderately Susceptible (MIC μg/mL)	Moderately Resistant (MIC μg/mL)	Resistant (MIC μg/mL)
Pyrazinamide	20–50 q.d. 40–80 b.i.w.	≤100	300	900	>900
Ethambutol	2–4 with 15 mg/kg dose; 4–6 with 25 mg/kg dose	≤2.0	4.0	8.0	≥16
Ethionamide	1–5	≤1.25	2.5	5.0	>10
Streptomycin, amikacin, kanamycin, capreomycin	35–45[a]	≤2.0	4.0	8.0	≥16

[a]Using the 2- and 6-hour postdose concentrations and linear regression, the C_{max} value (end of infusion concentration) can be calculated. Because time is needed for drug distribution, peak concentrations should not be drawn at the end of infusion because they will be falsely high.
MIC, minimal inhibitory concentration; q.d., once daily; b.i.w., twice weekly.

fourth drug to accompany isoniazid, rifampin, and PZA in short-course regimens, the overall relapse rate was lower when streptomycin rather than EMB was used as the fourth drug: relapse rate was approximately 6% in the streptomycin-containing regimens compared with 9% for the EMB-containing regimens (32). The indications for initiating empirical streptomycin or another aminoglycoside therapy include a high prevalence of initial drug resistance, very extensive disease, or malabsorption or inability to deliver oral drugs (32). Capreomycin is principally used for patients with multidrug-resistant TB who are also resistant to the aminoglycosides and/or are intolerant to them, although many of the adverse reactions between aminoglycosides and capreomycin are similar.

The recommended daily dose of streptomycin, kanamycin, and amikacin for TB for an adult is 15 mg/kg for persons 55 years of age or younger and with normal renal function. For those older than 55 years or weighing less than 50 kg, the usual daily dose is 750 mg (32). For a twice- or thrice-weekly regimen, the recommended dose for the

TABLE 51.2. DOSING OF PYRAZINAMIDE, ETHAMBUTOL, ETHIONAMIDE, AND AMINOGLYCOSIDES FOR TUBERCULOSIS

Drug	Daily Dose (mg/kg) [Maximal Dose (g)]	Twice-Weekly Dose (mg/kg) [Maximal Dose (g)]	Thrice-Weekly Dose (mg/kg) [Maximal Dose (g)]
Pyrazinamide	Children and adults: 15–30 mg/kg (2 g)	Children and adults: 50–70 mg/kg (4 g)	Children and adults: 50–70 mg/kg (3 g)
Ethambutol	Children and adults: 15–25 mg/kg (2.5 g)	Children and adults: 50 mg/kg	Children and adults: 25–30 mg/kg
Ethionamide	Children: 15–20 mg/kg; adults: 500–1,000 mg in divided doses		
Streptomycin[a] i.m. or i.v. (149)	Children: 20–30 mg/kg (1 g); adults: 15 mg/kg (1 g)[b]	Children and adults: 25–30 mg/kg (1.5 g)	Children and adults: 25–30 mg/kg (1.5 g)
Amikacin/kanamycin	Children: 15–30 mg/kg; adults: 15 mg/kg	After bacteriologic conversion, dose can be reduced to 2 to 3 times weekly	After bacteriologic conversion, dose can be reduced to 2 to 3 times weekly
Capreomycin (i.m. or i.v.)	Children: 15–30 mg/kg; adults: 15 mg/kg (1 g)	After bacteriologic conversion, dose can be reduced to 2 to 3 times weekly	After bacteriologic conversion, dose can be reduced to 2 to 3 times weekly

[a]Dose of streptomycin in intermittent therapy varies widely from 1,000 mg two or three times weekly to approximately 1,600 mg twice weekly. When used with other potent drugs such as isoniazid, rifampin, or pyrazinamide with or without ethambutol, higher dosing may not be required.
[b]For persons older than 55 years or weighing less than 50 kg, the maximal daily dose is 750 mg.
i.m., intramuscular; i.v., intravenous.
Adapted from American Thoracic Society and Centers for Disease Control and Prevention. Treatment of tuberculosis and tuberculosis infection in adults and children. *Am J Respir Crit Care Med* 1994;149:1359–1374 and Centers for Disease Control and Prevention, Division of Tuberculosis Elimination. *Core curriculum on tuberculosis.* Atlanta: CDC, 1994.

aminoglycosides is 25 mg/kg. For patients with renal insufficiency, the initial loading dose is 5 to 7.5 mg/kg with subsequent reduced doses guided by estimated or calculated creatinine clearance and by serum drug levels. Because serum level determination for kanamycin or streptomycin typically requires a referral laboratory, amikacin may be preferred for patients with decreased renal function because laboratory determination of amikacin levels is more widely available. Amikacin, kanamycin, and capreomycin are approved for use by the U.S. Food and Drug Administration for intravenous use. Although streptomycin is only approved for intramuscular use, it has been given intravenously under an investigational protocol with no overall prohibitive adverse effect (32,128).

Mechanism of Resistance

In general, resistance to aminoglycosides may result from alteration in uptake, bacterial enzymatic modification of the aminoglycoside molecule, and/or alteration in the ribosome binding sites (129). The first two types of mechanisms have not been described for the mycobacteria. Because of structural similarities and differences (Fig. 51.7), *M. tuberculosis* cross-resistance occurs between amikacin and kanamycin (130) but not between amikacin/kanamycin compared with streptomycin (131). In *M. tuberculosis*, resistance to amikacin and kanamycin may result from an A → G substitution at position 1400 of the 16S ribosomal RNA gene (*rrs*) (132,133). Streptomycin resistance may be owing to mutations in either the *rpsL* locus encoding the S12 ribosomal protein or two separate regions of the *rrs* gene (134–137). Thus, alteration of either the 16S rRNA binding site or the S12 ribosomal protein, components of the 30S ribosomal subunit, results in the inability of aminoglycosides to disrupt translation of bacterial mRNA, resulting in antibiotic resistance. Alternative mechanisms of resistance such as alteration in uptake or permeability may account for the aminoglycoside-resistant strains that do not carry mutations in either *rpsL* or *rrs* because aminoglycoside-modifying enzymes have not been found in *M. tuberculosis* (136).

Adverse Reactions and Drug Interactions

The major toxicities associated with the aminoglycosides are (a) cochlear (auditory) toxicity, (b) vestibular toxicity, and (c) nephrotoxicity (Table 51.3). In general, amikacin or kanamycin is relatively more ototoxic. Streptomycin is associated with significantly more disabling vestibular toxicity than the other aminoglycosides or capreomycin (32). However, such toxicities are extremely uncommon when used for 2 months on an intermittent schedule in relatively young persons without prior renal or eight-nerve dysfunctions (32). Significantly rarer adverse effects of aminoglycosides include fever, rash, neuromuscular blockade, hypokalemia, and hypomagnesemia.

The incidence of ototoxicity varies widely depending on the population being studied and the method used to diagnose such abnormalities but is likely to be approximately 3% to 10% for either cochlear or vestibular toxicity (reviewed in reference 129). Interestingly, the damage may be fairly isolated to either the cochlear or vestibular component, or rarely to both. The mechanism(s) for the cochlear toxicity is unclear, although the target site is considered to be the outer hair cells of the organ of Corti (138). Individual variations in sensitivity to the ototoxic effects of aminoglycosides are well documented. This observation mirrors the finding that genetic predisposition may be the greatest risk factor for aminoglycoside-induced cochlear toxicity (139,140). In contrast, no genetic predispositions to aminoglycoside-induced vestibular or renal toxicity are known. Recently, Wang et al. (141) showed in an isolated outer hair cell toxicity assay that sera from patients with aminoglycoside-induced hearing loss were significantly more toxic than sera from patients with normal hearing or minimal hearing loss. In addition, the percentage of damaged outer hair cells was significantly higher when streptomycin had been treated with sera or a serum protein fraction from patients with hearing loss than sera or serum protein fraction from a control group. These important findings suggest that sera from individuals with cochlear sensitivity to aminoglycoside antibiotics may metabolize these drugs to cochlear toxic compound(s). Although serum aminoglycoside concentrations were also considered to be a

TABLE 51.3. MONITORING FOR TOXICITY

Drug	Recommended Monitoring Tests
Pyrazinamide	Baseline measurements: uric acid, hepatic enzymes Repeat tests if indicated, e.g, signs and symptoms of joint or liver toxicity
Ethambutol	Baseline and monthly tests: visual acuity, color vision
Ethionamide	Baseline hepatic enzymes, repeat tests if indicated Baseline and periodic thyroid function tests
Streptomycin, kanamycin, amikacin, capreomycin	Baseline hearing/vestibular examination, serum blood urea nitrogen and creatinine, and serum potassium and magnesium Repeat tests monthly or if indicated

risk factor for ototoxicity (142), more recent data suggest that high peak serum concentrations are well tolerated if the interval between doses is increased. For example, Hudson and Sbarbaro (143) noted only a 9% to 10% incidence of ototoxicity when streptomycin at doses of 27 mg/kg were given twice weekly. Aminoglycoside-induced cochlear dysfunction is generally considered to be irreversible. The early detection of auditory damage may be difficult because high-frequency hearing loss usually occurs before any sense of hearing loss and thus may not be detectable based on patient complaints or bedside assessment. Injury to the type I hair cells of the ampullar cristae by aminoglycosides is the mechanism of the vestibular toxicity. Signs and symptoms of vestibular toxicity include nausea, vomiting, vertigo, and nystagmus (129).

The proximal renal tubule cells may accumulate aminoglycosides, accounting for the nephrotoxicity associated with aminoglycosides. The mechanism of renal toxicity is hypothesized to be the inhibition of intracellular phospholipases in the proximal tubule. The renal insufficiency is typically characterized by nonoliguric decrease in glomerular filtration rate occurring after at least a week of therapy. Risk factors for aminoglycoside-induced nephropathy include volume depletion, advanced age, coadministration of other nephrotoxic agents such as the nonsteroidal antiinflammatory drugs, poorly understood genetic predisposition, and liver disease (144). An increased trough serum concentration is widely considered a risk factor, and although it may itself hasten renal insufficiency, it is more likely to be a reflection of decreased glomerular filtration rate. Baseline and periodic surveillance of urinalysis, blood urea nitrogen levels, and creatinine values is indicated (32).

Capreomycin can affect the renal tubular cells, resulting in wasting of potassium, calcium, and magnesium. As with the aminoglycosides, capreomycin may also cause nephrotoxicity and its maintenance doses need to be reduced for patients with renal insufficiency (145,146). Although no rigorous comparisons have been made, it is the clinical impression that older patients experience less renal and eight-nerve toxicity with capreomycin than with amikacin or kanamycin (113).

REFERENCES

1. Mitchison DA. Basic concepts in the chemotherapy of tuberculosis. In: Gangadharam PRJ, Jenkins PA, eds.*Mycobacteria. II. Chemotherapy*. New York: Chapman and Hall, 1998:15–50.
2. Steele MA, Des Prez RM. The role of pyrazinamide in tuberculosis chemotherapy.*Chest* 1988;94:842–844.
3. Yeager RL, Munroe WGC, Dessau FI. Pyrazinamide (Aldinamide) in the treatment of pulmonary tuberculosis.*Am Rev Respir Dis* 1952;65:523–546.
4. Conte JE, Golden JA, Duncan S, et al. Intrapulmonary concentrations of pyrazinamide.*Antimicrob Agent Chemother* 1999; 43:1329–1333.
5. Ellard GA, Humphries MJ, Gabriel M, et al. Penetration of pyrazinamide into the cerebrospinal fluid in tuberculous meningitis.*Br J Med* 1987;294:284–285.
6. Malone RS, Fish DN, Spiegel DM, et al. The effect of hemodialysis on isoniazid, rifampin, pyrazinamide, and ethambutol.*Am J Respir Crit Care Med* 1999;159:1580–1584.
7. Conte JE, Lin E, Zurlinden E. High-performance liquid chromatographic determination of pyrazinamide in human plasma, bronchoalveolar lavage fluid, and alveolar cells.*J Chromatogr Sci* 2000;38:33–37.
8. Heifets LB. Antimycobacterial drugs.*Semin Respir Infect* 1994; 9:84–103.
9. McDermott W, Tomsett R. Activation of pyrazinamide and nicotinamide in acidic environments *in vitro.Am Rev Tuberc* 1954;70:748–754.
10. Heifets LB, Lindholm-Levy PJ. Pyrazinamide sterilizing activity *in vitro* against semidormant *Mycobacterium tuberculosis* bacterial populations.*Am Rev Respir Dis* 1992;145:1223–1225.
11. Heifets LB, Iseman MD. Radiometric method for testing susceptibility of mycobacteria to pyrazinamide in 7H12 broth.*J Clin Microbiol* 1985;21:200–204.
12. Heifets LB. Drug susceptibility testing in mycobacteriology. In: Heifets LB, ed.*Clinical mycobacteriology*. Philadelphia: WB Saunders, 1998:641–656.
13. Heifets LB, Lindholm-Levy PJ. Is pyrazinamide bactericidal against *Mycobacterium tuberculosis? Am Rev Respir Dis* 1990; 141:250–252.
14. Heifets L. Susceptibility testing of *Mycobacterium tuberculosis* to pyrazinamide.*J Med Microbiol* 2002;51:11–12.
15. Zhang Y, Permar S, Sun Z. Conditions that may affect the results of susceptibility testing of *Mycobacterium tuberculosis* to pyrazinamide.*J Med Microbiol* 2002;50:42–49.
16. Heifets L, Sanchez T. New agar medium for testing susceptibility of *Mycobacterium tuberculosis* to pyrazinamide.*J Clin Microbiol* 2000;38:1498–1501.
17. Crowle AJ, Dahl R, Ross E, et al. Evidence that vesicles containing living, virulent *Mycobacterium tuberculosis* or *Mycobacterium avium* in cultured human macrophages are not acidic. *Infect Immun* 1991;59:1823–1831.
18. Sturgill-Koszycki SP, Schlesinger P, Chakraborty P, et al. Lack of acidification in *Mycobacterium* phagosomes produced by exclusion of the vesicular proton ATPase.*Science* 1994;263:678–681.
19. Heifets L, Higgins M, Simon B. Pyrazinamide is not active against *Mycobacterium tuberculosis* residing in cultured human monocyte-derived macrophages. *Int J Tuberc Lung Dis* 2000;4:491–495.
20. Heifets LB. Antimicrobial agents: pyrazinamide. In: Yu VL, Merigan TC, Barriere SL, eds. *Antimicrobial therapy and vaccines*. Baltimore: Williams & Wilkins, 1999:668–676.
21. Crowle AJ, Salfinger M, May MH. 1,25 (OH)$_2$-vitamin D$_3$ synergizes with pyrazinamide to kill tubercle bacilli in cultured human macrophages. *Am Rev Respir Dis* 1989;129:542–552.
22. Konno K, Feldmann FM, McDermott W. Pyrazinamide susceptibility and amidase activity of tubercle bacilli. *Am Rev Respir Dis* 1967;95:461–469.
23. Heifets LB, Flory MA, Lindholm-Levy PJ. Does pyrazinoic acid as an active moiety of pyrazinamide have specific activity against *Mycobacterium tuberculosis? Antimicrob Agents Chemother* 1989; 33:1252–1254.
24. Speirs RJ, Welch JT, Cynamon MH. Activity of n-propyl pyrazinoate against pyrazinamide-resistant *Mycobacterium tuberculosis*: investigations into mechanism of action of and mechanism of resistance to pyrazinamide. *Antimicrob Agent Chemother* 1995;39:1269–1271.
25. Zhang Y, Scorpio A, Nikaido H, et al. Role of acid pH and deficient efflux of pyrazinoic acid in unique susceptibility of *Mycobacteria tuberculosis* to pyrazinamide. *J Bacteriol* 1999; 181:2044–2049.

26. Zimhony O, Cox JS, Welch JT, et al. Pyrazinamide inhibits the eukaryotic-like fatty acid synthetase I (FASI) of *Mycobacterium tuberculosis*. *Nat Med* 2000;6:1043–1047.
27. Boshoff HI, Mizrahi V, Barry CE. The effects of pyrazinamide on fatty acid synthesis by whole mycobacterial cells and purified FAS-I. *J Bacteriol* 2002;184:2167–2172.
28. Zhang Y, Telenti A. Genetics of drug resistance in *Mycobacterium tuberculosis*. In: Jacobs WR, Hatfull GF, eds. *Molecular genetics of mycobacteria*. Washington, DC: ASM Press, 2000: 235–254.
29. East African/British Medical Council. Results at 5 years of a controlled comparison of a 6-month and a standard 18-month regimen of chemotherapy for pulmonary tuberculosis. *Am Rev Respir Dis* 1977;116:3–8.
30. East African/British Medical Research Council. Controlled clinical trial of four short-course regimens of chemotherapy for two durations in the treatment of pulmonary tuberculosis. Second report. *Tubercle* 1980;61:59–69.
31. Santha T, Nazareth O, Krishnamurthy MS, et al. Treatment of pulmonary tuberculosis with short course chemotherapy in South India—5 year follow-up. *Tubercle* 1989;70:229–234.
32. Iseman MD. Tuberculosis chemotherapy, including directly observed therapy. A clinician's guide to tuberculosis. Philadelphia: Lippincott Williams & Wilkins, 2000:271–321.
33. Bass JB, Farer LS, Hopewell PC, et al. Treatment of tuberculosis and tuberculosis infection in adults and children. American Thoracic Society and the Centers for Disease Control. *Am J Respir Crit Care Med* 1994;149:1359–1374.
34. Controlled trial of 2,4, and 6 months of pyrazinamide in 6-month, three-times weekly regimens for smear-positive pulmonary tuberculosis, including an assessment of a combined preparation of isoniazid, rifampin, and pyrazinamide: results at 30 months. *Am Rev Respir Dis* 1991;143:700–706.
35. East and Central African / British Medical Research Council. Controlled clinical trial of 4 short-course regimens of chemotherapy (three 6-month and one 8-month) for pulmonary tuberculosis. *Tubercle* 1986;67:5–15.
36. Singapore Tuberculosis Service/British Medical Research Council. Long-term follow-up of a clinical trial of six-month and four-month regimens of chemotherapy in the treatment of pulmonary tuberculosis. *Am Rev Respir Dis* 1986;133:779–783.
37. Mitchison DA, Nunn AJ. Influence of initial drug resistance on the response to short-course chemotherapy of pulmonary tuberculosis. *Am Rev Respir Dis* 1985;133:423–430.
38. American Thoracic Society, Centers for Disease Control and Prevention. Targeted tuberculin testing and treatment of latent tuberculosis infection. *Am J Respir Crit Care Med* 2000;161 [Suppl]:S221–S247.
39. Chapuis L, Ji B, Truffot-Pernot C, et al. Preventive therapy of tuberculosis with rifapentine in immunocompetent and nude mice. *Am J Respir Crit Care Med* 1994;150:1355–1362.
40. Lecoeur HF, Truffot-Pernot C, Grosset JH. Experimental short-course preventive therapy of tuberculosis with rifampin and pyrazinamide. *Am Rev Respir Dis* 1989;140:1189–1193.
41. American Thoracic Society Update. Fatal and severe liver injuries associated with rifampin and pyrazinamide for latent tuberculosis infection, and revisions in American Thoracic Society/CDC recommendations—United States, 2001. *Am J Respir Crit Care Med* 2001;164:1319–1320.
42. Berning SE, Cherry TA, Iseman MD. Novel treatment of meningitis caused by multidrug-resistant *Mycobacterium tuberculosis* with intrathecal levofloxacin and amikacin: case report. *Clin Infect Dis* 2001;32:643–646.
43. Scorpio A, Zhang Y. Mutations in *pncA*, a gene encoding pyrazinamidase/nicotinamidase, cause resistance to antituberculous drug pyrazinamide in tubercle bacillus. *Nat Med* 1996;2:1–6.
44. Sreevatsan S, Pan X, Zhang Y, et al. Mutations associated with pyrazinamide resistance in *pncA* of *Mycobacterium tuberculosis* complex organisms. *Antimicrob Agents Chemother* 1997;41: 636–640.
45. Hirano K, Takahashi M, Kazumi Y, et al. Mutation in *pncA* is a major mechanism of pyrazinamide resistance in *Mycobacterium tuberculosis*. *Tuber Lung Dis* 1998;78:117–122.
46. Scorpio A, Lindholm-Levy P, Heifets L, et al. Characterization of *pncA* mutations in pyrazinamide-resistant *Mycobacterium tuberculosis*. *Antimicrob Agents Chemother* 1997;41:540–543.
47. Chang S-J, Thibert L, Sanchez T, et al. *pncA* mutations as a major mechanism of pyrazinamide resistance in *Mycobacterium tuberculosis*: spread of a monoresistant strain in Quebec, Canada. *Antimicrob Agent Chemother* 2000;44:528–532.
48. Boshoff HIM, Mizrahi V. Expression of *Mycobacterium smegmatis* pyrazinamidase in *Mycobacterium tuberculosis* confers hypersensitivity to pyrazinamide and related amides. *J Bacteriol* 2000;182:5479–5485.
49. Pilheu JA, DeSalvo MC, Koch O. Liver alterations in antituberculosis regimens containing pyrazinamide. *Chest* 1981;80: 720–724.
50. Zierski MB, Bek E. Side effects of drug regimens used in short-course chemotherapy for pulmonary tuberculosis. A controlled clinical study. *Tubercle* 1980;61:41–49.
51. van der Kooi K, Mottet J-J, Regamey C. Isoniazid is not always the cause of hepatitis during treatment of tuberculosis. *Clin Infect Dis* 1994;19:987–988.
52. Centers for Disease Control and Prevention. Fatal and severe hepatitis associated with rifampin and pyrazinamide for the treatment of latent tuberculosis infection—New York and Georgia, 2000. *MMWR Morb Mortal Wkly Rep* 2000;50: 289–291.
53. Horn DL, Hewlett D, Alfalla C, et al. Limited tolerance of ofloxacin and pyrazinamide prophylaxis against tuberculosis. *N Engl J Med* 1994;330:1241.
54. Ridzon R, Meador J, Maxwell R, et al. Asymptomatic hepatitis in persons who received alternative preventive therapy with pyrazinamide and ofloxacin. *Clin Infect Dis* 1997;24: 1264–1265.
55. Koumbaniou C, Nicopoulos C, Vassiliou M, et al. Is pyrazinamide really the third drug of choice in the treatment of tuberculosis? *Int J Tuberc Lung Dis* 1998;2:675–678.
56. Ellard G, Haslam R. Observations on the reduction of the renal elimination of urate in man caused by the administration of pyrazinamide. *Tubercle* 1976;57:97–103.
57. Hong Kong Tuberculosis Treatment Services/British Medical Research Council. Adverse reactions to short-course regimens containing streptomycin, isoniazid, pyrazinamide, and rifampicin in Hong Kong. *Tubercle* 1976;57:81–95.
58. Jain A, Mehta VL, Kulshrestha S. Effect of pyrazinamide on rifampicin kinetics in patients with tuberculosis. *Tuber Lung Dis* 1993;74:87–90.
59. Karlson AG. The *in vitro* activity of ethambutol (dextro-2,2'-[ethylenediimino]-di-1-butanol) against tubercle bacilli and other microorganisms. *Am Rev Respir Dis* 1961;4:905–906.
60. Karlson AG. Therapeutic effect of ethambutol (dextro-2,2'-(ethylenediimino)- di-1-butanol) on experimental tuberculosis in guinea pigs. *Am Rev Respir Dis* 1961;84:902–904.
61. Thomas JP, Baughn CO, Wilkinson RG, et al. A new synthetic compound with antituberculous activity in mice: ethambutol (dextro-2,2'-[ethylenediimino]-di-1-butanol). *Am Rev Respir Dis* 1961;83:891–893.
62. Lewis ML. Antimycobacterial agents: ethambutol. In: Yu VL, Merigan TC, Barriere SL, eds. *Antimicrobial therapy and vaccines*. Baltimore: Williams & Wilkins, 1999:643–650.
63. Liss RH, Letourneau RJ, Schepis JP. Distribution of ethambu-

tol in primate tissues and cells.*Am Rev Respir Dis* 1981;123: 529–532.

64. Varughese A, Brater DC, Benet LZ, et al. Ethambutol kinetics in patients with impaired renal function. *Am Rev Respir Dis* 1986;134:34–38.

65. Forbes M, Kuck NA, Peets EA. Effect of ethambutol on nucleic acid metabolism in *Mycobacterium smegmatis* and its reversal by polyamines and divalent cations. *J Bacteriol* 1965;89: 1299–1305.

66. Forbes M, Kuck NA, Peets EA. Mode of action of ethambutol. *J Bacteriol* 1962;84:1299–1305.

67. Cheema S, Asotra S, Khuller GK. Ethambutol induced leakage of phospholipids in *Mycobacterium smegmatis*. *Int Res Commun Sys Med Sci Biochem* 1985;13:178–186.

68. Takayama K, Armstrong EL, Kunugi KA, et al. Inhibition by ethambutol of mycolic acid transfer into the cell wall of *Mycobacterium smegmatis*.*Antimicrob Agents Chemother* 1979;16: 240–242.

69. Paulin LG, Brander EE, and Poso HJ. Specific inhibition of spermidine synthesis in *Mycobacteria* spp by the dextro isomer of ethambutol. *Antimicrob Agents Chemother* 1985; 28:157–159.

70. Takayama K, Kilburn JO. Inhibition of synthesis of arabinogalactan by ethambutol in *Mycobacterium smegmatis*. *Antimicrob Agents Chemother* 1989;33:1493–1499.

71. Mikusova K, Slayden RA, Besra GS, et al. Biogenesis of the mycobacterial cell wall and the site of action of ethambutol. *Antimicrob Agents Chemother* 1995;39:2484–2489.

72. Chopra I, Brennan P. Molecular action of anti-mycobacterial agents. *Tuber Lung Dis* 1998;78:89–98.

73. Belanger AE, Besra GS, Ford ME, et al. The embAB genes of *Mycobacterium avium* encode an arabinosyl transferase involved in cell wall arabinan biosynthesis that is the target for the antimycobacterial drug ethambutol. *Proc Natl Acad Sci U S A* 1996;93:11919–11924.

74. Wolucka BA, McNeil MR, deHoffmann E, et al. Recognition of the lipid intermediate for arabinogalactan/arabinomannan biosynthesis and its relation to the mode of action of ethambutol on mycobacteria. *J Biol Chem* 1994;269:23328–23335.

75. Khoo KH, Douglas E, Azadi P, et al. Truncated structural variants of lipoarabinomannan in ethambutol drug-resistant strains of *Mycobacterium smegmatis*—inhibition of arabinan biosynthesis by ethambutol. *J Biol Chem* 1996;271:28682–28690.

76. Khoo KH, Tang JB, Chatterjee D. Variation in mannose-capped terminal arabinan motifs of lipoarabinomannans from clinical isolates of *Mycobacterium tuberculosis* and *Mycobacterium avium* complex. *J Biol Chem* 2001;276:3863–3871.

77. Telenti A, Philipp WJ, Sreevatsan S, et al. The *emb* operon, a gene cluster of *Mycobacterium tuberculosis* involved in resistance to ethambutol. *Nat Med* 1997;3:567–570.

78. Cole ST, Eiglmeier K, Parkhill J, et al. Massive gene decay in the leprosy bacillus. *Nature* 2001;409:1007–1011.

79. Besra GS, Khoo KH, McNeil MR, et al. A new interpretation of the structure of the mycolyl-arabinogalactan complex of *Mycobacterium tuberculosis* as revealed through characterization of oligoglycosylalditol fragments by fast-atom bombardment mass spectrometry and ¹H-nuclear magnetic resonance spectroscopy. *Biochemistry* 1995;34:4257–4266.

80. Brennan PJ, Nikaido H. The envelope of mycobacteria.*Annu Rev Biochem* 1995;64:29–63.

81. Alcaide F, Pfyffer GE, Telenti A. Role of *embB* in natural and acquired resistance to ethambutol in mycobacteria. *Antimicrob Agents Chemother* 1997;41:2270–2273.

82. Escuyer VE, Lety MA, Torrelles JB, et al. The role of the *embA* and *embB* gene products in the biosynthesis of the terminal hexaarabinofuranosyl motif of *Mycobacterium smegmatis* arabinogalactan. *J Biol Chem* 2001;276:48854–48862.

83. Gangadharam PRJ, Pratt PF, Perumal VK, et al. The effects of exposure time, drug concentration, and temperature on the activity of ethambutol versus *Mycobacterium tuberculosis*. *Am Rev Respir Dis* 1990;141:1478–1482.

84. Liss RH. Bactericidal activity of ethambutol against extracellular *Mycobacterium tuberculosis* and bacilli phagocytized by human alveolar macrophages. *S A Med J* 1982;62:15–19.

85. Heifets LB, Iseman MD, Lindholm-Levy PJ. Ethambutol MICs and MBCs for *Mycobacterium avium* complex and *Mycobacterium tuberculosis*.*Antimicrob Agents Chemother* 1986;30: 927–932.

86. Suo J, Cheng C-E, Lin TP, et al. Minimal inhibitory concentrations of isoniazid, rifampin, ethambutol and streptomycin against *M. tuberculosis* strains isolated before treatment of patients in Taiwan. *Am Rev Respir Dis* 1988;138:999–1001.

87. Ethambutol [Editorial]. *Tubercle* 1966;47:292–295.

88. Albert R, Sbarbaro JA, Hudson L, et al. High-dose ethambutol: its role in intermittent chemotherapy—a six-year study. *Am Rev Respir Dis* 1976;114:699–704.

89. Bobrowitz ID. Ethambutol-isoniazid versus streptomycin-ethambutol-isoniazid in original treatment of cavitary tuberculosis. *Am Rev Respir Dis* 1974;109:548–553.

90. Bobrowitz ID, Robins DE. Ethambutol-isoniazid versus PAS-isoniazid in original treatment of pulmonary tuberculosis. *Am Rev Respir Dis* 1967;96:428–438.

91. Doster B, Murray FJ, Newman R, et al. Ethambutol in the initial treatment of pulmonary tuberculosis: U.S. Public Health Service Tuberculosis Therapy Trials. *Am Rev Respir Dis* 1973; 107:177–190.

92. Lees AW, Allan GW, Smith J, et al. Ethambutol plus isoniazid compared with rifampicin plus isoniazid in antituberculosis continuation treatment. *Lancet* 1977;1:1232–1233.

93. Hong Kong Chest Service/British Medical Research Council. Controlled trial of 6-month and 8-month regimens in the treatment of pulmonary tuberculosis: the results up to 24 months. *Tubercle* 1979;60:201–210.

94. Hong Kong Chest Service/British Medical Research Council. Five-year follow-up of a controlled trial of five 6-month regimens of chemotherapy for pulmonary tuberculosis. *Am Rev Respir Dis* 1987;136:1339–1342.

95. Combs D, O'Brien R, Geiter L. USPHS tuberculosis short-course chemotherapy trial 21: effectiveness, toxicity, and acceptability—the report of final results. *Ann Intern Med* 1990;112: 397–406.

96. Pablos-Mendez A, Raviglione MC, Laszlo A, et al. Global surveillance for antituberculosis-drug resistance, 1994–1997. World Health Organization–International Union against Tuberculosis and Lung Disease Working Group on Anti-Tuberculosis Drug Resistance Surveillance. *N Engl J Med* 1998;338:1641–1649.

97. Lety MA, Nair S, Berche P, et al. A single point mutation in the *embB* gene is responsible for resistance to ethambutol in *Mycobacterium smegmatis*. *Antimicrob Agent Chemother* 1997;41:2629–2633.

98. Sreevatsan S, Stockbauer KE, Pan X, et al. Ethambutol resistance in *Mycobacterium tuberculosis*: critical role of *embB* mutations. *Antimicrob Agents Chemother* 1997;41:1677–1681.

99. Belanger AE, Inamine JM. Genetics of cell wall biosynthesis. In: Hatfull GF, Jacobs WR, eds. *Molecular genetics of mycobacteria*. Washington, DC: ASM Press, 2000:191–202.

100. Adel A. Ophthalmological side-effects of ethambutol. *Scand J Respir Dis* 1969;69:54–58.

101. Joubert PH, Strobele JG, Ogle CW, et al. Subclinical impairment of colour vision in patients receiving ethambutol. *Br J Clin Pharmacol* 1986;21:213–216.

102. Rabinovitz M, Pitlik SD, Halevy J, et al. Ethambutol-induced thrombocytopenia. *Chest* 1982;81:765–766.

103. Bobrowitz ID. Ethambutol in pregnancy. *Chest* 1974;66:20–24.
104. Lewit T, Nebel L, Terracina S, et al. Ethambutol in pregnancy: observations on embryogenesis. *Chest* 1974;66:25–26.
105. Gugler R, Allgayer H. Effects of antacids on the clinical pharmacokinetics of drugs. *Clin Pharmacokinet* 1990;18:210–219.
106. Rist N, Grumbach F, Libermann D. Experiments on the antituberculosis activity of alpha ethylthioisonicotinamide. *Am Rev Tuberc* 1959;79:1–5.
107. Quemard A, Laneelle G, Lacave C. Mycolic acid synthesis: a target for ethionamide in mycobacteria? *Antimicrob Agent Chemother* 1992;36:1316–1321.
108. Heifets LB, Lindholm-Levy PJ, Flory M. Comparison of bacteriostatic and bactericidal activity of isoniazid and ethionamide against *Mycobacterium avium* and *Mycobacterium tuberculosis*. *Am Rev Respir Dis* 1991;143:268–270.
109. Heifets L. Qualitative and quantitative drug-susceptibility tests in mycobacteriology. *Am Rev Respir Dis* 1988;137:1217–1222.
110. Banerjee A, Dubnau E, Quemard A, et al. *inhA*, a gene encoding a target for isoniazid and ethionamide in *Mycobacterium tuberculosis*. *Science* 1994;263:227–230.
111. Fattorini L, Iona E, Ricci ML, et al. Activity of 16 antimicrobial agents against drug-resistant strains of *Mycobacterium tuberculosis*. *Microb Drug Resist* 1999;5:265–270.
112. Baulard AR, Betts JC, Engohang-Ndong J, et al. Activation of the pro-drug ethionamide is regulated in mycobacteria. *J Biol Chem* 2000; 275:28326–28331.
113. Iseman MD, Madsen LA. Drug-resistant tuberculosis. *Clin Chest Med* 1989;10:341–353.
114. Berning SE, Peloquin CA. Antimycobacterial agents. In: Yu VL, Merigan TC, Barriere SL, eds. *Antimicrobial therapy and vaccines*. Baltimore: Williams & Wilkins, 1999:650–654.
115. Waksman SA, Schatz AI. Present status of streptomycin therapy. *Lancet* 1946;66:77–78.
116. Edson RS, Terrell CL. The aminoglycosides. *Mayo Clin Proc* 1999;74:519–528.
117. Peloquin CA. Antituberculosis drugs: pharmacokinetics. In: Heifets LB, ed. *Drug susceptibility in the chemotherapy of mycobacterial infections*. Boca Raton, FL: CRC Press, 1991:59–88.
118. McHenry MC, Wagner JG, Hall PM, et al. Pharmacokinetics of amikacin in patients with impaired renal function. *J Infect Dis* 1976;134:S343–S348.
119. Purohit P, Stern S. Interactions of a small RNA with antibiotic and RNA ligands of the 30S subunit. *Nature* 1994;370:659–662.
120. Peterson AA, Hancock REW, McGroarty EJ. Binding of polycationic antibiotics and polyamines to lipopolysaccharides of *Pseudomonas aeruginosa*. *J Bacteriol* 1985;164:1256–1261.
121. Heifets LB, Lindholm-Levy PJ. Comparison of bactericidal activities of streptomycin, amikacin, kanamycin, and capreomycin against *M. avium* and *M. tuberculosis*. *Antimicrob Agents Chemother* 1989;33:1298–1301.
122. Wolinsky E, Steenken W. Effect of streptomycin on the tubercle bacillus. The use of Dubos and other media in tests for streptomycin sensitivity. *Am Rev Tuberc* 1947;55:281–288.
123. Ho YI, Chan CY, Cheng AF. *In vitro* activities of aminoglycosides-aminocyclitols against mycobacteria. *J Antimicrob Chemother* 1997;40:27–32.
124. Lounis N, Ji B, Truffot-Pernot C, et al. Which aminoglycoside or fluoroquinolone is more active against *Mycobacterium tuberculosis* in mice? *Antimicrob Agents Chemother* 1997;41:607–610.
125. Donald PR, Sirgel FA, Venter A, et al. The early bactericidal activity of amikacin in pulmonary tuberculosis. *Int J Tuberc Lung Dis* 2001;5:533–538.
126. Medical Research Council. Streptomycin treatment of pulmonary tuberculosis. *BMJ* 1948;2:769–782.
127. Fox W, Sutherland I, Daniels M. A five-year assessment of patients in a controlled trial of streptomycin in pulmonary tuberculosis. *Q J Med* 1954;23:347–366.
128. Peloquin CA, Berning SE. Intravenous streptomycin [Letter]. *Ann Pharmacother* 1993;27:1546–1547.
129. Gilbert DN. Aminoglycosides. In: Mandell GL, Bennett JE, Dolin R, eds. *Principles and practice of infectious diseases*. Philadelphia: Churchill Livingstone, 2000:307–336.
130. Allen BW, Mitchison DA, Chan YC, et al. Amikacin in the treatment of pulmonary tuberculosis. *Tubercle* 1983;64:111–118.
131. Tsukamura M, Mizuno S. Cross-resistance relationships among the aminoglycoside antibiotics in *Mycobacterium tuberculosis*. *J Gen Microbiol* 1975;88:269–274.
132. Alangaden GJ, Kreiswirth BN, Aouad A, et al. Mechanism of resistance to amikacin and kanamycin in *Mycobacterium tuberculosis*. *Antimicrob Agents Chemother* 1998;42:1295–1297.
133. Prammananan T, Sander P, Brown BA, et al. A single 16S ribosomal RNA substitution is responsible for resistance to amikacin and other 2-deoxystreptamine aminoglycosides in *Mycobacterium abscessus* and *Mycobacterium chelonae*. *J Infect Dis* 1998;177:1573–1581.
134. Cooksey RC, Morlock GP, McQueen A, et al. Characterization of streptomycin resistance mechanisms among *Mycobacterium tuberculosis* isolates from patients in New York City. *Antimicrob Agents Chemother* 1996;40:1186–1188.
135. Nachamkin I, Kang C, Weinstein MP. Detection of resistance to isoniazid, rifampin, and streptomycin in clinical isolates of *Mycobacterium tuberculosis* by molecular methods. *Clin Infect Dis* 1997;24:894–900.
136. Riska PF, Jacobs WR, Alland D. Molecular determinants of drug resistance in tuberculosis. *Int J Tuberc Lung Dis* 2000;4:S4–S10.
137. Sreevatsan S, Pan X, Stockbauer KE, et al. Characterization of *rpsL* and *rrs* mutations in streptomycin-resistant *Mycobacterium tuberculosis* isolates from diverse geographic localities. *Antimicrob Agent Chemother* 1996;40:1024–1026.
138. Hutchin T, Cortopassi G. Proposed molecular and cellular mechanism of aminoglycoside ototoxicity. *Antimicrob Agent Chemother* 1994;38:2517–2520.
139. Fischel-Ghodsian N, Prezant TR, Chaltraw WE, et al. Mitochondrial gene mutation is a significant predisposing factor in aminoglycoside ototoxicity. *Am J Otolaryngol* 1997;18:173–178.
140. Pandya A, Xia X, Raduaabazar J, et al. Mutation in the mitochondrial 12S rRNA gene in two families from Mongolia with matrilineal aminoglycoside ototoxicity. *J Med Genet* 1997;34:169–172.
141. Wang S, Bian Q, Liu Z, et al. Capability of serum to convert streptomycin to cytotoxin in patients with aminoglycoside-induced hearing loss. *Hearing Res* 1999;137:1–7.
142. Gatell JM, Ferran F, Araujo V, et al. Univariate and multivariate analyses of risk factors predisposing to auditory toxicity in patients receiving aminoglycosides. *Antimicrob Agents Chemother* 1987;31:1383–1387.
143. Hudson LD, Sbarbaro JA. Twice weekly tuberculosis chemotherapy. *JAMA* 1973;223:139–143.
144. Bertino JS, Booker LA, Franck PA, et al. Incidence of and significant risk factors for aminoglycoside-associated nephrotoxicity in patients dosed by using individualized pharmacokinetic monitoring. *J Infect Dis* 1993;167:173–179.
145. Garfield JW, Jones JM, Cohen NL, et al. The auditory, vestibu-

lar and renal effects of capreomycin in humans. *Ann N Y Acad Sci* 1966;135:1039–1046.

146. Lehmann CR, Garrett LE, Winn RE, et al. Capreomycin kinetics in renal impairment and clearance by hemodialysis. *Am Rev Respir Dis* 1988;138:1312–1313.

147. American Thoracic Society and Centers for Disease Control and Prevention. Treatment of tuberculosis and tuberculosis infection in adults and children. *Am J Respir Crit Care Med* 1994;149:1359–1374.

148. Centers for Disease Control and Prevention, Division of Tuberculosis Elimination. *Core curriculum on tuberculosis.* Atlanta: CDC, 1994.

149. Van Scoy RE, Wilkowske CJ. Antimycobacterial therapy. *Mayo Clin Proc* 1999;74:1038–1048.

FLUOROQUINOLONES AS ANTITUBERCULOSIS AGENTS

KARL DRLICA
TAO LU
MUHAMMAD MALIK
XILIN ZHAO

The fluoroquinolones are broad-spectrum antibacterial agents that block DNA replication and kill bacterial cells. In the past decade, their use with respiratory infections has steadily increased, owing in part to the development of resistance to traditional antibiotics. In the mid-1980s, one member of the class, ofloxacin, showed activity against tuberculosis (1). Although it was clear that resistance would arise from therapy with the fluoroquinolones (1,2), ofloxacin and ciprofloxacin were used a few years later in New York City for cases of multidrug-resistant (MDR) tuberculosis. In a matter of months, patients were found harboring strains of *Mycobacterium tuberculosis* that had become resistant to these compounds (3). When resistant isolates were recovered and examined *in vitro*, some quinolones (e.g., sparfloxacin) were more effective than others (e.g., ciprofloxacin) at blocking mutant growth even after normalization to effects with susceptible cells (4,5). It appeared that fluoroquinolone structure could be manipulated to obtain compounds having enhanced activity against resistant mutants. Investigational C-8-methoxy fluoroquinolones (Fig. 52.1) were soon found to be exceptionally active against resistant mutants (5,6), and strategies were formulated for restricting mutant selection (7–9).

During the 1990s, two C-8-methoxy fluoroquinolones (moxifloxacin and gatifloxacin) were developed commercially for use against gram-positive pathogens. As expected, these agents exhibited excellent activity against resistant mutants of *Streptococcus pneumoniae* and *Staphylococcus aureus* (10,11), raising the hope that mutant selection could be severely restricted (8,12). Moxifloxacin and gatifloxacin also had exceptional activity with *M. tuberculosis* if assessed by a mutant selection criterion (13). However, when examined for activity in cultured cells (14) or in animal models

(discussed later), the C-8-methoxy compounds were not lethal enough to be spectacular antituberculosis agents. Thus, successful use of fluoroquinolones with tuberculosis will probably require finding appropriate combination therapies.

MECHANISM OF FLUOROQUINOLONE ACTION

Bacteriostatic Action

With most bacteria, DNA gyrase and DNA topoisomerase IV are the intracellular targets of the fluoroquinolones (reviewed in references 15,16). These two enzymes act by transiently breaking DNA and passing a region of duplex DNA through the break (17); the fluoroquinolones trap a reaction intermediate containing enzyme and broken DNA. Formation of drug–enzyme–DNA complexes inhibits DNA replication (18–21) and transcription (22), in both cases by blocking polymerase movement (20,23). This property of the drug–enzyme–DNA complexes explains how quinolones inhibit cell growth.

Several bacterial pathogens, including *M. tuberculosis*, lack a gene encoding DNA topoisomerase IV, as indicated by examination of genomic nucleotide sequences (24). The absence of topoisomerase IV may contribute to the long doubling time of *M. tuberculosis* because in other bacteria this enzyme plays an important role in both the elongation and decatenation phases of DNA replication (25). It also makes gyrase the only fluoroquinolone target in *M. tuberculosis*.

Crystal structures are available for portions of eukaryotic topoisomerase II (26,27), bacterial GyrA protein (28), and bacterial GyrB protein (29). If we assume that the eukaryotic structure is representative, the GyrA subunits are seen as forming dimers through two contact regions, one termed the DNA gate and the other the exit gate. Each GyrA sub-

K. Drlica, T. Lu, M. Malik, and X. Zhao: Public Health Research Institute, Newark, New Jersey.

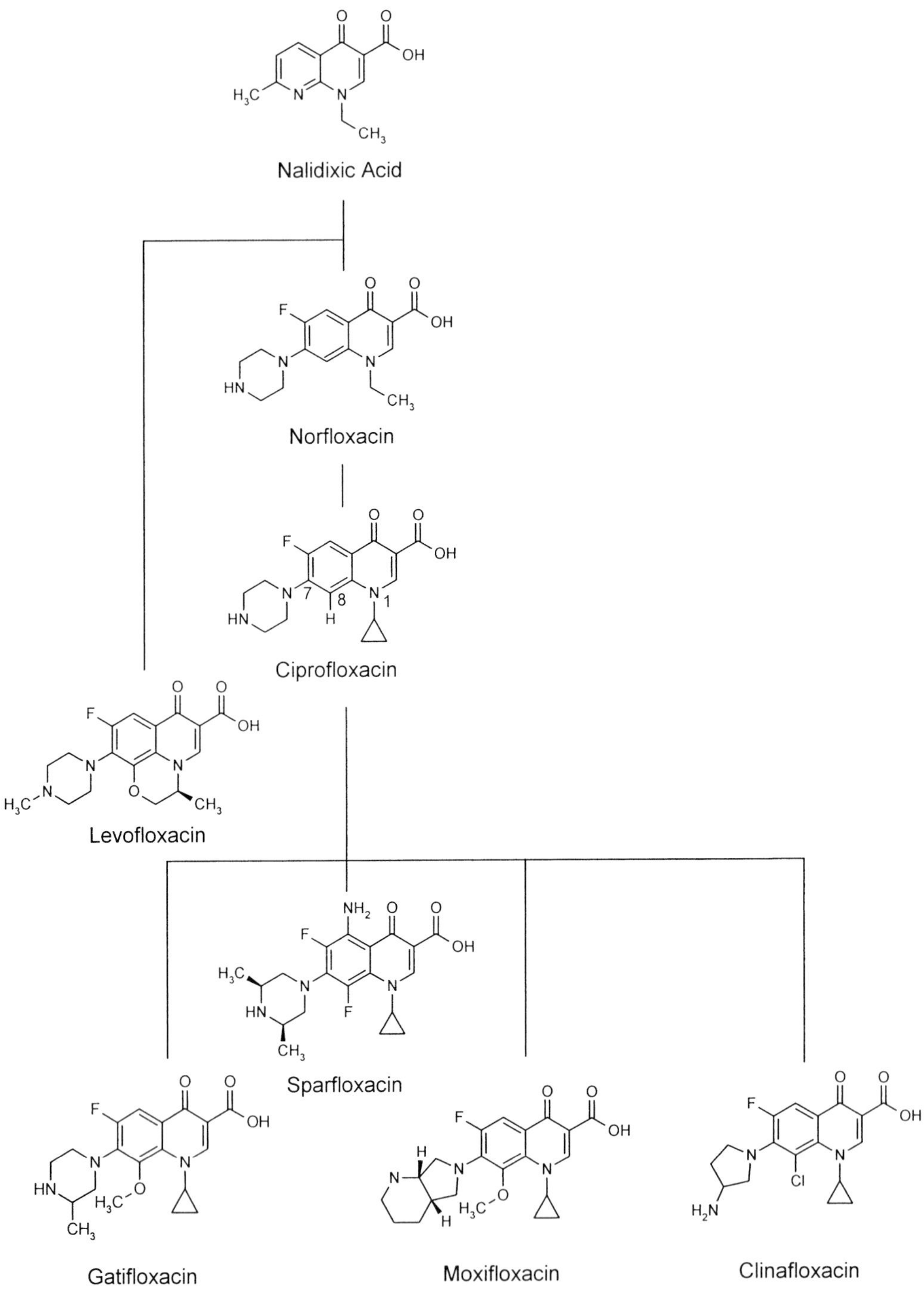

FIGURE 52.1. Fluoroquinolone structure. For reference, the ring atoms of ciprofloxacin are numbered.

unit also interacts with a GyrB subunit. A general scheme for DNA strand passage can be envisioned (Fig. 52.2) (30). First, one portion of duplex DNA, the gate or G segment, binds to a surface of a GyrA dimer that is stabilized by binding to GyrB subunits. The gyrase subunits may assemble on the DNA, or perhaps more often, the DNA passes through

the GyrB clamp (discussed later) to reach the GyrA surface [Fig. 52.2(c)] (31). Gyrase cleaves both strands of the G segment, while the protein portion of the DNA gate is closed ([Fig. 52.2(d)] cleavage occurs even when the gate is locked by protein cross-linking) (32). Adenosine 5'-triphosphate (ATP) binding to GyrB promotes dimerization and forma-

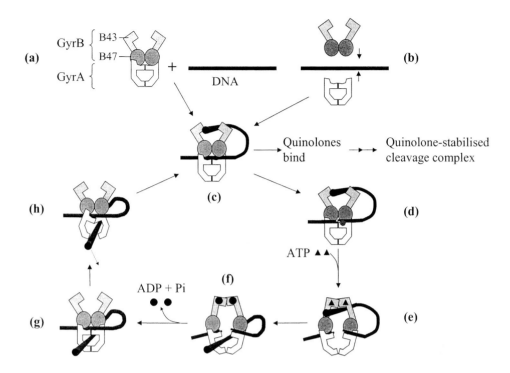

FIGURE 52.2. DNA strand passage catalyzed by DNA gyrase. *a:* The 43- and 47-kd regions of GyrB, along with the 64-kd region of GyrA are shown as a tetramer. The 33-kd C-terminal domains of GyrA are omitted for clarity, as is the DNA wraparound gyrase. Supercoiling occurs when gyrase either binds a G segment of DNA *(a)* or assembles onto the G segment *(b)*. The resulting complex *(c)* is a substrate for quinolone binding. The ternary complex *(c)* cleaves DNA to form a cleavage complex *(d)*. Adenosine 5′-triphosphate *(ATP)* binds to the 43-kd domains of GyrB, causing them to close and capture the T segment of DNA *(e)*. The T segment is transported through the break in the G segment and into the bottom cavity of gyrase *(f)*. The break in the G segment is religated *(g)*, and the T segment is then released from the bottom cavity through the exit gate in the enzyme *(h)*. The exit gate closes, resetting the enzyme for a new round of supercoiling. Between capture of the T segment and resetting of the enzyme, ATP is hydrolyzed and adenosine 5′-diphosphate *(ADP)* is released. [The figure, adapted from Heddle JG, Barnard F, Wentzell L, et al. The interaction of drugs with DNA gyrase: a model for the molecular basis of quinolone action. *Nucleosides Nucleotides Nucleic Acids* 2000;19:1249–1264, was provided by Dr. J.G. Heddle (John Innes Centre, Norwich, U.K.).]

tion of a protein clamp that captures a second region of DNA, the transport or T segment [Fig. 52.2(e)] (31). The DNA gate opens, and the T segment passes through [Fig. 52.2(f)]. The G segment of DNA is then rejoined [Fig. 52.2(g)], and the T segment passes through the exit gate of the GyrA protein [Fig. 52.2(h)]. The ATP-operated clamp of the GyrB protein reopens on ATP hydrolysis. Gyrase can act processively by remaining attached to the G segment and drawing T segments repeatedly into the GyrB clamp after each round of ATP hydrolysis.

The major resistance alleles alter amino acids 90 and 94 in the GyrA protein of *M. tuberculosis* (33). These amino acids, which correspond to amino acids 83 and 87 in the *Escherichia coli* protein, are located in α-helix 4 on a surface where DNA is thought to bind (28) (Fig. 52.3). One hypothesis is that the quinolones interact with this helix immediately after DNA has bound. Gyrase then introduces two staggered, single-strand breaks into the DNA, and the

quinolones prevent religation of the breaks. Since gyrase is covalently bound to the 5′ ends of the DNA, it is trapped as a ternary complex by the drug. Removal of the drug allows gyrase to reseal the DNA break, thereby restoring the ability to replicate DNA.

Although our understanding of fluoroquinolone action comes largely from work with *E. coli*, the topoisomerases are highly conserved. Thus, most of the conclusions drawn from *E. coli* studies apply broadly. For example, the chromosomal DNA cleavage and rapid inhibition of DNA synthesis that are characteristic of quinolone action are observed with *Mycobacterium smegmatis* (34). Moreover, the activity of gyrase purified from *M. tuberculosis* is inhibited by fluoroquinolones unless the enzyme is obtained from a resistant mutant (35). As mentioned previously, another common feature is the location of resistance mutations in homologous regions of mycobacterial and *E. coli* gyrase (33,36). One difference is that the *M. tuberculosis* GyrA

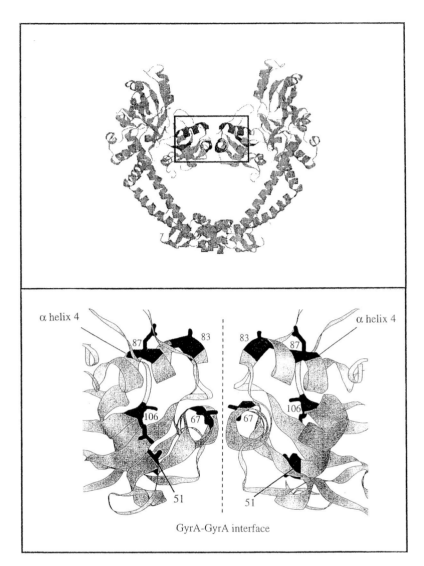

α helix 4

α helix 4

GyrA-GyrA interface

FIGURE 52.3. Structure of DNA gyrase GyrA59 dimer. Ribbon representation (generated in Ras-Mol) of the GyrA59 fragment (28), courtesy of J.G. Heddle (John Innes Centre, Norwich, U.K.) is shown. **Top:** The entire GyrA59 dimer; **bottom:** an enlargement of the boxed region in the **top**. Amino acids that change to confer quinolone resistance are indicated in black and by the amino acid numbers (numbering is according to *Escherichia coli* GyrA structure). Amino acid 51 is in helix 2, amino acid 67 is in helix 3, and amino acids 83 and 87 are in helix 4. (Adapted from Friedman SM, Lu T, Drlica K. A mutation in the DNA gyrase A gene of *Escherichia coli* that expands the quinolone-resistance-determining region. *Antimicrob Agents Chemother* 2001;45: 2378–2380.)

protein contains an alanine at the position equivalent to 83 in the *E. coli* protein. In most bacteria, that position is occupied by a serine or threonine; substitution of a hydrophobic amino acid is associated with resistance (37,38). Thus, many wild-type mycobacterial gyrases exhibit reduced sensitivity to fluoroquinolones (Table 52.1). This change may relate to the absence of topoisomerase IV because the position equivalent to amino acid 83 in *E. coli* is also altered in two other species that lack topoisomerase IV, *Helicobacter pylori* and *Treponema pallidum* (39,40).

Bactericidal Action

Two findings with *E. coli* indicate that the lethal action of fluoroquinolones is distinct from their ability to block growth. First, one fluoroquinolone can exhibit more bacteriostatic activity than another and yet be less lethal (6). Second, inhibition of protein synthesis prevents older quino-

lones, such as nalidixic acid, from killing cells but not from blocking DNA replication. We have proposed that cell death during short-term treatment is owing to the release of double-stranded DNA breaks from drug–enzyme–DNA complexes (41) (Fig. 52.4). Release is thought to occur in two ways: one that is blocked by inhibitors of RNA or protein synthesis and one that is not. In the first mode, newly made protein is likely to be involved in quinolone action. However, no specific suicide protein has yet been identified. The second mode is postulated to arise from dissociation of gyrase subunits from the drug–enzyme–DNA complexes (15,41).

Extended exposure to quinolones, such as that used to measure minimal bactericidal concentration, is likely to elicit secondary events that may include lethal filamentation (19,42). Such events, which may be quite important clinically, probably stem from rapid inhibition of DNA replication rather than from release of breaks from com-

TABLE 52.1. FLUOROQUINOLONE-RESISTANT ALLELES IN THE GYRA PROTEIN OF MYCOBACTERIA

Species GyrA Codon:	75	88	90	91	94	126	MIC[b]	Ref.
Tuberculosis group								
Mycobacterium tuberculosis								
TN1626	A	G	A	S	D	A	ND	36
Single mutants	S	A,C	V	P	A,G,L,N,Y	E		36
H37Ra		G	A	S	D		0.3	61
Single mutants		C	V	P	H			33,61
Double mutant			V	P				61
Double mutant			V		G			61
H37Rv		G	A	S	D		0.5	37,93
Single mutants			V		N			93
Erdman		G	A	S	D		≤1	33
Single mutants			V					33
Clinical isolate		G	A	S	D			4
Single mutants		C	V	P	A,G,H,N,Y			4,33,74,93,94
Mycobacterium bovis bacille Calmette–Guérin		G	A	S	D		0.5	5,37
Single mutants			V		N			5,33
Double mutant			V		N			5
Mycobacterium kansasii		G	A	S	D		0.5	37
Mycobacterium leprae		G	A	S	D		ND	37
Mycobacterium fortuitum (3rd biovar)		G	A	S	D		0.13	37
Mycobacterium smegmatis		G	A	S	D		0.5	37
Single mutants		A,C	V		A,G,H,N,Y			36,57,95
Double mutant			V		G			95
GyrA Ser-90 group								
Mycobacterium fortuitum		G	S	S	D		0.06	37
Mycobacterium peregrinum		G	S	S	D		0.25	37
Mycobacterium aurum		G	S	S	D		0.03	37
Highly resistant group								
Mycobacterium avium		G	A	S	D		16	37
Mycobacterium intracellulare		G	A	S	D		4	37
Mycobacterium marinum		G	A	S	D		4	37
Mycobacterium chelonae		G	A	S	D		2	37
Mycobacterium abscessus		G	A	S	D		32	37

[a]Amino acid abbreviations are A (alanine), C (cysteine), D (aspartic acid), G (glycine), H (histidine), N (asparagine), P (proline), V (valine), Y (tyrosine). For resistant mutants, only the amino acid changes from wild type are listed. Amino acid numbers are assigned according to those of *Mycobacterium tuberculosis*.
[b]Determined for ciprofloxacin and expressed in micrograms per milliliter.
MIC, minimal inhibitory concentration; ND, not determined.

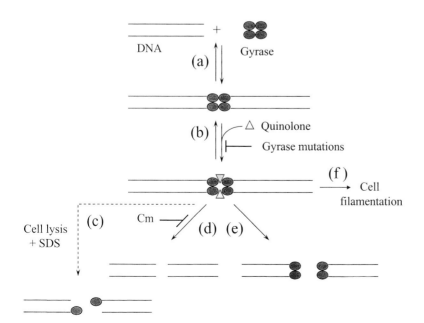

FIGURE 52.4. Scheme for bacteriostatic and bactericidal action of fluoroquinolones. Gyrase and DNA interact (*a*) to form complexes, and quinolones reversibly trap the complexes (*b*). Resistance mutations interfere with complex formation. Cell lysis in the presence of an ionic detergent such as sodium dodecyl sulfate *(SDS)* releases DNA fragments in which the GyrA protein is covalently bound to the 5′ ends of DNA (*c*). Complexes become lethal lesions in two ways. *d:* A suicide protein releases double-strand DNA breaks from the complexes; chloramphenicol *(Cm)* inhibits this pathway. *e:* The gyrase subunits dissociate to release double-strand DNA breaks. Complex formation may also lead to cell filamentation (*f*), which is expected to be a lethal event.

plexes because the minimal bactericidal concentration can be quantitatively similar to minimal inhibitory concentration (MIC) (43); release of breaks requires higher quinolone concentrations (41). Thus, formation of drug–enzyme–DNA complexes leads to cell death in several ways. Understanding and improving each of these lethal activities is likely to be of major importance in developing new quinolones.

Three features of lethal action have been observed with mycobacteria that are also characteristic of effects seen with other bacteria. First, chloramphenicol, an inhibitor of protein synthesis, partially inhibits fluoroquinolone lethality (5,34). Second, C-8-methoxy and C-8-halogen moieties enhance lethal activity (5,11,14). Third, mycobacteria exhibit the paradoxical loss of lethal activity seen when very high drug concentrations are tested (5,11). Thus, studies of fluoroquinolone lethality with model organisms, i.e., *E. coli*, should be applicable to *M. tuberculosis*.

FLUOROQUINOLONE EFFICACY IN ANIMAL MODELS

Mice have served as the main animal model for studying fluoroquinolone activity. The compounds are generally administered orally after mice are infected with either *M. avium-intracellulare* complex or *M. tuberculosis*, usually by intravenous injection or intranasal inoculation. Survival of animals, reduction in splenomegaly, lesions on lungs, and mycobacteria [colony-forming units (CFUs)] recovered from tissues (spleen, lungs, liver, and blood) are then measured as end points.

In general, *in vivo* efficacy reflects *in vitro* potency in terms of rank order of compounds. Gatifloxacin, moxifloxacin, and sparfloxacin are currently the most active compounds, with the number of CFUs from the spleen generally being lower after treatment with moxifloxacin than with sparfloxacin (44,45). However, differences seen *in vitro* are not always observed in mice (46,47). For example, with some isolates, the MIC of gatifloxacin is lower (0.031 µg/mL) than that of moxifloxacin (0.125 µg/mL), but in mice, the two compounds show similar potency when *M. tuberculosis* is recovered from lungs and spleen (45). In another example, clinafloxacin, which has an MIC range similar to that of moxifloxacin and sparfloxacin, shows little effect against *M. tuberculosis* under conditions in which the other two compounds prevent mortality, reduce splenomegaly, lower the development of gross lung lesions, and depress the recovery of mycobacteria from spleen (44).

When mouse models are used to compare antituberculosis compounds, the fluoroquinolones show intermediate activity. For example, rifampicin and isoniazid often display more activity than levofloxacin, ofloxacin, sparfloxacin, clinafloxacin, and gatifloxacin (44,46–49). Aminoglycosides

(amikacin, streptomycin, isepamicin, and kanamycin) fall between sparfloxacin and levofloxacin/ofloxacin when CFUs from the spleen and lungs are assayed (47). The macrolide roxithromycin is more effective than levofloxacin against *M. avium* when tested with infected mice, resulting in a 0.7-log reduction of CFUs from the blood when the same dose of levofloxacin allows CFUs to increase by 0.2 log (50). Thus, currently used fluoroquinolones are not particularly noteworthy for their activity in mice.

Efficacy can be improved by combining fluoroquinolones with other drugs. For example, a combination of moxifloxacin and isoniazid is significantly more effective than either compound alone, with the difference being more striking in the lung than the spleen (48). In another example, several combinations involving moxifloxacin or gatifloxacin are more effective than either fluoroquinolone by itself (45), but combinations are not always more effective. With *M. avium-intracellulare* complex–infected mice, a combination of levofloxacin and roxithromycin was only marginally better than roxithromycin alone (50), whereas with *M. tuberculosis*, ethambutol contributes little to combinations containing gatifloxacin (45); we recently found that ethambutol interferes with the lethal activity of fluoroquinolones *in vitro* (T. Lu, unpublished observations, 2003). To date, combinations of gatifloxacin or moxifloxacin with isoniazid and rifampicin are among the most promising (45).

Because the pharmacokinetics of the compounds differ, efforts have been made to adjust doses to mimic those used in humans. For example, daily doses of 50 mg/kg sparfloxacin and 200 mg/kg ofloxacin/levofloxacin with mice are thought to model those used clinically. In this situation, sparfloxacin is comparable with levofloxacin and is more effective than ofloxacin (47,49). In another example, 2 weeks after infection and initiation of treatment, 100 mg/kg moxifloxacin, in combination with isoniazid, rifampin, and pyrazinamide, is less bactericidal than 150 mg/kg streptomycin combined with the three other nonquinolone antituberculosis agents (51). After 6 months of therapy, however, followed by an additional 3 months without treatment to allow for relapse, the percentage of culture-positive mice was lower with the moxifloxacin-containing regimen than with the streptomycin-containing one (51). Thus, moxifloxacin seems to be at least as effective as streptomycin. It may even be more effective because the equivalent human dose of moxifloxacin is approximately four times that used in the mouse experiment (51).

CLINICAL EFFICACY OF FLUOROQUINOLONES

The fluoroquinolones were first reported to be active against tuberculosis in a study of patients carrying drug-resistant *M. tuberculosis* (1). These patients were treated with ofloxacin, along with agents to which resistance had arisen. Approximately 80% of the patients showed a decrease in culture positivity after a low daily dose (300 mg). The dose was subsequently increased to 800 mg, also in combination with other agents (52,53). The development of quinolone resistance, which is discussed in the next section, argues that the agent has a suppressive effect. However, the use of combination therapy (54) makes it difficult to ascribe a clear effect to the presence of the quinolone.

The fluoroquinolones are occasionally suggested for latent tuberculosis and prophylaxis. Data are scant, but one counterexample exists. When a patient treated with ciprofloxacin for 4 years for a nontuberculosis disease became immunocompromised, tuberculosis was reactivated (55). Thus, ciprofloxacin may not be effective for latent tuberculosis. With respect to prophylaxis, a combination of pyrazinamide and ciprofloxacin seems to be only marginally effective (56).

FLUOROQUINOLONE RESISTANCE

Resistance is associated with treatment failure (1,52). Because strains resistant to one fluoroquinolone have reduced susceptibility to all quinolones, resistance serves as a disincentive for the pharmaceutical industry to seek more effective derivatives; resistance makes the fluoroquinolone class a nonrenewable resource. Experiments described below suggest that our best hope for preserving the compounds is to avoid low doses and marginally effective derivatives. In a subsequent section, we point out why pharma-

cokinetic mismatches should be avoided during combination therapy.

Effect of Fluoroquinolone Concentration on Selection of Resistant Mutants

The recovery of bacterial colonies from fluoroquinolone-containing agar plates depends strongly on drug concentration (7,36). As the concentration increases, the fraction of input cells recovered as colonies drops sharply and plateaus (Fig. 52.5). With *M. tuberculosis*, mutants recovered at low concentration exhibit changes in GyrB. At higher fluoroquinolone concentrations, a variety of GyrA variants becomes prevalent. Eventually, a concentration is reached at which no mutant is recovered even when more than 10^{10} cells are applied. At that point, a second sharp drop in colony recovery is observed. The second-drop concentration, which corresponds to the MIC of the most resistant, single-step mutant (57), has been termed the mutant prevention concentration (MPC) (7).

Low concentrations of fluoroquinolones that have smaller C-7 moieties, such as ciprofloxacin, select variants of *M. tuberculosis* that lack changes in either GyrA or GyrB (36). The molecular basis for this low-level resistance, which is more pronounced with *M. smegmatis*, has not been established (36). With *M. smegmatis*, some of the nongyrase mutants express unselected resistance to ampicillin and chloramphenicol (36), suggesting that changes occurred in either drug efflux or drug uptake that apply to many agents. Increasing selective pressure on *M. smegmatis* leads to the

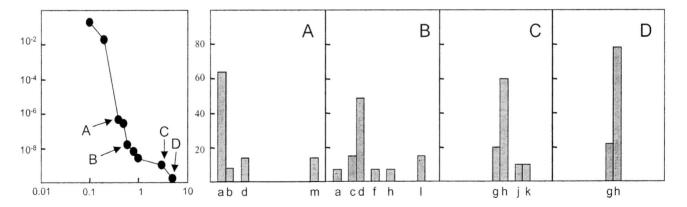

FIGURE 52.5. Effect of fluoroquinolone concentration on the spectrum of resistance alleles recovered with *Mycobacterium tuberculosis*. Mutants were recovered from sets of agar plates containing ciprofloxacin **(left)**. Nucleotide sequence analysis was performed on DNA from mutants obtained at fluoroquinolone concentrations indicated by *arrows*. **Right:** The prevalence of the various alleles. *Bars on right* indicate the percentage represented by each allele [in each panel **(A–D)**, nine to 15 mutants were examined]. GyrA variants are indicated by the following letters: a, non-*gyrA* mutants; *b*, A74S; *c*, G88A; *d*, A90V; *f*, D94A; *g*, D94Y; *h*, D94G; *j*, G88C; *k*, D94L; *l*, D89N; *m*, A126E. (Adapted from data presented in Zhou J-F, Dong Y, Zhao X, et al. Selection of antibiotic resistance: allelic diversity among fluoroquinolone-resistant mutations. *J Infect Dis* 2000;182:517–525.)

recovery of a variety of GyrA mutants; however, GyrB variants are generally not obtained.

Many bacterial species other than mycobacteria have both gyrase and topoisomerase IV as quinolone targets. In such cases, the concentration at the second sharp drop in mutant recovery is determined by formation of ternary complexes with the secondary target. When the cellular consequences of the complexes are similar for the two targets, as is the case for C-8-methoxy fluoroquinolones with *S. pneumoniae* (10), the first and second drops in mutant recovery occur at similar concentrations. Then the plateau is reduced to an inflection point (7,10).

Gyrase-Mediated Resistance

Resistant variants of the GyrA protein have alterations that occur in a stretch of amino acids called the quinolone-resistance determining region. For *E. coli*, the region extends from codons 51 to 106 (58,59), with major resistance changes located at codons 83 and 87. As pointed out previously, these two amino acids are part of α helix 4 (Fig. 52.3). Resistance at codon 83 is acquired by substitution of a hydrophobic amino acid, such as leucine and phenylalanine, for serine or threonine. Position 87 tends to be aspartic or glutamic acid. Resistance is associated with changes to asparagine, tyrosine, glycine, or histidine, often after mutation has occurred at position 83. In *M. tuberculosis*, amino

acid 90 (equivalent to 83 of *E. coli*) is alanine. This alanine is suspected of being responsible for wild-type *M. tuberculosis* having lower susceptibility to quinolones than mycobacterial species that have a serine at position 90 (*Mycobacterium fortuitum*, *Mycobacterium peregrinum*, and *Mycobacterium aurum* (37) (Table 52.1). When gyrase is purified from *M. smegmatis*, which is one of the Ala-90 species, it is found to be only 2% as sensitive to ciprofloxacin as gyrase purified from *E. coli* (60); MIC is 33 times higher. Thus, the sensitivity of purified gyrase parallels bacterial susceptibility, a feature also seen with resistant variants of *M. tuberculosis* (35). Because slow-growing mycobacteria probably contain only one drug target, second-step mutations also map in gyrase (5,61).

The identity of the most resistant, first-step mutant depends on fluoroquinolone structure. With *M. smegmatis*, a C-8-methoxy compound having a C-7-ring ethyl at the N position selects for a GyrA Gly to Cys change at position 89, whereas a compound having the ethyl group at a carbon adjacent to the ring nitrogen is less discriminating (Fig. 52.6). Apparently Cys-89 interferes more with fluoroquinolone binding when an ethyl group is attached to the C-7 piperazinyl ring nitrogen than when the ethyl is bound to a ring carbon. These data are consistent with the C-7 fluoroquinolone ring binding to gyrase near the N terminus of α helix 4, whereas the remainder of the quinolone attaches more toward the C terminus (Fig. 52.7). Such an orienta-

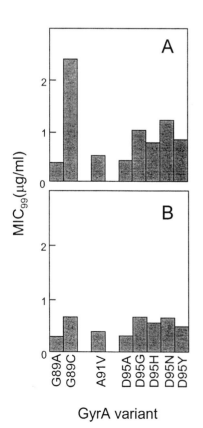

FIGURE 52.6. Effect of GyrA variation on susceptibility to fluoroquinolones. The minimal inhibitory concentration (for 99% of the cells) was determined for two structurally similar fluoroquinolones with the indicated fluoroquinolone-resistant mutants of *Mycobacterium smegmatis* (the changes in the GyrA variants are indicated by standard amino acid abbreviations with the letter preceding the number indicating the wild-type amino acid and the letter following the number representing the variant.) *A*: Fluoroquinolone PD161144, which has an ethyl group attached to the C-7 ring nitrogen. *B*: Fluoroquinolone PD161148, which has its ethyl group attached to a C-7 ring carbon adjacent to the nitrogen. (Adapted from data presented in Sindelar G, Zhao X, Liew A, et al. Mutant prevention concentration as a measure of fluoroquinolone potency against mycobacteria. *Antimicrob Agents Chemother* 2000;44:3337–3343.)

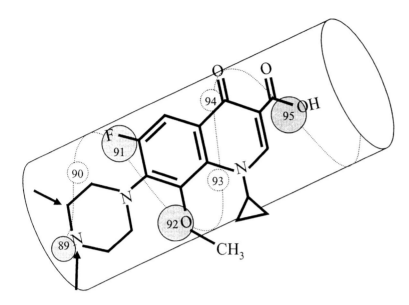

FIGURE 52.7. Orientation of fluoroquinolones and GyrA α helix 4. α Helix 4, adapted from the crystal structure of the breakage–reunion domain of the GyrA protein of *Escherichia coli* (28), is drawn parallel to the long axis of the fluoroquinolone. Amino acid numbers represent positions in the *Mycobacterium smegmatis* GyrA protein. *Arrows* indicate position of ethyl group. (Adapted from Sindelar G, Zhao X, Liew A, et al. Mutant prevention concentration as a measure of fluoroquinolone potency against mycobacteria. *Antimicrob Agents Chemother* 2000; 44:3337–3343.)

tion would explain why in *E. coli* a mutation at position 81 confers resistance to fluoroquinolones but not to nalidixic acid (62), a compound that lacks a C-7 ring. The effect of ethyl positioning is more pronounced when a methoxy group is at position C-8 (57), which supports the idea that the methoxy group affects quinolone positioning on gyrase (63).

Resistance mutations in *gyrB* have not been studied as extensively as those in *gyrA*. With *M. tuberculosis*, the Asn-510 to Tyr change predominates (Table 52.2). Because a conformational change occurs in GyrB on fluoroquinolone binding (64), available crystal structures are not readily interpreted in terms of GyrB drug binding sites.

TABLE 52.2. GYRB-MEDIATED RESISTANCE IN *MYCOBACTERIUM TUBERCULOSIS*

Amino Acid Change[a]	No. (%) of Mutants Recovered	Ref.
G481C	1 (2)	36
I497L	3 (5)	36
N510Y	47 (76)	36
N510T	1 (2)	36
N510D	2 (3)	36
N510K	2 (3)	36
T511I	2 (3)	36
T511N	1 (2)	36
E512D	1 (2)	36
E512V	2 (3)	36

[a]Amino acid abbreviations are C (cysteine), D (aspartic acid), E (glutamic acid), G (glycine), I (isoleucine), K (lysine), L (leucine), N (asparagine), T (threonine), V (valine), and Y (tyrosine). In each set, the first amino acid is that found in wild-type cells for the number indicated, and the second amino acid is found in the mutant.

Nongyrase-Mediated Resistance

Nongyrase mutants are characteristically recovered among mycobacteria when the cells are challenged with low concentrations of fluoroquinolone (36). Some *M. tuberculosis* isolates, when challenged with a second round of fluoroquinolone treatment, acquire additional determinants at approximately ten times the frequency observed with wild-type cells (J. Zhou, unpublished observation, 2002). Thus, the enrichment of nongyrase mutants could accelerate the development of resistance. A similar phenomenon is seen with *M. smegmatis*. However, an additional class of mutant is found in which susceptibility to ampicillin and chloramphenicol is lower by approximately twofold, and in this class, the frequency for selection of additional fluoroquinolone resistance determinants is unchanged. These nongyrase mutants have not been characterized in molecular terms.

It is commonly assumed that some nongyrase, fluoroquinolone-resistance mutations are involved in drug efflux. Indeed, many bacteria have efflux systems that lower fluoroquinolone susceptibility, and low-level resistance mutations often behave as if they up-regulate genes encoding efflux pumps. Two principal efflux systems are present in gram-positive bacteria. Both fall in the major facilitator family, a group of proteins characterized by 12 to 14 transmembrane helices and utilization of proton motive force as an energy source. One type is called the Bmr (bacillus multidrug resistance)-NorA (fluoroquinolone resistance) group; the other is termed the QacA (quaternary ammonium compound export) group. Some staphylococci also produce the Smr (small multidrug resistance) pump that contains only four transmembrane helices. Efflux systems in *M. tuberculosis* are poorly understood. One putative efflux mutant has an MIC for fluoroquinolones that is approximately one-fourth that observed with *gyrA* mutants, and it exhibits decreased accumulation of radioactive norfloxacin (61).

More is known about *M. smegmatis* efflux, although it is not clear which statements also apply to *M. tuberculosis* because *M. smegmatis* is normally a saprophytic organism. Two efflux genes have been identified in *M. smegmatis*. One, initially called *mtp*, is homologous to several different ATP-binding cassette transporters (65). ATP-binding cassette transporters are members of a large family of multisubunit proteins that import or export a variety of molecules using the energy of ATP hydrolysis as the driving force (reviewed in reference 66). The *mtp* gene is overexpressed in a ciprofloxacin-resistant strain (65), and high-level resistance created by stepwise challenge is associated with mutant accumulation of only a third as much fluoroquinolone as wild-type cells when assayed by measurement of ciprofloxacin fluorescence (67). In this ciprofloxacin-resistant clone, a phosphate-specific transporter is amplified (68), and when the *pstB* gene is disrupted, the MIC for ciprofloxacin drops from 64 to 8 μg/mL (69). Disruption of the *pstB* gene in a wild-type background reduces phosphate uptake and renders the cells twice as susceptible to ciprofloxacin (68). It has been argued that *mtp* represents an amplification of the *pst* operon (69).

The other efflux gene that has been studied, *lfr* (low-level fluoroquinolone resistance), lowers ciprofloxacin susceptibility through increased expression when cloned onto a plasmid (70). The *lfr* gene has been cloned, and sequence analysis indicates that the protein is related to a member of the major facilitator family of membrane efflux pumps (other related members are QacA of *S. aureus*, TcmA of *Streptomyces glaucescens*, and ActII and Mmr of *Streptomyces coelicolor*). These genes increase the MIC for compounds such as ethidium bromide, acriflavine, and cetyl trimethylammonium bromide (CTAB); their action is inhibited by energy uncouplers such as carbonyl cyanide m-chlorophenylhydrazone (CCCP). Preliminary experiments suggest that overexpression of the Lfr protein may increase the frequency at which subsequent resistance determinants are acquired (70), and hybridization experiments indicate that homologs to *lfr* are present in the genome of *M. tuberculosis* (70).

Another type of nongyrase resistance is represented by *mfpA* (71). This gene, originally cloned from *M. smegmatis*, decreases fluoroquinolone susceptibility when present on a plasmid in *M. smegmatis* and *M. bovis* bacille Calmette–Guérin (BCG). *M. smegmatis* strains deficient in the gene exhibit a small increase in fluoroquinolone susceptibility (71). Because efforts to demonstrate an efflux phenotype were unsuccessful, attention has focused on amino acid sequence similarities between MfpA and McbG, a plasmid-encoded protein found in *E. coli*. This protein is thought to help protect gyrase from attack by microcin B17, a plasmid-encoded bacteriocin. Another of these gyrase-protecting proteins, Qnr, is thought to be responsible for conferring plasmid-borne fluoroquinolone resistance in gram-negative bacteria (72,73).

Clinical Resistance to Fluoroquinolones

In general, clinical isolates of fluoroquinolone-resistant *M. tuberculosis* behave as first-step laboratory mutants. Most of the resistant clinical strains have alterations at GyrA codon 94, although a few have changes at positions 88 and 90 (3,4,33,74). Thus, a single mutation appears to be sufficient to cause resistance. Although extensive surveillance work has not been performed to assess the prevalence of fluoroquinolone resistance, at least one report shows that resistance sharply increased after it was recommended that quinolones be used as antituberculosis agents: in the Philippines, the prevalence of fluoroquinolone resistance in a hospital-based study was four times higher among isolates collected from 1995 to 2000 than among those obtained from 1989 to 1994 (75). The prevalence of ciprofloxacin- and ofloxacin-resistance is now at 27% and 35%, respectively. During the comparison periods, MDR tuberculosis showed little increase, whereas fluoroquinolone-resistance among isolates that showed no other resistance exhibited a 17-fold increase. Clearly, use of the compounds is not being restricted to MDR cases.

We also expect to see fluoroquinolone resistance increase in other countries. For example, in Spain, 6% of the isolates already have an MIC for ofloxacin that is 2 μg/mL or greater, and an enthusiasm for use of the compound has been expressed (76). Two patient types are likely to contribute to the development of resistance: those who attain abnormally low serum levels of antituberculosis agents (77) and those who have weakened defense systems owing to human immunodeficiency virus infection or chemotherapy (78). In both types, large bacterial populations are more likely to develop, which then increases the probability that resistant mutants will be present. As expected, such patients tend to acquire resistance *de novo* (53).

The experiences in the Philippines and Spain do not bode well for the fluoroquinolones as antituberculosis agents; if major changes are not made, the new agents moxifloxacin and gatifloxacin will succumb to resistance. We present a framework for considering dosing strategies that stress preventing the development of resistance.

MUTANT RESTRICTION STRATEGIES

Mutant Selection Window

The efficacy of an antimicrobial agent is related to two parameters: its potency with a particular pathogen, generally measured as the MIC, and the exposure the pathogen receives in the host (79). The two are combined by approximating the length of time serum levels are above the MIC, the area under the time-concentration curve that is above the MIC, or the ratio of the maximal concentration (C_{max}) to the MIC. For fluoroquinolones, the empirical pharmacodynamic indices area under the time-concentration

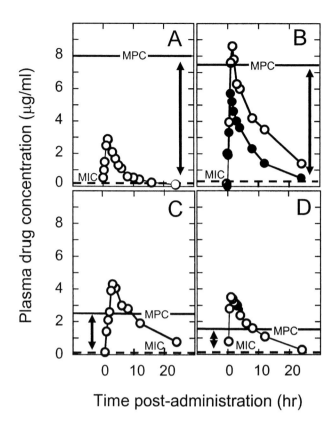

FIGURE 52.8. Mutant selection window. Pharmacokinetic profiles are shown for ciprofloxacin (750 mg) (*A*), levofloxacin (500 mg, *filled circles*; 750 mg, *open circles*) (*B*), moxifloxacin (400 mg) (*C*), and gatifloxacin (400 mg) (*D*). Values for the minimal inhibitory concentration (*MIC*) and mutant prevention concentration (*MPC*) are indicated for a clinical isolate of *Mycobacterium tuberculosis* (13). *Double-headed arrows* indicate mutant selection window.

curve/MIC and C_{max}/MIC are related to favorable patient outcome with some pathogens (80).

The MIC-based pharmacodynamic approach is designed to suppress the growth of susceptible cells, since as monotherapy a compound at concentrations greater than the MIC will selectively enrich mutants unless other factors are considered. One of those factors is the host defense system, which probably plays a major role in removing resistant mutants. Indeed, it may be the main reason that the development of resistance in a given patient is rarely seen with pathogens other than *M. tuberculosis* and *Pseudomonas aeruginosa*. Nevertheless, resistance does arise often enough to render compounds ineffective, even when the microbe is highly susceptible (e.g., penicillin and *S. pneumoniae*). To suppress the development of resistance, higher values of area under the time-concentration curve/MIC, derived from clinical studies, have been recommended (80). However, those values may be below that required to block resistance with large numbers of patients.

An alternative strategy for directly attacking mutants was suggested by examination of the effect of fluoroquinolone

concentration on mutant selection with mycobacteria (7). Resistant mutants are selected within a specific concentration window. The lower limit of the window can be approximated as the concentration that blocks the growth of 99% of the cells (MIC_{99}). The upper limit is the MIC of the most resistant mutant, a concentration called the MPC. The concentration range between MIC_{99} and MPC is termed the mutant selection window (9,81), which is quite broad for *M. tuberculosis* (Fig. 52.8).

The selection window idea leads to a straightforward dosing strategy to restrict the selection of a resistance: dose to maintain relevant concentrations above MPC throughout therapy. To determine whether a particular compound and dose are likely to restrict the selection of resistance, MPC is compared with serum drug concentration (12) (refinement is expected to come from the use of drug concentrations at the site of infection and from correction for factors such as protein binding that may sequester or inactivate the compound). Data for ciprofloxacin and levofloxacin with *M. tuberculosis* are shown in Figure 52.8. Serum concentrations for both compounds fall inside the mutant selection window for considerable periods of time, and they never exceed the MPC. The same is true for other commonly used antituberculosis compounds, as illustrated by the ratio the MPC to C_{max} being greater than 1 (Table 52.3). Thus, all these agents are expected to readily select resistant mutants when used as monotherapy. By the mutant selection criteria, the C-8-methoxy fluoroquinolones are unusual: gatifloxacin and moxifloxacin are the only compounds that have an MPC/C_{max} ratio that is less than 1 (Table 52.3; Fig. 52.8).

Although the C-8-methoxy fluoroquinolones are superior to the older compounds with respect to the maintenance of concentrations above the MPC, their long half-lives could be detrimental for infrequent dosing because their concentrations would be in the window for long periods. Short half-life compounds would drop below the window quickly and stop applying selective pressure. These monotherapy considerations are important even when the compounds are intended to be used in combination therapy because the prevalence of *M. tuberculosis* with resistance to the other compounds in the regimen is likely to increase.

A second factor in the development of resistance is mutation frequency. This parameter varies with resistance allele and drug concentration. For gyrase mutations, it is approximated by the level of the plateau seen in Fig. 52.5. For quinolones with mycobacteria, resistant mutants are recovered at a frequency of approximately 10^{-7} to 10^{-8}.

Combination Therapy

When the concentration of a compound cannot be maintained above the MPC (Table 52.3), it is necessary to use combinations of agents having different intracellular targets. Clinical experience shows this to be the case (82). Sev-

TABLE 52.3. POTENCY OF ANTITUBERCULOSIS AGENTS AGAINST *MYCOBACTERIUM TUBERCULOSIS*[a]

Antibiotic	MIC$_{99}$	MPC	Dose[b]	C$_{max}$	MPC/C$_{max}$	Ref. for C$_{max}$
Rifampicin	0.02	>80	600	9.5	>8	96
Streptomycin	0.2	>320	1000	34	>9	97,98
Isoniazid	0.06	20	250	7.6	2.6	96
Capreomycin	2.0	160	1000	33	4.8	98
Kanamycin	1.5	>800	500	21	>38	99
Cycloserine	14	70	750	35	2	100
Fluoroquinolones						
Ciprofloxacin	0.15	8.0	750	4.4	1.8	101
Levofloxacin	0.2	7.5	500	5.7	1.3	102
Moxifloxacin	0.037	2.5	400	4.5	0.55	103
Gatifloxacin[c]	0.03	1.5	400	3.7	0.41	104
Sparfloxacin	0.075	2.5	200	1.4	1.8	105
PD161148	0.07	1.5	—	NA	—	

[a]Experiments were performed with clinical isolate TN6515 (106). Data from Dong Y, Zhao X, Kreiswirth B, et al. Mutant prevention concentration as measure of antibiotic potency: studies with clinical isolates of *Mycobacterium tuberculosis*. *Antimicrob Agents Chemother* 2000;44:2581–2584.
[b]Recommended by manufacturer in milligrams.
[c]Experiments were performed with PD135432, which is identical to gatifloxacin.
C$_{max}$, maximal drug concentration; MIC, minimal inhibitory concentration (in micrograms per milliliter); MPC, mutant prevention concentration (in micrograms per milliliter); NA, not available.

eral factors indicate that combination therapy will probably be required for C-8-methoxy fluoroquinolones even though their concentrations do exceed MPC. First, the half-lives are too short to ensure that serum concentrations will be greater than the MPC throughout therapy. Second, the large number of bacilli present during infection, sometimes on the order of 10^9 (83), makes it likely that resistant mutants will be present spontaneously. Third, C-8-methoxy fluoroquinolones are not bactericidal enough to quickly eradicate the pathogen.

Pharmacokinetics are important for restricting the development of resistance with combination therapy because mismatches can allow the occurrence of periods equivalent to monotherapy (8). A clinical experiment using human immunodeficiency virus–positive patients with tuberculosis (84) illustrates this point. In one arm of a two-drug combination protocol, drug concentration decreased to less than the MIC later for isoniazid than for rifampicin. Thus, no period equivalent to rifampicin monotherapy was expected to occur. In the other arm of the experiment, the concentration of rifapentine, a long-lived derivative of rifampicin (84), decreased to less than the MIC after that of isoniazid. In this case, a period equivalent to rifapentine monotherapy was extensive. Rifampicin/rifapentine-resistant mutants were obtained from patients only in the second arm. We have suggested that efforts should be made to superimpose pharmacokinetic profiles so that no agent in the combination therapy will be above its MIC, while the concentration of the other agents is below (9).

The long half-lives of moxifloxacin and gatifloxacin make it difficult to combine these agents with compounds such as rifampicin and isoniazid without creating substantial periods of fluoroquinolone monotherapy (Fig. 52.9).

Gatifloxacin has the shorter half-life, suggesting that it may fit slightly better than moxifloxacin with the other agents. As shown in Figure 52.9, rifapentine has a much longer half-life than either fluoroquinolone. Thus, combining rifapentine with moxifloxacin or gatifloxacin would reduce the frequency at which fluoroquinolone resistance develops,

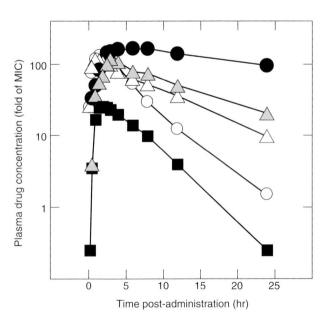

FIGURE 52.9. Pharmacokinetics of compounds potentially used in combination with fluoroquinolones. Serum concentrations after administration of approved doses of rifampicin (*filled squares*), isoniazid (*open circles*), rifapentine (*filled circles*), moxifloxacin (*shaded triangles*), and gatifloxacin (*open triangles*).

but at the expense of rifapentine resistance. Efforts are now needed to find antituberculosis compounds that will be good pharmacokinetic matches.

EFFECT OF FLUOROQUINOLONE STRUCTURE ON ACTION AND RESISTANCE

In the past three decade, approximately 10,000 quinolones have been synthesized. Approximately a dozen have entered clinical practice. The need for good efficacy and low human toxicity has served as strong selective forces, and the evolution of the compounds can be seen (85). Two separate lines have shown activity with *M. tuberculosis* (refer to Figure 52.1 for structures). One is represented by levofloxacin and the other by ciprofloxacin (moxifloxacin and gatifloxacin have evolved from ciprofloxacin). In this final section, we consider the influence of several aspects of structure on quinolone efficacy.

N-1 Substituents

Addition of a cyclopropyl group at position N-1 distinguishes ciprofloxacin from the earlier compound norfloxacin. This addition has a significant effect on lethal action with *E. coli*: ciprofloxacin kills cells in which protein synthesis has been halted, whereas norfloxacin does not (86). We have speculated that lethal action by quinolones in the absence of protein synthesis is owing to dissociation of the gyrase subunits after the enzyme is trapped on DNA by the quinolone. That would be equivalent to the release of double-strand breaks (41). How the cyclopropyl group stimulates such a process is unknown. However, it is probably relevant to mycobacteria because chloramphenicol, an inhibitor of protein synthesis, partially inhibits the lethal action of fluoroquinolones in *M. bovis* BCG (5).

Attachment of a *tert*-butyl at position N-1 has also received attention, particularly with *M. avium* (87). Compounds with a *tert*-butyl group have as much, or more, bacteriostatic activity than cyclopropyl derivatives. Lethal action has not been investigated. The levofloxacin-ofloxacin group also has a moiety attached to position N-1 (Fig. 52.1). Whether this accounts for the ability of levofloxacin to kill *S. aureus* in the absence of protein synthesis (88) is not known. In general, the bactericidal potency of levofloxacin is intermediate to ciprofloxacin and the C-8-methoxy derivatives discussed later (11).

C-8 Substituents

Early studies that combined computational methods with bacteriostatic assays indicated that C-8-methoxy and C-8-halogens improve fluoroquinolone action against *M. avium* (89). At about the same time, we noticed that sparfloxacin (C-8-F) has more bacteriostatic activity than

ciprofloxacin (C-8-H) against resistant mutants of *M. tuberculosis* (4,5). Because sparfloxacin and ciprofloxacin have structural differences other than substituents at the C-8 position, we investigated paired C-8-halogen, C-8-methoxy, and C-8-H fluoroquinolones. The methoxy moiety improved bacteriostatic and bactericidal activity with wild-type cells of *M. bovis* BCG (5), *M. smegmatis* (11,57), and *M. tuberculosis* (5,14).

The effect of the C-8-methoxy group was much more striking when *gyrA* resistance mutants were examined. With *M. bovis* BCG, enhancement of bacteriostatic activity was approximately tenfold; the improvement in lethal activity was also striking (5). As expected, the C-8-methoxy group increased effectiveness against clinically resistant isolates of *M. tuberculosis*, both in liquid culture and human macrophages (5,14). In general, the methoxy group enhances activity more than C-8-halide moieties (11).

The question of how C-8 substituents affect fluoroquinolone activity has been addressed mainly with *E. coli* (63). When the effect of *gyrA* resistance mutations on the presence of a C-8-methoxy group was examined, the alleles fell into two categories. One group was located in α helix 4 of the GyrA protein and one was located outside the helix. The protective effect of mutations mapping in the helix was decreased substantially by the C-8-methoxy group, whereas that was not the case for those mapping outside the helix. These data are consistent with α helix 4 being part of a quinolone binding site, a conclusion that is also suggested by mutations in the helix conferring the greatest reduction in susceptibility. We speculate that substitution of Leu or Trp for Ser-83 and Asn, Gly, His, or Tyr for Asp-87 may confer quinolone resistance by making the microenvironment of α helix 4 less electron rich and less able to bind quinolone. C-8-methoxy or C-8-halogenated fluoroquinolones may then increase sensitivity by partially restoring electron richness to the region.

Substitution of proline for alanine at codon 84 generates a helix mutant that behaves like cells containing nonhelix mutations (63). Unlike other substitutions that confer resistance, a proline is expected to disrupt helix structure. Thus, it is not surprising that the effect of an Ala-84 to Pro change differs from the mutations at positions 83 and 87. Perhaps perturbation of the helix between positions 83 and 87 alters the alignment between the putative quinolone-binding sites at those amino acids.

C-8-Br and C-8-H compounds are indistinguishable when tested for bacteriostatic activity with wild-type *M. bovis* BCG, but the C-8-Br is clearly more effective against a first-step gyrase mutant. That explains why the Br-containing derivative is better than its C-8-H control at restricting resistance (5): enhanced activity against mutants lowers MPC (36,57). We currently believe that enhanced attack of mutants is the reason why gatifloxacin and moxifloxacin show such low values for MPC with *M. tuberculosis* (Table 52.3).

C-7 Substituents

A variety of ring structures has been added to the C-7 position. The most characterized is the piperazinyl ring. For *M. avium*, small alkyl groups added to the ring improve bacteriostatic activity, with optimal activity being found when one or two methyl groups are present (87). A similar observation was found for *M. smegmatis* with both wild-type cells and gyrase mutants (57). The relative effect of these features on intracellular drug concentration and drug–gyrase–DNA complex formation is unknown. C-7 ring structure has not been examined systematically for effects on lethal action. It could have a significant effect if we are correct about the orientation of quinolones on gyrase (Fig. 52.6) because that would mean that the C-7 rings point toward each other from separate subunits. Addition to the rings might then create repulsive forces that would weaken gyrase subunit interactions. Whether changes in the C-7 moieties influence gyrase subunit dissociation is not known.

SUMMARY

Work with ofloxacin and levofloxacin shows that fluoroquinolones can be part of an effective treatment for tuberculosis in some patients. However, the relatively weak killing power of the fluoroquinolones has relegated them to second-line status. Expanded use, particularly with MDR cases in which other members of the combination therapy are neither highly effective nor pharmacokinetically well matched, is likely to lead to an increasing prevalence of fluoroquinolone resistance. New C-8-methoxy derivatives exhibit greater lethality, at least *in vitro* and enhanced activity against resistant mutants. Whether the currently available compounds moxifloxacin and gatifloxacin are active enough to prevent the development of resistance remains to be established. If not, their application and the application of the older quinolones must be very carefully controlled to avoid widespread resistance.

The long half-lives of the new fluoroquinolones may pose a serious problem for use in combination therapy. We have already seen how long a half-life can be associated with increased development of resistance for rifapentine (discussed in reference 8). Although the C-8-methoxy fluoroquinolones have the advantage of achieving concentrations greater than the MPC, formulating a suitable combination may be a formidable challenge.

The broad spectrum of fluoroquinolone action poses another problem for their use as antituberculosis agents because long-term use is likely to have a profound effect on other patient flora. For example, resistant members of other species may be selectively enriched, particularly among gram-positive organisms. Low potency fluoroquinolones, such as levofloxacin and ciprofloxacin, readily select resistant mutants of *S. aureus* (90) and *S. pneumoniae* (10,12,91,

92). The reverse situation can also occur; resistant tuberculosis can arise during fluoroquinolone treatment for another disease (74). Thus, the use of broad-spectrum agents can have effects beyond their intended purpose. It is likely that more effective compounds can be designed. The challenge is to keep resistance from becoming so extensive that new derivatives are useless owing to cross-resistance.

REFERENCES

1. Tsukamura M, Nakamura E, Yoshii S, et al. Therapeutic effect of a new antibacterial substance ofloxacin (DL8280) on pulmonary tuberculosis. *Am Rev Respir Dis* 1985;131:352–356.
2. Rastogi N, Ross B, Dwyer B, et al. Emergence during unsuccessful chemotherapy of multiple drug resistance in a strain of *Mycobacterium tuberculosis*. *Eur J Clin Microbiol Infect Dis* 1992;11:901–907.
3. Sullivan EA, Kreiswirth BN, Palumbo L, et al. Emergence of fluoroquinolone-resistant tuberculosis in New York City. *Lancet* 1995;345:1148–1150.
4. Xu C, Kreiswirth BN, Sreevatsan S, et al. Fluoroquinolone resistance associated with specific gyrase mutations in clinical isolates of multidrug resistant *Mycobacterium tuberculosis*. *J Infect Dis* 1996;174:1127–1130.
5. Dong Y, Xu C, Zhao X, et al. Fluoroquinolone action against mycobacteria: effects of C8 substituents on bacterial growth, survival, and resistance. *Antimicrob Agents Chemother* 1998;42:2978–2984.
6. Zhao X, Xu C, Domagala J, et al. DNA topoisomerase targets of the fluoroquinolones: a strategy for avoiding bacterial resistance. *Proc Natl Acad Sci U S A* 1997;94:13991–13996.
7. Dong Y, Zhao X, Domagala J, et al. Effect of fluoroquinolone concentration on selection of resistant mutants of *Mycobacterium bovis* BCG and *Staphylococcus aureus*. *Antimicrob Agents Chemother* 1999;43:1756–1758.
8. Drlica K A strategy for fighting antibiotic resistance. *ASM News* 2001;67:27–33.
9. Zhao X, Drlica K Restricting the selection of antibiotic-resistant mutants: a general strategy derived from fluoroquinolone studies. *Clin Infect Dis* 2001;33[Suppl 3]: S147–S156.
10. Li X, Zhao X, Drlica K Selection of *Streptococcus pneumoniae* mutants having reduced susceptibility to levofloxacin and moxifloxacin. *Antimicrob Agents Chemother* 2002;46:522–524.
11. Lu T, Zhao X, Li X, et al. Enhancement of fluoroquinolone activity by C-8 halogen and methoxy moieties: action against a gyrase resistance mutant of *Mycobacterium smegmatis* and a gyrase-topoisomerase IV double mutant of *Staphylococcus aureus*. *Antimicrob Agents Chemother* 2001;45:2703–2709.
12. Blondeau J, Zhao X, Hansen G, et al. Mutant prevention concentrations (MPC) for fluoroquinolones with clinical isolates of *Streptococcus pneumoniae*. *Antimicrob Agents Chemother* 2001;45:433–438.
13. Dong Y, Zhao X, Kreiswirth B, et al. Mutant prevention concentration as a measure of antibiotic potency: studies with clinical isolates of *Mycobacterium tuberculosis*. *Antimicrob Agents Chemother* 2000;44:2581–2584.
14. Zhao B-Y, Pine R, Domagala J, et al. Fluoroquinolone action against clinical isolates of *Mycobacterium tuberculosis*: effects of a C8-methoxyl group on survival in liquid media and in human macrophages. *Antimicrob Agents Chemother* 1999;43:661–666.

15. Drlica K, Zhao X DNA gyrase, topoisomerase IV, and the 4-quinolones. *Microbiol Mol Rev* 1997;61:377–392.

16. Drlica K, Hooper DC Mechanisms of quinolone action. In: Hooper DC, ed. *The quinolone antimicrobials.* Washington, DC: American Society for Microbiology *(in press).*

17. Champoux JJ. DNA topoisomerases: structure, function, and mechanism. *Annu Rev Biochem* 2001;70:369–413.

18. Snyder M, Drlica K DNA gyrase on the bacterial chromosome: DNA cleavage induced by oxolinic acid. *J Mol Biol* 1979;131: 287–302.

19. Goss W, Deitz W, Cook T. Mechanism of action of nalidixic acid on *Escherichia coli.* II. Inhibition of deoxyribonucleic acid synthesis. *J Bacteriol* 1965;89:1068–1074.

20. Wentzell L, Maxwell A The complex of DNA gyrase and quinolone drugs on DNA forms a barrier to the T7 DNA polymerase replication complex. *J Mol Biol* 2000;304:779–791.

21. Hiasa H, Yousef D, Marians K. DNA strand cleavage is required for replication fork arrest by a frozen topoisomerase-quinolone-DNA ternary complex. *J Biol Chem* 1996;271:26424–26429.

22. Manes SH, Pruss GJ, Drlica K. Inhibition of RNA synthesis by oxolinic acid is unrelated to average DNA supercoiling. *J Bacteriol* 1983;155:420–423.

23. Willmott CJR, Critchlow SE, Eperon IC, et al. The complex of DNA gyrase and quinolone drugs with DNA forms a barrier to transcription by RNA polymerase. *J Mol Biol* 1994;242: 351–363.

24. Cole ST, Brosch R, Parkhill J, et al. Deciphering the biology of *Mycobacterium tuberculosis* from the complete genome sequence. *Nature* 1998;393:537–544.

25. Hiasa H, Marians KJ. Two distinct modes of strand unlinking during theta-type DNA replication. *J Biol Chem* 1996;271: 21529–21535.

26. Berger JM, Gamblin SJ, Harrison SC, et al. Structure and mechanism of DNA topoisomerase II. *Nature* 1996;379: 225–232.

27. Fass D, Bogden CE, Berger JM. Quaternary changes in topoisomerase II may direct orthogonal movement of two DNA strands. *Nat Struct Biol* 1999;6:322–326.

28. MoraisCabral JH, Jackson AP, Smith CV, et al. Crystal structure of the breakage-reunion domain of DNA gyrase. *Nature* 1997;388:903–906.

29. Wigley DB, Davies GJ, Dodson EJ, et al. Crystal structure of an N-terminal fragment of the DNA gyrase B protein. *Nature* 1991;351:624–629.

30. Wang JC. Moving one DNA double helix through another by a type II DNA topoisomerase: the story of a simple molecular machine. *Q Rev Biophys* 1998;31:107–144.

31. Williams N, Howells A, Maxwell A. Locking the ATP-operated clamp of DNA gyrase: probing the mechanism of strand passage. *J Mol Biol* 2001;306:969–984.

32. Williams NL, Maxwell A. Locking the DNA gate of DNA gyrase: investigating the effects on DNA cleavage and ATP hydrolysis. *Biochemistry* 1999;38:14157–14164.

33. Takiff H, Salazar L, Guerrero C, et al. Cloning and nucleotide sequence of the *Mycobacterium tuberculosis gyrA* and *gyrB* genes, and characterization of quinolone resistance mutations. *Antimicrob Agents Chemother* 1994;38:773–780.

34. Drlica K, Xu C, Wang J-Y, et al. Fluoroquinolone action in mycobacteria: similarity with effects in *Escherichia coli* and detection by cell lysate viscosity. *Antimicrob Agents Chemother* 1996;40:1594–1599.

35. Onodera Y, Tanaka M, Sata K. Inhibitory activity of quinolones against DNA gyrase of *Mycobacterium tuberculosis. J Antimicrob Chemother* 2001;47:447–450.

36. Zhou J-F, Dong Y, Zhao X, et al. Selection of antibiotic resistance: allelic diversity among fluoroquinolone-resistant mutations. *J. Inf. Dis.* 2000;182:517–525.

37. Guillemin I, Jarlier V, Cambau E. Correlation between quinolone sensitivity patterns and sequences in the A and B subunits of DNA gyrase in mycobacteria. *Antimicrob Agents Chemother* 1998;42:2084–2088.

38. Guillemin I, Sougakoff W, Cambau E, et al. Purification and inhibition by quinolones of DNA gyrases from *Mycobacterium avium, Mycobacterium smegmatis* and *Mycobacterium fortuitum* bv. *peregrinum. Microbiology* 1999;145:2527–2532.

39. Fraser C, Norris S, Weinstock G, et al. Complete genome sequence of *Treponema pallidum,* the syphilis spirochete. *Science* 1998;281:375–388.

40. Tomb J, White O, Kerlavage A, et al. The complete genome sequence of the gastric pathogen *Helicobacter pylori. Nature* 1997;388:539–547.

41. Chen C-R, Malik M, Snyder M, et al. DNA gyrase and topoisomerase IV on the bacterial chromosome: quinolone-induced DNA cleavage. *J Mol Biol* 1996;258:627–637.

42. Piddock L, Walters R. Bactericidal activities of five quinolones for *Escherichia coli* strains with mutations in genes encoding the SOS response or cell division. *Antimicrob Agents Chemother* 1992;36:819–825.

43. Chow R, Dougherty T, Fraimow H, et al. Association between early inhibition of DNA synthesis and the MICs and MBCs of carboxyquinolone antimicrobial agents for wild-type and mutant [*gyrA nfxB(ompF) acrA*] *Escherichia coli* K-12. *Antimicrob Agents Chemother* 1988;32:1113–1118.

44. Ji B, Lounis N, Maslo C, et al. *In vitro* and *in vivo* activities of moxifloxacin and clinafloxacin against *Mycobacterium tuberculosis. Antimicrob Agents Chemother* 1998;42:2066–2069.

45. Alvirez-Freites E, Carter J, Cynamon M. *In vitro* and *in vivo* activities of gatifloxacin against *Mycobacterium tuberculosis. Antimicrob Agents Chemother* 2002;46:1022–1025.

46. Ji B, Lounis N, Truffot-Pernot C, et al. *In vitro* and *in vivo* activities of levofloxacin against *Mycobacterium tuberculosis. Antimicrob Agents Chemother* 1995;39:1341–1344.

47. Lounis N, Ji B, Truffot-Pernot C, et al. Which aminoglycoside or fluoroquinolone is more active against *Mycobacterium tuberculosis* in mice? *Antimicrob Agents. Chemother* 1997;41:607–610.

48. Miyazaki E, Miyazaki M, Chen J, et al. Moxifloxacin (Bay12-8039), a new 9-methoxyquinolone, is active in a mouse model of tuberculosis. *Antimicrob Agents Chemother* 1999;43:85–89.

49. Klemens SP, Sharpe C, Rogge M, et al. Activity of levofloxacin in a murine model of tuberculosis. *Antimicrob Agents Chemother* 1994;38:1476–1479.

50. Bermudez L, Kolonoski P, Young L. Roxithromycin alone and in combination with either ethambutol or levofloxacin for disseminated *Mycobacterium avium* infections in beige mice. *Antimicrob Agents Chemother* 1996;40:1033–1035.

51. Lounis N, Bentoucha A, Truffot-Pernot C, et al. Effectiveness of once-weekly rifapentine and moxifloxacin regimens against *Mycobacterium tuberculosis* in mice. *Antimicrob Agents Chemother* 2001;45:3482–3486.

52. Yew W, Kwan S, Ma W, et al. In vitro activity of ofloxacin against *Mycobacterium tuberculosis* and its clinical efficacy in multiply resistant pulmonary tuberculosis. *J Antimicrob Chemother* 1990;26:227–236.

53. Yew W, Chan C, Hau C, et al. Outcomes of patients with multidrug-resistant pulmonary tuberculosis treated with ofloxacin/levofloxacin-containing regimens. *Chest* 2000;117:744–751.

54. Singla R, Gupta S, Gupta R, et al. Efficacy and safety of sparfloxacin in combination with kanamycin and ethionamide in multidrug-resistant pulmonary tuberculosis patients: preliminary results. *Int J Tuberc Lung Dis* 2001;5:559–563.

55. Lalonde R, Barkun J. Prolonged ciprofloxacin therapy fails to prevent reactivation tuberculosis. *Clin Infect Dis* 1998;27: 913–914.

56. Stevens J, Daniel T. Chemoprophylaxis of multidrug-resistant tuberculosis infection in HIV-uninfected individuals using ciprofloxacin and pyrazinamide. *Chest* 1995;108:712–717.

57. Sindelar G, Zhao X, Liew A, et al. Mutant prevention concentration as a measure of fluoroquinolone potency against mycobacteria. *Antimicrob Agents Chemother* 2000;44: 3337–3343.

58. Yoshida H, Bogaki M, Nakamura M, et al. Quinolone resistance-determining region in the DNA gyrase *gyrA* gene of *Escherichia coli. Antimicrob Agents Chemother* 1990;34: 1271–1272.

59. Friedman SM, Lu T, Drlica K. A mutation in the DNA gyrase A gene of *Escherichia coli* that expands the quinolone-resistance-determining region. *Antimicrob Agents Chemother* 2001;45: 2378–2380.

60. Revel-Viravau V, Truong QC, Moreau N, et al. Sequence analysis, purification, and study of inhibition by 4-quinolones of the DNA gyrase from *Mycobacterium smegmatis. Antimicrob Agents Chemother* 1996;40:2054–2061.

61. Kocagoz T, Hackbarth CJ, Unsal I, et al. Gyrase mutations in laboratory-selected fluoroquinolone-resistant mutants of *Mycobacterium tuberculosis* H37Ra. *Antimicrob Agents Chemother* 1996;40:1768–1774.

62. Cambau E, Borden F, Collatz E, et al. Novel *gyrA* point mutation in a strain of *Escherichia coli* resistant to fluoroquinolones but not to nalidixic acid. *Antimicrob Agents Chemother* 1993;37: 1247–1252.

63. Lu T, Zhao X, Drlica K. Gatifloxacin activity against quinolone-resistant gyrase: allele-specific enhancement of bacteriostatic and bactericidal activity by the C-8-methoxy group. *Antimicrob Agents Chemother* 1999;43:2969–2974.

64. Kampranis S, Maxwell A. Conformational changes in DNA gyrase revealed by limited proteolysis. *J Biol Chem* 1998;273: 22606–22614.

65. Banerjee S, Misra P, Bhatt K, et al. Identification of an ABC transporter gene that exhibits mRNA level overexpression in fluoroquinolone-resistant *Mycobacterium smegmatis. FEBS Lett* 1998;425:151–156.

66. Fath M, Kolter R. ABC transporters: bacterial exporters. *Microbiol Rev* 1993;57:1005–1017.

67. Banerjee SK, Bhatt K, Rana S, et al. Involvement of an efflux system in mediating high level of fluoroquinolone resistance in *Mycobacterium smegmatis. Biochem Biophys Res Commun* 1996; 226:362–368.

68. Bhatt K, Banerjee S, Chakraborti P. Evidence that phosphate specific transporter is amplified in a fluoroquinolone resistant *Mycobacterium smegmatis. Eur J Biochem* 2000;267:4028–4032.

69. Banerjee SK, Bhatt K, Misra P, et al. Involvement of a natural transport system in the process of efflux-mediated drug resistance in *Mycobacterium smegmatis. Mol Gen Genet* 2000;262: 949–956.

70. Takiff HE, Cimino M, Musso MC, et al. Efflux pump of the proton antiporter family confers low-level fluoroquinolone resistance in *Mycobacterium smegmatis. Proc Natl Acad Sci U S A* 1996;93:362–366.

71. Montero C, Mateu G, Rodriguez R, et al. Intrinsic resistance of *Mycobacterium smegmatis* to fluoroquinolones may be influenced by new pentapeptide protein MfpA. *Antimicrob Agents Chemother* 2001;45:3387–3392.

72. Martinez-Martinez L, Pascual A, Jacoby G. Quinolone resistance from a transferrable plasmid. *Lancet* 1998;351:797–799.

73. Tran J, Jacoby G. The mechanism of plasmid-mediated quinolone resistance. In: *40th Interscience Conference on Antimicrobial Agents and Chemotherapy,* 2000.

74. Perlman D, ElSadr W, Heifets L, et al. Susceptibility to levofloxacin of *Mycobacterium tuberculosis* isolates from patients with HIV-related tuberculosis and characterization of a strain with levofloxacin monoresistance. *AIDS* 1997;11:1473–1478.

75. Grimaldo E, Tupasi T, Rivera A, et al. Increased resistance to ciprofloxacin and ofloxacin in multidrug-resistant *Mycobacterium tuberculosis* isolates from patients seen at a tertiary hospital in the Philippines. *Int J Tuberc Lung Dis* 2001;5:546–550.

76. Casal M, Ruiz P, Herreras A, et al. Study of the in vitro susceptibility of *M. tuberculosis* to ofloxacin in Spain. *Int J Tuberc Lung Dis* 2000;4:588–591.

77. Elliott A, Berning S, Iseman M, et al. Failure of drug penetration and acquisition of drug resistance in chronic tuberculosis empyema. *Tuber Lung Dis* 1995;76:463–467.

78. Telzak E, Chirgwin K, Nelson E, et al. Predictors for multidrug-resistant tuberculosis among HIV-infected patients and response to specific drug regimens. *Int J Tuberc Lung Dis* 1999; 3:337–343.

79. Craig W Pharmacokinetic/pharmacodynamic parameters: rationale for antibacterial dosing of mice and men. *Clin Infect Dis* 1998;26:1–12.

80. Thomas J, Forrest A, Bhavnani S, et al. Pharmacodynamic evaluation of factors associated with the development of bacterial resistance in acutely ill patients during therapy. *Antimicrob Agents Chemother* 1998;42:521–527.

81. Zhao X, Drlica K. Restricting the selection of antibiotic-resistant mutants: measurement and potential uses of the mutant selection window. *J Infect Dis* 2002;185:561–565.

82. Fox W, Elklard G, Mitchison D. Studies on the treatment of tuberculosis undertaken by the British Medical Research Council Tuberculosis Units, 1946–1986, with relevant subsequent publications. *Int J Tuberc Lung Dis* 1999;3:S231–S279.

83. Canetti G. The J. Burns Amberson Lecture: present aspects of bacterial resistance in tuberculosis. *Am Rev Respir Dis* 1965;92: 687–703.

84. Vernon A, Burman W, Benator D, et al. Acquired rifamycin monoresistance in patients with HIV-related tuberculosis treated with once-weekly rifapentine and isoniazid. *Lancet* 1999;353:1843–1847.

85. Lu T, Malik M, Drlica-Wagner A. C-8-methoxy fluoroquinolones. *Res Adv Antimicrob Agents Chemother* 2001;2: 29–41.

86. Smith JT, Lewin CS. Chemistry and mechanisms of action of the quinolone antibacterials. In: Andriole VT, ed. *The quinolones.* Academic Press: San Diego, 1988:23–82.

87. Klopman G, Fercu D, Renau T, et al. N-1-*tert*-butyl-substituted quinolones: in vitro anti-*Mycobacterium avium* activities and structure-activity relationship studies. *Antimicrob Agents Chemother* 1996;40:2637–2643.

88. Lewin C, Smith J. Bactericidal mechanisms of ofloxacin. *J Antimicrob Chemother* 1988;22[Suppl C]:1–8.

89. Klopman G, Fercu D, Li J-Y, et al. Antimycobacterial quinolones: a comparative analysis of structure-activity and structure-cytotoxicity relationships. *Res Microbiol* 1996;147:86–96.

90. Acar J, Goldstein F. Trends in bacterial resistance to fluoroquinolones. *Clin Infect Dis* 1997;24:S67–S73.

91. Davidson R, Cavalcanti R, Brunton J, et al. Resistance to levofloxacin and failure of treatment of pneumococcal pneumonia. *N Engl J Med* 2002;346:747–750.

92. Tillotson G, Zhao X, Drlica K. Fluoroquinolones as pneumococcal therapy: closing the barn door before the horse escapes. *Lancet Infect Dis* 2001;1:145–146.

93. Alangaden GJ, Manavathu EK, Vakulenko SB, et al. Character-

ization of fluoroquinolone-resistant mutant strains of *Mycobacterium tuberculosis* selected in laboratory and isolated from patients. *Antimicrob Agents Chemother* 1995;39:1700–1703.

94. Cambau E, Sougakoff W, Besson M, et al. Selection of a *gyrA* mutant of *Mycobacterium tuberculosis* resistant to fluoroquinolones during treatment with ofloxacin. *J Infect Dis* 1994;170:479–483.

95. Revel V, Cambau E, Jarlier V, et al. Characterization of mutations in *Mycobacterium smegmatis* involved in resistance to fluoroquinolones. *Antimicrob Agents Chemother* 1994;38:1991–1996.

96. Acocella G, Nonis A, Perna G, et al. Comparative bioavailability of isoniazid, rifampin, and pyrazinamide administered in free combination and in a fixed triple formulation designed for daily use in antituberculosis chemotherapy. II. Two-month, daily administration study. *Am Rev Respir Dis* 1988;138:886–890.

97. Acocella G, Conti R, Luisetti M, et al. Pharmacokinetic studies on antituberculosis regimens in humans. *Am Rev Respir Dis* 1985;132:510–515.

98. Black HR, Griffith RS, Peabody AM. Absorption, excretion and metabolism of capreomycin in normal and diseased states. *Ann N Y Acad Sci* 1966;135:974–982.

99. Cabana B, Taggart J. Comparative pharmacokinetics of BB-KS and kanamycin in dogs and humans. *Antimicrob Agents Chemother* 1973;3:478–483.

100. Zitkova L, Tousek J. Pharmacokinetics of cycloserine and terizidone. *Chemotherapy* 1974;20:18–28.

101. Israel D, Gillum G, Turik M, et al. Pharmacokinetics and serum bactericidal titers of ciprofloxacin and ofloxacin following multiple oral doses in healthy volunteers. *Antimicrob Agents Chemother* 1993;37:2193–2199.

102. Chien S-H, Rogge M, Gisclon L, et al. Pharmacokinetic profile of levofloxacin following once-daily 500 mg oral or intravenous doses. *Antimicrob Agents Chemother* 1997;41:2256–2260.

103. Sullivan JT, Woodruff M, Lettieri J, et al. Pharmacokinetics of a once-daily oral dose of moxifloxacin (Bay 12-8039), a new enantiomerically pure 8-methoxy quinolone. *Antimicrob Agents Chemother* 1999;43:2793–2797.

104. Nakashima M, Uematsu T, Kosuge K, et al. Single- and multiple-dose pharmacokinetics of AM-1155, a new 6-fluoro-8-methoxy quinolone, in humans. *Antimicrob Agents Chemother* 1995;39:2635–2640.

105. Montay G. Pharmacokinetics of sparfloxacin in healthy volunteers and patients: a review. *J Antimicrob Chemother* 1996;37 [Suppl A]:27–39.

106. Bifani P, Mathema B, Liu Z, et al. Identification of a W variant outbreak of *Mycobacterium tuberculosis* via population-based molecular epidemiology. *JAMA* 1999;282:2321–2327.

107. Heddle JG, Barnard F, Wentzell L, et al. The interaction of drugs with DNA gyrase: a model for the molecular basis of quinolone action. *Nucleosides Nucleotides Nucleic Acids* 2000;19:1249–1264.

PHARMACOKINETIC CONSIDERATIONS AND DRUG–DRUG INTERACTIONS IN TUBERCULOSIS TREATMENT

WILLIAM J. BURMAN

The pharmacokinetic behavior of the first-line antituberculosis drugs has been well described, and the technical ability exists to accurately measure the concentrations of these drugs. The association between drug concentrations (pharmacokinetics) and drug activity, either toxicity or efficacy, is called pharmacodynamics. Tuberculosis therapy generally uses weight-based doses, but situations have been identified in which these standard doses may be inappropriate. For example, patients with renal failure have marked differences in the pharmacokinetics of particular drugs (ethambutol, aminoglycosides), necessitating dose adjustments. Furthermore, the antituberculosis drugs are involved in many drug–drug interactions (1,2), although much more often causing changes in the concentrations of other drugs than being substantially affected themselves. Abnormal pharmacokinetics has also been hypothesized to be an important cause of treatment failure and relapse (3,4).

The pharmacokinetics of specific antituberculosis drugs is provided in detail in the chapters on drug classes. This chapter reviews general principles of the pharmacokinetics and pharmacodynamics of the antituberculosis drugs, reviews their drug–drug interactions, and discusses the possible use of therapeutic drug monitoring.

OVERVIEW OF THE PHARMACOKINETICS OF ANTITUBERCULOSIS DRUGS

The dose forms and basic pharmacokinetic parameters of the antituberculosis drugs are shown in Table 53.1. It is important to point out that the actions of these drugs on *Mycobacterium tuberculosis* differ markedly, and these differences have a greater effect on dosing frequency than do the pharmacokinetic properties (5). Some drugs, such as isoni-

azid, rifampin, and the aminoglycosides, produce prolonged suppression of mycobacterial growth after a dose (postantibiotic effect) (6,7), whereas other drugs, such as paraaminosalicylic acid (PAS) or thiacetazone (8), only suppress growth while the concentration of drug is greater than the *in vitro* minimal inhibitory concentration (MIC). Despite having short serum half-lives, drugs having prolonged postantibiotic effect can be dosed infrequently (twice or thrice weekly) (9–11), whereas those having little or no postantibiotic effect must be dosed often enough to keep the serum concentration greater than the MIC (e.g., twice daily for PAS) (12).

Further discussion of drug–drug interactions and dosing changes in special clinical situations are structured into sections on absorption, renal clearance, and hepatic metabolism.

ABSORPTION AND INTERACTIONS INVOLVING ABSORPTION

Effect of Food

The aminoglycosides and capreomycin are so poorly absorbed that parenteral administration is required. The other antituberculosis drugs are, in general, well absorbed. Dosing with food has variable effects (Table 53.2); many drugs are not affected, some (e.g., isoniazid) have modest decreases in absorption, and some have substantial increases in absorption (e.g., rifapentine and PAS) when given with food. The clinical significance of these changes are uncertain, although they have been the basis for recommendations ranging from taking all medications on an empty stomach (37) to administering all doses of rifapentine-containing therapy with a high-fat meal (38).

The continued uncertainty regarding the advisability of dosing antituberculosis drugs with food relates to the lack of knowledge of the pharmacodynamics of these medications. For example, food substantially decreases the maximal concentration of isoniazid (by 51%) but has relatively

W. J. Burman: Division of Infectious Diseases, University of Colorado Health Sciences Center; Infectious Diseases Clinic, Denver Public Health, Denver, Colorado.

TABLE 53.1. KEY PHARMACOKINETIC PROPERTIES OF ANTITUBERCULOSIS DRUGS[a]

Drug	Forms Available	Major Route of Metabolism	Half-Life (hr)	Average C_{max} (μg/mL)[b]
Isoniazid	Tablet, suspension, injection	Hepatic (*N*-acetyltransferase)	Fast acetylator: <2; slow acetylator: 2–4	2–8
Rifampin	Capsule, injection	Hepatic (deacetylation)	2–4	4–12
Rifabutin	Capsule	Hepatic (CYP 3A)	32–67	0.2–0.6
Rifapentine	Tablet	Hepatic (deacetylation)	14–18	10–20
Pyrazinamide	Tablet	Hepatic (deamidase)	2–10	30–60
Ethambutol	Tablet	Renal	2–4	1–4
Streptomycin	Injection	Renal	2–6	25–40
Amikacin (kanamycin)	Injection	Renal	2–3	35–40
Capreomycin	Injection	Renal	4–6	20–45
Levofloxacin	Tablet, injection	Renal	6–8	6–8
Moxifloxacin	Tablet, injection	Hepatic (glucuronidation, sulfate conjugation)	12	2–6
Cycloserine	Tablet	Renal	10	15–25
Paraamino salicylic acid	Granules (injection in Europe)	Renal, hepatic (acetylation)	1	20
Ethionamide	Tablet	Hepatic (not well characterized)	3	1.5

[a]Drugs, forms of drugs available, major route of metabolism, half-life, estimated C_{max} (with dose used in daily therapy.
[b]For standard dose used in daily therapy.

little effect on the total extent of absorption (12% decrease, as expressed by the area under the concentration-time curve) (13). If the antimycobacterial activity of isoniazid is dependent on achieving a high peak serum concentration, then dosing with food could substantially decrease its activity, whereas if isoniazid's activity is related to maintaining a concentration above a threshold for a critical time period, then dosing with food may have no effect or even a beneficial effect (by delaying the absorption and producing more prolonged concentrations above the threshold).

Pharmacodynamic studies of treatment of conventional bacterial infections have identified antimicrobial agents of both types. The activity of the aminoglycosides is maximized by achieving peak serum concentrations much greater than the minimal inhibitory concentration, so using high doses infrequently (at intervals much greater than the serum half-life) produces the best balance of efficacy and toxicity. Conversely, activity of the β-lactam antibiotics (e.g., the penicillins) is dependent on maintaining the drug concentration above the inhibitory concentration of the pathogen for as much of the dosing interval as possible; high peak levels do not add to the activity of β-lactam drugs. Existing data do not allow a definitive assessment of how the antituberculosis drugs fit into this paradigm of antimicrobial pharmacodynamics. For isoniazid, data from trials of once-weekly therapy with isoniazid and streptomycin demonstrate that time over a threshold concentration is more closely associated with clinical efficacy than is peak serum concentration (39).

Discussions about dosing antituberculosis drugs with food must also take into account two critical clinical realities: the importance of direct observation of therapy and

the management of common, bothersome side effects. The most common cause of treatment failure and relapse with self-administered therapy is nonadherence, not modest changes in pharmacokinetics that may occur when doses are ingested with food (40,41). Directly observed therapy relies on ingestion of all medications in the regimen together and is facilitated by having directly observed doses be as infrequent as possible. Although a strict interpretation of the effects of food might dictate that isoniazid be given on an empty stomach and rifapentine with food, the advantage of the combination of the once-weekly isoniazid and rifapentine regimen is to facilitate directly observed therapy. Separating the dose of isoniazid from the dose of rifapentine would run counter to the central purpose of this regimen.

Bothersome side effects are common with currently available tuberculosis treatment regimens (42). Nausea, occasionally with vomiting, is common during the initial four-drug phase of therapy (43). Successful management of these common, bothersome side effects is a critical aspect of a successful tuberculosis control program. Splitting the dose of a medication into several smaller doses is an appealing way to manage ingestion-related side effects but precludes directly observed therapy. Switching to medications other than the first-line drugs may compromise the effectiveness of the regimen. Therefore, proper management of bothersome side effects plays an important, if largely unrecognized role in tuberculosis treatment. Many patients obtain some relief from ingestion-related side effects by taking medications with food. Some programs also incorporate food into directly observed therapy visits as an incentive for adherence.

TABLE 53.2. EFFECTS OF FOOD AND ANTACIDS ON THE ABSORPTION OF ANTITUBERCULOSIS DRUGS

Drug (Ref.)	Effect of Food	Effect of Antacids (or Other Divalent Cations, Iron, Sucralfate)	Clinical Implications
Isoniazid (13–17)	Decreased C_{max} (9%–61%); less effect on AUC (decreased 9%–43%)	0%–19% decrease in AUC	Administer on an empty stomach, if possible
Rifampin (15,18–20)	Decrease in C_{max} (15%–36%) and AUC (4%–23%)	No significant change in serum concentrations	Administer on an empty stomach, if possible
Rifabutin (21,22)	No significant effect	No effect from antacids in chewable didanosine	May be given with food
Rifapentine (23)	Increased C_{max} (50%) and AUC (46%)	Unknown	May be given with food
Pyrazinamide (15,24)	Delayed T_{max}; no effect on AUC	No significant effect	May be given with food or antacids
Ethambutol (25–27)	Delayed T_{max}; 16% decrease in C_{max} but minimal effect on AUC	28% decrease in C_{max} and 10% decrease in AUC	May be given with food; do not coadminister with antacids
Levofloxacin (28,29)	No significant effect	Large decreases in C_{max} and AUC	Do not coadminister with di- and trivalent cations including antacids
Moxifloxacin (30–33)	No significant effect	Large decreases in C_{max} and AUC	Do not coadminister with di- and trivalent cations including antacids
Cycloserine (34)	Decreased C_{max} with high-fat meal but no change in AUC	No effect	May be given with food
Ethionamide (35)	No significant effect	No effect	Administering with food may improve tolerability
Paraaminosalicylic acid granules (36,49)	Increased C_{max} (50%) and AUC (70%)	16%–18% decrease in C_{max} and AUC	Administering with food may improve tolerability

AUC, area under the serum concentration–time curve; C_{max}, peak (maximal) serum concentration; T_{max}, time from drug ingestion to peak (maximal) serum concentration.

These considerations point out the need to consider more than pharmacokinetic data in formulating advice about food and tuberculosis therapy. It may be optimal to start by dosing all medications together on an empty stomach. However, if patients have difficulty with ingestion-related side effects, dosing with food is preferable to splitting doses or changing to second-line medications. For some drugs, such as ethionamide or PAS, ingestion-related side effects are so common that it may be preferable to start therapy by dosing with meals. It may be difficult to convince patients who have had an initial severe ingestion-related side effect to continue to take that medication.

Effects of Other Medications on Absorption

The absorption interaction that clearly affects the efficacy of therapy is the dramatic interaction between the fluoroquinolone antibiotics and several di- and trivalent cations. Both peak concentration and area under the time-concentration curve of levofloxacin and moxifloxacin are decreased substantially when administered with Fe^{2+}, Mg^{2+}, and AL^{3+} (31–33). Therefore, administration of antacids (including the antacid-containing chewable formulation of didanosine) (16), sucralfate, and iron supplements (including vitamins containing iron) should be separated from doses of fluoroquinolones by at least 2 hours. The effect of antacids is clearly mediated through the magnesium and aluminum cations, not their effect on gastric pH (33,44). As a result, medications other than antacids, such as H-2 antagonists (e.g., ranitidine), can be used with antituberculosis therapy for the patient who requires therapy for acid-peptic disease. Notably, milk products and calcium supplements do not decrease absorption of levofloxacin or moxifloxacin (45,46).

The absorption of rifampin can be substantially decreased by ingredients in medications that are administered at the same time. This was most clearly shown for a microbiologically inactive ingredient of an early formulation of PAS (47). This effect is the likely explanation for the inadequate absorption of rifampin from some combined formulation products containing rifampin and other first-line antituberculosis medications (e.g., isoniazid, pyrazinamide) (48,49). The combined formulation products available in the United States and Europe (Rifamate and Rifater) have adequate absorption characteristics, but products from other countries should not be used unless proven to have adequate bioavailability.

Parenteral Forms of Antituberculosis Medications

Patients occasionally present with severe, overwhelming tuberculosis or an inability to take oral medications owing to gastrointestinal problems (50). In such situations, parenteral forms of tuberculosis therapy can be life saving. Isoniazid, rifampin, the fluoroquinolones, and the aminoglycosides can all be given intravenously or intramuscularly (Table 53.1). Of the aminoglycosides, amikacin is the most useful for severely ill patients because it is generally available in acute-care hospitals and active against a very high proportion of *M. tuberculosis* isolates (51).

METABOLISM OF TUBERCULOSIS DRUGS

Renally Excreted Drugs

Renal insufficiency and tuberculosis frequently overlap. Renal tuberculosis can cause renal insufficiency (52,53). In developed countries, the more common association is that renal insufficiency is an immunosuppressive condition, increasing the likelihood of progression from latent to active tuberculosis. Several studies estimate that rates of active tuberculosis are ten to 25 times more common among patients on dialysis than among the general population (54,55).

The antituberculosis drugs eliminated primarily by the kidneys are the aminoglycosides (and capreomycin), ethambutol, levofloxacin, cycloserine, and PAS. There are no known drug interactions at the level of the kidney involving these drugs. The pharmacokinetic issues involving the renally excreted drugs are those of dose adjustments for patients with varying degrees of renal insufficiency and those on dialysis. The aminoglycosides and capreomycin, as nephrotoxins, should be avoided if at all possible in persons with renal insufficiency. However, when treating multidrug-resistant tuberculosis, use of the aminoglycosides or capreomycin may have to be considered, despite the possibility of nephrotoxicity.

Dosing recommendations for the antituberculosis drugs in the setting of renal insufficiency are shown in Table 53.3.

Fortunately, the three most important agents in the treatment of drug-susceptible tuberculosis (isoniazid, rifampin, and pyrazinamide) are predominantly metabolized by the liver. Isoniazid and rifampin can be used in standard doses, and pyrazinamide requires only a modest dose adjustment in the presence of severe renal insufficiency. The recommendations in Table 53.3 for dosing of renally excreted drugs are based on relatively small studies and should be used with close clinical monitoring for both toxicity and to ensure the efficacy of therapy. Although there is controversy about the overall role of therapeutic drug monitoring in tuberculosis treatment, therapeutic drug monitoring is recommended when dosing potentially toxic, renally excreted drugs in the setting of renal insufficiency. Serum concentrations of ethambutol, the aminoglycosides, and cycloserine are available through reference laboratories and should be obtained among patients being treated with these drugs who have substantial renal insufficiency.

TABLE 53.3. DOSE ADJUSTMENTS OF ANTITUBERCULOSIS DRUGS FOR RENAL INSUFFICIENCY AND RENAL REPLACEMENT THERAPY[a] (E.G., DIALYSIS, HEMOFILTRATION)

Drug (Refs.)	Estimated Creatinine Clearance			Renal Replacement Therapy	
	>50	10–49	<10	Hemodialysis	Peritoneal Dialysis
Pyrazinamide (56)	No change	No change	15–25 mg/kg/d or 25–35 mg/kg thrice weekly	25–35 mg/kg after dialysis	25–35 mg/kg thrice weekly
Ethambutol[b] (56)	Normal dose	15–20 mg/kg thrice weekly	15 mg/kg thrice weekly	15–25 mg/kg thrice weekly	15–25 mg/kg thrice weekly
Streptomycin, amikacin, capreomycin[b]	500 mg/d	Use an alternative, nonnephrotoxic drug, if at all possible		750 mg twice or thrice weekly	750 mg twice or thrice weekly
Levofloxacin (57,58)	Normal dose	500 mg every 48 hr	500 mg every 48 hr	500 mg after dialysis	500 mg every 48 hr
Moxifloxacin	Normal dose	No adjustment necessary		Not evaluated	Not evaluated
Cycloserine[b] (59)		250–500 mg every 24 hr	250 mg every 24 hr	250–500 mg after dialysis	15 mg/kg after dialysis
Paraaminosalicylic acid (59)		No standard recommendations		4 g twice daily	4 g twice daily

[a]e.g., dialysis, hemofiltration.
[b]Therapeutic drug monitoring is highly recommended for patients with impaired renal function who require treatment using ethambutol, aminoglycosides (capreomycin), and cycloserine.

Hepatically Metabolized Drugs

Hepatic disease is also common among persons with active tuberculosis. Although hepatic involvement is very common in disseminated forms of tuberculosis (60,61), it rarely causes marked impairment of hepatic function (62). However, for several reasons, persons with preexisting hepatic disease are at increased risk of active tuberculosis. Alcohol abuse is common among persons with tuberculosis (63), probably because of its association with homelessness and other situations in which exposure to tuberculosis occurs (64). In addition, in many urban areas, injection drug use is associated with tuberculosis, and such patients often have chronic viral hepatitis (63). Finally, chronic hepatitis B is endemic in areas of the world, such as Southeast Asia, with high rates of tuberculosis (65). Therefore, the clinician treating tuberculosis will frequently face questions about the use of hepatically metabolized and potentially hepatotoxic drugs among persons with preexisting liver disease.

Metabolism of hepatically metabolized drugs, such as isoniazid and the rifamycins, is diminished among persons with severe liver disease (3). It might seem prudent to avoid all potentially hepatotoxic drugs in this situation, but this risks failure of tuberculosis treatment because the three most potent drugs can cause hepatotoxicity. Furthermore, most patients with preexisting liver disease will tolerate standard tuberculosis treatment regimens, with careful monitoring for hepatotoxicity (9,66). Among persons with severe hepatic disease, one may wish to avoid the standard regimen containing all three first-line drugs with the potential for hepatotoxicity (isoniazid, rifampin, and pyrazinamide). The most important potent of these drugs, and probably the least hepatotoxic, is rifampin, and therefore, a regimen such as rifampin, ethambutol, and a fluoroquinolone is an option for a patient with severe liver disease (66).

Although serum concentrations of hepatically metabolized drugs are increased in persons with hepatic dysfunction, there are no guidelines for dose adjustments in this situation. In part, this reflects the paucity of pharmacokinetic data among persons with active tuberculosis and significant liver disease. Furthermore, there is no simple test, analogous to serum creatinine, that provides an accurate indicator of the rate of hepatic metabolism of drugs. Finally, there is no clear relationship between serum concentrations of the hepatically metabolized drugs and the chance of toxicity. In general, standard doses of isoniazid, rifampin, and pyrazinamide are used for patients with liver disease, with careful clinical and laboratory monitoring for toxicity.

Mechanisms of Drug Interactions Involving Hepatic Metabolism

The rifamycins and, to a lesser extent, isoniazid cause many clinically relevant drug–drug interactions. Much less often, antituberculosis drugs are affected by other medications. Table 53.4 lists the common drug interactions and suggests clinical management strategies. The length of the list is intimidating, but some general principles can help the clinician to anticipate and manage drug–drug interactions among patients with tuberculosis (see later) (Table 53.5).

The locus of these drug interactions is the liver (and, to a lesser extent, the wall of the gut) among enzymes that metabolize exogenous substances such as drugs. The most important set of enzymes is the cytochrome P-450 family of enzyme systems, and most interactions are related to a specific member of this enzyme family, cytochrome P-450 3A (CYP 3A). However, drug interactions can involve other hepatic enzymes; for example, rifampin's effect on glucuronosyltransferase mediates the interaction with steroid hormones, like those contained in oral contraceptives (71).

Drugs can affect the cytochrome P-450 system in two ways: inhibition or induction (Table 53.6). Induction of cytochrome P-450 results in an increased synthesis of the enzyme, leading to an increase in the metabolism of target drugs and a decrease in their concentrations. Enzyme induction may, therefore, result in loss of clinical efficacy of a drug metabolized by that system. The rifamycins are all inducers of CYP 3A, although there are substantial differences in their potency as inducers (72). Rifampin and rifapentine are potent CYP 3A inducers and, therefore, have a greater potential for drug interactions; rifabutin is less potent and may be used in place of rifampin to decrease to a manageable level the magnitude of a problematic drug interaction.

Inhibition of a cytochrome P-450 enzyme system blocks the metabolism of target drugs, hence increasing their concentrations and potentially causing toxicity. Isoniazid is a relatively potent inhibitor of several cytochrome P-450 isozymes (CYP 2C9, CYP 2C19, CYP 2E1) (73), but has minimal effect on CYP 3A (74). Because CYP 2C9, CYP 2C19, and CYP 2E1 metabolize fewer drugs than CYP 3A, isoniazid has fewer interactions than the rifamycins. The most well-documented interactions owing to isoniazid are with phenytoin and carbamazepine (75,76). It is important to point out that rifampin affects phenytoin and has the opposite effect (decreasing its concentrations). When both isoniazid and rifampin are used, the effects of rifampin on other drugs generally predominates (77).

Rifabutin is metabolized in part by CYP 3A (78) (in addition to being an inducer of that enzyme) and, as such, can be affected by inducers and inhibitors of CYP 3A. Rifabutin concentrations can be increased to potentially toxic levels when administered with CYP 3A inhibitors [e.g., ritonavir, clarithromycin (79,80)] and decreased to potentially ineffective levels by CYP 3A inducers [e.g., efavirenz (69)]. Guidelines are available for managing the complex drug–drug interactions involving rifabutin among patients with human immunodeficiency virus (HIV) infection (81,82).

TABLE 53.4. CLINICALLY SIGNIFICANT DRUG–DRUG INTERACTIONS INVOLVING THE RIFAMYCINS AND ISONIAZID

Drug Class	Drugs Whose Concentrations Are Substantially Decreased by the Rifamycins	Comments
Antiinfectives	Human immunodeficiency virus-1 protease inhibitors (saquinavir, indinavir, nelfinavir, amprenavir, ritonavir, lopinavir/ritonavir, atazanavir)	Can be used with rifabutin; ritonavir, at doses of 400–600 mg twice daily, probably can be used with rifampin
	Nonnucleoside reverse-transcriptase inhibitors (efavirenz, nevirapine, delavirdine)	Delavirdine should not be used with any rifamycin; doses of nevirapine (67) and efavirenz (68) may need to be increased if given with rifampin; no dose increase needed if given with rifabutin (69)
	Macrolide antibiotics (clarithromycin, erythromycin)	Azithromycin has no significant interaction with rifamycins
	Doxycycline	May require use of an alternate drug or drug combination
	Azole antifungal agents (ketoconazole, itraconazole)	Itraconazole and ketoconazole concentrations may be subtherapeutic with any of the rifamycins; fluconazole can be used with rifamycins, but the dose may need to be increased
	Atovaquone	Consider alternate form of *Pneumocystis carinii* treatment or prophylaxis
	Chloramphenicol	Consider an alternative antibiotic
	Mefloquine	Consider alternate form of malaria prophylaxis
Hormone therapy	Oral contraceptives	Women with reproductive potential on oral contraceptives should be advised to add a barrier method of contraception when on a rifamycin
	Tamoxifen	May require alternate therapy
	Levothyroxine	Monitoring of serum thyroid-stimulating hormone recommended, may require increased dose of levothyroxine
Narcotics	Methadone	Rifampin use may require methadone dose increase; rifabutin infrequently causes methadone withdrawal
Anticoagulants	Warfarin	Monitor prothrombin time; may require two- to threefold dose increase
Immunosuppressive agents	Cyclosporine, tacrolimus	Rifabutin may allow concomitant use of cyclosporine and a rifamycin
	Corticosteroids	Monitor clinically; may require two- to threefold dose increase (70)
Anticonvulsants	Phenytoin, lamotrigine	Therapeutic drug monitoring recommended; may require dose increase
Cardiovascular agents	Calcium channel antagonists	Clinical monitoring recommended; may require change to an alternate drug
	β-blockers	Clinical monitoring recommended; may require dose increase or change to an alternate drug
	Angiotensin-converting enzyme inhibitors (e.g., enalapril), angiotensin receptor antagonist (e.g., losartan)	Monitor clinically, may require a dose increase or use of an alternate drug
	Digoxin (among patients with renal insufficiency), digitoxin	
	Antiarrhythmics (e.g., quinidine, mexilitine)	
Theophylline	Theophylline	Therapeutic drug monitoring recommended; may require dose increase
Oral hypoglycemics	Sulfonylurea drugs (e.g., glyburide)	Therapeutic drug monitoring recommended; may require dose increase
		Monitor blood glucose; may require dose increase or change to an alternate drug
Hypolipidemics	Simvastatin, fluvastatin	Monitor hypolipidemic effect; may require use of an alternate drug
Psychotropic drugs	Antidepressants (nortriptyline, buspirone)	Therapeutic drug monitoring recommended; may require dose increase or change to alternate drug
	Neuroleptic agents (haloperidol, quetiapine)	Monitor clinically; may require a dose increase or use of an alternate drug
	Benzodiazepines (e.g., diazepam)	Monitor clinically; may require a dose increase or use of an alternate drug

Isoniazid Interactions

Drug Class	Drugs Whose Concentrations Are Substantially Decreased by Isoniazid	Comments
Anticonvulsants	Phenytoin, carbamazepine	Therapeutic drug monitoring recommended; may require dose increase or change to alternate drug
Psychotropic drugs	Benzodiazepines (diazepam, triazolam)	Monitor clinically; may require a dose increase or use of an alternate drug

TABLE 53.5. PRINCIPLES FOR ANTICIPATING AND MANAGING DRUG–DRUG INTERACTIONS IN TUBERCULOSIS TREATMENT

Rifampin probably causes more clinically significant interactions than any other drug; check for possible interactions every time rifamycin-containing tuberculosis treatment is started

Many rifampin interactions have been described, and many more have not yet been evaluated; check a regularly updated reference for drug interactions and look for possible as well as documented interactions

Ask patients to bring in all concurrent medications and to check with the tuberculosis care provider before starting any new medications during treatment

Some drug interactions can be managed by monitoring the effect of the drug and/or its serum concentrations and adjusting the dose of the affected drug; other interactions require a change in therapy

Rifabutin has less effect on drugs other than rifampin; some drug interactions can be managed by using rifabutin in place of rifampin (e.g., human immunodeficiency virus-1 protease inhibitors, cyclosporine)

If a drug dose is increased to compensate for the effect of a rifamycin, it will probably have to be decreased again when the rifamycin is discontinued

Communicate with the primary care provider

Principles for Anticipating and Managing Drug Interactions in Patients Being Treated for Tuberculosis

The first and most important step in anticipating and managing drug interactions is to recognize the need to evaluate for a possible interaction. Because of the breadth and potency of rifampin as an enzyme inducer and the number of drugs metabolized by those enzyme systems, rifampin is probably the cause of more clinically significant drug interactions than any other drug. Therefore, tuberculosis care providers must be particularly vigilant about checking for drug interactions. Evaluating for possible drug interactions requires an accurate accounting of all medications that a patient is taking. Because patients often have difficulty remembering medication names, doses, and dosing frequencies, it is helpful to ask that all medications, prescription and nonprescription, be brought to a clinic appointment.

Many drug–drug interactions involving the rifamycins have been described, but the list in Table 53.4 is surely incomplete. As new drugs are developed and approved, new interactions are identified. Therefore, the tuberculosis care provider needs to have access to a regularly updated source of information on drug interactions. Second, it is important to look for possible as well as documented interactions. Studies to evaluate for possible interactions with rifampin have not

been performed for all drugs on the market. Any drug known to be metabolized by CYP 3A or glucuronidation should be presumed to have an interaction with rifampin.

The management of a drug–drug interaction depends on the action of the drugs and the magnitude of the change in concentrations. Drugs, such as warfarin, having a very narrow therapeutic window require close monitoring and dose adjustment [the dose may have to be doubled or tripled to compensate for the effect of rifampin (83,84)]. The magnitude of the interaction may allow compensation by dose adjustment in some cases; in others, the decrease in serum concentrations related to rifampin is so great that it cannot be ameliorated by dose adjustment. For example, concentrations of most of the HIV-1 protease inhibitors are decreased by 80% to 90% when given with rifampin (37), and it is not possible to increase the dose high enough to compensate for this marked decrease. Some of these interactions can be managed by substituting rifabutin for rifampin. Again, using the example of HIV-1 protease inhibitors, rifabutin results in no change or modest decreases in their concentrations that either require no dose adjustment [e.g., nelfinavir (85), amprenavir (86)] or a modest dose increase [e.g., indinavir (74)]. Finally, there are a few drugs [delavirdine (87), itraconazole (88), ketoconazole] whose concentrations are markedly decreased by any of the currently approved rifamycins. These drug interactions will either require an

TABLE 53.6. SUMMARY OF METABOLIC DRUG INTERACTIONS INVOLVING THE CYTOCHROME P-450 SYSTEM CYP 3A

Mechanism	Examples	Effect of Inducer/Inhibitor on Other Drugs	Clinical Effect
Induction of CYP 3A	Rifampin > rifapentine > rifabutin, nevirapine	↓ Serum concentrations	↓ Efficacy
Inhibition of CYP 3A	Ketoconazole ≥ ritonavir > indinavir, amprenavir > nelfinavir, delavirdine > saquinavir	↑ Serum concentrations	↑ Toxicity

alternative agent [e.g., fluconazole (89) instead of itraconazole] or use of nonrifamycin regimen to treat tuberculosis. This is a complex decision because nonrifamycin regimens are less effective for curing tuberculosis; consultation with an expert in the field is suggested.

CASE PRESENTATION

A 38-year-old woman was brought to clinic by a family member with a 3-day history of somnolence. She had completed standard short-course treatment for drug-susceptible pulmonary and pleural tuberculosis 10 days earlier. She had an uneventful treatment course with appropriate clinical, microbiologic, and radiographic response. Her medical history was notable for heroin abuse, treated with methadone maintenance therapy. On examination, she was very somnolent but awoke to tactile stimulation; there were no focal neurologic deficits. On further discussion with the methadone program staff, her daily dose had been increased from 40 to 70 mg because of withdrawal symptoms occurring soon after she started tuberculosis therapy. After completion of tuberculosis treatment, the inductive effect of rifampin was no longer present, the equivalent to a substantial increase in methadone dose. Her methadone dose was decreased to 40 mg per day, and her somnolence resolved.

This case illustrates the need to account for drug interactions at the other end of tuberculosis treatment when stopping therapy. If the dose of a medication has been changed (increased in the case of rifampin interactions, decreased in the case of isoniazid interactions) to compensate for a drug interaction, it will probably have to be readjusted within 1 to 2 weeks of the interacting tuberculosis drug being stopped. Finally, it also illustrates the importance in anticipating and managing drug interactions and of ongoing close communication with other care providers.

THERAPEUTIC DRUG MONITORING IN TUBERCULOSIS TREATMENT

Overview of Therapeutic Drug Monitoring

Therapeutic drug monitoring is the measurement of drug concentrations (generally in the blood) and then adjustment of the dose of a drug to achieve a concentration that is thought to produce the desired effect and has a relatively low probability of causing toxicity. Therapeutic drug monitoring is most useful for drugs having a narrow therapeutic window (the range of concentrations that have efficacy and yet infrequently cause toxicity), such as warfarin. The requirements for therapeutic drug monitoring are given in Table 53.7.

Therapeutic drug monitoring is not relevant to most patients with drug-susceptible tuberculosis treated with first-line drugs using directly observed therapy. Despite tenfold differences in serum concentrations of isoniazid and rifampin among such patients, the outcomes of therapy are excellent; 95% or more are cured with a single course of therapy. However, some have suggested that abnormal pharmacokinetics are responsible for a significant proportion of the patients who fail such treatment or relapse after completing a course of therapy (3,4). For example, Kimerling et al. (3) reported that isoniazid concentrations were low in 68% of patients with treatment failure or relapse, and 64% had low rifampin concentrations. In addition, some studies suggest that patients with HIV-related tuberculosis have lower than expected concentrations of antituberculosis drugs (90), leading to suggestions for therapeutic drug monitoring in this population (91).

The occurrence of drug–drug interactions suggests a role for therapeutic drug monitoring, although the need for doing so would be infrequent because the concentrations of the antituberculosis drugs are seldom significantly changed as a result of drug–drug interactions (they more often cause

TABLE 53.7. REQUIREMENTS FOR THERAPEUTIC DRUG MONITORING

Requirement	Applicability for Tuberculosis Treatment
Technical capability to measure drug concentrations in a timely manner	Available at reference laboratories in developed countries
Efficacy and toxicity cannot be easily monitored using simple laboratory tests (e.g., the prothrombin time for warfarin) or clinical data (e.g., blood pressure and pulse for β-blockers)	No widely available rapid marker of treatment efficacy
Substantial interpatient differences in drug concentrations that cannot be accurately predicted using commonly available information (such as the estimated creatinine clearance)	Five to tenfold differences in serum concentrations of first-line drugs
Knowledge of the association between drug concentrations and their effects, efficacy, and toxicity (the therapeutic range)	Largely unknown
Dose adjustments based on measurements of drug concentrations are feasible and likely to be tolerated	True for some drugs but may not be for others (e.g., ethionamide, paraaminosalicylic acid)
Clinicians will use drug concentrations appropriately	Not well studied
Therapeutic drug monitoring will be cost-effective	Not well studied

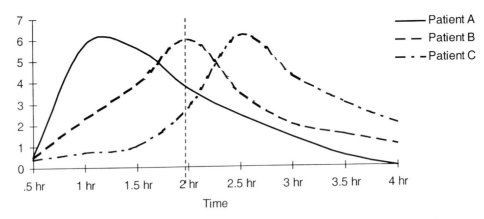

FIGURE 53.1. The effect of differences in absorption rate on the estimate of maximal concentration (C_{max}) by a single 2-hour postdose sample. In this hypothetical example, all patients have the same C_{max} (6 μg/mL) but substantially different 2-hour concentrations (2.8, 6.0, and 3.7 μg/mL) because of differences in the rate of absorption. The result is a substantial underestimation in the average C_{max} (3.5 μg/mL). This is a significant problem with drugs having variable absorption rates and short serum half-lives, such as isoniazid, rifampin, and ethambutol.

changes in the concentrations of other drugs). Finally, the second-line drugs have a narrower therapeutic index than the first-line drugs. Therefore, some have suggested routine therapeutic drug monitoring among patients being treated with second-line drugs, whether because of infection with a drug-resistant strain or because of toxicity from first-line drugs.

Although these situations could be used to target therapeutic drug monitoring to high-risk patients whom it may benefit, there are many practical problems in so doing. Although there is the technical capability to measure drug concentrations accurately, the interpretation of these results is difficult. First, most of the antituberculosis drugs have relatively short serum half-lives and significant variability in the time to maximal concentration (T_{max}). As a result, sparse sampling schemes in which serum concentrations are measured at one or two time points may misclassify patients. Figure 53.1 shows the effect of differences in T_{max} on the estimation of the maximal concentration (C_{max}) when only one time point is assessed. Even among human volunteers evaluated under ideal conditions, this effect can be substantial, ranging from 50% for isoniazid (13) to 30% for rifampin (18). It is likely that this problem of variations in T*max* affecting the estimate of C_{max} is even greater among patients with active tuberculosis evaluated under treatment conditions (e.g., in which drugs may be administered after meals, there is a higher incidence of concomitant illnesses that may affect pharmacokinetics). This problem can be obviated by measuring three or more time points, but this would be expensive and difficult to perform in most treatment programs.

The fundamental problem of using therapeutic drug monitoring in tuberculosis treatment is the lack of knowledge about the pharmacodynamics of these drugs (relationship between serum concentrations and clinical effect, either microbiologic efficacy or toxicity). As shown in Table 53.8, clinical evidence suggests relationships between dose and outcome (efficacy or toxicity), but there has been little

TABLE 53.8. RELATIONSHIP BETWEEN DOSE OF THE FIRST-LINE DRUGS AND CLINICAL EVENTS IN TUBERCULOSIS TREATMENT

	Relationship Between Serum Concentrations and Clinical Outcomes	
Drug	**Efficacy**	**Toxicity**
Isoniazid	Only with once-weekly therapy	Higher levels have been associated with neuropathy but no clear relevance when using supplemental vitamin B_6
Rifampin	Decreased efficacy with 450-mg dose but insufficient data to create target range	Only with high doses (≥900 mg given once weekly)
Rifabutin	No difference in efficacy of 300 and 150 mg (daily)	Increases at high doses (>600 mg/d) or when 300 mg is used with 3A4 inhibitors but insufficient data to create target range
Ethambutol	Efficacy decreases at doses of <25 mg/kg, insufficient data to create target range	Increases at doses of >15 mg/kg
Pyrazinamide	Very few data	Increases at doses of 40 mg/kg/d

research to establish relationships between serum concentrations and efficacy. In response to the lack of clinically validated therapeutic ranges, some have used the range of concentrations achieved in normal volunteers as the "normal range." However, it is not at all clear that drug concentrations lower than those achieved in healthy volunteers are subtherapeutic and that such a normal range is an adequate surrogate for a clinically validated therapeutic range. Indeed, recent pharmacokinetic studies suggest that patients being treated for active tuberculosis commonly have serum concentrations of first-line drugs lower than those in healthy volunteers (92).

Studies purporting to show that low drug concentrations are common causes of treatment failure or relapse have had major methodologic problems, the most prominent being the lack of sampling from patients who were cured of tuberculosis (controls) (3,4). In a recent large study including controls, there were no significant differences between the C_{max} or area under the time-concentration curve of isoniazid or rifampin among controls versus patients with treatment failure or relapse treated with a standard twice-weekly regimen (93). Although several potent risk factors for treatment failure or relapse were identified, such as the presence of cavitation and 2-month culture positivity, pharmacokinetic parameters of isoniazid and rifampin were not predictive of treatment outcome. Surely at extreme values, pharmacokinetic parameters must be associated with efficacy and toxicity, but this study demonstrates that there are no clear relationships in the range of concentrations achieved in the majority of patients. The implication of these findings is that the first-line drugs have broad therapeutic ranges allowing efficacy with low rates of toxicity, despite the tenfold differences in serum concentrations that are seen with standard weight-based dosing. Indeed, that is the reason these drugs and the current doses were chosen as first-line therapy.

A more compelling rationale can be made for therapeutic drug monitoring for selected second-line drugs, such as cycloserine, ethionamide, PAS, and the aminoglycosides. These agents are inherently less active than the first-line drugs and have appreciable toxicity at doses required to achieve microbiologic efficacy. However, it is not clear that routine therapeutic drug monitoring is indicated for these drugs. The recent success of treating multidrug-resistant tuberculosis in a pilot program in Peru suggests that choosing regimens based on accurate *in vitro* susceptibility tests and ensuring that treatment is given as directly observed therapy are the two key elements in the successful treatment of multidrug-resistant strains, not therapeutic drug monitoring (94).

There are also concerns about the practical aspects of therapeutic drug monitoring in the setting of outpatient tuberculosis treatment. It is challenging to obtain multiple, well-timed samples and ensure proper specimen storage and handling in any routine clinical care setting. The expense of therapeutic drug monitoring is considerable because multiple drugs must be measured at multiple time points to adequately characterize pharmacokinetic parameters. Finally, experience with drugs for which therapeutic drug monitoring is well established demonstrates that errors in sampling and interpretation are very common. In a study of therapeutic drug monitoring of anticonvulsants, only 14% of the serum concentrations were obtained appropriately (95).

RECOMMENDATIONS FOR THERAPEUTIC DRUG MONITORING IN TUBERCULOSIS TREATMENT

Therapeutic drug monitoring has a very limited role in tuberculosis treatment. Given the potency and tolerability of the first-line drugs, standard weight-based dosing of these drugs is very successful, even in higher risk groups, such as those with HIV-related tuberculosis. Therefore, therapeutic drug monitoring should be restricted to situations in which highly abnormal concentrations might be expected, such as ethambutol concentrations in severe renal insufficiency. Whether therapeutic drug monitoring will help in the management of treatment failure has not been demonstrated, although it can be considered in the rare patient failing directly observed therapy. The occurrence of relapse is more likely to be related to factors other than pharmacokinetics (96), and routine therapeutic drug monitoring is not recommended for such patients. Therapeutic drug monitoring is probably not helpful in most patients requiring treatment with second-line drugs. Targeted use, however, may be beneficial. Examples of such situations include the patient on prolonged aminoglycosides (longer than 3 to 4 months) and patients requiring cycloserine therapy (because there is clinical evidence of a relationship between concentrations and neuropsychiatric toxicity of this drug).

ACKNOWLEDGMENT

This work was supported in part by the Tuberculosis Trials Consortium of the Centers for Disease Control and Prevention.

REFERENCES

1. Baciewicz AM, Self TH. Isoniazid interactions. *South Med J* 1985;78:714–718.
2. Venkatesan K. Pharmacokinetic drug interactions with rifampin. *Clin Pharmacokinet* 1992;22:47–65.
3. Kimerling ME, Phillips P, Patterson P, et al. Low serum antimycobacterial drug levels in non-HIV-infected tuberculosis patients. *Chest* 1998;113:1178–1183.
4. Mehta JB, Shantaveerapa H, Byrd RP Jr, et al. Utility of rifampin blood levels in the treatment and follow-up of active pulmonary tuberculosis in patients who were slow to respond to routine directly observed therapy. *Chest* 2001;120:1520–1524.
5. Burman WJ. The value of *in vitro* drug activity and pharmacoki-

netics in predicting the effectiveness of antimycobacterial therapy: a critical review. *Am J Med Sci* 1997;313:355–363.

6. Dickinson JM, Mitchison DA. Suitability of rifampicin for intermittent administration in the treatment of tuberculosis. *Tubercle* 1970;51:82–94.

7. Dickinson JM, Mitchison DA. Observations *in vitro* on the suitability of pyrazinamide for intermittent chemotherapy of tuberculosis. *Tubercle* 1970;51:389–396.

8. Dickinson JM, Mitchison DA. *In vitro* studies on the choice of drugs for intermittent chemotherapy of tuberculosis. *Tubercle* 1966;47:370–380.

9. Cohn DL, Catlin BJ, Peterson KL, et al. A 62-dose, 6-month therapy for pulmonary and extrapulmonary tuberculosis: a twice-weekly, directly observed, and cost-effective regimen. *Ann Intern Med* 1990;112:407–415.

10. Hong Kong Chest Service/British Medical Research Council. Controlled trial of 6-month and 9-month regimens of daily and intermittent streptomycin plus isoniazid plus pyrazinamide for pulmonary tuberculosis in Hong Kong: the results up to 30 months. *Am Rev Respir Dis* 1977;115:727–734.

11. Hong Kong Chest Service/British Medical Research Council. Controlled trial of four thrice-weekly regimens and a daily regimen all given for 6 months for pulmonary tuberculosis. *Lancet* 1981;1:171–174.

12. Peloquin CA, Berning SE, Huitt GA, et al. Once-daily and twice-daily dosing of p-aminosalicylic acid granules. *Am J Respir Crit Care Med* 1999;159:932–934.

13. Peloquin CA, Namdar R, Dodge AA, et al. Pharmacokinetics of isoniazid under fasting conditions, with food, and with antacids. *Int J Tuberc Lung Dis* 1999;3:703–710.

14. Melander A, Danielson K, Hanson A, et al. Reduction of isoniazid bioavailability in normal men by concomitant intake of food. *Acta Med Scand* 1976;200:93–97.

15. Zent C, Smith P. Study of the effect of concomitant food on the bioavailability of rifampicin, isoniazid, and pyrazinamide. *Tuber Lung Dis* 1995;76:109–113.

16. Gallicano K, Sahai J, Zaror-Behrens G, et al. Effect of antacids in didanosine tablet on bioavailability of isoniazid. *Antimicrob Agents Chemother* 1994;38:894–897.

17. Hurwitz A, Schlozman DL. Effects of antacids on gastrointestinal absorption of isoniazid in rats and man. *Am Rev Respir Dis* 1974;109:41–47.

18. Peloquin CA, Namdar R, Singleton MD, et al. Pharmacokinetics of rifampin under fasting conditions, with food, and with antacids. *Chest* 1999;115:12–18.

19. Siegler DI, Bryant M, Burley DM, et al. Effect of meals on rifampicin absorption. *Lancet* 1974;2:197–198.

20. Khalil SAH, El-Khordagui LK, El-Gholmy Z. Effect of antacids on oral absorption of rifampin. *Int J Pharm* 1984;20:99–106.

21. Narang PK, Lewis RC, Bianchine JR. Rifabutin absorption in humans: relative bioavailability and food effect. *Clin Pharmacol Ther* 1992;52:335–341.

22. Sahai J, Narang PK, Hawley-Foss N, et al. A phase I evaluation of concomitant rifabutin and didanosine in symptomatic HIV-infected patients. *J Acquir Immune Defic Syndr* 1995;9:274–279.

23. Owens RC Jr, Keung AC, Gardner S, et al. Pharmacokinetic and food effect evaluation of rifapentine in subjects seropositive for the human immunodeficiency virus. Presented at the 37th Interscience Conference on Antimicrobial Agents and Chemotherapy. Toronto, Ontario, Canada, 1997(abst A-2).

24. Peloquin CA, Bulpitt AE, Jaresko GS, et al. Pharmacokinetics of pyrazinamide under fasting conditions, with food, and with antacids. *Pharmacotherapy* 1998;18:1205–1211.

25. Peloquin CA, Bulpitt AE, Jaresko GS, et al. Pharmacokinetics of ethambutol under fasting conditions, with food, and with antacids. *Antimicrob Agents Chemother* 1999;43:568–572.

26. Ameer B, Polk RE, Kline BJ, et al. Effect of food on ethambutol absorption. *Clin Pharmacy* 1982;1:156–158.

27. Mattila MJ, Linnoila M, Seppala T, et al. Effect of aluminum hydroxide and glycopyrronium on the absorption of ethambutol and alcohol in man. *Br J Clin Pharmacol* 1978;5:161–166.

28. Lehto P, Kivisto KT. Effect of sucralfate on absorption of norfloxacin and ofloxacin. *Antimicrob Agents Chemother* 1994;38:248–251.

29. Lehto P, Kivisto KT, Neuvonen PJ. The effect of ferrous sulphate on the absorption of norfloxacin, ciprofloxacin, and ofloxacin. *Br J Clin Pharmacol* 1994;37:82–85.

30. Lettieri J, Vargas R, Agarwal V, et al. Effect of food on the pharmacokinetics of a single oral dose of moxifloxacin 400mg in healthy male volunteers. *Clin Pharmacokinet* 2001;40:19–25.

31. Stass H, Kubitza D. Effects of iron supplements on the oral bioavailability of moxifloxacin, a novel 8-methoxyfluoroquinolone, in humans. *Clin Pharmacokinet* 2001;40:57–62.

32. Stass H, Schuhly U, Moller JG, et al. Effects of sucralfate on the oral bioavailability of moxifloxacin, a novel 8-methoxyfluoroquinolone, in healthy volunteers. *Clin Pharmacokinet* 2001;40:49–55.

33. Stass H, Bottcher MF, Ochmann K. Evaluation of the influence of antacids and H2 antagonists on the absorption of moxifloxacin after oral administration of a 400mg dose to healthy volunteers. *Clin Pharmacokinet* 2001;40:39–48.

34. Zhu M, Nix DE, Adam RD, et al. Pharmacokinetics of cycloserine under fasting conditions and with high- fat meal, orange juice, and antacids. *Pharmacotherapy* 2001;21:891–897.

35. Auclair B, Nix DE, Adam RD, et al. Pharmacokinetics of ethionamide administered under fasting conditions or with orange juice, food, or antacids. *Antimicrob Agents Chemother* 2001;45:810–814.

36. Peloquin CA, Zhu M, Adam RD, et al. Pharmacokinetics of para-aminosalicylic acid granules under four dosing conditions. *Ann Pharmacother* 2001;35:1332–1338.

37. Burman WJ, Gallicano K, Peloquin C. Therapeutic implications of drug interactions in the treatment of HIV-related tuberculosis. *Clin Infect Dis* 1999;28:419–430.

38. Tam CM, Chan SL, Lam CW, et al. Rifapentine and isoniazid in the continuation phase of treating pulmonary tuberculosis: initial report. *Am J Respir Crit Care Med* 1998;157:1726–1733.

39. Tuberculosis Chemotherapy Centre, Madras. A controlled comparison of two fully supervised once-weekly regimens in the treatment of newly diagnosed pulmonary tuberculosis. *Tubercle* 1973;54:23–45.

40. Ormerod LP, Prescott RJ. Inter-relations between relapses, drug regimens and compliance with treatment in tuberculosis. *Respir Med* 1991;85:239–242.

41. Edsall J, Collins JG, Gray JAC. The reactivation of tuberculosis in New York City in 1967. *Am Rev Respir Dis* 1970;102:725–736.

42. Furin JJ, Mitnick CD, Shin SS, et al. Occurrence of serious adverse effects in patients receiving community-based therapy for multi-drug-resistant tuberculosis. *Int J Tuberc Lung Dis* 2001;5:648–655.

43. Terra M, Burman W, Breese P, et al. Streptomycin vs. ethambutol as the fourth drug in highly intermittent, directly observed tuberculosis treatment. *Am J Respir Crit Care Med* 2001;163 [Suppl]:A498 (abst).

44. Nix DE, Watson WA, Lener ME, et al. Effects of aluminum and magnesium antacids and ranitidine on the absorption of ciprofloxacin. *Clin Pharmacol Ther* 1989;46:700–705.

45. Neuvonen PJ, Kivisto KT. Milk and yoghurt do not impair the absorption of ofloxacin. *Br J Clin Pharmacol* 1992;33:346–348.

46. Stass H, Wandel C, Delesen H, et al. Effect of calcium supple-

ments on the oral bioavailability of moxifloxacin in healthy male volunteers. *Clin Pharmacokinet* 2001;40:27–32.

47. Boman G, Lundgren P, Stjernstrom G. Mechanism of the inhibitory effect of PAS granules on the absorption of rifampicin: adsorption of rifampicin by an excipient, bentonite. *Eur J Clin Pharmacol* 1975;8:293–299.

48. Buniva G, Pagani V, Carozzi A. Bioavailability of rifampicin capsules. *Int J Clin Pharmacol Ther Toxicol* 1983;21:404–409.

49. Cavenaghi R. Rifampicin raw material characteristics and their effect on bioavailability. *Bull Int Union Tuberc Lung Dis* 1989;64:36–37.

50. Koestner JA, Jones LK, Polk WH, et al. Prolonged use of intravenous isoniazid and rifampin. *DICP* 1989;23:48–50.

51. Ho YI, Chan CY, Cheng AF. In-vitro activities of aminoglycoside-aminocyclitols against mycobacteria. *J Antimicrob Chemother* 1997;40:27–32.

52. Wisnia LG, Kukolj S, Lopez de Santa Maria J, et al. Renal function damage in 131 cases of urogenital tuberculosis. *Urology* 1978;11:457–461.

53. Kennedy AC, Burton JA, Allison ME. Tuberculosis as a continuing cause of renal amyloidosis. *BMJ* 1974;3:795–797.

54. Andrew OT, Schoenfeld PY, Hopewell PC, et al. Tuberculosis in patients with end-stage renal disease. *Am J Med* 1980;68:59–65.

55. Chia S, Karim M, Elwood RK, et al. Risk of tuberculosis in dialysis patients: a population-based study. *Int J Tuberc Lung Dis* 1998;2:989–991.

56. Malone RS, Fish DN, Spiegel DM, et al. The effect of hemodialysis on isoniazid, rifampin, pyrazinamide, and ethambutol. *Am J Respir Crit Care Med* 1999;159:1580–1584.

57. McMullin CM, Brown NM, Brown IM, et al. The pharmacokinetics of once-daily oral 400 mg ofloxacin in patients with peritonitis complicating continuous ambulatory peritoneal dialysis. *J Antimicrob Chemother* 1997;39:829–831.

58. Lameire N, Rosenkranz B, Malerczyk V, et al. Ofloxacin pharmacokinetics in chronic renal failure and dialysis. *Clin Pharmacokinet* 1991;21:357–371.

59. Malone RS, Fish DN, Spiegel DM, et al. The effect of hemodialysis on cycloserine, ethionamide, para- aminosalicylate, and clofazimine. *Chest* 1999;116:984–990.

60. Hill AR, Premkumar S, Brustein S, et al. Disseminated tuberculosis in the acquired immunodeficiency syndrome era. *Am Rev Respir Dis* 1991;144:1164–1170.

61. Sahn SA, Neff TA. Miliary tuberculosis. *Am J Med* 1974;56:494–505.

62. Essop AR, Posen JA, Hodkinson JH, et al. Tuberculosis hepatitis: a clinical review of 96 cases. *Q J Med* 1984;53:465–477.

63. Centers for Disease Control and Prevention. *Reported tuberculosis in the United States, 1998*. Atlanta: CDC, 1999.

64. Burman WJ, Reves RR, Hawkes AP, et al. DNA fingerprinting with two probes decreases clustering of *Mycobacterium tuberculosis*. *Am J Respir Crit Care Med* 1997;155:1140–1146.

65. Barry M, Craft J, Coleman D, et al. Clinical findings in Southeast Asian refugees. *JAMA* 1983;249:3200–3203.

66. Saigal S, Agarwal SR, Nandeesh HP, et al. Safety of an ofloxacin-based antitubercular regimen for the treatment of tuberculosis in patients with underlying chronic liver disease: a preliminary report. *J Gastroenterol Hepatol* 2001;16:1028–1032.

67. Robinson P, Lamsom M, Gigliotti M, et al. Pharmacokinetic interaction between nevirapine and rifampin. Presented at the International Conference on AIDS, Geneva, 1998, 60623.

68. Benedek IH, Joshi A, Fiske WD, et al. Pharmacokinetic interaction between efavirenz and rifampin in healthy volunteers. Presented at the 12th World AIDS Conference. Geneva, Switzerland, 1998, 42280.

69. Benedeck IH, Fiske WD, White SJ, et al. Pharmacokinetic interaction between multiple doses of efavirenz and rifabutin in healthy volunteers. Presented at the 36th Annual Meeting of the Infectious Diseases Society of America, Denver, 1998, 461.

70. McAllister WA, Thompson PJ, Al-Habet SM, et al. Rifampicin reduces effectiveness and bioavailability of prednisolone. *BMJ* 1983;286:923–925.

71. Reinach B, de Souse G, Dostert P, et al. Comparative effects of rifabutin and rifampicin on cytochromes P450 and UDP-glucuronosyl-transferases expression in fresh and cryopreserved human hepatocytes. *Chem Biol Interact* 1999;121:37–48.

72. Li AP, Reith MK, Rasmussen A, et al. Primary human hepatocytes as a tool for the evaluation of structure-activity relationship in cytochrome P450 induction potential of xenobiotics: evaluation of rifampin, rifapentine, and rifabutin. *Chem Biol Interact* 1997;107:17–30.

73. Self TH, Chrisman CR, Baciewicz AM, et al. Isoniazid drug and food interactions. *Am J Med Sci* 1999;317:304–311.

74. Indinavir pharmacokinetic study group. Indinavir (MK 639) drug interactions studies. *XI International Conference on AIDS*. Vancouver, Canada, 1996, MoB174.

75. Miller RR, Porter J, Greenblatt DJ. Clinical importance of the interaction of phenytoin and isoniazid: a report from the Boston Collaborative Drug Surveillance Program. *Chest* 1979;75:356–358.

76. Valsalan VC, Cooper GL. Carbamazepine intoxication caused by interaction with isoniazid. *BMJ* 1982;285:261–262.

77. Kay L, Kampmann JP, Svendsen TL, et al. Influence of rifampin and isoniazid on the kinetics of phenytoin. *Br J Clin Pharmacol* 1985;20:323–326.

78. Battaglia R, Pianezzola E, Salgarollo G, et al. Absorption, disposition and preliminary pathway of 14C-rifabutin in animals and man. *J Antimicrob Chemother* 1990;26:813–822.

79. Sun E, Heath-Chiozzi M, Cameron DW, et al. Concurrent ritonavir and rifabutin increases risk of rifabutin-associated adverse events. Presented at the XI International Conference on AIDS. Vancouver, Canada, 1996, MoB171.

80. Shafran SD, Singer J, Zarowny DP, et al. A comparison of two regimens for the treatment of Mycobacterium avium complex bacteremia in AIDS: rifabutin, ethambutol, and clarithromycin versus rifampin, ethambutol, clofazimine, and ciprofloxacin. *N Engl J Med* 1996;335:377–383.

81. Centers for Disease Control and Prevention. Prevention and treatment of tuberculosis among patients infected with human immunodeficiency virus: principles of therapy and revised recommendations. *MMWR Recomm Rep* 1998;47:1–58.

82. Centers for Disease Control and Prevention. Updated guidelines for the use of rifabutin or rifampin for the treatment and prevention of tuberculosis among HIV-infected patients taking protease inhibitors or nonnucleoside reverse transcriptase inhibitors. *MMWR Morb Mortal Wkly Rep* 2000;49:185–189.

83. Casner PR. Inability to attain oral anticoagulation: warfarin-rifampin interaction revisited. *South Med J* 1996;89:1200–1203.

84. Romankiewicz JA, Ehrman M. Rifampin and warfarin: a drug interaction. *Ann Intern Med* 1975;82:224–225.

85. Kerr BM, Daniels R, Clendeninn N. Pharmacokinetic interaction of nelfinavir with half-dose rifabutin. *Can J Infect Dis* 1999;10[Suppl B]:21B(abst).

86. Polk RE, Brophy DF, Israel DS, et al. Pharmacokinetic Interaction between amprenavir and rifabutin or rifampin in healthy males. *Antimicrob Agents Chemother* 2001;45:502–508.

87. Borin MT, Chambers JH, Carel BJ, et al. Pharmacokinetic study of the interaction between rifabutin and delavirdine mesylate in HIV-1 infected patients. *Antiviral Res* 1997;35:53–63.

88. Smith JA, Hardin TC, Patterson TF, et al. Rifabutin decreases itraconazole plasma levels in patients with HIV-infection. Presented at the 2nd National Conference on Human Retroviruses, Washington, DC, 1995.

89. Trapnell CB, Narang PK, Li R, et al. Increased plasma rifabutin levels with concomitant fluconazole therapy in HIV-infected patients. *Ann Intern Med* 1996;124:573–576.

90. Sahai J, Gallicano K, Swick L, et al. Reduced plasma concentrations of antituberculous drugs in patients with HIV infection. *Ann Intern Med* 1997;127:289–293.

91. Peloquin CA. Using therapeutic drug monitoring to dose the antimycobacterial drugs. *Clin Chest Med* 1997;18:79–87.

92. Peloquin C, Benator D, Hayden K, et al. Low rifapentine, rifampin, and isoniazid plasma levels are not predicted by clinical and demographic features. *Am J Respir Crit Care Med* 2001; 163:A498(abst).

93. Weiner M, Burman W, Vernon A, et al., and the Tuberculosis Trials Consortium. Low isoniazid concentrations associated with outcome of TB treatment with once-weekly isoniazid and rifapentine. *Am J Respir Crit Care Med* 2003;167:1341–1347.

94. Farmer P, Kim JY. Community based approaches to the control of multidrug resistant tuberculosis: introducing "DOTS-plus." *BMJ* 1998;317:671–674.

95. Schoenenberger RA, Tanasijevic MJ, Jha A, et al. Appropriateness of antiepileptic drug level monitoring. *JAMA* 1995;274:1622–1626.

96. Tuberculosis Trials Consortium. Once-weekly rifapentine and isoniazid versus twice-weekly rifampin and isoniazid in the continuation phase of therapy for drug-susceptible pulmonary tuberculosis: a prospective, randomized clinical trial among HIV-native persons. *Lancet* 2002;360:528–534.

PHARMACOGENOMICS OF TUBERCULOSIS

CARL N. KRAUS
CLIFTON BARRY III

Chemotherapy of bacterial infectious diseases relies on delivering the most effective antimicrobial agent at the optimal dose without causing toxicity to the patient undergoing treatment. The optimal dose of an antibiotic in any individual patient depends on factors such as the efficiency with which that individual absorbs, distributes, and clears the drug being used as well as the efficacy of the drug against the particular strain of pathogen causing the infection. The reality of clinical practice is such that the actual dose given to one patient is largely the same as that given to every other patient, barring adjustments for weight, age, disease severity, or comorbid illness. In addition, it is assumed that the minimal inhibitory concentration for the particular strain of bacteria infecting a specific individual is an average value of previously tested strains. Further, we assume that individuals absorb, distribute, metabolize, and excrete a given antibiotic at an average rate. Toxicity is likewise handled empirically; an individual is assumed to have an average tolerance and then monitored for adverse consequences, with sometimes harmful results. Pharmacogenomics is the science of replacing the assumption of average behavior relating to bacterial sensitivity, host pharmacokinetics, and host toxicities with specific information based on genomic DNA sequences of both the host and the bacterium. This information can reveal the actual drug sensitivity of the particular agent causing disease, the actual drug levels achievable in the infected individual, and the actual risk of an adverse event of chemotherapy. Pharmacogenomics is therefore the knowledge-based tailoring of therapy to each individual patient and each individual pathogen (1–5).

The concept of individual variation among humans in response to therapy or environmental effectors is not new. Glucose-6-phosphate dehydrogenase deficiency was first documented by Pythagoras in 510 B.C. who recognized

that fava bean ingestion was dangerous only for a small subset of individuals who developed hemolytic anemias (6). The first "proof of principle" that individual inherited metabolic variations may have important clinical significance was the recognition by Garrod in 1902 that there existed variability in some general detoxifying enzymes in an autosomal recessive fashion (7). This disorder, now referred to as alkaptonuria, can have significant arthritic sequelae. That these variations could be measured and understood at a population level was first demonstrated in 1932 by Snyder who observed autosomal recessive inheritance of the ability to taste phenylthiourea (8). Although these inborn differences in metabolism are relatively extreme, more subtle defects in regulation or expression levels of some pathways combine to create an almost infinite spectrum of individual human phenotypes that in many cases only show up when an individual is subjected to the stress of infection and chemotherapy.

Contemporary tuberculosis (TB) chemotherapy relies on multiple drugs given simultaneously in an empirically determined regimen that largely resulted from studies in mice (9–12). The role of individual variation in response to therapy has not been assessed, although it is widely known and accepted that the disease of as many as 15% of all patients who undergo chemotherapy will not be cured and that of those whose disease is cured, approximately 5% will relapse with active disease within a year of completing even the ideal recommended 6-month course of four antibiotics (13). In addition, as many as 13% of patients undergoing TB chemotherapy will experience adverse effects of this extremely lengthy therapy (14). A fraction of the treatment failures (nonresponders and relapses) will occur because the infecting strain of tubercle bacillus has developed genotypic resistance to the antitubercular agents used, another fraction will fail because of poor compliance with the regimen, and another fraction will fail because of poor pharmacokinetics or pharmacodynamics of the drugs in these patients. Selecting drug regimens based on individual strain and host

C. N. Kraus and C. Barry III: Tuberculosis Research Section, National Institute of Allergy and Infectious Diseases, National Institutes of Health, Rockville, Maryland.

genotypes can maximize the likelihood that an individual patient will have a positive outcome after anti-TB chemotherapy. It can also minimize the risk that an individual patient will experience an adverse effect from these therapies.

Multidrug-resistant TB has risen worldwide and now accounts for more than two million cases per year (15). For patients who harbor resistant organisms, therapy becomes even more problematic because many second-line agents require parenteral administration and have additional associated toxicities. Understanding why patients fail to respond to therapy and tailoring therapy to individuals can be expected to lead to less frequent emergence of drug resistance by avoiding exposure of the organism to subtherapeutic doses of antituberculars. Avoiding adverse events of drug treatment would also decrease the chance that patients will terminate therapy prematurely, another factor that can lead to the emergence of drug resistance.

With the mapping of the human genome (16) and the TB genome (17), we can evaluate TB-specific and host-specific factors that have direct impact on clinical drug efficacy. Thus, we are now in a unique position to bridge the gap between genomics and clinical pharmacology. This will allow more efficacious, less toxic, and potentially shorter drug regimens for the treatment of TB.

BACTERIAL FACTORS THAT INFLUENCE THE OUTCOME OF TUBERCULOSIS CHEMOTHERAPY

Despite the fact that *Mycobacterium tuberculosis* as a species exhibits a very low rate of synonymous mutation in its genome (18), there are convincing reasons to believe that this organism has acquired genetically encoded differences that have important ramifications for its interaction with the human host. For example, an outbreak of TB in a clothing factory in a rural area of the United States in 1995 resulted in the isolation of a strain (dubbed CDC1551) characterized as hypervirulent (19). This characterization was based on a much larger than expected number of skin test conversions but not with an increase in the actual number of cases of active TB. Subsequently, it was established that although this strain induces a more significant immune response from the host, it is in fact attenuated for virulence (at least in animal models) (20). The complete genome sequence of this strain was recently published (21), and the results support the contention that there is a large number of polymorphic gene loci among clinical isolates of *M. tuberculosis*.

Although the functional significance of these polymorphisms has not been established with certainty, other strains, such as HN878, isolated from a prison outbreak in Texas, have a much more lethal effect on infected mice than either CDC1551 or typical laboratory strains (22).

Although the genotypic basis for this hyperlethality remains imprecise, the phenotype appears to be mediated by the interaction of lipid components of the mycobacterium with the murine innate immune system. It stands to reason that this phenotypic hyperlethality in mice will have important functional consequences for humans infected with similar strains. It is also reasonable to expect that humans infected with such strains may have higher bacillary loads, prove more difficult to treat, and may therefore be at higher risk of relapse or the development of drug resistance. There is already substantial documentation that some families of related isolates (such as the W or Beijing family) may be overrepresented in isolates of *M. tuberculosis* that develop multidrug resistance, suggesting that some adaptation of this family directly affects therapeutic outcome (23–26).

Although there still remains considerable work to be done regarding the precise genes that contribute to various therapeutic outcomes, it is quite clear that such genes exist and their elucidation will provide an important tool for the pharmacogenomic evaluation of individual patients. Such evaluations might lead, for example, to extending the duration of therapy for patients infected with strains known to be difficult to eradicate.

Although strain variation selected by coevolution with the human host still remains largely exploratory and experimental, strain variation that is selected by drug pressure has been well studied and carefully documented. Determination of the molecular mechanism of action of most of the front-line antimycobacterial agents has allowed not only improved understanding of the mechanisms of action of these agents but also the basis for genotypic identification of resistant strains (27–29). In some cases, such as rifampicin resistance, the genetic basis for resistance has been determined experimentally and validated clinically (30). In other cases, such as isoniazid resistance, the molecular mechanism of action and genetic basis for resistance remain controversial (31). Despite ambiguity with respect to some agents, progress has been made in identifying the genetic correlates of drug susceptibility. Because multidrug resistance with respect to TB therapy refers only to resistance to the two most effective anti-TB drugs isoniazid and rifampicin, significant progress has been made with respect to diagnosing this dual resistance at the genetic level. In one study in a high TB incidence community in South Africa, sequence information relating to only three codons, two in *rpoB* and one in *katG* could successfully identify 90% of multidrug-resistant cases (32).

Although rifampicin and isoniazid have been the most thoroughly explored anti-TB agents in terms of genetic alterations associated with clinical resistance, the mechanism of action and clinically useful genetic markers of drug resistance have been identified for pyrazinamide and ethambutol, the two less active components of standard multidrug therapy (28,33–35). Among second-line anti-TB agents, the mechanisms of aminoglycosides, ethionamide, and fluoroquinolones are clear and some genetic markers are available for detection (36–38). In short, many of the drug resistance–associated genetic alleles are at a stage suitable for pharmacogenetic exploitation.

Current diagnostic techniques used to genotype *M. tuberculosis* for drug resistance have relied on direct gene sequencing after polymerase chain reaction (PCR) amplification, heteroduplex analysis, or single-strand conformational polymorphism analysis (39). Although these techniques are useful, they have limitations in that only a small number of resistance-determining alleles can be analyzed and that the technical sophistication necessary to conduct PCR and gel electrophoretic analysis is often beyond the capabilities of typical clinical laboratories (40). High-density oligonucleotide arrays have been applied to the problem of determining rifampicin resistance among *M. tuberculosis* isolates (41,42). Sequencing using moderate-density, solid-phase arrays has been used successfully in determining rifampicin resistance alleles (43). More exciting has been the successful immobilization of both the PCR process and allele-specific detection through arrays of primers that amplify known drug-related polymorphisms (44). These "TB microchips" have been shown to be capable of detecting more than 30 mutant variants of rifampicin-resistant alleles in approximately 1.5 hours (45,46).

Although these approaches are also technically challenging to carry out reproducibly, the techniques are amenable to producing standardized, automated portable platforms that would reduce the impact of variable skill levels in the clinical laboratory. Although rifampicin resistance is currently the only real example in which the relationship between bacterial genotype and clinically significant resistance has been evaluated in this fashion, the capacity clearly exists to apply this technology broadly. Importantly, these tools are also increasingly being used in the developing world where the need is most acute (47).

HOST FACTORS INVOLVED IN SUSCEPTIBILITY TO TUBERCULOSIS

The first investigation suggesting the existence of an inherited predisposition to TB infection examined twins at risk of the disease and was performed in the middle of the past century. These studies revealed a significantly higher concordance of TB infection among monozygotic (65% to 85%) than dizygotic (25% to 28%) twins (48,49). In Lubeck, Germany, in 1926, an accidental mix up of vaccine and challenge strains led to the inoculation of 251 children with a virulent strain of *M. tuberculosis*. Of these children, 31% of the children died, 50% developed radiographically confirmed disease, and 19% had no evidence of disease (50). This tragic episode in the history of medicine underscores the marked variability of individual susceptibility to the development of TB disease after infection.

In fact, human infection with *M. tuberculosis* results in one of two outcomes: 40% of the time, uncontrolled bacterial replication will lead to active disease, and the remaining 60% of the time, the host controls the infection and an asymptomatic or latent disease develops and is maintained as long as the individual's immune system remains uncompromised (51,52). In immunocompetent individuals, approximately 10% of such latent infections will ultimately reactivate and cause clinically significant disease, and the remaining 90% experience no apparent ill consequences of this cryptic bacterial state other than conversion to purified protein derivative (PPD) sensitivity (53,54). For every symptomatic or latent case of TB, there are also many apparently highly exposed individuals that never convert to PPD positivity nor develop active disease (55–57). Bacille Calmette–Guérin vaccination can confer PPD sensitivity but even in as many as 40% of individuals vaccinated with bacille Calmette–Guérin, no tuberculin sensitivity results (58,59). This is also clear at a population level in which some groups have been shown to be at increased risk of both susceptibility to infection and progression to active disease. African Americans, for example, were found to be more readily infected by *M. tuberculosis* than whites in a nursing home population in Arkansas (60).

Since these original studies, many specific heritable factors, including elements of both the innate and acquired immune response, have been implicated in susceptibility to the development of TB. Genetic factors associated with human infection have identified associations between both major histocompatibility complex genes and non–major histocompatibility complex genes. The human leukocyte antigen (HLA) class II DR2 serotype, which includes multiple HLA alleles, has been associated with the development of active TB in geographically diverse populations from India, Indonesia, Russia, and Mexico (61–64). The development of tuberculoid leprosy, caused by the closely related leprosy bacillus, has likewise been correlated with major histocompatibility complex genotype. In this case, alleles that encode an arginine at particular positions in the HLA-DRB1 peptide-binding region have been associated with increased susceptibility (65). Recently, Goldfeld et al. (66) examined a large cohort of Cambodian patients and identified a strong association of TB susceptibility with the presence of a particular DQB1*0503 allele. Other, less clearly defined HLA associations have also been documented, including a relative decrease in HLA-B18 and relative increase in HLA-A2 in patients with TB (67). HLA-DR2 appears to also have strong influence on host susceptibility, with a higher frequency among patients with TB (68).

Non-HLA host variations also play a role in host susceptibility to TB. The best examples are provided by the landmark studies investigating the role of interferon gamma (IFN-γ) and interleukin (IL)-12 receptor deficiencies and susceptibility to mycobacterial disease. Mutations in the IFN-γ receptor have been shown to predispose to infection with atypical mycobacteria and *Salmonella* organisms in Maltese children (69,70) and with bacille Calmette–Guérin infection in a Tunisian (71). IFN-γ or IFN-γ receptor–deficient mice have also been shown to be hypersusceptible to mycobacterial disease (72,73). Immunity to mycobacterial disease is severely compromised in patients with IL-12 receptor deficiencies (74,75).

Several other polymorphisms in genes of unknown functional impact on human TB have also been identified including polymorphisms in the IL-1 gene complex, the vitamin D receptor, the IL-10 promoter, and the tumor necrosis factor-α promoter. However, the evaluation of many of these polymorphisms in a single, well-characterized population with pulmonary TB and PPD-positive controls suggests that many of these associations are ethnic specific.

For example, polymorphisms in noncoding regions of the natural resistance–associated macrophage protein 1 (Nramp1) were evaluated among patients with and without TB in West Africa (76). Early studies had shown that susceptibility to infection in the mouse was associated with a nonconservative Gly-105 to Asp-105 substitution within a predicted transmembrane functional domain of Nramp (77). Later studies suggest, however, that Nramp1 is of limited importance in containment by the immune system in Nramp1-deficient mice (78). The Gambian study evaluated more than 800 individuals, half with and half without confirmed pulmonary TB. They found four polymorphisms in the *Nramp1* gene that appeared to be associated with susceptibility to TB in this population (odds ratio >4.0). However, the study by Delgado et al. (79) evaluated 358 Cambodian patients with TB and 108 PPD-positive controls and found that two of these polymorphisms were, in fact, associated with resistance in this population, whereas two others had no association with disease susceptibility.

Observations that vitamin D metabolism activates TB-infected macrophages and inhibits intracellular growth led investigators to evaluate the potential role of vitamin D receptor polymorphisms in the risk of TB acquisition in more than 200 Gujarati Asians (80). There was no significant independent association with any of the polymorphisms and TB susceptibility. However, two of three polymorphisms evaluated appeared to be associated within the context of 25-hydroxycholecalciferol deficiency. In contrast, one of the associations was found to be associated with resistance in The Gambia (81) and no association was found between these polymorphisms and TB susceptibility or resistance in India (82) or Cambodia (79). Mannose-binding protein polymorphisms have also been associated with disease susceptibility (83). Three mutant alleles in patients with TB were six times more common than in control subjects. Thus, many of the non-HLA associations identified to date appear to be influenced by ethnicity and their significance in TB susceptibility or resistance remains unclear.

Presumably, there are also genetic factors that predispose a host to initial infection with *M. tuberculosis* after exposure. Although these have been more difficult to assess because patient exposure cannot be ascertained with certainty, recent studies suggest that elements of the innate immune response directly affect the susceptibility of a host to development of a delayed-type hypersensitivity response signifying nonprogressive infection. In a survey of 55 anonymous healthy volunteers, monocytes isolated from 22 of these donors demonstrated a significant ability to kill *M. tuberculosis in vitro* (S. Matsumoto, F. A. Sher, C. E. Barry III, unpublished data, 2002). All the donors whose monocytes were highly effective in killing *M. tuberculosis* lacked any detectable T-cell response to PPD. Although these donors may have been exposed to *M. tuberculosis*, the efficiency of their innate immune response prevents even a viable subclinical infection from developing. This result is significant because it suggests that a subset of the human population has an unidentified innate immune mechanism rendering them at very low risk of primary infection.

Host factors not only play a role in determining disease susceptibility but also disease manifestations. The site of infection with TB directly affects prognosis and therapeutic choice. Patients with meningeal involvement require regimens with good penetration through the blood–brain barrier and usually prolonged courses of treatment. Investigators at Case Western Reserve University showed that polymorphisms in the IL-1 locus can influence site of infection and PPD status, with a larger proportion of subjects with the IL-1Ra A2(−)/IL-1β (+3953) A1(+) haplotype having pleural involvement and subjects with the IL-1Ra A2(+) allele having a depressed delayed-type hypersensitivity response to PPD (84).

HOST FACTORS INVOLVED IN DETERMINING THE EFFICACY AND TOXICITY OF TUBERCULOSIS CHEMOTHERAPY

One of the most clearly recognized pharmacogenomic factors that influence the response to therapy and toxicity in TB therapy are polymorphisms in *N*-acetyltransferase (NAT). The genetic diversity of these enzymes has marked influence on isoniazid metabolism resulting in either toxic levels in patients who are slow acetylators and more likely to live at lower latitudes near the equator or subtherapeutic levels in the patients who are fast acetylators and more commonly live at higher latitudes (85). Isoniazid is metabolized by hepatic and enteric NAT2 to acetyl isoniazid and then subsequently hydrolyzed to isonicotinic acid and acetylhydrazine. There exist numerous polymorphisms of this gene that determine the rate of acetylation. The major genotypes have recently been grouped into three metabolic phenotypes: fast acetylators, intermediate acetylators, and slow acetylators. These phenotypes are population specific, with a large proportion of whites, blacks, and South Indians having the fast acetylator phenotype (approximately 50%) and a large proportion of Chinese, Japanese, and Eskimos having the slow acetylator phenotype (approximately 80% to 90%) (86). Although NAT2 polymorphisms have not yet been associated with therapeutic outcomes in patients receiving daily supervised treatments, it is not clear how this may affect treatment failure, the development of drug resistance, or the rate of sputum conversion.

The major toxicities associated with isoniazid include hepatitis, neuropathy, and a lupus-like syndrome. Although there does not yet seem to be a link between acetylator status and therapeutic outcome, toxicity is associated with acetylhydrazine (87). Toxicity is largely associated with competition for acetylation by monoacetylhydrazine with isoniazid. Monoacetylhydrazine reaches higher levels in the slow acetylator phenotype owing to enhanced competition for enzyme binding. Fast acetylators are less likely to encounter this difficulty because of the high throughput of drug through NAT2. Hepatotoxicity is age related with a 2.5% to 3.5% risk of events after the age of 50. Two large studies, one American and one European, estimate the total risk of hepatotoxicity at approximately 0.6% (88). Adverse hepatic drug events such as mild elevation of transaminases occur in 8% to 10% of individuals (89).

Rifampicin, the other important drug in TB therapy, facilitates its own elimination by inducing the microsomal cholinesterases and B esterases involved in deacetylation to desacetylrifampicin (90). Conversion to the desacetyl form increases bile excretion, resulting in a net decrease in bioavailability over time. The effect can be quite significant, resulting in a halving of the initially achieved serum concentrations and markedly decreasing the half-life of the drug (91).

Rifampicin also has potential hepatotoxic effects, with an approximate incidence of 1.11% based on a metaanalysis of more than 1,200 patients (88). This value holds greater uncertainty because in TB, it is not usually provided as monotherapy, whereas isoniazid treatment of latent *M. tuberculosis* is standard of care. Rifampin, unlike isoniazid, is also a potent inducer of multiple phase I and II metabolic enzymes. More than 40% of currently available medications are metabolized by the phase I CYP 2D6 pathway and many other rifampicin-induced enzymes such as CYP 1A2, CYP 2C, and CYP 3A play key roles in determining the rate of metabolism of multiple other medications, from antihypertensives to lipid-lowering agents. Interindividual variations of rifampicin related P-450 induction are clearly present but are not currently used in a clinical setting (92). Phase II enzymes, such as glucuronosyltransferase, sulfotransferase, and P glycoproteins are also induced by rifampicin. Induction of these proteins can lead to the loss of efficacy of multiple drugs if not considered by the prescribing clinician.

Pyrazinamide metabolism occurs through both ring hydroxylation at the 5 position and deamidation to form pyrazinoic acid or 5-hydroxypyrazinoic acid. Studies of specific inhibitors in rats have identified xanthine dehydrogenase as the relevant enzyme for hydroxylation (93). Microsomal deamidation to pyrazinoic acid, however, not hydroxylation, appears to be the rate-limiting step (94). A subgroup of patients with renal insufficiency or xanthine oxidase deficiency can have significantly altered clearance rates for this drug (95,96).

Pyrazinamide toxicities are associated with hepatitis, rash, and nongout polyarthralgias. Pyrazinoic acid, the major metabolite of pyrazinamide, inhibits the renal tubular secretion of uric acid causing hyperuricemia. Arthritic events can be present in as many as 40% of patients receiving the drug. Although hyperuricemia can be related to slow or fast urate excreters, the presence of excess pyrazinoic acid owing to slow metabolism would enhance these renally associated adverse events.

Ethambutol is metabolized initially to an aldehyde by alcohol dehydrogenase and then to its dicarboxylic acid by aldehyde dehydrogenase (97). It is mostly excreted unchanged in the urine with toxicities related to drug dose and renal insufficiency with no direct association as of yet to enzyme polymorphisms.

Of greatest interest to clinical care has been the recent evaluation of rifampicin/pyrazinamide for the treatment of latent TB infection. Investigators (98) evaluated more than 1,500 human immunodeficiency virus–positive individuals over a 6-year period and found that the use of rifampicin/pyrazinamide on a daily basis for 8 weeks was as efficacious and safe as the standard 12-month isoniazid monotherapy. These results were soon generalized and non–human immunodeficiency virus–infected patients were treated with the same regimen reported in an article in *Morbidity and Mortality Weekly Report* describing 21 cases of hepatotoxicity (five fatal) from February through August 2001 (99). The study investigators more recently described a non–human immunodeficiency virus–positive, incarcerated population that did well on this 2-month regimen, albeit at a lower and less frequent dosing schedule (100). There was no direct evaluation yet reported of potential genetic influences that may have contributed to these adverse events. The episode does, however, underscore the need for further understanding and evaluation of host–drug–pathogen interactions to minimize the potential for such toxic events.

ROLE OF PHARMACOGENOMICS IN THE NEW MILLENNIUM

From both a social and an economic perspective, it is clear that efforts to eradicate TB are well worth the investment. Meeting the current World Health Organization goal of providing adequate directly observed therapy, short course to India alone is estimated to prevent six million deaths, cure 25 million individuals, and save more than $27 billion over the next two decades (15). These figures pale next to the potential benefit of worldwide TB elimination. Shortening the course of TB treatment regimens will be instrumental in reaching this goal. This will necessitate the evaluation and introduction of new anti-TB agents into clinical practice, a need underscored by the rise of multidrug-resistant TB worldwide. Regretfully, pharmaceutical interest is limited because of the small global market, which is estimated at approximately $440 million annually with the current estimated cost for bringing a new drug to market at $500 to $800 million (101). Owing to the economic status of the population afflicted with TB, the market for TB therapeutics is not likely to change dramatically in the future.

Approximately 80% of drugs fail approval at some point during clinical trials evaluation. The time, effort, and cost of these drug evaluations are a major disincentive to the pursuit of novel antiinfectives, not to mention anti-TB agents. From the standpoint of clinical evaluation of new drugs, pharmacogenomics promises to dramatically reduce the size of the trial necessary to validate efficacy because diagnostic uncertainties can be eliminated [e.g, is the

pathogen drug resistant? does the host have a predisposition for ADME (drug *a*bsorption, *d*istribution, *m*etabolism, or *e*xcretion) problems?] (Fig. 54.1). Conclusions drawn from clinical trials are typically generalizable only to the screened population, the rifampicin/pyrazinamide evaluation being a prime example of this belief. The greater the generalization is from a trial, the more patients are needed for enrollment with greater diversity as well as trial duration and ultimately cost for trial management and subject follow-up. By genetically screening both patient and pathogen, the subject number can theoretically decline as well as study duration, cost, and likelihood of failure with the given population screened (102). Decreasing the cost and reducing adverse events may make it practical for more companies to invest in drugs with niche markets with challenging diagnostic and marketing problems such as TB.

Pharmacogenomics will affect not only the cost of drug discovery and development but also the fundamental process of drug selection and utilization. Pharmacogenomics will facilitate a shift from the simple clinical empiricism, now considered the standard in infectious disease care, to a system of precision therapeutics using molecular tools based on a detailed understanding of drug–microbe–host interactions.

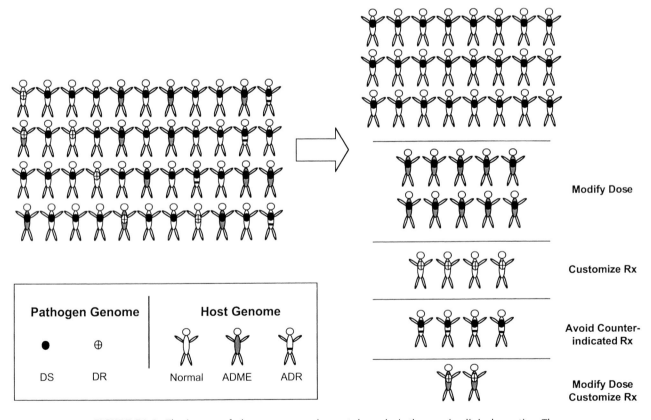

FIGURE 54.1. The impact of pharmacogenomics on tuberculosis therapy in clinical practice. The ability to rapidly genotype the bacteria will determine drug-susceptible or drug-resistant infection. The ability to rapidly genotype the host will identify individuals with defects in ADME (drug *a*bsorption, *d*istribution, *m*etabolism, or *e*xcretion) or those individuals at risk of an adverse drug reaction. Patients can be immediately stratified into the appropriate therapy group.

Because there is a limited number of genes central to drug disposition in the human host, evaluation of such genes will not require disease-specific research, only a disease- and drug-specific understanding of the relevant pharmacology (103). Rare side effects can be minimized by preidentification of patient populations at risk of adverse events. Specific genetic polymorphisms will be used to guide selection of the optimal drug regimen for each patient, taking into consideration disease severity, age, comorbid conditions, and immunologic status. Polymorphisms in both the bacterial and host genome will determine the appropriate duration of therapy to achieve a lasting cure. Conceptually, all these benefits have already been recognized by industry, which has dramatically increased the investment in pharmacogenomics subsidiaries (104).

Pharmacogenomics in a broad sense will also have a direct impact on the ability to accurately diagnose TB. The mainstay of TB diagnostics is microscopic evaluation of smears prepared from patient sputum, an insensitive and technically challenging technique that is time-consuming and error prone. Speciation of mycobacteria other than TB is unavailable in many parts of the world and performed routinely only by advanced laboratories for the most part with sophisticated PCR-based techniques. New technologies for implementing the principles of pharmacogenomics will include miniaturized "lab-on-a-chip" techniques that take advantage of advances in micromanufacturing and microdetection (Fig. 54.2). Not only do these require small sample volumes (and minimal handling), but construction

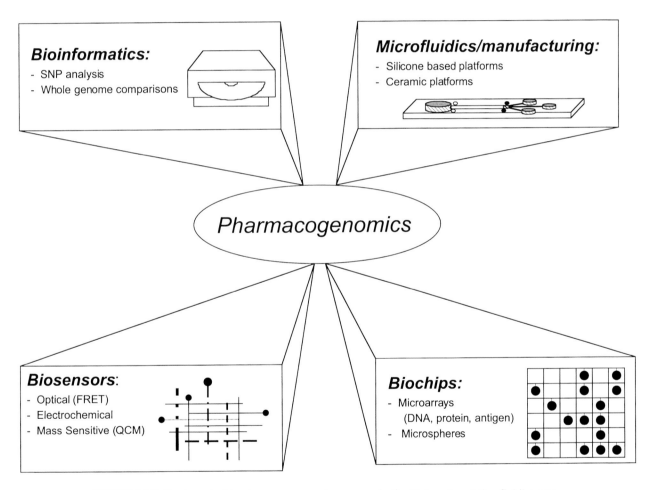

FIGURE 54.2. Tools central to pharmacogenomic progress in the 21st century. Microfluidics manufacturing is the biologic analog of the microchip revolution at the end of the past century and will provide the enabling technology for lab-on-a-chip pharmacogenomic analysis. Micromanufacturing uses diverse substrates (from silicone to ceramics) that markedly enhance the ability to manipulate extremely small volumes of fluids and biomolecules. DNA, protein, antigen, and antibody biochips will serve as the new template for clinical queries, eliminating interlaboratory variations and maximizing diagnostic accuracy. New biosensor technologies will be essential for detecting the minute quantities of material manipulated on chip. With adequate miniaturization, such technologies can serve as important diagnostic tools for the clinician in the field. Data generated from genome sequencing of more pathogens will inform multiple bioinformatic systems, allowing data mining of both host and pathogen genes related to drug disposition, virulence, pathogenicity, and host response.

of such tools is now taking place with a prominent emphasis on eliminating interoperator differences. For direct detection of genomically relevant targets, significant enhancements in detection sensitivity must occur. Coupling *in situ* PCR with array-based sequence detection strategies for drug-susceptibility assessment has already been discussed. Standard detection methods and sample handling techniques must be replaced with miniaturized on-chip analytical techniques with highly sensitive detection strategies and sophisticated bioinformatics capabilities (105–108). Advanced optical phenomenon, such as fluorescent resonance energy transfer have already begun to be applied in techniques such as molecular beacon analysis (109). Coupling such optical technologies directly with molecular recognition of target molecules, whether antibodies, nucleic acids, drugs, or metabolites, is a problem similar to recreating signal transduction phenomenon in intact cells (110,111). There are now examples of membrane-anchored recognition systems that directly couple molecular recognition and optical signal generation (112). Similar highly sensitive and specific detection systems are currently being applied with the goal of developing a field-portable, battery-operated diagnostic platform capable of detecting multiple pathogens, including TB (B. Swanson, K. Grace, C. E. Barry III, unpublished data, 2002).

Because only a minority of patients infected with TB will develop active disease, pharmacogenomics has still another application. Typically, development of a delayed-type hypersensitivity reaction to PPD after exposure to an index case signals that an individual has been infected but does not reveal the likelihood that active disease will result. Current standard of care suggests that all such cases receive prophylactic chemotherapy, which decreases the risk of disease development but exposes the host to unnecessary toxicity risks. Knowledge of an individual's genotype with regard to genes associated with disease susceptibility would limit the number of individuals subjected to the risk of prophylactic isoniazid therapy to just those who would benefit from such treatment.

Infectious disease clinicians of the 21st century will have at their disposal the tools to tailor therapy to the specific individual afflicted with a specific pathogen. Knowledge- and technology-based approaches to diagnosis, therapy, and toxicity management will replace empirical clinical practice. Low-cost, field-portable devices will penetrate even low-income, disease-endemic countries and bring modern medicine and technology to the places where it is most urgently needed.

REFERENCES

1. Pillans PI. Increasing relevance of pharmacogenetics of drug metabolism in clinical practice. *Intern Med J* 2001;31:476–478.
2. Kalow W. Pharmacogenetics in biological perspective. *Pharmacol Rev* 1997;49:369–379.
3. Lu AY. Drug-metabolism research challenges in the new millennium: individual variability in drug therapy and drug safety. *Drug Metab Dispos* 1998;26:1217–1222.
4. Wolf CR, Smith G, Smith RL. Science, medicine, and the future: pharmacogenetics. *BMJ* 2000;320:987–990.
5. Ensom MH, Chang TK, Patel P. Pharmacogenetics: the therapeutic drug monitoring of the future? *Clin Pharmacokinet* 2001;40:783–802.
6. Rusnak JM, Kisabeth RM, Herbert DP, et al. Pharmacogenomics: a clinician's primer on emerging technologies for improved patient care. *Mayo Clin Proc* 2001;76:299–309.
7. Mancinelli L, Cronin M, Sadee W. Pharmacogenomics: the promise of personalized medicine. *AAPS Pharm Sci* 2000; 2:E4.
8. Wieczorek SJ, Tsongalis GJ. Pharmacogenomics: will it change the field of medicine? *Clin Chim Acta* 2001;308:1–8.
9. Grosset J, Truffot C, Fermanian J, et al. [Sterilizing activity of the main drugs on the mouse experimental tuberculosis]. *Pathol Biol (Paris)* 1982;30:444–448.
10. Grosset J. Bacteriologic basis of short-course chemotherapy for tuberculosis. *Clin Chest Med* 1980;1:231–241.
11. Horsburgh CR Jr, Feldman S, Ridzon R. Practice guidelines for the treatment of tuberculosis. *Clin Infect Dis* 2000;31: 633–639.
12. Mitchison DA. Role of individual drugs in the chemotherapy of tuberculosis. *Int J Tuberc Lung Dis* 2000;4:796–806.
13. Bass JB Jr, Farer LS, Hopewell PC, et al. Treatment of tuberculosis and tuberculosis infection in adults and children. American Thoracic Society and The Centers for Disease Control and Prevention. *Am J Respir Crit Care Med* 1994;149: 1359–1374.
14. A Hong Kong Tuberculosis Treatment Services/Brompton Hospital/British Medical Research Council Investigation. *Tubercle* 1974;55:1–27.
15. Cegielski JP, Chin DP, Espinal MA, et al. The global tuberculosis situation. Progress and problems in the 20th century, prospects for the 21st century. *Infect Dis Clin North Am* 2002; 16:1–58.
16. Venter JC, Adams MD, Myers EW, et al. The sequence of the human genome. *Science* 2001;291:1304–1351.
17. Cole ST, Brosch R, Parkhill J, et al. Deciphering the biology of *Mycobacterium tuberculosis* from the complete genome sequence. *Nature* 1998;393:537–544.
18. Sreevatsan S, Pan X, Stockbauer KE, et al. Restricted structural gene polymorphism in the *Mycobacterium tuberculosis* complex indicates evolutionarily recent global dissemination. *Proc Natl Acad Sci U S A* 1997;94:9869–9874.
19. Valway SE, Sanchez MP, Shinnick TF, et al. An outbreak involving extensive transmission of a virulent strain of *Mycobacterium tuberculosis*. *N Engl J Med* 1998;338:633–639.
20. Manca C, Tsenova L, Barry CE 3rd, et al. *Mycobacterium tuberculosis* CDC1551 induces a more vigorous host response *in vivo* and *in vitro*, but is not more virulent than other clinical isolates. *J Immunol* 1999;162:6740–6746.
21. Fleischmann RD, Alland D, Eisen JA, et al. Whole-genome comparison of *Mycobacterium tuberculosis* clinical and laboratory strains. *J Bacteriol* 2002;184:5479–5490.
22. Manca C, Tsenova L, Bergtold A, et al. Virulence of a *Mycobacterium tuberculosis* clinical isolate in mice is determined by failure to induce Th1 type immunity and is associated with induction of IFN-alpha /beta. *Proc Natl Acad Sci U S A* 2001;98: 5752–5757.
23. Agerton TB, Valway SE, Blinkhorn RJ, et al. Spread of strain W, a highly drug-resistant strain of *Mycobacterium tuberculosis*, across the United States. *Clin Infect Dis* 1999;29:85–95.
24. Moss AR, Alland D, Telzak E, et al. A city-wide outbreak of a

multiple-drug-resistant strain of *Mycobacterium tuberculosis* in New York. *Int J Tuberc Lung Dis* 1997;1:115–121.

25. Niemann S, Richter E, Rusch-Gerdes S, et al. Double infection with a resistant and a multidrug-resistant strain of *Mycobacterium tuberculosis*. *Emerg Infect Dis* 2000;6:548–551.

26. van Rie A, Warren RM, Beyers N, et al. Transmission of a multidrug-resistant *Mycobacterium tuberculosis* strain resembling "strain W" among noninstitutionalized, human immunodeficiency virus-seronegative patients. *J Infect Dis* 1999;180: 1608–1615.

27. Gillespie SH. Evolution of drug resistance in *Mycobacterium tuberculosis*: clinical and molecular perspective. *Antimicrob Agents Chemother* 2002;46:267–274.

28. Somoskovi A, Parsons LM, Salfinger M. The molecular basis of resistance to isoniazid, rifampin, and pyrazinamide in *Mycobacterium tuberculosis*. *Respir Res* 2001;2:164–168.

29. Riska PF, Jacobs WR Jr, Alland D. Molecular determinants of drug resistance in tuberculosis. *Int J Tuberc Lung Dis* 2000;4 [Suppl]:S4–S10.

30. Mokrousov I, Filliol I, Legrand E, et al. Molecular characterization of multiple-drug-resistant *Mycobacterium tuberculosis* isolates from northwestern Russia and analysis of rifampin resistance using RNA/RNA mismatch analysis as compared to the line probe assay and sequencing of the rpoB gene. *Res Microbiol* 2002;153:213–219.

31. Slayden RA, Barry CE 3rd. The genetics and biochemistry of isoniazid resistance in mycobacterium tuberculosis. *Microbes Infect* 2000;2:659–669.

32. Van Rie A, Warren R, Mshanga I, et al. Analysis for a limited number of gene codons can predict drug resistance of *Mycobacterium tuberculosis* in a high-incidence community. *J Clin Microbiol* 2001;39:636–641.

33. Suzuki Y, Suzuki A, Tamaru A, et al. Rapid detection of pyrazinamide-resistant *Mycobacterium tuberculosis* by a PCR-based in vitro system. *J Clin Microbiol* 2002;40:501–507.

34. Ramaswamy SV, Amin AG, Goksel S, et al. Molecular genetic analysis of nucleotide polymorphisms associated with ethambutol resistance in human isolates of *Mycobacterium tuberculosis.Antimicrob Agents Chemother* 2000;44:326–336.

35. Belanger AE, Besra GS, Ford ME, et al. The embAB genes of *Mycobacterium avium* encode an arabinosyl transferase involved in cell wall arabinan biosynthesis that is the target for the antimycobacterial drug ethambutol. *Proc Natl Acad Sci U S A* 1996;93:11919–11924.

36. DeBarber AE, Mdluli K, Bosman M, et al. Ethionamide activation and sensitivity in multidrug-resistant *Mycobacterium tuberculosis*. *Proc Natl Acad Sci U S A* 2000;97:9677–9682.

37. Alberghina M, Nicoletti G, Torrisi A. Genetic determinants of aminoglycoside resistance in strains of *Mycobacterium tuberculosis*. *Chemotherapy* 1973;19:148–160.

38. Zhou J, Dong Y, Zhao X, et al. Selection of antibiotic-resistant bacterial mutants: allelic diversity among fluoroquinolone-resistant mutations. *J Infect Dis* 2000;182:517–525.

39. Drobniewski FA, Wilson SM. The rapid diagnosis of isoniazid and rifampicin resistance in *Mycobacterium tuberculosis*—a molecular story. *J Med Microbiol* 1998;47:189–196.

40. Fluit AC, Visser MR, Schmitz FJ. Molecular detection of antimicrobial resistance. *Clin Microbiol Rev* 2001;14:836–871.

41. Gingeras TR, Ghandour G, Wang E, et al. Simultaneous genotyping and species identification using hybridization pattern recognition analysis of generic *Mycobacterium* DNA arrays. *Genome Res* 1998;8:435–448.

42. Troesch A, Nguyen H, Miyada CG, et al.*Mycobacterium* species identification and rifampin resistance testing with high-density DNA probe arrays. *J Clin Microbiol* 1999;37:49–55.

43. Head SR, Parikh K, Rogers YH, et al. Solid-phase sequence scanning for drug resistance detection in tuberculosis.*Mol Cell Probes* 1999;13:81–87.

44. Strizhkov BN, Drobyshev AL, Mikhailovich VM, et al. PCR amplification on a microarray of gel-immobilized oligonucleotides: detection of bacterial toxin- and drug-resistant genes and their mutations. *Biotechniques* 2000;29:844–848, 850–852, 854.

45. Mikhailovich V, Lapa S, Gryadunov D, et al. Identification of rifampin-resistant *Mycobacterium tuberculosis* strains by hybridization, PCR, and ligase detection reaction on oligonucleotide microchips. *J Clin Microbiol* 2001;39:2531–2540.

46. Mikhailovich VM, Lapa SA, Gryadunov DA, et al. Detection of rifampicin-resistant *Mycobacterium tuberculosis* strains by hybridization and polymerase chain reaction on a specialized TB-microchip. *Bull Exp Biol Med* 2001;131:94–98.

47. Caws M, Drobniewski FA. Molecular techniques in the diagnosis of *Mycobacterium tuberculosis* and the detection of drug resistance. *Ann N Y Acad Sci* 2001;953:138–145.

48. Comstock GW. Tuberculosis in twins: a re-analysis of the Prophit survey. *Am Rev Respir Dis* 1978;117:621–624.

49. Kallman FJ, Reisner D. Twin studies on the significance of genetic factors in tuberculosis. *Am Rev Tuberc* 1943;47: 549–574.

50. Levin M, Newport M. Inherited predisposition to mycobacterial infection: historical considerations. *Microbes Infect* 2000;2: 1549–1552.

51. Manabe YC, Bishai WR. Latent *Mycobacterium tuberculosis*—persistence, patience, and winning by waiting. *Nat Med* 2000;6: 1327–1329.

52. Flynn JL, Chan J. Tuberculosis: latency and reactivation. *Infect Immun* 2001;69:4195–4201.

53. Marks GB, Bai J, Simpson SE, et al. Incidence of tuberculosis among a cohort of tuberculin-positive refugees in Australia: reappraising the estimates of risk. *Am J Respir Crit Care Med* 2000;162:1851–1854.

54. Comstock GW, Edwards PQ. The competing risks of tuberculosis and hepatitis for adult tuberculin reactors. *Am Rev Respir Dis* 1975;111:573–577.

55. Stead WW. Variation in vulnerability to tuberculosis in America today: random, or legacies of different ancestral epidemics? *Int J Tuberc Lung Dis* 2001;5:807–814.

56. Stead WW. The origin and erratic global spread of tuberculosis. How the past explains the present and is the key to the future. *Clin Chest Med* 1997;18:65–77.

57. Stead WW. Perspective: a molecular approach to tuberculosis control—an idea that might work. *J Infect Dis* 1997;176: 547–548.

58. Johnson H, Lee B, Doherty E, et al. Tuberculin sensitivity and the BCG scar in tuberculosis contacts. *Tuber Lung Dis* 1995;76: 122–125.

59. Moreno S, Blazquez R, Novoa A, et al. The effect of BCG vaccination on tuberculin reactivity and the booster effect among hospital employees. *Arch Intern Med* 2001;161:1760–1765.

60. Stead WW, Senner JW, Reddick WT, et al. Racial differences in susceptibility to infection by *Mycobacterium tuberculosis*. *N Engl J Med* 1990;322:422–427.

61. Brahmajothi V, Pitchappan RM, Kakkanaiah VN, et al. Association of pulmonary tuberculosis and HLA in south India. *Tubercle* 1991;72:123–132.

62. Bothamley GH, Beck JS, Schreuder GM, et al. Association of tuberculosis and *M. tuberculosis*-specific antibody levels with HLA. *J Infect Dis* 1989;159:549–555.

63. Khomenko AG, Litvinov VI, Chukanova VP, et al. Tuberculosis in patients with various HLA phenotypes. *Tubercle* 1990;71: 187–192.

64. Rajalingam R, Mehra NK, Jain RC, et al. Polymerase chain

reaction–based sequence-specific oligonucleotide hybridization analysis of HLA class II antigens in pulmonary tuberculosis: relevance to chemotherapy and disease severity. *J Infect Dis* 1996;173:669–676.

65. Zerva L, Cizman B, Mehra NK, et al. Arginine at positions 13 or 70-71 in pocket 4 of HLA-DRB1 alleles is associated with susceptibility to tuberculoid leprosy. *J Exp Med* 1996;183: 829–836.

66. Goldfeld AE, Delgado JC, Thim S, et al. Association of an HLA-DQ allele with clinical tuberculosis. *JAMA* 1998;279: 226–228.

67. Rajalingam R, Mehra NK, Mehra RD, et al. HLA class I profile in Asian Indian patients with pulmonary tuberculosis. *Indian J Exp Biol* 1997;35:1055–1059.

68. Sriram U, Selvaraj P, Kurian SM, et al. HLA-DR2 subtypes & immune responses in pulmonary tuberculosis. *Indian J Med Res* 2001;113:117–124.

69. Dorman SE, Holland SM. Interferon-gamma and interleukin-12 pathway defects and human disease. *Cytokine Growth Factor Rev* 2000;11:321–333.

70. Newport MJ, Huxley CM, Huston S, et al. A mutation in the interferon-gamma-receptor gene and susceptibility to mycobacterial infection. *N Engl J Med* 1996;335:1941–1949.

71. Jouanguy E, Altare F, Lamhamedi S, et al. Interferon-gamma-receptor deficiency in an infant with fatal bacille Calmette–Guerin infection. *N Engl J Med* 1996;335: 1956–1961.

72. Cooper AM, Dalton DK, Stewart TA, et al. Disseminated tuberculosis in interferon gamma gene-disrupted mice. *J Exp Med* 1993;178:2243–2247.

73. Kamijo R, Le J, Shapiro D, et al. Mice that lack the interferon-gamma receptor have profoundly altered responses to infection with bacillus Calmette–Guerin and subsequent challenge with lipopolysaccharide. *J Exp Med* 1993;178:1435–1440.

74. Altare F, Durandy A, Lammas D, et al. Impairment of mycobacterial immunity in human interleukin-12 receptor deficiency. *Science* 1998;280:1432–1435.

75. Aggarwal B, Puri RK. *Human cytokines: their role in disease and therapy.* Cambridge, MA: Blackwell Science, 1995.

76. Bellamy R, Ruwende C, Corrah T, et al. Variations in the NRAMP1 gene and susceptibility to tuberculosis in West Africans. *N Engl J Med* 1998;338:640–644.

77. Vidal SM, Malo D, Vogan K, et al. Natural resistance to infection with intracellular parasites: isolation of a candidate for BCG. *Cell* 1993;73:469–485.

78. North RJ, LaCourse R, Ryan L, et al. Consequence of Nramp1 deletion to *Mycobacterium tuberculosis* infection in mice. *Infect Immun* 1999;67:5811–5814.

79. Delgado J, Baena A, Thim S, et al. Ethnic-specific genetic associations with pulmonary tuberculosis are ethnic specific. *J Infect Dis* 2002;186:1463–1468.

80. Wilkinson RJ, Llewelyn M, Toossi Z, et al. Influence of vitamin D deficiency and vitamin D receptor polymorphisms on tuberculosis among Gujarati Asians in west London: a case-control study. *Lancet* 2000;355:618–621.

81. Bellamy R, Ruwende C, Corrah T, et al. Tuberculosis and chronic hepatitis B virus infection in Africans and variation in the vitamin D receptor gene. *J Infect Dis* 1999;179:721–724.

82. Selvaraj P, Narayanan PR, Reetha AM. Association of vitamin D receptor genotypes with the susceptibility to pulmonary tuberculosis in female patients & resistance in female contacts. *Indian J Med Res* 2000;111:172–179.

83. Selvaraj P, Narayanan PR, Reetha AM. Association of functional mutant homozygotes of the mannose binding protein gene with susceptibility to pulmonary tuberculosis in India. *Tuber Lung Dis* 1999;79:221–227.

84. Wilkinson RJ, Patel P, Llewelyn M, et al. Influence of polymorphism in the genes for the interleukin (IL)-1 receptor antagonist and IL-1beta on tuberculosis. *J Exp Med* 1999; 189:1863–1874.

85. Weber WW. Populations and genetic polymorphisms. *Mol Diagn* 1999;4:299–307.

86. Parkin DP, Vandenplas S, Botha FJ, et al. Trimodality of isoniazid elimination: phenotype and genotype in patients with tuberculosis. *Am J Respir Crit Care Med* 1997;155:1717–1722.

87. Peretti E, Karlaganis G, Lauterburg BH. Acetylation of acetylhydrazine, the toxic metabolite of isoniazid, in humans. Inhibition by concomitant administration of isoniazid. *J Pharmacol Exp Ther* 1987;243:686–689.

88. Steele MA, Burk RF, DesPrez RM. Toxic hepatitis with isoniazid and rifampin. A meta-analysis. *Chest* 1991;99:465–471.

89. Scharer L, Smith JP. Serum transaminase elevations and other hepatic abnormalities in patients receiving isoniazid. *Ann Intern Med* 1969;71:1113–1120.

90. Burman WJ, Gallicano K, Peloquin C. Comparative pharmacokinetics and pharmacodynamics of the rifamycin antibacterials. *Clin Pharmacokinet* 2001;40:327–341.

91. Acocella G. Clinical pharmacokinetics of rifampicin. *Clin Pharmacokinet* 1978;3:108–127.

92. Branch RA, Adedoyin A, Frye RF, et al. *In vivo* modulation of CYP enzymes by quinidine and rifampin. *Clin Pharmacol Ther* 2000;68:401–411.

93. Yamamoto T, Moriwaki Y, Suda M, et al. Effect of BOF-4272 on the oxidation of allopurinol and pyrazinamide *in vivo*. Is xanthine dehydrogenase or aldehyde oxidase more important in oxidizing both allopurinol and pyrazinamide? *Biochem Pharmacol* 1993;46:2277–2284.

94. Lacroix C, Hoang TP, Nouveau J, et al. Pharmacokinetics of pyrazinamide and its metabolites in healthy subjects. *Eur J Clin Pharmacol* 1989;36:395–400.

95. Yamamoto T, Higashino K, Kono N, et al. Metabolism of pyrazinamide and allopurinol in hereditary xanthine oxidase deficiency. *Clin Chim Acta* 1989;180:169–175.

96. Lacroix C, Tranvouez JL, Phan Hoang T, et al. Pharmacokinetics of pyrazinamide and its metabolites in patients with hepatic cirrhotic insufficiency. *Arzneimittelforschung* 1990;40:76–79.

97. Breda M, Benedetti MS, Bani M, et al. Effect of rifabutin on ethambutol pharmacokinetics in healthy volunteers. *Pharmacol Res* 1999;40:351–356.

98. Gordin F, Chaisson RE, Matts JP, et al. Rifampin and pyrazinamide vs isoniazid for prevention of tuberculosis in HIV-infected persons: an international randomized trial. Terry Beirn Community Programs for Clinical Research on AIDS, the Adult AIDS Clinical Trials Group, the Pan American Health Organization, and the Centers for Disease Control and Prevention Study Group. *JAMA* 2000;283:1445–1450.

99. Update: fatal and severe liver injuries associated with rifampin and pyrazinamide for latent tuberculosis infection, and revisions in American Thoracic Society/CDC recommendations—United States, 2001. *MMWR Morb Mortal Wkly Rep* 2001;50: 733–735.

100. Chaisson RE, Armstrong J, Stafford J, et al. Safety and tolerability of intermittent rifampin/pyrazinamide for the treatment of latent tuberculosis infection in prisoners. *JAMA* 2002;288: 165–166.

101. The Global Alliance for TB Drug Development (GATB). Economics of TB drug development, 2001.

102. Fijal BA, Hall JM, Witte JS. Clinical trials in the genomic era: effects of protective genotypes on sample size and duration of trial. *Control Clin Trials* 2000;21:7–20.

103. Ledley FD. Can pharmacogenomics make a difference in drug development? *Nat Biotechnol* 1999;17:731.

104. Persidis A. The business of pharmacogenomics. *Nat Biotechnol* 1998;16:209–210.

105. Jain KK. Applications of biochip and microarray systems in pharmacogenomics. *Pharmacogenomics* 2000;1:289–307.

106. Jain KK. Post-genomic applications of lab-on-a-chip and microarrays. *Trends Biotechnol* 2002;20:184–185.

107. Searls DB. Bioinformatics tools for whole genomes. *Annu Rev Genomics Hum Genet* 2000;1:251–279.

108. Searls DB. Using bioinformatics in gene and drug discovery. *Drug Discov Today* 2000;5:135–143.

109. Tyagi S, Marras SA, Kramer FR. Wavelength-shifting molecular beacons. *Nat Biotechnol* 2000;18:1191–1196.

110. Epstein JR, Lee M, Walt DR. High-density fiber-optic genosensor microsphere array capable of zeptomole detection limits. *Anal Chem* 2002;74:1836–1840.

111. Wang J. From DNA biosensors to gene chips. *Nucleic Acids Res* 2000;28:3011–3016.

112. Song X, Shi J, Swanson B. Flow cytometry-based biosensor for detection of multivalent proteins. *Anal Biochem* 2000;284:35–41.

Tuberculosis, Second Edition, edited by William N. Rom and Stuart M. Garay. Published by Lippincott Williams & Wilkins, Philadelphia, 2004

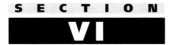

SECTION

VI

PREVENTION AND CONTROL

55

THE TUBERCULIN SKIN TEST AND TREATMENT OF LATENT TUBERCULOSIS INFECTION

JOSEPH H. BATES

TUBERCULIN SKIN TEST

In 1882, Robert Koch read a paper before the Berlin Physiological Society describing the discovery of the tubercle bacillus. Soon afterward, Koch set out to develop a cure for the disease, and his approach was to stimulate the development of specific host resistance. He observed that when a second injection of viable organisms was given to a guinea pig already infected with a subcutaneous focus of tuberculosis produced by a previous injection of *Mycobacterium tuberculosis*, the animal showed healing at the site of the second focus (1). This specific resistance attracted great interest and came to be called the Koch phenomenon.

The fluid medium in which tubercle bacilli had grown was designated by Koch as *lymph* and afterward as *tuberculin*—a substance that he thought might provide a cure for the disease. Afterward, tuberculin was thought of as any material, other than living tubercle bacilli, that contained tuberculoprotein or degradation products of the proteins that were able to elicit hypersensitive reactions. The tuberculin that enjoyed the most widespread use was called Koch's Old tuberculin. It was prepared by taking a liquid medium in which tubercle bacilli had been grown, sterilizing it with heat, producing a bacteria-free filtrate, and then concentrating it by evaporation to one-tenth of its original volume.

In the early part of the 20th century, the developing knowledge relating to foreign protein hypersensitivity as seen with anaphylaxis, the Arthus phenomenon, serum sickness, and asthma stimulated many investigations regarding the role of hypersensitivity in infectious diseases. A major work in this area was published in 1907 by von Pirquet (2), setting out a detailed study of vaccinal hypersensitivity as begun by Jenner many years before. He followed this work by developing a simple and safe cutaneous test for

hypersensitivity to *M. tuberculosis* by the application of tuberculin to a scarified area of skin. He demonstrated that if a tuberculous child was inoculated with a solution of Koch's Old tuberculin, a papule 5 to 20 mm in diameter appeared at the site and then gradually disappeared over a period of 8 days or longer (3,4). He introduced the word *allergy* to designate this changed or altered state because children who were not infected with tubercle bacilli were found to have a negative response to the "allergy test."

These observations by von Pirquet were of great importance because before this time and for several years afterward, the use of tuberculin was controversial. It was held by some as a strong remedy for all forms of disease and by others as both dangerous and useless for either diagnosis or treatment. Tuberculin gradually lost favor as a therapeutic modality, and its value to test for allergy to tuberculosis gained in recognition. It came to be used in patients with the aim of discriminating between the various forms of tuberculosis or for use in judging prognosis. This use led to the first quantitative method of tuberculin testing, considering a reaction positive if its diameter exceeded a particular size (usually 5 mm) and giving successive tests using increasing doses to determine the lowest degree of tuberculin dilution that elicited a positive reaction. Moro (5) incorporated tuberculin into an ointment that could be rubbed into the skin, and this procedure was modified and used widely for many years as a "patch test." This led to the intradermal injection of tuberculin, as introduced by Mantoux (6) in 1910, and this method has stood the test of time because the intradermal injection of 0.1 mL of a carefully prepared solution of test material is the most accurate way to perform the tuberculin test. Today, the Mantoux test is the most widely used procedure for administration of tuberculin, but multiple-puncture devices (MPDs) are also in common use. The MPDs can deliver the test material into the skin through a solution placed on the skin or wet-coated on the points (tines) of the device just before administration (7). In other instances, the test material is allowed to dry on the points before packaging. There are various types of MPDs

J. H. Bates: Department of Epidemiology, University of Arkansas College of Public Health; Deputy State Health Office, Arkansas Department of Health, Little Rock, Arkansas.

containing from four to nine points, and they can be coated with Koch's Old tuberculin or a purified protein derivative (PPD) of tuberculin. The MPDs can deliver varying amounts of test material into the skin depending on the skin texture, thickness and moisture, time of contact, and actual technique of administration, and therefore its reproducibility does not compare favorably with that of the Mantoux method.

PREPARATION OF STANDARDIZED TUBERCULIN

Several types of tuberculin have been prepared including Koch's Old tuberculin and PPD of tuberculin. Landi (8) provided a detailed account of the techniques required to produce these and other tuberculins. Over time, PPD has come to be the skin test material used most commonly worldwide. The final product is termed *tuberculoprotein* and can be stored in powder form or solubilized in a phosphate buffer as a concentrated PPD solution. The International Standard Tuberculins are in the custody of the International Laboratory for Biological Standards, Statens Seruminstitut, Copenhagen, Denmark. The standard for PPD used for humans prepared by Seibert and Glenn (9,10) has been identified as PPD-S. It was adopted as the International Standard by the World Health Organization in 1951 (11).

INTERPRETATION OF TUBERCULIN SKIN TEST

The tuberculin skin test indicates whether sensitivity owing to a past or present mycobacterial infection exists in a person. In studies of large population groups, reactivity ranges from none to very strong reactions, with all intermediate-sized gradients observed. Because a positive reaction is elicited after only a dose of a fraction of a microgram, it is most unusual for a generalized unfavorable reaction to occur, even in the most sensitive individual.

The most common dose of tuberculin used is 5 tuberculin units, equivalent to the activity of 0.1 μg of the standard PPD-S. After this dose is injected intradermally into a sensitive subject by the Mantoux method (usually on the dorsal side of the forearm), infiltration of the injection site with mononuclear cells can be demonstrated after several hours. The inflammatory reaction increases progressively over a period of 1 to 4 days, producing a persistent erythema and induration at the site. The key cells involved are lymphocytes and monocytes, but polymorphonuclear granulocytes are also present. There may be considerable variation in the rate of development of a positive reaction. In persons tested for the first time, the reaction usually develops more slowly and does not peak until approximately 72 hours after the test dose is injected, but among subjects tested repeatedly, the reaction is accelerated and may peak

at 24 hours or so; this point was first described by Mantoux (12). In the best of circumstances the reaction should be read at 24, 48, and 72 hours, but in most cases, this is not possible and the 48-hour reading is the one most commonly taken. The extent of induration should be measured in two diameters at right angles and the average of these values recorded as the result. Although the technique of digital palpation to detect induration is commonly used, this method may not identify the margins of the indurated area very well. Bearman et al. (13) studied the variability of readings among experienced workers and found marked variation among the most experienced readers. Sokal (14) found that this type of error could be reduced using a ballpoint pen, drawing a line beginning 1 to 2 cm away from the margin of the skin test reaction and moving slowly toward its center, exerting moderate pressure against the skin. When the ballpoint reaches the margin of the indurated area, resistance to further movement is noted, and this point is designated as the outer margin of induration. The procedure is repeated from the opposite side and the distance between the opposing lines is measured.

Furcolow (15) performed a series of investigations testing PPD reactions in patients with tuberculosis and their contacts and in nontuberculous patients. A small dose of tuberculin was sufficient to elicit a positive reaction in almost all the patients with tuberculosis. When much higher doses were used, many of the persons not reacting to the lower dose showed positive reactions. These observations were extended by Edwards and Palmer (16) who tested patients with culture-proven tuberculosis who were on treatment and recovering from tuberculosis, patients having pulmonary infection with *Mycobacterium kansasii* (photochromogenic organisms), and healthy U.S. Navy recruits. All subjects were tested with PPD-S and with a tuberculin prepared from a strain of *M. kansasii* designated as PPD-Y. The results of these skin test observations are shown in Figure 55.1. The reactions to PPD-S in patients with tuberculosis and the reactions to PPD-Y in patients infected with *M. kansasii* give a normal probability frequency curve. When PPD-Y is given to patients with tuberculosis, the most common reaction is a positive response, although not as positive as when PPD-S is used.

Then healthy naval recruits were tested with PPD-S, PPD-Y, and a third antigen (PPD-B) prepared from an organism now designated as *Mycobacterium avium-intracellulare complex*. Most recruits gave negative or weak reactions to all three antigens, but a number did react positively to PPD-B, and much fewer reacted to PPD-Y or PPD-S. These data are shown in Figure 55.2. It is probable that many of the individuals with large reactions to PPD-B and weak reactions to PPD-S and PPD-Y were showing nonspecific hypersensitivity to the PPD-S and PPD-Y skin test material owing to shared antigens among these three species. Since these reports, it has become well recognized that infection with various nontuberculous mycobacteria

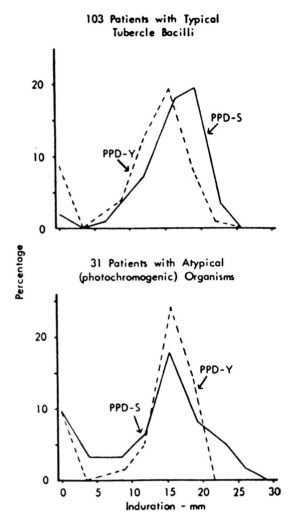

FIGURE 55.1. Frequency curves of sizes of reactions to purified protein derivative (*PPD*)-Y and PPD-S for patients with proven tuberculosis and proven pulmonary infection caused by *Mycobacterium kansasii.*

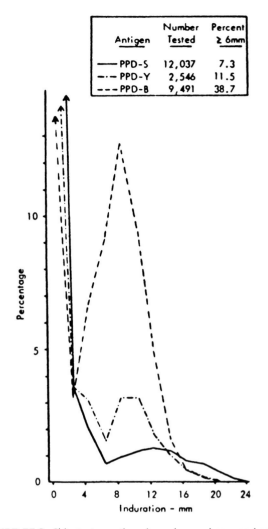

FIGURE 55.2. Skin test reaction sizes observed among healthy U.S. Navy recruits tested with antigens obtained from *Mycobacterium tuberculosis* [purified protein derivative (*PPD*-S)], *Mycobacterium kansasii* (PPD-Y), and *Mycobacterium avium-intracellulare complex* (PPD-B).

may produce skin test responses to PPD-S that fall within the same size range as those found for some patients with proven tuberculosis. This nonspecific sensitivity owing to nontuberculous mycobacteria is especially common among persons residing in the southeastern region of the United States, although it may be noted in any geographic area. A similar type of cross-reaction may be produced in bacille Calmette–Guérin–vaccinated persons.

Observations of stable patients with culture-proven tuberculosis reported by Furcolow et al. (17) showed that 99% of 468 patients had positive PPD skin test reactions, and these observations were confirmed by others over the next two decades (18). Stead (19) pointed out that approximately 20% of newly admitted patients seen in a general hospital with positive sputum cultures and 30% of debilitated elderly and other very ill patients gave negative responses. It is now well recognized that false-negative reac-

tions are predictable in patients who have advanced human immunodeficiency virus (HIV) infection or overwhelming disease and in patients with uremia or sarcoidosis or on chemotherapy for serious malignant disorders. In a few patients, no definite cause for the false-negative reaction can be found. The use of other antigens to accompany the tuberculin skin test to evaluate for anergy is theoretically attractive, but these companion antigens have not been carefully standardized and may not be readily available, and their use adds cost and complexity to patient care without clear evidence of benefit.

Boosting of waned tuberculin sensitivity can occur when the skin test is applied repeatedly over time (20). These reactions are more common among the elderly and persons of any age living in geographic locations where nontuberculous mycobacterial infections are common. Among some older adults, the boosting effect may not be observed until a third or fourth sequential test is done (21). Among the elderly, it is appropriate to consider an increase of 15 mm or more of induration after a negative skin test reaction as a true conversion (22). Boosting is controlled by using a two-step procedure for all persons having sequential skin testing such as persons entering long-term care facilities, employees of health care institutions, and prison workers. Those persons with a negative initial test result are immediately retested, and the second test result is recorded as the baseline reading. The two-step process is recommended for employees older than 35 years of age and for those who have had prior bacille Calmette–Guérin vaccination. An increase in induration of 10 mm or more within a 2-year period is classified as a conversion to a positive test result among persons younger than 35 years old. For those age 35 and older, the increase required to be considered a conversion is 15 mm or more.

The Centers for Disease Control and Prevention have advised that the size of the induration from the Mantoux test used to define a positive reaction be adjusted according to the test situation (23). Table 55.1 provides a summary of the recommended guidelines for interpretation of skin test results.

As an alternative to tuberculin skin testing to assess cell-mediated immune reactivity to mycobacterial infection, the measurement of whole-blood interferon levels has been evaluated in a U.S. population survey. The results suggest that for persons being screened for latent tuberculosis infection, the interferon gamma assay is comparable with the skin test (24). This assay has some advantages over the skin test because it requires only a one patient visit, does not give a booster effect, is not subject to reader subjectivity regarding the test result, and measures the response to several mycobacterial antigens concurrently. The value of this test

for screening for latent tuberculosis infection as it is used in a nonresearch setting is yet to be determined.

TREATMENT OF LATENT TUBERCULOSIS INFECTION

Treatment of latent tuberculosis infection is the administration of a chemotherapeutic agent or agents for the purpose of preventing tuberculosis infection from progressing to disease. If a person who is taking isoniazid inhales living tubercle bacilli, in some instances, an antituberculosis drug or drugs may be given to prevent infection; it is reasoned that the organisms that are inhaled will be killed by the antimicrobial agent before infection can become established. Prevention of infection in this way is uncommon. but when used for this purpose, it is termed *primary chemoprophylaxis*. When tubercle bacilli establish infection, the host usually contains the infection and a positive tuberculin reaction is the only evidence of infection, even though the organisms may remain viable and enclosed within granulomatous, fibrotic lesions. These viable but dormant organisms have the potential to become metabolically active at a future date, producing active disease. Treatment used in this way is a major component of the tuberculosis control program in the United States, but this approach has not been adopted for use worldwide because some control programs depend on bacille Calmette–Guérin vaccination at an early age and for others, the financial resources are not adequate to fund this approach (25,26).

The possible use of isoniazid for the prevention of tuberculosis was stimulated by the observations of Lincoln who reported that isoniazid therapy of tuberculosis in children prevented the development of miliary and meningeal tuberculosis, complications that were sometimes seen during treatment with other drugs. Although no adequate controlled trials have been designed to test the effectiveness of primary prophylaxis in humans, many excellent trials involving more than 125,000 subjects have been done to evaluate the effectiveness of treating latent infection. The results indicate that isoniazid given to tuberculin reactors can reduce the risk of active tuberculosis by as much as 90% in those who complete a full course of treatment, and in children the reduction in risk approaches 100% (27–29).

The results of these trials vary widely, from a reduction in tuberculosis of 25% in Tunisia to 92% among Dutch naval personnel. Some reasons for this variation are the amount of medication actually taken and the duration for which it was given (26,28). Protection is most marked during the medication period. However, it persists after treatment; it persisted through the observation period of the various trials, and among Alaskan villagers, protection persisted for as long as 19 years (30,31). Isoniazid also can be effective in preventing reactivation of previously untreated tuberculosis disease; a number of controlled trials involv-

TABLE 55.1. RECOMMENDED GUIDELINES FOR INTERPRETATION OF SKIN TEST RESULTS

Size of Induration (mm)	Situations in which Test Result Is Considered Positive
<5	Never
≥5	Persons with HIV infection, persons in close contact with an infectious patient with tuberculosis, persons whose chest radiograph is consistent with healed tuberculosis
≥10	Intravenous drug abusers known to be HIV seronegative, persons with medical conditions known to be at risk of developing tuberculosis, persons born in countries with high tuberculosis prevalence, persons from high-risk communities, persons who are medically underserved, and residents of long-term care facilities
≥15	All others

HIV, human immunodeficiency virus.

ing more than 35,000 subjects have been reported (26,32,33). Among those for whom the medication was given for at least 1 year, the reduction in tuberculosis owing to isoniazid was 66%, and the reduced risk persisted throughout the observation period. Giving isoniazid to persons with healed tuberculosis who previously received adequate chemotherapy provides no additional protection. Isoniazid given to symptom-free, tuberculin-positive persons who are seropositive for HIV reduces the risk of tuberculosis and increases the time to development of symptomatic HIV disease and acquired immunodeficiency syndrome (34). Fear that isoniazid given alone for prophylaxis might allow the emergence of tubercle bacilli resistant to isoniazid has not been substantiated.

The usual therapy regimen is isoniazid at 300 mg daily in a single dose (10 mg/kg daily for children) for 9 months (35). Treatment for 9 months is also advised for persons with HIV infection or other major forms of immunosuppression and for those with stable, abnormal-appearing chest radiographs suggestive of past tuberculosis. For persons who are at high risk of tuberculosis whose adherence to therapy is in doubt, supervised therapy is indicated when possible, and if resources to provide daily supervised therapy are not adequate, an alternative to daily treatment is isoniazid given twice weekly at a dose of 15 mg/kg.

Alternative regimens of short duration are useful in circumstances in which a longer treatment period is not a reasonable expectation. Rifampin given daily for 4 months is indicated when isoniazid cannot be used. Rifampin together with pyrazinamide given daily for 2 months may be used in selected conditions when it is urgent to give treatment and when a period of treatment for longer than 2 months is not possible. However, this drug combination has been found to present a substantial risk for hepatotoxicity, and persons receiving this regimen should have liver function tests done twice monthly. Rifabutin, a rifamycin highly active against *M. tuberculosis*, can be used for patients taking protease inhibitors as treatment for HIV infection, but the dose must be adjusted downward. Counseling from a person expert in the use of these inhibitors is advised before the antituberculosis therapy is begun.

Isoniazid therapy carries with it the risk of side effects. The most important toxic effects are on the liver. The drug is well tolerated by most persons, particularly children, but 2% to 3% of adults older than age 50 develop chemical evidence of liver injury, and this can lead to clinical hepatitis if the drug is not stopped promptly. Despite this concern, fatal cases continue to occur, especially among minority women (36). Factors that can increase the risk of isoniazid hepatitis are alcohol or drug abuse, previous hepatitis, simultaneous use of hepatotoxic drugs, and the postpartum state. These risks for toxicity together with some deaths generate dispute among experts over balancing the risks and benefits in low-risk populations that has not been resolved (37). Several analyses compar-

TABLE 55.2. CRITERIA FOR DETERMINING THE NEED FOR PREVENTIVE THERAPY FOR PERSONS WITH A POSITIVE TUBERCULIN REACTION BY CATEGORY AND AGE GROUP

Category	Age (yr)	
	<35	≥35
With risk factor[a]	Treat all ages if reaction to 5 TU of PPD is >10 mm (or ≥5 mm and patient is a recent contact, is HIV infected, or has radiographic evidence of old TB)	
No risk factor		
High-incidence group[b]	Treat if PPD reaction is >10 mm	Do not treat
Low-incidence group[c]	Treat if PPD reaction is >15 mm	Do not treat

[a]Risk factors include human immunodeficiency virus infection, recent contact with an infectious person, recent skin test conversion, abnormal-appearing chest radiograph, intravenous drug abuse, and some medical risk factors.
[b]High-incidence group includes foreign-born persons; medically underserved, low-income populations; and residents of long-term care facilities.
[c]Lower or higher cutoff points may be used to identify positive reactions, depending on the relative prevalence of *Mycobacterium tuberculosis* infection and nonspecific cross-reactivity in the population.
PPD, purified protein derivative; TB, tuberculosis; TU, tuberculin unit.

ing the risk of hepatotoxicity with the benefit of preventing tuberculosis have been reported, with conflicting conclusions (38–41). As shown in Table 55.2, the Centers for Disease Control and Prevention have provided guidelines for determining how the use of therapy can be given to minimize the risks of toxicity and yet benefit those at highest risk (42). These criteria advise against prophylaxis in low-risk populations. Stead et al. (29) found that hepatitis developed in 4.5% of elderly nursing home residents treated with isoniazid for a new infection.

Resistance of the infecting strain of *M. tuberculosis* to isoniazid essentially precludes the use of this drug in preventive treatment. In situations in which infection with an isoniazid-resistant strain is deemed likely, prophylaxis should be provided with another drug or drugs to which the organism is known to be sensitive.

REFERENCES

1. Koch R. Fortsetzung der Mittheilung uber ein Heilmittel gegen tuberculose. *Dtsch Med Wochenschr* 1891;17:101–102.
2. von Pirquet CE, *Klinische Studien uber Vakzination and Vakzinale Allergie.* Leipzig: Deuticke, 1907.
3. von Pirquet CE. Tuberkulindiagnose durch Cutane Impfung. *Berl Klin* 1907;24:644.
4. von Pirquet CE. Die Diagnostische Wert der kutanen Reaction bei der Tuberculose des Kindersalters auf Grund von 100 Sektionen. *Wiener Klin Wochenischr* 1907;20:1128.

5. Moro E. Ueber line diagnostisch verwertbare Reaktion der haut auf Eiribung mit. Tuberkulinsalbe. *Munch Med* 1908;55:216–218.
6. Mantoux C. L'intradermo-reaction a la tuberculin et son interpretation clinique. *Presse Med* 1910;18:10–13.
7. Heaf H. The multiple puncture tuberculin test. *Lancet* 1951;2:151–153
8. Landi S. Production and standardization of tuberculin. In: GP Kubica, LG Wayne, eds.*The mycobacteria (part A)*. New York: Marcel Dekker, 1984:505–535.
9. Seibert FB, Glenn JT. The isolation and properties of the purified protein derivative of tuberculin. *Am Rev Tuberc* 1934;30:713–720.
10. Seibert FB, Glenn JT. Tuberculin purified protein derivative; preparation and analysis of a large quantity for standard. *Am Rev Tuberc* 1941;44:1–25.
11. World Health Organization. *Expert Committee on Biological Standardization, fifth report (WHO Technical Report Series, no. 56)*. Geneva: World Health Organization, 1952:6.
12. Mantoux C. La voie intradermique en tuberculinotherapie, *Presse Med* 1912;20:146–148.
13. Bearman JE, Kleinman H, Glyer VV, et al. A study of variability in tuberculin test reading. *Am Rev Respir Dis* 1964;90:913–919.
14. Sokal JE. Measurement of delayed skin test responses. *N Engl J Med* 1975;293:501–502.
15. Furcolow ML. Quantitative studies of the tuberculin reaction. I, Titration of tuberculin sensitivity and its relation to tuberculous infection. *Public Health Rep* 1941;56:1082.
16. Edwards LB, Palmer CE. Epidemiologic studies of tuberculin sensitivity. I. Preliminary results with purified protein derivatives prepared from atypical acid-fast organisms. *Am J Hyg* 1958;68:213–231.
17. Furcolow MI, Hewell B, Nelson WE. Quantitative studies of the tuberculin reaction. III. Tuberculin sensitivity in relation to active tuberculosis. *Am Rev Tuberc* 1942;45:504–520.
18. Johnston W, Saltzman HA, Bufkin JH, et al. The tuberculin test and the diagnosis of clinical tuberculosis. In: *Veterans Administration–Armed Forces: transactions of the 18th Conference on the Chemotherapy of Tuberculosis*. Washington, DC: VA Department of Medicine and Surgery, 1959:155–159.
19. Stead WW. The face of tuberculosis. *Hosp Pract* 1969;4:62–68.
20. Thompson NR, Glassroth J, Snider DE, et al. The booster phenomenon in serial tuberculin testing. *Am Rev Respir Dis* 1979;119:587–597.
21. Vanden Brande P, Demedts M. Four stage tuberculin testing in elderly subjects induces age-dependent progressive boosting. *Chest* 1992;101:447–450.
22. Stead WW, To T. The significance of the tuberculin skin test in elderly persons. *Ann Intern Med* 1987;107:837–842.
23. Centers for Disease Control. Screening for tuberculosis and tuberculous infection in high-risk populations and the use of preventive therapy for tuberculosis infection in the United States. Recommendations of the Advisory Committee for Elimination of Tuberculosis. *MMWR Recomm Rep* 1990;39:1–12.
24. Mazurek GH, Lo Bue PA, Daley CL, et al. Comparison of a whole-blood interferon γ assay with tuberculin skin testing for detecting latent *Mycobacterium tuberculosis* infection. *JAMA* 2001;286:1740–1747.
25. McDermott W, Raffel S, Canetti G, et al. Chemoprophylaxis of tuberculosis. *Am Rev Respir Dis* 1959;80:1–21.

26. Ferebee SH. Controlled chemoprophylaxis trials in tuberculosis. A general review. *Adv Tuberc Res* 1970;17:28–106.
27. International Union Against Tuberculosis Committee on Prophylaxis. Efficacy of various durations of isoniazid preventive therapy for tuberculosis. Five years follow-up in the IUAT trial. *Bull WHO* 1982;60:555–564.
28. Hsu KHK. Thirty years after isoniazid. Its impact on tuberculosis in children and adolescents. *JAMA* 1984;251:1283–1285.
29. Stead WW, To T, Harrison RW, et al. Benefit-risk considerations in Preventive treatment for tuberculosis in elderly persons. *Ann Intern Med* 1987;107:843–845.
30. Horowitz O, Magnus K. Epidemiologic evaluation of chemoprophylaxis against tuberculosis. Twelve years follow-up of a community-wide controlled trial with special reference to sampling method. *Am J Epidemiol* 1974;99:333–342.
31. Comstock GW, Baum C, Snider DE. Isoniazid prophylaxis among Alaskan Eskimos. A final report of the Bethel isoniazid studies. *Am Rev Respir Dis* 1979;119:827–830.
32. Krebs A, Farer LS, Snider DE, et al. Five years follow-up of the IUAT trial of isoniazid prophylaxis in fibrotic lesions. *Bull Int Union Tuberc Lung Dis* 1979;54:65–69.
33. Falk A, Fuchs GF. Prophylaxis with isoniazid in inactive tuberculosis. *Chest* 1978;73:44–48.
34. Pope JW, Jean SS, Hi HI, et al. Effect of isoniazid prophylaxis on incidence of active tuberculosis and progression of HIV infection. *Lancet* 1993;342:268–272.
35. International Union Against Tuberculosis Committee on Prophylaxis. Efficacy of various durations of isoniazid preventive therapy for tuberculosis: five years of follow-up in the IUAT trial. *Bull WHO* 1982;60:555–564.
36. Snider DE, Caros GJ. Isoniazid-associated hepatitis deaths: a review of available information. *Am Rev Respir Dis* 1992;145:494–497.
37. Comstock GW. Prevention of tuberculosis among tuberculin reactors: maximizing benefits, minimizing risks. *JAMA* 1986;256:2729–2730.
38. Fitzgerald JM, Gafini A. A cost effectiveness analysis of the routine use of isoniazid prophylaxis in patients with a positive Mantoux skin test. *Am Rev Respir Dis* 1990;142:848–853.
39. Jordan TJ, Lewis E, Reichman LB. Isoniazid preventive therapy for tuberculosis. Decision analysis considering ethnicity and gender. *Am Rev Respir Dis* 1991;144:1357–1360.
40. Rose DN, Schecter CB, Silver AL. The age threshold for isoniazid chemoprophylaxis for low-risk tuberculin reactors. *JAMA* 1986;256:2709–2713.
41. Centers for Disease Control and Prevention. The use of preventive therapy for tuberculosis infection in the United States. Recommendations of the Advisory Committee for Elimination of Tuberculosis. *MMWR Recomm Rep* 1990;39:9–12.
42. Centers for Disease Control and Prevention. Recommendations for the management of persons exposed to multidrug-resistant tuberculosis. *MMWR Recomm Rep* 1992;41:59–71.

FURTHER READING

Centers for Disease Control and Prevention. Targeted tuberculin testing and treatment of latent tuberculosis infection. *MMWR Recomm Rep* 2000;49:1–51.

TUBERCULOSIS TRANSMISSION AND CONTROL IN HOSPITALS AND OTHER INSTITUTIONS

EDWARD A. NARDELL
KENT A. SEPKOWITZ

TUBERCULOSIS AS AN AIRBORNE INFECTION

Scientists of antiquity, including Aristotle and the ancient Persians, considered tuberculosis (TB) a contagious disease. This view predominated through the Middle Ages and into the 17th century, when cities in Italy and Spain began to require reporting of all cases of TB and the burning of a consumptive's personal belongings after death. The great physicians of the time, including Valsalva and Morgagni, were so convinced that TB was contagious that they refused to perform autopsies on persons who died of the disease (1,2).

However, by the late 19th century, the notion that TB was in fact not contagious gained sway. In 1882, Williams, of the Brompton Hospital for Consumption in London, published a study that served as the basis of many future statements. He insisted that TB was not transmissible, pointing to the hundreds of workers caring for thousands of patients across the decades, none of whom had developed TB. Supported by additional reports from large sanitoria in Europe and the United States (1), this view entered the standard medical texts of the day until the 1930s. For example, Fishberg, an eminent pulmonologist, wrote that it was not dangerous for "healthy adults to be coughed at by patients suffering from pulmonary or laryngeal tuberculosis" (3).

In Thomas Mann's *Magic Mountain*, set at the outbreak of World War I, visitors and staff at the International Sanitarium Berghof in Davos, Switzerland, freely interacted with essentially untreated TB patients without apparent fear of infection (4). Most adults in Europe at that time would have been already infected with TB early in life and were, therefore, not fully vulnerable to new infection. Clusters of cases in families such as the Brontës gave rise to the notion that TB might be hereditary, not infectious. Although there had long been theories implicating "bad air" as the cause of various maladies, from the time microbes were first recognized as pathogens until 1935, only direct person-to-person contact, including direct droplet spread, was considered an important mode of contagion. Airborne spread, meaning spread well beyond immediate close contact, was discounted as unlikely for any disease. This belief was championed by Charles Chapin (5), the influential health officer of Providence, RI, whose 1910 monograph *Sources and Modes of Infection* stated:

> Bacteriology teaches that former ideas in regard to the manner in which diseases may be airborne are entirely erroneous; that most diseases are not likely to be dust-borne, and they are spray-borne for only 2 or 3 feet, a phenomenon which after all resembles contact infection more than it does aerial infection as ordinarily understood.

In fairness to Chapin, he hedged by saying "most diseases," specifically allowing the possibility that TB might be airborne. After all, Koch had isolated the tubercle bacillus from sputum not many years earlier, and Klein had by then infected guinea pigs by exposure in the ventilating shaft of Brompton Hospital. In the 1930s, public health posters in the United States and Great Britain contained messages such as "Do not spit without remembering that TB is spread by this means." Although sputum containing Koch's bacilli was recognized as a potential vehicle for transmission, the mechanism by which it might be infectious was not yet understood. Sputum hygiene, not air hygiene, was the order of the day, with spittoons common fixtures in public places. Fomites, such as on shared bottles, eating utensils, and bed-

E. A. Nardell: Department of Medicine, Harvard Medical School; Department of Pulmonary Medicine, The Cambridge Hospital, Cambridge, Massachusetts.

K. A. Sepkowitz: Department of Medicine, Weill Medical College of Cornell University; Infection Control, Memorial Sloan–Kettering Cancer Center, New York, New York.

ding were suspect, as was house dust that might be contaminated by sputum. Another 1930s public health poster from England warned, "Dry sweeping sends dust into the air that may contain tubercle germs." Wet mopping was recommended instead. The misconception that hospital ward dust might spread TB persists to this day in some high-prevalence countries. However, dust particles are far too large to reach the vulnerable alveolar portion of the lung.

In 1935, a Harvard sanitary engineer, William Firth Wells, challenged Chapin, arguing that measles was airborne and could be controlled with germicidal ultraviolet irradiation. In 1931, Wells (6) had developed his air centrifuge, allowing him to sample air for bacteria and leading to his 1934 paper, "On Air-borne Infections: II. Droplets and Droplet Nuclei." Droplet nuclei, the dried residua of larger respiratory droplets, he argued, were light enough to remain aloft by room air currents until inhaled or exhausted and were also capable of carrying pathogenic microbes to the deepest reaches of the lung. He had been commissioned by the Massachusetts Department of Public Health to use his air centrifuge to investigate the possibility that workers in textile mills were becoming ill by inhaling contaminated aerosols used to keep down dust. Wells was accompanied in this investigation by a Harvard medical student, Richard Riley, who actually wrote the paper describing their success in recovering the same bacteria from stagnant water, ward air, and sick workers. In his 1955 text, *Airborne Contagion and Air Hygiene*, Wells (7) credited Richard Riley for "the basic distinction between infective droplet nuclei and germ laden dust." However, according to Riley, it was Wells alone who made the brilliant leap from human infection caused by artificially generated droplet nuclei in textile mills to person-to-person transmission through cough- and sneeze-generated droplet nuclei.

Table 56.1 lists some of the properties of droplet nuclei–borne infections compared with those spread by larger respiratory droplets.

The history of airborne infection is intimately linked with ultraviolet germicidal irradiation (UVGI), initially used to prove that infection was airborne by interrupting it and later used as a promising public health intervention, analogous to water disinfection to reduce waterborne infections. In 1942, Wells et al. (8) published the results of using upper room UVGI to interrupt measles transmission in day schools in two suburbs of Philadelphia. Although the results were striking, future attempts to replicate the experiment failed. They had chosen just the right setting, affluent suburbs where children were driven to and from school and returned to single-family homes. Transmission interrupted in school was less likely to occur elsewhere. They concluded that the two subsequent experiments had failed because transmission occurred outside school, in crowded tenements in an experiment conducted in the Southall district of London and on school buses in rural upstate New York. An important lesson was learned, however. Unlike potable water, where central or end user disinfection is possible, it is inconceivable to disinfect air centrally or in the countless sites where airborne transmission might occur. To be effective, any form of air disinfection must be selectively applied to infections spread predominantly as droplet nuclei and only in those settings where the main sites of transmission can be included in the intervention. Despite the 1942 measles study and other evidence, in 1946, the American Public Health Association stated (9): "Conclusive evidence is not available at present that the airborne mode of transmission is predominant for any particular disease."

A decade would pass before Riley demonstrated that TB is unequivocally airborne. Wells had conceived of the definitive experiment, but it was ultimately Riley who actually did the study in Baltimore between 1958 and 1962 when Wells was near the end of his life. In an essay written just months before his death in 2001, Riley (10) relates some of the previously untold details of this remarkable 4-year experiment. A six-bed hospital ward was renovated so that exhaust air passed through guinea pig exposure chambers located in a penthouse above the ward (Fig. 56.1) (11). Guinea pigs had previously been shown to be so susceptible to TB that they become infected when a single inhaled droplet nucleus reached the alveolus, as seen in Figure 56.2 (12). Hundreds of guinea

TABLE 56.1. DROPLET NUCLEI VERSUS RESPIRATORY DROPLETS

Droplet Nuclei Transmission (Airborne Infection)	Respiratory Droplet Transmission (An Extension of Direct Contact)
1–5 μm-diameter particles (dried residua of larger particles)	>100 μm-diameter particles
Remain suspended indefinitely	Settle out within 1 m of the source
Alveolar deposition	Upper airway deposition
Contain few microbes	Contain many microbes
UVGI susceptible in air	UVGI resistant on surfaces
Examples: tuberculosis, measles	Examples: staphylococcus, respiratory syncytial virus

UVGI, ultraviolet germicidal irradiation.

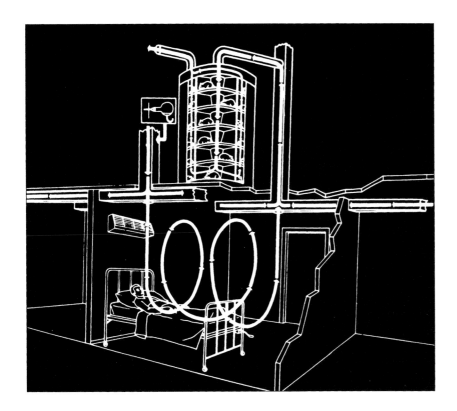

FIGURE 56.1. Schematic diagram of a hospital unit, ventilation ducts, and guinea pig exposure chamber unit used in aerosol transmission experiments. (From Riley RL, Wills FW, Mills CC, et al. Air hygiene in tuberculosis: quantitative studies of infectivity and control in a pilot ward. *Am Rev Tuberc Pulmonary Dis* 1957; 75:420–431, with permission.)

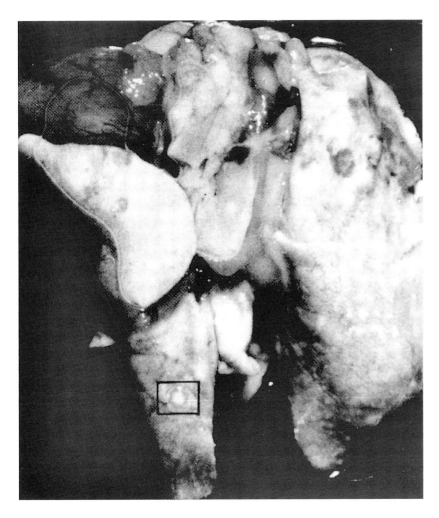

FIGURE 56.2. A guinea pig lung containing a single tubercle from an animal that had a positive tuberculin test. (From Riley RL. Aerial dissemination of pulmonary tuberculosis. The Burns Amberson lecture. *Am Rev Tuberc Pulmonary Dis* 1957;76:931–941, with permission.)

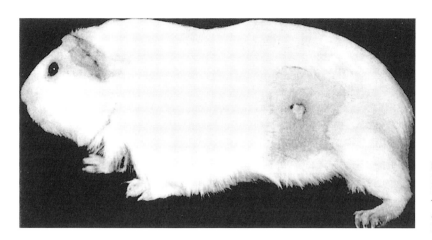

FIGURE 56.3. Positive tuberculin test in a guinea pig indicating transmission of infection. (From Riley RL. Aerial dissemination of pulmonary tuberculosis. The Burns Amberson lecture. *Am Rev Tuberc Pulmonary Dis* 1957;76:931–941, with permission.)

pigs breathed air from the ward, essentially serving as a quantitative air sampler. Tuberculin skin test conversion of the guinea pigs (Fig. 56.3) indicated infection. The only connection between the patients and the guinea pigs was the ward air. The experiment not only proved that TB was an airborne infection but showed that patients varied greatly in infectiousness, drug-resistant cases appeared to be less infectious, and treatment greatly curtailed transmission. During the second 2 years of the experiment, 50 of the total 63 guinea pigs infections were attributed to 107 smear-positive patients; however, 15 of the drug-susceptible infections were attributed a single patient with laryngeal TB (13). Table 56.2 indicates the relative infectiousness of the sputum smear–positive patients on the ward, considering that 100% infections caused by untreated, drug-susceptible cases.

Note that this study was done before the availability of rifamycins, so drug resistance refers primarily to isoniazid, streptomycin, and paraaminosalicylic acid resistance. The relative infectiousness of patients with multidrug-resistant (MDR) TB, i.e., resistance to at least isoniazid and rifamycin, has not yet been studied in a similar manner.

TABLE 56.2. RELATIVE INFECTIOUSNESS OF PATIENTS[a]

No. of Patients	No. of Guinea Pigs Infected	Relative Infectiousness of Patients (%)
Susceptible TB		
61 untreated	29	100
29 treated	1	2
Drug-resistant TB		
6 untreated	14	28
11 treated	6	5

[a]All smear-positive patients, relative to the amount of time on the ward.
TB, tuberculosis.

This study also showed that concentrations of infectious TB organisms in ward air were extremely low, averaging one in more than 10,000 ft³ of air. This has important implications for air disinfection, as discussed later in this chapter.

Tuberculosis Risk for Health Care Workers

In 1994, after the devastating outbreaks in U.S. urban hospitals (14), the Centers for Disease Control and Prevention (CDC) issued a revision of the guidelines, which organized an institution's response according to three categories (15). These include, in decreasing order of priority, administrative, environment, and personal protective equipment (particulate respirators), discussed in detail later (15). After initial balking by hospitals and workers who considered the measures costly, cumbersome, and unproved, the guidelines were effectively adopted. Coincident with much greater attention to infection control and the use of more effective treatment, the rate of TB infection and disease among health care workers (HCWs) decreased dramatically in all U.S. hospitals across all occupations.

In 1997, the Occupational Safety and Health Administration (OSHA) proposed creating a TB standard that would place TB with hepatitis B and human immunodeficiency virus (HIV) as the only infections with a specific federally enforceable rule. The proposal generated a tremendous debate; many physicians thought that the current approach to TB control, based on the 1994 revision of the TB control guidelines and simple common sense, appeared to be effective during the 1990s. Supporters of the OSHA rule emphasize that TB continues to pose an occupational risk to HCWs, just as beryllium poses a risk to miners and repetitive stress to office workers, thus, a federal guideline to protect at-risk workers must be developed to prevent cost-conscious hospital administrators from cutting corners.

As noted previously, administrative measures, particularly triage and placement of suspect cases into isolation, are considered the most important element in protecting

HCWs and other institutional workers. Recognition of the contribution of the unsuspected case led to exuberant approaches to isolation often resulting in ten to 30 patients isolated for each case of TB diagnosed. With practice and an increased understanding of the myriad presentations of TB among the HIV infected, clinicians became better able to select those patients truly at high risk of TB. In the most practiced institutions at the height of the resurgence, the "rule-out ratio" was as low as 7:1, i.e., seven suspect cases isolated, of which one actually had TB. That ratio appears to be as low as possible with current diagnostic tools. However, the appearance of a rapid, sensitive, and specific test for TB disease could reduce overisolation quickly. In addition to the resource waste inherent in overisolation, there are unpublished, anecdotal reports that patients isolated for TB receive inferior medical care while in isolation.

In addition to improving early placement of patients in isolation, administrative measures call for institution of an effective institutional TB control program (15). In most medical centers, infection control and the employee health service are charged with this task. Infection control typically ensures that all cases of suspected or proven TB are reported and tracked and that delays in placement in isolation are quantified and addressed. In addition, they ensure that any exposed HCWs are informed and sent to the employee health service for evaluation and treatment, if appropriate.

The employee health service is charged with the task of monitoring employees for tuberculin conversion. Regular 6- to 12-month testing of hospitals with thousands of employees can be a cumbersome task, particularly given the need to see each individual twice to complete the test. The two-step method, although important in avoiding false skin test conversions and unnecessary treatment (16,17), requires employees to make three or four visits to the employee health service to complete skin testing. Although computer-based tracking programs will allow an employee health service to maintain current records, employee compliance with tuberculin skin testing is now, as ever, the main obstacle to identifying new conversion. As TB case rates in the United States continue to decrease and occupational infection further recedes as a perceived risk to worker safety, the task of serial testing will become even more difficult.

The inherent problems in basing a hospital-wide program on a test as difficult to administer and interpret as the tuberculin skin test requires a thorough understanding of local TB rates as well as the prevalence of tuberculin skin test positivity in both HCWs and general communities. Approximately 5% of the U.S. population is tuberculin positive. Many series of HCWs have shown higher rates, although most reported studies have been conducted in the context of an outbreak. In general, purified protein derivative prevalence in urban hospitals, with higher numbers of workers from TB-endemic countries, is more than 20% to 30%, with a lower prevalence in community hospitals. A multicenter study of skin test conversions among HCWs in

low- and high-risk institutions, conducted by the CDC, identified an annual risk of infection of approximately 1%, which is considered high (18). However, conversion rates were highest among foreign-born and bacille Calmette–Guérin–vaccinated workers, regardless of occupational exposure. There was also evidence of household and community transmission to workers, unrelated to their work exposure (16,19–21).

An ongoing debate revolves around the relative contribution of community versus occupational exposure to tuberculin conversion in HCWs. Before the outbreaks in the United States in the late 1980s and early 1990s, a CDC-led study had concluded that community-based exposure predominated (22). This was reflected by an association between HCW conversion rate and socioeconomic status or place of residence reflected by zip code, but no demonstrable association between job category and risk of conversion. In this report, the CDC found "no correlation between patient exposure or job classification and the prevalence of significant (PPD) reactions" (22).

During the nosocomial TB outbreaks associated with the 1985 to 1992 resurgence, numerous workers became infected and developed disease, and some died, although almost all deaths were associated with concomitant HIV infection or MDRTB (20). Despite this, few studies demonstrated occupational risk outside the outbreak setting. An often-quoted study from St. Louis reported that zip code of residence was the most significant risk for tuberculin conversion (23), whereas in Atlanta, despite high rates of TB in the hospital, rates of purified protein derivative conversion correlated with socioeconomic status and not job description (24).

In contrast, reports from New York City (25) and Montreal (21) suggested that occupation was indeed associated with risk of conversion and that those with high rates of patient contact were at higher risk. Because of the uncertainties of the tuberculin test and the difficulty knowing where patients and workers are at a given time, the issue remains unsettled. The CDC, however, believes strongly that community exposure is the dominant risk for tuberculin conversion in U.S. workers outside an outbreak setting. This assumption informs the recently updated guidelines for control of TB in health care settings.

Health Care Workers at Special Risk

Pathologists are at risk of both inoculation TB ("prosector's wart") and inhalation of bacilli during dissection (26,27). Meade (28) demonstrated a marked decrease in tuberculin conversions among medical students, from 81% to 4%, when autopsies on tuberculous patients were discontinued.

Autopsies performed on patients not suspected of having TB continue to cause spread. In one report, an elderly man with progressive small cell lung cancer died of respiratory failure, presumably because of his tumor (29). No precautions were taken during the autopsy, which disclosed disseminated TB. Eight (14.5%) of 55 exposed employees, including several pathologists, developed tuberculin conversions, and two developed active disease.

Several reviews have ranked infections occurring among laboratory workers (30,31). Pike (30) found 194 reported cases of laboratory-acquired TB, including four fatal cases, making TB the sixth most common occupationally acquired infection among laboratory workers in that study. Infection may occur by either accidental aerosolization with inhalation or inadvertent inoculation. Collins and Grange (31) noted that most series placed the risk of development of active TB by the laboratory worker to be two to nine times higher than that of the general population.

Malasky et al. (32) demonstrated the risk for pulmonary physicians who perform bronchoscopy or work in intensive care units (ICUs). They compared the tuberculin conversion rates of pulmonary fellows-in-training with those of infectious disease fellows-in-training. Over 3 years, 14 training programs provided information. Conversion was higher among pulmonary fellows-in-training [seven of 62 (11%) versus one of 42 (2.4%)]. Because infectious disease and pulmonary fellows-in-training are expected to spend equal amounts of time with patients with TB, the higher proportion of tuberculin conversion was ascribed to probable exposures during bronchoscopy or during time spent in ICUs.

Fagen (33) published a report of conversion rates among medical students by sending a survey to the deans of all 126 American medical schools; responses were obtained from 101 and annual conversion rates from 75. The mean annual conversion rate for all schools was 1.8% (range, 0% to 12%).

Blumberg et al. (34) evaluated the rates of tuberculin skin test conversion over a 5-year period among house staff in Atlanta. Documented conversions occurred for 52 (2.4%) of 2,144 house staff. Conversion rates decreased after the first 6 months from 5.98 to 1.09 per 100 person-years worked over the next 4.5 years ($p < 0.001$). Analysis demonstrated graduation from a foreign medical school and being part of the house staff of a department of medicine were risks for tuberculin conversion.

Development of a policy to both protect HIV-infected HCWs and maintain their safety is a complex challenge. The unique susceptibility of HIV-infected persons to TB infection and disease has been demonstrated both in U.S. studies and the ongoing public health disaster occurring in Africa where high rates of HIV infection and latent and community TB have resulted in an exponential increase in TB cases. In the United States, potent antiretrovirals have improved overall immune function, improving the sensitivity of the tuberculin skin test. This in turn enhances the usefulness of ongoing surveillance. That said, even HCWs with excellent responses to antiretrovirals may be at increased risk of nosocomial TB. Therefore, hospitals must

place into effect deliberate safeguards to limit potential exposure. One such measure, restricting HIV-infected HCWs from working on HIV specialty wards, may be difficult to enforce. However, informed, self-imposed restrictions should be encouraged. If workers choose to work with patients at risk of TB, an emphasis on early isolation, effective negative pressure rooms, and well-fitting respirators is likely to preserve both worker safety and worker confidentiality.

Although smear-positive pulmonary disease is most often the source of a nosocomial outbreak, both smear-negative disease and extrapulmonary TB have caused nosocomial spread. In a case of a patient with a tuberculous psoas abscess, 59 (13.4%) of 442 exposed employees tuberculin converted and nine cases of active TB occurred (35). Five days after incision and drainage of the patient's abscess, local irrigation was given every 8 hours with a Water Pik (Teledyne, Los Angeles, CA) oral hygiene appliance; irrigation was continued for the next 10 days, when the patient died.

In developing countries, occupational TB also has become a source of intense concern. HIV-endemic areas, including Malawi, Côte d'Ivoire (36), and South Africa (37), report a substantial increase in cases of TB among workers, many of whom die of the disease: 25% in a series from Malawi. Cases of TB among HCWs have tripled over the past 10 years in Ethiopia (38). In areas of lower TB incidence, such as Thailand, direct patient contact was a risk for a reactive purified protein derivative (39). In Brazil, medical students and chemical engineering students had identical rates of tuberculin skin test reactivity at the start of school, but at graduation, medical students had four times the prevalence (40). Serbia and Estonia also have reported increased rates of active TB among HCWs (41).

The World Health Organization and the CDC have published guidelines for the prevention of tuberculosis in resource-limited settings (http://www.who.int/gtb/publications/healthcare/PDF/WHO99-269.pdf). This document emphasizes the importance of inexpensive administrative (early isolation) and environmental (natural ventilation) controls rather than more costly interventions such as negative air pressure rooms or expensive respirators.

Homeless Shelters, Jails, and Other Institutional Settings

TB has long been associated with those persons on the fringe of society and therefore with institutions, such as shelters, jails, and prisons. At the beginning of the 1985 to 1992 resurgence in the United States, Nardell et al. (42) reported an outbreak of drug-resistant cases among the homeless of Boston, associated primarily with one large shelter. The outbreak was remarkable because it challenged the current belief that most chronic TB in low-prevalence areas resulted from reactivation, not new infection. The occurrence of case after case of cavitary TB in homeless adults in Boston, all with the same isoniazid- and streptomycin-resistance pattern, was at first hard to reconcile. Phage typing (a predecessor of molecular fingerprinting) provided further evidence that the drug-resistant cases were clonally related, consistent with new transmission occurring in the shelter. Moreover, in seven of 25 cases, there was documented prior tuberculin positivity or active disease, leading to another unorthodox conclusion—that exogenous reinfection occurred in these cases and presumably in many other cases for whom past medical records were unavailable. Since then, shelter-associated TB has been widely reported. In New York City, for example, approximately half of homeless men are infected with TB, a figure that has not yet decreased with the decline in TB in that city over the past decade (43). In Los Angeles, using both molecular and traditional epidemiologic methods, Barnes et al. (44) identified three shelters as the source of transmission for 70% of a cohort of 79 TB cases among the homeless of that city. Control options for the homeless are limited to early identification, removal, effective treatment of communicable TB cases, skin testing and treatment of newly infected staff, and environmental controls, such as less crowding (e.g., avoidance of bunk beds), better ventilation, and use of additional air disinfection (e.g., ultraviolet air disinfection) (45,46). Directly observed therapy is often not sufficient to achieve cure in homeless patients because of mental illness and substance abuse. Long-term hospitalization in a therapeutic milieu has long been used with success in Massachusetts (47,48). Treatment of latent infection among the homeless has been tried using incentives, but success has been limited owing to transience, substance abuse, and mental illness.

The situation in jails is similar to that in shelters—a transient high-risk population, and similar approaches have been suggested (49). In some municipal jails, the rate of TB has been high enough that miniature chest x-rays have been found to be cost-effective in screening new entrants, a technique not recommended for most of the population (50,51). Prisons are quite different from jails in that the length of stay is longer, allowing time for better screening and for supervised treatment of infection and active disease (52,53). Prisons played an important role in the spread of MDR-TB in upstate New York in the early 1990s (54).

If TB in prisons remains a problem in the United States and other low-prevalence countries, it is a brewing disaster in many high-prevalence countries. In the former Soviet Union, for example, a growing epidemic of MDR-TB is focused in the prisons but is gradually making its way into the general population of the entire region, including bordering low-prevalence countries such as Finland as thousands of prisoners are released each month (55).

CONTROL OF TUBERCULOSIS IN HEALTH CARE AND OTHER INSTITUTIONS: THE RATIONAL APPLICATION OF PATIENT ISOLATION, BUILDING VENTILATION, AIR FILTRATION, ULTRAVIOLET AIR DISINFECTION, AND PERSONAL RESPIRATORS

As already discussed, the apparent success of current TB infection control practices has been attributed largely to administrative controls, i.e., the prompt recognition and isolation of patients with known or suspected infectious TB. This approach has been especially effective under relatively high-risk conditions in which staff have been motivated by skin test conversions or nosocomial disease occurring in their institution to sustain a state of heightened awareness and where diligent triage and isolation of patients are rewarded by identifying sufficient numbers of potentially infectious cases to reinforce good practice (20). However, as indicated in the previous section, for the past decade, the number of TB cases in the United States has been decreasing and is the lowest ever recorded. Because other conditions with similar symptoms (chronic cough, fever, weight loss, and lung infiltrates) are not decreasing, this means that an increasing percentage of patients isolated for possible TB will not have the disease. This is good news in many ways, but as patient after patient isolated to rule out TB turns out not to have the disease, adherence to protocols is likely to decline, setting the stage for missing cases when they do present. The following example taken from a health department investigation of a hospital exposure illustrates what may be an increasingly common situation in the future:

> In a community hospital in a low-prevalence state, routine TB skin testing of the ICU staff revealed several definite conversions, including a nurse whose chest x-ray showed a small infiltrate. She was asymptomatic and smear negative, but a sputum culture grew *M. tuberculosis*. Expanded testing of all ICU staff and others who frequented the ICU revealed a total of 23 definite skin test conversions, including eight nurses, three nurses' aides, five respiratory therapists, and two physicians. A minister and a computer technician who visited the ICU regularly were among those infected, as was a nurse who worked in the ICU for only a few months and tested positive on starting a new job. No other active cases resulted. The nurse with active TB was thought not to be the source of the conversions because she was smear negative, had no cough, and her husband and children were skin test negative. There were no known TB patients in the ICU during the period when the infections were likely to have occurred, and public health records revealed no cases in the area served by the hospital that might have been responsible. The source case was assumed to have been an ICU patient who died with undiagnosed TB. The records of all ICU patients with abnormal chest x-rays during that period were reviewed. Three elderly patients who had died with abnormal chest x-rays were considered suspi-

cious for active TB, and their time in the ICU could account for most or all of the staff infections. One patient who was thought to have died of biopsy-proven lung cancer had a for-malin-fixed tissue specimen tested for TB by polymerase chain reaction, and it was positive. However, the pleural biopsy of one of the other two patients also tested positive for TB by polymerase chain reaction, although the histology was nonspe-cific. Nucleic acid extracted from both specimens had the same spoligotype fingerprint pattern. At this point, it is not possible to say which, if either, of the patients was the source of trans-mission and which might have been another secondary case. All three suspected patients had been in single-bed ICU cubi-cles with negative pressure capacity, but none was turned on because TB was not suspected in these critically ill, compli-cated patients. Personal respiratory protection was not in use for the same reason. Conversely, the hospital's practice of rou-tine annual skin testing of ICU staff uncovered this outbreak before the ICU nurse became symptomatic and possibly con-tagious. Although ventilation rates were adequate, less trans-mission might have resulted had there been additional air dis-infection in each cubicle, for example, by upper room UVGI.

Such exposures are unlikely to be common, especially if cases continue to decrease, but they will be increasingly dif-ficult to prevent as case rates decrease in an aging popula-tion presenting with more and more complex medical prob-lems. Unless rapid, highly sensitive and specific tests for active TB are developed, our current triage and isolation strategy alone is unlikely to offer sufficient protection in the future. Until better diagnostic tests are available, improved ways to prevent transmission from unsuspected cases will be needed. Greater emphasis on general air disinfection is one approach, as detailed in the following sections.

Low Probability of Tuberculosis Infection in Most Institutions: Implications for Control by Air Disinfection

The concentration of infectious droplet nuclei under the real-life conditions of Riley's experimental TB ward, where most of the six patients had been started on the best avail-able chemotherapy, averaged one in more than 10,000 ft^3 of air. Although low, 8 hours per day exposure to such con-centrations over 3 years would, by calculation, explain the high rates of infection experienced by student nurses in the prechemotherapy era (12). However, for most workers in most institutions today, exposure to even one infectious TB patient is unlikely. For those who are exposed to a patient with TB of average infectiousness, moreover, the probabil-ity of inhaling even a single infectious droplet nucleus is usually small. Many workers have inherited some innate resistance to TB, which means that not every inhaled droplet nucleus causes infection. Therefore, although a sin-gle inhaled droplet nucleus may be sufficient to cause TB infection in a highly susceptible host, under the low-preva-lence conditions extant today in most health care facilities in the United States, the risk of infection for workers

appears to be low, determined by a series of low-probability events.

Given the importance of the chance appearance of an unsuspected case of TB, greater attention should be devoted to maintaining vigilance for TB so that infectious cases are not inadvertently placed in congregate settings and to start-ing treatment promptly. Recall that in Riley's air sampling study, patients on chemotherapy infected only a small frac-tion of the guinea pigs compared with untreated patients (Table 56.2). Although patients are believed to remain infectious for as long as 2 weeks on effective chemotherapy, and respiratory isolation is necessary during that time, rela-tively few people should be entering isolation rooms, and the risk of spread is already greatly reduced before any envi-ronmental interventions are applied. Compared with the importance of triage and isolation of infectious cases, the details of isolation (e.g., the exact number of room air changes in isolation rooms, the possibility that a puff of iso-lation room air might escape, the differences in filtration efficiency of various personal respirators) probably consti-tute relatively minor determinants of risk. In high-risk insti-tutions, however, where TB patients are regularly admitted, MDR-TB is prevalent, and bronchoscopy and other aerosol-generating procedures are performed, environmen-tal interventions and effective respirator use may have a greater role in protecting HCWs (56). In both low- and high-risk settings, however, greater emphasis should be placed on general ventilation and other methods of addi-tional air disinfection throughout facilities to reduce trans-mission, such as upper room germicidal irradiation and high-efficiency particulate air (HEPA) filtration, to prevent transmission from unsuspected sources.

A recent study in Canadian hospitals focusing on set-tings considered at relatively high-risk of TB transmission found higher rates of skin test conversion in those facilities where patient rooms had lower levels of general ventilation, but there was no increased risk associated with inadequate levels of ventilation in TB isolation rooms (Table 56.3) (57). This study contrasts with the CDC prospective study that found little risk associated with patient care, but it should be noted that the Canadian study targeted high-risk facilities, whereas the CDC study did not.

Building Ventilation

Public buildings in industrialized countries are constructed with mechanical heating, ventilation, and air conditioning (HVAC) systems that usually condition and recirculate most of the returned air, exhausting some fraction of it and replacing it with outside air to control odors, carbon diox-ide buildup, and air contaminants such as smoke. Because developers, architects, and engineers are most familiar with these technologies, it is understandable that increased ven-tilation is often proposed to reduce airborne disease trans-mission in buildings (15). However, recommended build-

TABLE 56.3. RISK FACTORS FOR TUBERCULIN SKIN TEST CONVERSION IN CANADIAN HOSPITALS

Risk Factor	Adjusted Odds Ratio	CI (95%)
Respiratory therapist	6.1	3.1–12.0
Nursing	4.3	2.7–6.9
Housekeeping	4.2	2.3–7.6
<2 air changes per hour (nonisolation patient rooms)	3.4	2.1–5.8
Physiotherapy	3.3	1.5–7.2
Inadequate ventilation (isolation rooms)	1.0	0.8–1.3

CI, confidence interval.

ing ventilation rates are not designed for infection control. Higher rates recommended to control infectious agents have been based largely on clearance rates for contaminants when the source is not continuous. As the following discussion indicates, protection provided by ventilation is usually limited. Greater protection usually requires additional air disinfection by UVGI or HEPA filtration.

Building Ventilation with Outside Air: Quantitative Considerations

With a uniform concentration of particles and uniform mixing of incoming air, 63% of the air and airborne organisms will be removed with each air change. However, under more realistic conditions, when there is an uneven distribution of infectious particles and uneven mixing of fresh air with contaminated air, less than 63% of air and airborne particles are flushed out with each air change. The true decreases per air change that have been measured are in the range of 20% to 60%.

Another consequence of the fact that infectious particles are unevenly evenly distributed in air is that some exposed individuals may inhale multiple infectious doses and others inhale none during the same period. Mathematical models of airborne infection have been developed to describe the impact of ventilation on the transmission of airborne infectious diseases (58,59). In these models, the incidence of infection (λ) at time t is a function of the prevalence (Pr) of infectious cases at time t, the average pulmonary ventilation rate per person (p), the duration of the exposure (d), the outdoor air ventilation rate (v), and the number of doses of airborne infection added to the air per unit time by each infectious person (q).

Assuming that the number of infectious cases is constant, the cumulative incidence (CI) of infection is:

$$CI = S(1 - e^{-\lambda t}) = S(1 - e^{-Pr \cdot q \cdot p \cdot d/v})$$

In this expression, the incidence rate (λ) is equivalent to the total number of doses per unit volume of air per unit time. Note that the terminology used in this expression, the Wells–Riley equation, reflects current epidemiology convention and differs slightly from that used to describe the probability of airborne infection in earlier

publications (60). Dividing through the equation by S yields an expression for the fraction infected among those exposed, or the probability of infection ($1 - e^{-Pr \cdot q \cdot p \cdot d/v}$). Plotting the probability of infection as function of ventilation with outside air (v) in volume per unit of time for various values of Pr, q, p, or d, generates a family of logarithmic decay curves. Figure 56.4 (60a) shows two examples of such curves derived from two actual TB exposures reported in the literature (58,61). The two labeled points

The Effect of Ventilation on the Probability of Infection

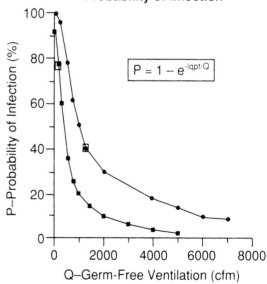

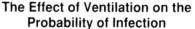

FIGURE 56.4. Two different examples of extensive transmission are represented. In both cases, I was 1 and p was assumed to be 0.353 ft³/min, a constant. The other transmission factors for the exposures reported by Nardell and Catanzaro were q = 13 and 250 quanta per hour (qph), t = 9,600 and 150 minutes, and Q = 1,450 and 150 ft³/min (cfm). (Modified from Riley RL, Nardell EA. Controlling transmission of tuberculosis in health care facilities: ventilation, filtration, and ultraviolet air disinfection. In: *Plant technology and safety management series, no. 1.* Oakbrook Terrace, IL: The Joint Commission on Accreditation of Healthcare Organizations, 1993:25–31.)

ICU and office building reflect the probability of infection $(1 - e^{-\text{Pr} \cdot q \cdot p \cdot d/v})$ at the actual ventilation rate (v) for each exposure, as indicated on the graph. Assuming that all other factors (Pr, q, p, d, and S) remain constant, the curves represent the theoretical probability of infection predicted for increasing or decreasing ventilation (v) above or below the actual values. Although plotted on the same axes, the curves cannot be compared directly with one another because the actual ventilation rate per occupant and the room air changes resulting from the ventilation rate in each exposure were very different. The purpose of their juxtaposition is to illustrate one circumstance, the ICU exposure, where actual room total outdoor air ventilation was well below recommended levels and where easily achievable increases in ventilation from the actual value are predicted to result in substantial decreases in risk. The actual exposure conditions result in a data point high up on the vertical limb of the curve where small changes in ventilation result in large changes in risk. In contrast, in the office building, ventilation was only slightly below national standards, and achievable increases are relatively modest and, therefore, result in a smaller decrease in risk. In this case, the actual data point is near the bottom of the vertical limb of the curve where each additional infection averted requires a larger and larger increase in ventilation. A simple way to think of the relationship between risk of infection and ventilation is that each doubling of ventilation reduces the *remaining* risk by approximately half. The ICU exposure was brief (2.5 hours during a bronchoscopy and intubation) but intensive (i.e., q estimated at 250 infectious doses generated per hour), during which ten of 13 (80%) exposed persons were infected. Ventilation was so low [150 ft³/min (cfm)] that it would be realistic to double it and even double that value again and again, resulting in protection of almost all the exposed susceptible occupants. However, the office building exposure was longer (30 days) but much less intensive (q estimated at 13 infectious doses generated per hour), resulting in infection of 27 (40%) of 67 exposed workers. In this case, increasing ventilation from the existing 15 cfm outdoor air per occupant (1,450 cfm) to the currently recommended 20 cfm would be possible but is predicted to protect only a few of the 27 workers infected. Even doubling ventilation to 2,900 cfm (30 cfm per occupant, highly unusual for an office building) would have protected only approximately half of those infected, according to the equation.

Building ventilation is often limited by design (e.g., capacity of blowers, ducts), comfort (e.g., noise, drafts), and economic consideration (e.g., cost of conditioning outside air). Whereas an isolation room or ICU may be designed to have 12 or more air changes per hour, many congregate settings are not. Still, the relationship described between ventilation and airborne infection holds within the limits of the assumptions used in the above equation (uniform air mixing, equal susceptibility). For these reasons, in congregate indoor settings where airborne transmission is likely, it is desirable to consider supplementing ventilation with other means of air disinfection, such as air filtration or UVGI. The air disinfecting effects of these alternative measures have been equated to ventilation and air disinfection purposes only and called equivalent ventilation, that is, when 63% of airborne infectious particles are removed by filtration or inactivated by UVGI, they have produced one equivalent air change. Obviously, neither particle filters nor UVGI removes carbon dioxide nor replaces oxygen so equivalency is limited to air disinfection. Ventilation is still required to serve its usual functions.

Air disinfection by filtration or UVGI follows the same logarithmic relationship described for ventilation. This is a fundamental relationship for all disinfecting processes in which a particular percentage of a population of organisms is inactivated with each exposure. One well-mixed air change (produced by ventilation, filtration, or UVGI) inactivates approximately 63% of airborne organisms, and a second air change inactivates approximately 63% of what remains, and so on, producing a logarithmic decay curve. However, because filtered air is recirculated, it may be possible to achieve higher levels of equivalent air changes at lower cost than outdoor air ventilation because heating and cooling costs are less. Like ventilation, air filtration requires mechanical air flow and may also be limited by occupant comfort (noise and drafts). It should be stated that safety need not depend entirely on air disinfection in the case of high-risk situations such as bronchoscopy or mechanical ventilation. Had there been appropriate respiratory protection in addition to better air disinfection during the ICU procedures, for example, it is likely that no one would have been infected.

Tuberculosis Transmission Patterns: Adjacent Space and Recirculation

Building ventilation, natural or mechanical, serves not only to dilute the concentration of droplet nuclei in air but also to transport infection within rooms and buildings. Within spaces contiguous to the infectious patient, natural air currents (drafts) and forced air movement normally rapidly disperse and dilute airborne droplet nuclei to extremely low average concentrations. However, even at low concentrations, infections will occur if the duration of exposure is long enough or if enough people are exposed.

Despite a natural inclination not to be "coughed on" by the patient with active TB, immediate proximity to the coughing TB patient is likely to increase the risk of infection only transiently while the concentration of droplet nuclei is elevated, but the risk quickly decreases as droplet nuclei rapidly disperse within the available space. With some exceptions, epidemiologic patterns of TB transmission in developed countries rarely implicate transient exposures as important, pointing instead to relatively long exposures and to the clinical characteristics of source patients as the critical factors. The distinction often blurs because persons exposed at close proximity are usually breathing air in the same room as the source patient for some period. The anecdotal experience that many nurses and physicians with frequent but brief exposures to patients with active TB in TB clinics, for example, remain uninfected over entire careers supports Riley's estimates of extremely low average concentrations of droplet nuclei, normally requiring prolonged cumulative contact time for transmission, as documented by the experience of student nurses decades earlier (12,62,63). However, surveys of large populations using molecular epidemiology are finding clear linkages between cases of TB in which there has been no prolonged contact, supporting a subtle but inescapable conclusion of the Wells–Riley equation that however small the risk to the individual from brief exposures is, if enough people breath air with an infectious TB patient, even in public places, sporadic infections must occur, accounting for some part of the background rate of tuberculin positivity found in the community (64).

The role of air currents as a mode of TB transmission in a hospital was demonstrated by a TB outbreak where proximity to the room of the source patient appeared to have been the predominant transmission factor (65). As discussed in the section on transmission from extrapulmonary TB, the patient had a soft-tissue abscess that was ultimately diagnosed as TB. Investigation later showed that air flowed out of the patient's room into the corridor owing to a malfunction of the ventilation system. Fifty-eight other patients were exposed over 3 days in rooms off the same corridor. Infection rates ranged from 67% across the hall from the source patient to 37%, 29%, 10%, and 0% as the distance from the source increased. The other rooms were found to be pressure neutral with respect to the corridor. Air currents generated by personnel and other factors apparently carried droplet nuclei down the corridor, their concentration becoming progressively more dilute. As is usually the case, the cause of this unusual exposure was multifactorial, but the main reason was that the case was not suspected. Had TB been suspected, the abscess would not have been irrigated, the patient would have been placed in an effective isolation room, and therapy would have begun.

Mechanical ventilating systems have facilitated transmission throughout buildings, as in the office building already mentioned. In a South Florida clinic treating HIV-infected patients, a case–control epidemiologic investigation found that the highest risk of infection was simply being in the buildings for 40 hours per week (66). Because the HVAC system recirculated droplet nuclei, exposure was nearly universal and barely dependent on proximity to the source patients. Because air in most health care facilities is recirculated, patients not suspected of having TB in almost any area can contribute to infection throughout the

building. Although air from isolation rooms is routinely exhausted directly to the outside (with substantial energy loss), single-pass, nonrecirculating ventilation for entire buildings is prohibitively expensive for all but some specialized facilities. Air disinfection within ducts using UVGI or HEPA filters is a less expensive, highly effective way to permit safe air recirculation (67). Effective air disinfection within rooms, corridors, and common areas using upper room UVGI also helps to prevent the recirculation of infectious droplet nuclei at the same time that it prevents in-room transmission.

Patient Isolation: Directional Airflow, Negative Pressure, and Anterooms

Negative-pressure isolation uses directional airflow from low- to high-risk areas to protect persons in areas adjacent to potentially infectious source patients. To produce directional airflow, room air is exhausted at a rate greater than air intake through the ventilation system, so the necessary make-up air is drawn from adjacent, low-risk areas. The negative pressure generated in isolation rooms relative to adjacent areas is normally extremely small and difficult to measure. Demonstrating that the direction of airflow around doors is into rooms is what really matters, and this is readily monitored with a smoke stick or wisp of cotton. Note that it is possible to have air entering under the door but exiting over it, so that checking airflow direction in several locations is recommended. Unless rooms are sealed, however, it is not uncommon for air pressure fluctuations outside (through leaky windows) or elsewhere inside the building to negate the small gradients in pressure, sometimes reversing the direction of airflow (68). Directional airflow can also reverse over time as ventilation system filters become clogged, fan belts slip, or as a result of building renovations. Some leakage from negative-pressure isolation rooms normally occurs owing to the turbulence generated by opening and closing doors. Experiments using tracer gases in model isolation rooms have shown that the transfer of contaminated air between adjacent negative-pressure rooms off the same corridor can actually be enhanced by greater negative pressure (69). The greater the negative pressure in isolation rooms is, the greater the probability is that air invariably leaked into a common corridor from one room as doors open and close will be entrained by another room. Although properly functioning anterooms can minimize isolation room leakage, they add yet another level of complexity and cost and may negatively affect patient care by making personal contact between patient and caregiver more difficult. The effect of respiratory isolation on quality patient care has yet to be fully evaluated. This is especially important because of the relatively large number of patients who must be isolated as suspects but who are found not to have TB. Patients suspected of having TB are likely to be isolated for a relatively long time because it is often easier to prove that patients have TB than to show that they do not have the disease.

Practical Considerations for Effective Ventilation: Room Air Mixing and Maintenance of Mechanical Systems

As important as the numbers of room air changes or cubic feet per minute of outdoor air ventilation is the adequacy of air mixing within the room so that appropriate dilution and removal of droplet nuclei are achieved. Unfortunately, the location of ventilation diffusers and exhaust ducts is often determined by aesthetic and architectural factors other than the efficiency of room air mixing. Moreover, in forced-air systems that commonly serve both heating and cooling functions, diffuser locations that encourage air mixing during one cycle (i.e., cooling from ceiling diffusers) often encourage stagnation during the other cycle (i.e., heating from ceiling diffusers). Because room air mixing is essential for effective air disinfection by all three engineering modalities (dilutional ventilation, filtration, and UVGI), health care facilities should be encouraged to evaluate and upgrade their ventilation systems not only to meet the current requirements for outdoor air but also to provide optimal air mixing within rooms. Air mixing within rooms is considered in greater detail where UV air disinfection is discussed.

According to building engineers, faulty maintenance is more often the cause of inadequate ventilation than a poor original design (68). Maintenance programs in health care facilities should be upgraded and supplemented by performance testing to evaluate the adequacy of ventilation, including assessment of directional airflow and room air mixing during both heating and cooling cycles. For many facilities, performance testing will require outside consultation. Because TB is transmitted throughout health care facilities, optimal ventilation system performance should not be limited to isolation and procedure rooms but should include entire buildings. Although effective isolation of newly identified sources is desirable, the current disproportionate attention to isolation in health care facilities diverts attention from air disinfection in corridors, common areas, and other potentially more important sites of transmission from patients with unsuspected TB. As discussed later, deployment of upper room UV air disinfection in patient rooms and common areas can supplement the protection of ventilation, and deployment in corridors can prevent transmission between rooms in a way analogous to negative-pressure ventilation (70,71).

In summary, current federal guidelines to prevent TB transmission in health care facilities acknowledge what was known and clearly stated by the National Tuberculosis Association more than 25 years ago, that patients with unsuspected TB present the greatest risk of transmission; yet the same guidelines focus almost entirely on the known

or suspected TB patients in isolation rooms. The guidelines do recommend increased surveillance so that fewer cases are missed, but with existing diagnostic tests, there appear to be limits to our ability to detect TB amid the many other causes of cough, fever, weight loss, and lung infiltrates (72). Although earlier detection should help, the current focus on the engineering of isolation rooms diverts attention and resources from other areas where transmission from undiagnosed patients occurs.

Effective, well-engineered ventilation throughout facilities, with good room air mixing, should prevent the kind of widespread transmission that has been associated with substandard ventilation. Within the limits of practicality, however, the protection provided by optimal building ventilation alone is usually incomplete (58). It is not possible to specify a number of air changes to prevent TB transmission. However, the standard ventilation recommendations of the American Society of Heating, Refrigeration, and Air Conditioning Engineers and American Institute of Architects should provide a good baseline level of protection (see websites for latest updates) (72,73). For isolation and procedure rooms, directional airflow from adjacent corridors helps to contain droplet nuclei, but negative-pressure isolation is often difficult to achieve and expensive to maintain. Anterooms can help to maintain respiratory isolation but are expensive and may impair patient care. Both air filtration and upper room UVGI can supplement ventilation as means of air disinfection and patient isolation.

AIR FILTRATION MACHINES

In view of the practical limitations of building ventilation alone to prevent TB transmission, engineers have turned to fan- or blower-driven room air filtration devices, supplementing ventilation with "equivalent" air changes for infection control and patient isolation. HEPA filters can reliably remove particles in the size range of droplet nuclei (1 to 5 μm diameter). Many air filtration devices are on the market, but few have been subjected to rigorous, independent testing of their ability to clear airborne particulates under field conditions. Some of the devices incorporate UVGI air disinfection and filtration, but there is no rational basis to use both technologies in the same unit because HEPA filters remove 99.97% of particulate larger than 0.3 μm in diameter, leaving no microorganisms to kill by irradiation. Irradiation of filter surfaces is ineffective and unnecessary. Some devices use intensive UV alone as a means of air disinfection. If properly designed, such devices should easily inactivate whatever tubercle bacilli pass through them. A convincing demonstration of the efficacy of duct irradiation against virulent TB was the second 2 years of the Baltimore Veterans Administration

Hospital study in which none of the guinea pigs breathing irradiated ward air was infected, whereas another colony of animals breathing unirradiated ward air became infected at approximately the same rate as the guinea pigs during the first 2 years (62). The main advantage of UV over HEPA filtration in ducts or air disinfection devices is that a bank of UV tubes offers less resistance to airflow, permitting the use of smaller, quieter blowers. The National Jewish Center for Immunology and Respiratory Disease in Denver, which for decades has treated some of the nation's most drug-resistant TB cases, attributes its remarkable staff safety record of its TB unit over the past 10 years to the use of a unique high-volume, ceiling-mounted UV air disinfection system for isolation rooms (74). Although any added air disinfection is likely to be beneficial, there is a danger that portable, plug-in devices may be considered "quick fixes" for what is an exceedingly complex problem. Here are several questions to consider before investing in portable (or stationary) air filtration equipment to reduce the spread of TB:

1. Is the volume of air movement sufficient to substantially reduce the risk of infection? Because TB can be transmitted by extremely low concentrations of infectious droplet nuclei, large volumes of air must be filtered to substantially reduce the risk of transmission. This same limitation applies to building ventilation. A reasonable goal would be at least ten or more effective, equivalent air changes per hour in addition to the actual outdoor air changes produced by the HVAC system.
2. Is room air mixing adequate to prevent air stagnation? Although many such devices agitate room air, there is a possibility of refiltering much of the same air repeatedly, primarily in the immediate vicinity of the device.
3. Are the noise levels and drafts created by the machine tolerable for patients and staff?
4. Is the device constructed to prevent leakage around filters when the device is moved or the filter is changed?
5. Is there a convenient way to know whether the device is working properly? A pressure gauge reflecting the pressure differential across the filter is useful, but it must be monitored regularly by someone who understands what it means. We have seen large room fan filtration units in a homeless shelter whose obtrusive, loud rumble reassured operators but were providing absolutely no benefit because their filters were full, and airflow had all but stopped.

Fan filtration devices have been used to create effective negative-pressure isolation rooms by recirculating HEPA-filtered air from the room through a duct to an anteroom. For some institutions, a retrofit isolation room of this type may be far preferable to the costs of construction and operation of standard negative-pressure isolation rooms using 100% exhaust to the outside (75,76).

UPPER ROOM ULTRAVIOLET GERMICIDAL IRRADIATION

After widespread enthusiasm for the use of UVGI air disinfection in the 1930s and 1940s, interest and usage waned because of concerns over its efficacy and safety, lack of familiarity with the technology, and the widespread use of chemotherapy for TB and immunization for some of the common respiratory viruses. However, UVGI is again of interest not only because of its potential efficacy, low cost, and ease of application but also because it can be used throughout high-risk institutions, wherever transmission is likely (70). Despite the historical controversy, the use of UVGI is supported by more scientific evidence of efficacy for TB than exists for room ventilation, air filtration, or the use of particulate respirators to prevent TB transmission (62,67,70,71,76–82). This is not to suggest that the other technologies are not effective but simply that they have not been studied as thoroughly for the control of TB or other airborne organisms. The scientific evidence supporting the use of UVGI can be divided into three components: (a) evidence of susceptibility of airborne tubercle bacilli to UV radiation, (b) evidence of sufficient convective air mixing between the upper and lower parts of rooms to achieve effective room air disinfection, and (c) evidence that UVGI is safe for room occupants.

Susceptibility of Airborne Tubercle Bacilli to Ultraviolet Radiation

There have been numerous studies of the efficacy of UVGI (254 nm UV) in killing or inactivating a wide range of microorganisms. However, many of these studies have been done on culture plates, which is a very different environment than organisms suspended in air. In general, airborne organisms are more susceptible to UV than are organisms on surfaces where they can be protected by a thin layer of fluid. Airborne organisms may also be metabolically different than organisms growing in culture. Riley et al. (82) used an apparatus pictured in Figure 56.5 to determine the susceptibility of aerosolized virulent *M. tuberculosis*. The susceptibility was reported as a Kethley Z value, whose units are cumbersome to use. Recall, however, that when 63% of organisms are removed by any means, we speak of one equivalent air change, by analogy to the effects of ventilation. Translated into equivalent air changes per hour, just 1 $\mu W/cm^2$ of 254 nm UV inactivates tubercle bacilli at a rate equivalent to 15 air changes per hour. That is, if an entire room could be irradiated at 1.0 $\mu W/cm^2$, the result would be an inactivation rate for tubercle bacilli equivalent to 15 air changes per hour of ventilation. As discussed later, people in the lower room cannot be exposed for very long at 1 $\mu W/cm^2$, and an hour of exposure is much longer than desirable to kill tubercle bacilli. However, if a much larger

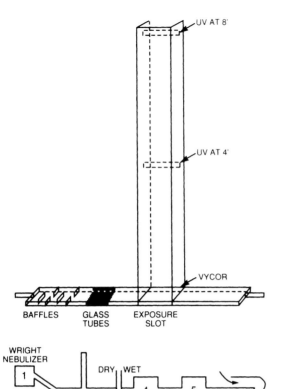

UV dose is used in the upper room, organisms can be rapidly killed there, whereas occupants in the lower room remain unaffected. At 50 μW/cm^2, a realistic intensity in the upper room within 1 m of a UV fixture, it takes just 12 seconds at 50% humidity to achieve a 90% reduction of airborne tubercle bacilli. Unfortunately, in a test apparatus, and possibly in rooms, humidity greater than 80% greatly reduces the efficacy of UVGI for a given dose (81).

Convective Room Air Mixing and Ultraviolet Efficacy

Actual room experiments using *Serratia marcescens*, which are approximately seven times more susceptible to UV radiation than are tubercle bacilli, produced equivalent air changes in the lower part of the room that were often in excess of 50 per hour and sometimes in excess of 100 per hour, but these very high equivalent air changes required excellent convective room mixing (78–80,82). These experiments showed that the most effective means of producing increased convective air mixing in rooms was the temperature gradient between the upper and lower parts of the room (Fig. 56.6). Fans were also effective in improving air mixing (79,80) (Fig. 56.7). The latter experiment also illustrated the relatively small benefit of increased UV dose in the absence of air mixing. Using bacille Calmette–Guérin organisms artificially aerosolized into a 200-ft^2 room, Riley et al. (82) found that a single 17-W UV fixture added the equivalent of ten room air changes to a room with only natural ventilation, where convective mixing was encouraged by radiator heating (Fig. 56.8). The latter experiment has been used as a dose guide for the current application of upper room UVGI.

FIGURE 56.5. Top: Apparatus used to expose aerosolized bacteria to ultraviolet (*UV*) radiation of known intensity. **Bottom:** Block diagram shows train of apparatus for producing a bacterial aerosol, exposing it for a known period of time to UV radiation of known intensity, under conditions of known temperature, humidity, and particle size. (Modified from Riley RL, Kaufman JE. Effect of relative humidity on the inactivation of airborne *Serratia marcescens* by ultraviolet radiation. *Appl Microbiol* 1972;23:1113–1120.)

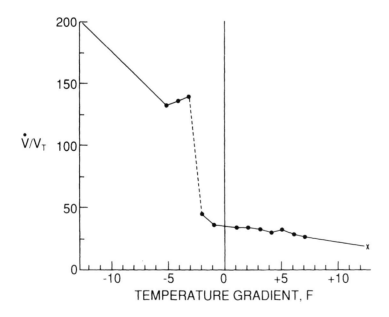

FIGURE 56.6. Calculated rate of air exchange between upper and lower zones (V/V$_T$) in air changes per hour as a function of temperature gradient between upper and lower parts of the room (°F) with ultraviolet radiation on, ceiling fans off. (Modified from Riley RL, Permutt S, Kaufman JE. Room air disinfection by ultraviolet irradiation of upper room air. *Arch Environ Health* 1971;23:35–40.)

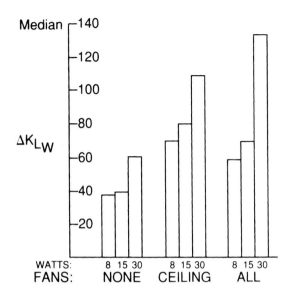

FIGURE 56.7. Effect of fans (one low-velocity ceiling paddle fan and two high-velocity floor blowers) and ultraviolet (UV) wattage on germicidal effect of UV, where K_{LW} represents equivalent air turnovers. (Modified from Riley RL, Permutt S. Room air disinfection by ultraviolet irradiation of upper air—air mixing and germicidal effectiveness. *Arch Environ Health* 1971;22: 208–219.)

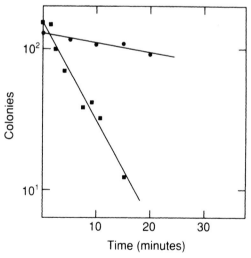

FIGURE 56.8. Disappearance of bacille Calmette–Guérin from room air with and without upper room air ultraviolet (*UV*) irradiation, using one suspended fixture with a 17-W tube. UV added the equivalent of ten air changes per hour to the two air changes per hour produced by natural ventilation and die-away of organisms. (Modified from Riley RL, Knight M, Middlebrook G. Ultraviolet susceptibility of BCG and virulent tubercle bacilli. *Am Rev Respir Dis* 1976;113:413–418.)

Based on the known susceptibility of tubercle bacilli to UV radiation, there is little doubt that radiation of the upper room air with one 30-W tube per 200 ft^2 is more than adequate to provide increases in equivalent air changes in the lower part of the room far in excess of anything that could be achieved by practical forms of mechanical ventilation, provided there is adequate convective exchange between the upper and lower parts of the room. There is also little doubt that adequate convective exchange can be produced by rather simple measures, but how often the convective exchange is adequate is completely unknown. There is very little information about the magnitude of room convective air exchanges because there have been very few studies of the problem. The problem has not been studied because of a mistaken emphasis on the sensitivity of the organism to UV radiation and the implicit assumption that the effectiveness of UV radiation of the upper air would be significantly increased if we could increase the intensity of the irradiation. It seems more likely that an optimal distribution of simple, fairly low wattage fixtures in the upper part of the room would be highly effective in decontaminating the lower room air under conditions in which the convective exchange is great. Without knowledge of the convective air exchange, adequate radiation of the upper part of the room might lead to a marked increase in equivalent air changes in the lower part with a significant reduction in droplet nuclei or, when convective exchange is minimal, might produce only a slight benefit. This degree of uncertainty is an unattractive feature of UV air disinfection as it is carried out today, although similar uncertainty about room air mixing applies as well to air disinfection by dilutional ventilation and room air filtration. To overcome this problem in a hospital setting, there will need to be much closer cooperation between ventilation engineers and the proponents of UVGI. The problem of convective air exchange is within the domain of the engineers and great strides in upper room air disinfection await the interest of engineers in this fascinating problem.

Safety of Upper Room Ultraviolet Air Disinfection

UVGI uses a narrow band (95% 253.7-nm wavelength) of the UV portion (200 to 400 nm) of the electromagnetic spectrum to inactivate airborne pathogens. Short-wavelength UV irradiation (253.7 nm, UV-C) is rapidly lethal for airborne bacteria at intensity levels easily achieved in the upper part of the room, above people's heads, but it is safe for occupants at the much lower intensity levels permitted in the occupied part of the room. Longer wavelength UV-A and UV-B have a much greater penetrating capacity than does UV-C, and long-term exposure to the intensive, longer wavelength UV in sunlight has been associated with skin cancer and cataracts. UV-C has more energy than UV-B and would in theory be more damaging to tissues than UV-B were it not almost completely (95%) absorbed by the outer, dead layer of the stratum corneum (83) (Table 56.4). Accidental direct exposure to high-intensity UV-C can cause temporary, painful, but superficial irritation of the eyes (photokeratoconjunctivitis) or skin erythema. Eye irritation is transient owing to the normally rapid turnover of the corneal epithelium (84). Painters and maintenance personnel have experienced photokeratoconjunctivitis caused by accidental direct UV-C exposure after working in the upper part of a room without first turning off the UV fixtures. Because UV-C does not penetrate the cornea, it does not reach the lens to cause cataracts. Intensive, direct skin exposure can cause erythema and could cause a mild to moderate "sunburn" in sensitive individuals. Prolonged high-intensity UV-C irradiation of hairless mice has produced skin cancers, but at the low-level, 8-hour exposures permitted for people in the lower part of a room (6 mJ/cm²), Forbes and Urbach (85) and Sterenborg (86) estimated that human skin cancer would require more than 300 years of exposure!

Although systemic immunosuppression has been induced by UV-B irradiation of mice, the UV dose required was relatively large compared with potential UVGI exposures in the lower part of a room (87). Moreover, the immunosuppressive effect presumably requires UV penetration to the cellular level, readily achieved with more penetrating UV-B in mice owing to their relatively thin epidermis but unlikely in thicker skinned humans with low-level, low-penetrating UV-C exposure. There is no evidence of systemic immunosuppression in humans from UV-C exposure. Activation of HIV in cell cultures exposed to UV-B or UV-C has been reported, and concerns have been raised that pulsed UV actinotherapy and sunbathing could be an important activation factor for HIV-infected persons (88,89). If true, the effect should be discernible epidemiologically, given the numbers of HIV-infected persons under observation and the wide range of sun exposure geographically and among individuals. This has not been observed, nor have patients treated with UV-A for psoriasis had evidence of clinical or laboratory progression in their HIV infections (90,91). By comparison with ordinary outdoor exposures to the more intense and penetrating UV-A and UV-B in sunlight, the low levels of UV-C permitted in the lower part of a room should pose no significant added risk, whereas it should offer substantial protection from TB infection, a well-established hazard for HIV-infected persons (83) (Table 56.4).

Current exposure safety guidelines for UV-C are based on a combination of animal data and voluntary human exposures using eye irritation as the end point (92). The exposure limit for 254 nm UV is 6.0 mJ/cm² over any 8-hour period. If eye exposure were continuous (i.e., 8-hour stare time), this threshold would be reached at an intensity of 0.2 µW/cm². Unfortunately, for years, this intensity has been widely promulgated as the upper limit of acceptable UV intensity at eye level. However, occupant movement within rooms, angles of incidence of UV rays reflected from ceilings, and shielding by brows and eyelids all greatly reduce true UV exposure to the cornea, the same factors that ordinarily prevent photokeratoconjunctivitis outside from exposure to UV-B in sunlight. In unpublished studies using a personal UV monitor, Yasui et al. found that patients occupying rooms with eye-level intensities of as much as 2.0 µW/cm² (i.e., ten times the 8-hour limit for continuous eye exposure) have had no eye complaints and register total UV 8-hour exposures of only 20% to 30% of the 6.0 mJ/cm² limit. This indicates that actual eye exposure is far from continuous. For more than 50 years, upper room UVGI has been used safely in hospitals, clinics, jails, and shelters around the country without injuries more serious than an occasional, transient eye irritation from accidental direct exposure. In more than 15 years of experience using upper room UV throughout a 350-bed shelter for the homeless in Boston and in our long-term TB treatment unit, there have been no complaints of adverse effects.

PARTICULATE RESPIRATORS TO PREVENT TUBERCULOSIS TRANSMISSION

Particulate respirators work by filtering contaminants (droplet nuclei containing TB) out of the air. By reducing the fraction of droplet nuclei reaching the lungs, particulate

TABLE 56.4. SKIN: APPROXIMATE *IN VITRO* TRANSMISSION (PERCENTAGE)

Depth (µm)	Layer	254 nm	296 nm	365 nm
0	Surface	100	100	100
10	Stratum corneum	42	50	80
20		18	25	64
30	Viable layer	5	15	50
50		0.4	6	31
70		0.03	2	19

Modified from Bruls WAG. Transmission of human epidermis and stratum corneum as a function of thickness in the ultraviolet and visible wavelengths. *Photochem Photobiol* 1984;40:485–494.

respirators achieve benefits that should be proportional to the risk at hand. Thus, in high-risk exposure settings the benefit of a respirator may be great, but in low- or negligible-risk settings, they may be of little or no benefit and may divert attention from other more effective TB control practices. Respirators are divided into two categories: negative pressure and positive pressure. With a negative-pressure respirator, the wearer inhales, creating negative pressure in the space between the respirator and the face and drawing air through filtration material into the lungs. The creation of negative pressure within the respirator is the device's Achilles' heal because it creates the potential for leakage of contaminants between the face and respirator (face seal leakage). Positive-pressure respirators blow air into the space between the face and respirator, and the potential for inward air leakage is much less. As in the case of respiratory isolation for infection control, the use of particulate respirators assumes that the potential sources of TB transmission within health care facilities are identifiable, whereas experience and many published reports, old and new, suggest that unsuspected TB patients pose the greater risk (61,70,72,93,94). Unless respirators are used by workers caring for all patients, an unacceptable option, they would not have been useful for the majority of TB patients responsible for reported exposures in hospitals. The use of respirators to prevent TB transmission remains among the most contentious issues in this field. There are no data to show that the efficacy of any respirator program in preventing TB transmission. Two cost-effectiveness analyses (95,96) calculated the cost of preventing a single case of TB, based on the current HEPA respirator recommendations. Survey data from 159 Veterans Affairs facilities in the United States resulted in cost estimates of $7 million per case of TB prevented, and $100 million per life saved (95). At a 700-bed university teaching hospital in Virginia with 47 TB isolation rooms, the cost estimate to prevent a single TB case ranged from $1.3 million under optimal conditions to $18.5 million if respirator use was suboptimal and more workers than necessary were exposed (96). Although some may regard it unethical to consider the economic cost of lowering risks for workers, another view holds that it would be more unethical not to consider cost because the large sums of money spent on respirators would be unavailable for other, potentially more cost-effective interventions. Whereas the broad application of high-efficiency, personal respiratory protection appears to result in expenditures well out of proportion with the risk, selective use of less costly respirators of sufficient efficacy by those at greatest risk pushes the cost efficacy analysis back toward an acceptable balance. A more recent survey of the cost of N-95 respirators and a fit testing program for four urban and one rural community hospital are more reasonable, although not inexpensive (97). The projected median annual cost of N-95 respirators was approximately $62,000, with almost another $20,000 needed for a fit testing program.

In view of both the potential utility and the inherent limitations of personal respirators to prevent TB transmission and the cost considerations just discussed, efforts to better tailor the application of respirators of various efficiencies to specific TB risks are essential. Fennelly and Nardell (56) published a model that takes into consideration levels of risk, levels of ventilation, and the utility of various levels of respiratory protection. Until data are available to support or refute the cost-effectiveness of specific applications, the following recommendations should serve as a compromise position between views that at one extreme would require full respiratory protection for large numbers of hospital workers and at the other would greatly limit the respirator requirement to demonstrably high-risk settings where environmental controls are lacking.

Respirators are currently recommended for three specific health care settings: isolation rooms, high-risk procedure rooms, and the transport of potentially infectious patients by closed vehicles (15). As noted, patients on therapy in isolation rooms are unlikely to be the most important sources of transmission. Relatively few persons should be exposed, and, by necessity, many suspect patients in isolation do not have TB. Identifying high-risk persons before transport in a closed vehicle poses a problem similar to isolation, but these individuals are not on therapy, so respiratory protection is appropriate. The use of effective respirators during high-risk procedures is not controversial, especially in institutions where MDR-TB is common. Institutions should be given greater freedom to establish an appropriate level of respiratory protection for workers, based on community and institutional data on risk, as detailed in current CDC guidelines (15). The selection of respirators is discussed in detail.

Much of the controversy over respirator use was quieted when the National Institute of Occupational Safety and Health revised its certification procedure and established N-95 respirators as the appropriate level of respiratory protection for health care facilities (98). N-95 respirators come in a variety of shapes and sizes, are relatively inexpensive, and are only slightly more uncomfortable than surgical masks. Unfortunately, the National Institute of Occupational Safety and Health recommends and OSHA requires that all respirators must be fit tested as part of a respirator program, even though there is growing (as yet unpublished) evidence that the fit testing of disposable respirators does not correlate with greater protection. Ironically, new models of disposable respirators are becoming available that fit most workers without fit testing. Workers who cannot be fitted to any negative-pressure respirator are required to use a positive-pressure respirator at even greater cost, inconvenience, and potential interference with work. Finally, hospitals are complex institutions where patients, physicians, nurses, students, volunteers, visitors, and countless ancillary personnel interact. Neither limiting access to patients in isolation nor supplying effective respiratory protection to all those who should have legitimate access to these patients is entirely satisfactory.

Respirator Selection

From an industrial hygiene perspective, there are three factors to consider in respirator selection: (a) the nature of the hazard, (b) the potential for leakage around the respirator, and (c) the efficiency of the filter material. As already emphasized, a broader perspective on respirator use includes a number of other parameters, including the practical consequences for both workers and their patients and the likelihood that respirators will be in use when the hazard is at hand.

This discussion deals with respirators for HCWs. The selection of a mask for a potentially infectious patient is an entirely different matter. Masks on patients are stigmatizing and should be used only for those patients unable or unwilling to cover coughs or sneezes with a hand or tissue. Any barrier at the mouth, including a hand or tissue, serves to trap some of the relatively large respiratory droplets that would otherwise evaporate into droplet nuclei. No ordinary mask or respirator can contain the force or volume of air expelled in vigorous coughing. For the purpose of stopping large respiratory droplets, neither fit nor filtration efficiency is critical. When masking the patient is necessary, an ordinary tied or cup surgical mask will suffice. When masks become wet with secretions, they could in theory become effective atomizers when the patient coughs. However, testing N-95 respirators found no significant reaerosolization of bacteria with simulated violent coughing or sneezing (99).

Risk Assessment: Tuberculosis Versus Multidrug-Resistant Tuberculosis

The nature of the hazard is of particular importance in respirator selection. For atmospheres of modest risk (i.e., drug-susceptible TB), the requirements for respiratory protection need not be as strict as for exposure to atmospheres where inadequate protection might result in substantial morbidity or mortality (i.e., MDR-TB). In the former case, infection of a HCW is not desirable but is usually treatable. In the latter case, there is no proven preventive treatment, and even treatment of active disease is fraught with hazards. Unfortunately, the presence of MDR-TB is often not known or suspected at the time of the initial clinical contact. Fortunately, MDR-TB has been a regional phenomenon in the United States, and its incidence has been declining. Globally, however, MDR-TB is increasing in many parts of the world, a phenomenon that will be reflected in TB cases among the foreign born. If exposure to MDR-TB is a rational concern in an institution, use of powered air purifying respirators is justified for all aerosol-generating procedures. Ideally, respirator choices should be institution and region specific, based in part on the prevalence of MDR-TB.

Face Seal Leakage

Face seal leakage represents the entrance of air between the respirator and the face of the HCW. This represents the most important variable degrading the protectiveness of respirators (100–102). Face seal leakage is affected by a number of factors including match between size of the face piece and facial size, facial hair, poor respirator positioning, incorrect placement of head straps, facial oils, perspiration leading to slippage, and damage to the respirator.

In theory, face seal leakage can be minimized by two components of a respirator program: training on proper respirator usage and fit testing. Quantitative fit testing is possible for nondisposable respirators, but only qualitative fit testing applies to disposable personal respirators and is required by OSHA before respirator selection. As already noted, there is growing evidence that qualitative fit testing disposable respirators is relatively ineffective. There are also new models of disposable N-95 respirators that appear to fit well without fit testing. Many respirators can and should also be fit checked at the time of each use. Given the limited availability of respirator sizes and the inability to quantitatively fit test personal respirators, the potential for significant face seal leakage exists. Estimates for face seal leakage for personal respirators range from 10% to 20%. In addition, filter leakage and respirator deterioration owing to repeated usage are of concern. In contrast, positive air pressure respirators and line respirators can be quantitatively fit tested and have an estimated face leakage rate of only 2%, a fivefold greater level of protection compared with negative-pressure respirators (92).

Efficiency of Respirator Filtration

The reduction of transmission of TB particles through filter material is accomplished by the impaction of particles on the fibers of the material or by electrostatic attraction. Five factors affect leakage of aerosols through a filter: (a) the filtration characteristics of each type of filter, (b) size distribution of the aerosol, (c) linear velocity through the material, (d) filter loading, and (e) electrostatic charges on the filter or aerosol. There are no field trial data demonstrating that personal respiratory protection of any kind is effective in preventing TB transmission. However, as with ventilation, air filtration, and UV irradiation, basic principles can be applied in the absence of data. The ability of respirators to protect workers from particular airborne hazards is well established. To the extent that personal respirators can reduce the number of inhaled droplet nuclei, they should reduce the chance of infection. A respirator that is only 80% efficient against droplet nuclei is not useless if it is worn at the time of exposure. An 80% efficient respirator is equivalent in protective value to increasing ventilation five times or a fivefold reduction in the duration of exposure. Given the engineering difficulties of even doubling ventilation and the administrative difficulty of reducing exposure time, the benefits of less than fully efficient respirators cannot be dismissed. It is important to recognize that as part of a full infection control program, respirators need not be 100% efficient to be useful. In the example of transmission associated with bronchoscopy cited in the discussion of ventilation, correcting deficient ventilation would have reduced the number of persons infected from ten to two or three. Together with the improved ventilation, a respirator that was only 80% efficient (combined face seal leakage and filtration) would have been nearly fully protective against the most infectious case of TB on record (61). At very dilute particulate concentrations, increments in respirator filtration efficiency, as with increased ventilation, add increasingly small increments to protection (56).

CONCLUSIONS

To the extent that diagnosis, treatment, administrative controls, and effective environmental precautions substantially reduce the already low risk of transmission from patients with known or suspected TB, respirators may add only marginally to worker protection. In high-risk settings (high exposure or MDR-TB), respirator benefits are likely to be more important. The cost-effectiveness of individual interventions to prevent TB infections should be assessed for institutions at different levels of TB risk, including the risk of MDR-TB. A range of respirator options should be available, depending on the estimated risk of TB, with HEPA and positive-pressure respirators reserved for high-risk procedures, especially in areas where MDR-TB is prevalent. Institutions caring for TB patients that have demonstrable safety records using their own combinations of administrative, environmental, and personal respirator protection should not be required to meet arbitrary federal standards for which no evidence of efficacy exists.

REFERENCES

1. Sepkowitz KA. Tuberculosis and the health care worker: a historical perspective. *Ann Intern Med* 1994;120:71–79.
2. Dufault P. Tuberculosis infection among nurses and medical students in sanatoriums and general hospitals. *N Engl J Med* 1941;224:711–715.
3. Fishberg M. *Pulmonary tuberculosis*, 4th ed. Philadelphia: Lea & Febiger, 1932.
4. Mann T. *The magic mountain.* New York: Alfred A. Knopf, 1924.
5. Chapin CV, eds. Infections by air. In: *Sources and modes of infection.* New York: John Wiley & Sons, 1910.
6. Wells W. On air-borne infection: II. Droplets and droplet nuclei. *Am J Hyg* 1934;20:611–618.
7. Wells W. *Airborne contagion and air hygiene.* Cambridge, MA: Harvard University Press, 1955.
8. Wells WF, Wells MF, Wilder TS. The environmental control of epidemic contagion: I. An epidemiologic study of radiant disinfection of air in day schools. *Am J Hyg* 1942;35:97–121.
9. Subcommittee for the Evaluation of Methods of Control of Airborne Infections. Present status of the control of airborne infections. *Am J Public Health* 1947;37:13–22.
10. Riley RL. What nobody needs to know about airborne infection. *Am J Respir Crit Care Med* 2001;163:7–8.
11. Riley R, Wells W, Mills C, et al. Air hygiene in tuberculosis: quantitative studies of infectivity and control in a pilot ward. *Am Rev Tuberc Pulmonary Dis* 1957;75:420–431.
12. Riley RL. Aerial dissemination of pulmonary tuberculosis. The Burns Amberson Lecture. *Am Rev Tuber Pulmonary Dis* 1957;76:931–941
13. Riley R, Mills C, O'Grady F. Infectiousness of air from a tuberculosis ward—ultraviolet irradiation of infected air: comparative infectiousness of different patients. *Am Rev Respir Dis* 1962;84:511–525.
14. Menzies D, Fanning A, Yuan L, et al. Tuberculosis among health care workers. *N Engl J Med* 1995;332:92–98.
15. CDC. Guideline for preventing the transmission of *Mycobacterium tuberculosis* in health-care facilities, 1994. Centers for Disease Control and Prevention. *MMWR Recomm Rep* 1994;43:1–132.
16. Cauthen GM, Snider DE Jr, Onorato IM. Boosting of tuberculin sensitivity among Southeast Asian refugees. *Am J Respir Crit Care Med* 1994;149:1597–1600.
17. Rivera P, Fella P, Hale M, et al. Two-step tuberculin skin testing (TST) is practical and necessary for screening all new employees. *Am J Infect Control* 1995;23:352–356.
18. Panlilio AL, Burwen DR, Curtis AB. Tuberculin skin testing surveillance of health care personnel. *Clin Infect Dis* 2002;35:219–227.
19. Menzies R, Vissandjee B, Rocher I. The booster effect in two-step tuberculin testing among young adults in Montreal. *Ann Intern Med* 1994;120:190–198.
20. Blumberg HM, Watkins DL, Berschling JD, et al. Preventing the nosocomial transmission of tuberculosis. *Ann Intern Med* 1995;122:658–663.
21. Greenaway C, Menzies D, Fanning A, et al. Canadian Collaborative Group in nosocomial Transmission of Tuberculosis. Delay in diagnosis among hospitalized patients with active tuberculosis—predictors and outcomes. *Am J Respir Crit Care Med* 2002;165:927–933.
22. Snider DE Jr, Cauthen GM. Tuberculin skin testing of hospital employees: infection, "boosting," and two-step testing. *Am J Infect Control* 1984;12:305–311.
23. Bailey TC, Fraser VJ, Spitznagel EL, et al. Risk factors for a positive tuberculin skin testing among employees of an urban, Midwestern teaching hospital. *Ann Intern Med* 1995;122:580–585.
24. Larsen NM, Biddle CL, Sotir MJ, et al. Risk of tuberculin skin test conversion among health care workers: occupational vs community exposure and infection *Clin Infect Dis* 2002;35:796–801.
25. Louther J, Rivera P, Feldman J, et al. Risk of tuberculin conversion according to occupation among health care workers at a New York City hospital. *Am J Respir Crit Care Med* 1997;156:201–205.
26. Lundgren R, Norrman E, Asberg I. Tuberculosis infection transmitted by autopsy. *Tubercle* 1987;68:147–150.
27. Templeton G, Illing L, Young L, et al. The risk of transmission of *Mycobacterium tuberculosis* at the bedside and during autopsy. *Ann Intern Med* 1995;15:955–956.

28. Meade G. The prevention of primary tuberculous infections in medical students: the autopsy as a source of primary infection. *Am Rev Tuberc* 1948;58:675–683.

29. Kantor HS, Poblete R, Pusateria SL. Nosocomial transmission of tuberculosis from unsuspected disease. *Am J Med* 1988;84: 833–838.

30. Pike RM. Laboratory-associated infections: incidence, fatalities, causes and prevention. *Annu Rev Microbiol* 1979;33:41–66.

31. Collins C, Grange J. Tuberculosis acquired in laboratory and necropsy rooms. *Commun Dis Public Health* 1999;2:161–167.

32. Malasky C, Jordan T, Potulski F, et al. Occupational tuberculous infections among pulmonary physicians in training. *Am Rev Respir Dis* 1990;142:505–507.

33. Fagen MJ Poland G. Tuberculin skin testing in medical students: a survey of U.S. Medical schools. *Ann Intern Med* 1994;120:930–931.

34. Blumberg HM, Sotir M, Erwin M, et al. Risk of house staff tuberculin skin test conversion in an area with a high incidence of tuberculosis. *Clin Infect Dis* 1998;27:826–833.

35. Hutton MD, Stead WW, Cauthen GM, et al. Nosocomial transmission of tuberculosis associated with a draining abscess. *J Infect Dis* 1990;161:286–295.

36. Kassim S, Zuber P, Wiktor SZ. Tuberculin skin testing to assess the occupational risk of *Mycobacterium tuberculosis* infection among health care workers in Abidjan, Cote d'Ivoire. *Int J Tuberc Lung Dis* 2000;4:321–326.

37. Wilkinson D Gilks CF. Increasing frequency of tuberculosis among staff in a South African district hospital: impact of the HIV epidemic on the supply side of health care. *Trans R Soc Trop Med Hyg* 1998;92:500–502.

38. Eyob G, Gebeyhu M, Goshu S, et al. Increase in tuberculosis incidence among the staff working at the Tuberculosis Demonstration and Training Centre in Addis Ababa, Ethiopia: a retrospective cohort study (1989–1998). *Int J Tuberc Lung Dis* 2002; 6:85–88.

39. Do AN , Limpakarnjarat K, Uthaivoravit W, et al. Increased risk of *Mycobacterium tuberculosis* infection related to the occupational exposures of health care workers in Chiang Rai, Thailand. *Int J Tuberc Lung Dis* 1999;3:377–381.

40. Silva VM, Cunha AJ, Oliveira JR, et al. Medical students at risk of nosocomial transmission of *Mycobacterium tuberculosis*. *Int J Tuberc Lung Dis* 2000;4:420–426.

41. Kruuner A, Danilovitsh M, Pehme L, et al. Tuberculosis as an occupational hazard for health care workers in Estonia. *Int J Tuberc Lung Dis* 2001;5:170–176.

42. Nardell E, McInnis B, Thomas B, et al. Exogenous reinfection with tuberculosis in a shelter for the homeless. *N Engl J Med* 1986;315:1570–1575.

43. Schluger NW, Huberman R, Holzman R, et al. Screening for infection and disease as a tuberculosis control measure among indigents in New York City, 1994–1997. *Int J Tuberc Lung Dis* 1999;3:281–286.

44. Barnes PF, Yang Z, Pogoda JM, et al. Foci of tuberculosis transmission in central Los Angeles. *Am J Respir Crit Care Med* 1999;159:1081–1086.

45. Nardell EA. Tuberculosis in homeless, residential care facilities, prisons, nursing homes, and other close communities. *Semin Respir Infect* 1989;4:206–215.

46. Brickner P, Vincent R, Nardell E, et al. Ultraviolet upper room air disinfection for tuberculosis control: an epidemiological trial. *J Healthcare Safety Compliance Infect Control* 2000;4: 123–131.

47. Etkind S, Boutotte J, Ford J, et al. Treating hard-to-treat tuberculosis patients in Massachusetts.*Semin Respir Infect* 1991;6: 273–282.

48. Singleton L, Turner M, Haskal R, et al. Long-term hospitaliza-tion for tuberculosis control. Experience with a medical-psychosocial inpatient unit. *JAMA* 1997;278:838–842.

49. Stead WW. Special problems in tuberculosis. Tuberculosis in the elderly and in residents of nursing homes, correctional facilities, long-term care hospitals, mental hospitals, shelters for the homeless, and jails. *Clin Chest Med* 1989;10:397–405.

50. Puisis M, Feinglass J, Lidow E, et al. Radiographic screening for tuberculosis in a large urban county jail. *Public Health Rep* 1996;111:330–334.

51. Jones TF, Schaffner W. Miniature chest radiograph screening for tuberculosis in jails: a cost-effectiveness analysis. *Am J Respir Crit Care Med* 2001;164:77–81.

52. Stead WW. Undetected tuberculosis in prison. Source of infection for community at large. *JAMA* 1978;240:2544–2547.

53. Snider DE Jr, Hutton MD. Tuberculosis in correctional institutions. *JAMA* 1989;261:436–437.

54. Valway SE, Greifinger RB, Papania M, et al. Multidrug-resistant tuberculosis in the New York State prison system, 1990–1991. *J Infect Dis* 1994;170:151–156.

55. Holden C. Stalking a killer in Russia's prisons. *Science* 1999; 286:1670.

56. Fennelly K, Nardell E. The relative efficacy of respirators and room ventilation in preventing occupational tuberculosis. *Infect Control Hosp Epidemiol* 1998;19:754–759.

57. Menzies D, Fanning A, Yuan L, et al. Hospital ventilation and risk for tuberculous infection in Canadian health care workers. Canadian Collaborative Group in Nosocomial Transmission of TB. *Ann Intern Med* 2000;133:779–789.

58. Nardell E, Keegan J, Cheney S, et al. Airborne infection: theoretical limits of protection achievable by building ventilation. *Am Rev Respir Dis* 1991;144:302–306.

59. Riley E, Murphy G, Riley R. Airborne spread of measles in a suburban elementary school. *Am J Epidemiol* 1978;107:421–432.

60. Riley RL, Wells WF, Mills CC, et al. Air hygiene in tuberculosis: quantitative studies of infectivity and control in a pilot ward. *Am Rev Tuberc Pulmonary Dis* 1957;75:420–431.

60a. Riley RL, Nardell EA. *Plant technology and safety management series, no. 1.* Oakbrook Terrace, IL: The Joint Commission on Accreditation of Healthcare Organizations, 1993.

61. Catanzaro A. Nosocomial tuberculosis. *Am Rev Respir Dis* 1982; 123:559–562.

62. Riley RL, Mills CC, O'Grady R, et al. Infectiousness of air from a tuberculosis ward—ultraviolet irradiation of infected air: Comparative infectiousness of different patients. *Am Rev Respir Dis* 1962;84:511–525.

63. Sultan L, Nyka C, Mills C, et al. Tuberculosis disseminators—a study of the variability of aerial infectivity of tuberculosis patients. *Am Rev Respir Dis* 1960;82:358–369.

64. Small PM, Hopewell PC, Singh SP, et al. The epidemiology of tuberculosis in San Francisco. A population-based study using conventional and molecular methods. *N Engl J Med* 1994; 330:1703–1709.

65. Hutton DM, Stead WW, Cauthen GM, et al. Nosocomial transmission of tuberculosis associated with a draining abscess. *J Infect Dis* 1990;161:286–295.

66. Calder RA, Duclos P, Wilder MH, et al. *Mycobacterium tuberculosis* transmission in a health clinic. *Bull Int Union Tuberc Lung Dis* 1991;66:103–106.

67. Riley R, Nardell E. Clearing the air: the theory and application of ultraviolet air disinfection. *Am Rev Respir Dis* 1989;139: 286–294.

68. Lindberg P. Improving hospital ventilation systems for tuberculosis infection control. Joint Commission: 1993 *Plant Technology and Safety Management (PTSM) Series* Oakbrook Terrace, IL: The Joint Commission on Accreditation of Healthcare Organizations. 1993;No. 1:19–23.

69. Keene JH, Sansone EB. Airborne transfer of contaminants in ventilated spaces. *Lab Anim Sci* 1984;34:453–457.
70. Riley R. Ultraviolet air disinfection: rationale for whole building irradiation. *Infect Control Hosp Epidemiol* 1994;15:324–325.
71. Riley RL, Kaufmann JE. Air disinfection in corridors by upper air irradiation with ultraviolet. *Arch Environ Health* 1971;22:551–553.
72. Scott B, Schmid M, Nettlman MD. Early identification and isolation of inpatients at high risk for tuberculosis. *Arch Intern Med* 1994;154:326–330.
73. ASHRAE. *Indoor air quality position document*. Atlanta: American Society of Heating, Refrigerating and Air Conditioning Engineers, 2001.
74. Iseman MD. A leap of faith. What can we do to curtail intrainstitutional transmission of tuberculosis? *Ann Intern Med* 1992;117:251–253.
75. Marier RL, Nelson T. A ventilation-filtration unit for respiratory isolation. *Infect Control Hosp Epidemiol* 1993;14:700–705.
76. Nardell E. Fans, filters, or rays? Pros and cons of the current environmental tuberculosis control technologies. *Infect Control Hosp Epidemiol* 1993;14:681–685.
77. Macher JM. The use of germicidal lamps to control tuberculosis in health care facilities. *Infect Control Hosp Epidemiol* 1993;14:723–728
78. Riley R, Permutt S, Kaufman J. Room air disinfection by ultraviolet irradiation of upper room air. *Arch Environ Health* 1971;23:35–40.
79. Riley R, Permutt S. Room air disinfection by ultraviolet irradiation of upper air—air mixing and germicidal effectiveness. *Arch Environ Health* 1971;22:208–219.
80. Riley R, Permutt S, Kaufman J. Convection, air mixing, and ultraviolet air disinfection in rooms. *Arch Environ Health* 1971;22:200–207.
81. Riley RL, Kaufman JE. Effect of relative humidity on the inactivation of airborne *Serratia marcescens* by ultraviolet irradiation. *Appl Microbiol* 1972;23:1113–1120.
82. Riley R, Knight M, Middlebrook G. Ultraviolet susceptibility of BCG and virulent tubercle bacilli. *Am Rev Respir Dis* 1976;113:413–418.
83. Bruls W. Transmission of human epidermis and stratum corneum as a function of thickness in the ultraviolet and visible wavelengths. *Photochem Photobiol* 1984;40:485–494.
84. Sliney D, Grandolfo M, eds. *Ultraviolet radiation and the eye*. New York: Plenum Press, 1990:237–242.
85. Forbes P, Urbach F. Experimental modifications of carcinogenesis I. Fluorescent whitening agents and shortwave ultraviolet irradiation. *Food Cosmet Toxicol* 1974;13:335–337.
86. Sterenborg H. The dose-response relationship of tumorigenesis

by ultraviolet radiation of 254 nm. *Photochem Photobiol* 1988;47:245–253.
87. Jeevan A, Kripke M. Alteration of the immune response to *M. bovis* BCG in mice exposed chronically to low dose of UV irradiation. *Cell Immunol* 1990;130:32.
88. Zmudzka B, Beer J. Activation of human immunodeficiency virus by ultraviolet radiation. *Photochem Photobiol* 1990;52:1153.
89. Zmudzka B, Miller S, Jacobs M, et al. Medical UV exposures and HIV activation. *Photochem Photobiol* 1996;64:246–263.
90. Zmudzka BZ, Beer JZ. Ultraviolet therapy and patients with HIV infection. *Arch Dermatol* 1998;134:1025–1026.
91. Akaraphanth R, Lim HW. HIV, UV and immunosuppression. *Photodermatol Photoimmunol Photomed* 1999;1:28–31.
92. National Institute for Occupational Safety and Health. *Criteria for a recommended standard for occupational exposure to ultraviolet radiation*. Cincinnati: National Institute for Occupational Safety and Health, 1972.
93. Mathur P, Sacks L, Auten G, et al. Delayed diagnosis of pulmonary tuberculosis in city hospitals. *Arch Intern Med* 1994;154:306–310.
94. Lin-Greenberg A, Anez T. Delay in respiratory isolation of patients with pulmonary tuberculosis and human immunodeficiency virus infection. *Am J Infect Control* 1992;20:16–18.
95. Nettleman MD, Fredrickson M, Good NL, et al. Tuberculosis control strategies: the cost of particulate respirators. *Ann Intern Med* 1994;121:37–40.
96. Adal KA, Anglim AM, Palumbo CL, et al. The use of high-efficiency particulate air-filter respirators to protect hospital workers from tuberculosis. A cost-effectiveness analysis. *N Engl J Med* 1994;331:169–173.
97. Kellerman SE, Tokars JI, Jarvis WR. The costs of healthcare worker respiratory protection and fit testing programs. *Infect Control Hosp Epidemiol* 1998;19:629–634.
98. National Institute of Occupational Safety and Health. *Respiratory protective devices* (42 CFR part 84). Cincinnati: National Institute for Occupational Safety and Health, 1995.
99. Qian Y, Willeke K, Grinshpun SA, et al. Performance of N95 respirators: reaerosolization of bacteria and solid particles. *Am Ind Hyg Assoc J* 1997;58:876–880.
100. Chen CC, Lehtimaki M, Willeke K. Aerosol penetration through filtering face-pieces and respirator cartridges. *Am Ind Hyg Assoc J* 1992;53:566–574.
101. Hinds WC, Kraske G. Performance of dust respirators with facial seal leaks: experimental. *Am Ind Hyg Assoc J* 1989;48:836–841.
102. Chen CC, Ruuskanen J, Pilacinski W, et al. Filter and leak penetration characteristics of a dust and mist filtering facepiece. *Am Ind Hyg Assoc J* 1989;51:632–639.

THE ROLE OF INTERNATIONAL ORGANIZATIONS IN GLOBAL TUBERCULOSIS CONTROL

RICHARD J. O'BRIEN

Historically, two international organizations have played pivotal roles in promotion of tuberculosis (TB) control globally through promulgation of technical standards and guidelines, provision of technical and material assistance to national TB control programs (NTPs), training of NTP staff, and research activities in support of control programs. These are the International Union Against Tuberculosis and Lung Disease (IUATLD), a nongovernmental organization based in Paris, and the World Health Organization (WHO). More recently, major foundations, including the Bill and Melinda Gates Foundation and the Rockefeller Foundation, began to provide large amounts of funding in support of specific projects and activities, including targeted support for research aimed at the development of new tools and support for the creation of novel mechanisms and organizations to further TB control and set the stage for TB elimination. These organizations include private-public sector partnerships, such as the Global Alliance for TB Drug Development (TB Alliance).

This chapter presents brief historical perspectives of the IUATLD and WHO and details those activities that have led to the establishment of the global TB control strategy popularly known as DOTS (*d*irectly *o*bserved *t*herapy, *s*hort course). It describes the development of the Stop TB Partnership, a global coalition of countries, donor agencies, and technical and research organizations that have developed a global plan for the coordination of control activities, and concludes with a summary of the work of selected foundations supporting TB control and the recently established TB Alliance.

INTERNATIONAL UNION AGAINST TUBERCULOSIS AND LUNG DISEASE

The IUATLD is the oldest international, health-related nongovernmental organization, with its roots tracing back

to the first international conference on internal medicine in Paris in 1867. Subsequently, a series of meetings led to the establishment of an international coordinating bureau in Berlin 1902, with representation from national voluntary TB organizations charged with the planning of international TB meetings that were held every 4 years. After the bureau's offices were destroyed during World War I, the organization was officially established as the International Union Against Tuberculosis in 1920 and based in Paris. In 1986, its name was changed to the IUATLD to reflect increasing interest in other lung diseases, notably asthma, acute respiratory infection in children, and smoking-related lung disease.

The Early Years

In its early years of existence, the IUATLD's focus was on the TB problem in the member associations' own countries, largely in North America and Europe, and its activities were primarily devoted to the organization of international meetings and the publication of its journal *The Bulletin of the International Union Against Tuberculosis*. By the early 1960s, as the TB epidemic came under control in those countries, the IUATLD began to focus on TB in developing countries. These activities were supported by funding from its more affluent members and evolved into the IUATLD's Mutual Assistance Programme, which was formally established in 1961. The purpose of this program was to provide both technical and material support to NTPs in developing countries. Specific activities included strengthening the leadership of NTPs, the organization of training workshops and provision of educational materials, NTP staff travel to both regional and international meetings, and operational research projects to address NTP deficiencies and evaluate innovative approaches to providing TB services. During the first 15 years of its existence, the Mutual Assistance Program conducted these activities in 18 low-income countries in Africa, Asia, and Latin America, with the majority of

R. J. O'Brien: Research and Evaluation Branch, Division of Tuberculosis Elimination, Centers for Disease Control and Prevention, Atlanta, Georgia.

support coming from Canada, The Netherlands, and MIS-EREOR, a German charitable organization.

By the mid-1970s, several changes had occurred in TB control that redirected the IUATLD's efforts to focus more specifically on the establishment of effective NTPs in a limited number of countries. These changes included decreased support from many constituent organizations that began to focus on other respiratory health problems as TB rates decreased greatly in industrialized countries, withdrawal of support for TB control by the WHO with its new emphasis on the establishment of primary health care (see later), and technical advances in TB diagnosis and treatment together with a realization that widespread use of bacille Calmette–Guérin vaccination had little impact on reducing the TB epidemic.

Despite these changes, the IUATLD was able to maintain its focus and contribute significantly to the development of model NTPs in developing countries, largely owing to the efforts of two outstanding personalities, Annik Rouillon and Karel Styblo. As Executive Director of the IUATLD, Annik Rouillon was tireless in advocating for support for IUATLD activities and for TB control in low-income countries. Switzerland and Norway, together with continued Dutch support, became the IUATLD's primary donors.

Building the Scientific Basis for Effective Tuberculosis Control

Certainly, the IUATLD's most outstanding contribution to TB control was that of Karel Styblo in establishing highly effective NTPs, beginning with his work in Tanzania. Using guidelines promulgated in a 1974 WHO Expert Committee Report on Tuberculosis, Styblo began working with the government of Tanzania in 1977 to establish a countrywide TB program that had a strong central unit for supervision and training but provided diagnostic and treatment services that were integrated into the general health services. Diagnosis was based on sputum acid-fast bacillus (AFB) smear examination of "TB suspects," i.e., persons with a chronic cough and other symptoms of TB presenting to health services. Treatment was ambulatory and used the regimen in general use at that time for low-income countries, 12 months of isoniazid and thiacetazone, supplemented with streptomycin for the first 2 months of treatment. Unfortunately, the initial results were disappointing with high rates of nonadherence and cure rates of less than 40%.

Undaunted, Styblo persuaded the Tanzanian program to adopt two major changes: provision of rifampin-based, short-course therapy using rifampin, isoniazid, pyrazinamide, and streptomycin for the first 2 months, followed by 6 months of isoniazid and thiacetazone. In multicenter clinical trials in East Africa conducted under the auspices of the British Medical Research Council and the leadership of Wallace Fox and Denis Mitchison, this regimen had been shown to be highly effective. For use in Tanzania, patients were hospitalized for the first 2 months where treatment could be easily supervised. The remainder of treatment was self-administered, with patients given monthly supplies of drug until completion of treatment. After a highly successful pilot study in one region of the country in 1982, this treatment strategy was gradually expanded and was countrywide by 1986. The success rate improved significantly, with cure rates of 75% or greater. Unfortunately, despite sustained success in achieving high cure rates, the anticipated impact of effective TB control in reducing TB transmission and leading to a reduction in TB incidence was not seen in Tanzania. The advent of human immunodeficiency virus (HIV) and acquired immunodeficiency syndrome (AIDS) has had a devastating effect on the TB situation in a number of sub-Saharan African countries, including Tanzania, seriously threatening the continued success of TB control.

With the successful implementation of the program in Tanzania, the essential elements of an effective NTP in a developing country were evaluated and firmly established: (a) government commitment to provide adequate staff and treatment facilities; (b) passive case finding based on sputum smear examination of persons with suspected TB; (c) administration of a standardized, short-course therapy regimen, with directly observed therapy (DOT) at least for the first 2 months [and whenever rifampin was administered to provide full protection against the emergence of multidrug-resistant (MDR) TB]; (d) a secure supply of high-quality drugs and diagnostic reagents, and (e) a system of recording and reporting with quarterly analysis of the outcome of treatment for all newly diagnosed smear-positive cases using standard definitions ("cured" as documented by sputum AFB smear negativity during the last 2 months of treatment, "treatment completed" without bacteriologic confirmation, "died," "lost" to follow-up, and "transferred" out of the health jurisdiction). Informed readers will recognize these as the elements of the DOTS strategy that has been adopted and successfully promulgated by WHO (see later).

In addition to these basic strategies, another essential element was incorporated into the program: systematic training and monitoring conducted by staff at the central unit with close scrutiny paid to the quarterly reports of newly registered patients with newly diagnosed AFB smear–positive pulmonary TB and cohort analysis of treatment outcome. Finally, two additional standardized regimens were used: the nonrifampin-containing, 12-month regimen for most newly diagnosed patients with extrapulmonary TB and AFB sputum smear–negative pulmonary TB patients and an 8-month, rifampin-containing retreatment regimen for patients failing the initial regimen for new smear-positive cases. With the advent of HIV, ethambutol replaced both streptomycin and thiacetazone, and the 12-month regimen has been gradually abandoned. The retreatment regimen used rifampin, isoniazid, pyrazinamide, and ethambutol for 3 months, supplemented with streptomycin for the first 2 months, and then rifampin, isoniazid, and ethambutol for 5 months. In the absence of rifampin resistance that was essentially nonexistent in Tanzania, this regimen was highly effective in curing failure and relapse patients, many of whom had either initial or acquired resistance to isoniazid and thiacetazone.

Subsequently, under Styblo's leadership, the IUATLD assisted in the implementation of similar collaborative programs in a number of other countries, including Mozambique, Benin, Nicaragua, and Malawi, providing evidence that effective NTPs could be established in the most difficult of circumstances, including civil war. In the late 1980s, with assistance from the World Bank, Chris Murray teamed with Rouillon and Styblo to conduct a cost-effectiveness analysis of TB control based on data from these collaborative programs. Their work found TB treatment of AFB smear–positive patients under these programs to be among the most cost-effective of all available health interventions in low-income countries, including childhood immunization and oral rehydration for diarrheal illness. This work was among several of the more important factors that has led to a significant rebirth of interest and investment in global TB control that began in the early 1990s and greatly accelerated as the 20th century came to a close.

Keeping the Faith

Although its role in provision of direct technical assistance to NTPs has somewhat lessened with the subsequent involvement of a large number of other donor organizations and countries in global TB control under the Stop TB Partnership (see later), the IUATLD continues to play an essential role in global TB. Beginning in the mid-1990s, the IUATLD began to organize yearly World Tuberculosis Conferences that for several preceding decades had been held every 4 years. In addition to the scientific program, the conference provides an opportunity for a large number of individuals interested in global TB control to meet and plan coordinated activities. The IUATLD now has a new journal, the *International Journal for Tuberculosis and Lung Disease* that has become in a short time the preeminent biomedical journal for the publication of articles of interest to those working in this field. It has continued a long-established tradition of conducting training courses for national program managers and has developed a number of high-quality technical manuals that are freely available on the IUATLD website. Notable among these are monographs on the epidemiology of TB and on the scientific basis for TB control. Continuing a tradition of active engagement in research studies, the IUATLD has also established a clinical trials program for the conduct of programmatically relevant therapy trials through NTPs in Africa and Asia. Finally, through changes in its constitution, the IUATLD has

moved from an organization of constituent members of national TB associations to one that includes individual members that have been given an increasing voice in its work.

WORLD HEALTH ORGANIZATION

Early Activities

Soon after the establishment of the WHO in 1947, TB was given the highest priority, with a focus on bacille Calmette–Guérin vaccination that was the only widely available control measure at that time. With the advent of effective multidrug treatment for TB by the early 1950s, increased attention was given to case finding and treatment, although the optimal treatment regimen of isoniazid and paraaminosalicylic acid, with streptomycin for the initial portion of therapy, was too expensive for widespread use in developing countries. The availability of thiacetazone as an inexpensive replacement for paraaminosalicylic acid in the late 1950s made effective treatment more widely available, and WHO resources assisted in the establishment of vertical TB control programs in high-incidence countries with strong central units providing training and supervision down to the delivery level. With time, however, it became evident that such programs were unable to cope with the large number of patients in need of diagnostic and treatment services and that integration with general health services was needed. Based on operational research conducted by the British Medical Research Council in India, a model for such integration was developed. This emphasized the establishment of diagnostic and treatment services in the general health services with logistics, training, and supervision remaining the responsibility of a central TB program. The organizational principles for this model of TB control were laid out in the 1974 WHO Expert Committee report mentioned previously.

Unfortunately, the application of these principles for the establishment of effective TB control programs in low-income countries was the exception rather than the rule. Most countries could not or would not provide sufficient support to establish and manage efficient programs. The increased emphasis that the WHO placed on primary health care, beginning in the late 1970s, further weakened support for effective TB control programs. As the disease continued to wane in industrialized countries, interest in the global TB problem continued to lessen. By the late 1980s, the staff of the WHO's Tuberculosis Unit had dwindled to two professionals and one secretary.

Rebuilding: The Global Epidemic Rediscovered

Beginning in the late 1980s, the situation began to change dramatically, as interest in the global TB problem was reawakened. There were several major factors related to this reversal. As noted earlier, Styblo's demonstration that effective TB control in high-incidence countries was possible and the related finding that this intervention was among the most cost-effective of health interventions available in low-income countries provided strong evidence to help to convince funding agencies to invest in TB control. The WHO Tuberculosis Unit was reinvigorated with the appointment of a new director, Dr. Arata Kochi, in 1988. Under Kochi, the Unit issued a series of reports that quantified the unappreciated extent of the global burden of TB morbidity and mortality, resulting in the figures that are commonly mentioned today: eight million new cases and two million deaths per year, largely occurring among adults in their most productive ages. At the same time, TB began its resurgence in several industrialized countries, notably in the United States where outbreaks of MDRTB led to heightened public interest and concern.

It was perhaps in the area of advocacy and public education that the WHO Tuberculosis Unit was initially most successful. In 1991, the World Health Assembly called attention to the global problem, affirmed the principles of TB control as formulated earlier, and established the global targets of 70% detection of new, AFB smear–positive cases and 85% cure of detected cases by the year 2000. The Tuberculosis Unit began to issue a series of annual reports generally timed for release on World TB Day on March 24, commemorating Robert Koch's announcement in 1882 of his discovery of the tubercle bacillus. In the 1993 report, the Director General of the WHO declared TB to be a global public health emergency. The 1994 report provided data to indicate that, compared with AIDS and other tropical diseases, global funding for TB control was seriously deficient, especially considering the extent of the burden of disease.

Packaging and Promoting Directly Observed Therapy, Short Course

However, it was the 1995 report with its red wheel on the cover that was most noteworthy. This wheel had the word "stop" spelled out in lowercase letters with an outstretched hand signaling WHO's intention to halt the epidemic. When the wheel was rotated 180 degrees, the word changed to "dots" and the hand offered TB medications. The message was that DOTS was needed to stop the TB epidemic. In the following year's report, the WHO declared DOTS to be the public health breakthrough of the decade. Although it took the organization some time to resolve confusion over the term DOTS, in the end, declaring that the acronym referred to the strategy of comprehensive TB control rather than the narrow element of direct observation of treatment, it has become among the most successfully marketed terms for a health intervention in history. There was ensuing rapid acceptance of the DOTS strategy and successful implemen-

tation and expansion in a number of countries, with notable success in China and subsequently India, two countries that contain more than 40% of the global TB burden. Today, virtually all national health ministries advocate the DOTS strategy as their countries' TB control policy.

As increased publicity lead to greater worldwide interest in TB, funding for WHO and national TB control programs began to increase. This enabled staff in what had now become the WHO Global Tuberculosis Programme to increase activities in technical support to national programs as well as undertake a variety of surveillance activities and support applied and operational research aimed at the development of new control tools and the improvement of existing control programs. Most notable of the surveillance activities was the initiation of systematic surveillance for drug resistance and routine reporting of case finding and program performance based on treatment outcome of patients treated under DOTS programs. By 1997, 102 countries had adopted the DOTS strategy, an increase from only 19 countries in 1993. However, DOTS coverage was low, with only an estimated 35% of the world's TB patients living in areas with DOTS services. Although remarkable progress had been made, it was becoming apparent that the pace of change was too slow to have the anticipated impact. A sense of urgency grew from a meeting in London in 1998 when the WHO convened an *ad hoc* committee to review the constraints to DOTS expansion. At that meeting, the WHO announced that its 2,000 global targets would not be met and identified 16 key countries where progress was notably suboptimal.

Stop TB Partnership: Renewed Commitment

As the decade drew to a close, the remarkable progress of the Global Tuberculosis Programme and the WHO's leadership role in global TB control were threatened by a major internal reorganization as the leadership of the WHO changed. This reorganization resulted in the dissolution of the Global Tuberculosis Programme and the splitting of its functions throughout a new communicable disease program. Fortunately, a small unit, the Stop TB Initiative, was created that preserved the visibility of TB within the organization. The Stop TB Initiative was the indirect result of a movement that was conceived by several North American institutions in 1996 to develop a global TB plan that would describe the roles and responsibilities of the various global agencies, institutions, and governments interested in TB control. It also was spurred by a closely related activity funded by the George Soros Open Society Institute to calculate the costs of implementing effective TB control worldwide (the global TB investment plan).

A series of meetings coordinated by the Stop TB Initiative led to the proposal for the development of a partnership agreement to be adopted by both high-burden countries and donor countries and institutions outlining the specific activities to be undertaken jointly in support of DOTS expansion globally. In March 2000, the WHO convened a meeting in Amsterdam on TB and sustainable development attended by ministers of health and finance from the 20 countries that contribute 80% of the world's TB cases. The resulting Amsterdam Declaration to Stop TB that was adopted by the meeting participants called on all interested parties to join the Stop TB Initiative and bring all available resources to bear on TB control. The meeting also reset the date for meeting the global case finding and treatment targets to 2005. Subsequently, a series of meetings led to the development of the Global Plan to Stop TB that included a formal structure (Fig. 57.1) and governance for the Stop TB Partnership. This plan was formally adopted at the first Stop TB Partners Forum held in Washington, DC, in October 2001, a meeting attended by representatives of more than 120 organizations committed to global TB control.

The Stop TB Coordinating Board serves as the governing body of the Partnership. The Board is constituted to reflect the major interests of the Stop TB Partners, representing science, policy makers, financial donors, TB program managers, the private sector, civil society, and those concerned with advocacy and communications. The Board members represent their respective countries, regions, or organizations. The Board acts to support Stop TB partners according to agreed policy and strategy, to approve the work plan and budget of the Stop TB Secretariat, to mobilize adequate resources for partner activities, to coordinate and promote advocacy and social mobilization, and to review the progress of the implementation of the Global Plan. The Secretariat that is housed within the WHO is intended to carry out the mandates of the Board and assist the partners in their key activities. It serves to coordinate activities of its

partners in three important areas: information and communication, investment mechanisms, and coordination and mobilization. It also manages the Global TB Drug Facility (see later).

Many of the coordinated activities are carried out through the Stop TB Working Groups. Currently, there are three working groups dealing with programmatic issues and three with new tools development. The largest of these is the DOTS Expansion Working Group that focuses on assistance to the 22 highest burden countries in the context of the "Expanded DOTS Framework for Effective Tuberculosis Control" (Table 57.1). It is housed within the newly formed Stop TB Department that in effect reestablished the former Global Tuberculosis Programme. Each of these countries has developed a medium-term DOTS implementation plan that is technically sound, takes into consideration national health structures, and specifies outside collaborating partners for specific activities. Important in these activities is the identification of budget and resource gaps and outside institutions and agencies that are able to meet these needs. Several collaborative initiatives have developed in support of the aims of this working group. Notable among these is the TB Coalition for Technical Assistance, funded by the U.S. Agency for International Development, with membership currently limited to the WHO, IUATLD, the Centers for Disease Control and Prevention, American Lung Association, American Thoracic Society, and the Royal Netherlands Tuberculosis Control Association. The Tuberculosis Coalition for Technical Assistance aims to substantially improve and expand the capacity of the U.S. Agency for International Development to respond to the global TB epidemic by providing state-of-the-art, context-appropriate, technically sound and cost-effective consultation and technical assistance to high-incidence countries and U.S. Agency for International Development

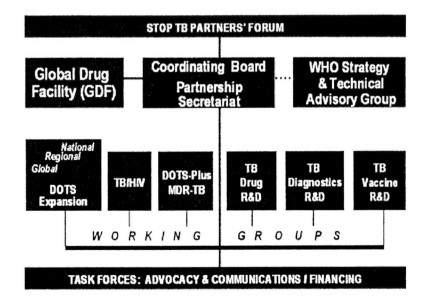

FIGURE 57.1. Stop TB Partnership framework.

TABLE 57.1. EXPANDED DIRECTLY OBSERVED TREATMENT, SHORT COURSE FRAMEWORK FOR EFFECTIVE TUBERCULOSIS CONTROL

Essential elements of directly observed treatment, short course

1. Sustained political commitment to increase human and financial resources and make tuberculosis control a nationwide activity and an integral part of the national health system.
2. Access to quality assured tuberculosis sputum microscopy for case detection among persons presenting with symptoms of tuberculosis, screening of individuals with prolonged cough by sputum microscopy, and special attention to case detection among human immunodeficiency virus–infected persons and other high-risk groups, e.g., persons in institutions.
3. Standardized chemotherapy to all confirmed cases of tuberculosis under proper case management conditions including direct observation of treatment; proper case management conditions imply technically sound and socially supportive treatment services.
4. Uninterrupted supply of quality-assured drugs with reliable drug procurement and distribution systems.
5. Recording and reporting system enabling outcome assessment of each patient and assessment of the overall program performance.

Basic operations for directly observed treatment, short course implementation

1. Establish a national tuberculosis program with a central unit.
2. Prepare a program development plan based on a systematic review of the current situation, with detailed information on budget, sources of funding, and responsibilities.
3. Prepare a program manual that includes the structure of the program, job descriptions, case definitions, detailed instructions on case finding/diagnosis and treatment, instructions for monitoring and reporting, and plans for drug distribution, stock keeping, and supervision.
4. Establish a recording and reporting system using the standardized format and definitions.
5. Plan and initiate a training program.
6. Establish a microscopy services network with a system for training and quality control.
7. Establish treatment services that include provision of directly observed treatment.
8. Secure a regular supply of drugs and diagnostics materials.
9. Design a plan of supervision.

Additional key operations

1. Information, education, communications, and social mobilization.
2. Involving private and voluntary health care providers.
3. Economic analyses and financial planning.
4. Operational research that is program based and problem solving.

Adapted from Stop TB, World Health Organization. An expanded DOTS framework for effective tuberculosis control. *Int J Tuberc Lung Dis* 2002;6:378–388.

missions, and complement and enlarge on existing global TB control efforts through the Stop TB Partnership and the DOTS Expansion Working Group.

The other two program-oriented working groups address specific problems that threaten TB control: the HIV/AIDS epidemic and the spreading problem of MDRTB. The association between TB and HIV is well known, and the spreading HIV epidemic is threatening the modest gains in TB control in a number of countries, particularly those in sub-Saharan Africa that have seen rates of TB increase four-fold and more. It has become evident that the DOTS strategy has had little impact on stemming the tide of HIV-associated TB in these settings. Although calls have been issued for closer collaboration between NTPs and AIDS control programs to address this problem, it is only in the past year or two that progress is being made. In part, this stems from the move to provide AIDS care, including antiretroviral medications, to AIDS patients in low-income countries. In addition, low-cost interventions to prevent opportunistic infections, including TB, have been shown to be effective in some settings, providing new incentives for persons to be tested for HIV infection. The purpose of the TB/HIV Working Group is to implement an expanded strategy for TB control in populations with a high HIV prevalence that consists of interventions against both TB (intensified case finding and cure and TB preventive therapy) and interventions against HIV (condoms, sexually transmitted disease treatment, needle exchange, and antiretroviral therapy). The Working Group and its partners are actively promoting close collaboration between NTPs and AIDS control programs in these activities. The Working Group has issued several important documents outlining the strategy and specific technical approaches to program implementation.

The DOTS-Plus Working Group that focuses on MDRTB aims to approve, conduct, and oversee pilot projects based on its technical guidelines and to improve access to second-line TB drugs for these projects. In 1998, after several years of sometimes acrimonious debate about the wisdom of allocating resources for treatment of patients with MDRTB when expansion of basic DOTS programs remained an urgent priority, the WHO and several of its partners, including the Harvard Partners in Health group, conceived DOTS-Plus, a strategy for the management of MDRTB. Based on the principle that these programs could only be implemented in areas where DOTS has been firmly and successfully established, several pilot projects are underway to evaluate the strategic approaches. One of the outstanding questions is whether drug susceptibility testing must be available for all suspected MDRTB patients or whether a standardized regimen of second-line drugs based on the prevailing susceptibility patterns of patients who fail standard treatment and retreatment might suffice. A notable accomplishment of this group, assisted by Médecins Sans Frontières, was reducing the cost of second-line drugs by more than 90%. Under the DOTS-Plus Working Group, the Green Light Committee was established to review applications for these concessionally priced second-line drugs in the context of DOTS-Plus demonstration projects. This entire effort has greatly benefited from the provision of a large grant from the Bill and Melinda Gates Foundation to the Harvard group for collaborative activities with the Peruvian NTP.

Three working groups are focusing on the development and assessment of new tools for TB control: drugs, diagnostics, and vaccines. The Working Group on TB Drug Development is housed within the Global Alliance for TB Drug Development, whose activities are described later. The Working Group on Diagnostics is coordinated by the United Nations Development Programme, World Bank, WHO Special Programme for Research and Training in Tropical Diseases and is closely related to the Programme for Research and Training in Tropical Diseases TB Diagnostics Initiative whose aim is to exploit technical advances in basic research to develop new diagnostic tests that are appropriate for use in low-income countries. The TB Diagnostics Initiative partners with industry, academic researchers, and national and local health officials to facilitate and accelerate the development of priority diagnostic tools by working jointly with industry to facilitate commercial development of necessary tools. Priorities are the development of low-cost diagnostics to supplement or replace sputum smear microscopy, with an emphasis on tests with increased sensitivity to improve the diagnosis of AFB smear–negative pulmonary TB and tests for the rapid diagnosis of rifampin-resistant TB.

The Working Group on New Vaccines builds on previous WHO efforts in defining a global research strategy for TB vaccine research and development and fosters partnerships among the different players in the public and private sectors. Its activities include defining a global vaccine research strategy, facilitating and coordinating vaccine

development efforts among academia, industry, and regulators, on the one hand, and the public health community as representatives of the end-user communities, on the other, supporting vaccine development approaches that are neglected by industry, promoting innovative partnerships to propel vaccine development and availability, and assisting in the conduct of clinical trials in developing countries. Important partners in this effort are the National Institutes of Health National Institute of Allergy and Infectious Disease that has developed the "Blueprint for TB Vaccine Development" and the Tuberculosis Vaccine Collaboration Program of the Sequella Global Tuberculosis Foundation.

The Global TB Drug Facility (GDF) is a mechanism to expand access to and availability of high-quality TB drugs to facilitate global DOTS expansion. By securing the timely supply of drugs for both NTPs and nongovernmental organizations that are implementing control programs, the GDF complements other activities designed to improve coverage and quality of global TB control. Insecure financing and shortages of TB drugs are frequent and serious in many parts of the world and have hampered DOTS expansion. Although poor drug supply is not unique to TB control, its impact may be especially severe. Drugs are essential to TB prevention and cure; inadequate and erratic supply can contribute to the emergence of MDRTB. Ensuring an uninterrupted supply of quality drugs through the GDF will free human and financial resources to address management, service delivery, training, supervision, and other services essential for scaling up DOTS. Initially begun with financial support from the Canadian International Development Agency, the GDF seeks to raise $250 million that it estimates is required to provide drugs to NTPs to treat ten million TB patients and achieve the year 2005 objectives. Through direct procurement mechanisms, the GDF has obtained standard first-line TB drugs and fixed-dose combinations at costs that are 30% less than those obtained through usual tender mechanisms. By mid-2002, 23 countries had been approved for GDF support and 11 of these had received drugs from the GDF.

Finally, DOTS expansion is benefiting from the newly created Global Fund to Fight AIDS, Tuberculosis, and Malaria. Spurred by a growing recognition of the extent and impact of HIV/AIDS, TB, and malaria, the leaders of the G8 countries that met in Okinawa in July 2000 announced year 2010 global targets for reduction in mortality from these three diseases. In response, the WHO organized an advocacy forum in Winterthur, Switzerland, in October 2000 that called for a new, global public-private partnership leading to strengthened cooperation, increased coordination, and greater investments aimed at these three diseases, with an overall goal of improving health outcomes. In April 2001, the U.N. Secretary General issued a call to action for the creation of a global fund to fight HIV/AIDS. Subsequently, declarations and financial commitments were issued, and by mid-2002, these contributions and pledges totaled $2 billion, a significant amount but still far short of the estimated need of $10 billion per year. The Global Fund to Fight AIDS, Tuberculosis, and Malaria was legally established as a foundation under Swiss law and issued its first call for proposals in early 2002. In April, the first grants were announced, which included an initial $54 million for direct support for TB control in 14 counties, including three with a focus on both HIV and TB. It is expected that this amount and the number of recipient countries will increase significantly in the next several years.

PRIVATE–PUBLIC PARTNERSHIPS AND NEW TOOLS FOR ELIMINATION

Foundation Support for Tuberculosis Research

Historically, the little funding available for TB research was provided by governments and nongovernmental organizations. As the 20th century ended, a new paradigm was created as the Bill and Melinda Gates Foundation was established. With an endowment of approximately $23 billion, the Foundation is actively supporting projects and research efforts aimed at improving global public health, with a focus on infectious diseases, including TB. The Foundation has provided $60 million for the development of new TB tools, specifically new diagnostics ($10 million to the WHO Special Programme for Research and Training in Tropical Diseases TDR), vaccines ($25 million to Sequella Global Tuberculosis Foundation), and drugs ($25 million to the TB Alliance).

Global Alliance for Tuberculosis Drug Development

It has been three decades since a major, new TB drug has been approved for use in the United States. The greatest impediment to new drug development has been the high cost and lengthy process of development coupled with the relatively small market, both domestic and global, for TB medications. In recognition of this problem, the Rockefeller Foundation, together with National Institutes of Health and several members of the Stop TB Partnership, organized a major meeting on the topic that was held in Cape Town, South Africa, in February 2000. The meeting brought together scientists, public health officials, TB experts, and representatives of pharmaceutical companies and donor organizations interested in TB to discuss the science of TB drug discovery and development and ways in which the process of drug development might be accelerated. The meeting concluded by its participants pledging through the Cape Town Declaration to work together on a number of activities, the most important being the creation of a global alliance that would provide leadership, raise funds, advo-

cate, and coordinate efforts in various sectors and settings to improve health equity by developing and delivering a simple and affordable TB treatment in endemic countries this decade.

Subsequently, a business consultant group was contracted to assist representatives of the signatories of the Cape Town Declaration to develop a structure and a business plan for the organization. In September 2000, the TB Alliance was established as a tax-exempt foundation in the United States, and the following month it was launched by the Director General of the WHO at a health research meeting in Bangkok. By then, it had received pledges of support from the Rockefeller and Gates foundations. During the following year, the TB Alliance opened offices in New York, Brussels, and Cape Town.

The mission of TB Alliance is to accelerate the discovery and/or development of cost-effective new drugs that would achieve one or more specific goals: shorten or simplify treatment of active TB, provide a more effective treatment of MDRTB, and/or improve the treatment of latent TB infection. The TB Alliance functions as a lean research and development organization, outsourcing drug research and development projects and moving drug compounds along the development line to achieve regulatory approval and bring them to market at affordable prices for those in greatest need. The TB Alliance pursues a social mission by employing the best practices of the private sector and by drawing on resources from both the public and private realms. One of its unique strengths was the establishment of a stakeholders association, consisting of those individuals and organizations that provided the impetus for its establishment as well as representatives from developing nations, governments, nongovernmental organizations working on TB, foundations, and other significant contributors to the fight against TB. This group plays an important role in the governance and support of the organization by being represented on the Board of Directors and being the body that nominates candidates for Board membership. In this role, the association can ensure that the TB Alliance remains true to its mission.

During the first year of its existence, the TB Alliance established its Scientific Advisory Committee, which issued its first call for proposals and, after a careful review of selected full proposals, recommended several for funding in June 2001. The projects include both infrastructure building (e.g., support for experimental studies of compounds of interest to the TB Alliance, developing regulatory standards to facilitate drug approval, and enhancing the capacity for high-quality clinical trials in developing countries) and several specific new compounds and compound series in early preclinical development. The TB Alliance also seeks to partner with industry, and in February 2002 announced its first agreement with Chiron Corporation to in-license and further develop the novel drug PA-824 and its analogs. The TB Alliance also issued two major documents, the "Scientific

Blueprint for TB Drug Development," which outlines in great detail the process of TB drug discovery and development, and the "Economics of TB Drug Development." The later report is a rigorous, authoritative source of information on the potential market for new TB drugs, detailed costs of TB drug development, potential financial and social returns on investment, and options for funding and conducting drug development. The report provides data required for informed investment decisions by industry, foundations, government organizations, and world health and financial organizations.

CONCLUSION

Through the leadership of the IUATLD and the WHO, the global TB problem now is receiving unprecedented attention. DOTS, a highly effective technical control strategy, has been developed and adopted worldwide. The strategy has been expanded to address the related problems of HIV infection and MDRTB that are threatening effective TB control in many countries. The adoption of the Global Plan to Stop TB and the establishment of the Stop TB Partnership by virtually all the governments and agencies working on TB provides for planning and coordination of global control activities and rational resource allocation at a time when financial support for TB is dramatically increasing. The related initiatives of foundations to support applied research will help to guarantee that new diagnostic, treatment, and prevention tools become available to make possible accelerated progress toward control and eventual elimination of this ancient scourge.

SUGGESTED READINGS

Cegielski JP, Chin DP, Espinal MA, et al. The global tuberculosis situation. Progress and problems in the 20th century, prospects for the 21st century. *Infect Dis Clin Am* 2002;16:1–58.

Enarson DA. Principles of IUATLD collaborative tuberculosis programmes. *Bull Int Union Tuberc Lung Dis* 1991;66:195–200.

Raviglione MC, Pio A. Evolution of WHO policies for tuberculosis control, 1948–2001. *Lancet* 2002;395:775–780.

Rouillon A. The mutual assistance programme of the IUATLD. Development, contribution, and significance. *Bull Int Union Tuberc Lung Dis* 1991;66:159–172.

Stop TB, World Health Organization. An expanded DOTS framework for effective tuberculosis control. *Int J Tuberc Lund Dis* 2002;6:378–388.

WEBSITES

Bill and Melinda Gates Foundation: www.gatesfoundation.org

Global Alliance for TB Drug Development: www.tballiance.org

International Union Against Tuberculosis and Lung Disease: www.iuatld.org

Additional International Union Against Tuberculosis and Lung Disease teaching materials: www.tbrieder.org

Stop TB Partnership and Secretariat: www.stoptb.org

World Health Organization Stop TB Department: www.who.int/gtb

United Nations Development Program–World Bank, World Health Organization Special Programme for Research and Training in Tropical Diseases: www.who.int/tdr/diseases/tb

Tuberculosis, Second Edition, edited by William N. Rom and Stuart M. Garay. Published by Lippincott Williams & Wilkins, Philadelphia, 2004

.

BACILLE CALMETTE–GUÉRIN: EFFICACY AND IMMUNITY

ANDRÉ L. MOREIRA

Tuberculosis is estimated to kill approximately two million people worldwide annually (1). Despite improved disease control and effective antituberculous therapy, the global incidence of tuberculosis is not declining. Therefore, effective vaccination for tuberculosis is a world priority. Immunization with the bacille Calmette–Guérin (BCG) is still the only vaccine available against tuberculosis.

The history of BCG begins in 1908 when Albert Calmette and Camille Guérin began their work with a strain of *Mycobacterium bovis* isolated from a cow that had tuberculous mastitis. *M. bovis* is the most frequent agent of tuberculosis in cattle. The French investigators began subculturing the organism every 3 weeks on a glycerinated beef-bile-potato medium. In 1921, after 13 years and 230 subcultures, they noticed that the *M. bovis* BCG had lost its virulence for animals (2,3). At that time, BCG was given orally as a vaccine to children with a high risk of developing tuberculosis, such as children of a parent with the disease. They observed that only 3.9% of the children given BCG died of tuberculosis compared with an expected mortality of 32.6% from tuberculosis (4). Since then, more than one billion children in more than 182 countries throughout the world have been vaccinated with BCG. The vaccine is relatively safe and inexpensive to produce. However, its efficacy in controlled clinical trials is notoriously variable in protecting vaccinated persons from developing pulmonary tuberculosis.

In this chapter, the latest experimental studies on the mechanism of action of BCG vaccination in animals is reviewed and correlated with the results of human clinical trials.

VACCINE PRODUCTION

Before one can discuss efficacy and immunity to BCG vaccination, one must understand basic principles of vaccine production and safety. Early BCG strains were propagated in hundreds of laboratories using culture methods routine to the particular laboratory. This method of cultivation continued into the 1960s, when such repeated subculturing was discovered to have resulted in BCG strains that differed markedly. Heterogeneous *in vitro* characteristics such as the appearance of the colonies (spreading versus nonspreading), viability on culture medium (5), biochemical composition and activity (6–8), drug resistance (9), and immunogenicity in animals and humans (5,10,11) have been found among currently available vaccines. In 1950, the World Health Organization issued the first in a series of recommendations for BCG production. In 1982, responsibility for the international quality control of BCG vaccines was given to the Statens Seruminstitut in Copenhagen, Denmark. Three parent strains (Glaxo, Tokyo, and Pasteur) now account for more than 90% of the vaccines used worldwide. The Pasteur strain of BCG currently serves as the international reference strain of the vaccine (12). In the United States, the U.S. Food and Drug Administration set the standards for the production of BCG vaccines.

BCG vaccines must be freeze-dried preparations of live bacilli from a primary or secondary seed lot of a BCG strain identified by complete historical records. Estimates of the total bacillary mass by opacity and dry weight; viability as determined by oxygen uptake, germination rate, or colony counts; and heat stability must be documented. In addition, production lots must be incapable of producing disease in guinea pigs (13), an animal that is highly sensitive to tuberculosis.

VACCINE SAFETY

The original BCG strain was given as an oral vaccine to newborns within the first 10 days of life. The oral route of vaccination was soon abandoned because most of the infants failed to show tuberculin skin test conversion, which was thought to correlate with the development of protective immunity. Higher doses of the vaccine also were required for oral immunization, causing an unacceptably high inci-

A. L. Moreira: Department of Pathology, New York University School of Medicine; Department of Pathology, New York University Medical Center, New York, New York.

dence of side effects. Administration of the vaccine by the subcutaneous method produced large abscesses; therefore, the intradermal method was chosen as the best technique for BCG vaccination because it caused only superficial abscesses (14). Today, BCG is considered one of the safest vaccines available. Complications are rare and include regional suppurative adenitis and osteitis. In a large study of adverse effects after vaccination with BCG, only 5% of vaccinees reported adverse reactions. Abscess at the site of the injection was the most commonly reported complication. Lymphadenitis occurred in approximately 1% of the study population (15).

Regional lymphadenitis may occur within the first 5 months after vaccination. In these patients, *M. bovis* BCG can be cultured from approximately 5% of the lesions (16). A prospective survey of two million infants vaccinated between 1979 and 1981 found the risk of lymphadenitis to be 0.025 per 1,000 (17).

The World Health Organization recommends drainage and direct instillation of an antituberculosis drug into the adherent or fistulated lymph nodes as treatment for BCG lymphadenitis. Systemic treatment with antituberculosis drugs is ineffective (18).

Osteitis is a rare complication of BCG vaccination (17). Osteitis most commonly develops within 4 to 144 months of vaccination. The most frequent site affected is the epiphysis of the long bones, particularly in the legs. Antituberculosis therapy, coupled in some cases with surgical curettage and débridement, usually results in healing of the skeletal lesions.

The most serious complication of BCG vaccination is disseminated BCG disease. Although rare, disseminated BCG disease is usually fatal. Disseminated disease is most frequently seen in children with concomitant immunodeficiencies, such as severe combined immunodeficiency syndrome and chronic granulomatous disease. Most cases of disseminated BCG infections occur within the first 6 months of vaccination. Treatment of disseminated BCG disease is similar to the treatment of active tuberculosis, with one exception: Pyrazinamide is not used in the therapeutic regimen because all BCG strains are resistant to this antibiotic. Even when treated with potentially effective chemotherapeutic agents, many patients with disseminated BCG infection die, particularly if the patient has demonstrable underlying immunosuppression.

BACILLE CALMETTE–GUÉRIN VACCINATION AND TUBERCULIN SKIN TEST

Much has been said about the relationship of BCG vaccination, development of delayed-type hypersensitivity reaction to purified protein derivative (PPD), and protection from tuberculosis. Tuberculin reactivity is discussed in more detail elsewhere in this book. In summary, tuberculin reac-

tivity usually develops after vaccination with BCG. Sensitivity appears as early as 10 days after vaccination with maximal responses observed by 12 weeks (19). After BCG vaccination, it is not possible, on an individual basis, to distinguish between a tuberculin skin test reaction caused by virulent mycobacterial infection or by vaccination itself (20). Therefore, the use of the purified protein derivative skin test as a diagnostic tool for tuberculosis is impaired in BCG-vaccinated persons.

Although tuberculin sensitivity occurs after BCG vaccination and a positive reaction suggests the existence of immune cells capable of recognizing mycobacterial antigens, there is poor correlation between tuberculin reactivity and protection against active tuberculosis (21,22).

CLINICAL TRIALS FOR VACCINE EFFICACY

Many controlled trials testing the efficacy of BCG vaccine in humans have been carried out (23). The estimates of vaccine efficacies found in each study vary from no protection to approximately 80% protection of vaccinees from developing pulmonary tuberculosis. To simplify the discussion, the variability of BCG efficacy in human clinical trials is discussed in the light of the results of two metaanalysis studies. Metaanalysis is the statistical analysis of a collection of studies for the purpose of integrating the findings; data from clinical trials and case–control studies are combined to increase the statistical power for comparing end points such as vaccine efficacy, risk of disease after exposure, behavioral characteristics, and disease.

Clemens et al. (24) reviewed eight major controlled trials of BCG efficacy, focusing on the methodologic and statistical approaches used in each trial. The published reports of the trials were compared based on (a) the unbiased allocation of study participants to either the vaccine or control group (such random allocation would ensure equal susceptibility to tuberculosis in both groups); (b) the equal follow-up and surveillance of the two study groups for symptoms of tuberculosis; (c) the unbiased detection of tuberculosis in vaccinated and unvaccinated persons. The equal frequency of diagnostic tests in the vaccine and control groups and the interpretation of clinical information in a manner blinded to vaccination status would minimize "detection bias." Following these criteria, the investigators concluded that the major source of bias in the trials was in the detection and diagnosis of tuberculosis. Systematic chest radiographic surveys of all study participants with blinded reading of the films were done in only three of the trials: in North American Indians (25), in children in Chicago (26), and in England (23). The efficacy of BCG vaccine in these trials was 75% to 80%.

The statistical precision of each of the trials was estimated. Studies with the greatest statistical precision reported the higher vaccine efficacies. Trials demonstrating little or no protection after BCG vaccination had wider confidence intervals, thus less statistical precision. From these qualitative analyses, Clemens et al. (24) concluded that BCG can confer protection against tuberculosis and that the disparate results found in the controlled trials may have resulted, at least in part, from methodologic differences in the studies.

In another metaanalysis, Colditz et al. (27) included studies if there were vaccinated and concurrent control groups and if vaccine efficacy was measured by the detection of at least one case of tuberculosis during the study. A numerical ranking score was assigned to each study using the following criteria: (a) the inclusion in the report of a description of the vaccine strain, dose, and route of administration; (b) the number of participants lost to follow-up during the study; (c) equal surveillance for tuberculosis in the vaccinated and control groups; and (d) the quality of the diagnostic confirmation of tuberculosis. Studies were added to the analysis in the order of their relative score. When data from the prospective clinical trials were used, the protective effect of vaccination decreased because studies with lower ranking scores were included in the analysis. Including seven clinical trials that used random allocation of participants to receive or not to receive the vaccine (23,28–33), they observed a combined protective effect of 63%. If six studies that used less stringent alternative or systematic allocation schemes (25,26, 34–37) were added, the protective effect decreased to 51%. Data from ten case–control studies of BCG efficacy (38–47) showed similar results; that is, the number of cases of tuberculosis was reduced by at least 50% after BCG vaccination.

Many different BCG strains have been used in both clinical trials and case–control studies of vaccine efficacy. Whereas a rigorous analysis of the effects of individual strains on BCG efficacy was not possible, a significant protective effect of vaccination was seen across many study designs, populations, and strains. Colditz et al. (27) concluded that many different strains were able to confer some degree of protection. The use of nonlyophilized vaccines in earlier prospective studies and the changes that have occurred in vaccine strains over time raise questions as to the comparability of the vaccine strains evaluated for efficacy and those available today. The issue of differences in vaccine strains remains controversial despite the current analysis.

The compilation of the global data on BCG using metaanalysis has provided some insight into the true efficacy of the vaccine. However, applying the results of the analysis to public health practice should be done with caution. Because the variability in protection afforded by BCG is so great and the reasons for this variation are unknown, estimates of vaccine efficacy in populations cannot be directly translated to equal protective effects in an individual person.

PROTECTIVE IMMUNITY AFTER VACCINATION: LESSONS FROM ANIMAL MODELS

Immunity to tuberculosis and the mechanism of action of BCG vaccination on the immune response to tuberculosis have been investigated in many animal models. A role for cell-mediated immunity in protection against tuberculosis was demonstrated by experiments in which mice given T lymphocytes from BCG-vaccinated animals were more resistant to tuberculosis. These mice were shown to have decreased numbers of *Mycobacterium tuberculosis* bacilli in the lungs and spleens when they were later challenged with *M. tuberculosis* (48). Passive transfer of sera from BCG-vaccinated animals (rabbits) did not confer protection against challenge of animals with virulent *M. tuberculosis* (49). Recently, molecularly engineered mice with a knockout of B lymphocytes contained an aerosol challenge with virulent *M. tuberculosis* as well as control mice (50). Although specific antimycobacterial antibodies seem to play a role in opsonization and phagocytosis of *M. tuberculosis*, their role in protective immunity *in vivo* is not clearly defined (51–53).

The effect of BCG vaccination on the immune response to mycobacterial antigens has been investigated in more detail in the murine model because of the availability of immunologic reagents. To understand the effect of BCG vaccination on individual components of the immune system, experiments were designed in which mice were first infected with BCG by the intravenous or subcutaneous route. After a few weeks of infection, lymphocytes were harvested from spleens or regional lymph nodes of the BCG-infected animals. The lymphocytes then were tested *in vitro* for their response to mycobacterial antigens. In this setting, BCG vaccination enhances cell-mediated immunity by boosting lymphocytic proliferation (54,55) and the production of cytokines, which indicate T-cell activation. BCG vaccination also promotes an effective immune response by priming lymphocytes to produce cytokines, such as interferon-gamma (INF-γ) and interleukin-2 (IL-2) (54–58). IFN-γ plays a central role in the control of mycobacterial infections *in vivo* (59,60).

The effect of BCG vaccination on the immune response seems to be dose dependent but independent of the route of BCG administration (57). A low dose of the vaccine is associated with the generation of an exclusive cell-mediated immune response, favoring the production of IFN-γ, whereas higher doses of the vaccine induce a mixed response with production of IFN-γ and IL-4, which is associated with the appearance of a humoral response and reduced ability to transfer delayed-type hypersensitivity to mycobacterial antigens (57). Levy et al. (61) studied the effect of BCG vaccination on the modulation of the infection by *M. tuberculosis in vivo*. In these experiments, animals were first vaccinated with BCG and later challenged with *M. tuberculosis*. They observed that BCG vaccination does not prevent infection by *M. tuberculosis* itself or prevent the establishment of a primary focus of infection (61). These findings were confirmed by Smith et al. (62), who found that the number of organisms recovered from the lung, spleen, and lymph nodes of BCG vaccinated guinea pigs was not significantly different from the number isolated from unvaccinated animals until 14 days after challenge. After 2 weeks, vaccinated animals showed fewer organisms in the spleen and no evidence of dissemination of bacilli to lobes of the lungs not infected at the time of challenge. The enhanced resistance to tuberculosis offered by BCG vaccination was associated with the recruitment of activated lymphocytes to the site of infection. This finding was later confirmed by other investigators (63–66). These data suggest that vaccination with BCG does not protect against infection itself but rather increases resistance by preventing uncontrolled multiplication and dissemination of *M. tuberculosis* from the primary foci of infection to other parts of the lung and body.

There are two theories to explain the lack of protection against *M. tuberculosis* infection by BCG vaccination: (a) the intracellular nature of the parasite and (b) the expression of immunity in the pulmonary parenchyma.

M. tuberculosis is a facultative intracellular parasite. It means that the organism can live outside cells and inside cells. After aerosol exposure, *M. tuberculosis* is phagocytosed by resident alveolar macrophages. These cells supposedly migrate to regional lymph nodes where they present antigens to T lymphocytes and initiate a specific immune response to the invading pathogen. However, the influx of activated lymphocytes into the site of infection occurs 2 to 3 weeks after infection. This lag in recruitment of specific immunity may work in favor of the tuberculous bacilli by allowing them to proliferate unrestrictedly and establish a primary focus of infection.

The pulmonary tissue is designed for gas exchange. Therefore, any interference with its normal structures will result, in part, in disruption of gas exchange. The lungs have many physiologic mechanisms to ensure sterility of the pulmonary alveoli, including the ciliated tracheobronchial epithelium and mucous production, which are effective in preventing larger particles (>10 μm) from reaching the alveolar sacs. However, *M. tuberculosis* is disseminated as airborne particles of less than 5 μm in diameter and can be deposited directly into the alveolar sacs, bypassing the physiologic barrier.

It was believed that the pulmonary tissue had immunosuppressive properties to protect its environment from the deleterious effects of inflammation. That concept is changing. The immune response in the lungs is better understood from models of inflammatory diseases affecting the upper airway, such as asthma and viral infections (67). In these models, immune expression is centered in epithelial cells, the first cells to enter in contact with antigens and allergens. Epithelial cells, when in contact with allergens, coordinate the expression of adhesion molecules and chemoattractants

with that of underlying endothelial cells, so that leukocytes can efficiently and quickly migrate through the tissue. IFN-γ appears to be a potent and specific coordinator of this event (67,68). IFN-γ signaling initiates the expression of genes that favor recruitment of immune cells such as intercellular adhesion molecule-1, genes involved in antigen presentation and processing such as transporter and antigen processor-1, and other genes responsible for further amplification of the immune response. Therefore, an inflammatory response in the upper airway can be established efficiently.

The role of epithelial cells in the immune response to mycobacterial antigens has not been clearly demonstrated; however, *M. tuberculosis* can infect type II pneumocytes (69–71) leading to the expression of chemokines by the infected cells (70). The expression of immunity in the alveolar sac is, however, poorly understood. Orme (64) showed that IFN-γ messenger RNA is expressed in the pulmonary parenchyma early during the course of *M. tuberculosis* infection, as measured by the reverse transcriptase polymerase chain reaction. The origin of the cytokine is unknown at this point but most likely arises from "innate" immunity. Orme (64) observed that mice unable to mount a specific immune response, such as transgenic mice that recognize only a peptide from ovalbumin, are able to control an aerosol challenge of *M. tuberculosis* for the first 3 weeks of infection, similar to immunocompetent (control) mice. Subsequently, mycobacteria grow unrestrictedly in the lungs of the transgenic mice. Control mice, however, mount a specific immune response to mycobacteria, and the growth of the organism is restricted after the first few weeks of infection. Whether BCG vaccination can enhance the production of IFN-γ by an innate immune response in the pulmonary parenchyma in the early stages of *M. tuberculosis* infection is unknown, but one can infer from the data in the literature that this is not the case. North et al. (66) showed that BCG vaccinated mice expressed specific immunity in the lung slightly earlier than unvaccinated mice, and at day 20 after infection had a tenfold reduction in the number of virulent bacilli in the lung compared with unvaccinated mice. The enhanced control of the multiplication of *M. tuberculosis* was associated with a reduction in the size of granulomas and prolonged survival curves. In that same study, variation in the route of infection (aerosol versus intravenous route) with the virulent *M. tuberculosis* modulated outcome. North et al. (66) observed that mice challenged by the aerosol route with *M. tuberculosis* died of the infection faster than mice infected by the intravenous route, regardless of their vaccination status. This suggests that, independent of the state of memory immunity to mycobacteria generated by BCG vaccination, the primary site of infection, alveolar macrophages in the aerosol challenge and blood monocytes in the intravenous challenge, are able to modulate the expression of immunity in the lung. Similar results were observed by Cooper et al. (72), who observed that, despite efficient control of *M. tuberculosis* in the spleens and livers of immunized mice, the growth of *M. tuberculosis* in the lungs of BCG-vaccinated mice eventually reached similar levels as those observed in unvaccinated control mice, confirming that the expression of immunity is regulated differently in the lungs.

If BCG vaccination cannot protect against the initial infection, then at which point during *M. tuberculosis* infection does BCG interfere? In all these studies using experimental models, vaccination induces a state of resistance to tuberculosis manifested by a significant reduction in the number of virulent bacteria in the infected organs. The reduction in bacterial load varies from a 0.7- to a 2-log reduction. The highest reduction rate is seen in the guinea pig models (65). BCG vaccination is associated with a reduction of hematogenous seeding of *M. tuberculosis* from the lungs to other organs (73) and induces a reduction in the size of the granulomas in the lungs and other organs of infected animals (63–66,73–76). In the guinea pig model, smaller granulomas are also associated with a reduction in necrosis (73,76). Therefore, vaccination reduces inflammation and destruction of tissue. Preservation of pulmonary function is associated with prolonged survival in experimental models of infection (65,73).

The mechanism by which BCG vaccination induces an increased resistance to *M. tuberculosis* is not clearly defined, but many components of the immune system have been implicated in this protective role against tuberculosis. The protective role of CD4 T lymphocytes in resistance to tuberculosis is undoubtedly well established (53,77–79). In fact, passive transfer of CD4 T cells from immune mice to naive mice can confer resistance to tuberculosis (80). However, questions remain concerning the effect of BCG vaccination on the quality of generated CD4 memory T cells and the persistence of this population of cells (81). The resistance conferred by BCG vaccination wanes when vaccinated mice are allowed to age before challenge with virulent bacteria (82).

The role of CD8 T cells on BCG vaccination–induced resistance, however, is not clear (53,79,83). CD8 lymphocytes appear to be important in resistance to *M. tuberculosis* infection but not in the control of BCG infection (53,84), suggesting a differential role of this T-cell subset in the control of virulent and nonvirulent strains of mycobacteria. Interest in the role of CD8 T lymphocytes in the control of mycobacterial infection has emerged in recent years and is a highly active subject of study (79,83).

RECOMBINANT BACILLE CALMETTE–GUÉRIN VACCINES

Owing to the experience with BCG vaccination in animal models and human beings, the immunostimulatory properties of BCG (85–88), and the demonstrable positive effect

of vaccination with this bacterium in conferring resistance to tuberculosis, new strategies are being pursued to improve the efficacy of BCG. An exciting approach comes with the development of techniques that allow genetic manipulation of the bacterium by transforming BCG in a vehicle for the expression of foreign genes (85). Recombinant BCG may be used as a carrier to deliver antigens and other biologically active molecules directly into the site of infection. These recombinants can be used to test new improved vaccines but may also be useful tools to dissect the mechanism of immunity against mycobacteria. Many potential recombinant BCG vaccines have been created using this technique in an attempt to create vaccines for human immunodeficiency virus infection (89,90), Lyme disease (91), and leishmaniasis (92). An exciting report from Horwitz et al. (76) showed that a preparation of recombinant BCG secreting a 30-kd major secretory protein from *M. tuberculosis* proved more effective than the parental BCG in reducing bacillary load in *M. tuberculosis*–infected guinea pigs. The 30-kd major secretory protein of *M. tuberculosis* induced protective immunity against an aerosol challenge with virulent *M. tuberculosis* (93). However, vaccination with the purified protein offered levels of protection similar to those with BCG itself (93). The combination of a live vaccine such as BCG with additional *M. tuberculosis* antigen improved the efficacy of BCG. Vaccination with the recombinant BCG secreting the 30-kd protein also reduced tissue injury because it resulted in smaller tuberculous lesions in the lungs, spleens, and livers of vaccinated guinea pigs compared with animals vaccinated with the parental BCG strain (76).

The role of cytokines as immune adjuvants has been investigated in mycobacterial infections. Recombinant cytokines such as IL-2 + IL-12 when admixed with culture filtrate proteins from *M. tuberculosis* as a vaccine against tuberculosis showed protection similar to that of BCG alone (74).

The role of cytokines in generating more effective memory T cells has been further evaluated in experiments in which recombinant BCG that secretes murine cytokines was used as a vaccine for tuberculosis. The secretion of cytokines by BCG did not impair the viability of the bacilli because all recombinants showed similar growth rates *in vitro* and *in vivo* (94). In addition, the cytokines secreted by the recombinant BCG were biologically active (73,85,94). Mice were vaccinated by the subcutaneous route with recombinant BCG secreting murine cytokines such as IL-2, IFN-γ, and tumor necrosis factor (TNF)-α. A recombinant BCG carrying only the plasmid was used as control. After aerosol infection with *M. tuberculosis*, the recombinant BCG that secreted murine cytokines offered the same protection as the parental BCG in controlling the growth of *M. tuberculosis* in the lungs and spleens of infected mice. However, a differential effect among the cytokines was noted when the granulomatous response to an aerosol challenge with *M. tuberculosis* was analyzed. At 12 weeks post-infection, the lungs of unvaccinated controls contained an extensive inflammatory infiltrate composed of macrophages, lymphocytes, and neutrophils within the alveolar spaces consistent with a pneumonic process, in addition to coalescent granulomas, which occupied approximately 80% of the parenchyma. The size of the granulomas was reduced by 50% in animals vaccinated with parental BCG. Vaccination with BCG secreting IL-2 or BCG secreting IFN-γ resulted in significantly smaller granulomas than those seen in mice vaccinated with the parental BCG (75). The area of the lungs occupied by granulomas in the BCG/IFN-γ–vaccinated mice was approximately 30% and 20% for those vaccinated with BCG/IL-2. Vaccination with the recombinant BCG that secretes TNF-α resulted in larger granulomas than observed in animals vaccinated with the parental BCG (75). Immunohistochemical analysis of the granulomas in these experiments showed that despite the differences in the size of the pulmonary lesions, there was no difference in the composition of the granulomas in relation to the ratio of CD4/CD8 positive lymphocytes in the tissue. There was no difference in the expression of T-cell activation markers such as CD 25 (IL-2 receptor), CD69 (early activation marker), CD80, and CD82. These results suggest that the composition of the immune response at the site of sensitization (vaccination site) can modify the overall status of immunity and resistance to a given antigen (systemic immunity expressed at the site of infection). The results obtained from experiments using recombinant BCG preparations indicate that the efficacy of BCG vaccine can be modified.

Resistance to tuberculosis offered by BCG vaccination can be separated into two effects. One is restriction of growth of *M. tuberculosis* and the second is reduction in inflammation at the primary site. Thus, modifications in the antigenic component of the vaccine and modifications in the immune response to the vaccine itself may generate memory T cells that will give rise to a more efficient, less inflammatory immune response. Cytokines of the Th1 type are better candidates for priming memory T cells than the inflammatory cytokines such as TNF-α. Whether recombinant BCG will become an affordable alternative to the traditional BCG vaccination needs to be evaluated because the cost of vaccination is an important consideration in the developing countries.

CORRELATION BETWEEN CLINICAL TRIALS AND ANIMAL MODELS

Results from metaanalysis studies suggest that BCG vaccination offers at least 50% protection from acquiring tuberculosis (27). How can we reconcile these data with the fact that in animal models, BCG vaccination does not prevent infection but rather induces resistance and prolonged survival by reducing pulmonary lesions and hematogenous spread? In most animal models, the end point of analysis is the development of disease. Therefore, the protocols of experimental infection are optimized for that purpose, i.e., 100% infection rate. Experiments in which animals would be exposed to *M. tuberculosis* in a similar fashion to that in nature would have prohibitive costs. Under natural conditions, only 10% of individuals exposed to *M. tuberculosis* develop clinical pulmonary tuberculosis. In human beings, infection is a fine balance between the number of infecting organisms, the virulence of a given organism, and the host response to infection. Therefore, modification of resistance to infection by more efficient BCG preparations can theoretically shift the balance between exposure and disease.

In the metaanalysis studies, the influence of other factors on BCG efficacy were tested, e.g., age at vaccination. Vaccine efficacy was greater in children and decreased with increasing age. The protective effect was 85% at birth and decreased to 52% for those vaccinated at 20 years of age. It was not possible in the metaanalysis studies to evaluate the duration of protection after BCG vaccination. Long-term surveillance of vaccinees is hampered by increasing losses to follow-up over time and the decreases in tuberculosis incidence in most countries over the past several decades.

Experiments aimed at the effect of aging on resistance to tuberculosis after BCG vaccination have been carried out in mice. The half-life of memory T cells to *M. tuberculosis* indeed is influenced by age. BCG-vaccinated mice infected with *M. tuberculosis* several months after vaccination are less resistant to tuberculosis compared with recently vaccinated ones (82). How the pool of memory T cells is lost in human or animal models is still a subject of speculation. A more stringent analysis of the effects of age on vaccine efficacy was not possible in the metaanalyses owing to the lack of available data on BCG vaccination in adults.

Is it possible that the lack of effect of BCG vaccination in adults can be explained solely based on loss of effective or memory T cells? Another aspect to be considered when analyzing the lack of effect of BCG vaccination in the adult population comes from data from the Chingleput trial in India (29). Vaccination with BCG in that population offered minimal protection in vaccinees aged 0 to 14 years; however, more adult vaccinees had tuberculosis than did the unvaccinated control subjects (29). In a BCG vaccine trial carried out in Malawi, significantly higher rates of pulmonary tuberculosis were reported among BCG scar–positive persons (95). Does BCG vaccination fail to protect adults from developing tuberculosis? Does BCG vaccination exacerbate tuberculosis? Experiments in animal models suggest the latter. Based on the information that an effective immune response can control tuberculosis in the majority of people exposed to the bacilli, attempts have been made to improve the immune response to tuberculosis. In experimental models, *M. tuberculosis*–infected mice have been treated with different preparations of immune stimulants including purified proteins from *M. tuberculosis* (75,96,97), recombinant cytokines (75), and recombinant BCG–secreting murine cytokines (75). In all these studies, further stimulation of the ongoing immune response to *M. tuberculosis* led to no modification in the bacterial load in the lungs of infected animals (75,96,97). However, postexposure vaccination or immune stimulation of *M. tuberculosis*–infected mice led to exacerbation of the inflammatory infiltrate in the lungs, leading to more tissue destruction (morbidity) and an increased mortality rate (75,96,97). In fact, the exacerbation of tuberculous lesions after exposure to products of *M. tuberculosis* was demonstrated by Koch in 1908 (Koch's phenomenon). Therefore, it is possible that vaccination of adults with BCG may lead to exacerbation of subclinical (undiagnosed) tuberculous infection. Vaccination of adults with BCG or other vaccine preparations must be approached carefully. One must ensure that the target population does not carry subclinical infection with *M. tuberculosis.*

Another possible explanation for the lack of effect of BCG vaccination in the adult population comes from epidemiologic studies of BCG vaccination suggesting that the geographic location of the study and the incidence of active tuberculosis in the study control group had the strongest associations with BCG efficacy. Geography might be a surrogate for factors such as the prevalence of nontuberculous mycobacterial infections, climate, dietary factors, or the genetic susceptibility of individual populations (27). The hypothesis that environmental mycobacterial exposure may modify the immune response to BCG vaccination has been investigated. Orme (53) suggested that repeated exposure of BCG-vaccinated mice to dead *Mycobacterium avium* impairs resistance to tuberculosis by reducing the pool of memory T cells. Others suggested that environmental mycobacteria, such as *M. avium* and soil isolates from a region in Malawi in which BCG vaccination has no effect against pulmonary tuberculosis, can block the sensitizing effect of BCG (98,99). The same saprophytic mycobacteria do not affect sensitization of mice to subunit vaccines (99). In human beings, exposure to fast-growing saprophytic mycobacteria is, however, associated with a reduced risk of developing tuberculosis (98). Even BCG itself in large doses fails to protect mice from a challenge with *M. tuberculosis* by inducing a Th2-type immune response (57).

The interplay of exposure to different mycobacteria in the protective immune response to tuberculosis is an important area of investigation that will enable us to better understand the complex immune response to *M. tuberculosis.*

Metaanalyses also showed that BCG vaccination had a protective effect of 78% against disseminated tuberculosis and a 71% protective effect from death caused by tuberculosis. There was a protective effect of 64% against tuberculous meningitis. These data correlate nicely with the results of studies of animal models of infection, wherein vaccination has consistently led to a reduction in inflammation and

destruction of tissue. This is especially true for models of tuberculous meningitis. The pathogenesis and severity of tuberculous meningitis is directly related to the inflammatory response generated by the bacterium. Virulent strains, such as *M. bovis* Ravenel, induce severe meningitis with leukocytosis and high levels of the cytokine TNF-α in the cerebrospinal fluid, whereas less virulent strains such as BCG strain Montreal do not. The virulence of the latter could be accentuated when the bacterium expressed TNF-α (recombinant BCG secreting murine cytokine) (100). In addition, treatment of infected animals with a combination of antibiotics and an antiinflammatory drug, such as thalidomide, which reduces TNF-α production, led to increased survival of rabbits infected intracisternally with *M. bovis* Ravenel (101).

Given the complexity of the immune response to intracellular pathogens and the relationship of *M. tuberculosis* (a very well adapted pathogen) with the host cells and tissues, BCG vaccination is still a promising aid in the fight against tuberculosis. Recent scientific advances in the fields of microbiology, immunology, and genetics have highlighted many important factors necessary for understanding of the pathogenesis of mycobacterial infections and for protection against the diseases that they cause. Continued research on the basic and clinical aspects of BCG vaccination are key to efficient control of tuberculosis worldwide.

ACKNOWLEDGMENT

I acknowledge that some of the material on the epidemiology of BCG vaccination discussed in this chapter was a modification of what had been written by Dr. Robin E. Huebner in the first edition of this book. I am grateful to Dr. Jerry Waisman, Dr. Ann Marie Nelson, and Dr. Brian A. West for their invaluable comments and help in editing this chapter.

REFERENCES

1. Dye C, Scheele S, Dolin P, et al. Consensus statement. Global burden of tuberculosis: estimated incidence, prevalence, and mortality by country. WHO Global surveillance and monitoring project. *JAMA* 1999;282:677–689.
2. Grange JM, Gibson J, Osborn TW. What is BCG? *Tubercle* 1983;64:129–139.
3. Gardner LV. The history of the R1 strain of tubercle bacillus. *Am Rev Tuberc* 1932;25:577–590.
4. Calmette A. *La vaccination preventive contra la tuberculosis.* Paris: Masson et Cie, 1927.
5. Gheorghiu M, LaGrange PH. Viability, heat stability and immunogenicity of four BCG vaccines prepared from four different BCG strains. *Ann Immunol* 1983;134C:125–147.
6. Minnikin DE, Parlett JH, Magnusson M, et al. Mycolic acid patterns of representatives of *Mycobacterium bovis* BCG. *J Gen Microbiol* 1984;130:2733–2736.
7. Abou-Zeid C, Smith I, Grange J, et al. Subdivision of daughter

strains of bacille Calmette–Guérin (BCG) according to secreted protein patterns. *J Gen Microbiol* 1986;132:3047–3053.

8. International Union against Tuberculosis. Phenotypes of BCG-vaccines seed lot strains: results of an international cooperative study. *Tubercle* 1978;59:139–142.

9. Hesselberg I. Drug resistance in the Swedish/Norwegian BCG strain. *Bull WHO* 1972;46:503–507.

10. Grange JM, Gibson JA. Strain to strain variation in the immunogenicity of BCG. *Dev Biol Stand* 1986;58:37–41.

11. Nyboe J, Bunch-Christensen K. Assay in man of different BCG products. *Bull WHO* 1966;35:645–650.

12. Milstien JB, Gibson JJ. Quality control of BCG vaccine by WHO: a review of factors that may influence vaccine effectiveness and safety. *Bull WHO* 1990;68:93.

13. *Fed Reg* 1985;50:50159–50166.

14. Rosenthal SR. Routes and methods of administration. In: *BCG vaccine: tuberculosis–cancer.* Littleton, MA: PSG Publishing, 1980:146–175.

15. Turnbull FM, McIntyre PB, Achat HM, et al. National study of adverse reactions after vaccination with bacilli Calmette–Guerin. *Clin Infect Dis* 2002;34:447–453.

16. Lotte A, Wasz-Hockert O, Poisson N, et al. BCG complications. *Adv Tuberc Res* 1984;21:107–193.

17. Lotte A, Wasz-Hockert O, Poisson N, et al. Second IUATLD study on complications induced by intradermal BCG-vaccination. *Bull Int Union Tuber Lung Dis* 1988;63:47–59.

18. World Health Organization. *BCG vaccination of the newborn. Rationale and guidelines for country programmes* (WHO/TB/86.147). Geneva: World Health Organization, 1986.

19. Stewart CJ. Skin sensitivity to human, avian and BCG PPDs after BCG vaccination. *Tubercle* 1968;49:84–91.

20. Snider DE. Bacille Calmette–Guérin vaccinations and tuberculin skin tests. *JAMA* 1985;253:3438–3439.

21. Comstock GW. Identification of an effective vaccine against tuberculosis. *Am Rev Respir Dis* 1988;138:479–480.

22. Hart PD'A, Sutherland I, Thomas J. The immunity conferred by effective BCG and vole bacillus vaccines in relation to individual variations in tuberculin sensitivity and to technical variations in the vaccines. *Tubercle* 1967;48:201–210.

23. Hart PD, Sutherland I. BCG and vole bacillus vaccines in the prevention of tuberculosis in adolescence and early adult life. *BMJ* 1977;2:293–295.

24. Clemens JB, Chuong JJH, Feinstein AR. The BCG controversy: a methodological and statistical reappraisal. *JAMA* 1983;249:2361–2369.

25. Aronson JD, Aronson CF, Taylor HC. A twenty-year appraisal of BCG vaccination in the control of tuberculosis. *Arch Intern Med* 1958;101:881–893.

26. Rosenthal SR, Loewinsohn E, Graham M, et al. BCG vaccination against tuberculosis in Chicago. A twenty-year study statistically analyzed. *Pediatrics* 1961;28:622–641.

27. Colditz GA, Brewer T, Berkey C, et al. Efficacy of BCG in the prevention of tuberculosis: meta-analysis of the published literature. *JAMA* 1994;271:698–702.

28. Vandiviere HM, Dworski M, Melvin I, et al. Efficacy of bacillus Calmette–Guerin and isoniazid-resistant bacillus Calmette–Guerin with and without isoniazid chemoprophylaxis from day of vaccination. *Am Rev Respir Dis* 1973;108:301–313.

29. Tripathy SP. Fifteen-year follow-up of the Indian BCG prevention trial. *Bull Int Union Tuberc Lung Dis* 1987;62:69–72.

30. Aronson JD. Protective vaccination against tuberculosis with special references to BCG vaccination. *Am Rev Tuberc* 1948;58:275–281.

31. Coetzee AM, Berjak J. BCG in the prevention of tuberculosis in an adult population. *Proc Mine Med Officers Assoc* 1968;48:41–53.

32. Ferguson RS, Simes AB. BCG vaccination of Indian infants in Saskatchewan. *Tubercle* 1949;30:5–11.

33. Rosenthal SR, Loewinsohn E, Graham M, et al. BCG vaccination in tuberculous households. *Am Rev Respir Dis* 1961;84:690–704.

34. Comstock GW, Woolpert SF, Livesay VT. Tuberculosis studies in Muscogee County, Georgia. Twenty-year evaluation of a community trial of BCG vaccination. *Public Health Rep* 1976;91:276–280.

35. Comstock GW, Livesay VT, Woolpert SF. Evaluation of BCG vaccination among Puerto Rican children. *Am J Public Health* 1974;64:283–291.

36. Frimodt-Moller J, Acharyulu GS, Kesava Pillai K. Observations on the protective effect of BCG vaccination in a south Indian rural population: fourth report. *Bull Int Union Tubercle Lung Dis* 1973;48:40–49.

37. Levine MI, Sackett MF. Results of BCG immunization in New York City. *Am Rev Tuberc* 1946;53:517–532.

38. Wunsch-Filho V, de Castilho EA, Rodrigues LC, et al. Effectiveness of BCG vaccination against tuberculosis meningitis: a case-control study in Sao Paulo, Brazil. *Bull WHO* 1990;68:69–74.

39. Miceli I, De Kantor IN, Colaiacovo D, et al. Evaluation of the effectiveness of BCG vaccination using the case-control method in Buenos Aires, Argentina. *Int J Epidemiol* 1988;17:629–634.

40. Rodrigues LC, Gill ON, Smith PG. BCG vaccination in the first year of life protects children of Indian subcontinent ethnic origin against tuberculosis in England. *Int J Epidemiol* 1991;45:78–80.

41. Young TK, Hershfield ES. A case-control study to evaluate the effectiveness of mass neonatal BCG vaccination among Canadian Indians. *Am J Public Health* 1986;76:783–786.

42. Houston S, Fanning A, Soskolne CL. The effectiveness of bacillus Calmette–Guérin (BCG) vaccination against tuberculosis: a case-control study in Treaty Indians, Alberta, Canada. *Am J Epidemiol* 1990;131:340–348.

43. Packe GE, Innes JA. Protective effect of BCG vaccination in infant Asians: a case-control study. *Arch Dis Child* 1988;63:277–281.

44. Putrali J, Sutrisna B, Rahoyoe N, et al. A case-control study of effectiveness of vaccination in children in Jakarta, Indonesia. Proceedings of the Eastern Regional Tuberculosis Conference of IUAT, 1983, Jakarta, Indonesia. 1983:194–200.

45. Myint TT, Win H, Aye HH, et al. Case-control study on evaluation of BCG vaccination of newborn in Rangoon, Burma. *Ann Trop Paediatr* 1987;7:159–166.

46. Camargos PAM, Guimaraes MDC, Antunes CMF. Risk assessment for acquiring meningitis tuberculosis among children not vaccinated with BCG: a case-control study. *Int J Epidemiol* 1988;17:193–197.

47. Sirinavin S, Chotpitayasunondh T, Suwanjutha S, et al. Protective efficacy of neonatal bacillus Calmette–Guérin vaccination against tuberculosis. *Pediatr Infect Dis J* 1991;10:350–365.

48. Lefford MJ. Induction and expression of immunity after BCG immunization. *Infect Immun* 1977;18:646–653.

49. Smith DW. Protective effect of BCG in experimental tuberculosis. *Adv Tuberc Res* 1985;22:66–73.

50. Johnson CM, Cooper AM, Frank AA, et al. *Mycobacterium tuberculosis* aerogenic rechallenge infections in B cell-deficient mice. *Tuber Lung Dis* 1997;78:257–261.

51. Glatman-Freedman A, Casadevall A. Serum therapy for tuberculosis revisited: reappraisal of the role of antibody-mediated immunity against *Mycobacterium tuberculosis*. *Clin Microbiol Rev* 1998;11:514–532.

52. Teitelbaum R, Glatman-Freedman A, Chen B, et al. A mAB recognizing a surface antigen of *Mycobacterium tuberculosis*

enhances host survival. *Proc Natl Acad Sci U S A* 1998; 95:15688–15693.

53. Orme IM. The search for new vaccines against tuberculosis. *J Leukoc Biol* 2001;70:1–10.

54. Zlotta AR, Drowart A, Van Vooren JP, et al. Evolution and clinical significance of the T cell proliferative and cytokine response directed against the fibronectin binding antigen 85 complex of bacillus Calmette–Guerin during intravesical treatment of superficial bladder cancer. *J Urol* 1997;157:492–498.

55. Murray PJ, Aldovini A, Young RA. Manipulation and potentiation of antimycobacterial immunity using recombinant bacilli Calmette–Guerin strains that secrete cytokines. *Proc Natl Acad Sci U S A* 1996;93:934–939.

56. O'Donnell MA, Aldovini A, Duda RB, et al. Recombinant *Mycobacterium bovis* BCG secreting functional interleukin-2 enhances gamma interferon production by splenocytes. *Infect Immun* 1994;62:2508–2514.

57. Power CA, Wei G, Bretscher PA. Mycobacterial dose defines the Th1/Th2 nature of the immune response independently of whether immunization is administered by the intravenous, subcutaneous, or intradermal route. *Infect Immun* 1998;66: 5743–5750.

58. Mason CM, Dobard E, Shellito J, et al. CD4+ lymphocyte responses to pulmonary infection with *Mycobacterium tuberculosis* in naïve and vaccinated BALB/c mice. *Tuberculosis (Edinb)* 2001;81:327–334.

59. Cooper AM, Dalton DK, Stewart TA, et al. Disseminated tuberculosis in IFN-gamma gene-disrupted mice. *J Exp Med* 1993;178:2243–2248.

60. Flynn JL, Chan J, Triebold KJ, et al. An essential role for interferon-gamma in resistance to *Mycobacterium tuberculosis* infection. *J Exp Med* 1993;178:2249–2254.

61. Levy FM, Conge GA, Pasquier JF, et al. The effect of BCG vaccination on the fate of virulent tubercle bacilli in mice. *Am Rev Respir Dis* 1961;84:28–36.

62. Smith DW, McMurray DN, Wiegeshaus EH, et al. Host-parasite relationships in experimental tuberculosis. IV. Early events in the course of infection in vaccinated and nonvaccinated guinea pigs. *Am Rev Respir Dis* 1970;102:937–949.

63. Orme IM. Progress in the development of new vaccines against tuberculosis. *Int J Tuberc Lung Dis* 1997;1:95–100.

64. Orme IM. Immunology and vaccinology of tuberculosis: can lessons from the mouse be applied to the cow? *Tuberculosis (Edinb)* 2001;81:109–113.

65. Orme IM, McMurray DN, Belisle JT. Tuberculosis vaccine development: recent progress. *Trends Microbiol* 2001;9: 115–118.

66. North RJ, Lacourse R, Ryan L. Vaccinated mice remain more susceptible to *Mycobacterium tuberculosis* infection initiated via the respiratory route than via intravenous route. *Infect Immun* 1999;67:2010–2012.

67. Holtzman MJ, Morton JD, Shornick LP, et al. Immunity, inflammation, and remodeling in the airway epithelial barrier: epithelial-viral-allergic paradigm. *Physiol Rev* 2002;82:19–46.

68. Look DC, Keller BT, Rapp SR, et al. Selective induction of intracellular adhesion molecule-1 by interferon-gamma in human airway epithelial cells. *Am J Physiol* 1992;263:L79–L87.

69. Bermudez LE, Goodman J. *Mycobacterium tuberculosis* invades and replicated within type II alveolar cells. *Infect Immun* 1996; 64:1400–1406.

70. Lin Y, Zhang M, Barnes PF. Chemokine production by a human alveolar epithelial cell line in response to *Mycobacterium tuberculosis*. *Infect Immun* 1998;66:1121–1126.

71. Bermudez LE, Sangari FJ, Kolonoski P, et al. The efficiency of the translocation of *Mycobacterium tuberculosis* across a bilayer of epithelial and endothelial cells as model of the alveolar wall

is a consequence of transport within mononuclear phagocytes and invasion of alveolar epithelial cells. *Infect Immun* 2002; 70:140–146.

72. Cooper AM, Callahan JE, Keen M, et al. Expression of memory immunity in the lung following re-exposure to *Mycobacterium tuberculosis*. *Tuber Lung Dis* 1997;78:67–73.

73. McMurray DN. Guinea pig model of tuberculosis. In: Bloom BR, ed. *Tuberculosis. Pathogenesis, protection, and control*. Washington, DC: ASM Press, 1994:135–148.

74. Baldwin SL, D'Souza C, Roberts AD, et al. Evaluation of new vaccines in the mouse and guinea pig model of tuberculosis. *Infect Immun* 1998;66:2951–2959.

75. Moreira AL, Tsenova L, Aman MH, et al. Mycobacterial antigens exacerbate disease manifestations in *M. tuberculosis* infected mice. *Infect Immun* 2002;70;2100–2107.

76. Horwitz MA, Harth G, Dillon BJ, et al. Recombinant bacillus Calmette–Guerin (BCG) vaccines expressing the *Mycobacterium tuberculosis* 30-kDa major secretory protein induce greater protective immunity against tuberculosis than conventional BCG vaccines in a highly susceptible animal model. *Proc Natl Acad Sci U S A* 2000;25:13853–13858.

77. Caruso AM, Serbina N, Klein E, et al. Mice deficient in CD4 T cells have only transiently diminished levels of IFN gamma, yet succumb to tuberculosis. *J Immunol* 1999;162:5407–5416.

78. Scanga CA, Mohan VP, Yu K, et al. Depletion of CD4+ T cells causes reactivation of murine persistent tuberculosis despite continued expression of interferon-gamma and nitric oxide synthase 2. *J Exp Med* 2000;192:347–358.

79. Flynn JL, Chan J. Immunology of tuberculosis. *Annu Rev Immunol* 2001;19:93–129.

80. Orme IM. Characteristics and specificity of acquired immunologic memory to *Mycobacterium tuberculosis* infection. *J Immunol* 1988;140:3589–3593.

81. Orme IM. The kinetics of emergence and loss of mediator T lymphocytes acquired in response to infection with *Mycobacterium tuberculosis*. *Infect Immun* 1987;138:293–298.

82. Brooks JV, Frank AA, Keen MA, et al. Boosting vaccine for tuberculosis. *Infect Immun* 2001;69:2714–2717.

83. D'Souza CD, Cooper AM, Frank AA, et al. A novel nonclassic beta2-microglobulin-restricted mechanism influencing early lymphocyte accumulation and subsequent resistance to tuberculosis in the lung. *Am J Respir Cell Mol Biol* 2000;23:188–193.

84. Bloom BR, Fine PEM. The BCG experience: implications for future vaccines against tuberculosis. In: Bloom BR, ed. *Tuberculosis. Pathogenesis, protection, and control*. Washington, DC: ASM Press, 1994:531–558.

85. Murray PJ, Young RA. Secretion of mammalian proteins from mycobacteria. In: Parish T, Stoker NG, ed. *Methods in molecular biology, vol 101: mycobacteria protocols*. Totowa, NJ: Humana Press, 1998:275–284.

86. Engers HD, Bergquist R, Modabber F. Progress on vaccines against parasites. *Dev Biol Stand* 1996;87:73–84.

87. Boulanger D, Warter A, Sellin B, et al. Vaccine potential of a recombinant glutathione S-transferase cloned from *Schistosoma haematobium* in primates experimentally infected with a homologous challenge. *Vaccine* 1999;17:319–326.

88. Ota MO, Vekemans J, Schlegel-Haueter SE, et al. Influence of *Mycobacterium bovis* bacillus Calmette–Guerin on antibody and cytokine responses to human neonatal vaccination. *J Immunol* 2002;168:919–925.

89. Aldovini A, Young RA. Humoral and cell-mediated immune responses to live recombinant BCG-HIV vaccines. *Nature* 1991;351:479–482.

90. Stover CK, de la Cruz VF, Fuerst TR, et al. New use of BCG recombinant vaccines. *Nature* 1991;351:456–460.

91. Langermann S, Palaszynski S, Sadziene A, et al. Systemic and

mucosal immunity induced by BCG vector expressing outer-surface A of *Borrelia burgdorferi*. *Nature* 1994;372:552–555.

92. Connell ND, Medina-Acosta E, McMaster WR, et al. Effective immunization against cutaneous leishmaniasis with recombinant bacilli Calmette–Guerin expressing the *Leishmania* surface proteinase gp63. *Proc Natl Acad Sci U S A* 1993;90: 11473–11477.

93. Horwitz MA, Lee BW, Dillon BJ, et al. Protective immunity against tuberculosis induced by vaccination with major extracellular proteins of *Mycobacterium tuberculosis*. *Proc Natl Acad Sci U S A* 1995;92:1530–1534.

94. Moreira AL, Tsenova l, Murray PJ, et al. Aerosol infection of mice with recombinant BCG secreting murine IFN-gamma partially reconstitutes local protective immunity. *Microb Pathog* 2000;29:175–185.

95. Ponninghaus JM, Fine PE, Sterne JA, et al. Efficacy of BCG vaccine against leprosy and tuberculosis in northern Malawi. *Lancet* 1992;339:636–639.

96. Turner J, Rhoades ER, Keen M, et al. Effective preexposure tuberculosis vaccines fail to protect when they are given in an immunotherapeutic mode. *Infect Immun* 2000;68:1706–1709.

97. Turner OC, Roberts AD, Frank AA, et al. Lack of protection in mice and necrotizing bronchointerstitial pneumonia with bronchiolitis in guinea pigs immunized with vaccines directed against the hsp60 molecule of *Mycobacterium tuberculosis*. *Infect Immun* 2000;68:3674–3679.

98. Fine PE, Floyd S, Stanford JL, et al. Environmental mycobacteria in northern Malawi: implications for the epidemiology of tuberculosis and leprosy. *Epidemiol Infect* 2001;126:379–387.

99. Brandt L, Feino Cunha J, Weinreich OA, et al. Failure of the *Mycobacterium bovis* BCG vaccine: some species of environmental mycobacteria block multiplication of BCG and induction of protective immunity to tuberculosis. *Infect Immun* 2002;70:672–678.

100. Tsenova L, Bergtold A, Fredman VH, et al. Tumor necrosis factor alpha is a determinant of pathogenesis and disease progression in mycobacterial infection in the central nervous system. *Proc Natl Acad Sci U S A* 1999;96:5657–5662.

101. Tsenova L, Sokol K, Fredman VH, et al. A combination of thalidomide plus antibiotics protects rabbits from mycobacterial meningitis-associated death. *J Infect Dis* 1998;177: 1563–1572.

TUBERCULOSIS VACCINE SCIENCE

PETER ANDERSEN
BRIGITTE GICQUEL
KRIS HUYGEN

At the beginning of the 20th century, Camille Guérin and Albert Calmette initiated their attempts to produce a tuberculosis (TB) vaccine from a strain of *Mycobacterium bovis*. In the first studies from 1921 to 1927, bacille Calmette–Guérin (BCG) was shown to have protective efficacy against TB in a study on children (1). Today, more than three billion people have received this vaccine, and although it is still the most widely used vaccine globally, its benefits and drawbacks are still discussed. This discussion include elements such as safety aspects, loss of sensitivity to tuberculin as a diagnostic reagent, and, in particular, the fact that while helping to end the TB epidemic in Europe, this vaccine has been less successful in the developing world. Since the disappointing outcome of the large trial in Chingleput, India (2), an improved TB vaccine offering efficient and consistent protection has been an international research priority.

Exploiting the recent progress made in vaccine technology, several novel methods for improving or substituting the existing BCG vaccine have appeared over the past decade. Deciphering the total *Mycobacterium tuberculosis* genome sequence (3) and the rapid advances in genomics and proteomics have had a dramatic impact on the study of TB and, in particular, on the development of new TB vaccines. Advances in molecular biology and genomics have made manipulation of the genome easier and have resulted in the identification of numerous novel antigens. At the same time, progress in immunology has changed the way we look at vaccination and new technologies (e.g., DNA vaccines, recombinant vectors, new adjuvants) have matured to the stage where their efficacy in animal models is proven and their use in humans can be envisaged. Today, the TB vaccine field uses a wide range of novel vaccine technologies such as protein

subunit vaccination with one or a few defined products administered in optimized adjuvant formulations, DNA vaccine technology, viral delivery systems, attenuated mycobacterial vaccines, and various combinations of these delivery systems in prime boost regimens. Several promising experimental vaccines showing protective efficacy at the level of the standard BCG vaccine have been described (4). However, to develop a novel vaccine strategy superior to BCG, fundamental immunologic mechanisms responsible for protection and reasons explaining the failure of BCG still need to be fully resolved (for a discussion of potential reasons for the failure of BCG, see references 5,6). Of interest in this regard has been the development of animal models (and new vaccines) designed to test the situations hypothesized to have led to failure in BCG vaccination or that are likely to arise in the course of testing new vaccines in humans. Only a few years ago, it was generally accepted that clinical trials of new TB vaccines would not take place for at least a decade. However, the first trials are now ready to start (7) and within the next couple of years will move TB vaccine research from the laboratory into the clinic.

TARGETING THE IMMUNE SYSTEM IN TUBERCULOSIS VACCINE DEVELOPMENT

The acquired cellular immune response to *M. tuberculosis* is complex and involves multiple cellular subsets: CD4 and CD8 T cells and unconventional T cells such as $\gamma\delta$ T cells and double-negative $\alpha\beta$ T-cell subsets all play a role. However, in animal models, a key role for CD4 T cells in acquired resistance against TB is generally accepted and Th1 cells and interferon gamma (IFN-γ) are the major effectors that lead to macrophage activation, phagosomal acidification, and release of reactive nitrogen and oxygen intermediates. Consequently, the CD4 T-cell subset has been the major target for new experimental TB vaccines, and IFN-γ has been widely used as a correlate of protective immunity and for screening novel antigens of relevance for

P. Andersen: Department of TB Immunology, Statens Serum Institute, Copenhagen, Denmark.

B. Gicquel: Unit of Mycobacterial Genetics, The Pasteur Institute, Paris, France.

K. Huygen: Department of Mycobacterial Immunology, Pasteur Institute of Brussels, Brussels, Belgium.

TB vaccine development (8–10). However, it is clear that caution is needed when using IFN-γ as a single criterion for the selection of vaccine antigens (11), and increasing IFN-γ during vaccination is not necessarily associated with enhanced protection (12,13). Although the relative importance of different T-cell subsets is still debated (14), it has become increasingly clear in recent years that CD8 T cells are also very important players in the host defense against TB infections (15). CD8 cells have been implicated in the immune response both during the primary infection (16,17) and in the more chronic phase of infection in which an important role for this subset in the prevention of the reactivation of latent disease was suggested in a recent study (18). The CD8 subset is the main target for a number of novel vaccination strategies using DNA and viral vector systems (discussed in detail later) and a combination of both CD4 and CD8 T-cell subsets may be necessary to obtain optimal protection (19,20).

The search for nonprotein antigens from *M. tuberculosis* is an area of intense research, and, in particular, the lipid moieties recognized by αβ double-negative subsets in the context of CD1 molecules have attracted much interest (21,22). Although direct evidence of the role of these subsets in acquired immunity to TB is still lacking, inclusion of these molecules in novel vaccines could provide the link between innate and adaptive immunity needed for an optimal future TB vaccine (23,24). A crucial point of particular concern in the development of vaccines is the induction of long-lived immunologic memory. Long-term protection induced by most current vaccines seems to be mediated by humoral immune responses. In contrast, for diseases that are controlled by cell-mediated immune responses such as TB, human immunodeficiency virus, and malaria, there are no currently available uniformly effective vaccines. T-cell memory is maintained by a population of differentiated T cells, and major gaps still exist in our knowledge of the factors responsible for the induction and maintenance of this population (for an overview, see reference 25). In this regard, it is worth mentioning that BCG generally works well and protects against childhood manifestations of TB, but as children reach adolescence, the incidence of TB increases and protection by BCG is no longer detectable (26,27). Therefore, the immune response induced by BCG might be efficient for only 10 to 15 years. The ability of different vaccine delivery systems to maintain immunologic memory (28), and detailed understanding of these differences is fundamental for our attempts to develop a vaccine better than BCG.

GENOMICS, PROTEOMICS, AND VACCINE DESIGN

The *M. tuberculosis* genome contains approximately 4,000 different open reading frames, which potentially encode the same number of proteins. The completion of the *M. tuber-*

culosis genome (3) has greatly accelerated TB vaccine development and made it much easier to identify molecules expressed by the pathogen. Even a fragment of protein sequence is usually enough to identify a specific open reading frame. The task of subsequently pulling the gene out of the gene library, cloning it, and expressing it is a relatively simple task. This has meant that the number of recombinant antigens available for testing as vaccine candidates has increased from less than ten 8 years ago to many hundred purified reagents today. Likewise, progress in translating the genome information into proteins expressed has resulted in two-dimensional electrophoresis proteomic maps comprising more than 1,500 spots and, to date, the identification of several hundreds of proteins (29,30). Although the vast information from genomics and proteomics is a major step forward, the rational identification of vaccine candidates still lacks parameters that define protective antigens, and refining the selection of candidate antigens for further evaluation is therefore a priority. Containment of *M. tuberculosis* in the granuloma creates a physical microenvironment that has not been characterized in detail but nutrient limitation, low pH, hydrolytic enzymes, reactive nitrogen and oxygen species, and reduced oxygen tension are believed to be important factors (31). One approach is to study the proteome from bacteria grown inside the macrophage or under conditions mimicking the intracellular milieu and identify the components up-regulated under these growth conditions (32,33). *In vitro* low oxygen culture models have therefore recently been used by different laboratories to study the events that allow *M. tuberculosis* to survive in the granuloma and to identify proteins that are differentially expressed by the bacteria in this metabolic state. The 16-kd small heat shock protein or α-crystallin homolog (HspX, Rv2031c) (34) was the first protein identified as highly expressed under low oxygen conditions, and recently a large number of proteins was found to be up-regulated under similar conditions (33). Antigens that play a role as virulence factors are always considered lead candidates in vaccine design and expected to be up-regulated by the pathogen during infection. The latest development in the identification of virulence genes is signature-tagged mutagenesis, which has been used to generate panels of insertion mutants with varying levels of attenuation (35,36). The method allows an easy identification of the mutated virulence genes responsible for the attenuation, and the gene products can subsequently be tested as vaccines.

In the postgenomic era, bioinformatic tools have provided a number of novel possibilities to accelerate antigen discovery. Antigens secreted by *M. tuberculosis* have, for a number of years, attracted much interest as a source of potentially protective antigens responsible for the high efficacy of live vaccines (37,38). The general export pathway in prokaryotes mediates protein translocation across the cytoplasmic membrane by means of an NH_2-terminal secretory signal peptide, and a recent study pointed to 52 proteins as most likely secreted based on searching the genome (39).

Another selection criterion may be to focus on proteins that are absent from or expressed at low levels in BCG and therefore may contain important protective T-cell antigens in *M. tuberculosis* that are not primed by a BCG vaccination (40–43). These antigens have been suggested as attractive vaccine candidates to supplement BCG vaccination, and molecular techniques have revealed 16 DNA segments representing 129 open reading frames that are absent from various strains of BCG. Another possibility is to search the genome for gene families related to known immunodominant antigens and thereby potentially find other proteins of relevance to human infection. For example, the antigen ESAT-6 is broadly and strongly recognized by both CD4 and CD8 T cells from TB-infected individuals and protective in animal models (11,44,45). Searching the complete genome, several genes that share size, genomic organization, and as much as 35% homology have been identified (46), and so far a surprising number of the molecules encoded by these genes has been demonstrated to be strongly recognized by the immune system (47), thus demonstrating that a postgenomic antigen discovery program may be a very rational way to rapidly identify interesting vaccine antigens. Approximately 9% of the coding capacity of the *M. tuberculosis* genome is allocated to the PE and PPE gene families, whose names are derived from the Pro-Glu (PE) (n = 99) and Pro-Pro-Glu (PPE) (n = 68) motifs near their N terminus (3). The function of these proteins is unknown, but most PE and PPE proteins (the so-called PE-PGRS and PPE-MLS families) carry variable copies of tandem repeats of amino acid sequence motifs in their C-terminal regions. This gene family has been shown to contain targets for the immune system such as Mtb39a and Mtb41 (48,49) and represent with the large number of closely related genes an abundant source of potentially interesting antigens.

The approaches described previously start with the bacteria as the launch point for identifying candidate vaccine antigens. However, the alternative is to screen the complete genome in a completely nonbiased way for epitopes that will be recognized by the human immune system. The approach relies on computer algorithms to identify T-cell epitopes that bind the human major histocompatibility complex (MHC) most strongly and also promiscuously (i.e., to more than one MHC allele) (50). Vaccines developed with this approach would potentially have to go straight to clinical trials because immune recognition in the animal models normally used for TB vaccine testing such as mice and guinea pigs (with the possible exception of human leukocyte antigen transgenic mice) would not be expected.

ANIMAL MODELS FOR TUBERCULOSIS VACCINE EVALUATION

How to choose the most promising candidate vaccine to enter in clinical trials is an important question widely debated in the scientific community. Because there is still no good *in vitro* correlate of protective immunity, the current approach is the evaluation of experimental vaccines in animal challenge studies. TB in various animal models manifests itself differently, and different models have therefore been used in a stepwise fashion depending on cost or to model particular aspects of human disease such as granuloma formation or caseous necrosis. The mouse has the most extensively studied immune system of any animal, and manipulation and evaluation of the immune response in this species are routine. Currently, most TB vaccines are screened in the mouse model first because it is cost-effective and the immune response primed by the vaccine can be thoroughly characterized. Mice are, however, relatively resistant to *M. tuberculosis* infection, and granulomas in the mouse rarely progress to necrosis, caseation, or liquefaction as observed in humans. The mouse is therefore more suited for an initial comparative screening than detailed long-term studies of selected vaccines. Guinea pigs have the advantage of being highly susceptible to TB, even more susceptible than humans, and develop severe lesions in their lungs similar to those observed in human disease. For this reason, they have been the favored model for TB research for decades and have allowed a detailed study of the vaccine activity and ability to control the different phases of disease: implantation, bacillemia, and progressive disease with cavitation (51). Now that immunologic reagents such as cytokines and antibodies have started to emerge (52), this model will become even more valuable for TB vaccine research. Vaccine efficacy in these models has traditionally mostly been assessed by reduction of bacterial numbers during the initial phase of logarithmic growth (53). Compared with these original observations, recent data suggest that there is no direct correlation between the level of protection monitored by bacterial numbers in the organs at early time points and the further development of clinical disease measured as weight loss and prolonged survival (54). Furthermore, longer-term infections mimic better the situation in humans in whom disease is often only apparent months or years after infection and are therefore becoming more widely used, despite the increased costs involved. The model that most closely resembles human disease is nonhuman primates, and as candidate vaccines with high efficacy are developed and human trials of these vaccines become a reality, the need for supporting data in primate models has increased. In this regard, cynomolgus monkeys are probably the models closest to human disease with a chronic, slowly progressive, localized form of pulmonary TB (55). That the final result in animal models is crucially dependent on the model chosen (51) was, however, recently emphasized by the observation that two species of macaque differ greatly in the protective effect of the current BCG vaccine (56). Cynomolgus monkeys vaccinated with BCG were almost completely protected against pathology and had greatly reduced numbers of bacteria in their lungs compared with nonvaccinated animals. In contrast, rhesus monkeys had severe pathology in the lungs, with cavitations, caseous necrosis, and bacterial loads that were not significantly different from unvaccinated animals.

Even though our understanding of the pros and cons of different TB animal models has increased in the past decade, most human vaccination and disease still occur under conditions very different from the standard animal models. BCG works efficiently in some clinical trials (70% to 80% efficacy), and therefore it might be difficult for a candidate vaccine to be better under those circumstances. However, through the development of animal models that mimic real-life conditions for the target population in question, novel vaccines can be compared in models in which BCG is impaired and in which possible reasons for the failure of this vaccine could be addressed. Three such models are currently being evaluated in TB vaccine research:

1. Animals previously sensitized with environmental mycobacteria. This model aims to test vaccines in situations relevant to BCG failure. It has long been suggested that sensitization to mycobacteria from the environment may inhibit the efficacy of BCG vaccination (57). Recent work in mice and cattle has shown that exposure to environmental mycobacteria block completely BCG multiplication and thereby protective activity (58,59). However, the data from the mouse model demonstrate that the immune responses generated by this sensitization were not sufficient to efficiently protect against later infection with *M. tuberculosis*. In contrast, a subunit vaccine was not inhibited by prior sensitization, indicating that such vaccines could be deployed in areas where BCG vaccination has been ineffective (58).
2. Animals previously vaccinated with BCG. This model is developed as a consequence of the fact that most of the world population that would be the target for a novel efficient TB vaccine already are and probably also in the future would be vaccinated with BCG. Therefore, novel vaccines are tested as booster vaccines after prior BCG vaccination instead of as a replacement for BCG. Following this line of reasoning, Brooks et al. (60) recently demonstrated that midlife boosting with a vaccine based on antigen 85A (Ag 85A) in adjuvant resulted in levels of protection in the lungs of boosted mice comparable with those of young BCG-vaccinated mice, whereas BCG activity had waned in mice receiving BCG alone (60).
3. Animals latently infected with *M. tuberculosis*. Only 5% to 10% of TB-infected individuals progress directly to active TB; the majority carries the infection in a latent or chronic form and may reactivate disease decades later (61). The first successful efforts to develop animal models to address this important problem was the Cornell model based on initial intravenous TB infection followed by chemotherapy treatment that reduces the

infectious load and establishes a low-level chronic infection (62). In this model, neither immunization with killed *Mycobacterium vaccae* nor the BCG vaccine altered the rate of relapse to active disease (63). This model has been the subject of renewed interest from several laboratories in which both the influence of model modifications and the importance of cellular subsets have been studied (18,64). Lowrie et al. (65) recently presented the first evidence from animal models to support a potential role of postexposure vaccination or immunotherapy in TB by demonstrating that HSP60 DNA vaccines administered to infected mice lead to accelerated bacterial clearance (see DNA Vaccines section).

Several vaccines have by now been demonstrated to be efficacious in various animal models. However, it is clear that the outcome of vaccine testing in animal models is greatly influenced by the choice of model (for an overview, see reference 66). It therefore becomes crucial to compare the efficacy of the lead candidate vaccines in standardized animal models. A vaccine that, in addition to being protective in the standard models, confers protection in animal models in which BCG has failed to provide protection, such as the rhesus macaques (56) or some of the novel mouse models mentioned previously, should receive the highest priority for further development.

SUBUNIT VACCINES

The subunit and DNA vaccine approach is based on the assumption that a few antigens are sufficient to induce and maintain a protective immune response. The development of subunit vaccines has benefited tremendously from the sequencing of the TB genome, and the accelerated identification of novel antigens has resulted in the identification of defined antigens protective in animal models (Table 59.1). To include antigens that give rise to beneficial responses and exclude potential detrimental components is the ultimate advantage provided by subunit vaccines, but, in addition, the safety profile and possible incorporation of a TB subunit vaccine in existing childhood vaccines make the subunit approach attractive. Attempts to develop a subunit vaccine against TB date back to the early attempts in the 1950s and 1960s in which different cell wall fractions from *M. tuberculosis* administered in oil emulsions were shown to protect against subsequent challenge at levels equal to or even superior to live BCG (67). However, demonstrations that these vaccines induced primarily a short-lived, nonspecific immune response (68) owing to the presence of immunostimulatory components from the mycobacterial cell wall such as muramyl dipeptide and trehalose dimycolate (69) led to the belief that only immunization with live mycobacteria induced efficient acquired immunity to TB.

TABLE 59.1. TUBERCULOSIS VACCINE CANDIDATE ANTIGENS WITH PROVEN EFFICACY IN ANIMAL MODELS

Antigen	Molecular Mass[a]/Sanger Identification	Delivery System	Ref.
MTB8.4	8.4 kd/Rv1174c	Subunit/DNA	153
ESAT-6	9.9 kd/Rv3875	Subunit/DNA	11,82,116
MPT63	13.7 kd/Rv1926c	DNA	116
MPT64	22.4 kd/Rv1980c	DNA	112
MPT83	19.9 kd/Rv2873	DNA	116
Ag85B	30.7 kd/Rv1886c	Subunit/DNA	73,82
Ag85A	31.7 kd/Rv3804c	DNA	54,100,106,108
PstS-1	36.0 kd/Rv0934	Subunit/DNA	154,155
PstS-3	35.8 kd/Rv0928	DNA	156
MTB39	39.1 kd/Rv1196	DNA	49
MTB41	41.4 kd/Rv0915c	DNA	48
hsp60	55.9 kd/Rv3417c	DNA	99,157
hsp70	66.8 kd/Rv0350	DNA	153

[a]The predicted mass was calculated from the amino acid sequence of the corresponding open reading frame but adjusted if an N-terminal signal sequence was suggested.

It was suggested that proteins secreted by living bacilli in the phagosome would be available for processing and presentation to the immune system at an early stage of infection and thereby that vaccines based on these antigens would result in accelerated recognition of infected macrophages and efficient protection (37,38). In 1991, Andersen et al. (38) defined a short-term culture filtrate enriched in secreted antigens from *M. tuberculosis* and found that it contained only minimal amounts of proteins released from the cytoplasm. Hubbard et al. (70) subsequently reported the protective effect in mice of vaccination with culture-filtrate proteins prepared from log-phase *M. tuberculosis* cultures, whereas Pal and Horwitz (71) published similar observations in guinea pigs. Both of these two early studies used incomplete Freund adjuvant (IFA) as an adjuvant for their protein preparations. In 1994, Andersen (72) reported long-lived, protective responses equivalent to those induced by BCG vaccination, using a vaccine based on short-term culture filtrate in cationic lipid vesicles made from dimethyl-dioctadecylammonium bromide and demonstrated that the protection was transferable by CD4+ T cells. These initial observations from different laboratories initiated extensive antigen discovery programs that aimed to identify key antigenic molecules in culture filtrates. Some of the first antigens purified from culture filtrate and tested as vaccine were the components of the 30- to 33-kd Ag 85 complex and the 38-kd phosphate-binding protein (73,74). In particular, the Ag 85A and B components and the low molecular mass antigen ESAT-6 have been demonstrated to promote significant levels of immunity in a number of studies from independent laboratories (Table 59.1). Even a single epitope derived from ESAT-6 was found to confer efficient protection comparable with the protection afforded by BCG in the C57BL/6 mouse

model of TB infection (11). Recently, Olsen et al. (75) continued this work by the development of a subunit vaccine consisting of a fusion protein of Ag 85B and ESAT-6. This vaccine induced levels of protection superior to that of the single components in mice, and promoted a very efficient memory immune response. Coler et al. (76) recently described a new promising molecule, Mtb 8.4, isolated from culture filtrate. This low molecular mass antigen, in combination with the adjuvant IFA, induced not only the expected CD4 response but also CD8 cells and protection in the mouse model.

Adjuvants for Subunit Vaccines

For a disease such as TB, which requires cellular immunity, the choice of adjuvant is important. Adjuvants allow the immune system to store antigen for prolonged periods, thus providing a continued stimulus for memory cells and the initial stimuli for recruitment and differentiation of T cells. Currently used adjuvants for human vaccines (e.g., aluminum salts) are only used in vaccines that generate a humoral response (e.g., diphtheria, tetanus, hepatitis B vaccines) and induce a predominant Th2 response (12,77). The protective efficacy of different TB vaccines tested so far has correlated with the Th1/Th2 balance of the response primed by the vaccine, and aluminium-adjuvanted vaccines have been shown to be counterproductive (12,78). Adjuvants that are currently being evaluated for TB subunit vaccines include IFA (79,80), polylactide microspheres (81), dimethyl-dioctadecylammonium bromide cationic lipid vesicles (72), as well as the nontoxic lipid A derivative monophosphoryl lipid A (54,82). Of importance for later clinical trials, with the exception of IFA, these adjuvants are characterized by a low toxicity and either have been tested or are under testing in humans. Current efforts are focused on the dissection of the cytokine networks involved in the action of adjuvants leading to the development of a Th1 response protective against TB. In a series of studies, it was demonstrated by specific cytokine neutralization that both interleukin (IL)-6 and IL-12 participate in the induction of a type 1 protective T-cell response and protective immunity by a dimethyl-dioctadecylammonium bromide adjuvant TB subunit vaccine (83,84). Importantly, however, it also became clear that subsequent supplementation of subunit vaccines by these key cytokines may result in increased T cell–dependent IFN-γ but not necessarily higher efficacy of the vaccines (13). Along the same line, chitin particles (*N*-acetyl-D-glucosamine polymer) were recently tested as adjuvant for the mycobacterial antigen Ag 85B (85). In this study, it was demonstrated that chitin particles induced a clear-cut Th1 response, whereas BCG down-regulate the Th1 response by stimulating a prostaglandin E_2 synthesis. However, a balanced Th1/Th2 response may, in fact, be what is needed to circumvent excessive immunopathology at the site of infection. It is clear that the granulomatous reaction is beneficial and serves to wall off the site of infection, as demonstrated in intercellular adhesion molecule-1 knockout mice that succumbed with widespread tissue necrosis and no organized granulomatous tissue (86). Induction of too strong Th1 responses (e.g., by mixing IL-12 into the vaccines) may, conversely, result in exaggerated responses and mortality owing to consolidation of lung tissues by lymphocytic granulomas (54) and caseous necrosis (87). Although several adjuvants have been reported to enhance Th1 responses, it has been difficult to find any adjuvant that efficiently facilitates class I–restricted CD8 responses, although some reports have emphasized the potential of immune-stimulating complexes in this regard (88). In the light of the importance of this subset for immunity against TB, research in this field should be pursued.

DNA VACCINES

The general principle of genetic vaccination using naked bacterial plasmid DNA is surprisingly simple, yet a major breakthrough in this technology was only made during the past 10 years. In a seminal paper from 1990, Wolff et al. (89) reported that injection into muscle cells of naked plasmid DNA encoding the bacterial enzyme β-galactosidase could lead to direct gene transfer to the muscle cell and subsequent synthesis of the enzyme by that cell (89). In 1992, Tang et al. (90) demonstrated that plasmid injection elicited an immune response, and the next year Ulmer et al. (91) were the first to report on protective efficacy of DNA vaccination against an infectious disease, i.e., influenza A (91). Since then, DNA vaccines have been reported to

induce protective immunity in numerous animal models of parasitic, viral, and bacterial diseases (92). These DNA vaccines offer several potential advantages, including ease of preparation, stability, relatively low cost, and safety for immunocompromised patients. Several clinical trials are currently being performed in the field of cancer, allergy, human immunodeficiency virus, and malaria (93).

In a DNA vaccine, the gene for an antigen is inserted into a bacterial plasmid vector, pDNA is amplified in transformed bacteria, and the purified plasmid DNA encoding the immunogen is injected into an immunocompetent host. Cellular targets are mainly muscle cells (intramuscularly immunization) and keratinocytes (epidermal gene gun immunization), but bacterial DNA also gets into professional antigen-presenting cells present in and attracted to the injected sites. Once inside the cell, the plasmid translocates to its nucleus in a way that is not completely understood. Transcription of the coding information is driven by a strong eukaryotic promoter such as the promoter of the first immediate early antigen (IE1) of cytomegalovirus.

The methylation pattern of injected plasmid DNA remains of a bacterial nature (methylated adenosines) as long as 19 months after injection, indicating that no replication occurs in the eukaryotic host (94). Furthermore, sequence homology with eukaryotic sequences is minimal, and as a result of these two factors, the risk of homologous recombination and mutagenic or potentially carcinogenic integration is very low. Random integration may take place, but at chances less than one copy per 150,000 nuclei (95).

Stimulation of the Immune System

DNA vaccination is an easy method for generating strong humoral and cellular immune responses. The priming of the immune response involves professional antigen-presenting cells (dendritic cells, Langerhans cells) that endocytose DNA into acidic vesicles for subsequent transport to the nucleus (96). Cross-priming after uptake by dendritic cells of apoptotic bodies originating from transfected muscle cells and keratinocytes is also very important in the initiation of the immune response. Bacterial DNA has inherent adjuvant properties and triggers production of costimulatory cytokines by these antigen-presenting cells through its interaction with a specific Toll-like receptor, i.e., TLR9 (97). The particular motif in bacterial DNA that interacts with mouse TLR9 is a six-base DNA consisting of an unmethylated CpG dinucleotide flanked by two 5′ purines and two 3′ pyrimidines: GACGTT (98). For humans, the optimal sequence is slightly different: GTCGTT. The major costimulatory cytokines induced are IL-12, which stimulates natural killer cells to produce IFN-γ and favors the development of the Th1 subset, and IL-6, which stimulates B cells, favors antibody production, and also plays a role in T-cell differentiation (98). DNA vaccines stimulate both the exogenous (MHC class II restricted) and the endogenous (MHC class I restricted) antigen presentation pathway. It is particularly this class I–restricted presentation, resulting in strong CD8$^+$-mediated immune responses, that is a hallmark of DNA vaccines and that makes them particularly attractive as vaccine formulations against intracellular viruses, parasites, and bacteria. After DNA vaccination, antigenic material is generated from within the host cell and endogenous processing can take place in much the same way as after infection with intracellular pathogens. As such, DNA vaccines mimic the infection with live pathogens, in contrast to vaccines based on protein antigens or killed pathogens that are preferentially processed through the exogenous presentation pathway that generates MHC class II–restricted CD4$^+$ responses.

DNA Vaccination against Tuberculosis

The number of preclinical studies on DNA vaccination against mycobacterial infections has increased enormously over the past years. (For a complete list, search the DNAvaccine.com website.)

In 1996, Tascon et al. (99) and Huygen et al. (100) were the first to document on the value of naked DNA vaccination in TB, using plasmid DNA encoding a 65-kd heat shock protein from *Mycobacterium leprae* and the 32-kd mycolyltransferase or Ag 85A from *M. tuberculosis*, respectively. Subsequently, various degrees of immunogenicity and prophylactic efficacy against TB have been reported (mostly in C57BL/6 mice) with DNA vaccines encoding a number of antigens (Table 59.1). Whereas most DNA vaccines tested so far encode secreted or surface-exposed mycobacterial proteins, some laboratories have focused on cytoplasmic proteins such as the 65-kd heat shock protein (99) and the MTB39 protein (49) (belonging to the PPE family) that are found predominantly in bacterial lysates. Strong humoral and Th1-biased cellular immune responses can be induced with some of these DNA vaccine candidates, particularly when administered by the intramuscular route (101). Robust (nanogram levels) antigen-specific IFN-γ responses but very little IL-4 or IL-5 can be detected in spleen cell culture supernatants from DNA-vaccinated mice, and antibody isotypes reflect this Th1 bias. Strong CD8$^+$-mediated cytotoxic T lymphocyte responses can also be induced with these DNA vaccines. Interestingly, the epitopic repertoire for both CD4$^+$ and CD8$^+$ T cells is broadened by DNA vaccination compared with infection with live *M. tuberculosis* or vaccination with BCG (102–104), suggesting that antigenic processing may be slightly different.

The value of DNA vaccines in the immunotherapy of TB is a controversial matter. *M. tuberculosis*–infected BALB/c mice given four doses of plasmid DNA encoding hsp65 of *M. leprae* demonstrated a rapid and spectacular decline in live bacteria in the spleen and lungs as long as 5 months later (65). Conversely, the Ag 85A DNA vaccine known to induce protective immunity and prevent long-

term necrosis in guinea pigs failed to protect mice when given in an immunotherapeutic model in mice infected earlier by aerosol with *M. tuberculosis* (105). Interestingly, in the latter experiment, the Ag 85A DNA vaccine had no effect on the course of infection in the lungs but did reduce significantly the bacterial load in the spleen. Also, hsp65 DNA vaccination given at the end of an 8-week chemotherapy course was capable of completely preventing the reactivation of bacterial growth after immunosuppressive corticosteroid injection in the Cornell model of reactivation (65).

So far, all preclinical TB DNA vaccines have been tested in the mouse, with the exception of one report in guinea pigs by Baldwin et al. (54), who reported that vaccination with DNA encoding Ag 85A can prevent the onset of caseating disease, which is the hallmark of the aerogenic infection model in this species. Survival was prolonged in Ag 85A DNA–vaccinated guinea pigs but still not at the level of BCG-vaccinated animals.

Mechanism of Action and Modulation of Efficacy of DNA Vaccines

DNA vaccines induce strong CD4$^+$- and CD8$^+$-mediated immune responses, but the relative importance of these compartments in protection conferred by the vaccine may differ according to the antigen and the mouse strain used. Thus, the Ag 85A DNA vaccine (effective in B6 mice) is essentially a CD4$^+$ vaccine that significantly decreases the bacterial replication in the lungs and prolongs the survival of *M. tuberculosis*–infected β$_2$-microglobulin knockout mice (which lack functional CD8$^+$ T cells) but fails to protect CD4 knockout mice (106). This is further corroborated by the fact that epidermal gene gun immunization with Ag 85A DNA vaccine is not protective, although this immunization route can induce strong CD8$^+$-mediated cytotoxic T-lymphocyte responses (101). Conversely, adoptive transfer studies in hsp65 DNA–vaccinated BALB/c mice have shown that the most potent protective T cell is a CD8$^+$/CD44^{hi} cell population that produces IFN-γ and is cytotoxic (107).

DNA vaccines offer the advantage that they can be formulated to target specific cell compartments for antigen processing. Plasmids encoding a secreted form of the protein by fusing it to the signal sequence of human tissue plasminogen activator are generally more immunogenic both for B and T cells than plasmids encoding a mature form (108–110). Transient transfection experiments *in vitro* have shown that plasmids encoding a secreted form show higher expression levels than plasmids encoding nonsecreted proteins, and this is probably the most important factor involved in the increased immunogenicity (109). Better availability of the released antigen to professional antigen-presenting cells may also be of importance. The effect of the tissue plasminogen activator leader sequence is most pronounced for weakly immunogenic constructs or when DNA is used at suboptimal doses or at low-dose number (108). This may explain why some authors have failed to observe differences between DNA encoding secreted and mature protein forms (111). Secreted forms are targeted to the endoplasmic reticulum where they are glycosylated on their asparagine residues, but this glycosylation does not influence their immunogenicity (D. L. Montgomery and K. Huygen, unpublished results, 1998).

A specific way to increase MHC class I presentation is by tagging DNA constructs to ubiquitin, which will result in proteins that are targeted preferentially to the proteasome system. The mycobacterial culture filtrate proteins MPT64 and ESAT-6 were expressed as chimeric proteins fused to one of three variants of the ubiquitin protein (UbG, UbA, and UbGR). Immunization with plasmids expressing the UbA and UbGR fusion shifted the host response toward a stronger Th1-type immunity, which was characterized by low or absent specific antibody levels, a lower number of IL-4–producing cells, and a higher number of IFN-γ–producing T cells. However, despite these higher IFN-γ levels produced *in vitro*, these ubiquitinated constructs did not provide a better protective response *in vivo* that the nonubiquitinated tissue plasminogen activator–fused antigens (112).

A limiting factor for DNA vaccines is the transfection efficacy and the amount of actual protein synthesized. It is estimated that injection of microgram doses of DNA results in production of only nanogram doses of protein. Complexation of DNA in cationic lipids (113) and intramuscularly immunization combined with muscle electroporation (114) can increase the efficacy of immunization. Coimmunization with a plasmid-expressing granulocyte-macrophage colony-stimulating factor can enhance the T-cell immunity of DNA vaccines encoding Ag 85B or MPT64 approximately twofold, but this is not sufficient to improve the efficacy of this vaccination against an aerosol challenge with *M. tuberculosis* (115).

Finally, multisubunit vaccination by coimmunization with different DNA vectors may result in a greater degree of protection, as indicated by reduced colony-forming unit counts, and as much as sevenfold prolonged survival times after high-dose aerosol challenge (116,117).

RECOMBINANT POXVIRUSES AND *SALMONELLA* AS VACCINE CARRIERS

Recombinant poxviruses induce the whole spectrum of immune responses to coexpressed microbial antigens, ranging from strong antibody and CD4+ T-cell responses to the consistent generation of CD8+ T cells. They can be used both as tools to dissect CD8+ T-cell responses and as candidate vaccines capable of inducing a balanced CD4+/CD8+ T-cell response (118). Vaccinia virus has been widely used and has a well-defined safety profile in humans. In addition,

these vaccines are temperature stable and can be administered orally. Compared with naked DNA vaccines, which encode only one particular antigen, recombinant viruses and bacteria have the disadvantage of being complex vectors with some intrinsic antigenicity and hence limited possibility for homologous boosting. Injection of recombinant vaccinia virus–expressing Ag 85A and Ag 85B from *M. tuberculosis* in B6 mice induced significant Th1-type spleen cell cytokine secretion, particularly when the genes were expressed as a fusion with the tissue plasminogen activator signal sequence (118). These recombinant vaccinia virus were also used to infect monocyte-derived macrophages that could subsequently be used as target cells for analyzing CD8+-mediated cytotoxic T lymphocyte responses in human BCG vaccines and TB-infected individuals (119–121). Vaccination of B6 mice with recombinant vaccinia viruses expressing the 19- and 38-kd glycolipoproteins significantly reduced the bacterial counts in the lungs of *M. tuberculosis* H37Rv–infected mice (122).

Recently, recombinant attenuated *Salmonella typhimurium* has been evaluated as a vaccine carrier strain for TB antigens (123). A *Salmonella* strain, which secretes ESAT-6 via the hemolysin secretion system of *Escherichia coli*, was tested, and a single dose was found to reduce numbers of tubercle bacilli in the lungs throughout the course of TB infection. A combined prime boost vaccination with DNA vaccines did not considerably enhance protection compared with the recombinant *Salmonella* alone.

HETEROLOGOUS PRIME BOOST WITH DIFFERENT VECTOR SYSTEMS

A different approach to vaccine design relies on two different vaccines for priming and boosting immune responses, and this strategy recently demonstrated potential in animal models of various diseases (124,125). In TB, a successful prime boost immunization regimen was recently reported with ESAT-6 or MPT63 (126). In this study, an immune response to the two antigens was primed by naked DNA immunization followed by boost with recombinant modified vaccinia virus Ankara. This combination resulted in increased numbers of CD4+ and CD8+ IFN-γ–producing cells and levels of protection equivalent to BCG in an experimental challenge model. This strategy can also be adapted to boost BCG-induced immunity, and human trials using modified vaccinia virus Ankara–expressing Ag 85A as a booster for immune responses in humans have recently started (127). Reversing the order, BCG can also be used to boost an immune response primed by a DNA vaccination. Sequential immunization with mycobacterial Ag 85B–expressing DNA and *M. bovis* BCG was more effective than BCG immunization alone in protecting B6 mice against an aerosol *M. tuberculosis* infection (128). Depletion of the CD8+ T cells impaired this protection in their spleens but not in their lungs, suggesting that the improved efficacy was partially mediated by CD8$^+$ T cells. This was somewhat surprising because Ag 85B has been reported not to contain K^b or D^b restricted epitopes (106).

Very recently, DNA priming and heterologous boosting with modified vaccinia virus Ankara encoding Ag 85A was described to confer protection against *M. tuberculosis* infection in the lungs of BALB/c mice equivalent to that obtained with BCG (129). Also, boosting of DNA primed Th1-type immune response with protein in adjuvant can result in better immunogenicity and efficacy of the vaccine (104).

LIVE MYCOBACTERIAL VACCINES

Currently, this field is developing along two parallel tracks: building on BCG by improving its immunogenicity and decreasing residual virulence and developing a better vaccine based on rational attenuation of *M. tuberculosis*.

Building on Bacille Calmette–Guérin

BCG was not initially isolated as an avirulent isolate, but during the initial passaging of *M. bovis* on media with ox bile (which acts as a detergent to disperse clumps of bacilli), mutations accumulated, leading to bacilli that are more resistant to this culture condition and attenuated in various animal models. The genetic alterations responsible for these changes were completely unknown until recently when comparative genomic analysis of BCG and *M. bovis* identified mutations and deletions in more than 100 genes, which explains why BCG has not reverted (41,130,131). One region, RD1, is missing in all BCG strains but is present in all *M. bovis* and *M. tuberculosis* strains (41,130,131). The RD1 region might contain some of the genes involved in virulence or regulators of virulence genes. However, *M. tuberculosis* virulence genes identified so far have been located outside this region. Recent studies have shown that the inactivation of genes involved in the synthesis of cell wall constituents results in attenuated strains (35,36,132–134), and BCG may therefore progressively have accumulated mutations that modify the cell wall, leading to its attenuation and altered colony morphology. A combination of mutations is probably responsible for the attenuation of BCG, each of these mutations having a partial effect on virulence. Calmette distributed BCG to many laboratories where it was grown in a number of different culture conditions. This resulted in BCG daughter strains that share major characteristics but also differ by the presence of additional mutations and deletions. These differences result in the presence or absence of several antigens, different immunogenicity in animal models, and a variable number of side effects observed after vaccination (135). It has been speculated that reintroduction of a number of genes missing from BCG might result in strains with increased immunogenicity and expressing an enriched antigen repertoire. Experiments

are currently underway in a number of laboratories to test this hypothesis. Horwitz (136) recently reported that a recombinant BCG overexpressing Ag 85B induces protective immunity against TB superior to that induced by the parental BCG strains from which they were derived. In this study, the gene coding for Ag 85B from *M. tuberculosis* was cloned into a shuttle vector and transferred into BCG. BCG expresses a form of Ag 85B highly homologous to that produced by *M. tuberculosis* (it differs by only two amino acids), and the somewhat surprising activity of this strain is hypothesized to result from the high level of expression of the antigen in the recombinant strain, which carries several copies of the Ag 85B gene. Whatever the reason, this is the first recombinant BCG vaccine that has been reported to give higher levels of protection than BCG in the guinea pig model.

It has been speculated that BCG can be improved by engineering the bacilli to stimulate a more efficient immune response. Like the immune responses observed after infection with other pathogens, inoculation of BCG represses some and induces other molecules involved in innate and acquired immune responses. Recent studies with microarrays confirmed previous experiments (137) and showed that IL-12 expression from phagocytes is repressed (138). The integration of genes coding for cytokines, chemokines, soluble receptors, antagonists of molecules inhibiting responses such as transforming growth factor β (139) or costimulatory molecules into BCG may potentially enhance its immunogenicity (140). In a study by Murray (141), BCG strains secreting IL-2, IFN-γ, or granulocyte-macrophage colony-stimulating factor were constructed and antigen-specific proliferation and cytokine release were found to be enhanced in splenocyte cultures derived from mice immunized with the recombinant strains compared with the parental strain of BCG.

As described previously, MHC class I–restricted CD8 T-cell responses are believed to be important in TB infection, and BCG has been engineered to increase antigen presentation by this pathway. Recombinant BCG producing listeriolysin from *Listeria monocytogenes* was constructed to allow mycobacterial antigens to be released from BCG-containing phagosomes and into the cytoplasm for MHC class I presentation (142). Although the addition of listeriolysin did not allow the release of BCG from phagosomes, an increased class I presentation of cophagocytosed proteins was observed in mice immunized with recombinant listeriolysin-producing BCG.

New Attenuated Vaccines Based on *Mycobacterium tuberculosis*

Vaccines derived from the "human strain" by rational attenuation might lead to vaccines that express essential antigens that are missing in BCG. The progress in efficient genetic tools to manipulate mycobacteria (143,144) allows the introduction of precise mutations into the genome of *M.*

tuberculosis and the use of random mutagenesis with a transposable element to generate libraries of mutants. Mutants with the desired phenotype can then be isolated and characterized. In the latter approach, animal models and *in vitro* cell cultures can be used to screen for mutants with attenuated phenotypes. Sequencing the regions flanking the transposon can identify the gene inactivated by the transposon and responsible for the attenuation of the mutant. This sequence can then be compared with the sequences of the entire *M. tuberculosis* genome and with the genomes of other living organisms in data banks. The identification of genes with similar sequences and identified functions will allow the prediction of the functions impaired in the mutant. Such an approach was used to screen libraries of mutants obtained by signature-tagged transposon mutagenesis. This method generates libraries of mutants by randomly inserting transposons, each containing a unique tag to make it possible to distinguish between different mutant strains. Groups of mutants containing different tags were used to inoculate mice. Mutants that do not persist are recognized by the absence of their tags in the bacilli collected from organs after infection. This approach led to the discovery of 13 new virulence loci (35). Four of them are clustered and are involved in the synthesis of phthiocerols and phthiocerol dimycocerosates (35,36). Mutants impaired in the synthesis of these lipids or their transport across the cell wall are avirulent and protect guinea pigs from a challenge with *M. tuberculosis* in the low-dose aerosol model as efficient as BCG (B. Gicquel, unpublished data, 2002).

M. tuberculosis mutants can also be constructed by allelic replacement, giving rise to auxotrophic strains impaired for the synthesis of purines, leucine, methionine, isoleucine, tryptophan, and proline. The disruption of genes in these biosynthetic pathways also leads to attenuation in other pathogens (145). The inactivation of *purC* resulted in an avirulent strain that cannot persist in mice or in *in vitro* cultured macrophages (146). The *purC* mutant provided some protection in guinea pigs but lower than that observed after BCG immunization (146). The inactivation of the leucine or methionine pathways in BCG resulted in attenuated strains that protected both mice and guinea pigs against a virulent challenge with *M. tuberculosis* (147,148). The *leu* BCG was found to be completely attenuated and does not even replicate and kill SCID mice (148). The authors suggest that such an highly attenuated auxotrophic BCG vaccine could play a role as a vaccine in immunocompromised individuals. Very recently, *Trp* and *pro* auxotrophic *M. tuberculosis* strains were constructed and evaluated (149). These strains are attenuated in SCID mice and provide protection in C57BL/6 mice. The protective efficacy of these strains in guinea pigs remains to be studied.

As dealt with in detail earlier in this chapter, there has been considerable interest in genes coding for exported proteins from *M. tuberculosis*. One of them, *erp*, codes for a protein with repeat sequences. The inactivation of this gene resulted in an attenuated mutant unable to replicate in cultured macrophages, mice, and guinea pigs (150). In contrast to the auxotroph *purC* mutant, the erp mutant persists in the animal for at least 2 months without replicating.

SUMMARY

Vaccination campaigns against potentially fatal viral diseases for which treatment does not exist have to be continued until eradication of the disease (e.g., the small pox campaign). After complete eradication, the vaccination program can stop if no disease reservoirs exist. Vaccination against bacterial diseases for which an efficient treatment exists (such as TB) is a different issue in which the long-term benefits of vaccination need to be modeled from the economic and global health perspective (151). For TB, however, the antibiotic regimen used to treat this disease is very demanding, including three different antibiotics and a treatment that lasts for 6 months and requires medical follow-up. Thus, although efficient treatment exists, it is very difficult to implement it in many Third World countries. Furthermore, resistant strains have emerged and are a serious concern, particularly in Eastern Europe where 14% of primary TB isolates are multidrug resistant (152). Consequently, although treatable in most cases, TB will not be eliminated without an efficient vaccine.

An ideal vaccine against TB should be safe and stable and provide life-long complete protection against disease and infection after a single administration. None of the vaccines described in this chapter fulfills these criteria, but in a practical sense, candidates that fall short in one or more of these characteristics would still be very valuable and cost-effective tools in the global fight against TB. For a TB vaccine to be used widely in the Third World, an additional concern is cost. The very limited yearly health care budget in many developing countries may preclude or delay the use of advanced and expensive vaccine technologies (e.g., prime boost or multicomponent subunit vaccines) even if they are highly efficacious. Therefore, in addition to resolving the scientific uncertainties surrounding the development of a TB vaccine, the future challenge is to convert promising laboratory vaccines into affordable technologies for worldwide dissemination.

REFERENCES

1. Calmette A, Plotz H. Protective inoculation against tuberculosis with BCG. *Am Rev Tuberc* 1929;19:567–572.
2. Fifteen year follow up of trial of BCG vaccines in south India for tuberculosis prevention. Tuberculosis Research Centre (ICMR), Chennai. *Indian J Med Res* 1999;110:56–69.
3. Cole ST, Brosch R, Parkhill J, et al. Deciphering the biology of *Mycobacterium tuberculosis* from the complete genome sequence. *Nature* 1998;393:537–544.
4. Andersen P. TB vaccines: progress and problems. *Trends Immunol* 2001;22:160–168.

5. Smith D, Wiegeshaus E, Balasubramanian V. An analysis of some hypotheses related to the Chingelput bacille Calmette–Guerin trial. *Clin Infect Dis* 2000;31[Suppl 3]:S77–S80.

6. Fine PE. Bacille Calmette–Guerin vaccines: a rough guide. *Clin Infect Dis* 1995;20:11–14.

7. Brennan MJ, Fruth U. Global Forum on TB Vaccine Research and Development. World Health Organization, June 7–8, 2001, Geneva. *Tuberculosis* 2001;81:365–368.

8. Covert BA, Spencer JS, Orme IM, et al. The application of proteomics in defining the T cell antigens of *Mycobacterium tuberculosis*. *Proteomics* 2001;1:574–586.

9. Skjot RL, Oettinger T, Rosenkrands I, et al. Comparative evaluation of low-molecular-mass proteins from *Mycobacterium tuberculosis* identifies members of the ESAT-6 family as immunodominant T-cell antigens. *Infect Immun* 2000;68:214–220.

10. Alderson MR, Bement T, Day CH, et al. Expression cloning of an immunodominant family of *Mycobacterium tuberculosis* antigens using human CD4(+) T cells. *J Exp Med* 2000;191:551–560.

11. Olsen AW, Hansen PR, Holm A, et al. Efficient protection against *Mycobacterium tuberculosis* by vaccination with a single subdominant epitope from the ESAT-6 antigen. *Eur J Immunol* 2000;30:1724–1732.

12. Lindblad EB, Elhay MJ, Silva R, et al. Adjuvant modulation of immune responses to tuberculosis subunit vaccines. *Infect Immun* 1997;65:623–629.

13. Leal IS, Smedegard B, Andersen P, et al. Failure to induce enhanced protection against tuberculosis by increasing T-cell-dependent interferon-gamma generation. *Immunology* 2001; 104:157–161.

14. Mogues T, Goodrich ME, Ryan L, et al. The relative importance of T cell subsets in immunity and immunopathology of airborne *Mycobacterium tuberculosis* infection in mice. *J Exp Med* 2001;193:271–280.

15. Flynn JL, Chan J. Immunology of tuberculosis. *Annu Rev Immunol* 2001;19:93–129.

16. Serbina NV, Liu CC, Scanga CA, et al. CD8+ CTL from lungs of *Mycobacterium tuberculosis*-infected mice express perforin *in vivo* and lyse infected macrophages. *J Immunol* 2000;165:353–363.

17. Flynn JL, Goldstein MM, Triebold KJ, et al. Major histocompatibility complex class I-restricted T cells are required for resistance to *Mycobacterium tuberculosis* infection. *Proc Natl Acad Sci U S A* 1992;89:12013–12017.

18. van Pinxteren LA, Cassidy JP, Smedegaard BH, et al. Control of latent *Mycobacterium tuberculosis* infection is dependent on CD8 T cells. *Eur J Immunol* 2000;30:3689–3698.

19. Serbina NV, Lazarevic V, Flynn JL. CD4(+) T cells are required for the development of cytotoxic CD8(+) T cells during *Mycobacterium tuberculosis* infection. *J Immunol* 2001;167: 6991–7000.

20. Orme IM. Characteristics and specificity of acquired immunologic memory to *Mycobacterium tuberculosis* infection. *J Immunol* 1988;140:3589–3593.

21. Gumperz JE, Brenner MB. CD1-specific T cells in microbial immunity. *Curr Opin Immunol* 2001;13:471–478.

22. Moody DB, Sugita M, Peters PJ, et al. The CD1-restricted T-cell response to mycobacteria. *Res Immunol* 1996;147:550–559.

23. Ulrichs T, Porcelli SA. CD1 proteins: targets of T cell recognition in innate and adaptive immunity. *Rev Immunogenet* 2000; 2:416–432.

24. Shen Y, Zhou D, Qiu L, et al. Adaptive immune response of Vgamma2Vdelta2+ T cells during mycobacterial infections. *Science* 2002;295:2255–2258.

25. Kaech SM, Wherry EJ, Ahmed R. Effector and memory T-cell differentiation: implications for vaccine development. *Immunol Nat Rev* 2002;2:251–262.

26. Colditz GA, Berkey CS, Mosteller F, et al. The efficacy of bacillus Calmette–Guerin vaccination of newborns and infants in the prevention of tuberculosis: meta-analyses of the published literature. *Pediatrics* 1995;96:29–35.

27. Hart PD, Sutherland I. BCG and vole bacillus vaccines in the prevention of tuberculosis in adolescence and early adult life. *BMJ* 1977;2:293–295.

28. Lima KM, Bonato VL, Faccioli LH, et al. Comparison of different delivery systems of vaccination for the induction of protection against tuberculosis in mice. *Vaccine* 2001;19:3518–3525.

29. Rosenkrands I, King A, Weldingh K, et al. Towards the proteome of *Mycobacterium tuberculosis*. *Electrophoresis* 2000;21: 3740–3756.

30. Jungblut PR, Schaible UE, Mollenkopf HJ, et al. Comparative proteome analysis of *Mycobacterium tuberculosis* and *Mycobacterium bovis* BCG strains: towards functional genomics of microbial pathogens. *Mol Microbiol* 1999;33:1103–1117.

31. Fenton MJ, Vermeulen MW. Immunopathology of tuberculosis: roles of macrophages and monocytes. *Infect Immun* 1996; 64:683–690.

32. Lee BY, Horwitz MA. Identification of macrophage and stress-induced proteins of *Mycobacterium tuberculosis*. *J Clin Invest* 1995;96:245–249.

33. Rosenkrands I, Slayden RA, Crawford J, et al. The hypoxic response of *Mycobacterium tuberculosis* studied by metabolic labeling and proteome analysis of cellular and extracellular proteins. *J Bacteriol* 2002;184:3485–3491.

34. Yuan Y, Crane DD, Barry CE 3rd. Stationary phase-associated protein expression in *Mycobacterium tuberculosis*: function of the mycobacterial alpha-crystallin homolog. *J Bacteriol* 1996; 178:4484–4492.

35. Camacho LR, Ensergueix D, Perez E, et al. Identification of a virulence gene cluster of *Mycobacterium tuberculosis* by signature-tagged transposon mutagenesis. *Mol Microbiol* 1999;34:257–267.

36. Cox JS. Complex lipid determines tissue-specific replication of *Mycobacterium tuberculosis* in mice. *Nature* 1999;402:79–83.

37. Orme IM. Induction of nonspecific acquired resistance and delayed-type hypersensitivity, but not specific acquired resistance in mice inoculated with killed mycobacterial vaccines. *Infect Immun* 1988;56:3310–3312.

38. Andersen P, Askgaard D, Ljungqvist L, et al. Proteins released from *Mycobacterium tuberculosis* during growth. *Infect Immun* 1991;59:1905–1910.

39. Gomez M, Johnson S, Gennaro ML. Identification of secreted proteins of *Mycobacterium tuberculosis* by a bioinformatic approach. *Infect Immun* 2000;68:2323–2327.

40. Mattow J, Jungblut PR, Schaible UE, et al. Identification of proteins from *Mycobacterium tuberculosis* missing in attenuated *Mycobacterium bovis* BCG strains. *Electrophoresis* 2001;22: 2936–2946.

41. Behr MA, Wilson MA, Gill WP, et al. Comparative genomics of BCG vaccines by whole-genome DNA microarray. *Science* 1999;284:1520–1523.

42. Gordon SV, Brosch R, Billault A, et al. Identification of variable regions in the genomes of tubercle bacilli using bacterial artificial chromosome arrays. *Mol Microbiol* 1999;32:643–655.

43. Mahairas GG, Sabo PJ, Hickey MJ, et al. Molecular analysis of genetic differences between *Mycobacterium bovis* BCG and virulent *M. bovis*. *J Bacteriol* 1996;178:1274–1282.

44. Pathan AA, Wilkinson KA, Klenerman P, et al. Direct *ex vivo* analysis of antigen-specific IFN-gamma-secreting CD4 T cells in *Mycobacterium tuberculosis*-infected individuals: associations with clinical disease state and effect of treatment. *J Immunol* 2001;167:5217–5225.

45. Ravn P, Demissie A, Eguale T, et al. Human T cell responses to the ESAT-6 antigen from *Mycobacterium tuberculosis*. *J Infect Dis* 1999;179:637–645.

46. Berthet FX, Rasmussen PB, Rosenkrands I, et al. A *Mycobacterium tuberculosis* operon encoding ESAT-6 and a novel low-molecular-mass culture filtrate protein (CFP-10). *Microbiology* 1998;144:3195–3203.

47. Skjot RLV, Agger EM, Andersen P. Antigen discovery and tuberculosis vaccine development in the post-genomic era. *Scand J Infect Dis* 2001;33:643–647.

48. Skeiky YA, Ovendale PJ, Jen S, et al. T cell expression cloning of a *Mycobacterium tuberculosis* gene encoding a protective antigen associated with the early control of infection. *J Immunol* 2000;165:7140–7149.

49. Dillon DC, Alderson MR, Day CH, et al. Molecular characterization and human T-cell responses to a member of a novel *Mycobacterium tuberculosis* mtb39 gene family. *Infect Immun* 1999;67:2941–2950.

50. De Groot AS, Bosma A, Chinai N, et al. From genome to vaccine: in silico predictions, *ex vivo* verification. *Vaccine* 2001;19:4385–4395.

51. Smith D, Wiegeshaus E, Balasubramanian V. Animal models for experimental tuberculosis. *Clin Infect Dis* 2000;31[Suppl 3]:S68–S70.

52. Klunner T, Bartels T, Vordermeier M, et al. Immune reactions of CD4- and CD8-positive T cell subpopulations in spleen and lymph nodes of guinea pigs after vaccination with bacillus Calmette Guerin. *Vaccine* 2001;19:1968–1977.

53. Wiegeshaus EH, McMurray DN, Grover AA, et al. Host-parasite relationships in experimental airborne tuberculosis. 3. Relevance of microbial enumeration to acquired resistance in guinea pigs. *Am Rev Respir Dis* 1970;102:422–429.

54. Baldwin SL, D'Souza C, Roberts AD, et al. Evaluation of new vaccines in the mouse and guinea pig model of tuberculosis. *Infect Immun* 1998;66:2951–2959.

55. Walsh GP, Tan EV, dela Cruz EC, et al. The Philippine cynomolgus monkey (*Macaca fasicularis*) provides a new non-human primate model of tuberculosis that resembles human disease. *Nat Med* 1996;2:430–436.

56. Langermans JA, Andersen P, van Soolingen D, et al. Divergent effect of bacillus Calmette-Guerin (BCG) vaccination on *Mycobacterium tuberculosis* infection in highly related macaque species: implications for primate models in tuberculosis vaccine research. *Proc Natl Acad Sci U S A* 2001;98:11497–11502.

57. Palmer CE, Long MW. Effects of infection with atypical mycobacteria on BCG vaccination and tuberculosis. *Am Rev Respir Dis* 1966;94:553–568.

58. Brandt L, Feino Cunha J, Weinreich Olsen A, et al. Failure of the *Mycobacterium bovis* BCG vaccine: some species of environmental mycobacteria block multiplication of BCG and induction of protective immunity to tuberculosis. *Infect Immun* 2002;70:672–678.

59. Buddle BM, Wards BJ, Aldwell FE, et al. Influence of sensitisation to environmental mycobacteria on subsequent vaccination against bovine tuberculosis. *Vaccine* 2002;20:1126–1133.

60. Brooks JV, Frank AA, Keen MA, et al. Boosting vaccine for tuberculosis. *Infect Immun* 2001;69:2714–2717.

61. Lillebaek T, Dirksen A, Baess I, et al. Molecular evidence of endogenous reactivation of *Mycobacterium tuberculosis* after 33 years of latent infection. *J Infect Dis* 2002;185:401–404.

62. McCune RM, Tompsett R, McDermott W. The fate of *Mycobacterium tuberculosis* in mouse tissues as determined by the microbial enumeration technique. II. The conversion of tuberculosis infection to the latent state by the administration of pyrazinamide and companion drug. *J Exp Med* 1957;104:763–802.

63. Dhillon J, Mitchison DA. Effect of vaccines in a murine model of dormant tuberculosis. *Tuber Lung Dis* 1994;75:61–64.

64. Scanga CA, Mohan VP, Joseph H, et al. Reactivation of latent tuberculosis: variations on the Cornell murine model. *Infect Immun* 1999;67:4531–4538.

65. Lowrie DB, Tascon RE, Bonato VL, et al. Therapy of tuberculosis in mice by DNA vaccination. *Nature* 1999;400:269–271.

66. Smith DW. Protective effect of BCG in experimental tuberculosis. *Adv Tuberc Res* 1985;22:1–97.

67. Ribi E, Larson C, Wicht W, et al. Effective nonliving vaccine against experimental tuberculosis in mice. *J Bacteriol* 1966;91:975–983.

68. Anacker RL, Barclay WR, Brehmer W, et al. Duration of immunity to tuberculosis in mice vaccinated intravenously with oil-treated cell walls of *Mycobacterium bovis* strain BCG. *J Immunol* 1967;98:1265–1273.

69. Masihi KN, Brehmer W, Azuma I, et al. Stimulation of chemiluminescence and resistance against aerogenic influenza virus infection by synthetic muramyl dipeptide combined with trehalose dimycolate. *Infect Immun* 1984;43:233–237.

70. Hubbard RD, Flory CM, Collins FM. Immunization of mice with mycobacterial culture filtrate proteins. *Clin Exp Immunol* 1992;87:94–98.

71. Pal PG, Horwitz MA. Immunization with extracellular proteins of *Mycobacterium tuberculosis* induces cell-mediated immune responses and substantial protective immunity in a guinea pig model of pulmonary tuberculosis. *Infect Immun* 1992;60:4781–4792.

72. Andersen P. Effective vaccination of mice against *Mycobacterium tuberculosis* infection with a soluble mixture of secreted mycobacterial proteins. *Infect Immun* 1994;62:2536–2544.

73. Horwitz MA, Lee BW, Dillon BJ, et al. Protective immunity against tuberculosis induced by vaccination with major extracellular proteins of *Mycobacterium tuberculosis*. *Proc Natl Acad Sci U S A* 1995;92:1530–1534.

74. Vordermeier HM, Coombes AG, Jenkins P, et al. Synthetic delivery system for tuberculosis vaccines: immunological evaluation of the *M. tuberculosis* 38 kDa protein entrapped in biodegradable PLG microparticles. *Vaccine* 1995;13:1576–1582.

75. Olsen AW, van Pinxteren LA, Okkels LM, et al. Protection of mice with a tuberculosis subunit vaccine based on a fusion protein of antigen 85b and esat-6. *Infect Immun* 2001;69:2773–2778.

76. Coler RN, Campos-Neto A, Ovendale P, et al. Vaccination with the T cell antigen Mtb 8.4 protects against challenge with *Mycobacterium tuberculosis*. *J Immunol* 2001;166:6227–6235.

77. Yip HC, Karulin AY, Tary-Lehmann M, et al. Adjuvant-guided type-1 and type-2 immunity: infectious/noninfectious dichotomy defines the class of response. *J Immunol* 1999;162:3942–3949.

78. Elhay MJ, Andersen P. Immunological requirements for a subunit vaccine against tuberculosis. *Immunol Cell Biol* 1997;75:595–603.

79. Coler RN, Skeiky YA, Vedvick T, et al. Molecular cloning and immunological reactivity of a novel low molecular mass antigen of *Mycobacterium tuberculosis*. *J Immunol* 1998;161:2356–2364.

80. Dhiman N, Khuller GK. Immunoprophylactic properties of 71-kDa cell wall-associated protein antigen of *Mycobacterium tuberculosis* H37Ra. *Med Microbiol Immunol (Berl)* 1997;186:45–51.

81. Dhiman N, Khuller GK. Protective efficacy of mycobacterial 71-kDa cell wall associated protein using poly (DL-lactide-co-glycolide) microparticles as carrier vehicles. *FEMS Immunol Med Microbiol* 1998;21:19–28.

82. Brandt L, Elhay M, Rosenkrands I, et al. ESAT-6 subunit vaccination against *Mycobacterium tuberculosis*. *Infect Immun* 2000;68:791–795.

83. Leal IS, Florido M, Andersen P, et al. Interleukin-6 regulates the phenotype of the immune response to a tuberculosis subunit vaccine. *Immunology* 2001;103:375–381.

84. Leal IS, Smedegard B, Andersen P, et al. Interleukin-6 and inter-leukin-12 participate in induction of a type 1 protective T-cell response during vaccination with a tuberculosis subunit vaccine. *Infect Immun* 1999;67:5747–5754.

85. Shibata Y, Honda I, Justice JP, et al. Th1 adjuvant *N*-acetyl-D-glucosamine polymer up-regulates Th1 immunity but down-regulates Th2 immunity against a mycobacterial protein (MPB-59) in interleukin-10-knockout and wild-type mice. *Infect Immun* 2001;69:6123–6130.

86. Saunders BM, Frank AA, Orme IM. Granuloma formation is required to contain bacillus growth and delay mortality in mice chronically infected with *Mycobacterium tuberculosis*. *Immunology* 1999;98:324–328.

87. Ehlers S, Benini J, Held HD, et al. Alphabeta T cell receptor-positive cells and interferon-gamma, but not inducible nitric oxide synthase, are critical for granuloma necrosis in a mouse model of mycobacteria-induced pulmonary immunopathology. *J Exp Med* 2001;194:1847–1859.

88. Le TT, Drane D, Malliaros J, et al. Cytotoxic T cell polyepitope vaccines delivered by ISCOMs. *Vaccine* 2001;19:4669–4675.

89. Wolff JA, Malone RW, Williams P, et al. Direct gene transfer into mouse muscle in vivo. *Science* 1990;247:1465–1468.

90. Tang D, Devit M, Johnston SA. Genetic immunization is a simple method for eliciting an immune response. *Nature* 1992;356:152–154.

91. Ulmer JB, Donnelly JJ, Parker SE, et al. Heterologous protection against influenza by injection of DNA encoding a viral protein. *Science* 1993;259:1745–1749.

92. Donnelly JJ, Ulmer JB, Shiver JW, et al. DNA vaccines. *Annu Rev Immunol* 1997;15:617–648.

93. *Abstract Book Keystone Symposium on Genes-Based Vaccines: Mechanisms, Delivery and Efficacy*, Breckenridge, 2002.

94. Wolff JA, Lutdke JJ, Ascadi G, et al. Long-term persistence of plasmid DNA and foreign gene expression in muscle cells. *Hum Mol Genet* 1992;1:363–369.

95. Nichols WW, Lewith BJ, Manam SV, et al. Potential DNA vaccine integration into host cell genome. *Proc Natl Acad Sci U S A* 1995;772:30–39.

96. Tonkinson JL, Stein CA. Patterns of intracellular compartmentalization, trafficking and acidification of 5′-fluorescein labeled phosphodiester and phosphorothioate oligodeoxynucleotides in HL60 cells. *Nucleic Acids Res* 1994;22:4268–4275.

97. Hemmi H, Takeuchi O, Kawai T, et al. A Toll-like receptor recognizes bacterial DNA. *Nature* 2000;408:740–745.

98. Klinman DM, Yi A-K, Beaucage SL, et al. CpG motifs present in bacterial DNA rapidly induce lymphocytes to secrete IL-6, IL-12 and IFN-γ. *Proc Natl Acad Sci U S A* 1996;93:2879–2883.

99. Tascon RE, Colston MJ, Ragno S, et al. Vaccination against tuberculosis by DNA injection. *Nat Med* 1996;2:888–892.

100. Huygen K, Content J, Denis O, et al. Immunogenicity and protective efficacy of a tuberculosis DNA vaccine. *Nat Med* 1996;2:893–898.

101. Tanghe A, Denis O, Lambrecht B, et al. Tuberculosis DNA vaccine encoding Ag85A is immunogenic and protective when administered by intramuscular needle injection, but not by epidermal gene gun bombardment. *Infect Immun* 2000;68:3854–3860.

102. Zhu XJ, Stauss HJ, Ivanyi J, et al. Specificity of CD8(+) T cells from subunit-vaccinated and infected H-2(b) mice recognizing the 38 kDa antigen of *Mycobacterium tuberculosis*. *Int Immunol* 1997;9:1669–1676.

103. Denis O, Tanghe A, Palfliet K, et al. Vaccination with plasmid DNA encoding mycobacterial antigen 85A stimulates a CD4+ and CD8+ T-cell epitopic repertoire broader than that stimulated by *Mycobacterium tuberculosis* H37Rv infection. *Infect Immun* 1998;66:1527–1533.

104. Tanghe A, D'Souza S, Rosseels V, et al. Increased immunogenicity and protective efficacy of a tuberculosis DNA vaccine encoding Ag85 following protein boost. *Infect Immun* 2001;69:3041–3047.

105. Turner J, Rhoades ER, Keen M, et al. Effective preexposure tuberculosis vaccines fail to protect when they are given in an immunotherapeutic mode.*Infect Immun* 2000;68:1706–1709.

106. D'Souza S, Denis O, Scorza T, et al. CD4+ T cells contain *Mycobacterium tuberculosis* infection in the absence of CD8+ T cells in mice vaccinated with DNA encoding Ag85A. *Eur J Immunol* 2000;30:2455–2459.

107. Bonato VLD, Lima VMF, Tascon RE, et al. Identification and characterization of protective T cells in hsp65 DNA-vaccinated and *Mycobacterium tuberculosis* infected mice. *Infect Immun* 1998;66:169–175.

108. Baldwin SL, D'Souza CD, Orme IM, et al. Immunogenicity and protective efficacy of DNA vaccines encoding secreted and non-secreted forms of *Mycobacterium tuberculosis* Ag85A. *Tuber Lung Dis* 1999;79:251–259.

109. Li Z, Howard A, Kelley C, et al. Immunogenicity of DNA vaccines expressing tuberculosis proteins fused to tissue plasminogen activator signal sequences.*Infect Immun* 1999;67:4780–4786.

110. Montgomery DL, Huygen K, Yawman AM, et al. Induction of humoral and cellular immune responses by vaccination with M-tuberculosis antigen 85 DNA. *Cell Mol Biol* 1997;43:285–292.

111. Martin E, Kamath AT, Triccas JA, et al. Protection against virulent *Mycobacterium avium* infection following DNA vaccination with the 35-kilodalton antigen is accompanied by induction of gamma interferon-secreting CD4+ T cells. *Infect Immun* 2000;68:3090–3096.

112. Delogu G, Howard A, Collins FM, et al. DNA Vaccination against tuberculosis: expression of a ubiquitin-conjugated tuberculosis protein enhances antimycobacterial immunity. *Infect Immun* 2000;68:3097–3102.

113. D'Souza S, Denis O, Rosseels V, et al. Improved tuberculosis DNA vaccines by formulation in vaxfectin. *Infect Immun* 2002;70:3681–3688.

114. Tollefsen S, Tjelle TE, Schneider J, et al. Improved cellular and humoral immune responses against *Mycobacterium tuberculosis* antigens after intra-muscular DNA immunisation combined with muscle electroporation. *Vaccine* 2002;20:3370–3378.

115. Kamath AT, Hanke T, Briscoe H, et al. Co-immunization with DNA vaccines expressing granulocyte-macrophage colony-stimulating factor and mycobacterial proteins enhances T-cell immunity, but not protective efficacy against *M. tuberculosis*. *Immunology* 1999;96:511–516.

116. Morris S, Kelley C, Howard A, et al. The immunogenicity of single and combination DNA vaccines against tuberculosis. *Vaccine* 2000;18:2155–2163.

117. Delogu G, Li A, Repique C, et al. DNA vaccine combinations expressing either tissue plasminogen activator signal sequence fusion proteins or ubiquitin-conjugated antigens induce sustained protective immunity in a mouse model of pulmonary tuberculosis. *Infect Immun* 2002;70:292–302.

118. Malin AS, Huygen K, Content J, et al. Vaccinia expression of *Mycobacterium tuberculosis*-secreted proteins: tissue plasminogen activator signal enhances expression and immunogenicity of *M. tuberculosis* Ag85. *Microbes Infect* 2000;2:1677–1685.

119. Smith SM, Malin A, Atkinson SE, et al. Characterisation of human *Mycobacterium bovis* BCG reactive CD8+ T-cells. *Infect Immun* 1999;67:5223–5230.

120. Smith SM, Klein MR, Malin AS, et al. Human CD8+ T cells specific for *Mycobacterium tuberculosis* secreted antigens in tuberculosis patients and healthy BCG-vaccinated controls in the Gambia. *Infect Immun* 2000;68:7144–7148.

121. Smith SM, Brooks R, Klein MR, et al. Human CD8+ CTL spe-

cific for the mycobacterial major secreted antigen 85A. *J Immunol* 2000;165:7088–7095.

122. Zhu X, Venkataprasad N, Ivanyi J, et al. Vaccination with recombinant vaccinia viruses protects mice against *Mycobacterium tuberculosis* infection. *Immunology* 1997;92:6–9.

123. Mollenkopf HJ, Groine-Triebkorn D, Andersen P, et al. Protective efficacy against tuberculosis of ESAT-6 secreted by a live *Salmonella typhimurium* vaccine carrier strain and expressed by naked DNA. *Vaccine* 2001;19:4028–4035.

124. Estcourt MJ, Ramsay AJ, Brooks A, et al. Prime-boost immunization generates a high frequency, high-avidity CD8(+) cytotoxic T lymphocyte population. *Int Immunol* 2002;14:31–37.

125. Schneider J, Gilbert SC, Hannan CM, et al. Induction of CD8+ T cells using heterologous prime-boost immunisation strategies. *Immunol Rev* 1999;170:29–38.

126. McShane H, Brookes R, Gilbert S, et al. Enhanced immunogenicity of CD4+ T-cell responses and protective efficacy of a DNA-modified vaccinia virus Ankara prime-boost vaccination regimen for murine tuberculosis. *Infect Immun* 2001;69:681–686.

127. Unknown. New TB vaccine trials begin. *Trends Immunol* 2002;23:11.

128. Feng CG, Palendira U, Demangel C, et al. Priming by DNA immunization augments protective efficacy of *Mycobacterium bovis* bacille Calmette–Guerin against tuberculosis. *Infect Immunol* 2001;69:4174–4176.

129. McShane H, Behboudi S, Goonetilleke N, et al. Protective immunity against *M. tuberculosis* induced by dendritic cells pulsed with both CD8+ and CD4+ T cell epitopes from antigen 85A. *Infect Immun* 2002;70:1623–1626.

130. Brosch R. Comparative genomics of the mycobacteria. *J Med Microbiol* 2000;290:143–152.

131. Mahairas GG. Molecular analysis of genetic differences between *Mycobacterium bovis* BCG and virulent *M. bovis*. *J Bacteriol* 1996;178:1274–1282.

132. Dubnau E, Chan J, Raynaud C, et al. Oxygenated mycolic acids are necessary for virulence of *Mycobacterium tuberculosis* in mice. *Mol Microbiol* 2000;36:630–637.

133. Glickman MS, Cox JS, Jacobs WR Jr. A novel mycolic acid cyclopropane synthetase is required for cording, persistence, and virulence of *Mycobacterium tuberculosis*. *Mol Cell* 2000;5:717–727.

134. Yuan Y, Zhu Y, Crane DD, et al. The effect of oxygenated mycolic acid composition on cell wall function and macrophage growth in *Mycobacterium tuberculosis*. *Mol Microbiol* 1998;29:1449–1458.

135. Ten Dam HG. *BCG vaccination in: tuberculosis*. New York: Marcel Dekker, 1993.

136. Horwitz MA. Recombinant bacillus Calmette–Guerin (BCG) vaccines expressing the *Mycobacterium tuberculosis* 30-kDa major secretory protein induce greater protective immunity against tuberculosis than conventional BCG vaccines in a highly susceptible animal model. *Proc Natl Acad Sci U S A* 2000;97:13853–13858.

137. Nigou J, Zelle-Rieser C, Gilleron M, et al. Mannosylated lipoarabinomannans inhibit IL-12 production by human dendritic cells: evidence for a negative signal delivered through the mannose receptor. *J Immunol* 2001;166:7477–7485.

138. Nau GJ, Richmond JF, Schlesinger A, et al. Human macrophage activation programs induced by bacterial pathogens. *Proc Natl Acad Sci U S A* 2002;99:1503–1508.

139. Marshall BG. Enhanced antimycobacterial response to recombinant *Mycobacterium bovis* BCG expressing latency-associated peptide. *Infect Immun* 2001;69:6676–6682.

140. Shankar P, Schlom J, Hodge J.W. Enhanced activation of rhesus T cells by vectors encoding a triad of costimulatory molecules (B7-1, ICAM-1, LFA-3). *Vaccine* 2001;20:744–755.

141. Murray PJ. Manipulation and potentiation of antimycobacterial immunity using recombinant bacille Calmette–Guerin strains that secrete cytokines. *Proc Natl Acad Sci U S A* 1996;93:934–939.

142. Hess J. *Mycobacterium bovis* bacille Calmette–Guerin strains secreting listeriolysin of *Listeria monocytogenes*. *Proc Natl Acad Sci U S A* 1998;95:5299–5304.

143. Bardarov S. Conditionally replicating mycobacteriophages: a system for transposon delivery to *Mycobacterium tuberculosis*. *Proc Natl Acad Sci U S A* 1997;94:10961–10966.

144. Pelicic V. Efficient allelic exchange and transposon mutagenesis in *Mycobacterium tuberculosis*. *Proc Natl Acad Sci U S A* 1997;94:10955–10960.

145. Levine MM, Hone MD, Stoker BAD, et al. *New and improved vaccines against typhoid fever in: new generation vaccines*. New York: Marcel Dekker, 1990.

146. Jackson M. Persistence and protective efficacy of a *Mycobacterium tuberculosis* auxotroph vaccine. *Infect Immun* 1999;67:2867–2873.

147. Chambers MA, Williams A, Gavier-Winden D, et al. Identification of a *Mycobacterium bovis* BCG auxotrophic mutant that protects guinea pigs against *M. bovis* and hematogenous spread of *Mycobacterium tuberculosis* without sensitization to tuberculin. *Infect Immun* 2000;68:7094–7099.

148. Guleria I, Teitelbaum R, McAdam RA, et al. Auxotrophic vaccines for tuberculosis. *Nat Med* 1996;2:334–337.

149. Smith DA. Characterization of auxotrophic mutants of *Mycobacterium tuberculosis* and their potential as vaccine candidates. *Infect Immun* 2001;69:1142–1150.

150. Berthet FX. Attenuation of virulence by disruption of the *Mycobacterium tuberculosis* erp gene. *Science* 1998;282:759–762.

151. Bishai DM, Mercer D. Modeling the economic benefits of better TB vaccines. *Int J Tuberc Lung Dis* 2001;5:984–993.

152. World Health Organization/TB. *Anti-tuberculosis drug resistance in the world*. Geneva: WHO, 1997.

153. Lowrie DB, Silva CL, Colston MJ, et al. Protection against tuberculosis by a plasmid DNA vaccine. *Vaccine* 1997;15:834–838.

154. Falero-Diaz G, Challacombe S, Banerjee D, et al. Intranasal vaccination of mice against infection with *Mycobacterium tuberculosis*. *Vaccine* 2000;18:3223–3229.

155. Zhu XJ, Venkataprasad N, Thangaraj HS, et al. Functions and specificity of T cells following nucleic acid vaccination of mice against *Mycobacterium tuberculosis* infection. *J Immunol* 1997;158:5921–5926.

156. Tanghe A, Lefèvre P, Denis O, et al. Immunogenicity and protective efficacy of tuberculosis DNA vaccines encoding putative phosphate transport receptors. *J Immunol* 1999;162:1113–1119.

157. Silva CL, Bonato VL, Lima VM, et al. Characterization of the memory/activated T cells that mediate the long-lived host response against tuberculosis after bacillus Calmette–Guerin or DNA vaccination. *Immunology* 1999;97:573–581.

TUBERCULOSIS ELIMINATION IN THE UNITED STATES

MICHAEL F. IADEMARCO
KENNETH G. CASTRO

From 1953, when national reporting of U.S. incident tuberculosis (TB) cases was first fully implemented, through 1984, the number of cases reported to the Centers for Disease Control and Prevention (CDC) decreased from 84,304 to 22,255. This average annual decline of 5% to 6% was only interrupted by a transient increase in 1980, which has been attributed to cases arising from a large influx of refugees from Southeast Asia (1). This consistent decline from 1953 through 1984 led to optimism that TB could be eliminated from the United States. In 1987, the Secretary of the U.S. Department of Health and Human Services called for the establishment of an Advisory Committee (now Council) for the Elimination of Tuberculosis (ACET), whose purpose would be to provide recommendations for eliminating TB as a U.S. public health problem. In 1989, the ACET published a strategic plan for the elimination of TB in the United States, establishing a goal of TB elimination (defined as a case rate of less than one per one million population) by the year 2010.

However, in the midst of this planning, it became apparent that something was amiss: A remarkable reversal had occurred in the long-standing trend of decreasing TB cases. From 1985 through 1992, reported cases increased 20.1%, from 22,201 to 26,673; this represented a 13% increase in the case rate, from 9.3 per 100,000 population to 10.5 per 100,000 population. Based on an extrapolation of the trend in cases observed from 1980 through 1984, one can posit that approximately 52,000 excess cases of TB occurred from 1985 through 1992 (3). These increases, which included outbreaks of drug-resistant TB that resulted in many illnesses and deaths, resulted in the mobilization of resources to improve TB prevention and control activities. Subse-

quently, from 1992 through 2001, the number of reported TB cases in the United States decreased 40% (4). This chapter discusses the factors associated with the increase in TB cases, the impact of public health actions intended to reverse the epidemic, and future challenges for the prospects of elimination.

FACTORS ASSOCIATED WITH THE TUBERCULOSIS EPIDEMIC IN THE UNITED STATES

The stagnation in the declining TB cases and case rate in 1985 and the subsequent epidemic peaking in 1992 was primarily influenced by five factors (5). First, U.S. health care professionals experienced a gradually decreasing capacity to identify, appropriately treat, and prevent cases of TB, probably the result of the decades of decreasing TB case rates. This was compounded in 1972 by the shift of federal support away from categorical block grants for public health funding to state and big city governments (6–9).

Second, the concurrent epidemic of acquired immunodeficiency syndrome and an increasing number of persons infected with human immunodeficiency virus (HIV) placed a significant number of persons at greatly increased risk of progressing to TB disease if infected with *Mycobacterium tuberculosis*. A substantial body of evidence linking the epidemics of TB and HIV has accumulated (10–14). HIV infection has both an amplifying and accelerating effect on the natural history of TB; it is often prevalent among populations with *M. tuberculosis* infection, and *M. tuberculosis* infection tends to rapidly progress to active TB disease among persons with HIV infection.

Third, the TB epidemic coincided with the immigration of many persons from countries with a high prevalence of *M. tuberculosis* infection, reflecting the commonality of TB throughout parts of the world (4,15–17). The country of origin for persons with TB was first reported uniformly in

M. F. Iademarco: Division of Tuberculosis Elimination, National Center for HIV, STD, and TB Prevention, Centers for Disease Control and Prevention; School of Medicine and Rollins School of Public Health, Emory University, Atlanta, Georgia.

K. G. Castro: Division of Tuberculosis Elimnation, Centers for Disease Control and Prevention, Atlanta Georgia.

1986, at which time 4,925 cases (22% of all reported cases) occurred in persons born outside the United States. From 1986 to 1992, there was a continuous increase in the number of TB cases reported in foreign-born persons and in the proportion of cases accounted for by foreign-born persons: In 1992, 7,270 cases (27%) occurred in foreign-born persons. Cases in foreign-born persons accounted for approximately 60% of the increase in cases reported in the United States from 1986 to 1992. By 2001, 7,865 cases, or 50% of all TB patients for whom birthplace is known, were in foreign-born persons.

Fourth, adverse social conditions and inadequate infection control practices in health care settings have been postulated as contributing factors in the recent increase in TB by facilitating increased active transmission of *M. tuberculosis* (18,19). Poverty, crowded housing, homelessness, substance abuse, and incarceration in correctional facilities all contribute to the creation of environments that facilitate the transmission of TB (20–26). Concomitantly, a health care infrastructure lacking appropriate infection control practices and having inadequate access to care may cause delayed diagnosis and treatment of persons with TB, which, in turn, prolongs infectiousness and increased transmission. An indicator of recent transmission of *M. tuberculosis* is the occurrence of TB outbreaks. During the recent TB epidemic, several outbreaks occurred in a variety of settings, including health care facilities, correctional institutions, shelters for homeless persons, long-term care facilities, substance abuse treatment centers, residential facilities, and schools (8,27–56).

Fifth, increased transmission as a result of inappropriate treatment led to an increase in the number of persons infected with drug-resistant strains of *M. tuberculosis*, which are more complicated and costly to treat. Outbreaks of drug-resistant cases greatly strained the existing public health infrastructure, created great public concern, and brought significant attention to the national TB epidemic. Although affecting the entire country, the scope and nature of the epidemic varied across the country, indicating that there were different operative combinations of these contributing factors in different regions.

RESPONSE TO THE EPIDEMIC AND ASSOCIATED REVERSAL IN TREND

A decision to address the problem and a comprehensive strengthening of TB control activities, including the availability of large, sustained increases in TB-specific federal and local support, is credited with reversing the TB case rate, from 10.5 per 100,000 population in 1992 to 5.6

[1]http://www.harlemtbcenter.org/
[2]http://www.nationaltbcenter.edu/
[3]http://www.umdnj.edu/ntbcweb/tbsplash.html

per 100,000 population in 2001 (4,57–60). One of the pivotal TB control activities that brought about these fundamental changes was an enhancement of the national TB surveillance system, which provided information that allowed the CDC to better monitor and target groups at increased risk of TB disease through the collection of data on the patient's history or risk of coinfection with HIV, substance abuse, homelessness, residence in long-term care or correctional facilities, type of provider, type of drug regimen, drug resistance, the use of directly observed therapy, and completion of therapy. Another important intervention was an expanded capability of local health departments to investigate TB outbreaks with the assistance of state governments and the CDC, especially in congregate and institutional settings. In addition, an unprecedented number of evidence-based public health TB guidelines have been published since 1992 (61–79), coupled with extensive education, communication, and training efforts, all pursued through expanded collaborations with partners such as the American Lung Association, the American Thoracic Society, the Infectious Diseases Society of America, the International Union Against Tuberculosis and Lung Disease, the National Coalition for the Elimination of Tuberculosis, the Royal Netherlands Tuberculosis Association, the World Health Organization (WHO), and the U.S. Agency for International Development (59). The creation and consistent support of three national TB model centers has been a cornerstone of this effort (Charles P. Felton National Tuberculosis Center at Harlem Hospital[1], 2002; Francis J. Curry National Tuberculosis Center[2], 2002; New Jersey Medical School National Tuberculosis Center[3], 2002).

From 1992 through 2001, TB case rates declined every year. This trend has been associated with an increase in activities essential for TB control. These activities include increasing the percentage of those persons diagnosed with TB who are started on an appropriate four-drug regimen (from 41% to 79%, 1993 to 2001), are given only directly observed therapy (from 22% to 50%, 1993 to 1999), and complete treatment in less than 1 year (from 64% to 80%, 1993 to 1999) (4). These were accomplished along with high rates of reporting (80) and recognition of the obligation of the United States to contribute to global TB control (59). In addition, there have been substantial improvements in the rates of HIV testing (from 46% to 63% in persons aged 25 to 44 years old and from 30% to 49%, in persons of all ages, from 1993 to 2000) and a decrease in the rates of TB and HIV coinfection if HIV tested (from 29% to 17% in persons aged 25 to 44 years old and from 15% to 9% in persons of all ages, from 1993 to 2000), and in the numbers of cases with drug resistance (from 1,564 to 859 isolates resistant to at least isoniazid and from 485 to 142 isolates resistant to at least isoniazid and rifampin, from 1993 to 2001).

CHOICE BETWEEN ELIMINATION AND CYCLES OF NEGLECT

In this era of renewed optimism for TB elimination, there have been two recent milestones. The ACET issued a revised TB elimination plan (76) and the Institute of Medicine (59) published *Ending Neglect: The Elimination of Tuberculosis in the United States.* The fundamental challenge is whether as a nation we will take decisive action to eliminate TB in the United States or fall again into the cycle of neglect and resurgence that has characterized the history of U.S. TB control efforts. It has long been acknowledged that as the numbers of persons with TB decrease, there are an accompanying complacency and lack of political will required to provide long-term, sustainable support (9,19,59). Therefore, after 9 years of decline in the TB case rate from 1993 to 2001, the United States is at a crossroads. Of concern is the fact that the percentage decrease in the number of cases from 2000 to 2001 was only 2.4%, whereas from 1993 to 2000, the annual rate of decrease averaged 5.9 (range, 3.7% to 7.5%). Although one instance does not constitute a trend, the 2001 aggregate estimate may be the harbinger of stagnation in our efforts toward elimination. Even if the overall trend from 1993 continues, elimination will not be achieved for the next several decades (59). The most compelling argument favoring efforts to eliminate TB was advanced by the ACET in declaring the following: "Because eliminating TB from the United States will have widespread economic, public health, and social benefits, committing to [TB elimination] will also fulfill an obligation to persons throughout the world who have this preventable and curable disease." Furthermore, in 1999, one decade after the publication of the original strategic plan, the ACET reaffirmed its call for the elimination of TB in the United States (76).

CHALLENGES AND NEXT STEPS

In attempting to prevent another cycle of neglect, to accelerate the decline in TB, and to proceed at a reasonable pace toward elimination, we must avoid the substantial risk of renewed complacency in the face of declining TB cases in the United States This is especially important in the setting of the current global TB emergency (81). However, the opportunity to eliminate TB in the United States is threatened by several converging factors: (a) the persistence and growth of the global TB epidemic; (b) the retreat of TB into high-risk populations at the margins of society; (c) the limitations of current control measures, the need for new diagnostic tests and treatments, and the absence of a highly effective vaccine; and (d) changes in the health care system that make the current context of TB

elimination very different from that of a decade ago (59,76,82).

To end the cycle of neglect that has characterized TB control in the United States, the Institute of Medicine report *Ending Neglect: The Elimination of Tuberculosis in the United States* recommended an aggressive strategy to (a) maintain control of TB; (b) accelerate the decline in TB incidence; (c) develop new tools for TB diagnostics, treatment, and prevention; (d) increase efforts in the United States to help fight the global epidemic; and (e) mobilize and sustain public support for TB elimination, and track progress (59). As a first step toward addressing these issues, the CDC prepared a response to the Institute of Medicine's report (82) that outlines goals and objectives that will move us toward the elimination of TB (Table 60.1). In addition, the Federal Tuberculosis Task Force has drafted a more comprehensive response that incorporates the role and responsibilities of other federal agencies involved in TB-related activities, such as the U.S. Food and Drug Administration, the National Institutes of Health, the Agency for Health Care Policy and Research, the Federal Bureau of Prisons, the Health Care Financing Administration, U.S. Agency for International Development, the Occupational Safety and Health Administration, the Department of Veterans Affairs, the Department of Housing and Urban Development, and the U.S. Marshall Service (T. Durden, personal communication, 2002).

ELIMINATION IN LOW INCIDENCE AREAS

In 2002, the CDC published the ACET's recommendations to address TB in low-incidence areas (83). In 2001, 23 states had TB incidence rates less than or equal to the ACET year 2000 interim objective of 3.5 cases per 100,000 population. This rate is defined as low incidence (2,4). Health departments in low-incidence states and those in low-incidence regions within other states need distinctive, area-specific strategies for maintaining the skills and resources required for finding increasingly rare TB cases, containing outbreaks, and ending transmission (83). The capacity for conducting all the essential components of a TB prevention and control program must be retained at local, state, and national levels; failure to do so increases the risk of additional outbreaks and a new TB resurgence. In low-incidence areas, it is especially important to have an adequate public health infrastructure and creative integration of resources, some of which until now have not played a key role in TB control. Further operational research will help to determine the most efficient control measures. Eventually, with a series of local successes in eliminating TB, low incidence will be attainable in all states, and the nation will profit from the lessons learned in the current low-incidence states. In parallel, these efforts need to recog-

TABLE 60.1. RESPONSE OF THE CENTERS FOR DISEASE CONTROL AND PREVENTION TO ENDING NEGLECT: THE ELIMINATION OF TUBERCULOSIS IN THE UNITED STATES: SUMMARY OF GOALS AND OBJECTIVES

Goal I: Maintain control of tuberculosis (TB)
  Objectives
    A. Maintain and enhance local, state, and national public health surveillance for TB.
    B. Support the infrastructure needed for laboratory-based identification and treatment of TB.
    C. Ensure that patient-centered case management and monitoring of treatment outcomes are the standard of care for all patients with TB.
    D. Develop community partnerships and strengthen community involvement in TB control.
    E. Improve the timely investigation and appropriate evaluation and treatment of contacts with active TB disease and latent TB infection.
    F. Ensure appropriate care for patients with multidrug-resistant TB and monitor their response to treatment and treatment outcomes.
    G. Ensure that health care facilities maintain infection-control precautions.
    H. Develop improved engineering and personal protective techniques to prevent TB transmission.
    I. Improve TB control in foreign-born populations entering or residing in the United States.
    J. Educate the public and train health care providers to maintain excellence in TB services.
Goal II: Accelerate the decline
  Objectives
    A. Increase the capacity of TB control programs to implement targeted testing and treatment programs for high-risk persons.
    B. Promote the appropriate regionalization of TB control activities in high, intermediate, and low TB incidence areas of the United States.
    C. Characterize circulating *Mycobacterium tuberculosis* strains using DNA fingerprinting methods.
    D. Develop national, state, and local capacity to respond to outbreaks of TB.
Goal III: Develop new tools
  Objectives
    A. Develop a coordinated plan for TB research.
    B. Develop new methods to diagnose persons with latent TB infection and to identify infected persons who are at high risk of developing active TB.
    C. Develop and assess new drugs to improve TB treatment and prevention.
    D. Develop a new and effective TB vaccine.
    E. Develop and implement a program of research on behavioral factors related to TB treatment and prevention. Rapidly transfer findings from research studies into practice.
Goal IV: Increase involvement in global efforts
  Objectives
    A. Provide leadership in public health advocacy for TB prevention and control.
    B. Provide technical support and build capacity for implementation of directly observed treatment, short course, especially in those countries that contribute significantly to the U.S. TB burden.
    C. Develop models for the diagnosis and treatment of patients with multidrug-resistant TB.
    D. Provide technical, programmatic, and research support aimed at reducing the incidence of TB as an opportunistic disease in countries with a high human immunodeficiency virus burden.
Goal V: Mobilize and sustain support
  Objectives
    A. Develop and implement a health communications campaign focusing on the resources and support needed to eliminate TB.
    B. Help communities foster nontraditional, multisectoral, public-private partnerships to improve the effectiveness of their communications activities, with particular attention to culturally appropriate materials.
    C. Support the development of state- or area-specific TB elimination plans that contain communications activities to build support for TB elimination.
Goal VI: Track progress toward elimination
  Objectives
    A. Develop innovative analyses for examining surveillance data to help focus elimination efforts.
    B. Develop novel indicators of progress in elimination.
    C. Conduct periodic evaluations of TB program performance at federal, state, and local levels.
    D. Conduct an annual progress review.

TB, tuberculosis.
From CDC. *CDC's response to ending neglect: the elimination of tuberculosis in the United States.* U.S. Department of Health and Human Services, 2002.

nize the movement toward managed care and address the formulation of model contractual language for assessing comprehensive TB services (84).

INTERSECTION BETWEEN TUBERCULOSIS IN THE FOREIGN-BORN AND THE GLOBAL EPIDEMIC

The proportion of TB cases among persons born outside the United States has increased since the CDC began collecting these statistics in 1986. In 2001, this proportion reached 50%. This is no different from the trend in many other industrialized countries where, in some cases, the proportion is significantly greater than 50% (85–89). In the United States, five countries (Mexico, the Philippines, Vietnam, China, and India) account for 45% of the foreign-born TB, although local epidemiologic profiles vary. The elimination of TB in the United States will not be possible without adequate control of TB throughout the world. To address this problem, the United States is significantly and materially involved in the global effort to control TB through a number of efforts, including the WHO's Stop TB Partnership. In collaboration with the U.S. Departments of State and Defense and international partners and donors, the CDC and other Department of Health and Human Services agencies are directly providing technical assistance and financial support to improve the capacity of national TB control programs, with the following priorities. First, the CDC is committed to assisting countries that are the source of most of the U.S. foreign-born TB patients (e.g., Mexico, the Philippines, Vietnam). Second, the CDC is working to expand the implementation of the WHO TB control strategy in high-burden countries. Third, it is critical to mitigate HIV-related TB, especially in sub-Saharan Africa. The CDC's Global AIDS Program and the multinational Global Fund to Fight AIDS, TB, and Malaria are tangible efforts to address these dual epidemics. Fourth, we must control and prevent multidrug-resistant TB in countries identified by the WHO as having high rates of resistance (90,91).

DEVELOPMENT OF NEW TOOLS

An acknowledgment of the need to develop new tools to facilitate the control and eventual elimination of TB has prompted a renewal of interest in TB-related research. The tools currently available for TB control and prevention are effective but are labor intensive and frequently underused (Fig. 60.1). Therefore, improvements in these tools and the development of new tools are urgently needed (59,92). In

---

[4]http://www.niaid.nih.gov/dmid/tuberculosis
[5]http://www.niaid.nih.gov/dmid/tuberculosis

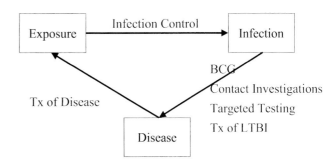

FIGURE 60.1. Existing tuberculosis interventions for prevention, control, and eventual elimination. Social mobilization and partnerships (e.g., community-based organizations, human immunodeficiency virus management and care, correctional and immigrant services, and medical services) are essential to effective interventions. Research and development of new tools are needed for diagnostic tests, safe and effective vaccine(s), and shorter regimens for the management of latent tuberculosis infection and tuberculosis disease. *BCG*, bacille Calmette–Guérin.

response to these needs, research efforts toward developing such tools are underway in epidemiology (including statistical modeling), biology, molecular biology, immunology, diagnosis, treatment, preventive therapy, behavioral studies, and operational research into factors associated with improvements in TB program management. The National Institutes of Health have increased their funding for TB research and are currently supporting investigator-initiated research, small business innovation research, training, and, increasingly, international collaborations (National Institutes of Health Tuberculosis Research Activities[4], 2002). An important development with far-reaching research potential was the recent sequencing of the genome of *M. tuberculosis* (93).

Historically, the CDC has been the lead U.S. agency for the conduct of clinical trials to evaluate TB treatments. However, the conduct of U.S. Public Health Service trials in TB had come to a virtual standstill after Study 21, an evaluation of 6-month, short-course treatment that began in 1981 (94). It was not until 1995, when the CDC and investigators at academic medical centers, health departments, and Veterans Affairs hospitals (comprising the CDC Tuberculosis Trials Consortium) initiated U.S. Public Health Service Study 22, a randomized trial to evaluate once-weekly rifapentine and isoniazid in the continuation phase of treatment. The findings demonstrated the efficacy of once-weekly treatment during the continuation phase of anti-TB therapy for selected TB patients (95) and have been used to update TB treatment recommendations being issued jointly by the CDC, American Thoracic Society, and Infectious Disease Society of America (79).

In 1998, the ACET recommended renewed efforts toward development of new, safe, and effective vaccines for TB (61). A 20-year Blueprint for Vaccine Development was published (National Institutes of Health Tuberculosis Research Activities[5], 2002). In 2001, the CDC established the Tuberculosis Epidemiological Studies Consortium, composed of 22 collaborative research groups, each consisting of a formal partnership between an academic institution and a state or metropolitan TB control program. In 2001, the National Institute of Allergy and Infectious Diseases of the National Institutes of Health issued its Global Health Research Plan for HIV/AIDS, Malaria, and Tuberculosis (National Institutes of Health Tuberculosis Research Activities[6], 2002). In 2000, a nongovernmental organization was formed as a partnership of industry, government, academia, private foundations, and the WHO to develop the Global Alliance for TB Drug Development (96). Optimally, these efforts will result in the development of new tools, including new drugs and an effective vaccine for TB elimination.

SOCIAL MOBILIZATION AND PUBLIC HEALTH ADVOCACY

The Institute of (59) report *Ending Neglect* concludes with the following thought:

> As has been demonstrated in the past century of control efforts, social mobilization is critical to sustaining tuberculosis control programs. Moreover, the tuberculosis control community must pay as much attention to social mobilization efforts as it pays to the technical, medical, and scientific issues.

As a result of increased attention, unparalleled since the early part of the 20th century, there has been a significant and measurable growth in interest in TB. These advocacy efforts are challenged by the fact that a majority of persons who contracts TB can be counted among the marginalized aspects of societies, not only complicating their access to health care and the preventive benefits of public health, but simply because of their propensity to have little voice in guiding our nation's decisions on health priorities. Therefore, bringing persons with TB and their views to the forefront is a necessary step to raise awareness of the problem and to address unmet needs. This can only happen through active partnership with and mobilization of communities with persons at high risk of TB, health care professionals (private and public), industry, media, and policy makers (71,76). In addition, the elimination of TB is necessarily tied to increased and sufficient financial resources to accomplish the requisite tasks (59,82). A recent report published by the National Coalition for the Elimination of Tuberculosis (97) posited:

> Resurgence is again a threat. Given the huge resources required to re-establish control in the 1990s, the prudent action now is to provide the funding needed to accelerate progress toward eliminating tuberculosis in the U.S. The alternative is to allow people in this country and around the world to suffer unnec-

essarily from this terrible, yet preventable and treatable, disease.

Furthermore, U.S. engagement and significant participation in broad global efforts to improve health are necessary to reap global TB control.

Specific objectives and action steps are outlined in the Global Plan to Stop Tuberculosis, published by the WHO-hosted Stop TB partnership (98). This document describes the ubiquitous nature of TB and its global toll in illness and death, along with its socioeconomic impact and acknowledges that "threats to effective tuberculosis control are threats to global health." The crucial role of advocacy at the global, national, and local levels is described. The agreed-on mission of this global partnership consists of four parts

> to ensure that every tuberculosis patient has access to effective diagnosis, treatment, and cure; to stop the worldwide transmission of tuberculosis; to reduce the inequitable social and economic toll of tuberculosis; and to develop and implement new preventive, diagnostic, and therapeutic tools and strategies to eliminate tuberculosis.

It has become increasingly clear that the successful elimination of TB necessitates going beyond technical remedies and must include socioeconomic interventions aimed at improving the overall welfare of individuals and communities.

SUMMARY

Eliminating TB from the United States will require (a) sustained and increased efforts such as those that have been initiated over the past several years; (b) continued support to rebuild and update the country's health care infrastructure and prevent it from deteriorating again; (c) the maintenance of an effective surveillance system to enable rapid identification of changes in disease trends and to adjust our prevention and control strategies accordingly; (d) continued epidemiologic studies to improve our understanding of the dynamics of TB transmission and to use the data to model effective interventions; and (e) research for the development of new diagnostic tests, therapeutics, and a safe and effective vaccine. To succeed in eliminating TB, we must build an expanding coalition of governmental and nongovernmental partners to increase the impact of our prevention and control activities. Because persons with TB are commonly afflicted with other health or social problems, the efforts of TB control programs should ideally facilitate referrals and access to other needed services, such as HIV treatment and care, drug rehabilitation services, and correctional and immigrant/refugee health services. We must also establish priorities for activities and increase their efficiency. With adequate attention to the problem and resources, there is a reasonable probability that the elimination of TB in the United States will eventually be achieved.

---

[6]http://www.niaid.nih.gov/dmid/tuberculosis

ACKNOWLEDGMENT

We acknowledge Samuel W. Dooley and Dixie E. Snider who coauthored this chapter in the first edition of this textbook, forming the foundation of this chapter. Original contributions from these authors have been retained in the current chapter. Also, we would like to acknowledge and thank Ann Lanner for editorial assistance.

REFERENCES

1. Rieder HL, Cauthen GM, Kelly GD, et al. Tuberculosis in the United States. *JAMA* 1989;262:385–389.
2. CDC. A strategic plan for the elimination of tuberculosis in the United States.*MMWR Morb Mortal Wkly Rep* 1989;38[Suppl 3]:1–25.
3. Cantwell MF, Snider DE Jr, Cauthen GM, et al. Epidemiology of tuberculosis in the United States, 1985 through 1992. *JAMA* 1994;272:535–539.
4. CDC. *Reported tuberculosis in the United States, 2001*. Washington, DC: U.S. Department of Health and Human Services, 2002.
5. Bloom BR, Murray CJ. Tuberculosis: commentary on a reemergent killer. *Science* 1992;257:1055–1064.
6. Binkin NJ, Vernon AA, Simone PM, et al. Tuberculosis prevention and control activities in the United States: an overview of the organization of tuberculosis services. *Int J Tuberc Lung Dis* 1999;3:663–674.
7. Leff DR, Leff AR. Tuberculosis control policies in major metropolitan health departments in the United States. VI. Standard of practice in 1996. *Am J Respir Crit Care Med* 1997;156:1487–1494.
8. Snider GL. Tuberculosis then and now: a personal perspective on the last 50 years.*Ann Intern Med* 1997;126:237–243.
9. Stone R. Tuberculosis rebounds while funding lags. *Science* 1992;255:1064.
10. Corbett EL, Steketee RW, ter Kuile FO, et al. HIV-1/AIDS and the control of other infectious diseases in Africa. *Lancet* 2002;359:2177–2187.
11. Mukadi YD, Maher D, Harries A. Tuberculosis case fatality rates in high HIV prevalence populations in sub-Saharan Africa. *AIDS* 2001;15:143–152.
12. Girardi E, Raviglione MC, Antonucci G, et al. Impact of the HIV epidemic on the spread of other diseases: the case of tuberculosis. *AIDS* 2000;14[Suppl 3]:S47–S56.
13. Glynn JR. Resurgence of tuberculosis and the impact of HIV infection. *Br Med Bull* 1998;54:579–593.
14. Telzak EE. Tuberculosis and human immunodeficiency virus infection. *Med Clin North Am* 1997;81:345–360.
15. CDC. Tuberculosis among foreign-born persons who had recently arrived in the United States–Hawaii, 1992–1993, and Los Angeles County, 1993. *MMWR Morb Mortal Wkly Rep* 1995;44:703–707.
16. Talbot EA, Moore M, McCray E, et al. Tuberculosis among foreign-born persons in the United States, 1993–1998. *JAMA* 2000;284:2894–2900.
17. World Health Organization. *Global tuberculosis control* (WHO Report 2000, WHO/CDS/TB/2000.275). Geneva: WHO, 2000.
18. Brudney K, Dobkin J. Resurgent tuberculosis in New York City. Human immunodeficiency virus, homelessness, and the decline of tuberculosis control programs. *Am Rev Respir Dis* 1991;144:745–749.
19. Reichman LB. The U-shaped curve of concern. *Am Rev Respir Dis* 1991;144:741–742.
20. Gandy M, Zumla A. The resurgence of disease: social and historical perspectives on the `new' tuberculosis. *Soc Sci Med* 2002;55:385–396.
21. Kvale G. Tackling the diseases of poverty. *Lancet* 2001;358:845–846.
22. Barr RG, Diez-Roux AV, Knirsch CA, et al. Neighborhood poverty and the resurgence of tuberculosis in New York City, 1984–1992. *Am J Public Health* 2001;91:1487–1493.
23. Bock NN, McGowan JE Jr, Blumberg HM. Few opportunities found for tuberculosis prevention among the urban poor.*Int J Tuberc Lung Dis* 1998;2:124–129.
24. Reyes H, Coninx R. Pitfalls of tuberculosis programmes in prisons.*BMJ* 1997;315:1447–1450.
25. Barclay DM III, Richardson JP, Fredman L. Tuberculosis in the homeless.*Arch Fam Med* 1995;4:541–546.
26. Landesman SH. Commentary: tuberculosis in New York City—the consequences and lessons of failure. *Am J Public Health* 1993;83:766–768.
27. CDC. Outbreak of multidrug-resistant tuberculosis at a hospital—New York City, 1991. *MMWR Morb Mortal Wkly Rep* 1993;42:427–424.
28. CDC. Drug-susceptible tuberculosis outbreak in a state correctional facility housing HIV-infected inmates—South Carolina, 1999–2000. *MMWR Morb Mortal Wkly Rep* 2000;49:1041–1044.
29. Beck-Sague C, Dooley SW, Hutton MD, et al. Hospital outbreak of multidrug-resistant *Mycobacterium tuberculosis* infections. Factors in transmission to staff and HIV-infected patients. *JAMA* 1992;268:1280–1286.
30. Bergmire-Sweat D, Barnett BJ, Harris SL, et al. Tuberculosis outbreak in a Texas prison, 1994. *Epidemiol Infect* 1996;117:485–492.
31. Comer WJ Jr, Felix R. Re: "Risk factors for transmission of *Mycobacterium tuberculosis* in a primary school outbreak: lack of radical difference in susceptibility to infection." *Am J Epidemiol* 1995;142:666–668.
32. Conover C, Ridzon R, Valway S, et al. Outbreak of multidrug-resistant tuberculosis at a methadone treatment program. *Int J Tuberc Lung Dis* 2001;5:59–64.
33. Curtis AB, Ridzon R, Novick LF, et al. Analysis of *Mycobacterium tuberculosis* transmission patterns in a homeless shelter outbreak. *Int J Tuberc Lung Dis* 2000;4:308–313.
34. Daley CL, Small PM, Schecter GF, et al. An outbreak of tuberculosis with accelerated progression among persons infected with the human immunodeficiency virus. An analysis using restriction-fragment-length polymorphisms. *N Engl J Med* 1992;326:231–235.
35. Di Perri G, Cruciani M, Danzi MC, et al. Nosocomial epidemic of active tuberculosis among HIV-infected patients. *Lancet* 1989;2:1502–1504.
36. DiStasio AJ, Trump DH. The investigation of a tuberculosis outbreak in the closed environment of a U.S. Navy ship, 1987. *Mil Med* 1990;155:347–351.
37. Edlin BR, Tokars JI, Grieco MH, et al. An outbreak of multidrug-resistant tuberculosis among hospitalized patients with the acquired immunodeficiency syndrome. *N Engl J Med* 1992;326:1514–1521.
38. Frieden TR, Sherman LF, Maw KL, et al. A multi-institutional outbreak of highly drug-resistant tuberculosis: epidemiology and clinical outcomes. *JAMA* 1996;276:1229–1235.
39. Griffith DE, Hardeman JL, Zhang Y, et al. Tuberculosis outbreak among healthcare workers in a community hospital. *Am J Respir Crit Care Med* 1995;152:808–811.
40. Hoge CW, Fisher L, Donnell HD Jr, et al. Risk factors for trans-

mission of *Mycobacterium tuberculosis* in a primary school out-break: lack of racial difference in susceptibility to infection. *Am J Epidemiol* 1994;139:520–530.

41. Ikeda RM, Birkhead GS, DiFerdinando GT Jr, et al. Nosocomial tuberculosis: an outbreak of a strain resistant to seven drugs. *Infect Control Hosp Epidemiol* 1995;16:152–159.

42. Jereb JA, Burwen DR, Dooley SW, et al. Nosocomial outbreak of tuberculosis in a renal transplant unit: application of a new technique for restriction fragment length polymorphism analysis of *Mycobacterium tuberculosis* isolates. *J Infect Dis* 1993;168: 1219–1224.

43. Jereb JA, Klevens RM, Privett TD, et al. Tuberculosis in health care workers at a hospital with an outbreak of multidrug-resistant *Mycobacterium tuberculosis. Arch Intern Med* 1995;155:854–859.

44. Kenyon TA, Ridzon R, Luskin-Hawk R, et al. A nosocomial outbreak of multidrug-resistant tuberculosis. *Ann Intern Med* 1997; 127:32–36.

45. Luby S, Carmichael S, Shaw G, et al. A nosocomial outbreak of *Mycobacterium tuberculosis.J Fam Pract* 1994;39:21–25.

46. Mohle-Boetani JC, Miguelino V, Dewsnup DH, et al. Tuberculosis outbreak in a housing unit for human immunodeficiency virus-infected patients in a correctional facility: transmission risk factors and effective outbreak control. *Clin Infect Dis* 2002;34: 668–676.

47. Nivin B, Nicholas P, Gayer M, et al. A continuing outbreak of multidrug-resistant tuberculosis, with transmission in a hospital nursery. *Clin Infect Dis* 1998;26:303–307.

48. Penman AD, Kohn MA, Fowler M. A shipboard outbreak of tuberculosis in Mississippi and Louisiana, 1993 to 1994. *Am J Public Health* 1997;87:1234.

49. Ridzon R, Kenyon T, Luskin-Hawk R, et al. Nosocomial transmission of human immunodeficiency virus and subsequent transmission of multidrug-resistant tuberculosis in a healthcare worker. *Infect Control Hosp Epidemiol* 1997;18:422–423.

50. Shannon A, Kelly P, Lucey M, et al. Isoniazid resistant tuberculosis in a school outbreak: the protective effect of BCG. *Eur Respir J* 1991;4:778–782.

51. Sundberg R, Shapiro R, Darras F, et al. A tuberculosis outbreak in a renal transplant program. *Transplant Proc* 1991;23:3091–3092.

52. Valway SE, Sanchez MP, Shinnick TF, et al. An outbreak involving extensive transmission of a virulent strain of *Mycobacterium tuberculosis. N Engl J Med* 1998;338:633–639.

53. Wenger PN, Otten J, Breeden A, et al. Control of nosocomial transmission of multidrug-resistant *Mycobacterium tuberculosis* among healthcare workers and HIV-infected patients. *Lancet* 1995;345:235–240.

54. Ridzon R, Kent JH, Valway S, et al. Outbreak of drug-resistant tuberculosis with second-generation transmission in a high school in California. *J Pediatr* 1997;131:863–868.

55. Valway SE, Greifinger RB, Papania M, et al. Multidrug-resistant tuberculosis in the New York State prison system, 1990–1991. *J Infect Dis* 1994;170:151–156.

56. Dooley SW, Villarino ME, Lawrence M, et al. Nosocomial transmission of tuberculosis in a hospital unit for HIV-infected patients. *JAMA* 1992;267:2632–2634.

57. Chaulk CP, Moore-Rice K, Rizzo R, et al. Eleven years of community-based directly observed therapy for tuberculosis. *JAMA* 1995;274:945–951.

58. Frieden TR, Fujiwara PI, Washko RM, et al. Tuberculosis in New York City—turning the tide. *N Engl J Med* 1995;333:229–233.

59. Institute of Medicine (U.S.). *Ending neglect: the elimination of tuberculosis in the United States.* Washington, DC: National Academy of Science, 2000.

60. McKenna MT, McCray E, Jones JL, et al. The fall after the rise: tuberculosis in the United States, 1991 through 1994. *Am J Public Health* 1998;88:1059–1063.

61. CDC. Development of new vaccines for tuberculosis. Recommendations of the Advisory Council for the Elimination of Tuberculosis (ACET). *MMWR Recomm Rep* 1998;47:1–6.

62. CDC. Essential components of a tuberculosis prevention and control program. Recommendations of the Advisory Council for the Elimination of Tuberculosis. *MMWR Recomm Rep* 1995;44: 1–16.

63. CDC. Guidelines for preventing the transmission of Mycobacterium tuberculosis in health-care facilities, 1994. *MMWR Recomm Rep* 1994;43:1–132.

64. CDC. Initial therapy for tuberculosis in the era of multidrug resistance. Recommendations of the Advisory Council for the Elimination of Tuberculosis [published erratum appears in *MMWR Morb Mortal Wkly Rep* 1993;42:536]. *MMWR Recomm Rep* 1993;42:1–8.

65. CDC. Laboratory practices for diagnosis of tuberculosis—United States, 1994. *MMWR Morb Mortal Wkly Rep* 1995;44: 587–590.

66. CDC. Nucleic acid amplification tests for tuberculosis. *MMWR Morb Mortal Wkly Rep* 1996;45:950–952.

67. CDC. Performance evaluation program for *Mycobacterium tuberculosis* drug-susceptibility testing process. *MMWR Morb Mortal Wkly Rep* 1994;43:17–18.

68. CDC. Preventing and controlling tuberculosis along the U.S.-Mexico border. *MMWR Recomm Rep* 2001;50:1–27.

69. CDC. Prevention and treatment of tuberculosis among patients infected with human immunodeficiency virus: principles of therapy and revised recommendations. Centers for Disease Control and Prevention. *MMWR Recomm Rep* 1998;47:1–58.

70. CDC. Progress toward the elimination of tuberculosis—United States, 1998. *MMWR Morb Mortal Wkly Rep* 1999;48:732–736.

71. CDC. Recommendations for prevention and control of tuberculosis among foreign-born persons. Report of the Working Group on Tuberculosis among Foreign-Born Persons. Centers for Disease Control and Prevention. *MMWR Recomm Rep* 1998;47:1–29.

72. CDC. Screening for tuberculosis and tuberculosis infection in high-risk populations. Recommendations of the Advisory Council for the Elimination of Tuberculosis. *MMWR Recomm Rep* 1995;44:19–34.

73. CDC. Targeted tuberculin testing and treatment of latent tuberculosis infection. American Thoracic Society. *MMWR Recomm Rep* 2000;49:1–51.

74. CDC. The role of BCG vaccine in the prevention and control of tuberculosis in the United States. A joint statement by the Advisory Council for the Elimination of Tuberculosis and the Advisory Committee on Immunization Practices. *MMWR Recomm Rep* 1996;45:1–18.

75. CDC. Tuberculosis control laws—United States, 1993. Recommendations of the Advisory Council for the Elimination of Tuberculosis (ACET) [erratum appears in *MMWR Morb Mortal Wkly Rep* 1993;42:983.]. *MMWR Recomm Rep* 1993;42:1–28.

76. CDC. Tuberculosis elimination revisited: obstacles, opportunities, and a renewed commitment. Advisory Council for the Elimination of Tuberculosis (ACET). *MMWR Recomm Rep* 1999;48: 1–13.

77. CDC. Update: nucleic acid amplification tests for tuberculosis. *MMWR Morb Mortal Wkly Rep* 2000;49:593–594.

78. CDC. Updated guidelines for the use of rifabutin or rifampin for the treatment and prevention of tuberculosis among HIV-infected patients taking protease inhibitors or nonnucleoside reverse transcriptase inhibitors. Centers for Disease Control and Prevention. *MMWR Morb Mortal Wkly Rep* 2000;49: 185–189.

79. American Thoracic Society/Centers for Disease Control and Prevention/Infectious Disease Society of America. Treatment of tuberculosis. *Am J Respir Crit Care Med* 2003;167:603–662.

80. Curtis AB, McCray E, McKenna M, Onorato IM. Completeness and timeliness of tuberculosis case reporting. A multistate study. *Am J Prev Med* 2001;20:108–112.
81. Tuberculosis: a global emergency. *World Health Forum* 1993;14:438.
82. CDC. *CDC's response to ending neglect: the elimination of tuberculosis in the United States.* Washington, DC: U.S. Department of Health and Human Services, 2002.
83. CDC. Progressing toward tuberculosis elimination in low-incidence areas of the United States—recommendations of the Advisory Council for the Elimination of Tuberculosis. *MMWR Recomm Rep* 2002;5:1–16.
84. Miller B, Rosenbaum S, Stange PV, et al. Tuberculosis control in a changing health care system: model contract specifications for managed care organizations. *Clin Infect Dis* 1998;27:677–686.
85. Long RS. The epidemiology of tuberculosis among foreign-born persons in Alberta, Canada, 1989–1998: identification of high risk groups. *Int J Tuberc Lung Dis* 2002;6:615–621.
86. Cowie RL, Sharpe JW. Tuberculosis among immigrants: interval from arrival in Canada to diagnosis. A 5-year study in southern Alberta. *CMAJ* 1998;158:599–602.
87. Eriksson M, Bennet R, Danielsson N. Clinical manifestations and epidemiology of childhood tuberculosis in Stockholm 1976–95. *Scand J Infect Dis* 1997;29:569–572.
88. MacIntyre CR, Plant AJ, Yung A, et al. Missed opportunities for prevention of tuberculosis in Victoria, Australia. *Int J Tuberc Lung Dis* 1997;1:135–141.
89. Raviglione MC, Sudre P, Rieder HL, et al. Secular trends of tuberculosis in western Europe. *Bull World Health Organ* 1993;71:297–306.
90. Dye C, Williams BG, Espinal MA, et al. Erasing the world's slow stain: strategies to beat multidrug-resistant tuberculosis. *Science* 2002;295:2042–2046.
91. Espinal MA, Laszlo A, Simonsen L, et al. Global trends in resistance to antituberculosis drugs. World Health Organization-International Union against Tuberculosis and Lung Disease Working Group on Anti-Tuberculosis Drug Resistance Surveillance. *N Engl J Med* 2001;344:1294–1303.
92. Miller B, Castro KG. Sharpen available tools for tuberculosis control, but new tools needed for elimination. *JAMA* 1996;276:1916–1917.
93. Cole ST, Brosch R, Parkhill J, et al. Deciphering the biology of *Mycobacterium tuberculosis* from the complete genome sequence. *Nature* 1998;393:537–544.
94. Combs DL, O'Brien RJ, Geiter LJ. USPHS Tuberculosis Short-Course Chemotherapy Trial 21: effectiveness, toxicity, and acceptability. The report of final results. *Ann Intern Med* 1990;112:397–406.
95. The Tuberculosis Trials Consortium. Rifapentine and isoniazid once a week versus rifampicin and isoniazid twice a week for treatment of drug-susceptible pulmonary tuberculosis in HIV-negative patients. *Lancet* 2002;360:528–534.
96. Pablos-Mendez A. Working alliance for TB drug development, Cape Town, South Africa, February 8, 2000. *Int J Tuberc Lung Dis* 2000;4:489–490.
97. White paper National Coalition for the Elimination of Tuberculosis. TB Elimination: The Federal Funding Gap. American Lung Association, Washington, DC. http://www lungusa org/press/legislative/leg032102 html 2002.
98. Stop TB Partnership. *The global plan to stop tuberculosis* (WHO/CDS/STB). Geneva: WHO, 2001.

Tuberculosis, Second Edition, edited by William N. Rom and Stuart M. Garay. Published by Lippincott Williams & Wilkins, Philadelphia, 2004

INDEX

Note: Page numbers followed by *f* indicate an illustration; page numbers followed by *t* indicate a table.

dendritic. *See* Dendritic cells
Antiretroviral therapy. *See also* Highly active
antiretroviral therapy
drug interactions with, management of,
816
interactions of, with tuberculosis drugs,
677–678, 695–696, 695*t*, 718–720,
719*t*
isoniazid, 751
rifamycins, 763
Antisense RNA methods, for virulence
studies, 141
Aortic aneurysm, 431, 515, 517
Aortography, in aneurysms, 517
Apaf-1 protein, in apoptosis regulation, 310
Aphonia, in laryngeal tuberculosis, 478
Apoptosis, 309–320
definition of, 309
fate of cells in, 311–312, 315
infection and, 312
of lymphocytes, 317
of macrophages, 136, 217, 312–317
in absence of T lymphocytes, 313
Fas in, 314
fate of, 315
in granuloma homeostasis, 316–317
in host defense, 316–317
microbicidal effects of, 314
morphology of, 309, 310*f*
in presence of T lymphocytes,
315–316
purinergic receptors in, 314
regulation of, 314
tuberculosis susceptibility and, 315
tumor necrosis factor in, 313–314
mechanisms of, 309, 312, 311*f*
microbicidal effects of, 314
morphology of, 309, 310*f*
vs. necrosis, 309
regulation of, 310–311
rifampin in, 761
Apoptotic bodies, fate of, 311–312, 315
Appendicitis, *Mycobacterium avium-*
intracellulare complex, 692
Appendix, tuberculosis of, 526, 526*t*
Arabinin, as ethambutol target, 778–779
Arabinofuran, 118, 119*f*, 778–779
Arabinogalactan, in cell wall
assembly of, 124–126, 125*f*
position of, 115–116, 116*f*
structure of, 118, 119*f*
Arabinosyltransferases, as ethambutol
targets, 779
Arachnoiditis, tuberculous, 451, 566–567
ARDS. *See* Respiratory failure
L-Arginine, in nitric oxide synthase
production, 227
Arterial blood gases
in miliary tuberculosis, 435
in respiratory failure, 369
Arthralgia, from pyrazinamide, 777
Arthritis
Mycobacterium avium-intracellulare
complex, 692
Mycobacterium kansasii, 698
nontuberculous mycobacterial, 654

osteoarthritis, vs. osteoarticular
tuberculosis, 581
rheumatoid
vs. osteoarticular tuberculosis, 581
pulmonary tuberculosis in, 375
tuberculous, 578, 580–582
Arthus reaction, in tuberculid, 600
Articular tuberculosis. *See* Osteoarticular
tuberculosis
Artificial pneumothorax, therapeutic,
639–640, 640*f*
Artists, with tuberculosis, 3–11, 9*t*–10*t*
Arylamine *N*-acetyltransferase
in isoniazid inactivation, 744
in isoniazid resistance, 748
polymorphisms of, 826–827
Ascites
in hepatobiliary tuberculosis, 437–438
in miliary tuberculosis, 431*f*
in pericarditis, 510
in peritonitis, 531–532
Asia. *See also* China; Southeast Asia
tuberculosis in
China, 14*t*, 15*t*, 17
HIV infection and, 665–666
in immigrants, 34–35, 34*f*, 37*t*, 39
Southeast, 14*t*, 15*t*, 16, 19, 20*f*
Asialoglycoprotein type 2 receptor, on
dendritic cells, 270
Aspartate aminotransferase, in hepatobiliary
tuberculosis, 538
Aspergilloma, in cavities, 327, 333
hemoptysis in, 367, 645
radiography in, 418, 419*f*
Asphyxiation, in hemoptysis, 367
Atlantoaxial tuberculosis, 573
Atypical mycobacterial infections. *See*
Nontuberculous mycobacterial
infections
Auramine O, 166, 166*t*, 167*f*, 332, 332*f*
Autonephrectomy, in genitourinary
tuberculosis, 551, 553, 555*f*
Autopsy, tuberculosis transmission in,
847–848
Autotolerance, dendritic cells in, 275–276
Azithromycin
for *Mycobacterium avium-intracellulare*
complex infections, 693–694
for nontuberculous mycobacterial
infections
osteoarticular, 584
pulmonary, 657, 658*t*
prophylactic, for *Mycobacterium avium-*
intracellulare complex infections,
696–697
Azotemia, in genitourinary tuberculosis,
551, 552

B
Bacille Calmette–Guérin. *See also* Bacille
Calmette–Guérin vaccine
antibodies to, in central nervous system
tuberculosis, 449
for bladder cancer, systemic
dissemination in, 551
Brazil, 76

Connaught, 76, 77*f*
dendritic cell interactions with, 279
genome of, 68, 71, 76, 77*f*, 77*t*, 78
heat shock protein repressors in, 147
in host resistance studies, 194–195
identification of, 171
infection with, dissemination of, 429
mutations of, 893
Pasteur, 71, 76
PE proteins of, 70*f*
phenotypic differences in, 75
phospholipase inhibitor effects on, 217
RD1 region of, 76, 78
resistance in, 195, 795*t*
strains of, 76, 875, 893
uptake of, in Peyer patches, 526
virulence of
DNA microarray analysis for, 143
Erp in, 153
19-kd protein in, 152
Mas in, 153
PcaA in, 154
PurC, 148
Bacille Calmette–Guérin vaccine, 875–884
accidental infections from, 193
administration routes for, 875–876
animal models for, 877–881, 886
for central nervous system tuberculosis,
458
complications of, 601–602, 621
cutaneous lesions from, 601–602, 601*f*
development of, 875
duration of protection from, 886
efficacy of, 71, 621
animal models of, 877–881
clinical trials of, 876–877, 880–881
geographical factors in, 881
molecular studies of, 56–57
epidemiologic effects of, 19
genetic diversity in, 75–76
historical aspects of, 875, 885
in HIV infection, 621, 633, 681
immunoassay in, vs. latent tuberculosis,
189–190
improvement of, 71, 893
for infant with infected mother, 633
for miliary tuberculosis, 439
oral administration of, 875–876
Pasteur strain of, 875
for pediatric patients, 621
postexposure, 111
production of, 875
recombinant, 879–880
safety of, 875–876
single-gene comparisons of, 76
vs. subunit vaccines, 888–890, 889*t*
testing of, mouse models for, 242
tuberculin skin test results in, 178,
614–615, 876
whole-genome comparisons of, 76, 77*f*,
77*t*, 78
Bacillemia, in intestinal infections, 526
Bacilluria, 550–551
Bacillus subtilis
genome of, 137–138
sigma factors of, 145

pharmacokinetics of, 781, 810*t*
potency of, 802*t*
susceptibility testing of, 172*t*, 173*t*
toxicity of, monitoring for, 784*t*
Capsule-like layer, of cell wall, 115–117, 116*f*
Carboxymycobactin, synthesis of, MbtB in, 149
Carcinoma
  bronchiogenic, tuberculosis and, 373–374, 418–418, 419*f*
  squamous cell, laryngeal tuberculosis with, 480
Cardiac arrhythmias, in pericarditis, 510
Cardiac tamponade
  in lymphadenopathy, 491
  in pericarditis, 514–515
Cardiomegaly, in pericarditis, 511
Cardiomyopathy, in pericarditis, 515
Cardiovascular tuberculosis. *See also* Pericarditis, tuberculous
  aortic aneurysms, 431, 515, 517
  endocarditis in, 431, 517–518
  myocarditis in, 431, 518
Carpal tunnel syndrome, 579
Carson, James, on artificial pneumothorax, 639–640
Caseation. *See also* Ghon foci and Ghon complex
  in granulomas, 254, 255*f*
  in hepatobiliary tuberculosis, 540, 542
  in intestinal tuberculosis, 527
  in lymphadenopathy, 491–492
  in meningitis, 446
  in miliary tuberculosis, 428, 429
  in myocardial tuberculosis, 518
  in osteoarticular tuberculosis, 581
  pathology of, 323, 324*f*
  in pediatric patients, 611
Case definition, of tuberculosis, 31–32, 32*t*
Case finding, vs. tuberculin skin test screening, 615
Case management system, 723
Caspases, in apoptosis, 217, 309–310, 311*f*
Catalases
  KatG as, 739–743, 742*f*, 745, 746*t*, 747, 749–750
  in *Mycobacterium tuberculosis* identification, 170
  in virulence, 150–151
Catarrhal pattern, of reactivation tuberculosis, 351
Cathepsins, destructive effects of, 136
Catheter-related infections, nontuberculous mycobacterial, 655
Cauda equina syndrome, in Pott disease, 567
Cavitation
  drug activity within, 774*f*
  healing of, 355
  in HIV infection, 671
  in miliary tuberculosis, 432*f*
  in primary tuberculosis, 327, 327*f*, 396, 397*f*
  in reactivation tuberculosis, 354–355
CCAAT/enhancer binding protein-β, 287

in HIV coinfection, 302, 304–305, 304*f*, 305*f*
CCL chemokines, in dendritic cell migration, 273
CD1 proteins, 257, 258*f*, 263–267
  actions of, 264–266, 264*t*
  antigen interactions with, 263–264, 264*t*
  genes of, 263
  inhibition of, 265
  isoforms of, 263
  structures of, 263
  T lymphocyte types and, 265
CD11b, in phagocytosis, 207
CD14, in phagocytosis, 205
CD48, on dendritic cells, 273
CD54, on dendritic cells, 273
CD58, on dendritic cells, 273
CD62L, in dendritic cell migration, 274
CD80, on dendritic cells, 273
CD86, on dendritic cells, 273
CD91, in apoptosis, 311–312
CD205 (DEC-205, lectin), on dendritic cells, 270, 272, 277
CD207 (langerin), in dendritic cells, 270, 277
CDC1551 strain. *See Mycobacterium tuberculosis*, CDC1551 strain of
Cefoxitin
  for *Mycobacterium abscessus* infections, 659
  for nontuberculous mycobacterial infections
    osteoarticular, 583
    pulmonary, 658*t*
Cell(s), programmed death of. *See* Apoptosis
Cell-mediated immune response, 251–262. *See also* Cytokines; Dendritic cells; Granuloma(s); T lymphocytes
  in early infection, 252, 253*f*, 254, 255*f*
  in HIV coinfection, 667–668
Cellulitis
  nontuberculous mycobacterial, 655
  tuberculous, 599
Cell wall, 115–134
  N-acetylglucosamine in, 118, 120*f*–121*f*, 122
  N-acetylmuramic acid in, 118, 120*f*–121*f*, 122
  arabinogalactan in
    assembly of, 124–126, 125*f*
    position of, 115–116, 116*f*
    structure of, 118, 119*f*
  arabinomannan in, 115, 116*f*, 130
  core structure in, 117–118, 117*f*, 119*f*
  decaprenyl phosphate in, 122–123, 122*f*
  decaprenylphosphoryl-D-arabinose in, 119*f*, 123
  decaprenylphosphoryl-D-mannose in, 123
  dimycocerosate in
    structure of, 127, 128*f*
    synthesis of, 129–130, 129*f*
  dTDP-rhamnose in, 119*f*, 122
  geranyl diphosphate-mannose in, 123
  glucan in, 130
  layers of, 115, 116*f*

lipoarabinomannan in. *See* Lipoarabinomannan
lipomannan in, structure of, 118, 120*f*
methyl-branched fatty acids in, 129–130, 129*f*
mycolic acids and mycolates of
  position of, 115–116, 116*f*
  structures of, 118, 119*f*
  synthesis of, 123–124
noncovalently bound lipids in
  structures of, 126–128, 126*f*–129*f*
  synthesis of, 129–130, 129*f*
overview of, 115–117, 116*f*
peptidoglycans in
  assembly of, 124, 124*f*
  structure of, 117–118, 117*f*
phosphatidylinositol mannosides in, 130
uridine 5'-diphosphate-galactofuranose in, 119*f*, 122
virulence factors of, 151–154
Centers for Disease Control
  drug regimen recommendations of, 716, 716*t*
  drug resistance statistics of, 37
  nucleic acid amplification assay recommendations of, 179
  proportion susceptibility test method of, 172, 172*t*
  surveillance system of, 31, 32*t*, 33
  tuberculosis elimination activities of, 901, 902*t*, 903–904
  tuberculosis transmission prevention guidelines of, 846–847
Central nervous system nontuberculous mycobacterial infections, 692
Central nervous system tuberculosis, 445–464. *See also* Meningitis
  abscess in, 241, 451
  antibody and antigen tests in, 449–450
  case study of, 446–447
  cerebrospinal fluid examination in, 447
  clinical manifestations of, 446–447, 447*t*
  diagnosis of, 447–450, 449*f*
  epidemiology of, 445
  historical aspects of, 445
  in HIV infection, 457–458
  microbiology of, 447–448
  in miliary tuberculosis, 431
  neurologic signs in, 447, 447*t*
  nucleic acid amplification tests in, 450
  pathogenesis of, 445–446
  pathology of, 341–342, 341*f*, 446
  prevention of, 458
  prognosis for, 456–457, 457*f*
  radiography in, 448–449, 448*f*, 449*f*
  risk factors for, 445
  sequelae of, 456–457
  of spinal cord, 451
  stages of, 447, 447*t*
  treatment of, 452–456, 453*t*, 454*f*
  tuberculomas in, 341, 431, 450–451, 451*f*
  types of, 341
Centrifugation, for specimen preparation, 165–166

in rapid diagnosis, 178–179
in smear-negative, culture-positive
tuberculosis, 362–363
Nursing, drug transmission in, 631–632
Nursing homes, tuberculosis in, 23, 40,
378–379

O

Occupational Safety and Health
Administration, tuberculosis
standard of, 846
Occupational tuberculosis
cutaneous, 594
in dentists, 485
in health care workers. *See* Health care
workers, tuberculosis in
in miners, 92–93
prevention of, building ventilation for,
850–854, 851*f*
Ocular nontuberculous mycobacterial
infections, 692
Ocular tuberculosis, 465–473
choroidal, 469–472, 470*f*–472*f*
conjunctival, 466, 467*f*
corneal, 467
diagnosis of, 471, 473
Eales disease, 472–473
eyelid, 465
histopathology of, 471–472, 472*f*
history of, 465
in HIV infection, 472
lacrimal system, 465
neuroophthalmic, 468–469
orbital, 468, 468*f*
retinal, 473
scleral, 467
uveal, 469, 469*t*
Odynophagia
in oral tuberculosis, 484
in pediatric patients, 611
Ofloxacin
efficacy of, 105, 105*f*, 721, 797
for multidrug-resistant tuberculosis, 679,
732–733
for *Mycobacterium avium-intracellulare*
complex infections, 694
in pediatric patients, 619*t*
in pregnancy, 631
resistance to, 800
Ophthalmopathy, in pituitary tuberculosis,
589
Optic nerve
ethambutol toxicity to, 780
tuberculosis of, 468–469
Optic neuritis
from ethambutol, 473
from isoniazid, 474
Oral cavity, tuberculosis of, 484–485
Orbital tuberculosis, 468, 468*f*
Organomegaly
in congenital tuberculosis, 632
in hepatobiliary tuberculosis, 537–538
in miliary tuberculosis, 429, 431*f*
in *Mycobacterium avium-intracellulare*
complex infections, 692, 693
in *Mycobacterium genavense* infections,
699

Orificial tuberculosis, 595*t*, 598
Oropharynx, tuberculosis of, 484–485
Orthopnea, in pericarditis, 510, 511*t*
Orthostatic hypotension, in adrenal
tuberculosis, 587
Orwell, George, 3
Osteitis, in bacille Calmette–Guérin
vaccination, 876
Osteoarthritis, vs. osteoarticular
tuberculosis, 581
Osteoarthropathy, in reactivation
tuberculosis, 354
Osteoarticular nontuberculous
mycobacterial infections, 583–584,
584*t*, 654–655
Mycobacterium avium-intracellulare
complex, 692
Mycobacterium kansasii, 698
Osteoarticular tuberculosis, 577–586
clinical presentation of, 578–580
diagnosis of, 580–582
differential diagnosis of, 581
epidemiology of, 577–578
in HIV infection, 578
lichen scrofulosorum in, 595*t*, 600, 600*f*
osteomyelitis, 485, 578–579
in pediatric patients, 580, 613
of peripheral joints, 578
Poncet disease, 580
radiography in, 581–582
risk factors for, 578
spinal. *See* Pott disease
tenosynovitis, 579
treatment of, 582–583, 582*t*, 583*t*
Osteomyelitis
Mycobacterium avium-intracellulare
complex, 692
Mycobacterium haemophilum, 699
Mycobacterium kansasii, 698
nontuberculous mycobacterial, 583–584,
654
tuberculous, 485, 578–579
Osteopontin, action of, 292
Osteoporosis
in osteoarticular tuberculosis, 581
in tenosynovitis, 579
Otitis media, tuberculous, 480–482, 481*f*
Otolaryngologic tuberculosis. *See* Head and
neck tuberculosis
Otologic tuberculosis, 480–482, 481*f*,
482*f*
Otorrhea, in otologic tuberculosis, 481
Ototoxicity, of aminoglycosides, 784–785
Outbreaks
in Canadian Indians, 193
CDC1551 strain, 55
C strain, 55–56, 56*f*
due to ventilation malfunction, 853
in HIV infection, 718
in homeless shelters, 848–849
nosocomial, 33
in primate colonies, 245
W strain, 55
Outer electron-dense layer, of cell wall, 115,
116*f*, 130
Ovary, tuberculosis of. *See* Females,
genitourinary tuberculosis in

Oxygen
molecular, in nitric oxide synthase
production, 227
reactive. *See* Reactive oxygen
intermediates
OxyR, in antioxidant gene activation,
744–745

P

Pain
in adrenal tuberculosis, 587
in cervical spinal tuberculosis, 572
in genitourinary tuberculosis, 552
in hepatobiliary tuberculosis, 437
in intestinal tuberculosis, 528, 528*t*
in laryngeal tuberculosis, 478
in *Mycobacterium avium-intracellulare*
complex infections, 692
in *Mycobacterium genavense* infections,
699
in oral tuberculosis, 484
in osteoarticular tuberculosis, 578, 580
in pericarditis, 510, 511*t*
in peritonitis, 532
in pleural tuberculosis, 500
in Pott disease, 567
in primary tuberculosis, 349
in reactivation tuberculosis, 353
in thyroid tuberculosis, 590
Palate, tuberculosis of, 484–485
Palmar ganglion, compound, 579
Pancreas, tuberculosis of, 326, 326*f*,
526–527
Pancreatitis, *Mycobacterium avium-
intracellulare* complex, 692
Pancytopenia, in miliary tuberculosis, 435
Panniculitis, in erythema nodosum, 601
Pannus
in corneal tuberculosis, 467
in osteoarticular tuberculosis, 581
Papillary conjunctivitis, hypertrophic, 466
Papilledema, in central nervous system
tuberculosis, 447
Papillomacular bundle, ethambutol toxicity
to, 473
Papillomatosis
in laryngeal tuberculosis, 479
in warty tuberculosis, 596
Papulonecrotic tuberculids, 595*t*, 599–600,
599*f*
Paraaminosalicylic acid
for central nervous system tuberculosis,
452
dosage for, in kidney failure, 813*t*
drug interactions with, 811*t*
food interactions with, 811*t*
historical aspects of, 714
interactions with, 734
monitoring of, 819
for multidrug-resistant tuberculosis, 679
for pediatric patients, 619*t*
pharmacokinetics of, 810*t*
for Pott disease, 568, 571
in pregnancy, 631
susceptibility testing of, 172*t*, 173*t*
Paracentesis, in peritonitis, 532–533
Paradoxical pulse, in pericarditis, 510, 511*t*